P9-CDJ-238

MAYO CLINIC
FAMILY HEALTH BOOK

MAYO CLINIC
FAMILY HEALTH BOOK

Scott C. Litin, M.D.
Editor in Chief

Third Edition

HarperResource
An Imprint of HarperCollins*Publishers*

Mayo Clinic Family Health Book provides reliable, practical, comprehensive, easy-to-understand information on issues relating to good health. Much of its information comes from physicians, research scientists and other health care professionals at Mayo Clinic. This book is intended to supplement the advice of your personal physician, whom you should consult about your individual medical condition. *Mayo Clinic Family Health Book* does not endorse any company or product. MAYO, MAYO CLINIC, MAYO CLINIC HEALTH INFORMATION and the Mayo triple-shield logo are marks of Mayo Foundation for Medical Education and Research.

HarperCollins books may be purchased for educational, business or sales promotional use. For information, please write: Special Markets Department, HarperCollins Publishers, Inc., 10 East 53rd Street, New York, NY 10022.

Layout and production by Mayo Clinic Health Information, Rochester, Minn.

Stock photography for lifestyle photos from Artville, Digital Stock, Digital Vision Ltd., © Isabelle Rozenbaum/PhotoAlto, PhotoDisc and Stockbyte. The individuals pictured in these lifestyle photos are models, and the photos are used for illustrative purposes only. There is no correlation between the individuals portrayed and the condition or subject being discussed.

Library of Congress Cataloging-in-Publication Data

Mayo Clinic family health book/Scott C. Litin, editor in chief.—3rd ed.
p. ; cm.
Includes index.
ISBN 0-06-000250-6
1. Medicine, Popular. I. Title: Family health book. II. Litin, Scott C. III. Mayo Clinic.
[DNLM: 1. Medicine—Encyclopedias—English. 2. Medicine—Popular Works. WB 120 M473 2003]
RC81 .M473 2003
613—dc21

2002027349

Printed in the United States of America

Third Edition

04 05 06 07 QW 10 9 8 7 6 5 4 3

Foreword

All of us at Mayo Clinic are pleased and proud to recommend the book that you're holding. This new and revised edition of *Mayo Clinic Family Health Book* contains updated information on more than 1,000 diseases and disorders, along with important advice on preventive care for maintaining good health.

Mayo Clinic has always based its medical practice on meeting the unique needs of each patient and empowering individuals to make decisions concerning their health care. In 1932, Dr. Charles H. Mayo stated, "The object of all health education is to change the conduct of individual men, women and children by teaching them to care for their bodies well." With this educational mission, and the institution's depth and breadth of medical knowledge, experience and expertise, Mayo Clinic occupies an unparalleled position as a source of health information. Since 1983, Mayo Clinic has published reliable and easy-to-understand health information for millions of consumers through award-winning newsletters, books and online services. Revenue from these publishing activities supports Mayo Clinic programs, including medical education and research.

Mayo Clinic comprises more than 45,000 physicians, scientists, nurses and other support personnel at its three major locations in Rochester, Minn., Jacksonville, Fla., and Scottsdale, Ariz., and its regional community-based health care practices.

On behalf of all of the individuals who make up Mayo Clinic's extended family of health care professionals, thank you for selecting this latest edition of *Mayo Clinic Family Health Book.*

Denis A. Cortese, M.D.

President and Chief Executive Officer
Mayo Foundation

Hugh C. Smith, M.D.

Chair, Rochester Board of Governors

George B. Bartley, M.D.

Chair, Jacksonville Board of Governors

Victor F. Trastek, M.D.

Chair, Scottsdale Board of Governors

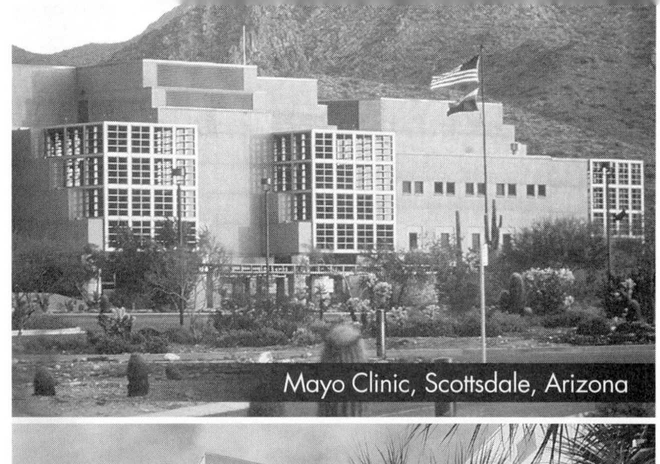

Mayo Clinic, Scottsdale, Arizona

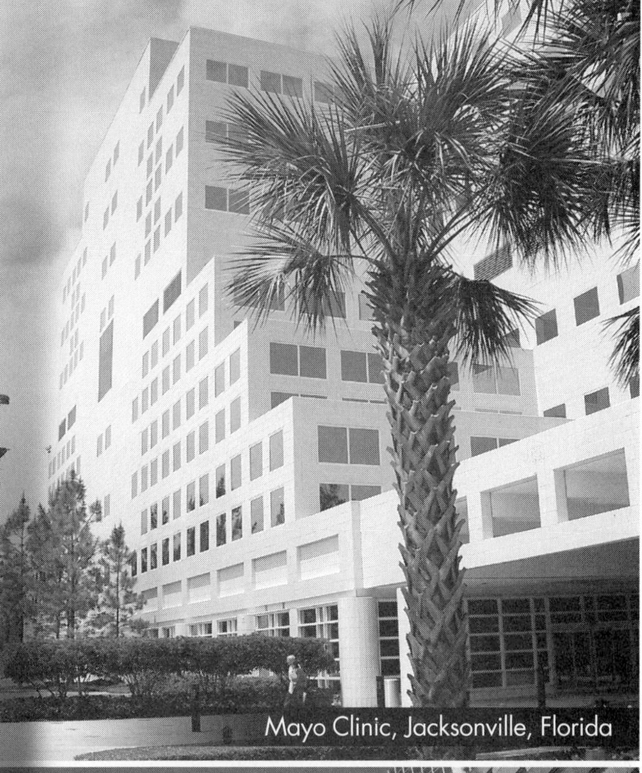

Mayo Clinic, Jacksonville, Florida

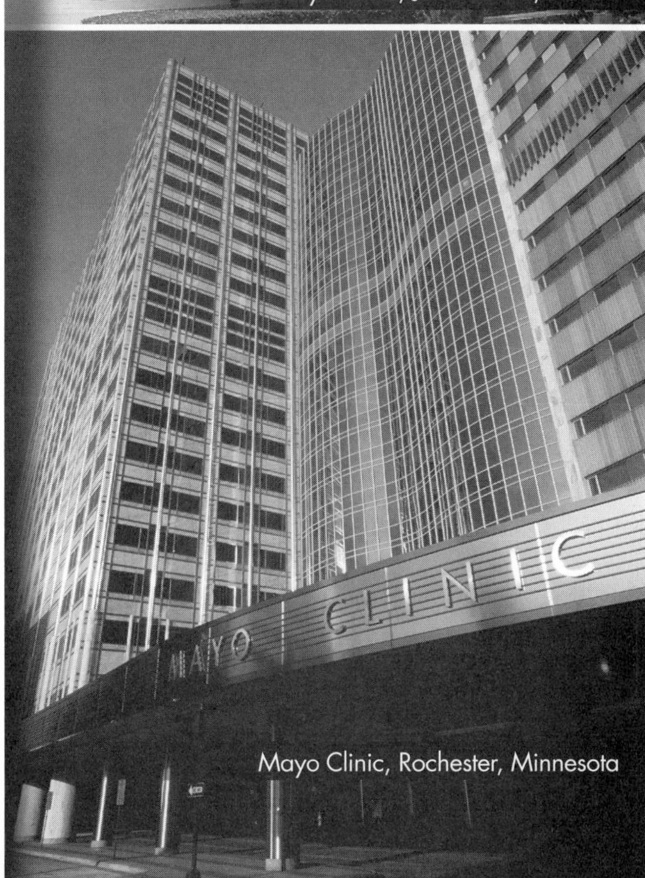

Mayo Clinic, Rochester, Minnesota

Editorial Staff

Editor in Chief	Scott Litin, M.D.
Associate Editor	Kenneth Berge, M.D.
Managing Editor	Karen Wallevand
Copy Editor	Mary Duerson
Proofreaders	Miranda Attlesey Donna Hanson Judith Shuster
Creative Director	Daniel Brevick
Art Directors	Brian Fyffe Stewart Koski Paul Krause Christopher Srnka
Illustrator	Kent McDaniel
Medical Illustrators	Stephen Graepel John Hagen Michael King M. Alice McKinney
Photographers	James Bambenek Mary Frantz Elman Hanken Joseph Kane Richard Madsen Carol Sparrow Randy Zeigler
Editorial Research Manager	Deirdre Herman
Editorial Research Librarians	Anthony Cook Michelle Hewlett
Contributing Writers	Rachel Bartony Lee Engfer Rebecca Gonzalez-Campoy Regina Martinez Stephen Miller Anne O'Connor Susan Rodsjo Robin Silverman
Editor in Chief, Books/Newsletters	Christopher Frye
Indexer	Cohen & Carruth Inc.
HarperCollins Publishers	Leah Carlson-Stanisic, Design Manager Penelope Haynes, Senior Production Editor Karen Lumley, Senior Production Manager Donna Ruvituso, Executive Managing Editor Toni Sciarra, Senior Editor

Assistant Editors

Robert Albright, D.O., Nephrology
Charles Beatty, M.D., Otorhinolaryngology
W. Mark Brutinel, M.D., Pulmonary Medicine
Helmut Buettner, M.D., Ophthalmology
Jane Carlon, M.D., Radiology
April Chang-Miller, M.D., Rheumatology
Maria Collazo-Clavell, M.D., Endocrinology
Wyatt Decker, M.D., Emergency Medicine
Paul Friedman, M.D., Cardiovascular Diseases
Lawrence Gibson, M.D., Dermatology
Philip Hagen, M.D., Preventive Medicine
Roger Harms, M.D., Obstetrics and Gynecology
Jay Hoecker, M.D., Pediatrics
Robert V. Johnson, M.D., Neonatology
Pamela Karnes, M.D., Medical Genetics
John E. King, M.D., Gastroenterology and Hepatology
Keith Kramlinger, M.D., Psychiatry
Leo Kupp, D.D.S., Dental Specialties
Edward Laskowski, M.D., Physical Medicine and Rehabilitation
James Li, M.D., Allergy
David P. Martin, M.D., Anesthesiology/Pain Clinic
Timothy Moynihan, M.D., Oncology
Jennifer K. Nelson, R.D., Nutrition
Todd Nippoldt, M.D., Endocrinology
Donald Novicki, M.D., Urology
Ronald Petersen, M.D., Neurology
S. Vincent Rajkumar, M.D., Hematology
Deborah Rhodes, M.D., Internal Medicine/Breast Clinic
Robert Sheeler, M.D., Family Medicine
Sheldon Sheps, M.D., Hypertension
Michael Stuart, M.D., Orthopedics
Jerry Swanson, M.D., Neurology
Paul Takahashi, M.D., Internal Medicine/Geriatrics
Zelalem Temesgen, M.D., Infectious Diseases
Donald Williams, Ph.D., Psychology

Additional Contributors

Administration and Legal Counsel
Rick Colvin
Richard Edwards
Sara Gilliland
Daniel Goldman, J.D.
James Hale Sr.
David E. Larson, M.D.
Kathleen Meyerle, J.D.
Vicki Moore
Steven Stenhaug

Anatomy
Stephen Carmichael, Ph.D.
Wojciech Pawlina, M.D.

Anesthesiology
Keith Berge, M.D.

Cardiovascular Diseases
Thomas Allison, Ph.D.
John Bresnahan, M.D.
Brooks Edwards, M.D.
Raymond Gibbons, M.D.
David Holmes Jr., M.D.
Stephen Kopecky, M.D.
Thomas Kottke, M.D.
Thom Rooke, M.D.
Ray Squires, Ph.D.
Lois Thorkelson, R.N.
Douglas Wood, M.D.
R. Scott Wright, M.D.

Chaplain Services
Warren Anderson, M.Div.

Dental Specialties
Kevin Reid, D.M.D.
Phillip Sheridan, D.D.S.
Victoria Zook

Dermatology
Jayne Feind
Henry Randle, M.D.
Randall Roenigk, M.D.
Donna Whipple
Patricia Witman, M.D.

Ears, Nose and Throat
Ann Anderson
Christopher Bauch, Ph.D.
David Fabry, Ph.D.
Ray Gustafson, M.D.
Kathryn Kerst
AnnaMary Peterson
Jon Shallop, Ph.D.

Emergency Services
Julia Rosekrans, M.D.

Endocrinology
Bart Clarke, M.D.
Donald Hensrud, M.D.
Pasquale Palumbo, M.D.

Family Medicine
John Bachman, M.D.
Joseph Furst, M.D.
John Wilkinson, M.D.

Gastroenterology and Hepatology
David Ahlquist, M.D.
Albert Czaja, M.D.
Eugene DiMagno, M.D.
Mark V. Larson, M.D.
Edward Loftus Jr., M.D.
Jean Perrault, M.D.
Johnson Thistle, M.D.
William Tremaine, M.D.

Hematology
Stephen Ansell, M.D.
Angela Dispenzieri, M.D.
Michelle Elliott, M.D.
Morie Gertz, M.D.
Thomas Habermann, M.D.
C. Christopher Hook, M.D.
William Nichols Jr., M.D.
Luis Porrata, M.D.
Rajiv Pruthi, M.D.
Ayalew Tefferi, M.D.

Hospice Program
Ann Bartlett, R.N.

Human Resources
M. Kim Bryan, J.D.

Hypertension
Gary Schwartz, M.D.

Infectious Diseases
Abinash Virk, M.D.

Internal Medicine
Brent Bauer, M.D.
Darryl Chutka, M.D.
Alan Duncan, M.D.
J. Taylor Hays, M.D.
Richard Hurt, M.D.
Ruth E. Johnson, M.D.
Mark Liebow, M.D.
Paul Mueller, M.D.
Robert Orenstein, D.O.
Gregory Poland, M.D.
Sandhya Pruthi, M.D.
Lynne Shuster, M.D.
Janet Vittone, M.D.
Dietlind Wahner-Roedler, M.D.

Laboratory Medicine and Pathology
Robert Kisabeth, M.D.
Carol Reynolds, M.D.

Literary Agent
Arthur Klebanoff

Mayo Medical Ventures
Aleta Capelle
Elizabeth Davies
Richard Dietman
Michelle Felten
Marne Gade
Carol Gunderson
Mary Hines
Kevin Kaufman
Joey Keillor
Mary Ann Kemp
Vonda LaChance
Laura Long
Carol Olson
Rozella Pearson
Jill Pepelnjak
Gary E. Peterson
S. Rebecca Roberts
Daniel Simmons
Beverly Steele
Jill Thompson-Riese
Richard Van Ert

Media Support Services
Nancy Moltaji

Medical Genetics
Dusica Babovic-Vuksanovic, M.D.

Neurology
Andrea Adams, M.D.
J. Eric Ahlskog, M.D.
Allen Aksamit, M.D.
Patty Atkinson, M.D.
Raymond Auger, M.D.
James Bower, M.D.
Robert Brown Jr., M.D.
Jeffrey Buchhalter, M.D.
Charles Harper Jr., M.D.
B. Mark Keegan, M.D.
David Kimmel, M.D.
Paola Sandroni, M.D.
Michael Silber, M.D.
Joseph Sirven, M.D.
Elson So, M.D.
Guillermo Suarez, M.D.

Nutrition
Jenny Buccicone, R.D.
Sara DiCecco, R.D.
Nancy Kaufman, R.D.
Diane L. Olson, R.D.
Jennifer Rogers, R.D.
Charla Schultz, R.D.
Jacalyn See, R.D.

Obstetrics and Gynecology
Ann Craighead, R.N.
Susan Crawley, R.N.
Charles Field, M.D.
Margaret Gadient, R.N.
Mary Gallenberg, M.D.
Andrew Good, M.D.
Lori Hoefs, R.N.
Thomas Kastner, M.D.
Elizabeth LaFleur, R.N.
Linda Letts, R.N.
Dawn E. Nelson, R.N.
Kirk Ramin, M.D.
Jerelyn Sehl, R.N.
Cheryl Stuhldreher, R.N.
Ann Teske, R.N.
Eunice Wicks, R.N.

Oncology
Steven Alberts, M.D.
Donna Betcher, R.N.
Harry Long, M.D.
Randolph Marks, M.D.
Scott Okuno, M.D.
Paula Schomberg, M.D.

Ophthalmology
George Hohberger, M.D.

Orthopedics
Peter Amadio, M.D.
James Graham, D.P.M.
William Shaughnessy, M.D.
Thomas Shives, M.D.

Pediatrics
William Barbaresi, M.D.
Daniel Broughton, M.D.
Robert Jacobson, M.D.
Patricia Simmons, M.D.
Jill Swanson, M.D.
Robert Voigt, M.D.

Pharmacy Services
Tracy Berg, R.Ph.
Todd M. Johnson, Pharm.D.
Joseph Kostick, R.Ph.

Physical Medicine and Rehabilitation
Timothy Madson, P.T.
Jeffrey M. Thompson, M.D.
Gudni Thorsteinsson, M.D.

Psychiatry and Psychology
Ted Laska
Terry Schneekloth, M.D.
Lloyd Wells, M.D.

Pulmonary Medicine
Eric Edell, M.D.
Paul Scanlon, M.D.

Radiology
E. Meredith James, M.D.
Gary Miller, M.D.
Kristie Nelson
Steven Williams

Rheumatology
Audrey Nelson, M.D.

Sleep Center
Peter Hauri, Ph.D.
Timothy Morgenthaler, M.D.
Eric Olson, M.D.

Social Services
Mary Ely

Speech Pathology
Jack Thomas

Surgery
Dudley Davis, M.D.
Richard Devine, M.D.
John Donohue, M.D.
Michael Ebersold, M.D.
Fredric Meyer, M.D.
Christopher Moir, M.D.
Thomas Orszulak, M.D.
Mickel Prieto, M.D.
Geoffrey Thompson, M.D.
Jonathan van Heerden, M.D.

Urology
Deborah Lightner, M.D.
David Patterson, M.D.

Preface

Innovations in the field of medicine continue to hold great promise. Advances in technology and diagnostic and surgical techniques, and the development of new medications, are providing doctors and scientists with ever-more-powerful tools for diagnosing and treating disease. Today more than ever, all people have a better chance of living a longer, healthier life.

However, medical advances alone can't guarantee good health. You still play a crucial role in determining your future health and wellness. Even more important than the ability to treat disease is the ability to prevent it. And that's where your actions can pay off the most. Healthy lifestyle habits, such as exercising daily, eating well and seeing your doctor at appropriate times, are still your best bet for enjoying a long and productive life.

Mayo Clinic Family Health Book is based on the premise that knowledge is essential in maintaining good health. The third edition of *Mayo Clinic Family Health Book* was created by revising and rewriting much of the information in the previous edition and adding new chapters and sections. It's our hope that this fully updated third edition will serve not only as a reference during times of illness but also as a guide in helping you and your family adopt healthy lifestyle practices. We believe that the more you know about how your body functions — and potential threats to its health — the better equipped you are to live well. Within this book, you'll find practical and easy-to-understand information to help you remain productive and make educated decisions regarding your health.

The information provided in this book isn't a substitute for seeing a doctor. No book can replace the advice of a physician who has evaluated your overall health. The intent of this book is to help you better understand various diseases, disorders, tests and treatments so that you can communicate more effectively with your doctor and the two of you can work together to manage your health.

Mayo Clinic Family Health Book is based on the expertise of hundreds of Mayo Clinic health care professionals and the advice they give their patients day in and day out. A special thanks goes out to many Mayo Clinic staff members who took time from their busy schedules to offer their advice and guidance as we prepared this new edition. Thank you also to David Larson, M.D., and David Swanson for their enormous efforts as editor in chief and managing editor, respectively, of the previous editions of *Mayo Clinic Family Health Book.*

This book could not have been completed without the dedication and efforts of two people in particular, Managing Editor Karen Wallevand and Associate Editor Kenneth Berge, M.D.

A final thank you goes to my wife, Jolene, my daughter, Cassie, and my son, Sam. They have taught me the true meaning and importance of the word family.

To one and all, my sincere gratitude for a job well-done.

Scott C. Litin, M.D.
Editor in Chief

Contents

How to Use This Book

The information in this book is organized into six parts, as well as a 40-page color section, comprehensive glossary, resources section and index. To use the book efficiently, you may find it helpful to understand how the information is arranged.

Part I: Living Well

Good habits are key to healthy living. Part I contains practical guidance on topics such as nutrition, exercise, weight control, stress, and use of tobacco, alcohol and other drugs. The information in this part is intended to help you make healthy lifestyle changes and to understand the potential consequences of behaviors that are risks to your health.

Part II: Common Conditions and Concerns Through Life's Stages

Each chapter in this section addresses a different stage of life, beginning with infancy and progressing to late adult years. If you want to understand more about normal life changes or certain health problems that you might encounter in your children, your parents or yourself, this is the place to look.

Part III: Making Sense of Your Symptoms

Many times it's easy to figure out what's causing certain signs or symptoms you're experiencing. For example, sneezing, a sore throat and a runny nose are often associated with a common cold. Other times, though, it can be more difficult to make sense of what your body is telling you. This special section is intended to help you better identify possible causes of certain signs or symptoms.

Part IV: First Aid and Emergency Care

No one is immune to injury or a medical emergency. This special section offers comprehensive information on many minor injuries as well as major health emergencies that you could face at any time.

Visual Guide

This special section contains 40 pages of color illustrations depicting human anatomy and many common diseases and disorders.

Part V: Diseases and Disorders

In this comprehensive section, we discuss both common and rare health conditions. It's here that you can find detailed information about a specific ailment. Each disease or disorder often begins with a listing of common signs and symptoms, followed by a description of the condition and information on how it's often diagnosed. Treatment also is discussed and, when appropriate, information is provided on prevention. Most entries are organized in the format shown on the opposite page.

Part VI: Tests and Treatments

This section can give you a better understanding of the tests commonly used to evaluate your health and identify disease. It also reviews common forms of treatment, including use of medication, surgery and complementary and alternative therapies. In addition, it includes information on various methods to manage pain that may accompany chronic conditions.

Glossary and Resources

At the end of the book is a glossary that contains a comprehensive list of medical, anatomic and health care terms. The glossary is followed by a list of health organizations that may offer additional information on various health concerns.

Index

The detailed index at the end of the book makes it easy for you to access specific topics within the text. The index includes both medical and lay terminology.

Name of disease

Pneumonia

Key signs and symptoms

Signs and symptoms
- Coughing
- Shortness of breath
- Pain in the chest (pleurisy)
- Chills
- Fever

Basic description of the disease

Pneumonia is an inflammation of the tissues of your lungs. Rather than being one specific infection, however, what your doctor calls pneumonia may actually have more than 50 different causes. The results range from a mild condition to a life-threatening illness.

Pneumonia can result from bacteria, such as pneumococci or streptococci, a virus, such as influenza, or a chemical irritant. To make pneumonia more easily understood, the many varieties can be classified into various subtypes.

Community-acquired pneumonia
Community-acquired pneumonia gets its name from the way it's transmitted — in the community at large rather than in a hospital. Common causes include pneumococci and mycoplasma. The influenza virus also can cause pneumonia.

Hospital-acquired pneumonia
This type of pneumonia is acquired in the hospital. The number of potential infecting agents is generally much greater with hospital-acquired pneumonia than with community-acquired pneumonia.

Aspiration pneumonia
Aspiration pneumonia results from bacteria being breathed into the lungs. Usually, this occurs when the contents of your stomach enter your lungs after you've vomited. It can also occur with diseases that interfere with swallowing.

Pneumonia caused by opportunistic organisms
Pneumonia is more likely to strike people with impaired immune systems. Organisms that aren't harmful in healthy people can be extremely dangerous in people with diseases such as AIDS, sickle cell anemia and other conditions that impair the immune system. Medications that suppress your immune system, such as corticosteroids or certain types of chemotherapy for cancer, also increase your risk of opportunistic infections.

Informative illustration

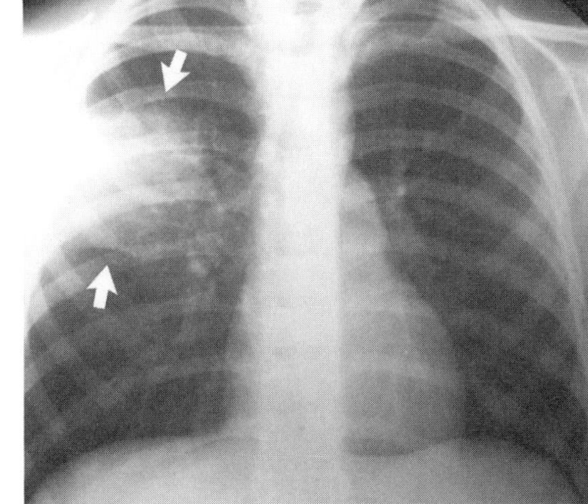

This chest X-ray reveals pneumonia in the upper lobe of the lung (see arrows).

How the disease is diagnosed

Diagnosis
Signs and symptoms of pneumonia vary depending on the type and extent of infection. At first, pneumonia may appear to be a cold or it may develop as a complication of a cold. A fever typically accompanies most types, as does a cough. The cough may be dry or it may produce colored or bloody sputum.

Using a stethoscope, your doctor may detect distortions in the sounds of your breathing that suggest the presence of infection. Chest X-rays also may help identify the location and extent of the infection.

Potential consequences

How serious is pneumonia?
Pneumonia is common, occurring in more than 1 in every 100 people annually. The seriousness of this disorder depends largely on its cause and your overall health.

A healthy person generally has sufficient defense mechanisms to be able to resist or control the invading organism. Susceptibility of pneumonia is increased among individuals whose defense mechanisms are impaired by aging, a chronic illness, alcoholism or the use of immunosuppressant drugs. In older adults and people weakened by another disease, pneumonia can be fatal.

Information on treatment

Treatment
The treatment your doctor recommends depends on the cause of the pneumonia — whether it's a bacterium, virus or other agent — and the severity of your symptoms. If the cause is bacterial, you'll likely receive an antibiotic.

The choice of antibiotic is determined by several factors, including the specific bacteria causing the infection. Hospitalization may be necessary in severe cases.

Information on prevention

PREVENTION TIP

You can reduce your risk of one type of pneumonia with the pneumococcal vaccine. It protects against a common form of the disease that results from the pneumococcus bacteria. For more information on the vaccine, see page 15.

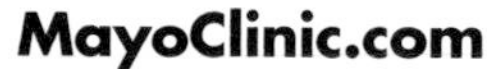

MayoClinic.com

For additional information regarding your health and well-being, visit our Web site, MayoClinic.com, at *www.MayoClinic.com.* In the ever-changing health care environment, MayoClinic.com can provide you with continually updated information about healthy living and disease as well as advances in diagnosis and treatment.

MayoClinic.com is a trusted source for health information whether you have a newly diagnosed condition, are facing a major treatment decision or simply need a healthy recipe for dinner.

As in this book, MayoClinic.com provides trustworthy, practical and easy-to-understand information to help you live well and take charge of your health.

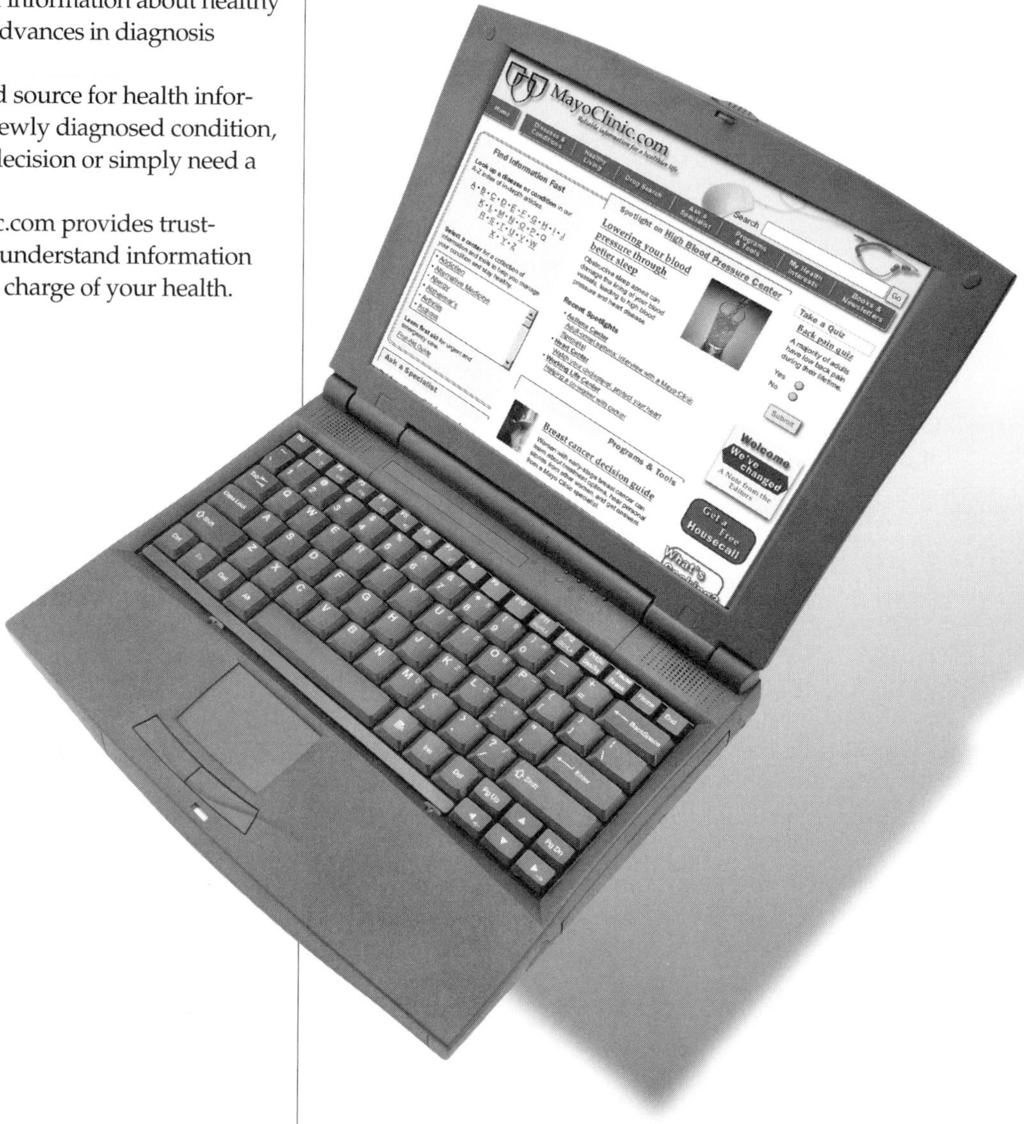

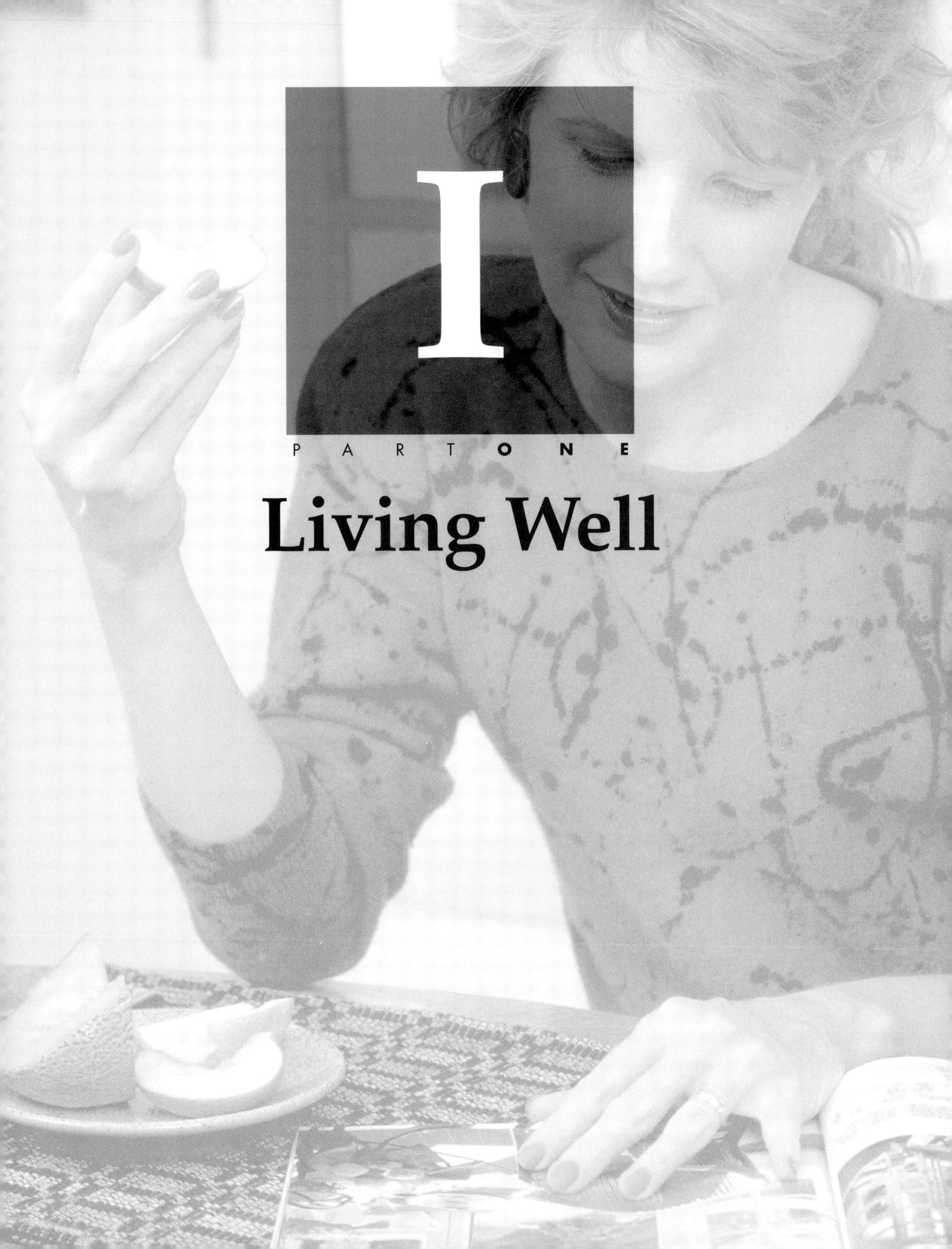

I

PART ONE

Living Well

CHAPTER 1 PART I

Getting Immunized

Prevention is crucial to good health. It's far better to prevent a disease than to treat it. One of the best ways to protect yourself and your family from many diseases is to get vaccinated. *Immunization*, another term for vaccination, is the best line of defense against diseases such as measles (rubeola), mumps, tetanus, hepatitis and polio. Immunization stimulates your body's natural defense mechanisms to resist infectious disease, destroying the virus before you become sick.

Thanks to vaccines, many infectious diseases that were once common in the United States are now rare or nonexistent. Parents no longer have to fear that their children will die of or become disabled by diphtheria, whooping cough (pertussis) or measles. Children don't have to keep away from water fountains and swimming pools to avoid getting polio.

Since coming into widespread use during the 20th century, immunizations have saved billions of lives around the world. However, despite the availability of vaccines, many people remain underimmunized. One reason for this is that some parents have concerns about the safety and risks of vaccines. These concerns are often the result of incorrect information.

How Vaccines Work

Every day, your body is threatened by bacteria, viruses and other germs. When a disease-causing microorganism enters your body, your immune system mounts a defense, producing proteins called antibodies to fight off the invader. The goal of your immune system is to neutralize or destroy the foreign invader, rendering it harmless and preventing you from getting sick.

Understanding immunity

Your body's immune system fights off foreign invaders and protects you from disease in the following two ways:

Post-exposure immunity

Post-exposure immunity develops after you've been exposed to a certain organism. Your immune system puts into play a complex array of defenses to prevent you from getting sick again from that type of virus or bacteria.

Exposure to a foreign invader (antigen) activates the production of certain white blood cells in your body called B cells (B lymphocytes). B cells produce plasma cells, which in turn produce a huge number of antibodies designed specifically to fight that particular invader. These antibodies circulate in your body's fluids, and the next time that invader enters your body, the antibodies recognize it and destroy it. Once your body produces a particular antibody, it can rapidly resume production of more if needed.

In addition to the work of B cells, white blood cells called macrophages confront and destroy foreign invaders. The macrophages "process" the invaders, figuring out if they present a threat. If your body encounters a germ that it has never been exposed to before, information about the germ is relayed to white blood cells called helper T cells. These cells aid in the development of other infection-fighting cells, including memory T cells.

Once you've been exposed to a specific virus or bacterium, the next time you encounter it, antibodies and memory T cells go to work. They immediately react to the organism, attacking it before disease can develop. Your immune system can recognize and effectively combat thousands, if not millions, of different organisms.

Vaccine immunity

Vaccine immunity results from injection of a vaccine. The vaccine

Vaccine Immunity

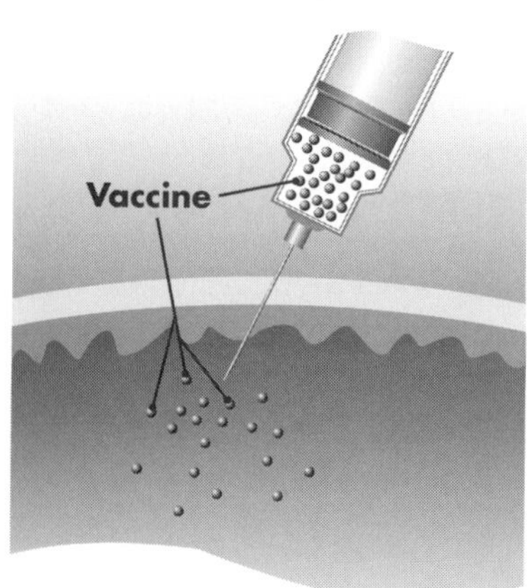

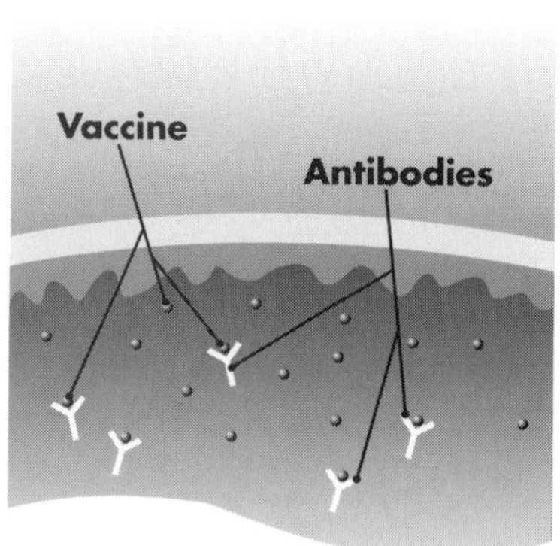

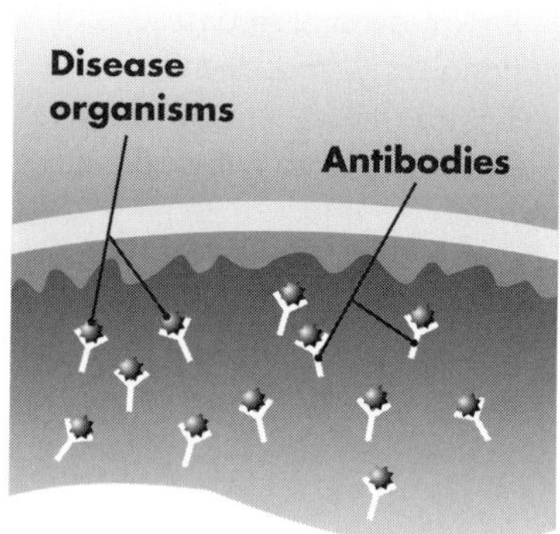

A vaccine with dead or harmless forms of a virus, bacteria or other organism is injected into an individual (left). The vaccine stimulates the immune system to produce antibodies against the organism (center). In any subsequent exposure to this germ, the antibodies attack and stop the infection (right).

triggers your immune system's infection-fighting ability and memory without exposure to the actual disease. A vaccine contains a killed or weakened form or derivative of the infectious germ. When given to an individual who's healthy, the vaccine triggers an immune response. The vaccine makes your body think that it's being invaded by a specific organism, and your immune system goes to work to destroy the invader and prevent it from infecting you again.

If you're exposed to a disease for which you've been vaccinated, the invading germs are met by antibodies prepared to destroy them. The immunity you develop following vaccination is similar to the immunity acquired from natural infection. For some diseases, the vaccine may be better at creating immunity than a natural infection would be. And vaccines can be administered without the risk of the serious effects of disease.

Several doses of a vaccine may be needed for a full immune response. Some people fail to build immunity to the first doses of a vaccine but often respond to later doses. In addition, the immunity provided by some vaccines, such as tetanus and pertussis, isn't lifelong. Because the immune response may decrease over time, you may need another dose of a vaccine (booster shot) to restore or increase your immunity.

Types of vaccines

Vaccines are prepared in several different ways. For each type, the goal is the same — to stimulate an immune response without causing disease.

Live weakened

Some vaccines, such as those for measles, mumps and chickenpox (varicella), use live viruses that have been weakened (attenuated).

Killed or inactivated

Other vaccines use inactivated (killed) bacteria or viruses. The inactivated polio vaccine (IPV) is made this way.

Toxoid

Some types of bacteria cause disease by producing toxins that invade the bloodstream. Toxoid vaccines, such as those for diphtheria and tetanus, use bacterial toxins that have been rendered harmless.

Acellular and subunit

Acellular and subunit vaccines are made by using only part of the virus or bacteria. The hepatitis and *Haemophilus influenzae* type b (Hib) vaccines are made in this way.

Benefits of Vaccines

Because many vaccine-preventable diseases are now uncommon in the United States, some people feel less urgency about getting themselves or their children immunized. Few people have ever seen a case of diphtheria, polio or tetanus. Some may feel that cleanliness and sanitation are enough to prevent disease.

If you wonder if it's necessary to keep up with immunizations, the answer is yes. Many infectious diseases that have virtually disappeared in the United States can reappear quickly. The germs that cause the diseases still exist and can be acquired by people who aren't protected by vaccination. As travelers unknowingly carry disease from one country to another, a new outbreak in the United States may be only a plane trip away. From a single entry point, an infectious disease can spread quickly among unprotected individuals.

The persistent threat of disease is just one reason public health officials recommend vaccinations. Vaccines provide a number of benefits to individuals, communities and the world population.

? Question and Answer

Won't breast-feeding provide my child with natural immunity? Is vaccination necessary?

Proteins in a mother's milk do offer protection against some infections, such as colds, ear infections and diarrhea. This immunity generally lasts for only a month to about a year. And even a child who is breast-fed doesn't acquire immunity from his or her mother against a number of serious contagious diseases, such as whooping cough (pertussis).

Safety

Many people have questions and concerns about vaccine safety. A common fear is that vaccines may trigger serious side effects or even cause disease. Parents may worry after hearing or seeing reports about a severe "reaction" that occurs shortly after a child's immunization visit and is ascribed to a side effect or complication of the vaccine. Such stories about immunization fears frequently circulate on the Internet.

In fact, vaccines are extremely safe. Before they can be used, they must meet strict safety standards set by the Food and Drug Administration (FDA). Meeting these standards requires a lengthy development process of up to 10 years followed by three phases of clinical trials.

Once vaccines are licensed and made available to the general public, the FDA and the Centers for Disease Control and Prevention (CDC) continue to monitor their safety. Furthermore, vaccines are subject to ongoing research, review and refinement by doctors, scientists and public health officials.

Your chances of being harmed by a disease are far greater than your chances of being harmed by a vaccine used to prevent disease.

Effectiveness

Vaccines are highly effective. Most childhood vaccines are effective in 85 percent to 99 percent or more of children who receive them. For example, a full series of measles vaccine protects 99 of 100 children from measles, and a polio vaccine series protects 99 of 100 children from polio.

In some instances a vaccine provides only partial immunity. It doesn't prevent the disease, but it often lessens the duration of the illness and the severity of the symptoms.

> **? Question and Answer**
>
> **Are there times when my child shouldn't be vaccinated?**
>
> In a few circumstances, immunization should be postponed or avoided. Talk to your doctor if you're unsure if your child should be vaccinated.
>
> Immunization may be inappropriate if a child:
>
> - Has had a serious or life-threatening reaction to a previous dose of that vaccine
> - Has a known, significant allergy to a vaccine component, such as chicken eggs or gelatin
> - Has a medical condition, such as AIDS, leukemia or cancer, that has compromised the child's immune system and could allow a live virus vaccine to cause illness
>
> Immunizations may need to be deferred to a later date if a child:
>
> - Has a moderate to severe illness
> - Has taken steroid medications in the last 3 months
> - Has received a transfusion of blood or plasma or been given blood products within the past year
>
> Immunization shouldn't be delayed because a child has a minor illness, such as a common cold, an ear infection or mild diarrhea. The vaccine will still be effective, and it won't make your child sicker.

A reduction in suffering and disability

In addition to being potentially fatal, many infectious diseases can cause permanent harm. Polio can cause paralysis. Meningitis can cause deafness. Measles can cause brain damage and death. Hepatitis can cause liver damage. Vaccines prevent these serious complications.

One example is the *Haemophilus influenzae* type b (Hib) vaccine. Before the vaccine became available in 1987, the bacteria caused about 20,000 serious infections in American infants and children each year. Hib meningitis killed 600 children annually and left many survivors with deafness, seizures or mental retardation. By 2000, immunization had reduced the incidence of Hib disease by 99 percent.

Protection of community health

Immunizing protects not only your or your child's health but also the health of your community. In any community there are a small number of people who shouldn't be vaccinated — for example, individuals who are allergic to an ingredient in a vaccine or who have a condition that precludes certain vaccinations. These people depend on others not passing disease on to them.

If 95 percent of the people in a community are immunized, unprotected individuals are much less likely to be exposed to the germ, so they have a smaller chance of becoming infected. This is called herd immunity.

Eradication of disease worldwide

Immunization protects more than one city, one country and one generation. Its benefits can extend across the world and into the future. The long-term goal of an immunization program is to completely eliminate a disease. At least in one instance, this goal has

Estimated Incidence* of Invasive Hib Disease, 1987-2000

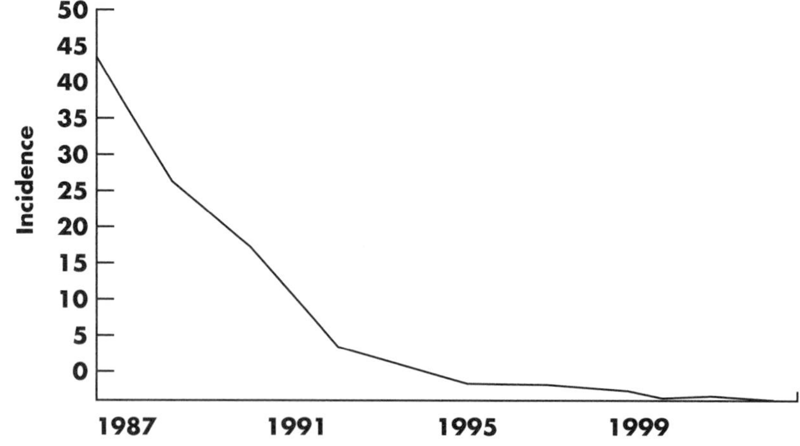

*Rate per 100,000 children <5 years of age

Source: Centers for Disease Control and Prevention

Between 1987 and 2000, the number of Haemophilus influenzae type b (Hib) cases in the United States declined by 99 percent, thanks to the Hib vaccine.

become a reality. The worldwide eradication of smallpox is a success story of modern medicine.

Smallpox was devastating to humankind for centuries. It spread in epidemics and killed as many as 60 percent of its victims. The disease caused severe headache, fever and a red, blistering rash that often left disfiguring scars on its survivors. Up to one-third of people with the disease were blinded from corneal infection.

At the end of the 18th century, Edward Jenner, an English physician, discovered that inoculating individuals with cowpox virus — a virus that's similar to smallpox but usually harmless — prevented them from getting smallpox. Campaigns were launched in the United States and in Europe to immunize people against smallpox. In 1967, the World Health Organization (WHO) launched a global campaign to eliminate smallpox. The last reported case occurred in 1977, signaling the end of one of the deadliest and most feared diseases in history. As a result, smallpox vaccination is no longer necessary. However, the United States does have some vaccine in storage should the smallpox virus ever be used as a weapon of bioterrorism.

The success of the smallpox immunization campaign has encouraged global efforts to eradicate other infectious diseases. Polio has been wiped out from the Western Hemisphere, and the number of cases worldwide has dropped dramatically. Within the United States, vaccines have reduced the incidence of measles by 99 percent and Hib disease by 98 percent. The incidence of diphtheria in the United States dropped from 206,000 cases and 15,520 deaths in 1921 to only 1 reported case in 1999. For future generations, such diseases could become a thing of the past.

Vaccine Additives

In addition to the killed or weakened microorganisms that make up vaccines, small amounts of other substances may be added to enhance the immune response, prevent contamination and stabilize the vaccine against temperature variations and other conditions. Vaccines may also contain small amounts of materials used in the manufacturing process, such as gelatin.

One additive that has received much attention recently is a preservative called thimerosal, which is a derivative of mercury. Thimerosal has been used in medical products since the 1930s and in small amounts in some vaccines to prevent bacterial contamination. No evidence shows that children have been harmed by such mercury use in vaccines. Nonetheless childhood vaccines are now made without thimerosal or with only trace amounts.

Side Effects of Vaccines

Although vaccines are considered very safe, like all drugs they aren't completely free of side effects. Most side effects are minor and temporary, such as a sore arm, a mild fever or swelling at the injection site. Serious reactions, such as a seizure or high fever, are very rare. According to the Centers for Disease Control and Prevention (CDC), serious side effects occur on the order of 1 per thousand to 1 per million of doses. The risk of death from a vaccine is so slight that it can't be accurately determined. When any serious reactions are reported, they receive careful scrutiny from the Food and Drug Administration and the CDC.

Some vaccines have been blamed for chronic illnesses, such as autism or diabetes. But decades of vaccine use in the United States provides no reliable evidence that vaccines cause chronic illness. Researchers have on occasion reported a link between vaccine use and chronic illness. But when other researchers have tried to duplicate those results — a test of good scientific research — they haven't been able to do so.

The belief that vaccines cause autism stems from an article published in 1998 by a group of researchers in Great Britain who reported a link between autism and the measles-mumps-rubella (MMR) vaccine. Since then many other studies have refuted that report, finding no evidence that any vaccine increases the risk of autism or any other behavioral disorder.

Similarly, reports have surfaced in the media and on the Internet linking vaccines to sudden infant death syndrome (SIDS), diabetes, cancer and other serious conditions. No reliable scientific evidence backs up any of these claims.

Weighing the risks and benefits

The consequences of acquiring a disease that can be prevented by immunization are far greater than serious side effects that may result from vaccine use. For example, if your child gets mumps, the risk of developing encephalitis, a

Signs of a Severe Reaction

After vaccination, watch for any unusual conditions, such as a serious allergic reaction, high fever or behavior changes. Signs and symptoms of a serious allergic reaction include difficulty breathing, hoarseness or wheezing, hives, paleness, weakness, a fast heartbeat, dizziness and swelling of the throat. If you think that you or your child may be experiencing a severe reaction, call your doctor or go to the emergency department immediately.

brain inflammation that can cause permanent, serious brain damage, is 1 in 300. For measles the risk is 1 in 2,000. In contrast, the risk of contracting encephalitis from the mumps and measles vaccines is less than 1 in 1 million. If a child gets serious Hib disease, the chances of death are 1 in 20. The vaccine for Hib disease, meanwhile, hasn't been associated with any serious adverse reactions.

You're the final arbiter in deciding what vaccines your child receives. If you have concerns, talk with your child's doctor, who can help you weigh the benefits and risks of immunization.

Well-Child Immunization Schedule

The following chart lists the recommended routine childhood immunizations. Vaccine guidelines for children change fairly often as new vaccines are developed, recommendations on timing and dosages are revised and more combination vaccines are created. Your health care professional will have the latest guidelines.

Health insurance usually covers most of the cost of immunizations. A federal program called Vaccines for Children provides free vaccines to children who lack health insurance coverage and to other specific groups of children. Ask your doctor about it.

Recommended Ages for Routine Childhood Vaccinations

Vaccine ▼ Age ▶	Birth	1 mo.	2 mos.	4 mos.	6 mos.	12 mos.	15 mos.	18 mos.	24 mos.	4-6 yrs.	11-12 yrs.	13-18 yrs.
Hepatitis B (Hep B)[1]	1st	2nd			3rd							
Diptheria, tetanus, pertussis (DTaP)			1st	2nd	3rd		4th			5th		
Haemophilus influenzae type b (Hib)			1st	2nd	3rd	4th						
Inactivated polio vaccine (IPV)			1st	2nd	3rd					4th		
Measles, mumps, rubella (MMR)						1st				2nd		
Chickenpox, or varicella (VZV)						1st						
Pneumococcal conjugate (PCV-7)			1st	2nd	3rd	4th						

Additional Vaccines for High-Risk Children

Vaccine	Birth	1 mo.	2 mos.	4 mos.	6 mos.	12 mos.	15 mos.	18 mos.	24 mos.	4-6 yrs.	11-12 yrs.	13-18 yrs.
Pneumococcal polyvalent (PPV-23)[2]												
Hepatitis A (Hep A)[3]												
Flu (influenza)[4]												

Denotes age range for indicated dose

Any dose not given at the recommended age should be given at a subsequent visit to a health care professional when indicated and feasible. Talk to your child's doctor for the latest information.

1. Infants born to mothers who are actively hepatitis B-positive or mothers whose hepatitis B status is unknown should receive the first dose of vaccine within 12 hours of birth. Infants whose mother is not actively hepatitis B-positive should receive the first dose by age 2 months.
2. Pneumococcal polysaccharide vaccine (PPV-23) is recommended in addition to pneumococcal conjugate vaccine (PCV-7) for certain high-risk groups.
3. Hepatitis A vaccine is recommended for use in selected areas and for certain high-risk groups.
4. Flu (influenza) vaccine is recommended annually for children age 6 months and older with certain risk factors — including but not limited to asthma, heart disease, sickle cell disease and diabetes. The vaccine also is encouraged for healthy children aged 6 to 23 months and others wishing to obtain immunity.

Source: Advisory Committee on Immunization Practices (February 2002).

Childhood Immunizations

Many of the most familiar diseases of childhood — chickenpox, measles, mumps — are highly infectious ailments that can be passed easily from person to person. Fortunately, many of them can be prevented through immunization. For more information on many of the diseases that follow, see Chapter 20, "Infectious Diseases."

Chickenpox (varicella)

Chickenpox (varicella) is a common childhood disease. It can also affect adults who aren't immune. More children in the United States die of this disease than of any other vaccine-preventable disease.

The chickenpox virus is spread by breathing in infected droplets or by direct contact with fluid from the rash, which is the best-known sign of the disease. The rash begins as superficial spots on the face, chest, back and other areas of the body. The spots quickly fill with a clear fluid, rupture and turn crusty.

Recommendation
Children should receive one dose of the chickenpox vaccine between 12 and 18 months of age or at any age after that if they haven't had the disease. People who don't receive the vaccine until 13 years of age or older require two doses 4 to 8 weeks apart.

Diphtheria

Diphtheria is a bacterial infection that spreads from person to person through airborne droplets. It causes a thick covering (membrane) in the back of the throat and can lead to severe breathing problems, paralysis, heart failure and death. The disease is rare in the United States.

Recommendation
The diphtheria vaccine typically is given in combination with the tetanus and pertussis vaccines (a DTaP shot). Immunization should begin when a child reaches 2 months of age. A child should receive five shots in the first 6 years of life and continue to receive boosters of tetanus-diphtheria toxoid (Td), adult type, every 10 years beginning at age 11 or 12.

German measles (rubella)

German measles (rubella), a disease that spreads through the air, is typically a mild infection that causes rash and slight fever. However, if a woman gets rubella during pregnancy, she may have a miscarriage, or the baby could be born with severe birth defects.

Recommendation
Usually, two doses of the combination

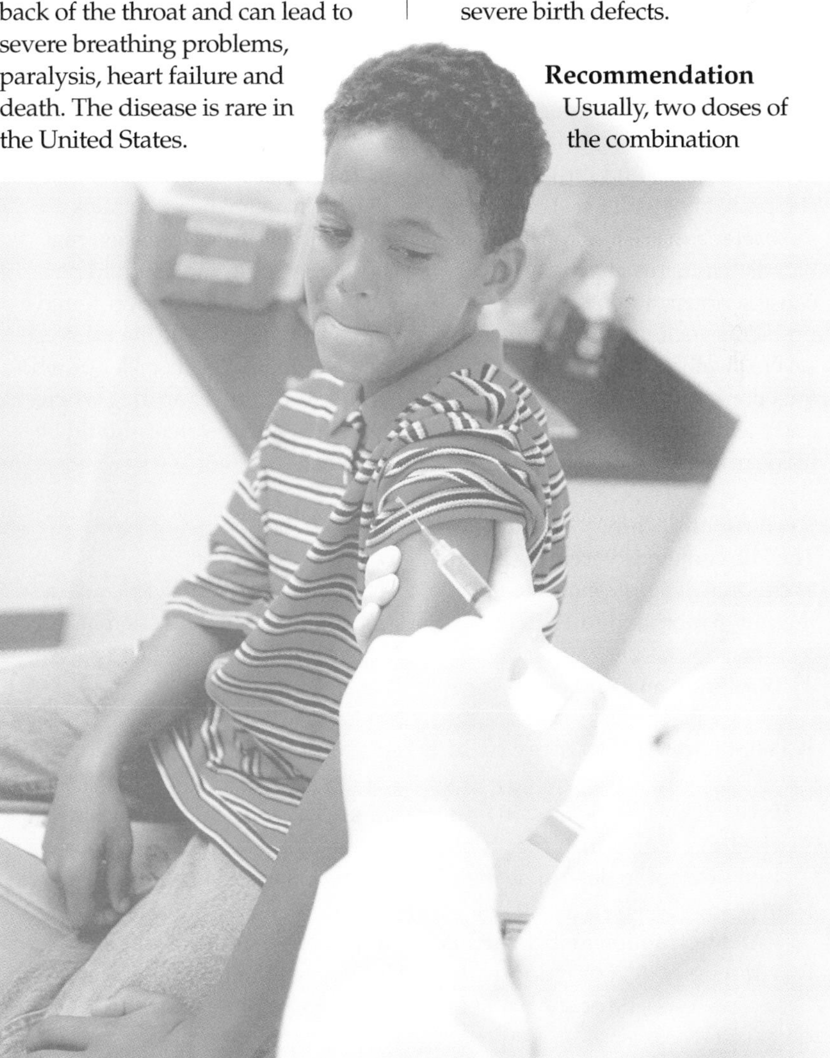

Minimizing the Trauma of Shots

Most kids dread getting a shot. Here are a few tips to help ease your child's fear and discomfort:

- Be honest. Children who know in advance that they're going to get a shot tend to do better than kids who aren't told beforehand. On the day of the appointment, tell your child that he or she will feel a little prick like a tiny bee sting and that it will hurt for only a few seconds but it will help prevent him or her from getting a bad sickness.
- Hold your child and talk with him or her while the shot is being given.
- Teach your child to focus on other things during the vaccination process.
- Give reinforcement afterward: "You did a really good job."

measles-mumps-rubella (MMR) vaccine are given, the first at ages 12 months to 15 months and the second at ages 4 to 6 years. In the event this schedule isn't followed, girls should receive the live weakened (attenuated) vaccine before their first period to avoid the risk of contracting rubella during pregnancy. Live attenuated vaccines aren't recommended for pregnant women or some individuals with immune systems impaired from diseases such as human immunodeficiency virus (HIV), AIDS or cancer. After receiving this vaccine, women should avoid pregnancy for 30 days.

Haemophilus influenzae type b disease

Haemophilus influenzae type b (Hib) disease is primarily a childhood illness, but it can also affect some adults. It's caused by bacteria that spread from person to person through the air. If the bacteria stay in a child's nose and throat, he or she probably won't get sick. But if the bacteria move into the lungs or bloodstream, this infection can cause serious and potentially fatal problems, including pneumonia, severe swelling in the throat and infections of the blood, joints, bones and membrane around the heart (pericarditis).

Recommendation
The Hib conjugate vaccine is given to children at ages 2 months, 4 months, 6 months and 12 to 15 months. The vaccine typically is given at the same time as other vaccines. Children over 5 years of age usually don't need Hib vaccine. But some older children and adults with special health conditions should receive it. Such people include those with sickle cell disease, human immunodeficiency virus (HIV), AIDS or no spleen, and those who have undergone a bone marrow transplant or cancer treatment.

Hepatitis A

Hepatitis A is a liver disease caused by the hepatitis A virus. It's usually spread by eating or drinking contaminated food or water or by close personal contact.

Recommendation
The two-dose series of the hepatitis A vaccine is recommended for children who live in a state, county or community where the rates of hepatitis A are at least twice the national average (typically Western states). In addition, children who live in an area where the rates are greater than the national average but not twice as high should be considered for vaccination. Children who have chronic liver disease or a clotting factor disorder or who will be traveling to an area where hepatitis A is prevalent should be vaccinated.

Hepatitis B

The hepatitis B virus can cause a short-term (acute) illness marked by loss of appetite, fatigue, diarrhea, vomiting, jaundice and pain in muscles, joints and the abdomen. More rarely it can lead to long-term (chronic) liver damage (cirrhosis) or liver cancer.

The virus is spread through contact with the blood or other body fluids of an infected person. This can happen by having unprotected sex, sharing needles when injecting illegal drugs, or during birth, when the virus passes from an infected mother to her baby. However, over one-third of people who have hepatitis B in the United States don't know how they got it.

Recommendation
The hepatitis B vaccine is given to children in three doses — at birth to 2 months, at least 1 month later (1 to 4 months of age) and then at 6 to 18 months. The hepatitis B vaccine is usually given at the same time as other vaccines.

Measles (rubeola)

Measles (rubeola) is primarily a childhood illness, although adults also are susceptible. It's the most contagious human virus known. The measles virus is transmitted through the air in droplets, such as from a sneeze.

Signs and symptoms include fever, cough, sneezing, runny nose, eye irritation and a sore throat. Measles can lead to an ear infection, pneumonia, seizures, brain damage and death.

Recommendation
A live, weakened measles vaccine is given to children at 12 to 15 months of age, usually in combination with mumps and rubella vaccines (MMR). A second dose is given at 4 to 6 years of age. If the immunization schedule is missed, older children and adults can be safely inoculated with a live vaccine.

Children who have leukemia or another severe illness and are receiving radiation, steroid or antimetabolite therapy shouldn't be

? **Question and Answer**

What should I do if my child misses a vaccination?

If your child falls behind on immunizations, catch-up immunization schedules can address the problem. Make an appointment with your child's doctor to determine the vaccinations your child needs and when he or she should receive them.

An interruption in the schedule usually doesn't require a child to start a series over or redo any doses. Until your child receives the entire vaccine series, he or she won't have maximum possible protection against diseases.

PREVENTION TIP

Some vaccines cause minor, temporary side effects, such as a mild fever or sore arm. To minimize these effects, you can take acetaminophen (Tylenol, others) before or after vaccination. Follow the label instructions for the correct dose. You can also use an ice pack on the injection site to reduce redness and swelling.

vaccinated. In general, vaccines made from live, attenuated viruses or bacteria are not given to people whose immune systems are impaired because of the small chance that the weakened virus in the vaccine could cause disease.

Meningococcal disease

Meningococcal disease is caused by the bacterium *Neisseria meningitidis*. Serious complications of the disease include blood infection (septicemia) and meningitis, an infection of the brain and spinal cord coverings. Meningococcal disease can result in deafness, nervous system problems, seizures, strokes, mental retardation and death.

Meningococcal disease is most common in infants under 1 year of age and in people with certain medical conditions. In addition, first-year college students, particularly those who live in dormitories, are at increased risk of getting the disease.

Recommendation

The vaccine isn't routinely recommended for children, but it's offered to students before they start college so that they can reduce their risk of getting meningococcal disease. Some colleges are now requiring or at least recommending the vaccine.

Mumps

Mumps is a childhood disease that can also occur in adults. Mumps is caused by a virus that's acquired by inhaling infected droplets. The disease causes fever, headache, fatigue and swollen, painful salivary glands. It can lead to deafness, meningitis and inflammation of the testicles or ovaries, with the possibility of sterility.

Recommendation

Typically, two doses of a combined measles-mumps-rubella (MMR) vaccination are given, the first at ages 12 to 15 months and the second at 4 to 6 years of age. Adult females who receive the immunization should avoid pregnancy for 30 days afterward. Use of this vaccine has markedly decreased the incidence of mumps in the United States.

Pneumococcal disease

Pneumococcal disease is the leading cause of bacterial meningitis and ear infections among children under 5 years old. It also causes blood infections and pneumonia. Children under age 2 are at the highest risk of the most serious consequences of this disease.

Pneumococcal disease is caused by *Streptococcus pneumoniae* bacteria. The bacteria spread from person to person through physical contact or by inhaling infected droplets. Because many strains of the bacteria have become resistant to several antibiotics, the disease can be difficult to treat.

Recommendation

Pneumococcal conjugate vaccine (PCV) can help prevent serious pneumococcal disease. It can also prevent one cause of ear infections. The vaccine is given to all children in four doses between ages 2 and 15 months. It's also recommended for children between ages 2 and 5 years who haven't had pneumococcal vaccine and are at high risk of the disease. This includes children without a spleen and children who have sickle cell disease, chronic heart or lung disease, human immunodeficiency virus (HIV), AIDS or other diseases that may affect the immune system, such as cancer or diabetes. Children who take medications that affect the immune system, such as chemotherapy or steroids, also should be vaccinated.

In addition to PCV, pneumococcal polysaccharide vaccine (PPV) is recommended for certain high-risk

? Question and Answer

Does my child need a flu shot?

The flu (influenza) vaccine, which is updated every year, is safe for children 6 months or older. The vaccine is encouraged for healthy children aged 6 to 23 months. Children at high risk of getting the flu also should be vaccinated against the disease. Children are at high risk if they:

- Have asthma or another chronic lung condition
- Have cardiovascular disease
- Are taking a medication that suppresses their immune system
- Have sickle cell disease, human immunodeficiency virus (HIV), AIDS, diabetes, chronic kidney disease, chronic metabolic disease

If your child isn't at high risk of getting the flu but lives with someone who is — an individual with chronic lung or cardiovascular disease or a compromised immune system — you may want to have your child vaccinated. That way the child will be less likely to infect others. You also may get the flu vaccine for your child, just to reduce the chance that your child will get the flu.

individuals. A first dose may be given as early as age 2 years, and a second dose may be recommended 5 years later. In children at highest risk of severe pneumococcal infection, the second dose may be recommended after 3 years if the revaccination would take place before the child has reached age 10.

Polio

Polio is caused by a virus (poliovirus) that enters the body through the mouth. Polio affects the brain and spinal cord, often resulting in paralysis or death. Polio vaccination began in the United States in 1955.

No polio cases have been reported in this country for more than 20 years, but the disease is still common in some parts of the world, and the virus could be brought into the United States. For that reason getting children vaccinated against polio continues to be important.

There are two types of polio vaccines:

- Oral polio vaccine (OPV) contains a weakened version of the live poliovirus. OPV is taken by mouth in liquid form.
- Inactivated polio vaccine (IPV) contains the chemically killed virus. IPV is given by multiple injections.

Recommendation

In the United States, only IPV is used. It's given in four doses, at ages 2 months, 4 months, 6 to 18 months and at about age 5 years. This last one is a booster dose. OPV is used in countries where polio epidemics still occur. Although both vaccines work well, OPV provides better protection against epidemics. However, because OPV contains live poliovirus, it can cause polio in very rare instances — 1 case per 2.4 million doses. For that reason, and because the risk of getting polio in the United States is now low due to high vaccination rates, OPV is no longer used in the United States. The IPV polio shot can't cause polio.

> **? Question and Answer**
>
> **Is it safe to give multiple vaccines at once? Isn't that a lot for a child's immune system to handle?**
>
> Some immunizations for children are given in a mixed shot, such as those for measles, mumps and rubella (MMR) and those for diphtheria, tetanus and pertussis (DTaP). In addition, the recommended schedule for immunizing children involves giving up to four vaccines at the same time.
>
> Many parents worry that the baby's immune system will be overloaded, with damaging effects. But a child isn't harmed by receiving more than one immunization at a time. Consider that every day children survive exposure to many different germs. For example, a strep throat infection exposes a child to more than 100 different antigens.
>
> A large number of studies show that simultaneous immunization with multiple vaccines is convenient, safe and effective. Giving several vaccinations at once means fewer office visits, which saves time and money for parents and may be less traumatic for the child. It also helps meet the goal of immunizing children as early as possible to protect them during the vulnerable early months of their lives.

Tetanus

Tetanus causes painful tightening of the muscles, usually all over the body. It can be difficult to open your mouth (lockjaw) or swallow. Tetanus isn't a contagious disease. The tetanus bacteria enter the body through deep or dirty cuts or wounds.

Recommendation

The tetanus vaccine typically is given in combination with those for diphtheria and pertussis (DTaP vaccine). Immunization should be started when a child reaches 2 months of age and is given in a series of five shots in the first 6 years of life.

Starting at age 11 or 12, people should continue to get vaccinated every 10 years with the adult form of the tetanus-diphtheria (Td) toxoid vaccine.

Whooping cough (pertussis)

Whooping cough (pertussis) is a disease that causes severe coughing spells, making it hard for infants and toddlers to eat, drink or even breathe. The word *pertussis* is from the Latin word for "cough." These coughing spells can last for weeks and can lead to pneumonia, seizures, brain damage and death. Severe whooping cough primarily occurs in children younger than 2 years and is contracted by inhaling infected droplets, often coughed into the air from an adult with a mild case of the disease.

Recommendation

The DTaP immunization combines vaccines for diphtheria, tetanus and pertussis. It's given as a series of five shots beginning when the infant is 2 months old and continuing to between ages 4 and 6. The DTaP vaccine is a better-tolerated version of an older vaccine called DTP. The *a* stands for "acellular," meaning that only specific parts of the pertussis bacteria are used in the vaccine.

The older pertussis vaccine contained whole, killed pertussis bacteria. This vaccine was associated with a higher incidence of reactions such as persistent crying and high fever. DTP is no longer used in the United States.

Flu (Influenza) Shots

Flu (influenza) vaccine protects against influenza types A and B viruses. Type C is less common and usually causes only a mild illness. Therefore it isn't included in the vaccine.

Because influenza viruses change (mutate) often, the influenza vaccine is updated each year to ensure it's as effective as possible. The Food and Drug Administration consults with disease experts worldwide 6 to 9 months before flu season to decide which strains of the virus will be used to make a particular year's vaccine. This decision is based on which viruses are most likely to circulate in the United States during the upcoming flu season.

The vaccine is made from highly purified, egg-grown viruses that have been inactivated. Because the viruses in the vaccine are killed, you can't get influenza from the vaccine. The vaccine is given as one injection, usually into the upper arm muscles. Children under 9 years of age receive the vaccine the first time as two shots, 1 month apart. It takes about 2 weeks for the vaccine to protect you, and the protection may last up to a year. Getting immunized doesn't guarantee that you won't get the flu, but if you do get it, the illness should be less severe and there's less risk of hospitalization or death due to influenza complications. Because the virus changes so rapidly, you need a new shot each year.

The vaccine may cause some soreness at the injection site. A small percentage of people run a slight fever and have minor generalized muscle aches 6 to 24 hours after immunization. These symptoms may last 1 or 2 days.

Severe reactions are rare. Because of the possibility of having another allergic reaction, people who have had a serious allergic reaction to chicken eggs or to a previous dose of flu vaccine should talk to their doctor about whether they can be immunized. If you're pregnant, wait until after your third month before being vaccinated, although the vaccine is considered safe at any stage of pregnancy.

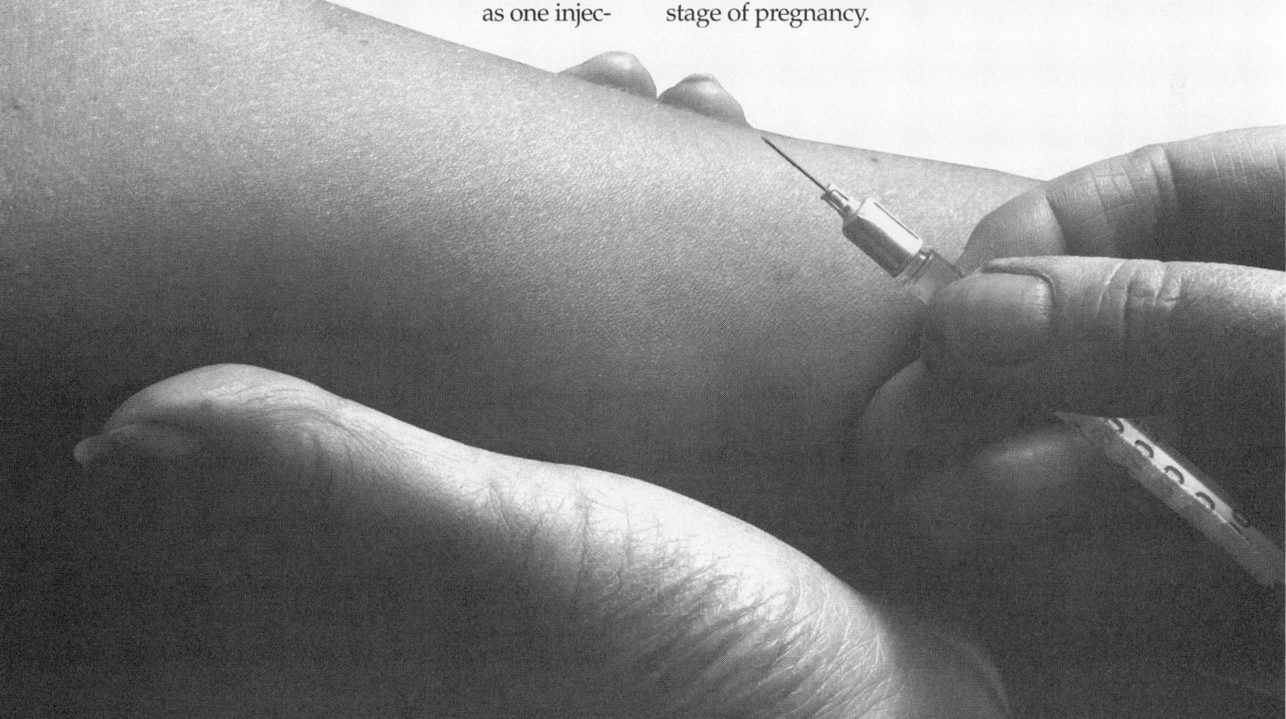

Adult Immunizations

Many adults believe that the need for immunization ends with childhood. They assume that the vaccines they received as children will protect them for the rest of their lives. This is partly true, but:

- Some adults were never vaccinated as children.
- Newer vaccines weren't available when some adults were children.
- Immunity can decrease over time.
- With age you become more susceptible to infectious diseases, such as pneumonia and the flu.

Each year 20,000 or more Americans die of diseases that could've been prevented by routine adult vaccinations. Often the reason is lack of awareness that the shots are needed. A number of vaccines are recommended for adults. The ones you may need depend on your health, medical history and risk of exposure to various illnesses.

Chickenpox (varicella)

Chickenpox (varicella) is a viral disease that spreads from person to person by inhaling infected respiratory droplets from the air or by physical contact with fluid from the chickenpox rash. The illness is much more serious in adults than in children.

Recommendation
If you've never had chickenpox or been vaccinated against the disease, consider getting the two-dose varicella immunization series. But don't get immunized if you've had a serious allergic reaction to gelatin or the antibiotic neomycin, both ingredients in the vaccine.

Flu (influenza)

Flu (influenza) is a highly contagious viral respiratory disease that spreads through the air. It's different from the common cold or the so-called stomach flu. It's a disease caused by one of three types of viruses — influenza A, B and C. People most at risk of developing serious complications from the disease are older adults and individuals with weakened immunity. Influenza causes at least 10,000 deaths a year in the United States.

Recommendation
Adults age 50 and older and individuals at high risk should get an annual vaccination. However, anyone can request vaccination to reduce the risk of getting the flu. You may be at increased risk of complications if you:

- Are living in a long-term-care facility or nursing home, no matter what your age
- Have a serious, long-term health condition, such as heart disease, lung disease (including asthma), metabolic disease (including diabetes), kidney disease or anemia
- Have an impaired immune system because of the human immunodeficiency virus (HIV), AIDS or other diseases that affect the immune system, or because of medications that weaken the immune system, such as steroids or chemotherapy
- Will be pregnant during the flu season
- Are a health care or public safety worker who provides care or service to people at high risk
- Live with people at high risk

Hepatitis A

Hepatitis A is a liver disease caused by the hepatitis A virus. It's usually spread by eating or drinking contaminated food or water or by close personal contact.

Recommendation
The two-dose series of the hepatitis A vaccine is recommended for people who live in or will be traveling to places where the disease is prevalent. This vaccination is also recommended for people who have chronic liver disease, have a clotting factor disorder, use illegal drugs or are male and homosexual. Some food handlers or food service workers and child care center workers may want to be vaccinated. The vaccination isn't recommended if you're hypersensitive to alum or 2-phenoxyethanol, a preservative.

A combination hepatitis A and B vaccine is available for adults who are at high risk of being exposed to both viruses. It's given in three doses, which is less than the five doses needed if the two vaccines are given separately.

Hepatitis B

Hepatitis B is a viral liver disease that's spread by infected blood, sexual contact and prenatal exposure. More than one-third of all cases have no known risk factor. The disease can result in liver damage or liver cancer.

Recommendation
The vaccination, administered in three doses, is recommended for the following groups:

- Adolescents who haven't been vaccinated
- Health care workers and public safety workers who might be exposed to blood and body fluids
- People who inject illegal drugs
- Sexual partners of people with hepatitis B
- People who are sexually active with multiple partners
- Men who have sex with other men
- People on kidney dialysis
- Certain international travelers

A combination hepatitis A and B vaccine is available for adults who are at high risk of being exposed to both the hepatitis A and hepatitis B viruses. It's given in three doses, which is less than the five doses needed if the two vaccines are given separately.

Lyme disease

Lyme disease is a bacterial infection spread by the bite of an infected deer tick. The disease is most common in northeastern and north central United States and in parts of California.

A vaccine — Lymerix — was developed for the disease but was pulled off the market in 2002 by its manufacturer, who cited low demand for the product. Other vaccines may eventually be developed. If you live in an area where Lyme disease is a concern, talk to your doctor about what prevention methods may be appropriate for you.

Measles, mumps and rubella

Measles, mumps and rubella (German measles) are infectious viral diseases that can cause serious complications in adults. The viruses are spread from person to person through airborne droplets that are inhaled.

Recommendation
Anyone 18 years of age or older who was born after 1956 and does not have documentation showing that they have had either measles, mumps or rubella or the vaccines for those diseases should be immunized. One or two shots are recommended, especially for people who are in college, in a health care pro-

fession or are traveling in a foreign country. The vaccination isn't recommended for people who are pregnant, have an impaired immune system or are allergic to the antibiotic neomycin. After receiving the immunization, women should avoid pregnancy for 30 days.

Meningococcal disease

Meningococcal disease is caused by *Neisseria meningitidis* bacteria. It can cause blood infection (septicemia) and meningitis, an infection of the brain and spinal cord coverings. Meningococcal disease can result in deafness, nervous system problems, seizures, strokes, mental retardation and death.

Recommendation

Vaccination for meningococcal disease isn't routinely recommended for the general population. It's recommended for at-risk people during an outbreak, for someone who has a compromised immune system because of lack of a functioning spleen, and for travelers to countries where meningococcal disease is a concern. Because first-year college students, particularly those who live in dormitories, are at increased risk of getting the disease, they should consider getting vaccinated before starting college.

Pneumococcal disease

Pneumococcal disease is a serious bacterial infection that can cause pneumonia, bloodstream infections, ear infections, sinusitis and meningitis. The disease is most serious in older adults and individuals who are chronically ill.

Recommendation

Adults age 65 and older should get the pneumococcal polysaccharide

Adult Immunization Recommendations

Vaccine	Recommendation
Chickenpox, or varicella (VZV)	Two-dose series for any adult who hasn't had chickenpox or been vaccinated against it.
Flu (influenza)	Every year for people age 50 and older and others at high risk.
Hepatitis A (Hep A)	Two-dose series for travelers and people in high-risk groups.
Hepatitis B (Hep B)	Three-dose series for high-risk groups, health care workers and others who might be exposed to infected blood or body fluids.
Measles, mumps, rubella (MMR)	One or two doses for adults who were born after 1956 and don't have proof of previous immunization or infection.
Meningococcal	One dose for people with a compromised immune system and for travelers to certain countries. First-year college students are at increased risk of meningococcal disease and should consider vaccination.
Pneumococcal polysaccharide vaccine (PPV-23)	Age 65 and older or adults of any age with a medical condition that increases the risk of infection. People with health problems and those who received their first shot before age 65 may need a second shot.
Tetanus-diphtheria (Td) toxoid	Booster every 10 years for most people, and as soon as possible after getting a deep or dirty wound.

Who Should Avoid Live Vaccines?

Live, weakened (attenuated) vaccines usually are derived from the naturally occurring germ. They're made by passing the virus or bacteria through cell cultures over time until the germ's disease-causing ability has deteriorated. Live attenuated vaccines can infect people, but they typically don't cause serious disease. These vaccines include:

- Measles vaccine
- Mumps vaccine
- Rubella vaccine
- Chickenpox (varicella) vaccine

There's a very slight risk that live attenuated vaccines could cause disease if a person's immune system is weakened. For this reason, live attenuated vaccines aren't recommended for certain groups of people, including pregnant women and people with an impaired immune system. Women who get a live attenuated vaccine are advised to avoid pregnancy for 1 to 3 months afterward.

Check with your doctor before getting one of these vaccines if you:

- Have human immunodeficiency virus (HIV), AIDS or another disease that affects your immune system
- Are being treated with drugs that affect the immune system, such as steroids, for 2 weeks or longer
- Have any kind of cancer
- Are receiving treatment for cancer with chemotherapy or radiation
- Recently had a blood transfusion or received other blood products
- Have tuberculosis

vaccine (PPV). It's also recommended for adults of any age who:

- Have a chronic, high-risk medical condition, such as diabetes or heart, lung or kidney disease
- Have an impaired immune system
- Have had their spleen removed
- Live in a nursing home or long-term-care facility
- Have received an organ transplant

People age 65 and older who are generally healthy may need only one shot. Those who received their first shot before age 65 may need a 5-year booster shot. You can get a pneumococcal vaccination any time of the year, but it's often convenient to get it when you receive your flu shot.

Tetanus and diphtheria

Tetanus, also known as lockjaw, is a bacterial infection that develops in contaminated wounds. Diphtheria is primarily a bacterial throat infection spread by breathing infected droplets from the air.

Recommendation

It's reasonable for adults to get a tetanus-diphtheria (Td) toxoid booster shot every 10 years. If you have a deep or dirty wound, you may need a booster shot if your last Td vaccination was more than 5 years ago. If you've never had a tetanus shot, you may need a three-dose series. ■

CHAPTER 2 PART I

Eating Right

Whether you eat to live or live to eat, you no doubt take some interest in food. It's one of the great pleasures of life and a life-giving essential. Food is so important that from the beginning of recorded history, it has formed the basis for rituals in every society.

The food you eat is the source of energy and nutrition for your body. Getting enough food is rarely a problem for most Americans, but good nutrition can be a challenge. Many chronic diseases, including cardiovascular disease, diabetes, osteoporosis and cancer, are in part caused by eating too much of the wrong foods and not enough of the right ones.

According to the U.S. Surgeon General, dietary factors and physical inactivity contribute to more than 300,000 deaths each year. The number of people who are overweight is increasing, especially among children. Being overweight increases your risk of developing several diseases.

For these reasons, eating well and maintaining a healthy weight are crucial components of a healthy lifestyle. The decisions you make every day about selecting and preparing food affect how you feel and how well you'll live in the years ahead. To feel good, ward off disease and perform at a peak level, you need to eat a nutritionally balanced diet.

Contrary to popular opinion, eating more healthfully doesn't have to require drastic changes in your diet. To eat well, you don't have to give up your favorite foods or spend a lot of time poring over new recipes, scrutinizing labels and searching out exotic foods. For most people, a few small changes can make a big difference in their health.

This chapter provides an overview of the basics of good nutrition, as well as the recommended dietary guidelines for all Americans. It looks at a number of healthy eating plans and discusses the role of diet in preventing and managing certain diseases. By applying the principles outlined in this chapter to your daily eating habits, you should be able to maintain a healthy weight, keep your energy up and get the nutrients you need.

Nutrition Basics

No single food provides all of the nutrients that your body needs to meet its energy needs. Eating a variety of foods ensures that you get the nutrients and other substances associated with good health.

A healthy diet is one that emphasizes vegetables, fruits, whole grains and lean sources of protein, including dried beans, fish, low-fat dairy products and lean meats. Such foods optimize nutrition and help promote a healthy weight. Simply by eating more plant-based foods — grains, fruits, vegetables and legumes — you can add more variety and health-enhancing nutrients to your diet.

Nutrition isn't the only reason to add variety. Choosing among many flavors, colors and textures in food also boosts your satisfaction and pleasure. If, for example, your fruit choice is limited to bananas, you're missing out on the sensual delights of other fruits — blackberries, kiwis and mangoes, to name a few.

Learning more about how your body uses the nutrients that different foods provide can help you better understand how eating patterns affect your health.

Key nutrients

Every day your body requires a certain amount of energy to function properly. Energy is provided by the major nutrients in foods — carbohydrates, proteins and fats. Other components of food are needed in much smaller amounts. These include essential amino acids, fatty acids, minerals and vitamins. Each food component has a different function in the regulation, growth and repair of your body's cells.

Carbohydrates

Carbohydrates are your body's main energy source — the primary fuel for your cells. Carbohydrates are starches or sugars. Starches — which are found primarily in bread, rice, pasta, cereals, fruits and vegetables — are known as complex carbohydrates. Sugars — found in fruits, milk and foods made with sugar, such as candy and other sweets — are called simple carbohydrates. Digestion changes complex carbohydrates into simple sugars, the fuel your body uses.

Approximately 55 percent to 65 percent of your daily calories should come from carbohydrates. Try to get most of them from complex carbohydrates. Cane or beet sugar (sucrose) and corn syrup (which contains fructose) make up a considerable portion of the average American diet. Unlike complex carbohydrates and simple sugars found in milk and fruits, they contain no significant nutrients.

Fiber

Fiber is the part of plant foods that your body doesn't absorb. The two types of fiber are soluble and insoluble. Fiber-rich foods usually contain both kinds. Some foods are higher in soluble fiber. These include citrus fruits, strawberries, apples, legumes, oatmeal and oat bran. Insoluble fiber is found in wheat bran, whole-grain breads, pasta, cereals and many vegetables. Whole grains that haven't had their bran removed — such as whole-wheat flour — are better sources of fiber than are refined grains, such as white flour.

Soluble fiber may help lower blood cholesterol and blood sugar levels. Insoluble fiber holds on to water and provides bulk to stool, helping to prevent constipation.

You need 20 to 35 grams of fiber each day. Most people eat about half this amount.

Protein

Your body needs protein to make and maintain tissues such as muscles and organs. Protein is composed of building blocks called amino acids. Your body naturally produces some — but not all — amino acids. Those that must be obtained from the foods you eat are called essential amino acids.

You can get protein from a variety of sources. Grains and vegetables supply small amounts of protein. A plant-based diet that includes a wide variety of grains, legumes, vegetables, nuts and seeds can meet your daily protein needs. Meat, seafood, poultry, eggs, soy products and dairy products are the richest sources of protein. You don't need to eat large amounts to obtain essential amino acids. About 12 percent of your daily calories should come from protein.

Fat

Fat is your most concentrated energy source. Some fat in your diet is necessary for your body to function properly. Too much fat, however, can have a negative effect on your health.

Fat is a natural component of various foods, and it comes in different forms. It's found in foods of animal origin, such as meat, poultry and fish, and in foods of vegetable origin, such as avocados and olives.

Chemists classify fat according to the molecular structure of its building blocks, called fatty acids. Those that your body can't make are termed essential. They must be supplied by the foods you eat. Other types of fatty acids are saturated and unsaturated. Unsaturated fat is further subdivided into monounsaturated and polyunsaturated.

Many foods contain a mixture of fatty acids in various proportions. For example, although olive oil is termed a monounsaturated fat, it also contains small proportions of both saturated and polyunsaturated fatty acids.

Try to limit total fat to no more than 30 percent of your daily calories and saturated fat to no more than 10 percent of your daily calories.

Saturated fat

Saturated fat is usually solid or waxy at room temperature. It's less likely to turn rancid, which is why it's used in many processed foods that must withstand long storage times. Foods high in saturated fat include butter, cheese, whole milk, cream, chocolate, coconut oil, palm oil, lard and solid shortenings. Meat — including beef, pork and lamb — can be high in fat, most of it saturated. In poultry, most of the fat is found in the skin.

Polyunsaturated fat

Polyunsaturated fat is usually liquid at room temperature and in the refrigerator. Foods high in this type of fat include vegetable oils, such as safflower, corn, sunflower, soy and cottonseed oils.

Monounsaturated fat

Monounsaturated fat is liquid at room temperature but begins to solidify in the refrigerator. Foods high in monounsaturated fat are olive, peanut and canola oils, avocados and most nuts.

Trans fat

Trans fat comes from adding hydrogen to vegetable oil through a process called hydrogenation. This makes the fat more solid and less likely to spoil. Hydrogenated fat is a common ingredient in commercial baked goods and other processed foods. Most margarines and shortenings also are high in trans fat.

Water

Water seems so ordinary that you may forget how vital it is to health. Water plays an important role in nearly every major body function. It regulates body temperature,

Fat and Blood Cholesterol

Different types of dietary fat have different effects on blood cholesterol. Your total blood cholesterol level can be divided into two major parts: low-density lipoprotein (LDL) cholesterol — commonly referred to as the "bad" cholesterol — and high-density lipoprotein (HDL) cholesterol — commonly referred to as the "good" cholesterol. LDL cholesterol is deposited in your arteries, narrowing them and increasing your risk of cardiovascular diseases, such as a heart attack. HDL cholesterol removes cholesterol deposits from your artery walls, reducing your risk of cardiovascular disease.

Saturated fat raises your total blood cholesterol level, primarily by increasing LDL cholesterol. Monounsaturated fat tends to lower LDL cholesterol while keeping your HDL cholesterol from dropping. Polyunsaturated fat tends to reduce your total blood cholesterol level, but at the expense of the protective HDL cholesterol. The effects of trans fat are less clear. It's thought to have adverse effects on blood fats, increasing LDL cholesterol and decreasing HDL cholesterol.

Effects of Fats on Blood Cholesterol Levels

Type of fat	Total cholesterol	LDL cholesterol	HDL cholesterol
Saturated fat	increases	increases	no effect
Monounsaturated fat	lowers	lowers	protects
Polyunsaturated fat	lowers	lowers	lowers

In your daily diet, consume mainly monounsaturated fats, such as olive or canola oil. Avoid or limit saturated fats and trans fats. Most saturated fat comes from foods such as meat and dairy products.

carries nutrients and oxygen to cells and removes wastes. Water also cushions joints and helps protect organs and tissues.

Most adults need to drink six to eight glasses of water daily for proper hydration. Some circumstances call for more water, such as when you're sweating on a hot day, exercising vigorously or breastfeeding. Young children and adults of advanced age may not sense thirst, so it's important to offer them beverages regularly.

You can meet part of your water requirement with fluids such as milk, juice and soup. Beverages containing caffeine or alcohol can have a dehydrating effect and shouldn't count toward your daily water intake.

To increase your consumption of water:

- Take water breaks instead of coffee breaks.
- Bring bottled water when traveling, and keep a bottle with you at work.
- Drink a glass of water with meals and snacks.
- Substitute sparkling water for alcoholic drinks at social gatherings.

Vitamins

Vitamins are essential to life. They play a role in many body functions. Vitamins enable your body to process proteins, carbohydrates and fat. Certain vitamins also help produce blood cells, hormones, genetic material and nervous system chemicals. Your body is unable to synthesize adequate amounts of most vitamins, so you need to get them from the foods you eat.

The 14 essential vitamins are divided into two categories: fat-soluble and water-soluble.

Fat-soluble

The fat-soluble vitamins are A, D, E and K. They're stored in body fat. Vitamins A and D are also stored in the liver, and reserve supplies may last as long as 6 months. Reserves of vitamin K, however, may be sufficient for only a few days, and the supply of vitamin E is somewhere in between. Because they're stored, excess fat-soluble vitamins can accumulate in your body to toxic levels. Your body is especially sensitive to too much of vitamins A and D.

Water-soluble

The water-soluble vitamins include C, choline, biotin and the seven B vitamins. They're stored in the body to a lesser extent than fat-soluble vitamins.

Some people believe that water-soluble vitamins are harmless, even when taken in large amounts, but this isn't always true. Consuming excessive amounts of some water-soluble vitamins, including vitamins B-6, folic acid (B-9), niacin (B-3) and C, can have adverse effects.

Minerals

Your body also needs 16 minerals to function properly. Major minerals (macrominerals) include calcium, magnesium, phosphorus, potassium, sodium and chloride. Calcium, phosphorus and magnesium are important in the development and health of your bones and teeth. Sodium, potassium and chloride, known as electrolytes, help regulate the water and chemical balance in your body. Potassium is also a major component of muscle.

Your body needs smaller amounts of the remaining minerals, known as trace minerals (microminerals). These include iron, iodine, zinc, copper, fluoride, selenium and manganese, among others.

For young children, teenage girls and women of childbearing age, it's especially important to get adequate iron to allow for growth and

Vitamin D

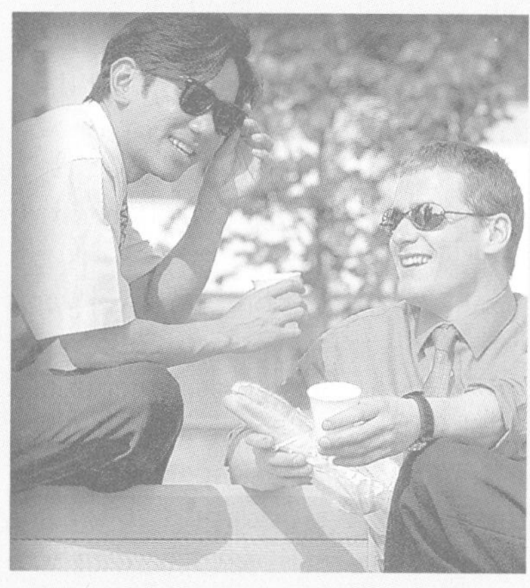

Calcium is essential for strong bones, but to enhance the amount of calcium that reaches your bones, you also need vitamin D.

Your body makes vitamin D from two sources — sunlight and food. Most of the vitamin D in your body results from sun exposure. When you're exposed to ultraviolet light rays, a chemical in your skin is converted into a form of vitamin D. Your liver and kidneys then change it into an active form that your body can use.

Egg yolks and fatty fish such as herring, mackerel and salmon naturally contain vitamin D. Several food products are fortified with vitamin D, such as milk and some breakfast cereals.

Some people don't get enough vitamin D, either due to lack of exposure to sunlight or to not eating foods that contain the vitamin. In addition, with age, the skin becomes less efficient at synthesizing vitamin D and the body less able to absorb it from food.

If you don't eat foods that contain vitamin D or you rarely spend time outdoors, you may want to consider taking a vitamin D supplement to meet your daily requirement. Individuals age 70 and under shouldn't take more than 400 international units (IU) a day unless their doctor prescribes more. For people older than age 70, the recommended amount is 600 IU a day.

Although excessive sun exposure isn't healthy for your skin, a little bit of sun — about 15 minutes a day — can be good for your bones.

Vitamin and Mineral Supplements

You can get your entire daily requirement of vitamin C by eating an orange — or by taking a vitamin C tablet. So which is better? In most cases, the orange. The best way to get the vitamins and minerals you need is through food, not supplements.

Many American adults take vitamin supplements regularly. Some people regard them as essential food replacements. Others see them as harmless insurance.

A daily multivitamin and mineral supplement that supplies close to 100 percent of the dietary recommendations isn't harmful, and it could be beneficial if your diet doesn't contain a wide variety of foods. But supplements can't provide other important elements in food.

Before taking any supplement other than a standard multivitamin and mineral supplement, check with your doctor or a registered dietitian. It's also important that you not take more than the recommended amount. Many nutrients can be harmful if taken in large amounts.

Benefits of food

Whole foods provide a number of benefits that you can't find in a pill:

- *Whole foods are complex.* They contain a variety of the nutrients your body needs. An orange, for example, provides not only vitamin C but also beta carotene, calcium and other nutrients.
- *Whole foods provide fiber.* Fiber is important for digestion and may help prevent heart disease, diabetes and constipation.
- *Whole foods contain phytochemicals.* Fruits and vegetables contain substances called phytochemicals, such as lycopene or flavonoids. Phytochemicals are naturally occurring compounds that plants produce to protect themselves against bacteria, viruses or fungi. Unlike vitamins and minerals, phytochemicals have no known nutritional value. But they may help protect against a variety of diseases, including cancer, heart disease, osteoporosis and diabetes.

Who needs supplements?

For most people, a healthy diet provides adequate vitamins and minerals. However, a vitamin or mineral supplement may be appropriate if:

- *You're age 65 or older.* As you get older, health problems may lead to a poor diet, making it difficult for you to get the vitamins and minerals you need. In addition, your body may not be able to absorb vitamins B-6, B-12 and D as well as it used to, making supplementation more necessary. There's also evidence that a multivitamin may improve your immune function and decrease your risk of some infections as you age.

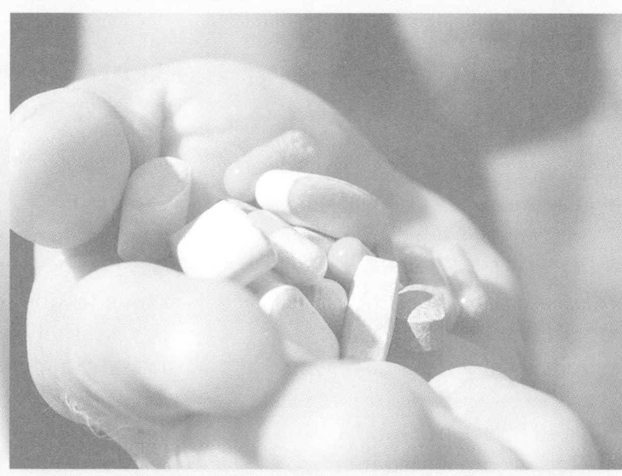

- *You're a postmenopausal woman.* For some women, it can be difficult to obtain the recommended amounts of calcium and vitamin D without supplementation. Both calcium and vitamin D supplements have been shown to protect against osteoporosis.
- *You don't eat well.* If you don't eat the recommended five servings a day of fruits and vegetables, taking a multivitamin supplement may be reasonable. However, your best course of action would be to adopt better eating habits.
- *You're on a very low-calorie diet.* If you eat fewer than 1,000 calories a day, you may benefit from a vitamin and mineral supplement.
- *You smoke.* Tobacco decreases the absorption of many vitamins and minerals, including vitamin B-6, vitamin B-12, vitamin C, folate and niacin.
- *You drink alcohol excessively.* Excessive alcohol use can impair digestion and absorption of thiamin, folate and vitamins A, D and B-12. Altered metabolism also affects minerals such as zinc, selenium, magnesium and phosphorus.
- *You're planning to become pregnant, are pregnant or are breast-feeding.* During these times, you need more of certain nutrients especially folic acid — the synthetic form of folate. Folic acid helps prevent neural tube defects such as spina bifida in the fetus. Iron supplements taken during pregnancy can help prevent anemia in the mother.
- *You eat a special diet or have a chronic condition.* If your diet has limited variety because of intolerance or a food allergy, you may benefit from a vitamin and mineral supplement. If you're a vegetarian who eliminates all animal products from your diet, you may need additional vitamin B-12 and zinc. If you don't eat dairy products and don't get 15 minutes of sun exposure each day, you may need to supplement your diet with calcium and vitamin D.

Some chronic medical conditions can increase your need for a variety of nutrients while impairing your appetite or the way your body handles nutrients. In these cases, special supplements may be necessary.

development and prevent diseases such as iron deficiency anemia. Foods high in iron include:

- Shellfish, such as shrimp, clams, mussels and oysters
- Lean meats, especially beef, and organ meats, which are also high in cholesterol
- Turkey, dark meat
- Sardines
- Spinach and other dark leafy greens
- Dried beans, peas and lentils
- Cereals with added iron
- Enriched and whole-grain breads

Calories

A calorie is a measure of energy. When carbohydrates, protein and fat are burned (metabolized) in the body, they produce energy, which is measured in a unit known as the kilocalorie. The kilocalorie — commonly referred to as calorie — is used to express both the energy provided by food and the energy your body needs to function. It's defined as the amount of energy required to raise the temperature of 1 kilogram (2.2 pounds) of water by 1 degree Celsius (1.8 degrees Fahrenheit).

People's energy needs vary considerably with their activity level, body size, sex and age. The average adult requires about 1,900 calories a day. An older, petite, sedentary woman may need only about 1,600 calories a day, and a young, physically active man may need 2,800 calories or more daily.

The term *empty calories* is often applied to sugar and alcohol. They contribute energy (calories) but no other essential nutrients, such as vitamins or minerals. Consuming sugar and alcohol on occasion in small amounts is OK, as long as you eat a variety of other foods to provide essential nutrients. But too many daily calories from sugar and alcohol can undermine your efforts to maintain a healthy weight.

Body composition

The phrase, "You are what you eat," is true. The same ingredients that make up foods — water, protein, fat and carbohydrates — are the primary components of the human body.

Water

Water is a major component of body tissues made of protein, such as muscles and organs, and of the body's carbohydrate stores. Water makes up about 40 percent of body weight for very obese people and about 70 percent of body weight for very lean individuals.

Protein

Tissues composed of protein — muscles and vital organs — function as the machinery of your body. These protein structures make up about 30 percent to 60 percent of body weight.

Carbohydrates

Carbohydrates are stored in the liver and muscles in the form of glycogen. Glycogen makes up about 1 percent to 5 percent of your body weight.

If you switch from a normal diet to a very low-calorie or a very low-carbohydrate diet, you may lose 3 or 4 pounds within a day or two. Such weight loss, however, comes from a reduction of glycogen and water — not fat.

Fat

Unlike protein and carbohydrates, fat is an extremely concentrated form of reserve energy that contains little water. In an individual with a healthy weight, 15 percent to 20 percent of body weight is fat. In an extremely obese person, as much as 50 percent of body weight is fat.

These discrepancies in stored fat are the result of the way our bodies work. If you eat more food than your body can use or too many high-fat foods, your body stores the extra energy as fatty tissue. If you eat less food than your body needs, you lose fatty tissue.

Body fat primarily serves as a fuel reserve, but it also provides padding and insulation. In women, body fat also produces small amounts of estrogen, which helps protect against bone loss and osteoporosis.

A Healthy Balance

Eating well doesn't have to be complicated. Unless you need a special diet for a specific health problem, the best approach is to follow national dietary recommendations.

Nutrition Professionals

If you feel that you need help in getting essential nutrients and developing a healthier diet, talk to a registered dietitian (R.D.). Registered dietitians are registered with the American Dietetic Association. To obtain this credential, a person must earn an undergraduate degree in a 4-year program in food science and nutrition at an accredited college or university, complete 6 to 12 months of training in practical aspects of dietetics and pass a national examination. In addition, registered dietitians must complete 75 hours of professional education every 5 years.

Other professionals also may be helpful in dealing with nutrition-related questions. Some doctors have a particular interest in nutrition. Home economists are often a good source of information on meal planning and food preparation.

Unfortunately, the term *nutritionist* is sometimes used by people who have no credible nutritional training and who may be selling dietary supplements or weight-loss schemes. Some of these people may even display a diploma or certificate that means very little.

These recommendations have evolved over the years to keep pace with scientific knowledge as experts have developed a better understanding of how diet influences general health and helps prevent disease.

National dietary recommendations incorporate the best judgment of nutrition professionals, based on current knowledge. The recommendations are intended for healthy individuals over age 2. They include the concepts of variety, balance and moderation in food choices.

Eat more vegetables, fruits and grains

Eating a variety of vegetables, fruits and grains — especially whole-grain foods — is the basis of healthy eating. Fruits, vegetables and grains are low in calories and fat and provide essential vitamins and minerals, fiber and phytochemicals important for good health.

Most people, including children, don't eat enough fruits and vegetables. Try to eat five servings of fruits and vegetables a day — at least two servings of fruit and at least three servings of vegetables.

Fruits contain little or no fat and provide fiber and a variety of vitamins and minerals. In addition, fruits contain phytochemicals that can reduce your risk of cardiovascular disease and some cancers. Vegetables also contain vitamins, minerals, fiber and phytochemicals. They're also low in calories and virtually fat-free.

All grains and foods made from grains — cereals, bread, rice and pasta — are rich in complex

Healthy Additions

Here are some tips on easy ways to incorporate more fruits, vegetables and whole grains into your diet:

Fruits

- Keep a bowl of fruit on the kitchen counter or table for snacks.
- Add fresh or dried fruit to breakfast cereals.
- Replace the oil in baked goods with thick fruit purees such as applesauce, mashed bananas and prunes.
- Use fruit sauces as toppings on desserts and pancakes.
- Instead of drinking soda pop, use 100 percent fruit juice mixed with sparkling water.

Vegetables

- Keep ready-to-eat, raw vegetables handy in a clear container in the front of your refrigerator for snacks or meals on the go.
- Eat a variety of salad greens, including arugula, chicory, collards, dandelion greens, kale, mustard greens, spinach and watercress.
- Stir-fry vegetables with a small portion of poultry, seafood or meat.
- Add ½ cup of shredded carrots to spaghetti sauce.
- Top a baked potato with 1 cup of steamed vegetables.

Whole grains

- For breakfast, choose high-fiber cereals, such as bran flakes, shredded wheat and oatmeal.
- Substitute whole-wheat toast or multigrain muffins for bagels and pastries.
- Make sandwiches with whole-grain breads or rolls.
- Expand your grain repertoire with foods such as kasha, brown rice, wild rice, bulgur and wheat berries.
- Use rice or barley in soups, stews, casseroles and salads.

Nutrient Notables

The fruits and vegetables listed below are the best sources of vitamin A (carotenoids), vitamin C, folate and potassium. Many other fruits and vegetables are high in nutrients and add variety to your diet.

Sources of vitamin A

- Orange vegetables, including carrots, sweet potatoes, pumpkin, winter squash
- Dark leafy greens, such as spinach, collards, turnip greens
- Orange fruits, such as mango, cantaloupe, apricots
- Tomatoes, sweet red peppers

Sources of vitamin C

- Citrus fruits and juices, kiwi fruit, strawberries, cantaloupe, papaya
- Broccoli, peppers, tomatoes, cabbage, potatoes with skin, brussels sprouts
- Dark leafy greens, such as romaine lettuce, turnip greens, spinach

Sources of folate

- Dried beans and peas
- Oranges, orange juice
- Dark leafy greens, such as spinach, mustard greens, romaine lettuce
- Green peas

Sources of potassium

- Tomatoes, tomato products
- White or sweet potatoes, winter squash
- Cooked greens, such as spinach
- Bananas, orange and grapefruit juices, dried fruits, such as apricots and prunes
- Dried beans and lentils

Source: Dietary Guidelines for Americans, 2000

carbohydrates and provide a variety of nutrients. Despite a common misconception that breads and pasta are fattening, these foods are relatively low in fat and calories, unless you add high-fat spreads, dips or sauces.

Aim for at least six servings of grains each day. When possible, choose whole grains because they contain more fiber than refined grains do. Whole grains haven't had their most nutrient-packed parts — the endosperm, germ and bran — removed by milling. Different whole-grain foods differ in nutrient content, so eat foods made from a variety of them — such as whole-wheat bread, brown rice and oatmeal.

Reduce fat and cholesterol

Reducing fat and cholesterol doesn't mean eliminating them altogether. Too little fat in the diet can deprive you of essential nutrients. Focus on reducing your consumption of foods high in fat, especially saturated fat. Select foods made from monounsaturated fats, such as olive and canola oil.

Even though monounsaturated and polyunsaturated fats have few adverse effects on blood fats, it's still important to consume them in moderation. Eating lots of fat of any type adds excess calories.

Foods that are high in cholesterol tend to raise blood cholesterol. Even so, high blood cholesterol levels are most often due to a diet high in saturated fat rather than one high in cholesterol.

Aim for a total fat intake of no more than 30 percent of calories, with 10 percent or less from saturated fat. For example, if you consume 2,000 calories a day, your upper limit on total fat will be 65 grams, with 20 grams or less of saturated fat. To reduce fat in your diet, eat fewer foods high in saturated fat. Limit meat, butter, cheese, whole milk and cream in your diet, as well as foods made from chocolate, solid shortenings, and palm and coconut oils.

Try to keep your daily cholesterol intake to less than 300 milligrams. Animal foods — including meat, poultry, fish, milk and milk products — contain cholesterol. Concentrated sources of cholesterol include organ meats, such as liver, and egg yolks.

Limit sugar and salt

Foods containing sugars added during processing or preparation generally provide calories but few vitamins and minerals. High-sugar foods also promote tooth decay. For these reasons, dietary guidelines recommend that you limit foods and beverages containing added sugars.

In the United States, the No. 1 source of added sugars is nondiet soft drinks. Other major sources include candies, cakes, cookies, fruit drinks and dairy desserts, such as ice cream. Don't let soft drinks or other sweets crowd out foods that you need to maintain good health.

Salt (sodium chloride) is the main source of sodium in foods. Many studies have shown that high levels of sodium are associated with high blood pressure. Most Americans

Good Fat

One type of fat, called omega-3 fatty acids, may have a protective effect against heart disease, particularly sudden death from heart attack. This type of fat is thought to help lower your triglyceride level. Triglycerides are a type of blood fat. Omega-3 fatty acids may also lower blood pressure slightly.

Foods containing omega-3 fatty acids are part of a healthy diet, but the typical American diet has few of them. The best sources of omega-3 fatty acids are flaxseed and fatty, cold-water fish, such as salmon, mackerel, sardines, herring, bass, shark, swordfish, tuna and trout. Other foods containing this type of fat include walnuts and soybean and canola oils.

Health experts recommend eating fish twice a week. However, fish oil supplements generally aren't recommended. You can incorporate flaxseed into your meals by sprinkling the small, reddish-brown, ground or cracked seeds over salads, soups and cereal. Flaxseed is also rich in fiber, an essential fatty acid called alpha linolenic acid, and lignans, substances that may help prevent certain types of cancer.

Forms of Sugar

Sugar travels under many disguises, depending on how it's formed and processed. A food is likely to be high in sugar if one of the following names appears first or second in the list of ingredients, or if several of these names are listed:

- Brown sugar
- Corn sweetener
- Corn syrup
- Dextrose
- Fructose
- Fruit juice concentrate
- Glucose
- High-fructose corn syrup
- Honey
- Invert sugar
- Lactose
- Maltose
- Malt syrup
- Molasses
- Raw sugar
- Sucrose
- Syrup
- Table sugar

consume too much salt. Healthy children and adults need only a small amount of salt daily. The recommended daily limit of sodium is 2,400 milligrams, the amount found in about 1 teaspoon of salt.

Only small amounts of sodium occur naturally in foods. Most of the sodium you eat is added during food processing or preparation.

To limit sodium, choose and prepare your foods carefully. Check labels on processed foods. Frozen dinners, soups, packaged mixes, cereals, cheese, salad dressings and sauces may be high in sodium. When preparing meals, flavor the food with herbs, spices or fruits instead of salt.

Limit alcohol

Alcoholic beverages supply calories but few nutrients. Alcoholic beverages are harmful when consumed in excess, and some people should not drink them at all.

If you drink alcoholic beverages, do so in moderation. This is generally defined as no more than one drink a day for women and two drinks a day for men. One drink is defined as 12 ounces of beer, 5 ounces of wine or 1.5 ounces of 80-proof distilled spirits. Drink alcohol with meals to slow its absorption, and don't drink before or while driving.

Some individuals shouldn't drink any alcohol. This includes pregnant women and individuals with liver disease or other medical conditions sensitive to alcohol. In addition, people using certain medications shouldn't consume alcohol.

Eat moderate-sized portions

With the trend toward larger portions, many Americans have a distorted view of appropriate serving sizes. Knowing and controlling food portions can help you maintain a healthier diet, whether or not you're trying to lose weight. To practice moderation, avoid eating too much or too little of any one food. By avoiding large portions of certain foods, you're able to eat a wider variety of foods during a meal.

Try these other suggestions for reducing food portions:

- Serve food on plates instead of putting serving bowls on the table.
- Serve main dishes on a smaller plate.
- When eating out, ask for a take-home container. Save part of the meal for another time.
- Skip second servings.
- Don't feel as though you have to clean your plate.

Food Labels

Food labels can serve as an important guide to better nutrition. Food labels have several parts, including the ingredients list and Nutrition Facts label. The ingredients list tells you what's in the food, listed in descending order by weight. The Nutrition Facts label contains information pertaining to serving size, total fat and daily values of various nutrients.

You can use the Nutrition Facts label to see if a food is a good source of a particular nutrient. Or you can compare labels to see, for example, which brand of frozen dinner is lower in saturated fat or which breakfast cereal contains more fiber.

Nutrition labeling is required for almost all foods. Voluntary information for commonly eaten raw fruits, vegetables and seafood also is available in most grocery stores. This information may be provided in a brochure, pamphlet, sign or poster.

Nutrition labeling is also voluntary for single-ingredient raw meat and poultry products. Ground beef and chicken parts, for example, aren't required to have a nutrition label. However, processed products such as corned beef, hot dogs and frozen entrees with meat must have nutrition labeling on each package.

Nutrition Facts
Serving Size 6 Wafers (28 g)
Servings Per Container About 10

Amount Per Serving	
Calories 130	Calories from Fat 40
	% Daily Value*
Total Fat 4.5 g	**7%**
Saturated Fat 1 g	**4%**
Polyunsaturated Fat 0 g	
Monounsaturated Fat 1.5 g	
Cholesterol 0 mg	**0%**
Sodium 130 mg	**5%**
Total Carbohydrate 20 g	**7%**
Dietary Fiber 3 g	**13%**
Sugars Less than 1 g	
Protein 3 g	
Vitamin A 4% •	Vitamin C 0%
Calcium 0% •	Iron 6%
Phosphorus 10%	

* Percent Daily Values are based on a 2,000-calorie diet. Your daily values may be higher or lower depending on your calorie needs:

		Calories: 2,000	2,500
Total Fat	Less than	65 g	80 g
Sat. Fat	Less than	20 g	25 g
Cholesterol	Less than	300 mg	300 mg
Sodium	Less than	2,400 mg	2,400 mg
Total Carbohydrate		300 g	375 g
Dietary Fiber		25 g	30 g

Label components

Each food label contains information pertaining to:

Serving size
The serving size is based on the amount of the labeled food people normally eat and is listed in both household and metric measures. Check the serving size to see if the amount you normally eat is similar to the serving size on the label. If you eat more, then the number of calories and nutrients you get from that item will be higher. A figure indicating the servings per container also is included so that you can calculate the calories and nutrients in the whole product.

Total fat
Each label includes total fat in each serving. You can use this information to add up the amount of fat you eat.

For a 1,600-calories-a-day diet — recommended for older adults and most women — limit total fat to 53 grams and saturated fat to 13 grams (g). For a 2,200-calories-a-day diet — recommended for active women and most men — limit total fat to 73 g and saturated fat to 24 g. These guidelines can help you keep fat at less than 30 percent of your daily calories.

Nutrients
Each label lists amounts of the following nutrients in a single serving of the food: fat, cholesterol, sodium, carbohydrate, dietary fiber, sugars, protein, vitamins A and C, calcium, iron and phosphorus. Some labels list other nutrients as well.

Percent Daily Value
The Percent Daily Value column tells you how much of the recommended daily amount of a nutrient one serving contains, based on a diet of 2,000 to 2,500 calories a day. Use the figures to compare products and to tell which food is higher or lower in nutrients.

Nutrient claims

Some food labels also contain standardized claims, such as "low-fat" and "high in fiber." Claims involving nutrient content are defined and regulated by the Food and Drug Administration. The accompanying chart defines some of the common claims. In addition to claims such as "light" or "lean," sometimes health claims are made that link foods or food components with a reduced risk of certain chronic diseases.

Nutrient Claims on Food Labels

Food term	What it means
Light or "lite"	*For fat:* Contains 50 percent less fat than a comparable product *For calories:* Contains 33 percent fewer calories than a comparable product *and* contains fewer than 50 percent of calories from fat *For sodium:* Contains at least 50 percent less sodium than a comparable product
Reduced	Contains at least 25 percent less of a nutrient than a comparable product
Free	Contains none or "inconsequential" amounts of the nutrient, such as fat, saturated fat, cholesterol, sodium, sugar or calories
Low	*For fat:* Contains 3 grams (g) or fewer *For cholesterol:* Contains 20 milligrams (mg) or fewer *and* no more than 2 g of saturated fat *For saturated fat:* Contains 1 g or less *For sodium:* Contains 140 mg or fewer *For calories:* Contains 40 calories or fewer
High	Contains at least 20 percent of the recommended daily value for a nutrient, such as fiber or vitamin C, based on a 2,000-calories-a-day diet
Good source	Contains 10 percent to 19 percent of the recommended daily value for a nutrient, based on a 2,000-calories-a day diet
Healthy	Must be low in fat, saturated fat and sodium and must provide at least 10 percent of the recommended daily value for vitamin A, vitamin C, calcium, iron, protein or fiber
Lean	Meat, poultry, seafood or game meat that has, per 3 oz., less than 10 g of total fat, less than 4.5 g of saturated fat and less than 95 mg of cholesterol
Extra lean	Meat, poultry, seafood or game meat that has, per 3 oz., less than 5 g of total fat, less than 2 g of saturated fat and less than 95 mg of cholesterol

Is There an Ideal Diet?

Many people yearn for — and spend a lot of time and money seeking — the perfect eating plan. This ideal diet would result in excellent health, providing energy, strength and resistance to disease. It would delay aging and keep you at your ideal weight.

Does such an eating plan exist? Probably not. Your nutritional needs differ at different stages of life, and they may change if you have a chronic disease. Everyone has unique genetic tendencies toward diseases, so food components such as salt or fats pose different risks to different people. Food intolerances and allergies also affect what kinds of foods you eat. In addition, your culture, family background, religious and moral beliefs and the cost and availability of food all affect your food choices. People like different foods and prepare the same foods in different ways.

Although there really isn't one perfect diet for everyone, some general principles for choosing foods apply to most people. A healthy eating plan can be created in many ways. These plans are often portrayed in the shape of a pyramid with the foods that should be eaten most forming the base. Probably the most familiar pyramid is the Food Guide Pyramid established by the U.S. Department of Agriculture (USDA).

In addition to the USDA pyramid, nutrition and health professionals have developed several other food pyramids to reflect other healthy eating patterns. Pyramids have also been formulated for young children and for individuals over age 70.

The various food guide pyramids that follow have much in common, and you can use any of them as a basis for eating well. They're consistent with current nutritional recommendations, and they follow the same premise of variety, portion control and moderation in eating.

One difference is that the USDA Food Guide Pyramid includes recommended servings in each food group based on age, sex and level of activity. Serving sizes are specifically defined. This is especially useful if you're trying to lose weight.

To see how far your diet is from those recommended by the pyramids, keep a food diary for several days. Then compare how much of your diet comes from the bottom of the pyramid and how much comes from the top. If you're top-heavy, work your way to the bottom by making small, gradual changes, such as eating more vegetables, fruits and whole grains and limiting fats and sweets.

USDA Food Guide Pyramid

The three food groups at the base of the USDA Food Guide Pyramid are grains, fruits and vegetables. Eating a variety of these foods is the basis of healthy eating. Starchy foods aren't fattening unless you cook them with added fat or top them with butter, cream or rich sauces.

The middle of the pyramid contains the milk and cheese group and the meat and beans group. These foods contribute protein, calcium, iron and zinc to your diet. Eat moderate amounts of these foods. Choose skim or low-fat dairy products whenever possible. Eat legumes more frequently and eat lean cuts of meat and poultry without skin. Prepare them without added fat.

The small tip of the pyramid includes fats, oils and sweets. These are foods such as salad dressings, cooking oils, butter, margarine, sugar, soft drinks, candy and most desserts. Foods in this section provide calories but have little nutritional value. Eat them sparingly.

Combine foods from each major group in the pyramid however you like. For example, you might make a meal of tortillas from the grains group and beans from the meat and beans group. Eating three balanced meals a day — rather than one or two — may help you to control snacking.

USDA Food Guide Pyramid

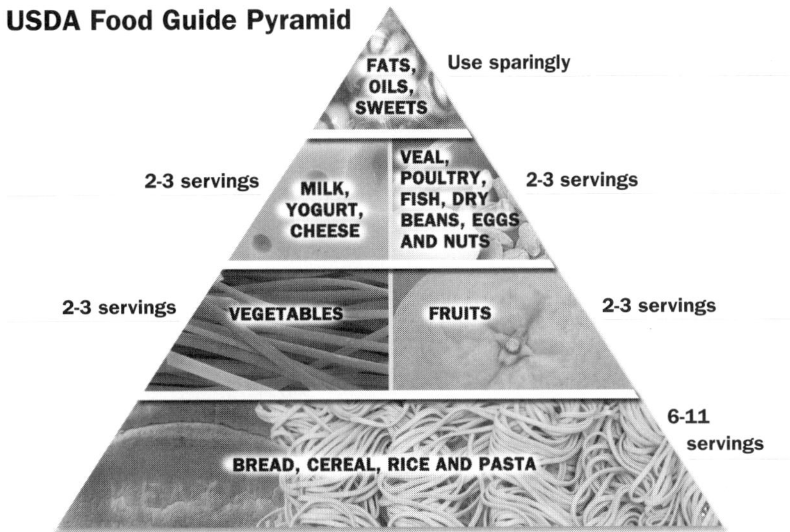

Source: U.S. Department of Agriculture, 2000

How Much Should I Eat?

	Children ages 2 to 6 years, women, some older adults	Older children, teenage girls, active women, most men	Teenage boys, active men
Calories per day	About 1,600	About 2,200	About 2,800
Servings per day			
Grains group	6	9	11
Vegetable group	3	4	5
Fruit group	2	3	4
Milk group	2 or 3*	2 or 3*	2 or 3*
Meat and beans group	2, for a total of 5 oz.	2, for a total of 6 oz.	3, for a total of 7 oz.
Fat			
Total fat	53 grams (g)	73 g	93 g
Saturated fat	13 g	24 g	31 g

*The number of servings depends on your age. Older children and teenagers — those ages 9 to 18 — and adults over age 50 need three servings daily. Others need two servings daily. The recommended number of milk group servings for pregnant or lactating women is the same as for nonpregnant women.

Source: Dietary Guidelines for Americans, 2000

If you need to avoid all foods from one or more of the food groups, make sure to get enough nutrients from other food groups. For example, if you don't consume milk products because of lactose intolerance or for another reason, choose other foods that are good sources of calcium.

Mediterranean Diet Pyramid

Because the Mediterranean Diet Pyramid is based on a cultural eating pattern, it includes a more limited range of foods than does the USDA Food Guide Pyramid.

The Mediterranean Diet Pyramid reflects traditional eating patterns in Greece, Crete and southern Italy. The value of this eating style came into focus in the 1950s and 1960s, when studies showed that Greek men were the least likely to develop heart disease among men from seven countries that participated in the study, including the United States.

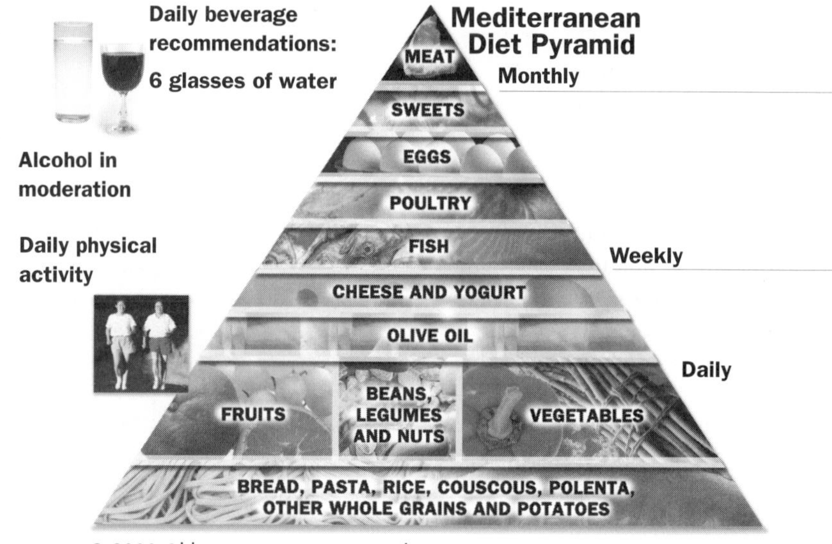

The Mediterranean eating plan emphasizes fresh fruits and vegetables, grains of all types and legumes such as beans, lentils and peas. Mediterranean dishes are also enhanced with olive oil, a monounsaturated fat that appears to help protect against heart disease. Wine, in moderation, is part of this pyramid, because red wine with meals is a Mediterranean tradition.

Asian Diet Pyramid

The Asian Diet Pyramid also reflects a cultural eating pattern. It emphasizes grains, including rice, noodles, breads, millet and corn, as well as fruits, vegetables, legumes, nuts and seeds. As in the Mediterranean diet, fat in the Asian pyramid comes largely from vegetable oils high in monounsaturated fat, such as

Sizing Up a Serving

Keep an eye on serving sizes as you prepare and eat meals. The number of servings that are appropriate for you depends on your age, sex and activity level.

For some foods, the number of recommended servings a day might seem high, but some of the serving sizes may be smaller than what you usually eat or what you see on food labels. For example, many people eat two slices of bread in a meal, which equals two servings. On food labels, one serving of cooked rice or pasta often is 1 cup, but on the USDA Food Guide Pyramid, one serving of these foods is only 1/2 cup.

If you follow the suggested number of servings, in the recommended amounts, you'll help control your caloric intake.

Grains group
- 1/2 cup (3 ounces) cooked cereal, rice or pasta
- 1 ounce ready-to-eat cereal (check the label for the serving size)
- One slice whole-wheat bread
- 1/2 bagel, English muffin or hamburger bun
- Six small crackers (saltine size)

Vegetable group
- 1 cup (2 ounces) raw leafy green vegetables
- 1/2 cup (3 ounces) other vegetables, cooked or raw
- One medium potato
- 6 fluid ounces vegetable juice

Fruit group
- One medium orange, apple, banana or pear
- 12 grapes
- 1/2 cup (3 ounces) chopped, cooked or canned fruit
- 1/4 cup (1 1/2 ounces) raisins
- 6 fluid ounces fruit juice

Milk, yogurt and cheese group
- 1 cup (8 fluid ounces) low-fat or fat-free milk or yogurt
- 1 1/2 ounces natural cheese, such as cheddar
- 2 ounces processed cheese, such as American
- 2 cups (16 ounces) low-fat or fat-free cottage cheese

Meat, poultry, fish, dry beans, eggs and nuts group
- 2 to 3 ounces cooked lean meat, fish or skinless poultry
- 1/2 cup (3 1/2 ounces) cooked legumes or dried beans
- One egg
- 2 1/2-ounce soy burger
- 2 tablespoons peanut butter
- 1/4 cup (1 ounce) seeds
- 1/3 cup (1 ounce) nuts
- 1/2 cup (4 ounces) tofu

peanut oil. The Asian Diet Pyramid contains limited dairy products, considering them optional and to be eaten only in low-fat forms.

A major difference between the Mediterranean and Asian pyramids and the USDA pyramid is their distinction between plant and animal proteins. The Asian and Mediterranean pyramids group plant-based proteins — soybeans, beans and nuts — separately from animal proteins found in meat, poultry, eggs and dairy products. Red meat is recommended infrequently — a few times a month or less — and poultry and eggs are recommended weekly.

Latin American Diet Pyramid

The Latin American Diet Pyramid is based on traditional healthy eating patterns in Latin American regions, including Mexico, Central America and South America. The diet emphasizes food from plant sources, especially maize (corn) and potatoes, as well as fruits, vegetables, grains, beans, nuts and seeds. In this diet, a variety of fruits and vegetables and whole grains are eaten at main meals. Fish, shellfish, plant oils (corn, soybean, olive), dairy products and poultry can be eaten once a day, and red meat, sweets and eggs are limited to once a week or less.

The pyramid places daily physical activity at the base to promote healthy weight, fitness and well-being.

Vegetarian Diet Pyramid

There are many vegetarian eating plans. At the very least, most exclude red meat. Others omit all animal flesh, including chicken and fish. Some vegetarians don't eat eggs or milk products. The most strict vegetarians (vegans) eat only grains, legumes, fruits, vegetables, nuts and seeds and products made from these foods.

If you don't eat any animal products, it becomes more challenging

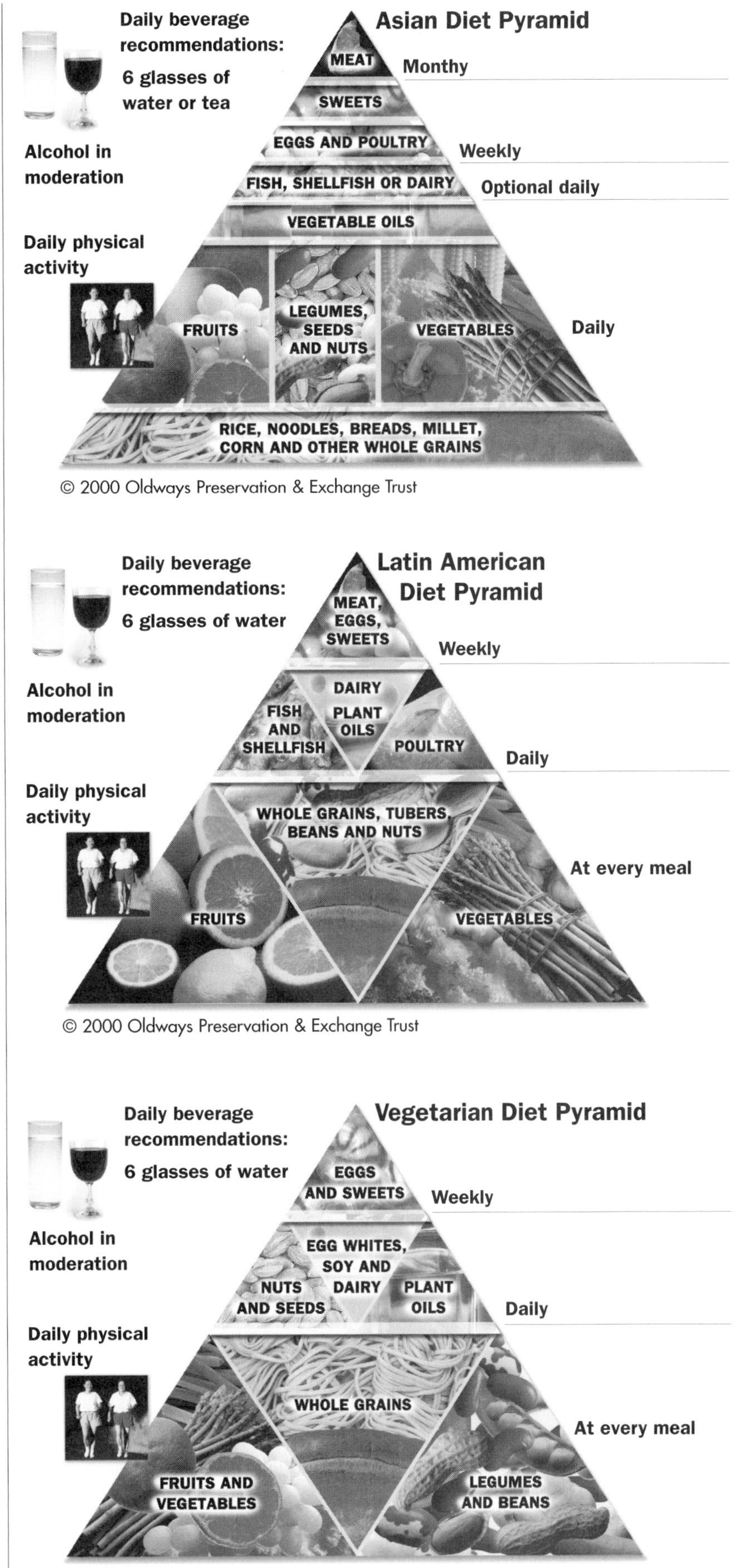

to meet daily recommendations for essential amino acids from protein as well as requirements for calcium, iron, zinc and vitamins B-12 and D. The Vegetarian Diet Pyramid can help in making good food choices.

This pyramid specifies whole grains and puts them at the same level as fruits and vegetables, which are to be eaten at every meal. Daily choices include moderate amounts of nuts and seeds, egg whites, soy milk and dairy products, as well as plant oils. Eggs and sweets are at the top of the pyramid and should be eaten once a week or less. The vegetarian pyramid also recommends at least six glasses of water each day.

Mayo Clinic Healthy Weight Pyramid

Like other dietary pyramids, the Mayo Clinic Healthy Weight Pyramid focuses on vegetables, fruits and grains as the basis for a healthy diet. The emphasis is on nutritious foods that contain a small number of calories in a large amount of food. In addition to helping you stay well, this pyramid is designed to help you lose weight. The Mayo Clinic Healthy Weight Pyramid is discussed in more detail in Chapter 3, "Controlling Your Weight."

Diet and Disease

Some factors that affect your risk of disease are beyond your control, such as age and family history. But what you may not realize is how much you can control your disease risk. A healthy lifestyle — including eating well, not smoking, being physically active and maintaining a healthy weight — can improve, or even eliminate, significant risk factors for several important chronic conditions. By following the dietary recommendations outlined in this chapter, you can reduce your risk of disease and improve the quality of your life.

Some chronic diseases, such as celiac disease, liver disease and kidney disease, require you to follow a specialized diet. For some of these conditions, dietary changes can be lifesaving. If you need to follow a special diet, it's important to work with a registered dietitian initially to develop an appropriate eating plan.

To help prevent diseases, it's not necessary that you follow a specialized diet, but it's important that you eat a healthy diet.

Coronary artery disease

High blood cholesterol can lead to accumulation of fatty deposits (plaques) in the arteries that feed your heart (coronary arteries), narrowing the arteries and increasing your risk of heart attack or stroke.

A low-fat, low-cholesterol diet can help reduce your blood cholesterol level and minimize your risk of coronary artery disease. Limit saturated fat to less than 10 percent of your total calories, and total fat to no more than 30 percent of daily calories. In addition, try to keep your daily consumption of cholesterol to less than 300 milligrams.

Heart-healthy foods that can help lower blood cholesterol and reduce plaques include:

- High-fiber foods
- Fish, especially salmon, mackerel and herring
- Soy products, such as soybeans, tofu, tempeh, miso, soy milk and soy flour

Love Those Legumes

The term *legume* refers to a large family of plants whose seeds develop inside pods and are usually dried for ease of storage. Legumes include beans, peas and lentils. Because legumes are high in protein, these plant foods make an excellent substitute for animal sources of protein.

Selecting legumes
Look for these common legumes in your supermarket:

- White or navy beans
- Lima beans
- Pinto and black beans
- Black-eyed peas
- Split peas
- Brown lentils
- Chickpeas (garbanzos)

Ethnic markets often have less common legumes. Indian markets, for example, usually offer a good selection of lentils, including pink and orange ones. Purchase legumes that have been recently dried. Look for legumes of a uniform size that will cook evenly.

Storing legumes
Store legumes at room temperature. After purchase, place them in tightly covered jars away from heat, light and moisture. They'll keep well for up to 1 year.

Cooking legumes
Carefully sort legumes before using them. Bags of legumes may include a few small stones or fibers that you'll want to remove before cooking.

Beans and other large dried legumes, such as chickpeas and black-eyed peas, require pre-soaking overnight or for about 6 to 8 hours before cooking. This rehydrates them for more even cooking. Split peas and lentils don't require pre-soaking. You can also purchase legumes that are precooked and canned.

To incorporate legumes into everyday meals:

- Feature beans, peas or lentils in soups, stews or casseroles.
- Add chickpeas or black beans to salads.
- Use pureed beans as the basis for dips and spreads.

- Foods rich in antioxidants — vitamins C, E and A (carotenoids)
- Foods rich in folate or fortified with folic acid (the synthetic form of folate) and vitamins B-6 and B-12

High blood pressure

Left untreated, high blood pressure can damage your arteries and increase your risk of stroke and heart disease. Limiting sodium and alcohol and maintaining a healthy weight can help prevent or reduce high blood pressure. In recent years, the role of diet in treating and preventing high blood pressure has drawn more attention.

Studies indicate that a diet rich in fruits, vegetables and low-fat dairy products can help lower your blood pressure. An eating guide based on these principles is called Dietary Approaches to Stop Hypertension, or the DASH diet.

The benefits of the DASH diet are improved even further by reducing sodium in your diet. Limiting sodium to less than 2,000 milligrams (mg) a day is generally recommended. The average American consumes 4,000 to 6,000 mg of sodium a day. People who have certain forms of liver, heart and kidney disease may be advised to restrict their sodium intake even more.

For a detailed discussion of DASH, see page 744.

Cancer

Researchers continue to evaluate and clarify the role that diet and nutrition play in the development of cancer. Evidence suggests that about one-third of the cancer deaths in the United States each year are related to dietary factors. Thus, your dietary choices, along with not smoking and getting regular physical activity, can help reduce your risk of cancer.

Eating more fruits and vegetables is one of the most important things you can do to protect against cancer. The American Cancer Society

Caffeine and Your Health

As you probably realize when you stumble into the kitchen for that first cup of morning coffee, caffeine is a stimulant. It affects people in different ways. For some, it may cause a temporary rise in blood pressure or irregular heartbeats. But moderate use of caffeine — for example, two or three cups of coffee a day — poses little health risk for most people.

Coffee, tea, chocolate and many kinds of soft drinks contain varying amounts of caffeine. Some medications also contain caffeine. If you're concerned about your caffeine intake, ask your doctor for advice.

Approximate Caffeine Content

	Milligrams of caffeine
Regular coffee	
Brewed, drip method, 6 oz.	105
Brewed, percolator method, 6 oz.	75
Instant (1 rounded tsp., dry), 6 oz.	60
Espresso, 1 oz.	50
Decaffeinated coffee	
Brewed, drip or percolator method, 6 oz.	2
Instant (1 rounded tsp., dry), 6 oz.	2
Espresso, 1 oz.	5
Regular tea	
Brewed for 3 minutes, 6 oz.	35
Instant (1 rounded tsp., dry), 6 oz.	25-35
Green, 6 oz.	25
Bottled, 12 oz.	15
Decaffeinated tea	
Brewed for 5 minutes, 6 oz.	1-5
Soft drinks, 12 oz.	
Mountain Dew	55
Mellow Yellow	50
Colas, regular or sugar-free	35-50
Unsweetened baking chocolate, 1 oz.	60
Dark, milk, semisweet and sweet chocolate, 1 oz.	5-20
Unsweetened powdered cocoa, 1 tbsp.	10
Chocolate milk, 8 oz.	10
Cocoa beverage, 8 oz.	5
Chocolate syrup, 1 oz.	5
Chocolate pudding, ½ cup	5-10
Chocolate ice cream, ½ cup	2
Medications	
No-Doz, maximum strength	200
Vivarin	200
No-Doz, regular strength	100
Excedrin	65
Vanquish	33
Anacin	32
Excedrin PM	0

recommends that most of the foods you eat come from plant sources. In addition to fruits and vegetables, these include grains — especially whole grains — beans and other legumes. The society also calls for limiting your intake of high-fat foods, particularly those from animal sources.

Eating more plant foods leaves less room for foods that might increase your risk of cancer — such as fatty meats. High-fat diets are associated with a higher risk of colon, prostate and endometrial cancers. In addition, excess calories from fat can lead to obesity, another risk factor for several cancers.

Avoiding or limiting alcohol may reduce your risk of various cancers, including those cancers of the mouth, esophagus, pharynx, larynx, liver and breast.

For more information on cancer and nutrition, see Chapter 19, "Cancer."

Diabetes

There's no specific diabetes diet. The basic nutritional guidelines for people with diabetes are the same as those outlined earlier in this chapter, with greater emphasis on eating meals at regular times. The American Diabetes Association recommends that individuals with diabetes work with a registered dietitian to develop a meal plan based on food preferences, lifestyle and health concerns, such as weight or blood cholesterol levels.

More than 90 percent of adults with diabetes have type 2 diabetes (formerly called adult-onset or non-insulin-dependent diabetes). Being overweight is the greatest risk factor for this form of diabetes. Eating plenty of whole grains, vegetables, fruits and legumes can make it easier to limit calories and lose weight. The fiber in these foods may also help lower your blood sugar.

If you have diabetes, you're at higher risk of developing cardiovascular disease, so it's important to limit fat in your diet, particularly saturated fat.

Sugar isn't forbidden if you have diabetes. Simple carbohydrates, such as table sugar, honey, jelly, fruit juice and candy, affect blood sugar about the same as complex carbohydrates, such as bread, rice and potatoes. It's the total amount of carbohydrates in your diet, rather than the source, that matters most.

Sugar may not interfere with blood sugar control as long as you substitute a sugary food for a starchy food that contains an equal amount of carbohydrates. Keep in mind, though, that it's a good idea to limit the amount of high-sugar foods you eat because they're often high in fat and contain unwanted calories.

For more information on diabetes and nutrition, see Chapter 32, "Endocrine System."

Antioxidants and Disease Prevention

Antioxidants are substances that protect your body's cells from the damaging effects of toxic molecules called free radicals. Free radicals may contribute to diseases, including cardiovascular and lung disease, cataracts and cancer. Important antioxidants include vitamins C, E and A (carotenoids), such as beta carotene. Other types of antioxidants, called flavonoids and polyphenols, are found in brewed tea (especially green tea), red wine and chocolate.

Despite the health benefits of vitamins C and E and beta carotene, current evidence is conflicting and too weak to recommend taking antioxidants in supplement form. More scientific study is needed to establish the safety and benefits of antioxidant supplements. Instead, nutrition experts recommend that you get antioxidants in your daily diet.

The following foods are good sources of antioxidants:

Vitamin C
- Green peppers and sweet red peppers
- Collards
- Broccoli
- Spinach
- Tomatoes
- Potatoes
- Strawberries
- Oranges and their juice
- Grapefruit and their juice

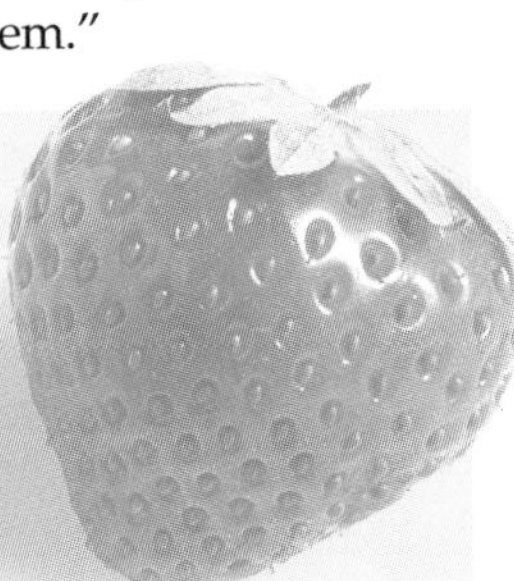

Vitamin E
- Vegetable oils and products made with them
- Wheat germ
- Nuts and seeds
- Fortified cereals

Vitamin A

Vitamin A (carotenoids) are found in deep yellow, dark green and red vegetables and fruits such as:
- Carrots
- Winter squash
- Sweet potatoes
- Spinach
- Broccoli
- Green peppers and sweet red peppers
- Tomatoes and tomato products
- Papaya
- Cantaloupe
- Mango
- Apricots
- Watermelon

Osteoporosis

About one in four women develop osteoporosis following menopause. For both women and men, risk increases with age. Osteoporosis is characterized by a reduction in bone mass, causing your bones to become thin, fragile and prone to fracture.

Consuming adequate amounts of calcium helps prevent osteoporosis. The recommended intake for men and women between ages 19 and 50 is 1,000 milligrams (mg) a day. For men and women over age 50, 1,200 mg a day is recommended. Many people consume barely half the daily recommended amount of calcium.

Because of differences in absorption, calcium found in fiber-rich vegetables often isn't absorbed as well as that found in dairy products. If you eat a high-fiber diet, be sure to include other food sources high in calcium.

In general, it's best to get as much calcium as you can from your diet. But if you can't get the recommended amount from food, supplements can help make up the difference. Discuss taking a dietary supplement with your doctor, particularly if you're a woman past menopause.

Celiac disease

Celiac disease, also called celiac sprue or nontropical sprue, is a digestive disease caused by an intolerance to gluten, a protein found in wheat, barley, rye and possibly oats. For affected individuals, gluten triggers an immune system response that damages the small intestine and prevents absorption of some nutrients in food.

Avoiding foods that contain gluten is the treatment for celiac disease. Although it may sound simple, doing so can be challenging. Products made from gluten-containing grains such as wheat, barley, rye and oats are staples of American and European diets. Wheat breads of all kinds contain gluten, as do most baked goods, cereals and pasta. In addition, many processed foods contain small amounts of emulsifiers, thickeners and other additives derived from these grains and must be avoided.

Rice, potatoes and corn don't contain gluten, and foods made from these ingredients are acceptable. Plain meats, fish, poultry, eggs, dairy products, vegetables and fruits also don't contain gluten.

Even trace amounts of gluten can cause severe damage to the intestines. Strict diet compliance can control the disease and prevent life-threatening complications. Regular checkups with your doctor and a registered dietitian also are an important part of treatment.

Kidney stones

Kidney stones (renal lithiasis) are fairly common. A kidney stone is a mineralized deposit that forms on the inner surface of your kidney and passes into the lower urinary tract.

A diet that's high in protein may increase your risk of some types of kidney stones. If you don't drink enough fluids, especially water, you may be more likely to develop kidney stones. In many cases, you can prevent kidney stones by making a few changes in your diet.

The most important thing you can do to lower this risk is to drink lots of water. Drinking extra fluids dilutes urine, making it less likely that crystals will develop. If you have a history of kidney stones, your doctor will probably recommend that you drink about 3½ quarts (14 cups) of fluid each day. Although most liquids count, water is best. Lemonade also is a good choice. The citrate in lemonade helps prevent some stones from forming.

If you tend to form calcium stones in your kidneys, your doctor may recommend restricting foods rich in oxalates. These include meats — especially organ meats, such as liver — beets, chocolate, coffee, rhubarb, cooked spinach,

Chocolate: A Healthy Food?

Not surprisingly, studies show that chocolate is one of the most craved foods. And it may not be just the sweet, rich taste or the melt-on-your-tongue consistency that accounts for its power to captivate. To researchers, chocolate's appeal is a combination of its nutrients and chemical composition, as well as its fat and sugar.

Chocolate contains high levels of antioxidant flavonoids, which are plant-based compounds also present in black tea and some fruits and vegetables. These antioxidants help limit the negative effects of low-density lipoprotein (LDL) cholesterol, the "bad" blood cholesterol. Reducing the effects of LDL cholesterol may help protect against clogging of the arteries (atherosclerosis) that can lead to heart disease and stroke.

The darker the chocolate, the higher it's likely to be in flavonoids. In addition, dark chocolate contains other antioxidants called catechins, which are thought to help prevent heart disease and boost your immune system. Even the fat in chocolate isn't as bad as it could be. More than half the saturated fat is stearic acid, which doesn't raise blood cholesterol.

If you crave chocolate, it's OK to indulge occasionally. There's room in a healthy diet for chocolate, and it may even have some benefit. But before you indulge your sweet tooth too much, remember that moderation remains the rule. Chocolate is high in sugar, fat and calories.

strawberries, tea and wheat bran. People bothered by calcium stones used to be told to avoid foods with a high calcium content. But studies have shown that dairy foods and other high-calcium foods actually might help prevent some calcium stones.

It's not clear if calcium supplements increase or reduce your risk of calcium stones. It's generally best to talk to your doctor before taking any supplements.

Kidney failure

Kidney (renal) failure may result from diseases such as diabetes, high blood pressure, kidney stones, infection, injury or exposure to toxins. The kidneys lose their ability to filter fluids and waste from blood, causing dangerous levels of these substances to accumulate in your body.

If you have acute kidney failure, you'll probably be placed on a diet high in carbohydrates and low in protein, potassium and fluid to prevent excess fluids and wastes from accumulating in your blood while your kidneys heal. A sudden rise in potassium levels could impair your heart's function and may be life-threatening. If you're on dialysis, you may need more protein, and your intake of fluids, phosphorus, sodium and potassium may be restricted.

Chronic kidney failure has many nutritional implications. Eating a diet low in protein may ease symptoms of nausea, vomiting and lack of appetite. A low-protein diet may also help slow progression of the disease and preserve kidney function.

You may need to curtail the amount of water you drink to reduce fluid accumulation. If your kidney disease is associated with high blood pressure, you may need to restrict salt in your diet as well as the amount of liquid that you drink. Your doctor may direct you to limit your consumption of foods high in potassium and phosphorus.

Liver disease

Advanced liver disease can result in an increased amount of ammonia in your blood, retention of fluid in your abdomen (ascites) and fatigue. Several dietary measures can help relieve these problems. It's important to work closely with your doctor and dietitian to develop an appropriate eating plan.

Some protein is broken down into ammonia, so your doctor may suggest that you decrease dietary protein. Instead of eating a whole day's worth of protein in one sitting, divide it into several meals throughout the day. It's usually better to eat four to six meals a day rather than two or three.

It's also important to make sure you're getting adequate calories. If you have high blood pressure or fluid retention, you may need to limit your sodium intake.

Food Safety

Another important aspect of healthy eating is keeping the food you eat safe from food-borne illness caused by microorganisms such as bacteria, viruses and parasites.

Food-borne illness

Food-borne illness, often referred to as food poisoning, is a gastrointestinal infection caused by eating contaminated food. The food may contain harmful bacteria, toxins, parasites, viruses or chemical contaminants. Bacteria such as campylobacter, salmonella, *Escherichia coli (E. coli)* and listeria, and Norwalk-like viruses are among the most common causes of food-borne illness.

Many common foods can contain large numbers of bacteria. Perishable foods such as fresh fruits and vegetables, salads, eggs, meats, poultry, fish, shellfish and milk products are most susceptible to bacterial contamination. Seafood also is a leading cause of food-borne illness.

Getting Adequate Calcium

Getting plenty of calcium in your diet is important for growth and maintenance of healthy bones and teeth throughout life. Adolescents and adults over age 50 have an especially high need for calcium. At younger ages, people are growing. At older ages, they begin to lose calcium from bone.

Sources of calcium include:

- *Milk or milk products.* Skim or low-fat milk, low-fat yogurt and cheese are especially high in calcium. If you're lactose intolerant, try lactose-free or lactose-reduced milk. Lactaid and other lactose-reduction treatments are available as chewable tablets that you take with a meal that contains lactose.
- *Fish and vegetables.* Canned fish with soft bones included, such as salmon and sardines, is a good source of calcium. Dark leafy greens, such as collards and turnip greens, also contain calcium.
- *Calcium-enriched products.* These include breakfast cereal with added calcium, orange juice with added calcium, tofu made with calcium sulfate and soy milk with added calcium.
- *Calcium supplements.* Calcium carbonate is the preferred supplement because the rate of calcium absorption is comparable to that of milk. Avoid calcium supplements made from bone meal, dolomite or oyster shell. These products are often advertised as natural calcium, but they may contain toxic substances such as lead, mercury and arsenic.

Eating even a small portion of an unsafe food can make you sick. Common signs and symptoms are loss of appetite, nausea, vomiting, diarrhea and abdominal pain. Signs and symptoms may appear within a half-hour of eating the food, or they may not develop for up to 3 weeks.

In most people, the discomforts of food-borne illness pass within a few hours. For some people, however, food poisoning may be life-threatening. This is especially true for infants, pregnant women, older adults and people in poor health or with a weakened immune system.

Preventing food-borne illness

Food and water supplies in the United States are generally safe and are subject to inspection and regulation. But it's impossible to keep the entire food supply completely free of potentially dangerous bacteria. For this reason, you're the final line of defense against food hazards.

How do you make sure that the food you eat is safe? The following steps can help prevent food-borne illness in your home:

Wash your hands, utensils and food surfaces often

Wash your hands with warm, soapy water before and after handling or preparing food, especially raw meat, poultry, fish, shellfish and eggs. Then use hot, soapy water to wash the utensils, cutting board and other surfaces you used.

You can wash an acrylic cutting board in your dishwasher. Disinfect a wooden cutting board with a solution of 2 teaspoons of household bleach mixed with 1 quart of water. Flush the board thoroughly after applying the bleach. Replace cutting boards when they become worn or have hard-to-clean grooves.

In addition, always wash your hands after using the bathroom, changing diapers or playing with pets.

Keep raw foods separate from ready-to-eat foods

When shopping, preparing food or storing food, keep raw meat, poultry, eggs, fish and shellfish away from other foods. This prevents cross-contamination from one food to another. Store raw foods in containers in the refrigerator so that the juices don't drip onto other foods.

Cook foods to a safe temperature

Uncooked and undercooked animal foods are potentially unsafe. The best way to tell if meat, poultry or egg dishes are cooked to a safe temperature is to use a food thermometer. Cook fish and shellfish until the outside is opaque. Fish should flake easily with a fork.

Heat sauces, soups and gravies to a boil. If you marinate meat or poultry, don't serve the unused marinade unless it has been cooked at a rolling boil for several minutes. Reheat leftovers thoroughly. Don't eat raw or partially cooked eggs or unpasteurized milk products. Drink only pasteurized juices.

Refrigerate perishable foods promptly

Refrigerate or freeze perishable foods within 2 hours of purchasing or preparing them. If the temperature is above 85 F, refrigerate them within 1 hour. Freeze fresh meat,

Fish and Sushi

Fish is an important part of a healthy diet. It's a lean source of protein, and it contains heart-healthy omega-3 fatty acids. Eating fish regularly may protect you against coronary artery disease and some cancers.

But you also need to be careful about your fish choices. In some locations, sushi is a popular way to prepare fish. Sushi refers to a Japanese dish of small cakes of cold rice flavored with vinegar, sugar and salt, typically garnished with raw fish, other types of seafood and vegetables. Raw fish may harbor parasites that can cause gastrointestinal disease or reactions ranging from hives to shock.

Some fish may also contain environmental toxins, particularly polychlorinated biphenyls (PCBs) and methyl mercury. Heed the warnings from your state's department of natural resources or your local health department about unsafe fish.

Here are some guidelines when eating fish:

- Only eat sushi fish that was fresh frozen. Freezing raw fish can kill the parasites. Ask the provider if the fish was frozen.
- If you're breast-feeding, pregnant or planning to become pregnant, avoid shark, swordfish, king mackerel and tilefish. In addition, avoid serving these fish to children.

  These fish contain the highest levels of mercury, which may harm an unborn baby's developing nervous system. Limit other varieties of fish to no more than 12 ounces of cooked fish a week. Choose shellfish or smaller, younger fish, such as perch or stream trout.
- At the market, look for fresh fish with clear eyes that bulge slightly, firm and shiny flesh that springs back when pressed, bright pink or red gills, no slime and no discoloration. The fish shouldn't have a strong fishy smell.
- Remove visible fat and skin before cooking. Broil the fish on a rack or grill so that the fat drips away.
- Vary the fish you eat to limit exposure to possible contaminants.
- Cook fish and seafood thoroughly and wash your hands, cutting boards and utensils with soap and water after coming in contact with fish.

poultry, fish and shellfish that can't be used in a few days. Thaw meat, poultry, fish or shellfish in the refrigerator, microwave or in cold water that's changed every 30 minutes. Cook the food immediately after thawing. Use refrigerated leftovers within 3 to 4 days.

Follow safety instructions
Read the label on food products and follow the safety instructions, such as "Keep refrigerated" and "Safe-handling suggestions."

Serve foods safely
Keep hot foods hot — 140 F or above — and cold foods cold — 40 F or below. Harmful bacteria can grow rapidly in the danger zone between these temperatures. Avoid letting food sit out on the table after meals. When serving large quantities of food, bring out small batches at a time. Throw out any leftovers that have been at room temperature more than 2 hours or in hot weather more than 1 hour.

When in doubt, throw it out
If you aren't sure if a food has been prepared, served or stored safely, discard it. A food that has been left at room temperature too long may contain bacteria that can't be destroyed by cooking. Don't taste food that you're unsure about — just throw it out. Even if it looks and smells fine, it may not be safe to eat.

Discard foods that are moldy. Hard cheese can be an exception. Trim off the mold by cutting deeply and outward from the unmoldly area.

Recommended Safe-Cooking Temperatures

160 F	Ground meat, chops, roasts, pork, egg dishes
165 F	Ground poultry, casseroles, leftovers, stuffing
170 F	Poultry breasts, well-done meats
180 F	Whole poultry, legs, thighs, wings

PREVENTION TIP

Food-borne illness is especially serious for pregnant women, young children, older adults and people with a weakened immune system. Individuals at high risk should take extra precautions by avoiding the following foods:

- Unpasteurized juices and ciders
- Unpasteurized milk and milk products
- Soft cheeses — such as feta, brie and Camembert — blue-veined cheese and unpasteurized cheese
- Raw sprouts
- Raw or rare meat and poultry
- Raw fish and shellfish
- Raw eggs and egg products
- Pâtés

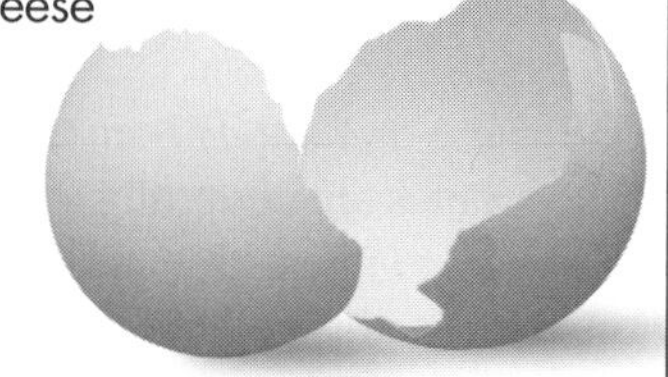

Ensuring safe drinking water

America's drinking water is among the safest in the world, and most people don't have to worry about the quality of their water. But water-treatment equipment sometimes can break down, or other unforeseen problems can occur. The Environmental Protection Agency (EPA) requires city or other public health officials to notify you if your water doesn't meet safety standards or if required monitoring isn't being done.

Even though water may look, smell and taste pure, it can contain substances that can make you ill. Conversely, chemicals used to purify water supplies may add unpleasant tastes or odors, but are safe if used properly.

Here are some general precautions regarding water safety:

- Don't drink water of unknown safety. Water from streams or lakes should be considered contaminated. Carry your own bottled water, or purify stream or lake water before using it for drinking or cooking. A variety of portable water filtration devices are available for this purpose. Or you can boil it for about 10 minutes.
- If you're unsure about your water supply, put it to the test. County or city health officials can tell you about potential contaminants and help you find individuals or certified testing laboratories to sample and analyze your water and interpret the results.
- If your water supply comes from a private well or groundwater source, such as a lake or stream, you're responsible for ensuring that your water is safe. Have your water tested annually or any time that you notice a change in color or odor.
- If your drinking water meets EPA standards, you generally don't need a home water filter. If you decide to buy one, follow the suggested maintenance steps. ■

CHAPTER 3 PART I

Controlling Your Weight

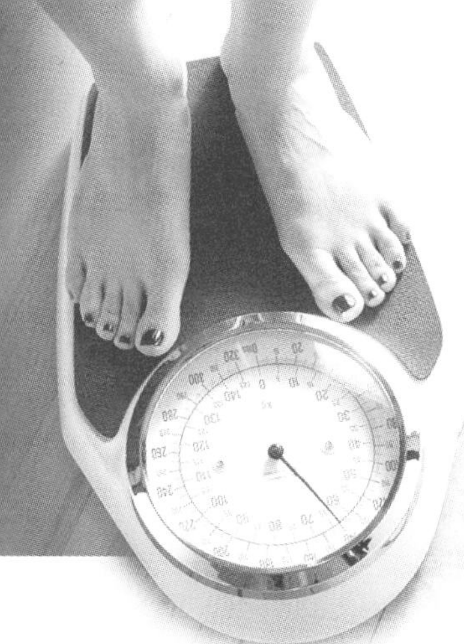

The majority of Americans weigh more than they should. In fact, obesity has reached epidemic proportions in the United States. More than half the population is overweight, and one in four adults are considered obese. Childhood obesity also is at an all-time high.

With the easy availability of calorie-dense foods, the bombardment by commercial messages urging you to eat and the prevalence of sedentary work and leisure activities, it's easy to pack on pounds.

After a certain point, body fat can interfere with your health. The more your weight increases, the more problems you'll face in staying healthy and living longer. Excess weight can lead to heart disease, diabetes and high blood pressure, among other conditions.

Improving your health over the long term is the most important reason for reaching and maintaining a healthy weight. Along with that, you'll likely feel better physically, feel better about yourself and have more energy.

Losing weight is hard. There's no quick, easy fix. But despite the challenges, you aren't doomed to be overweight.

This chapter offers strategies for losing weight gradually by changing your eating and activity habits. These long-term changes in your lifestyle can lead to successful weight loss and better health.

Is Your Weight Healthy?

How much should you weigh? For more than 50 years, insurance companies have related weight to health risk, and consumers and health experts have struggled with the concept of acceptable weight.

Traditionally, *overweight* was defined as weighing more than the healthy weight listed in the height-weight tables developed by life insurance companies. But weight charts don't take into consideration how much of your weight is fat or where on your body you're carrying that fat — both important factors in predicting associated health risks. For example, athletes often are overweight by weight table standards because of increased muscle development or a large bone structure. But they're not carrying too much fat.

A combination of three more-accurate measurements — body mass index (BMI), waist measurement and personal and family medical history — can give you a better idea of what shape you're in.

Body mass index

The first step in determining if your weight is healthy is to figure out your body mass index (BMI). Weigh yourself and have your height measured. Then determine your BMI by using the chart on the next page.

BMI considers weight in relation to height. The BMI ranges shown are for adults. They're not exact ranges of healthy and unhealthy weights, but show that health risk increases with higher weight levels. BMI doesn't consider your individual makeup and factors such as being big boned or highly muscular, but it is an improvement over height-weight tables.

A BMI of 19 to 24.9 is desirable. If your BMI falls within this healthy range, there's generally no health advantage to your losing weight. A BMI of 25 to 29.9 suggests that you're overweight. If you have a BMI of 30 or more, you're considered obese.

The further your BMI is above the healthy range, the higher your weight-related health risks. If your BMI is 25 or more, losing weight may improve your health and reduce your risk of weight-related diseases. If your BMI falls below 18.5, you're probably underweight. Ask your doctor to assess your weight and health.

Waist circumference

Your waist circumference measurement indicates where most of your fat is located. People who carry most of their weight around their waist are often referred to as apples. Those who carry most of their weight below their waist — in their thighs, hips and buttocks — are known as pears.

Generally, it's better to have a pear shape than an apple shape. Extra weight around your waist puts you at higher risk of heart disease, diabetes and some cancers. The pear distribution of body fat is determined largely by heredity, and the apple distribution is affected more by environment.

To measure your waist, find the highest point on each of your hips and measure across your abdomen just above those points.

- For women, a waist measurement of 35 inches or more is associated with higher health risks.
- For men, a waist measurement of 40 inches or more is associated with higher health risks.

Excess abdominal fat may place you at greater risk of health problems, even if your BMI is about right. If your BMI is 24 or higher and your waist circumference exceeds healthy guidelines, the risk is even greater.

Personal and family medical history

Your personal medical history and family medical history provide additional information about your risk of developing weight-related health problems.

If you answer yes to any of the following questions, you're likely to benefit from weight loss if you're overweight (BMI 25 to 29.9) or obese (BMI 30 or higher):

- Do you have a personal or family history of high blood pressure, diabetes, heart disease, sleep apnea, osteoarthritis or high blood fats (cholesterol and triglycerides)?

Body Mass Index (BMI)

	Healthy		Overweight					Obese				
BMI	**19**	**24**	25	26	27	28	29	30	35	40	45	50
Height	**Weight in pounds**											
4′10″	91	115	119	124	129	134	138	143	167	191	215	239
4′11″	94	119	124	128	133	138	143	148	173	198	222	247
5′0″	97	123	128	133	138	143	148	153	179	204	230	255
5′1″	100	127	132	137	143	148	153	158	185	211	238	264
5′2″	104	131	136	142	147	153	158	164	191	218	246	273
5′3″	107	135	141	146	152	158	163	169	197	225	254	282
5′4″	110	140	145	151	157	163	169	174	204	232	262	291
5′5″	114	144	150	156	162	168	174	180	210	240	270	300
5′6″	118	148	155	161	167	173	179	186	216	247	278	309
5′7″	121	153	159	166	172	178	185	191	223	255	287	319
5′8″	125	158	164	171	177	184	190	197	230	262	295	328
5′9″	128	162	169	176	182	189	196	203	236	270	304	338
5′10″	132	167	174	181	188	195	202	209	243	278	313	348
5′11″	136	172	179	186	193	200	208	215	250	286	322	358
6′0″	140	177	184	191	199	206	213	221	258	294	331	368
6′1″	144	182	189	197	204	212	219	227	265	302	340	378
6′2″	148	186	194	202	210	218	225	233	272	311	350	389
6′3″	152	192	200	208	216	224	232	240	279	319	359	399
6′4″	156	197	205	213	221	230	238	246	287	328	369	410

Source: Adapted from National Institutes of Health Clinical Guidelines on the Identification, Evaluation, and Treatment of Overweight and Obesity in Adults, 1998

- Have you gained at least 10 pounds as an adult?
- Do you smoke cigarettes, overeat, have more than one alcoholic drink a day or lead an inactive lifestyle?

Assessing your weight

If your BMI is 25 or greater, your waist circumference equals or exceeds the healthy guidelines, or you answered yes to at least one of the personal and family history questions, you're likely to benefit from losing weight. Discuss your weight with your doctor during your next checkup.

If you're obese, even a modest weight loss may improve your health. Studies of more than 200 severely obese people found that those who lost 10 percent to 20 percent of their body weight and kept it off for 3 years reduced their risk of some diseases by 25 percent to 75 percent.

If your extra weight is all around your waist, taking 2 inches off your waist may lower your blood pressure and reduce your risk of many diseases.

Your Weight and Your Health

Obesity is a chronic disease that develops from the interaction between genes and the environment. Researchers' understanding of how and why people become obese is incomplete, but it involves a combination of factors. What is known is that weight and health are intimately connected. Obesity has direct links to serious diseases that can shorten your life.

Risk factors for becoming overweight

Weight is largely determined by how you balance your intake of calories with the energy you burn in everyday activities. If you consume more calories than you burn, you gain weight. Overeating and lack of physical activity are the main causes of being overweight. But many other factors contribute to this condition.

Aging and Body Fat

Your body composition changes as you age. Muscle mass decreases slowly after ages 30 to 35 and more rapidly after age 55. Translated into what your scale tells you, if you weigh 10 pounds more at age 65 than you did at 30, you may actually be carrying 15 to 20 pounds more fat.

The distribution of fat also changes with age. As you get older, body fat tends to shift from the face, arms, legs and neck to the trunk and abdomen — hence the appearance of the spare tire or love handles.

For women, menopause can play a role in midlife body changes. During the years leading up to menopause, you begin to produce less estrogen, a process that's associated with weight shifting to the middle. And, as you age, you may either gain weight or have more trouble staying at the same weight.

For both men and women, as you grow older your body becomes less able to handle the load when you overeat, and you're more likely to store the excess as fat. One solution is to eat smaller meals.

An excellent way to deal with age-related weight changes is to exercise. Aerobic exercise helps you burn calories, and strength-training exercises increase muscle mass and strengthen bones. See Chapter 4, "Keeping Active," for detailed information about aerobic exercise and strength training.

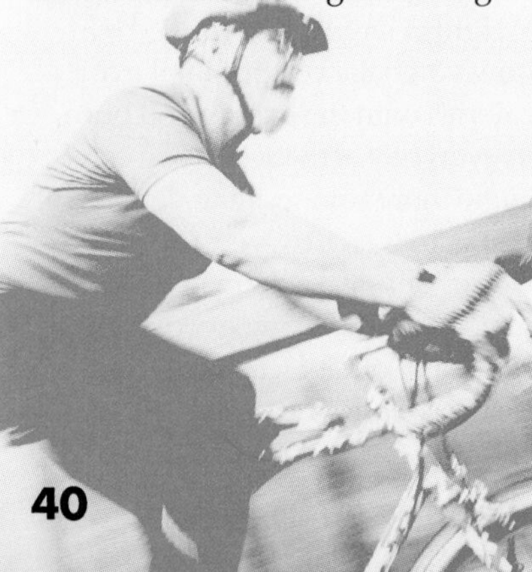

Genetics
Genes play a part in how your body balances calories and energy. If one or both of your parents are overweight, your chances of being overweight increase by 25 percent to 30 percent. Your genes also affect the amount of body fat you store and how that fat is distributed. But your genetic makeup doesn't guarantee that you'll be overweight.

Diet
Regular consumption of high-fat foods, such as fast foods, contributes to weight gain. High-fat foods are dense in calories. Loading up on soft drinks, candy and desserts also promotes weight gain. Such foods and beverages are high in sugar and calories.

Inactivity
Sedentary people are more likely to gain weight because they burn fewer calories through physical activity.

Psychological factors
Some people overeat to cope with problems, such as stress, anxiety or depression.

Sex
Men have more muscle and less fat than do women. Because muscle burns a greater number of calories than fat, men expend up to 20 percent more calories than do women, even at rest. For women, achieving and maintaining a healthy weight may be a tougher challenge.

Age
As you get older, you gradually lose muscle, and fat accounts for a greater percentage of your weight. Less muscle mass leads to a decrease in the rate at which your body uses calories. The result is a reduction in calorie needs. If you don't decrease your caloric intake with age, you'll likely gain weight.

Pregnancy
After each pregnancy, a woman's weight tends to increase an average of 4 to 6 pounds over her pre-pregnancy weight.

Medications
Side effects of some medications — corticosteroids and tricyclic antidepressants, in particular — can contribute to weight gain.

Quitting smoking
Some smokers gain weight after quitting. This may be partially due to nicotine's ability to raise the rate at which your body burns calories (metabolic rate). When smokers quit, they burn fewer calories, and they tend to eat more because their senses of taste and smell improve.

Medical problems
Endocrine and metabolic disorders contribute to only a small percentage of cases of obesity. Less than 5 percent of all cases of obesity can be traced to a medical cause such as low thyroid function or other hormonal imbalances. A low metabolic rate is rarely a cause of obesity.

Dangers of being overweight

Regardless of how a person becomes overweight, the condition can ultimately be a matter of life and death. Overweight and obese people are more likely to develop a number of potentially serious health problems.

Studies show that your risk of certain diseases and disorders increases as your body mass index increases. In addition, your overall risk of death increases with obesity.

High blood pressure
When you have excess body fat, you tend to retain sodium. To dilute the extra sodium, your body holds on to more water. This increases the volume of your blood, and eventually the pressure inside your arteries builds up. The excessive force makes your heart work harder.

Excess weight is often associated with an increase in heart rate and a reduction in the capacity of blood vessels to transport blood. These two factors can also increase blood pressure and may lead to the bursting of a blood vessel in the brain (hemorrhagic stroke).

Diabetes
Obesity is a leading cause of type 2 diabetes (formerly called adult-onset or noninsulin-dependent diabetes). Excess fat makes your body resistant to insulin, the hormone that helps transport sugar (glucose) from your blood into individual cells. If your body is resistant to insulin, your cells can't get the sugar they need for energy.

Coronary artery disease
With increased weight, there's an increased risk of coronary artery disease. Coronary artery disease typically results from the buildup of fatty deposits (plaques) in the arteries that feed your heart. Over time, these deposits can narrow your heart's arteries, so less blood flows to your heart. The diminished blood flow can cause chest pain (angina). Complete blockage can lead to a heart attack.

Stroke
The accumulation of plaques in arteries that feed the brain can lead to a stroke. When an artery leading to your brain becomes narrowed, a blood clot can form in the artery, interrupting blood flow to your brain. The result is an ischemic stroke. Being overweight or obese increases risk of an ischemic stroke, even in the absence of high blood pressure and diabetes.

Abnormal blood fats
A diet high in saturated fats can lead to obesity as well as to elevated levels of low-density lipoprotein (LDL or "bad") cholesterol and reduced levels of high-density lipoprotein (HDL or "good") cholesterol. Obesity is also associated with high levels of another type of blood fat, triglycerides.

Over time, some of these blood fats can contribute to the buildup of fatty deposits in arteries throughout your body. This condition is called atherosclerosis, and it puts you at risk of coronary artery disease and stroke.

Osteoarthritis
This joint disorder most often affects the knees, hips and lower back. Excess weight puts extra pressure on these joints and wears away the cartilage that protects them, resulting in joint pain and stiffness.

Sleep apnea
Obstructive sleep apnea is a serious condition that causes you to stop breathing for short periods during sleep. The upper airway becomes blocked intermittently during sleep, resulting in lower blood oxygen levels and subsequent drowsiness during the day. Sleep apnea can also cause heart failure. Most people with sleep apnea are overweight. The more overweight an individual is, the more severe his or her sleep apnea tends to be.

Cancer
Several types of cancer are associated with being overweight. In women, these include cancers of the breast, uterus, colon and gallbladder. Overweight men have a higher risk of colon and prostate cancer.

Gallstones
Gallstones are more common in people who are overweight, although it's not clear how being overweight results in gallstones.

Physical discomfort
As fat accumulates, it crowds the space occupied by your organs. Some obese people can't sit comfortably because of fat in their abdomen. In a seated position, an obese person may have limited ability to breathe.

Social and emotional consequences
In a country that tends to equate thinness with beauty, intelligence and success, overweight adults may experience psychological stress, reduced income and discrimination.

Benefits of modest weight loss

The good news is that you don't have to lose a lot of weight to enjoy health benefits. Modest losses of just 10 percent to 20 percent of your body weight can lower your blood pressure, reduce your risk of cardiovascular disease and stroke, improve control of diabetes, improve symptoms of osteoarthritis and sleep apnea and lower your risk of cancer.

The amount of weight you need to lose to improve your health may be much less than what you may feel you need to lose to be thin or achieve an "ideal" appearance.

The first goal in dealing with being overweight is to achieve and maintain a healthier weight. For example, if you weigh 200 pounds and are obese by BMI standards, start by trying to lose 10 to 20 pounds (5 percent to 10 percent of your weight). Talk to your doctor about setting a realistic weight-loss goal.

How to Lose Weight

If you've struggled with your weight, you likely know that both losing weight and keeping it off can be very difficult. Many diets promote temporary weight loss, but they may also encourage unhealthy eating habits, and their long-term effects are often minimal.

Healthy weight loss is weight loss that's slow and steady. Aim to lose no more than ½ to 2 pounds a week.

A good weight-loss plan has three components — a healthy diet, regular physical activity and the right attitude.

A healthy diet

What you eat and how much you eat play key roles in managing your weight. Learn to enjoy a variety of healthy foods.

To lose weight and keep it off, eat moderate amounts of nutrient-rich, low-fat, low-calorie foods. Decreasing calories doesn't mean decreasing the taste or satisfaction of food or increasing preparation time. You can lower your calorie intake by eating foods that are tasty, healthy and practical.

Eat the right mix of foods

To help guide your daily food choices, Mayo Clinic doctors and nutrition experts developed the Mayo Clinic Healthy Weight Pyramid. The pyramid is a tool to help you eat a balanced, nutritious diet while achieving a healthy weight. It illustrates the types and amounts of food you need to eat every day from each of five key food groups.

The triangular shape of the pyramid shows you where to focus when selecting foods that can help promote healthy weight. The most important foods — vegetables and fruits — form the foundation of the pyramid.

The pyramid emphasizes lower-calorie foods that help you feel full. It provides all of the nutrients you need. Unlimited fruits and vegetables make it high in vitamins, minerals, fiber and plant nutrients called phytochemicals. The diet is low in fat, saturated fat, cholesterol and sodium, and it provides adequate protein and calcium.

Mayo Clinic's pyramid is different from the USDA Food Guide Pyramid in these ways:

- It emphasizes weight management.
- It places vegetables and fruits at its foundation as opposed to grains — breads, cereals and starches — because vegetables and fruits are very low in calories and high in health-enhancing properties. It's suggested that you eat at least four servings of vegetables and at least three servings of fruit each day, but you're allowed to eat virtually unlimited amounts of both. If you fill up on these healthy foods, you'll leave less room for foods with fewer nutrients and more calories.
- It emphasizes healthy choices within each of five food groups. That's because not all foods within a group provide the same health benefits, even though they may contain the same number of calories. For example, with carbohydrates, it's best to select brown rice or whole-grain pasta and breads because whole grains are higher in fiber, vitamins and minerals than white refined rice, pasta and breads.
- Daily physical activity is located in the middle of the pyramid to emphasize its central role in both managing weight and improving health.

Vegetables

Vegetables are low in calories and virtually fat-free while providing a variety of vitamins, minerals and, in most cases, fiber. In addition, vegetables contain phytochemicals, substances that can reduce your risk of cardiovascular disease and cancer. Some vegetables belong within the carbohydrates group instead of the vegetable group because they're high in starch, contain more calories than typical vegetables and function more like a carbohydrate in your body. These include corn, potatoes, sweet potatoes and winter squash.

Fruits

Fruit plays an important role in eating well. Along with few calories and little or no fat, fruit also contains vitamins, minerals, fiber and phytochemicals. Fresh and frozen fruits are best because they're bulkier and lower in energy density than canned fruits, fruit juices and dried fruits. Foods that are lower in energy density have fewer calories relative to their volume.

The 'Mayo Clinic Diet' Myth

Various versions of the so-called Mayo Clinic Diet have surfaced over the years. The problem is, there is no Mayo Clinic Diet. The origin of these mythical diets is unknown.

No one-size-fits-all diet that pushes grapefruit or eggs or promises to rapidly peel off pounds is approved by Mayo Clinic. For some individuals, such diets can be dangerous.

Instead of relying on "miracle diets," take stock of your current eating and exercise habits. A healthy diet combined with physical activity is the best approach for safe, effective weight loss. Think long term and work on changes in your food selections and exercise habits that you can maintain for life.

Carbohydrates

Carbohydrates include grain products such as cereal, bread, rice and pasta. These foods provide a variety of nutrients and are generally low in fat and calories. It's often other ingredients added to grain products or creamy sauces served with them that add calories and fat.

The best grains are whole grains because they're higher in fiber, vitamins and minerals. Choose brown rice, whole-grain pasta and breads that contain whole-wheat or whole-grain flour as their primary ingredient.

Protein/Dairy

The foods in the protein/dairy group usually provide most of the protein in your diet. Because many animal-based protein sources are high in fat and saturated fat, the Mayo Clinic Healthy Weight Pyramid emphasizes plant-based sources of protein, such as beans, peas and lentils, and low-fat or fat-free dairy products. Dairy products

Mayo Clinic Healthy Weight Pyramid

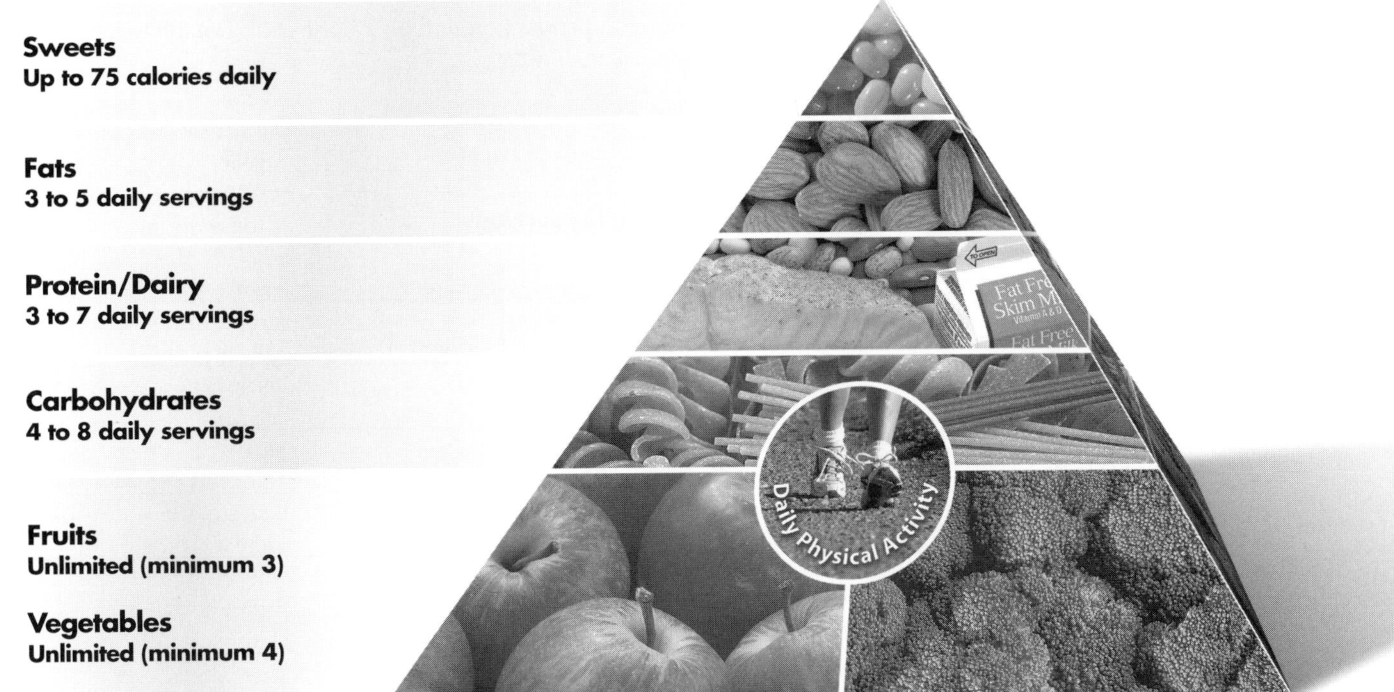
Sweets
Up to 75 calories daily
Fats
3 to 5 daily servings
Protein/Dairy
3 to 7 daily servings
Carbohydrates
4 to 8 daily servings
Fruits
Unlimited (minimum 3)
Vegetables
Unlimited (minimum 4)
Daily Physical Activity

 See your doctor before you begin any healthy weight plan.

are good sources of calcium, and milk is fortified with vitamin D.

Fats
Because ounce for ounce fat has more than twice the calories of carbohydrates and protein, reducing the fat in your diet is an important way to cut calories. Cook foods with little or no oil or other fats. When needed, use monounsaturated fat, such as olive or canola oil.

Sweets
The sweets group includes candies, desserts and other processed sweets. You can eat foods in this group in amounts up to 75 calories a day. Once you get used to a diet that emphasizes fruits, vegetables and grains, you may not miss sweets.

Choose foods low in energy density

The Mayo Clinic Healthy Weight Pyramid emphasizes foods that are low in energy density. Energy density is the number of calories in a given volume of food. Low energy-dense foods, such as vegetables, have a large volume and weight but not many calories. What makes foods low in energy density is water and fiber. Foods with a low energy density contain a lot of both. Foods with high energy density, such as fat and table sugar, contain a large number of calories in just a small amount of the food.

By choosing foods low in energy density, you won't go hungry. You'll feel full and satisfied, so it's harder to eat large amounts of calories. This promotes weight loss. It also leaves room in your eating plan for some of your favorite energy-dense foods, such as chocolate, in small quantities.

Pay attention to calories

To lose weight, you need to consume fewer calories than you burn. The number of calories you need each day depends on several factors, including your age and activity level.

The Mayo Clinic Healthy Weight Pyramid suggests these starting calorie goals:

Men
If you weigh:
- 250 pounds or less: 1,400 calories a day
- 251 to 300 pounds: 1,600 calories a day
- 301 pounds or more: 1,800 calories a day

Women
If you weigh:
- 250 pounds or less: 1,200 calories a day
- 251 to 300 pounds: 1,400 calories a day
- 301 pounds or more: 1,600 calories a day

Over time, your calorie needs may change based on health risks, how much weight you lose and your goals and preferences. Calories can be adjusted to the next higher level if you're too hungry or you've reached your target weight.

Servings and Serving Sizes

The number of servings to choose from each food group depends on your daily calorie goal. The following chart lists the number of servings recommended for various calorie levels:

	Starting calorie goals			
	1,200	**1,400**	**1,600**	**1,800**
Food group	**Recommended number of daily servings**			
Vegetables	4 or more	4 or more	5 or more	5 or more
Fruits	3 or more	4 or more	5 or more	5 or more
Carbohydrates	4	5	6	7
Protein/Dairy	3	4	5	6
Fats	3	3	3	4

Food group	**Average serving size**
Vegetables	2 cups leafy or 1 cup solid
Fruits	½ cup sliced or one medium piece
Carbohydrates	½ cup grain or cereal or one slice bread
Protein/Dairy	½ cups beans, 3 oz. fish, 1 cup skim milk or 1 ½ to 2 oz. meat or hard cheese
Fats	1 tsp. oil or 2 tbsp. nuts

Check product labels to learn how much of the food is considered a serving and how many calories and grams of fat are in the food. Many items sold as single portions actually provide two or more servings.

Cutting calories to below 1,200 a day if you're a woman or 1,400 a day if you're a man usually doesn't provide enough food for you to be satisfied in the long term. These calorie levels also make it difficult for you to get some of the nutrients you need for good health, such as folate, magnesium and zinc.

Find healthy ways to satisfy your appetite

Losing weight doesn't mean that you have to deprive yourself of pleasure or go hungry. Try these tips to help curb your appetite.

- *Eat three meals a day.* Eating regular meals and snacks prevents the famine-then-feast cycle. If you start with a breakfast that includes a high-fiber cereal, whole-grain bread and fresh fruit, you're more likely to eat less later in the day.
- *Eat only when you're hungry.* By responding only to physical signals to eat, you may be less apt to eat in response to stress or boredom.
- *Eat slowly.* Savoring the flavors and textures of food can enhance satisfaction. Eating slowly also allows your brain to receive the signal that you've eaten and you're full.
- *Ride out the urge.* Food cravings generally pass within minutes, maybe even seconds. Distract yourself with an activity unrelated to food until the desire to eat passes.
- *Start small.* If you always finish what's in front of you, start with half the amount of food you usually eat. You may find smaller servings more satisfying. To make less food seem like more, serve your main course on a smaller plate.

Regular physical activity

Studies show that people who want to optimize weight loss — and keep it off — must do more than transform their eating habits. They need to make physical activity and exercise a part of their daily routine. To stay fit and maintain a healthy weight, you need to keep active.

The goal of exercise to promote weight loss is to burn calories, but it has many other benefits as well. Physical activity promotes loss of body fat and development of muscle. Muscle uses more calories than fat does. So the more muscle mass your body has, the more calories it'll burn, even when you're at rest.

The best way to lose body fat is through steady aerobic exercise — activities that increase your breathing and heart rate, such as walking, bicycling, jogging and swimming. Regular aerobic exercise is best, but any extra movement helps burn calories. Activities such as mowing the lawn or taking the stairs instead of the elevator at work help with weight management.

The ultimate goal should be at least 30 minutes of moderate to vigorous physical activity on most or preferably all days of the week. Start slowly and gradually build up your time and intensity level and stick to it.

If you're obese — particularly if you're unfit and have health problems — check with your doctor before starting an exercise program.

For more information about developing an exercise program, see Chapter 4, "Keeping Active."

The right attitude

Anyone who has tried to lose weight knows that this is more challenging than it sounds. To make lasting changes, you need to address your habits, emotions, needs, thinking and the behaviors that made you overweight in the first place.

Part of being successful is to plan how you'll incorporate changes into your lifestyle. This takes concentration, time and effort — and then a firm commitment. In addition, some people need to address psychological issues, such as depression or an eating disorder, before they can lose weight.

No one can make you lose weight. In fact, increased external pressure — often from people close to you — may make matters worse. Likewise, trying to lose weight to satisfy someone else rarely works either. Make diet and exercise changes that you want for yourself.

Research indicates that a number of tools and tips are effective in helping change attitudes and behaviors:

Make a commitment

Focus on all of the good things about losing weight, such as having more energy and improving your health. Then look at the negatives, such as finding the time to exercise. Look for creative solutions to overcome any negatives and then commit yourself to losing weight.

Make lifestyle changes a priority

As you're planning to launch new weight-related lifestyle changes, try to resolve other problems in your life. It takes a lot of mental and physical energy to change habits. Don't set yourself up for failure by trying to make lifestyle changes when you're distracted by other major issues, such as marital or financial problems.

Set small, realistic goals

Remember that you're in this for the long haul. You're making lifestyle changes, and the goals you write down are your first steps in that direction. Anything you undertake too intensely or too vigorously will quickly become uncomfortable, and you're more likely to give it up. Don't set a weight goal that's unrealistic.

Focus on the positive

Rather than dwelling on what you can't eat, focus on what you can. Discover new tastes and activities.

Know your habits

To become aware of your eating behaviors, ask yourself if you tend to eat when you're bored, angry, tired, anxious, depressed or socially pressured. Assess your eating style and shopping and cooking techniques. Were you taught to always clean your plate? Do you eat fast? Do you eat while watching TV? See if any patterns emerge and identify possible triggers for eating.

Have a plan

Work out a strategy to gradually change the habits and attitudes that may have undermined past efforts to lose weight. Choose a definite start date. Determine a realistic eating plan that factors in plenty of water, vegetables and fruits. Consider how often and how long you'll exercise. When and where will you do it? How will it fit into your schedule? What are the potential roadblocks in your plan, and how will you deal with them?

Willpower vs. Self-Control

Some people think that they can achieve a healthy weight if they exert enough willpower. But that just sets you up to fail when your willpower cracks. Try focusing on self-control rather than willpower. Self-control is, "Ice cream is my problem food, so I'm not going to keep it in the house." Willpower is, "I'm going to keep buying ice cream, but I won't eat it." Self-control means planning for success ahead of time.

If you like sweets, consider finding a way to occasionally fit them into your diet without destroying your overall eating plan. You may be surprised to discover that just knowing it's all right to allow yourself a treat now and then can make it easier to say no.

Metabolism and Weight

Metabolism is the complex biochemical process by which the food you eat is converted into the energy your body needs to function. The nutrients you eat — carbohydrates, proteins, fats and others — combine with oxygen to release energy resulting in heat, carbon dioxide, water and waste products. The energy created is used for muscular activity and for essential chemical processes in the body. The heat helps maintain body temperature.

The amount of energy your body uses at rest is called the basal metabolic rate (BMR). This rate is expressed in calories.

The number of calories you burn daily depends not just on your BMR but also on how much you exercise and on your body's muscle-to-fat ratio. All activity, not just strenuous exercise, helps boost your calorie burn.

The more muscle and the less fat you have, the more calories you burn. That's one reason experts recommend strength training as a way to build muscle mass. It's also why men — who typically have more lean muscle than do women and therefore burn more calories — tend to lose weight faster and gain it more slowly.

Many people who've had difficulty losing weight blame it on slow metabolism. In fact, very few people burn fewer calories at rest than they should according to estimates based on their height, weight and age. Because people who weigh more have more muscle as well as fat, overweight people have a higher metabolic rate, contrary to popular belief.

Chronic dieting probably has little permanent effect on your metabolism, but taking in fewer calories does mean you have less energy to burn. You may feel sluggish if you severely restrict your calories.

Avoid your food triggers
Store food out of sight and don't keep junk food around. Practice substituting healthy food for unhealthy food. Distract yourself from your desire to eat with something positive, like calling a friend.

Plan ahead for unusual circumstances
Think of effective strategies for keeping your commitment while at work, on vacation, at parties and during the holidays. For example, envision yourself at a party taking a small portion of a few items or taking only fresh fruits and vegetables. Mentally rehearse this plan.

Keep a record
In addition to keeping track of your weight and food intake, keeping an activity diary can help you be physically active and discover any behaviors that you may need to improve. Track other important health parameters, such as blood pressure and cholesterol levels.

Draw on support from others
Ultimately, only you can help yourself lose weight, and you have to take responsibility for your own behavior. But that doesn't mean that you have to do everything alone. Ask for support from your spouse, family and friends.

It may be helpful to talk to a weight-loss specialist or others trying to lose weight who can help you think of food and exercise in a new light. Group programs such as Weight Watchers, Take Off Pounds Sensibly (TOPS) or Overeaters Anonymous can support your efforts, giving you eating plans and reinforcement from others on the same path.

Don't give up
No matter how prepared you are, you'll occasionally overeat or eat foods you're trying to avoid. Rather than letting a setback derail your efforts, accept that the setback happened and get back on track. Don't expect to be perfect — and never give up.

Failure of the Fads

Americans spend billions of dollars yearly on weight-loss programs and products, looking for the magic cure that will help them shed pounds quickly and painlessly. Fad diets have been around for decades, and new ones surface regularly.

Fad diets promise quick and easy weight loss. Unfortunately, people often find that whatever pounds they drop come right back, in part because they get tired of avoiding bread or loading up on grapefruit or feeling hungry while existing on very few calories.

Some of the popular diets in circulation today include:

Low-calorie liquid diets
Low-calorie liquid diets like Medifast and Optifast are prescribed under medical supervision as an intervention for seriously overweight people. They're not intended as a long-term solution because they restrict calories to about 800 a day.

Meal replacements
Meal replacements include Slim-Fast, which is an over-the-counter product. The plan suggests that you replace one to two meals with the drink, then eat a healthy, balanced third meal that's low in fat and calories.

The Atkins diet
Robert Atkins, M.D., believes that carbohydrates promote insulin pro-

duction, which leads to weight gain and other health risks. The Atkins diet, therefore, limits carbohydrates to 20 to 40 grams a day initially. Most grains, beans, fruits, breads, pastas and vegetables are excluded. He says you can eat as much meat, eggs, cheese, butter and cream as you want.

Without enough dietary carbohydrates, your body begins to burn its stored carbohydrates for energy — which releases a lot of water weight. Your body also starts burning some fat. Burning fat without carbohydrates also creates byproducts called ketones that build up in your bloodstream. Ketones are processed through your kidneys before they're eliminated. Ketones suppress appetite, but they also cause fatigue and nausea. The long-term health effects of this diet are unknown. Because the diet excludes so many foods, supplements are needed.

The Zone diet

The Zone diet is based on the belief that the key to successful weight loss is a diet in which every meal has a carbohydrate-to-protein ratio of 4 to 3. For overweight people, a caloric ratio of 40 percent carbohydrate, 30 percent protein and 30 percent fat is recommended. The diet's goal is to sustain a specific ratio of insulin and glucagon, regulators of carbohydrate metabolism.

However, there's little evidence that metabolism can be manipulated through such dietary changes. People will lose weight if they follow the prescribed diet in the book because it's low in total calories and emphasizes fruits and vegetables.

The Sugar Busters diet

When you consider that on average Americans consume nearly 3 pounds of sugar a week, the premise of the Sugar Busters diet — "Cut sugar to trim fat" — might seem worthwhile. But the concept, which lumps in whole foods such as potatoes, corn and carrots with refined sugars found in cakes, candies and sodas, goes too far.

Cutting back on sugar is only one aspect of healthy dietary changes. Without making any other nutritional changes, and particularly by permitting the intake of saturated fat and decreasing beneficial vegetables, this diet is unlikely to help you lose weight — or at least keep it off over the long term.

The grapefruit diet

Many versions of the grapefruit diet exist — even one that's erroneously called the Mayo Clinic Diet. All of these plans require you to eat half a grapefruit before every meal to reap the benefits of the fruit's so-called fat-burning enzymes. Calories typically are limited to fewer than 800 a day. Grapefruit has no fat, is low in calories and sodium and is packed with vitamin C. But very low calories — and deficits in protein, fiber and several important vitamins and minerals — can make such a diet unhealthy and dangerous for some people.

The blood type diet

The blood type diet provides a detailed list of foods that you

Tips for Parents of an Overweight Child

Parents play a crucial role in helping children who are obese feel loved, control their weight and develop healthy habits.

Take advantage of every opportunity to build your child's self-esteem. Overweight children are at increased risk of low self-esteem because of the social emphasis on appearance and being slim. Don't be afraid to bring up the topic of health and fitness, but do be sensitive that a child may view your concern as an insult. Talk to your kids directly, openly and without being judgmental.

In addition, consider the following advice:

- *Be a role model.* Make sure your own lifestyle doesn't encourage overeating and inactivity in your kids. Don't order french fries if you don't want your kids ordering them. Don't buy Oreos if you don't want your kids sneaking them from the cookie jar.
- *Make eating an activity in itself.* Your family should take care not to eat while watching television, riding in a car or walking through the kitchen. Sit down to eat, enjoy the meal and then get up and do something else.
- *Don't reward with food.* Don't reward your children with snacks. Find alternative ways of celebrating, such as taking a walk, going to the bowling alley, playing a game of cards or going on a bike ride.
- *Limit television, video and computer time.* There's a clear link between television time — especially when combined with eating — and obesity. Children shouldn't have televisions in their bedrooms, and all kids should limit television, video game and computer time not related to homework to no more than an hour or two a day.
- *Focus on positive goals.* Help your child focus on achieving positive goals such as being able to bike for more than 20 minutes without getting tired or keeping up with other kids when running laps in physical education class.
- *Take small steps as a family.* Make sure changes are subtle and involve the whole family. For example, take a family walk in the evenings, have fruit for dessert rather than banning desserts altogether and don't pick up fast food as frequently.

Nonprescription Weight-Loss Products

Diet products sold without a prescription promise to help you shed pounds by raising your metabolism or suppressing your appetite. Side effects from these products, though, can be dangerous.

People tend to regard over-the-counter drugs and herbal products less seriously than prescription medications and often take too much or mix them with other drugs. In addition, because the manufacturing of herbal products isn't regulated by the Food and Drug Administration (FDA), you can't be sure what you're getting.

Nonprescription diet products can't help you with anything beyond short-term, temporary weight loss, if that. These products are usually more harmful than helpful.

Here's a look at some of the more popular over-the-counter diet preparations and what they will and won't do for you.

Ephedrine

One of the most popular nonprescription weight-loss products is Metabolife, an herbal dietary supplement. Similar products are Metabolite and MetaboMax. The main ingredient in all of these is ephedrine, which is derived from ephedra (ma-huang). Ephedrine is used to treat asthma. It's also used to make the street drug methamphetamine, commonly known as speed. Chemically, there's only a slight difference between methamphetamine and ephedrine. This drug can suppress your appetite slightly, but it can also cause high blood pressure, heart rhythm irregularities, insomnia, nervousness, tremors, seizures, heart attack, stroke and death.

Chitosan

Chitosan is a dietary supplement made from chitin, a starch found in the skeletons of shrimp, crab and other shellfish. Because chitosan isn't digested, it passes through your intestinal tract unabsorbed, so it adds no calories. The chemical nature of chitosan makes it bind with some of the fatty foods you eat, removing some of this fat from your body rather than allowing it to be absorbed. However, one study found no more weight loss from chitosan than from a placebo.

Hydroxycitric acid

A common ingredient in herbal weight-loss products, hydroxycitric acid (HCA) comes from a plant native to

should eat or avoid, depending on your blood type. The premise is that each blood type has its own unique antigen marker that reacts in negative ways with certain foods. There's no scientific evidence that diets should be based on blood type.

The cabbage soup diet

What could be simpler? Eat as much cabbage soup as you want for 7 days, and you'll lose 10 to 15 pounds. Other foods, too, are prescribed during the weeklong program, including potatoes, fruit juices and some vegetables. The only problem is that cabbage soup proponents report feeling lightheaded and weak because the diet is too low in protein, vitamins and complex carbohydrates.

Others

Countless other fad diets are touted. Many of them advise reducing carbohydrate intake and include few, if any, fruits, vegetables and grains.

The bottom line is, be wary of diets that promise a quick fix or that sound too good to be true. Although traditional recommendations for weight management — eating a variety of vegetables, fruits and grains and being physically active daily — may seem boring, they generally lead to improved health and permanent weight loss.

When You Need More Help

It's best to lose weight through a healthy diet and regular physical activity. Some people, though, have physical limitations that keep them from exercising. Others need extra help reducing their calorie intake. If you're among those who can't seem to lose weight on your own and your excess weight is causing health problems, medications or surgery may help.

Prescription weight-loss drugs aren't for people who just want to lose a few pounds for cosmetic reasons. They're for people with a body mass index (BMI) of 30 or higher or for those with a BMI of 27 or greater who have health problems that may improve with weight loss. Surgery may be the next best step if you're extremely obese.

Medications

Prescription medications for weight loss are appropriate for moderately overweight and obese people who have health complications related to weight and who are enrolled in a weight management program that emphasizes healthy nutrition and physical activity. Drugs should be viewed only as a tool to help make

India, *Garcinia cambogia*. Popular brand names of this herb include Citrus Slim, Citrimax and CitriLean. A study in the *Journal of the American Medical Association* reported that the herb is ineffective for weight loss.

5-hydroxytryptophan
Sold under names such as Natrol, Natural Balance and Solaray, 5-hydroxytryptophan (5-HTP) products contain a contaminant linked to a rare and potentially deadly blood disorder. Chemically, 5-HTP is closely related to L-tryptophan, a dietary supplement banned in 1990 after researchers found the same contaminant that has since been discovered in some 5-HTP products.

Appetite suppressants
Appetite suppressants, such as Dexatrim and Acutrim, may contain the ingredient phenylpropanolamine (PPA) — a stimulant used in cough and cold medicines that has been linked to an increased risk of stroke.

The FDA warns consumers to avoid use of products containing PPA. Even if Dexatrim and Acutrim remove PPA, making them safer to use, you still have to control your appetite once you stop taking these products. Otherwise it's likely that you'll gain back the weight that you lost.

Pyruvate
Pyruvate is a popular weight-loss supplement that, according to some people, may have a slight effect in helping you shed pounds. Pyruvate, in the form of pyruvic acid, is formed in the body during digestion of carbohydrates and protein. It's also in several foods, such as red apples, cheese and red wine. Pyruvate seems safe, but its claims of boosting metabolism, decreasing appetite and aiding in weight loss remain unproved.

Herbal laxatives and diuretics
Herbal laxatives and diuretics cause you to lose water, and thus weight, but not fat. Laxatives and diuretics can lower your potassium levels, causing heart and muscle problems. In addition, if you use laxatives too often, your bowels can become dependent on them.

Caffeine
A few studies indicate that in people who exercise and eat a low-fat diet, consuming large amounts of caffeine or other stimulants may slightly enhance weight loss. But taken in large doses, caffeine can cause jitters, irritability, insomnia and high blood pressure. And if combined with other stimulants, such as ephedrine, the side effects may be more serious.

changes in diet, not as the solution to the problem.

If you're among those who can benefit from weight-loss medication, you'll likely need to take it indefinitely. Many studies show that when such drug treatment is stopped, much or all of the excess weight returns. The dilemma with taking the drugs indefinitely is that the most commonly used prescription drugs are so new that possible long-term effects are unknown.

Even if you qualify for weight-loss drug therapy, a drug may not work for you. Studies suggest that if you don't lose at least 4 pounds within the first month on a particular medication, it's probably not going to help you.

Weight-loss medications include:

Sibutramine
Sibutramine (Meridia) makes you feel full more quickly. Although this drug generally helps you lose more weight than you could through diet and exercise alone, it's no magic bullet. In a 1-year study, sibutramine users lost an average of only 7 to 10 pounds more than people who simply followed a low-calorie diet and took a placebo pill. Side effects can include increased blood pressure, headache, dry mouth, constipation and insomnia.

Orlistat
Orlistat (Xenical) inhibits the absorption of fat by blocking the action of the enzyme lipase in your digestive tract. Lipase breaks down dietary fat so that your body can absorb it. Orlistat can prevent absorption of up to 30 percent of dietary fat. Unabsorbed fat is eliminated in the stool. Orlistat may also improve weight loss by discouraging you from eating excessive fat.

Side effects associated with the drug include oily and frequent bowel movements. The average weight loss with orlistat is modest and similar to what you could expect with sibutramine. Because orlistat blocks absorption of some nutrients, including fat-soluble vitamins, your doctor will likely recommend that you also take a multivitamin.

Surgery

Generally, surgery for weight loss is reserved for people who are severely overweight and who have health problems as a result. Before you consider surgery, make sure that you've made every effort to exercise and change your eating habits and adjust any lifestyle factors that contributed to your weight gain. If you do have surgery, its success will depend in part on your commitment to carefully follow the guidelines given to you about food choices and exercise.

A surgeon will evaluate you as a candidate for weight-loss surgery. Surgery may be considered if your body mass index is above 40 or if you have weight-related health problems. Candidates for surgery usually are evaluated by a variety of medical professionals, including an internist, a dietitian and a psychologist.

Since the 1950s, when surgery for obesity was first performed, doctors have used various techniques to achieve weight loss. Today, the most common operations fall into one of two categories: vertical banded gastroplasty and gastric bypass.

Vertical banded gastroplasty

Vertical banded gastroplasty uses a band of staples to create a small pouch at the top of your stomach, where food enters from your esophagus. Using a surgical stapler, the surgeon partitions your stomach into upper and lower sections. The upper pouch is small and empties into the lower pouch, which is the remainder of your stomach. The dime-sized opening where the upper pouch empties into the rest of your stomach is wrapped with a piece of nonexpandable plastic. This banding of the opening between the upper stomach pouch and the rest of the stomach helps prevent the opening from expanding.

Initially, the upper pouch can hold only about 1 or 2 ounces of food, though this can later expand to several ounces. After the operation, you're able to eat only small portions of food at a time without experiencing discomfort or nausea.

Gastric bypass

Gastric bypass is the surgical procedure most often recommended for weight loss. During this procedure, a surgeon staples your stomach all the way across the top, leaving a tiny pouch. The surgeon then cuts the small intestine and sews a part of it directly onto the upper pouch. This redirects the food so that it bypasses most of your stomach and the first section of your small intestine. Food flows directly into the middle section of your small intestine, limiting absorption of calories.

This surgery does double duty. It reduces what you can eat, and it reduces the calories your body absorbs. Even though food never enters the lower part of your stomach, the stomach continues making digestive juices that flow into your small intestine. This procedure appears to be most effective.

When used appropriately, weight-loss surgery can result in dramatic improvements in weight and health. In the first 1 to 2 years after this operation, most people lose 50 percent to 60 percent of their excess weight. Generally, individuals who follow dietary and exercise recommendations keep most of that weight off long term.

However, weight-loss surgery does have side effects. Rapid weight loss can result in fatigue, dry skin and temporary hair loss. A hernia or weakness, which may require surgical repair, can develop at the site of your incision. In addition, if you eat too much or too fast, you'll experience nausea, vomiting, sweating and shakiness, called dumping syndrome. Over time, you'll be able to increase your food intake.

Surgery for weight reduction isn't a miracle procedure. Though you can expect to lose weight and keep it off, you still need to eat healthy foods and remain active. ■

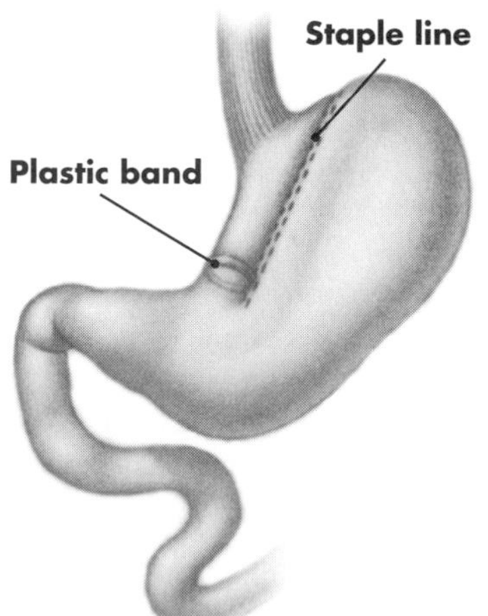

Vertical banded gastroplasty divides your stomach into upper and lower sections. The upper pouch holds only 1 to 2 ounces of food, so you feel full sooner. Food is released into the lower section through a small opening surrounded by a plastic band that helps prevent expansion of the opening.

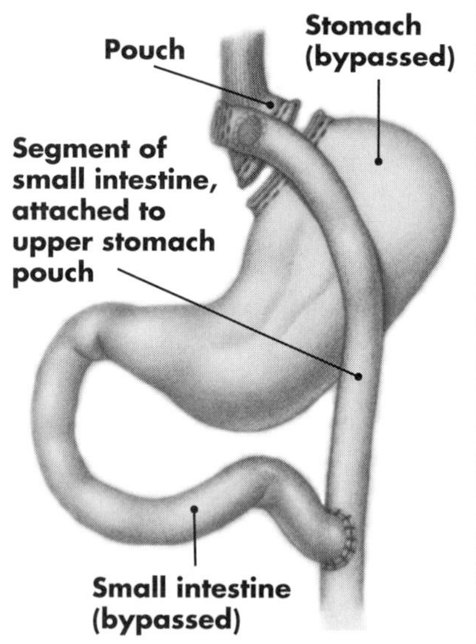

Gastric bypass creates a small pouch at the top of your stomach and a bypass around most of your stomach and part of your small intestine.

CHAPTER 4 PART I

Keeping Active

Modern society seems to conspire against physical activity. With our cars, computers, TVs and countless labor-saving devices, it's easy to get through each day with little physical exertion. Yet our bodies are designed to move. And it's important that they do.

Regular physical activity results in a number of health benefits. Adding more physical activity to your day doesn't mean that you have to become a marathon runner or head to the gym each morning. Simple modifications to your lifestyle can go a long way toward improving your health. For many years the common belief was that you had to exercise vigorously if you wanted to become physically fit and improve your health. But studies show that even light activity is good for your health — and it's definitely better than doing nothing at all. And moderate physical activity on a regular basis gives you most of the health benefits of rigorous exercise, according to the Centers for Disease Control and Prevention and the National Institutes of Health.

Fitness Pays

The decision to become more active is an investment in yourself, your family and your future. For a modest time investment, the rewards are enormous.

Along with eating well, physical activity is the key to improving your overall health and preventing illness. People who are physically active can often perform at a level comparable with that of an inactive person who's 10 to 20 years younger. Regular physical activity can help you control your weight, improve your coordination and balance, reduce muscle aches and pains and avoid insomnia. It may also prevent, delay or control the following diseases and conditions, among others:

High blood pressure

Physical activity is critical to efforts to prevent or control high blood pressure. Activity challenges your heart, which is a muscle. With exercise your heart becomes stronger and can pump more blood with less effort. The result is less pressure on your arteries.

Abnormal blood fats

Daily physical activity can reduce your low-density lipoprotein (LDL) cholesterol level and increase your high-density lipoprotein (HDL) cholesterol level. LDL cholesterol is commonly referred to as the bad cholesterol, and HDL cholesterol as the good cholesterol. Regular activity also helps reduce triglycerides, another type of blood fat (lipid).

Diabetes

Physical activity lowers the amount of a sugar (glucose) in your blood. Diabetes is characterized by blood sugar levels that are too high. If you have or are at risk of diabetes, daily activity combined with a healthy diet can help keep your glucose levels under control.

Coronary artery disease and stroke

Coronary artery disease is damage to the arteries that supply blood to your heart. The damage typically results from narrowing of the arteries (atherosclerosis), which may stem from a variety of factors, including high blood pressure, diabetes, smoking or high cholesterol. Complete blockage of the arteries can cause a heart attack.

Physical activity helps prevent coronary artery disease — and reduces your risk of having a heart attack — by helping you achieve and maintain a healthy weight and control diabetes, elevated cholesterol and high blood pressure.

Physical activity also helps reduce your risk of stroke by preventing or slowing the narrowing of the arteries that supply blood to the brain. Blockage of these arteries can cause a stroke.

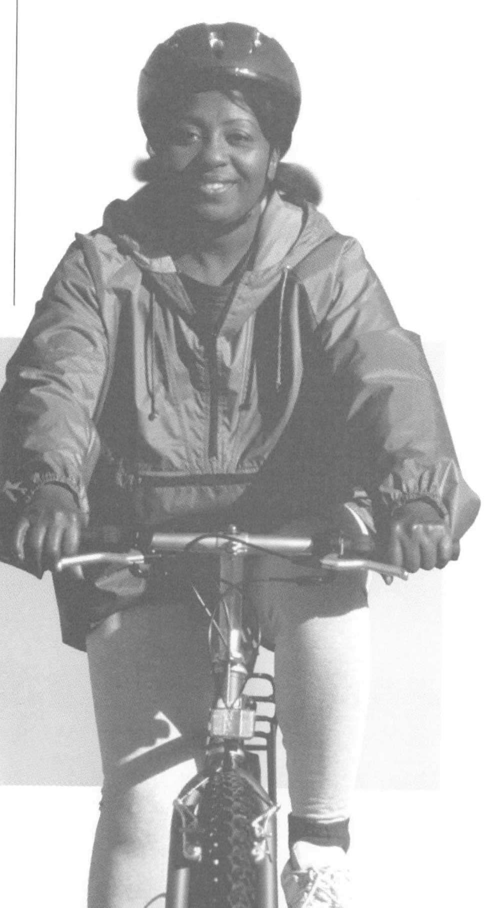

Physical Activity vs. Exercise

The terms *physical activity* and *exercise* are often used synonymously, but there is a difference between the two. Physical activity refers to any body movement that burns calories, such as mowing the lawn, walking up stairs, making the bed or walking your dog. Exercise is a more structured form of physical activity. It involves a series of repetitive movements designed to strengthen or develop some part of the body and improve your heart and lung capacity — your cardiovascular fitness. Exercise includes walking, swimming, bicycling and many other activities.

Both physical activity and exercise are valuable to your health. The important thing is to keep moving, whether or not the activity is structured.

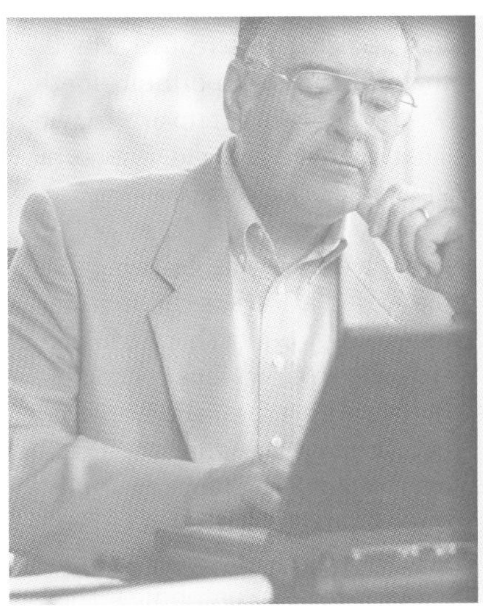

Are You at Risk?

If you sit most of the day, chances are you're not physically fit. People who are fit generally can:

- Carry out daily tasks without fatigue and have ample energy to enjoy leisurely pursuits
- Walk a mile or climb a few flights of stairs without becoming winded or feeling leg fatigue
- Carry on a conversation during light to moderate exercise, such as brisk walking

Signs of being not fit (deconditioned) include feeling tired most of the time, being unable to keep up with others your age, avoiding physical activity because you know you'll quickly tire and becoming short of breath or fatigued after walking a short distance.

Osteoporosis
Women and men who perform strength training and weight-bearing activities, such as walking, have a better chance of avoiding osteoporosis, a bone-thinning disease. Osteoporosis is more common in women than in men.

Arthritis
If you have arthritis, appropriate exercises to maximize the range of motion and strength of muscles surrounding your joints may reduce pain and injury. Physical activity can also improve your energy level and help you control your weight, which is important because excess weight places unnecessary stress on your joints.

Cancer
Staying active may reduce your risk of some cancers, including cancers of the colon, rectum, prostate, breast, kidney and lining of the uterus (endometrium). Activity may reduce cancer risk by helping prevent obesity, a risk factor for many types of cancer.

Regular physical activity reduces cancer risk in other ways, too. For example, it may cut your risk of colorectal cancer by stimulating movement through your bowel and reducing the time your colon is exposed to harmful substances that may cause cancer.

And for breast and prostate cancer, regular physical activity may act on hormone levels in a way that reduces your risk.

Depression and anxiety
Studies indicate that aerobic exercise and strength training help relieve symptoms of depression. When you exercise, your body releases chemicals called endorphins, which are your body's natural painkillers. Endorphins also help relieve stress and anxiety.

Everyday Fitness

For many people, lack of physical activity simply may be a matter of time. You don't doubt that activity is good for you, but you just can't seem to set aside time in your day to be active. You're not alone. Despite the proven benefits of physical activity — and the risks of inactivity — more than two-thirds of American adults don't get the recommended amount of physical activity. Medical and fitness organizations generally recommend partaking in at least 30 minutes of light to moderate physical activity most, if not all, days of the week.

If you have trouble carving 30 minutes out of your day for a specific activity, such as walking or bicycling, try another approach.

No Such Thing as Too Old

Even if you've never exercised before, it's never too late to incorporate more physical activity into your life. In one study, participants who averaged 87 years of age when they began an activity program increased their muscle strength by more than 110 percent, their walking speed by 12 percent and their stair-climbing power by 28 percent. Another study found that even frail adults in their 90s benefited from a program of strength training.

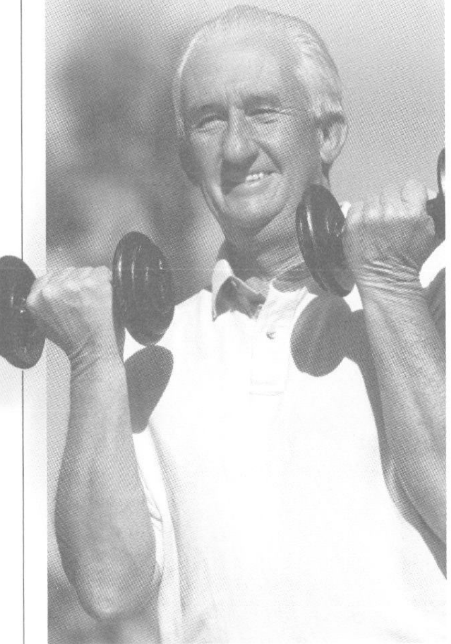

On the Move

Here are some suggestions for incorporating more activity into your everyday life:

- Instead of sitting and talking with a friend, go for a walk together.
- Walk or bike to a nearby store instead of driving.
- Listen to music and dance your way through housecleaning.
- Use a push lawn mower instead of a motorized or riding mower.
- Wash your car by hand instead of using the automatic carwash.
- Rake leaves, prune bushes, spend time in the garden.
- Play with your kids instead of watching them play.
- When watching television, pedal a stationary bike, walk on a treadmill, stretch or lift free weights.
- Hide your remote control and get up to change the channel.
- Park farther away from work or the shopping mall.
- Walk around the mall a couple of times.
- Avoid drive-throughs. Park the car and walk in.
- Climb the stairs instead of using the elevator.
- Do stretching exercises at your desk.
- Take a break from what you're doing and walk around.

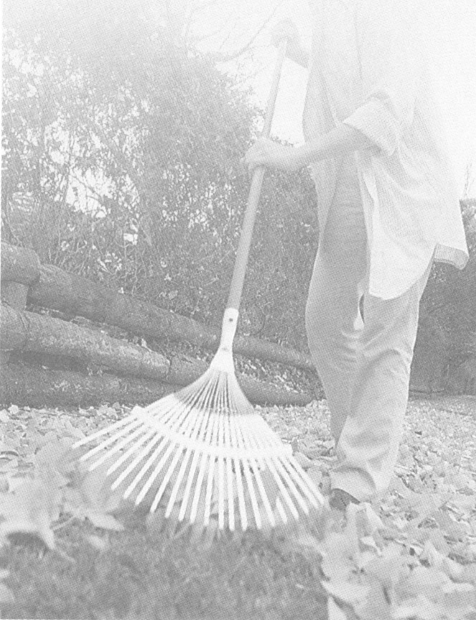

Incorporate more physical activity into the things you already do. This "lifestyle activity" approach is like snacking on exercise. Do a smidgen of activity in the morning. Have two or three more servings later in the day, and perhaps one in the evening. Over the course of the day, 5 or 10 minutes of activity here and there add up. So how do you get your exercise servings? Park your car at the far end of the parking lot and walk. Take the stairs instead of the elevator. Every move counts — and the more, the better.

The key is attitude. You have to want to get out of the habit of sitting and embrace new, more active habits. Pick something you like to do. Make a date to go dancing every Friday. Go walking with a friend. Ride a bike with your grandchild.

This approach works. In one study, researchers divided 235 sedentary men and women into two groups. One group did traditional, structured exercise for 20 to 60 minutes, 3 to 5 days a week. The other group incorporated moderate-intensity lifestyle activities such as brisk walking or stair climbing into their day. After 24 months, both groups had similar improvements in blood cholesterol, blood pressure, percentage of body fat and cardiovascular fitness. The structured exercisers gained the most cardiovascular fitness, but the moderate-intensity group benefited significantly.

Doing something is better than nothing, and consistency is more important than intensity. It's the total amount of activity that counts, not great exhibits of endurance. Think of physical activity as an ongoing part of your day.

Family Fitness

A great way to integrate fitness into your daily life is to make it a family affair. Family exercise builds healthy bodies — and healthy families. Look for fun, creative activities that provide an opportunity for the whole family to get up and moving. That might be going to the zoo, biking together or going bowling.

Although some children get enough exercise just by being kids, many don't. Today's children are increasingly out of shape compared with those of previous generations. Between 12 percent and 21 percent of children in the United States are overweight — a number that has more than doubled in the last 20 years.

Many factors contribute to the increase in childhood obesity. The biggest culprit is television, followed closely by video games and computers. Spending time in front of a screen encourages a sedentary lifestyle. To make matters worse, only 25 percent of school-age children take physical education courses, meaning that fewer kids get exercise at school.

Studies show that active children are healthier, stronger, more flexible and have greater endurance and lung capacity. In addition, they perform better in school, are more mentally alert, sleep better, are sick less often and bounce back more quickly when they do catch a bug.

Equally important, children who exercise regularly are more likely to grow up to be fit, lean adults, with better posture and sleep habits.

Teaching healthy habits

Parents play a key role in their children's attitudes toward physical activity. As a parent you help them make good decisions about nutrition and exercise.

When your family does active things together, you teach your kids healthy habits that can last a lifetime. Research shows that children are about six times more likely to be active when both parents exercise.

Exercising together also provides good family time. The sheer pleasure of doing something fun together eases conflicts, tensions and pressures. Family fun time breaks up the

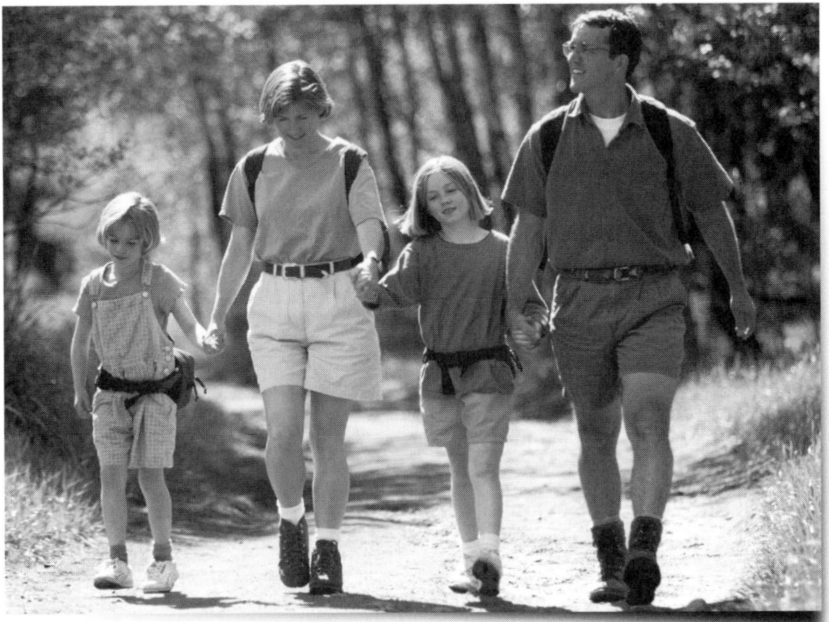

routine of seeing one another only at the breakfast table before dashing off to your separate days. Structured family activities also help control disruptive behavior.

The earlier you start adding fitness to your family routine, the more readily the kids will accept it as a normal part of family life. A child who grows up taking after-dinner walks with mom or dad accepts the walks as family routine.

Getting the ball rolling

How can you nurture an active child? How do you get a 3-year-old interested in exercise? And what about your 12-year-old who's embarrassed to be seen with you? Getting kids of any age to be active doesn't have to be a tough sell. Consider the following steps:

Limit television, computer time and video games

Many studies have found a direct relationship between childhood obesity and hours of television watching. As hours of viewing increase, so does weight.

Sitting in front of a computer or playing games is just as sedentary. Set a limit on these activities, such as 1 to 2 hours a day or 10 TV programs a week. Don't let your child have a television in his or her bedroom.

Plan a family activity three times a week

A family activity could be a trip to the playground, a driveway game of basketball, a bike ride or just a family stretch time. Spur-of-the-moment activities can be fun, but if you set aside a certain time of the day or week when your family can be together, you're more likely to accomplish your goal. Plan for at least three family activities a week.

Emphasize activity, not exercise

Your family activity doesn't have to be a structured exercise program — the object is just to get the kids moving. Free-play activities such as playing hide-and-seek, tag or jump-rope can be great for burning calories and improving fitness.

Make your activity fun and varied. A lot of kids' games involve exercise by nature.

Do things your children like

Engage your children in physical activities related to their interests and abilities. For example, if a child is artistic, go on a nature hike to collect leaves and rocks that he or she can use in a collage. If a child likes

Making Exercise Fun

Be creative when choosing activities. Every family is different. Do whatever gets your kids pumped. Start with the ideas below, then add some of your own.

- Don't just go for a walk. Take the kids on an adventurous treasure hunt.
- Don't just run. Run like a gorilla. Fly like a bee. Walk like a spider. Hop like a bunny. Stretch like a cat.
- Play fast-moving games such as tag, Simon says or kickball.
- Build a fort.
- See who can pull the most weeds in the vegetable garden or who can collect the most litter in the neighborhood.
- Plot the mileage of each family hiking and biking trip on a map of the United States to see how far your outings would have taken you if you had traveled in one direction.
- Plan family vacations around hiking, skiing, snorkeling or camping. Take along a ball or Frisbee for rest stops.
- Organize neighborhood volleyball or baseball games or sledding or skating parties.

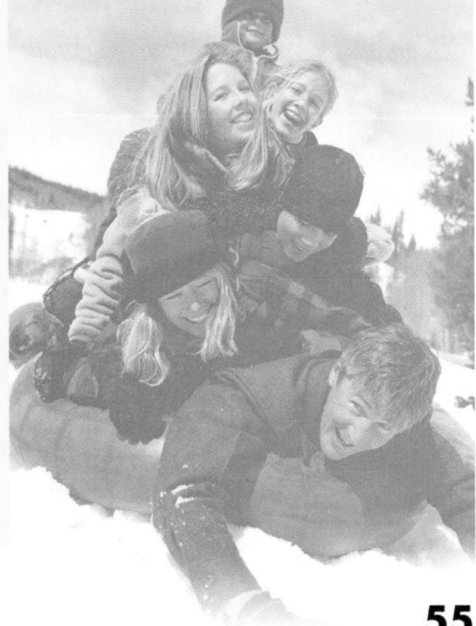

to climb, head for the nearest neighborhood jungle gym or climbing wall. If a child likes to read, walk to the neighborhood library.

Promote physical education
If you're concerned about the lack of physical education opportunities at your child's school, work with your local PTA, school board or school administrators to improve the offerings in your district. If your child is in child care, make sure the program offers at least 20 minutes of physical activity each day.

Participating in sports

Sports offer many benefits. On the physical side, participants experience improved fitness, coordination and weight control. Sports also offer meaningful lessons in social and psychological development, such as interacting with others, following directions and dealing with setbacks and defeat. Children who participate in sports tend to have better body image and self-esteem.

To help your child find the right sport, expose him or her to a variety of athletic activities. Let him or her try team sports like softball or soccer, as well as sports that offer an opportunity for more individual participation, such as tennis, running or golf.

If your child shows interest in a sport, consider the time commitment, cost, characteristics of the sport and your child's physical maturity level. You can help by being positive and encouraging. Emphasize effort and improvement over winning or personal performance. And keep the sport in perspective. It's important to be supportive, but don't become overly invested in whether your child wins or loses.

And if your kids show no interest whatsoever in sports, don't worry. A healthy lifestyle doesn't have to include organized sports. What's more important is that your child be involved in some form of physical activity.

A Personal Fitness Program

Daily activity is good. However, for maximum health benefits, a structured fitness program is best. The program need not be very strenuous. But the activity needs to be regular, and it should be moderately challenging.

A fitness program takes time to show results. Don't expect to whip yourself into shape overnight. By gradually increasing the duration and intensity of your activity, you can improve your overall fitness in 8 to 12 weeks.

Identify your goals

Tailor your fitness program to your needs, abilities, schedule and other personal factors. Develop a routine that works best for you and your lifestyle. If your program is so difficult that you're rarely able to do it, or your workout is so long that you can't seem to fit it into your schedule more than once or twice a week, you probably won't stick with it.

What do you want to gain from your program? Be specific. Are you 55 and concerned about warding off a heart attack? Are you 75 and want to enjoy more recreational activities and prolong your independence? Do you want to lose weight? Relieve your stress? Lower your blood pressure? Maybe you just want to feel better.

Keep your expectations realistic. If you have short, thick legs, your fitness program isn't going to give you a ballet dancer's body. What you can expect is an increased level of fitness and more energy.

Plan your activities

An optimal fitness program incorporates activities designed to meet three basic goals: improved aerobic capacity, strength and flexibility. Each activity session should begin

? Question and Answer

Should I consult a doctor before starting a fitness program?

If you're healthy and you don't have a family history of cardiovascular disease, you can probably begin moderate exercise without a medical examination, even if you haven't been active for many years. However, check with your doctor in these situations:

- You have a family history of heart-related problems before age 55.
- You have heart, lung, liver or kidney disease.
- You have high blood pressure, high cholesterol, diabetes, arthritis, osteoporosis or asthma.
- You smoke.
- You're significantly overweight.
- You're unsure of your health status.

Also see your doctor if you become lightheaded, if you have discomfort in your chest during exercise or if you become short of breath from only mild exertion.

If you're taking medications, you might also ask your doctor if they require adjustment or pose any problems related to exercise. For example, if you have diabetes, exercise can lower your blood sugar level. As a result, you may need a lower amount of insulin or other diabetes medication.

with a warm-up period and end with a cool-down and stretching.

Aerobic exercises

Aerobic means "with oxygen," as opposed to *anaerobic*, meaning "without oxygen." Aerobic activities involve continuous motion as you repeatedly contract muscle. Aerobic activities increase your breathing and heart rate, improving your cardiovascular fitness — the health of your heart, lungs and circulatory system. Anaerobic exercises work muscle groups, but they don't provide as much cardiovascular benefit.

From a health standpoint, aerobic exercise is about as close as you can get to a "magic potion." Besides making your heart more efficient, aerobic exercise can help you lose weight, ease stress, boost your immune system and reduce your risk of certain diseases. Aerobic exercise also improves your stamina and muscle health, making it easier for you to do everyday tasks such as household chores and climbing stairs.

Moderate-paced walking, bicycling, running, cross-country skiing and swimming are examples of aerobic exercises.

Strength exercises

Strength (resistance or strength-training) exercises build your muscle strength and endurance, which in turn can improve your posture, balance and coordination. To increase strength, an exercise must involve resistance to muscle contractions. In other words, your muscles have to push or pull against some force, such as when you lift weights.

In general, people who aren't active lose about 10 percent of their lean muscle mass each decade after age 30. Strength training can help slow and prevent or even reverse this process. Because strength exercises also strengthen bones, they protect against the bone-thinning disease osteoporosis. In addition, these exercises support your joints, cut your risk of injury and increase your metabolism, which helps keep your weight in check.

Two excellent ways to build lean muscle mass are working out with free weights (dumbbells or barbells) and using weight machines. Workouts with free weights simulate some moves made in everyday life. Some newer weight machines also emphasize stabilization of the body during exercise, and they permit more natural body movement arcs than do older machines.

For some people, though, lifting weights is difficult or isn't recommended because of an injury or a condition such as arthritis. If you're concerned that free weights or weight machines may not be good for you, talk to your doctor, a physical therapist or a certified athletic trainer. You may be able to do strength training if you stick to light weights and don't overdo it.

You can build strength in other ways too. The following exercises strengthen specific muscle groups. Include some of these exercises in your fitness routine at least twice a week. If you're out of shape, begin with 5 repetitions each and try to build to 25 repetitions.

Abdominal Exercises

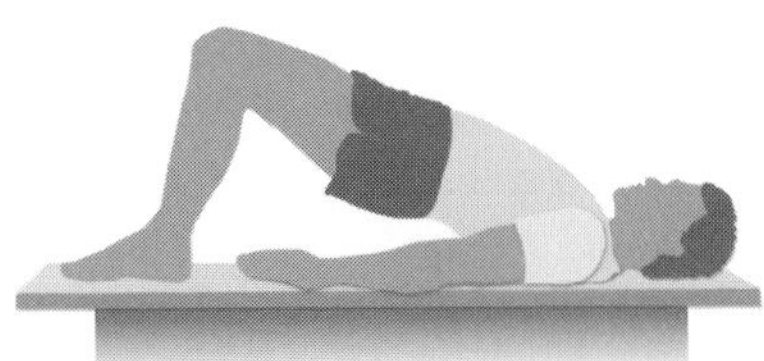

Lie on a firm surface with your feet flat, about shoulder width apart. Raise your buttocks off the mat, keeping a level line from your knees to your hips. Keep your shoulders, head and neck relaxed and on the surface. Hold the position until you're fatigued and can no longer keep your knees and hips in a straight line. Relax and repeat.

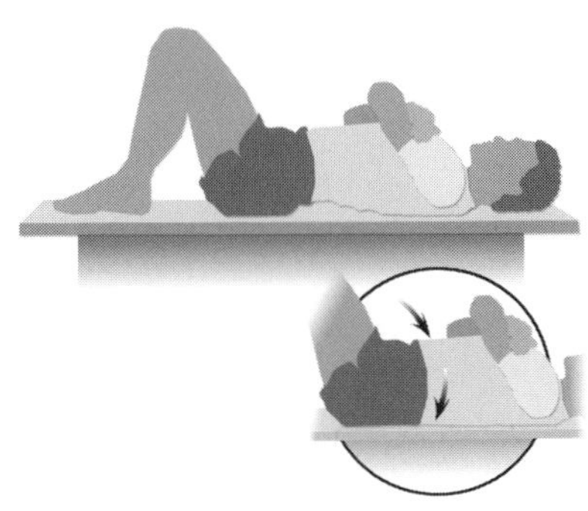

Lie on a firm surface with your knees bent. Flatten the small of your back against the surface and concentrate on tightening your abdominal muscles. Relax and repeat.

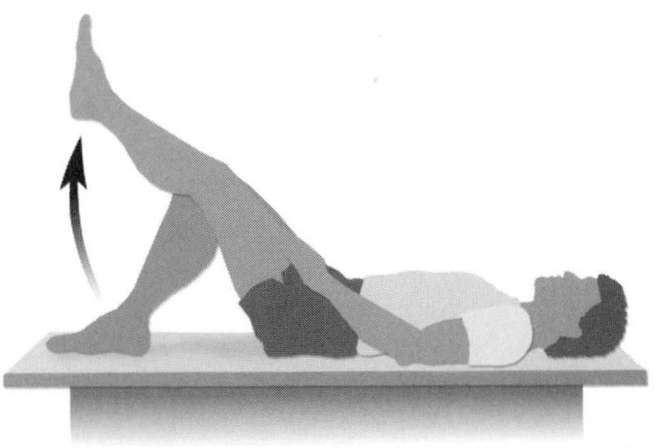

Lie on a firm surface. Bend your right knee and keep your left knee straight. Hold your abdominal muscles tight and slowly raise and lower your left leg. Relax and repeat. Reverse legs.

Back Exercises

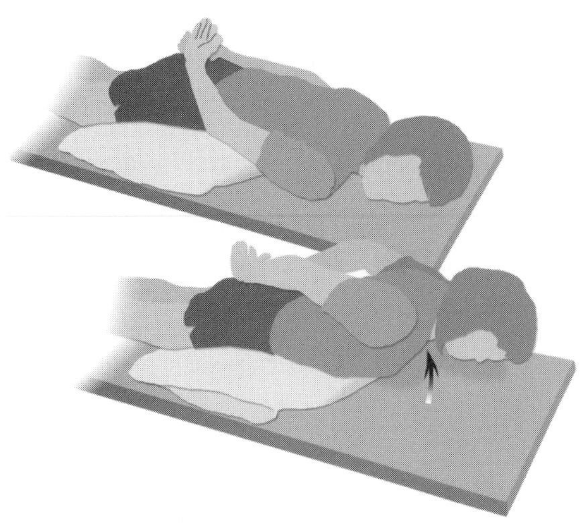

Lie facedown over a large pillow. Position the pillow under your navel to keep your spine in a neutral position. Place your hands behind your hips. Pulling your shoulder blades together, raise your head and chest. Keep your neck relaxed. Return to the starting position and repeat.

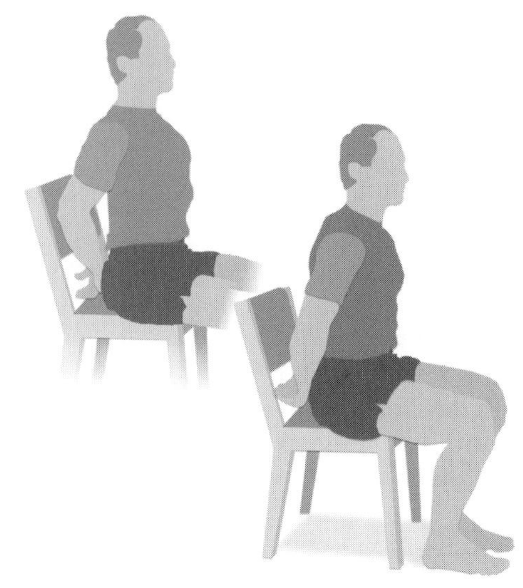

Sit upright in a chair. Put your hands on your hips or behind your back and pull your shoulder blades together. Relax and repeat.

Chest and Arm Exercises

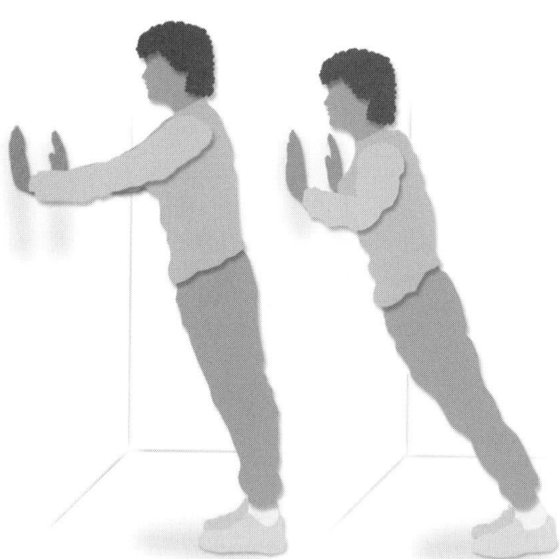

Stand facing a wall, far enough away from it so that you can place your palms on the wall with your elbows slightly bent. Keeping your heels flat on the floor, slowly bend your elbows and lean toward the wall, supporting your weight with your arms. Straighten your arms and return to a standing position. Repeat. As you build strength, try standing farther from the wall.

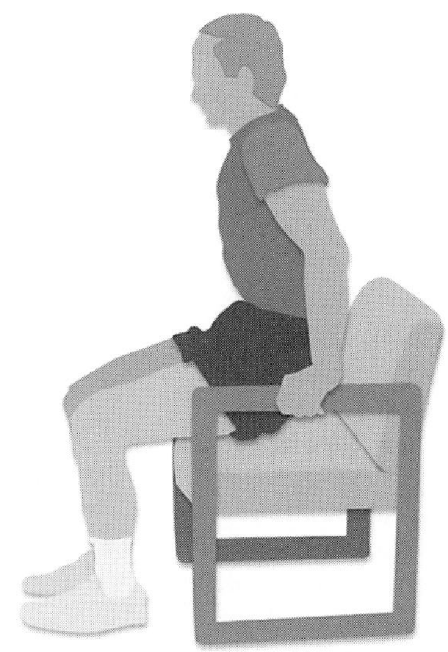

Sit in a sturdy chair that has arms, with your feet firmly on the floor. Place your hands on the arms. Push your body up off the surface of the chair using your arms only, not your feet. Relax and repeat.

Leg Exercises

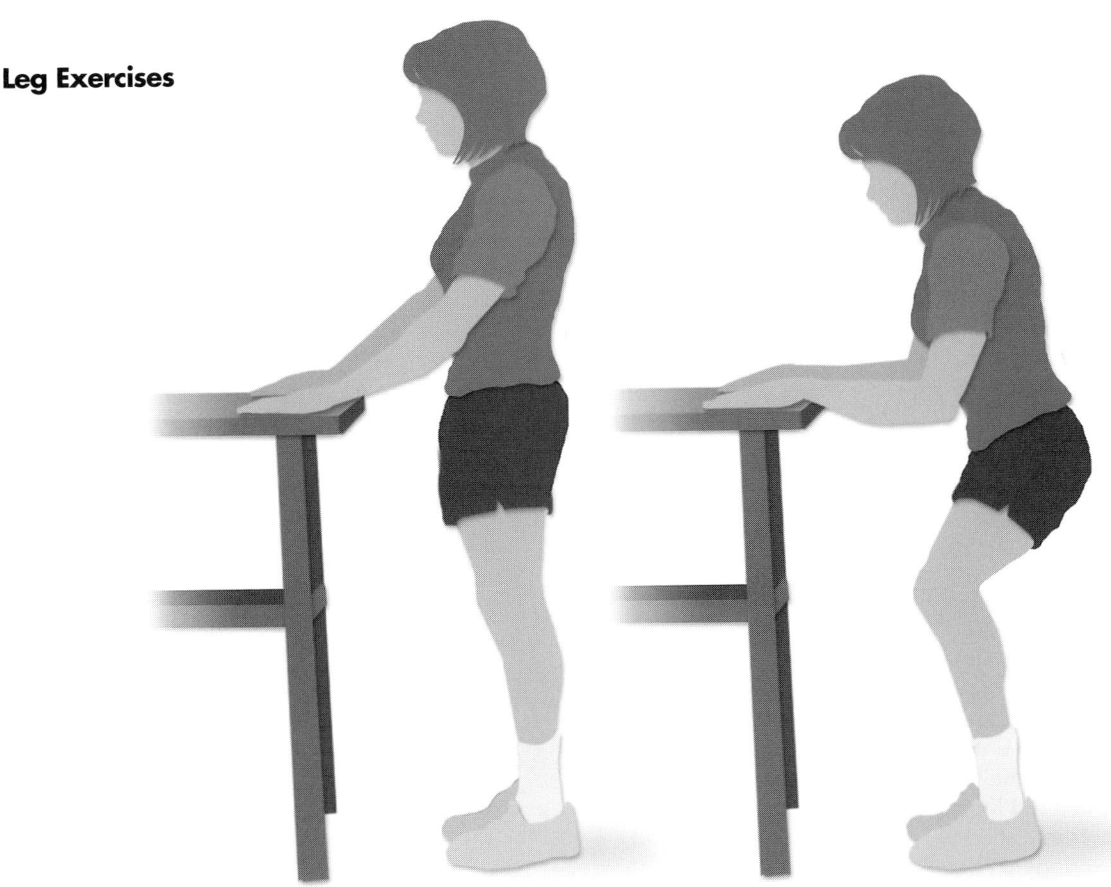

Stand with your feet flat on the floor, slightly more than shoulder width apart. Keeping your back straight and looking straight ahead, slowly lower your hips downward and backward as you bend your knees to between 30 degrees and 60 degrees. Pause for a moment and return to your starting position. Repeat. To maintain balance, lightly hold on to a table or countertop.

Stand with your feet flat on the floor. Hold on to the back of a sturdy chair. Slowly raise your heels and stand on tiptoe. Hold the position for a few seconds. Then slowly lower your heels and repeat.

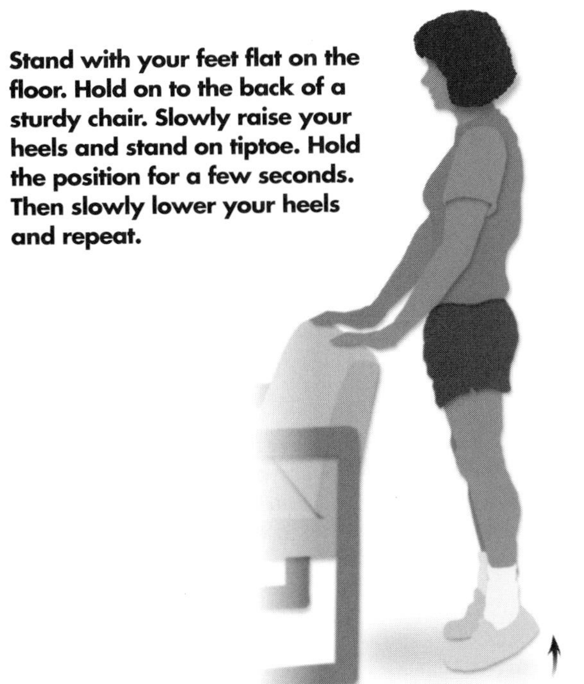

Stand with your feet flat on the floor. Hold on to a table or the back of a sturdy chair. Without moving your spine, slowly bend one knee so that your foot lifts up behind you. Hold the position. Slowly lower your foot. Repeat with the other leg.

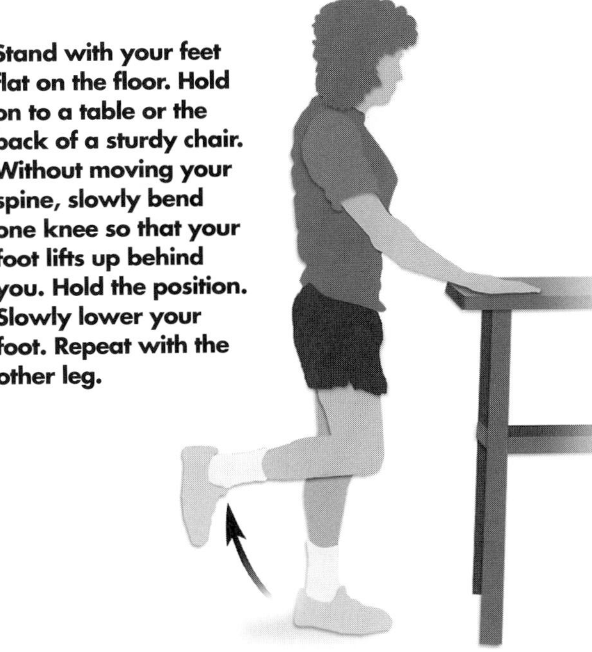

Stretching and flexibility exercises

Regular, careful stretching can help you limber up, feel younger and reduce risk of injury. Flexibility is a "use it or lose it" function. You need to regularly flex your muscles and move your joints through their full range of motion to prevent muscles from shortening and tightening.

Everyone has a different genetic set-point for flexibility. No matter what your level, though, you can become more flexible.

Stretching exercises get the blood flowing, literally warming up your muscles and getting them ready to work out. At the close of a period of activity, stretching your muscles helps them cool down and retain their flexibility. Basic stretches to improve your flexibility focus on the body's major muscle groups, including your calf muscles, thigh muscles, lower back muscles, neck and shoulders.

Following are some stretching exercises that you can do before and after you exercise. Stretch slowly, holding a position for 30 to 60 seconds and then slowly release the stretch.

Never bounce, and stretch only until you feel a noticeable pull — not pain. Do at least three repetitions of each stretching exercise.

Calf Stretch

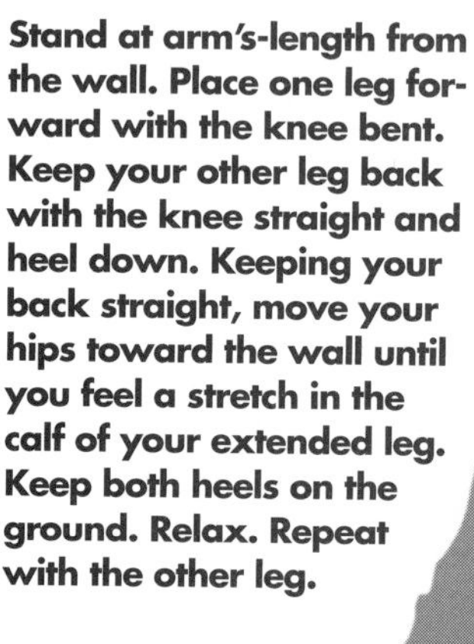

Stand at arm's-length from the wall. Place one leg forward with the knee bent. Keep your other leg back with the knee straight and heel down. Keeping your back straight, move your hips toward the wall until you feel a stretch in the calf of your extended leg. Keep both heels on the ground. Relax. Repeat with the other leg.

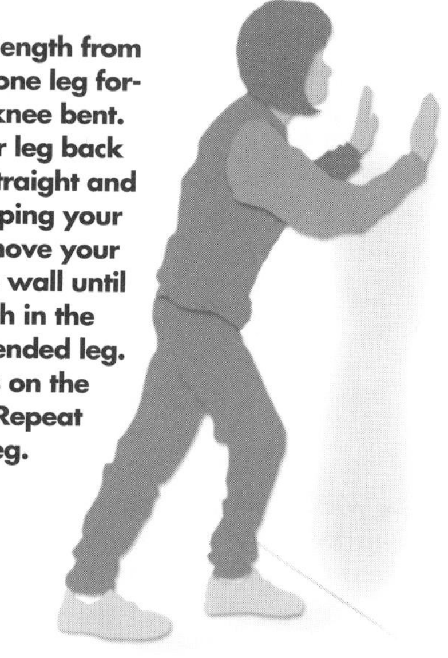

Lower Back Stretch

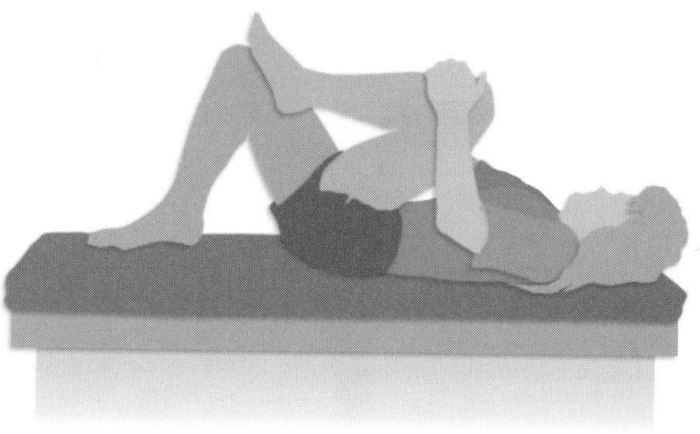

Lie on a firm surface with your knees bent and feet flat. Pull your left knee toward your shoulder with both hands. If you have knee problems, pull from the back of your thigh. Relax. Repeat with your other leg.

Upper Thigh Stretch

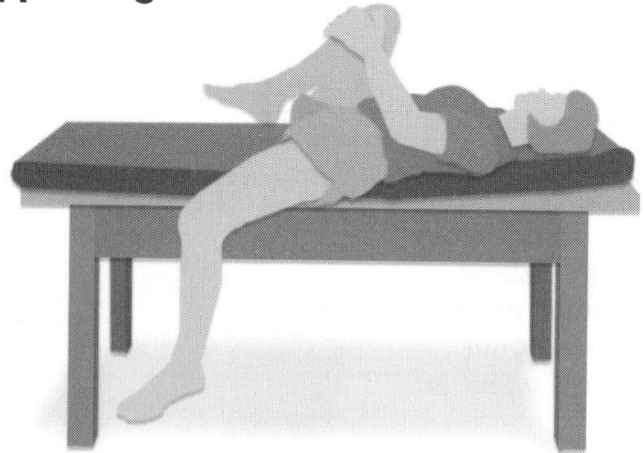

Lie on your back on a table or firm bed, with one leg and hip as safely near the edge as possible. Grasp the knee of the other leg with both hands and pull it toward your chest until your lower back flattens against the table. If you have knee problems, pull from the back of your thigh. Then relax your straight leg so that it hangs over the edge. Relax. Repeat with the other leg.

Chest Stretch

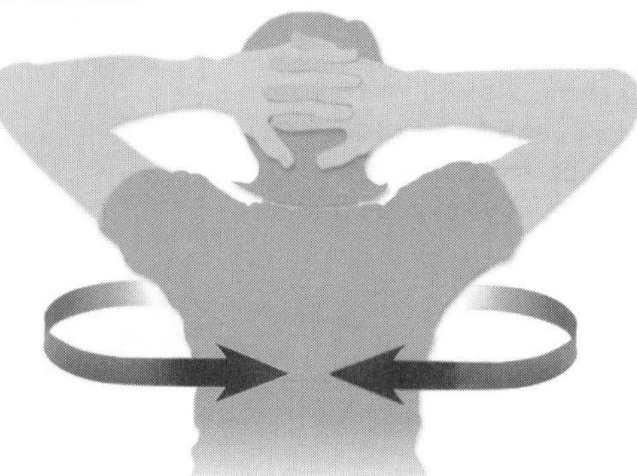

Clasp your hands behind your head. Pull your elbows gently back by pinching your shoulder blades together while inhaling deeply. Breathe normally while holding the position. Relax and repeat.

Common Types of Exercise

The choices are endless when it comes to physical activity. No single form of exercise or piece of equipment is best. Select an activity or activities that fit your personality and lifestyle. Do you like to exercise alone or in a group? Do you like to be outdoors or to stay inside?

In the following pages, we discuss some of the most common physical activities. These are just starting points for a world of physical activity.

Walking

A brisk walk is a simple and cost-free means of improving your physical fitness. It requires no special skills, equipment, lessons or other participants. If you've been inactive and are a bit out of shape, a program of walking could be just the challenge you need.

Walking, like other forms of aerobic exercise, can help increase the efficiency of your heart and lungs, allowing you to do more work with less effort. It can improve muscle tone and help shape muscles in your legs, hips, buttocks and abdomen.

Walking can also be a valuable part of a weight-loss program. On average, a brisk 1-hour walk burns about 250 to 350 calories, depending on your weight and level of fitness.

Regular walking can help prevent some age-related diseases. Walking increases bone density and may lower the risk of osteoporosis and lessen the pain of arthritis. Walking improves balance and coordination, so walkers are less prone to injury from falls.

A Walking Program

The following chart outlines how to gradually increase the pace and intensity of your walking program:

Week of program	Distance in miles	Time in minutes per mile
1-2	1-2	15-30
3-4	2-2½	13-25
5-6	2½-3	13-20
7-8	3-4	13-20
9-10	4-5	13-20

Does the Shoe Fit?

A good pair of walking shoes is important in preventing injury. The shoes should be supportive and comfortable:

- ***Toe box.*** A toe box helps prevent calluses on the tops and sides of your toes. Look for one that's rounded and roomy.
- ***Exterior.*** A good shoe exterior provides comfort and durability. Look for leather or other sturdy materials.
- ***Interior.*** A good interior offers comfort and protection. Look for a padded heel counter to reduce chafing, a padded tongue and ankle to protect the front of your foot, and a smooth, absorbent lining. Check for removable insoles that you can air out or replace.
- ***Heel counter.*** A heel counter stabilizes your foot through its forward roll and keeps it from rolling from side to side. For more support look for a heel counter that extends all around the side of the shoe toward the arch. A padded one reduces chafing.
- ***Rocker shape.*** The rocker shape provides flexibility and proper heel strike. Look for a natural heel-to-toe curve. The heel should be slightly beveled upward in the back.
- ***Insole.*** The insole, also called a sock liner, adds a measure of cushioning and support.

Lightweight walking shoes provide less support and durability. More rigid shoes last longer. Some people prefer to wear running shoes for walking because of the cushioning. That's fine, as long as the shoe fits well.

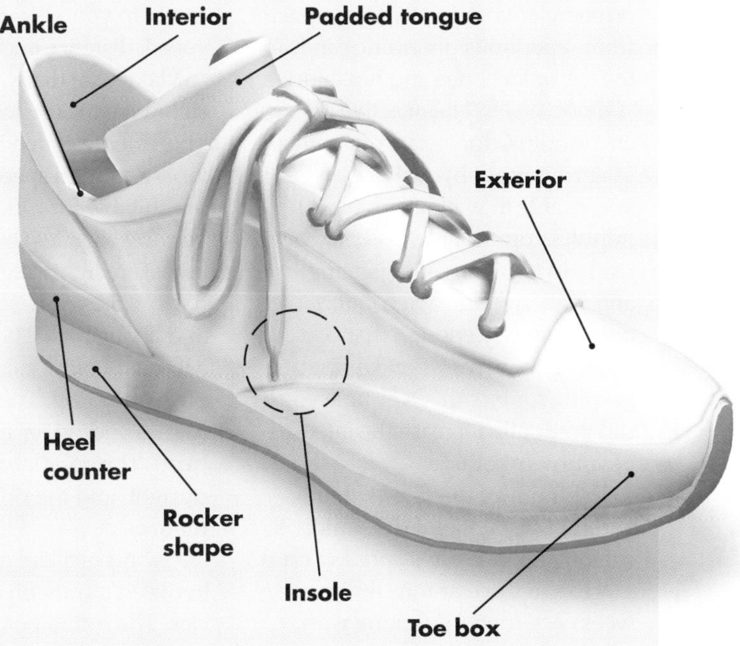

Walking can also be a tonic for the mind. It can help you unwind at the end of a busy day or after a difficult task. Get your spouse or a friend to join you, and it's a chance to connect with others.

Start out slowly and increase the duration and pace of your workout over a period of 4 to 6 weeks. Begin by walking on flat ground. When that becomes too easy, look for gentle hills to increase the intensity of your workout. Many people find that it helps to establish a routine, such as walking at the same time each day. Vary your route to keep it interesting.

Running

Many people enjoy running and find that it fits well into a busy schedule. If you run at a pace of about 8 miles an hour, you'll burn twice as many calories as you do when you walk at a pace of 4 miles an hour. This means you can be more efficient with your exercise time. Other people like the excitement of running in 5-kilometer, or longer, races.

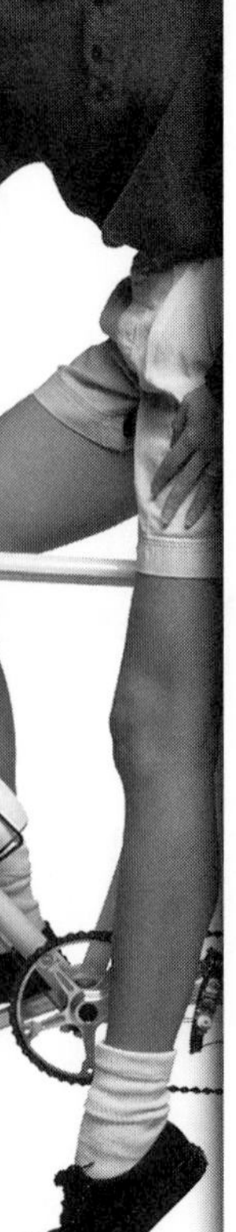

But running isn't for everybody. If you have a heart or lung condition, talk to your doctor about whether it's an appropriate exercise for you. Running can also be hard on some of your joints. The impact from repetitious pounding can lead to foot, ankle, knee and hip injuries.

If you haven't been active for several months, don't start out with a long run. Begin by walking. When you're able to walk 2 miles in 30 minutes comfortably, you may be ready to try alternating jogging and walking. Run at a comfortable pace — slowly enough that you can carry on a conversation without gasping for breath. Over time you can gradually increase the intensity of your workout.

To minimize the risk of injury and muscle and joint discomfort, run on alternate days and don't run more than three or four times a week. Alternating running with low-impact activities such as biking or swimming lessens the risk of overload injuries and works your muscles in different ways. Remember to warm up and cool down. Allow 5 to 10 minutes before and after your workout for walking and stretching.

Bicycling

As the old cliche has it, "You never forget how to ride a bicycle." This is more or less true, and bicycling is a great way to get aerobic exercise. With bicycling, as with any form of aerobic exercise, schedule regular workouts. Select a time of day to cycle that works for you. For example, if managing stress is a goal, a ride after work may relax you for an evening at home. Include a warm-up and cool-down period, and stretch your muscles before and after you cycle.

Don't challenge yourself by setting the gears to make pedaling hard, producing a strain resembling that of a hard run. This doesn't work your heart and lungs effectively and puts excessive strain on your knees. Pedaling more rapidly at all times — even while going downhill — helps make your ride an aerobic activity. A pedaling rate of 80 to 100 revolutions a minute is generally ideal. Cycle computers can help you keep track of this, plus speed, distance and elapsed time.

Make sure that you have the right bike to suit your needs. Some bikes are designed for smooth surfaces and high speeds, and others are suitable for rough terrain. Touring bicycles (racing or road bikes) are lightweight and have narrow tires, low-slung handlebars and about 18 to 21 gear settings. Mountain bicycles are designed for off-road riding. They have sturdier frames and wider tires with more tread. The handlebars are more upright, and the riding posture is more erect.

Hybrid bicycles are a cross between mountain and racing bicycles. The riding posture is more upright, and the tire width is midway between road and mountain bike tires. Hybrid bikes often have 21 speeds. Those with shock absorbers built into the front wheel struts and seat posts provide added comfort on uneven surfaces.

Make sure the bike fits you well. When you're seated on a bicycle with your foot on the pedal lowest to the ground, your leg should be not quite fully extended. You should be able to reach the handlebars, work the brakes and shift gears while keeping your eyes on the road. When straddling a racing bicycle with your feet on the ground, there should be 1 to 3 inches of clearance between you and the crossbar. For a mountain or hybrid bicycle, the clearance should be 3 to 6 inches.

Always wear a helmet when riding a bicycle. This helps protect you from serious head injury should you fall or be in an accident.

Exercise machines

Each type of exercise machine has something unique to offer. Some machines exercise your lower body only, and others build upper body strength or aerobic capacity. The following devices can build both strength and aerobic capacity:

Stationary cycle

A stationary cycle builds leg strength and cardiovascular capacity and is an excellent choice for both beginning and serious exercisers. Some cycles have moving handlebars that provide an upper body workout as well. If you have knee problems, be sure the cycle's resistance can be adjusted to a low setting and that your seat height is set appropriately.

If you have low back problems, you might want to use a recumbent cycle, in which you sit in a chair-like seat with pedals in front of you rather than below the seat.

Rowing machine

A rowing machine offers a good aerobic workout by putting your entire body in action. It helps strengthen your back, shoulders, stomach, legs and arms. Proper technique is important to avoid back strain.

Treadmill
A treadmill builds leg strength and aerobic capacity. Most treadmills offer an adjustable degree of incline to simulate walking or running up hills. You can adjust speed for walking or running. Higher-horsepower models generally run more smoothly and are more durable.

Stair climber
A stair climber helps tone and strengthen your hips, buttocks, thighs, hamstrings, calves and lower back and provides an effective aerobic workout. Compared with running, a stair climber causes less wear and tear on your ankles and knees. However, the device can aggravate certain knee problems.

A stair climber may consist of a moving flight of stairs (like walking up a down escalator) or independent steps that move up and down at various rates or heights.

Cross-country ski machine
A cross-country ski machine offers a good overall workout, but some people find it hard to master. It requires some practice in learning to move your arms and legs in rhythmic opposition.

Elliptical trainer
An elliptical trainer provides a total upper and lower body workout and aerobic conditioning. The device is similar to a cross-country ski machine, but the leg-and-arm action is elliptical — up and down at an angle — rather than back and forth. It's easier to master than the cross-country ski machine.

Swimming and water workouts

Water exercise is as close as you can get to a zero-impact aerobic workout. Water's buoyancy supports

How Many Calories Does It Burn?

The chart below shows approximately how many calories you burn while performing various activities for 1 hour. Calorie expenditure varies widely depending on the exercise, intensity level and individual. For example, a trained athlete may exercise with greater economy of motion and expend less energy.

Activity	Average calories used in 1 hour	
	120- to 130-lb. person	**170- to 180-lb. person**
Aerobics class	290-575	400-800
Backpacking	290-630	400-880
Badminton	230-515	320-720
Basketball		
Game	400-690	560-960
Nongame	170-515	240-720
Bicycling		
Outdoor	170-800	240-1,120
Stationary	85-800	120-1,120
Bowling	115-170	160-240
Canoeing	170-460	240-640
Dancing	115-400	160-560
Golfing (walking and carrying or pulling bag)	115-400	160-560
Handball	460-690	640-960
Hiking	170-690	240-960
Jogging		
5 mph (12 min./mile)	460	640
6 mph (10 min./mile)	575	800
Racquetball	345-690	480-960
Rope skipping	345-690	480-960
Rowing	170-800	240-1,120
Running		
7 mph (9 min./mile)	690	960
8 mph (7½ min./mile)	745	1,040
10 mph (6 min./mile)	860	1,200
Skating, ice or roller	230-460	320-640
Skiing		
Cross-country	290-800	400-1,120
Downhill	170-460	240-640
Soccer	290-690	400-960
Squash	345-690	480-960
Stair climbing	230-460	320-640
Swimming	230-690	320-900
Tennis	230-515	320-720
Volleyball	170-400	240-560
Walking		
2 mph (30 min./mile)	150	210
3 mph (20 min./mile)	200	275
4 mph (15 min./mile)	250	340

Shopping for Exercise Equipment

Most health clubs and many workplaces have exercise machines. Or you can purchase exercise equipment to use at home. Before buying home fitness equipment, carefully consider your situation. If you've made physical activity a habit, then the investment is probably worth it. If you're still exploring various activities and haven't established a routine, you may want to wait before buying equipment.

In general, you get what you pay for when you purchase an exercise machine. The low-priced models may be unstable, uncomfortable and even unsafe. Look at the warranty — it's usually one sign of quality. Make sure the equipment is solidly built, with no exposed cables or chains. Look for a machine that operates smoothly and is comfortable to use. A comfortable seat is critical for cycles and rowing machines. Before buying a machine, try out various types at a dealer or fitness center.

your weight and significantly reduces stress on your joints, bones and muscles. Water pressure also helps reduce swelling. Swimming or water exercises are a good choice if you have arthritis or an injury or disability that prevents you from doing other forms of exercise, are recovering from illness or surgery or are pregnant or overweight.

For individuals who run or walk regularly, swimming is a good cross-training activity. Indoor swimming is also a good option for bad weather days. You can also do strengthening exercises in water. Water provides resistance as you move through it. Walking in water works the leg and abdominal muscles. While in the water, you can use barbells, weighted boots, paddles and webbed gloves if you want extra resistance.

Even if you fear deep water or don't like to swim, you can try a water workout in the shallow end of the pool. Simply walking in shallow water provides significant aerobic benefits. Most water aerobic classes are taught in the shallow end of the pool. Such classes often are offered by organizations such as health clubs, YMCAs, YWCAs and medical centers.

Weightlifting

Lifting free weights or using weight machines strengthens muscles and joints and helps maintain bone density. But weightlifting doesn't improve aerobic fitness.

When beginning a weightlifting program, get advice and instruction from a qualified instructor, such as a physical therapist, athletic trainer or fitness specialist. Many gyms and health clubs have such an adviser on staff. This person can help you design a program that fits your fitness level, abilities and goals yet is varied enough to keep you interested. Correct technique is most important. Take time to learn from a qualified fitness professional, not just your friends.

Weightlifting for muscle toning and overall fitness is different from strength training for a particular sport or activity. Each requires a unique set of exercises tailored to your overall goal and fitness needs.

It's best to start with conservative amounts of resistance to minimize the risk of injury. Begin with a weight that you can lift comfortably 12 to 15 times in a row, and avoid working the same muscle group on consecutive days. For example, if you exercise your biceps and triceps on Monday, wait until Wednesday before repeating these exercises.

Typically, increases in strength are noticeable after 4 to 6 weeks of regular lifting. Improvement in muscle shape and size takes longer, perhaps 6 to 16 weeks. Three workouts a week will build muscle, and two a week will maintain the strength you've gained.

Getting and Keeping Going

Once you've come up with some reasonable goals and developed a workable plan, the next — and perhaps the biggest — challenge is to do it! Starting a fitness program takes initiative. Sticking with it takes commitment. Here are some tips to help you get and stay on track:

Begin gradually
Rome wasn't built in a day, and you're not going to zip from strolls around the block to a marathon overnight. Don't overdo it. If your body isn't accustomed to vigorous exercise, your joints, ligaments and muscles are more vulnerable to injury. Establish a suitable pace and intensity level.

Plan a logical progression
If you're out of shape or have unstable joints from injury or arthritis, start by improving your muscle strength and flexibility. Build strength by exercising the weakest parts of your body. When you're ready to add aerobic exercise, start at a comfortable level, such as walking slowly for 5 to 10 minutes. Gradually increase the duration and speed each time you exercise.

Schedule exercise appointments
A written plan might encourage you to stay on track, and an exercise diary or log helps chart your progress. Schedule an exercise appointment just as you would a golf game or meeting. An exercise log is also helpful in establishing the habit of physical activity. Try to exercise at least 30 minutes most, if not all, days of the week.

Once you've been at it awhile, a typical session might include a 5-minute warm-up, 30 minutes of aerobic activity and 5 to 10 minutes to cool down and stretch. And every 2 or 3 days, include 10 to 20 minutes of strength exercises. At first this may seem quite time-consuming. But once you're in the habit, it won't seem like a strain on your schedule. You may even look forward to the break from work and other obligations. And remember, you don't have to do your activities all at one time. A good night of dancing is an exercise session all in itself.

Make it fun

Boredom is a major reason people quit exercising. To keep exercise interesting and combat boredom:

- Listen to music while exercising. Music makes you daydream, which makes time pass more quickly.
- Watch television, read or listen to books on tape while using a treadmill.
- Exercise with a friend. You can chat and encourage each other to keep going.
- If you like the social interaction of a group setting, join an aerobics class or a golf league.

Include variety

Alternating between different types of activities (cross-training) reduces your chance of injury from overusing a specific muscle or joint. You might walk one day, bicycle the next and swim later in the week. Doing different types of exercise also reduces boredom.

Don't be afraid to try a new sport. There are many physical activities that you might enjoy. How about taking tennis or cross-country skiing lessons? Or check out activities such as tai chi or yoga.

Be flexible and forgiving

If you're traveling or too busy on a certain day to do your full workout, it's OK to adapt your exercise program to accommodate your schedule. If you have a cold or the flu, it's better for your body to take a few days off. If you fall off your fitness program for some reason, don't lose hope. It happens to everyone. Just get going again and gradually return to your previous fitness level.

Set goals

Reaching a goal gives you encouragement. Start with simple, realistic goals, such as walking 3 or 4 days a week. You're more likely to quit in frustration if you bite off more than you can chew.

Once you've been exercising for awhile, consider increasing your goals. For example, your new goal might be to walk for 30 minutes 6 days a week, to complete a 5-kilometer run or to bicycle 10 miles. Change your goals to keep things interesting and to advance to the next level of fitness.

Track your progress

Keep a record of your progress. An exercise log helps you see what you've accomplished and helps determine your goals for the future.

Reward yourself

When you reach a goal, treat yourself. If a gold star doesn't do the trick, buy yourself a new CD or go out for the evening. Equally important, work on developing internal rewards that come from feelings of accomplishment, self-esteem and control of your own behavior. Savor the good feelings that being active gives you.

Preventing Injury

Most injuries that occur during physical activity result from the "terrible toos" — too much, too hard, too fast, too soon, too long.

For example, a novice runner who struggles to complete 5 miles the first day out will feel aches and pains. And a couch potato who comes to life for the annual company softball game is an excellent candidate for a sprain or some other painful injury.

Warm up

Warming up prepares your body for exercise and helps you avoid muscle stiffness, soreness and injury. Muscles that have been inactive are "cool." One way to warm them up is to start off with a low-intensity aerobic exercise, such as a slow to moderate walk. This gradually increases your heart rate (pulse), body temperature and blood flow to your muscles.

Another way to warm up is to slowly and gently stretch your muscles. This increases flexibility and helps to maximize the range of motion around your joints. To avoid a pulled muscle that can result from stretching, it's often best to walk for at least 3 to 5 minutes before stretching. If you only have time to stretch once during an exercise session, it's best to do it right afterward, when your muscles are warmer and more elastic. See page 60 for examples of common warm-up and cool-down stretches.

Exercise at the appropriate intensity

The intensity of a workout refers to how hard you work when you exercise. Moderate-intensity exercise improves your cardiovascular fitness. But your workout shouldn't be too strenuous. Going full tilt doesn't provide many additional fitness benefits and may put you at increased risk of muscle or joint soreness or injury.

The following three measurements and tests can help you gauge whether you're exercising at the right intensity level to achieve cardiovascular fitness:

Heart rate

The more intense your aerobic exercise, the higher your heart rate (pulse) will be. When you exercise as hard as you can, your heart beats

Calculating Your Target Heart Rate

Here's how to determine your target heart rate for aerobic exercise. The following example is based on a 40-year-old individual:

1. Figure your maximum heart rate by subtracting your age from 220:
   220 - 40 = 180

2. Calculate 50 percent and 80 percent of your maximum heart rate:
   180 x 0.5 = 90
   180 x 0.8 = 144

3. The resulting two figures give you the range in which your target heart rate falls:
   90 to 140 beats a minute

at its maximum rate. Most people should exercise at a level that puts their heart rate at 50 percent to 80 percent of their maximum. This is called the target heart rate.

To determine if you're within your target range, take your pulse while you're exercising. Place two fingers on the inside edge of your wrist, press gently and feel for your pulse. Count your pulse for 10 seconds and multiply the number you get by six.

Some medications, such as beta blockers, slow the heart rate and may invalidate the use of the target heart rate. To gauge the intensity of a workout, individuals on these medications need to rely more on their perceived exertion rather than on an actual heart rate.

Perceived exertion scale

Another way to gauge the intensity of your exercise is to use the perceived exertion scale. Perceived exertion is the total amount of physical effort you experience during a physical activity, taking into account all sensations of exertion, physical stress and fatigue.

For an activity to produce health benefits, you need to exert a moderate to somewhat strong effort — a 3 or 4 on the perceived exertion scale. A 0 rating indicates a minimal level of exertion, such as sitting comfortably in a chair. A 10 corresponds to maximum effort, as when jogging up a steep hill.

Talk test

The third method, the talk test, is the simplest. While you're exercising, you should be able to carry on a short conversation without being short of breath. If you can't do this, you're probably pushing too hard and need to slow your pace.

Drink plenty of water

Water helps maintain your normal body temperature and cools working muscles. To help replenish lost fluids, drink water before and after your activity. Don't rely on thirst to tell you when you need a drink. During exercise your thirst mechanism is suppressed.

Use pain relievers with caution

If you're taking pain relievers, it's easier to overexert and damage your muscles, ligaments or tendons without realizing it.

Perceived Exertion Scale

10	Very, very strong
9	Very difficult
8	More difficult
7	Very strong
6	Stronger
5	Strong
4	Somewhat strong
3	Moderate
2	Weak
1	Very weak
0	Nothing at all

Cool down

Immediately after your aerobic exercise, allow your heart rate to gradually return to normal by spending 3 to 5 minutes in a low-intensity activity, such as slow walking. This also helps prevent blood from pooling in your legs, which may cause dizziness.

Stretching after exercise also is important. It helps to keep your muscles limber and prevents muscle soreness and stiffness. You can use the same stretching exercises you used to warm up.

Take precautions in hot weather

When exercising in the heat, it's important to take precautions to avoid heat stress (see page 396). On hot days, more blood circulates through your skin to dissipate heat. As a result, less blood is available for your muscles, so your heart rate during exercise will be higher than on cool days. To compensate, decrease the intensity of your exercise to keep your heart rate within your target range.

On hot days, exercise outside early in the morning or later in the evening, when it's cooler. If possible, do your exercise in the shade, indoors or in a pool. Drink water before and after exercising. If you plan to exercise for more than 30 minutes, stop and drink water every 15 to 20 minutes.

Proper attire also is important. Wear lightweight, loose-fitting clothes made of fabrics that breathe and that wick moisture away from your body. White fabrics reflect sunlight and are cooler on sunny days. A light-colored hat or cap also will help.

Take precautions in cold weather

In extremely cold, windy weather, exposed skin can freeze in a short time, a condition called frostbite. If you exercise in extreme cold, protect exposed skin as much as possible. As with warm-weather exercising, make sure you drink

Be Aware of Warning Signs

If you experience any of the following signs or symptoms during exercise, stop and consult your doctor:

- Chest pain or tightness
- Dizziness or faintness
- Pain in an arm or your jaw
- Severe shortness of breath
- Bursts of very rapid or slow heart rate
- An irregular heartbeat
- Excessive fatigue
- Severe joint or muscle pain

Moderate activity shouldn't cause discomfort. Your breathing will be faster, and you'll feel like you're working, but you shouldn't feel pain or be exhausted.

plenty of fluids. Your body needs water in cold weather too.

Dress for the conditions. Dressing in layers is the best strategy in the cold. This provides added insulation and allows you to add or shed layers as appropriate. "High-tech," lightweight fabrics keep you warmer and drier and are more resistant to wind and water than are old-fashioned cotton sweats.

In extremely cold or windy conditions, wear a soft scarf or cold-air mask over your mouth and nose. In addition, try to breathe through your nose because your nose warms, filters and humidifies the air before it enters your lungs.

Polypropylene glove liners can help keep your hands drier and warmer inside your gloves or mittens. In addition, be sure to wear a hat — most heat loss is through the head.

Treat an injury

If you sprain an ankle or twist a knee, don't ignore it and just hope that it'll get better. See a doctor and follow his or her recommendations. Allow the injury time to heal before testing it too vigorously.

Activity and Chronic Illness

There was a time when people with certain chronic medical conditions were told to avoid physical activity for fear it would make their condition worse. But research has shown that physical activity actually can improve the health of people with many chronic illnesses.

Some chronic conditions, such as arthritis, asthma, diabetes and cardiovascular disease, can't be cured. However, many can be effectively managed with healthy lifestyle choices, medications and other treatments. If you have a chronic condition, talk to your doctor about a physical activity program that's appropriate for you.

Arthritis

Although pain and stiffness may discourage you from being active, the only way to keep your joints functioning their best is to move them and strengthen the muscles that support them. Exercising can also help control your weight, reduce pain and injury, and improve your energy level and ability to accomplish daily tasks.

Any movement, no matter how little, can help. Take part in low-impact activities that place less stress on your joints. Water exercises such as swimming and water walking are ideal because water's buoyancy takes weight off your joints.

Other low-impact activities include biking and cross-country skiing. Strengthening exercises are important, too. If you can't lift weights, try more gentle forms of resistance training, such as strength exercises that you do with a chair or against a wall.

As with all physical activity, start out slowly and gradually increase the amount of time and the intensity level. Take breaks when you feel you need to.

Asthma

Exercise is a common trigger of asthmatic symptoms, a condition called exercise-induced asthma. You're more prone to exercise-induced asthma if you have asthma due to allergies. Signs and symptoms of exercise-induced asthma include coughing, wheezing, chest tightness and shortness of breath.

Just because you have asthma doesn't mean you have to be inactive. In fact, it's best if you're active. Regular exercise strengthens your heart and lungs and helps you lose weight so that you can breathe more easily.

Here are some tips for exercising with asthma:

- To help prevent symptoms, inhale a fast-acting bronchodilator medication 15 to 30 minutes before exercising.
- Before beginning vigorous activity, warm up for 5 to 10 minutes with light activity and stretching, to help open your airways.
- Choose activities that are less likely to trigger asthma symptoms. Swimming is a good choice. Some sports, such as distance running, soccer and basketball, are more likely to trigger symptoms.
- Choose activities that involve short or intermittent periods of exercise, such as golf, volleyball or softball.
- Be aware that cold-weather activities, such as skiing or ice hockey, are more likely to cause wheezing. If you do exercise in cold weather, wear a face mask to warm the air you breathe. Don't exercise in subzero temperatures.
- Try to exercise in an environment that doesn't aggravate your condition. For instance, if there's a high pollen count, exercise indoors.

Diabetes

Exercise can help you manage your diabetes by lowering blood sugar and increasing insulin efficiency. It also helps prevent or delay the development of complications that can result from diabetes, such as high blood pressure and coronary artery disease. In addition, exercise helps control weight, an important factor for many people with the most common form of diabetes, called type 2 (formerly called adult-onset or noninsulin-dependent) diabetes.

Try to exercise at least 30 minutes a day most days of the week. Aerobic activities are generally best. Plan your activities to fit your mealtimes and medication dosage, and check your blood sugar before and after exercising. If it's below 100 milligrams per deciliter (mg/dL), you may need to eat a snack before you exercise to avoid low blood sugar. You shouldn't exercise if your blood sugar level is above 300 mg/dL.

If you've lost some of the feeling in your feet due to diabetic neuropathy, talk to your doctor about appropriate forms of exercise. You may want to avoid exercises such as walking, running or aerobics. Swimming or bicycling may be better choices.

High blood pressure

Physical activity is critical to controlling high blood pressure. Regular activity makes your heart stronger, so it doesn't have to work as hard to pump blood. Exercise also helps promote weight loss. Increased weight can contribute to high blood pressure.

Regular physical activity can lower your blood pressure by about the same amount as many blood pressure medications — 5 to 10 millimeters of mercury. This may even be enough to prevent your having to take medication. If you're taking medication, exercise can help your medication work more effectively.

Consistency is more important than intensity. Try to get at least 30 minutes of moderately intense activity most, if not all, days of the week. Aerobic activity has the greatest effect on blood pressure.

Coronary artery disease

If you have coronary artery disease, exercise is important. Regular exercise can help prevent a heart attack by reducing pressure on damaged arteries and reducing buildup of cholesterol-containing plaques. When plaques form in an artery, they narrow the passageway for blood flow and can lead to formation of a blood clot.

If you've had a heart attack, regular exercise helps to reduce the risk of a second heart attack. Many people worry that they'll have a heart attack during exercise. The chances of that happening are small. Most heart attacks occur during rest, not activity. To minimize health risks and maximize exercise benefits:

- See your doctor. Before you begin a regular exercise program, have a physical examination and talk with your doctor about the best way to get started.
- Exercise regularly. Cardiovascular risk increases if you alternate intense workouts with weeks or months of inactivity.
- Warm up and cool down. This reduces stress on your heart and risk of muscle strain.
- Wait 2 to 3 hours after a large meal before exercising. Digestion increases blood flow to your digestive system and away from your heart.
- Listen to your body. If you experience heart palpitations, lightheadedness or pain in your chest, jaw or arm, stop and seek immediate medical attention.

Osteoporosis

Regular exercise helps maintain, and may even increase, bone density. It also strengthens muscles. Strengthening your muscles and bones helps to improve your balance, which can reduce the risk of falls and, therefore, fractures associated with osteoporosis.

Because of the varying degrees of osteoporosis and the risk of fracture, ask your doctor or a physical therapist for advice on exercises that are safe and appropriate for you. Walking is often an ideal weight-bearing activity because you can do it anywhere with minimal risk of injury.

Strength training may include use of free weights, weight machines, resistance bands or water exercises. These exercises strengthen muscles and bones and help slow bone mineral loss. Back-strengthening exercises, such as gentle back arches, help strengthen back and abdominal muscles.

Avoid high-impact exercises that place excessive stress on your bones, such as tennis or running. Also avoid rowing machines, which require deep forward bending that could lead to a vertebral fracture.

Chronic pain

A common misconception is that exercise increases pain. Not so — exercise can help reduce it. When you're inactive, you become deconditioned — you lose muscle tone and strength, and your cardiovascular system works less efficiently. Regular physical activity builds stronger muscles, bones and joints, which can help reduce pain.

In addition, during physical activity your body releases chemicals called endorphins that can block pain signals from reaching your brain. The more endorphins you produce on your own, the less you need to rely on external forms of pain management, such as medications. These natural pain-relieving chemicals also help alleviate anxiety and depression, conditions that can make pain more difficult to control.

Your fitness program should be tailored to your specific condition. Talk with your doctor or a physical therapist about activities that may be beneficial for you. ■

CHAPTER 5 PART I

Managing Stress

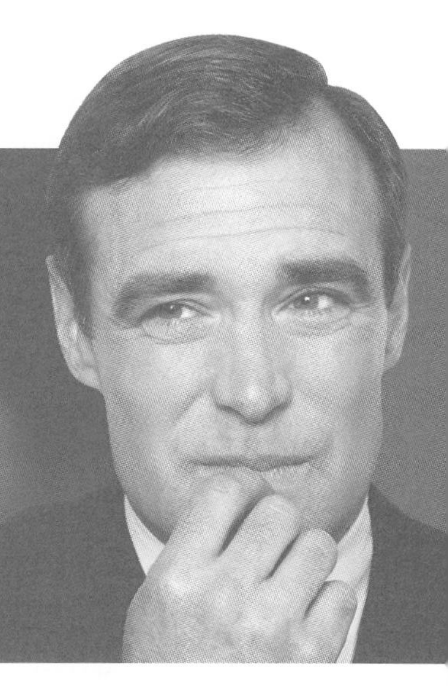

Heavy workloads, a demanding family life, aging parents — these situations and countless others can lead to stress. Stress is something that most people know well and experience often. It's unavoidable. Stress comes from events that you consider to be positive — a job promotion, vacation or marriage — as well as from negative events — the loss of a job, a divorce or the death of a loved one. It's your personal response to situations and circumstances that causes you to feel pressure. In short, stress is a normal part of daily life.

Understanding Stress

Stress isn't just an outside force. Rather, it's your physiologic response to specific stimuli (stressors). Your stress response mobilizes bodily systems so that they can help you adapt to the constant demands and changes in your life.

Long workdays, too little sleep and information overload are among the leading sources of stress. However, situations that create stress are as unique as you are. Your personality, genes and past experiences — your overall ability to cope — influence how you deal with stressful situations. Missing the bus, standing in line at the store or getting a parking ticket may not bother you, but another person may find these situations extremely stressful.

Whatever the cause of your stress, the thing to remember is that when environmental demands exceed your ability to cope, it creates stress, and stress can produce symptoms and lead to illness.

Stress can be short term (acute) or long term (chronic), and the effects of stress can accumulate over time. Acute stress commonly is a reaction to an immediate or perceived threat. In such cases, you respond with an alarm reaction that readies your body for an emergency. Chronic stress is often related to situations that aren't short lived, such as relationship problems, loneliness or financial worries.

When you experience stress — especially severe stress — a physical response occurs to meet the energy demands of the situation. Your heart beats faster, your breathing quickens, and your blood pressure rises. In addition, your blood sugar rises, and blood flow to your brain and large muscles increases. After the threat passes, your body relaxes again. You may be able to handle an occasional stressful event, but when it happens regularly, the effects multiply and compound over time.

Stress and Health

Many of the physical reactions that accompany stress can damage your long-term health by contributing to physical or emotional illness. Stress may be a factor in many illnesses, from headaches to heart disease. Stress may aggravate an existing health problem. Or it may trigger an illness if you're already at risk of that particular condition.

The Fight-or-Flight Response

When stress is intense, as in a perceived threat, a phenomenon called fight or flight occurs. Your pituitary gland, which is located at the base of your brain, secretes hormones that regulate many body processes. When you perceive danger, this gland increases the secretion of a hormone called adrenocorticotropic hormone, which causes your adrenal gland to produce and release other hormones. These hormones — adrenaline (epinephrine) and cortisol — immediately cause your pulse to quicken, your muscles to tense and your blood pressure to increase. These responses prepare your body to fight the danger or flee.

To increase blood to your large muscles, your heart begins to beat faster, and your blood pressure increases abruptly. Blood is directed away from your stomach and skin to your muscles. Your body also releases potential sources of energy into your bloodstream in the form of blood sugars and fat. And it secretes certain chemicals that make it easier for your blood to clot in case of an injury.

Your nervous system also moves into action by causing the pupils in your eyes to dilate so that you can see better if lighting is poor and by tensing your facial muscles, possibly to make you look more menacing. Perspiration increases to keep your body cool, and respiration accelerates to increase oxygen in your blood. All of these changes prepare your body for an emergency, real or perceived.

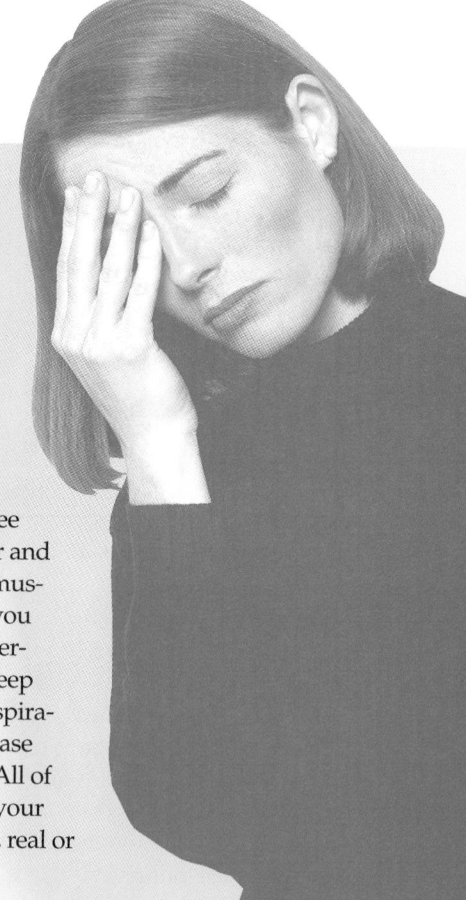

Suppresses the immune system

The hormone cortisol produced during the stress response may suppress your immune system, increasing your susceptibility to infectious disease. Studies suggest that the risk of bacterial infections such as tuberculosis and group A streptococcal disease increases during stress. Stress may also make you prone to upper respiratory viral infections such as a cold or the flu.

Increases risk of cardiovascular disease

During acute stress your heart beats quickly, which makes you more susceptible to heart rhythm irregularities and a type of chest pain called angina. What's more, if you're a "hot reactor," acute stress may add to your risk of a heart attack. Hot reactors exhibit extreme increases in heart rate and blood pressure in response to daily stress. These surges may gradually injure your coronary arteries and heart. Increased blood clotting from persistent stress also can put you at risk of a heart attack or stroke.

Worsens other illnesses

Other relationships between illness and stress aren't as clear-cut. However, stress may worsen your symptoms if you have any of the following conditions:

Asthma
A stressful situation can make your airways overreactive, precipitating an asthma attack.

Gastrointestinal problems
Stress may trigger or worsen symptoms associated with some gastrointestinal conditions, such as irritable bowel syndrome or nonulcer dyspepsia.

Chronic pain
Stress can heighten your body's pain response, making chronic pain associated with conditions such as arthritis, fibromyalgia or a back injury more difficult to manage.

Mental health disorders
Stress may trigger depression in people who are prone to the disorder. It may also worsen symptoms of other mental health disorders, such as anxiety.

? Question and Answer

Is there such a thing as good stress?

Stress may result from positive or negative situations. Stress brought on by a positive cause provides a feeling of excitement and opportunity. For example, stress often helps athletes perform better in competition. Other examples of positive stress include a new job or the birth of a child.

Negative causes of stress occur when you feel out of control or under constant or intense pressure. You may have trouble concentrating, or you may feel alone. Family, finances, isolation and health problems are common negative causes of stress.

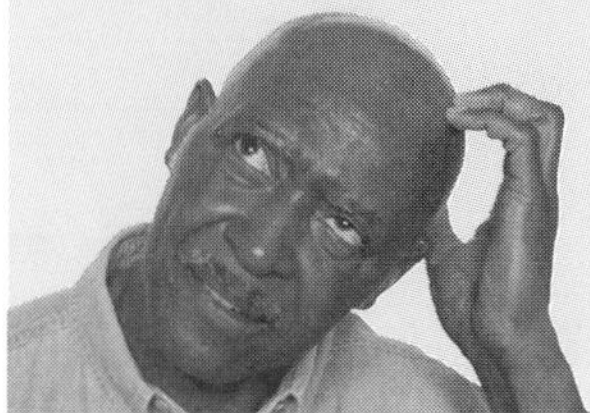

Stress Myths

Understanding the truth about stress will help you better cope with this common problem. Here are several myths that surround stress:

Myth: No stress is best
Fact: Everyone needs some stress in life to keep things interesting. The real issue is finding the right balance. Managed stress can help you to be productive and happy. Poorly managed stress, though, can hurt and even kill you.

Myth: Stress is everywhere, so there's nothing you can do about it
Fact: This isn't true. When you take steps to manage your life, stress doesn't have to overwhelm you. Set priorities, address small tasks first and then make your way to the complex ones. When you don't prioritize, all of your problems seem to have equal weight, making you feel as though stress is everywhere.

Myth: One size fits all for stress reduction
Fact: Because everyone's different, what works to reduce stress for you is as individual as you are.

Myth: If you don't have symptoms, you must not be stressed
Fact: Just because you don't seem to have symptoms of stress doesn't mean you're not under stress. You may not recognize the symptoms, or you may be taking medications that mask them. Such medications can deprive you of signs warning you to ease up.

Myth: Only major stress symptoms cause problems
Fact: Not so. This implies "minor" symptoms such as headache and stomach ailments can be ignored. These "minor" symptoms may actually be early warning signs that you need to better manage stress in your life.

Recognizing Stress

You may not recognize that you're under stress. Your first indications that your body and brain are feeling pressured may be associated symptoms of stress — headache, insomnia, upset stomach, digestive changes. An old nervous habit such as nail biting may reappear. Instead of recognizing these symptoms as signs of stress, you may at first interpret them as an illness.

The presence of stress may also become apparent through psychological changes. The most common one is increased irritability with people close to you. You may also feel more cynical, pessimistic or resentful. Many stressed people report a sense of being victimized, misunderstood or unappreciated. You may find that things that you would normally enjoy seem burdensome. Some people become anxious, reclusive or prone to crying or laughing. Others engage in inappropriate behavior. Occasionally, these changes are so gradual that you or those around you don't recognize them until your health or relationships change.

Coping with Stress

You can deal with stress in many ways. You may talk about your problems with others, listen to some music to help you relax, or sit in a warm bathtub or hot tub at the end of the day. Much of this you do without really thinking about it. Most of the time you may do pretty well in getting through life's crises as they arise. However, there are probably times when you could do better. The following strategies can help you better manage stress.

Signs and Symptoms of Stress

Physical	Psychological	Behavioral
Headache	Anxiety	Overeating or loss of appetite
Grinding teeth	Irritability	Impatience
Tight, dry throat	Feeling of impending doom	Being argumentative
Clenched jaws	Depression	Procrastination
Chest pain	Slowed thinking	Increased use of alcohol or drugs
Shortness of breath	Racing thoughts	Increased smoking
Pounding heart	Feeling of helplessness	Withdrawal or isolation
High blood pressure	Feeling of hopelessness	Neglecting responsibility
Muscle aches	Feeling of worthlessness	Poor job performance
Indigestion	Feeling of lack of direction	Burnout
Constipation or diarrhea	Feeling of insecurity	Poor personal hygiene
Increased perspiration	Sadness	Change in religious practices
Cold, sweaty hands	Defensiveness	Change in close relationships
Fatigue	Anger	
Insomnia	Hypersensitivity	
Frequent illness	Apathy	

Identify your stressors

The first step in learning to manage stress is to identify what's causing it. Not everyone responds to events the same way.

For instance, a so-called workaholic may be thought by others to be working into an early grave, when in fact that person feels more in control when taking on extra challenges at work. For this person, work itself may be a form of stress management, and the unstructured time of a vacation or "relaxation" at home may actually be a greater source of stress.

Your stress may be linked to external factors, such as:

- Work
- Family
- Community
- Environment
- Unpredictable events

Stress can also come from internal factors, such as:

- Unrealistic or high expectations
- Perfectionism
- Worry
- Negative attitudes and feelings
- Irresponsible behavior
- Poor health and health habits

Once you identify the sources of your stress, you might not be able to avoid them, but you'll at least know what's causing your symptoms. That in itself may be a benefit by making you feel more in control.

Practice tolerance

As a part of your overall strategy to better manage stress, try to become more tolerant — of yourself and of situations over which you have no control. You need to understand and accept that changes are constant and that changes — losses and events over which you may have little control — will continue to occur, like it or not.

Interpersonal Conflicts

Often life's hurdles revolve around dealing with interpersonal conflicts. The three most typical types of interpersonal conflicts are marital conflicts, family conflicts and job-related conflicts.

Marital conflicts

Couples often enter into a relationship with unrealistic expectations. An overly romantic view of marriage fosters this tendency. Instead of realizing that they're marrying ordinary human beings with strengths and weaknesses, some people tend to idealize their mates and expect nothing less than perfection.

Over the course of a marriage, couples typically face a series of predictable transitions. Adjustments to having children, changing jobs, losing parents and changing sexual needs all present challenges. If the marriage is to flourish, the couple must communicate and resolve inevitable conflicts effectively.

A marriage counselor often can bring troublesome issues to light and foster communication so that a couple can recognize and deal with stress in their marriage.

Family conflicts

A family is a complex network of relationships. Each member has a different relationship with each other member in the family. These differences may be a reflection of age, birth order, sex, personality type or a combination of several such factors. Each of these relationships, in turn, affects the rest of the family unit.

Problems within a family are often brought to the surface when one member is showing signs of a problem — for example, trouble in school, substance abuse or inappropriate sexual behavior. These occasions may reveal a pattern of behavior that everyone is contributing to, such as spending too little time with one another, and that everyone in the family needs to help change. Family therapists often help identify specific problems that all family members can work on.

Job-related conflicts

Interpersonal conflicts in the workplace present a multitude of issues. Competition can develop among co-workers. Conflict may stem from an individual's desire for power and control, changes in the workplace or differences in people's work habits.

Problems often result from a lack of proper communication among co-workers and between management and employees.

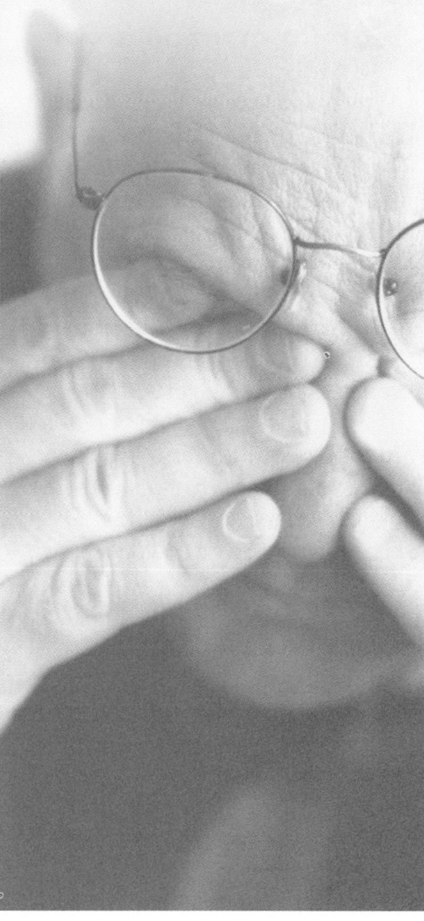

Getting Professional Help

You don't need to handle all of your problems alone. Help from a counselor, psychiatrist, psychologist or clergyperson may be just what you need in order to handle stress. Many people believe that seeking outside help is a sign of weakness, which adds to their sense of inadequacy, hopelessness or anger. But it takes strength to realize that you need help and good judgment to seek it. If you need assistance finding someone who can help you, ask your doctor, local health organization or employer for recommendations.

With professional guidance, you may be able to determine if what you're feeling is stress or an illness. If you're experiencing physical or psychological symptoms that affect your ability to work, play or find pleasure in life, they may be a signal of something more than stress.

If you're like most people, you're more understanding of other people's distress than of your own. You may think that you should always feel happy. As long as you believe this, you're bound to be disappointed. Accepting that you'll always experience a certain degree of stress, and that this is normal, is helpful in managing stress.

Learn to manage anger

Anger management is an important technique for reducing stress. Anger can significantly increase and prolong stress if you remain angry for an extended period. Anger can even trigger a heart attack. Learning to manage anger is a lot like learning to manage stress. Here are some suggestions to help you get started:

Identify your anger triggers
Once you know what sets you off, plan ahead for how you'll avoid becoming angry when you're in such a situation.

Identify symptoms of emerging anger
What do you do when you start to get angry? Do you clench your teeth? Do your shoulders begin to tense up? Do you feel your heart begin to beat faster? Does your face flush? Read these signs and symptoms like a caution light — a warning that you're getting angry.

Respond to your symptoms
When you find yourself becoming angry, take a short timeout. Count to 10, take a few deep breaths, look out a window — anything to buy time so that your brain can catch up with your emotions and you can think before you act.

Take time to cool down
Before you confront a person or situation that has made you angry, find a way to release some of your emotional energy. Go for a walk, clean the house or run. And don't hit the send button on that angry e-mail you just wrote.

Don't bottle up your anger
If your anger stems from what someone said or did, talk directly to that person. Don't verbally attack the person with accusations. Deal only with this episode and approach it from the perspective of how you feel instead of what the person did.

Find release valves
Look for creative ways to release the energy produced by your anger. These might include listening to music, painting, dancing or writing in your journal.

Seek advice
If you find yourself becoming angry often, confide in people who care about you, such as family members or friends. Ask them to help you brainstorm possible coping solutions or find a medical professional who can help you.

Practice positive thinking

Positive self-talk is another effective way to cope with stress. Self-talk is the endless stream of thoughts that run through your head every day.

These automatic thoughts can be positive or negative. Some are based on logic and reason. Others may be misconceptions that you formulate from lack of adequate information. The goal of positive self-talk is to weed out the misconceptions and challenge them with rational and positive thoughts. Studies indicate that a positive, hopeful attitude can help manage stress, but a negative attitude can aggravate it.

How can you learn positive self-talk? The process is simple, but it takes time and practice. Throughout the day, stop and evaluate what you're thinking. And find a way to put a positive spin on your negative thoughts. One reasonable rule about self-talk is this: Don't say to yourself anything you wouldn't say to someone else.

Develop an action plan

Once you've identified your stressors and have accepted that they exist, it's time to address them. Some stressors are under your control; others aren't. Concentrate on events that you can change. For example, if your busy day is a source of stress, ask yourself if it's because you tend to squeeze too many things into your day or because you aren't organized. Here are some tips that may help:

Plan your day
Planning your day can help you feel more in control of your life. Keep a schedule of your daily activities so that you're not faced with conflicts or last-minute rushes to get to an appointment or activity on time.

Managing Your Time

Often, stress is a result of too much to do and too little time. Or it may stem from procrastination. Setting priorities and practicing some simple time management skills may go a long way toward depressurizing your day.

1. Dump all of your tasks onto a master list. Include everything you have to do, large and small. You may have 50 items. Mark key dates and deadlines for big projects on your calendar.
2. Each day, list 5 to 10 items that you want to accomplish that day.
3. Divide your daily list into three levels — A, B and C:
   - *A* items are the two or three tasks that you must do. These tasks are both important and urgent and probably will take the most energy. Do them first or when your energy level is the highest.
   - *B* items are important but not urgent. These activities will help you move toward your long-range goals.
   - *C* items are routine stuff, but things that you must do today. Can you delegate any of these?

If you're still having problems getting the right things done, analyze how you spend your time for several days. You may be wasting time on unimportant things or things that aren't on your list.

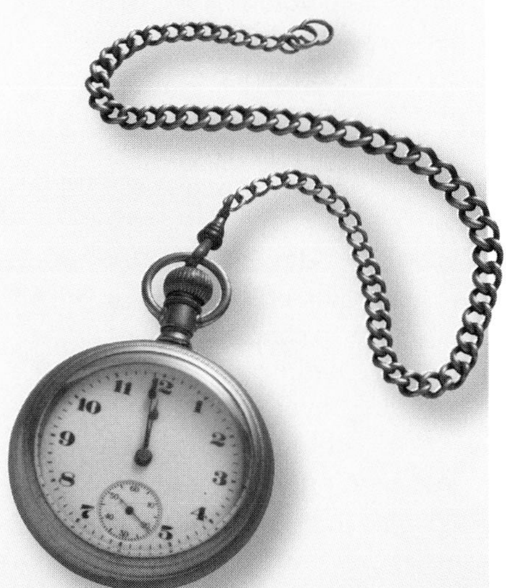

Simplify your life
Prioritize, plan and pace yourself. Simplify your life by cutting out some activities or delegating tasks. Keep your house, car and personal belongings in working order to prevent untimely, expensive and stressful repairs.

Get organized
Organize your home and work space so that you don't have to spend time looking for things you've misplaced.

Take occasional breaks
Periodically during the day, take time to relax, stretch or walk.

Get adequate sleep, stay physically active and eat well
A healthy body helps promote good mental health. Sleep helps you tackle problems with renewed vigor. Physical activity helps burn off stress-related tension. A balanced diet provides you with energy to handle daily stress.

Discuss your concerns
Talking with a trusted friend helps to relieve stress and may put events in perspective.

Remember what's important
Decide on your priorities and concentrate on the things of most importance to you.

Get away
Take a break from your normal routine and enjoy a change of scenery or a different pace.

Enjoy a good laugh
It's healthy to spend time with people who have a positive outlook, take themselves lightly or have a sense of humor. Laughter helps reduce or relieve tension.

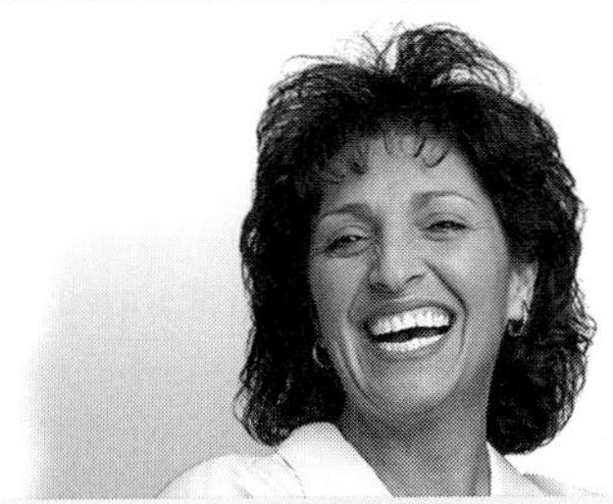

Turning Negatives Into Positives

Here are some examples of typical negative mental messages and how you can give them a positive twist:

Negative thought	Positive thought
I've never done it before.	It's an opportunity to learn something new.
It's too complicated.	Let's look at it from a different angle.
I don't have the resources.	Necessity is the mother of invention.
There's not enough time.	Let's re-evaluate some priorities.
There's no way it'll work.	I can make it work.
I don't have the expertise.	I'll find people who can help me.
It's good enough.	There's always room for improvement.
It's too radical a change.	Let's take a chance.

Experiment with relaxation techniques

Relaxation is more than watching television or taking a break from work. True relaxation is positive and satisfying — a feeling of peace of mind. Seek out activities that give you pleasure, be it physical activity, art, music or some other hobby, and try to devote at least 30 minutes to these activities every day.

Other techniques that can lessen the discomfort and duration of stress include progressive muscle relaxation, visualization and relaxed breathing.

Progressive muscle relaxation

Progressive muscle relaxation is a technique that involves relaxing a series of muscles one at a time.

1. Sit or lie in a comfortable position and close your eyes. Allow your jaw to drop and your eyelids to relax, but don't squeeze your eyelids shut.
2. Mentally scan your body, starting with your toes and working slowly up through your legs, buttocks, torso, arms, hands, fingers, neck and head. Focus on each part individually.
3. Tighten the muscles in one area of your body, hold them for a count of five and then relax them. Imagine the tension melting away from your muscles. Then move on to the next area.

Visualization

Also known as guided imagery, visualization involves lying quietly and picturing yourself in a pleasant and peaceful setting.

1. Allow thoughts to flow through your mind, but don't focus on any of them. Tell yourself that you're relaxed and calm, that your hands are heavy and warm — or cool if you're hot — that your heart is beating calmly.
2. Breathe slowly, regularly and deeply.
3. Once you're relaxed, imagine yourself in a favorite place or in a spot of beauty and stillness.
4. After 5 or 10 minutes, rouse yourself gradually.

With practice you'll be able to imagine your favorite place or spot of great beauty and stillness and trigger the relaxation response in your body.

Relaxed breathing

Another form of relaxation focuses on deep, relaxed breathing. Rehearse it throughout the day so that it becomes natural and you can apply it when you feel stressed.

1. Lie on a bed or couch or sit in a chair.
2. Place your feet slightly apart and rest your hands on your abdomen or in your lap.
3. Slowly inhale while counting to four, allowing your abdomen to rise about 1 inch — you should feel the movement with your hand. Don't pull up your shoulders or move your chest.
4. As you breathe in, imagine the warmed air flowing into all parts of your body.
5. Pause 1 second after inhaling.
6. Slowly exhale and count to four. As you exhale, your abdomen will slowly fall.
7. As air flows out, imagine your tension also flowing out.
8. Pause 1 second after exhaling.
9. Repeat 5 to 10 times.

If it's difficult to make your breathing regular, take a slightly deeper breath, hold it for a second or two and let it out slowly through pursed lips for about 10 seconds. Repeat this once or twice.

How to succeed

No matter what steps you take to manage stress, two simple reminders can help you be successful: practice and be patient.

Practice

The steps you're taking may be new to you. In fact, at first you may feel uncomfortable doing them. Work on your coping skills daily until they come naturally. You want to get to the point that you can use them anytime, anywhere.

When you're practicing relaxation techniques, get comfortable — loosen tight clothing and remove your shoes and belt if need be.

Be patient

Don't worry about how well you're doing and don't expect to see immediate benefits. It takes time and practice for stress management skills to become automatic. Keep working at it. ■

PREVENTION TIP

For information on additional methods of relaxation, see Chapter 43, "Complementary and Alternative Medicine."

CHAPTER 6 PART I

Addressing Risky Behaviors

Research indicates that your health in later life depends more on your lifestyle choices than on your genes. And the sooner you adopt healthy habits, the greater is your chance of living to a ripe old age.

What are your health trouble spots — activities or habits that increase your risk of disease? For some people, the answer may be inactivity and an unhealthy diet. For others, trouble spots may be activities that have a more rapid and direct negative impact on health. These activities — commonly referred to as risky behaviors — include tobacco use, excessive use of alcohol, drug abuse and unsafe sex.

If you aren't involved in any of these activities, don't start. If you are, it's not too late to change. Addressing risky behaviors can add years to your life.

Tobacco Use

Smoking is the single largest preventable cause of premature death and disability in the United States. Yet nearly 50 million Americans smoke — that's more than 25 percent of the adult population. Each day more than 3,000 people under the age of 18 start smoking.

Doctors frequently see patients whose serious medical conditions are related to smoking. Medical care for smoking-related illnesses in the United States costs billions of dollars annually. The indirect costs of smoking are equally astounding. Fire started by cigarettes causes significant property damage. Higher insurance premiums and taxes needed to fund disability benefits for people who are ill as a result of smoking also are part of the cost.

Consider these facts:

- Smoking is responsible for nearly one in five deaths in the United States.
- Approximately 10 million people in the United States have died of smoking-related illnesses since the first U.S. Surgeon General's report on smoking and health was issued in 1964.
- Each year, more Americans die of smoking-related diseases than from alcohol, AIDS, drug abuse, car accidents, fire, suicide and murder — combined.
- On average, smokers die 10 to 12 years earlier than nonsmokers do. Smokers between the ages of 35 and 70 have death rates three times higher than have nonsmokers of the same age.

Smoking and disease

The popularity of the cigarette is a 20th-century phenomenon. The number of cigarette smokers skyrocketed in the early 1900s following the introduction of new mass production technology combined with highly effective advertising campaigns. Before long, reports of a connection between smoking and the incidence of diseases such as lung cancer began to appear.

Today, tobacco use is recognized as a major risk factor in many diseases. This should come as no surprise. Cigarette smoke contains more than 4,000 chemicals, including 63 carcinogens and trace amounts of such poisons as cyanide, arsenic and formaldehyde. In addition, carbon monoxide in cigarette smoke displaces oxygen from your red blood cells, which robs your tissues of oxygen.

The delicate tissues of the mouth, throat and voice box (larynx) are affected by repeated exposure to cigarette smoke. After the smoke passes through your mouth, your lungs retain 70 percent to 90 percent of the compounds you inhale. A few puffs on a cigarette reduce the effectiveness of the cilia inside your bronchial tubes. Cilia are tiny, hairlike bodies that normally work like brooms to sweep foreign particles out of your lungs. Smoking just one cigarette can slow the sweeping actions of the cilia for almost an hour.

Regular smoking virtually paralyzes the cilia, leaving your lungs exposed to billions of tiny particles from cigarette smoke. With the cilia largely inactive, tar from the cigarette smoke begins to build up and damage lung tissues. When cooled inside your lungs, the tar forms a brown sticky layer on the lining of breathing passages. This layer contains the tar and other chemicals that can cause cancer.

Cancer

Smoking is a major risk factor for cancers of the mouth, larynx, pharynx, esophagus, lung, stomach, pancreas, kidney, urinary bladder and cervix.

Here are some other sobering statistics:

- A smoker is twice as likely to develop cancer as is a person who doesn't smoke, and a heavy smoker is four times more likely to develop cancer than is a nonsmoker.
- Lung cancer has long been the leading cause of cancer deaths in American men, and in 1987 it surpassed breast cancer as the leading cause of cancer deaths in American women.
- Overall, smoking accounts for at least 30 percent of all cancer deaths.

Chronic obstructive pulmonary disease

Smoking is also the major cause of chronic lung diseases such as chronic obstructive pulmonary disease (COPD). This disease includes lung disorders such as emphysema and chronic bronchitis.

More than 80 percent of deaths from COPD are related to cigarette smoking. In fact, a smoker is 10 times more likely to die of COPD than is a nonsmoker.

In addition to paralyzing or destroying the cilia in your lungs, tobacco smoke irrevocably damages or destroys the tiny air sacs (alveoli) in your lungs in which carbon dioxide is exchanged for oxygen. When these air sacs are

Attention Women Smokers

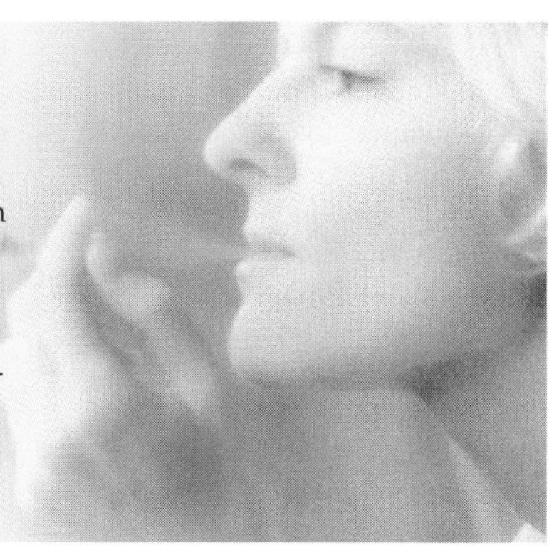

Women who smoke have additional risks to consider:

- Female smokers older than age 35 who use birth control pills are at high risk of heart attack, stroke and blood clots in the legs.
- Female smokers have an increased risk of developing osteoporosis, a disease that makes bones brittle.
- Women who smoke during pregnancy are more likely to have a miscarriage, stillbirth or a baby with a low birth weight. Studies also show a direct relationship between smoking during pregnancy and risk of sudden infant death syndrome.

injured, your body is less able to transport adequate levels of oxygen to your vital organs. Eventually, as you struggle for each breath, COPD often becomes fatal.

Cardiovascular disease

Cardiovascular disease includes conditions such as high blood pressure, coronary artery disease and stroke. The single most important health effect of smoking may be its role in developing cardiovascular disease.

Nicotine in tobacco smoke acts on your adrenal glands, causing them to secrete hormones that temporarily increase your blood pressure and your heart rate. The carbon monoxide from tobacco smoke binds to hemoglobin in your blood, taking the place of valuable oxygen and reducing the amount of oxygen available to your tissues and organs.

Carbon monoxide may have a direct effect on the heart muscle itself, on your blood vessels and perhaps even on the clotting of your blood. Smoking may increase the clumping (clotting) action of certain blood cells (platelets), and it decreases the ability of the arteries to dilate when they need to do so. The mechanism is complex, but smoking is also a contributing factor to the accumulation of cholesterol in arteries (atherosclerosis). This may explain why smoking is also associated with stroke. Smoking contributes to other circulatory problems as well.

Here are some statistics about tobacco use and risks to your heart:

- Almost 180,000 Americans die each year of cardiovascular disease caused by smoking.
- The risk of heart disease is 70 percent higher among smokers.
- Thirty-five percent of smoking-related deaths from heart disease occur before age 65.
- A smoker is two times more likely to die of a heart attack than is a nonsmoker, and the risk is even higher for heavier smokers.
- A smoker who has had a heart attack and continues to smoke is six times more likely to have a second heart attack than is one who stops smoking.

Why smokers smoke

Increased knowledge of the hazards of smoking, along with increased smoking restrictions or bans, has had a deterring effect on smokers. More than 40 million Americans identify themselves as former smokers. The number of men who smoke has declined substantially, from one-half of the adult men in 1965 to about one-quarter today. Among women, there isn't much decline. As a result, the numbers of male and female smokers are now about equal.

The reasons people start smoking or refuse to quit are rarely simple. Some smokers report that their cigarettes offer them a surge of energy, especially to wake them up in the morning or keep them awake at other times. Nicotine acts as a stimulant with an adrenaline-like effect. Your heart rate and blood pressure increase while you're smoking.

Some smokers note that cigarettes calm them down when they're under stress. In addition, a cigarette gives them something to do with their hands if they're nervous or even gives them a sense of security.

Nicotine in tobacco is an addictive drug that leads to an addictive response. The degree of addiction depends to some degree on how much and how long the smoker has smoked. The addiction most smokers experience is both psychological and physical. For some, regular use of cigarettes in many life situations has convinced them that they can't cope with life without smoking.

Nicotine can be as addictive as alcohol, heroin or cocaine. The central element of addiction is loss of control. Nicotine controls your behavior by making you feel good, so you want to use it more. You may want to quit, but you can't or won't, even when you know tobacco is harmful to your health.

You may be dependent on nicotine if you experience one or more of the following characteristics:

- You've made a serious but unsuccessful attempt to stop or reduce the amount of tobacco you use.
- Your attempts to stop have led to withdrawal symptoms, such as craving tobacco or feelings of anxiety, irritability, frustration or anger. Other signs and symptoms include trouble concentrating or sleeping and an increase in

appetite with possible weight gain.

- You continue to use tobacco even when you have a serious health problem, such as heart or lung disease, that you know is made worse by tobacco use.
- You develop a "tolerance" for tobacco. You may notice that a certain number of cigarettes daily produces less effect than it used to and that you need to smoke more to achieve a desired effect.

Teenage smoking

Most cigarette smokers start early in life. Among smokers born since 1935, more than 80 percent started smoking before age 21, and more than half started before age 18. Today, a million teenagers begin smoking each year. An increasing number of them are female. Even though smoking has generally declined since the mid-1960s, an increasing number of teenagers smoke. This group continues to be a major target for advertising by the tobacco industry. And more recently, college campuses have been the target of widespread promotion.

It has been well documented that a high percentage of teenagers who smoke are in families in which one or both parents smoke. Cigarette smoking among teenagers also seems to be connected to peer pressure. In a survey of 3,000 junior high students, the most likely predictor of whether a boy or girl smoked was having friends who smoked.

Education doesn't appear to be an effective deterrent to smoking among teenagers. Nine of every 10 teenagers surveyed believed that smoking was harmful to their health. And 85 percent of those who smoked said that they didn't plan to be smokers for more than 5 years. Most of the teenagers who took up smoking had been adamantly against smoking in their younger years. Parents who continue to smoke with no visible ill effects can have a substantial influence. In such situations teenagers' concerns about smoking diminish, and many take up smoking.

Cigarette alternatives

Contrary to popular belief, using other types of tobacco products or cigarette alternatives endangers your health just as much as smoking regular cigarettes.

Light cigarettes

Cigarette companies have implied over the years that so-called light cigarettes — those that are low-tar, low-nicotine — are safer and cause fewer health risks. However, features such as ventilated filters don't reduce your exposure to harmful chemicals in tobacco. Smokers addicted to nicotine will get their fix of nicotine, regardless. They may compensate for the diluted smoke by taking more frequent puffs, inhaling more deeply or simply smoking more cigarettes. Those who smoke light cigarettes may actually end up taking in as much or more tar and nicotine as they would with regular cigarettes. They may also inhale more carbon monoxide and other dangerous chemicals.

Furthermore, switching to low-tar, low-nicotine cigarettes doesn't decrease your risk of lung cancer, emphysema, heart attack or other diseases. In fact, smokers of light cigarettes may be at increased risk of certain types of disease because they inhale more chemicals or smoke more cigarettes.

Cigars

Since 1993, cigar use in the United States has increased nearly 50 percent. Much of the increased use of cigars comes from adults with higher levels of income and education. Evidence also suggests that many new cigar users are teenagers and young adult males.

Unlike cigarettes, cigars vary in size and appearance. And whereas cigarettes are made from blends of tobacco, cigars are made primarily of a single tobacco. Like cigarette smoking, the health risks from cigar smoking increase with the number of cigars a person smokes each day.

Although many cigar smokers don't fully inhale smoke into their lungs, they're still exposed to smoke in their oral cavity, as well as to the secondhand smoke in the smoking environment. Considering that cigar smoke contains as many poisonous chemicals as cigarette smoke, cigar smokers are at risk of the same smoking-related illnesses. Cigar smokers and cigarette smokers have similar risk levels of cancers of the mouth, throat and esophagus. And cigar smokers are still 4 to 10 times more likely to die of cancers of the lung and larynx than are nonsmokers.

Pipes

Studies on the risks of lung or heart disease in people who smoke only a pipe compared with people who smoke only cigarettes or cigars are limited. However, pipe smoking is associated with cancers of the lip and mouth and clearly increases the level of carbon monoxide in your blood. And there's enough evidence available on the dangers of tobacco use to recommend that you become a nonsmoker — regardless of the type of smoking — to minimize your risk of cancer, heart disease and lung disease.

Spit tobacco and snuff

Spit tobacco (chewing tobacco) is usually sold in loose leaf form or compressed in a plug. Users generally place spit tobacco between their cheek and gum and keep it there for several hours. Nicotine is absorbed into the bloodstream through the cheek lining. Snuff is powdered tobacco. A small amount is placed between the lower lip and the gum.

In recent years, there's been an increase in the use of spit tobacco and snuff. The number of young males using spit tobacco grew 10 times between 1970 and 1990. Spit tobacco and snuff have been thought to be a safe alternative to cigarette smoking. But they're not safe at all. Studies show that smokeless tobacco can produce a high level of nicotine in the blood. The consequence of regular use is long-term nicotine dependence and its associated health risks.

Health risks include cancers of the oral cavity and throat, particularly where tobacco is held in the mouth. Frequently, a white, leathery patch forms at the place in your mouth where you hold tobacco. This condition, called leukoplakia, is precancerous.

Spit tobacco and snuff can cause swollen, bleeding gums and lead to the loss of teeth. They can also cause an increased heart rate, higher blood pressure and even an irregular heartbeat.

The bottom line is, no smoke is safe smoke, and no tobacco use is safe.

Secondhand smoke

More than 50,000 Americans die each year of exposure to secondhand (passive) smoke. As a result, most states have enacted laws limiting smoking in public places.

The Environmental Protection Agency (EPA) has classified environmental tobacco smoke as a group A carcinogen that's responsible for more than 3,800 cases of lung cancer in nonsmokers each year. Other group A carcinogens include asbestos, radon and benzene.

Inhaling secondhand smoke causes your heart to beat faster, your blood pressure to increase and the level of carbon monoxide in your blood to rise. Side-stream smoke from a burning cigarette contains twice as much tar and nicotine as does inhaled smoke, three times more of a cancer causing compound called 3,4-benzpyrene, five times more carbon monoxide and possibly 50 times more ammonia.

The deadly effects of secondhand smoke are far-reaching and clear:

- In the United States, 27 percent of homes with children age 6 and younger allow smoking, affecting 9 to 12 million children.
- Children exposed to secondhand smoke are at greater risk of developing asthma, ear infections, pneumonia and bronchitis.
- Infants and children regularly exposed to secondhand smoke are hospitalized 7,500 to 15,000 times each year for treatment of respiratory tract infections.
- Approximately 3,000 nonsmokers die each year of lung cancer as a result of secondhand smoke.
- About 40,000 nonsmokers die each year of cardiovascular disease as a result of secondhand smoke.

Health issues related to secondhand smoke are so grave that all parents should quit or smoke only outdoors — if for no other reason than the health of their children and to encourage their children not to start smoking themselves.

How to stop smoking

Most smokers understand that tobacco use is hazardous to their health. What many beginning smokers fail to understand, however, is that smoking also is an addiction that involves chemicals that affect emotions and behavior.

Because nicotine is an addictive drug, quitting smoking can be very difficult. In fact, most people fail in their first attempt. If you don't succeed the first time, don't stop trying.

Develop a stop plan

Becoming smoke-free is a result of planning and commitment, not

Coping with a Lapse

A lapse usually occurs when an ex-smoker is placed in a situation in which he or she would have smoked in the past but currently lacks a plan to cope without a cigarette or is unable to resist when someone who offers one.

Lapses happen. It may be one puff or it may be days of smoking. The thing to remember is a lapse doesn't mean failure. And it doesn't mean you should stop trying to quit. Millions of ex-smokers experienced lapses before they were finally able to maintain a smoke-free lifestyle.

Here are some tips for how to get back on track so that a lapse doesn't become a return to regular smoking:

Stop what you're doing

Stop smoking and throw all of your cigarettes away. Take a break or go for a walk and give yourself time to think. Call a friend or professional to help you get back on track.

Assess and learn

If you're kicking yourself for having a cigarette, stop. Take this opportunity to catch your breath, assess what happened and make a new plan. By looking at what happened, you can learn about the risks you faced and modify your approach to quitting.

Get back on track

Return to being smoke-free. Review your stop-smoking plan and figure out where you can strengthen and improve.

If your lapse occurred over several days, you may want to use nicotine replacement products to manage renewed signs of withdrawal. Follow your original plan regarding how much and how often to use this medication. If you have questions, consult your doctor.

luck. It helps to develop a stop plan that combines various strategies, or plans of action, for:

- Coping with symptoms of nicotine withdrawal
- Surviving urges to smoke
- Gaining social support and guidance, when necessary

Don't expect to find a ready-made stop plan that you simply adopt as your own. No one plan works for everybody. Build a stop plan you feel comfortable with and that fits your lifestyle. Choose various techniques and tools that you feel suit your needs. These become your strategies to stop smoking.

Generally, stop plans combine several strategies. Studies show that using more then one strategy increases your chance of becoming smoke-free.

Experiment with and adapt strategies to achieve a combination that you feel comfortable with.

For the first week, keep it simple and be flexible. If you're using your stop plan but feel something isn't working, revise your plan.

You may experience physical withdrawal symptoms for 3 to 10 days. When these symptoms begin to lessen, you may still have an impulse to smoke at those times you usually would light up, such as after a meal or when getting behind the wheel of your car.

For some ex-smokers, periodic urges to smoke may come and go for months to years. However, the intensity and duration of these urges invariably grow smaller with the passage of time.

Stop strategies

Your doctor is a valuable resource as you develop your stop plan and work to become smoke-free. Following are some important strategies to help you stop smoking.

Self-help

The self-help method involves working on your own to quit smoking. It involves using health resources to plan and maintain your efforts. Resources may include publications and Internet sites sponsored by national health organizations, such as the American Cancer Society or the American Lung Association.

A self-help strategy is important for building motivation and confidence. The knowledge you gain helps you handle cravings and avoid high-risk situations to smoke.

Group support

For some people, the support of a group is critical for success in stopping. The group, headed by a group leader, meets regularly in an organized treatment program. These programs generally offer multiple sessions over at least a 2-week period, with each session lasting 20 to 60 minutes. The sessions focus on problem-solving and skills training to stop smoking. They provide you with the social support of others dealing with similar problems.

Public health departments in many communities and on college campuses offer smoking cessation programs. Some businesses offer

Medications to Help You Quit

You have several choices of medications to help you stop smoking. Here are some of the nicotine replacement and non-nicotine options currently available:

Nicotine patch

A nicotine patch (Nicoderm) delivers a steady dose of nicotine into your bloodstream through your skin. Most nicotine patch products are available without a prescription. Nicotine patches are used daily for 6 to 12 weeks and have been shown to be very effective, but they're not a magic cure.

Skin irritation often occurs after several weeks of use. After you remove the patch, apply hydrocortisone cream over the area of affected skin to help relieve the irritation. Apply the patch to a different site each day to reduce skin irritation.

Nicotine nasal spray

Nicotine nasal spray (Nicotrol) delivers nicotine into the bloodstream through the lining of your nose. Among nicotine replacement products, it provides the most rapid relief of withdrawal symptoms. The nasal spray is available only with a doctor's prescription.

This nasal spray can cause a hot, peppery feeling in your nose, along with coughing and sneezing, watering eyes and throat irritation. These side effects usually improve within the first week of use. If you experience prolonged side effects, talk with your doctor.

Nicotine inhaler

A nicotine inhaler (Nicotrol) resembles a short cigarette with a plastic mouthpiece. However, the nicotine isn't inhaled. Rather, it's puffed, which allows nicotine to be absorbed into your bloodstream through the lining of your mouth. The nicotine inhaler is available only with a doctor's prescription.

You may feel irritation in your mouth or throat. Drink water to relieve any soreness or dryness. Talk with your doctor if you experience other problems.

Nicotine gum

Nicotine polacrilex (Nicorette) is a gum-like resin that delivers nicotine into your bloodstream through the lining of your mouth. There are two forms of

smoking treatment clinics for their employees.

Individual counseling
As the name implies, the individual counseling method involves working one-on-one with a trusted doctor, psychologist, nurse or counselor for professional advice and support. Trained professionals allow you to express your feelings, your fears of not being able to stop or problems with family or friends. They help you gain coping skills, overcome obstacles and learn to live as a nonsmoker. You can contact your counselor when you experience withdrawal symptoms or need help in handling the urge to smoke.

Cold turkey
Cold turkey is the most frequently used method to stop smoking. It's a sudden, decisive break from cigarettes. On a chosen day, you stop smoking completely with little or no reduction beforehand. Cold turkey isn't something you do on a whim. It requires preparation, emotionally and physically, to withstand the strong desire to smoke. Some form of medication is usually recommended for smokers who use this method.

Medication
Medication helps ease the withdrawal symptoms of nicotine addiction until the worst effects are over. It also allows you to focus on other concerns, such as changing behaviors that lead to smoking. Remember, though, that any medication you decide to use is only an aid. You still need to be psychologically ready to quit. You and your doctor can decide which medication is right for you.

Two basic types of medication are used: non-nicotine medications designed to reduce nicotine cravings and nicotine replacement products. Nicotine replacement products deliver nicotine to your brain via the bloodstream without smoking. As your nicotine dependence weakens, you gradually decrease the use of the medications. The gradual reduction of your nicotine replacement dose reduces the chance of withdrawal. Nicotine replacement products come in a variety of forms, including a patch, nasal spray, inhaler or gum.

What to expect when you stop

Immediately after quitting, you may feel more hungry, tired and short-tempered than usual. You may have strong cravings for a cigarette and find it difficult to concentrate and maintain your focus. You may also have trouble sleeping and experience a temporary increase in coughing.

Nicotine withdrawal symptoms are the result of your body's clearing itself of the nicotine. Most of the nicotine will be gone within 3 days, but your body's desire for it may continue much longer.

Increased hunger and improvement in your senses of taste and smell may indirectly result in modest weight gain. Quitting doesn't

Nicorette: One contains 2 milligrams (mg) of nicotine, and the other contains 4 mg. The gum is available at pharmacies without a prescription.

When it's used properly, nicotine gum gradually releases nicotine. The goal is to use just enough to maintain your nicotine level and hold in check any withdrawal symptoms. Bite into the nicotine gum a few times and then park it between your cheek and gum in order to maximize nicotine absorption.

You can use nicotine gum daily in decreasing amounts for several weeks while you slowly break your desire to reach for a cigarette. Once you feel comfortable in your smoke-free behavior, you can taper off the gum within 3 to 6 months after you stop smoking.

Don't eat or drink anything while using the gum. Nicotine that's swallowed won't be effective and may cause heartburn or nausea.

Non-nicotine medication
The medication bupropion (Zyban) doesn't contain nicotine, and it isn't addictive. Bupropion is a medication developed to treat depression. For the treatment of depression, it's marketed under the name Wellbutrin.

Bupropion raises the level of a chemical in your brain called dopamine, the same chemical released by nicotine. Thus, bupropion helps replicate the feel-good response you get from smoking. This medication is only available with a doctor's prescription.

The most common side effects include dry mouth, headache, difficulty sleeping, decreased appetite and nausea. To lessen stomach symptoms, bupropion may be taken with food unless otherwise instructed. If you experience side effects, talk with your doctor before deciding to stop the medication. If you have a history of seizures, serious head trauma or previous stroke, don't take this drug. As with all medications, if you're pregnant or breast-feeding, talk with your doctor before starting bupropion.

Many new medications for treating nicotine addiction and tobacco use are under study. These include both nicotine replacement medications and other non-nicotine medications. Medications are an important aid in treating nicotine addiction. But they're only effective when used by smokers who are motivated to quit smoking and who've developed a thorough plan for quitting.

mean that you'll automatically gain weight, however. Some people lose weight after quitting smoking.

Here are some tips to guard against a major weight gain:

- Drink a glass of water before every meal.
- Eat more slowly so that you don't have second helpings.
- If you usually have dessert, substitute low-calorie fruit, a small piece of plain cake or a cookie for a rich dessert. Low-fat frozen yogurt makes a great dessert too.
- Leave the table as soon as you're finished eating.
- If you miss having something in your mouth, chew sugarless gum or snack on foods such as carrots, pickles or celery.
- Find things to keep your hands busy that don't involve food. Try gardening or another hobby.
- Control the urge to eat when you're not truly hungry. Do other things when the urge strikes. This will reduce your caloric intake, and you won't feel deprived.
- Exercise daily.

These suggestions are by no means complete, nor are they suitable for everyone. Test them to find out what works for you. You might find that recording your progress is helpful. Make a list of which techniques work for you.

Tension and irritability are common withdrawal symptoms. Find ways to help you relax when you get tense. Take a walk or a shower, or soak in the bathtub. Breathe deeply and slowly, as though you're inhaling a cigarette, and repeat this several times.

The benefits of quitting

Within a few days of quitting smoking, you'll begin to notice some changes in your body. Your senses of smell and taste may improve. You may breathe easier, and your smoker's cough will begin to disappear, although you may still cough and bring up mucus for a while. You may also notice an improvement in your stamina.

Even more lasting and important benefits of quitting smoking begin almost immediately. Within 24 hours, the levels of carbon monoxide and nicotine in your system will decrease significantly. The effects of smoking on bronchitis will begin to reverse from the very first day you quit. Although the effects of emphysema are irreversible, breathing is made easier, and progression of the disease is slowed.

By the end of your first nonsmoking year, your risk of heart attack will decrease by half, and by 5 years it'll be almost the same as that of individuals who have never smoked. The American Cancer Society believes that quitting smoking immediately decreases your chances of esophageal or pancreatic cancer. Within 7 years, your risk of bladder cancer will drop to that of a nonsmoker. And after 10 to 15 years of not smoking, your statistical risk of getting cancer of the lung, larynx or mouth will approach that of people who have never smoked.

Just as importantly, by stopping smoking you have taken control over a very important part of your life. You'll feel better about yourself and your abilities. In addition, those around you will benefit from not inhaling smoke from your cigarettes. You'll also rid yourself of the unpleasantness associated with smoking — bad breath, yellow teeth and smelly clothing and hair. And you'll set the right example for your children, grandchildren and friends.

Alcohol Abuse and Alcoholism

Many people who choose to drink alcohol are able to limit their consumption to amounts that cause no harmful health or social consequences. Millions of other people, though, use alcohol excessively and suffer adverse consequences. According to the National Institute on Alcohol Abuse and Alcoholism, more than 13 million Americans abuse alcohol.

Alcohol abuse and alcoholism are major social, economic and public health problems. In the United States alone, the annual cost of lost productivity and health care expenses related to alcoholism is estimated to be more than $150 billion.

It's important to keep in mind that alcoholism is a disease. In fact, alcoholism is the third largest killer in the United States, ranking behind heart disease and cancer. If traffic fatalities and death certificate diagnoses related to alcohol use were included in the statistics, alcoholism would be recognized as the nation's No. 1 killer.

Controversy persists over what levels of drinking are problematic or unhealthful. The importance of distinguishing between alcohol abuse and alcoholism is chiefly related to treatment approaches.

What's alcohol abuse?

Drinking problems in individuals who don't have all of the characteristics of alcoholism are often referred to as alcohol abuse, harmful use of alcohol or problem drinking.

People who abuse alcohol engage in repeated excessive drinking that can result in physical, psychological or social problems. They may continue to consume alcohol despite knowing that doing so generally poses problems. However, these individuals aren't dependent on alcohol and don't have impaired control over its use.

Teenagers can develop drinking problems in just months. Overall, alcohol consumption among high school students is decreasing, as it is among adults. However, use of alcohol is still high and often increases dramatically during the 10th and 11th grades. In addition, more adolescent girls are drinking.

According to the National Highway Traffic Safety Administration, each year in the United States more than 2,000 young people between the ages of 15 and 20 die in alcohol-related car accidents. Alcohol is also often implicated in other causes of death in teenagers, including drownings, fires and suicides.

Binge drinking among teenagers also is a problem in high school and on college campuses. Consuming six or more glasses, cans or drinks of alcohol in one sitting constitutes binge drinking.

What's alcoholism?

Alcoholism is a chronic, progressive and often fatal disease. The condition involves a preoccupation with alcohol and impaired control over its use. You may continue to abuse alcohol despite serious adverse health, personal, work-related and financial consequences. Alcoholism may involve a physical dependence on the drug alcohol. Genetic, psychological and social factors all contribute to the addiction.

Signs and symptoms

Most alcoholics deny they have a problem. Other signs and symptoms of alcoholism include:

- Drinking alone or in secret
- Forgetting conversations or commitments
- Making a ritual of having drinks before, with or after dinner and becoming annoyed when this ritual is disturbed or questioned
- Losing interest in activities and hobbies that used to bring pleasure
- Irritability as usual drinking time nears, especially if alcohol isn't available
- Keeping alcohol in unlikely places at home, at work or in the car
- Gulping drinks, ordering doubles, becoming intoxicated intentionally to feel good or drinking to feel "normal"
- Having legal problems or problems with relationships, employment or finances

Each of these may be continuous or periodic. It's the physical dependence (addiction) to alcohol — demonstrated by tolerance and withdrawal symptoms — and compulsive behavior related to its use that usually distinguish alcoholics from problem drinkers.

Causes

Alcohol addiction occurs insidiously as excessive use of alcohol alters the balance of some brain chemicals, causing a strong desire for more. These chemicals include:

- Gamma aminobutyric acid (GABA), which inhibits impulsiveness
- Glutamate, which excites the nervous system
- Norepinephrine, which is released in response to stress
- Dopamine, serotonin and opioid peptides, which are responsible for pleasurable feelings

Excessive, long-term drinking can deplete or increase levels of some of these chemicals, causing the body to crave alcohol to restore good feelings or to avoid negative ones.

Psychological factors also can lead to excessive drinking. Having friends or a close partner who drinks regularly, but who may not abuse alcohol, could lead to excessive drinking on your part. It may be difficult for you to distance yourself from these enablers or at least from their drinking habits.

In addition, social and cultural factors can contribute to the addiction process. The glamorous way that the advertising industry and the entertainment media portray alcohol use sends messages that it's OK to drink excessively.

Alcohol Myths

There has never been a shortage of myths about alcoholism.

Myth: *Older adults don't become alcoholics.*
Fact: Older adults aren't immune to alcoholism, although the disease is less prevalent in those age 65 or older.

Myth: *A drink can warm you up.*
Fact: Alcohol dilates your blood vessels and may give you a sensation of warmth, but only temporarily. Increased heat loss through your skin actually decreases your body temperature when you drink alcohol. Consequently, the risk of serious, even fatal, low body temperature (hypothermia) is increased if you drink alcohol in a cold environment.

Myth: *When drunk, you reveal your true personality.*
Fact: Alcohol may permit traits to surface that you suppress when sober, and excessive drinking can distort your personality. But your true personality is revealed when you're sober.

Myth: *Strong black coffee can help you sober up.*
Fact: Coffee neither increases the rate at which your liver processes alcohol nor changes your blood alcohol levels. The initial lift that coffee provides may lead you to believe that you're reasonably alert and sober when, in fact, you're not.

Risk factors

Continued alcohol use over time can produce a physical dependence on alcohol. However, drinking by itself is just one of the risk factors that contribute to alcoholism. Other risk factors include:

- *Age.* People who begin drinking at an early age — in their teens or earlier — are at a higher risk of becoming alcoholics.
- *Genetics.* Your genetic makeup may cause imbalances in one or more of several brain chemicals and increase your risk of alcohol dependency.
- *Sex.* Men are more likely to become alcoholics than are women. But the incidence of alcoholism among women has increased in the past 30 years.
- *Family history.* The risk of alcoholism is higher for people who had a parent or parents who abused alcohol.
- *Emotional disorders.* Depression or anxiety places you at a greater risk of abusing alcohol to temporarily block out the turmoil.

How alcohol affects your body

Alcohols are a group of compounds, many of which are ingredients in perfumes, extracts, tinctures, paints and other products. Alcohols are essential to many manufacturing processes.

The form of alcohol in the beverage you drink is ethyl alcohol (ethanol), a colorless liquid that in its pure, undiluted form has a biting or burning taste. It's produced by the fermentation of sugars that occur naturally in grains, such as barley, and in fruits, such as grapes.

When you drink alcohol, it depresses your central nervous system by acting as a sedative or tranquilizer. In some people, the initial reaction may be stimulation, but as drinking continues, sedative effects occur. By depressing the controlling centers of your brain, alcohol relaxes you and reduces your inhibitions. The more you drink, the more sedated you become.

Initially, alcohol affects areas of thought, emotion and judgment. Eventually, alcohol can impair your speech and muscle coordination and produce sleep. Taken in large enough quantities, alcohol can be lethal. It can cause life-threatening coma by severely depressing vital centers of your brain.

The principal site for alcohol absorption is your small intestine, although very small amounts are absorbed in your mouth and esophagus and only slightly more is absorbed in your stomach. The rate at which the alcohol is absorbed depends on whether you've recently eaten. If your stomach is empty, alcohol is usually quickly absorbed. Food in your stomach or small intestines, especially solid and fatty foods, slows the emptying of your stomach and the absorption of the alcohol into your bloodstream.

Once alcohol has been absorbed, it's quickly transported throughout your body to wherever there's water, including inside individual cells. This distribution accounts for the intoxicating effects of alcohol. Taking a drink on a full stomach spreads the metabolism of that drink over a longer period of time and results in a lower concentration of alcohol in your blood.

Nearly all of the alcohol is burned as fuel for your body, although small amounts are lost in your urine and from the lungs. It's the alcohol in the air you exhale that's measured in breath tests to determine the amount of alcohol in your body. The level of alcohol in your exhalations closely reflects the concentration of alcohol in your blood.

Alcohol dilates the blood vessels nearest your skin to produce an initial feeling of warmth, although this is only temporary. Your pulse rate increases, and you produce more urine because of increased fluid intake and the action of the alcohol on your kidneys. Alcohol also stimulates your stomach to secrete acid.

Your body uses alcohol just as it uses other food, metabolizing it in the liver to produce heat and energy. The food value of alcohol is limited because it provides no vitamins, minerals or proteins. Alcoholics often have deficiencies in nutrients. Doctors once thought that liver damage common among alcoholics, such as fatty liver and cirrhosis, was related to the effect of alcohol on nutritional status. Today, it's known that the toxic effect of alcohol can harm the liver directly.

Alcohol intoxication

How much food you've eaten and how recently you've eaten aren't the only factors that affect how you respond to alcohol. Your sex, age, size and body fat also play important roles. Drinking equal amounts of alcohol may have a greater effect on a woman than on a man. Women generally are smaller and have a higher percentage of body fat than do men. They may also metabolize alcohol less efficiently than do men. Older adults also are more susceptible to the effects of alcohol than are younger people.

The intoxicating effects of alcohol relate to the concentration of alcohol, which in turn reflects levels present in your blood and brain. Most states define legal intoxication as a blood alcohol concentration of at least 0.08 or 0.10 percent. Even at concentrations much lower than the legal limit, many people lose some coordination and reaction time.

Health effects of excessive alcohol use

Drinking excessive amounts of alcohol produces several harmful effects on your brain and nervous system. Excessive use of alcohol can also damage your liver, pancreas and cardiovascular system and cause other illnesses.

Brain and nervous system disorders

Alcohol abusers and alcoholics, as well as occasional or first-time drinkers, may forget all or part of what occurred during the time they were drinking. This temporary loss of memory is referred to as a blackout. Some excessive drinkers have problems with short-term memory that may persist for several weeks after stopping drinking. However, memory usually improves with abstinence.

Excessive alcohol use can leave you exhausted in the morning, even after a full night's sleep. This morning fatigue is caused by the sedating effect of alcohol that interferes with your brain's ability to produce an adequate amount of deep, dreaming sleep, called rapid eye movement (REM) sleep.

If you're an alcoholic and are deficient in nutrients, particularly thiamin, you may be affected by a neurologic disorder called Wernicke-Korsakoff syndrome. This condition consists of two separate disorders — Wernicke's syndrome and Korsakoff's syndrome. These often occur together in alcoholics.

The first symptom of Wernicke's syndrome is often weakness and paralysis of your eye muscles, which may result in double vision. Later on you may not be able to stand or walk without help. Korsakoff's syndrome involves severe amnesia, particularly loss of recent memory. If you have both syndromes, you may experience episodes in which you forget your identity, become disoriented and have hallucinations.

Treatment for Wernicke-Korsakoff syndrome is straightforward: thiamin supplements and abstinence from alcohol. The effects of this disorder, usually aren't completely reversible.

Gastrointestinal disorders

Alcohol can irritate the mucous lining of your stomach and produce gastritis. This also may cause severe retching and vomiting that can tear the upper part of your stomach and the lower part of your esophagus. These tears, called Mallory-Weiss tears, can bleed.

Persistent drinking can interfere with the absorption of the B vitamins, particularly folate and thiamin, as well as other nutrients. Most of these problems will improve if you stop drinking.

Other alcohol-induced problems, such as liver damage, hepatitis and dilated veins of the esophagus (esophageal varices), may require immediate medical attention. Damage caused by alcohol-induced cirrhosis of the liver tends to be progressive. When alcohol reaches your liver, enzymes metabolize it. A healthy liver can process alcohol at a rate of about 50 calories an hour. This is equivalent to about 1 ounce of 40 percent alcohol in about an hour. If your liver becomes overwhelmed by larger amounts of alcohol, the alcohol will remain in your blood until your liver can process it. In alcoholics, both acute and chronic inflammation of the pancreas (pancreatitis) may develop.

Cardiovascular system disorders

A drink of alcohol temporarily reduces blood pressure. But if you consume alcohol excessively, it can increase your blood pressure. Similarly, although some reports indicate that moderate daily drinking may prevent one type of heart trouble, the harmful effects of excessive use of alcohol clearly outweigh any potential benefits.

One or two alcoholic drinks a day, or up to 1 ounce of ethyl alcohol, may reduce your risk of coronary artery disease. This protective effect may be due, in part, to changes in blood fats. People who regularly consume alcohol have increased levels of high-density lipoprotein (HDL) cholesterol. This "good" cholesterol may inhibit narrowing of the arteries (atherosclerosis).

However, a condition called alcoholic cardiomyopathy frequently develops in people who use alcohol excessively. This disease injures and destroys the heart muscle and

Are You at Risk?

Some disorders have manifestations that make a diagnosis easy. Alcoholism, however, often defies easy classification because its characteristics vary greatly from one problem drinker or alcoholic to the next.

To cope with this difficulty, Mayo Clinic has developed the Self-Administered Alcoholism Screening Test (SAAST). Based in part on the Michigan Alcoholism Screening Test, the SAAST consists of 37 questions. In use since 1972, the test can identify 95 percent of alcoholics ill enough to be hospitalized.

The test aims to identify behavior patterns, medical signs and symptoms and consequences of drinking in the alcoholic. Here's a sample of questions from the test:

1. Do you have a drink now and then?
2. Do you feel you're a normal drinker (that is, you drink no more than average)?
3. Have you ever awakened the morning after drinking the previous evening and found that you couldn't remember a part of the previous evening?
4. Do close relatives ever worry or complain about your drinking?
5. Can you stop drinking without a struggle after one or two drinks?
6. Do you ever feel guilty about your drinking?
7. Do friends or relatives think you're a normal drinker?
8. Are you always able to stop drinking when you want to?
9. Have you ever attended a meeting of Alcoholics Anonymous (AA) because of your drinking?
10. Have you gotten into physical fights when drinking?

If your responses match four or more of those listed below, you may be at risk of alcoholism: 1. yes 2. no 3. yes 4. yes 5. no 6. yes 7. no 8. no 9. yes 10. yes

produces symptoms that range from an irregular heartbeat (arrhythmia) to heart failure.

Sexual disorders

Alcohol abuse can cause impotence in men. In women, it can disrupt menstruation.

Cancer

Following cardiovascular disease, cancer is the next leading cause of death among alcoholics. Individuals who drink excessive amounts of alcohol have a rate of cancer higher than that of the general population, especially cancer of the voice box (larynx), esophagus, stomach and pancreas.

Diabetes complications

Alcohol prevents the release of sugar (glucose) from your liver and increases the risk of low blood sugar (hypoglycemia). This is dangerous if you have diabetes and are taking insulin to control your blood sugar level.

Recognizing an alcoholic

How can you tell if you, a friend or a family member is an alcoholic? Anyone with a drinking problem can be an alcoholic. Alcoholism knows no social or economic bounds. Many people with alcoholism are highly regarded and pass for years among friends and associates as healthy and normally functioning people. Alcoholism strikes young and old, men and women, rich and poor and people of all races.

Medical professionals recognize alcoholism as a disease. Nevertheless, many people in this country have been slow to accept alcoholism as a disease and still believe that an alcoholic is someone who has disgraced himself or herself because of personal weakness.

Because of the lingering social stigma that surrounds alcoholism, many alcoholics see themselves as weak and bad people. Some may rationalize the problems that are brought on by their alcoholism, such as a broken marriage or a lost job, as the consequence of bad luck or something caused by others. This burden of shame and blame is one of the greatest stumbling blocks to an alcoholic's recovery.

In fact, alcoholism is a treatable disease. A step toward recognizing if you or someone you know may have a drinking problem is to evaluate the drinking patterns. Indications of alcoholism include:

PREVENTION TIP

If you drink alcohol daily or almost daily and you're scheduled for surgery, advise your doctor of your alcohol use beforehand. Otherwise, you may experience withdrawal symptoms while in the hospital, which could affect your recovery. Knowledge of your drinking habit allows your doctor to take precautions before surgery to prevent unwanted side effects.

Denial

Believing that your problems are caused by factors other than drinking, even when the consequences of drinking behaviors are clearly evident, is a sign of alcoholism. Rather than admitting the problem, an alcoholic often becomes defensive, gets angry, blames others and continues to drink without seeking help.

Increased tolerance

Tolerance to the effects of alcohol is an early sign of alcohol dependence. The need to drink more than the usual amount of alcohol to feel its effects is evidence of increased tolerance. Alcoholics may appear sober even after consuming more alcohol than would intoxicate moderate drinkers.

But beware. No matter how much tolerance you seem to develop, your liver is still unable to metabolize pure alcohol at a rate faster than approximately 1 ounce of 40 percent liquor an hour. Using tolerance as a measure of how much to drink is unsafe.

Withdrawals and delirium tremens

If your body is dependent on alcohol and you suddenly stop drinking, you're likely to experience physical and psychological withdrawal symptoms. These signs and symptoms include:

- Hand tremors
- An increase in pulse, blood pressure and body temperature
- Nausea, diarrhea and other gastrointestinal discomfort
- Insomnia

Generally, these signs or symptoms last 3 to 7 days, although some may last for weeks. With delirium tremens (DTs), more dangerous withdrawal signs and symptoms can occur:

- Delirium
- Confusion
- Aggression
- Vivid hallucinations
- Severe tremors
- Paranoid ideas
- Seizures

These signs and symptoms often last 3 to 5 days, sometimes longer, and usually require urgent medical evaluation and treatment in a hospital setting.

Your doctor can help you deal with withdrawal symptoms. For some individuals who want to stop drinking, a hospital-based detoxification program can be helpful and may be necessary.

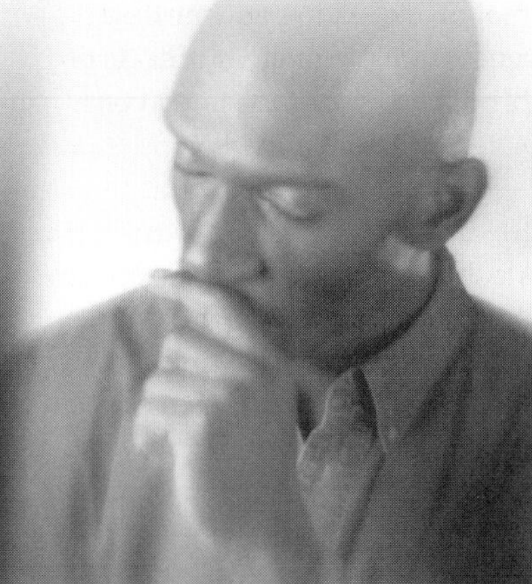

Treating alcohol abuse and alcoholism

Most people with alcohol problems who enter treatment do so reluctantly, usually under pressure from their family, employers or friends. In some cases, health or legal problems motivate them to seek help. Such pressure to seek treatment is often necessary because many people who have a drinking problem use denial, enabling them to believe they don't need help.

Acknowledging the problem

People who have a drinking problem often build a protective shell by developing strategies, both conscious and unconscious, to avoid being confronted. Denial may be so profound that an alcoholic may genuinely not recognize the extent of his or her problem. One of the first goals of treatment is to penetrate personal defenses that have developed over the years.

Blaming the person with alcoholism for the illness only feeds that person's feeling that no one understands him or her. It's important to understand that an alcoholic is someone who has been made ill by a disease.

Intervention

The pre-treatment phase is crucial for family members, friends, employers and other people concerned about someone who has a drinking problem. The chances of recovery increase if the person who has a drinking problem can be confronted with the seriousness of the negative consequences of his or her drinking.

There's no ideal person or persons to confront an alcoholic or alcohol abuser. Confrontation facilitated by a professional knowledgeable about alcoholism and alcohol abuse can result in sparing family members, including the person with a drinking problem, years of suffering and destruction of relationships. An employer or an authority figure that the alcoholic or alcohol abuser respects also may be appropriate. Sometimes, the best person to intervene is a recovering alcoholic.

There's no ideal time or place for a confrontation. However, don't confront an alcoholic or alcohol abuser when the person is drunk or drinking. Pick a time when he or she is sober or in the process of getting sober.

In a kind but candid way, tell the alcoholic or alcohol abuser to get help or be prepared to suffer the consequences, such as being fired, divorced or faced with a driving under the influence (DUI) conviction. Don't let the person deny your concerns about his or her drinking. And don't try to bail him or her out of trouble or offer another chance. An escape from the consequences of drinking is usually interpreted as permission to drink again.

Addressing the needs of family members

Drinking problems usually impair relationships in the family and workplace. If unaware of the true nature of alcoholism and alcohol abuse and of the need for specialized treatment for someone who has a drinking problem, the family continues to become increasingly distraught and traumatized.

Families may experience psychological, marital, parental, economic, physical and spiritual problems as the disease of alcoholism progresses. By directing their attention toward the alcoholic or alcohol abuser, families may neglect these other issues. Families commonly use denial to cope as readily as the person who has the drinking problem. It often becomes the family's major defense mechanism in attempting to deal with the unending series of crises that the alcoholic or alcohol abuser poses, which saps their energies and morale.

Family members often respond to the havoc in their lives with anger, sarcasm, emotional outbursts or depression. Although blame is understandable, it's

Alcoholics Anonymous and Al-Anon

The Fellowship of Alcoholics Anonymous was formed in 1935. As a self-help group of recovering alcoholics, Alcoholics Anonymous (AA) offers a sober peer group as an effective model of how you can achieve total abstinence.

The AA program is built around the Twelve Steps (see page 90), which are straightforward suggestions for men and women who choose to lead sober lives. The Twelve Steps aren't requirements for membership but rather are guides for people who choose to live their lives sober. As guides to recovery, the Twelve Steps help alcoholics accept their powerlessness over alcohol. They stress the necessity for honesty about the past and present.

Recovery in AA is based on accepting the unique experience of each alcoholic. Through listening and sharing stories, alcoholics learn that they're not alone. There are no fees for membership, only a willingness to remain sober.

In the mid-1950s, family members of recovering alcoholics formed a complementary self-help group called Al-Anon. This group is designed for people who are affected by someone else's alcoholism. In sharing their stories, Al-Anon members gain a greater understanding of how the disease affects the entire family, not just the alcoholic. Al-Anon also accepts the Twelve Steps of AA as the principles by which participants are to conduct their lives. It emphasizes how members need to learn detachment and forgiveness if they too are to be free of the disease.

In many communities, Alateen groups are available to provide support for teenage children of alcoholics.

The 12 Steps of Alcoholics Anonymous

The Twelve Steps of Alcoholics Anonymous (AA) are at the heart of the program of personal recovery. They describe the experience of the founding members of AA:

1. We admitted we were powerless over alcohol — that our lives had become unmanageable.
2. We came to believe that a Power greater than ourselves could restore us to sanity.
3. We made a decision to turn our will and our lives over to the care of God as we understood Him.
4. We made a searching and fearless moral inventory of ourselves.
5. We admitted to God, to ourselves and to another human being the exact nature of our wrongs.
6. We were entirely ready to have God remove all these defects of character.
7. We humbly asked Him to remove our shortcomings.
8. We made a list of all persons we had harmed and became willing to make amends to them all.
9. We made direct amends to such people wherever possible, except when to do so would injure them or others.
10. We continued to take personal inventory and when we were wrong promptly admitted it.
11. We sought through prayer and meditation to improve our conscious contact with God as we understood Him, praying only for knowledge of His will for us and the power to carry that out.
12. Having had a spiritual awakening as the result of these steps, we tried to carry this message to alcoholics and to practice these principles in all our affairs.

counterproductive in dealing with alcoholism or alcohol abuse. Family members must learn why the person who has a drinking problem behaves as he or she does. With guidance, family members can learn how to avoid enabling and rescuing the alcoholic or alcohol abuser. Instead, they need to react constructively and establish a climate for positive responses.

Countless alcoholics and problem drinkers are recovering today simply because their families chose to start the process of recovery, often by entering treatment programs for family members, such as Al-Anon (see page 89).

Treatment programs

A wide range of treatments is available to help with alcohol problems. Treatment is tailored to the individual and may involve evaluation, brief intervention, counseling, an outpatient program, a residential program or an inpatient program.

The first step in treatment is to determine whether you're alcohol dependent. If you haven't lost control over your use of alcohol, your treatment may involve reducing your drinking. If you're dependent on alcohol, cutting back is ineffective and inappropriate. Abstinence must be a part of your treatment goal.

Alcohol abuse

For people who aren't physically dependent on alcohol but still experience the adverse effects of drinking, the goal of treatment is prevention of alcoholism by a screening procedure or brief interventions.

Screening

Two major types of screening are used. One is designed for people who seek medical care for problems unrelated to alcohol use or those who participate in random alcohol testing programs. It's also used for drivers who are stopped at random for testing of their breath to measure alcohol amount.

The other type of screening program involves people who've been identified as possibly having a drinking problem. Hospital-based programs screen patients admitted for traumatic injuries. Court-mandated programs screen adolescents or adults arrested for violent crimes or drivers who have positive results on a breath or blood alcohol test. Employee assistance programs screen employees with impaired performance.

Brief interventions
Brief interventions usually involve alcohol abuse specialists who establish a specific treatment plan with an individual identified as having an alcohol problem. These interventions may include many components:

- Direct feedback
- Contracting and goal setting
- Behavior modification
- Use of written material such as self-help manuals
- Counseling
- Follow-up care extending over multiple visits to a treatment center

Alcoholism

Treatment for alcoholism typically takes place in an outpatient setting with services for all stages of recovery. However, residential or inpatient care is still the most appropriate treatment if you have serious concurrent medical or psychiatric problems or if you're living in an environment that won't support your recovery.

The most common residential alcoholism treatment programs in the United States are based on an approach that includes abstinence, individual and group therapy, participation in Alcoholics Anonymous (AA), educational lectures, activity therapy and use of recovering lay counselors and multiprofessional staff. Many of today's outpatient services include these same components.

Here's what you might expect from a typical treatment program:

Detoxification and withdrawal
If you arrive at the facility intoxicated or are a heavy, chronic drinker, treatment may begin with a program of detoxification that may take 3 to 7 days. You may be given medications to prevent delirium tremens (DTs) or other withdrawal symptoms. Then you enter either a residential treatment program or outpatient treatment program, depending on your needs.

Acceptance of the illness
Effective treatment is impossible unless you accept that you're addicted to alcohol and unable to control your drinking. The admission of powerlessness over alcohol is an act of letting go of the alibis and excuses that once supported your abuse of alcohol. This is one of the most important steps to recovery.

Medical assessment and treatment
Common medical problems related to alcoholism are high blood pressure, elevated blood sugar and liver and heart disease. A doctor may review your health status and take steps to treat any complications.

Abstinence
Most treatment programs for alcoholism require abstinence from alcohol and drugs.

Recovery
Education about the disease of alcoholism, the damage it does to the body, the problems it causes and the experience of recovery is a critical part of treatment. During this phase, most programs include daily classes, group therapy, individual counseling, recreational therapy and an introduction to the principles of AA. Psychological support and additional medical care also may be provided, if needed.

Some of the trained staff involved in recovery programs may be recovering alcoholics themselves who are able to share their experiences and serve as role models.

Psychological support and psychiatric treatment
A psychologist or psychiatrist may provide an assessment and assist with individual counseling and support. Sometimes, emotional symptoms of alcoholism may mimic psychiatric disorders, or an alcoholic may have an accompanying psychiatric illness. If you have a psychiatric illness, such as major depression, this condition also needs to be treated to facilitate recovery.

Medication
Medications can be used in combination with other therapies to treat alcoholism. Some medications help you to achieve abstinence and increase long-term recovery. Others reduce the desire to drink and the craving for alcohol. An alcohol-sensitizing drug called disulfiram (Antabuse) may be a strong deterrent. Disulfiram won't cure alcoholism nor can it remove the compulsion to drink. But if you drink alcohol, the drug produces a severe physical reaction that includes flushing, nausea, vomiting and headache.

Naltrexone (ReVia), a medication that blocks the narcotic high, also reduces the urge to drink in recovering alcoholics. Unlike disulfiram, naltrexone doesn't cause an adverse reaction within a few minutes of taking a drink. It may produce side effects, though, particularly liver damage.

Several other medications for alcoholism are in the testing phase to determine their safety and effectiveness.

Continuing support
Aftercare programs and AA can help recovering alcoholics abstain from alcohol, manage relapses and cope with lifestyle changes.

Drug Abuse

The abuse or misuse of addicting drugs is an increasing public health issue in this country. Drug abuse doesn't involve only those substances considered illegal. It occurs if you take any drug inappropriately — for purposes other than for what it's intended or in a manner or quantity other than directed. Nicotine and alcohol, discussed earlier, also are addicting substances.

Most of the millions of people who take prescription medications don't abuse them. However, many misuse them, sometimes out of ignorance and carelessness.

People abuse drugs — prescription or illegal — for various reasons. Mind-altering psychedelics produce effects that alter the way you experience reality. Stimulants such as amphetamines give a temporary sensation of increased energy and lifted spirits. Painkillers (analgesics) reduce the sensation of pain and induce drowsiness. And sedative drugs create a feeling of relaxation. To achieve such effects is a frequent motivation for misuse.

The drugs to which you can become addicted include:

- *Cannabis compounds.* These compounds are found in marijuana and hashish.
- *Hallucinogens.* These include the drugs lysergic acid diethylamide (LSD) and phencyclidine (PCP).
- *Designer drugs.* These include synthetic compounds such as Ecstasy, which has both amphetamine-like and hallucinogenic effects.
- *Opiates and opioids.* These include narcotic painkillers produced naturally from opium or made synthetically. They include heroin and the prescription medications morphine, codeine and methadone.
- *Central nervous system depressants.* These include barbiturates and benzodiazepines. Benzodiazepines include prescription tranquilizers such as diazepam (Valium), alprazolam (Xanax), lorazepam (Ativan), clonazepam (Klonopin) and chlordiazepoxide (Librium).
- *Central nervous system stimulants.* These include amphetamines and cocaine.
- *Inhalants.* Some people become addicted to substances found in glue, paint and solvents.

PREVENTION TIP

Avoid alcohol when you take tranquilizers. If you drink alcohol while taking tranquilizers, it can cause drowsiness, intoxication, impaired memory or even death. Taken together, these two depressant drugs cause hundreds of fatal drug overdoses each year.

Abuse of medications

Millions of Americans abuse prescription and nonprescription medications, sometimes with tragic results. Hospital emergency rooms report that approximately the same percentage of drug emergencies are due to misuse of legal medications as to misuse of illegal drugs. The abuse of prescription drugs, especially painkillers and tranquilizers, is widespread. Frequently, a person is able to maintain a dependence on prescription medications by obtaining prescriptions from multiple doctors.

Many people misuse over-the-counter drugs as well. Aspirin, cough medicines, laxatives, diet pills, nasal sprays and numerous other medications can be abused if taken in higher doses or more frequently than recommended.

Addiction to tranquilizers

Addiction to tranquilizers — anti-anxiety and sleep-inducing medications — is a major drug problem in this country. Although it's not clear how many people are addicted to tranquilizers, as many as 10,000 emergency room visits a year are related to misuse of tranquilizers, and every year thousands of people enter drug treatment centers for the same reason.

Tranquilizers such as diazepam (Valium), alprazolam (Xanax) and chlordiazepoxide (Librium) — all part of a family of drugs named benzodiazepines — are typically prescribed for a limited time to help alleviate nervousness or tension caused by the stress of everyday life or associated with an emotional disorder. Sleeping aids such as flurazepam (Dalmane) and temazepam (Restoril) also are part of this family.

Problems can arise when people use the drugs too long, too often or at too high a dosage.

Another issue related to the abuse of benzodiazepines is the mistaken belief that they're not addicting. When they first became available, many people used them instead of barbiturates, another family of sedatives, which carry a higher risk for overdosage and toxicity.

However, benzodiazepines have been found to have strong addictive potential. In fact, virtually all of the medications in the benzodiazepine group can cause physical and psychological addiction if used at a high dosage or over a prolonged time.

Addiction to painkillers

The ideal painkiller (analgesic) would be one that furnishes sufficient pain relief, produces a minimum of side effects, acts promptly, prevents development of increased tolerance and is nonaddicting. Unfortunately, there is no such ideal painkiller.

Analgesics can be divided into addictive and nonaddictive types. The first group includes opiates and opioids, such as morphine and methadone. The second group includes nonopioids such as aspirin and acetaminophen.

The strongest painkillers are opiates and opioids. Opiates are narcotic drugs derived from the opium plant. Opioids are synthetic nar-

Pregnancy and Drug Abuse

Many drugs pass through the placenta and reach the fetus. The first trimester of pregnancy generally is the stage at which the fetus is most sensitive to drugs in the mother's body.

Many women who smoke marijuana during their pregnancy deliver premature babies or babies who have a low birth weight. Women who use tranquilizers and amphetamines while pregnant may have a baby born with congenital malformations. Taking barbiturates, opiates and cocaine while pregnant may cause fetal addiction.

If you use marijuana when breast-feeding, the drug may pass through your breast milk to your baby.

cotic substances with the same properties.

Morphine, a frequently used opiate for treating severe pain, is usually prescribed for only short periods because it can be addictive if used inappropriately and for longer than the pain is present. The opiate codeine is often used in combination with non-narcotic drugs such as acetaminophen (Tylenol, others) and cough suppressants.

People who are most likely to develop an addiction to narcotic analgesics are those with chronic pain. To help people with chronic pain avoid developing a drug dependency, treatment usually includes multidisciplinary therapies for managing pain.

Abuse of illegal drugs

The term *street drugs* is often used to describe illegal drugs because the drugs often are sold on the street. Many people abuse illegal drugs by using them "recreationally" in an attempt to relax, experience euphoria, enhance sexual activity or heighten the senses. Some athletes use street drugs to try to improve their athletic performance.

Whatever their intended use, illegal drugs can be extremely hazardous to your health not only because of their nature but also because of the unknown potency of the drug and risk of contamination with other dangerous substances. Most of these drugs are highly addictive.

Marijuana

The most popular illegal drug in the United States is marijuana. Studies suggest that a significant percentage of high school seniors have smoked marijuana and that some students smoke it every day.

The hemp plant *(Cannabis sativa)*, from which marijuana is derived, contains more than 400 chemicals, including tetrahydrocannabinol (THC). The THC in marijuana is what causes its effect on mood and is probably responsible for the hunger that many people experience after using marijuana.

Marijuana cigarettes are made from the leaves and tops of the plant. The amount of THC varies from plant to plant and from cigarette to cigarette. Hashish, a more powerful derivative drug prepared from the resin of the hemp plant, contains far greater concentrations of psychoactive THC.

If you smoke marijuana, THC is quickly absorbed from your lungs into your bloodstream and rapidly distributed to most tissues and organs of your body. To eliminate THC, your liver converts the substance into waste products (metabolites). The rate at which they're cleared from your body is slower than that of many other psychoactive drugs. If you smoke marijuana regularly and then stop, THC can be found in your urine for more than 4 weeks after use.

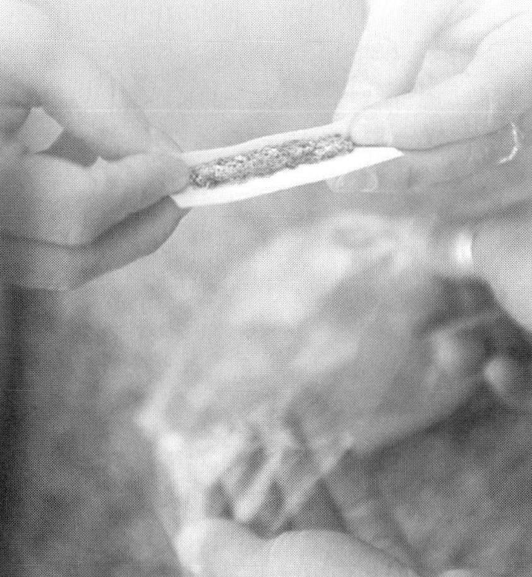

The effects of marijuana are almost immediate. Your heart rate increases by as much as 50 percent, depending on the potency of the marijuana. People with a poor blood supply to the heart may have chest pains. High doses of marijuana may produce many of the same behavioral effects as severe alcohol intoxication. Although the high may subside, many of the negative effects may linger for up to 6 hours after you smoke marijuana. These include difficulty in performing functions that require concentration, rapid reactions and physical coordination.

Chronic marijuana smokers show evidence of decreased lung capacity and chronic bronchial irritation. Marijuana may also contain the fungus aspergillus. Studies suggest that serious lung infections can result from inhaling this organism. Because chronic marijuana smoking may impair your body's immune system, your lungs may be more susceptible to aspergillus and other infectious agents.

Clinical testing suggests that marijuana may negatively affect your reproductive system, possibly causing irregular menstrual cycles in women and a temporary loss of fertility in both men and women. Some studies have suggested that there may be a significant relationship between use of marijuana during pregnancy and premature birth.

Although often misunderstood and misrepresented to the public, marijuana is a drug of dependence. Regular use often results in the same type of drug dependence described for other substances.

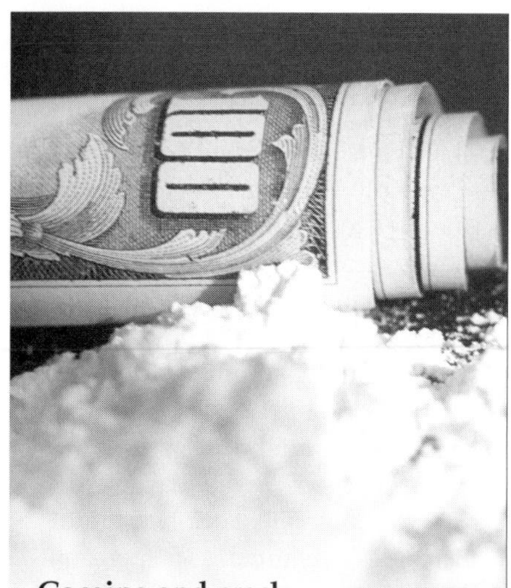

Cocaine and crack

Cocaine was once referred to as the champagne of drugs, in part because it was an expensive drug preferred by the wealthy. Today, it's one of the most widely used illegal drugs in this country. Cocaine is popular with drug users because it leads to a sense of euphoria. These effects are the basis of the profound psychological dependence associated with the drug.

The signs and symptoms of cocaine use include dilation of the pupils, increased heart rate and breathing and a slight rise in body temperature. These effects are mostly of short duration. They reach their peak about 15 to 20 minutes after you inhale the drug through your nose (snort it) in the form of a powder and last about an hour.

Unwanted effects of chronic use of cocaine include a persistent restlessness, anxiety and sleeplessness. Another problem associated with inhaling cocaine is a mildly stuffy or runny nose. Long-term use can cause ulcers on the mucous membranes of your nose and even a hole (perforation) in your nasal septum. In addition, people who chronically abuse cocaine may develop paranoid hallucinations, called cocaine psychosis, which may involve the senses of smell, taste, touch or sight.

Smoking cocaine (free-basing) creates a faster and more intense high. In freebase form, the drug can cause confusion, slurred speech and anxiety.

Crack cocaine also is smoked and has essentially the same effect as freebase cocaine. Both forms are extremely addictive. Crack's name comes from the sound of burning "rocks" of cocaine. It produces an intense high in a matter of seconds. A profound low may follow, leaving the chronic abuser despondent and desperate for more. Short-term physical effects of crack are increased heart rate and increased blood pressure.

Cocaine can overwork your heart, forcing it to beat too fast and too powerfully. As your heart tires, it becomes susceptible to irregularities in its rhythm that can be life-threatening. Cocaine can also induce coronary artery spasm, a sudden narrowing of the arteries leading to your heart. Such spasms can cause a blood clot to form. If the clot completely blocks the flow of blood to your heart, it can cause a heart attack, dangerous heartbeat irregularities or sudden death.

Injecting cocaine by means of shared needles increases the risk of exposure to human immunodeficiency virus (HIV), infectious hepatitis and other diseases that can be passed by sharing nonsterile needles or contaminated solutions.

Hallucinogens

Hallucinogenic drugs were widely used in the 1960s and early 1970s. The popularity of such drugs diminished during the next 20 years, but some observers report a renewed interest in the use of hallucinogens. The most common hallucinogens used today are lysergic acid diethylamide (LSD) and phencyclidine (PCP).

LSD

Hallucinogens were popular because they produced a vivid perception of changes in sensation, depth perception, passage of time and body image. Some users reported experiencing a mixing of the senses. Under the influence of LSD, one could seemingly hear colors or see sounds.

LSD can also cause powerful negative experiences, referred to as bad trips, in which the user has an overwhelming sense of fear, perhaps of being abandoned, going insane or dying. In some instances, abusers have had no comprehension of their limitations and have died because they tried to fly out of windows or walk on water.

Another effect of hallucinogenic drugs is the production of sustained altered mental states that can last 8 hours or more. Flashbacks also may occur days or weeks after the conclusion of the initial trip, in which the user re-experiences previous effects even though he or she hasn't ingested any more of the drug.

LSD and similar drugs increase heart rate and blood pressure, dilate the pupils and cause sleeplessness, tremors and loss of appetite. Heavy, long-term use of hallucinogens can cause impaired memory, an abbreviated attention span and difficulty with abstract thinking.

PCP

This powerful hallucinogen, sometimes referred to as angel dust, was once used by veterinarians to sedate large animals. But the drug so disturbed and bewildered the animals before it put them to sleep that veterinarians abandoned its use. From this use came other street names for the drug, such as *hog* and *horse tranquilizer*.

In contrast to its effect in animals, PCP taken in very small doses by humans causes a loss of inhibition and induces a state of general euphoria. Other effects include increased heart rate and breathing, sweating, flushing of the skin and increased body temperature. It may also cause some unsteadiness.

But what makes the drug especially dangerous is its unpredictability. Almost any dose may result in destructive, violent behavior. When users have turned violent or acted in bizarre ways, they've been known to lose all control. Additional signs and symptoms include muscle rigidity, loss of concentration, vision disturbances, speech impairment, convulsions, delirium, fear of isolation and paranoia. PCP has been known to induce a toxic psychosis that resembles schizophrenia.

Ecstasy

Ecstasy is a club drug that's gaining in popularity. Also called MDMA (short for methylenedioxymethamphetamine), the drug is most often used at large, organized all-night parties, called raves, and at rock concerts and clubs — thus the name *club drug*. Studies show that this amphetamine derivative causes brain damage that can last at least 2 weeks after stopping its use. Ecstasy injures brain neurons involved with regulating mood, emotion, learning, memory, sleep and pain.

Methamphetamine

Methamphetamine (meth) is a powerful stimulant that's also gaining popularity among drug abusers. It comes in many forms and can be smoked, injected, ingested orally or snorted. Users may feel an intense sensation (rush) or a long-lasting high, depending on how it's taken.

Effects of methamphetamine use include insomnia, increased activity, decreased appetite, anxiety, psychotic behavior and violent behavior.

Narcotics

Narcotics (opioids and opiates) generally are prescribed to relieve severe pain. But the medications often are obtained illegally. Heroin is a narcotic. Given in low doses over short periods, narcotics aren't addictive, but in large doses taken over time, they're highly addictive.

Side effects, especially when taken in high doses, include decreased respiration, a drop in blood pressure, dizziness, nausea, sweating, general weakness and a depressed sex drive. When a narcotic is injected using a shared needle, users sometimes acquire diseases or disorders such as AIDS, hepatitis, blood infection (septicemia) congested lungs and pneumonia. Taking a narcotic with other sedatives can cause death.

Oxycodone (OxyContin), a prescription pain reliever, is the latest opioid to become a popular street drug with a high market value. Its effects are more intense when the long-acting tablets are chewed.

Drugs and sports performance

When you exercise, your nervous system is stimulated naturally. This stimulation boosts production of hormones, including adrenaline (epinephrine). These hormones increase the amount of blood your heart pumps, resulting in increased blood to your muscles, release of sugar (glucose) from the liver and release of fatty acids from body fat to fuel your muscles.

These effects are important to anyone who's exercising. The increased blood flow ensures that your muscles receive a constant supply of oxygen and nutrients, and potentially toxic waste products produced by the accelerated metabolism are more quickly removed.

To further improve their athletic performance, some athletes turn to drugs. The abuse of anabolic steroids and other drugs by athletes is now often front-page news. The problem is international in scope, involving professional and amateur athletes in a wide range of sports.

An elevated level of awareness of the problem has led to more drug testing of athletes. Some who require a drug for a medical disorder are even banned from using that drug during competition because it may artificially boost performance. In addition to putting an athlete's future in jeopardy, sports performance drugs cause health risks.

Anabolic steroids

A group of drugs used by some athletes are androgenic-anabolic steroids. Because these drugs are closely related chemically to natural male hormones, anabolic steroids mimic the effects of the male sex hormone testosterone. They increase the buildup of muscle tissue.

Anabolic steroids have several legitimate medical uses. They may be used to treat skeletal and growth disorders and certain types of anemia, as well as to offset the negative effects of irradiation and chemotherapy. But when the drugs are used over a prolonged period, they can cause serious side effects. An overload of anabolic steroids can lead to jaundice and liver failure.

Another potential liver problem is peliosis hepatis. In this condition the liver develops blood-filled cysts that can rupture. Liver failure can result. There's also the potential for formation of liver tumors. In addition, anabolic steroids may increase blood pressure and decrease levels of high-density lipoprotein (HDL) cholesterol — the "good" cholesterol. Studies suggest that anabolic steroids may also cause heart damage.

Anabolic steroids can lead to reduction in sperm production, decrease in the size of the testicles and reduction in the amount of sex hormones produced, resulting in a diminished sex drive. In female athletes the drugs may reduce production of the female sex hormones estrogen and progesterone, inhibit development of eggs and ovulation, reduce breast size and disrupt the menstrual cycle.

All of these changes are reversible when use of anabolic steroids is discontinued. However, female athletes sometimes find that male secondary sex characteristics, such as an increase in facial hair or a deepening of the voice, persist after they stop using anabolic steroids.

Other undesirable effects in both men and women include changes in overall hair-growth patterns, acne, an increased thinning or loss of hair and, possibly, increased aggressiveness.

Sympathomimetic amines
Some professional and world-class athletes have admitted using sympathomimetic amines, a class of stimulant drugs that mimic the natural effects of a stimulated sympathetic nervous system. These drugs can increase alertness and physical endurance and delay the onset of fatigue.

This class of drugs includes ephedrine and its derivatives (pseudoephedrine and phenylpropanolamine), which are often used as decongestants in cold and hayfever preparations. Ephedrine is also an ingredient in many asthma medications.

Psychomotor stimulant drugs
The psychomotor stimulant drugs most often abused are amphetamines (amphetamine, dextroamphetamine and methamphetamine) and methylphenidate (Ritalin).

Amphetamines have a limited role in medicine but are used in the treatment of hyperactive children and narcolepsy. Street names for the illegal use of these drugs include speed, dexies, greenies and pep pills. Amphetamines are usually taken orally, but chronic abusers often prefer to inject them because this method produces a more immediate and stronger effect.

The effects of psychomotor stimulants are similar to those of sympathomimetic amines. They increase heart rate, respiration and blood pressure and generally heighten the activity of the sympathetic nervous system. These drugs also affect the brain, so the user feels more alert, confident and perhaps even euphoric. Consequently, psychomotor stimulants may improve athletic performance, more through psychological than physical effects. Apart from increasing endurance, the benefits of these stimulants on athletic performance are limited or even negative.

Getting High Off of Inhalants

Some people inhale various substances that can give them a high. One common prescription inhalant is called amyl nitrite, or "poppers." This drug is a vasodilator that relaxes smooth muscle in small blood vessels, causing them to expand and lower blood pressure. It's usually prescribed for treating angina pectoris. But people inhale amyl nitrite because it produces an intense and immediate high and seems to intensify sexual orgasm. The effects are short-lived, lasting only minutes. Amyl nitrite isn't physically addictive, but it's not free of side effects. Users often suffer headaches, dizziness, an accelerated heart rate, nasal irritation and coughing spells. Headaches seem to be the one side effect that can persist long after use.

Other substances people inhale that don't require a prescription include a category of volatile inhalants sold as room deodorizers. These generally contain butyl nitrite and isobutyl nitrite. Butyl nitrite is thought to intensify a sexual experience. Other inhalants that some people use include:

- Solvents
- Glue
- Paint
- Nitrous oxide

The physical risks from inhaling these substances range from an irregular heart beat (cardiac arrhythmia) to liver and kidney impairment.

How to recognize drug abuse and addiction

Drug abuse occurs if you take any drug other than as directed — whether for a different reason or in another manner or quantity. Abuse of drugs may lead to an addiction (drug dependence). Drug abuse or drug dependence can cause health problems that range from physical to psychological, mild to severe, and reversible to permanent — or even fatal.

Compulsive use of a drug, or loss of control over its use, suggests addiction. The state of addiction includes both psychological dependence and physical dependence, causing a need to take the drug again.

Psychological dependence occurs when the desire or need for a drug evolves into a preoccupation with it. The abuser needs the drug to feel better. A person who abuses drugs may develop a tolerance, so he or she needs more and more of the substance to achieve the desired effects.

Physical dependence has occurred when withdrawal symptoms appear shortly after discontinuing use of the drug. These may become severe and possibly life-threatening, sometimes requiring immediate medical attention. Examples of these signs and symptoms include agitation, tremors, anxiety, insomnia, depression, convulsions and hallucinations.

Recognizing early signs and symptoms of addiction can be difficult. They vary from drug to drug and person to person. However, people who are addicted to one or more drugs usually exhibit changes in their behavior that may gradually affect personal relationships and work performance. Their behavior may be erratic and their mood unpredictable, alternating between periods of exhilaration or agitation and exhaustion or lethargy. Irritability is another sign. Some addicted individuals no longer sleep well, and others may crash and sleep for long periods. They may lose their interest in eating or experience unexplained weight loss.

Changes in personality and behavior — such as spending

increasing amounts of time away from home, behaving differently in class or at work or constantly demanding or needing money — also may suggest drug dependence.

Other possible clues to drug abuse are bloodshot eyes, dilated pupils and a dazed or expressionless appearance. Individuals abusing hallucinogens may appear distracted and have to be spoken to several times before responding, or they may gaze at an object without reason for long periods. Other drugs may produce excessive sweating or flushed skin. An unexplained rash or an irritated nostril or runny nose may be a sign that someone has been using an opiate.

However, many drug dependent individuals appear normal, even to close friends.

Treating drug addiction

Treatment of drug addiction typically involves steps to help the person withdraw from using the drug, followed by counseling and attending self-help groups to help him or her resist using the addictive drug again.

Withdrawal therapy

The goal of withdrawal therapy (detoxification) is for the person to stop taking the addictive drug as quickly and safely as possible. Detoxification may involve gradually reducing the dose of the drug or temporarily substituting other substances with less severe side effects.

For some people it may be safe to undergo withdrawal therapy on an outpatient basis. Other people may require placement in a hospital or residential treatment center.

Withdrawal from different types of drugs produces different side effects and requires different approaches.

Depressants

Minor side effects of withdrawal may include restlessness, anxiety, sleep problems, rapid heartbeat, high blood pressure, low-grade fever and sweating. More serious signs and symptoms include hallucinations, whole-body tremors, seizures, profuse sweating and vomiting. The most serious stage of withdrawal may include delirium and is potentially life-threatening. Withdrawal therapy may involve gradually scaling back the amount of the drug you've been using.

Stimulants

Side effects of withdrawal typically include depression, excessive sleepiness, fatigue, headache, irritability and an inability to concentrate. In some cases, signs and symptoms may include suicide attempts, paranoia and impaired contact with reality (acute psychosis). Treatment during withdrawal is usually limited to emotional support from your family, friends and doctor. Your doctor may recommend medications to treat paranoid psychosis or depression.

Narcotics

Side effects of withdrawal of narcotics such as heroin, morphine and codeine can range from relatively minor to severe. The mild symptoms may include anxiety and drug cravings. Severe reactions include sleeplessness, acute psychosis, rapid pulse, rapid breathing, high blood pressure, abdominal cramps, vomiting, diarrhea and weakness.

If you're withdrawing from heroin, your doctor may give you methadone to reduce the craving for heroin and to gently ease you off it.

Staying clean

After detoxification, therapies such as counseling, treatment programs and self-help group meetings can help you stay off of drugs.

Counseling

Individual or family counseling with a psychiatrist, psychologist or addiction counselor may help you resist the temptation to resume using addictive drugs. Behavioral therapy can help you develop ways to cope with your drug cravings, strategies to avoid drugs and prevent relapse and ideas on how to deal with a relapse, if it occurs. Counseling may involve discussions related to your job, legal problems or relationships with family and friends. Family members also may receive counseling to help them develop better communication skills and be more supportive.

Treatment programs

Treatment programs generally include educational sessions and individual, group and family counseling. They're available in various settings — outpatient, residential and inpatient.

Self-help programs

Self-help programs use the 12-step program first developed by Alcoholics Anonymous. Self-help groups exist for people addicted to drugs such as cocaine, sedatives and narcotics. The message is that addiction is a chronic disorder with a danger of relapse and that ongoing maintenance treatment — which may include medications, counseling and attending self-help group meetings — is necessary to prevent a relapse. Your doctor or counselor can help you locate a self-help group. Or you can find listings for self-help groups in the telephone book, at the library and on the Internet.

Unsafe Sex

Sexually transmitted diseases (STDs) are on the increase in the United States. To avoid them, it's important that you understand what puts you and your family and friends at risk of contracting STDs. Most STDs are treatable, but some, such as AIDS, have no cure. Most people with AIDS will eventually die of the disease.

Preventing sexually transmitted diseases

Sexually transmitted diseases include chlamydial infections, gonorrhea, genital herpes, venereal warts, syphilis and the human immunodeficiency virus (HIV), which causes AIDS. Many of these can be acquired during a single sexual encounter. Although HIV can also result from shared use of contaminated needles or, rarely, a blood transfusion, its main mode of transmission is sexual contact. The virus is present in semen and vaginal secretions and can enter a person's body through small tears in the vaginal, penile or rectal tissues, which can occur during sexual activity.

None of these infections is spread through casual contact such as handshaking, talking, sitting on a toilet seat or living in the same house with an infected person. The microorganisms that cause STDs, including HIV, all die quickly once they're outside the body.

Entering into a monogamous relationship

The only sure ways of preventing a sexually transmitted disease are through sexual abstinence or a mutually monogamous relationship with an uninfected person. If you or your partner has several sexual partners — either heterosexual or homosexual — you'll be at high risk of contracting disease.

Using condoms

Use of a condom during sexual intercourse doesn't eliminate the risk of acquiring or transmitting a sexual disease, but it can significantly reduce the risk. The key is correct and consistent condom use.

A condom, also known as a prophylactic or a rubber, is a thin sheath that covers an erect penis. Condoms can be purchased over-the-counter at drug stores, discount stores and convenience stores and are available in various thicknesses, colors and shapes. They may be lubricated or unlubricated, have a plain end or a reservoir end, and have a smooth, ribbed or corrugated texture.

When purchasing condoms, look for packages that mention STD protection and check the expiration date on the package. Condoms sometimes are made of animal membrane, but pores in this type of natural material may allow HIV to pass through. Latex condoms are recommended instead.

Condoms should be stored at room temperature until needed. To be effective, a condom must be undamaged, applied to the erect penis before any genital contact and kept snugly in place until it's removed on completion of sexual activity. Extra lubrication — even with lubricated condoms — can help prevent a condom from breaking. Use only water-based lubricants. Oil-based lubricants can cause a condom to break down.

After intercourse of any kind, the proper way to remove the condom is to hold on to it tightly at the rim and pull out slowly while the penis is still hard, to prevent spillage. If you mistakenly put a new condom on inside out and it doesn't unroll easily, don't flip it over because there may be semen in it. Use another.

A female condom is available that also can help reduce the risk of contracting a sexually transmitted disease. The availability of a female condom gives many women more control over their personal health. Most forms of female-directed contraception, such as the pill or diaphragm, don't protect against STDs. However, studies indicate that use of a spermicide decreases the frequency of gonorrhea and chlamydial infections. Using a spermicide in conjunction with a diaphragm also may help kill bacteria.

Avoiding certain sexual practices

Various sexual practices carry different degrees of risk of contracting a sexually transmitted disease. Receptive (passive) anal intercourse is the riskiest behavior for acquiring HIV because it may damage the anal and rectal membranes and allow the virus to enter the bloodstream. The passive partner is at much higher risk of contracting HIV than is the active partner, although gonorrhea and syphilis can be acquired from infection in the passive partner's rectum. Most studies have focused on male homosexuals, but heterosexual anal sex involves similar risks.

Heterosexual vaginal intercourse, particularly with multiple partners, also carries a risk of contracting HIV. The virus is believed to be more easily transmitted from the man to the woman than vice versa. This type of sex is how most other STDs are transmitted or acquired.

Oral sex also is a possible means of transmission of HIV, gonorrhea, herpes, syphilis and other STDs. Accepting the penis in the mouth (fellatio) with ejaculation and swallowing of semen is the most common cause of throat gonorrhea. Oral contact with the clitoris and vaginal opening (cunnilingus) is a frequent method of transmission of the herpes virus. Activities that involve only skin-to-skin contact, such as hugging, massage and mutual masturbation, with no exposure to body fluids, shouldn't spread disease.

Common sexually transmitted diseases

Sexually transmitted diseases result from bacteria, viruses and other organisms transmitted through sexual contact. For more information on the specific diseases and their treatment, see Chapter 20, "Infectious Diseases."

Gonorrhea

Gonorrhea is caused by the bacterium *Neisseria gonorrhoeae*. In the United States, almost 500,000 cases of gonorrhea are reported each year. It's most common in individuals 15 to 29 years old.

In men, the first symptoms generally appear between 2 days and 2 weeks after exposure to the bacteria. First, you'll experience a tingling sensation in the passageway that carries urine through the penis (urethra). A few hours later, urination becomes painful, and a milky penile discharge is noted. As the infection progresses, urethral pain becomes worse and large amounts of creamy, pus-like discharge are produced.

In women, symptoms may not appear for 1 to 3 weeks, if at all. The infection usually affects the cervix and other reproductive organs as well as the urethra. You may develop frequent, urgent and painful urination and a pus-like discharge from the vagina or urethra. In about 50 percent of women, the only signs and symptoms are a slight increase in vaginal discharge and some inflammation, which may be evident only on physical examination. The symptoms are often so mild that many women don't realize they have the infection. In many cases, the only suggestion that a woman may have gonorrhea is the knowledge that someone she had sex with has developed the disease.

In both sexes, rectal gonorrhea may result from anal intercourse with an infected person or from the infection spreading from one's own genital area. It may cause some discomfort in the anal area and a rectal discharge, but in many cases no symptoms are noted. Oral sex can produce pharyngeal gonorrhea, resulting in a sore throat, pain on swallowing and redness of the throat and tonsils. If the infection spreads to the eye, it can cause a red, inflamed eye (conjunctivitis).

Gonorrhea is an acute infection that can become chronic if not treated. In men, gonorrhea may lead to inflammation of a sperm-holding duct connected to the back of the testis (epididymis). In women, it can spread to the uterus and fallopian tubes, causing pelvic inflammatory disease, which may result in infertility.

Gonorrhea can also spread through the bloodstream to cause infection in other parts of the body, such as joints. Because gonorrhea is contagious, it's important that you abstain from sexual contact until your infection is eliminated.

Chlamydia

Another sexually transmitted infection in men and women is caused by the bacterium *Chlamydia trachomatis*. This organism may be transmitted by either vaginal or anal sex.

Touching your eye with a hand that's moistened with infected secretions can cause an eye infection, and a mother can pass the infection to her child during delivery. *Chlamydia trachomatis* is the most common cause of blindness worldwide.

In many cases, especially in women, symptoms of chlamydial infection may be minimal or nonexistent. When symptoms are present, they're often similar to those of gonorrhea. In men, chlamydia may cause a burning sensation during urination and a discharge from the urethra. The symptoms are milder than those caused by gonorrhea and may appear 1 to 3 weeks after exposure to the bacteria.

Women may experience burning urination, a thin vaginal discharge or lower abdominal pain. But many don't realize they have the disease until informed by a sexual partner. In men, untreated chlamydial infections can cause inflammation of the urethra and epididymis. In women, they can lead to urethral infection and inflammation of the cervix, fallopian tubes and other pelvic organs.

All sexual partners of an infected person must be treated, even if they have no symptoms. Otherwise they may pass the disease back and forth.

Syphilis

Syphilis is a complex disease caused by the bacterium *Treponema pallidum*. Although once very prevalent, this disease has become less common among heterosexual people, compared with gonorrhea and chlamydia. But recently, the incidence of syphilis has increased in poor, urban areas of the United States and in people with AIDS.

Usually transmitted by sexual contact, the organism gains entrance to the body through minor cuts or abrasions in the skin or mucous membranes. The disease can also be transmitted by infected blood and from a mother to her unborn child during pregnancy (congenital syphilis).

Syphilis has three active stages. In the primary stage, painless sores appear on the genitals, the genital area, the rectum or the mouth from 10 days to 6 weeks after exposure. Pain may occur if the sores become infected with other bacteria.

The second stage begins anytime from a week to 6 months after the first stage. A red rash may appear on any surface of the body, including the palms of the hands and soles of the feet. Lesions sometimes appear on the lips, mouth, throat, genitals and anus. During this stage, the lesions on the skin and mucous membranes are extremely infectious. You may also have flu-like symptoms, such as headache and aching in the bones and joints. An intermediate period called latent syphilis follows. During this period no symptoms are present.

Don't Delay

If you suspect that you may have a sexually transmitted disease (STD), see your doctor right away. The sooner you get tested and begin treatment — if necessary — the less chance of serious complications developing and the healthier you and your partner will be.

The last stage, known as tertiary syphilis, includes widespread infection that may affect any of the internal organs, including your bones, heart and brain.

Syphilis can be cured if a diagnosis is made early and the infection is treated appropriately. If it's not, the disease can lead to many complications and even death.

Genital herpes

Genital herpes is caused by the herpes simplex virus type 2 (HSV-2). It's transmitted by vaginal or anal sex. The virus enters the body through tiny tears or abrasions in the skin or mucous membranes. It can infect the eyes by contact with a contaminated finger. It affects both men and women.

The initial symptom of genital herpes is pain or itching of the skin around the involved area. This stage is known as the prodromal period and begins 2 to 7 days after exposure to the virus. Anytime from a few hours to several days after the prodromal stage, sores begin to appear. In women they erupt in the vaginal area, external genitals, buttocks and anus. In men, they're on the penis, scrotum, buttocks, anus and thighs. Sores may be present but invisible inside the cervix in women and the urethra in men.

While the sores are present, it may be painful to urinate. They begin as small, tender, red bumps and become blisters within a few days. Then the blisters rupture, becoming ulcers that ooze or bleed. After 3 to 4 days, scabs form and the ulcers heal. You may experience pain and tenderness in the genital area until the infection clears. During the first outbreak, you may experience flu-like symptoms, as well as swollen lymph nodes in the groin.

There's no cure or vaccine for herpes. The virus remains dormant in the infected areas and periodically reactivates, causing symptoms. The disease is very contagious whenever sores are present.

Herpes generally doesn't cause any other serious permanent complications besides the sores. However, newborn infants can become infected as they pass through the birth canal of mothers with open sores, which may result in brain damage, blindness and death. This infection is more common in infants of mothers who are having their first outbreak of active herpes infection at the time of delivery. The rate of herpes infection in newborns is increasing as the rate of genital herpes in women increases.

Venereal warts

Venereal warts (genital warts) are caused by the human papillomavirus (HPV). Venereal warts affect both men and women and are easily transmitted through sexual contact. Individuals with an impaired immune system and pregnant women are particularly susceptible.

Venereal warts may develop from 3 weeks to 3 months after exposure to the virus. In men, they usually appear near the tip of the penis and sometimes on the shaft or scrotum. In women, they may appear on the vaginal lips, inside the vagina, on the cervix or around the anus. HPV can also cause cervical lesions and is a major cause of cervical cancer.

Venereal warts generally aren't serious, although they're contagious. However, women with cervical lesions caused by HPV have a higher risk of cervical cancer and should have a Pap test annually.

HIV and AIDS

AIDS is a chronic, life-threatening condition caused by the human immunodeficiency virus (HIV). By damaging or destroying the cells of your immune system, HIV interferes with your body's ability to effectively fight off viruses, bacteria and fungi that cause disease. This makes you more susceptible to many infections your body would normally resist.

The virus and the infection itself are both known as HIV. The term *acquired immunodeficiency syndrome* (AIDS) refers to later stages of HIV infection. HIV is most commonly spread by sexual contact with an infected partner. Untreated women with HIV can also pass the infection to their babies during pregnancy, delivery or later through their breast milk.

The Centers for Disease Control and Prevention estimates that 900,000 Americans are living with HIV and AIDS. Symptoms vary depending on the phase of the infection. When first infected with HIV, you may have no symptoms at all. It's often more common to develop a brief flu-like illness 2 to 6 weeks after being infected. But because the signs and symptoms of an initial infection — which may include fever, headache, sore throat, swollen lymph glands and rash — are similar to those of other diseases, you might not realize you've been infected.

Once the virus enters your body, it multiplies in your lymph nodes and slowly begins to destroy certain white blood cells that coordinate your immune system. You may remain symptom-free for 8 or 9 years. But the virus continues to multiply and destroy immune cells. Eventually, you may develop mild infections or chronic signs and symptoms such as swollen lymph nodes, diarrhea, weight loss, fever, cough and shortness of breath. During the last phase of HIV — which occurs approximately 10 to 11 years after infection — more serious symptoms may begin to appear. ■

CHAPTER 7 PART I

Caring for Your Teeth

Your teeth are among your most important assets. Attached to jaws driven by powerful muscles, your teeth enable you to chew your food into a form that aids digestion. Teeth, of course, also have a cosmetic dimension. Frequently, the first thing we notice about other people is their smile. Clean, healthy-looking teeth are a sign the world over of general good health. In the past, a healthy smile belonged only to the young because most people lost their teeth by middle age. Now, however, dental care, improved nutrition and good dental hygiene make it possible for most of us to keep our teeth for our entire lives.

Care of Your Teeth

Essential to maintaining a set of healthy teeth is a lifelong program of good dental hygiene — one that you begin early and practice consistently through the years. This includes brushing your teeth at least twice a day and flossing at least once a day. In addition, it may include reducing the number of times throughout the day in which you snack on sugary foods or sip sugary beverages. The more often you consume sugary substances, the more often you provide fuel for cavity-causing bacteria.

Tooth decay

Tooth decay, which results in cavities (caries), is more commonly a problem in children and young adults, but it can occur in adults of any age. Bacteria in your mouth are constantly in the process of forming dental plaque, a sticky, colorless film that can cling to your teeth. Oral bacteria in plaque feed on the sugars and starches in the foods and drinks you consume, converting them to various forms of acid. When acid-producing plaque clings to your teeth over long periods of time, the acid can progressively dissolve the outer layer on your teeth.

Start your child early on a program of regular brushing and flossing. Decay can begin as soon as your child's baby (primary) teeth begin to erupt. Never allow your infant to sleep with a bottle of fruit juice or milk. The sugar content of these beverages encourages decay. If your baby seems to require the soothing presence of a bottle at bedtime, offer a bottle of water.

Teach your toddler to brush his or her teeth in the morning and evening. Reinforce the habit by setting a good example. Make sure that all of your children brush with fluoride toothpaste and have regular dental checkups, beginning no later than age 3.

Periodontal disease

The principal cause of tooth loss in adults is periodontal disease. Periodontal disease is an infection of the gums and other tissues that support the teeth. The frequency of gingivitis, a mild form of periodontal disease, is high in all age groups — reportedly more than 85 percent in adults age 45 or older.

The frequency of periodontitis, a more serious form, increases with age (see page 708). Close to 50 percent of adults age 45 or older are thought to be affected. Advanced periodontitis can lead to loosening and eventual loss of teeth. However, you can prevent gum disease with proper daily care of your teeth.

The most frequent sign of gum disease is swollen gums that bleed easily, especially during brushing and flossing. Other signs and

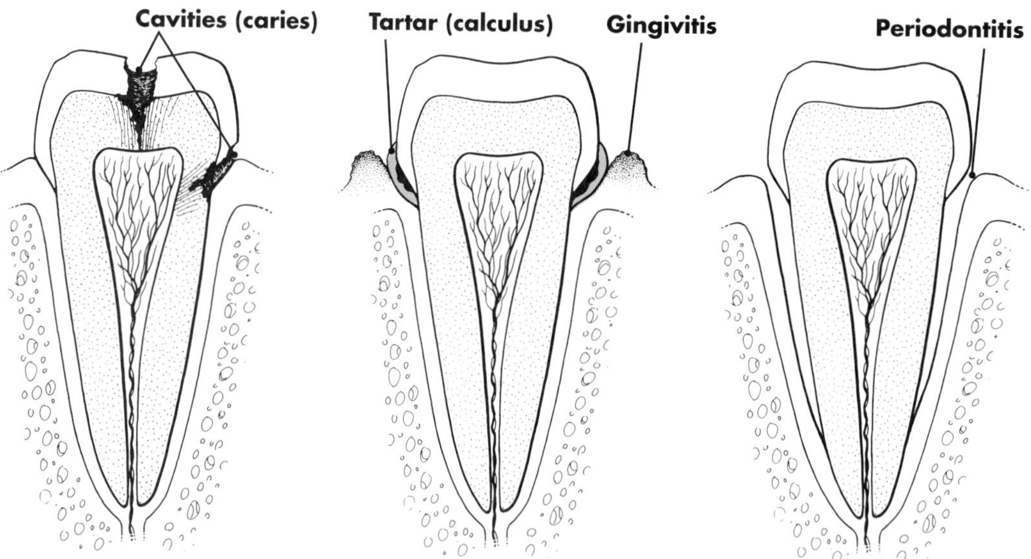

The principal cause of tooth loss is dental cavities (caries). The accumulation of tartar (calculus) can lead to gingivitis and, eventually, detachment of gums from the tooth (periodontitis) — another cause of tooth loss.

Sensitive Teeth

When your teeth become painful to certain stimuli — touch, cold, hot, air, sweet or sour foods or plaque — you may have what dentists call dentin hypersensitivity, or sensitive teeth. This condition is usually caused by enamel erosion or gum recession that exposes the root of the tooth. If you avoid sensitive areas during brushing, flossing, chewing or drinking because of discomfort, you need treatment. Failing to clean your teeth thoroughly because of sensitivity can lead to tooth and gum disease.

After determining the cause of your sensitive teeth, your dentist can treat the troubled area and recommend a maintenance program. This may include using a desensitizing toothpaste, applying a prescribed fluoride solution daily at home or having your dentist cover the exposed areas with bonding agents.

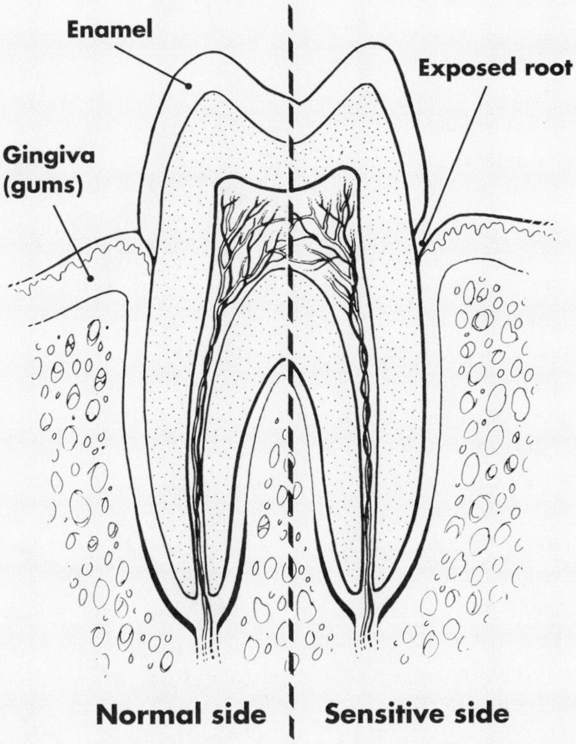

Recession of the gumline that exposes the root of a tooth can cause the tooth to be sensitive to stimuli such as cold and touch.

symptoms include bad breath, soft or tender gums, pus from the gumline — where the gum forms a collar around the tooth — shrinkage of the gum away from the tooth, a loose tooth and changes in the tooth position and bite.

Like tooth decay, the cause of periodontal disease is plaque. When plaque accumulates along the gumline, it irritates your gums, making them tender and likely to bleed. This condition is called gingivitis (see page 707).

If you don't remove the plaque daily by brushing and flossing, over time it can harden and form a difficult-to-remove substance called tartar (calculus). Chronic periodontal disease may develop if plaque and tartar spread beneath your gumline. With chronic bacterial irritation, gum tissue may begin to detach from the teeth, allowing pockets of infection to form. As plaque and tartar spread into the pockets and continue to irritate gum tissue, your gums may further detach from your teeth. This condition is called periodontitis. Eventually, infections in the dark, airless pockets can destroy the tissue and bone supporting your teeth. Untreated, periodontal disease can progress until your teeth loosen and fall out.

The best method for controlling plaque and tartar is to brush thoroughly and regularly. Brush your teeth at least twice each day, floss at least once a day and limit the amount of sugar you eat, particularly between meals.

Proper Flossing and Brushing

Good oral care depends more on brushing and flossing techniques than on use of any particular brand name or new, improved product. Rather than paying a premium price for a so-called anti-plaque or anti-tartar toothpaste, your best protection against disease is frequent brushing with a fluoride toothpaste and flossing.

Brushing and flossing are the best ways to remove bacteria and food particles before dental problems begin. Start by flossing your teeth once each day and brushing them at least twice a day — in the morning and before going to bed. Better yet, brush after each meal or snack. A complete cleaning with a fluoride toothpaste, toothbrush and dental floss should take 3 to 5 minutes. The proper order for cleaning is floss first, brush second. This order allows you to brush away food particles and bacteria loosened by the flossing.

Flossing

Take at least 18 inches of dental floss — unwaxed or waxed,

How to Floss and Brush

When flossing and brushing, proper technique is important.

To floss
Wrap waxed or unwaxed dental floss around the middle fingers of both hands, leaving 2 or 3 inches of floss between these fingers. For upper teeth, position the floss between the thumb of one hand and the index finger of the other, then insert it between your teeth and gently move it back and forth from the top to the bottom of your teeth. For lower teeth, it works best to position the floss between your index fingers.

To brush
Use a soft-bristle brush and minimal pressure. Begin with the outer surfaces of all of your teeth and the inner surfaces of your back teeth. Position your brush horizontally and brush back and forth gently with short — half-a-tooth-wide — strokes at the gumline. Next, brush vertically away from the gumline. To clean the inner surfaces of upper and lower front teeth, brush vertically, moving your toothbrush over both teeth and gums. To clean the junction between your teeth and gums, brush at a 45-degree angle (see insert), keeping the bristles angled against the gumline. Also brush the chewing surfaces with a gentle scrubbing motion and brush your tongue to freshen your breath.

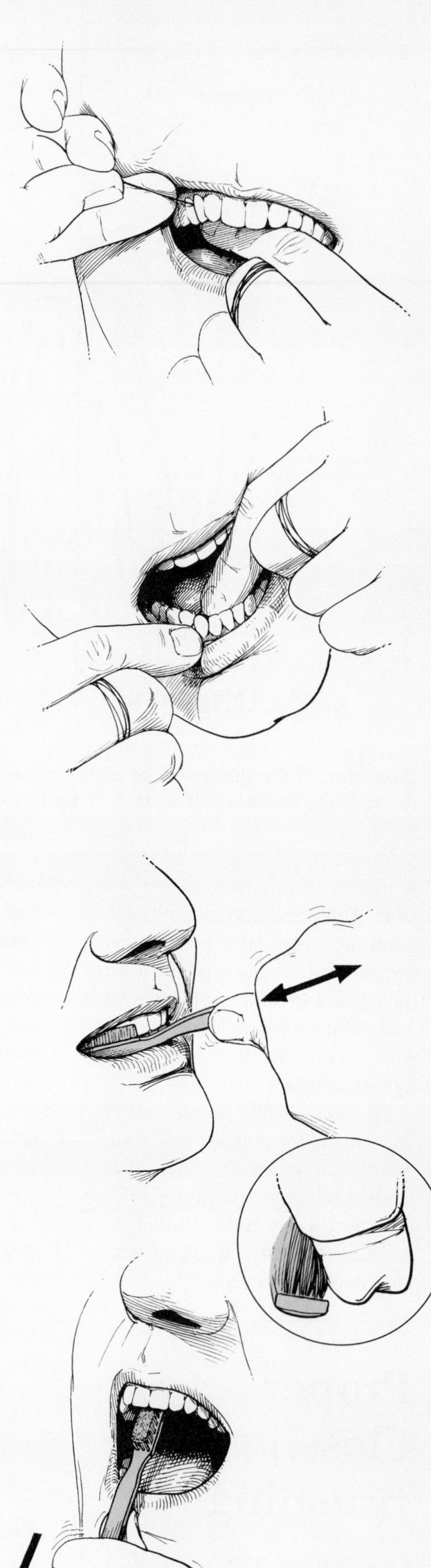

whichever is more comfortable for you — and wind most of it around the middle finger of one hand. Wind a turn or two around the middle finger of the other hand so that you have 2 to 3 inches of floss between these fingers.

Using a gentle sawing motion, work the floss between your teeth without snapping it into the gums. At the gumline, hold the floss taut, bend it into a C shape and scrape up and down on the side of each tooth. Each stroke should go slightly below your gumline until you feel resistance.

Don't be alarmed if your gums bleed the first few times you floss. If the bleeding continues each time you floss, consult your dentist. The problem may be improper flossing. Your dentist can demonstrate the proper technique.

Brushing

Brush your teeth at least twice daily, especially in the evening. To begin, put a small amount of fluoride toothpaste on your toothbrush and position the toothbrush horizontally on your teeth. To effectively clean the top and bottom surfaces of all teeth, move the brush back and forth horizontally and then vertically away from the gumline in a series of short, gentle strokes.

For surfaces adjacent to your gums, move the brush in short back-and-forth strokes or in a rotary motion over both teeth and gums. Positioning your toothbrush at an angle will help clean the junction between your teeth and gums more effectively. Also brush the chewing surfaces with a gentle scrubbing motion and brush your tongue to freshen your breath.

Toothpaste
With few exceptions most toothpastes have enough fluoride to protect your teeth against decay. But a growing awareness of dental health has led to a burgeoning array of specialty products. Gone are the

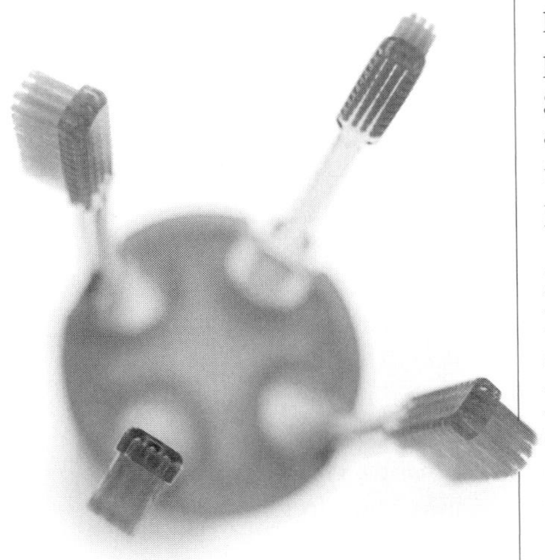

days when toothpastes promised only to prevent cavities. Now they also claim to fight plaque, control tartar, reduce sensitivity and more.

To clean and protect your teeth, what type of toothpaste do you really need? Here's an analysis of some popular claims:

Anti-plaque
Some products claim to remove plaque or kill bacteria that can cause plaque. But all toothpastes remove some plaque if you floss and brush well. Regardless of the product, you can't remove all plaque by brushing. Even if you use a plaque-fighting toothpaste, be sure to have regular checkups.

Tartar control
No toothpaste can remove tartar (calculus) below the gumline. That takes professional cleaning by a dental hygienist. Tartar is the white or yellowish deposit that plaque hardens into when mixed with minerals in saliva.

Anti-tartar toothpastes can help prevent a buildup of tartar on the teeth. Regular flossing and brushing remove plaque, leaving little plaque to harden into tartar. An anti-tartar paste may increase your teeth's sensitivity to cold. If so, change to a product without tartar control.

Baking soda
Baking soda is a mild abrasive and stain remover — but when wet it loses some of its stain-removing power. Some pastes contain hydrogen peroxide to help kill bacteria and loosen plaque. However, effective brushing with a fluoride toothpaste serves the same purpose.

Desensitizing
Desensitizing pastes contain chemicals that block the perception of pain in your teeth. Before using such a product, check with your dentist. Sometimes, sensitive teeth may be a sign of a problem that needs treatment, not coverup.

Extra whitening
Before using any kind of whitening gel or polishing cream, ask your dentist for advice. Whitening toothpastes contain ingredients such as peroxide bleach or papaya enzymes, which may be harsh on delicate gum tissue, especially if you have receding gums. Smokers' toothpastes also contain strong abrasives that may be harsh on gum tissue.

Natural
If you use a natural toothpaste product — most don't contain artificial ingredients such as a sweetener — be sure it has fluoride. Without it, natural pastes won't effectively fight decay.

Use of Fluoride

Several decades ago, scientists found that adding fluoride to drinking water with low levels of fluoride greatly decreased the number of cavities in children who drank the water. Today, the scientific evidence is conclusive: The addition of fluoride to drinking water and toothpaste helps to prevent cavities, particularly among children. Ingesting trace amounts of fluoride through drinking water is especially helpful during early childhood,

Selecting a Toothbrush

A toothbrush with soft, rounded-end or polished bristles is best for cleaning your teeth and gums. Stiff or hard bristles are more likely to injure gum tissues. The size and shape of the brush should allow you to reach every tooth. Brushes come in various sizes for children and for adults and with various configurations of bristles.

Remember that only the tips of the bristles do the cleaning, so there's no need to exert a great deal of pressure. Replace your toothbrush every 3 to 4 months, or sooner if the bristles become bent. Then you'll always be using bristles that are effective in brushing plaque, bacteria and sugars from the surface of your teeth and gums. Splayed bristles are a sign that it's past the time to replace your brush.

Electric toothbrushes with rotating or vibrating bristles to aid in plaque removal are a popular part of the toothbrush market. Some studies have shown that properly used electric toothbrushes remove plaque and improve gum tissue health better than do manual toothbrushes. In addition, an electric toothbrush may be easier to use if arthritis or dexterity problems make it difficult for you to brush properly. It also may be an effective tool for caregivers who brush the teeth of others.

Although an electric toothbrush may be more efficient, you can still achieve good oral hygiene with a properly used manual toothbrush — and often at a fraction of the cost of an electric toothbrush. If you have doubts about which brush to use for you and your family, ask your dentist for a recommendation.

when the teeth are developing. During a child's development, fluoride is incorporated into the enamel structure of the teeth and provides continuing protection.

Fluoride is inexpensive, safe and effective. Still, only half of our population drinks fluoridated water. If you have children and your municipal water supply isn't treated, ask about fluoridation for drinking water in your schools. If you don't have access to fluoridated water, whatever your age, you may want to ask your dentist about supplemental fluoride drops or tablets available by prescription. Children and older adults are most susceptible to tooth decay. For them, fluoride mouth rinses can be useful, as can topical fluoride treatments applied by a dentist.

In addition, you and your family should always brush with a fluoride toothpaste. Many fluoride toothpastes are available, including flavors formulated to appeal to children. Concentrated sources of fluoride, such as toothpastes and mouth rinses, aren't meant to be ingested. Ingestion of too much fluoride during the development of your child's teeth can result in fluorosis, a condition where the teeth develop with permanent splotches of varying shades of white.

A Dental Checkup

One of the most important steps in keeping teeth healthy is to visit your dentist regularly for a thorough checkup.

You and your children — beginning at age 3, or earlier if symptoms appear — should visit the dentist twice a year. You may need to see your dentist more frequently if certain conditions or problems exist.

People who have several cavities a year and who pay little attention to oral hygiene may need to see their dentist more often, for treatment and cleaning. Even individuals without natural teeth should see their dentist periodically. Your dentist will determine your examination schedule according to your specific needs.

Medical history

Before your dentist or hygienist asks you to "Open wide, please," he or she will probably ask a few questions about your general health. The answers can have a direct bearing on your treatment.

For example, certain kinds of heart conditions make people susceptible to an infection of the heart valves when their gums are manipulated, such as during a thorough dental cleaning or when a tooth is filled or extracted. These individuals should take an antibiotic medication before dental treatment. People who are allergic to penicillin can have a reaction when it's prescribed for tooth infections, and people with diabetes whose disease is poorly controlled can become ill after the stress of dental treatment.

Your dentist or dental assistant may also ask if you're on any medications so that your dentist doesn't prescribe medications that could cause harmful interactions.

Examination

A dentist typically examines both your mouth and teeth. In your gums and the soft tissues of your mouth, a dentist looks for signs of gingivitis, periodontitis and less common disorders such as leukoplakia, oral lichen planus or oral cancer (see Chapter 25, "Teeth and Mouth").

If you have dentures, your gums will be examined for signs of pressure and uneven wear, indicated by patches of thickened skin, soreness or reddened areas. Your dentist will also check your soft tissues, tongue and lips for lesions or other abnormalities.

A dentist examines each tooth using a dental explorer and a small

Dental Care and Heart Conditions

Among individuals with certain heart conditions, an infection in another part of the body, such as the mouth, can lead to a heart infection (endocarditis). However, most dental infections don't result in endocarditis.

People at greatest risk of this type of infection are those with damaged heart valves. Bacteria and other microorganisms found in the mouth can attach to tissues in areas of the heart where blood flow is turbulent — such as on defective or damaged heart valves — and multiply there.

Endocarditis can occur whenever bacteria circulate in the bloodstream. The organisms may enter your bloodstream during dental or surgical procedures, such as getting a tooth pulled or having your tonsils removed.

More often, though, endocarditis follows a minor gum injury or may be the result of poor dental hygiene. Endocarditis is a serious illness and can be fatal.

To lower the risk of endocarditis, people with heart valve problems should brush and floss their teeth daily and get regular checkups. These individuals should also take antibiotics before dental work.

Be sure to tell your dentist if you have a heart condition.

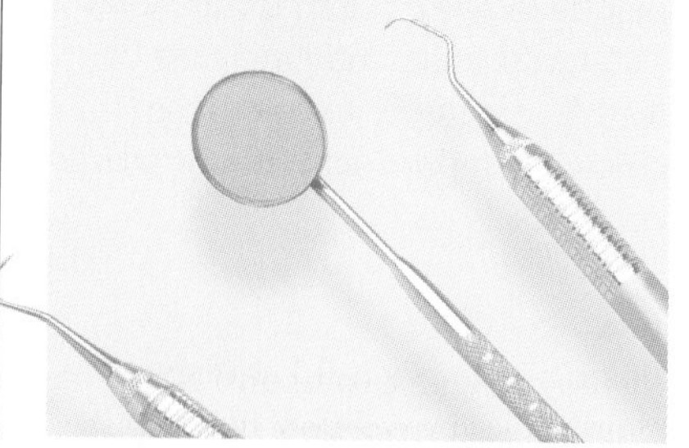

mirror. He or she looks for signs of decay, including discolored areas and small grooves (fissures) in the tooth enamel.

Existing fillings are checked for deterioration and for signs of new cavities around their edges. To measure signs of bone loss or gum disease, a dentist or hygienist inserts a periodontal probe around the base of each tooth.

X-rays

Almost all individuals who have been to a dentist have had dental X-rays taken. As in other medical fields, these X-rays are used to aid in diagnosing disease or injury. They're useful in identifying the presence and extent of dental cavities. An X-ray can detect decay in a tooth even when the enamel looks intact, particularly if the decay is hidden between teeth or is under the gumline.

X-rays can also help diagnose a tooth abscess, bone damage from periodontal disease, fractures of the jawbone and teeth and other abnormalities of the teeth and jaw. They also provide a status report on unerupted or impacted teeth.

A dental X-ray may be taken using traditional X-ray film or digital technology. To detect cavities, dentists use bitewing X-rays. A small piece of film is placed in your mouth, next to your teeth. You hold the film in place by biting down on the paper that covers the film. The X-ray machine is then aimed at the tooth, and the exposure is made. A digital image will be available immediately, and a film X-ray takes a few minutes to be developed. Either way, an X-ray image can help your dentist determine an appropriate course of action.

The amount of radiation used during a traditional X-ray is extremely small. The amount of radiation used to make a digital X-ray is even less. Still, no one should have more radiation exposure than necessary. Discuss with your dentist how often X-rays are necessary. As a precaution against excess radiation, your dentist should fit you with a lead apron that covers you from the chest to lower abdomen.

Cleaning

When your dentist or a dental hygienist cleans your teeth, his or her goal is to remove plaque and hardened plaque (tartar) accumulations. Tartar is a primary cause of gum diseases such as gingivitis and periodontitis. Tartar is most troublesome when it forms below the gumline.

Your dentist or hygienist can remove tartar in one of two ways. The traditional method involves scraping the deposits from your teeth with a sharp instrument

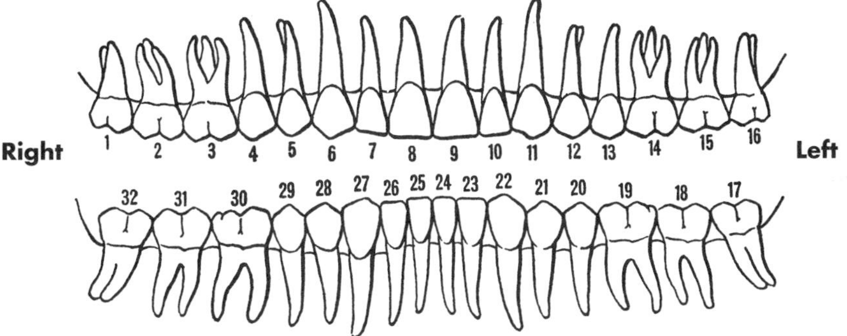

A permanent set of 32 teeth begins to erupt when a child is about 6 years old and is usually complete by age 12.

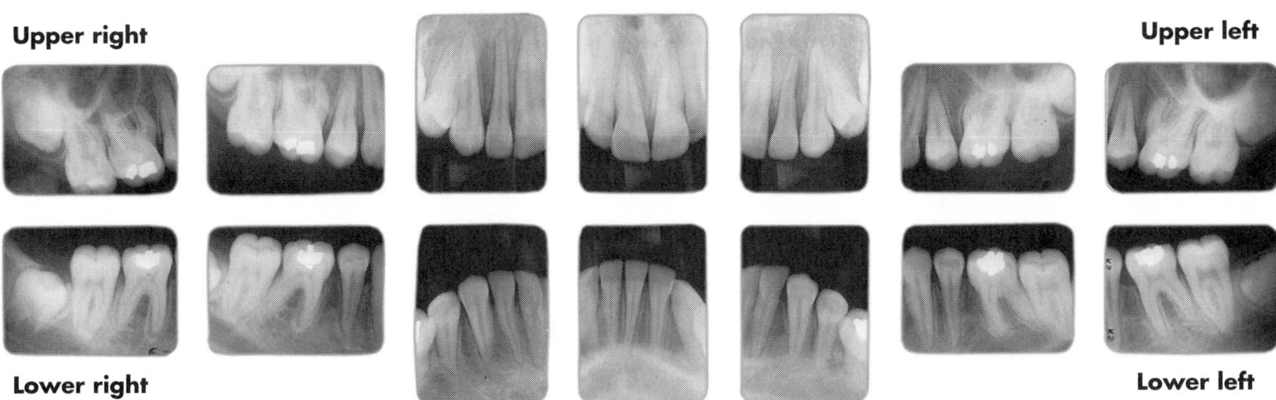

Dental X-rays are useful for diagnosing the presence and extent of cavities and other abnormalities of the teeth and supporting structures. Shown here is a set of full-mouth X-rays.

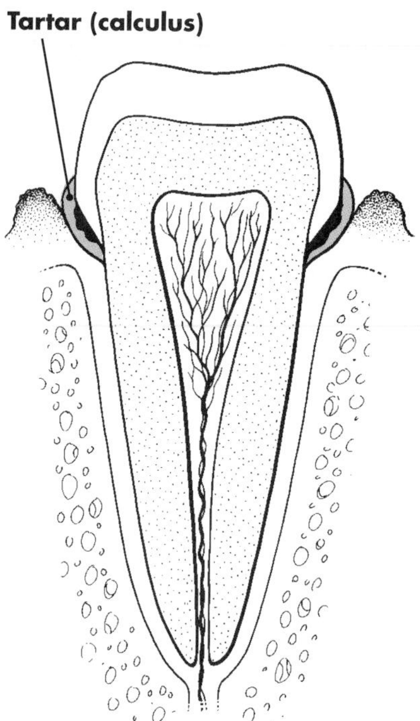

Tartar (calculus) is an accumulation of minerals and plaque on the surfaces of your teeth. When cleaning your teeth, your dental hygienist will remove the tartar — especially at or below the gumline — because it's a primary cause of gum disease.

known as a scaler. Another method involves use of an ultrasonic device that loosens the tartar through vibration. Whatever method is used, you may experience some gum bleeding. In some people, tartar develops quickly and must be removed every few months.

Once the tartar has been removed, the teeth are polished, which can be helpful in stain removal or in slowing plaque re-accumulation. Polishing is done with a special toothpaste applied by a device with rotating rubber heads. Dentists often finish children's checkups with an application of fluoride to help prevent tooth decay. ■

CHAPTER 8 PART I

Participating in Your Health Care

Years ago, people generally accepted a doctor's advice without question. But a one-way system of communication doesn't benefit you or your doctor. Better care results when you actively participate in your health care and work together with your doctor as a team.

Becoming more actively involved in your health can help you to live a healthier, more productive life. In addition to eating well and exercising, work with your doctor and other health care professionals to make sure that you receive recommended preventive health care and screening tests. If you have a medical condition, learn all that you can about it.

If you don't have a personal physician, take steps to find one. A primary care doctor can assess your current health, coordinate your care if you have significant or chronic health conditions and help you take preventive steps to avoid future disease.

Today's medical world is complex, but you're likely to have more options and resources than in the past. At least once each year, take stock of your health and your health resources.

Caring for yourself involves more than just going to the doctor. Read up on health care. In addition, find out if your employer offers programs that can help you achieve and maintain a healthy weight, stop smoking or improve your physical fitness.

Have a home medical kit with the basic items, such as a thermometer and medications. Keep doctors' telephone numbers and emergency numbers handy.

Keep a home medical file with test results from your doctor, diagnoses, names of medications, immunization records, dates of previous screening tests and a list of any allergies you may have. Know how your doctor's office works, who's on staff, which hospital he or she uses and where the emergency room is.

Medical Specialties

The American Board of Medical Specialties governs the primary medical specialties. In addition to the main specialties, some specialties have subspecialties. The various specialties and subspecialties include:

Specialties

Allergy and immunology
Anesthesiology
Colon and rectal surgery
Dermatology
Emergency medicine
Family practice
Internal medicine
Medical genetics
Neurologic surgery
Nuclear medicine
Obstetrics and gynecology
Occupational medicine
Ophthalmology
Orthopedic surgery
Otolaryngology
Pathology
Pediatrics
Physical medicine and rehabilitation
Plastic surgery
Preventive medicine
Psychiatry and neurology
Radiology
Surgery
Thoracic surgery
Urology

Subspecialties

Addiction psychiatry
Adolescent medicine
Aerospace medicine
Blood banking and transfusion medicine
Cardiac electrophysiology
Cardiovascular disease
Chemical pathology
Child and adolescent psychiatry
Clinical and laboratory immunology
Clinical and laboratory medicine
Clinical neurophysiology
Critical care medicine
Cytopathology
Dermatological immunology
Dermatopathology
Endocrinology, diabetes and metabolism
Forensic pathology
Forensic psychiatry
Gastroenterology
General vascular surgery
Geriatric medicine
Geriatric psychiatry
Gynecologic oncology
Hand surgery
Hematology
Immunopathology
Infectious disease
Maternal and fetal medicine
Medical microbiology
Medical oncology
Medical toxicology
Neonatal-perinatal medicine
Nephrology
Neuropathology
Nuclear radiology
Otology and neurotology
Pain management
Pediatric cardiology
Pediatric critical care medicine
Pediatric emergency medicine
Pediatric endocrinology
Pediatric gastroenterology
Pediatric hematology-oncology
Pediatric infectious disease
Pediatric nephrology
Pediatric otolaryngology
Pediatric pathology
Pediatric pulmonology
Pediatric radiology
Pediatric rheumatology
Pediatric surgery
Pulmonary disease
Reproductive endocrinology
Rheumatology
Sleep medicine
Sports medicine
Surgical critical care
Transplant medicine and surgery
Undersea medicine

Health Care Providers

Doctors, nurses and other medical professionals are part of the health care team. When you seek medical care, it helps to understand what each of these professionals does and the training he or she has.

Doctors

A doctor of medicine (M.D.) is ultimately responsible for delivering health care. Although the medical system relies on help from nurses and other professionals, final responsibility for your care falls on your doctor.

Becoming a medical doctor requires an undergraduate college degree, followed by successful completion of 4 years of medical school. Typically, medical students spend their first 2 years learning the foundations of medicine, including courses in human anatomy, physiology, biochemistry, human growth and development, microbiology and pharmacology.

The third and fourth years of medical school focus on an introduction to patient care. While continuing class work, medical students work with doctors in evaluating and treating patients. The main areas of medicine covered during these 2 years include:

- Internal medicine (medical care of adult patients)
- Neurology
- Surgery
- Pediatrics and adolescent medicine
- Obstetrics and gynecology
- Family medicine
- Psychiatry

Once a student earns a medical degree, he or she must complete a residency program of 3 or more years working in hospitals and outpatient clinics with experienced doctors. Typically, residents begin their training in a primary care specialty, such as internal medicine, family medicine or pediatrics, or in general surgery. A resident is eligible to apply for a state license to practice medicine once he or she has completed 1 year of an approved training program.

Doctors must annually renew their state license to practice. A state licensing board examines the credentials of and gives examinations to doctors applying to practice in that state.

The board also reviews patient or colleague complaints of inappropriate or unprofessional behavior by physicians. When necessary, this board may revoke a doctor's license if there's proof of misconduct.

A doctor who moves from one state to another must obtain a license in that new state. Often, the second state recognizes the credentials from the first state. However, some states require that doctors take and pass all of the qualifying examinations before receiving a license.

Once doctors complete a residency program, they're eligible to take an examination to be certified by the board in charge of their particular specialty.

Some physicians choose to narrow and deepen their focus in a particular area of medicine. Others choose to be generalists because they enjoy providing people with ongoing, comprehensive health care. Both types of doctors are necessary and can be certified by the board in charge of their particular specialty.

A primary care doctor looks out for your overall health and provides routine care for a variety of illnesses. When the usual treatments aren't successful, or to obtain a second opinion for a more complex problem, a primary care doctor often enlists the help of a specialist.

In some cases, the specialist also provides long-term care. If you have diabetes, for example, a diabetes specialist (endocrinologist) may become your main doctor. At other times, a specialist addresses a specific problem and recommends treatment options that a primary care physician can oversee.

A doctor's education doesn't end with obtaining a license or initial board certification. Doctors regularly attend continuing medical education courses to keep current with developments in their fields.

Some states require doctors to obtain a specific number of continuing education hours to keep their licenses. Medical boards that govern particular specialties also have continuing education requirements, which may be more stringent than those of the states.

? Question and Answer

What's the difference between an M.D. and a D.O.?

A D.O. is a doctor of osteopathy. An M.D. is a doctor of medicine. Both are full-fledged physicians.

Osteopathy is a recognized medical discipline that has much in common with conventional medicine. Similar to traditional physicians, doctors of osteopathy go through rigorous and lengthy training in academic and clinical settings. They're licensed to perform many of the same treatments as traditional doctors, including therapy and prescribing medications.

The difference between the two is that osteopaths may rely more on the use of manipulation to treat illness. With manipulation, doctors of osteopathy attempt to release pressure in the joints and align the spine and attached muscles to improve movement and flow of body fluids. Doctors of osteopathy often treat problems of the joints, muscles and tendons as well as certain types of headaches, breathing problems, digestive disorders and gynecologic complaints.

In addition to formal continuing education courses, doctors stay abreast of rapidly changing medical information by reading professional journals, attending conferences and interacting with their medical colleagues.

Nurses

Nurses support and assist doctors by helping them carry out treatment plans and evaluate results. They also often provide information to patients on managing health care problems at home.

There are different types of nurses. A registered nurse (R.N.) must complete specific coursework, typically leading to a college degree, and pass a state licensing examination. Some earn postgraduate degrees. A licensed practical nurse (L.P.N.) has less academic training than does an R.N. and isn't permitted to do all of the tasks allowed an R.N.

Most nurses are generalists. However, some specialize in a particular area of care, such as cardiology, pediatrics, psychiatry or surgery. Other specialized types of nurses include:

- Nurse anesthetist
- Nurse clinician
- Nurse educator
- Nurse midwife
- Nurse practitioner
- Occupational health nurse
- Public health nurse

These specialties require further education and board certification. In fact, nurse practitioners perform many of the same basic tasks that doctors do, examining and treating patients. In some states, they can write prescriptions on their own. In most other states, they may write prescriptions under the supervision of a doctor.

From the beginning of the nursing profession in the 1800s, nurses have focused on educating others about sound health practices. The goals of health education are to:

- Improve health and prevent complications
- Provide you with knowledge you need to make informed decisions
- Allay fears and anxieties
- Promote good health

Many nurses also conduct research and they may publish their results in professional journals, in addition to keeping up with new developments in nursing and medicine and attending professional conferences.

Other health care staff

In addition to doctors and nurses, many other people are vital to providing effective health care. Other types of health care professionals and skilled workers are listed here alphabetically with a description of what they do:

- *Attendants and orderlies* provide various basic services such as transporting people and helping nurses do basic care in health care facilities.
- *Audiologists* are specialists in the science of hearing. They evaluate hearing problems and assist in correcting them.
- *Emergency medical technicians (E.M.T.s)* offer emergency care, including life support, and transport sick and injured people to medical facilities.
- *Exercise physiologists* scientifically evaluate the effects of exercise on body functions and recommend healthy exercise programs.
- *Home health aides* help homebound people with activities of daily living such as dressing, grooming and eating. They also perform simple nursing tasks, such as changing bandages.
- *Laboratory technicians* perform tests and analyses on your blood, urine and other substances to help in diagnosing your condition and monitoring your progress.
- *Medical records personnel* keep health care files up-to-date and accessible.
- *Midwives* assist in prenatal care, attend to women in labor and assist in the delivery of babies.
- *Nurses' aides* carry out nonspecialized basic tasks in health care facilities, such as bathing and feeding people and making beds.
- *Occupational therapists* help you if you're injured or disabled to regain your ability to carry out everyday tasks. They also recommend possible physical modifications of your home, if necessary.
- *Opticians* grind and fit your eyeglass lenses and contact lenses.
- *Optometrists* test your vision and prescribe eyeglasses.
- *Pharmacists* formulate and dispense medications according to your doctor's prescriptions.
- *Physical therapists* help you if you're injured or disabled to regain lost physical functions, using techniques such as exercise, massage and ultrasound.
- *Physician assistants (P.A.s)* are trained in physical diagnosis and treatment, and they may specialize in a particular area of medicine. They work under the supervision of a doctor.
- *Podiatrists* treat injuries and other problems of the feet.
- *Psychologists* diagnose and treat mental health problems, using primarily counseling, testing and therapy.
- *Radiology technicians* help take and process X-rays, computerized tomography (CT) scans and other types of tests based on radiation.
- *Recreational therapists* use group activities including music and games to help people improve their communication skills or behavior patterns.
- *Registered dietitians (R.D.s)* help specify and modify eating habits to address your specific health condition.
- *Respiratory therapists* use respirators and other devices to improve your breathing ability and lung capacity.
- *Social workers* provide counseling about health-related and other problems an individual or family may be facing. They may also help with financing, care after

your hospital discharge and other needed services.
- *Speech therapists* treat disorders and injuries that affect a person's ability to speak, such as helping a child overcome a lisp or an adult regain speaking skills after a stroke.

Finding a Primary Care Doctor

A key step in preventive health and overall management of your health is developing an ongoing relationship with a primary care doctor who oversees all aspects of your health. Ideally, a primary care doctor is someone who knows you, your family health history and the conditions under which you live and work that may impact your health.

This person treats problems as they arise and makes sure you receive basic screening tests to prevent disease or catch it early when it can most easily be treated. Your primary care doctor also diagnosis and treats a variety of medical conditions and refers you to a specialist when you need to see one for a complex or unusual medical problem. He or she also makes sure that one treatment you're receiving doesn't conflict with another. This role is particularly important if you have long-term or multiple health problems that require consultations with various specialists.

A primary care doctor is usually a specialist in family practice, internal medicine, obstetrics and gynecology or pediatrics. A family doctor has training in almost every aspect of medicine, including obstetrics and pediatrics. An internist is a doctor who specializes in the diagnosis and treatment of health problems that occur in adults. A pediatrician specializes in diseases of children and adolescents.

The first step in finding a primary care doctor is to gather a list of names. Before you move into a new community, ask your current doctor for recommendations.

You can also obtain suggestions from other sources. One possible place to start is the Yellow Pages of your telephone directory. Doctors are typically listed by specialty and location.

You can also check with the American Medical Association (AMA) to get a list of doctors in your area. See page 1380 for information on how to contact the AMA. You can also ask your friends, colleagues and neighbors for recommendations.

Once you've compiled your list, contact each doctor's office for more information. Here are some questions that may help you make your selection:
- Is the receptionist's tone warm and friendly? Does this person answer your questions directly?
- What hospital does the doctor use?
- What are the office hours?
- Does the doctor accept your insurance plan?
- How and where would you get emergency care outside of normal office hours?
- How much time does the doctor allot for appointments?
- Will the doctor set up a brief get-acquainted appointment?

Second Opinions

There may come a time, especially if an illness develops, when you would like a second opinion before proceeding with a treatment recommended by your primary care doctor. In addition, some health insurance plans require a second opinion before agreeing to cover certain procedures.

Either you or your doctor can initiate the process of seeking a second opinion. A good personal physician should have no reservations about referring you to a specialist, when appropriate. Second opinions may also be useful when the diagnosis is clear, but the choice of treatments is less so.

A second opinion may also be in your best interest if:
- A condition for which you've received a diagnosis is serious
- The treatment your doctor advises is risky, experimental or controversial
- Major surgery appears necessary

If you'd like a second opinion to consider more options, tell your doctor so.

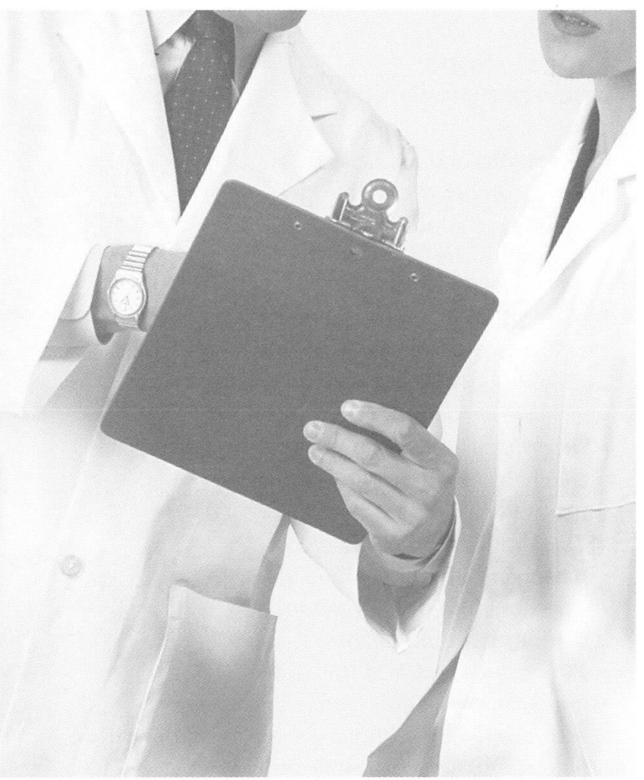

Developing a Good Relationship

The best medical care results from a partnership between you and your doctor. To make an accurate diagnosis or determine the best course of preventive care, your doctor needs information that only you can provide.

In turn, to treat a disease or keep from getting one, you need to follow your doctor's instructions. You each have important roles.

Here are some tips to help you receive the best care:

- Ask questions.
- Understand what your doctor and his or her staff are doing and why.
- If you have a disorder, ask about the diagnosis, including the name of the disorder, the prognosis and what to expect, and treatment recommendations.
- Follow up on your doctor's recommendations.
- Contact your doctor if you experience any unexpected events, discomfort or problems.

Expectations and responsibilities

Expectations and responsibilities also play an important role in developing a good relationship with your doctor.

Expectations of your doctor

When you see a doctor, you have certain expectations of your doctor, which he or she should provide:

- *Information.* You're entitled to as much information as you want about your illness.
- *Time.* You should be allowed a reasonable amount of time to ask questions and discuss concerns during an appointment.
- *Reasonable access.* You should be able to make an appointment to see your doctor within a reasonable amount of time. Some offices follow an "open access" policy — you can make same-day or next-day appointments.
- *Timely appointments.* You should be able to see your doctor within a reasonable amount of time once you arrive for your appointment. However, realize that he or she may be called away on occasion to address medical emergencies.

Gathering a Family History

In preparation for your medical examination, gather information about any childhood illnesses, accidents or operations.

It's important for your doctor to know about any genetic diseases in your family, such as Huntington's disease or sickle cell anemia. Parents can pass these ailments to their children, although not always to every child in each generation.

Similarly, many common diseases have apparent familial links. For example, if your father has heart disease, it doesn't necessarily mean that you'll also have heart disease. But your doctor should know about the history of this illness in your family so that he or she can watch for early signs and recommend preventive measures that may reduce other controllable risk factors.

To assemble a family history, make a list of any chronic diseases affecting your parents, grandparents, brothers, sisters, children and even aunts and uncles. Keep track of whether the diseases are on your mother's or father's side of the family. Such diseases include high blood pressure, diabetes, Alzheimer's disease, kidney disease, cardiovascular disease and cancers of the breast, uterus and colon. In addition, record any unusual diseases — even those that you don't believe are hereditary — and note if any immediate relatives died at a young age of an illness.

Provide this information to your primary care doctor for your medical record.

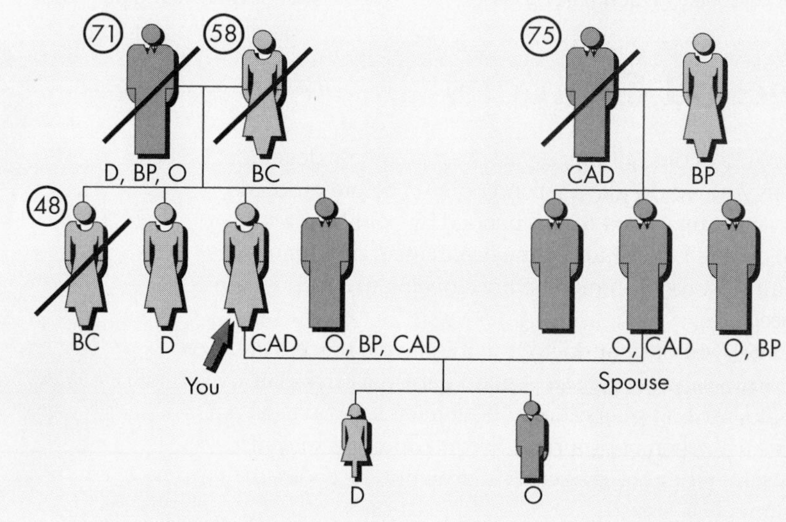

Here is an example of a family tree that charts a family medical history.

- *Emergency contacts.* Your doctor should give you information on how and where to go for care in case of an emergency, when he or she can't be reached.
- *Cost estimates.* You have a right to know about how much your care will cost.
- *Confidentiality.* Your condition and medical records are your and your doctor's business. For some conditions, such as certain infectious diseases, law requires that your doctor notify public health authorities.
- *Decision-making ability.* You have the right to participate in decisions about your care, based on your knowledge of your health or illness. This is called informed consent.

Responsibilities as a health care recipient

You also have certain responsibilities. Your doctor expects that you:

- *Be on time for office appointments.* If you must cancel, do so at least 24 hours in advance. This allows your doctor to see other patients during that appointment time. This provides better access for everyone, including you, the next time you need to see your doctor the same day that you call or the following day.
- *Provide information on medications.* Let your doctor know of all of the medications you're taking, including over-the-counter medicines, vitamins and supplements. List them or bring in the medication bottles. This allows your doctor to review and assess what you're taking, to make sure certain medications aren't causing symptoms or interacting with one another.
- *Know your own and your family's medical history.* Be prepared to discuss with your doctor your medical history and that of family members.
- *Answer questions accurately and completely.* This information helps your doctor better monitor your health, assess any health risks you may have and make the proper diagnosis, if one is needed.
- *Ask questions.* Your doctor is there to help you understand how to live healthfully and deal with disease. If you don't understand something, ask your doctor to clarify it for you until you do understand.
- *Follow treatment recommendations.* When your doctor prescribes a medication or another form of treatment, do what he or she recommends. Be patient — sometimes a treatment takes time to have an effect. However, if you experience any adverse effects or worsening symptoms, contact your doctor.

When to See a Doctor

Make an appointment to see your doctor if you have pain, shortness of breath or other symptoms indicating a medical problem. In addition, see your doctor on a regular basis for a preventive medical examination.

Regular preventive exams help your doctor assess your overall health and risk factors for disease. These checkups are important. Many diseases, such as diabetes, high blood pressure and some forms of cancer, don't cause any symptoms in their early stages but are detectable and, when found early, treatable.

How often you should get a medical checkup depends on your age, your health and your family medical history. The guidelines given here are for people who are generally healthy and have no symptoms of disease.

Basic physical examination

A physical examination generally includes a discussion of current symptoms and concerns, lifestyle habits and past health problems and a family history of certain health problems, along with a head-to-toe examination.

What to expect

During the exam, anticipate that your doctor or a nurse will likely:

- Check your height, weight, blood pressure and heart rate
- Check the inside of your mouth
- Examine your eyes, ears, nose and skin
- Feel for swollen lymph nodes in your neck, armpits and groin
- Listen for abnormal sounds from your heart, lungs or abdomen
- Feel for abnormalities or enlargements in your abdomen, especially your liver, spleen or kidneys
- Check your pulse in your neck, groin and feet
- Check reflexes

If you're a woman, your doctor may also perform a breast exam, a pelvic exam with a Pap test, and a digital rectal exam. These procedures are recommended when you become sexually active or turn age 18, whichever comes first.

If you're a man, your doctor may also examine your testicles for lumps or swelling and perform a digital rectal exam to examine your prostate gland.

Keep in mind your doctor may not check everything. If you have a specific problem — for example, you're losing weight for no apparent reason or you've noticed you're becoming increasingly short of breath — mention this to your doctor so that he or she can appropriately evaluate the problem.

When to have one

How often you need a complete physical exam depends on your sex, health history and risk factors for specific conditions and on your doctor's recommendations. Past recommendations often have suggested medical exams yearly. This often isn't necessary. A good rule of thumb would be to get a checkup at the following intervals. When you're having your first checkup, you and your doctor can discuss what fits your individual needs.

- Two times in your 20s
- Three times in your 30s
- Four times in your 40s
- Five times in your 50s
- Annually after age 60

Preventive Screenings

Regular preventive screening exams and tests are the best method for catching potential problems in the early stages, when the odds for successful treatment are the greatest. Preventive screening exams are often performed during regular physical examinations.

Which preventive screening exams and tests are appropriate for you? Only you and your doctor can make that decision. However, there are some general guidelines for preventive exams.

Following is a list of exams and tests generally recommended for women and men without symptoms or risk factors for a particular medical condition.

If you're older than age 50 or have one or more risk factors for a disease, your doctor may order additional tests or perform certain tests more frequently.

Recommended screenings

These are the tests you should undergo on a regular basis. The following tests are for both men and women:

Blood cholesterol test

A blood cholesterol test is actually several blood tests (serum lipids). A blood cholesterol screening measures total cholesterol as well as low-density lipoprotein (LDL or "bad") cholesterol, high-density lipoprotein (HDL or "good") cholesterol and triglycerides, another type of blood fat.

LDL cholesterol deposits fatty substances on your artery walls, and HDL cholesterol carries fatty deposits away from your arteries and to your liver for disposal. Problems occur when your LDL cholesterol deposits too much fat or when your HDL cholesterol carries away too little. This can lead to a buildup of cholesterol-containing fatty deposits (plaques) in your arteries, a condition called atherosclerosis.

What's the exam for?
It's to evaluate the levels of cholesterol and triglycerides (lipids) in your blood. Undesirable lipid levels raise your risk of heart attack and stroke.

When and how often should you have it?
Have a baseline cholesterol evaluation at age 20, then have it checked every 5 years if the levels are within normal ranges. If the readings are abnormal, you may have to have it checked more often.

Blood pressure measurement

Blood pressure is determined by the amount of blood your heart pumps and the resistance to blood flow in your arteries. The test measures systolic blood pressure — the peak pressure your heart generates when pumping blood out through your arteries — and diastolic blood pressure — the amount of pressure in the arteries when your heart is at rest between beats.

What's the exam for?
It's for early detection of high blood pressure. In general, the more blood your heart pumps and the narrower your arteries, the harder your heart must work to pump the same amount of blood. The longer that high blood pressure goes undetected and untreated, the higher your risk of heart attack, stroke, heart failure and kidney damage.

When and how often should you have it?
You'll likely have your blood pressure measured when you see a doctor for any reason. Have this test done at least every 2 years.

Colon cancer screening

A colon cancer screening involves one or more tests to look for precancerous cells or signs of cancer in your colon. The screening may take one of several forms. A barium X-ray and colonoscopy allow viewing of the full colon, which is desirable. Talk with your doctor about the goals and limitations of the following screening options:

- Fecal occult blood test
- Flexible sigmoidoscopy
- Barium X-ray
- Colonoscopy

A number of new tests to help identify cancer, such as specialized stool tests and those that use computerized tomography (CT) scans, are being evaluated. However, these tests aren't yet recommended for routine screening.

What's the exam for?
It's to detect cancer and precancerous growths (polyps) on the inside wall of the colon that may become cancerous. Many people skip colon cancer screening because of fear of embarrassment and discomfort. However, this screening could save your life by detecting growths before they turn cancerous or identifying cancer in its early stages when chances of a successful recovery are greatest.

When and how often should you have it?
For people with average risk, a colon cancer screening is recommended every 5 to 10 years, beginning after age 50. How often you should have a screening will depend on the test you receive, your doctor's recommendations and the results of the screening. If you're at high risk of colon cancer because of family history or other factors, your doctor may recommend beginning screenings before age 50.

Recommended Age-Specific Tests for Women

Test	Ages 20-39	Ages 40-50	Older than 50
Blood cholesterol test	Baseline at age 20, then every 5 years	Every 5 years	Every 5 years
Blood pressure measurement	Every 2 years	Every 2 years	Every 2 years
Clinical breast exam	Every 3 years	Annually	Annually
Colon cancer screening	Ask your doctor	Ask your doctor	Every 5-10 years
Dental checkup	Annually	Annually	Annually
Eye exam	Every 3-5 years	Every 3- 5 years	Every 1-3 years
Fasting blood sugar test	Ask your doctor	Baseline by age 45	Every 3 years
Mammogram	Ask your doctor	Baseline at age 40, then ask your doctor	Annually
Pap test	Every 1-3 years	Every 1-3 years	Every 1-3 years
Transferrin saturation test	Ask your doctor	Ask your doctor	Ask your doctor

Other Tests Women Should Consider

Test	Ages 20-39	Ages 40-50	Older than 50
Bone density measurement	Ask your doctor	Baseline at menopause	Ask your doctor
Full-body skin exam	Every 3 years	Every 2 years	Annually
Hearing test	Ask your doctor	Ask your doctor	Baseline by age 60
Hepatitis screening	Ask your doctor	Ask your doctor	Ask your doctor
Human immunodeficiency virus (HIV) and syphilis screening	Ask your doctor	Ask your doctor	Ask your doctor
Thyroid-stimulating hormone test	Ask your doctor	Ask your doctor	Ask your doctor

Recommended Age-Specific Tests for Men

Test	Ages 20-39	Ages 40-50	Older than 50
Blood cholesterol test	Baseline at age 20, then every 5 years	Every 5 years	Every 5 years
Blood pressure measurement	Every 2 years	Every 2 years	Every 2 years
Colon cancer screening	Ask your doctor	Ask your doctor	Every 5-10 years
Dental checkup	Annually	Annually	Annually
Eye exam	Every 3-5 years	Every 3-5 years	Every 1-3 years
Fasting blood sugar test	Ask your doctor	Baseline by age 45	Every 3 years
Transferrin saturation test	Ask your doctor	Ask your doctor	Ask your doctor

Other Tests Men Should Consider

Test	Ages 20-39	Ages 40-50	Older than 50
Full-body skin exam	Every 3 years	Every 2 years	Annually
Hearing test	Ask your doctor	Ask your doctor	Baseline by age 60
Hepatitis screening	Ask your doctor	Ask your doctor	Ask your doctor
Human immunodeficiency virus (HIV) and syphilis screening	Ask your doctor	Ask your doctor	Ask your doctor
Prostate-specific antigen (PSA) test and digital rectal exam	Ask your doctor	Ask your doctor	Annually
Thyroid-stimulating hormone test	Ask your doctor	Ask your doctor	Ask your doctor

Dental checkup

During a dental checkup, your dentist examines your teeth and gums and checks for growths on your tongue, lips and soft tissues.

What's the exam for?
It's to detect cavities and diseases such as periodontal disease. Your doctor also looks for lesions and other abnormalities in your mouth that could indicate cancer.

When and how often should you have it?
Have your teeth checked at least once a year or as your dentist recommends. Dental checkups should begin in childhood and continue throughout your adult life.

Eye exam

During an eye exam, an ophthalmologist or optometrist checks your vision and eye movement and looks for signs of disease.

What's the exam for?
It's to determine if you need corrective lenses and to identify if you may be at risk of diseases such as glaucoma, cataracts and age-related macular degeneration.

When and how often should you have it?
Have your eyes checked every 3 to 5 years until age 50, unless your eye doctor recommends more frequent checkups. After age 50, have your eyes checked every 1 to 3 years.

Fasting blood sugar test

This is a blood test that measures the level of sugar (glucose) in your blood following an 8-hour fast.

What's the exam for?
It's to check for high blood sugar levels, an indication of diabetes.

When and how often should you have it?
Have a baseline test by age 45. After age 50, have your blood sugar checked every 3 years. If you're at risk of diabetes because of family history or other factors, your doctor may recommend you be tested at a younger age and more frequently.

Transferrin saturation test

This is a blood test that measures the amount of iron bound to an iron-carrying protein (transferrin) in your bloodstream.

What's the exam for?
It's to detect hemochromatosis, a condition in which your body stores too much iron (iron overload). Excessive iron can damage your organs. In pregnant women and some infants, iron studies are done to make sure that iron levels aren't too low.

When and how often should you have it?
Ask your doctor. There's no agreement yet on whether or how often this test should be performed. Use of it should be tailored to your risks.

Additional recommended screenings for women

In addition to the basic screenings for all adults, women should get several other tests on a regular basis:

Clinical breast exam

This is a physical examination of your breasts and armpits that's typically part of a routine physical exam.

Your doctor looks for color changes, skin irregularities and changes in your nipples. Your doctor then feels for lumps and swollen lymph nodes.

What's the exam for?
It's to detect cancer and precancerous changes in your breasts.

When and how often should you have it?
Before age 40, have the exam at least every 3 years. After age 40, it's recommended that you have the exam annually.

Mammogram

In this screening exam, your breasts are compressed between plastic plates while a technologist takes X-rays of your breast tissue.

What's the exam for?
It's to detect cancer and precancerous changes in your breasts.

When and how often should you have it?
A baseline screening is generally recommended at age 40. Between ages 40 and 49, recommendations vary as to how often you should have a mammogram. Talk to your doctor. After age 50, have the test annually.

Pap test

In this test, your doctor inserts a plastic or metal speculum into your vagina. Then, using a soft brush, your doctor gently scrapes a few cells from your cervix, which are placed on a glass slide for laboratory analysis.

What's the exam for?
It's to detect cancer and precancerous changes in your cervical tissue.

When and how often should you have it?
An initial Pap test should occur at age 18 or with the beginning of sexual activity. Subsequent Pap tests are recommended every 1 to 3 years. After three consecutive annual Pap tests with normal results, you and your doctor may opt for less frequent testing. Ask your doctor about what's appropriate for you.

Additional screenings women should consider

Women should also consider having the health of their bones checked, especially after menopause:

Bone density measurement

This test involves a specialized X-ray scan of your lower back and hip region.

What's the exam for?
It's to detect osteoporosis, a disease involving loss of bone mass that can increase your risk of fractures.

When and how often should you have it?
Have a baseline exam following menopause, or earlier if you have a family history of osteoporosis or other risk factors. Repeat testing depends on the results of the baseline measurement and your doctor's recommendations.

Additional screenings men should consider

Men should also consider having the health of their prostate gland checked, especially after age 50:

Prostate-specific antigen test and digital rectal exam
During a digital rectal exam, your doctor inserts a lubricated gloved finger into your rectum and feels the prostate gland for any sores or lumps. The prostate-specific antigen (PSA) test is a blood test that measures the amount of a specific protein secreted by the prostate gland.

What's the exam for?
A digital rectal exam can detect noncancerous prostate enlargement (benign prostatic hyperplasia, or BPH) or prostate cancer.

A PSA test can detect prostate cancer. However, above normal PSA levels may stem from BPH or other noncancerous conditions as well.

When and how often should you have it?
Recommendations vary as to how often you should have a digital rectal exam and PSA test before age 50. Talk to your doctor.

After age 50, have a digital rectal exam and PSA test annually. If you're at low risk and you've established a pattern of low PSA levels and normal exams, your doctor may suggest spacing out your PSA tests to less frequent intervals.

Screenings for women and men to consider

Ask your doctor which of these may be appropriate for you:

Full-body skin exam
Your doctor examines your skin from head to toe, looking for moles or other growths that are irregularly shaped, have varied colors, are asymmetric or have grown or changed since the previous visit.

What's the exam for?
It's to check for skin cancer.

When and how often should you have it?
Have a full-body skin exam every 3 years in your 20s and 30s. Beginning at age 40, have the exam every 2 years, and after age 50, have it once a year.

Hearing test
During a hearing test, a doctor checks how well you recognize speech and sound at various volumes and frequencies.

What's the exam for?
It's to screen for hearing loss.

When and how often should you have it?
A baseline test is recommended by age 60, or earlier if you've been exposed to loud noises or suspect hearing loss.

Hepatitis screening
This is another blood test.

What's the exam for?
It's to screen for chronic hepatitis B or C. People with chronic hepatitis B or C are at greater risk of liver disease and liver cancer.

Questions to Ask

If your doctor recommends a test, ask the name of the test and its purpose. If you think you've had this test done recently, tell your doctor. You may not have to repeat it. Other questions you may want to ask, include:

- Why do I need this particular test?
- How accurate and reliable is the test?
- What happens if the test is positive? Or negative?
- Is the test invasive — it pierces the skin or enters the body — or non-invasive? If the test is invasive, what are the risks involved?
- How much does the test cost, and is it covered by insurance?
- What alternatives are available if I don't want this test?

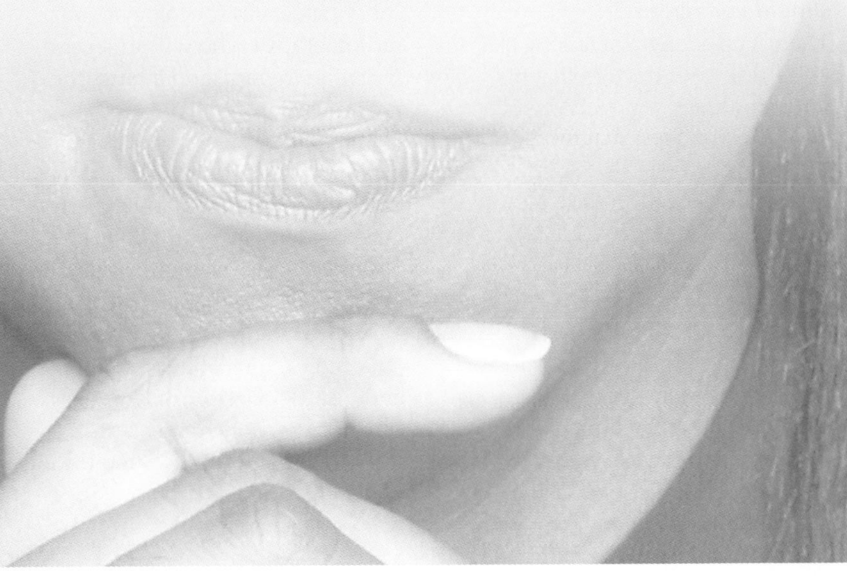

When and how often should you have it?
Your doctor may recommend this test if you have one or more risk factors for hepatitis.

HIV and syphilis screening
This involves two blood tests.

What's the exam for?
It's to screen for human immunodeficiency virus (HIV) and syphilis, infections that can lead to serious health problems. A positive test needs to be verified by a more sensitive blood test.

When and how often should you have it?
Your doctor may recommend this test if you have one or more risk factors for either condition.

Thyroid-stimulating hormone test
This is a blood test. Thyroid-stimulating hormone (TSH) is made by the pituitary gland in your brain. It stimulates your thyroid to produce its active hormone called thyroxine.

What's the exam for?
It's to detect if your thyroid is underactive (hypothyroidism), producing too little thyroxine, or overactive (hyperthyroidism), producing too much thyroxine.

When and how often should you have it?
There's no agreement among experts. Ask your doctor what fits your situation.

When to See a Specialist

At times, your primary care doctor may be uncertain about a diagnosis or about the best treatment for your problem. In this case, your doctor may refer you to a specialist.

Consulting another doctor with specific training in a certain area may be necessary and to your benefit if:

- You or your doctor would like a second opinion about your diagnosis or management options.
- You have a rare disease or unusual manifestations of a common disease.
- You need a special procedure or an operation.
- You aren't responding to therapy.
- Your disease is progressing especially rapidly or new complications are developing.
- You have significant symptoms that have persisted or progressed, and your doctor is unsure of the diagnosis.

Your personal physician may refer you to specialists he or she works with frequently. He or she may contact the specialist, brief the specialist about your case and schedule an appointment for you. Or you can locate a specialist on your own.

Before you see a specialist, put together a list of your questions. The specialist is likely to ask you about your medical history and may repeat some of the tests you already have undergone. Nevertheless, be sure a copy of your medical records reaches the specialist.

Often, areas of expertise overlap. For instance, if you've received a diagnosis of lung cancer, you may see one or more of the following: a lung (pulmonary) specialist, a cancer specialist (oncologist), a radiotherapist who will supervise radiation therapy and a lung (thoracic) surgeon.

Remember, medicine isn't an exact science. Different doctors — each highly qualified and experienced — may favor different options among the therapies available to treat a particular disease.

All treatments may be reasonable, but each will have advantages and disadvantages. Your primary care doctor can help you sort through the information and decide which treatment is best for you. ■

CHAPTER 9 PART I

Practicing Safety

A great deal of time, money, research and personal effort are invested each year in developing new ways to prevent disease. You, like millions of others, may be increasingly conscious of improving your diet, getting enough exercise and using other methods to help ensure your continued good health and that of your family.

All too often, though, people tend to overlook more obvious risks that pose a health danger. Nearly 1 in every 20 deaths in the United States result from accidents. Accidents are the most common cause of death in people younger than age 35. Half of all childhood deaths are due to accidents. On the highway, in the workplace and at home, accidents injure or disable tens of millions of Americans annually. Many of these accidents can be avoided.

The following pages offer various safety tips. This information isn't comprehensive, but it may alert you to potentially dangerous circumstances in your everyday life and during leisure activities.

Safety at Home

Every year, tens of thousands of Americans die of injuries sustained in their own homes. A few simple steps can often prevent accidental injuries and deaths.

Guns

If you keep a gun in your home, make sure that it's stored without ammunition, locked in a secure storage cabinet and out of the reach of children.

In addition, maintain the weapon carefully to prevent accidents due to malfunction. Periodically remove it from its place of storage and make sure that it's clean and working properly. Reacquaint yourself with the weapon's safety features and with its loading and unloading procedures.

More gun-related accidents occur in the home than anywhere else. Not far behind, though, are gun-related accidents in the workplace, on the highway and during recreation.

Fire

Fire is a leading cause of death and injury at home, not to mention a cause of extensive property damage. Most fires in homes result from carelessness. They often can be prevented with a few simple precautions and a little common sense.

Here are steps you can take to decrease the risk of personal injury and property damage from fires in your home:

Never smoke in bed

Careless smoking leads to the greatest number of deaths by fire in the United States. Keep cigarettes, cigars and pipes out of your bedroom and take care that they don't ignite a fire in furniture elsewhere in the home. When disposing of butts and ashes, be sure no embers remain.

Keep a fire extinguisher on hand

Have a fire extinguisher in the kitchen. You might also keep another one in the garage. Be sure members of your family know how to operate a fire extinguisher. Check the device annually.

Establish an escape plan

Be sure your home has adequate escape routes. If needed, purchase fire ladders or other means of escape from upstairs windows. Rehearse with your family procedures to follow in the event of a fire. Designate a family meeting place so that you can make sure everyone is accounted for. Keep stairways and halls uncluttered. Never padlock an exit door.

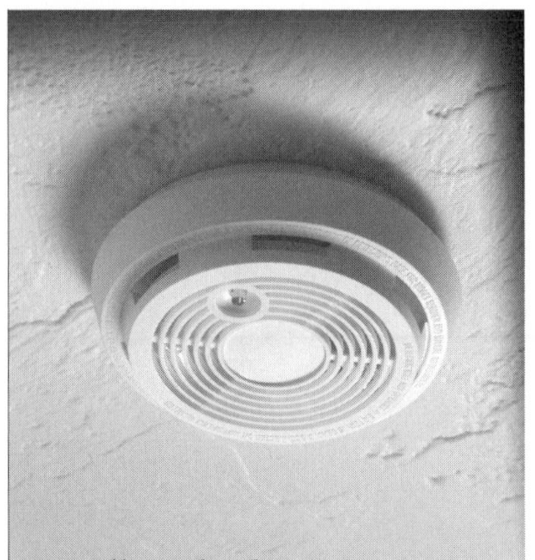

Install smoke detectors

Smoke detectors are valuable safety devices. Every home should be equipped with them. Locate your smoke detectors on the ceiling in the sleeping areas of your home and in areas where fires are most likely to start, such as the kitchen or garage. Make sure you have a smoke detector on each level of your home.

Place the smoke detector at least 6 inches from where the wall joins the ceiling. Avoid placing a detector in dead airspace, such as in a corner, where smoke may not reach it as quickly. Keep the detector away from shower areas because steam can set off a detector.

Test your smoke detector monthly to make sure that the batteries are good, and change the batteries at least once a year. If your smoke detectors are wired to your home electrical system, make sure they have backup batteries.

Be cautious of wood-burning stoves and space heaters

Be sure that the area around an open-flame space heater in your home is properly fireproofed. Building codes vary, but for most space heaters and wood-burning stoves, the walls around them must be a specified distance from the heater or stove or insulated with a fireproof material. The floor beneath and in front of the heater also must be insulated with a nonflammable material.

Keep kerosene or other freestanding heaters out of frequently used traffic paths in your home and away from hallways and stairways in particular. Many fires start when space heaters are knocked over, spilling fuel and igniting nearby furniture and surfaces.

Maintain electrical equipment
Make sure that the wiring in your home is up-to-date and in good order. If it isn't, hire a qualified electrician to make the necessary repairs. Don't overload wall outlets with adapters. Never increase the size of a fuse or circuit breaker as a means to sustain service of a line that's overloaded. If you don't increase the capacity of the wire in the line itself, it could heat up and start an electrical fire in the walls of your home.

Don't run extension cords across floors or under rugs or carpets. You can easily trip over exposed extension cords, especially at night. Over time, wear and tear on a cord beneath a carpet can damage the insulation and lead to overheating and a fire hazard.

Keep fireplaces and chimneys clean
Use a screen in front of your fireplace to prevent sparks from jumping out of the firebox, and never leave an open fire unattended.

Clean your chimney regularly and keep a chimney fire extinguisher on hand. If you vent a wood-burning stove into your chimney, clean the chimney twice a year. If a wood fire in your fireplace is only an occasional event, an every-other-year chimney cleaning may be sufficient. Have your chimney inspected for a buildup of creosote, a flammable resin that's a byproduct of wood fires. Don't postpone chimney repairs.

Remove flammable materials
As soon as you're done using rags or papers contaminated with paint remover or other chemicals, dispose of them safely. Don't leave them lying around in a garage or your basement. When such materials aren't disposed of properly, spontaneous combustion can occur, producing dangerous fumes and fire. Store newspapers, paper refuse and any other flammable trash away from heat sources.

Place paints and other household chemicals on a shelf that's both out of the reach of children and away from any risk of exposure to sparks and heat. Store matches out of the reach of children.

Carbon monoxide

Carbon monoxide is tasteless, odorless, colorless and deadly. Often referred to by its chemical formula, CO, this gas is produced by the incomplete combustion of carbon-based fuel. Many cookstoves, lamps, space heaters, furnaces, hot water heaters and engines produce carbon monoxide.

If the carbon monoxide level in a room or building becomes too high, you start breathing in an increasing amount of carbon monoxide. It begins to take the place of oxygen in your red blood cells. Too little oxygen and too much carbon monoxide prevent proper functioning of vital body organs and can cause death.

Causes of carbon monoxide poisoning
The risk of carbon monoxide poisoning is often greatest during cold weather. People typically seal and weatherstrip their homes as tightly as possible to conserve heat. But in doing so, they also decrease ventilation and increase the accumulation of indoor pollutants, such as carbon monoxide.

Carbon monoxide buildup is most likely to occur as a result of defective control valves or pilot lights on cooking or heating units such as furnaces and portable kerosene space heaters or inadequately ventilated flame-burning heaters and cookers.

Recreational vehicles, such as campers, also may have unvented ovens, stoves or flame-burning lamps that produce carbon monoxide. In addition, engine exhaust fumes may leak into pickup campers.

The signs and symptoms of carbon monoxide poisoning are vague. Headache, nausea, vomiting, fatigue and dizziness may occur but are easily confused with flu-like illnesses. When the concentration of carbon monoxide is very high, muscle paralysis and loss of consciousness may occur.

Be Cautious Around Fireworks

The brilliant illumination and resounding bangs and pops of fireworks provide thrills and excitement for young and old. But take care when using them.

When stored in your home, fireworks are a potential fire hazard. When put to use, they're even more dangerous. Potential risks include vision and hearing loss, burns to fingers and hands and the loss of fingers.

When using fireworks, be familiar with and obey laws that govern the purchase and use of fireworks in your state. Use fireworks outdoors only and in an open area on level ground. Stay a safe distance from them after they're lit and allow no horseplay when fireworks are being used. Never relight a dud. Douse it with water and discard it. Don't explode fireworks in a bottle, tin can or clay pot, and never tamper with or disassemble fireworks. Have a pail of water or hose on hand to douse the fireworks area when you're finished.

If you suspect carbon monoxide poisoning, get away from the source of the gas immediately. You may also want to see a doctor, especially if your symptoms are severe.

Preventing carbon monoxide poisoning

Purchase a carbon monoxide detector for your home. The detectors sound a warning when carbon monoxide levels in a home or other building exceed safe levels. Look for the code UL 2034 on the box. This indicates that the detector meets industry standards.

Make sure wood-burning stoves, space heaters, fireplaces and flame-burning appliances are properly installed, adjusted, operated and ventilated. Don't use ovens or gas ranges for heating and don't operate gas-powered vehicles in confined spaces, such as a garage or basement. Never burn charcoal inside your home, recreational vehicle or tent.

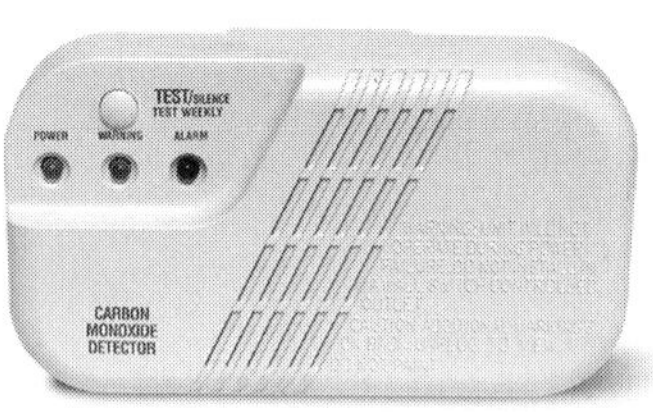

Other poisons

Small children are at special risk of poisoning. Their curiosity is boundless, and their bodies are small enough that relatively little poison can be harmful. In addition, small children tend to put whatever they find into their mouth.

Seemingly innocent products such as shoe polish, nail polish and nail polish remover can be hazardous. Make it a rule in your home that all hazardous items are to be kept in high cupboards, on high closet shelves or in locked cabinets. Designate such an area in your kitchen or utility room for household cleaners, another in your garage for garden or automotive poisons and another in your bathroom. Garden sheds, cellars and other areas where such goods may be stored require similar precautions.

Label All Poisons

If you store any poison in a container other than the one in which it was originally packaged, be sure to label the container clearly. The word *poison* should be prominently printed on it. Never use baby food jars or other familiar food containers to store poisons. Young children are likely to assume that they contain food and may help themselves.

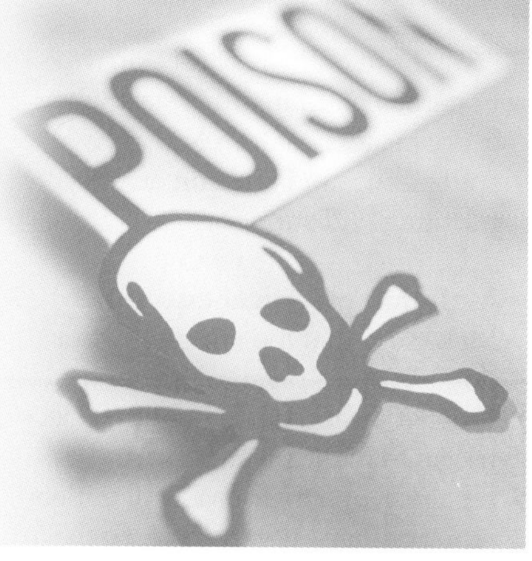

Household products

Common and potentially dangerous household poisons include:

- All products containing alcohol
- Cleaning products, especially those that contain chlorine bleach, ammonia and detergents
- Toilet and drain cleaners
- Paint and paint products such as turpentine and paint thinner
- Furniture and floor polishes
- Some cosmetics

Medications

Virtually all medications are poisonous, especially to a young child. Prescription medications, aspirin, acetaminophen (Tylenol, others), cough medicine, cold tablets and all other drugs must be stored on a high closet shelf or in a cabinet out of a child's reach. Also keep vitamins away from a child. Consumed in large quantities, they can be toxic.

Garden and garage items

Potentially dangerous garden and garage items include:

- All insecticides
- Mouse and rat pellets
- Weedkillers and flower, shrub and garden sprays and powders
- Fertilizers
- Farm chemicals
- Fuels and oils

Lawn Chemicals

Experts don't agree on the possible long-term health effects of exposure to lawn chemicals such as herbicides, pesticides and fertilizers.

The hundreds of chemicals used on lawns are registered with the Environmental Protection Agency (EPA). Registration by itself, though, doesn't ensure safety. The long-term health effects of some chemicals aren't known.

Two lawn chemical mainstays continue to receive scrutiny: diazinon and 2,4-D. Diazinon, an insecticide, has been banned by the EPA for use on golf courses and sod farms and is gradually being phased out. Its manufacture will end in 2003. The chemical is readily absorbed through skin and is toxic to birds. The herbicide 2,4-D, found in more than 100 landscaping and agricultural products, may be associated with a higher incidence of the cancer non-Hodgkin's lymphoma in dogs and, possibly, humans.

Recommendations

Be careful when using lawn chemicals. Wear waterproof gloves and shoes, a long-sleeved shirt, a breathing mask and protective goggles. Federal law requires you to follow instructions on pesticide labels. Many such chemicals are easily absorbed through skin and can be harmful if you inhale them.

Instead of relying on lawn chemicals, contact your local garden center, nursery or extension office to learn about nonchemical or low-chemical lawn care techniques.

Radon

The element uranium is found in soil and in rocks that contain granite, shale or phosphate. This means that uranium is also found in masonry building materials such as bricks and concrete.

As it decays, uranium releases a gas called radon. Generally, the gas is released in such small quantities that it's harmless. Sometimes, though, especially in the interior of some homes, radon can accumulate and reach a relatively high level. Radon decays to radioactive atoms that may attach themselves to dust particles and, when inhaled, may release small bursts of energy that can damage lung tissue and may increase a person's risk of lung cancer after many years of exposure.

Measuring radon

A commonly used measure of radioactivity in the United States is the curie. The Environmental Protection Agency urges you to take action if the average annual radon level in your home is 4 or more picocuries per liter of air. A picocurie is one-trillionth of a curie.

Several tests are available to measure radon levels. One is an alpha track detector. Available in hardware stores and supermarkets, this detector measures radon over several months to a year. Use at least two alpha track detectors in your home. Place one in the lowest level of your home that's a living area, such as a basement family room, and one in an upper living area, such as a bedroom. Follow the directions you receive with the testing device and return the device to the manufacturer as soon as the testing period ends. The manufacturer will send you the test results, usually within 2 weeks.

Reducing radon

If test results indicate that average radon levels in your home are more than 4 picocuries per liter of air, minor adjustments to your home may be recommended. Expensive remodeling is rarely required.

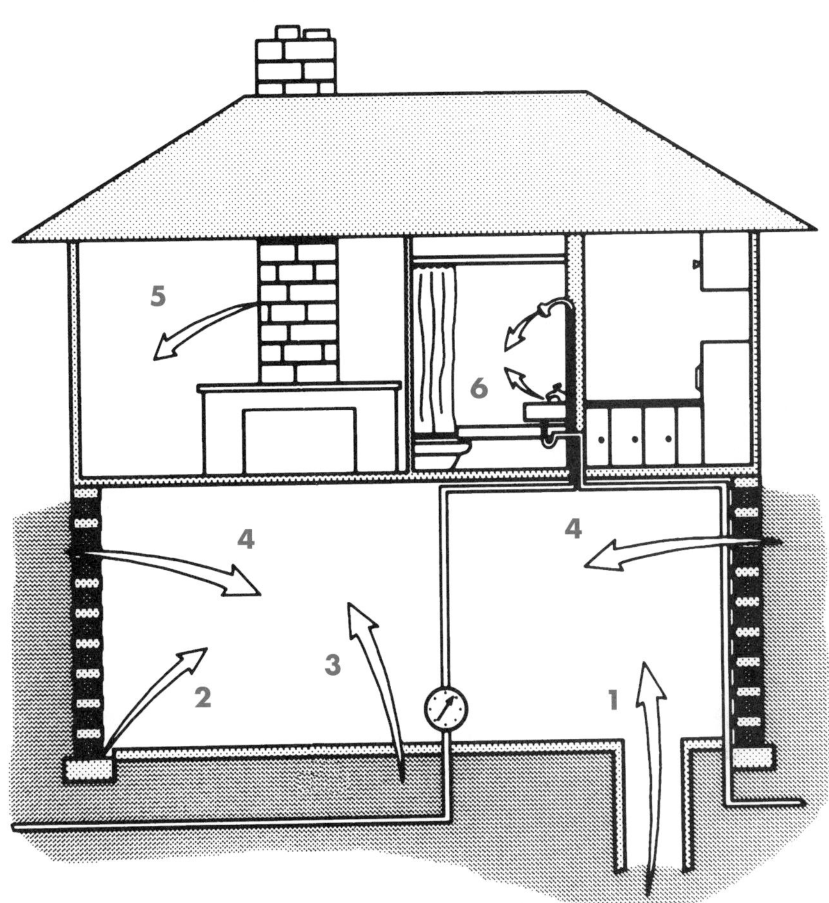

Here, in descending order of frequency, are the six most common routes by which radon can enter your home: (1) open sump pump, (2) gaps between wall-to-wall joints, (3) cracks in foundation floors and mortar joints, (4) pores in concrete blocks, (5) building materials and (6) water supply.

Try the following approaches:

- In the cellar or crawl space, cover large openings to the soil. Also cover sump pumps and vent them to the outside.
- Use a high-quality caulk that adheres to concrete to seal cracks and other openings in your basement floors and walls.
- Insulate the floor above any crawl space and keep vents open on all sides of your home to ventilate the basement or crawl space.
- If the radon reading is very high, you might consider installing a small fan that brings in fresh air. Another option is installation of an air-to-air heat exchanger. Retest your home after making changes to see if the radon level has decreased.

Drinking water

Many years ago, cholera, typhoid and other diseases caused by contaminated water left people worried about the safety of the water supply. Infectious disease is no longer a worry. Instead, the concern is about other contaminants — heavy metals, polychlorinated biphenyls (PCBs), pesticides and other chemicals.

Landfills, especially those in which hazardous wastes have been discarded, are potential sources of contamination. Outmoded or improperly maintained tanks at gas stations and fuel oil depots also may contaminate groundwater and wells. Industrial pollution or runoff

A Household Safety Checklist

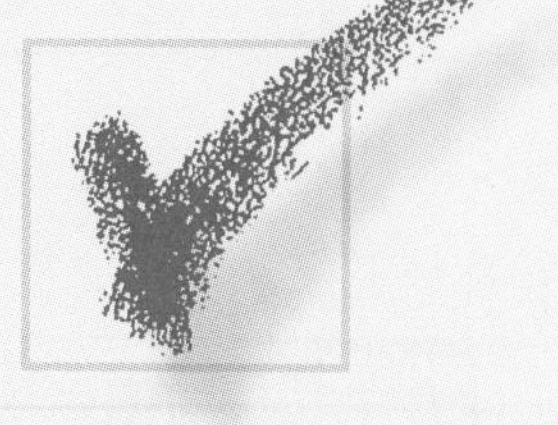

There's no such thing as an accident-free home. Accidents happen even to the most conscientious and careful people. However, you can decrease your risk of accident and injury at home by following these basic safety suggestions:

Kitchen

- *Clean up spills promptly.* Water, foods or other substances on a hard-surfaced floor can cause slips, falls and injuries.
- *Use a step stool to reach high shelves.* Don't stand on a chair or countertop.
- *Keep your kitchen knives stored out of the reach of children.* When using a knife to cut food, hold the food with your hand curled, not with your fingers extended.
- *Position pot and pan handles toward the back of the stove or counter.* If they protrude over the front, a careless movement or curious child could spill hot liquids or foods and cause a serious burn.
- *Keep grease and drippings away from open flames.* In case of a small kitchen fire, use salt, baking soda or a fire extinguisher to extinguish the flames. Don't throw water on the flames.
- *Unplug appliances not in use.* In particular, keep unused irons, toasters, food processors and coffee makers unplugged. Before washing or cleaning any electrical device, unplug it.
- *Store cleaning fluids and other chemicals in a high or locked cabinet.* Be sure that all poisons are safely stored and clearly marked.

Family and living rooms

- *Use a fire screen in front of a fireplace.* It prevents sparks from flying into the room.
- *Make sure no electrical cords cross the room.* They can trip you or, if worn, can cause a fire.
- *Keep drapery and window blind cords out of the reach of children.* Children may be tempted to play with the cords and can strangle themselves.
- *Regularly clean a humidifier.* Wash the water reservoir thoroughly on a regular schedule — at least once every 2 weeks when in use. Bacteria and fungi can grow in such moist environments and create a health hazard.

Bathroom

- *Don't use electrical appliances when you're wet.* This includes hair dryers and electric shavers. Electrical shock or death from electrocution can result.
- *Change all conventional bathroom outlets to ground-fault circuit interrupters.* Building codes in many states require them in new construction.
- *Use nonslip mats in and adjacent to the shower or bathtub.* They help prevent slips and falls. Grab rails also can prevent falls.
- *Never leave a baby or young child alone in the tub.* He or she can drown in only a small amount of water.
- *Keep all medicines safely out of the reach of children.* In addition, avoid discarding into the wastebasket razor blades, hypodermic needles or other potentially dangerous items.

Bedroom

- *Have a lamp within reach on your bedside table.* Turn it on when you get up at night, to avoid falling or running into something. Keep your glasses at hand too.
- *Keep medications out of reach.* This is especially true if young children visit your home.
- *Never smoke in bed.* Smoking in bed is particularly hazardous after drinking alcohol or when you're tired.
- *Unplug heating pads or electric blankets when they're not in use.* Left on, they can cause a fire.

Entrance and stairway

- *All stairs should be in good repair.* Replace broken or cracked stairs outside and within your home. Fasten carpeting on stairs securely. Every stairway should have a sturdy railing.
- *Maintain good lighting.* Make sure that the lighting in your hallways is bright. Place a switch at the bottom and top of each set of stairs.
- *Never leave objects on stairs.* Leaving an object on the stairs increases the risk of someone's stepping on it and falling. In addition, don't wax stairways or stair landings.

Utility room and basement

- *Maintain good lighting.* Install appropriate lighting fixtures near the washing machine and dryer, workbench and entrance areas.
- *Have your washing machine, dryer, furnace and hot water heater serviced regularly.* Make sure that your dryer is vented and that both the dryer and washing machine are grounded. Regularly clean out the lint tray in the dryer and replace the air filters in your furnace.
- *Keep detergents, cleaning products and chemicals out of the reach of children.* Try not to place these products in different containers. If you do, make sure to label them well.
- *Place a fire extinguisher in the basement or utility room.* Familiarize yourself with how to use it and check it periodically to make sure that it's fully charged.

from agricultural lands that have been treated with certain chemical fertilizers and pesticides may contaminate rivers, streams, lakes and groundwater.

The Environmental Protection Agency and local and state organizations are responsible for monitoring public water supplies. If your water comes from a well, test it every year for pollutants. If results indicate a problem, take steps to improve your water. A county public health official can provide guidance or put you in contact with the appropriate individual or agency.

Using bottled water may or may not be the answer. It's expensive, and often the water in bottles is no better than water from your tap. Boiling water is another option if your water is contaminated with bacteria, but this won't remove contaminants such as lead. Commercially available filters may help, although claims made for them sometimes exceed their actual usefulness.

Safety Outside the Home

Most accidents occur at home, but not far behind are accidents on the road, during recreation or at the workplace.

Safety on the road

Approximately 50,000 people die on the nation's roads and highways every year. Many more individuals are severely injured. This terrible toll is more often the result of alcohol or carelessness than it is of mechanical failure.

To help ensure your safety:

Always wear a seat belt

Seat belts save lives. Wear one every time you get into a car, even if you're traveling only a short distance. Most accidents occur within a few miles of home. Make sure your passengers wear seat belts too.

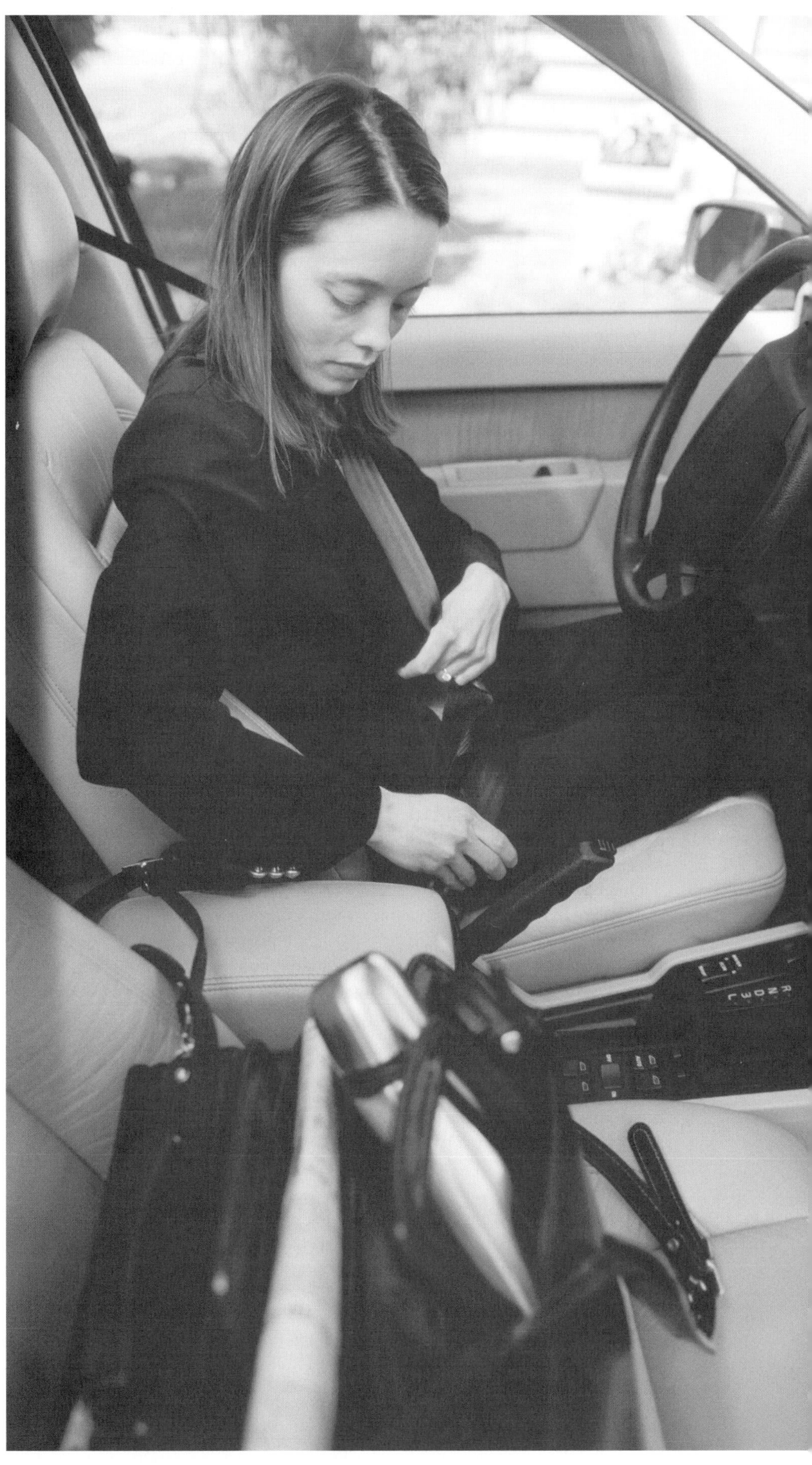

Place children in car seats
In most states, children who weigh less than 40 pounds must ride in specially designed car seats. Even if your state doesn't have this law, always buckle up your baby or young child when traveling by car. For more information on car and booster seats, see pages 165 and 201.

Get training
If you're operating a motorcycle, motorbike or all-terrain vehicle, consider taking a drivers' education course to learn how to operate the vehicle properly. Know the laws for that vehicle, and as with any motorized vehicle, don't drink and drive.

Drive defensively
Driving legally and sensibly isn't enough. If other drivers aren't capable or being careful, they can be the cause of an accident. Never assume that other drivers will drive responsibly. Driving defensively means that you're aware of other cars at all times and are prepared to take evasive action. Be prepared to react promptly if another driver suddenly makes an unexpected maneuver.

Don't follow other cars too closely. For every 10 miles per hour (mph) of speed, allow one car length between you and the car in front of you. At 50 mph, five car lengths or about 100 feet should separate you from the car ahead.

Make sure that your visibility is clear at all angles. Don't allow accumulation of objects to block your rear view. Learn where the blind spots are in your car.

Consider the weather
When it's snowing or raining or if visibility is reduced for any reason, slow down. If conditions become severe, don't travel until they improve. Be ready for the unexpected. In very cold weather, carry in your vehicle food, blankets and cold-weather clothing. Keep your gas tank as full as possible.

Don't drink and drive
Don't drive after consuming alcoholic beverages or when you've taken medications that make you drowsy or impair your reaction time. If you feel especially tired or ill, someone else should get behind the wheel.

Avoid distractions
Control the behavior of children in your car. Don't let the radio, an interesting conversation or a roadside attraction distract you from your driving.

Keep your car maintained
Service your car at the recommended intervals. Obeying proper maintenance schedules can help ensure that a mechanical failure won't cause a highway mishap.

Bicycle safety

Bicycling is a great form of recreation, but like most recreational activities, it's important to take steps to promote safety.

Wear a helmet
Three of four cyclists killed in cycle-related accidents die of head injuries. Wearing a helmet is a sensible precaution. Your helmet should have a durable outer shell and a polystyrene liner. Adjustable foam pads help ensure a proper fit at the front, back and sides, and the straps should hold it snug.

Ride with traffic
Wrong-way riders are much more likely to be involved in accidents with motor vehicles. In addition, all 50 states require cyclists to go with the traffic flow.

Follow traffic rules
Stop at stop signs. They're for bicycles as well as cars. Look both ways before proceeding. Before turning, always look back, signal and check for traffic.

Watch out for water
In wet conditions, braking ability is greatly decreased. Watch out for fallen wet leaves in the autumn. They can be slippery and hazardous.

Bicycle defensively
Make eye contact with other riders, drivers and pedestrians. Watch out for potholes, rubbish in your path and other hazards. Know your own reaction time and other skills. Beware of motorists who may be inclined to make a right turn into or in front of you.

Water and boating safety

The No. 1 rule of water safety is that everyone, young and old, should know how to swim. It's never too late to learn.

Swimming
If you have an outdoor pool, install a childproof fence around it and never let a child play or swim in it

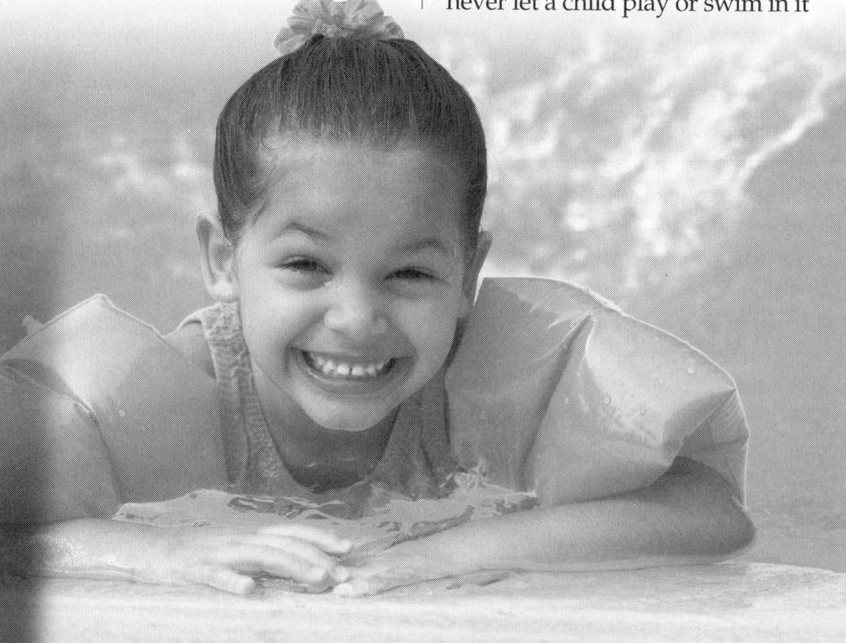

without adult supervision. In a pool or lake, it's a good idea not to swim alone, even if you're an excellent swimmer. Don't dive into the water without first checking its depth and looking beneath the surface for obstructions that may pose a risk. Don't go swimming if you've been consuming alcoholic beverages, a storm is threatening or boats or fishermen are operating in the immediate vicinity.

Flotation devices designed to be worn on the arms can be used for toddlers, but avoid flotation vests on toddlers. They can actually cause drowning.

Boating

When operating a boat or personal watercraft, always wear a personal flotation device (PFD), even if you're a good swimmer. Have as many PFDs on board as there are passengers. Don't overload your boat or personal watercraft and be sure that the operator is familiar with its workings and is qualified to drive it. When towing skiers, designate someone as a spotter to watch for downed skiers. Stay off the water in dangerous weather conditions. If your watercraft capsizes, stay with it until help arrives. Don't try to swim to shore.

Hiking and camping safety

The outdoors can be a wonderful place for exercise, fun and experiencing nature firsthand. Without proper consideration of the risks, however, a casual hike in the woods can be a dangerous or even life-threatening activity.

Recognize your limits

Suit your outdoor activity to your physical condition.

Plan ahead

If you're visiting an unfamiliar area, map your route in advance. Take the map with you and locate your position on it from time to time. Know the weather forecast and monitor changes as you travel. Let someone know where you're going and when you plan to arrive and return.

Dress for the occasion

Sturdy shoes are important for hiking. If you're hiking up a mountain, be prepared for climate changes. It'll probably be cooler or damper on top. Desert areas have unusually wide swings in temperature from midday to nighttime.

Carry appropriate equipment

Plan ahead and be sure that you have what you need for your outdoor adventure. Always carry first aid supplies when camping.

Be cautious around animals

If wild animals are acting oddly, rabies may be the cause, so stay clear of them. In addition, don't approach a young animal. A protective mother may be nearby. Don't keep food in your tent because it may attract unwanted animals. Rather, put it in a bag or pack and hang it from a nearby tree.

Don't drink the water

Never drink water from a stream or lake unless you've filtered or treated it as described below. Even if the water looks crystal clear, it may be contaminated with bacteria and parasites. In fact, drinking water from a rushing mountain stream is more likely to cause illness than is drinking from a placid lake because the parasites can't settle to the bottom.

You can make the water safe for drinking by using one of the following methods:

- Filtering it with a portable water filter, available at outdoor stores
- Boiling it for a minimum of 3 minutes
- Treating it with water purification tablets

Douse your campfire

Never risk the safety of other campers and animals by failing to drown your campfire.

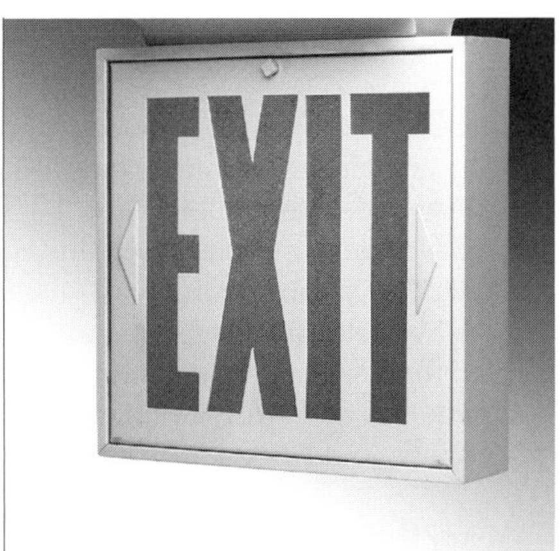

Hotel fire safety

Most hotels are safe from fire because they're protected by sprinklers and other precautions required by law. But the unexpected can happen. Therefore it's always good to take a few simple precautions:

- On arrival, find the two exits nearest your room. Determine where they go and make sure they're unlocked. Locate the fire alarm nearest your room.
- Once inside your room, familiarize yourself with its layout because if it were to become smoke filled, you wouldn't be able to see clearly. Review the hotel's fire safety information.
- If the fire alarm sounds, feel your door before you open it. If it's hot, don't open it. Instead, telephone for help. If your door is cool, open it slowly. Be alert for smoke and flames in the hall and go to the nearest exit. Take your room key with you. If smoke or flames block your exit, you may have to return to your room.
- If the fire is nearby and you're forced to stay in your room, telephone for help, turn off all air-conditioning and heating systems, and open your window slightly for ventilation. If smoke seeps into your room, soak sheets and towels with water and stuff them under and around the door to block out heat and smoke. Hold a wet washcloth over your face to keep cool and to filter out smoke particles.
- Never use elevators during a fire.

Safety in the workplace

In recent years, the Occupational Safety and Health Administration (OSHA) and state and local agencies have made important gains in eliminating hazards in the workplace. Yet potential dangers remain. Be on the alert for dangers and protect yourself and others by following safety guidelines.

Wear protective eyewear
If your job carries a risk of eye injury, your employer is required by law to provide you with protective glasses, and you're required to wear them. Wear them whenever you're operating machinery or are exposed to fumes or particles in the air that could endanger your eyes.

Wear protective ear devices
If your job carries a risk of ear injury, your employer is required by law to provide you with hearing protectors. Specially designed earmuffs are available. Some types close out the outside world. Others are fitted with earphones and a microphone that enable you to communicate with other workers.

Custom-molded earplugs or commercially available earplugs made of foam, plastic or rubber also effectively decrease your exposure to excessive noise. Cotton balls aren't adequate and can get stuck deep in your ear canal.

Take precautions around fumes, smoke, dust and gases
A wide variety of respiratory symptoms can result from exposure to toxic fumes, gases, dust particles and smoke in the workplace. A sampling of dangerous chemicals includes ammonia, cyanides, formaldehyde, acid fumes, hydrogen sulfide, diazomethane, halides, nitrogen dioxide, isocyanates, ozone, phosgene, phthalic anhydride and sulfur dioxide.

The processing of metals such as cadmium, chromium, nickel, beryllium, copper, magnesium and zinc can produce dangerous fumes. Dust diseases, including asbestosis (from asbestos), silicosis (from silica), byssinosis (from cotton) and miners' disorders such as black lung disease, generally result from long-term inhalation of dust particles.

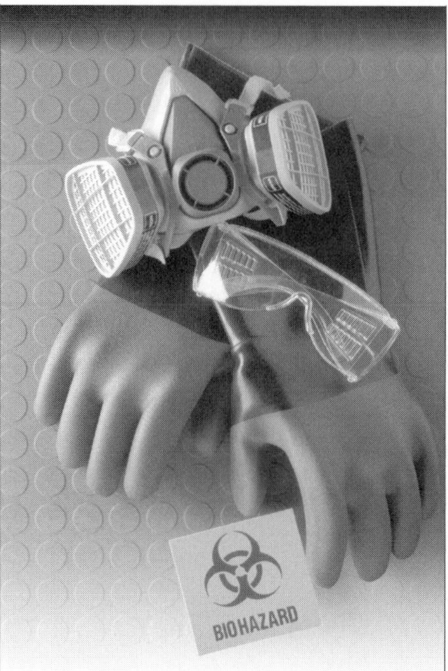

Workers who use high levels of heat, such as during welding, brazing, smelting, pottery making and furnace work, also are at risk of injury.

If your job involves any of these potential dangers, be sure to obey safety precautions posted in your workplace. Be especially careful if you handle hazardous materials. Wear proper clothing, an air-filtration mask, eyewear and other appropriate protection. Be sure the ventilation is adequate and make sure that you're familiar with the hazards of the substances with which you work.

If you're pregnant or trying to become pregnant, avoid any exposure to hazardous chemicals. If you suspect that you're at risk of exposure to dangerous smoke, fumes, dust or chemicals in your workplace, discuss the matter with your doctor. Many permanent respiratory ailments develop slowly as a result of industrial exposure over a period of years. Small exposures that may seem harmless can result in chronic disease.

Avoid alcohol, drugs and certain medications
Don't consume alcohol before or during work hours and never use illegal drugs. If you're taking medication that may make you drowsy, don't operate machinery.

Limit shift changes
If your job entails constant changing of shifts, your body will have more difficulty adjusting and readjusting as you get older. Some studies suggest that too-frequent shift changes over a lengthy period of time can put you at an increased risk of cardiovascular disease or peptic ulcer. In addition, fatigue can lead to injury and error in the workplace.

If you must rotate shifts:

- Work a shift for 3 weeks rather than rotating to a different schedule every week.
- Follow a sequence that goes day-evening-night. Research suggests that a more normal sleep pattern results when the shift sequence is day-evening-night rather than day-night-evening. ■

CHAPTER 10 PART I

Staying Healthy When Traveling

Each year, millions of Americans travel within the United States and abroad. Packing appropriate clothes and getting a passport and visa in order are activities that most travelers take for granted. Equally important, but often overlooked, is making sure you're properly immunized before traveling abroad, especially if you're traveling to a developing country. Also anticipate and plan for minor medical problems that could occur while traveling. About one in four people experience some type of illness or injury while traveling. Each year, a half million travelers need medical attention or require hospitalization.

Pre-travel Planning

If you're traveling, especially if you're going to a foreign country, it's important not to wait until the last minute to make all of your preparations. If you have a medical condition or if you may need vaccinations, it's especially important to see a doctor early. Follow these tips for a smoother trip:

Prepare 2 to 3 months ahead

As soon as you know your travel destinations, contact your doctor to see if you'll need any immunizations. Some immunizations require a series of vaccinations that you need to start several weeks to months before you leave. If you're planning to stay in a developing country for longer than 1 to 3 months, you may need to start your vaccinations 6 months before your departure.

If you have underlying health conditions such as heart disease, high blood pressure or diabetes, or you're disabled, discuss with your doctor any problems that you might anticipate and recommendations for dealing with them. If you take medication, you'll want to make sure that you take enough with you.

Talk to your doctor or pharmacist about advance filling of your prescriptions. Also talk to your doctor about what medications or medical supplies you should carry with you. All of this can be discussed with your primary doctor or with a travel medicine doctor.

Inquire about nearby medical facilities

Your travel guide or a travel medicine doctor may be able to supply you with information on hospitals near the destinations at which you'll be staying. The American embassy or consulate in the country you'll travel to also may be able to provide you with a list of hospitals and English-speaking doctors. Another reference for a list of medical facilities in the country to which you'll be traveling is the organization International Association for Medical Assistance to Travellers (see page 1383).

See your dentist

Don't let the excruciating pain of a toothache spoil your trip as you fly in a pressurized airplane cabin or bite into an unfamiliar delicacy. Have any needed dental work done before you leave.

Be aware of health precautions at your destination

High altitudes or severe air pollution, often a problem in large, foreign cities, can be a health risk for some individuals with chronic health conditions. Talk to your doctor about how to avoid or handle these situations.

Consider travel protection insurance

If you need medical care, most foreign doctors and hospitals won't bill your American insurance company directly. Rather, they'll require cash in advance or at least verification of your ability to pay for their services. You'll need to seek reimbursement when you return home.

Medicare doesn't pay for foreign medical services. Some travel protection insurance plans offer imme-

Travel Clinics

During the last decade, many travel clinics have been established across the United States. Services at travel clinics vary widely. Some offer vaccinations and informational handouts. Others offer comprehensive overviews on infectious diseases and other hazards you may encounter on a particular itinerary and detailed advice on how to minimize your risk of these illnesses. Some travel clinics are staffed with doctors trained in diagnosing and managing illness acquired while traveling in other countries.

In general, it's useful to see a travel medicine physician before any travel, but especially for prolonged travel — 4 weeks or more — to any country and before travel to Asia, Africa or Latin America. If you have a medical condition, it's particularly important that you see someone before you travel.

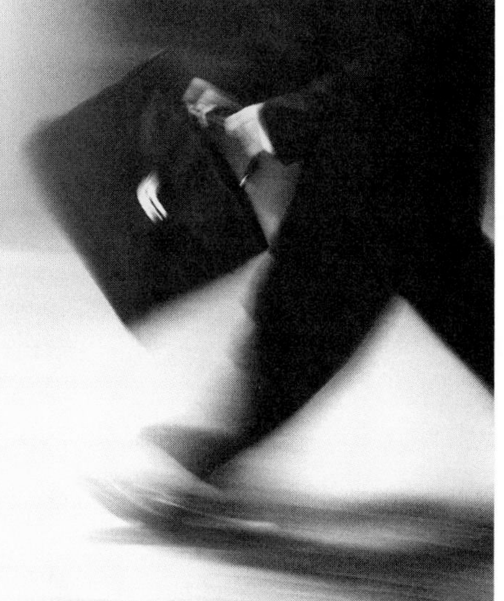

diate hospital deposit, emergency travel arrangements and, if necessary, emergency air evacuation. Ask your travel agent or insurance agent for detailed information.

Immunizations and Precautions

Many countries have immunization requirements that travelers must fulfill before entering. These are listed in the booklet *Health Information for International Travel*, updated regularly by the Centers for Disease Control and Prevention and published by the U.S. Government Printing Office.

You can also ask your doctor, your local travel clinic, local or state health department or the consulate or embassy of the country that you plan to visit about required immunizations.

Every adult and child should have up-to-date immunity against tetanus, polio, measles, mumps and rubella. Other immunizations you may need depend on the country you're visiting and perhaps the region of that country. For diseases in which a vaccine isn't available or isn't recommended, take precautions.

Generally, you're more likely to be exposed to an infectious disease in a rural area than in an urban one, particularly in less-developed countries. This is because water supply systems and sanitary conditions may not be as up-to-date in rural areas.

Diseases or conditions for which you may need to be vaccinated or take precautions include:

Cholera

Although a tourist's risk of acquiring cholera in affected areas is extremely low, travelers to areas with epidemic cholera should follow

A Medical Kit

When traveling abroad, it's a wise idea to take with you a list of past or present major illnesses, in addition to medications that you take and first aid supplies.

Medications

Make sure that you have an ample supply of medications that you or anyone in your family takes regularly. Prescriptions should be up-to-date. Keep prescription medications in their original pharmacy containers with the labels intact. This can help you avoid problems if security or customs officials check for illicit drugs.

Transport your medications and first aid kit in your carry-on luggage, in case your checked luggage is missing on arrival. An extra supply of essential medications kept in your checked luggage also is a good idea in case you stay longer than you anticipated or you lose your carry-on baggage. Be sure to include any special medications your doctor recommends, such as for motion sickness if that's a problem for you.

Taking a simple first aid kit with you is a sensible precaution. Supplies might include alcohol wipes, antiseptic cream, adhesive and gauze bandages, aspirin or acetaminophen, a thermometer, elastic wrap for sprains, insect repellent, sunscreen, lip balm, an antacid, a mild laxative and a decongestant. Also include sunglasses and a second pair of prescription glasses or contact lenses with more wetting and cleaning solutions than you would ordinarily use.

Medical records

In case of illness or an emergency, the doctor you consult on your trip will need to know something about your medical history. Carry a brief medical report in your wallet or a location where it's easily accessible. Make sure other members of your family or traveling group know where it is so that they can quickly and easily provide relevant information to any medical professional who may need it.

The medical information should include the following:

- Your name, address, telephone number, Social Security number and person to notify in case of an emergency.
- Your health status, including any chronic diseases you have or any allergies to medications, food or insects.
- Recent test results of any abnormalities for comparison in an emergency.
- A list of your medications and eyeglass or contact lens prescription for easier replacement. For medications, include the generic and brand names (if any) and the doses and frequency at which you take them. Also include typewritten copies of your prescriptions in case you lose your medication and need to have it refilled during your trip.
- Your immunization record, including dates you received your vaccines. Some countries require certificates of vaccination against diseases such as yellow fever.
- The name, address and telephone number of your primary care doctor.

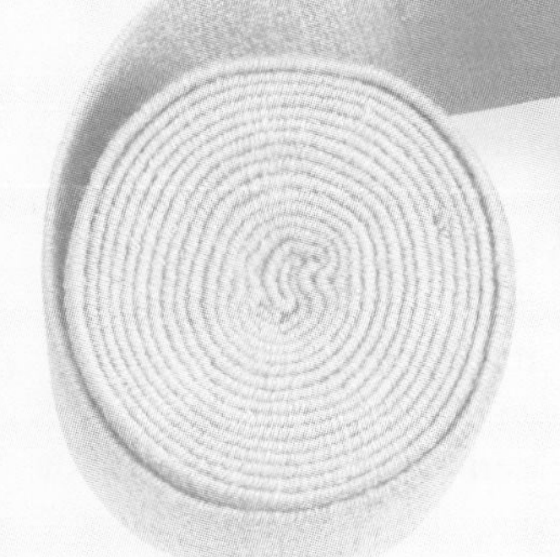

food and water precautions. The general rule, "Boil it, cook it, peel it, or forget it," can help prevent cholera.

If you're traveling to an area with cholera, don't consume:

- Unboiled or untreated water, or ice made from such water
- Food and beverages offered by street vendors
- Raw or partially cooked fish or shellfish
- Uncooked vegetables

Eat only foods that are cooked and hot or fruits that you peel yourself. Carbonated bottled water and carbonated soft drinks are usually safe if no ice is added.

A cholera vaccination protects approximately 50 percent of vaccinated individuals for 3 to 6 months. It generally isn't recommended or available in the United States. The vaccine also isn't a substitute for carefully watching what you eat and drink. If you develop severe watery diarrhea or diarrhea and vomiting during or within 1 week after travel to an area known to have cholera, seek immediate medical attention.

Hepatitis A

Vaccination for hepatitis A is recommended for all travelers to any area of the world where sanitation is poor. Hepatitis A is generally contracted from contaminated food or water or from contact with someone who's infected.

Hepatitis B

Get vaccinated for hepatitis B if you plan to travel for more than a month to an area where hepatitis B is prevalent, such as Southeast Asia, Africa, the Middle East, some islands in the Pacific, Haiti or the Dominican Republic, or if you're at high risk of the disease. People at increased risk include those handling blood or blood products, homosexuals, illicit drug users or individuals staying more than 6 months in a developing country.

Flu (influenza)

Individuals at high risk of serious illness from the flu (influenza) should be vaccinated before leaving the country. This includes older adults and individuals with a chronic illness. High-risk individuals should receive the influenza vaccine in the spring or summer months if traveling to the Southern Hemisphere, during the fall or winter months if traveling to countries in the Northern Hemisphere or anytime if traveling to the tropics.

Japanese encephalitis

Talk with your doctor about a vaccine for Japanese encephalitis if you're traveling to areas of Southeast Asia or the Indian Subcontinent, especially if you'll be traveling in rural areas or you're staying longer than 4 weeks. This vaccination series takes at least 2 to 6 weeks to complete, and it should be completed at least 10 days before you depart, in case side effects from the vaccination need attention.

Malaria

There's no vaccine against malaria, but effective preventive medications are available. In most countries of the world where malaria exists, resistance has developed to the medication chloroquine. Depending on the malaria endemic to the area you'll be traveling to, your doctor may prescribe chloroquine or another antimalarial medication such as mefloquine or primaquine.

You want to start taking this medication before you leave home and continue to take it during your travel and for a period of time after leaving the area. Discuss with your doctor possible adverse reactions to the medication. Your doctor will want to review your past and current medical history for any indications that you shouldn't take the medication.

Because malaria infection often mimics a flu-like illness or some other viral disease, be wary if you develop an illness with fever within 12 months after traveling to a malaria-prone area. Tell your doctor about your trip. A blood test can determine if you have the disease.

Other preventive measures include avoiding mosquito bites, which is how malaria is transmitted to humans. Stay in dwellings with screens on exterior doors and windows or sleep under mosquito netting. Spray rooms with insecticide and use mosquito repellent on exposed parts of your body and on your pillow at night. Effective repellents are those that contain DEET.

Avoid being outside between dusk and dawn. If you must be outside, wear protective clothing, apply repellents to exposed skin and move about as much as possible.

Measles

You may need the measles vaccine before going abroad if you previously had none or only one dose. If you were born before 1957, you're more than likely immune to measles and may not need the vaccine. In some situations, a blood test can be done to check your immunity to measles.

Meningitis

If you're traveling to regions such as sub-Saharan Africa where a certain type of meningitis — meningococcal meningitis — is prevalent, get the meningococcal vaccine. It's recommended before entry into Saudi Arabia for travelers going to Mecca during the annual hajj pilgrimage.

Plague

Vaccination against the plague consists of three injections, each given a month or more apart. It's given to people traveling to areas where the disease is still prevalent. This vaccine isn't available in the United States, and it's rarely advised for regular tourists.

Pneumonia

Several weeks before departure, adults age 65 and older and individuals with a chronic illness should receive the pneumococcal pneumonia vaccine if they haven't already been vaccinated. Once a person receives this vaccine, no further doses are generally necessary, with some exceptions.

If you had your first shot before age 65, you may need a 5-year booster shot. If you've had your spleen removed or you have another chronic illness that puts you at increased risk of pneumonia, you may need a repeat dose in 5 years.

Polio

For people who've had their childhood polio immunizations, a booster shot of the inactivated vaccine may be recommended for travel to some developing areas of the world, such as Africa, Asia, the Middle East and most areas of the former Soviet Union.

Rabies

If you plan to stay for more than a month in areas where rabies is common or you're likely to have extensive exposure to animals, you may want to acquire immunity to the disease before leaving by obtaining rabies vaccine doses.

Smallpox

Smallpox was eradicated as of 1977. Vaccination against the disease is unnecessary for travel.

Tetanus and diphtheria

A booster dose of adult tetanus-diphtheria (Td) toxoid is recommended every 10 years. Every child and adult should have up-to-date immunity at all times. If you have a contaminated wound and it has been more than 5 years since you last received a tetanus booster, get a booster dose.

Typhoid

If you're traveling to a country where typhoid is prevalent, your doctor may suggest that you receive a weakened live oral vaccine or an injectable vaccine. The oral vaccine is generally effective for up to 5 years, and the injectable vaccine is effective for 2 years.

In the United States, both the oral and the injectable vaccines are available. If you live in a country where typhoid is prevalent for an extended period of time, the oral or injectable vaccine should be repeated every 5 or 2 years, respectively, as long as you remain there.

Yellow fever

If you're traveling to certain areas of Africa and South America where yellow fever is widespread, get the live virus vaccine. This vaccine is available only at certain yellow fever vaccination centers. You also need to repeat the vaccination at least every 10 years.

Common Ailments of Travelers

Traveling can cause a variety of illnesses. Most often, the illness is related to a chronic condition. For example, individuals with circulatory problems are at increased risk of formation of a blood clot in a leg if confined to a tight space and unable to move for a considerable period, such as on a long airplane trip. A few conditions, though, tend to be fairly common during travel.

Altitude sickness

Signs and symptoms

- Headache
- Shortness of breath with mild exertion
- Fatigue
- Nausea
- Disturbed sleep
- Loss of appetite

Emergency signs and symptoms

- Severe breathing difficulty

Altitude sickness may occur when people who live in a low altitude make a trip to an altitude of more than 8,000 feet. It usually develops several hours after arriving at a high altitude. Skiers, hikers or others who travel to mountain slopes from lower elevations are often affected, especially if they fly into the high-elevation area.

How serious is altitude sickness?

Many people experience mild to moderate symptoms that generally resolve as the individual becomes adjusted to the change in altitude. However, symptoms can persist for several days. Rarely, some people experience a more severe form of altitude sickness that can produce severe breathing distress or severe brain illness. This is a medical emergency that can be fatal if not treated.

Treatment

Increasing intake of fluids and carbohydrates can help minimize the effects of mild altitude sickness. Rest is also helpful. For serious altitude sickness, get the affected person to a lower altitude and, if possible, provide him or her with oxygen.

Prevention

To avoid altitude sickness:

- *Allow time to adjust.* Rest a day after arriving to help you get used to the altitude.
- *Ascend slowly.* If possible, begin at an altitude below 6,000 feet.
- *Limit ascent.* Don't climb more than 3,000 feet a day or 1,000 feet if you're at 12,000 feet or above.
- *Take it easy.* Slow down if you're out of breath or tired.
- *Sleep at a lower altitude.* If you're above 11,000 feet during the day, sleep at 9,000 feet or lower if possible.

- *Avoid cigarettes and alcohol.* They worsen symptoms.
- *Consider medication.* Ask your doctor about acetazolamide (Diamox, Storzolamide) or other prescription medications that may prevent or lessen symptoms.

Jet lag

Signs and symptoms

- Fatigue, drowsiness
- Irritability
- Difficulty sleeping
- Loss of mental acuity
- Minor coordination problems

If you've ever traveled by air across several time zones, you're probably familiar with what it's like to experience jet lag — that dragged-out, out-of-sync feeling that can affect your pattern of eating, working, relaxing and sleeping. Jet lag results from the readjustment you demand of your body when traveling across time zones.

How serious is jet lag?

Flying eastward — and thus resetting your body clock forward — is often more difficult than flying westward and adding hours to your day. Flying north or south doesn't produce jet lag. Most people's bodies adjust at the rate of about 1 hour a day. If you pass through four time zones, for example, that means that your body may require about 4 days to re-synchronize its usual rhythms.

Prevention

To prevent jet lag or help reduce its effects:

Reset your body clock

Begin resetting your body's clock several days in advance of your departure by adopting a sleep-wake pattern similar to the day-night cycle at your destination. Or try setting your watch to the time of your destination while on the airplane so that you start thinking in terms of the new time.

Another strategy is to try to schedule your arrival at your destination at roughly your usual bedtime, according to the clocks in the time zone to which you're flying. Or try sleeping on the plane and plan to arrive at the hour you usually start your day. In these ways, you immediately begin to orient your body to the new time schedule.

Getting added sleep before departure also may help reduce jet lag. Alternatively, if you have an important event or meeting at your destination, get there 2 or 3 days in advance. That way, you won't be disadvantaged by jet lag.

Drink plenty of fluids and eat lightly

Drink extra liquids during your flight to avoid dehydration, but limit beverages with alcohol and caffeine. They increase dehydration and may disrupt your sleep.

Limit your intake of salty or fatty food. If you have a special diet, be sure to follow it. Many airlines offer special meals, but you'll need to make arrangements in advance.

Adjust your medication schedule

If you're on a regimen of medications, you may have to make adjustments as to when you take them to account for changes in time zones. Check with your doctor before leaving. If you have diabetes and are taking long-acting insulin, you may have to switch to regular insulin until you adjust to your new time change, food and activities. However, be sure to discuss the time change with your doctor.

Motion sickness

Signs and symptoms

- Restlessness that may progress to a cold sweat
- Dizziness
- Vomiting

Any type of transportation can produce motion sickness. You may experience motion sickness in a plane, on a boat, on a train or in a car.

Motion sickness results from increased activity of inner structures that control balance. The increased activity is often brought on by the motion of a vehicle. As soon as the motion stops, symptoms generally begin to improve.

How serious is motion sickness?

The illness isn't serious, but it can ruin a vacation. Some people find that the more they travel, the more their body adjusts to being in motion.

Prevention

If you're susceptible to motion sickness, try the following:

- In a ship, request a cabin in the middle, near the waterline.

Move Around

During a long trip, take time to stretch and walk. Extended sitting can put you at risk of a potentially fatal condition in which a blood clot forms in your leg, breaks loose and blocks an artery in your lung (pulmonary embolism).

Support hose also can help prevent clots or swelling of your feet and ankles during lengthy airline flights or train, bus or car trips. But avoid socks or stockings with tight elastic tops that constrict your legs and interfere with blood circulation.

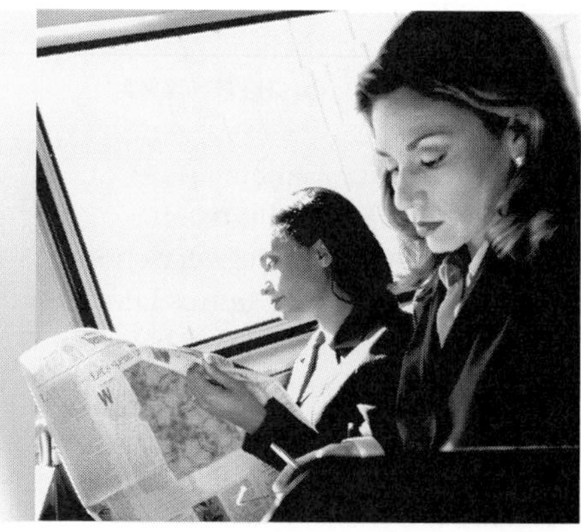

- On a plane, ask for a seat over the front edge of a wing.
- On a train, sit near a window and face forward.
- In an automobile, drive, or sit in the front passenger's seat.
- Keep your head still, rested against a chair back.
- Sleep or lie down.
- If you're on a boat, breathe plenty of fresh air.
- Avoid spicy foods and alcohol and don't overeat.
- Don't read.

Take an over-the-counter antihistamine such as meclizine (Bonine, Simply Motion) or dimenhydrinate (Dramamine, Calm-X) before you feel sick, unless your doctor advises otherwise. Expect drowsiness as a side effect.

Ask your doctor about the scopolamine patch (Transderm Scop). You need a prescription for this patch. You place the dime-sized patch behind your ear before you experience symptoms of motion sickness. One patch works for up to 3 days.

Traveler's diarrhea

Signs and symptoms

- Diarrhea
- Abdominal cramps

Traveler's diarrhea, turista, Montezuma's revenge, and Tut's tummy are familiar names for this common ailment of travelers. A trip to a foreign country by no means guarantees a bout with gastrointestinal discomfort. But if you travel to a country where the climate, social conditions or sanitary standards and practices are different from yours at home — particularly in developing nations — risk of traveler's diarrhea may be high.

Traveler's diarrhea may be attributed to a number of causes, including consuming food and drink that you're unaccustomed to, a difference in living habits and a change in the balance of bacteria that naturally live in your bowel. Usually, the problem is related to inadequate sanitation. Contaminated food and water may contain bacteria, viruses or parasites that cause diarrhea and abdominal cramps.

Replacing Lost Fluids

If you experience severe weakness after a bout of traveler's diarrhea, your body may have lost an excessive amount of fluids and minerals. If medical help is unavailable, prepare the following solution to help correct the problem. Mix 1/2 teaspoon of table salt (sodium chloride), 1/2 teaspoon of baking soda (sodium bicarbonate) and 4 tablespoons of table sugar (sucrose) in 1 quart of carbonated water. If carbonated water isn't available, bottled water or tap water boiled for 15 minutes is a suitable substitute. Drink the mixture over the course of the day, as a supplement to a clear liquid diet.

How serious is traveler's diarrhea?

Traveler's diarrhea most often begins abruptly while traveling or shortly after you return home. Usually, it's mild and subsides in 3 or 4 days, but you may not feel well for several more days. Sometimes, traveler's diarrhea can be more troublesome. If it's caused by organisms other than common bacteria, symptoms may be more severe, long-lasting and difficult to overcome. Medication is often needed to rid your body of the organism.

Treatment

If you do get traveler's diarrhea, drink plenty of safe liquids to replace lost fluids, salts and minerals. It's important not to get dehydrated. Orange, apple or other fruit juices are good for replacing lost potassium, but remember to avoid juices diluted with tap water. Broth, sweetened tea and soft drinks also are good for keeping up your strength.

As soon as you feel like eating again, start with fat-free, soft foods to avoid irritating your intestinal system. Bananas are a good source of potassium and can help slow diarrhea. Bland cereals, rice, gelatin, jellied consomme, simple puddings and soft-cooked eggs are other possibilities.

Some travelers take antibiotics as a preventive measure — even though public health experts discourage this — and other travelers pack the medications and take them only if symptoms develop. Most doctors recommend that you take only prescription drugs that relieve symptoms when they occur.

Paregoric or codeine and newer synthetic drugs such as loperamide (Imodium, Kaopectate) often ease cramps and diarrhea and can be taken orally. Although some authorities believe that these medications may prolong diarrhea and cramps, most people are pleased with the prompt relief the drugs offer. These medications shouldn't be taken if diarrhea is bloody.

Prevention

To reduce your risk of traveler's diarrhea when traveling to a foreign country, take the following precautions:

Talk to your doctor about preventive medications

No vaccines offer protection against traveler's diarrhea. You might consider taking bismuth subsalicylate (Pepto-Bismol, Bismate) tablets throughout your trip as a preventive measure. Doing so can decrease your risk of diarrhea.

Bismuth subsalicylate can turn your stools a dark charcoal color, so don't be alarmed if this occurs. In addition, talk with your doctor about use of bismuth subsalicylate, as well as other medications, should symptoms develop.

Watch what you drink

The first rule of thumb for avoiding diarrhea while traveling is to not drink the water unless it has been sterilized — whether it comes from a stream, a well or a tap. Bottled water may be safe, if it's factory bottled.

You can also purchase from camping stores a water-filter pump that removes many microorganisms. Check to see that the pump you're considering has a microfilter that prevents passage of parasites.

Iodine tablets or crystals, which you can also purchase at camping stores, kill most microbes. Be sure to follow the directions and allow the treatment to continue long enough before drinking the water. Drinking large amounts of water containing iodine isn't recommended.

At some of the newer resort hotels, you may be able to drink tap water if the water treatment system is up-to-date, but don't rely on it. Often, tourists will conscientiously avoid drinking water from the tap, only to come down with traveler's diarrhea from drinking beverages that contain ice.

If the water used to make ice isn't free of bacteria, when the ice melts into your drink, you'll be exposed to foreign bacteria.

Be careful of fruit juices because they often are diluted with tap water. Bottled wine, beer and carbonated soft drinks — without ice — are generally safe.

Be careful of what you eat

Cooked foods are usually safe, but don't eat raw foods — especially salads that contain lettuce or raw vegetables. Fruits and vegetables with a rind or skin that can be peeled immediately before you eat them usually are safe after careful washing. Avoid fruits and vegetables already peeled.

Eat in restaurants that have a reputation for safety. Don't eat foods from street vendors, and consume only foods, especially meat products, that are thoroughly cooked. If you're preparing your own meals, keep cold those items that can spoil. Even cooked food can be contaminated. Avoid unpasteurized milk and dairy products. ■

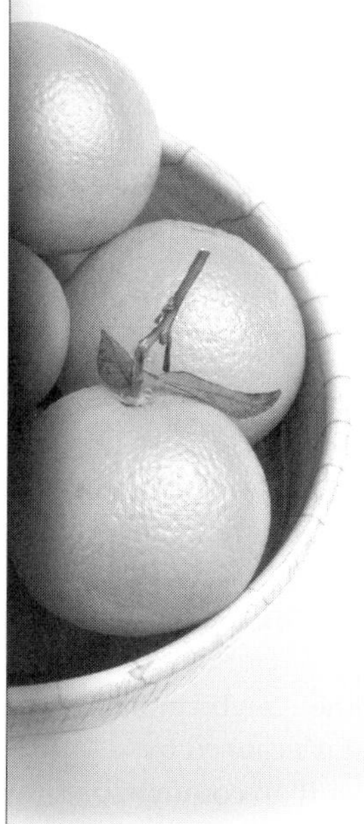

CHAPTER 11 PART I

Addressing End-of-Life Issues

One of life's few guarantees is that, someday, it will end. You may not know when or how you'll die, but you can prepare for your death. At the end of life, often many decisions need to be made, including medical and financial ones. Making these decisions while you're healthy and able to discuss your wishes with care providers and loved ones helps ensure that when you're dying and after your death, matters will be taken care of in the manner you prefer. This type of planning also helps to prevent disputes among loved ones.

Estate Planning

Whether you have a complex network of assets or you live simply, estate planning allows you to choose the individuals and organizations that you would like to benefit from your life of hard work. When you die, your assets are distributed. If you leave no indication of how you want your assets divided, state law decides for you. Now is the time to set up a formal plan to make your wishes known. With these issues settled, you're free to enjoy your final years without the stress of worrying about how your assets will be distributed after your death.

Assessing your estate

Before you begin to make plans for your estate, you need to take an inventory of what it entails. Your estate includes everything you own that conceivably has some value. Major items in your estate may include:

- A home
- Additional real estate
- Ownership interest in a business
- Life insurance
- Investments
- Retirement accounts
- Savings accounts
- Vehicles
- Other personal property

Drafting a will

The simplest way to ensure that your heirs get what you want them to have is to prepare a will. About half of all Americans, however, don't have wills in effect when they die. In these cases, a probate judge decides who gets what from an individual's estate. If you don't have any heirs and you don't leave a will, your state government may claim your money and property.

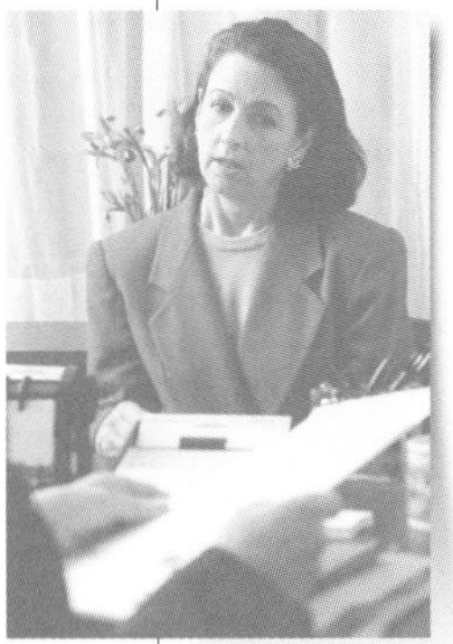

An attorney can be helpful in making sure your wishes are carried out. With an attorney you can draw up a will that describes your estate, names your beneficiaries and details what they're to receive and when they should receive it. You may make any other special provisions you wish and name a manager of your estate (personal representative).

Most wills go through probate court to some degree or another. The smaller your estate, the simpler that process is apt to be. It rarely takes longer than a year.

Preparing a living trust

Another way for you to dispense your estate to your heirs is to create what's called a revocable living trust. A living trust is a legal document created by a lawyer. It describes how you would like your estate distributed after you die and names a trustee to see to its execution.

The benefit of a living trust is that it allows your assets to be passed along to beneficiaries without going through the process of probate. In addition, you have the option of specifying how your property should be handled in the event that you become incapacitated.

Seeking estate counseling

No matter if your estate is simple and small or large and complex, it's often helpful to enlist the aid of an experienced attorney, certified public accountant, financial planner or other appropriate professional. Estate laws change frequently and are usually complicated. Someone with experience in financial and estate matters can help ensure that your heirs aren't left with a larger tax liability than necessary.

Long-Term-Care Insurance

Long-term-care insurance provides financial protection if you're unable to care for yourself because of a chronic illness, disability or cognitive impairment, such as Alzheimer's disease.

Long-term care is often very expensive and generally isn't covered by Medicare or involves substantial copayments. Medicaid typically requires beneficiaries to pay what they can before an individual can receive such benefits.

Long-term-care insurance is designed to help pay the cost of continued medical care, protecting your savings. This type of insurance generally covers a wide variety of services, from the cost of home health care to monthly nursing home payments. However, long-term-care insurance can be expensive, especially if you wait until you're older to purchase it. Buying the insurance when you're younger — such as in your 40s or 50s — and in good health, can prevent the insurance from being cost-prohibitive. Of course, then you have the expense of premiums over many years. Some experts feel that a good time for many people to buy this type of insurance is when they're in their 60s.

Long-term-care insurance isn't for everyone, but for many individuals it's worth considering. This type of insurance probably isn't the right choice if you have a limited income and few assets. Nor do you need it if you've saved enough to pay for long-term care, though you might still want to buy it to protect your assets.

Make certain that you understand exactly what the insurance covers and for how long. Many states give tax credits or tax deductions for costs of long-term-care insurance.

Funeral Costs

A traditional funeral and burial can cost thousands of dollars. For this reason, more Americans are setting aside money to cover the expenses of their eventual funeral. Or they're entering into contracts with funeral homes and prepaying for funeral packages. Nearly one out of three Americans over the age of 50 have prepaid some or all of their funeral expenses. Either approach will relieve some of the stress for loved ones when you die.

If you decide to purchase a funeral package — whether it's simply a cemetery plot or an entire package that includes a casket, vault and services — it's a good idea to shop around. There's nothing wrong with selecting a funeral home or a cemetery based on location, as long as it has a reputable standing in the community. But if you check at only one place, you may pay too much. Call or visit at least two funeral homes and cemeteries. The Federal Trade Commission's "Funeral Rule" requires funeral homes, though not cemeteries, to disclose their prices by telephone. Many will mail you their price lists.

If you're buying a package, be sure to get prices for the casket, the outer burial container — which is often required by cemeteries to prevent the ground from sinking — and the funeral home's general services, which may include:

- An initial consultation
- Copies of death certificates — you may need more than a dozen to settle matters such as insurance claims, social security issues and pension benefits
- Transportation of the body to the funeral home and burial site
- Preparation of the body for burial
- Use of the facilities for visitation or a memorial ceremony
- Other options, such as flowers, music or preparing obituary notices

An increasing number of people are choosing cremation over burial. Cremation can be less costly than a traditional funeral and burial. However, many costs and options are associated with cremation as well. The body must be cremated in a container, although not necessarily a casket. And many families choose to purchase a memorial spot for the urn containing the remains. Some cemeteries allow burial of the urn in a traditional plot, and others have urn gardens. Ask the facility providing the cremation services about various options and costs.

Advance Directives

With the advent of modern medications, surgical techniques and life-sustaining technologies, the field of medicine has become increasingly capable of prolonging the life and easing the pain of

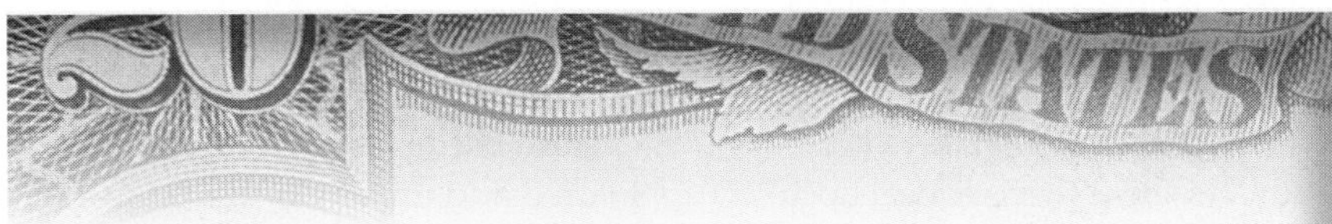

Gifting Your Assets

One way to ensure that your heirs and favorite charities or organizations get as much of your estate as possible is to gradually begin passing on your assets to them during your life. Doing so can also help to reduce your taxes. You can take several approaches:

- *Cash gifts.* You can give a gift of cash tax-free to anyone you choose. Beginning in 2002, the annual limit of $10,000 from one person to another or $20,000 from a couple to an individual began to increase. Your tax accountant can advise you on the current limits. You can pass any amount of money or property to your spouse while you're alive. However, this may increase the federal estate tax liability upon the death of the sole surviving spouse.
- *A bypass trust.* A bypass trust (also known as a credit shelter trust) can provide a surviving spouse with income during his or her life from a deceased spouse's estate while reducing or eliminating the heirs' estate tax after the death of that surviving spouse.
- *A charitable remainder unitrust.* A charitable remainder unitrust (CRUT) is created by giving a valuable asset, such as stock, to a charity. The charity in turn sells that asset and puts the funds into a trust that pays income to you for the rest of your life. At your death, the charity takes possession of the trust's assets.
- *A charitable lead trust.* A charitable lead trust (CLT) does exactly the opposite of a CRUT. Instead of you receiving income from a trust created from your assets, the charity receives the income. At your death, your heirs receive the assets of the trust.

seriously ill people. Sometimes, death due to natural failure of the heart, lungs or other organs can be postponed with life-prolonging measures.

Given these circumstances, one of the most important things that you can do with your doctor and your family is to have a frank discussion about how you wish to be treated if you can no longer communicate your desires.

Recent court decisions support the rights of people, particularly those with a prolonged illness, to live their final days as they choose. These decisions reflect society's evolving perspective that dying involves the whole person — not only the physical aspects but also the emotional and spiritual aspects.

If you're seriously ill or injured, the choice of whether to proceed with extraordinary lifesaving measures should be yours. When you're no longer able to communicate your wishes, an advance directive can guide your caretakers. An advance directive is a legal document that spells out the types of medical treatments and life-sustaining measures you do or don't want. Some advance directives allow for someone you've appointed to make medical decisions on your behalf.

An advance directive is generally used only if you lose mental capacity or suffer an injury or disease that impairs your ability to communicate. If you're over age 18 and are being admitted to a hospital, nursing home, hospice or home health care agency that receives Medicare funds, the institution is required by federal law to ask whether you have an advance directive. That information is documented in your record. The institution must also give you written information about your right, under state law, to accept or reject medical treatment. Whether or not you have an advance directive, federal law requires the institution to provide all individuals the same treatment options.

If you want to prepare an advance directive, your doctor or hospital staff can give you the necessary form and provide resources explaining the relevant state laws. You can also contact an attorney.

One of the most useful aspects of advance directives is that they provide an opportunity for individuals to discuss important matters with their family members before a life-threatening event. And if you ever do become seriously ill or injured and unable to communicate, this document can help relieve some of the anguish of family who would otherwise have to guess what medical treatment you would want.

Types of directives

The most common types of advance directives are living wills and durable powers of attorney for health care. The combination of a durable power of attorney for health care and a living will provides maximum personal participation in the face of many medical situations that require difficult decisions.

A living will

Living wills are usually written in general language because no one can anticipate all possible circumstances that may surround their death. Living wills may follow a standard format or be specific. For example, your living will might prohibit heroic procedures, but then your doctor has to make certain distinctions: Is the use of a respirator a heroic measure? What about a blood transfusion?

As new technologies develop and yesterday's heroic treatments become routine, the problem becomes increasingly complicated. For doctors, one of the biggest challenges is keeping patients and family members informed of ever changing life-sustaining technologies, and the personal impact of these treatments. It's a well-informed individual who's most likely to make thoughtful decisions about medical treatment.

To draft a living will, it's useful, but not essential, to get help from an attorney. It's also important to realize that all living wills have limitations because few people can predict their manner of death. You might consider stating in your living will your wish that extraordinary technological procedures not be used when your condition is terminal. But at what point is a condition considered terminal? In some states *terminal* is clearly defined, but in general this remains a subject of considerable debate.

A living will by itself carries only moral force in stating your preferences. To give legal authority to living wills, most states have passed statutes, often called natural death acts. In these states, the statutes interpret the extent of the authority and the legal force of the living will. The statutes aren't uniform among states. To ensure that your living

Health Care Services and Facilities

Near the end of life, there may come a time when it makes sense to get some extra help with day-to-day tasks. Or you may need extra help while you recover from an illness. There are several ways to receive this help, and it makes sense to think now about what you might want if someday you should need some assistance.

Options include:

- Home health care
- Assisted living
- Elder care
- Nursing homes

These options are discussed in detail in Chapter 16, "Adult Years."

will conforms to your state's requirements and will be followed, be familiar with the appropriate laws in your state before you prepare your living will, or let an attorney help you.

Once you've created a living will, review it periodically. Medical technology and your views and wishes may change. You have the option of revoking your living will and other advance directives at any time.

A durable power of attorney for health care

In addition to a living will, you may want to consider a document creating a durable power of attorney for health care. This document identifies the person you've selected to make health-related decisions for you should you become unable or unwilling to do so, giving this person legal authority to act on your behalf. Usually, the person is a spouse, family member or trusted friend.

This person, also called a proxy, helps ensure that your wishes aren't misinterpreted or ignored. And, unlike a living will, your proxy can respond specifically to the unique questions that your condition may create. When selecting someone to serve as your proxy, choose a person you trust and are comfortable with. He or she should fully understand your medical care philosophy and wishes and agree to serve in representing them. It also may be helpful, but not necessary, if this person lives close to you.

You need to be careful not to confuse a durable power of attorney for health care with a financial power of attorney. A financial power of attorney, also called a statutory short form power of attorney, allows a person you authorize to manage your money and property if you aren't able to do so.

What to address

It's impossible to predict exactly what issues will need to be addressed as you approach death. Therefore, it's not always clear what to include in an advance directive. However, the following health care scenarios are common and provide a guideline for discussions:

Discontinuing or withholding lifesaving treatment

Terminal illness may reach a point at which further treatment may only prolong the process of dying. At this point, you and your family, with help from your doctor and perhaps a religious adviser, may decide to stop further treatment except to ease pain and provide comfort.

You and your family may also decide in advance not to provide cardiopulmonary resuscitation (CPR) in the event you stop breathing or your heart stops beating.

Decisions that involve highly sensitive ethical matters often bring out differences of opinion among family members. For example, removing life-support systems may not present a dilemma for someone who sees the choice only in terms of death with dignity. For another relative, removing life-support systems may violate deep beliefs about the preservation of life. The best course of action isn't always obvious. This is why it's critical to communicate your feelings early and clearly to those whom you entrust with decisions about your care.

Some treatments also have a double effect that may need to be considered. For example, the primary effect of a narcotic such as morphine is to relieve pain, but a secondary effect of narcotics may be a decline in breathing ability, which can lead to death.

Artificial feeding

In addition to the use of CPR and ventilators to breathe, questions regarding use of other life-sustaining measures, such as nutritional support, may arise in the care of a person with a terminal illness.

Artificial feeding involves providing nourishment in a manner other than normal eating — usually by inserting into the stomach a tube that allows liquids to go directly into it. Occasionally, intravenous (IV) infusions are used for feeding. Several difficult questions arise in these situations: Is such feeding permanent? What will be the quality of life of the person? If feeding is discontinued, will the person experience thirst and hunger? Your caregiver can answer these questions.

Many difficult decisions can arise with a terminal illness. In making such decisions, unique factors must be weighed. Although there are few rules, each of us has our own framework of moral and ethical principles limited by legal boundaries that need to be considered.

Helpful Organizations

As you go about your day-to-day activities, it's difficult to think about the end of your life. It also can be difficult to discuss matters relating to your or a loved one's death and dying. However, there are organizations designed to help people with end-of-life issues.

For example, the Midwest Bioethics Center has put together a workbook with questions for people to consider, answer and discuss with family members. Its program, called Caring Conversations, is designed to help individuals and their families share meaningful conversations while making practical end-of-life decisions. The workbook covers everything from reflecting on personal relationships and religious beliefs to more specific, practical issues, such as whether you would ever want to refuse food, water or any other life-sustaining services. The workbook also goes over an advance directive in great detail and provides forms that may be of use to you in creating one. For more information on the center, see page 1384.

'Do Not Resuscitate' Orders

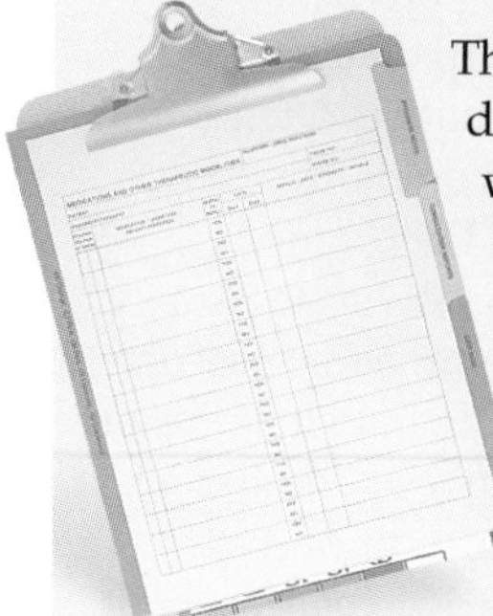

The directive "Do not resuscitate" (DNR) means that cardiopulmonary resuscitation (CPR) is not to be performed when a person's heart stops or he or she stops breathing. CPR is rarely appropriate for a patient with a terminal, irreversible illness when death is expected at any time.

The initials *DNR* are usually prominently displayed on the charts of patients in hospitals or nursing homes when it has been decided that CPR is not to be used. The decision to place DNR on the chart is made by the individual who is ill and his or her doctor. If the individual isn't competent or able to communicate, relatives, a doctor or someone who has been designated to make medical decisions for the person may make the decision. Sometimes, a request for a DNR order is part of a living will.

The decision whether to use CPR shouldn't have to be made in an emergency situation. This is the reason for making the decision early and making everyone who might be involved aware of it in advance. Placing DNR on a patient's chart doesn't imply that any lesser quality of care will be given. Individuals still are given adequate treatment for other conditions. For example, your doctor would still ask if you wanted to get antibiotics should an infection develop.

Organ Donation

Every year tens of thousands of people await organ transplants. Some are waiting for a donated cornea to help them see again. For others, the transplant is a matter of life and death, such as the donation of a heart or liver. But each year the number of organ donations fills only a fraction of the need.

The United Network for Organ Sharing (UNOS), the organization charged with organizing the sharing of organs, believes that the better people understand the donation process, the more willing they'll be to become a donor.

Who can donate?

Anyone, including newborns, can donate organs. There's no upper age limit. Older adults are often evaluated as donors. In addition, a medical illness doesn't necessarily mean that you can't donate your organs. At the time of death, the appropriate medical professionals will determine whether your organs are usable. Donation is acceptable to and even lauded by most religions.

Organ transplantation is less common at hospitals outside major medical centers. However, all hospitals are required by law to inform relatives of potential donors about UNOS, which was established in 1984 by the National Organ Transplantation Act. UNOS maintains an extensive computer network of individuals in need of donated organs.

The donation procedure

Some people have concerns about the donation procedure. They worry about disfigurement or if their care will be affected by their decision to donate.

Donation doesn't disfigure the body. Needed organs are removed surgically, in an operation similar to a gallbladder or appendix removal. When a person has stated a desire to be an organ donor after death, the procedure takes place only after all efforts to save the individual have been exhausted and death has been legally declared. The medical professionals who retrieve organs for transplantation aren't the same doctors who provide care for an ill person.

Organs that can be taken from one individual and transplanted into another include the heart, kidneys, pancreas, lungs, liver, intestines and eyes. Tissues that can be donated include skin, bone, heart valves and tendons.

Who receives the organs or tissues?

One myth that's difficult to dispel is that wealthy or famous people move to the top of the recipient list when they need a transplant. In reality, the organ allocation and distribution system is blind to wealth or social status. The length of time it takes to receive a transplant is governed by many factors, including blood type, length of time on the waiting list, severity of illness and other medical criteria.

UNOS doesn't consider factors such as race, sex, age, income or celebrity status when determining who receives an organ.

Becoming a donor

If you wish to be an organ donor, indicate that fact in an advance directive. In some states you can also make a notation on your driver's license indicating your preference. However, even if you take both of these steps, it's also crucial to discuss this issue with your family. Organ removal must happen shortly after death, and often family members don't have much time to make a decision on whether to donate a loved one's organs. Knowing the person's preference ahead of time can make the decision less difficult. ■

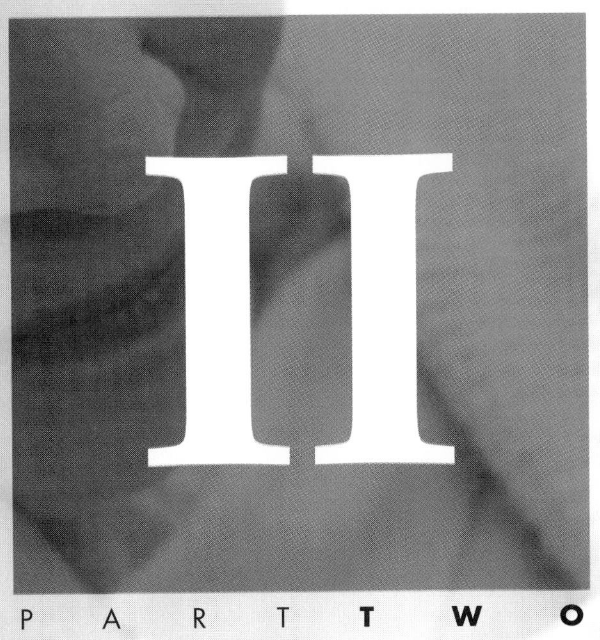

PART TWO

Common Conditions and Concerns Through Life's Stages

CHAPTER 12 PART II

Infant and Toddler Years

After 9 months of anticipation, the day finally arrives. Your daughter or son is born and takes her or his first breath. And so begins a new chapter in your life and the life of your child.

The first months of life are an exciting and challenging time, even for experienced parents, because every baby is different. Some babies nurse well from the beginning, and other babies seem to prefer feeding from a bottle. Some babies cry only when hungry, wet or tired, and other babies spend hours crying for no apparent reason. Some babies sleep through the night, and other babies prefer to take frequent catnaps.

As you and your baby adjust to being home together, life usually gets easier. During the first month, your baby may begin to fall into a somewhat predictable schedule of eating, sleeping and wetting diapers. This isn't to say that the schedule won't change. It frequently does during the first year of life. But among all of the changes, there's a newfound sense of predictability in what to expect from your baby during any given day.

The first year of life is a time of continuous and rapid change. Your baby will go from a diet of breast milk or formula to table food and even drinks from a cup. The young infant who spends a good part of each day sleeping becomes the 11-month-old who is active the whole day except for an afternoon nap. Your baby will progress from being able to sit up on his or her own to creeping and then to walking, which generally occurs between ages 9 and 16 months. You'll watch your baby evolve from communicating only by crying to cooing and squealing with pleasure when you walk into the room, and later to saying *mama* and *dada* and waving bye-bye.

Remember that not all babies develop at the same pace. If your baby doesn't reach a developmental milestone within the usual time frame, this doesn't necessarily mean that anything is wrong. Talk to your baby's doctor if you have concerns or questions about your baby's development.

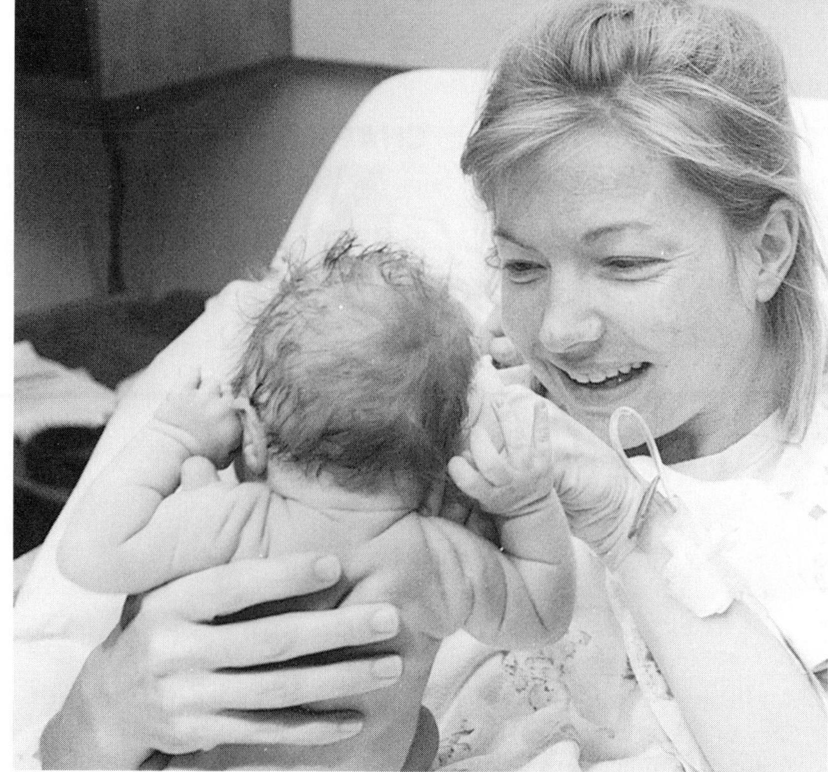

Getting acquainted with a minutes-old newborn is an especially joyous occasion.

Surviving the First Month

The first month of life is a period of adjustment and challenge for both the baby and parents. It can also be an exhausting time for parents, so take one day at a time. Here are some survival tips:

- Nap when your baby naps.
- Keep meal preparation simple.
- Let a few dust balls accumulate.
- Don't feel obligated to entertain all visitors.
- Accept offers of help with household tasks.
- Ask for assistance from family and friends, if you need help.

A Healthy Baby

During your baby's first year, it's natural to worry whether your baby is developing normally, even though serious abnormalities are uncommon. Many parents, especially first-time parents, have questions concerning their baby's weight, posture, skin color, vision, hearing, feeding, bowel movements, crying and sleeping.

Growth

The average newborn weighs between $5^1/_2$ and 10 pounds and is between 18 and 22 inches long. Within the first few days after birth, a baby will normally lose from 6 percent to 10 percent of its birth weight because of normal fluid loss.

By the time your baby is 1 month old, he or she probably has gained 1 to 3 pounds over his or her birth weight and grown 1 or 2 inches longer. Your baby will probably double his or her birth weight by the age of 4 to 5 months and triple it by the first birthday. Your baby's height will increase about 10 to 12 inches during the course of the year. The circumference of your baby's head will increase approximately 4 or 5 inches.

Posture and motor capabilities

The posture of your newborn simulates the fetal position. At birth, when placed on a firm surface, your baby can move his or her head from side to side. Unsupported, your baby's head will flop forward or backward. Support the head to prevent this. When held on an adult's shoulder, your newborn can lift his or her head. On his or her stomach, your baby may lie in a frog-like position or rolled in a ball. Your baby's fingers are balled into a fist.

At 1 month your baby's head still needs support, but he or she may hold the head steady for longer periods. Your baby can roll partway from back to side. When the infant's fingers are pried open, he or she can grasp a rattle but usually drops it right away.

By 4 months infants can sit with assistance and maintain good control of the head. When on his or her stomach, your baby may rock, rolling from side to side. Some infants at this age can roll from their stomach or side to the back, or transfer an object from one hand to the other.

Your baby may begin to crawl by 8 months. Some infants of this age can even stand when leaning against something. By the time many children have their first birthday, they're walking, although crawling still may be the preferred method of getting around. Your child may be capable of climbing and going down stairs or climbing out of the crib. Your child may also point with his or her index finger or take the covers off containers.

Apgar Score

Apgar scores are used to evaluate the general health of newborns at 1 minute and again at 5 minutes after birth. Five areas are assessed: heart rate, respiratory effort, muscle tone, response to stimulation, and color. Each area is rated on a scale of 0 to 2, and the numbers are totaled. The highest possible score is a 10.

A score of 8 to 10 indicates that the baby is in excellent condition. The heart rate is more than 100 beats a minute, the baby is breathing well and crying, is active, coughs or sneezes when the nose is suctioned, and has good skin color. Most newborns have a score of 7 to 9 and require nothing more than having mucus suctioned from the airway to improve their breathing. Newborns with a score of 4 or less at 1 minute after delivery require immediate assistance with their breathing. The heartbeat is slow or inaudible, the baby appears pale or even blue and reflex responses may be absent or depressed.

Skin color

Immediately after birth your baby's skin color may be dusky blue. This is the normal color for an infant before birth. During the first few minutes after birth, the normal increase of oxygen in their cardiopulmonary system causes infants of all races to become increasingly pinkish, especially their tongue, lips, palms and soles of the feet.

Some infants may be born with or soon develop jaundice, a yellowish discoloration of the skin and whites of the eyes. More than half of all full-term newborns and 80 percent of premature newborns who are otherwise healthy develop jaundice during the first few days of life. This is known as physiologic jaundice.

Jaundice isn't a disease but rather the result of the inability of the immature liver of an infant to fully metabolize bilirubin. Bilirubin is a molecule that forms when the body recycles red blood cells. Bilirubin in the skin gives it a yellowish tint.

It's common for jaundice to continue through the first week or two,

Question and Answer

When will my baby walk?

No one can answer this with precision. One child may walk as early as 9 months, and another may be content to crawl until 14 months or later.

Your new walker is amusing to watch. On plump feet that look flat because of baby fat, your child will toddle about with the toes turned out. Many babies are also bowlegged or knock-kneed. Virtually all of these characteristics are normal and disappear on their own.

Don't expect your new walker to be graceful. One minute your 1-year-old will be making his or her way across the room, and the next he or she will be lying in a heap on the floor. Falls can be frequent at first and usually are no real deterrent to the determined baby. Falls are part of learning to walk.

For the parent, however, they serve as a signal of things to come. A child who only weeks before had limited mobility now has discovered the ability to go where he or she wants to. By the time your explorer is 18 months old, he or she may be able to climb the stairs while holding your hand. By 2 years it's difficult to stop most children from traversing a steep stairwell. To prevent a dangerous fall, install a safety gate at the top and bottom of all staircases in the home.

especially in babies receiving breast milk. If jaundice develops or persists after the second week of life, it may be due to some other liver malfunction, a severe infection, an enzyme deficiency or abnormality of red blood cells. Jaundice present at birth or that appears within the first 24 hours may also be the result of several problems, including hemorrhage, an infection in the blood (sepsis) or a blood incompatibility between the baby and mother. If your baby's doctor is concerned about these possibilities, special blood tests may be done.

Most infants with physiologic jaundice require only observation. Generally, the condition is gone within 1 or 2 weeks. The severity of physiologic jaundice is often influenced by race. Asian and American Indian newborns are often affected more severely. Jaundice may be worse in babies who aren't eating well or in those having fewer bowel movements.

If your baby has a significantly increased amount of bilirubin, he or she may be placed under a high-intensity light, a procedure called phototherapy. Bilirubin absorbs light and is then converted into a form that can be excreted in the bile and urine. This treatment is continued until the amount of bilirubin has been reduced. Possible side effects of phototherapy include loose stools, rash and dehydration.

Vision

At birth your newborn's eyes are about three-fourths the size of what they'll be at adulthood. Your baby will probably keep his or her eyes shut much of the time. This doesn't mean that your baby can't see. From the moment of birth, your baby is capable of focusing on objects within 8 to 12 inches of his or her face. Infants are attracted to patterns more than to colors, and they enjoy faces. Infants are particularly interested in making eye contact and focusing on their mother's or father's face.

Many infants may have difficulty coordinating their eye movements during the initial months after birth. At times your baby may seem cross-eyed. In most cases this improves in the first few months.

Most newborns are unable to see nearby objects clearly. Some infants, particularly those born prematurely, are born nearsighted and unable to see clearly objects that are far away. As healthy infants grow, their eyes change, allowing them to see both near and far objects more clearly. In most infants, the ability to see things clearly progresses rapidly. By the time most children are 3 years old or even younger, they have 20/30 or 20/20 vision.

Sometimes a significant visual problem surfaces during infancy. As is often the case, the earlier the diagnosis, the better the chances that treatment will be successful. If you have any concerns about your baby's vision, talk to your baby's doctor (see page 157).

Hearing

Infants normally are born with a good sense of hearing. A healthy newborn blinks and startles in response to a loud sound and can distinguish differences in volume. Soft noises may produce something akin to a smile, and harsh or loud sounds may cause your newborn to cry. Your newborn may develop sound preferences, favoring a high-pitched voice such as his or her mother's over lower pitches.

Hearing is essential in the acquisition of speech and language. Even minor hearing loss can have a significant effect on your baby's ability to understand and to communicate. The loss may go undetected until the child is 18 to 24 months old, when it leads to speech problems. All newborns should be screened for hearing loss (see page 156).

Language

Your newborn's main method of communication is crying. Between 1 and 3 months, your baby's verbal repertoire is expanded with small throaty sounds, coos, squeals, chuckles, whimpers and vowel-like sounds such as *ooh, ah* and *ae*. Language comprehension is limited to responses to familiar voices.

Between 4 and 6 months is the babbling stage — complete with sighing, grunting, gurgling, laughing and crying differently for pain and hunger. Your child vocalizes for pleasure and displeasure.

Between 7 and 9 months your child repeats syllables, babbles in a singsong manner and may produce as many as 12 distinct sounds, particularly the *p, d, b* and *m* sounds. He or she may use different vowels. Your infant may use sounds as a means of play and may repeat the word *mama*. Toward the end of this period, you'll hear your baby imitating the intonation and speech sounds made by others. Your child will search for sources of sound, listen intently to speech and nonspeech sounds and recognize *dada*, *mama* and *bye-bye*. Your child may recognize his or her own name and is able to differentiate friendliness and anger from the tone of people's voices.

Between 10 and 12 months, the babbling may take on some of the melody of actual speech. Your child enjoys repeating sounds made by others. Considerable vocalization is used during play. Almost all of the consonant and vowel sounds are used. In some children the first words emerge during this period. Your child's comprehension also is improved by this time, and he or she can respond to names and simple requests and recognize the names of common objects and family members.

Nutrition

It's not uncommon for an infant to show little interest in feeding, particularly during the first couple of days after birth. By the end of the first week, most infants eat every 2 to 5 hours. A newborn is hungry at irregular intervals whether on a diet of breast milk or formula.

Feeding is still somewhat disorganized at 1 month. Babies may eat as often as every 2 to 3 hours during the day and one or more times in the night. Gradually over the course of the first month, the number of feedings over a 24-hour period may be reduced from 8 or 12 to 6 or 8. The length of feedings also is erratic. One day a breast-fed infant might want to nurse for 40 minutes at each breast, and the next day he or she may nurse for only 10 minutes.

By 2 weeks of age, your newborn may take in about 18 ounces of milk a day. By 1 month that may increase to about 25 ounces a day. The frequency of feedings depends on your baby's needs and the method of feeding. A baby between 1 and 3 months old probably will want between five and six feedings a day, eventually eating every 3 hours, except for a longer stretch at night. As the baby grows, the number of feedings is reduced. Typically, a 5-month-old is down to four or five feedings, and by 9 months the child may have only three milk feedings. Each baby's needs for growth are different, so follow your baby's cues to determine feeding frequency and volume.

Breast-feeding

A generation ago breast-feeding was not the norm for many American women. Today it has proved to be the ideal feeding method because of its nutritional and immunologic advantages and its emotional benefits.

Most breast-fed infants are offered an opportunity to nurse for feedings, although water itself is seldom needed unless the baby has a fever or diarrhea or is in a location of high heat. If an infant is feeding well, the amount of water in breast milk or formula is adequate.

Newborn Diet

Whether the source is breast milk or formula, the basic diet of a newborn includes the following components:

Calories

Calories are a measurement of the energy content of food. Everything we eat and much of what we drink contains calories. Human milk and standard formula usually have 20 to 30 calories per ounce: 9 percent to 15 percent come from protein, 45 percent to 55 percent from carbohydrates and 35 percent to 45 percent from fats.

Protein

Protein is essential for growth and for the repair of cells. Most of the major body organs are composed mainly of protein. If the body does not receive an adequate amount of protein, it begins to break down its muscles to supply protein for essential body needs. A human deprived of protein for a long enough period will develop lethargy, a distended abdomen and swelling.

Carbohydrates

Carbohydrates supply most of the body's energy needs. When the body doesn't receive enough carbohydrates, it compensates by using protein and fats for energy. Carbohydrates are stored in the liver and muscles. The infant's reserve is a fraction of that of the adult. Carbohydrates are necessary for your infant's health, even when he or she is ill.

Fats

Fats are a concentrated source of energy. They help protect body organs, vessels and nerves, provide insulation against changes in temperature, act as a vehicle for vitamin absorption and delay the time it takes for the stomach to empty, giving you a sensation of fullness. Unlike with some adults, infants and young children shouldn't be on a fat-restricted or low-fat diet.

Water

Water is essential for human life. Water accounts for 70 percent to 75 percent of your newborn's body weight, compared with only 60 percent to 65 percent of an adult's body weight. To remain healthy an infant must take in larger amounts of water per unit of body weight than an adult. The daily water requirement is between 10 percent and 15 percent of the infant's body weight. In an adult it's only 2 percent to 4 percent.

Fortunately, the water content of both breast milk and formula is high. Some formula-fed babies want water from a bottle between

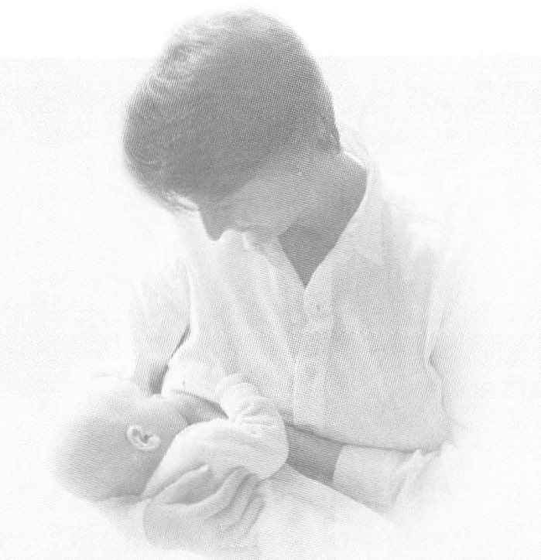

Minerals

Minerals are important to the structure and function of virtually every part of the body. For example, calcium and fluoride are necessary for the formation of strong bones and teeth, copper and iron are required for the production of red blood cells, and sodium is needed to maintain the water balance in the body.

Vitamins

Vitamins in minute amounts are needed for your organs to work properly. Vitamin A is important to eye health, and it keeps the linings of the bronchial, urinary and intestinal tracts healthy. Vitamin C is needed for bone, teeth and tissue development. Vitamin D is important to bone and teeth development.

the first time shortly after birth. Closeness between a mother and child is facilitated by breast-feeding, and the infant gets the health benefits of the mother's colostrum, a rich, lemon-colored breast liquid that's highly beneficial in protecting the baby against some diseases. In breast-feeding, frequent nonscheduled, lengthy feeding sessions are important in establishing a good milk supply.

Some women who decide to breast-feed need more flexibility than the method may allow, so they also introduce the infant to the bottle. If you want to supplement one or more breast-feedings a day with a bottle, you can pump your breasts and store the milk for later use. Have your baby's doctor or a lactation consultant demonstrate the proper procedure for pumping your breasts. Highly efficient breast pumps are now available to enable you to provide breast milk for your baby regardless of your circumstances or lifestyle.

Many parents prefer, and doctors recommend, a newborn be allowed to determine the schedule of feedings — at least to some degree. Many newborns are content to be fed every 4 hours, but others may demand more frequent feedings.

Even if your infant has been on a 3-hour feeding routine, the rules may suddenly change, and he or she may shorten the time between feedings. A parent should be prepared for some changes and unpredictability during the first months of life. There also may be periods of cluster ("bunch") feedings during which your baby may feed hourly for several hours.

It's important for a nursing mother to feel at ease while breast-feeding. Make sure you're comfortable, either lying down or sitting in a comfortable chair, preferably one with an armrest. Support the baby with his or her face held close to your breast. With the other hand you might want to support the breast so that the nipple is easily accessible to the infant's mouth. Allow your baby to finish feeding on one breast before you offer the other. Alternate which breast you offer first at each feeding to keep milk production even. Burp your infant after each feeding: Set the baby upright or against your shoulder and gently pat or rub his or her back until he or she burps.

Initially, a nursing mother may have tender nipples. Keep your nipples as dry as possible between feedings. Position your baby comfortably at your breast to help prevent cracked nipples. If soreness persists, call your baby's doctor or a lactation consultant.

If you're breast-feeding your baby, pay special attention to your own diet and habits. Eat a healthy diet that includes plenty of water. Be wary of taking any medication unless it's approved by your doctor. Avoid smoking and consume only a minimal amount of alcohol, if any.

Bottle-feeding

Although no infant formula can match all of the nutritional benefits of breast milk, it's an acceptable alternative. Infant formula is similar to breast milk and contains all of the nutrients your baby needs to develop and grow.

Most bottle-fed babies have their first feeding within 6 hours after delivery. A bottle-fed baby probably will need between six and nine feedings in a 24-hour period by the end of the first week of life.

The setting for bottle-feeding is similar to that for breast-feeding. A bottle should never be propped up against the infant. Rather the parent should take the time to hold the child closely during the feeding.

Making the Most of Feedings

Personal interaction is an important factor in your baby's development. Aside from providing the nutrients your baby needs to grow and develop, feeding time is an opportunity for you and your baby to get better acquainted. Your baby can learn about you, how the two of you relate and the security and love you provide.

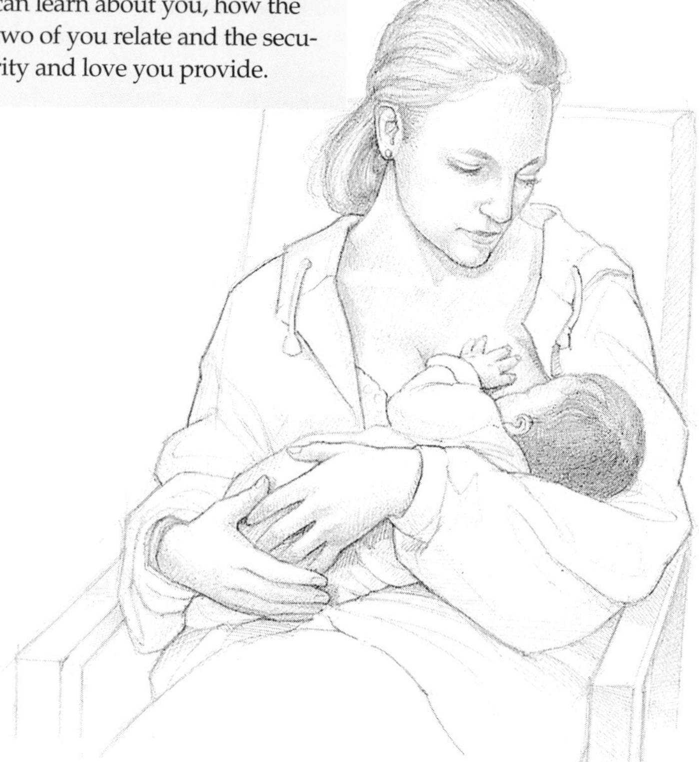

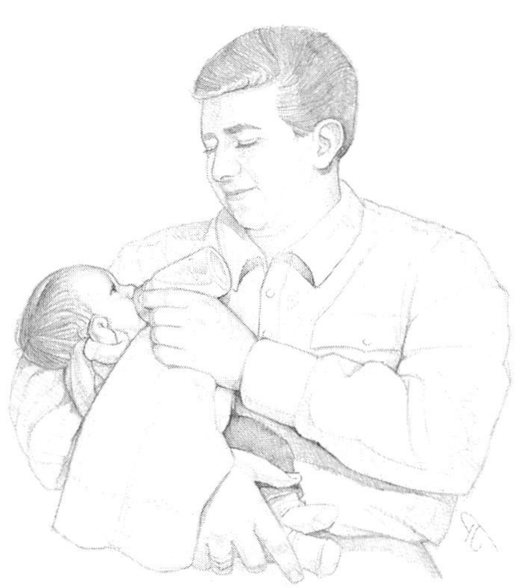

The formula should be warmed to body temperature, and the temperature tested by dropping a bit on your wrist. A word of caution: Don't warm the bottle in a microwave oven because the formula can become very hot and severely burn your infant. A bottle-feeding may last from 5 to 25 minutes, depending on the eagerness and sucking ability of the infant. Burp your baby after each feeding.

Solids

Parents always ask when they should offer their baby solids. This is a difficult question and one that has no shortage of opinions.

For several months the neuromuscular development of infants is geared toward sucking and swallowing liquids. The infant isn't ready to expand his or her diet until he or she has the ability to recognize a spoon and can swallow appropriately. This usually occurs around the age of 6 months. Before 4 to 6 months, your baby's gastrointestinal system may be unable to digest solids efficiently. In addition, your baby may be unable to sit up or hold his or her head erect for feedings.

From a nutritional standpoint, your baby gets everything he or she needs from breast milk or formula for the first 6 months. Some doctors, however, recommend starting babies on solids after 4 months. If your infant is nursing more often rather than less, your baby's doctor may also recommend an early introduction to solids.

Cereal

When it's time to offer your baby solids, many doctors recommend starting with a cereal. Single-grain cereal especially made for babies is often used as baby's first solid food because it's easy to digest. Mix 1 tablespoon of cereal with 4 or 5 tablespoons of formula or breast milk. Initially, babies generally respond better to solids if the solids are thin rather than thick. Put some food on the tip of a small spoon and place it in your baby's mouth. Don't be surprised if it comes back out. Many babies take time to adjust to this new taste and consistency. Be patient. Don't put solids in a bottle or a syringe-type feeder. The former can encourage your baby to overeat, and the latter can cause choking.

Pureed foods

After your baby is acquainted with cereal, your next step might be a pureed fruit or vegetable. At 8 months most infants are ready to try pureed meats, but breast milk or formula continues to provide ample amounts of protein.

Finger foods

After 8 months most babies are able to eat small pieces of table food. Toast, bits of cheese, pieces of scrambled egg, dry cereals, crackers, mashed potatoes and well-cooked pasta are good finger foods. Avoid foods that could choke your baby, such as hot dogs, grapes, popcorn, nuts, raisins and raw carrots.

Bowel movements

Infants usually have their first bowel movement within 24 hours after birth. Called a meconium stool, it's composed of intestinal secretions and amniotic fluid and is dark green. After your baby begins to drink breast milk or formula, the meconium stool changes to

Is Your Baby Getting Enough to Eat?

Many parents wonder whether their baby is getting enough to eat. The best answer to that question is to trust your baby. Babies are able to regulate their intake amazingly well. They'll eat as much as is needed, regardless of how much is left. When it's time to eat again, the baby will usually let you know.

If a baby doesn't get enough to eat, you'll soon know. He or she will cry until you offer more food. An infant who needs more food than is being given will awaken more often at night and will decrease rather than increase the time between feedings. You may even observe the baby chewing his or her fist more than usual.

The best early indication that your baby is receiving the necessary nourishment is weight gain. Keep in mind that some babies gain weight slowly, and others gain rapidly.

By the time your infant is between 6 and 8 months old, he or she may be eating 3 to 4 ounces — about 5 to 8 tablespoons — of solid food at each of three meals. A good diet for an infant of this age might include cereal and fruit for breakfast, cereal and fruit or vegetables for lunch and cereal, fruit and vegetables for supper. Although drinking patterns vary widely, many babies eating this diet reduce their milk consumption to about 16 ounces a day. Many babies also need a midmorning and midafternoon snack, which should be something nutritious such as fruit or yogurt.

In your baby's second 6 months, you may need to increase feedings with cereal to meet his or her needs for an adequate supply of iron. Sometimes, a baby's diet needs to be supplemented with vitamins and minerals. Consult your baby's doctor.

By his or her first birthday, your baby probably will be eating table food exclusively.

transitional stools, usually on the second or third day of life. These stools are usually greenish brown and may contain milk curds. After the passage of transitional stools, the stool resembles the bowel movement of an older infant.

By the end of the first week, most infants pass between three and five stools a day, although it's not uncommon for a baby, especially one that is breast-fed, to have more bowel movements each day. If your newborn goes for several days without having a bowel movement, don't panic. This doesn't necessarily mean that the baby is constipated (see page 170).

The stool of a breast-fed baby is odorless and mushy. The stool of a formula-fed baby has a characteristic fecal smell and is usually more formed. By 1 month most babies have three or four bowel movements a day, often after a feeding. However, some infants, especially some nursing babies, may not have one for 2 to 10 days. This is normal and not a cause for concern if the baby appears well.

Can You Spoil Your Baby?

If you're concerned about spoiling your newborn with too much love and attention, don't be. Responding to your baby's cry will not spoil him or her. Follow your instinct to respond to your baby's cries. Infants who are responded to consistently and quickly during the first 6 to 8 months of life cry less in later months than those left to cry. It seems that an important task for your infant to learn is that others will respond in a caring and predictable way. This helps your baby develop a strong trust in others and in self.

Crying

The amount a newborn cries, like many other aspects of development, varies. Some infants cry only when hungry or wet. Others cry more often.

On some days your baby may cry for 20 to 30 minutes four or five times — typically before eating, sleeping or having a bowel movement. On other days he or she may cry for hours. Crying usually peaks at about 6 weeks of age and tapers off by 3 or 4 months of age. In premature newborns the peak is typically 6 weeks after your due date.

What causes excessive crying during the first months of life? There's no easy answer to that question because every baby and every day are different. If your crying baby can't be consoled for more than a few moments by any method, your baby may have colic. For more information see page 172.

Trying to figure out what your baby is signaling with his or her cries is like being a detective. Hunger, discomfort, boredom, fear, loneliness, overstimulation or being overly tired are common reasons babies cry. Babies lack experience in reacting to the many new and confusing situations outside the womb. Although some make the transition easily, most need lots of cuddling and human contact day and night in those important first few months.

As the baby grows and matures, you'll begin recognizing different cries for different needs. You'll learn how to distinguish your baby's cries by trying different things and seeing what works and what doesn't. With time and familiarity, your understanding of your baby's needs will improve.

Sleeping

The average newborn spends more time sleeping than doing any other

Circumcision

Circumcision is a procedure in which the foreskin — the sheath of tissue covering the head of the penis — is removed. The practice has been performed since ancient times, and many parents today have their sons circumcised for religious or other reasons, including health and hygiene concerns.

Researchers have attempted to learn more about whether circumcision may prevent infection and certain types of cancer, but more studies are needed to clarify the medical pros and cons.

Like any minor surgery, circumcision poses some risk to the newborn. Local anesthesia may be used to lessen the pain for the baby. If you choose circumcision, it's usually done a few days after birth. An uncircumcised penis requires no special care beyond regular hygiene.

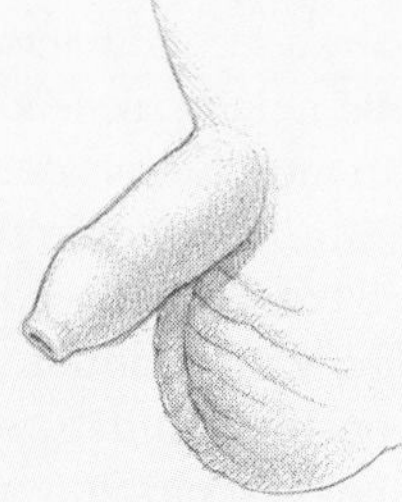

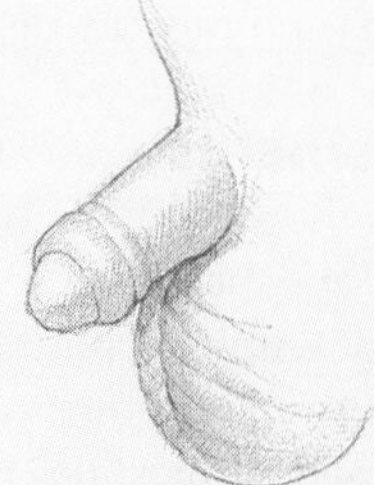

Before circumcision the foreskin of the penis extends over the end of the penis, or glans (left). After the brief operation, the glans is exposed (right).

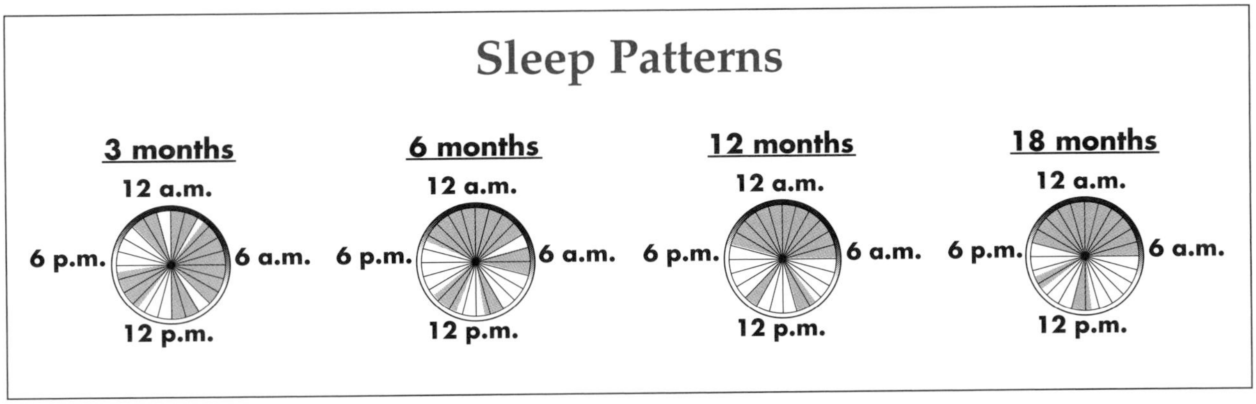

Sleep Patterns

3 months	6 months	12 months	18 months
12 a.m. / 6 a.m. / 12 p.m. / 6 p.m.	12 a.m. / 6 a.m. / 12 p.m. / 6 p.m.	12 a.m. / 6 a.m. / 12 p.m. / 6 p.m.	12 a.m. / 6 a.m. / 12 p.m. / 6 p.m.

asleep   awake

The sleep cycles of babies vary. This example shows how sleep is often erratic in the first months of life. With time, children generally settle into a routine.

activity. A newborn often has an alert period immediately after birth. After 1 to 2 hours of alertness, the baby sinks into a quiet sleep. During the next several days, most newborns sleep from 14 to 18 hours a day and are alert for only 30 minutes out of every 4 hours.

A 1-month-old baby spends most of the time sleeping, usually at least 14 hours a day. Generally, toward the end of the first month, parents observe that seven or eight daily sleep periods are reduced to three or four daily naps and a 5- or 6-hour block of sleep at night. Sleep patterns, however, are highly variable, and your baby may sleep more or less.

Sleep is divided into active and quiet sleep. Rapid eye movement (REM) sleep is when dreaming takes place. In the REM phase, the baby can be easily awakened. During this lighter sleep, babies may toss and turn, suck and gurgle. In the early months newborns have more of this lighter sleep than the quiet, deeper sleep. Deeper sleep, or quiet sleep, is referred to as non-REM sleep. As babies mature, they begin to have more quiet sleep like most adults have.

You'll also find that your infant is an active sleeper. Even though the baby is asleep, you may see his or her grimace, cry out, startle and move about without waking up.

By 6 months some babies are taking one or more daytime naps and may sleep 6 to 8 hours at a time. Be patient with your baby as he or she will reach this milestone of sleeping throughout the night on his or her own time. The time that this occurs varies from baby to baby. Throughout the first few years, there will be many nights of interrupted sleep from teething, illness or bad dreams.

An older infant is able to sleep through the night only when he or she no longer needs night feedings and has learned how to fall back to sleep without help. For more information on sleeping through the night, see page 172.

Newborn Screening Tests

Most states require routine screening for certain disorders that aren't apparent at birth. Screening tests for metabolic disorders, hearing loss and blood glucose levels are widely done. Early detection is important so that measures can be taken to prevent future health problems.

Your baby's doctor or the nursing staff at the hospital where your child is born will inform you of screening tests required or available in your state.

Metabolic disorders

Metabolic disorders, also called inborn errors of metabolism, occur when the body lacks the ability to properly use nutrients from food for normal growth and development. More than a thousand metabolic disorders exist.

Some metabolic disorders can be treated effectively if they're detected during an infant's first days or weeks after birth. If left untreated, these disorders can cause various problems, including mental retardation, cataracts and poor physical growth. To screen for metabolic disorders, a blood test is done. A few drops of blood are taken from your baby's heel. This is referred to as a heel stick.

Four metabolic disorders for which newborns are commonly tested are phenylketonuria, galactosemia, hypothyroidism and congenital adrenal hyperplasia.

Phenylketonuria

Phenylketonuria (PKU) is a congenital deficiency of a specific enzyme. Infants born with PKU are often normal at birth. The condition disrupts normal metabolism and may lead to developmental delays and IQ loss if the child's diet isn't carefully regulated beginning in early infancy. One in 12,000 babies born in the United States have PKU.

Although PKU can be detected as early as 4 hours after birth, most testing is done after the baby is at least 24 hours old because the test's accuracy depends on the baby's having eaten an adequate amount of protein. If your baby has PKU, a special diet will be prescribed. With early detection and treatment, normal development is possible.

Galactosemia

Galactosemia is an enzyme deficiency that affects the body's ability to metabolize galactose, one of the sugars normally present in milk. One in approximately 50,000 children are born with this inherited disorder which, if left untreated, can cause brain damage, cataracts and kidney and liver problems.

Symptoms associated with galactosemia include convulsions, lethargy, persistent jaundice, feeding difficulties and hypoglycemia.

Treatment involves a diet restricted in galactose content. When the diagnosis is made early, such medical problems can be prevented.

Hypothyroidism

Hypothyroidism is a deficiency in the production of thyroid hormone, which is essential for mental and physical growth and development.

Hypothyroidism occurs in about 1 in 4,000 births and is twice as common in females as males. Before screening became available, this disorder often went unrecognized. Symptoms such as sluggishness, constipation and poor growth may be absent or mild initially and then progress slowly.

If children with hypothyroidism are untreated, they're usually developmentally disabled and have short stature. Early treatment with thyroid hormone leads to normal growth and development.

Congenital adrenal hyperplasia

Congenital adrenal hyperplasia (CAH) blocks normal metabolism in many ways, resulting in a range of problems for approximately 1 in 15,000 newborns. Signs and symptoms may include vomiting, diarrhea, failure to gain weight and ambiguous genitals. Additional problems might include severely low sodium and dangerously high potassium levels in the blood.

A blood test in the first days of life can identify the condition before serious symptoms develop. Treatment is very effective and usually consists of cortisone-type medications and sometimes surgery.

Blood glucose

In the womb, an infant's blood sugar level remains normal because nutrition is being supplied from the placenta. After birth, a newborn must develop the ability to regulate its own blood sugar level.

Low blood sugar (hypoglycemia) occurs in some infants whose body is not yet able to regulate its own blood sugar levels. Infants whose mothers have diabetes are at greater risk of hypoglycemia because they're born with increased levels of insulin in their body.

Symptoms and signs may include jitters, lethargy, poor muscle tone and problems in feeding. Uncommon problems include difficulty breathing or seizures. The risk of seizures is of special concern because seizures caused by low blood glucose increase the risk of lasting neurologic or developmental problems.

A newborn's blood glucose level is commonly measured in the hours following birth to make certain that it's in the normal range. Feeding the baby breast milk, formula or glucose water usually helps return low levels to normal.

Hearing

Significant hearing loss in both ears affects approximately 1 to 3 out of 1,000 newborns. Infants at risk of hearing loss include those born with infections such as rubella (German measles), cytomegalovirus, syphilis and herpes, those who have head or neck injuries, severe jaundice, a family history of hearing loss during childhood and those born prematurely.

Hearing loss is a problem that may not be apparent at first and

Preventing Disease

Most of the medical care a newborn infant receives is geared toward the prevention of disease. Occasionally, bacteria in the birth canal cause serious eye infections in a newborn. Therefore, immediately after birth every newborn's eyes are protected with an antibiotic.

Usually, a dose of vitamin K is given after birth to prevent potential bleeding problems. Babies may receive the hepatitis B vaccine in the nursery, or later with other childhood immunizations, to protect them from any possible contact with hepatitis B, a viral infection that affects the liver. Several days after birth, routine screening tests will be performed for congenital problems.

It might be wise to continue to limit your newborn's visitors for a while after you leave the hospital. In particular, avoid crowds. Remember, colds and other illnesses that may be considered minor in an older baby pose greater risks during the first month of life.

All infants should be seen regularly by a doctor. Before you go home from the hospital, your baby's doctor will discuss this schedule with you. The first follow-up visit typically occurs within 2 weeks. Some pediatricians and family physicians recommend monthly visits during the first year of life. Others prefer to see the baby every 2 months, provided everything is going well, to monitor the baby's development and administer vaccinations. Read more about childhood vaccinations in Chapter 1, "Getting Immunized."

might go undetected until the child is 24 to 30 months of age, when concerned parents become aware that their child isn't developing normal speech. Hence, all newborns, including healthy babies, should be screened for hearing loss. Many hospitals now test the hearing of all babies while they're still in the nursery.

One simple, noninvasive screening test is the otoacoustic emissions (OAE) test. The OAE test measures sound waves generated in the inner ear (cochlea) in response to clicks or tone bursts. The waves are recorded, analyzed by a computer and interpreted by an audiologist.

However, none of the current hearing tests routinely used on newborns can detect slight hearing loss or minimal loss that will progress as the child grows. If hearing loss is suspected, your infant should have a follow-up hearing test between the ages of 3 and 6 months.

Certain types of hearing loss can be corrected. When the loss is due to ear infection, for example, antibiotics can treat the infection so that the ear can function normally. Surgery may correct congenital malformations of the ear.

Four types of hearing loss found in infants and children are:

Conductive hearing loss
Conductive hearing loss involves interference with the external ear's ability to receive sound or to transmit it from the external ear to the inner ear.

The most common causes are congenital abnormalities of the ear and ear infections. Often these problems can be treated with medication or surgery.

Sensorineural hearing loss
Sensorineural hearing loss results from abnormalities of the inner ear hair cells or of the auditory nerve. More than 50 percent of severe sensorineural hearing loss is hereditary. Other causes include severe jaundice, infection while in the uterus and medications. Sensorineural hearing loss is usually permanent.

Mixed hearing loss
Mixed hearing loss occurs when a child has both conductive and sensorineural hearing loss. This type of loss may be severe. Medication or surgery or both may restore a portion of the child's hearing loss.

Central auditory disorders
Central auditory disorders result from a problem in the central auditory nervous system, the ear's nerve linkage with the brain. Children with these disorders hear sound only as a jumble of noise.

Personality, Behavior and Development

Your newborn is a unique human being. From one healthy baby to the next, the variations are infinite. Part of the wonder of parenting is watching, recognizing and reinforcing the changes, development and behaviors as your infant's personality emerges.

Reflexes and responses

Your newborn's movements are governed by reflexes. Stroke its cheek, and the baby will likely root and try to suck. Prick the soles of its feet, and the knees and feet flex. Make a sudden noise, and your baby may startle.

All healthy babies are born with predictable reflexes that disappear in a predictable order as voluntary control of motor functions takes over.

The absence of a newborn's reflexes and responses may indicate a possible neurologic problem. Part of your newborn's hospital examination includes attempts to elicit various reflexes and responses.

Does Your Infant See Properly?

Some infants are born with partial or total loss of vision. Common causes include brain malformations, damage to the eyes due to infection, birth trauma, a significant loss of oxygen (hypoxia) and genetic diseases that affect either an eye or the nerves to the brain's vision center.

Although an important part of a newborn's initial physical examination includes a check for any apparent vision defects, it's not uncommon for some visual problems to go undetected during early infancy. Often the problem is discovered later by the parents when the child seems unusually clumsy.

You can watch for certain developmental signs to determine whether your baby's vision is indeed within the normal range. When your infant is between 4 and 6 weeks old, try the following test: Bring your face within 20 inches of your baby's. This should elicit a smile. By the time your infant is 3 months old, the baby should be able to visually follow a toy that is dangled in front of his or her face. The infant should also attempt to reach for a toy or rattle. A baby this age can see objects at least several feet away.

By the time your infant is 4 months old, his or her vision capabilities — the ability of the eye to distinguish color, adjust itself to various distances, see one image instead of two, perceive depth and orient itself to moving images — are near those of an adult. If you suspect that your baby's visual development is slow, consult your baby's doctor.

Reflexes and responses present in the newborn at birth are:

The startle reflex
The startle reflex (Moro's reflex) is one of the most frequent and dramatic newborn responses. It occurs when your infant hears a loud noise, has an abrupt change in position or is handled roughly.

The startle reflex causes an infant to arch his or her back and throw his or her head back. At the same time, he or she throws out his or her arms and legs and brings them abruptly back toward the body. The infant cries, then startles and then cries because of the startle. The startle reflex gradually disappears by the third month of life.

The grasp reflex
Stroking your infant sets off several responses. When you stroke the palm of his or her hand, your baby grasps your finger (palmar reflex). When you stroke the sole of your baby's foot, you'll see the toes turn downward, as if trying to grasp (plantar reflex). The palmar reflex disappears at about age 6 months.

Developmental Milestones

During the first 12 months of life, your baby works harder than at any other stage of his or her existence. In the course of this incredible first year, your infant goes from being totally dependent to walking, feeding himself or herself and even speaking a few words. Although every baby's developmental achievements are different, the following month-by-month milestones can be used as a general guide.

1st month — First smile
A momentous occasion during the early weeks of life is your baby's first smile. Although you'll often see a smile on your newborn, an infant generally doesn't have what is called a social smile until after the first month, usually by the eighth week.

2nd month — Voice recognition
By the second month of life, your baby can differentiate people from objects, with the former eliciting a much more immediate response. Your infant is beginning to recognize your voice. Thus you may find that the baby who screams when with a babysitter calms immediately when a parent enters the room and talks in a soothing voice.

3rd month — Independent play
An infant at 3 months can play for perhaps 10 or 15 minutes at a time, with minimal parental involvement. The infant at this age is more easily distracted and will even interrupt nursing to look at or listen to something that catches his or her attention. The baby will spend time staring at things — a picture, a mobile, his or her own hand.

4th month — Mirror play
A milestone during this period is your baby's behavior in front of a mirror. Hold him or her in front of the mirror and watch the infant smile. When the image smiles back, the baby will become very excited and begin to babble. It will puzzle him or her to see two of you, and he or she will repeatedly look back at you and then at the mirror.

5th month — Stranger anxiety
At 5 months your baby definitely knows the difference between his or her parents and strangers. For the first time, you may notice your baby is more cautious around strangers.

6th month — Finger foods
A 6-month-old infant is alert for half of his or her waking hours. By this age solid foods may be a part of his or her diet. Gone are the days when your baby was content to have you do all of the feeding. Now that the infant's dexterity is improved, he or she wants to pick up pieces of food and put them in his or her own mouth and anywhere else mood dictates.

The plantar reflex continues until 10 months of age.

The rooting and sucking reflexes

The rooting and sucking reflexes are two of your infant's important reflexes. Stroking the baby's cheek or lips produces the rooting reflex. The baby turns toward the stroking object and begins to root for the nipple. The sucking reflex is initiated once the nipple is taken into the baby's mouth.

Sucking and rooting reflexes usually diminish by the time the infant is 4 months old, although these reflexes can often be produced in a sleeping infant until the seventh month.

The tonic neck reflex

The tonic neck reflex is seen when your baby is on his or her back with his or her head turned to the side. The infant arches his or her body away from the face side, extends the arm on the face side and flexes the other arm and draws up the legs. This reflex is more prominent in the 2-month-old infant and

7th month — More mobility

Increased motor skills give the infant of 7 months a taste of freedom. At the same time that your baby longs to test his or her wings, however, he or she only wants to do it within sight of your reassuring presence. Don't be surprised if every time you leave the room your baby cries. The infant who has been content up until now to spend time in a playpen may suddenly rebel unless you're in the same room.

8th month — Separation anxiety

An 8-month-old baby is clearly attached to the parent providing most of his or her care. Separation anxiety often occurs at this age, and you may find that you can't leave the room without sending your baby into a panic. The baby who previously wasn't bothered by strangers suddenly may fear the next-door neighbor or even a grandparent. Or the infant may cry uncontrollably when the babysitter arrives, even when the caregiver is someone the baby knows. This reaction is a normal part of development and isn't something to be concerned about. Cuddle your child and reassure him or her that you will return soon. Always tell your infant that you're leaving and will return.

9th month — New games

An infant at 9 months is sophisticated enough to be bored. This is because his or her memory is more developed. Thus the infant is constantly searching for new stimulation, and the nightly game that has amused him or her for the past month suddenly has become uninteresting.

10th month — Imitation

A 10-month-old may begin to say no. Your child is also developing a sense of possession and may for the first time distinguish between baby's toys and those belonging to a sibling. You'll also notice how imitation plays a role in your infant's learning. During a meal the baby may offer you bits of food. Afterward he or she may attempt to wash your face and hands.

11th month — Testing authority

Although not always cooperative, your 11-month-old baby seeks your approval and will try to avoid your disapproval. Still, the infant can't avoid testing your authority. After you've put your son or daughter to bed, he or she may summon you every 5 minutes. At the same time, your every request is apt to be met with a resounding no. At this age, no sometimes means yes.

12th month — Temper tantrum

At 12 months some infants begin to have tantrums. Your eager eater may become picky. Bedtime problems are common at this age.

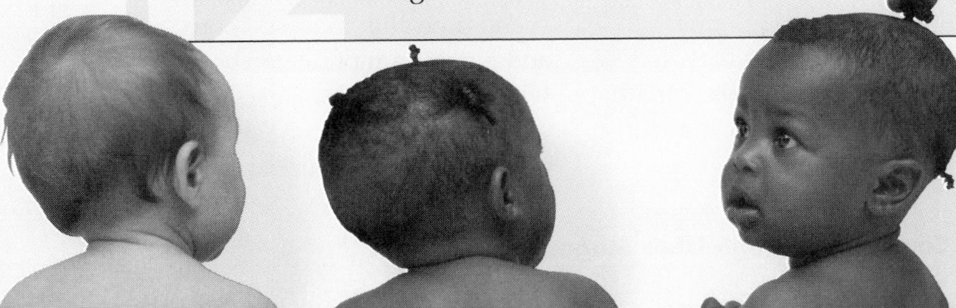

usually disappears by the sixth month.

The orienting response
The orienting response of your newborn is a response to a change in the environment. If, for example, the child hears or sees something new, he or she becomes more alert and less active. His or her head may turn toward the stimulus, and his or her heart rate increase. If the infant is adapting to a familiar stimulus, the heartbeat may slow.

The gag and blink reflexes
An infant is able to protect itself because of several responses and reflexes. Because of a strong gag reflex, your newborn is able to spit up mucus to help clear his or her windpipe. A strong blink reflex protects the newborn's eyes from glaring light. If a part of the infant's body is exposed to cold air, his or her entire body changes temperature, skin color appears mottled, limbs pull in close to the body to reduce the exposed surface, and he or she begins to shiver and cry in an attempt to stay warm.

Even though your newborn's reflexes will disappear — most of them during the first year of life — their usefulness seems to be more than short term. Studies indicate that your baby's brain stores information learned from these early reflexes.

Behavior

Your baby's sleeping, crying and eating patterns define your infant's behavior. A baby that sleeps easily, cries very little and eats predictably may be easier to care for. The irritable, fretful baby that feeds irregularly and sleeps little requires more attention. Normal infant behavior covers a wide range of patterns.

Your baby's behavior will influence how you parent. Initially, a newborn responds primarily to his or her immediate physical needs. But a newborn's emotional needs are equally important. Newborns need comforting and holding. They need the sound of your voice and the sight of your smile.

Prevailing wisdom used to be that a newborn could easily be spoiled. Babies were put on strict schedules and handled only when necessary. If a newborn cried for any reason other than hunger or a diaper change, the wails often were ignored. Experts now know that responsiveness is a better approach.

Research shows that the longer a parent takes to answer a baby's cry, the longer it takes to soothe the baby. Babies whose cries are answered quickly in the early months of their development may cry less often and for shorter periods in later months. Instead of becoming clingy toddlers, these babies are more likely to demonstrate healthy independence.

Rigid schedules have been cast aside in favor of flexible schedules that consider the needs of the baby and family. By observing what works and what doesn't, over time you'll discover many things about your baby's behavior. What does your baby enjoy? How much stimulation does your baby need? How can you help quiet your baby?

Parents often underestimate their baby's ability to calm down without help from mom or dad. Examples of such skills include sucking a finger or knuckle, listening to a repetitive noise or watching an interesting object. As your baby starts to demonstrate these skills, it's important to know when to intervene during a fussy spell and when to let your baby try to calm himself or herself down.

Bonding

Bonding between parent and child begins long before the baby is born or adopted. When parents-to-be first learn that they're expecting a child — whether through pregnancy or an adoption — they may begin to look through books for a name for their child. They may furnish a nursery. They hear their baby's heartbeat at a doctor visit or receive a photograph of the child they'll be adopting. They plan and dream, worry and hope. And finally they're rewarded with the arrival of the baby.

Bonding is the complex array of emotional ties and commitments that characterize the parent-child relationship. By the time a baby arrives, there's already a strong emotional link on the parents' part, a link that feels stronger for some parents than for others. Over the course of the next few months, the infant begins to develop an attachment to the person or people with whom he or she learns to associate protection, love and guidance.

Bonding begins immediately. Most babies have an alert period for 1 or 2 hours after the delivery, making it a particularly good time for parents and infant to become acquainted. The key isn't when bonding happens but that it does.

How does a parent bond with an infant? There's no easy recipe for bonding, just as there's no way to tell someone how to love. Bonding occurs during the day-to-day exchange of affectionate actions between parent and child.

A mother gently touches her infant, and that touch is pleasurable to the new baby. When the baby's cheek is touched, the infant turns toward the mother's face or toward the breast and begins to nuzzle and lick the nipple. This not only stimulates the production of milk but also is a powerful emotional stimulant. The baby gazes into the mother's eyes during breast- or bottle-feeding. The infant cries and the parent picks up the baby, strokes his or her cheek and speaks in a soft and soothing voice.

The importance of bonding is well recognized by hospitals and health professionals. Thus most hospitals encourage new parents to spend time with their newborn, and parents adopting newborns will enjoy doing the same.

If your infant is born prematurely or is seriously ill, your baby will probably be placed in an incubator and connected to machines to monitor vital signs. Initially, you may not be able to hold or even feed your infant. However, you'll still be encouraged to spend as much time as possible with your newborn. You can stroke the baby's skin, hold his or her tiny hand and soothe the crying with your voice. Even this limited contact is important and beneficial for both you and your baby.

It's not uncommon for parents to wonder before the baby arrives whether they'll be able to love this new person who is about to enter and change their lives. Even after birth or adoption, many a parent has looked at the new baby expecting to feel a rush of love and, instead, felt nothing or, worse, disappointment or even dislike.

Don't be too hard on yourself if you don't immediately fall in love with your infant. Parenting is never easy, and at times it can be downright trying. Love for your baby sometimes comes gradually. As you get to know each other, as you see the baby's eyes light up when you come into the room, or when the infant smiles at you for the first time, you'll soon find yourself loving your baby.

Sibling relationships

Much attention has been devoted to sibling rivalry — the hostilities and insecurities aroused in the older child by the birth of a sibling. But what about the infant and its relationship with big brother or sister?

Granted, life isn't always cozy for the infant with a sibling. This baby is apt to be poked and jabbed more than once, especially as he or she becomes more mobile. You have to monitor their play and make sure your infant isn't endangered.

On the positive side, watch your 5-month-old's delight when he or she is included in a game with an older sibling. Play with a sibling is so rewarding for the baby that he or she is sometimes willing to put up with a little roughness.

Besides the simple enjoyment of having a brother or sister to play with, your baby's mental and social development benefits from exposure to an older child. The infant learns self-protection, cooperation, imagination and how to get along with others. Moreover, the bond between your children is developed, and they gradually grow to love each other.

Don't feel guilty that your second and subsequent children don't get undivided attention, as did your first child. Remember, your first child didn't reap the benefits of an older brother or sister. There will be times when your baby actually prefers a brother or sister to you, or when a sibling's request that baby eat his or her cereal is quickly granted — whereas your efforts were met with resolute rejection.

Look for creative ways to involve older brothers or sisters in caring for the baby. Make a special effort to give your older children individual attention too. Encourage friends and family members to do the same. Your older children need to understand that you care about them as much as you care about the baby.

Be prepared for the "low point" in family relationships. It often occurs about 2 months after the baby's arrival. The novelty of a new baby is gone and so have your helpers. You may find it increasingly difficult to plan anything.

Discuss these common emotions with your partner, then persevere. Things will begin to fall into place again soon. This isn't to imply that relationships will always be smooth.

At around 9 months, some babies have trouble getting along with a sibling who only weeks before was an object of admiration. Babies this age are intent on battling their own insecurities and fears. An older sibling who loves to tease or assert authority is just too much sometimes. If this happens to your infant, don't worry. This stage will eventually pass.

General Care

For some parents caring for a newborn comes naturally. Others become anxious for fear of making a mistake or causing harm to their baby. Although there's no perfect approach to caring for a newborn, all parents can learn by their own experiences and the experience of others. Bathing, diapering, clothing, transporting and safety are some of the everyday issues all parents face.

Bathing

Bathing your infant can become one of the most rewarding routines of early parenthood. Your baby thrives on attention, touch and, eventually, the opportunity to play with you. Although not all infants will love the water from the first encounter, bathing can be a fun and special time for both of you.

Placing a tiny, slippery baby in an adult-sized bathtub can be awkward and uncomfortable for parents. Thus, many parents use a baby bathtub that can be placed in the kitchen sink or in the tub. Large bowls or wash basins also can be used. If you don't feel comfortable with a small tub, you can give the baby sponge baths initially. Many doctors recommend only sponge baths until the baby's navel is healed.

Never leave the baby unattended in the tub. It can be an extremely dangerous place if a baby is left alone, even if it contains only a small amount of water. All it takes is a second alone for a baby's head to become submerged. Don't allow yourself to be distracted by the doorbell or telephone. Let it ring.

Before you begin the bath, assemble everything you might need: soap, baby shampoo, a washcloth and towel, cotton balls, a clean diaper, an undershirt and a sleeper or nightgown. Fill the baby tub to a depth of only an inch or two, and before putting the baby in, touch the water with your elbow or wrist

Care of the Navel

The umbilical cord is a fetus's lifeline to its mother. During its 9 months in the uterus, the baby receives all of its nourishment through the blood vessels of the cord. At birth the connection is severed because it's no longer needed.

All that remains of the cord is a short stump, about an inch long. As the stump begins to wither and separate, the raw area is covered by a thin layer of skin, scar tissue forms, and usually the cord drops off within 12 to 15 days after birth.

Most of the time the care of the navel (umbilicus) is relatively easy. Many doctors advise parents not to cover the area because this may impede healing. The area around the cord should be kept clean and dry. When diapering the newborn, fold over the top of the diaper so that it doesn't cover the cord. This allows the cord to stay dry and prevents irritation.

Some doctors recommend sponge baths until the cord has dropped off. You may be advised to clean the area with a cotton ball dipped in plain water. Gently swab around the base of the cord to keep the area clean and to discourage infection.

A few days of crusted discharge or dried blood is normal until the cord falls off. Until the navel completely heals, infection is possible, although rare, because bacteria can enter the body through the opening. If your infant's navel area looks reddened or there's any discharge, call your baby's doctor.

Some babies develop small growths in this area, called umbilical granulomas. If your infant has a granuloma, the healing process is delayed. The area around the cord looks a dull red or pink, is moist and may emit an unpleasant-smelling discharge.

Initially, your child's doctor may recommend cleaning the area several times a day with alcohol. If the granuloma persists, he or she may seal (cauterize) the navel with silver nitrate.

to make sure it's comfortably warm but not hot.

Wash the baby's face with a soft, wet cloth but no soap. Use a cotton ball soaked in plain water to wipe around the baby's eyes. A shampoo is necessary only once or twice a week. Use a shampoo that's specially designed for infants. Wipe the suds off the scalp with a damp cloth. Don't pour water over the baby's face.

After the face is washed, soap the rest of the body. Most parents find it easier to soap the skin with their hand rather than a washcloth because the other hand is holding the baby. Wash the diaper area last. If the navel is still not healed, you may need to swab it with a cotton ball soaked in plain water. Try to keep bath time short because infants get chilly fast.

Neither lotion nor powder is necessary most of the time. Babies have delicate skin, and agents in lotions and powders that smell good can irritate sensitive skin. If your baby's skin is dry, choose an unscented lotion. If you choose to use powder, always keep it out of the baby's reach, and never dust it directly on him or her because the particles can irritate his or her lungs. Instead, apply some to your hand away from the baby and gently pat the powder on thinly.

As long as the baby's diaper area and face are thoroughly cleansed daily, infants probably need to be bathed with soap only once a week. If you wish to bathe your baby more often than that, use plain water. In winter, excess bathing tends to dry out a baby's skin.

Caring for the eyes and ears

During your baby's bath, wash around your infant's eyes with a soft washcloth or cotton ball and

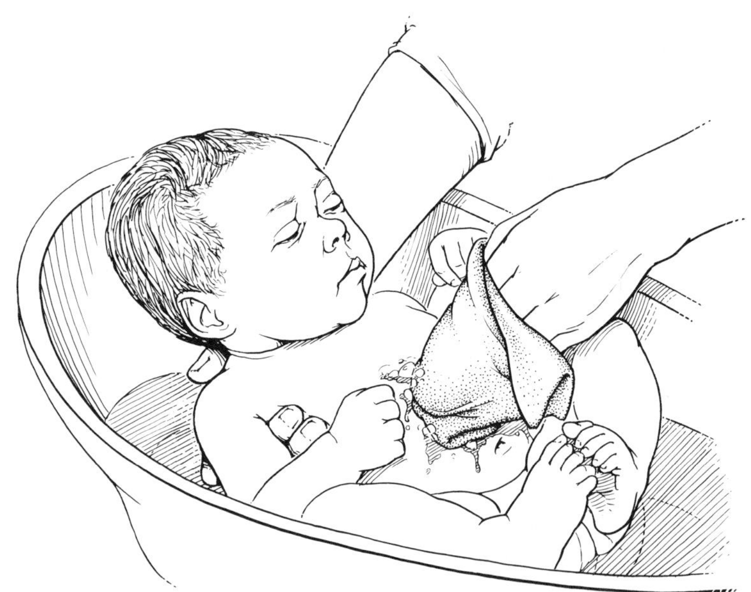

While bathing your newborn, support his or her head and torso with your wrist and hand to provide your baby both safety and a sense of security. Never leave your child unattended in the bath, even for a moment.

plain water. Don't use soap or any other cleanser because it'll irritate the baby's delicate eyes.

A newborn's eyes are bathed constantly by tears secreted by the tear glands. Many newborns develop a slight irritation of the eyes a few days after birth. This requires no treatment. If your baby's eyes are very red or pink, they may be infected, so call the baby's doctor.

Some newborns have a clear or white discharge from one or both eyes and may awaken with the affected eye glued shut. Usually, tears drain into the nose by the tear duct. In infants this duct is easily blocked, causing overflow of fluid from the eye. The blockage usually resolves in the first few months.

Treatment is only to clean the eye with plain water and a cotton ball, or if the blockage is persistent, your baby's doctor may prescribe antibiotics. If the problem continues, you may want to have your baby evaluated by an eye doctor.

Your baby's ears also are easy to care for. The outer ear is the only part you need to be concerned with during the baby's bath. Simply wash the ear with a soft cloth and mild soap. Don't be concerned about wax in the ear canal. Wax is formed in the ear canal for protection and normally comes out by itself. Don't try to remove the wax or insert anything into the ear for cleaning purposes. If an excessive amount of earwax makes it impossible for your baby's doctor to examine the child's ears, he or she will remove the wax with a special instrument. Any blood or discharge from your infant's ears should be reported to your baby's doctor.

Trimming of the nails

Trimming an infant's nails — especially for the first time — can be a bit of an adventure. Select a good pair of scissors. Ideally, the scissors should have blunt ends to prevent injury to a squirming baby. Small manicure scissors work well. Some parents prefer nail clippers.

Trimming a baby's nails while he or she is asleep is probably the preferred way because the infant is still. Another option is to enlist help and make this a two-person job. Have someone hold the baby's hands and feet steady while you do the trimming.

Diapers

Until your baby is toilet trained, you'll change many diapers. In general, neither cloth nor disposable diapers have been found to cause a higher incidence of diaper rash. But each baby is different, and yours may respond better to one type of diaper than the other.

When changing a baby who has had a bowel movement, use a disposable wipe or a washcloth with soap and water to clean the area thoroughly. A girl should be wiped from front to back to avoid getting stool bacteria into the urethra.

Disposable diapers

Disposable diapers are the choice of many parents because of their convenience. A disposable diaper is easy for even the most inexperienced parent to put on a baby. This type of diaper is pre-folded and secured around the baby with adhesive tape or Velcro-like strips.

Disposable diapers are convenient, but they're generally more expensive too. Another disadvantage is that they fill up your garbage and pose an environmental problem. In the United States,

Soft Spots

Every baby is born with soft spots (fontanels) on the top of its head. During birth it's necessary for the baby's relatively large head to move down a narrower birth canal. To do so the head must adapt itself to this smaller space. A completely formed skull couldn't do so. Thus, skull bones aren't tightly joined, and babies have spots on the top part of the skull where the bones haven't yet come together.

The size of fontanels varies. Generally, the larger they are, the longer they take to close. In some babies the bones come together by 9 months after birth. In others the process may take 2 years. The average is between 12 and 18 months.

New parents often are particularly concerned about soft spots. Some mothers are afraid to shampoo the infant's hair for fear they'll harm his or her brain. In fact, the baby's brain is well protected from normal handling by a tough, protective membrane over soft spots. Parents shouldn't be afraid of inflicting damage by simply touching the top of the baby's head.

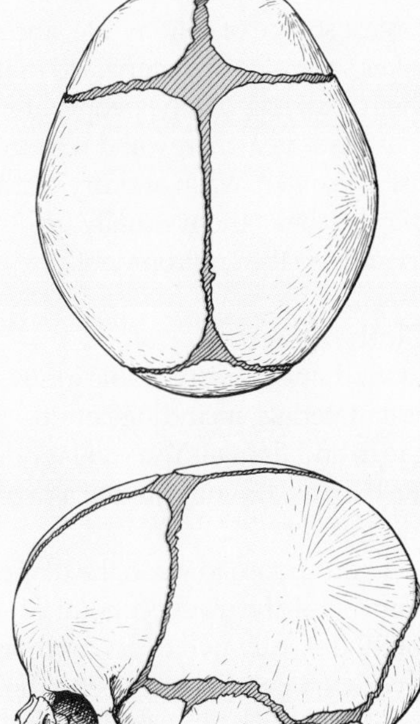

Your child's tiny skull consists of not one but several separate bones. During the first 1 to 2 years of life, these bones fuse to form a single protective bone mass. Until then there will be soft spots (fontanels) at the main junctures of the bones.

Is Your Baby Warm Enough?

How can you tell whether your baby needs extra clothing? Don't go by the warmth of your baby's hands. The hands aren't a good indicator of how warm a baby is because they tend to be cool even when the body is warm. The legs, arms and neck are better indicators. Your infant's face also can be a guide. If the infant is cold, the cheeks will lose all color. A cold baby is also more likely to be fussy.

disposable diapers are the third largest source of solid waste, and it takes several raw materials to make them. However, some people argue that the water, energy and resources used to make, wash and dry cloth diapers make them equally unfriendly to the environment.

Cloth diapers

Cloth diapers are available in several materials, including cotton, gauze and flannel. You can launder the diapers, or you can hire a diaper service.

If you choose to wash the diapers yourself — the most economical method — buy two dozen or more if you don't want to be tied to the washing machine every day.

You'll need a covered diaper pail partially filled with water to put used diapers in. Empty bowel movements into the toilet and rinse the diaper before putting it into the pail. Diapers should be machine washed with a mild soap or detergent and rinsed two or three times. Rinsing is important. A diaper containing soap residue can irritate your baby's skin.

If you hire a diaper service, the service will deliver clean diapers to your door and pick up the used ones, stored in a container. You may wish to compare the cost of a diaper service with the cost of disposable diapers. The difference might be slight. If your baby will be cared for in a child care center, check to see if it allows cloth diapers.

If you use cloth diapers, you can buy disposable diaper liners that help wick away moisture from the baby and make it easier to dispose of the solid waste before washing the diapers.

You can also find waterproof nylon shells with Velcro-type closures to hold the diaper in place. If you use diaper pins, slip two fingers between the baby and the diaper to avoid sticking him or her. Sometimes, it helps to soap the pin so that it slides through the diaper more easily.

Clothing

Comfort and convenience should be the important features of any newborn's wardrobe. In general, your newborn needs about one layer more of clothing than you have on. Make sure the material is soft, feels good to the touch and is loose enough for the baby to move about in without constraint. For your convenience and the baby's, the clothing should be easy to put on and take off. Also check to make sure clothing, especially sleepwear, is flame resistant.

In planning your infant's wardrobe, remember to buy larger sizes than your baby's age suggests. Most newborns can easily wear clothes made for a 3-month-old. Many 6-month-olds may be large enough to wear 9-month or even 12-month sizes. In the same vein, don't stock up on one particular size. Babies grow at an astonishing rate during the first year. Parents who buy too many clothes may end up with unused garments.

Nightgowns and stretchies

In the first 2 or 3 months, it's often easier to dress your baby the same during the day as you do at night. Knitted nightgowns and stretchies, which are usually made of a soft terry cloth or cotton, are perfect for sleep and wakeful periods. Because many babies virtually live in these clothes, you'll want to have several of each.

Once your infant begins to move around, you'll probably want to begin dressing him or her more for play and less for sleep. Jeans, cotton overalls with snaps along the legs and crotch, and knit pants and shirts are good choices.

When the weather is warm, sunsuits, shorts and T-shirts are appropriate.

Underclothes

Undershirts with a snap closing are usually easier to use on a very young baby. Unless the weather is extremely cold, a short-sleeved, medium-weight undershirt often is adequate.

Socks

Use socks when your child's clothing doesn't include foot coverings. Booties, while cute, aren't needed and often don't stay on. Shoes aren't necessary until the infant begins to walk.

Sweaters

During cool weather you may find that your baby needs a sweater for extra warmth over the stretchie. If you dress your baby in a sweater, make sure there's adequate room at the neck and that all of the buttons are sewn on securely.

Outerwear

A snowsuit, jacket or bunting is important if your infant will be taken out in cold weather. A warm hat also is important. The snowsuit or jacket should be lightweight, and the bunting needs to have a slot between the legs so that a car seat strap can be placed through it.

In the summer use a hat with a brim to cover your baby's face if he or she will be in the sun any length of time.

Bedding

Bedding should include flame-resistant fitted crib sheets and a mattress pad for protection. Crib blankets should be made of cotton or polyester. Cotton receiving blankets aren't particularly warm as a covering but are good for swaddling the infant to keep him or her from kicking off the covers.

Current precautions against sudden infant death syndrome (SIDS) recommend not putting your baby on its stomach to sleep. Also avoid putting your baby to sleep on sheepskin, waterbeds or thick layers of quilts and bedding. Plush toys should be left outside the crib.

Babies dressed in undershirts and nightgowns may not always need blankets. Studies have found that the incidence of SIDS goes down when precautions are taken. See page 172 for more information on SIDS.

Infant carriers and car seats

Safe places to keep your baby close by while you're at home are in a playpen, on a blanket placed on the floor or in an infant carrier. The safest place to keep your baby during a car ride is in an infant car seat.

Infant carriers

Infant carriers are inclined plastic seats that are useful for carrying an infant from one location to another. The seat is also a good place to put your awake baby when your arms are full. If you decide to use an infant carrier, make sure you always strap the infant into it. Keep the seat on the floor or a low table. Just a few slight rocking motions from the infant are enough to move the carrier off the edge of a countertop and bring baby crashing to the floor. Make sure that any seat you buy has a large enough base so that it won't tip easily once your baby becomes more active. Some car seats convert to serve as infant carriers, but not all infant carriers meet car safety standards.

Infant car seats

Not that long ago, parents assumed that the safest place for their baby during a ride in the car was in someone's arms. Today we know that a baby held in someone's arms is at increased risk of being severely injured or killed should an auto accident occur.

In the United States, it's required by law that infants and toddlers in cars be in a specially designed car safety seat. If you're preparing to welcome a baby into your home, a safety seat will be one of your most important purchases. Your baby shouldn't leave the hospital without a car seat. In fact, most hospitals won't allow parents to take an infant home unless they have a safety seat. Many hospitals or civic groups either rent or lend safety seats to parents of newborns.

A safety seat is designed to diffuse the forces of a crash over the child's entire body and to keep the child from being thrown out of the car or striking anything inside. Although no one can predict the outcome of an accident, an infant's chance of surviving even a serious accident is improved greatly when a safety seat is used properly.

Two types of safety seats are suitable for a newborn: an infant safety seat and a convertible car seat.

Infant safety seats

Infant safety seats are designed for babies weighing less than 20 pounds. They're equipped with either a three-point harness or five-point harness. A three-point harness fastens between the baby's legs, and a five-point harness comes from each side of the hips and over each shoulder to snap into a buckle below the crotch.

Because five-point harnesses help even the smallest of babies fit snugly inside a car seat, they provide more stability than do three-point harnesses.

The seat should be installed in the back seat with the baby facing the rear of the car. This position is crucial because during a crash, the back — the strongest part of the baby's body — absorbs the shock. Read both the owner's manual for your car and the safety seat manufacturer's instructions to determine the best placement.

Convertible car seats

A convertible car seat can be used from birth until the child's weight reaches the car seat's weight limit. This seat can be converted from the reclining, back-facing position to an upright and forward-facing position when the child is at least 1 year old and weighs more than 20 pounds.

When you shop for a convertible car seat, make sure you buy one that conforms to current federal motor vehicle safety standards. Seats manufactured before 1981 may not meet current standards.

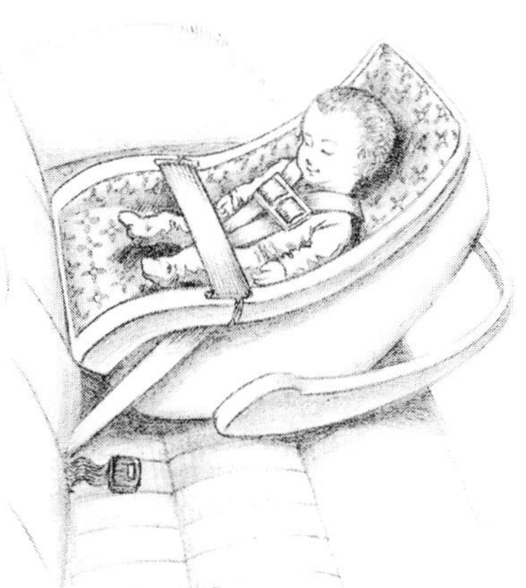

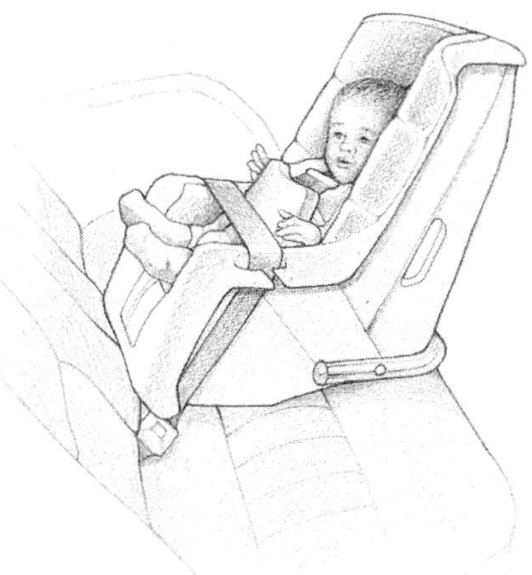

Infant safety seats (left) fit newborns best, but convertible car seats (right) can be used longer.

No matter what type of seat you purchase, it won't provide optimal protection unless it's used properly. Here are tips on proper use of car seats:

- Install the seat in the back seat of the car, preferably in the middle.
- Make sure the seat belt is fastened securely around the car seat.
- Adjust the harness straps so that they fit snugly and fasten all parts of the harness.
- If the seat has a top anchor strap, make sure it's installed.
- Don't install the car seat on a seat equipped with an air bag.
- Always use the car seat. Even if you're just going a block down the road, don't assume your baby will be safe unless he or she is securely fastened in the seat.

Home Safety

Making your home as safe as possible for your infant is especially important during the early months when your baby has no sense of danger. Your infant is particularly susceptible to injury in the home after he or she begins to crawl. It's up to you to make certain that your child's environment is as safe as possible.

Lead paint

For generations lead was used in plumbing pipes and paint. It was also used in typesetting, for sash weights in windows and in numerous other products. Many older homes were painted with lead-based paint.

Today we know that lead is poisonous. When ingested — whether in lead paint chips or in water tainted by lead pipes — lead can accumulate in a child's bone marrow, nerves and kidneys. Lead paint is present in an estimated 24 million U.S. homes where 4.4 million children younger than 6 years old live.

In many cases, lead poisoning produces no symptoms, but sometimes it causes irritability, weight loss, sluggishness, vomiting, constipation or abdominal pain. If you suspect lead poisoning in your child, consult your child's doctor. A blood test can determine the lead levels in your child's blood. If your child has lead poisoning, your doctor may recommend a change in your child's environment, diet or medication.

The best preventive approach is to inspect your home for potential sources of lead and eliminate them. Older homes should be checked to determine if any of the pipes are lead. Also beware of old lead toys or jewelry and fishing or curtain weights. Don't let your children play with them. Don't store juices in earthenware jars because the glazes may be lead based.

Crib

Since 1974, the federal government has required that the spaces between crib bars be no more than 2 3/8 inches. This precaution is important because it prevents an infant from getting his or her head stuck between the bars. If you're using an old crib, make certain that the bars are spaced in accordance with these specifications. Also make certain that the mattress fits the crib snugly because babies have been known to get their head caught in the space between the crib and the mattress, obstructing their breathing.

Make sure that any toys in the crib are soft, with no sharp edges that could hurt your baby. Remember to check stuffed animals for any loose buttons or parts that could find their way into a baby's mouth and cause choking.

As your baby grows older and begins to pull up on crib rails, be sure that the rails are positioned at their full height and the mattress is at its lowest position. The top of the rail should extend at least to the height of your baby's chest. Re-

Baby-Proofing Your Home

Your infant is particularly susceptible to injury in the home when he or she begins to crawl. It only takes a second for your baby to get into trouble, so it's important to be alert and to take extra safety measures.

- Never leave your infant unattended on a bed or table or in the bath.
- If you have stairs in your home, make sure you have gates at the top and bottom of all stairways.
- Cover your unused electrical outlets with protective covers.
- Keep pull cords for windows out of reach.
- Make sure that all cleaning solutions, insecticides and medications are stored well out of your infant's reach. If you don't have a high shelf or cupboard, you can buy locks that make it difficult for a child to open a cabinet.
- Keep plastic bags away from your baby. They can quickly smother a baby.
- Avoid scalds by lowering the temperature of the water heater in your dwelling.
- Keep kettles and pots on the back burners of stoves, if possible.
- Don't drink hot beverages or foods, such as coffee or soup, while holding your baby.
- Check your houseplants. Be familiar with the toxic plants in and around your home and make sure that they're well out of reach of your baby.

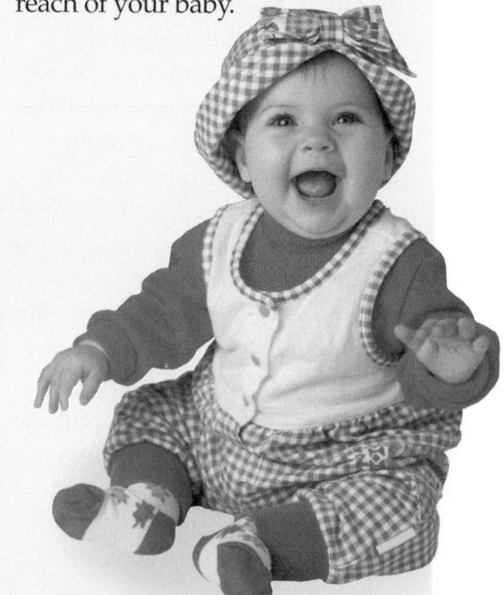

move bumper pads on which your baby might stand, enabling him or her to topple over a rail. To prevent strangling, don't string toys across the top of crib rails.

Toys

Always be on the lookout for toys that could be hazardous. Don't give your infant toys that contain small pieces that can be easily swallowed. Keep anything made of breakable material away from your baby. Avoid toys with sharp edges or loose buttons.

Most of the major toy companies indicate on the packages the age range for which a particular toy was designed. When you choose toys from a major company that are age appropriate for your newborn, you can feel relatively confident the toy is safe. Even so, examine the toy yourself to make sure nothing about it could hurt your baby.

Swings, jumpers and walkers

Swings, jumpers and walkers were all designed to give a baby increased mobility while freeing the parent to tend to other tasks. But they don't live up to their original intention. All of these "toys" need direct and attentive supervision because they can be dangerous.

By 4 months your baby is probably outgrowing an infant swing. A baby who can wiggle, scoot and shift can possibly topple out of a swing. Jumpers that hang on a doorway should always be positioned so that the baby's toes barely touch the floor. A baby in a jumper should always be supervised. Injuries can occur if the jumper falls or the baby pinches fingers between the jumper and door frame.

Walkers have caused countless injuries and shouldn't be used. Walkers are especially dangerous because their use can result in a severe accident, such as a fall down a flight of stairs. Many parents use child gates to help prevent such falls, but gates can unintentionally be left unlatched in the midst of a busy day.

Parents often believe that using a walker will speed a baby's walking abilities, but this simply isn't true. In fact, the use of a walker often robs the baby of time to crawl and learn to walk alone.

Common Conditions and Concerns

As a parent of a newborn, you'll spend many waking and sleeping hours worrying about your baby's health. You may have questions about blemishes on your baby's skin or have concerns if your baby is crying excessively. Birthmarks and excessive crying (colic) are two concerns you may ask your baby's doctor about. Some other common newborn health concerns include spitting up, teething, fever, ear infections, diarrhea and constipation.

Birthmarks

Birthmarks are common among newborns. Most are harmless and don't require treatment. Common birthmarks that can occur in newborns are salmon patches and hemangiomas.

Salmon patches

Often called stork bites or angel kisses, salmon patches are small, light pink, flat spots that appear on 30 percent to 50 percent of newborns. They're collections of small blood vessels (capillaries) close to the skin. Occurring most frequently on the eyelids, upper lip, area between the eyebrows, and back of the neck, salmon patches become more noticeable during crying bouts or when the temperature changes. Salmon patches often seem brighter in a child's first few months and then fade by 1 year of age. Those on the back of the neck often persist but usually aren't noticeable once the infant's hair grows.

Hemangiomas

Hemangiomas are noncancerous (benign) tumors made of newly formed blood vessels. Characteristically, hemangiomas are bright red, elevated, sharply demarcated lesions that may appear anywhere on the body.

Strawberry hemangiomas

Strawberry hemangiomas usually appear on the face, scalp, back or chest, but may be anywhere on the body. More common in girls, strawberry hemangiomas are seldom present at birth, but usually appear within the first 2 months of life.

Most strawberry hemangiomas grow rapidly, then remain at a fixed size and finally begin to disappear. Usually, no treatment is recommended, and they're no longer noticeable by the time a child is 9 years old. Strawberry marks developing on the face need closer observation for possible treatment. Some children with strawberry marks have some discoloration or a slight puckering of the skin after the mark is gone.

Cavernous hemangiomas

Cavernous hemangiomas are more deeply situated in the skin than are strawberry hemangiomas. They're typically a red-blue spongy mass made up of tissue filled with blood. The outcome of this type of lesion is hard to predict. Some disappear on their own. Depending on the location and size of the lesion, sometimes a steroid medication or laser treatment is helpful in treating it.

Port-wine stains

A port-wine stain is a flat hemangioma that consists of dilated capillaries. It often appears on the face. The size of the hemangioma varies. Occasionally, half the body surface may be affected. This is a permanent condition. Laser therapy has become the treatment of choice, but it's most successful on older children and adults.

Rashes

Rashes are common in infancy. The vast majority aren't serious and often can be managed at home. But a rash can be a sign of an infectious disease, such as chickenpox or measles. Have your baby examined by a doctor if you notice a rash that is purple, crusty and weepy or has blisters. Also call your child's doctor if the rash is accompanied by a fever.

Diaper rash

Most infants develop a diaper rash at some time or another. Diaper rash can have many causes. The typical diaper rash is the reaction of the newborn's sensitive skin to contact with moisture and irritants. This rash often goes away in a couple of days with exposure to air and more frequent diaper changes.

If your baby has diaper rash, change his or her diaper more often and gently wash the skin every time the diaper is changed. To clean the baby's bottom, use plain water, which is less irritating than baby wipes. If you've been putting plastic pants over the baby's diaper, stop using them until the rash disappears. Petroleum jelly, zinc oxide paste or lubricating cream can be applied to the rash several times a day. Mild rashes don't require ointment unless the skin is dry and cracked. Cornstarch or talcum powder shouldn't be used because they can worsen the condition.

If the rash is particularly persistent and severe, a 0.5 percent to 1 percent hydrocortisone cream can be used for a few days. For persistent diaper rash, many doctors recommend taking the baby's diaper off and exposing the affected area to air as frequently as possible.

If your baby's rash doesn't improve, it could mean the child has a yeast infection. The infection may appear on the buttocks and genitals as bright red spots that come together to form a solid red area with a scalloped border. This type of rash can be treated with an antiyeast cream or ointment and lots of airing.

If the rash is so severe that it interferes with your child's sleep, is a solid, bright red color, causes fever, results in blisters or boils, or drains pus, call your child's doctor.

Cradle cap

Cradle cap (seborrheic dermatitis) is a common problem that can occur at any age, but it's most common during infancy and again during adolescence. Cradle cap often begins during the infant's first month of life and may continue to be a problem throughout the first year. Its cause is unknown.

If your infant has cradle cap you probably first will notice dry, scaly patches on the scalp that give it a dirty appearance. A thick, yellow crust may form over the scales. You may notice some scaly patches around the hairline, eyebrows, eyelids, nose and behind the ears. Sometimes, the rash affects the entire body.

Cradle cap usually has a shorter course than many other rashes, and it responds to simple treatment. Without treatment it will go away over a period of a few months.

For cradle cap, avoid the temptation to wash your baby's hair frequently with baby shampoo. Once a week is often enough. After lathering, massage the scaly scalp with a soft toothbrush for a few minutes. If the scalp is very crusty, you can rub in mineral or baby oil an hour before you shampoo. If the rash is red and irritated, apply a 0.5 percent hydrocortisone cream, available without a prescription, once a week. Use of an antidandruff shampoo also may provide relief. A particularly stubborn case should be evaluated by your infant's doctor.

Drool rash

Many infants develop a rash on their cheeks and chin. The rash, which is caused by contact with food and regurgitated stomach contents, comes and goes. The only treatment generally required is cleansing the skin after a feeding. Placing a diaper under your infant's face during naps to absorb the drool or regurgitated material also may help.

Heat rash

Heat rash causes tiny pink bumps on the skin and usually occurs on the back of the neck and upper back. It's the result of blocked sweat glands. Typically, the rash occurs during hot, humid weather, although an infant who is overdressed or who has a fever may develop a heat rash at any time.

Treatment involves letting the skin dry on its own and dressing your infant in as few clothes as necessary. Use a fan while the child is sleeping. Cool rinses also may help.

Infantile eczema

Infantile eczema (atopic dermatitis) is a rough, red, patchy rash usually associated with extremely dry, sensitive skin. The most common areas for eczema are the cheeks and forehead. The problem may spread to the neck and behind the ears.

Eczema is more likely to occur in infants with a family history of allergies. These infants also have a tendency to develop asthma and seasonal allergies later in their lives. If your infant has eczema, you may first notice light red or tannish-pink patches of rough, scaly skin. The patches later become red (see the color illustration on page 436). The baby may seem restless or irritable due to itching. Occasionally, the rash begins to ooze and crust over. Infection of the skin may follow.

In some infants the rash can be traced to diet or a change in formula. Sometimes, the offender may be a laundry detergent, a fabric such as wool or excessive perspiration during hot weather. Rarely, eczema may be a symptom of a serious disease. Often the cause is hard to identify.

The main complication of eczema is infection of the lesions. Infants with eczema shouldn't be exposed to people with cold sores (herpes simplex).

To decrease the chance of more bacteria being introduced into the open skin, keep your baby's nails clipped as short as possible. If your baby will tolerate them, a pair of cotton mittens worn especially during sleep, which is when most of the scratching usually occurs, helps prevent further skin damage and infection.

Avoid temperature extremes. Most babies with eczema do better in a mild climate with moderate humidity because sweating seems to aggravate the rash. Avoid wool clothing and don't lay the baby on wool carpeting. Keep baths to a minimum and use bath oil to lubricate the dry skin.

If the eczema is particularly severe, your baby's doctor may recommend use of dressings soaked in a special solution to ease the redness and itching.

Corticosteroid lotions and creams can be applied after the dressing is removed. Antihistamines are often effective for controlling the itching. If your baby's lesions become infected, oral or topical antibiotics may be necessary. Most children outgrow infantile eczema by 3 to 5 years of age.

Milia

Milia are small white bumps or cysts on a newborn's face that resemble whiteheads. More than half of newborns have these little spots.

By the time the infant is 2 months old, the blocked skin pores generally open up and disappear. The bumps are harmless and don't need treatment.

Infant acne

About one-third of all infants develop acne, usually after the third week of life. The cause appears to be related to maternal hormones that cross the placenta before birth.

The presence of acne can be disturbing, but it's only temporary. In some infants the acne disappears within weeks. In others, it persists for up to 6 months. Generally, no treatment is necessary other than gently washing your baby's face daily with plain water and once or twice a week with a mild soap.

Thrush

Thrush is a mild yeast infection of the mouth that looks like whitish patches. The patches may be on the tongue and roof of the mouth and stuck to the inside of the cheeks. If the white spots don't come off when gently rubbed with a cotton swab, your baby may have thrush. Consult your baby's doctor.

Thrush in healthy newborns generally resolves on its own, but treatment with an antiyeast medication can hasten the process, particularly if the thrush is extensive. A breastfeeding mother also may need treatment if her nipples are sore.

An antiyeast cream may be necessary to treat diaper rash that can accompany thrush. Because yeast grows well on warm, moist skin, exposing infected areas to air will benefit both babies and mothers with thrush.

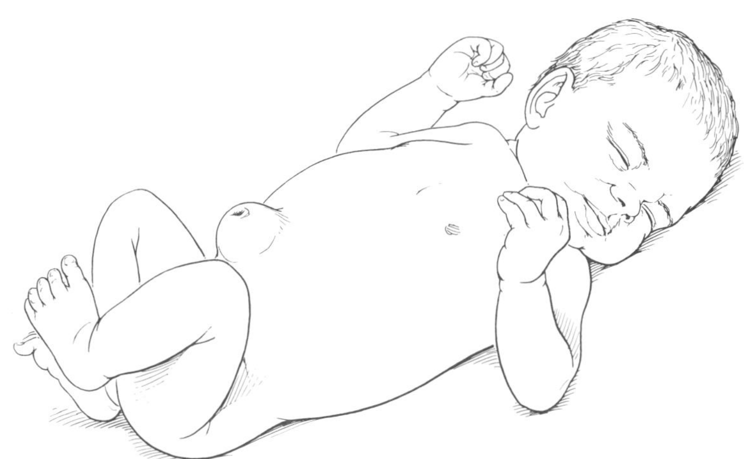

An umbilical hernia is caused by a failure of the ring around the navel to close. It results in a soft swelling that may protrude farther during coughing, straining and crying.

Umbilical hernia

An infant with an umbilical hernia has a soft bulge of tissue around the navel (umbilicus) that may protrude more when the baby cries, coughs or strains. It's caused by failure of the ring around the navel to close. As a result, a portion of the small intestine slips through the enlarged umbilical opening.

An umbilical hernia is more apt to occur in black infants and in those with a low birth weight. Unlike other hernias, umbilical hernias have little danger associated with them. Most infant umbilical hernias disappear by the time the baby is a year old. Surgery is rarely necessary unless the hernia becomes progressively larger, fails to heal by the time the child is 5 years old or causes an intestinal obstruction.

Spitting up and vomiting

Spitting up usually isn't a cause for concern, but vomiting may be.

Spitting up

Infants often spit up after a feeding. Spitting up is the gentle spilling of what's typically a small amount of milk from the baby's mouth. This shouldn't be confused with vomiting, during which the contents of the baby's stomach are ejected forcefully from its mouth.

One newborn may spit up after every feeding, and another may spit up only infrequently. The reason babies spit up isn't completely understood, but it's likely related to immature digestive systems. Unlike an older child or adult, the muscle between a baby's esophagus and the upper portion of the stomach isn't yet adept at holding contents in the stomach. Thus, any movement, even something as gentle as laying a child down, can cause the milk to be regurgitated.

Spitting up is messy for the parents, but it rarely signifies a serious problem. It gradually resolves by the time the child is between 6 months and a year old. Burping the baby after each feeding is important and can help reduce spitting up. Even though it may take a while, try to get the baby to burp after every feeding.

Immediately after a feeding, some babies do better sitting upright in an infant seat. Others spit up less when placed on their sides. Try to see if there's a position that works best for your child.

If your baby is a natural spitter, the problem may continue no matter what you do. If your baby seems healthy and is gaining weight, there's little cause for concern.

Vomiting

Vomiting can be the result of milk intolerance, or it can be a sign of another illness. Notify your baby's doctor if your infant vomits, but as long as the baby seems healthy and is gaining weight, there's probably no reason to be alarmed.

A newborn may vomit mucus, often streaked with blood, a few hours after birth. Typically, this is blood from the mother that the infant swallowed during delivery and is normal. Usually, this vomiting subsides after a few feedings. If it continues, it can signify an obstruction in the esophagus or intestines that warrants further evaluation. If your baby continues to have blood in vomit or is vomiting persistently, see a doctor as soon as possible.

Shaken Baby Syndrome

Shaken baby syndrome is a serious form of abuse that can cause severe head injury to a child and even death. It's caused by violent shaking of an infant or a child.

Often, the victims of shaken baby syndrome are children younger than 2 years old, but it can occur in children up to 5 years old. The abuse is often committed by an angry parent or caregiver who shakes a baby in an attempt to stop its crying, or as punishment. Shaken baby syndrome doesn't result from gentle bouncing or play.

Loose stools or diarrhea

The stool of a breast-fed newborn is naturally mushy. If the mother uses laxatives or eats food with laxative properties, the baby's stools may become even looser. Bottle-fed babies generally have firmer stools than do breast-fed babies.

If your baby has diarrhea during the first month, it may be caused by an infection. The stool is apt to be greenish and watery, and the curds normally found in the stool of a breast-fed newborn will be absent. There also may be an unpleasant odor.

If your newborn has persistent diarrhea, call your baby's doctor. If your baby has only a mild case of diarrhea, you may need to change the frequency or amount of your baby's feedings. Let your nursing baby continue to nurse, but don't be surprised if the baby wants less than usual. Occasionally, a prepared fluid solution to prevent dehydration may be suggested for a short time. If the diarrhea is more severe or your doctor thinks the baby is becoming dehydrated, he or she may need to be hospitalized.

Constipation

Don't be concerned if your baby misses a bowel movement or even goes for days without having one. The consistency of the stool indicates constipation, not the frequency of bowel movements. A baby who passes hard, pellet-like stools is constipated.

If your infant becomes constipated, it may be due to inadequate fluid or food intake. Constipation rarely occurs in breast-fed infants, but if it does, try more frequent feedings. For bottle-fed infants, increasing the amount of sugar or fluid in the formula should help alleviate the problem. Iron in your infant's formula usually doesn't cause constipation.

If constipation is present from birth, your baby's doctor may want to examine the infant's rectum to make sure there's no obstruction or congenital abnormality. Chronic constipation rarely indicates other problems, such as hypothyroidism.

Failure to gain weight

Babies undergo dramatic growth in the first days and months of life. The most common reason for slow weight gain is insufficient intake of milk. If you're breast-feeding, your baby's doctor or a lactation consultant may be able to suggest helpful changes in breast-feeding techniques or patterns. If you're bottle-feeding, sometimes a change in formula or an increase in the number of feedings will resolve the problem. Occasionally, failure to gain weight indicates medical problems that need further investigation.

Teething

Your baby will likely develop a first tooth between 5 and 9 months.

Most children have between six and eight teeth by the time they're a year old.

Many babies breeze through teething. Their only symptoms are increased drooling and an insatiable need to chew on things. For others the process is fraught with discomfort, daytime restlessness and crankiness. Your child may take to thumb sucking as never before, rub his or her gums and temporarily lose his or her appetite.

If your baby is among those with discomfort, try the following techniques:

- If your child allows, massage the swollen gum for a couple of minutes with or without a piece of ice. Some children voluntarily or involuntarily tend to bite your fingers in an attempt to relieve their discomfort.
- Offer your child a cold teething ring. You may also want to give your child some ice, an ice pop or a slice of frozen banana to gnaw on. Never tie a teething ring around your child's neck because it could cause strangulation.
- Don't use lotions or ointments designed to reduce teething pain. These not only are unnecessary but also may contain benzocaine, an agent that could numb the throat and cause your baby to choke. Many of these products also have a bitter taste, so your child may refuse to take them.
- If your child is uncomfortable, use acetaminophen (Tylenol, others) for a few days.

Fever

Fever in a newborn is defined as a rectal temperature of more than 101 F. Fever is the body's response to infection. Keep in mind that in the first few months of life, particularly in premature infants, an infection may not cause a fever. The key is how your baby acts. If he or she is more listless than normal, contact your baby's doctor. Also call the doctor if the fever is accompanied by a rash.

Febrile seizures

A seizure (convulsion) occurs as a result of abnormal activity in the brain's nerve cells. Typically, an infant having a seizure suddenly becomes unconscious, with his or her arms and legs held rigid. After a few seconds, the limbs and face may begin to twitch rhythmically.

The majority of childhood seizures are caused by fevers and are called febrile seizures. When seizures are recurrent and not related to fever, a child is said to have a seizure disorder.

A febrile seizure most often occurs in children between 6 months and 4 years of age who develop a sudden fever. Sometimes, a febrile seizure is the first indication that a child is ill. Febrile seizures occur in about 4 percent of children before the age of 4 years. Many children have no recurrence after the initial episode.

Febrile seizures typically are short — usually less than 5

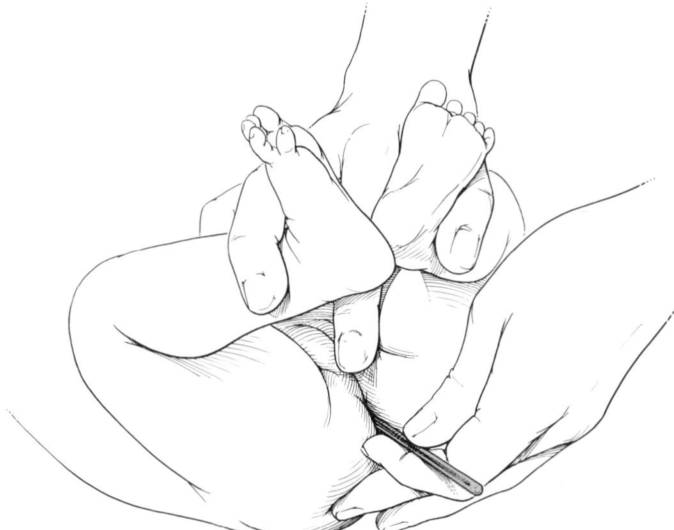

When you're taking a newborn's temperature with a rectal thermometer, insert the lubricated thermometer approximately 1 inch and hold it there for 3 minutes. Never let go of the thermometer while it's in your child.

? **Question and Answer**

Should I give my baby a pacifier?

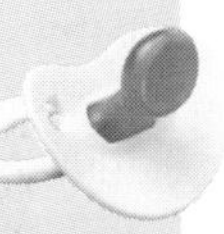

The answer to that question is somewhat controversial. Some doctors are adamantly against the use of pacifiers. Others believe that when pacifiers are used in moderation, they can be helpful for some babies who find comfort from sucking. Babies who suck on their fists, fingers or thumb may find a pacifier soothing.

Pacifiers shouldn't be introduced to breast-fed newborns until a nursing routine is well established.

If you give your infant a pacifier, the most important thing is to use it properly:

- Don't pop it into your baby's mouth every time it opens.
- Encourage your baby to go to sleep without the pacifier.
- Find other methods for calming your crying baby.
- Take the pacifier away as soon as your baby's need for extra sucking is gone, usually between 12 and 15 months of age.

minutes. It was once believed that a child who had a febrile seizure risked brain damage. This is rarely so. Seizures can be frightening for a parent, but in most cases the child is fine after the seizure.

If your infant with a fever has a seizure, these steps can help him or her avoid injury during the seizure:

- Place your child on his or her stomach or side, not on the back.
- Remove any hard or sharp objects near your child.
- Loosen tight or restrictive clothing that your child is wearing.
- Don't restrain or interfere with your child's movements.
- Don't attempt to put anything in your child's mouth.
- After the seizure is over and your baby is awake, notify your child's doctor. If you're unable to contact the doctor, take your baby to an urgent care center or a hospital emergency department for an examination.

Excessive crying (colic)

A colicky baby is one who's healthy and well-fed but has predictable periods of crying — usually at about the same time each day and most often in the evening — that may last for minutes or may continue for 2 or more hours. Colic occurs with equal frequency in male and female babies, firstborns and subsequent babies, and bottle-fed and breast-fed babies.

There are many theories as to the cause of colic, but the reasons for it remain unknown. Colicky spells usually begin within a few weeks of birth and usually disappear in the baby's third or fourth month. The baby can't be consoled for more than a few moments by any method. The crying has an effect on parent-child interaction and is a potential source of family disruption. A colicky baby is at greater risk of child abuse because overwhelmed parents may take out their frustration and anger on the crying child.

If your baby has colic, the weeks of crying can seem like an eternity. When you can't end the crying episodes by the usual consoling methods, you'll need to shift your tactics and concentrate on finding ways to survive the colicky weeks. Here are some suggestions:

- Rock your baby back and forth in a hammock motion.
- Try white noise. For example, turn on a vacuum cleaner, a hair dryer, radio static or any similar sound while rocking your baby.
- Go for a car ride.
- Put your crying baby in a sling or stroller and go for a brisk walk.
- Leave your baby with a supportive caregiver so that you can take a nap or get out of the house.
- If no one is available, lay the baby down for 5 or 10 minutes and do some on-the-spot stretching or vigorous exercises to re-energize yourself.

Although your attempts to console your baby may be unsuccessful, he or she still needs the reassurance of your presence. In addition, support from partner, family and friends is essential during this time.

If you're worried at any time that your baby is sick, or if you or others caring for your baby are starting to feel out of control with anger because of the excessive crying, bring your baby to the doctor's office or a hospital emergency department.

Sleep difficulties

Drooping eyelids, rubbing the eyes and inconsolable fussiness are the usual signs of fatigue in a baby. Many babies cry when they're put down for sleep, but if left alone, most will eventually quiet them-

Sudden Infant Death Syndrome

Sudden infant death syndrome (SIDS) is the sudden and unexplained death of an apparently healthy infant. Sometimes, the infant has had a slight cold recently. But more often than not, there are no signs that anything is wrong with the infant's health.

SIDS rarely occurs before 2 weeks or after 6 months of age, and the peak incidence is between the second and third months of life. Every year nearly 3,000 babies in the United States die of SIDS. Males are more likely to die of SIDS than females, and the syndrome seems to strike more often during cold weather.

Researchers studying this perplexing syndrome have noted that many of these children weren't really as healthy as they appeared to be. Some evidence now suggests that infants with SIDS may have had subtle abnormalities of the cardiac or central nervous system.

Although the cause remains elusive, doctors now know that certain infants may be at greater risk than others, although infants who aren't in this high-risk group also may die of this syndrome. Those at higher risk include premature or low-birth-weight babies, babies of smokers or drug users, babies who've had a sibling die of SIDS, babies who've stopped breathing and then have been resuscitated, and babies with low Apgar scores at birth.

Some conditions associated with a higher risk of SIDS are beyond your control. However, the following recommendations may help reduce the risk:

Sleep position
For the first 6 months, put your baby to sleep resting on his or her back, not the stomach. At the age when babies begin to move about in the crib while they sleep, par-

selves. It often takes 20 minutes of restlessness for a baby to fall asleep.

The following steps may help your baby learn how to fall asleep and get back to sleep if he or she awakes:

- Put your baby to bed drowsy but awake. A baby who habitually falls asleep in someone's arms may wake up in the night and not be able to fall asleep without being held.
- When your baby needs care or feeding in the night, use a soft voice and subtle body language to let the baby know it's nighttime, not playtime. Be businesslike and boring. Let your baby know this isn't the time for fun activities such as walking, rocking and playing.
- Think about your own sleep habits. When you awaken in the night, it takes a couple of minutes to find a comfortable position, settle in and fall back asleep. The same is true of your baby. Unlike you, however, one of the only comforting mechanisms your baby has is crying. Expect some crying as your baby tries to fall back to sleep.
- Make sure your baby is comfortable and safe. If you've made sure the crib and area around it are safe, you won't immediately become concerned about your baby's safety if you hear cries.
- Establish a bedtime routine — a winding down of the day's activities. You may want to turn off the television and have a quiet time 30 minutes before you put your baby to bed.

Ear infections

Middle ear infections (otitis media) are one of the most common illnesses affecting infants and young children. Seven of 10 children will have at least one middle ear infection by age 3. Although ear infections recur in one-third of these children, most children stop having multiple ear infections by the time they reach school age.

Ear infections often follow a cold, which causes fluid to build up behind a child's eardrum. The trapped fluid is an ideal breeding ground for bacteria or viruses that cause infection. In addition to an earache or a feeling of pressure and blockage in the ear, some children become irritable, lose their appetite or develop a fever. Some children may experience temporary hearing loss, but most ear infections don't result in permanent hearing loss.

Most ear infections clear on their own without antibiotics. But your child's doctor may prescribe antibiotics if the infection is severe or if your child has recurrent ear infections. If your child doesn't respond to antibiotics, your baby's doctor may recommend surgically inserting a small drainage tube into the eardrum to help prevent fluid buildup (see page 670).

Special Concerns

Most infants are born fully developed, healthy and ready to be taken home. Unfortunately, a few babies don't follow this pattern. Newborns requiring special care include premature babies, those with birth injuries, some congenital disorders or breathing difficulties, and babies born to drug-dependent mothers.

Premature babies

A baby born too soon hasn't had time for adequate development of body systems essential to life. Premature infants commonly need monitoring and systems support.

ents become concerned about maintaining a back-sleeping position. However, by the time your baby has learned to roll over from back to front or front to back, the risk of SIDS has already decreased.

Some babies have medical conditions that require sleeping on their stomach. If your baby's doctor recommends this position, it's usually best to follow that advice. Remember that sleeping tummy-down hasn't been shown to cause SIDS. It's only one of the factors that may increase the risk of the syndrome.

Bedding
Babies should sleep on a firm mattress. Avoid thick, fluffy padding under the baby, such as lambskin or quilts. Soft bedding materials may cause your baby to sink in and have difficulty breathing.

Diet
Breast-feeding may reduce the risk of SIDS.

Secondhand smoke
Provide a smoke-free environment for your baby. This measure is as important during your baby's first year of life as it was during pregnancy.

Room temperature
Your baby doesn't need a warmer environment than you do. If the temperature in the house is comfortable for you, it should be comfortable for your baby.

Electronic monitoring
Electronic monitoring of heart rate and breathing may be useful in dealing with some infants at high risk of SIDS. It's still uncertain whether electronic monitoring has any protective value. Babies have died suddenly and unexpectedly even while being monitored. If electronic monitoring is used, special training for the baby's caregivers is often required.

A premature baby is commonly defined as one born before 37 weeks of gestation. The word *premature* may concern some expectant parents because not long ago the survival rates for premature infants were much lower than those for full-term babies. However, recent advances in the care of low-weight, premature infants have greatly improved their chances of survival.

Risk factors

Many factors contribute to prematurity. Women who are undernourished, anemic or have had little or no prenatal care are more likely to give birth prematurely. A history of infertility, stillbirth and other premature births can increase the chance of premature birth, as can teenage pregnancy and smoking during pregnancy.

Often the stimulus for early labor comes from factors such as premature separation of the placenta, uterine abnormalities or a cervix that's too weak to bear the weight of the developing fetus. In addition, severe urinary tract infections in the mother may lead to a premature delivery. To reduce the likelihood of premature delivery, seek early and regular prenatal care.

Premature labor

If you go into premature labor, decisions involved in trying to stop your labor are complex. Your doctor can assess your health, the health of your baby, how your placenta and cervix are functioning, risks of infection and how far along you are in your pregnancy.

After taking these factors into consideration, your doctor can evaluate whether an attempt should be made to stop preterm labor and what these efforts might be. Interventions may include bed rest, intravenous fluids and medications to help you stop preterm labor. You may also be given antibiotics to prevent the risk of infection in both you and the baby.

Babies born after 23 weeks of gestation have a good chance of surviving with the help of newborn intensive care. As a rule, the longer the baby is in the womb, the better equipped it is to live outside with fewer complications and without long-term disabilities.

If your membranes have ruptured, a sample of amniotic fluid can predict the maturity of your baby's lungs and indicate whether there's infection in the amniotic fluid. If the membranes haven't ruptured, amniotic fluid can be collected by an amniocentesis test. If your baby's lungs aren't mature enough, you may be given steroids to enhance the maturation of the baby's lungs before birth.

Complications

One of the most serious and common complications of premature birth is underdeveloped lungs. A baby with breathing difficulty may require breathing assistance from a ventilator connected to a tube that's placed down the windpipe (trachea). The goal is to maintain adequate oxygen in the blood, blood circulation and nutrition while the baby's lungs mature.

Other problems associated with premature birth include heart problems, bleeding in the brain, pneumonia, low blood sugar concentration (hypoglycemia), anemia and infection.

The combination of very little body fat and immature skin prevents a premature infant from maintaining normal body heat. Babies born prematurely are taken to special units where they're placed under warmers or in incubators to help maintain normal body temperature.

Nutrition

Premature newborns often receive their initial nutrition intravenously. This is called total parenteral nutrition (TPN), which is used until the newborn is more stable and ready to start breast milk or formula feedings. Many premature infants haven't developed the sucking reflex or are too weak to suck. These infants may be fed through a tube inserted through their mouth and into their stomach. After these early feedings are well established, the infants begin feeding by breast or bottle. Antibodies in breast milk are important to premature babies.

Bonding

The trend today in neonatal nurseries is toward greater parental involvement. Parents are encouraged to spend time with their infant and to touch and caress him or her even when tubes, wires and other equipment make cuddling difficult. Whenever practical, parents are encouraged to feed the child and to change a diaper. Some parents bring books and read to their baby or play music.

Birth injuries

A birth injury is a trauma incurred by an infant during labor and delivery. Most often the injury occurs despite excellent obstetric care.

Certain conditions make the possibility of a birth injury more likely. Prematurity, an abnormal fetal position, prolonged pregnancy, an unusually large fetus and a small maternal pelvis are some conditions that can increase the risk of birth trauma.

Forceps sometimes are associated with birth injuries. Forceps are used to assist in difficult vaginal births. Forceps injuries generally are minor, involving facial or scalp abrasions. Often, forceps delivery is the safest way to end a labor that may threaten the health or life of the mother or child.

Another technique used to assist in difficult deliveries is vacuum extraction. In this method a rubber or plastic cap is placed on the head of the baby while the baby is in the birth canal. The doctor applies suction with a pump and then gently pulls on the instrument to help ease the baby down the birth canal. Newer methods that prevent excessive suction help protect the baby from injury.

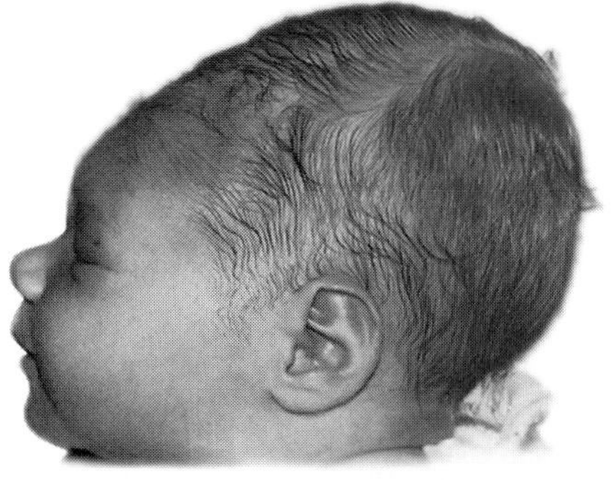

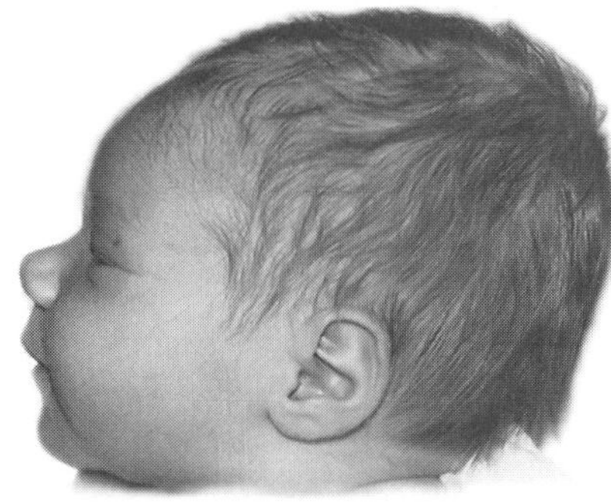

After traveling down the birth canal, a newborn commonly develops swelling of the scalp (left). The swelling isn't harmful and usually disappears in a few days when the baby's head assumes its normal shape (right).

Some common birth injuries include:

A swollen scalp

Swelling of the tissues of the scalp (caput succedaneum) occurs because of pressure on the head as it makes its way through the birth canal. The swelling usually disappears after a few days, and the baby's head soon assumes a normal shape.

A bruise under the scalp

A bruise under the scalp (cephalohematoma) is caused by slow bleeding. The swelling usually isn't visible until several hours after birth. This type of injury usually resolves within 2 weeks to 3 months. Treatment is rarely required.

A fractured collarbone

A fracture of the collarbone (clavicle) is the most frequent bone injury during labor and delivery, particularly when there's difficulty in delivering the shoulder. An infant with this injury is reluctant to move the arm on the affected side. The collarbone heals surprisingly quickly in an infant. Usually, the only treatment required is pain relief.

A dislocated nasal septum

Dislocation of the nasal septum, the cartilage between nasal passages, can cause the nose to appear asymmetric and flattened. The infant may have difficulty nursing and some problems breathing through its nose. Most nasal flattening resolves spontaneously. More severe flattening may require a minor procedure to reposition the dislocated septum.

Facial nerve palsy

Pressure over the facial nerve during labor or birth can cause weak-to-absent movement of a baby's facial muscles. The condition may involve an entire side of the infant's face. When the infant cries, the affected side of the face doesn't move, and the mouth is drawn to one side. The eye on the weak side can't close, and the corner of the mouth droops. Usually, improvement is rapid and complete.

Respiratory problems

At birth, a newborn must rapidly fill its lungs with air while at the same time clearing them of fluid. Simultaneously, the infant needs to increase the circulation of blood through its lungs.

A newborn must breathe without the lungs completely collapsing every time he or she exhales. Most full-term infants are able to accomplish this because the lungs have had time to develop fully and have enough of a liquid substance called surfactant. Surfactant helps reduce surface tension and prevents collapse of the lungs' small air spaces. However, many premature infants and even some full-term babies have problems breathing because their lungs initially lack surfactant.

Breathing problems in newborns include:

Respiratory distress syndrome

Respiratory distress syndrome (RDS) is characterized by difficulty breathing, breathing that's harsh and irregular with grunting, nasal flaring and perhaps a dusky blue skin color. RDS is a specific diagnosis that refers to a lack of surfactant. The severity of RDS correlates with the infant's gestational age and birth weight. The smaller and more premature the infant, the greater the chance he or she will have RDS. This disorder is rarely found in infants born at full term. Boys have this condition more often than girls, and white babies are affected more often than black babies.

RDS generally is recognized within minutes after birth. In some babies the distress at birth is so severe that resuscitation is necessary. Blood tests and an X-ray of the lungs can establish the diagnosis.

If your child is born with RDS, he or she will need to be in a newborn intensive care unit, where his or her vital signs will be monitored constantly. Nutrition and fluids may be given intravenously. Many infants with this condition require help in breathing. A breathing tube attached to a ventilator may be inserted down the mouth into the baby's trachea to provide assistance with breathing. Some babies are helped with a tube in the nose or a mask on the face to provide continuous positive airway pressure.

Infants with severe RDS may be given surfactant directly into their lungs. Other medications used in babies with RDS include diuretics to increase urine output and rid the body of extra water, corticosteroids to reduce inflammation in the lungs, bronchodilators to reduce wheezing and theophylline or caffeine to stimulate breathing.

The goal in caring for infants with respiratory distress syndrome is to keep them complication-free until the lungs have had time to develop. With the advent of special neonatal units and specially trained pediatricians (neonatologists), nurses and respiratory therapists, the mortality rate for infants with RDS has declined steadily.

Transient tachypnea

Transient tachypnea is a form of respiratory distress that can occur after an uneventful vaginal delivery or cesarean section and in both premature and full-term infants.

Infants born with this form of respiratory distress often have no signs of trouble other than rapid, shallow breathing. In some babies, the skin may have a bluish tinge, which can be alleviated with small amounts of inhaled oxygen.

Unlike infants with RDS, these infants rarely appear severely ill and most recover within 3 days. Treatment may include giving oxygen until the breathing improves, often within 12 to 24 hours. If the baby is breathing too fast to be fed orally, it may be necessary to use intravenous feeding. Usually, no other treatment is necessary.

Pneumothorax

Every infant is born with collapsed lungs. One of the miracles of birth is that within a few breaths the lungs inflate and the baby begins breathing. However, considerable pressure changes are needed to inflate the lungs that first time.

Occasionally, the lungs don't inflate evenly, and the pressure differences can cause a condition called pneumothorax, a condition that ruptures air sacs (alveoli) of the tiny lungs.

These ruptures allow air to leak out into the spaces between the thin membranes lining the lungs (pleurae) and the inner wall of the chest. This area is called the pleural space. If a small amount of air leaks, the infant will have shortness of breath, rapid or grunting breathing, and perhaps bluish lips and fingernail beds (cyanosis). If a large amount of air leaks, the infant may suddenly develop severe breathing difficulty.

Pneumothorax can be very serious if a lung collapses suddenly, but in most cases the leakage of air is small, and the air is reabsorbed on its own. Sometimes, no specific treatment is necessary. Pneumothorax may be treated by giving the infant extra oxygen to breathe for several hours. In the case of severe pneumothorax, the air that has leaked into the chest may need to be removed by inserting a tube into the space between the ribs (chest wall) and the lung.

Bronchopulmonary dysplasia

Breathing difficulties associated with premature birth generally improve within several days to weeks. Premature babies who still require assistance with ventilation or supplemental oxygen after a month are often described as having bronchopulmonary dysplasia (BPD).

Signs and symptoms of BPD include rapid breathing, wheezing, coughing and bluish lips and fingernail beds (cyanosis). BPD is often suspected in infants with RDS who don't recover quickly.

Babies with BPD need supplemental oxygen for an extended period and may need several medications. Most recover slowly over several months.

Drug withdrawal

The infant of a mother who took addicting drugs frequently during her pregnancy may go through withdrawal at birth. Drugs that can cause withdrawal in infants include narcotics (heroin, morphine, methadone), barbiturates (especially phenobarbital), prescription pain medications (analgesics), tranquilizers, sedatives, amphetamines and phencyclidine (PCP).

The infant may develop irritability, a high-pitched cry, sleeping and feeding problems, diarrhea, vomiting and convulsions. If the mother was addicted to barbiturates, withdrawal symptoms in the infant may not appear until 7 to 10 days after birth. The infant may also be at increased risk of problems due to poor intrauterine growth.

If withdrawal symptoms are mild, they're treated simply by providing a quiet, comforting environment, with swaddling, gentle handling and frequent feedings. If symptoms are severe, medications may be required. The smallest dose that will relieve the symptoms is given. After the newborn has had no symptoms for several days, the dose will be decreased until symptoms have disappeared without medication.

Central nervous system disorders

The central nervous system consists of the brain and spinal cord. Three important congenital disorders of the central nervous system are spina bifida, hydrocephalus and cerebral palsy.

Spina bifida

Spina bifida is a defect in the formation of a portion of the backbone and surrounding tissues. The defect can occur at any level but is most common at the base of the back. Approximately 1 in every 1,000 infants born in the United States have spina bifida.

Babies born with spina bifida typically have an outpouching of membranes covering the spinal cord (myelomeningocele) that causes a loss of neurologic control of the legs, bladder or bowel.

Surgery is performed soon after birth. The baby's back is closed to minimize the risk of infection and to preserve existing function to the spinal cord. More surgeries and other forms of medical treatment may be needed because of hydrocephalus and paralysis resulting from spina bifida.

Some children with spina bifida may have learning problems, but early intervention can help prepare them for school. Other children may experience problems with mobility and may need crutches, braces or wheelchairs.

Hydrocephalus

Hydrocephalus is an excessive accumulation of water in the brain due to an imbalance between the brain's production of cerebrospinal fluid (CSF) and its ability to absorb it. Sometimes, the cause is a blockage of the normal fluid pathways. Hydrocephalus in a young infant can result in an extremely large head. Hydrocephalus may affect as many as 1 in every 500 children.

The most obvious sign of congenital hydrocephalus is an abnormally large head. If the head of the fetus is so large that a vaginal delivery is impossible, the baby is delivered by Caesarean section. In some cases, the head may be normal at birth but then grow at an abnormally rapid rate.

Hydrocephalus may be detected during a routine prenatal ultrasound, but it's often discovered during infancy or early childhood. Computerized tomography (CT) or magnetic resonance imaging (MRI) is useful for differentiating hydrocephalus from other disorders and for finding the cause of the hydrocephalus.

The goal of treatment is to establish equilibrium between the production and the absorption of cerebrospinal fluid. Sometimes, medication is effective, but hydrocephalus often requires the surgical placement of a shunt system. This system diverts CSF from within the brain to another area of the body where it can be more readily absorbed. Shunts usually are needed for life. Complications may occur, such as mechanical failure of the shunt or infections.

Although hydrocephalus poses risks to both cognitive and physical development, with medical treatment many children live normal lives with few limitations.

Cerebral palsy

Cerebral palsy is one of the more common chronic health problems in children. It refers to abnormalities of motor control caused by injuries to the infant's brain during early development. The injury can occur before or during birth or during the first few months after birth.

Each year approximately 8,000 infants in the United States receive a diagnosis of cerebral palsy. There are many causes of cerebral palsy. One possible cause is inadequate circulation of blood in brain tissue. Abnormal brain growth and development early in the pregnancy is increasingly recognized as a cause of cerebral palsy. Injury to the brain during labor and delivery also can be a cause. Others include infection in or beside the brain, or bleeding in the brain. Often there's no obvious explanation.

Cerebral palsy isn't life-threatening, but it may require long-term care. There's no cure for cerebral palsy, but in some cases surgery may help reduce spasticity and resulting deformities. Treatment involves several techniques: aids such as braces and walkers to improve mobility, special education to help compensate for the child's motor difficulties and any learning disabilities, and early stretching exercises to help the muscles stay limber and prevent contractures. A contracture shortens the muscles or related tissues, making it difficult to flex the affected muscles.

Cerebral palsy is classified into the following four broad categories:

Spastic cerebral palsy

Spastic cerebral palsy is the most common type of this disorder. An infant with spastic cerebral palsy has an abnormal persistence of some newborn reflexes. A hyperactive grasp reflex leaves the infant's hands in a tight fist. As the infant grows, the limbs become more spastic and stiff.

All four limbs may be involved (spastic quadriplegia). When this occurs, there's often some degree of mental retardation as well.

Convulsions are more common. When the arms are affected to a lesser degree, the condition is called diplegia. Children with diplegia may acquire good use of their hands. Their intelligence is often normal or near normal, but they may have some difficulties drawing and writing.

Children with paralysis on one side of the body only (spastic hemiplegia) tend to have intelligence in the low-normal range, although some have average or above average intelligence.

Athetoid cerebral palsy

Athetoid (dyskinetic) cerebral palsy is characterized by uncontrolled, slow, writhing movements. These abnormal movements usually affect the hands, feet, arms or legs and, in some cases, the muscles of the face and tongue, causing grimacing or drooling. Children with this form of cerebral palsy may also have problems coordinating the muscle movements needed for speech.

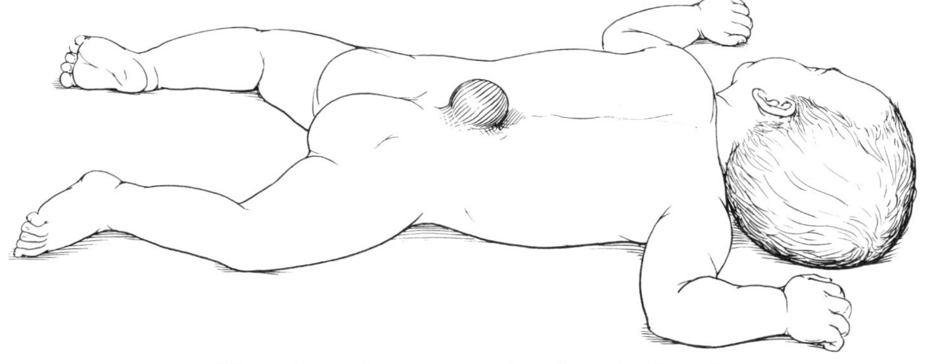

An outpouching of membranes covering the spinal cord (myelomeningocele) occurs in newborns with spina bifida.

Athetoid cerebral palsy affects about 10 percent to 20 percent of children with cerebral palsy.

Ataxic cerebral palsy

Ataxic cerebral palsy is rare. It affects balance and depth perception. Individuals with this form of cerebral palsy often have poor coordination and walk unsteadily with a wide-based stance, placing their feet unusually far apart. They may also have difficulty with quick or precise movements such as writing or buttoning a shirt.

Mixed forms

It's common for children with cerebral palsy to have more than one of the three previous forms. The most common mixed form includes spasticity and athetoid movements.

Congenital heart disorders

Approximately 1 of every 125 newborns are born with a congenital heart disorder. The heart defects range from mild to severe, with most cases being mild. The risk of having a baby with heart disease may be higher if you or other family members have had a baby with a birth defect.

The precise cause of a congenital heart disorder is rarely found. Genetic defects and certain viral infections during pregnancy may possibly be causes. Some chromosome abnormalities, such as the one that causes Down syndrome, are associated with heart defects. Infections such as German measles (rubella), contracted by the mother during the first 2 months of pregnancy, also increase the risk of congenital heart defects.

With recent advances in heart surgery, many of these heart defects can be successfully treated.

Ventricular septal defect

Ventricular septal defect (VSD) is the most common heart malformation, accounting for 20 percent to 25 percent of all congenital heart disease. An infant born with this condition has an opening between the lower chambers (ventricles) of its heart, causing increased blood flow under high pressure to the lungs.

Symptoms of VSD depend on the size of the defect. The problem may be discovered during a routine physical examination when a doctor detects a distinctive heart murmur. Babies born with large defects develop pulmonary hypertension, feeding difficulties, profuse perspiration, poor growth rates, recurrent pulmonary infections and cardiac failure in early infancy. Children with small defects may have no symptoms. Small ventricular septal defects may close on their own without treatment.

Treatment depends on the size of the defect. If medications are unsuccessful, an operation to close the defect may be done before the baby is a year old.

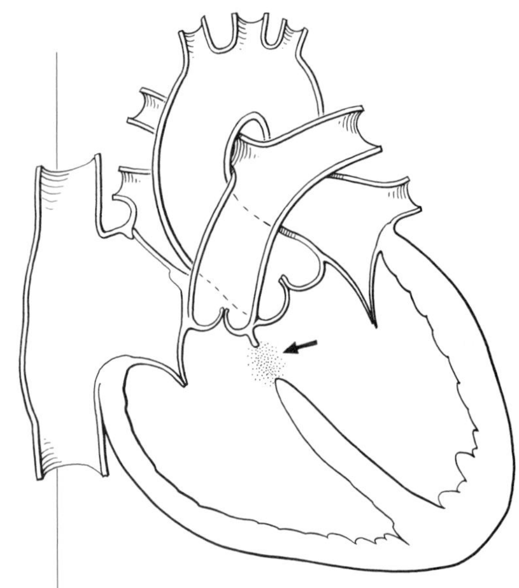

An unwanted opening between two of the chambers of the heart — ventricular septal defect (see arrow) — allows blood to flow under high pressure to the lungs. In many cases, the defect resolves itself, but in some instances surgical correction is required.

Atrial septal defect

Atrial septal defect (ASD) is an opening high in the heart between the upper chambers (atria), which produces abnormal blood flow. It's more common in female infants than in male infants, and it often occurs in children with Down syndrome. ASD accounts for 8 percent to 13 percent of congenital heart disease. Children with the condition frequently have no symptoms. Surgical closure is the recommended treatment. This is generally done around 4 years of age.

Patent ductus arteriosus

The ductus arteriosus is a vessel that leads from the pulmonary artery to the aorta while the infant is in the womb. This opening normally closes immediately after birth. When it doesn't, blood flows between the pulmonary artery and the aorta. Patent ductus arteriosus (PDA) accounts for 6 percent to 11 percent of cases of congenital heart disease.

In babies born prematurely, the ductus is less apt to close spontaneously. PDA occurs more often in female infants, in babies born at high altitude and in the offspring of women who had German measles (rubella) during the first 3 months of pregnancy.

When the ductus is small, often no symptoms are present. A large ductus will produce a heart murmur, pulmonary hypertension and growth restriction. In a premature infant, the ductus often closes spontaneously within weeks or months. In infants whose ductus fails to close, surgery may be necessary. This is most often done between the first and second years of life.

Constriction of the aorta

Constriction (coarctation) of the aorta results in increased blood pressure above the obstruction. Initially, no symptoms may be evident. Significant obstructions should be surgically relieved before 6 years of age to help prevent future complications. In severe cases, surgery may be necessary before then.

Aortic stenosis

Aortic stenosis is a narrowing of the valve through which blood leaves the heart to enter the aorta. Severe stenosis, which may be accompanied by breathing difficulties, is generally detected in early infancy. Mild or moderate stenosis may not present any noticeable symptoms, but during a routine physical examination a doctor may detect a heart murmur. The condition is more common in males.

Surgery is needed to treat severe stenosis. Children with mild or moderate obstruction should have periodic re-examinations because of the possibility of an increase in the obstruction.

Tetralogy of Fallot

Tetralogy of Fallot consists of a large ventricular septal defect, obstruction of blood flow from the heart's right ventricle to lung (pulmonary) arteries and a shift of the aorta to the right side of the heart. In addition, the right ventricle is enlarged. The result is decreased blood flow to the lungs.

The main sign of this disorder is a bluish cast to the skin (cyanosis). The manifestations of tetralogy of Fallot often begin slowly during the first year of life. Sometimes, the problem is apparent at birth.

The goal of treatment is to provide an increase in blood flow to the lungs. A heart operation is the usual treatment once your child is past infancy, but sometimes it's required sooner.

Pulmonary stenosis

Pulmonary stenosis is an obstruction in blood flow from the heart to the pulmonary artery. Mild or moderate obstruction may cause no symptoms. A newborn with a severe obstruction has a bluish cast to the skin and shows signs of heart failure. In severe cases, congestive heart failure can occur during the first month of life. Children with mild to moderate stenosis can lead a normal life, but they should have regular follow-up by a doctor. Those with more severe stenosis may require a procedure to open the valve.

Transposition of the great vessels

Transposition of the great vessels is a complex condition in which the two arteries arising from the heart are reversed. Blood returning to the heart from the body is pumped back to the body without passage through the lungs. Infants with this condition are often dusky blue (severely cyanotic) and must have immediate medical care. Several surgical procedures are available to treat the problem.

Congenital digestive and respiratory disorders

There are many congenital disorders of the digestive tract, some of which can cause partial or complete obstruction of passage of food or stool. The most common obstructions involve the first section of the small intestine (duodenum) or the lower portion of the gastrointestinal tract (rectum and anus).

Pyloric stenosis

Pyloric stenosis is a narrowing of the pylorus, the outlet of the stomach through which food and other stomach contents enter the small intestine. Although the precise cause is unknown, a family history of the condition may be a factor in its development. Pyloric stenosis occurs more often in males, affecting approximately 1 in 4,000 babies.

If your infant develops pyloric stenosis, the symptoms usually begin during the second or third week of life. The initial signs and symptom include regurgitation and possibly vomiting, at times forceful vomiting. After the signs and symptoms have been apparent for a week or so, the infant generally begins to vomit more forcefully (projectile vomiting). Rarely, the vomit will contain blood. Vomiting typically occurs during or shortly after a feeding, but it may be delayed for hours. After vomiting, the baby is hungry and wants another feeding.

An infant with pyloric stenosis has very small stools because little food is reaching the intestines. The baby may lose weight and become dehydrated. The infant's eyes may appear sunken, and the cheeks may be wrinkled. Infants with pyloric stenosis may appear uncomfortable but are not in great pain.

Pyloric stenosis usually can be diagnosed from the child's feeding history and from the identification of a pyloric mass on examination of the abdomen. An ultrasound examination is sometimes done. The condition usually requires an operation following rehydration with intravenous fluids. Within 6 hours after the operation, babies usually can resume oral feedings. The amount

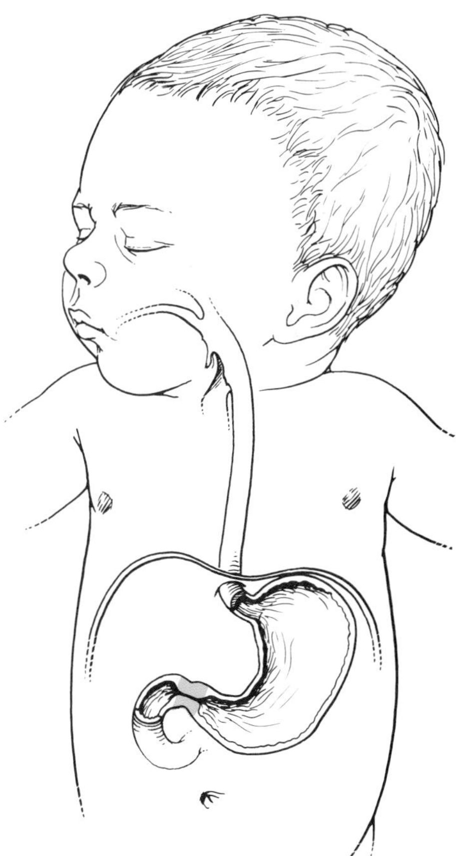

Pyloric stenosis is a narrowing of the outlet of the stomach (pylorus) through which stomach contents pass into the small intestine. The condition generally requires surgical treatment.

of the feeding is increased gradually. Most infants can go home about 2 days after the operation. A nonsurgical approach involving endoscopic balloon dilatation may be another option. The prognosis for an infant with pyloric stenosis is generally very good, depending on how early the diagnosis is made and the overall health of the infant.

Esophageal atresia

In an infant born with esophageal atresia, the tube leading from the throat to the stomach (esophagus) isn't properly connected. This condition can be accompanied by other disorders, which often involve the tube from the larynx into the lungs (trachea).

Signs and symptoms of esophageal atresia often are detected soon after birth. The infant may have an unusually large amount of secretions coming from its mouth, or it may choke, cough or turn blue when attempting to feed. Infants with this condition require surgery. If the underdeveloped segment is short, repair can be attempted immediately. If the segment is long, further growth of the esophagus may be necessary before attempting repair. In this event, a tube is temporarily placed through the abdominal wall into the stomach for feeding.

Biliary atresia

Biliary atresia is obstruction of the bile ducts. It affects an estimated 1 in 15,000 newborns. Infants with biliary atresia have persistent jaundice and an increased incidence of other abdominal abnormalities. The stools are pale to white, and the liver may be enlarged.

If an infant has biliary atresia, his or her doctor may recommend a procedure called the Kasai operation, which connects the liver to the small intestine, bypassing the malformed ducts. Children with biliary atresia often have persistent inflammation of the liver even after surgery. Some may ultimately require liver transplantation.

Intestinal atresia

Intestinal atresia involves an obstruction of the intestine that can occur anywhere in the intestines. A high obstruction is located just beyond the outlet of the stomach or in the upper small intestine. It causes vomiting, which tends to be persistent even when feedings have been discontinued. An infant with an obstruction in the lower small intestine or colon may have a distended abdomen, often accompanied later by vomiting. Vomiting of yellow-green material (bile) should always be investigated by a doctor.

An infant with an intestinal obstruction generally doesn't have a bowel movement, although meconium stools may pass during the first days of life if the obstruction is high in the small intestine. An obstruction may be complete or partial. When the baby has a partial obstruction, symptoms may not be immediately apparent.

Treatment depends on the type of obstruction. A complete obstruction requires prompt surgery to prevent severe complications. A partial obstruction may require surgery as well, but minor obstructions may not require surgery. With a prompt diagnosis and proper treatment, most infants recover from intestinal atresia completely.

Hirschsprung's disease

An infant born with Hirschsprung's disease gradually develops an abnormally large (dilated) colon. This condition, also called congenital megacolon, is due to a failure of the muscles of the colon to propel stool through the anus. Hirschsprung's disease accounts for about 25 percent of newborn intestinal obstruction.

Early signs may include a delay of or failure to pass meconium stool or have a bowel movement, vomiting and abdominal distention. Following a rectal examination, the baby may have a large bowel movement. Dehydration and weight loss also are common. Many infants with Hirschsprung's disease have alternating constipation and diarrhea.

Treatment for Hirschsprung's disease typically begins with an operation during which an opening on the outside of the abdomen (colostomy) is created so that the stool can pass into a disposable pouch. This is a temporary measure. The opening is closed during another operation in which the abnormal portion of the colon is removed — typically when the child is between 12 and 18 months old — and the colon rejoined. The treatment is highly successful in restoring normal bowel movements, although continued bouts of diarrhea or constipation can sometimes be a problem.

Imperforate anus

Congenital disorders of the anus and rectum are fairly common, occurring in 1 out of 5,000. Children born with anal and rectal problems have a higher incidence of other birth defects such as urinary tract disorders.

An infant born with an imperforate anus has an obstructed anal opening, preventing passage of stool. Imperforate anus is sometimes readily apparent on an examination or it may be suspected when a baby fails to pass a meconium stool within the first few days after birth.

Treatment depends on the location of the obstruction. If the anal opening is simply narrowed, an instrument can be used to dilate the opening. More typically, surgery is required. The higher the obstruction, the more major the surgical procedure. Some children require complete reconstruction of the anus. Others need a temporary opening on the outside of the body (colostomy) for the first 6 to 12 months of life.

Children with low anal obstruction generally do well after surgery and develop normal bowel control. When the obstruction is higher, there may be some uncontrolled passage of stool.

Diaphragmatic hernia

A diaphragmatic hernia occurs when an opening in the diaphragm enables some abdominal contents to pass into the chest cavity. In severe cases, the entire stomach and much of the intestines can displace the heart and lungs.

This condition typically is a life-threatening situation soon after birth and requires emergency surgery. A rare, later-appearing diaphragmatic hernia might be suspected in a baby who develops vomiting, severe colicky pain, discomfort after eating and constipation. Very rarely the condition causes only minimal symptoms and is discovered incidentally on a routine X-ray.

Omphalocele and gastroschisis

During normal fetal development, the abdominal organs initially develop outside the abdominal cavity and then move into the abdomen in an orderly fashion. In both omphalocele and gastroschisis, one or more of the abdominal organs (intestines, stomach, liver and spleen) remain outside the abdomen at birth.

When the organ or organs are contained in a protective envelope of tissue protruding through the umbilicus, the condition is called omphalocele. When they protrude through an opening beside the umbilicus, it's called gastroschisis. In this instance, the organs aren't protected by an envelope, and they may already be seriously damaged. With both conditions, surgery must be performed immediately and recovery can be slow.

Congenital emphysema

Congenital emphysema (infantile emphysema) occurs when a portion of a lung doesn't form properly. Air enters an infant's lungs but has trouble leaving. The affected part of the lung becomes overinflated, and air may leak out into the space around the lungs. In most cases, only one lobe is affected, usually an upper lobe.

Congenital lobar emphysema is almost always detected during the first 2 weeks of life. Signs and symptoms include persistent shortness of breath with wheezing and a bluish tinge to the lips and fingernail beds (cyanosis). In most cases, no cause can be identified. The infant's lungs may not have developed completely, or something may be obstructing the airway. A chest X-ray shows overinflation of the involved lobe of the lung and may reveal blockage of an air passage. If the baby's symptoms are severe, it may be necessary to remove the affected lobe.

Genetic Conditions

Whether your baby is born healthy or with a genetic disorder is determined by the interaction of the baby's genes (segments of DNA) and the environment in which the child develops. Genes determine many of your child's characteristics, which are passed from one generation to another. Usually this occurs uneventfully. Sometimes unexpected changes called genetic alterations (mutations) occur or are inherited from a parent.

Although most causes of genetic alterations are largely unknown, various environmental agents, such as radiation, viruses and chemicals, are among some of the factors that have been identified. For more information on genetics, see Chapter 18, "Genetics and Disease."

Other congenital disorders

Some children are born with a congenital disorder that's physically apparent. For example, features such as a small head, small ears, flat face and upward slanting eyes are characteristic of a child with Down syndrome.

Down syndrome

Down syndrome results from extra genetic material from chromosome number 21, creating three versions of this chromosome instead of the normal two. Down syndrome is the most common chromosomal disorder. An estimated 1 in every 800 to 1,000 infants are born with this condition.

A woman's chances of giving birth to a child with Down syndrome increases with age. For a 25-year-old woman, the chance of having a baby with this syndrome is 1 in 1,250. For a 35-year-old woman, the chance is 1 in 400, and for a 40-year-old woman, 1 in 100.

An infant born with Down syndrome may have a number of distinctive characteristics such as a small head, small ears, flat face and upward slanting eyes. The child's fingers often are relatively short, and the hands often have a single crease in the palms.

Infants born with Down syndrome may be of average size but then grow slowly and remain small. They have developmental delays that range from mild to severe. They also have an increased risk of congenital heart defects and gastrointestinal problems.

Babies with Down syndrome are at increased risk of problems such as respiratory infections, vision impairment, underactive thyroid and leukemia.

There's no specific treatment for Down syndrome. Heart or other associated conditions often can be repaired successfully with surgery. Many children with Down syndrome are happy, affectionate and easygoing. Many go to school, learn to read and write, find jobs and eventually live independent or semi-independent lives.

Upper extremity disorders

Sometimes, a baby is born with extra, missing or deformed hands, arms or fingers.

Total or partial absence of upper extremities
A child may be born without part of a finger, or in rare cases, an entire arm may be missing. As disheartening as this may be for parents, the child may actually do quite well. Just as with adults who are missing limbs, prosthetic limbs for infants and young children also are available. Once a baby with one arm is able to sit, a prosthesis usually can be fitted. Many such children do exceptionally well with no further treatment.

Polydactylism
Polydactyly is the presence of an extra finger or fingers, most commonly a fifth finger or an extra thumb. This problem is more common in black newborns. Frequently, the extra digit consists of only skin and soft tissue and can be removed easily. If the extra finger contains bone or cartilage, removal may also require surgery on adjacent structures and is usually performed after the infant is a few months old.

Syndactylism of the fingers
Syndactyly of the fingers is a webbing of the fingers. Because the bones in the fingers are of various lengths, the joints of the fused fingers don't line up and the fingers are difficult to use. The condition is corrected surgically. Without surgery, the child probably won't acquire significant use of the fingers.

Clubhand
Clubhand, a rare abnormality, is due to the absence of the bone on the thumb side of the forearm (radius) or the larger bone on the opposite side of the forearm (ulna). Treatment includes stretching the soft tissues of the arm during infancy. A later operation is necessary to reposition the bone, but retaining the new position can be a problem. Several operations may be necessary during childhood. Children with this condition also have a higher incidence of heart disease and blood problems.

Lower extremity disorders
A newborn's feet are proportionately longer and thinner than those of an older child, and the joints of the ankle and foot are extremely flexible. Often, normal feet may appear to be in abnormal positions.

In-toeing and out-toeing
In-toeing and out-toeing are common problems in which the foot or leg turns inward or outward. The condition is aggravated if the infant sleeps facedown. Both are usually positional or postural deformities that resolve spontaneously during growth and development. Treatment is rarely required.

Syndactylism of the toes
Syndactyly of the toes is a webbing of the toes. It's rarely more than a cosmetic problem. The scars and distortions of surgery may be more unsightly than the webbed toes. In contrast to webbed fingers, webbed toes usually function normally.

Clubfoot
Clubfoot occurs in approximately 1 of every 700 births. The term is used to describe several congenital foot abnormalities in which the foot is twisted out of shape or position. In most cases, the forefoot is twisted downward and inward, the arch is increased, and the heel is turned inward. About half of all infants with clubfoot have abnormalities in both feet.

Early treatment is essential and should begin soon after birth. The foot is manipulated to the normal position and then held there by a cast. This process is typically repeated every few days during the first 2 weeks of treatment and then at 1- to 2-week intervals. If this method is successful, corrective shoes may then maintain this position. If this method doesn't correct the problem, an operation, usually between 4 and 18 months of age, may be necessary.

Although the position of the corrected clubfoot may look relatively normal, the foot will never have completely normal contours, and the calf on the affected leg is often thinner than that on the normal leg. Orthopedic care throughout childhood is necessary for children born with clubfoot.

Extra toes
Extra toes can make it difficult to find shoes that fit. Most of the time the extra toes are surgically removed. The operation shouldn't be performed until the structures are large enough to be easily operated

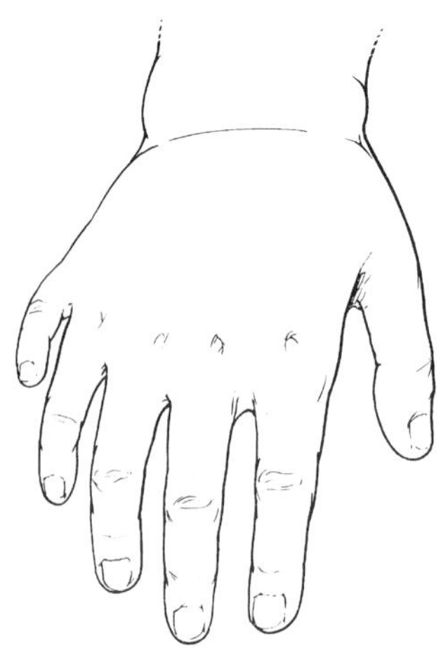

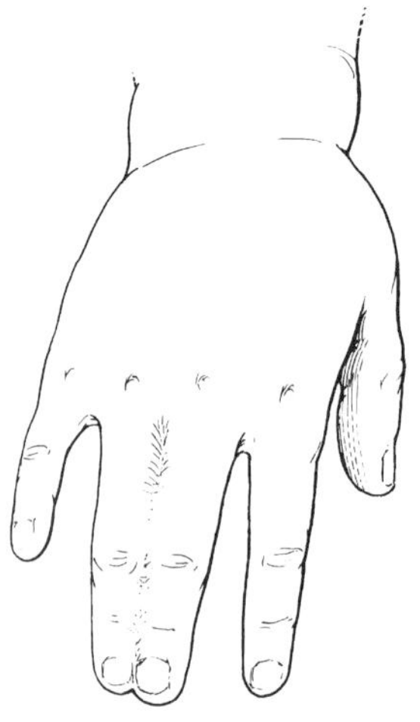

Both polydactylism, a congenital deformity of the hand in which the newborn has an extra finger, and syndactylism, webbing of the fingers, can be effectively treated surgically.

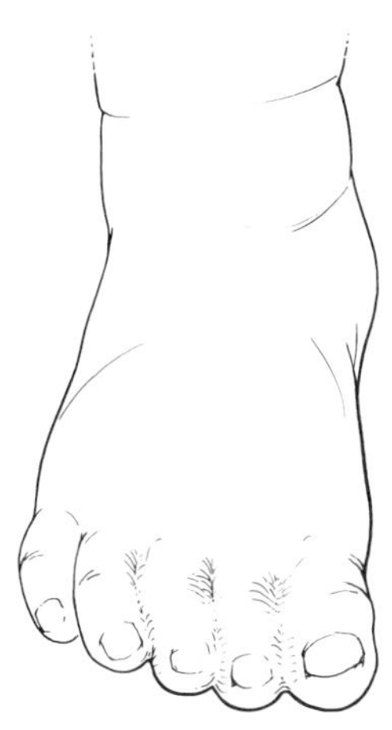

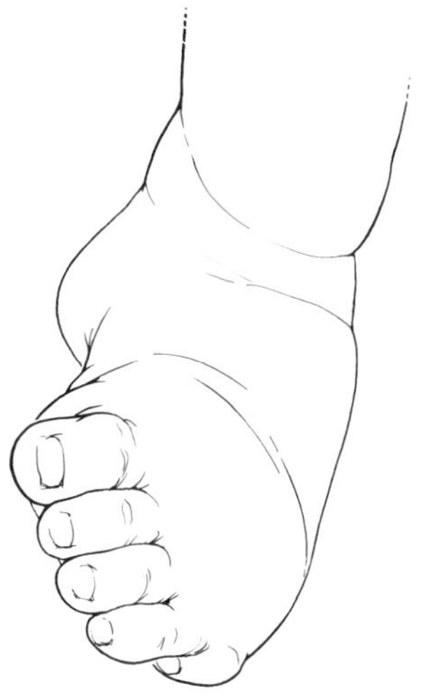

Webbing of the toes (syndactylism) is rarely more than a cosmetic problem, requiring no treatment. In contrast, clubfoot, in which the foot is twisted out of shape or position, requires therapy soon after birth.

on, yet it should be done before the child begins to walk and needs shoes.

Congenital hip dislocation

Congenital hip dislocation, also known as developmental dysplasia of the hip, is the result of abnormal development of the hip joint. The problem may be detected during initial examination at birth or in the first weeks to months of life.

A newborn with congenital hip dislocation is fitted with a brace or splint-like device to hold the head of the thighbone (femur) in the hip socket (acetabulum). This condition can be treated successfully immediately or shortly after birth.

Dwarfism

Dwarfism (skeletal dysplasia) may be due to several skeletal abnormalities, including disproportionate lengths of limbs and trunk. Sometimes, the infant's limbs are short initially. As the child grows, the trunk also becomes disproportionately short. Other problems may include hearing impairment and joint problems. There's no cure for the actual skeletal disorder, but many of the accompanying problems can be treated.

Treatment for dwarfism involves a combination of orthopedic techniques to maximize the child's mobility and function and, when possible, to correct malformations of the limbs and spine.

Funnel chest

Funnel chest (pectus excavatum) is a major indentation of the breastbone (sternum). The lower part of the bone is depressed toward the spine, and the chest has a funneled or hollow appearance.

This is usually a congenital problem, although rarely it's caused by rickets or a chronic airway obstruction. Some inherited muscle diseases also are associated with this condition.

Babies and children with funnel chest usually have normal lung function. Only rarely is heart function adversely affected. Surgery is recommended in severe cases with definite cardiac or respiratory abnormalities. Ideal candidates for treatment are children between the ages of 8 and 12. Successful treatment may result in the disappearance of the indentation. For mild to moderate cases, surgery often isn't necessary but may be performed for cosmetic reasons.

Lip and palate disorders

Cleft lip and cleft palate are separate birth defects that sometimes occur together. More than 5,000 infants in the United States are born with cleft malformations each year. Genetics seem to be more of a factor in cleft lip, with or without cleft palate, than in cleft palate alone.

An infant born with a cleft malformation, especially if only a cleft palate, has a higher incidence of other problems, including hearing impairment. An infant born with a cleft lip has a fissure or elongated opening where the upper lip failed to fuse. This can vary from a small notch at the top of the lip to a complete separation extending to the nose. If the palate is also cleft, the roof of the baby's mouth has failed to form properly.

With either or both conditions, the most immediate problem is

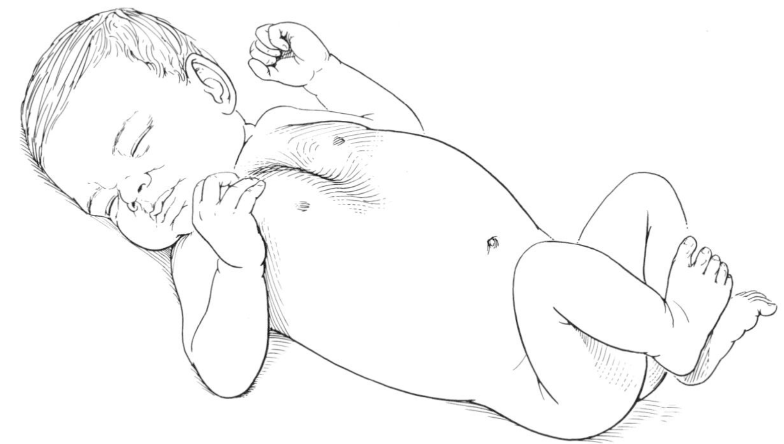

Funnel chest (pectus excavatum) is a congenital indentation of the chest. In severe cases, it can cause cardiac or respiratory problems. Mild cases generally don't require treatment.

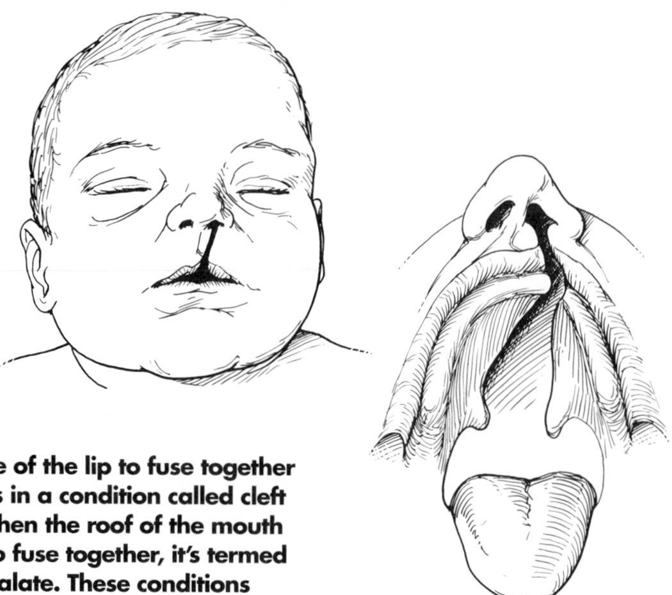

Failure of the lip to fuse together results in a condition called cleft lip. When the roof of the mouth fails to fuse together, it's termed cleft palate. These conditions require surgical correction.

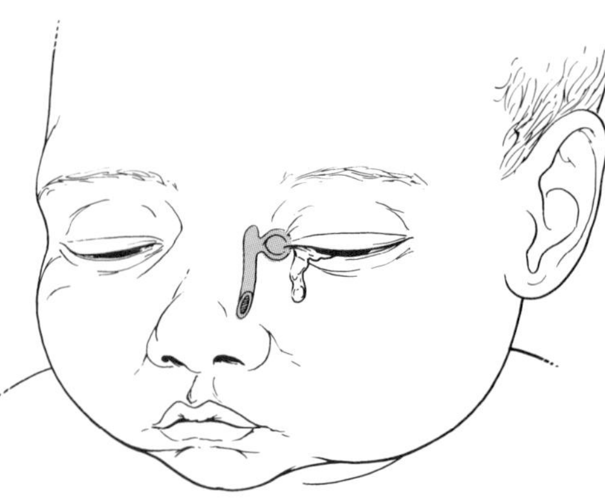

Persisting tears or a white or yellow discharge on the cheek of your infant may indicate an obstruction of the nasolacrimal duct.

feeding. Soon after birth, a specially designed prosthesis (obturator) can be fitted over the palate so that the baby can eat. Because the infant is growing rapidly, this device will have to be replaced every few weeks.

A baby with a cleft lip typically has an operation to close the lip at 1 or 2 months of age. Frequently, nasal widening is associated with cleft lip deformities. Closure of the cleft lip helps to narrow the base of the nose. A nasal operation usually is deferred until the child has reached adolescence. The cosmetic results depend on the severity of the malformation, the absence of infection and the surgeon's skill.

A cleft palate generally is closed within the first year of life to enhance normal speech development. The goals of surgery are to make it possible for the child to speak in a normal voice and to minimize nasal regurgitation. If a child doesn't have the operation by age 3, a prosthesis may be used to help the child develop better speech.

Complications of cleft lip or cleft palate include recurring ear infections, hearing loss, an excessive number of dental cavities and displacement of the teeth, requiring orthodontic correction. Some children continue to have speech problems even after surgery because of muscle problems in the palate.

Tear duct disorders

Congenital obstruction of the nasolacrimal duct results from incomplete development of the tear drainage system. Normally, tears and secretions from the eye drain from the tear ducts, which lead from two small openings at the inner corner of the eyelids into the nasal cavity. If this drainage system is partially or completely obstructed, tears can't drain from the eyes into the nose.

The problem usually becomes apparent within the first days or weeks after birth. A cold or exposure to wind or low temperature often aggravates the problem. The first sign a parent typically notices is the presence of tears in the baby's eyes, ranging from a pool of tears to tears spilling onto the baby's cheeks. There also may be some white or yellow discharge in the corners of the eyes and some crusting that glues the eyes shut while the baby sleeps.

Sometimes, infants with nasolacrimal duct obstruction develop inflammation in the duct area, causing the area to become swollen, red and tender. They may also have a fever and be irritable. The condition rarely harms the eyes, even when it persists for several months.

Treatment mainly involves cleansing the infant's lids with warm water and massaging the area between the infant's nose and the affected eye two or three times a day. Antibacterial drops or ointment may be used to prevent infection. If the condition persists throughout the first year, a doctor may need to surgically widen (dilate) the duct. Rarely is insertion of tubes or a reconstructive operation necessary.

Male genital conditions

The scrotum in a full-term newborn boy is relatively large. The scrotum may also look especially swollen after a breech birth. The scrotum of newborns with darker pigmentation usually is dark before the rest of the skin darkens during infancy. The foreskin in a newborn normally covers the end of the penis and should never be forced back. None of these characteristics is cause for alarm. Some genital conditions, however, do require treatment.

An undescended testicle

An undescended testicle is the absence at birth of one or both testicles from the scrotum. The testicle may be within the abdomen or be

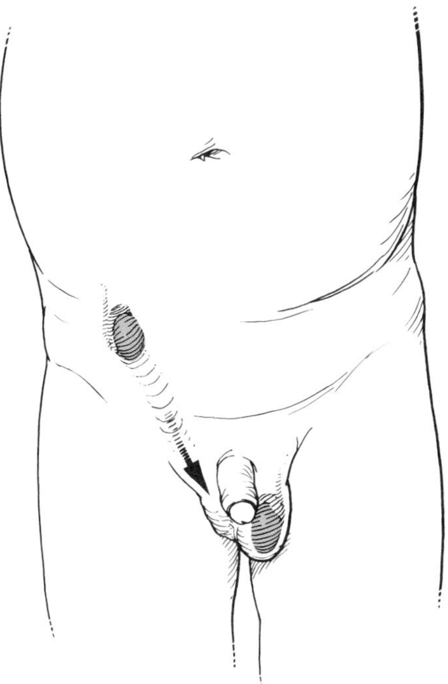

If one or both testicles fail to travel from the abdomen to the scrotum, the condition is termed undescended testicle.

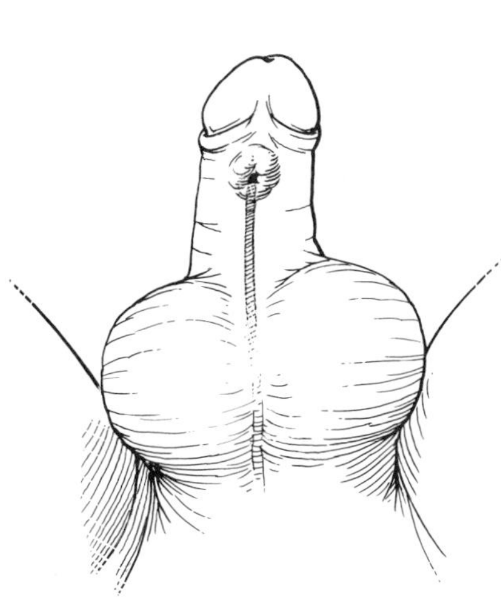

Hypospadias is a condition in which the urethral opening isn't located at its normal position at the end of the penis.

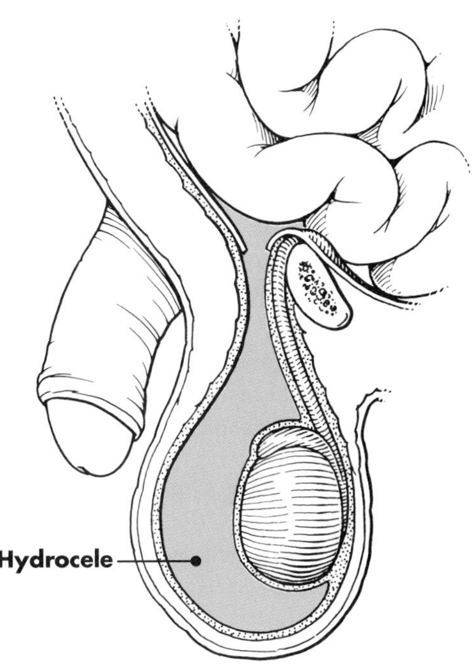

A common problem in newborns is an accumulation of fluid near the testicles, called a hydrocele.

absent altogether. The latter condition is rare and usually occurs in a child born with ambiguous sex characteristics.

About a month before birth, the testicles normally descend from an area near the kidney through a small opening in the abdominal muscles into their normal position in the scrotum. Approximately 1 in 125 boys are missing one or both testicles from the scrotum at birth. The incidence of undescended testicles is up to 17 percent in premature infants and up to 100 percent in infants weighing less than 2 pounds, because the testicles don't fully descend until after the seventh month of gestation.

In most cases, the testicle descends into the scrotum during the first few months of life, without any medical intervention. Sometimes, hormones are given to bring the undescended testicle into place. If it hasn't descended by the child's first birthday, it won't do so spontaneously, and the condition is commonly treated surgically.

Surgery is also important because often a boy with an undescended testicle has a hernia due to the failure of the opening in the abdominal muscles to close properly. In such cases, the intestines may slip through the muscle opening and become trapped. Often the operation can be done on an outpatient basis. Occasionally, a testicle has shrunk (atrophied) so severely that removal is indicated.

Left untreated, an undescended testicle might not produce sperm later in life, though if the other testicle functions normally it will produce enough sperm to maintain fertility. A boy born with an undescended testicle also has an increased risk of testicular cancer. Correction doesn't reduce this risk, but it does allow for better examination and earlier detection should a tumor develop.

Hypospadias

Hypospadias occurs in approximately 1 out of 330 newborns. In this congenital defect, the urethral opening isn't in its normal position near the end of the penis. In its mildest form, the opening is just on the underside of the glans. In its most severe form, it may be as far back as the scrotum. The more severe the degree of hypospadias, the more downward-curved the penis. This curving of the penis is called chordee.

Hypospadias is treated surgically. Circumcision shouldn't be done because the foreskin is used in the surgical repair. The more severe the condition, the greater the need for surgery because of urination and sexual problems. Unless the problem is corrected, the boy won't be able to stand while urinating and will have difficulty with sexual function later in life. The psychological consequences of having malformed genitals also are a factor in the consideration of surgery.

Many pediatric urologists believe the ideal age for surgery is during the first year, certainly before the child is toilet trained. A surgical procedure can bring the opening closer to the tip of the penis and also help straighten the penis.

Hydrocele

A hydrocele is an accumulation of fluid in the sheath around the testicle. Hydroceles may occur on one or both testicles. This condition is common in newborn boys. If the testicle can be examined easily and the amount of fluid remains constant, treatment is unnecessary. Small hydroceles usually disappear during the first year. However, if the sac changes size during the day, it may mean there's direct contact with the abdominal cavity, which generally requires surgery.

Female genital conditions

Hormonal changes in the mother before birth can cause changes in the breasts and genitals of her newborn daughter. Although these changes may be disturbing to new parents, they're generally temporary and often require no treatment.

Enlarged clitoris

The clitoris of the newborn girl is often enlarged, especially in premature babies, as a result of hormonal changes that affect the genital area. The size decreases after birth. If the clitoris seems unusually large, tests may be performed to confirm the child's sex.

Vaginal discharge

Vaginal discharge sometimes occurs in newborn girls. During the first 3 weeks, many mothers notice a thick, white discharge from the baby's vagina. Treatment is unnecessary.

Vaginal bleeding

Vaginal bleeding is sometimes a newborn girl's response to the absence of the maternal hormone estrogen after birth. This manifests as a few drops of blood from the vagina. Parents are understandably concerned to find blood in the diaper. This is a temporary condition.

Ambiguous genitals

Ambiguous genitals refers to the uncertain appearance of the baby's external sexual features. Sometimes, a female with normal ovaries who has been exposed to an excess of male hormones in the womb is born with male-like genitals (female pseudohermaphroditism). A male may be born with testicles but with ambiguous or completely female genitals (male pseudohermaphroditism). Some newborns have both ovaries and testicles and ambiguous genitals (true hermaphroditism). Causes of ambiguous genitals include tumors, chromosome abnormalities and hormone excesses or deficiencies.

When a newborn's sex is in question, only thorough testing and evaluation can establish the correct diagnosis, including the infant's sex. Ambiguous genitals is a serious problem that bears a significant impact on a child's future life and emotional health. Treatment may include hormone therapy and reconstructive surgery.

Enlarged Breasts

Enlarged breasts sometimes occur in girls or boys during the first 2 weeks of life because of the large amounts of maternal hormones that reach the baby before birth. Breast enlargement usually disappears in the first few months and is no cause for alarm.

Nipple disorders

Rarely, an infant is born with one or more extra (supernumerary) nipples. The nipples may occur with or without breast tissue and are usually located in the breast area.

Sometimes, the nipple doesn't have an areola — the darker pigment that surrounds a nipple. The condition occurs equally in males and females and may be associated with urinary problems.

Supernumerary nipples rarely present a medical problem, although they can respond to hormonal changes that occur during puberty, menstruation and pregnancy. When this happens, the nipples may enlarge and become painful. The presence of a third breast can be emotionally traumatic. Moreover, a supernumerary nipple is at the same risk as a normal nipple of developing disorders such as mastitis, abscesses and cancer. If your newborn has supernumerary nipples, they can be removed for cosmetic purposes.

An infant can also be born with the absence of a breast or nipple. Sometimes, the muscle underlying the breast also has failed to develop. When this occurs, nothing should be done during infancy or early childhood. An operation can be performed for cosmetic reasons when the child reaches puberty. ■

CHAPTER 13 PART II

Preschool to Preteen Years

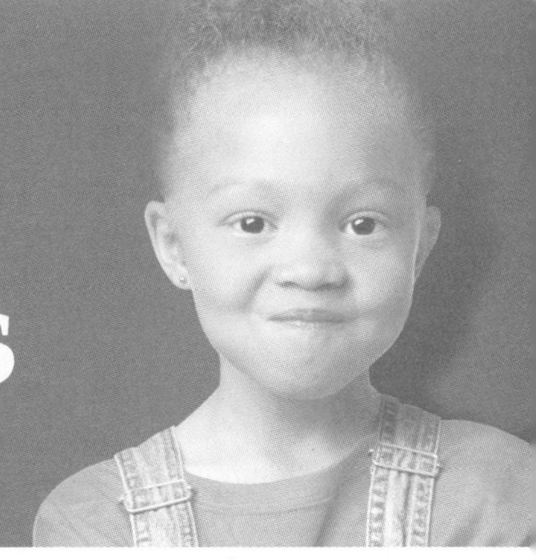

The years leading up to adolescence are exciting and challenging. During the preschool years, your child may sometimes be caught between wanting to "do it myself" and longing for the safety net that only you can provide. You'll probably have some anxieties during this time about issues as diverse as monsters hiding under the bed, toilet training and sibling rivalry. But you'll also enjoy seeing your child learn about communicating, socializing and becoming more self-reliant.

These years can be very satisfying for both you and your child as he or she develops his or her own personality and the relationship between the two of you grows.

Some amazing developmental changes occur during this time. For example, your 2-year-old, who proudly knows 50 words, becomes a 3-year-old who can carry on a conversation. Whether mastering the art of language or learning to use a new toy, preschoolers bring tremendous determination to acquiring new skills.

During the school-age years — from the time your child starts school until he or she becomes a teenager — your child will gradually become a citizen of a larger world. Peers and teachers are ever more influential as your child seeks greater independence from the family. More relationships will be formed outside the home.

Age 6 usually marks the start of your child's formal education. By then many children already have attended nursery school or child care, but starting kindergarten will be a whole new experience.

In school your child is required to adhere to the rules of an external authority and to devote more time to the work of learning. There's less time to play or to enjoy the informal learning that occurs in the preschool years.

At school your child is required to follow a rather fixed schedule. New rules extend the limit setting that you started in your child's preschool years.

Similar to younger children, school-age children are generally

Height and Growth Charts

Your doctor may use charts like this to assess your child's growth over time. Find your child's age on the bottom of the chart, and weight or height on the left side of the chart. The point where the two lines intersect indicates how your child compares in weight or height to others his or her age.

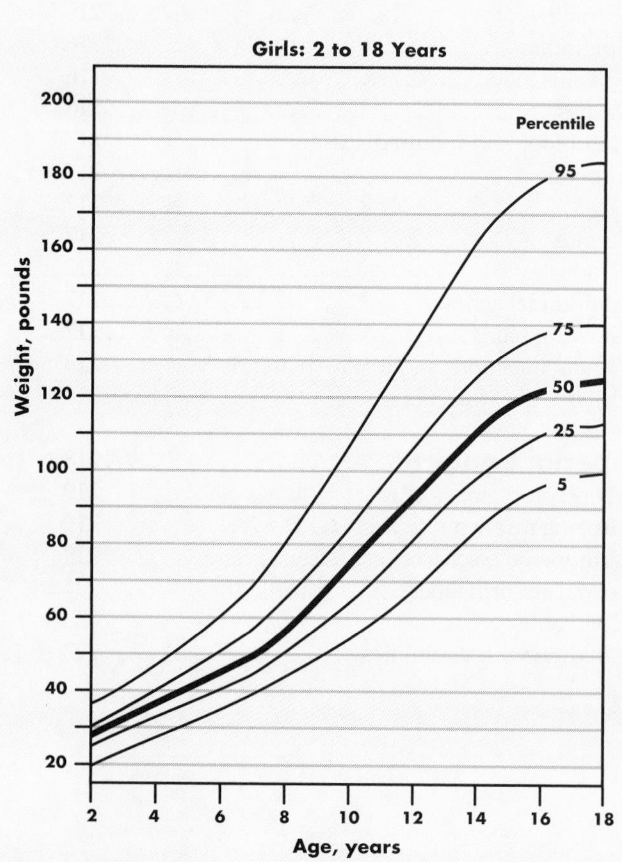

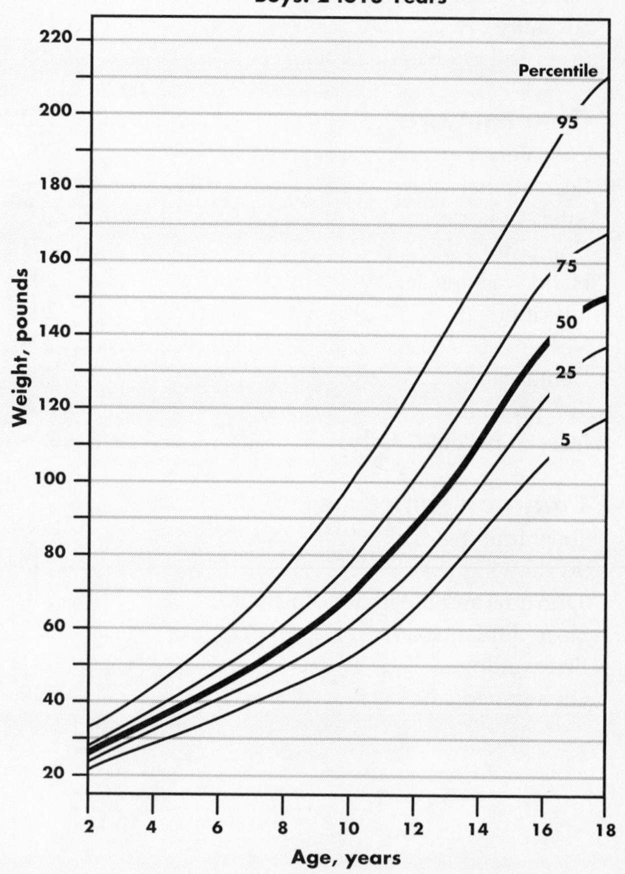

healthy, active and enthusiastic. Not surprisingly, it's often hard for them to control their energy and exuberance. If your child has deficits in vision and learning, these may become more apparent when he or she enters school.

Witnessing your child's achievements and integration into this wider world can be a great source of pride. At the same time, these new horizons may provoke anxiety for both you and your child.

As your child moves in directions that are new or unfamiliar or of which you don't approve, you may sense waning control. But you still have a crucial role to play in guiding your child through these years of development.

Growth and Development

During the preschool years and near the end of the preteen years, as your child is approaching adolescence, rapid changes occur in growth and development. In the middle, changes are often slow and steady.

Normal changes

The rapid weight gains during a child's first 2 years begin to level off around age 2. Your child's physical changes involve a transition from the plumpness of babyhood to the leaner body of a preschooler.

Although your son or daughter may not have a large vocabulary, he or she develops an increasing ability to understand language. This passive language lays the groundwork for the explosion of language between ages 2 and 3. Your child's communication may include reading and writing by age 5.

As your child becomes more mobile, safety becomes vitally important. Your preschooler will constantly explore by mouthing, touching, grabbing and climbing, with no curiosity left unsatisfied.

Between the ages of 6 and 12, your child will gain about 7 pounds a year and increase in height by approximately $2\frac{1}{2}$ inches a year. The growth of your child's head

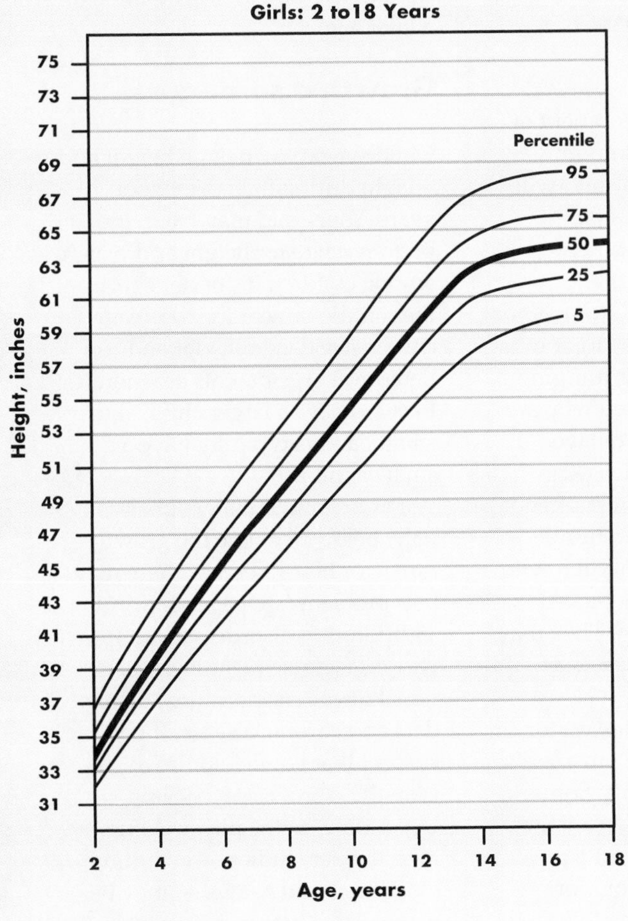

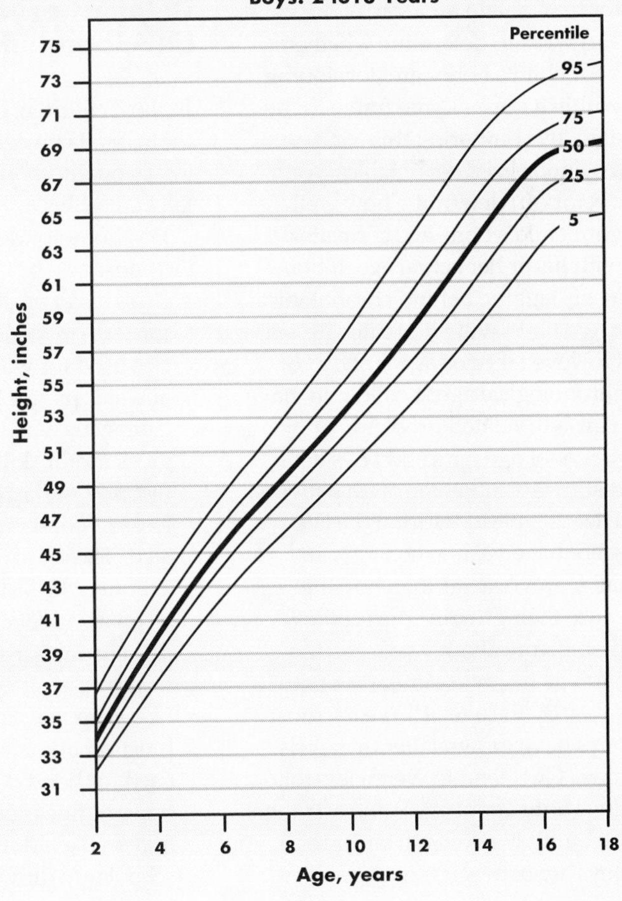

will slow down. This is the time when your child's brain has almost reached its adult size.

Your child's motor skills become more refined between the ages of 6 and 12. During this period, his or her running, jumping and throwing show steady improvement. To enhance this important process, continue to encourage your child to be physically active.

You and your child may enjoy tracking his or her progress on a growth chart at home. Your child's doctor may also keep watch of your child's height and weight. Abnormalities on your child's growth chart can provide early evidence of some serious diseases. For instance, when children develop chronic illnesses, their weight often stays the same or even decreases, and their height may not increase at the expected rate.

If you think your child seems unusually short or tall, you can ask his or her doctor about it. The doctor may obtain an X-ray of the hand and wrist to determine whether your child's bones are developing within a normal time frame (bone age). By comparing this X-ray with a standardized set of tables, your doctor can determine how well your child's bone age correlates with his or her actual age. If bone age is lagging behind chronological age, a child will often catch up. However, if bone age is ahead of chronological age, a child may have a growth-related problem.

School-age girls and boys have distinctly different growth patterns. There's a period during the late school-age years when girls are taller and heavier than boys because their growth spurt comes first. Before about 9 years of age, average height is similar for both sexes. By the age of 13 years, most boys have grown taller than girls have. Girls tend to weigh less than boys until about age 9 and after age 14, but they're often heavier than boys are between those ages.

Toward the end of the school-age years, children begin to grow at a dramatic but highly variable rate. This preadolescent growth spurt is a part of puberty, a sequence of changes that transforms a child into a young adult. The first stages of puberty generally begin at about age 10 in girls and age 12 in boys. For a discussion of normal growth and development during the teenage years, see page 226.

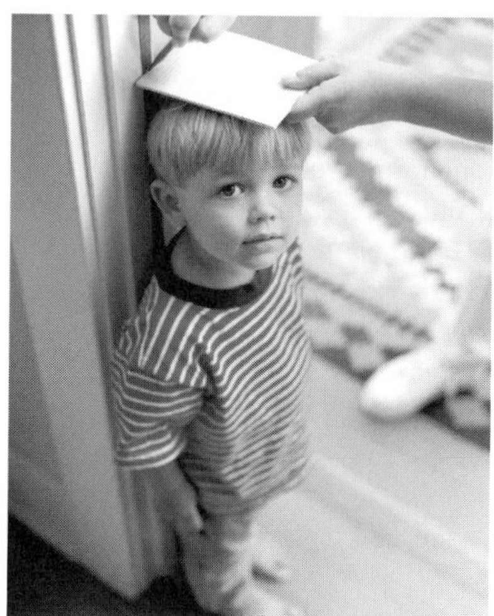

Delayed psychomotor development

In most children, development of motor skills proceeds smoothly. Occasionally, though, a child will fall behind his or her peers.

Psychomotor development includes:

- *Gross motor function.* Gross motor function involves the larger muscles used for walking, jumping and skipping. Children who are clumsy or who have delayed gross motor skills, such as an inability to skip or jump, often feel self-conscious and humiliated. These are the children who are often the last ones picked to be on an athletic team. They may develop a poor self-image as a result.
- *Fine motor function.* Fine motor function involves the muscles used for hand dexterity. Some types of fine motor dysfunction may make it difficult for a preschooler to draw or color or cause delay in learning to tie shoes. Some children show impairments in hand-eye coordination. Because of their problems with fine motor skills, these children often have difficulty when they enter school.

The cause for delayed psychomotor development is generally unknown, although it may run in families. If you suspect that your child may have a delay in psychomotor development, discuss your concerns with your doctor. Tests can determine if there's a problem.

If your child experiences a developmental delay in motor skills, he or she may lose an important area from which to draw for building self-esteem. As a parent, you need to preserve your child's sense of self-esteem by being understanding and patient with his or her progress. If you're impatient, even though your child ultimately will catch up, his or her self-esteem may suffer in the process. Most children do catch up and aren't impaired at a later age.

Growth disorders

Children vary widely in height and weight during their preschool years. Your child may fall in the bottom range for height and weight among children his or her age, in the middle or near the top. Your child's size generally depends on heredity. Large parents are more likely to have a larger child, and small parents typically have a smaller child.

If your child is either substantially below or above the growth range for his or her age, there may be a problem (see pages 188 and 189). Growth disorders result from various factors, including nutritional disorders, hormonal disorders and chronic disease. If you suspect that your child has a growth disorder, see a doctor. Depending on the physical findings, further studies — including blood tests and X-rays — may be necessary to determine the cause. Treatment depends on the specific problem. An obese child may be placed on a diet and exercise plan, whereas one who is malnourished may need high-calorie supplements and even hospitalization. Replacements of a deficient hormone may help children with growth disorders due to a hormone deficiency.

Nutritional disorders

Good nutrition contributes to normal growth. Malnutrition may result from insufficient food, an unbalanced diet, digestive problems, absorption problems or other medical conditions.

In the United States and other developed countries, malnutrition is uncommon. Severe cases of malnutrition may occur when a child has an associated chronic illness or disorder. Malnutrition can be the result of diseases such as cystic fibrosis or celiac disease, in which nutritional intake is normal but absorption of nutrients is not. The most common nutritional disorder in children in the United States is obesity.

Hormonal disorders

Sometimes, the pituitary or thyroid gland produces an insufficient or an excess amount of hormones, the result of which can be a growth disorder. These rare disorders include gigantism, dwarfism and hypothyroidism.

Chronic disease

Children with diseases such as congenital heart disease, chronic kidney failure or anemia may also have impaired growth.

Learning disorders

Children of normal or high intelligence can still have great difficulty in learning. Specific learning disabilities aren't disorders of seeing, hearing, emotions or overall mental capacity. Rather, they're often mental process disorders in acquiring or expressing knowledge — commonly referred to as cognitive learning disorders.

Factors Affecting Learning

Your child's ability to learn depends on complex mental processes that make learning possible. But overall health, emotional comfort and motivation are other important factors. Factors that can interfere with your child's ability to learn include:

Illness

Illness can leave a child tired and listless. This can interfere with learning, especially if the illness is chronic.

Emotions

If a child is depressed, worried or concerned about problems at home, learning can suffer. Worrying or daydreaming in school distracts the child from schoolwork.

Motivation

Lack of motivation also can be an impediment to learning. Your child needs to be motivated to learn in order to make full use of his or her capacities.

Cognitive learning disorders are more difficult to diagnose than are vision or hearing problems, and they often require consultation with specialists such as psychologists, developmental and behavioral pediatricians or child psychiatrists. Disorders of mental processing may include problems with remembering, recognizing patterns, focusing attention, writing, speaking and interpreting written words.

Various causes have been cited for learning disorders. Some of them stem from birth injuries. More commonly, however, they occur in children with normal health and intelligence. In some cases, they may be genetic. In other cases, there's evidence of disordered brain function, although no evidence of brain damage can be found.

Frequently, no specific cause for a child's learning disorder is found. Some experts in the field believe that in such instances the disorder may be due to developmental delays or slowing of the maturation process. Boys are affected more frequently than girls are.

A learning disorder can lead to chronic academic failure and to major social and emotional problems. Although children sometimes outgrow their learning disorder, this may occur too late to prevent severe limitation in future achievements and self-esteem. Early diagnosis and treatment can often minimize these consequences.

With special education and tutoring, many children can overcome their problem and perform much closer to their potential. They can achieve most academic and occupational goals if the appropriate teaching methods and motivation are found.

If your child has a learning disorder, you may not become aware of it until learning problems are recognized in the third or fourth grade. A thorough evaluation is essential for determining the specific disorder and ways to improve your child's education as soon as possible. Speech disorders, dyslexia and attention-deficit/hyperactivity disorder (ADHD) are examples of learning disorders.

Speech disorders

The critical period in a child's speech and language development is between ages 6 and 24 months. Occasional mispronunciations are

Stuttering

Stuttering typically begins between the ages of 2 and 5, while your child is mastering the basics of speech. In some children, stuttering first appears between ages 6 and 8, when school lessons include reading aloud and recitation, and often disappears by adolescence. Occasionally, older children develop the problem.

Two common characteristics of stuttering are repetition of sound, parts of words, whole words and phrases and prolongation or stretching of sounds or syllables. Examples of repetition are *b-b-b-bath*, *da-da-daddy* and *base-base-baseball*. An example of prolongation is *c----at*.

The causes of stuttering are only partially understood. Certain factors may promote tension of the muscles involved with speech and lead to stuttering. Stress, fatigue or excitement may trigger stuttering. Stuttering can run in families. Stuttering commonly isn't linked to intelligence or any measurable brain abnormality.

Occasional stuttering is common among children. These episodes usually disappear as speech and language develop, and they don't require attention.

Seek professional evaluation if your child becomes apprehensive about speaking, struggles with speech or begins to avoid sounds, words or speech altogether. A speech pathologist can help your child minimize his or her stuttering by reducing tension in his or her lips, tongue and jaw. A speech pathologist can also provide training skills to eliminate unnecessary, undesirable speech patterns.

As a parent, never label your child a stutterer. Try not to interrupt your child, show impatience or finish your child's sentences. Build your child's self-confidence by arranging quiet, one-on-one conversation and reading times.

normal up to about age 7 years, as long as your child's conversational speech is understood readily. About 5 percent of children have noticeable speech disorders by the time they start first grade.

Signs and symptoms

- Failure to use speech sounds correctly
- Speech that's hard to understand or scrambled
- Slow speech development
- Stuttering

In a majority of children with speech disorders, the cause of the speech problem is unknown and no physical cause is found. Types of speech disorders include difficulty in articulation, stuttered speech and voice problems.

Articulation problems refer to substituting one letter for another and leaving off the beginning and ending of words. Stuttering is difficulty in getting the words out in a smooth flow. Voice problems include too soft of a voice, a nasal voice or a loud, booming voice.

Your child may be normal physically, emotionally and intellectually but still have a speech disorder due to mental processing problems with spoken language. Your child may have difficulty receiving information and making sense of it. Sentences may come out scrambled or with one word substituted for another. The correct ordering of sounds may be impaired. Your child might be unable to tell the difference between two sounds or might have problems focusing on one specific sound or focusing on conversation while ignoring background noise.

Speech disorders can also result from conditions such as cerebral palsy, a cleft palate or lip, hearing loss or deafness, mental retardation, brain damage or autism.

Diagnosis

If you suspect that your child has a speech disorder, talk to your child's teacher or doctor. You may also need to seek help from a speech and language specialist. Most school systems offer these services. A speech pathologist will test your child's speech. He or she may use a game-like test with earphones to check for hearing loss or deafness in your child. In some instances, a complete physical and neurologic examination may be advised.

How serious are speech disorders?

With help from specialists — and from parents at home — many children with speech disorders are able to vastly improve their speech, but that doesn't mean they won't experience frustration. The social penalty can be costly if your child is taunted or rejected by other children at school. Early diagnosis and treatment are desirable before frustration and low self-esteem become problems.

Treatment

Children with speech disorders generally require speech therapy. This usually entails weekly sessions with a speech professional. Your child's speech therapist can explain how you can help at home.

Dyslexia

Dyslexia is a specific learning disability that primarily affects a child's ability to read. It's the most common learning disability in children. Dyslexia occurs in children with normal vision and normal intelligence. Children with dyslexia usually have normal speech, but they often have difficulty with reading and writing. The disorder is an impairment of the brain's ability to translate letters into their corresponding sounds.

Common signs of dyslexia include an inability to recognize letters and words on the printed page and a reading ability that's much below the expected level. Although the key factor of this reading disability is unknown, evidence shows that it may be associated with a malfunction of certain areas of the brain concerned with language. A family history of language disorders is frequently found. Dyslexia affects boys more often than girls. Approximately 10 percent to 15 percent of school-age children have this specific disorder.

Dyslexia is characterized primarily by a delay in the age at which a child begins to read. Most children are ready to learn this skill by age 6. Children with dyslexia often can't grasp the basics of reading in first or even second grade. Because a child with dyslexia has difficulty interpreting written language, reading is difficult.

The condition may also manifest itself by your child trying to read starting at the wrong end of the sentence, failing to see and hear similarities or differences in letters or words and being unable to sound out the pronunciation of an unfamiliar word. Children with dyslexia usually have difficulty with their ability to write.

Diagnosis

Reading achievement that's significantly below that expected for a child's age is the key sign of dyslexia. A diagnosis is generally made based on an evaluation of medical, cognitive, sensory processing (vision and hearing), educational and psychological factors.

A battery of specialized psychological tests may be performed to help diagnose the problem. An expert may analyze the process and quality of your child's reading skills. The results of these tests are used to plan treatment and track your child's progress.

Thorough vision, hearing and neurologic examinations also may be required to verify that your child's poor reading ability isn't due to another disorder. Dyslexia varies in severity from relatively mild to severe.

How serious is dyslexia?

If you have a child with a reading disability, you may find that his or her inability to read doesn't affect achievement in other school subjects, such as arithmetic. However, because reading is a skill basic to most other school subjects, a child with dyslexia is at a great disadvantage in most classes.

If untreated, the disorder may result in low self-esteem, behavioral problems, delinquency, aggression and withdrawal or alienation from friends, parents and teachers.

Treatment

Because there's no known way to correct the underlying brain malfunction, the primary form of treatment is generally remedial education. Psychological testing will help your child's teachers design a suitable remedial teaching program. Most important is frequent instruction by a reading specialist who uses both visual and phonic methods of teaching.

Techniques emphasizing many of the senses, including hearing, vision and touch, are used to improve reading. It's also important to provide emotional support and opportunities for achievement in areas other than reading.

If the reading disability is severe, your child may also benefit from several individual or small-group tutoring sessions each week. Progress is likely to be slow and laborious.

Children with milder forms eventually learn to read well enough to get through school and to be able to read newspapers. Those with severe forms may always have difficulty reading and may need to learn ways to bypass their reading problems, such as by using tape-recorded textbooks.

Attention-deficit/ hyperactivity disorder

Attention-deficit/hyperactivity disorder (ADHD) is another common learning disorder of childhood. Three percent to 5 percent of all children are affected by this condition. It typically begins in childhood and often continues into adolescence and adulthood. The key signs and symptoms of ADHD

Hyperactivity

Hyperactivity, or extreme overactivity, isn't a diagnosis or a separate disorder. Rather, it's a behavior that often accompanies other symptoms of attention-deficit/hyperactivity disorder (ADHD).

Children vary in their level of physical activity. In general, young children are active. Some youngsters are naturally much more active than others, and boys tend to be more active than girls. These variations in activity are normal.

However, a small percentage of children, more often boys than girls, are excessively active. Some seem to be in constant motion, and others are erratically active. These children aren't necessarily less coordinated or less intelligent than other children. The difference lies in how organized or purposeful their activity is and if it can be stopped when appropriate or on request.

Hyperactive children tend to act without consideration for results, punishment or other people's reactions. They can't direct their activity, and it's often difficult for parents or teachers to do so.

Contrary to some opinions, sugar alone doesn't cause or increase hyperactivity.

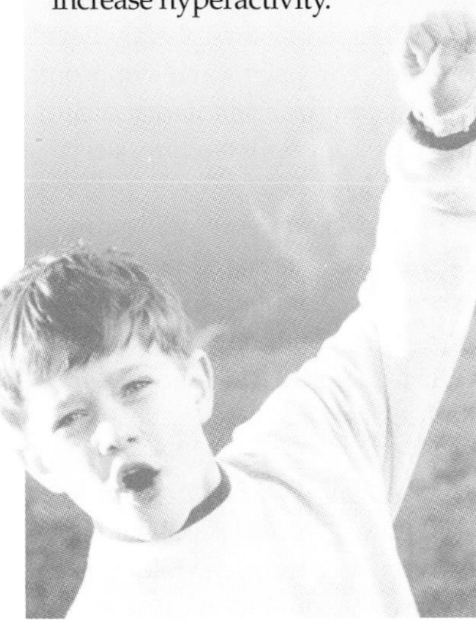

are difficulty paying attention and concentrating (inattention), difficulty staying still (hyperactivity), and difficulty controlling impulsive behavior (impulsivity).

The condition is also referred to as attention-deficit disorder (ADD), hyperkinesis and minimal brain dysfunction. Some children have ADD without hyperactivity.

As a result of this disability, your child may have problems with learning, following directions and remembering information. Your child's ability to learn depends on paying attention and remembering previous lessons and instructions.

Many sights, sounds, memories and other stimulating things compete for your child's attention. They can cause any child to have trouble paying attention. Most school-age children have the ability to focus their attention on a specific task and ignore distractions. Among children with ADHD, this ability is underdeveloped.

ADHD may not noticeably affect your child's intelligence or early development. It may become apparent only later as your child has increasing difficulty with learning after the second or third grade, when sitting still in class and paying attention become increasingly important.

Diagnosis
In making a diagnosis of ADHD, your doctor will likely want to observe your child's behavior and get a detailed history of early development. Early signs and symptoms may appear during infancy, including problems with feeding, sleeping and restlessness.

Physical and neurologic exams may be recommended to identify any sensory or neurologic disorders. Your child may also see specialists to partake in psychological and educational testing.

How serious is ADHD?
ADHD is a chronic problem that can continue through childhood and into adulthood. It can damage your child's self-esteem and confidence, generate rejection and ridicule by other children and cause academic and social failure. Treatment can help a child with learning, behavior control, friendships, social interactions and self-esteem.

Treatment
Your child may need remedial education to help with learning. Some children with ADHD also have behavioral problems that require specialized counseling for the child and parents. This is often provided by psychologists.

Treatment may focus on behavior modification techniques and restructuring home and school routines. Avoiding overstimulation and providing consistency can be effective for decreasing unacceptable behavior. Rewarding good behavior also is important.

Your child's doctor may prescribe medications to help focus your child's attention and reduce overactivity. Common medications are dextroamphetamine (Dexaspan, Dexedrine) and preparations of methylphenidate (Concerta, Ritalin).

In a hyperactive child, these medications often can improve attention. When the medication is carefully prescribed and the child's progress is followed closely by a doctor, the drug may be taken safely for as long as it's needed, even for years.

Some children experience side effects such as loss of appetite, nervousness, irritability and growth retardation. If your child experiences any of these signs or symptoms, discuss them with your child's doctor.

Taking Time for Yourself

Caring for a child with special needs can leave little time for the rest of the family. Even the most devoted parents need a break. However, because of your child's unique needs, you may be reluctant to leave him or her with a baby sitter.

Many communities recognize this need problem and have opened respite centers where parents can temporarily leave a special needs child with a caregiver experienced in caring for such children. If this type of option is provided in your community, consider taking advantage of it.

Mental disorders

Mental retardation and autism are examples of mental disorders in children. Although these conditions have no cures, resources are available to help parents and their children cope with them.

Mental retardation
Mental retardation can range from a slight slowness that makes school a struggle for the child to profound retardation that requires the child have constant care or supervision.

If your child has mental retardation, he or she will be slow in acquiring motor skills and language. Your child will also lack the social skills and emotional maturity appropriate to his or her age.

Mental retardation may be caused by inborn chromosomal or metabolic abnormalities such as Down syndrome or phenylketonuria (PKU). Other possible causes include prenatal German measles, toxoplasmosis and excessive alcohol use during pregnancy.

Mental retardation is different from most other disorders in that children with mental retardation don't catch up with their peers in development, and their disorders generally can't be treated.

With a learning disorder, an otherwise typical child may lag behind in a specific area of development.

With time and assistance from a specialist, this child has a good chance of catching up to others in his or her class. Some children have emotional or social immaturities stemming from a mental illness. Often, these can be treated.

How serious is mental retardation?

Mental retardation is generally evident before age 18 and often many years earlier. Mild forms of retardation may first become evident when your child begins school.

Children with mild retardation are able to learn academic skills but do so more slowly than the average child. Mild retardation often isn't diagnosed until a child begins school because it's then that he or she is compared with large numbers of peers and developmental differences become more apparent. Children with mild forms of mental retardation are often identified as educationally mentally disabled.

Children with moderate mental retardation may learn self-care skills such as dressing and using the toilet. They have limited ability to benefit from academic school programs but still profit greatly by attending school and may learn to perform certain simple jobs in a supervised setting.

Federal legislation guarantees an education to all developmentally disabled children in the United States. Community schools provide special education classes. Your child may spend part of the day in a class with other children with special needs and then attend a class or two with children who aren't disabled.

Children who are severely or profoundly retarded can learn minimal self-care skills such as using the toilet but require almost total supervision and care. These children often have limited communication skills.

Treatment

In the past, children with mental retardation were often institutionalized. Today, most of these children live at home or in group homes in their communities.

If your child is developmentally disabled, the goal of treatment is to help your child reach his or her potential, whatever that may be, and to enable him or her to cope as well as possible with limitations.

When a diagnosis of mental retardation is made in infancy, you and your baby can enroll in an infant stimulation program or an early childhood intervention program. Such programs offer multisensory stimulation in an attempt to facilitate emotional, intellectual and physical development. They also help you to understand more about your child's strengths and weaknesses and offer you support during what is usually an emotionally difficult time.

Every child needs friends. Despite the mainstreaming of developmentally disabled children with other children in schools, classmates don't always accept these children as friends. Thus, you as a parent must often take it upon yourself to plan social and recreational activities for your child.

Organizations for developmentally disabled children offer various activities, including summer camps. Such programs help your child both to become more comfortable in social situations and to increase his or her independence.

Autism

Autism is a severe mental illness of childhood. An autistic child may be extremely unresponsive to other people. He or she may communicate poorly, not want to cuddle and may even seem repulsed by physical contact. Autistic children fail to seek comfort when distressed, normally don't imitate adults in actions such as waving goodbye, and engage in virtually no social interaction.

An autistic child may exhibit repetitive body movements, such as hand flicking, hand twisting, spinning or headbanging. He or she may be fascinated by parts of objects, such as the spinning wheels of a toy car. The child may become upset over even the slightest change in his or her environment and may be unreasonably insistent on established routines.

Autism usually appears before a child is 3 years old. An autistic child may not speak or may mimic sounds made by others. He or she may have difficulty naming objects and may make bizarre facial expressions and gestures.

Autism has no single cause. And although it has no cure, many therapies and interventions have been developed to treat its signs and symptoms. The most effective treatments use a combination of special education, behavioral therapy and medication.

Personality and Behavior

The development of your child's personality is as important as his or her physical development. During the preschool years, issues may emerge that can affect the way your child behaves around you and other people. His or her psychological and social development proceed at a rapid clip. Impressive changes take place in his or her ability to reason, learn, act in a moral fashion, follow rules intelligently and interact with adults and other children. Many of these changes may seem surprising or even shocking to you as a parent, so it helps to have some understanding of the normal course of events.

Normal changes

Keep in mind that no child's behavioral development adheres to a strict schedule. Every child is different and develops according to his or her own schedule. If you think there's a problem with your child's development, consult your child's doctor.

During your child's early years, seek your child's company. Discuss

Smoothing the Stubbornness

At a young age, children go through a period when *no* is their favorite word. It doesn't matter what you say to the child, most of the time it will be met by an emphatic no. "Do you want to stay in the bathtub?" you ask your young daughter. "No," she answers. "Well, then, do you want to get out of the bathtub?" "No."

Stubbornness and tantrums are normal parts of childhood development. Although it may seem as though your child is purposely trying to provoke you, he or she isn't. This is simply one step down the long road toward independence.

Getting through this sometimes-difficult phase of development requires lots of patience and a good sense of humor. If you're the parent of a child in the thick of childhood stubbornness, remember that every parent goes through this and lives to laugh about it later.

The following tips may help make the road a little less bumpy:

- Don't take your child's negativism too seriously or too personally.
- Don't punish your child for saying no.
- Give your child choices: "Do you want to wear the red pants or the green pants?" Letting him or her choose will give your child a sense of freedom and control and make him or her more likely to cooperate. Be careful about asking a question with only one acceptable answer. For example, at bedtime, don't offer your child a choice between staying up and going to bed if you have no intention of letting him or her stay up.
- Give your child a transition time between activities. If, for example, your child is having fun but it's time to leave the playground, give him or her adequate time. "You can go down the slide three more times, and then we have to go home."
- Go easy on rules. Children this age aren't likely to follow a long list of house rules. Avoid arguing about unimportant things and decide which battles are really worth the struggle. Make sure that daily interactions with your child are weighted toward the positive, not the negative.
- Try to avoid saying no yourself. You want the child to see you as an agreeable person, someone he or she can imitate.

his or her interests and participate in activities, however mundane, together. The lines of communication that you keep open during these critical formative years may prove invaluable in later years as you help your child with behavior and personality issues.

Imagination

Preschoolers live part of their lives in a rich, imaginary world where anything is possible. Play during these years often revolves around pretending. Sometimes it's difficult for a child to know where pretending stops and reality starts.

For example, your 3-year-old may explain to you that he or she wasn't the one who broke your bottle of perfume but that it was a little green man with a yellow hat. Your child isn't lying, not in the true sense of the word. And you shouldn't punish your child or make him or her feel guilty for making up stories like this from time to time.

However, some children seem to live in their imaginations most of the day. If your child seems to be spending too much time with an imaginary friend whom he or she truly believes in, you might ask yourself if your child's real life is sufficiently interesting.

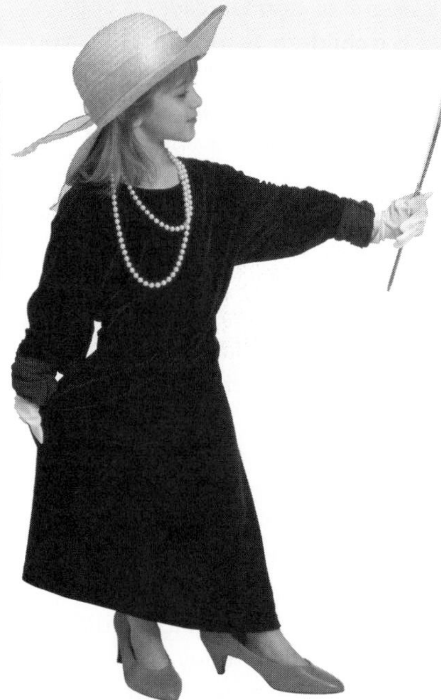

A child who lives in his or her own private dream world may need to spend more time with friends or may not be getting enough attention from his or her parents.

Increased independence

The increasing independence of your school-age child may stand in welcome contrast to the continual demands of your preschooler. Although it may be easy to allow your increasingly independent child to occupy himself or herself, an open and trusting relationship must be nurtured if it's to be maintained later during adolescence.

Social skills

During the preschool years, children tend not to conform. Social rules may be confusing to them. Behavior begins to change during the early school-age years. Children enjoy identifying with their peers and start understanding social situations. They often show a rigid conformity that makes them embrace each new social norm that they come to comprehend. You may have noticed that your child relishes some strict compulsion, such as never stepping on a crack in the sidewalk. This is one form of the child's temporary infatuation with arbitrary rules.

Thumb and Finger Sucking

All infants need to suck. Sucking on a thumb, finger or pacifier is common and helps soothe and calm most babies. By the time most children are 4, they've given up the practice, except when the issue has become a power struggle between parent and child or when it has become a deeply ingrained habit. Because thumb sucking during sleep is involuntary, it generally ceases when your child's sleep pattern matures.

Thumb or finger sucking in a preschool or school-age child isn't a serious problem. However, it makes your child appear babyish, which may subject him or her to ridicule from peers. Moreover, prolonged thumb or finger sucking can interfere with the normal alignment of the teeth, making orthodontic treatment necessary in later years.

If your child is younger than 4 and sucks his or her fingers or thumb, try to ignore or distract the child. Never punish, scold or pull your child's hand away from his or her mouth. These methods often make the problem worse.

In an older preschooler, you can appeal to vanity. Show your child how the thumb or finger is wrinkling and his or her teeth are beginning to protrude. Gently remind your child to stop thumb or finger sucking when you catch him or her in the act and offer praise when you notice he or she isn't doing it.

Toward the end of the school-age years, most children become more flexible about social roles and norms. They gradually learn to reconcile conflicting value systems, such as the ones at home and those at school. They come to recognize that compromise isn't necessarily a sign of weakness.

However, some degree of rigidity often remains. Eleven- and 12-year-olds are often extremely concerned about acting and dressing like their peers and not being out of the mainstream.

Moral behavior

Through the school-age years, children learn about moral behavior — how to distinguish between what's right and wrong. Your child must learn how to balance his or her needs and wants with the requirements of the family, school and society.

You can help your child develop a sense of duty, responsibility and realistic accomplishment. Encourage your child to assume a helpful role in the family. This may include assigning reasonable household chores such as setting the table. As your child accomplishes tasks you set, he or she will develop confidence in his or her abilities and a sense of responsibility regarding the tasks. This will also reinforce that he or she is an important part of the family.

Setting an example of moral behavior is also important. In addition, it's a good idea to limit and monitor your child's TV watching and to avoid or keep to a minimum his or her exposure to violence and inappropriate sexual behavior.

If you consistently specify what behavior you're rewarding or disciplining and explain why you're doing so, your child will be more likely to develop internal control of moral actions — a conscience. Less desirable are external controls, which influence behavior through fear of being caught or of displeasing parents.

Children who believe securely in their own worth tend to be more industrious, creative and successful at school. They're also better at resisting pressure to conform to their peers, which is especially important when peers demand that they participate with them in self-destructive behavior.

Peer pressure

Peers and siblings play important roles in the integration of your child into society. From their peers and siblings, children learn a great deal about competition and cooperation as well as about conformity and independence.

The influence of other children can rival or even exceed that of adults, partly because children play together as equals. It's easy for them to understand one another. Another child's perspective often provides an alternative to the prevailing wisdom that the child has been accustomed to hearing from his or her parents.

Parents and siblings may advocate different approaches than those of teachers and peers at school. Such conflict can pose problems for school-age children, who yearn to be liked and accepted by everyone. When sibling and peer norms conflict with those of adults, school-age children are often more inclined to follow their siblings and peers.

Elementary school is the first social world with which most children have to deal without direct help from their family. As school-age children become part of a peer group, new social traits become important to them, such as popularity and leadership. At this age, children are eager to be popular and don't want to be left out of the group.

Sibling relationships

Few things are as exasperating to parents as constant bickering among their children. Although these fights can make even easygoing parents wish they were raising an only child, fighting and competition between siblings is normal.

Problems between siblings include competition between a

Sharing

Around age 3, children learn the concept of sharing. Don't punish your child for refusing to share. However, encourage sharing and praise the child when he or she does.

In the same vein, many young children frequently grab toys away from a sibling or another child playing nearby. When this happens, take the toy away from the child and return it to the child who was using it. Always praise the child for asking to use a toy and for returning it on request.

young toddler and a newborn, physical aggression and incessant quarreling. Interestingly, on the days your children aren't fighting, they may be the best of friends.

Sibling rivalry

A certain amount of rivalry between siblings is normal, and it can help them learn how to interact fairly with other people. You don't necessarily need to be concerned if your children compete, roughhouse and bicker with each other. Despite the friction between them, most older siblings do contribute greatly to the education, socialization and support of younger siblings. Frequently, overt rivalry gives way to closeness by the end of the school-age years.

Sometimes, though, the discord between siblings can be severe. If so, you may want to seek family counseling to identify how the trouble started and how it can be stopped. The underlying cause of sibling antagonism may be a family problem such as marital strain. Without realizing it, parents can cast a child in a role that enmeshes him or her in a conflict between the mother and father, and the other siblings react according to their sympathies.

The birth of a sibling also can make a school-age child feel that his or her place in the family has been upset. Compared with a preschooler, a school-age child is usually better equipped to control his or her jealousy of a newborn sibling. Still, your school-age child may protest a decline in the amount of your attention that he or she receives by regressing to younger behavior.

It helps if you're sensitive to the school-age child's needs and reserve some time just for the two of you. School-age children often enjoy playing with and caring for "their" new baby. If concerns about your school-age child persist, talk to your child's doctor.

Fighting

Children must be taught that they can't kick, punch or bite each other. When your children physically fight, separate them immediately. Send them to separate rooms for a few minutes to calm down.

Quarrels

Help children learn the skills to settle their own arguments. When they do argue, try to ignore it and stay out of the argument, even if it means you have to go into another room. If they bring their argument to you, help them clarify the problem — but let them find the solution. When children settle an argument, praise them. Avoid showing favoritism.

Sexuality

Your preschool child has a natural sexual curiosity that manifests itself in various ways. Through the school-age years, your child will continue to define his or her sexuality. This process is a vital part of your child's larger task of discovering and deciding his or her identity. Your child may also make his or her first attempts to explore sexual activity before this period is over. Answer questions about sex directly and simply. Use anatomically correct language.

A preschooler

It's normal for children to explore their body and to do what feels good. Self-stimulation is one way a child's natural sexual curiosity is manifested. Boys typically pull at their penis, and girls rub their external genitalia.

Occasional masturbation is normal and nothing to worry about. A child stimulates himself or herself simply because it feels good. Some children masturbate because they're unhappy or experiencing and reacting to some stressful circumstances.

If your child masturbates, try not to get upset. Masturbation doesn't mean your child will grow up to be promiscuous or sexually deviant. It's not physically harmful, nor does it cause emotional problems, unless a parent overreacts and sends the message that sex is dirty and frightening.

Because it's difficult to stop a child from masturbating, it's best to simply accept it. However, you need to explain to your child that although it's all right to masturbate in the privacy of a bedroom or bathroom, other areas are off-limits. If your child suddenly starts masturbating in a social setting, try to distract him or her. If that fails, take your child aside and remind him or her that this is done only in the privacy of the bedroom or bathroom.

In addition to self-stimulation, many preschoolers are curious about their parents' body. A young child may want to touch a mother's breasts or a father's penis. Another child may be found half undressed, playing doctor with the child next door. These behaviors are normal.

Avoid showing shock or anger. Instead, stress that some activities are private and, although it's OK for your child to touch himself or herself, it's not OK for others, even friends, to touch them that way except for an examination by a doctor. Then point out that no other adult may touch him or her in that way either.

A school-age child

Most school-age children are already well on their way to reflecting the divergent sex roles that our society considers appropriate to men and women.

Perhaps you would prefer that your child feel free to express all aspects of his or her personality, including both masculine and feminine ones. However, you may notice how often your efforts are thwarted by the startling array of overt and subtle sex-stereotyping pressures from other relatives, peers, teachers, television and other media and society at large.

Regardless of your own attitudes, your school-age child may choose not to embrace the role assigned to his or her sex. A girl may be labeled a tomboy, and a boy a sissy. Society and the family may tend to put more pressure on boys than on girls to conform strictly to a narrow sex role. Traditionally, masculine behavior by girls is more often tolerated than is feminine behavior by boys.

If you're concerned that your school-age son is showing too much interest in playing with dolls or dressing up in girls' clothes, it's best to discourage him gently and not to show your anxiety. Be reassured, though, that a great many boys show varying degrees of masculinity as they mature. Sexuality and sex roles aren't static. They continue to evolve throughout childhood, adolescence and even adulthood.

Most school-age children devote most of their attention to peers of the same sex. Many even develop crushes on same-sex peers. However, it's also normal for them to explore the opposite sex tentatively. Curiosity and lack of understanding of social taboos are usually the reasons for their playing doctor.

During the school-age years, most school-age children continue to play occasionally with their own sex organs, as they did in infancy and the preschool years. Masturbation generally shouldn't be a cause for concern.

The onset of puberty provides a good opportunity to educate your child about sexual development, whether or not you've already done so. You can help prepare your child for the cascade of changes that his or her body will go through during the next few years. The goal is for the child to welcome these changes without shame or anxiety that they're occurring too quickly or too slowly.

In the late school-age years, children are most eager to conform. An obsession with "normality" coincides with the time when their body's development is diverging from that of their peers. Even children who are right in the middle of the spectrum of physical maturity often feel they're developing too rapidly or too slowly. You can help by reassuring your child that he or she fits well within the wide range of normal development.

Don't worry if your child's puberty starts a little earlier or later than that of his or her peers. This isn't a medical problem. However, your child may feel awkward and self-conscious about diverging from the average schedule. Be sensitive to these feelings.

At the same time, reassure your child that he or she is fine. It may help to stress that every child, including your child and each of his or her peers, is traveling along the same road toward adulthood and that everyone takes a different amount of time to arrive.

Fears and phobias

As your child grows, he or she will inevitably have certain fears, which will change with age. Such fears are normal and may even be necessary for psychological development.

Fear refers to the perception of a threat, whether actual or just a possibility. Fear is necessary for survival. For example, fear of a barking, snarling dog is normal. Your child perceives a real threat, and it's correct to be frightened and to try to avoid the danger.

However, a child who continues to be terrified of the friendly, tail-wagging cocker spaniel who lives next door has an irrational fear or phobia.

Fears vary from child to child, but some appear more commonly in certain age groups. For example, some children are afraid of a bath.

? Question and Answer

When is it a good time to talk with a child about the birds and the bees?

Your preschooler may be too young to understand how babies are made, but he or she isn't too young to learn about inappropriate touches. Explain that it's OK for your child to touch himself or herself in private but that it's not OK for others, even family or friends, to touch him or her that way except in special circumstances, such as during a doctor's examination.

A good time to begin talking about sex-related topics is when your child starts school. Pubertal changes generally begin at around age 11. Before your child reaches his or her early teens, your child should know about:

- The names and functions of male and female sex organs
- Puberty
- The menstrual cycle
- Sexual intercourse and pregnancy

The Schoolyard Bully

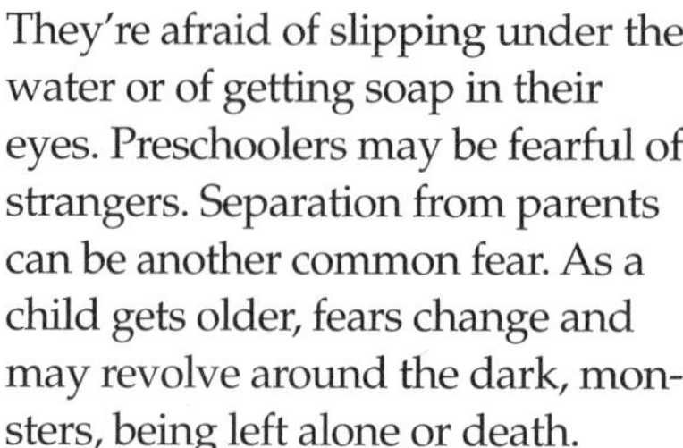

Bullying benefits no one. Bullies are more likely to have other behavioral problems at school and criminal records later in life. Victims are more likely to be depressed, have low self-esteem and miss school. In a survey conducted by the World Health Organization, 30 percent of children in grades 6 through 10 were involved in bullying, being bullied or both.

Children will tease one another and have their disagreements — that's not bullying. Bullying happens when the teasing and disagreements are intended to harm or disturb, occur repeatedly over time, victimize a less powerful child, or include name-calling, threats and spreading rumors.

Here are some suggestions on how to handle bullying:

- Teach your child to report incidents of bullying.
- Ask your child about being teased and whether he or she plays alone at recess.
- Teach your child to act confident because bullies look for victims who appear weak.
- Involve your child in activities that can help raise self-esteem, such as drama, music or sports.
- Ask to meet with your child's teacher and the parents of the bully.
- Ask for greater supervision at school.
- Find out whether your child's school has a no-tolerance policy toward bullying. If not, discuss with your child's teacher and school principal the possibility of creating one — it may reduce the chances of your child being either a bully or a victim.

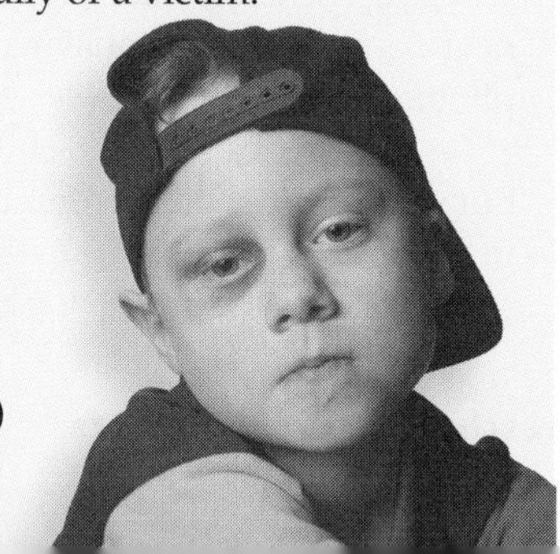

They're afraid of slipping under the water or of getting soap in their eyes. Preschoolers may be fearful of strangers. Separation from parents can be another common fear. As a child gets older, fears change and may revolve around the dark, monsters, being left alone or death.

If your child is going through a fearful time, try to be supportive and encouraging. Don't force your child to confront the object of the fear. Trying to make a child who's afraid of animals pet a dog will likely only complicate the situation.

Your reassurance in the form of a hug or kiss can be powerful medicine for a child who's afraid of the dark. A night light is often helpful.

Be creative in your quest for a solution. For instance, if your 3-year-old son is terrified that monsters are lurking in his dark room, initiate a nightly monster check. At bedtime every night, scour the room together in search of a monster. Once your son is reassured that no monsters are present, he'll likely go to bed and fall asleep. Within a few weeks, you'll no longer need to do the monster check.

This illustrates the years when magic seems real. You might also assign a stuffed bear the responsibility of staying awake all night to keep away monsters. In the morning, praise it for a job well done.

When your child conquers even a tiny part of his or her fear, praise him or her. Most fears resolve themselves in time. Those that don't or that hinder your child or family may require some counseling.

School phobia

School phobia — avoidance of school or refusal to go to school — may be a way of responding to overwhelming stress and situations a child can't control. School phobia is often an anxiety disorder distinguished by anxiety and a cycle of physical symptoms that get worse instead of better. The disorder seems to run in families and is most common in the early school grades. It affects boys and girls equally.

If your child is fearful and unable to cope with a situation at school, he or she may experience symptoms such as headache, stomachache, nausea, dizziness or hyperventilation. These are symptoms a child often has no conscious control over. Often, a child doesn't know exactly why he or she feels ill and finds it difficult to explain what's causing the discomfort.

Your child may be afraid of failing, being beat up by a school bully or being teased. Sometimes, children who've experienced the loss of a parent by death or divorce may fear that while they're at school another loss will occur.

Sympathy or nurturing the child for missing school likely will reinforce the physical symptoms. However, if the parent becomes angry, the child's anxiety is likely to increase, raising the stress level and worsening the physical symptoms.

Your child should be examined by a doctor to rule out a physical illness. If no physical problem can be found, consider having your child see a mental health professional, such as a psychiatrist, psychologist or counselor.

Among younger children, the problem can often be resolved by firmly expecting school attendance and providing emotional support for the child. Close cooperation between the parents and school personnel is essential. If the problem persists, or occurs among older children, evaluation and treatment by a mental health professional is often beneficial. Treatment for school phobia may include psychotherapy to help determine and manage the source of the anxiety and possibly medication to help treat the anxiety.

General Care

As a parent, you take many steps to help protect your child from disease and illness — getting your child vaccinated, taking him or her to the doctor when you're concerned about a high fever, and so on. Some everyday actions you do also are important to your child's health. These include everything from making sure your child is properly secured in a car to ensuring that he or she is building a foundation for a healthy diet.

Other common-sense habits also are health and life preserving. Don't smoke in the home. Make sure that firearms are kept locked and secured and the ammunition is stored separately. Use smoke and carbon monoxide detectors in the home. These behaviors and those that follow are all part of providing your child with the best possible care in everyday situations.

Car safety

Always buckle up your baby or young child in a specially designed car seat when traveling by car. For tips on the proper use of car seats for infants and toddlers, see page 165. Your child should ride in a car seat until he or she is 40 inches tall or has reached the car seat's weight limit. At that time, your child can switch from a car seat to a booster seat. Booster seats are recommended for children between the ages of 4 and 8. A booster seat helps to prevent severe abdominal and chest injuries in the event of a crash.

Booster seats come in two styles — with or without a high back. High-back booster seats can be used in any type of vehicle that has lap and shoulder belts. Booster seats without a high back should be used only in vehicles with headrests, to allow for proper positioning of your child's head and neck.

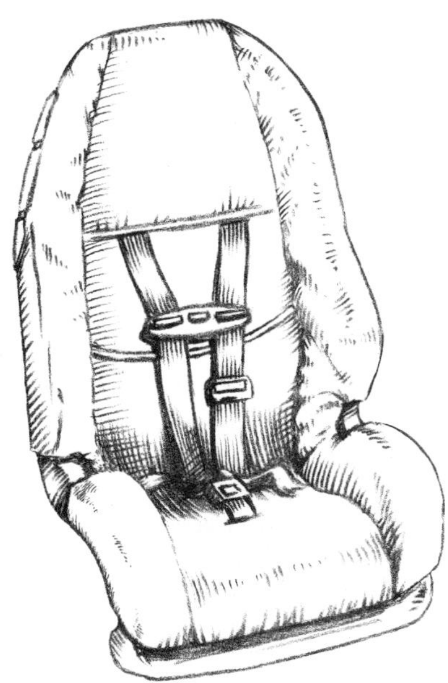

Booster seats are recommended for children between the ages of 4 and 8.

Both styles must be used with the vehicle's lap and shoulder belts.

Your child should use a booster seat until he or she is the right size to properly use the vehicle's lap and shoulder belts. Children are ready to use an adult safety belt when they can sit, without slouching, with their back against the vehicle seat and with their knees bent comfortably and completely over the seat's edge.

The shoulder strap shouldn't cross the neck. The shoulder and lap belts should both be worn. Children often put the adult shoulder strap behind them, leaving only the lap restraint functional. This doesn't provide adequate protection in case of an accident.

In vehicles with a front passenger air bag, children under age 12 should sit in the back seat. Even in vehicles that don't have a front passenger air bag, it's a good precaution to put young children in the back seat.

Recreational safety

Look for safe facilities for your child to use for supervised recreation. Backyards, playgrounds, parks and community centers are examples. Otherwise, children may choose to play in hazardous or poorly supervised places where the risk of injury is greater and, if an accident does occur, help is less available.

Organized sports such as youth baseball and soccer are excellent activities for school-age boys and girls. Look for programs that are supervised by adults and that emphasize discipline and team play rather than winning.

Biking, skateboarding and in-line skating are popular outdoor activities. However, participants in these activities are more likely to have accidents resulting in injuries to the head, back, knees, wrists and elbows. Wrist fractures are the most common serious injury related to these activities. Head injuries are the most life-threatening or potentially debilitating, which is why wearing a helmet is so important.

No matter what sport or

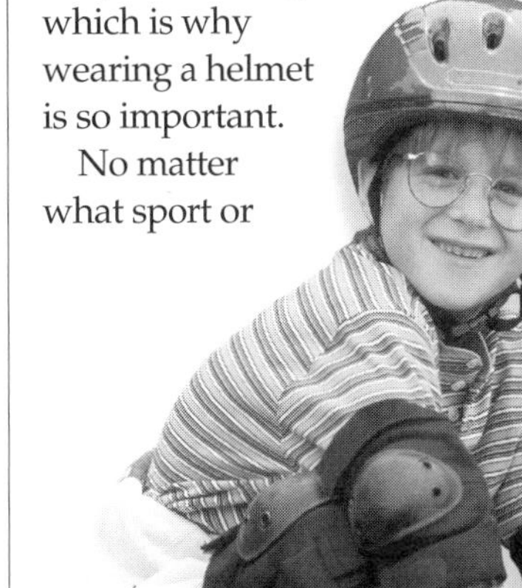

Why ► / ▼ What to wear	Cushion head blows	Prevent wrist injuries	Absorb impact	Prevent gravel burns
Helmet	✓		✓	
Wrist guards		✓	✓	✓
Knee and elbow pads			✓	✓

Children and Television

Children in the United States watch a lot of television. They spend approximately 4 hours each day watching television. This doesn't include time spent in front of the TV screen watching taped programs or playing video games. Although television can be educational and entertaining, healthier activities might be a better way to occupy your child's time. Children need to spend time socializing with their friends and family. Children need to be moving around and getting exercise. Too much time sitting in front of the television can contribute to childhood obesity.

Parents may also be concerned about programming and commercials that are sending out messages they don't want their children to be learning. For example, children may watch programming that doesn't show the consequences of drinking alcohol, smoking or using other drugs. Commercials advertise unhealthy foods targeted at children, such as candy, snacks and sugary cereals and beverages.

One area of special concern is the depiction of violence and its effect on children. According to many studies, exposure to media violence can make children more aggressive, and it can desensitize them to the abuse of others. Media violence may set the cultural norm for what a child considers acceptable behavior.

The following suggestions may help parents create a safer TV-viewing environment:

- *Set rules.* Establish limits on the amount and type of programming your child watches.
- *Watch television with your child.* Discuss issues that may come up during a show. For example, if both of you see a violent scene, ask your child to think about the feelings of the victim.
- *Learn about TV and video game ratings.* A TV-Y rating is assigned to shows or games designed for children of all ages, and a TV-Y7 rating means that the show or game contains mild fantasy violence or comedic violence more appropriate for children age 7 and older. Video games are rated EC (early childhood) for children age 3 and older, E (everyone) for children age 6 and older and T (teen) for users age 13 and older.
- *Use the v-chip.* The v-chip included in more recent TV models can be programmed to block inappropriate programs. An external v-chip box is available for televisions without the v-chip.

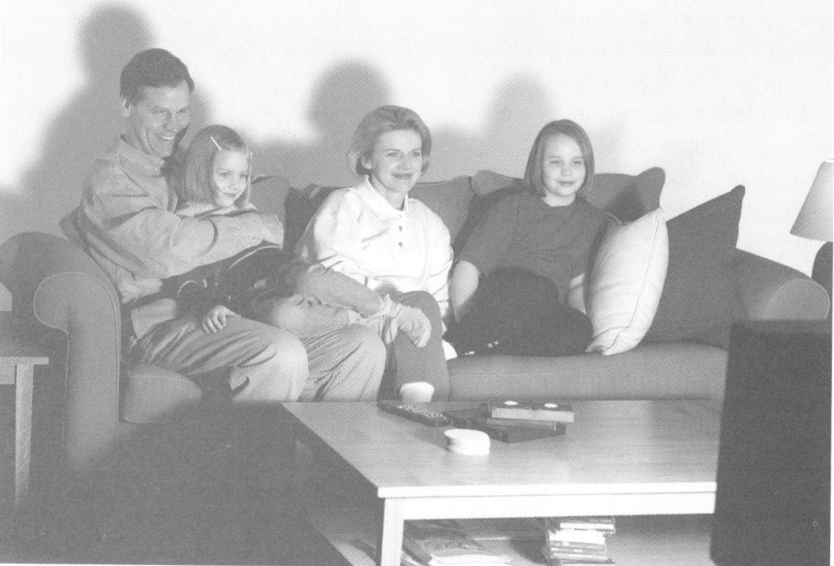

activity your child participates in, make sure that he or she uses appropriate protective gear. Doing so doesn't eliminate the risk of injuries, but it can lessen the frequency and severity of injuries.

Safety at home

Among children, the leading cause of death is accidents. Preschoolers, especially 2- and 3-year-olds, are particularly vulnerable to accidents in the home. Of course, you take certain precautions to ensure the safety of your baby. But when your child becomes mobile, move safety to the forefront of your mind and be alert to new dangers as the child's range increases.

As preschoolers grow, they'll be able to understand why they shouldn't stick their fingers in an electrical socket, put buttons in their mouth or play with matches. Even so, 4- and 5-year-olds do things that they know could hurt them. Even with an older child, never take chances with safety.

Common accidents in the home or during play include burns, drowning, poisoning, falls and choking. Although you can't prevent your child from getting bruises and bumps, safety measures may help reduce serious injury.

Burns

A child's skin is more sensitive than that of adults and can burn easily. If your child's skin comes in contact with hot (140 F or greater) tap water for just 3 seconds, he or she can get burned.

Here are some tips for minimizing the chances of a burn:

- Turn down the thermostat on your water heater to 120 F or less.
- Install smoke and carbon monoxide detectors on each floor of your home. Test them periodically.
- Never leave your child alone in your house.
- Keep matches out of your child's reach.
- When cooking, turn pot handles toward the back of the stove.

Avoid using front burners, if possible.
- Don't use place mats or tablecloths that your child can pull off the table because hot liquids placed on them could tumble onto the child.
- Never drink a hot beverage with a child on your lap or leave a hot beverage near the edge of a table, where your child might easily pull it off.
- Place electric outlet covers on all unused outlets. Avoid using long extension cords. Check all electric cords for defects.
- Keep out of a child's reach items such as a hot iron or curling iron.
- Have a fire extinguisher in your kitchen.

Drowning

A child loses consciousness after only 2 minutes under water. Many child drownings occur in residential swimming pools or bathtubs. To decrease the chance of drowning, follow these measures:

- Never leave a preschooler alone in the bathtub.
- Don't let your child swim in a pool without adult supervision.
- If you have an outdoor pool, install a childproof fence around it.
- Teach your child never to swim or go in the water without adult supervision.
- Always have your child wear a personal flotation device (PFD) when boating or around water. Set a good example by wearing a PFD yourself.

Poisoning

Poisoning is a common cause of accidents at home. Young children are especially vulnerable.

- Keep all medicine in a high or locked cabinet.
- Keep cleaning solutions out of the reach of children. If you must keep cleaning products in a low cupboard, install latches that make it impossible for your child to open the cupboard door.
- Don't store anything in the wrong container. For example, if you store paint thinner in a juice bottle, your child may take a drink, thinking it's juice.
- If you store toxic chemicals in the garage, keep them out of the reach of children.
- Many common houseplants are poisonous if eaten. You can obtain a list of these plants from your local poison control center. The safest approach is not to have a poisonous plant in your home. If you have one, keep it out of the reach of your child.
- Keep the number of the nearest poison control center next to your telephone and call the center immediately if you think your child has taken a poison.
- Keep ipecac syrup on hand to induce vomiting in case your child ingests something harmful. But never induce vomiting until you've been advised to do so by a poison control center official or your doctor. Some substances can cause more damage as they come back up the esophagus.

Falls

Falls are common during the preschool years. To protect your child from dangerous falls, follow these measures:

- If your child is still in a crib, keep the side rails up or consider moving your child to a bed. After a child reaches 2 years, a crib can become a danger if the child tries to climb in or out of it.
- Install gates at the top and bottom of each steep staircase in your home.
- Install a safety net or guard on outdoor decks or staircase openings where a young child could squeeze through.
- Make sure your windows are locked or have window guards.
- Don't put a child under age 6 in the top bunk of a bunk bed.
- Always supervise outdoor activity.
- Forbid the use of home trampolines when a parent isn't supervising. Don't allow more than one person on a trampoline at the

Safety Online

The Internet is a great tool for learning and entertainment, but it does present potential hazards, especially to children. Children may be exposed to material that depicts violence or explicit sex, lured by pedophiles or subjected to threatening or abusive messages in e-mail or bulletin boards.

If your child's use of the Internet causes you concern about his or her safety, here are signs to be aware of:

- Excessive online use, especially late at night
- Unsupervised time in a chat room that isn't moderated
- Lots of graphic files being downloaded
- Phone calls from strangers
- Face-to-face meetings with unfamiliar people

If you want to minimize the risks, consider the following suggestions:

- Tell your child never to give out personal information online, including credit card numbers and his or her name, telephone number and home address.
- Only allow use of supervised chat rooms run by a reputable server or site.
- Keep the computer in a common area of your home.
- Choose online services carefully. Some allow you to block out areas that you consider unsuitable for children. Or you can purchase filtering software.
- Learn more about the computer yourself. You can find bits of information indicating which Web sites have been accessed from your computer.
- Ask your child to sign an agreement that spells out your rules.

same time. Use a perimeter guard.
- Inspect playground and play equipment for safety. Serious accidents can occur at playgrounds. Before you let your child use play equipment, make sure that it's adequately maintained, with no rust, sharp edges or protrusions or loose nuts and bolts. The surface beneath swings or other playground equipment should not be concrete, asphalt or packed dirt but rather an energy-absorbing material such as loose sand or wood chips.

Choking

Young preschoolers will put anything into their mouth, which can cause choking. To help prevent a choking accident:

- Select toys appropriate for your child's age.
- Make sure your preschooler's toys don't have loose buttons or sharp edges.
- Avoid giving your child food that could get stuck in his or her throat. Such foods include whole hot dogs, popcorn, nuts, hard candy, peanut butter and raw carrots.
- Don't allow your child to eat food away from the table, especially while he or she is running.
- Secure drapery and window blind cords to windows.

Child care

Few issues are as important to working parents as that of child care. Finding quality child care can be challenging because all parents want the very best for their children. You'll want to find a dependable, loving caregiver and a clean, safe environment for your child.

Types of child care

Three types of child care settings are available:

- *Home child care.* Care is provided in the child's home. This option is the most convenient, but it may be more expensive.
- *Family child care.* Care is provided in the caregiver's home. This option is the most common form of child care for infants and toddlers. It provides a home-like atmosphere and limited group size. Regulations regarding how many children can be in a home setting, along with rules regarding safety, health, sanitation and fire codes, vary from state to state.
- *Child care center.* Care is provided outside of a caregiver's home in a child development center, child care center or nursery school. This option gives your child an opportunity to interact with a larger group of children. The number of child care centers is growing.

Searching for child care

If you're about to search for quality child care outside of your own home, here are things to look for:

- Make sure the child care provider is licensed by your state. This means that the provider has met certain standards and must comply with various health regulations. Family child care offered out of a private home may be less expensive, but the provider may not be licensed by the state. This means that the provider may not be monitored by state authorities.
- Visit several child care providers before you make your choice. Their operations should be open to parents at all times. Look for operations that allow parents to make unannounced visits. Such visits can serve to protect both the provider and the children. Be suspicious of any provider who requires a parent to call ahead before visiting.
- Interview the provider or director of the center. Ideally, the staff-to-child ratio at a child care center should be between 1 to 4 and 1 to 6, depending on the children's ages. The younger the children, the more staff required. Is a TV set present? If so, how often are the children allowed to watch it? TV viewing should be minimal and selective, if allowed at all. How is fighting between children handled? What education does the child care center have for or require of its teachers? Does the provider smoke? Are there any pets on the premises?
- Once you think you've decided on a provider, visit his or her facility again. Preferably, visit at a different time of day. Are the children happy and busy? Are there lots of things to do, or do the children appear to be at loose ends? Is the provider or staff warm, encouraging and willing to hug a crying child? Are there adequate sinks and toilets for the children? Make sure the playground is safe, with proper fences and equipment that's in good condition. In addition, check with your county child protective services office to see if the provider has ever been investigated.

Making the transition

Once you find a child care facility that's right for your child, take time to help your child adjust to it. Being apart from you can be painful and tearful, so plan to spend part of the first day with your child at the facility. This may be unnecessary for an older preschooler, particularly if he or she is outgoing and has spent time in the homes of friends.

For the first week or until your child adjusts, avoid rushing off in the morning. Stay for 5 or 10 minutes, until your child begins to interact with someone else. Then, rather than sneaking away while his or her back is turned, say good-bye and leave. You may find it helpful to let your child bring something from home, such as a favorite blanket or stuffed toy.

Child care and illness

Parents who have children in child care should expect them to pick up more colds and viruses than they would've if cared for at home. All young children get sick from time to time, but chances are that your child will have more bouts of illness during his or her time in child care. In part, this increase is because these common illnesses are so contagious. In addition, children are often contagious before the onset of symptoms, so a seemingly healthy child can infect many others. Thus, epidemics of childhood ailments in some centers are commonplace.

No practical measures can eliminate the spread of infection, but child care providers can help by washing their hands thoroughly after changing diapers and before handling food. They can also make sure that the children wash their hands before eating and after going to the bathroom. Sinks should be within children's reach. The room in which diapers are changed should be separate from the room in which food is prepared and eaten.

As a parent, you can help by not sending an ill child to child care. When is a child too sick to go? Each facility generally has its own rules, but most facilities won't let your child attend if he or she has a fever of more than 100.4 F, is vomiting or has diarrhea.

As to when your child can return to child care, it usually depends on how well he or she feels and whether the illness is contagious. Many cold symptoms persist for a week or more. Once the temperature is normal for 24 hours, your child can probably return to the facility even though he or she still has a slightly runny nose and minor cough. It's not practical to exclude a child from child care for the entire duration of a cold.

How Long Is My Child Contagious?

The following is a guide as to when a child who has had a contagious disease is no longer contagious:

Disease	No longer contagious
Chickenpox (varicella)	Generally after all sores are crusted, usually 7 days
Diarrhea	After stools form again
Head lice	After one treatment
Pinkeye (conjunctivitis)	24 hours after treatment begins if bacterial, longer if viral
Strep throat	24 hours after treatment begins

Hand washing

Hand washing is the best way to prevent the spread of infectious diseases. Many ailments, from the common cold to serious diseases such as an intestinal infection or liver inflammation (hepatitis), may be spread from person to person.

Good hand washing habits are important for your entire family. It's important to wash your own hands regularly and to show your children how to wash their hands properly. Both hands, including the palms and between the fingers, should be washed thoroughly with soap or detergent and water. Remind your children to wash their hands after using the bathroom, whether at home or in school.

Although access to soap and water may not always be available, make an effort to find a place where you can wash your hands. Encourage your child to wash for as long as it takes to sing the alphabet song. For a description of proper hand washing technique, see page 494.

Hand washing is critical in the following situations:
- Before preparing or eating food
- After blowing your nose, sneezing or coughing into your hand
- After handling uncooked meat or seafood
- After changing a diaper
- After playing with a pet
- After handling garbage
- After handling money

Nutrition

Some days it may seem as if your preschooler doesn't eat enough to keep an ant alive, and other days you can't keep him or her away from food. Such is a preschooler's appetite. Unlike an infant, who triples his or her weight during the first year and eats well, a preschooler's rate of growth slows considerably, as does his or her appetite. Some preschoolers are reluctant to try new foods or expand their food repertoire beyond three or four old favorites. By the time your child is of school age, his or her habits are well on the way to being established.

A preschooler's diet

When your child is 2 years old, he or she should be eating a variety of foods. Daily recommendations include:
- *Milk group (two servings).* Milk, cheese, cottage cheese and yogurt are excellent sources of calcium, which is necessary for building strong bones and teeth.

- *Meat group (two servings).* This group includes beef, poultry, lamb, fish, pork, liver, eggs, dried peas and beans and peanut butter. These foods are excellent sources of protein, which is necessary for the growth and repair of tissue cells.
- *Fruits and vegetables (five servings).* Give your child at least five servings a day from these food groups. To obtain an adequate amount of vitamin C, be sure that one or more servings are citrus fruit, berries, tomato, cabbage or cantaloupe.

  Also provide at least one serving of a green or yellow fruit or vegetable, all of which are excellent sources of vitamin A.
- *Grains (six servings).* This group includes whole-grain cereals, crackers, breads, rice and pasta.

These are the food groups necessary for a nutritionally balanced diet, but don't expect your preschooler to eat a completely balanced diet every day. When allowed to choose from a selection of nutritionally sound foods, most children tend to select diets that, over several days, offer the necessary balance. This may mean that one day your child might be eating a lot of peanut butter sandwiches, oranges and milk and the next day the menu is hamburgers, french fries and carrots.

Keep in mind that every child's energy needs are different. Your child isn't growing at the same rate he or she was as an infant, so it won't seem as if your child lives for the next meal. Your child doesn't need or want the quantities of food that he or she consumed with relish as an infant.

As your preschooler advances to the point where he or she can assume the same pattern of eating as that of older siblings or parents — a three-meal-a-day pattern — remember that snacking is acceptable. As parents, your role is to offer a variety of nutritious foods and to set a good example. Snacks are recommended for smaller preschoolers, who can't eat enough to satisfy their energy needs all at once. Small amounts of a variety of foods eaten frequently over the course of the day as a snack are healthy and normal. However, uncontrolled snacking can diminish your child's appetite for meals.

Food Guide Pyramid for Young Children

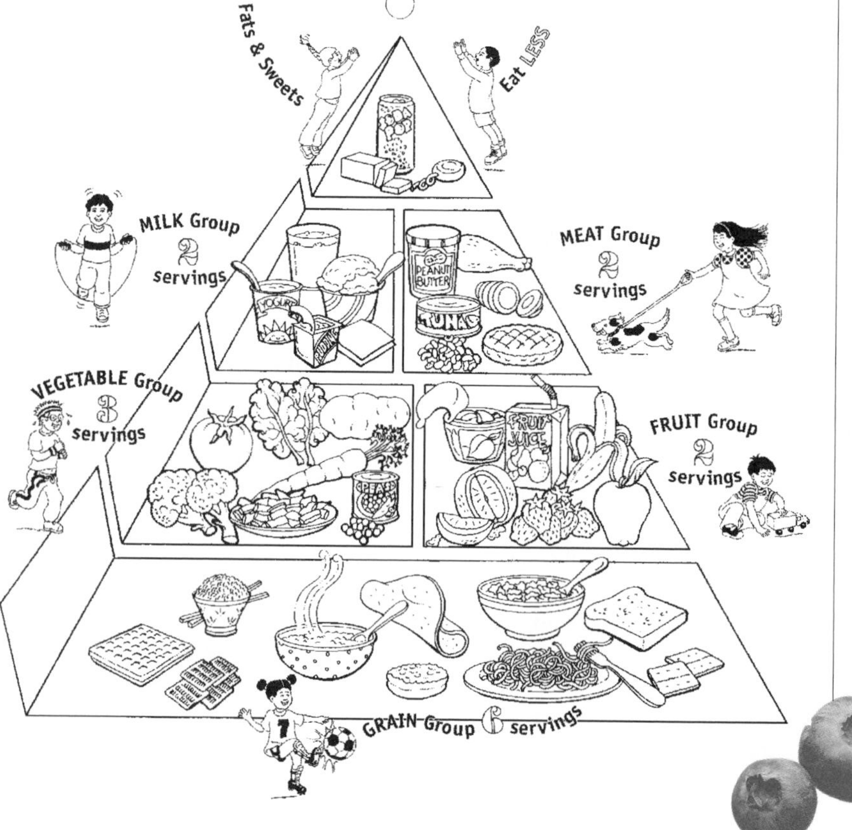
Fats & Sweets
Eat LESS
MILK Group
2
servings
MEAT Group
2
servings
VEGETABLE Group
3
servings
FRUIT Group
2
servings
GRAIN Group 6 servings

Source: U.S. Department of Agriculture, January 2000

Eating Well

Here are some tips for healthier eating for school-age children:

- *Reduce fat.* Use fat-free (skim) or low-fat (1 percent) milk. Instead of ice cream, serve ice milk, frozen low-fat yogurt or sherbet. Replace butter with margarine. Use ground beef with lower than 15 percent fat and low-fat ham. Bake or broil rather than fry foods. Rinse fried ground meat to reduce fat content.
- *Increase fiber.* Offer fresh fruits and vegetables regularly. Use whole-wheat flour when baking. Add low-fat granola, bran, rolled oats and cornmeal to quick breads.
- *Reduce sodium.* Reduce salt in recipes. Remove the saltshaker from the table. Serve soups that are lower in sodium. Look for snacks that are low sodium.
- *Reduce calories and sugar.* Use less sugar in recipes. Serve unsweetened fruit juice or fresh fruit whenever possible. Serve smaller portions of baked desserts.

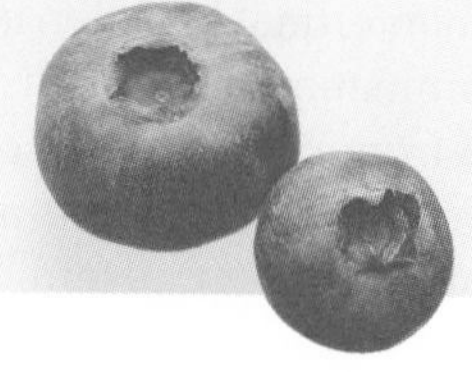

Remember that a balanced diet may also include desserts and fats such as butter, margarine, mayonnaise and oils. Dietary fat and cholesterol are important for your infant's growth. However, fats should be consumed in moderation after your child's second birthday.

A school-age child's diet

The school-age years are a good time to continue the healthy eating habits initiated during the preschool years. Equally important, promote regular physical activity to help maintain normal weight and physical fitness.

In general, the nutritional guidelines are similar for school-age children and adults. Have your school-age child eat a variety of foods that are lower in fat and higher in complex carbohydrates and fiber. At home, practice healthy eating habits to guide what your child learns about food choices.

Although you may be setting a good example at home, your child will be receiving conflicting messages from television, other media and friends. These outside influences become even stronger as your child matures, but so does your child's ability to make his or her own choices.

Help your child learn that breakfast is an important meal. It's worth getting the whole family up early enough to enjoy this meal together. After school, your child may need a snack. The amount and type of this snack should be controlled so that it tides your child over until supper but doesn't dull his or her appetite for the meal. A good choice is a piece of fruit, a whole-grain muffin or some low-fat yogurt.

A nutritional problem in some school-age children in the United States is iron deficiency anemia. However, your child will get enough iron, zinc and other essential minerals if he or she eats lean meats, whole grains, dried beans, fruits and vegetables. If your child is involved in vigorous physical activity, he or she will need more calories.

If heart disease or high cholesterol runs in your family, discuss this with your child's doctor, who will decide if your child's blood cholesterol and triglycerides (lipids) should be measured. If the value is high, your child may need to follow a diet that controls dietary fat and cholesterol.

If your child's lipid values are normal, it's important not to overdo a low-fat diet. Your school-age child is still growing and needs a balanced diet and adequate calories to grow to his or her full potential. For this reason, you don't want to impose too many dietary restrictions on your child.

As in the preschool years, feed your child in response to hunger but not in response to boredom or inappropriate behavior. When your child feels restless, encourage him or her to go outside and play rather than give more food. Remember, the best way to teach your child about good nutrition is by setting a good example in your own eating habits.

Obesity in Children

Obesity is more common during the first year of life, after age 5 or 6 and during adolescence than it is during the preschool years. Some medical disorders can cause obesity, but if your child is overweight, it's probably because he or she consumes more calories than necessary for growth and gets too little physical activity.

Not all children who are overweight are considered obese. Some children have larger-than-average body frames. These children tend to be stocky and look big, but they're not fat. A child is considered obese if he or she is more than 20 percent over what is considered his or her healthy weight.

Obesity is generally caused by a combination of factors. Heredity appears to play a role. If one or both parents are obese, their offspring are more likely to be overweight. In addition, overeating may be more common in households where family members are overweight than in households where family members aren't overweight. Lack of exercise also may be a factor. If your child is spending too many hours sitting in front of the television or computer, calories aren't being used and are turning to fat.

If your preschooler is obese, now is the time to do something, while you still have some control over what your child eats and how active he or she is. Once your child gets older and is more independent, modifying eating and exercise patterns is often much more difficult.

If you would like some assistance in developing a healthy diet for your child, consult your doctor or a dietitian. It's important to consider your child's nutritional needs and growth when making dietary changes. Don't use fad diets. They can be dangerous.

Of course, prevention is the best treatment. The time to be alert to obesity, especially if there's a family history of it, is when your child's eating and exercise habits are forming. Infant obesity has little correlation with adult obesity, but family eating habits may persist into adolescence and adulthood.

Sleeping

One way to help maintain your child's health is to encourage good sleeping habits. Establish with your child a regular sleep schedule with consistent wake and sleep times. An adequate amount of sleep gives your child energy and motivation. It can also enhance his or her learning abilities and decrease many behavioral problems.

Young children need plenty of sleep. Though sleep needs vary with each child, children between ages 2 and 5 generally require 10 to 12 hours of sleep to feel their best. This amount declines gradually to about 9 hours by the time they reach their teens. For information on sleep problems, see page 211.

Dental care

Some parents assume that a child has to be a certain age before dental hygiene becomes necessary. In fact, once your baby has a single tooth, you can begin a daily program of dental care.

Developing good habits early is key to preventive dental care. Encourage your child to brush his or her teeth every day. The technique might not be perfect, but it'll improve with time. Don't make teeth brushing a battle.

One by one, your child's permanent teeth will erupt during the school-age years. They replace the baby (primary) teeth at a rate of about four a year. Because permanent teeth need to last a lifetime, it's imperative to care for them well. Teach your child to brush his or her teeth after each meal. It's also a good time to demonstrate how to floss teeth.

Your child should begin to visit a dentist by age 3 years — sooner if the teeth appear abnormal or if he or she complains of a toothache. Schedule dental visits every 6 months or as your dentist recommends. When the permanent back teeth break through, your child's dentist may cover them with a brush-on sealant. This helps protect them against tooth decay.

Fluoride

If your water doesn't contain fluoride, your child's doctor or dentist may prescribe a fluoride supplement. From the time your child is 6 months until he or she is 10 years old, fluoride is an important deterrent to tooth decay.

Fluoride helps make your child's tooth enamel cavity resistant. Typically, your child consumes fluoride either in drinking water or in a supplement.

Diet

You can do your part to decrease the risks of tooth decay by limiting your child's consumption of sugary and starchy foods and sugary beverages. It's virtually impossible to keep children away from sweets altogether, but try to get them to avoid those that stick to the teeth or linger in your child's mouth.

Offer healthy snacks as treats. Vegetables and fruits not only help minimize cavities but also are nutritionally better for your child.

A combination of measures that include water fluoridation, sealants, brushing and flossing, good nutrition and regular visits to the dentist can help prevent dental cavities.

Sun protection

Protect your child's skin from the sun's ultraviolet (UV) rays. A child who experiences a severe, blistering sunburn may have a greater risk of developing skin cancer as an adult. Practice sun safety:

- Buy sunscreen designed for children that has a sun protection factor (SPF) of at least 15.
- Use sunscreen even on cloudy days. Clouds block only a small portion of UV rays.
- Limit your child's time at the pool or beach.
- If possible, keep your child out of the sun when UV rays are strongest. This is generally between 10 a.m. and 3 p.m.
- Dress your children in clothes made of tightly woven fabrics.

Insect repellents

When your child is outside, the following tips may help keep the insects away.

- Avoid using scented soaps or shampoos. Fragrances often attract insects.
- Avoid areas where insects may live, such as stagnant pools of water or gardens with blooming flowers.
- Don't dress your children in bright colors or flowery prints. They tend to attract insects. Wearing white can make it easier to find ticks.

When you're in an area that contains insects, use an insect repellent. The active ingredient in many insect repellent products is a chemical called DEET.

Although DEET is toxic if ingested or absorbed through the skin in large amounts, if used properly it doesn't present a health concern and is effective in repelling potentially disease-carrying mosquitoes and ticks.

However, follow these safety measures:

- Don't use repellents on infants younger than age 2 and use them sparingly on children ages 2 to 6.
- Use insect repellents that contain no more than 10 percent DEET. Read the label before purchasing the repellent.
- Never apply insect repellent on children's hands because they're likely to put their hands in their mouth or rub their eyes.
- Apply insect repellent to clothing rather than directly on the skin.

Common Concerns

As children age and move from one stage of growth and development to another, they'll experience various challenges and frustrations. Invariably these problems will pass, but proper coaching and reactions from parents can help.

Toilet training

Toilet training can be a difficult time in the lives of a child and his or her parents. But when handled properly, it can be simply one in a series of many milestones.

The first question most parents ask is, "When is the right time to attempt toilet training?" That's not an easy question to answer. One child's readiness for toilet training may be different from that of another. Some are toilet trained within 24 hours around age 2, and others still balk at the idea near their third birthday.

Generally, doctors advise not to train a child before 2 years, and many believe that even 2 years is too early. Unless a child appears extremely interested in being trained, most doctors usually advise waiting until between 2 and $2^{1}/_{2}$ years. Bladder control through the night comes later. Most children continue to wear underwear-type absorbent pants at night for several months afterward.

Signs your child is ready

No rule says that training will be successful immediately. Try it for a few days, and if your child clearly isn't interested or protests, put the plan off for a few weeks.

Some indications that your child may be ready for toilet training are:

- Your child uses bathroom words such as *potty*, *pee pee* or *poo poo*.
- Your child has watched others use the toilet.
- Your child indicates when he or she is wet or dirty and wants to be changed.
- Your child can briefly control his or her bowel and bladder.

Supplies

Once you determine that the time may be right, you'll need some supplies:

- A small potty chair that sits on the floor. Some children's toilet seats are designed to fit on a regular toilet, but many children prefer the floor type. A floor type not only allows the child to get on and off at will but also enables the child to push better because his or her feet are on the floor. Purchase the potty a few weeks before you're ready to begin training so that your child becomes familiar with it.
- Training pants, which are heavy, more absorbent underwear.
- Stickers, if you want to use tangible rewards in addition to your praise. Always reward your child for showing interest in using the toilet and not for what comes out when on the toilet. Your praise is the best reward you can give your child. Don't use food as a reward for using the toilet. But inexpensive, tangible rewards, such a stickers, are OK.

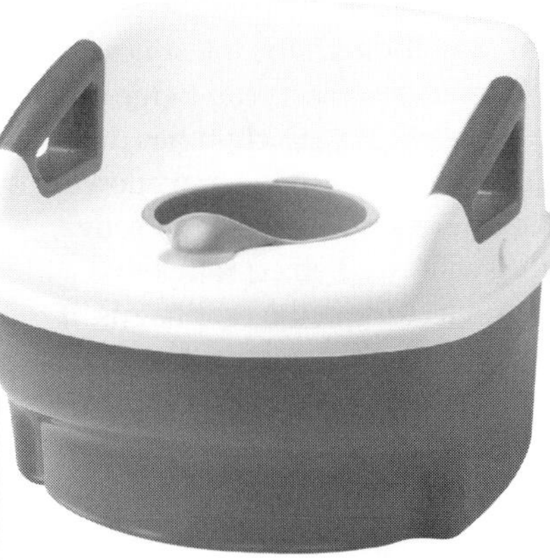

How to train your child

You can go about toilet training your child in various ways. No matter which one you ultimately choose, make sure that you don't turn the bathroom into a battleground.

Many doctors suggest allowing the child to become trained according to his or her own free will. This means no coercion whatsoever. Ask your child if he or she wants to sit on the potty. If the answer is no, don't pressure him or her. If your child sits a minute but doesn't do anything, let him or her get off the potty when ready. If your child urinates or has a bowel movement, be free with your praise. But when the inevitable "accident" occurs, don't scold or shame your toddler.

Other methods use similar principles but require more parental involvement. For example, take your child to the potty chair at appropriate intervals and ask him or her to pee pee. If your child is reluctant to cooperate, try entertaining him or her with books or games while he or she is seated on the potty chair. If your child doesn't urinate within 5 minutes, take him or her off the potty and try later. When your child does use the potty chair, offer praise.

For some children, bowel and bladder control occur simultaneously. Others achieve one before the other. In most cases, toilet training can be accomplished within 2 months. If not, it may be an indication that your child is too young, and you should probably try again in a few weeks or months.

If your child is older than $2^{1}/_{2}$ years and still isn't trained after 2 months of trying, he or she may be resisting toilet training. The most common cause of this resistance is too much parental pressure. Often, these children have been reminded too much or been forced to sit for long periods on the potty chair.

In trying to train a resistant child, shift the responsibility to him or her. Tell your child that you're not going to remind him or her to go to the bathroom and that he or she must decide when to go. Use positive reinforcement and incentives to reward your toddler for a day without wet or dirty pants. If your child has an accident, change him or her and then involve the toddler in cleaning up the mess. Don't punish or criticize. Try to be patient, however difficult that may be.

Several months after daytime control is achieved, try putting your child to bed without a diaper. Taking your child to the bathroom just before he or she goes to bed may hasten night training.

Putting Your Child to Sleep

The following tips may prevent your child from developing sleep problems or help your child overcome sleep difficulties:

- Don't sleep in the same room as your child.
- Don't entertain your child at night.
- Don't let your child nap more than 3 hours a day.

If your child is having difficulty falling asleep at night or sleeping through the night, try the following steps. Although this approach may leave you wide awake for a while, it should improve the situation within about 2 weeks. Remember, each child's needs vary.

- Put your child to bed awake, read a book, say good night and leave the room despite protests.
- Give your child a transition object, such as a favorite blanket or stuffed toy. Put on a recording of soothing music.
- If your child begins crying, don't go into his or her room immediately. Wait 15 or 20 minutes before checking on him or her. When you do go in, stay in the room for less than a minute.
- Don't turn on the light or pick up your child. Simply reassure him or her that everything is all right and that it's time for sleep.

The first night that you begin using this method, your child may cry for an hour, but generally the crying time will decrease each night. Some children awaken terrified. If your child's cries sound fearful rather than simply angry, go to him or her immediately. After you reassure your child, you may have to sit with him or her for a while. Don't play or talk.

Leaving the door open or using a night light also can work wonders. If you find your child crawling into bed with you at night, gently but firmly take him or her back to his or her bed. In the long run, this is better for you and your child.

Swallowing objects

Young children are naturally curious and are not averse to putting coins, safety pins, buttons, fruit pits and other things into their mouth. Keep these and other small objects out of reach.

In addition to a fondness for small objects, some children chronically ingest non-nutrient substances such as dirt, plaster, clay and ashes. This eating disorder, called pica, may occur during the first 2 years, when your child's natural curiosity compels him or her to sample everything. If your child persists with this practice, talk to your doctor. Pica may be a sign of an iron deficiency.

A watchful parent may be able to retrieve an object before it's swallowed. When your child swallows an object, it usually passes through the digestive system uneventfully. A good rule is that if a swallowed object passes into your child's stomach, it will usually pass the rest of the way through the intestines.

However, objects can lodge in the esophagus. If your child has difficulty with breathing or swallowing, or if he or she is spitting up saliva, the swallowed object may have become stuck in the esophagus. If this occurs, call for emergency help or go to the emergency department at your local hospital.

If your child stops breathing because of an obstruction, try the Heimlich maneuver (see page 344). Indications that an object may be stuck in your child's throat include chest pain, abdominal pain and vomiting.

If your child swallows a button battery, such as those found in watches, pocket calculators, cameras and hearing aids, contact your child's doctor right away or take your child to the emergency department of the hospital, even if no symptoms are present. Button batteries contain dangerous alkali fluids. If the battery gets lodged in the esophagus, the battery fluid can cause severe burns in only 2 hours.

Tantrums and breath holding

Few children make it through their toddler and preschool years without demonstrating temper tantrums. This stubborn, oppositional and defiant behavior is a natural part of moving from total dependence to a taste of independence.

Nothing is more exasperating than when your child decides to throw a temper tantrum. Any parent who has been through one knows that it doesn't take much to drive some youngsters to uncontrollable kicking, screaming, headbanging and even breath holding.

Often, in fact, the temper tantrum has nothing to do with you, but is your child's response to frustration. When a child reaches this point, he or she is out of control and beyond reason. Generally, a temper tantrum, once started, has to run its course.

Giving in is not the answer. If, for example, your child has a tantrum because you deny him or her a second cookie, you'll be sending the wrong message if you suddenly reverse your decision. Once the tantrum starts, giving your child a timeout is most helpful. Leave the room and try to ignore what's going on. Even if your child holds his or her breath, don't worry because this generally isn't harmful. As for any headbanging, children hate pain as much as adults. When things get too uncomfortable, they know it's time to quit.

When to return to your child is variable. Some parents find that their child finishes the tantrum on his or her own. Other children may need to be held for a moment before they can stop crying.

Although ignoring a tantrum is usually best, sometimes you must take other measures. Obviously, the child who decides to throw a tantrum in the middle of the supermarket can't be left there to kick and flail, nor should a child who is physically aggressive toward someone else or property be allowed to continue unchecked. Take the child to his or her room or separate your child from others until your child regains his or her composure.

Sleep difficulties

Crying uncontrollably at bedtime, waking up frequently during the night and getting out of bed and attempting to crawl in with mom and dad are common sleep problems among young children.

Sleep problems are a frequent complaint of parents. Whether the problem is temporary, intermittent or has been occurring for months, a child who's awake at night creates tired parents, not to mention a cranky child.

Causes of sleep difficulties vary, often depending on the age of your child. Common sleep problems that may interfere with your child's getting a good night's rest include:

- *Parental dependency*. If your child has always had problems sleeping through the night, you may have been too responsive to his or her night cries. Most infants awaken several times during the night but can put themselves back to sleep. If your child has learned that mom or dad will come rushing every time he or she cries, your child becomes dependent on a parent to get back to sleep. This can be a hard habit to break, especially with younger children.
- *Bed-wetting*. Bed-wetting (enuresis) is the most common reason children ages 3 to 15 wake up at night.
- *Nightmares*. Your child may have scary dreams that awaken him or her. The nightmares may be in response to stress or trauma that occurs during waking hours. Calmly reassure your child if he or she awakes after a nightmare.
- *Night terrors*. Night terrors are a condition in which a sleeping child awakens screaming, with no recollection of a nightmare. Sometimes the child may scream and still be asleep and unresponsive to your actions. Emotional tension increases night terrors. They generally occur between ages 3 and 5, and they tend to run in families.
- *Sleepwalking*. Sleepwalking is a condition in which a child is partially awake with open eyes and a dazed expression. He or she may sit up in bed, walk or do activities such as open doors, go to the bathroom or undress without being aware of what he or she is doing. If awakened, the child is often confused and disorientated. Sleepwalking tends to run in families and is most common in children ages 6 to 12. Gently guide your child back to bed without waking him or her. Keep doors and windows closed and locked and remove objects that your child could trip over.

Bed-wetting

"Mommy, Daddy, I wet my bed." Virtually every parent hears those words at one time or another, and many young children do on occasion have accidents during the night.

True bed-wetting (enuresis) is involuntary urination, mostly occurring at night, in a child age 5 or older. Usually, it doesn't indicate an emotional or physical problem. Children vary markedly in the age at which they're physiologically ready to stop wetting. Bed-wetting may be a problem if your child's bladder hasn't yet developed enough to hold urine through the night, or if your child hasn't learned how to recognize when his or her bladder is full, wake up and use the toilet.

If your child bed-wets and has never been totally dry for a year, the condition is known as primary enuresis. If your child starts wetting again after having been dry for at least a year, the condition is called secondary enuresis. This form of bed-wetting may develop temporarily in reaction to a stressful change in your child's development, such as the birth of a sibling or the first week of school.

Bed-wetting is much more common in boys than in girls, and it often runs in families. Your child may urinate during the first third of the night and remember nothing of the occurrence. Aside from wet pajamas, enuresis itself causes no direct impairment of your child's life, but a child who bed-wets is often afraid to attend sleepovers or go to camp.

Limiting your child's intake of liquids at bedtime is one way to make it easier for him or her to stay dry. Having your child urinate twice just a few minutes apart right before bedtime also may help, as might getting him or her up to go to the bathroom at night. Behavior modification techniques are often effective in eliminating enuresis. You may want to use wall charts with gold stars awarded for cooperating with bedtime routines. Enuresis is involuntary, so avoid rewarding dry nights and punishing wet ones.

If your child is motivated to stop wetting, alarm devices attached to a pad that awakens your child when the pad gets wet may help. Your child's doctor may prescribe medication, such as imipramine (Tofranil), desmopressin (DDAVP, Stimate) or oxybutynin (Ditropan), if your child is older and the problem persists.

In the case of secondary enuresis, have your child examined by a doctor to rule out any organic problems, such as urinary infection, seizure disorder or diabetes. Should the problem appear to be a reaction to stress, psychotherapy or family therapy may be helpful.

Although having to change bed linens repeatedly can be exasperating, try to express support for rather than anger toward your child. Doing so will not only help to enlist his or her cooperation but also prevent his or her losing self-esteem. Reward your child if he or she helps by getting into dry clothes and back to bed quickly.

Giving medicine

Many children resist taking medication. To sidestep such resistance, it helps to approach this task in a natural, matter-of-fact way. Explain that the medication needs to be taken and why. Apprehension on your part or the expectation of resistance can become a self-fulfilling prophecy.

It's generally best to avoid mixing medications with foods or drinks. If you do, make sure that the entire mixture is consumed. In addition, ask your pharmacist if the food or drink with which you mix the medication is compatible with the medication.

Don't try to get your child to take medication by promising a treat or, worse, telling him or her that the medication is candy. Children must learn to make a clear distinction between medicine and candy and to take all medications while supervised by an adult.

It's important to give medications exactly as prescribed — in the correct dose and at the correct interval. When your child begins to show signs of improvement, don't stop giving the medication unless specifically instructed to do so. Don't use remnants of old prescriptions.

Common Conditions

As many parents can attest, preschoolers do get sick with amazing frequency. Some months you seem to be caught in a revolving door between home and your doctor's office. No sooner is an ear infection cleared up than your child develops a cold. Before you know it, you're back to see your doctor.

Most parents are understandably concerned when their young child seems to fall prey to every virus that hits the block. In the back of your mind, you may wonder if something is wrong that's interfering with your child's ability to resist these infections.

Almost always such fears are groundless. If your child is active and gaining weight, there's probably nothing wrong with his or her health. It's a simple fact that young children are particularly susceptible to colds, ear infections and gastrointestinal viruses. Your child's immune system must be exposed to many viruses before it develops its own resistance.

School-age children gradually become less prone to common respiratory infections, such as colds. Most disorders of school-age children don't have serious consequences. At this age, children are extraordinarily resilient, and their young bodies easily recover from most common disorders.

Fever

An oral temperature of more than 99.5 F or a rectal temperature of more than 100.4 F is considered a fever. A fever is one of the body's ways of fighting infection.

Viral infections, strep throat and ear infections are the most common causes of fever in children. More serious illnesses also can cause fever, but fortunately they aren't common.

Although children tolerate most fevers quite well, high temperatures often provoke a great deal of anxiety for parents. If your child is responsive, continues to drink fluids and wants to play, there's probably nothing to worry about.

Contact your child's doctor or go to the emergency department if the fever is accompanied by considerable listlessness, severe headache, or persistent vomiting or stomachache. Also see a doctor if your child has a high fever that isn't responding to fever-reducing medication.

If you think your child will be more comfortable if you lower the fever, you can use acetaminophen (Tylenol, others) or ibuprofen (Advil, Motrin, others) to help reduce it. Extra fluids, minimal clothing and perhaps a sponge bath with tepid (not cold) water also may help. If you do bathe your child, be sure to stop the bath if he or she begins to shiver.

Don't use aspirin to reduce a fever in a child. Aspirin use in children has been linked to Reye's syndrome, a potentially life-threatening illness.

Some medical experts believe that reducing a low-grade fever blunts the body's immune response and may possibly prolong some illnesses.

Vomiting

Vomiting may or may not be associated with diarrhea. If your child is vomiting, avoid feeding him or her solid foods for about 8 hours. Your child may try to drink small amounts of clear liquids or suck on ice pops. If your child hasn't vomited for about 8 hours, you can try foods such as soda crackers, white bread or chicken soup.

See a doctor immediately if you see blood in vomit or note that your child has severe abdominal pain, has a swollen abdomen, is delirious or is difficult to awaken or exhibits signs of dehydration — no saliva or tears and absence of urination.

Diarrhea

Diarrhea is characterized by a change in one or more of the following stool patterns: frequency,

Immunizations

By age 6, your child should have completed the recommended schedule of childhood immunizations. Most states require that children have a documented, completed series of vaccinations before they enter kindergarten. For more information on childhood immunizations, see Chapter 1, "Getting Immunized."

Prevention of Diseases and Infestations

If you have a young child, you may have more colds and viral illnesses than your friends who don't have young children. Given the frequency with which young children contract these ailments and their high degree of contiguousness, this isn't a surprise. Infections that typically afflict families spread in various ways.

Respiratory infections such as colds most often spread through contact with secretions from the nose, mouth or eyes of an infected person. Toddlers are great at spreading colds because of their habit of touching and mouthing everything they come across.

Your child's sneeze can release potentially infectious agents into the air. Although colds are spread less commonly in this manner, the infectious particles contained in a sneeze or cough can travel up to 6 feet.

The sharing of combs, brushes and hats may contribute to the spread of ailments such as lice, ringworm and impetigo.

Although it's impossible to totally stop the spread of contagious disease and infestations within a family, you can take the following preventive steps:

- Wash your hands throughout the day and encourage your child to do likewise. This is particularly important before eating and after using the bathroom, blowing your nose or changing a diaper.
- Don't share combs, brushes and hats.
- Don't smoke around your child. Exposure to secondhand smoke increases both the frequency and the severity of your child's colds.
- After someone in your family has been ill, get him or her a new toothbrush and throw out the old one because it may contain bacteria that can cause reinfection.
- Use a disinfectant. Clean and disinfect bathrooms, the kitchen and diaper-changing areas frequently.
- Immunize your pets. It's likely your toddler and dog or cat will have frequent contact, so make sure your pet is immunized and wormed regularly.
- Cook foods thoroughly. To help prevent bacterial illness, cook eggs and meat thoroughly. And be sure that you carefully wash your hands and any object that comes into contact with uncooked food, particularly meat and eggs.

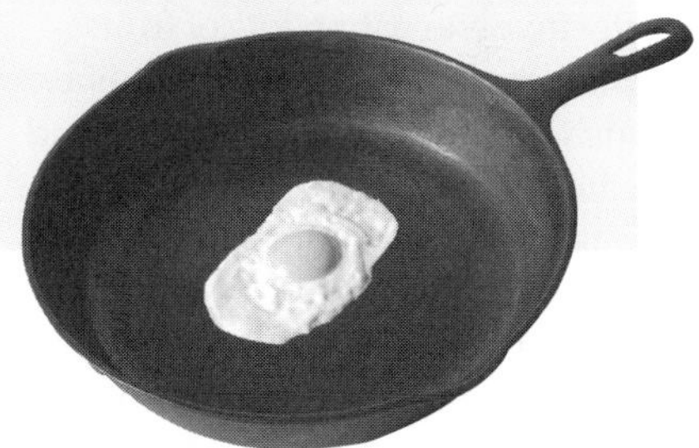

volume or content. Diarrhea is a common gastrointestinal disturbance, usually caused by a virus. Less commonly, diarrhea is the result of a bacterial or parasitic infection.

Mild diarrhea is the passage of a few mushy stools. Moderate or severe diarrhea is indicated by an increased frequency of bowel movements and stools that are more watery and, possibly, greenish. Dehydration is the main danger. The body can lose large amounts of fluid in the stools.

If your child has diarrhea, take steps to avoid dehydration by increasing your child's fluid intake. Water, juice, ice pops, broth and sport drinks are good choices. Don't use diet soda or diet juices. Commercially available oral electrolyte replacement solutions, such as Pedialyte or Lytren, provide excellent replacement of what the body loses with diarrhea. In addition, they help slow down the amount of fluid loss.

If your child isn't hungry, don't force food. If he or she wants to eat, offer a general diet and a lot of fluids. Foods that contain bulk — such as whole-grain cereal, fruits and vegetables — are good choices because they usually make the stool firmer. Diarrhea may last up to a week or a few weeks before bowel movements return to normal.

Some young children develop toddler's diarrhea. The child may have several days of loose stools that are foul smelling and runny. Some children are incredibly thirsty during this time.

Despite the diarrhea, a child with toddler's diarrhea usually is very active, appears healthy and doesn't have a fever. If the stool is tested for bacteria, it almost always is normal. This is because most cases of toddler's diarrhea are caused by viruses, such as the rotavirus.

It's unnecessary to call your doctor every time your child has a bout of diarrhea unless any of the following symptoms occur:

- Signs of dehydration — no wet diapers or urination for 8 hours, tearless crying, no saliva in the mouth
- A bowel movement every hour for more than 8 hours
- Blood, pus or mucus in the stool
- Severe abdominal pain or any abdominal pain lasting more than 12 hours
- Diarrhea that doesn't improve within 48 hours of dietary changes
- Mild diarrhea lasting more than a week

Constipation

Parents of young children are often overly concerned about their child's bowel movements. If your child doesn't have a daily bowel movement, you may incorrectly assume he or she is constipated. Although many people do have daily bowel movements, others may have a bowel movement only every second or third day.

The signs of constipation are the painful passage of stool, passage of a large, hard stool, an inability to pass stool even though the urge to defecate is strong, or going more than 3 days without having a bowel movement.

Constipation is often a result of not getting enough fiber or fluid in the diet. Constipation can also result from a child holding back passage of stool because it's inconvenient to go to the bathroom. Some children hold in the stool because a previous passage of a hard stool created a tear in the anal opening. It hurts when they try to have a bowel movement, so they try to avoid the pain.

Treatment for constipation generally involves eating lots of fruits and vegetables, foods high in fiber such as wheat breads, legumes and whole-grain cereals and drinking water and other fluids. In addition, encourage your child to sit on the toilet at regular intervals, perhaps after breakfast or supper. If this doesn't resolve the constipation, talk to your child's doctor.

Colds

The common cold is one of the most frequent illnesses of childhood. Preschoolers have an average of five to eight colds each year.

If your child constantly has a congested head, is sneezing and has a fever or sore throat, there are several possible causes. The most common cause of a constantly runny nose is simply a recurring cold.

Children older than 6 months often have recurring viral upper respiratory tract infections. A young child with a cold is generally sicker than are older children or adults with colds.

Fever may be an early sign of a cold. Irritability, restlessness and sneezing usually follow. A few hours later a clear liquid begins to drip from the nose, which gradually changes to a thick mucus that makes it difficult to breathe through the nose. The virus may irritate your child's throat and windpipe (trachea), causing a sore throat and cough. Other symptoms may include headache, lack of appetite and muscle aches.

What can you do for a cold? In general, there's little anyone can do to make your child better quickly. Usually, your child's temperature will return to normal in 1 to 3 days. Nose and throat symptoms generally disappear within a week. However, the cough may persist for 2 to 3 weeks.

Over-the-counter medications may relieve some of the symptoms, but they don't shorten the duration of the illness or prevent complications. Antibiotics are of no benefit for infections due to cold viruses. Antibiotics are taken to treat bacterial infections.

You can do some things to make your child more comfortable:

- *Clear mucus from the nose.* If your child is too young to blow his or her nose, remove mucus from the nose using a soft, rubber suction bulb. If your child is managing OK with breathing and eating, there's really no need for nasal suction.
- *Use saline nose drops.* If your child's nose is stuffed, try administering over-the-counter saline nose drops 15 to 20 minutes before meals and at bedtime. For a young child, tilt his or her head back and place three drops in each nostril. After waiting 1 minute, use a suction bulb to remove the loosened mucus. For an older child, put three drops in each nostril while he or she is lying faceup on the bed with his or her head over the side. After a moment, have your child blow his or her nose. This can be repeated several times in a row until the nose is cleared.
- *Give fever medicine.* If your child has aches or a fever of more than 102 F, you may give acetaminophen (Tylenol, others) or ibuprofen (Advil, Motrin, others). Never give your child aspirin. Aspirin use in children has been linked with Reye's syndrome, a life-threatening condition.
- *Use a humidifier or vaporizer.* If your child is congested or has a cough, use a cool mist humidifier or vaporizer to moisten the air. It may help your child breath easier. But make sure to keep the device clean to prevent the growth of bacteria and molds in it.

Ear infection

Middle ear infections (otitis media) are one of the most common illnesses affecting young children. The majority of children will have at least one middle ear infection by age 3. Although ear infections recur in one-third of these children, most children stop having multiple ear infections by the time they reach school age.

Ear infections often follow a cold that leads to fluid buildup behind a child's eardrum. This trapped fluid is an ideal breeding ground for bacteria or viruses that cause infection. In addition to having an earache or a feeling of pressure in the ear, your child may become irritable, lose his or her appetite, develop a fever and have trouble sleeping.

Most ear infections clear on their own without antibiotics. However,

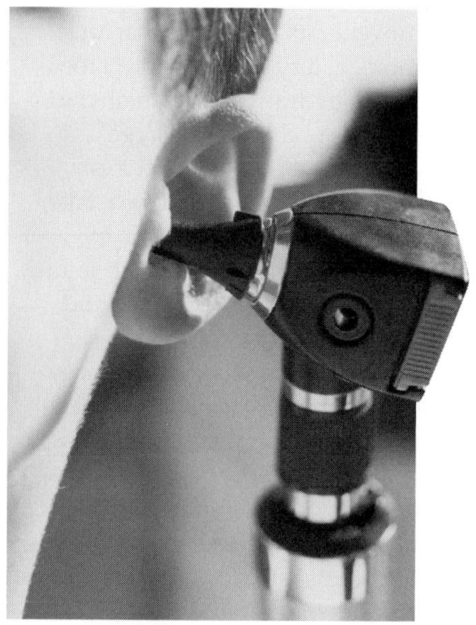

your child's doctor may prescribe antibiotics if the infection is severe or if your child has recurrent ear infections.

If your child doesn't respond to antibiotics, your child's doctor may recommend surgically inserting a small drainage tube into the eardrum to help prevent fluid buildup. For more information on ear infections, see page 668.

Strep throat

Strep throat is a common infection and is caused by the bacterium *Streptococcus pyogenes* (group A beta-hemolytic streptococcus). Often, a person with strep was exposed to someone else with the illness in the preceding 2 to 7 days.

Children ages 5 to 15 who are in a school classroom or some other group setting are most likely to get strep throat. The illness is generally spread by nasal or throat secretions. Less commonly, strep infection may be transmitted through food, milk or water contaminated with streptococci bacteria.

Common signs and symptoms of strep throat are a sore throat, red and swollen tonsils, swollen lymph glands in the front of the neck, fever, headache, muscle aches, abdominal pain and possibly vomiting.

Strep throat requires antibiotic treatment to prevent complications. For more information on strep throat, see page 491.

Croup

Croup is an inflammation of the voice box (larynx) and the airway just beneath it. Children with croup have a loud barking cough that may sound like the barking of a seal. Because of a narrowing of the airway, the voice becomes hoarse and breathing may become difficult. Croup is caused by a virus and is usually preceded by symptoms similar to those of a cold. Symptoms of croup are usually worse at night and may last from 5 to 7 days.

Children younger than 5 years are at greater risk of developing croup because their small airways are more susceptible to narrowing when swollen. Symptoms tend to be most pronounced in children younger than 3 years.

Most cases of croup aren't serious and can be treated at home. However, if your child has croup and develops stridor or other symptoms of airway distress, he or she should be seen by a doctor. Stridor is a harsh, high-pitched sound made when a child breathes in after a bout of coughing. For more information on croup, see page 491.

Pneumonia

Pneumonia refers to an infection or inflammation in the lungs. In young children it's often a passing illness that may remain undiagnosed and be regarded as a cold. Pneumonia can develop after a cold or the flu or on its own. It may result from a virus, a bacterium or another organism (see page 490).

Fever and a prominent cough are common warning signs. The cough may not produce phlegm in children as it does in adults. Rapid and labored breathing or respiratory distress also are signs of pneumonia. Treatment varies depending on the cause.

Tonsillitis

Tonsillitis is an infection and inflammation of the tonsils. It's common in preschool and school-age children. If your child has tonsillitis, his or her tonsils may become red and swollen and you may notice small patches of white discharge on them.

Sometimes, the adenoids, located in the back and upper part of the throat, will be swollen too — although you can't see them. Other signs and symptoms may include a sore throat, difficulty swallowing, fatigue, headache, fever, chills and sore and enlarged glands in the jaw and neck.

Warning Signs of Serious Illness

The following signs and symptoms may suggest a serious illness. If your child has any of these, call your doctor or go to the emergency department:

- A fever higher than 103 F
- A fever without an obvious cause (a cold or the flu) that lasts longer than 24 hours
- A fever that lasts more than 72 hours
- Lethargy or no drinking of fluids
- A stiff or painful neck
- Such severe pain that he or she doesn't want to be touched
- A sudden inability to walk
- Breathing difficulty
- Difficulty being awakened
- A convulsion
- Pain in the groin
- Blue lips
- Profuse drooling
- Persistent vomiting
- Purple or deep red spots on the skin
- Painful urination or lack of urine output accompanied by other signs of serious illness
- Bloody stools or urine

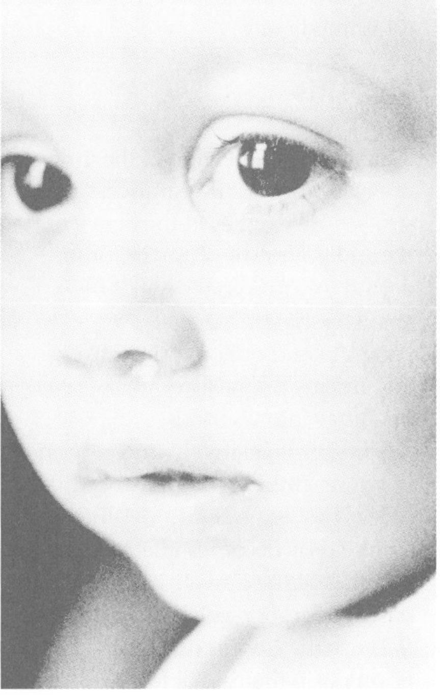

Surgery to remove your child's tonsils and possibly adenoids is generally considered only if the tonsillitis interferes with breathing or hearing, is recurrent or doesn't respond to antibiotics (see page 691). Antibiotics treat tonsillitis resulting from a bacterial infection.

Symptoms should disappear a few days after your child begins taking the medication. If the infection is resulting from a virus, no treatment is used aside from getting plenty of rest, drinking plenty of liquids and gargling with warm salt water to ease the symptoms.

Epiglottitis

Epiglottitis is an inflammation of the lid-like flaps of tissue and cartilage that cover your windpipe. It often occurs among children between the ages of 2 and 5 and is more common in boys than in girls.

Your child may have a sore throat, fever, difficulty swallowing and breathing and hoarseness. Epiglottitis usually results from a bacterial infection and may respond to treatment with antibiotics.

Epiglottitis causes severe inflammation and serious breathing difficulties and can cause death. If you suspect that your child has epiglottitis, have him or her seen by a doctor immediately.

Sinusitis

Sinusitis is an infection of the lining of one or more of the sinuses. The sinuses are cavities in the bones around your nose. They're connected to your nasal cavities by small openings. Normally, air passes in and out of your sinuses, and mucus drains through these openings into your nose.

Sinusitis is relatively uncommon in young children but may occur in older school-age children. When a sinus cavity becomes infected, nasal membranes also swell, causing nasal congestion or obstruction. Because the cavity can't drain, pus or mucus remains inside.

Sinus pain may result from the inflammation itself or from the pressure caused by built-up secretions in your sinus. For more on sinusitis, see page 687.

Rashes

Rashes can result from a variety of factors. Some of the most common include:

Chickenpox

Chickenpox (varicella) causes itchy red spots that quickly fill with a clear fluid to form blisters. The blisters eventually rupture and crust over. The initial rash tends to break out on the face, scalp, chest and back and may spread to the arms and legs (see the color illustration on page 436).

Spots continue to appear over 4 to 5 days, often accompanied by a fever, runny nose or cough. Your child is contagious until the rash crusts. It usually takes a 12- to 21-day incubation period after exposure to chickenpox before signs and symptoms appear. For most children, this period is 12 days.

Chickenpox occurs primarily in children, but adults who aren't immune can get it too. The incidence of chickenpox has declined since the development of a chickenpox vaccine. The vaccine is intended for children age 1 year or older and adults who haven't had the virus. For more information on chickenpox, see page 492. For more information on the chickenpox vaccine, see page 9.

Roseola

Roseola is a viral infection that typically affects children between 6 months and 3 years. It usually begins with a high fever lasting about 3 days. When the fever goes down, a rash appears on the trunk and neck lasting from a few hours to a few days.

The rash causes little discomfort and in most cases isn't serious. It disappears on its own without treatment, but acetaminophen (Tylenol, others) and tepid sponge baths can help relieve discomfort and fever. Occasionally, young children experience convulsions caused by the high fever (febrile seizure). Contact a doctor immediately if this happens. For more information on roseola, see page 497.

Fifth disease

Fifth disease is a common, mild infection in children. It's caused by a virus called human parvovirus B19. Doctors often refer to the illness as parvovirus infection.

The primary symptom of fifth disease is the appearance of bright red, raised patches on both cheeks, resembling slap marks (see the color illustration on page 436). A pink, lacy, slightly raised rash may also develop on the arms, trunk, thighs and buttocks. The rash may come and go for up to 3 weeks. Some children develop a slight fever and other mild, cold-like symptoms.

No specific treatment is recommended, but acetaminophen (Tylenol, others) may relieve the fever and discomfort. Pregnant women who suspect that they've been exposed to the virus should contact their doctor because there's a chance the fetus may develop serious complications.

Measles (rubeola)

Measles (rubeola) typically begins with a fever, often as high as 104 F to 105 F, a cough, sneezing, a sore throat and red, watery eyes. A red, blotchy rash appears on the face and behind the ears and spreads to the trunk, arms and legs. The rash may begin as fine, red spots that increase in size.

Sometimes, small, white spots may appear on the inside lining of the cheek. The rash usually lasts about a week, during which time it typically spreads from the forehead to the legs.

Measles occurs primarily in children, but adults are susceptible too. A vaccine to prevent measles has significantly reduced the incidence of this disease. For more information on measles, see page 496.

Hand-foot-and-mouth disease

Hand-foot-and-mouth disease is a mild but highly contagious disease primarily affecting preschool children. Symptoms of this viral infection include blister-like lesions on the tongue, mouth, hands and feet.

Children in child care centers are especially susceptible to outbreaks because the illness is spread by person-to-person contact. Meticulous hand washing can help prevent spread of the disease.

This illness isn't related to foot-and-mouth disease, which is a highly infectious viral disease of ruminant animals.

Impetigo

Impetigo is a common skin infection caused by streptococcal or staphylococcal bacteria that penetrates the skin through a cut, scratch or insect bite. The infection starts as a red sore that blisters briefly, oozes for a few days and forms a sticky crust. It usually appears on the face and is more common among young children (see color illustration on page 436).

The infection can easily spread to other people or other parts of your body just by scratching or touching the sores. Good hygiene can help prevent and limit the spread of impetigo. The sores and skin surrounding the infection should be kept clean. Trim your child's fingernails. If the infection spreads, your doctor may prescribe antibiotics to treat it.

Lice

Lice are tiny parasitic insects that cause intense itching. Head lice are often spread among children by direct contact or by clothing, combs and hairbrushes. They're commonly found on the scalp at the nape of the neck and over the ears. Small nits (eggs) that resemble tiny pussy willow buds attach to hair shafts.

Prescription and over-the-counter shampoos are available to remove lice. Make sure you read the directions carefully. Consult your doctor before using these products on children younger than 2 months or if you're pregnant. Infected children should be kept home until after the first shampoo treatment. A mixture of vinegar and water may be useful in dislodging nits, which must be manually stripped from hair shafts to prevent recurrence.

To prevent the spread of lice or reinfestation, wash sheets, clothing and hats with hot, soapy water and dry them at high heat, which kills the lice. Soak combs and brushes in very hot, soapy water for at least 5 minutes. Vacuum carpets, mattresses, pillows, upholstered furniture and car seats. For more information on lice, see page 501.

Scabies

Scabies is a contagious skin disease caused by tiny mites that burrow under the skin. The mites are almost impossible to see without a magnifying glass, but they make a characteristic burrow that looks like a thin, irregular pencil mark (see the color illustration on page 437).

The marks appear most often between the fingers, in the armpits, around the waist, along the insides of the wrists, on the back of the elbows, on the ankles and soles of the feet, around the breasts and genitals and on the buttocks. Itching is usually worse at night.

Scabies can spread from person to person in a family, child care setting or schoolroom. Bathing and over-the-counter preparations aren't effective in removing scabies. Consult a doctor for treatment.

Headaches

Headaches are more common during late childhood and early adolescence than during the preschool years. They rarely represent a serious problem. Usually, a headache is a sign that your child isn't getting enough fluids, food or sleep, or is experiencing stress. Headaches also are associated with many viral illnesses.

If your child frequently complains of headaches, even during times when he or she is otherwise well, consult a doctor. Migraines may be the culprit, especially if there's a family history of migraines. In children, this type of headache often is accompanied by light sensitivity and sleepiness. Recovery often follows within a few hours of the onset of the headache.

Abdominal aches

Stomachaches are common in children. Typically, the pains are nothing more than the result of eating something that doesn't agree with a child or the beginning of a bout with a gastrointestinal virus.

Sometimes, a child may complain of intermittent stomachaches or abdominal pain. These symptoms may relate to stress or fear concerning a social situation or school issue. In many children, the symptoms gradually disappear, but others have recurrent bouts of pain over many years.

Consult with your child's doctor if your child refuses to participate in day-to-day activities because of a stomachache or if the stomachache is accompanied by blood in the stool or vomit, persistent vomiting or diarrhea, or weight loss.

Growing pains

Many school-age children, particularly during the later years of this period, experience severe, recurrent limb pain. These pains may come on at any time, but they seem to occur most frequently in the evening, particularly after a day of strenuous activity.

Usually, these pains are located in the thighs or calves, and they last for an hour or two. The children are otherwise healthy, and the results of a physical examination and diagnostic tests are normal.

Although these pains probably aren't directly related to physical growth, the symptoms often are labeled growing pains. The pains have no known explanation and disappear over time without any lasting ill effects. The best treatment for growing pains is sympathy, understanding and the assurance that the symptoms don't represent a health problem.

To help alleviate some of the discomfort:

- Let your child use a warm (not hot) heating pad.
- Give recommended doses of acetaminophen (Tylenol, others) or ibuprofen (Advil, Motrin, others) for pain. Don't give aspirin unless advised by your doctor to do so.
- Call your child's doctor if the area becomes swollen, hot and tender, if your child develops a limp or an unexplained fever or if the pain persists more than a week or two.

Genital infections and irritation in girls

Genital infections in girls (vulvovaginitis) can occur both before and after puberty. The usual cause is inadequate bathing and toilet habits. A young girl may not wash her genitals adequately. Or she may wipe herself from back to front after bowel movements and inadvertently transport bacteria that live harmlessly in the intestines to the vaginal and urinary openings, where they can colonize.

Yeast, parasites, bacteria and irritants found in soaps and other toiletries can cause genital infections. Yeast infections are more common in girls who have entered puberty, have diabetes or have been taking antibiotics.

Your daughter's doctor may ask if she has had any vaginal discharge, itching or redness of the anus, vulva or vagina, or other infections. The doctor will likely examine the genital area and may take a sample of vaginal discharge to examine for bacteria, yeast and parasites.

Genital infections and irritation can often be prevented and treated by teaching your daughter about her genital area and showing her how to wipe from front to back. When she bathes, encourage her to wash her genital area and avoid taking bubble baths.

Her toilet paper and underpants should be white, not colored, because dyes can irritate the skin. Her underpants should also be all cotton and changed once a day. Discourage wearing clothing that increases moisture in the area, including attire such as tightfitting jeans and tights. Wearing a swimming suit for a prolonged period of time should be avoided.

For specific infections, treatment may involve taking oral antibiotics or applying a prescription cream to the genital area.

Urinary tract infection

Urinary tract infection occurs when bacteria enter the bladder via the channel leading from the bladder to the outside of the body (urethra). Under normal circumstances, these bacteria are rinsed out of the body during urination.

Urine itself has properties that inhibit the growth of bacteria. However, certain bacteria and anatomic abnormalities in the urinary system can increase the chance of a urinary tract infection.

Urinary tract infections are more common in girls than in boys. Usually, the infection is confined to the bladder, a condition called cystitis. Your child may feel as if she has to go to the bathroom constantly and may complain of pain with urination. The urine may be foul smelling.

A child who had been night trained may have episodes of bedwetting. Other signs and symptoms may include fever, vomiting and chills. In some cases, a child with a urinary tract infection has no signs or symptoms. Left untreated, a bladder infection can lead to a more serious kidney infection.

Urinary tract infections in girls can result from improper wiping after going to the bathroom. In some cases, dyes in bubble bathes may lead to a urinary tract infection. Other causes include genital abnormalities. Sometimes, urinary tract infections occur for no apparent reason.

Antibiotics are generally prescribed for a urinary tract infection. Some children who have recurrent urinary tract infections may need daily doses of an antibiotic for months or even years to keep their urine from getting infected.

After an infection, X-rays may be taken to determine whether urine is flowing from inside the bladder back to the kidneys (refluxing). When an abnormality, such as reflux, is responsible for the infections, surgery may be considered if antibiotic treatment isn't sufficient to control the problem.

Special Concerns

If you have special concerns about some aspect of your child's health or development, discuss them with your child's doctor or another health care professional. The following information is presented as a starting point in your effort to understand how you can best help your child.

Some children may have vision or hearing problems, physical disabilities, orthopedic disorders or sexual abnormalities. Others may exhibit signs of child abuse. Whatever their circumstances, every child in your care is counting on you to be informed about their condition and responsive to their needs.

Vision problems

The preschool years are crucial for the detection and successful treatment of many eye conditions. When detected in the preschool years, simple vision problems generally don't have an adverse effect on a child's learning. Sitting extremely close to the television or area of activity may be one indication of a vision problem. Others include squinting, eye rubbing, fatigue and headache.

Refraction abnormalities such as nearsightedness and farsightedness are the most common vision problems in children. A child with a refraction problem may seem to show a lack of interest in learning. A child who's farsighted may not want to look at books, and the one who is nearsighted may seem uninterested in activities more than a few feet away. These problems are usually easily corrected with prescription glasses.

Another condition that may be first noticed in early childhood is a misalignment of the eyes called strabismus (see page 640). Cross-eye is a type of strabismus. In some cases, one eye deviates only when your child is tired. In another form, both eyes deviate alternately.

The earlier the condition is discovered, the better the chances of improvement. If you feel your child's eyes may be misaligned, see your doctor. Early treatment can help prevent amblyopia, a condition in which the brain learns to ignore images from the weaker eye.

Hearing problems

In order to develop normal speech and language, a child must hear well. Even mild loss of hearing can interfere with your child's language development. The more severe the hearing loss, generally, the greater the learning problem.

Four types of hearing loss can occur in young children:

- Conductive hearing loss refers to an interference with the reception of sound from the external to the internal ear.
- Sensorineural hearing loss stems from abnormalities of the cochlear hair cells or the auditory nerve.
- Mixed hearing loss occurs when both conductive and sensorineural hearing loss are present.
- Central auditory disorders are the result of a dysfunction of the auditory center within the central nervous system.

Total deafness is often diagnosed within the first 6 months of life. If a child is partially deaf, however, the problem may not be detected until the child is 1 to 2 years old or older. At this point, your child may already have missed critical stages for language development and learning.

In the first 3 years of your child's life, look for the following warning signs that your child may have difficulty hearing:

- *1st year.* The child doesn't react to loud noises, doesn't imitate sounds or doesn't respond to his or her name.
- *2nd year.* The child doesn't play with his or her voice, doesn't imitate simple words, doesn't enjoy playing games, such as peekaboo or patty-cake, or isn't using two-word sentences to talk about or request things.
- *3rd year.* The child doesn't seem to understand "not now" and "no more" or can't follow simple directions.

The extent to which hearing loss influences your child's ability to learn depends on the severity of the loss, the range of frequencies affected, the age at which the loss occurs, how soon it's discovered and when treatment begins.

Some forms of hearing loss may be treated with medication. Others may require surgery, and still others may require a hearing aid. A hearing aid amplifies the hearing your child has and is considered the single most important tool toward allowing a hearing-impaired child to function normally. Techniques such as lip reading and sign language also may be beneficial, especially if the loss is more severe.

Orthopedic disorders

Beyond breaking a bone from time to time or pulling a muscle, most children don't have serious problems with their muscles, bones and joints. However, a wide range of growth patterns can occur in a preschool-age child. Flatfeet, pigeon-toe, bowlegs and knock-knee are all stages through which most children pass during the normal pattern of leg and foot development.

For example, your infant's toes tend to bend inward and the feet appear flat because of the abundance of baby fat in the arch. As the child ages, though, the arches gradually become visible by the age of 5. Likewise, legs are ordinarily slightly bowed from birth until about 2 years of age. Then your toddler's legs often overcorrect in the opposite direction, giving a knock-kneed appearance by age 3. Normally, legs straighten by 7 years of age.

Even when these variations continue through the school-age years, they seldom require treatment. Disease is rarely the cause.

Flatfeet

Your child's feet are flat if arches aren't apparent. There's no reason to be concerned about flatfeet in infants. Infants' baby fat always makes their feet look flat. However, if the arches don't become distinguished by age 5 years, your child may have flatfeet that are either flexible or fixed.

Flexible flatfeet look flat only when your child stands up. When he or she stands on tiptoe or the foot bears no weight, the arch is restored. Flexible flatfeet tend to run in families and are more common in Jewish and black people. The feet are mobile and painless and have excellent muscle strength.

Usually, flexible flatfeet don't require treatment. However, if the feet are extremely flat, your child's doctor may prescribe an arch support. Although this won't correct the problem, it can permit long walks and prevent foot strain.

Fixed or rigid flatfeet are cause for more concern because they may occur with congenital bone malformations. Your child's doctor will likely take X-rays to determine if this is the case. An operation may be appropriate if the condition isn't relieved by special footwear.

Pigeon-toe

In the condition called pigeon-toe, the toes turn inward. Most newborns are pigeon-toed as a holdover from their fetal position in the womb. They usually sleep with their toes pointed inward. Then, as they start to walk, their feet often turn inward to keep their balance and make up for conditions such as flatfeet, bowlegs and knock-knee.

The condition usually resolves spontaneously by age 5. If it persists, your child's doctor may watch your child standing and walking and also may take X-rays. He or she will check for the presence of diseases that can cause pigeon-toe, such as congenital bone malformations in which the bones of the thigh, shin, ankle or foot turn inward.

Sitting or sleeping on the inturned feet doesn't cause further deformity but may perpetuate the problem. If your infant's foot is flexible, your doctor may advise stretching exercises. If the foot is fixed, your child may need special shoes.

Encourage your child to sit and to walk with his or her toes straight ahead or turned slightly outward. Have your child sit cross-legged rather than with his or her knees together and the lower legs flat on the floor and pointing outward.

An underlying structural malformation, though uncommon, can be treated by putting the feet in casts and then in orthopedic shoes. Generations ago these treatments were commonly used. Today, doctors have learned that without correction, the malformation generally resolves spontaneously. If these measures don't work, an operation may be necessary, but a doctor usually won't advise such a surgery before your child is 9.

Knock-knee

When a child with knock-knee stands up, the knees touch each other but the ankles don't. Knock-knees are more common in girls than in boys, partly because their pelvis is wider. They occur more frequently in overweight children whose developing bones and joints are hard put to support their weight. Knock-knees also run in families.

A knock-kneed appearance can persist after age 4, but most children's legs straighten by age 7.

If the legs don't straighten or if the condition develops after your child is of school age, your child's doctor may perform tests to rule out diseases of the knee joint that can cause knock-knees, such as juvenile rheumatoid arthritis, rickets and infections. An unrecognized injury or developmental problem can cause asymmetrical knock-knees.

Children with severe knock-knees often have flatfeet, because the weight falls on the inner edge of the foot and ankle. If your child is overweight, this condition may strain the feet and require an arch support to relieve foot fatigue and

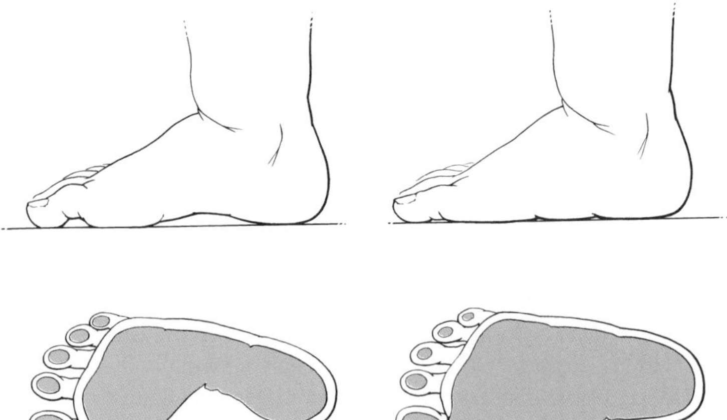

Flatfeet are feet that have little or no arch. Above at left (top and bottom) is a normal foot and footprint. If your child's foot and footprint more nearly resemble the illustrations at right, he or she has flatfeet.

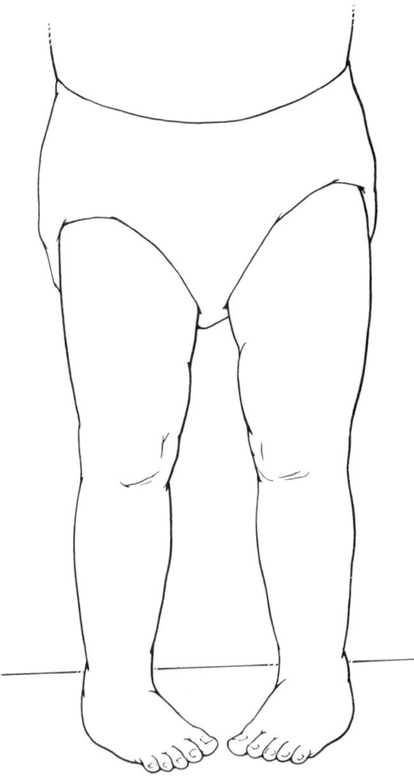

Newborns commonly arrive with pigeon-toe, in which the toes turn inward. Most often the condition resolves itself by age 5.

to prevent the inner border of the shoe from wearing.

A doctor may treat severe knock-knees with braces that are worn at night. Occasionally, an operation is needed, but not until the knees have had a chance to straighten on their own — after age 10 for girls and 12 for boys — but before growth is complete. However, in most cases the legs tend to straighten as your child grows, so treatment is seldom required.

Bowlegs

Legs are considered to be bowed if, when the ankles touch each other, the unbent knees don't. Legs are normally bowed at birth because of the way the fetus's legs are folded over each other in the cramped space of the womb. Legs often stay bowed for up to 2 years. If bowed legs persist or worsen after age 3, they should be examined by your child's doctor.

Sometimes, the legs merely appear bowed because of the distribution of the fat on your child's legs. When one leg is more bowed than the other, it may be due to an injury or a growth problem. Persistently bowed legs usually straighten without treatment by age 8. A doctor may prescribe braces worn at night to help correct the disorder. Surgical correction is a possibility if other measures fail.

In rare cases, bowlegs are caused by disorders such as rickets or Blount disease. In Blount disease, the shinbone curves out below the knee and isn't securely inserted into the knee. Severe problems of the knee joint may develop.

This disease tends to occur more often in children who are overweight, short or who walked at an early age. It's more common in girls than in boys. An operation on the upper part of the shinbone can correct it.

Sexual abnormalities

The onset of puberty occurs in both boys and girls in the later stages of the school-age years. In general, puberty is thought to be premature if it occurs before age 8 in girls and before age 9 in boys.

In girls, the first sign of puberty is generally the development of the breast bud (thelarche). The onset of menses (menarche) follows within several years. In boys, enlargement or growth of the testicles and penis is generally the first sign of puberty, to be followed by the appearance of pubic hair.

Several disorders concerning sexual development may occur during puberty, especially in girls:

Breast abnormalities

In girls, the development of the breast bud (thelarche) signals the onset of puberty. Breast development may be the only indication of

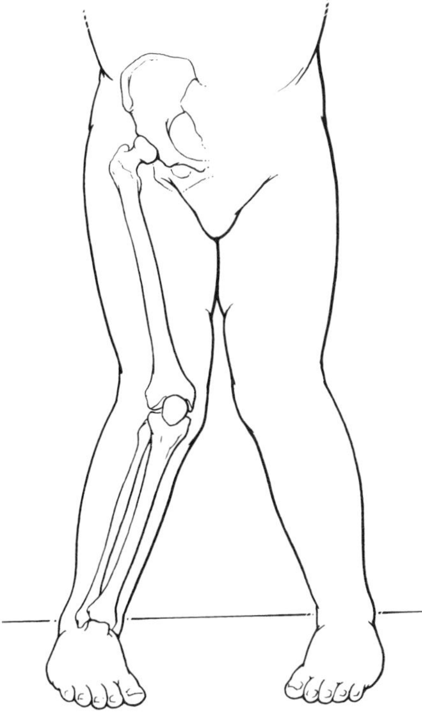

Knock-knees are the reverse of bowlegs. The knees are close together, but the ankles don't touch.

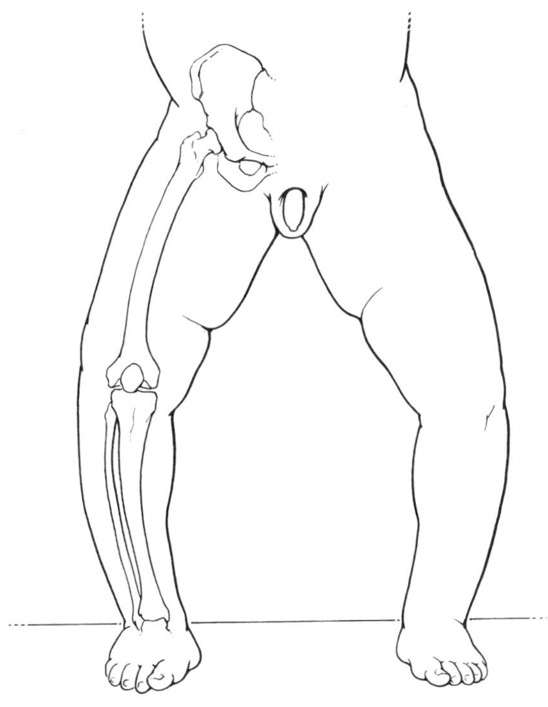

Most children are bowlegged as infants. If the legs are still bowed at age 3, consult your child's doctor.

Sexual Abuse

Sexual abuse of children involves an adult or older child forcing or persuading a child to participate in a sexual act.

Young people need affection. Depriving a child of healthy physical contact, such as hugging, may cause significant problems in a youngster's psychological development. Young children often seek physical contact with adults, but their need for affection shouldn't be mistaken for adult sexuality. Some adults inappropriately respond to this behavior by exploiting children for their own sexual gratification.

Children often seek some sexual contact with their peers. This usually is normal curiosity and experimentation. However, if your child describes an experience in which he or she was touched in an inappropriate way by an older child or an adult, take it seriously and take appropriate measures to prevent it from happening again.

Signs and symptoms

Indications of possible sexual abuse in a child include:

- Provocative or promiscuous sexual behavior
- Withdrawal from friends, family or school activities
- Unusually hostile or aggressive behavior

Sometimes, a doctor may identify evidence of trauma to the genital area or the presence of sexually transmitted infections. However, the absence of all of these signs and symptoms isn't necessarily proof that no abuse has occurred. In the vast majority of sexual abuse cases, there's no specific physical evidence of abuse.

How to respond

If you suspect that your child has been sexually abused, make sure that your child is safe from further harm. Take your child to his or her doctor or an emergency room at a hospital, preferably one that offers emergency and follow-up psychological support. The child will be checked and treated for any internal and external injuries, and the child may be tested for sexually transmitted diseases.

If the sexual abuse involved rape, handle it as a specific type of aggression against the child. This will help to minimize the sexual significance of the trauma and to prevent the child from experiencing lasting psychological effects. When you're in the presence of the child, it's best for you and the child's doctor not to dwell on the sexual nature of the assault. If you do, your child may become insecure and anxious, without clearly understanding what's going on.

Report the abuse to the proper authorities and have your child talk with a sensitive professional who's experienced at counseling victims of child abuse. This counseling is particularly important if the abuser was a family member or friend.

Don't keep the abuse a private or family matter. Most perpetrators are involved wit h several children. Seldom is the abuser a complete stranger to the child.

puberty for 6 months or so. It's not unusual for one breast to develop first and remain larger for months.

When the breasts start budding in girls younger than 8 years, this sign of early sexual maturation is called premature thelarche. Most often, premature thelarche occurs between the ages of 1 and 3 years. If it's not followed by the other signs of sexual maturity, such as hair growth in the genital area, the girl's puberty is considered to be premature and incomplete.

The budded breasts often flatten within a year, but they may persist until the normal onset of puberty. The condition is harmless and seldom affects the girl's growth. Supportive counseling is usually all that's necessary to help a young girl cope with her temporary difference from other girls. Consult your doctor for a full evaluation to differentiate premature thelarche from premature puberty.

Premature vaginal bleeding

Some school-age girls may have bleeding from the vagina before the expected age of menstruation. Consult your daughter's doctor if this occurs.

A doctor will first want to ascertain the source of the bleeding.

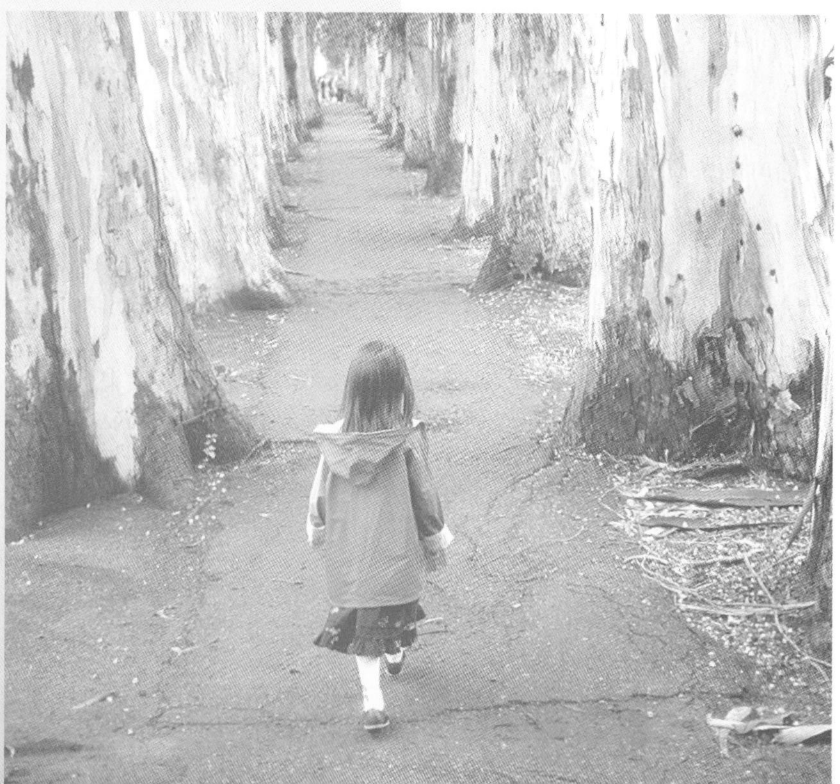

Often, the cause isn't the beginning of menstruation but another cause such as an inflammation of the genital and vaginal areas (vulvovaginitis), a genital tumor, trauma or a foreign body lodged in the vagina. In some cases, however, the cause is premature menstruation due to an early onset of puberty.

Premature adrenarche

Adrenarche refers to activity in the adrenal glands. Premature adrenarche occurs most often in girls between ages 5 and 8 years. It's often accompanied by rapid short-term growth. The armpits may sweat and grow hair. Pubic hair can develop (pubarche).

Your child's doctor may perform tests to determine if your daughter has other abnormalities of the adrenal glands, which in rare cases can cause premature adrenarche.

Premature puberty

Premature (precocious) puberty occurs much more commonly in girls than in boys but is rare. If you're concerned about premature puberty in your child, consult his or her doctor for a full evaluation.

Girls

In girls, premature puberty refers to the beginning of puberty before 8 years of age. The events of puberty may proceed as usual but start earlier than normal. In normal puberty (and usually in premature puberty), the breast buds appear first, then pubic hair appears and later menstruation begins, often with irregular cycles. Ovulation is uncommon but can occur.

Usually, no underlying cause can be determined. However, the condition is known to involve early maturation of one of the hormone-producing glands — the ovaries, pituitary or hypothalamus. Rarely, premature puberty results from a tumor of the brain or ovaries, so your child's doctor may initiate studies to rule out these possibilities. A doctor may also ask if your child has been exposed to or used any face creams or medications containing estrogens, which can also induce the disorder.

A potential long-term consequence of premature puberty is shorter height. It's usually associated with rapid short-term growth that stops earlier than normal.

Treatment for premature puberty may include psychological counseling for your child to help her deal with an appearance that's different from that of her peers. When puberty occurs very early, medication to change hormone balance may be considered to stop sexual development from progressing. Premature puberty shouldn't be minimized. However, it's reassuring that by about age 10 most of the girl's peers will have caught up with her in sexual maturity, and she probably won't feel so different anymore.

If your daughter undergoes puberty prematurely, it's important not to respond to her based on her physical appearance or to deny her hugs. Keep treating her like the little girl she is and advise her teachers to do the same.

Boys

In boys, premature puberty refers to the beginning of puberty before age 9. If your child develops signs of advanced sexual development at an early age, see your doctor. Signs generally include enlargement of the testicles and penis, appearance of pubic hair, deepening of the voice and accelerated growth.

Studies may be done to rule out a tumor of the brain and nervous system, adrenal gland or testes. An identifiable cause of the premature puberty is found in about half the boys who experience it.

Child abuse

Children of all ages can be abused. There are many ways children can be abused. Physical harm by beating or sexual assault is the most obvious form of abuse, but children left hungry in unsafe conditions or children who are emotionally abused with hurtful words are victims of child abuse as well.

Most often the abuser is related to the child and is involved in caring for the child. Parents who abuse their offspring come from all walks of life. Child abusers are male and female, and of all races, faiths, economic strata and political beliefs.

Abusive parents often tend to be lonely, angry and unhappy people who often are under stress with which they can't cope. Many of them were physically abused as children. Still, there's never a valid excuse for child abuse.

In dealing with child abuse, protection of the child is the most important objective. The goal of treatment of the entire family is for the majority of these families to remain intact and safe for the child, with the parents providing adequate care.

Abused children who are returned home without intervention run a significant risk of serious injury or even death.

Child abuse is a serious matter and everyone must help by reporting instances of suspected abuse or neglect. You can file a report by contacting professionals trained in dealing with suspected abuse.

Local social service agencies, law enforcement agencies or the child protective service office in your county can help. You may obtain further information and assistance by talking to doctors, counselors, clergy, school professionals or other professionals who deal with families having problems.

Parents who fear they have or may abuse their children are encouraged to contact these groups as well. In addition, many communities offer self-help groups such as Parents Anonymous.

Children with disabilities

The care of a child with a disability may require a combination of family support, social and academic adaptation, adjustments in the child's physical environment and, often, special medical care.

Permanent disabilities in children can include mental retardation, physical deformities such as the absence of a limb, or sensory defects such as blindness or deafness.

Whatever a child's limitations, it doesn't take him or her long to realize that he or she is different. Helping your child develop a sense of self-worth and an ability to get along in the world despite his or her differences is fundamental to the successful rearing of your child.

You can achieve this, in part, by helping your child become as self-sufficient as possible and by creating an environment in which he or she can develop to his or her full potential.

Few things are as traumatic as the birth of a child with a major disability. Some parents initially try to deny the reality of the situation, especially if the disability isn't apparent to others. It's normal to feel guilt, anger and fear about your ability to cope with a disabled child, as well as anxiety over your child's future.

If your child's handicap is severe, you may need to consider placement in a supervised living service at an early age. It used to be common to place severely retarded infants in institutions. Today, doctors know that infants and young children do better developmentally if they have a consistent parent figure in a nurturing home environment.

Still, parents of children with disabilities often come to the realization that they alone can't care for their child. Thus, the child may enter a facility equipped for children with special needs. Even so, you may want to attempt home care before considering placing your child in an alternative environment.

Coping strategies

If you're attempting to rear a child with disabilities at home, you can use the following coping strategies to make your child as happy and well adjusted as possible.

Treat all of your children alike

Some parents relax household rules for a disabled child, which only makes the child feel more different than he or she is. Rules should apply equally to all of the children in the family. Like his or her siblings, your disabled child should have certain responsibilities and should be punished for breaking the rules, provided that he or she is capable of understanding them.

Be aware of your attitude

Children are amazingly deft at compensating for a defect. For example, a child born without one hand becomes very proficient with the other hand and, having known nothing else, doesn't miss the absent hand. However, if you're embarrassed about the deformity, your child will sense these feelings and probably become self-conscious.

Don't neglect your other children

The care of a child with special needs can be so time-consuming that it becomes easy to ignore other family members. Try to set aside time each week to be alone with each child. Honestly answer your other children's questions about their brother or sister.

Accept your child's individuality

All children have strengths and weaknesses. When your child with special needs accomplishes something, no matter how small, praise him or her.

Don't isolate your child

All children need friends. It's normal to want to protect your child from a contagious illness and the potential cruelty of some children, but don't do it at the expense of your child's socialization. Schools now provide an education for all children within the community.

Previously, children with special needs went to one school together. Today, most public schools by law must provide special education classes for children with disabilities. And, in many cases, the children take classes with children in the mainstream student population. Mixing children with disabilities with the rest of the students can benefit everyone in the class.

Address special needs

A child's needs may range from a specially designed house and van to home care provided by a trained nurse or visits to a medical facility.

Accept help

Many community resources can help you meet the needs of your son or daughter. Some agencies offer financial help for qualifying parents who can't provide for their child's medical needs. Others offer services such as transportation, counseling, psychological evaluation, baby-sitting, child care and play activities.

Your child's doctor can be an excellent source of information about available community resources, for your child and for you. Public health nurses and social workers also know of local resources and are often a very useful source of information and support.

In addition, to support your child, don't be afraid to seek support for yourself. Parent support groups give parents a chance to express their common concerns and share information. In recent years, these groups have organized and become a force in influencing legislation that has expanded and improved opportunities for children with disabilities. ■

CHAPTER 14 PART II

Teenage Years

Adolescence is the period of transition between puberty and adulthood. It's a time of physical, emotional, psychological, social and mental growth. In chronological terms, the teenage years extend from ages 13 through 19. In biological terms, adolescence begins with puberty, the time when sexual reproduction first becomes a physical possibility.

Growth during these years is most apparent physically. Teenage boys and girls become taller and heavier, their body shape changes, and their facial features become more defined and mature.

Equally significant is the broadening of intellectual development, providing new insights and abilities to understand more complex matters. In addition, a teenager's psychological development helps integrate these multitude of changes into a better understanding of his or her physical and intellectual self.

Often, physical, intellectual and psychological developments occur at different rates and times. The differences can lead to anxiety, insecurity, conflict and other emotional hurdles.

During adolescence, the ongoing tug of war between parent and child begins to change. This struggle, which starts in infancy, involves the normal tension between the child's dependence on his or her parents and the need to be more independent.

Just as children are distinct from adults, so too are adolescents. Teenagers are no longer children but not yet adults. In the early teenage years, adolescents begin forging an identity that's separate from their parents. In contrast with younger age groups, they start to take responsibility for their own life and more is expected of them.

To ensure that a good relationship is maintained, it's crucial for both generations — parents and teenagers — to communicate with each other as openly as possible.

Growth and Development

Adolescence is the fastest period of growth and development, except for the first year of life. Growth occurs unevenly — relatively slow periods of change are interspersed with growth spurts.

Teenagers respond differently to these changes. Some teenagers feel frustrated or helpless, and others are excited about how their body is developing. Or the same teenager who felt frustrated one day may feel excited the next.

Normal growth changes

It's normal for growth to occur at different rates. Teenagers may feel insecure about being one of the shortest or tallest in the class. If your child is developing slower or faster than average, let him or her know that there's nothing to worry about. Show your love and provide reassurance by neither minimizing nor overdramatizing your child's concerns.

On average, the growth spurt begins at about age 10 in girls and 12 in boys, tending to reach its peak rate of change about 2 years later in both sexes. At the peak of the growth spurt, there's an increase in height of about 3 to 4 inches a year. Most boys grow faster than girls do. At the end of the growth spurt, adult height is nearly attained. If your child hasn't started an obvious increase in growth by age 15, consult your doctor.

Height isn't the only physical attribute that changes. As the spurt starts, fat collects on the buttocks and around the abdomen in both boys and girls. During the course of the spurt, boys accumulate mostly muscle and bone, and girls add more fat, particularly over their hips and in the breasts. The result is that fat makes up 25 percent of the total body weight in girls and between 15 percent and 20 percent in boys.

By the time of a girl's first menstrual period or the end of a boy's growth spurt, there's a distinct difference in contour between female and male bodies. The respective male and female sex hormones, along with family traits, account for most of the difference. These hormones are also responsible for secondary sex changes, which usually characterize puberty.

Sexual development

There's a wide range of normal ages when sexual maturation begins. The period of sexual maturation usually starts a couple of years later in boys than in girls. Sexual changes in girls begin anytime between ages 8 and 13. Sexual changes in boys start anytime between ages 9 and 14. If puberty starts outside the average age range, either earlier or later, consult your doctor.

Sexual changes in boys

The male body prepares for sexual maturity by producing more androgen hormones. Though these are commonly called male hormones, they're actually present in both sexes. These hormones, made mainly by the testicles, cause the physical changes of puberty.

One of the first changes in boys is the appearance of sparse, lightly pigmented pubic hair on the skin surrounding the base of the penis. The scrotum also enlarges and darkens. These changes are likely to be well under way before growth reaches its peak. Your son shouldn't be worried if he happens to develop some breast tissue about this time. Only rarely is this change due to any medical or hormonal problem. The breast enlargement usually disappears within a few months. If it persists or is particularly concerning, see your doctor.

The penis is able to become erect from infancy. But it's usually not until about 2 years after the start of puberty and 1 year after the penis starts to lengthen that it becomes capable of ejaculating semen for the first time. This may occur during masturbation, spontaneously during a sexual fantasy or during a nocturnal ejaculation.

Later, hair begins to appear under the arms and on the face. As the voice box (larynx) enlarges, the Adam's apple becomes more prominent. The voice also starts to have a deeper tone. Occasionally, the higher, younger voice may still be heard fleetingly when the voice cracks.

Throughout this period of sexual maturation, which usually lasts 4 or 5 years, the testicles continue to enlarge, and the penis gets longer and thicker. By the end of this period, the penis, testicles and pubic hair have fully developed, and mustache and beard hair have started to appear.

Sexual changes in girls

Sexual changes in girls result from an increase in hormones made in the ovaries and adrenal glands. The first visible change in females is either the beginning of breast development (breast budding) or the appearance of sparse, lightly pigmented pubic hair. Girls shouldn't worry if one breast starts developing before the other. Even when the breasts have fully developed, they're rarely exactly equal in size.

About a year after the breasts begin to develop, growth rate is likely to reach its peak. Within a year after the peak of a growth spurt, the menstrual period (menarche) may start. Take this opportunity to talk about sexuality with your daughter, including information on sexual intercourse and contraception.

There may be an intermittent increase in either white or yellow vaginal discharge during the months before onset of menstruation. It's also normal for the first few menstrual periods to occur irregularly. Within about a year, menstruation will usually become more regular. The average menstrual cycle includes a 3- to 7-day period about every 24 to 34 days.

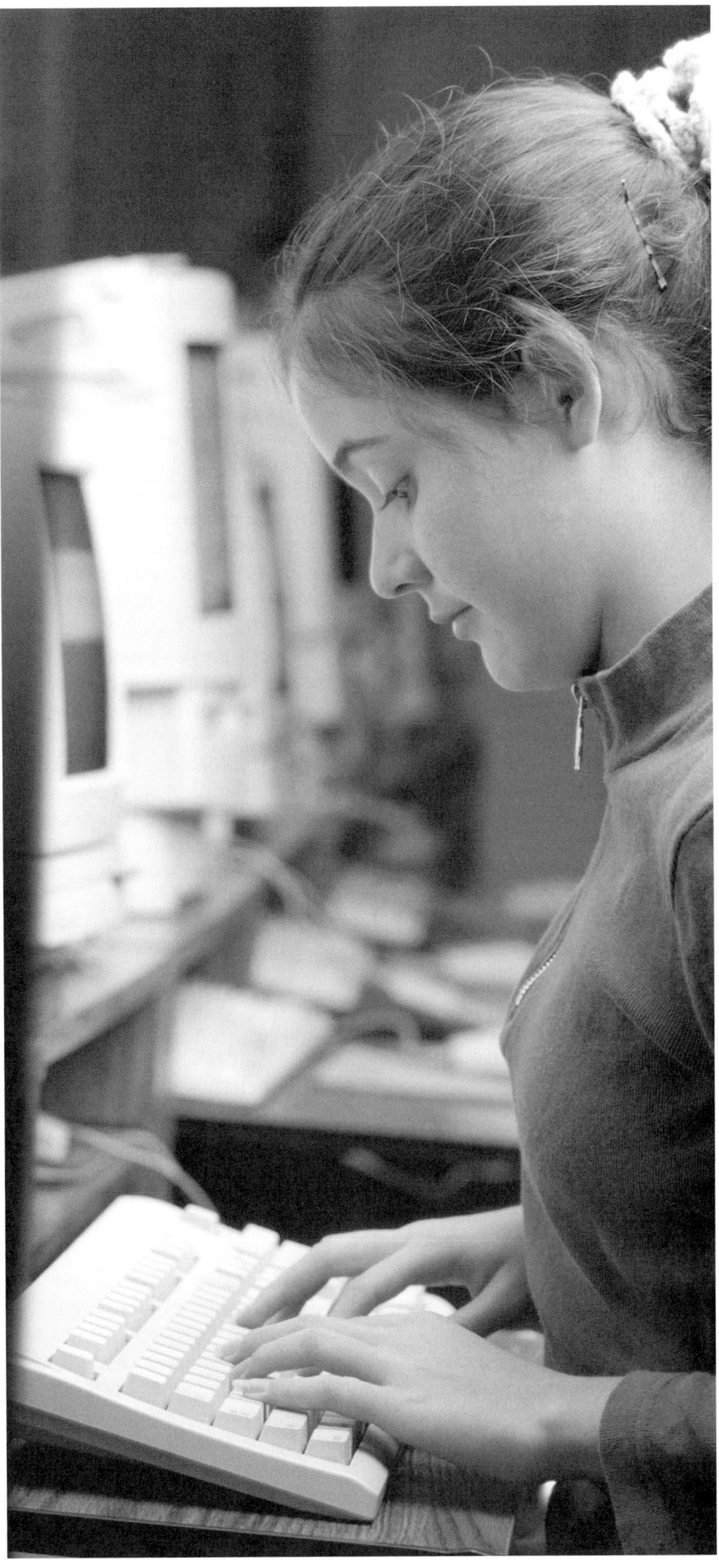

Painful menstruation (dysmenorrhea) is uncommon during the first few menstrual periods but may occur later in adolescence (see page 1076).

Physical changes include increasing height, breast growth, an increase in pubic and underarm hair, and deepening of the voice, though the voice doesn't change as much as that of a boy experiencing puberty. It usually takes 4 or 5 years to reach full body development.

There's a link between the timing of puberty and nutrition. Improvements in nutrition in recent decades are the principle explanation of why the onset of puberty occurs at younger ages in successive generations of young females in industrialized nations, such as the United States. Environmental factors may play a role as well.

Puberty also tends to start earlier in girls who have more body fat and later in those who are thin. Participating in some sports may delay puberty.

Intellectual development

During adolescence, the thinking process undergoes a gradual transformation from childhood into adulthood. Until about age 12, learning primarily involves understanding the logic of concrete things, objects that can be seen and felt. The next step in intellectual development is abstract thinking.

Throughout adolescence, children become increasingly adept at dealing with intangible ideas, including concepts that involve the past and the future. Newfound abilities allow an adolescent's thoughts to take wing, traveling through time, including speculating about what he or she and the surrounding world might become.

Along the way, this increase in powers of thought may blur some boundaries. Teenagers may feel that they're at the center of the universe, with the ability to do anything and everything. They may assume that others are thinking about them — positively or negatively — more than they really are. This feeling of being onstage can also make teenagers feel self-conscious, powerless or lost.

Teenagers may go through periods when at one moment they believe that everyone thinks as they do and the next moment that no one else in the world can understand their thoughts or feelings. Eventually, teenagers begin to realize that their thoughts are both distinct from and similar to those of others. They also realize that they really aren't the focus of everyone's attention.

Ultimately, abstract reasoning becomes more mature and comprehensive. Teenagers become capable of judging whether the relationships between two or more propositions are logical. They can solve increasingly complex problems. Teenagers become able to think scientifically, conceiving of hypotheses and of ways to test them. In addition, teenagers can also think reflectively. For example, your teenager can frame an argument for a discussion or debate and make judgments about an argument's strengths and weaknesses.

Maturation in a teenager's intellectual development changes the way he or she thinks about the world and how he or she behaves in response to it. Teenagers are able to discern much more clearly how past actions have affected what's happening now. They also become capable of predicting more accurately what implications their current actions or those of others will have for the future.

At this same time, teenagers begin to appreciate the cause-and-effect relationship between destructive behaviors, such as drug and alcohol abuse, and poor health. The health benefits of good nutrition and ample physical activity also may begin to make sense.

For the first time, you may notice your teenager's interest in discussing various serious subjects with his or her friends, family and teachers. Topics may involve love, morality, work, politics, religion and philosophy. Many teenagers spend a great deal of time wrestling with major questions, such as, "What's the purpose of life?"

Although a teenager will probably still be guided by parents, teachers and other adults, his or her decisions are made more independently. His or her decisions are also influenced by the thoughts and beliefs of peers.

Personality and Behavior

Much of an adolescent's psychosocial development involves coping with sexual development. Developing a distinct identity and becoming independent from parents also can be a struggle.

Adolescents basically go through three phases of psychosocial development: early, middle and late adolescence.

- *Early phase.* This phase starts at about age 13 or younger. In early adolescence, a teen's mental focus starts to shift from family to peers.
- *Middle phase.* The middle phase starts at around ages 15 to 17. This phase may involve outright conflicts over independence.
- *Late phase.* The late phase extends from the middle phase to age 19, or well into the 20s or even 30s in some individuals. By the end of late adolescence, independence is virtually secured, parental advice can be taken or not, and body image and gender role definition are established.

The process of going through these stages can be challenging. The diverse aspects of physical, psychological and social development aren't synchronized. Teenagers may alternate between childish and adult behaviors.

The gradual changes of these years enable your teenager to

develop a sense of who he or she is and to understand the nature of personal responsibility. Teenagers begin to understand that their actions and decisions have rewards or consequences. They begin to take an active role in making countless decisions about what to do and what not to do. Many times teenagers may prefer to seek the advice of an adult outside the family, such as a teacher or counselor.

Body image

Part of a teenager's maturation process is developing and accepting a realistic image of his or her body. If your teenager matures earlier or later than average — and many adolescents do — he or she may encounter trouble with peers and with his or her own body image. Difficulty with this image can manifest itself in eating disorders, particularly in girls. Peers and role models may influence your teenager's attitude toward his or her own body. It's important to listen to what children say about their body and to observe their behavior.

Common concerns

During maturation your teenager may:

- Feel uncomfortable with his or her physical self
- Be deeply concerned about whether his or her developing body is attractive
- Measure his or her body against that of his or her peers
- Fear that he or she is physically imperfect and develop anxiety

Some teens find it helpful to discuss these concerns with an understanding adult, whether it's a doctor, trusted teacher or parent.

Self-image

During adolescence, a teenager does a great deal of thinking about what kind of person he or she is and may become. He or she may muse, and then think seriously, about a career later in life. In early adolescence, your teenager may set career goals that are idealistic or unrealistically beyond his or her given talents and abilities. Later in adolescence, your teenager may set his or her sights more practically, considering careers that more immediately suit his or her abilities and interests. The merging of idle musings with practical planning is yet another part of the maturation process.

Because a teenager's psychosocial status is in flux, his or her role in society is extremely ambiguous. This presents complicated questions such as whether contraceptives should be prescribed to teenagers without parental consent. Generally, professionals in medicine, psychology and social work encourage teenagers to involve their parents in their psychosocial concerns. However, they won't reveal teenager's confidences unless they perceive a serious danger to the teen or others.

? Question and Answer

How do I offer reassurance to my teenagers who are struggling with their body image?

Offer some alternatives to our culture's beauty icons. Point out the number of people who succeed in life without "perfect" bodies. Focus on the numbers: There are 6 billion people in the world but fewer than 100 supermodels.

Express affection for your children often. Tell them that love doesn't depend on how tall they are or how much they weigh.

Increasing independence

In early adolescence, teenagers often start to experiment with new ways of behaving and dressing at home. At first a teen may seek some approval from family members before trying anything out on the outside world. As time goes by, your teenager may make a few tentative motions toward asserting his or her independence. Soon your teenager may become less interested in family activities and less willing to accept advice or criticism from family members. He or she may find more social comfort in a close relationship with a best friend of the same sex.

As your teenager starts to break away from family influence, he or she may pay more attention to peers. For some time, the peer group may even dominate your teenager's thinking and behavior. At first, the peer group is likely to be restricted to members of the same sex. Then it usually shifts to a mixed group. A peer group may provide a teenager with a sense of social status and security. In return, teenage cliques often demand conformity of behavior, attitudes and dress.

The struggle for independence is often most apparent in middle adolescence. Your teenager may start testing your controls and discipline. He or she may decide that your standards are unfair. A teenager may develop his or her own value system, or adopt that of his or her peer group, and challenge other authority.

Teenagers often delight in playing pranks and practical jokes. A teenager may also feel intense peer pressure to take risks that may pose dangers to himself or herself and others — for instance, experimenting with drugs, sex or vandalism. Some teenagers carry this activity even further into negative behavior. Rebellious acts taken too far can cause long-term trouble at home, at school and even with the law.

By late adolescence or early adulthood, teenagers often evolve another way of thinking about family. As a teenager becomes more comfortable with his or her own identity, he or she often starts to break free of the values of his or her peer group.

Achieving independence doesn't mean that your teenager cuts himself or herself off from others. Rather, your teenager has gained a foundation from education, family and community to allow him or her to start supporting himself or herself emotionally, socially and even financially. Part of this mature functioning is knowing when and how to use others for support. Your teenager may even be able to appreciate your values enough to seek your advice.

Parents often have a difficult time coping with the psychological changes in their adolescent children. But it's usually possible to achieve a delicate, ever-shifting balance between providing support and understanding while setting standards and limiting dangerous or harmful behavior.

When you disagree with what your teenager is doing, be firm without being harshly punitive. Respect your teenager's sincere efforts to achieve independence. Gradually, let go of the control that you've exerted over your teenager throughout childhood and trust that your teen will be guided by the self-control that you have helped to instill.

It's important to realize that parents are trying to make an adjustment from being providers and protectors to a less controlling role. The challenge that parents face is to relinquish involvement gracefully rather than abdicate their role.

Moral reasoning

Along with the psychosocial development of adolescence comes an evolution of standards. As teenagers move from childhood to adulthood, their moral standards may progress through more or less distinct phases. During each phase, a different type of moral reasoning predominates:

- *Influenced by self.* In early adolescence, children and young teens often evaluate situations in a self-centered or opportunistic manner. Judging if an action is moral may be based solely on whether the action will help or hurt them. The primary concern is avoiding punishment and gaining rewards for themselves.
- *Influenced by laws.* In middle adolescence, teenagers may become more motivated by conforming to legal standards. They start to realize that laws apply to everyone, including themselves. Accordingly, they may judge actions based on whether the actions are legal or illegal — not only on whether there's a risk of punishment.

  However, teenagers don't always obey the law. Many adolescents go through a phase of rebelling, testing the limits of authority and sometimes even breaking the law. Some may be asking to be disciplined, to experience tangible proof of the reality of the law. Ultimately, most teenagers progress beyond this testing phase.
- *Influenced by others.* By late adolescence or early adulthood, teenagers start caring more about how their actions affect others. Their moral concerns may now extend to rules of human behavior beyond the letter of the law. Teenagers may follow standards based on broad ethical principles that in some cases may be even more restrictive than the law. They start to view real-life moral conflicts in abstract terms. They can recognize everyday examples of justice, equality, honesty, responsibility, cooperation and reciprocity — and their opposites.

  Eventually, a teenager's standards evolve so that he or she becomes fully responsible for the morality of his or her actions. Ideally, teenagers develop their own detailed, individualized definitions of what society deems as right and wrong. They follow this internalized personal moral code relatively independently of the endorsement or disapproval of others. If they ever violate their principles, they feel guilty and experience self-condemnation.

The evolution of standards is intertwined with social interactions and intellectual development. Teenagers who participate in social activities have more opportunities to observe interactions. This experience may help them to form more mature moral judgments. However, neither social nor intellectual maturity necessarily guarantees the development of high moral standards.

Parents can encourage their teenagers' development of standards by the examples they set. Teenagers tend to develop more self-control and make more mature moral judgments when their parents have followed a certain style of child rearing. This style includes the following:

- Consistently disciplining, with reasoning and explanation
- Discussing how others feel about actions taken
- Promoting democratic family discussions, in which even young children can have their input

Common Conditions and Concerns

Adolescence has the reputation of being the healthiest of times, but many teenagers have significant health problems. Some diseases are more likely to appear during the teenage years. Adolescence is often a good time to establish habits for preventive care and examinations.

Routine examinations

As your teenager matures, he or she will be ready to assume increased responsibility for his or her own health. Ideally, your teenager should see his or her doctor alone at each office visit. Privacy is important because your teenager's concerns may be different from what you have in mind. Trust should be an important part of the relationship between your child and his or her doctor. Routine examinations provide teenagers an opportunity to seek professional guidance regarding their health-related concerns. Your teen's doctor will likely make the promotion of good health habits and healthy lifestyle behaviors a major focus of these medical visits.

Many teenagers are reluctant to discuss health-related concerns, such as acne, contraception, depression, drugs, being overweight, sexual practices, sexually transmitted diseases and getting along with parents and other adults. Doctors understand this reluctance. Often, it takes time, privacy and special skill for a doctor to draw out the teenager about his or her true concerns.

Although you may want to know everything that concerns your teenager, there are some health issues your child may not want to discuss with you. Continue to offer your support and let your child know that you're available to discuss any concerns that he or she has.

Checkups for teenagers offer an opportunity for early detection of chronic conditions that may pose health problems now or in adulthood. For example, the doctor will measure your teenager's blood pressure. As your teenager grows, his or her blood pressure will increase. This is normal. Because teenagers grow at varying rates, height tends to be a better determinant than age for deciding whether blood pressure is normal.

If your teenager has high blood pressure, early identification is important so that the doctor can intervene and help prevent complications.

Adolescent girls may be taught how to perform a monthly breast exam. If a teenage girl is sexually active, a doctor may perform a gynecologic exam and a Pap test to screen for cervical cancer.

Adolescent boys may be checked for a hernia, screened for testicular cancer and learn about testicular self-examination.

Let your teenager's doctor know about any diseases that run in the family. If your teenager has a chronic disease such as diabetes or asthma, a doctor can teach him or her how to manage the condition.

Nutrition

Energy requirements and nutrient requirements increase during adolescence. But busy teenagers with full school schedules, extracurricular activities and part-time employment may be eating on the go and not getting enough calories and all the nutrients they need. Tight schedules may lead to skipping some meals, especially breakfast, or to eating more frequently. Many teenagers eat a greater number of meals away from home, especially from fast-food restaurants and vending machines. This can lead to unhealthy eating habits. Overeating or restricting food consumption can make young people more vulnerable to eating disorders.

Greater independence from family and the desire to be accepted by peers often influence eating practices such as fad dieting, eating an unbalanced diet and indulging in alcohol. All of these factors put an adolescent at greater risk of inadequate nutrition. But this isn't true of all teens. Some families begin eating healthier because of the influence of their teens, who may follow vegetarian diets or other healthy eating practices. Vegetarian diets can be nutritionally adequate — even for teens — if they're appropriately followed and steps are taken to ensure consumption of essential nutrients.

Keep Up with Immunizations

By the time they reach their teens, most boys and girls have completed their childhood immunizations. But they still may need a few vaccinations. Adult-type combined tetanus-diphtheria (Td) toxoid should be given at age 11 or 12 and again every 10 years after that. A second measles-mumps-rubella (MMR) vaccine may be given around this time as well, if a teenager didn't receive it at an earlier age. Hepatitis B vaccination, a series of three shots, also is recommended for adolescents who haven't received the series. In addition, undergraduate college students should consider getting the meningococcal vaccine. It's especially recommended for first-year college students living in dormitories or resident halls because they're at increased risk of this serious bacterial disease.

For more information on vaccinations, see Chapter 1, "Getting Immunized."

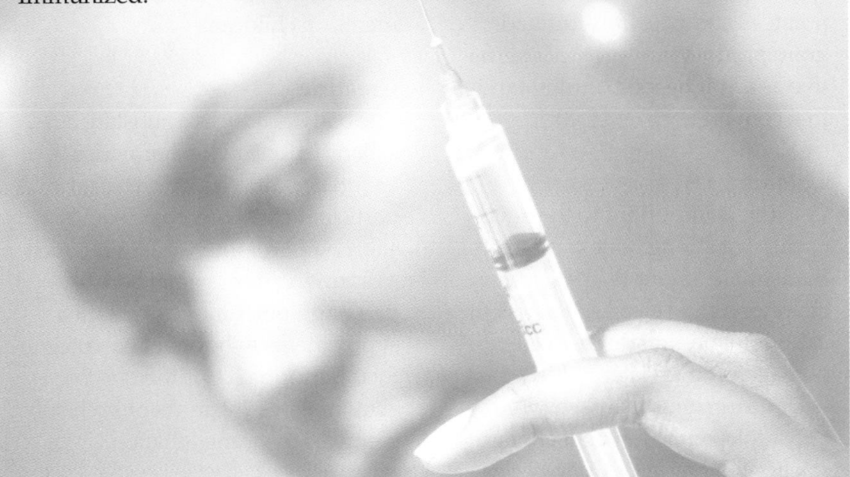

Parents have a crucial role in setting a good example and taking time to prepare and serve wholesome family meals. Get the entire family involved in meal planning and preparation. If family meals aren't possible because of different schedules, stock your kitchen with healthy, convenient snacks, such as fresh fruits and vegetables, fat-free yogurt, skim milk and whole-grain bread.

Nutritional status doesn't depend on one specific food choice but rather on the sum of food choices over several days and weeks. Even fast foods and desserts can be included in a healthy diet if you regularly eat a variety of foods from the various food groups.

Iron

Ample iron is essential during adolescence because of the expanding volume of blood in the body and an increase in muscle mass that teens experience as they grow. Extra iron is needed during growth spurts because it's important for muscle development and healthy red blood cells. Teenage girls especially need additional iron because of iron loss during menstruation.

A lack of iron in the diet can cause iron deficiency anemia. Signs and symptoms include pale skin, fatigue, lightheadedness and poor appetite.

To ensure an adequate supply of dietary iron, teenagers need to regularly eat iron-containing foods. These include meat, fish, poultry, eggs, legumes (peas and beans), potatoes and rice. Iron-fortified grain products are another alternative as are, if needed, multivitamins that contain iron.

Calcium

Calcium is important to the development of strong bones and teeth. Inadequate amounts of calcium in childhood may increase the risk of the bone-thinning disease osteoporosis common later in life.

Unfortunately, many children and adolescents don't get enough calcium in their diet. Only 14 percent of teenage girls and 35 percent of teenage boys are meeting recommendations for calcium consumption, which is 1,300 milligrams (mg) a day for children ages 9 through 18. One 8-ounce glass of milk provides 300 mg of calcium.

Dieting

Adolescents need certain nutrients and adequate calories to provide for their activity and growth. If they're not getting the nutrients they need, dieting may prevent teenagers from growing to their full height. Teenagers concerned about their weight should focus on healthy eating and increased exercise rather than on cutting calories.

If a serious weight problem is a concern, consult your teen's doctor or a registered dietitian. In youth, it's important to establish healthy patterns of eating and exercise. Children who are obese between ages 10 and 13 have an 80 percent chance of becoming an obese adult.

For more information on healthy eating, see Chapter 2, "Eating Right."

Young Athletes and Supplements

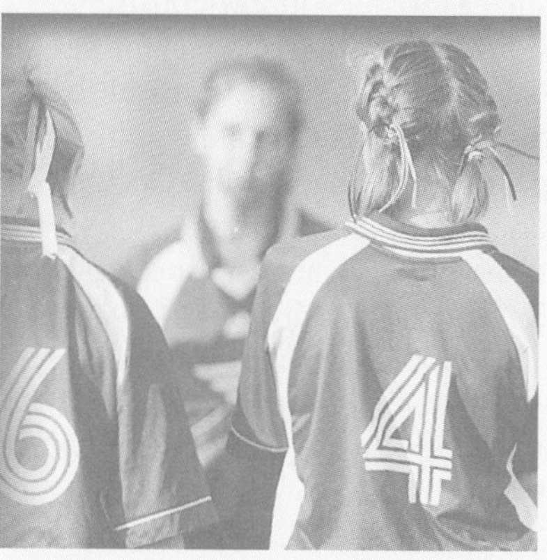

If your teenager is involved in sports, a balanced diet and an adequate intake of water is especially important for good performance. Supplements may claim to improve performance, but they may not be necessary, safe or legal.

Protein supplements

Most children get enough protein from their diet. This isn't difficult to do if they eat a variety of foods because protein is found in many foods, including cereal, beans, baked potatoes, nuts, cooked vegetables, milk and meat. Protein supplements aren't recommended for individuals with kidney disorders or diabetes. There's little known about the effect of protein supplements on children.

Creatine

The body produces a substance called creatine, which provides energy for muscles. Athletes who participate in sports that require short bursts of intense activity, such as sprinting or maximal bench pressing, sometimes use creatine supplements in hopes of enhancing their performance. Little is known about the possible risks of such supplements in young athletes.

Energy bars

Carbohydrates promote increased blood sugar levels. Athletes who participate in sports that require endurance, such as track or swimming, may eat energy bars containing mostly carbohydrates for energy. Plenty of water should be taken with an energy bar to help the body absorb the carbohydrates.

Sports drinks

During activity, your body loses salt in sweat. If too much salt is lost, the muscles can't function as well, and performance may decline. Sports drinks are helpful only if they contain elements such as sodium and potassium (electrolytes) to replenish salts lost in sweat. During activity that's less than 1 hour, these drinks don't appear to provide benefits, but they may offer benefits for activity of longer duration. Sports drinks may also be helpful in getting children to consume more fluids.

Exercise

Adolescents and young adults benefit greatly from a regular exercise routine. Regular exercise is good for overall health and helps control weight. Beginning good exercise habits as a teenager helps encourage healthy habits as an adult.

However, moderation is important. Excessive exercise can lead to injuries and, in females, menstrual abnormalities. Pain or swelling in the joints, a common complaint, is a sign of too much exercise or improper technique. Female athletes may experience discontinuation of menstrual periods (amenorrhea). When this occurs, a medical evaluation is important because the condition can increase a female's risk of bone thinning.

Injuries

Among American adolescents, injury is a major public health problem. Unintentional injuries are the leading cause of death among teenagers. Automobile accidents are the most common cause. Half the fatal accidents occur during evening hours, even though only about 20 percent of teenage driving is at night. Alcohol is often a factor. Seat belts could prevent many injuries and spare lives, but in spite of driver's education programs and state laws requiring their use, adolescents often fail to buckle up.

Athletic activities are leading causes of nonfatal injuries. Football is among the most hazardous. Knees and ankles are sites commonly injured, but head and neck injuries occur as well, despite advances in equipment.

Although less hazardous, participation in sports such as soccer and basketball can lead to injury, especially among boys. For girls, gymnastics poses the highest risk. For both, even sports such as cross-country running, swimming and tennis carry some risk. You can help minimize your teen's risk of injury by ensuring that he or she wears protective equipment designed for each sport he or she plays and gets appropriate physical conditioning.

Headaches

Recurrent headaches are common during late childhood and adolescence. They may be associated with a viral illness but rarely indicate a serious problem. Headaches may be related to factors such as stress, reaction to a medicine or food or a family history of migraines. If headaches occur frequently, come on suddenly without explanation, persist or get steadily worse, contact your child's doctor. Also contact your child's doctor if a headache follows a recent ear infection, toothache, strep throat or other infection.

Migraines usually occur for the first time in early adolescence, although they can also appear in young children and in adults. Migraines are repeated attacks of intense, throbbing head pain lasting at least an hour each episode. They're often accompanied by nausea, sensitivity to light and sometimes vomiting.

For more information on headaches, see page 554.

Vision problems

The rapid growth of adolescence also includes the eyes. Sometimes, a teenager's eyes change their shape as well as their size. As a result, problems with visual acuity often develop during adolescence. The most common problem is the development or worsening of nearsightedness (myopia), which can be easily corrected by prescription glasses or contact lenses.

Teenagers are also prone to injury-related vision problems. Most of these problems can be prevented by wearing protective goggles, masks or other headgear during sports.

If you suspect that your child has difficulty seeing or if your child complains of vision problems, consult your doctor or an eye specialist.

For more information on vision-related problems, see Chapter 23, "Eyes."

Hearing problems

Teenagers can develop a permanent high-frequency hearing loss that makes it more difficult for them to hear sounds higher than 4,000 hertz. The loss most often results from exposure to loud

Teens Behind the Wheel

Teenagers are less experienced drivers and more likely to take risks. Here are some safety tips if you have a teen driver in the house:

- *Limits.* Set limits for when your teenager can drive and who and how many people can be in the car. Also set limits if your teenager is a passenger. Most teenager passenger deaths occur when the automobile driver is a teenager.
- *Practice.* Provide supervised driving practice for your teenager under a variety of driving conditions, including nighttime and freeway driving.
- *Example.* Set a good driving example, such as always wearing your seat belt, obeying speed limits and being a defensive driver.
- *Safety.* Consider safety ratings when choosing a car for your teenager to drive.
- *Plan.* Offer a no-questions-asked backup plan so that your teenager can feel free to call anytime from anywhere if he or she needs a ride home. You'd rather have your teenager home safely than driving while intoxicated or riding with someone who's intoxicated.

noises, such as amplified music. To help prevent hearing loss, encourage your teen to reduce the music volume or to avoid excessively loud concerts.

If your teen is continually exposed to loud noises — for example, riding the subway train daily or working around heavy equipment — encourage him or her to wear earplugs. Ear protectors should be worn when using a firearm or being near someone who is.

For more information on hearing loss, see Chapter 24, "Ears, Nose and Throat."

Acne

Acne is a common problem and concern among teenagers. Three out of four teenagers have some acne. It usually starts around puberty and disappears by the end of the teenage years, but it can affect adults too. Medical attention and treatment with prescription drugs may be necessary if the acne is distressing, persistent or severe.

Acne occurs when the hair follicles of the skin become plugged with oil and dead skin cells. It can appear on the face, neck, chest, back, shoulders and scalp. Pimples result from inflammation of hair follicles. This inflammation is usually caused by overproduction of oil (sebum) by the sebaceous gland of each hair follicle. The oil can block the follicle and predispose it to bacterial infection and inflammation. When a pimple is plugged with white pus, it's called a whitehead. If this plug extends to the skin surface and is exposed to air, it turns black and is termed a blackhead.

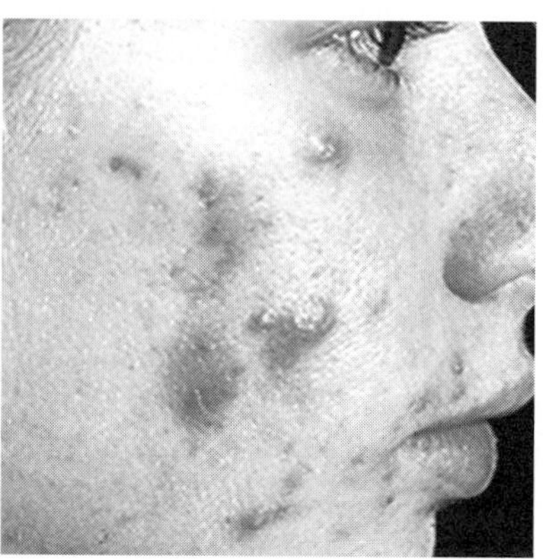

In both boys and girls, acne may be triggered by normal elevations of androgen hormones, which make the sebaceous glands produce extra oil. In girls, acne may worsen around the time of their menstrual periods.

For more information on acne, see page 1173.

Painful menstruation

Many females experience some pain on the first or second day of their period. For some, though, the pain is so severe that it disrupts normal daily activities. Painful menstruation (dysmenorrhea) is the leading cause of teenage girls and adult women missing work and school. It's most common in adolescence. The problem often subsides by the mid-20s or after pregnancy.

There are two types of dysmenorrhea: primary and secondary. Primary dysmenorrhea is pain occurring during menstruation, when the muscles of the uterus contract and the uterus sheds its lining. Secondary dysmenorrhea is pain caused by an underlying gynecological disorder, such as a fibroid tumor or sexually transmitted disease (STD).

Symptoms include general aching, pain in the lower abdomen possibly extending to the hips, lower back or thighs, nausea, vomiting and diarrhea. Soaking in a warm tub or exercising may help relieve the pain. For many women, prescription or over-the-counter nonsteroidal anti-inflammatory drugs (NSAIDs), such as ibuprofen (Advil, Motrin, others) or naproxen (Aleve, Naprosyn, others), are effective. These medications work better if taken early, when the menstrual cycle is starting, rather than waiting until cramps become more intense. Birth control pills also may be beneficial.

For more information on dysmenorrhea, see page 1076.

Urinary tract infections

Urinary tract infections may result when bacteria normally found in the colon colonize and enter the bladder via the channel leading from the bladder to the outside of the body (urethra). In adolescents who haven't had a urinary tract infection as children, the onset of infection frequently coincides with the onset of sexual activity.

The most common urinary tract infection is cystitis, inflammation of the bladder. Cystitis usually results when traces of stool contaminate the urethra. It can be caused by sexual intercourse, which can irritate the urethra. Signs and symptoms include urination that's frequent, urgent and painful, foul-smelling urine and a fever. If your adolescent has these signs and symptoms, he or she should see a doctor.

For more information on urinary tract infections, see page 940.

Infectious mononucleosis

Infectious mononucleosis is commonly referred to as mono or the kissing disease. Anyone can get mononucleosis, but its incidence is highest in teenagers.

The majority of cases of infectious mononucleosis are caused by the Epstein-Barr virus. Most people have been exposed to the Epstein-Barr virus by the time they're 35 but have built up antibodies. Although kissing can spread the virus, mono is more commonly spread by coughing, sneezing or sharing drinking glasses. It isn't highly contagious but can cause prolonged illness. The condition typically results in complete recovery.

Initial infection in children between ages 4 and 15 usually results in only mild signs and symptoms such as short-term fever and fatigue. In some instances, symptoms are minimal and the infection goes unrecognized. Later in adolescence and young adulthood, the virus may be a cause of a prolonged, exhausting illness.

Signs and symptoms include a fever that lasts several days, swollen glands, sore throat and fatigue. A blood test can indirectly check for evidence of the Epstein-Barr virus. Rest and plenty of fluids are the main treatments.

Most signs and symptoms ease within 10 days, but your teenager may still need another 2 to 3 weeks of rest before resuming normal activity — especially if his or her spleen is enlarged — and a couple more months to feel completely normal.

For more information on infectious mononucleosis, see page 494.

Growth disorders

Many growth disorders are diagnosed in childhood, but certain growth disorders appear during the teenage years:

Scoliosis

Scoliosis is a sideways (lateral) curvature of the spine that makes the spine look like an S or a C. The cause of most cases of scoliosis is unknown. The disorder can affect boys and girls, but adolescent girls are more likely to have serious scoliosis that requires treatment.

The onset of scoliosis is gradual and doesn't usually cause any pain. Screening for scoliosis is performed routinely at many schools. Some cases are too slight to need treatment. In other cases, treatment is needed with special braces or surgery. If untreated, scoliosis may cause permanent disability.

For more information on scoliosis, see page 981.

Osgood-Schlatter disease

Osgood-Schlatter disease is a painful inflammation of a tendon attachment point on the shinbone (tibia). It's common in young athletes, especially boys, during growth spurts.

Osgood-Schlatter is caused by overuse in activities that place repeated stress on the top of the shinbone, where the tendon of the kneecap inserts. The repeated pulling of the kneecap tendon causes the pain. The major symptom is knee pain, which is worsened by activity and relieved by rest.

Treatment involves resting and avoiding activities that place prolonged stress on the flexed knee. These include activities such as bicycle riding and playing basketball. Anti-inflammatory medications, such as ibuprofen (Advil, Motrin, others), also may be helpful. When growth of the affected bone ends, the pain usually subsides on its own.

Teenage Sexuality

Parents often feel perplexed and even threatened by their teenager's emerging sexuality. If you're the parent of a teenager, it's best for everyone if you can come to terms with your child's sexuality, show your trust and give him or her any help needed.

Your child may receive education about sex, family life and sexually transmitted diseases (STDs) at school. But don't rely on the school to explain all of the complexities of sexual relationships that you want your child to understand. No matter how awkward it may be for you, you have a responsibility to inform your child about the facts of life.

As parents, you are your child's primary sex educator. You may find it helpful to look through relevant materials and think through your answers ahead of time. In addition, books that you and your child can read together are invaluable for opening up a discussion. Avoid overloading your child with too much information, but do answer all of his or her questions honestly. If you don't know the answer to a particular question, tell your child that

Talking to Teens About Sex

Teaching your children about sex is most effective if you make it an ongoing discussion, beginning in the preschool and school-age years. During the teenage years, some new topics may come up.

- *Dating.* Some questions your teenager may have are: "When can I start dating?" "How will I know if I'm ready to have sex?" "Won't having sex help me keep my boyfriend or girlfriend?"
- *Abstinence.* Your teenager may be motivated to have sex because of peer pressure, curiosity or any number of other reasons. Tell your teenager that many teenagers decide to wait and that until he or she is ready, there are many other ways to express affection: intimate talks, long walks while holding hands, listening to music and dancing together, kissing, touching, hugging.
- *Date rape.* Date rape happens when someone your teenager knows forces him or her into sexual activity. Teach your children that no always means no. Let your child know that avoiding alcohol and drugs helps make him or her less vulnerable to be involved in date rape either as a victim or perpetrator. In addition, discuss use of date-rape drugs with your teen.
- *Sexual orientation.* Many young people wonder at some point whether they're gay, lesbian or bisexual. Let your child know that it's normal to have crushes on members of the same sex and that just having these feelings doesn't mean he or she is homosexual or bisexual. Stress that if your teen is gay, lesbian or bisexual, you won't reject him or her.

you'll look it up together. Sexual fantasies, masturbation, homosexuality, contraception, pregnancy and STDs are some topics your teenager may have questions about.

Emerging sexuality

Sexual feelings and fantasies normally increase during adolescence. Your teenager may find it difficult to deal with such feelings, particularly if they seem to conflict with the attitudes that he or she has been taught about sex. Friendships with members of the same sex and opposite sex will be influenced by these feelings and evolve during adolescence.

Friendships with the same sex
In early adolescence, your teenager's closest relationship outside the family is usually with a best friend of the same sex. At first, your teenager may retreat from his or her emergence as a sexual being into the safety of friendships with members of the same sex. At the same time, your teenager may be intrigued by sexual matters and frequently seek information about sex. Sometimes, the emergence of sexual feelings in early adolescence is expressed through telling dirty jokes.

When your teenager first becomes capable of sexual intercourse, he or she is probably years away from being emotionally prepared for this activity and its consequences.

Friendships in a peer group
In middle adolescence, your teenager starts feeling more aware of himself or herself as male or female. Your teenager may spend more time with a larger group of peers, a group within which a natural process of social experimentation occurs. Your teenager may become more interested in forming relationships with members of the opposite sex, but the choice may be influenced by his or her peer group's acceptance. Dating may start, as well as some sexual experimentation.

Your teenager may feel strong pressure from his or her peers to lose his or her virginity. Some teenagers react to this pressure, and to their own curiosity, by starting to have sexual intercourse at a very young age.

Friendships with the opposite sex
By late adolescence, your teenager may become more secure about his or her sexual identity. Your teenager may be ready to establish an intimate relationship that demands a different type of sharing and commitment. Your teenager may feel emotionally ready to have sexual intercourse with this person. But your teenager is unlikely to be prepared to become a parent and should know about various methods to prevent pregnancy and to reduce the risk of sexually transmitted diseases (STDs).

Sexual fantasies

Daydreaming is an important part of adolescence that can provide an outlet for expanding imaginations. Many daydreams have some sexual content. Your teenager may also have sexual fantasies at night. Sexual thoughts may be hypothetical experiences or memories of real-life experiences. It's normal to have sexual fantasies. Sexual fantasies may even be useful in the development of sexual identity because they allow exploration of sexual situations that would be inappropriate to act out.

Masturbation

Masturbation is stimulation of the genitals for sensual pleasure. Some teenagers feel guilty about masturbating because of old, unfounded myths — for example, that masturbation will cause you to go blind or to develop warts.

Your child may have started masturbation before adolescence. It provides a way for teenagers to release sexual tension, give themselves pleasure, savor sexual fantasies and even curb impulses to engage in inappropriate sexual activity with others. As long as your teenager doesn't masturbate publicly, there's nothing unusual, harmful or unacceptable about the practice.

Homosexuality

Some teenagers seek out members of their own sex. Openly homosexual teenagers may face rejection by some of their peers, teachers and family members. Teenagers having difficulty adjusting to their sexual orientation, or to others' reactions to it, may find psychotherapy or counseling helpful.

Sexually active male homosexuals are at risk of contracting sexually transmitted diseases (STDs), such as chlamydia, hepatitis B, gonorrhea, AIDS and syphilis. At even higher risk are those who've experimented with several sexual partners. Using a condom during sex can reduce, though not eliminate, the risk of getting infected.

Sexual activity

Teenagers who've had sexual intercourse at least once are considered sexually active. Many teenagers begin having sex in their mid- to late teens. Studies indicate that more than half of all 17-year-olds have had intercourse. The average age of first intercourse for girls is 17. For boys, it's 16.

Male and female adolescents tend to report different reactions to their first experience of sexual intercourse. Girls tend to say they felt scared, guilty, worried, embarrassed and curious. Boys, on the other hand, usually report feeling excited, thrilled, satisfied, happy and mature.

A wide range of dating patterns is normal. Teenagers may not date at all in junior high or high school, or they may have one high school sweetheart. The most common pattern is two or three close emotional commitments as a teenager, one after the other. Typically, during the course of each relationship, neither partner dates others and, if sexual activity is part of the relationship, has no other sexual partners.

About 20 percent of sexually active high school students have had four or more sexual partners. These individuals are at a higher risk of acquiring sexually transmitted diseases (STDs).

Contraception

Sexually active teenagers who don't use contraception have a 90 percent chance of getting pregnant within 1 year. If your teenager is considering sexual intercourse, encourage some method of birth control. Both boys and girls should know what types of birth control are available.

One type of birth control is hormonal contraception. This includes oral contraceptives (the pill). Another type is the barrier method. This includes the condom (rubber) or diaphragm. The choice of methods may be affected by motivation to avoid pregnancy and access to medical care.

Each type of birth control has its advantages and disadvantages. Condoms provide the most protection from infection compared with other forms of contraception. Condoms may not be as good as other methods, though, in preventing pregnancy. It's common for many individuals to use both condoms and another method of birth control, such as oral contraceptives. Ultimately, the best way to protect against STDs and pregnancy is abstinence.

For more information on preventing pregnancy, see page 1061.

Teenage pregnancy

The United States has the highest rate of teenage pregnancy of any Western industrialized nation. Nearly 1 million American teenage girls become pregnant each year, and about half those pregnancies end in live births. Despite a steady decline in teenage pregnancy and birth rates, 4 out of 10 girls in the United States get pregnant at least once before age 20. One-half of teenage pregnancies occur within 6 months of becoming sexually active.

Most teenage pregnancies are unplanned or unwanted. Poverty, lack of education about birth control, misinformation about birth control, having a mother who became pregnant as a teen and denial of the risks of becoming pregnant are several factors that may contribute to the risk of teenage pregnancy.

Raising a child is a serious responsibility. Most teenagers aren't ready, emotionally or financially, to make the necessary commitment. Just as an adult father should participate in caring for and supporting his child, so too should a teenage father. But often a teenage mother ends up having to raise her child under difficult circumstances, without help from the child's father.

Sexually transmitted diseases

More than 25 diseases can be spread through sexual activity. One-fourth of the 15 million new cases of sexually transmitted diseases (STDs) each year occur in teenagers. Chlamydia and gonorrhea are the most common sexually transmitted diseases among teenagers. Young women are biologically more susceptible than young males to chlamydia, gonorrhea and human immunodeficiency virus (HIV). The rate of new infections with herpes and human papillomavirus (HPV) is typically highest during the late teens and early twenties.

Teenagers and young adults are at high risk of STDs because they're less likely to use condoms consistently and more likely to have more than one partner and have a partner who's been sexually active with others. Most adolescents' decision-making and communication skills are still developing and may not keep pace with their sexual activity. Lack of adequate sex education also may play a role.

Pregnancy Myths

Don't assume that your teenager knows everything about getting pregnant. Here are some common pregnancy myths:

Myth: You can't get pregnant the first time.
Fact: It can take only one episode of sexual intercourse to become pregnant, even if it's your first time.

Myth: You can't get pregnant if the penis is pulled out before ejaculation.
Fact: Fluid-carrying sperm commonly leaks out of the penis before and after ejaculation.

Myth: You can't get pregnant during your period.
Fact: Chances of pregnancy may be reduced during menstruation, but it's possible to get pregnant at anytime.

Myth: You can't get pregnant if you douche.
Fact: Flushing the vagina with water or another liquid doesn't prevent pregnancy.

Each type of STD is caused by a different infectious agent. The risk of catching a sexually transmitted disease increases with multiple sexual partners. Signs and symptoms don't accompany all STDs. When no signs or symptoms are present and if sexual partners aren't aware of an infection, the infection is more likely to be passed on.

Sexually active teens should see a doctor regularly to be tested and examined for common STDs. Whenever one is diagnosed, it's important for all sexual partners to be examined and treated. In all cases, abstaining from sexual contact is important until the infection is successfully treated.

Most STDs can be treated with medications. Various antibiotics are available to kill the bacteria that cause some of them. AIDS, which is caused by a virus, is an exception. While medication can slow progression of the disease, there's no cure. Other diseases, such as herpes or HPV, may recur in spite of being treated. HPV is the leading cause of cervical cancer. Routine Pap tests are important in early detection of cervical cancer.

The longer treatment is delayed, the more difficult a sexually transmitted disease is to control and the greater the risk of complications. For instance, repeated bouts of pelvic inflammatory disease can leave a young woman incapable of getting pregnant.

Not participating in sexual activity (abstinence) is the most effective way to avoid STDs. For teens who are sexually active, steps to minimize risk include using a condom and being selective about their sexual partners. Condoms are usually effective — although not foolproof — at blocking the spread of infectious agents, provided they're used correctly. When a condom and contraceptive foam are used together, they offer added protection against pregnancy and the spread of STDs.

For more information on sexually transmitted diseases, see Chapter 6, "Addressing Risky Behaviors," and Chapter 20, "Infectious Diseases."

Special Concerns

Adolescence is often regarded as a turbulent phase, but studies show that most teenagers don't go through the turmoil and rebellion often associated with this stage in life. For some adolescents, though, the teenage years can be especially challenging.

Rebellious behavior

A child who previously has been obedient and calm may become moody, inconsistent, unpredictable and even rebellious in adolescence. Your adolescent may argue with you about a range of issues, large and small. They can include everything from what to wear and when to take out the garbage to when to come home at night and whether to engage in sexual activity.

A certain amount of teenage rebellion, risk taking and testing of authority is normal. It may be an essential stage in the adolescent's process of separating from parents and developing a personal identity. However, most teenagers don't rebel greatly.

Rebellion can be seen as part of the process by which adolescents define their identity. They may take an action merely to see what reactions it provokes in the people around them. This is why you shouldn't just give up on your rebellious teenager. Intervene when his or her behavior exceeds limits

Conduct Disorders

It's normal for teenagers to act out and test authority. But a persistent disregard for the norms and rules of society can have serious consequences. If your child has demonstrated at least three of the following behaviors over 6 months, he or she should be evaluated by a mental health professional because he or she may have a conduct disorder:

- Stealing
- Constant lying
- Truancy
- Starting fires
- Breaking into homes, offices or cars
- Destroying others' property
- Displaying physical cruelty to animals or humans
- Forcing others into sexual activity
- Starting fights
- Using weapons in fights

Often children with a conduct disorder have underlying problems that have been overlooked or ignored, such as depression or attention-deficit/hyperactivity disorder (ADHD).

Appropriate treatment is important. One goal of treatment is to help the adolescent realize and understand the effects of his or her behavior on others. Treatment may include behavior therapy and psychotherapy. Children with accompanying depression or ADHD may be treated with medications in addition to psychotherapy.

you have set. Eventually, a teenager will learn from the consequences of the behavior and work toward the establishment of his or her own boundaries.

Mild rebellion is common and even normal in early and middle adolescence. By late adolescence, most teenagers are on their way to developing a sense of perspective. They have become better able to delay gratification, compromise on conflicting demands and set limits.

If rebellious behavior becomes more self-destructive or lingers into late adolescence, consult your doctor or a mental health professional. Family problems may be causing or worsening the rebellion. Therapy involving the whole family may help alleviate these problems.

If your teenage child is rebellious, hold your ground. Keep stating your concerns and setting reasonable limits. Don't threaten punishments that you won't carry out. In most cases, with your firm handling, your teenager will outgrow this rebellious phase without any lasting damage to himself or herself or others.

Beliefs and behaviors usually change by the time a teen grows up and starts a family. Your child is likely to return to the viewpoints and standards learned from you during childhood. With this in mind, try to prevent rifts during your child's adolescence that will stand in the way of a later reunion.

As a parent, you remain the greatest influence on your teenager's beliefs and behavior, even more than his or her peers. Even when your child appears to be disagreeing with everything you say, he or she needs you to hold and defend your own reasonable and consistent view of the world.

School problems

Problems in school can occur for a variety of reasons. While also evident in school-aged children from kindergarten on, such problems can become more serious during the teenage years.

Learning disabilities

A learning disability can cause a teenager to perform poorly in school, regardless of intelligence. Though often diagnosed in the earlier school years, a learning disability sometimes doesn't come to light until a child has reached his or her teens.

Attention-deficit/hyperactivity disorder

One half of the children with attention-deficit/hyperactivity disorder (ADHD) continue to have symptoms as adolescents and adults. About 80 percent of children who are on medication need to continue treatment into their teenage years. ADHD is a mental disorder that can cause additional stress and frustration during the teenage years, when academic and social demands increase.

Failure to pay attention to details, excessive distractibility, inability to organize and impulsiveness can interfere with learning. Coping strategies such as using a daily planner for assignments and appointments, keeping a routine and setting aside a quiet time and place to do homework may be helpful.

Participation in extracurricular activities such as sports, drama and debate teams can offer an outlet for excess energy and an opportunity to make friends. Keep in touch with your teen's teachers about how he or she is doing.

Chronic illness

If your teenager has had a chronic illness through childhood and adolescence, such as asthma or cystic fibrosis, he or she may need to miss school during acute episodes of the disease. Too often, these absences put your child at risk of school failure. Your child may need extra encouragement and support to make up the missed schoolwork. As parents, don't support frequent school absences for minor physical complaints. Work with your child's doctor, teachers and school nurse. Together, you can help minimize absences.

School phobia

Avoidance of school or refusal to attend school may be a way of responding to overwhelming stress and situations that an adolescent can't control. School phobia most often appears when a student first begins school. If the problem persists in an older child, evaluation and treatment by a mental health professional is often beneficial.

Truancy

Truancy may start with cutting an occasional class and then escalate into prolonged absences. Truancy can result from conflicts within the family, parental expectations that are too high, lack of parental attention and peer pressure to drop out. Truants are often rebellious teenagers who are in trouble not only at school but also at home and elsewhere.

Sometimes, truancy can be reversed with an educational plan that emphasizes behavior management and involves the family, school and medical personnel. Individual and family psychotherapy also may help. If the teenager still doesn't attend school regularly, it may be possible to work out an educational alternative such as work-study and independent study programs.

School failure

School failure can result from truancy. It's difficult for your child to know what's going on in class if he or she doesn't attend. Some schools automatically drop students who've been absent more than a certain amount of time. A host of other problems can be involved in school failure. Future employment opportunities for high school dropouts are limited, so it's important to prevent school failure.

Depression

It was once thought that only adults got depressed, but researchers are finding that children and teenagers are prone to the same types of depression as adults. The incidence of major depression in children and teenagers peaks during adolescence. Unfortunately, depression in this age group often isn't recognized and treated. Below are some facts to consider:

- Depression may occur in as many as one in eight teenagers in the United States.
- If a child or teenager has an episode of depression, he or she has a greater than 50 percent chance of having another episode in the next 5 years.
- Two-thirds of children with mental illness don't get the treatment they need.
- Suicide is the third leading cause of death for 15- to 24-year-olds and the sixth leading cause of death for 5- to 15-year-olds.
- The rate of suicide for 5- to 24-year-olds has tripled since 1960.

Recognizing depression in children and teenagers can be challenging because its signs and symptoms may easily be attributed to a growing phase or hormonal changes. Many behaviors associated with depression in young people are common reactions in children and teenagers. For example, almost all teenagers argue with their parents or teachers or refuse to do chores from time to time. The criteria used to make a diagnosis of depression include the number, duration and severity of signs and symptoms.

Risk factors

During the teenage years, girls become twice as likely as boys to experience depression. A family history of depression also may be a risk factor. Other risk factors include the following:

- Experiencing significant stress
- Being the victim of abuse or neglect
- Experiencing the death of a parent or other loved one
- Breaking up with someone
- Having a chronic illness, such as diabetes
- Experiencing other trauma
- Having a behavioral disorder

Treatment

If you think your child may be depressed, arrange for him or her to see a doctor or mental health professional. Professional treatment can help your child regain hope that things can get better and that his or her problems will be overcome. Treatment may involve medication, psychotherapy or a combination of the two.

Although opinions differ on which form of treatment to use first, growing evidence shows that the best approach for most young people has been a combination of medication and a form of psychotherapy called cognitive-behavioral therapy. A combined approach is especially helpful for severe depression.

A Depression Checklist for Parents

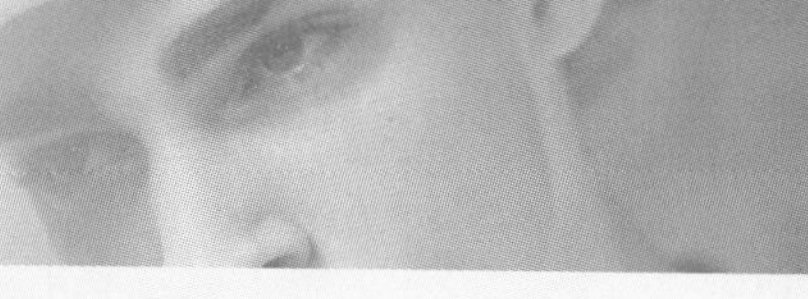

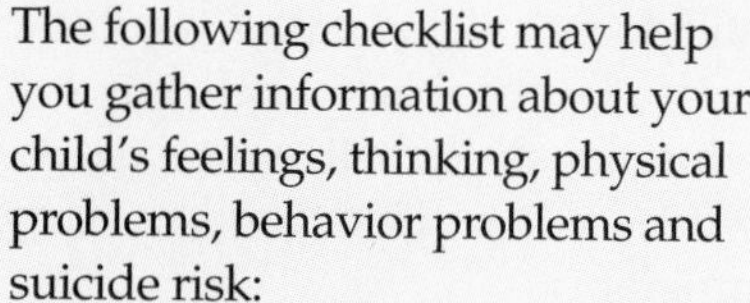

The following checklist may help you gather information about your child's feelings, thinking, physical problems, behavior problems and suicide risk:

Feelings

Does your child demonstrate:

- Sadness
- Emptiness
- Hopelessness
- Guilt
- Worthlessness
- Lack of enjoyment in everyday pleasures

Thinking

Does your child have trouble:

- Concentrating
- Making decisions
- Completing schoolwork
- Maintaining grades
- Maintaining friendships

Physical problems

Does your child complain of:

- Headache
- Stomachache
- Lack of energy
- Sleeping problems — too much or too little
- Weight or appetite changes — gain or loss

Behavior problems

Is your child:

- Irritable
- Not wanting to go to school
- Wanting to be alone most of the time
- Having difficulty getting along with others
- Cutting classes or missing school
- Dropping out of sports, hobbies or other activities
- Drinking alcohol or using drugs

Suicide risk

Does your child talk or think about:

- Suicide
- Death
- Other morbid subjects

If your child experiences five or more of these signs or symptoms for at least 2 weeks, he or she may be experiencing depression or another mental illness. Write down how long the signs and symptoms last, how often they occur and give examples. This information will help a doctor or therapist better understand your child's emotional state. Address suicide concerns immediately.

Medication

In the past, doctors were reluctant to prescribe antidepressants to children and teenagers because of the lack of evidence available concerning the safety and effectiveness of these drugs on young people. But recent studies indicate that when used on a short-term basis, some newer antidepressants, especially selective serotonin reuptake inhibitors (SSRIs), are safe and effective.

SSRIs include the medications citalopram (Celexa), fluvoxamine (Luvox), fluoxetine (Prozac), paroxetine (Paxil) and sertraline (Zoloft). More research is needed to evaluate their long-term effectiveness in children and teenagers. Often, antidepressants are combined with psychotherapy. Some studies suggest that this combined approach can be more effective than when antidepressants are used alone.

Generally, antidepressants are a first choice of treatment among doctors when the child or teenager:

- Has severe symptoms that likely won't respond well to psychotherapy
- Doesn't have immediate access to psychotherapy
- Has psychosis or bipolar disorder
- Has chronic depression or recurring episodes

Even after the symptoms of depression have subsided, it's generally recommended to continue taking the medication for several months to help prevent a recurrence. When it's time to stop taking the drug, your child's doctor will slowly taper off the medication over a period of weeks or months. If depression recurs — especially during the tapering off period or shortly thereafter — it's usually necessary to resume the medication.

Psychotherapy

Certain types of short-term psychotherapy, especially cognitive-behavioral therapy, have been shown to relieve symptoms of depression in children and

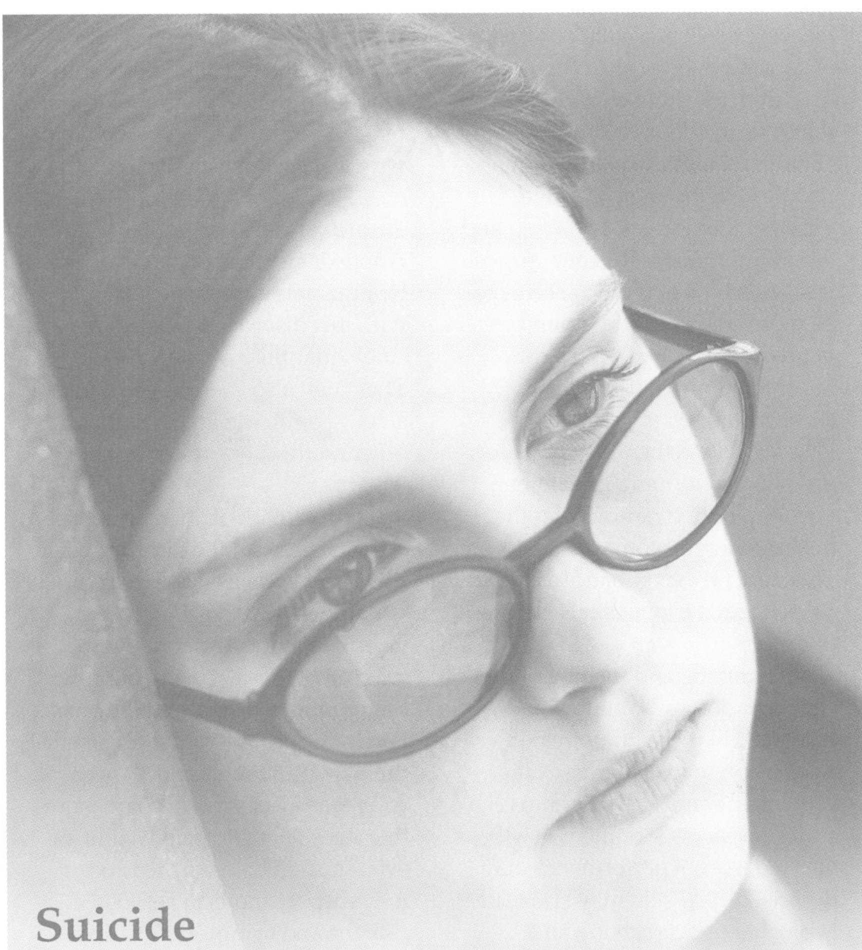

Suicide

Sometimes, depressed teenagers' lives become so painful that they feel they have nothing to live for. Most adolescents who attempt suicide are depressed. Other suicides may be motivated by triggers such as the breakup of a relationship, the death of a friend or family member, psychological problems within the family, chronic physical illness, drug abuse or physical or sexual abuse. There are many reasons why teenagers attempt suicide. Sometimes, they give no warning, and the attempt can't be predicted.

The rate of suicide among 5- to 24-year-olds in the United States has tripled since 1960. Suicide is the third leading cause of death among adolescents. When teenage boys attempt suicide, they're more likely to use guns and be successful in killing themselves. In contrast, teenage girls more often use drugs, which may not be lethal.

Because depressed adolescents often feel that their family doesn't understand them, make a special effort to bridge this communication gap. Your hopes and dreams for your child's happiness, strength and success shouldn't stand in the way of your accepting his or her revelations of depression. Ask your child how he or she really feels — and then listen. Ask how long the mood lasts and how intense it is. You can help by offering your support and concern. You can also reassure your child that he or she will not feel this way forever. Most episodes of depression eventually end. A teenager who's experiencing deep depression for the first time may not recognize or believe that it will end.

If your child confides that he or she has considered suicide, take it seriously and seek a psychiatric evaluation for him or her immediately. Even if you think you know with certainty that your child isn't really going to kill himself or herself, it's a cry for help that deserves to be heeded.

teenagers. When a child or teenager is depressed, he or she often has distorted, negative views, which reinforce the depression. Cognitive-behavioral therapy helps young people develop more positive views of themselves, the world and their life situation. Research suggests this type of therapy seems to be more effective than group or family therapy. It can also work faster than other forms of psychotherapy.

Sometimes a therapist may recommend continuing psychotherapy for a period of time after the depressive symptoms are gone. This may further enhance a child's or teenager's coping skills, decreasing relapse.

Recognizing and treating depression is important. Children and teenagers living with untreated depression may experience other problems. Family relationships can suffer, social development may be affected, school performance may decline. Depression may also lead to alcohol or drug abuse, and depressed children and teenagers may be at risk of suicide. Fortunately, if depression in children and teenagers is quickly identified and treated, its duration, severity and risk of complications can be reduced.

Eating disorders

Many teenagers are preoccupied with the way their body looks. Most teenage girls, and some teenage boys, may occasionally go on a diet for a few weeks to lose weight. If dieting becomes an obsession, it may be a sign indicating a potential eating disorder.

Eating disorders are more common during adolescence and early adulthood but can occur in childhood or midlife. Although eating disorders occur in both sexes, teenage girls and young women are more likely than teenage boys and young men to develop an eating disorder. Anorexia nervosa and bulimia nervosa are two types of eating disorders. Variations of these disorders include binge eating without purging, purging without binge eating and anorexic behavior with less severe weight loss.

Anorexia nervosa

Anorexia nervosa is characterized by unusual eating habits. People with this disorder typically eat only small quantities of a few foods. They may also exercise compulsively, vomit, use laxatives or take other medications to control their weight.

One hallmark of anorexia nervosa is that a girl with the disorder perceives her body as fat even if she's very thin. Often lacking body fat, girls with anorexia nervosa don't have much development of breasts, thighs or a waistline, and they maintain the appearance of younger children. If your daughter isn't overweight and her growth chart shows that she's failing to gain weight, or even starting to lose it, her doctor may suspect anorexia nervosa.

Signs and symptoms of anorexia include weight loss (sometimes severe), failure to maintain body weight at or above a minimally normal weight, intense fear of gaining weight, menstrual changes or the absence of menstruation and preoccupation with exercise and academic achievement.

For more information on anorexia nervosa, see page 1233.

Bulimia nervosa

Bulimia nervosa involves uncontrolled eating (bingeing) and then throwing up or using laxatives (purging) to avoid weight gain. Unfortunately, bulimia nervosa doesn't always send clear-cut signals. Depending on the frequency and timing of the binges and purges, some teenagers with bulimia maintain their normal weight, whereas others lose or even gain weight. An estimated 1 percent to 4 percent of females have bulimia nervosa in their lifetime.

Signs and symptoms of bulimia include an unhealthy focus on body shape and weight, recurrent episodes of binge eating, uncontrollable eating behavior, a binge followed by efforts to prevent weight gain — such as self-induced vomiting, using laxatives or other medications, or excessive exercise.

For more information on bulimia nervosa, see page 1233.

Tobacco use

Some teenagers don't even consider the health risks associated with smoking, or they overestimate their ability to stop once they start. Many teenagers believe that they can stop smoking anytime they choose. The reality is that among high school seniors who smoke from one to five cigarettes a day, 70 percent will still be smoking 5 years later. More than half those who smoke in high school have already tried unsuccessfully to stop.

Teenagers start smoking earlier than many parents realize. Ten percent of current adult smokers began when they were between 9 and 10 years old, and half the teenagers who start to smoke begin by 14 years of age. The earlier a child begins smoking, the greater the chance that he or she will become a heavy smoker as an adult. In addition, teenagers who smoke tobacco are more likely to experiment with marijuana and other illegal drugs.

Here are some strategies parents might try to keep their adolescent from smoking:

- *Set a personal example of not smoking.* If you as a parent smoke, one of the best reasons to stop is for the sake of your children. Parents teach best by example.
- *Talk with your children.* Ask whether their friends smoke. The risk of your child smoking is 13 times higher if his or her best friends smoke. Most teenagers smoke their first cigarette with a friend who already smokes.
- *Learn what your children think about smoking.* Ask them to read this information so that you can discuss it together.

- *Help your child explore ways to deal with peer pressure.* Use nonjudgmental questions and rehearse with them how they could handle tough situations.
- *Encourage your teenager to enjoy maximal energy and health.* The active, vivacious lifestyles portrayed in many cigarette advertisements are actually more representative of nonsmokers. People who smoke have colds and other respiratory infections more frequently.
- *Note the social repercussions.* Individuals who smoke often have bad breath, and smoking makes their hair and clothes smell. Smoking can also produce a chronic cough and makes skin wrinkle prematurely.
- *Work with your schools.* Become active in community stop smoking programs.

For more information on tobacco use, see page 78.

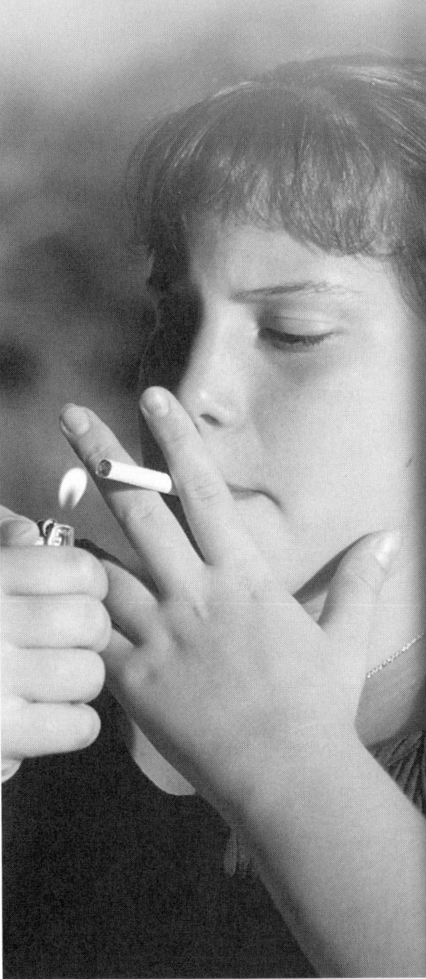

Alcohol abuse

Most young people try alcoholic beverages during their teenage years. Alcohol is widely available, and many adolescents drink excessively. Although it may take years for many adults to develop alcohol dependence, teenagers often become addicted within months. Alcohol use by itself or with other drugs can harm your child's normal growth and development and is associated with safety risks.

Alcohol use among teenagers increases dramatically during the 10th and 11th grades. Each year in the United States, more than 2,000 young people between the ages of 15 and 20 die in alcohol-related motor vehicle accidents, and many more are left disabled. Alcohol is also often implicated in other teenage deaths, including drownings, suicides and fires.

For young people, the likelihood of addiction depends on the influence of parents, peers and other role models, susceptibility to advertising, how early in life they begin to use alcohol, a psychological need for alcohol and genetic factors that may predispose them to addiction.

Look for these signs in your child:

- Loses interest in activities and hobbies
- Appears anxious or irritable
- Has difficulties in relationships with friends or joins a new crowd
- Receives lower grades in school

To prevent teenage alcohol use, set a good example regarding alcohol use. Talk to your children about alcohol use and discuss both the legal and medical consequences of drinking.

For more information on alcohol abuse and alcoholism, see page 84.

Drug abuse and addiction

Just like an adult who may drink to feel more comfortable at a party, an adolescent may take a drug to relax and join the crowd. But drug use is a counterproductive strategy. Social interactions are more successful when one is really one's self, rather than some other personality induced by a drug. Drugged people often withdraw socially and may become depressed. Likewise, depressed adolescents may abuse more drugs in a vain effort to improve their mood.

For most adolescents, experimentation with drugs starts with alcohol or tobacco. Because alcohol and cigarettes are legal for adults, they're easily accessible to teenagers.

Nearly 80 percent of high school seniors in the United States have had one alcoholic drink, and more than half have smoked during their lifetime. Next may come smoking marijuana. Almost half the high school seniors in the United States have used marijuana in their lifetime. Fortunately, relatively few teenagers graduate to trying harder drugs or using marijuana heavily or regularly over prolonged periods.

The teenage years should include the evolution of independence, increase in knowledge and formation of a sexual identity, among other processes. All this may be daunting enough when your adolescent child is cleareyed. However, if your child has an alcohol or drug addiction, the challenges of adolescence can be overwhelming.

Peer pressure and learning problems at school may make teenagers more likely to abuse drugs. Conversely, drug abuse can dampen an adolescent's motivation to do well in school. Drugs can impair the learning process, causing memory loss and shortening the attention span. Drug-abusing teenagers compromise their future outside of school too. They may get into legal trouble for abusing illegal drugs, selling them or stealing to get enough money to buy them.

Drugs can disrupt the process by which your teenager develops a secure identity. They can also mar judgment and self-control. They release inhibitions and can make it

Question and Answer

How can I know if my teenager is using drugs?

These clues are only possible indications that your teenager is using drugs:

- *School.* Your child suddenly exhibits a dislike of school and looks for excuses to stay home. Contact school officials to see if your child's attendance record matches what you know about his or her attendance. An A or B student who suddenly begins to fail courses or receives only minimally passing grades may be using drugs.
- *Physical health.* Listlessness and apathy are possible indications of drug use.
- *Appearance.* Appearance is extremely important to adolescents. A warning sign of drug use can be a sudden lack of interest in clothing or appearance.
- *Personal behavior.* Teenagers enjoy privacy. However, be wary of exaggerated efforts to bar you from their bedroom or keep you from knowing where they go with their friends.
- *Money.* Sudden requests for more money without a reasonable explanation for its use may be an indication of drug use.

Adolescents need to know that there's an open line of communication with their parents. Even in the face of your child's reluctance to share feelings, continue to express an interest in listening to your child talk about his or her experiences.

easier for your child to do things that he or she wouldn't normally consider doing, including sexual activity.

Most seriously, drug abuse raises the risk of death during adolescence. The three leading killers of teenagers — accidents, murder and suicide — are more prevalent among drug abusers.

In addition, when adolescents share needles and syringes used to do drugs intravenously, they're at high risk of getting AIDS and hepatitis.

The most effective way to discourage your teenage child from abusing drugs is to gear your message to his or her level of intellectual and moral development. Particularly in early and middle adolescence, your child may be less impressed by the long-term health effects of these substances than by their immediate social consequences.

Even more important than delivering an antidrug message is to set a good example. Addictive behavior often repeats itself in successive generations of a family. There may be a genetic component, but learning by the example of others also may play a role. If your child is abusing drugs and others in your family have struggled with alcoholism or drug addiction, early education and intervention can help break this cycle. Helping to build your child's self-confidence can help him or her to resist peer pressure to use drugs and alcohol.

Inhalant abuse

Kids don't need to take drugs to get high. There are more than 1,000 types of inhalants that kids may abuse, including gasoline, paint thinners, aerosol sprays, nail polish remover and household cleaners.

Sniffing inhalants offers an inexpensive alternative to illicit drugs, and inhalants are readily available. Kids can also huff — soak rags in inhalants and press the rags to their mouth. Another option is bagging — inhaling fumes from chemicals poured into a plastic bag.

Inhalants may produce a quick, powerful high. Inhalant abuse can start in grade school and continue throughout adolescence. About 17 percent of American teenagers report using inhalants at least once in their life.

When children sniff, huff or bag, they may ingest a host of toxic chemicals — butane, propane, fluorocarbons, nitrites and more. Chronic abusers are at risk of weight loss, muscle weakness, lack of coordination and addiction. Other possible effects include damage to the brain, heart, kidneys and liver. Inhalant abuse can be deadly.

People who abuse inhalants often look and act like they're intoxicated with alcohol. Immediate manifestations include:

- Excitation that's followed by drowsiness
- Lightheadedness
- Dizziness
- Loss of inhibitions
- Increased irritability
- Insomnia
- Hallucinations
- Disruptive behavior

Unfortunately, adults often fail to recognize inhalant abuse. Parents and doctors may be more concerned about their children's use of alcohol, nicotine and illegal drugs, such as marijuana. Preventing inhalant abuse starts with spotting clues to the problem.

The Consumer Product Safety Commission suggests the following as possible signs of inhalant abuse:

- An unusual breath odor or chemical odor on clothing
- Slurred or disoriented speech
- Drunk, dazed or dizzy appearance
- Signs of paint or other products on the face or fingers
- Red or runny eyes or nose
- Spots or sores around the mouth
- Nausea or loss of appetite
- Anxiety, excitability, irritability or restlessness
- Sitting with a pen or marker near the nose

- Constantly smelling clothing sleeves
- Hiding rags, clothes or empty containers of the potentially abused products in closets and other places

Tell your children about the risks and that even experimentation is dangerous. Make sure that your child's doctor, teachers, counselors and coaches know about inhalant abuse so that they can reinforce the danger of it and recognize potential signs of trouble. Open discussion can prevent a tragedy.

Sexual abuse

Sexual abuse can occur in adolescence as well as earlier in childhood. It can include a spectrum of unacceptable behavior from fondling to rape. Sexual abuse is any act of sexual contact forced on one person by another.

Rape usually involves force or the threat of force. However, rape also includes situations in which the victim is unable to give consent because of being drunk, drugged, mentally ill or developmentally disabled. Almost half the reported rape victims are adolescents. Most sexual abuse of teenagers involves girls, but the rate of assaults on boys may be increasing.

Incest is sexual contact between close relatives. It can occur between a teenager or younger child and a member of the family. The perpetrator can be anyone perceived to be a family member, even if that person isn't related to the adolescent by blood or marriage. Examples may include the boyfriend of an adolescent's mother or a foster parent. Even when it doesn't involve blood relatives or any threat of force, incest is a betrayal of trust.

Sexual abuse can be devastating, hostile and dehumanizing. Sexual abuse often causes major psychological trauma that has lasting effects on the victim's self-worth and identity. This is especially true for adolescents, who are still figur-

Online Safety

During the teenage years, parents generally allow their children to do more things on their own. Sexual predators may take advantage of this unsupervised time to befriend unsuspecting children. Teenagers socializing in online chat rooms and discussion groups may innocently become friends with and be lured into meeting a sexual predator. Although the Internet is a great tool for learning, make sure your children are aware of the potential dangers.

For more information about children and safety on the Internet, see page 203.

Abusive Dating Relationships

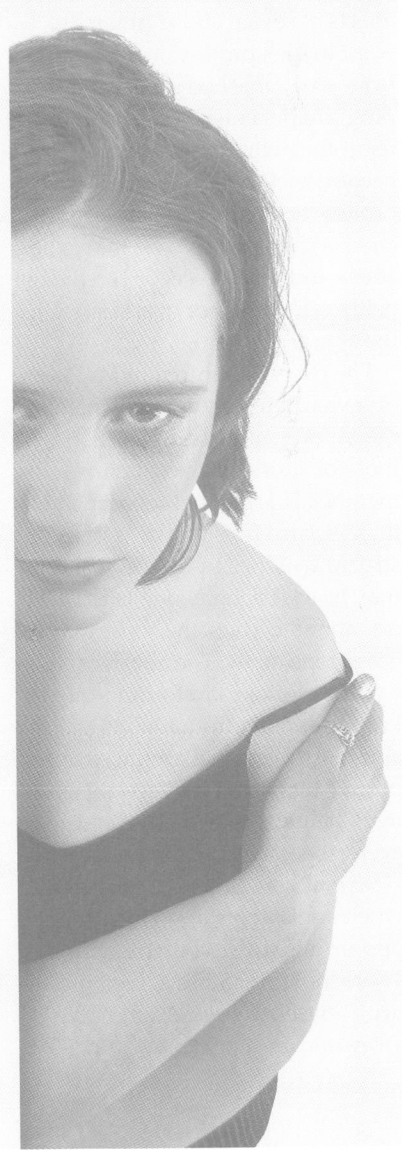

It's estimated that a third of all teenage girls are involved in abusive dating relationships. Is your daughter at risk? Consider the warning signs:

- Increasingly distant from family and friends
- Unexplained injuries or an explanation that doesn't make sense
- Lost interest in school or dropping grades
- Moody or depressed
- Suddenly uninterested in her appearance
- Involved with a boyfriend who's verbally or physically abusive
- Involved with a boyfriend who demonstrates a violent temper
- Involved with a boyfriend who calls constantly and appears possessive

If you suspect abuse, talk with your daughter immediately. With the information you've gathered, get her actively involved in developing a plan to end the violence.

If you have reason to believe that your daughter's boyfriend is going to hurt her in a specific situation, take steps to protect her.

ing out who they are, including their sexual identity. If rape is a teenager's first sexual experience, future sexual adjustment may be difficult.

Following sexual abuse, the victim may go through rapid mood swings, feeling alternately degraded, angry, guilty and helpless. The victim may be plagued for a long time by fears, nightmares and disturbed sleep. The victim's relationships with peers and consensual sexual partners may suffer. Fearing retaliation from the attacker, the victim may not report the abuse, act withdrawn and develop ritualistic behavior as a defense.

Counseling can help the victim and family to cope with long-term effects of sexual abuse. You may want to seek professional guidance from an established sexual abuse program or center. Some parents reject their children who have become victims, while others overprotect them. You can help your child come to terms with the sexual abuse and then proceed with life by neither denying nor overreacting to the abuse.

The psychological ramifications of sexual abuse by a family member can be even more complex than those of abuse by a non-family member. Fearing that reporting these occurrences will disrupt the structure of the family, the victim may be too frightened to tell anyone about it. Thus, the abuse may occur repeatedly. The abusive relative may invoke family authority to keep the victim from reporting the abuse. As the abuse continues unreported, the victim may feel increasingly helpless, ashamed, guilty and even responsible.

Serious consequences can occur when adolescents don't have the opportunity to disclose the abuse. These individuals are at high risk of drug abuse, promiscuity, running away or even suicide. ■

CHAPTER 15 PART II

Pregnancy and Childbirth

Pregnancy is one of life's most treasured times for many women. As they anticipate their baby's birth, many women eat better, exercise more and pay better attention to their health than ever before. But however short 9 months may appear to some, it can seem very long if the pregnancy is difficult or the outcome uncertain.

Fortunately, there has never been a better time to have a baby. Pregnancy will always involve risks to mother and baby, but medical advances have taught us much about how to minimize those risks and how to better deal with the unavoidable problems. With proper care and regular visits to your doctor, chances are you and your baby will be strong and healthy.

Preparing for Pregnancy

Before attempting to become pregnant, it's a good idea to see your doctor for a thorough medical history and physical examination. This is important because many conditions that are initially without symptoms can complicate pregnancy. Diabetes, high blood pressure, pelvic tumors and anemia are just a few common conditions that can be detected easily during a comprehensive general examination.

If your doctor discovers a health problem, in most cases it doesn't mean that you can't have a child. But you'll want to have the problem under control before attempting pregnancy. Some pregnant women with chronic diseases such as diabetes may be best cared for by a pregnancy specialist (obstetrician) who specializes in high-risk pregnancies.

A pre-pregnancy physical is also a good time to ask questions of your doctor or discuss concerns you may have. A particular disease or genetic abnormality may run in your family. Or maybe you're older than 35 and worried about the possibility of having a child with Down syndrome or another birth defect. Maybe you've been pregnant before and had a problem, such as miscarriage, and you're worried about a recurrence. A frank discussion with your doctor can provide helpful information about your chances of having a healthy baby.

During your pre-pregnancy physical, your doctor will likely prescribe folic acid. Whenever possible, women should take folic acid from at least 1 month before conception through the first 3 months of pregnancy. Folic acid has been shown to prevent birth defects in early fetal development (neural tube defects).

Before conception is also a good time to re-examine your lifestyle. If you're overweight and want to lose weight, do it before you become pregnant. Pregnancy isn't the time to begin a diet. If you smoke, quit. Women who smoke during pregnancy tend to have babies with lower birth weight than do nonsmokers, and these babies may have developmental problems. In addition, smokers have a higher incidence of miscarriages and stillbirths.

Don't use alcohol or illegal drugs during pregnancy. If you take medication — prescription or over-the-counter — ask your doctor about whether you may continue to take it before you try to become pregnant.

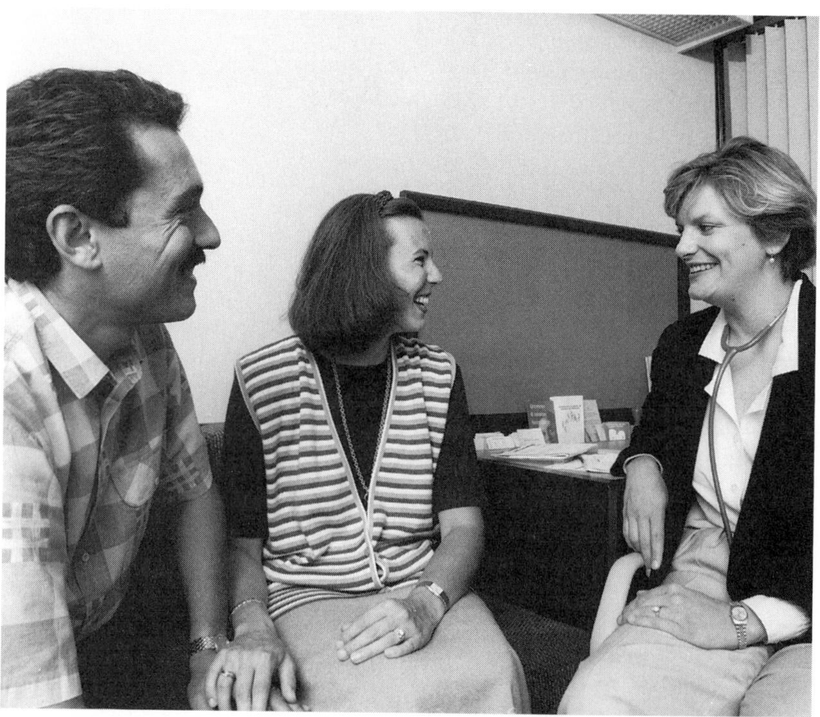

Taking time to get acquainted with your doctor and to ask questions and discuss concerns is an important part of prenatal visits.

Prenatal Care

One of the most important things you can do for you and your baby is to arrange for prenatal care as soon as you suspect that you're pregnant. By the time most women call for an appointment with a doctor, they already know they're pregnant — a home pregnancy test was positive, and they're starting to experience signs and symptoms of pregnancy. If your pregnancy hasn't been confirmed, you can have this done at your doctor visit.

Many doctors advise that you seek prenatal care as soon as you've missed a period, especially if you're trying to conceive. At the very latest, wait no longer than two missed periods before seeing a doctor.

During your first visit, you may be asked to fill out a detailed health form. Your doctor will also ask questions about your family health history and overall health to determine if you might have pre-existing conditions that could cause problems or that require special measures during the pregnancy.

In order to try to pinpoint when your baby will be born (its due date), it's important to determine when you conceived, so your doctor will ask you when you had your last menstrual period. The due date is only an approximation, however. Few babies are born on the precise date they're expected. It's perfectly normal for a baby to be born anywhere from 2 weeks before to 2 weeks after the due date.

After taking your medical history, the next step of the first prenatal visit is often a physical examination and a pelvic examination. After this initial pelvic examination, another usually isn't done until late in the pregnancy, and then only to determine if labor is imminent. Blood and urine tests are generally done during the first visit.

Your doctor or another member of his or her health care team will likely also discuss important issues of pregnancy with you, such as nutrition, weight gain, exercise and signs of potential complications. Most doctors see their pregnant patients every 4 to 6 weeks for the first 7 months, once or twice during the eighth month and then weekly.

After the initial visit, regular visits usually begin with your weight and blood pressure measurements. You may also be asked to submit a urine sample for testing. Your doctor will want to know if you're having any problems.

After about 10 to 12 weeks' gestation, an exciting part of the visit is listening to your baby's heartbeat, which can be detected with a Doppler instrument. Your doctor may also feel your abdomen to determine whether the baby is growing properly.

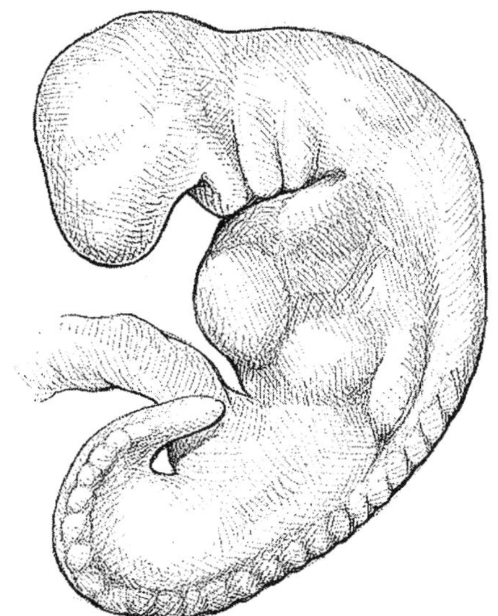

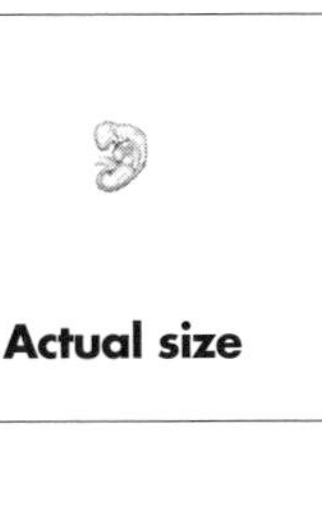

Actual size

Four weeks following conception, an embryo is no longer microscopic but is still less than a quarter inch in length. Growth is rapid during the fourth week. The embryo triples in size.

Pregnancy Tests

The earliest way to know for sure if you're pregnant is to have a pregnancy test. By 4 days of age, a fertilized egg begins to secrete a hormone called human chorionic gonadotropin (HCG). This hormone spreads into the body's tissues. Initially, it can be detected in the blood and shortly thereafter in the urine.

Most home pregnancy tests are conducted with a sample of urine, because urine can be easily obtained at home. Many types of urine tests are used to detect the presence of HCG. Most depend on a reaction between the HCG and an anti-HCG antibody. A second reaction indicates if the first reaction took place. Often, that's a color change.

Most home pregnancy tests are easy to use and quite accurate if you follow the instructions carefully and correctly. Most involve a stick that's placed in the stream of urine for a few seconds. After a specified amount of time — usually just a few minutes — a color change occurs on the stick if you're pregnant. With some brands, a dark ring indicates pregnancy.

How accurate are pregnancy tests?

Keep in mind that any pregnancy test, whether done at home or in a doctor's office, is more accurate if you use your first urine of the day. In addition, its accuracy depends on the timing of the test and how closely you follow the instructions. A test taken on the first day of your missed period is likely to be about 90 percent accurate. You'll get a more accurate reading — about 97 percent accurate — if you wait another week to take the test.

If the test is performed in the very early days of pregnancy, it may indicate you're not pregnant when in fact you are. This is called a false-negative test result. This type of result can occur because early in pregnancy the levels of HCG may be low enough to go undetected. For this reason, a negative result from a pregnancy test is less reliable than a positive result.

If your test result is negative but you have symptoms or signs of pregnancy, try the test again a week later or consult your doctor. If the result is positive, see your doctor for prenatal care. To confirm that you're pregnant, your doctor may get a blood sample for an HCG blood test.

Pregnancy and Nutrition

The best time to start thinking about good nutrition is before you plan to become pregnant. Then you can be sure that your baby will have all of the essential nutrients from the moment of conception. Improvements that you make in your own diet can also spark a healthful change for the family.

Nutrition risk factors

If you have a history of good eating habits, you begin your pregnancy with optimal amounts of most of the nutrients needed for your baby's tremendous growth and development. A history of chronic dieting, skipping meals, fasting or eating a limited variety of foods can put you and your baby at nutritional risk. Other factors that put you at increased risk of poor nutrition include using cigarettes, alcohol or illegal drugs, carrying more than one baby and being significantly underweight or overweight at the time of conception.

Extremely poor eating habits before or during pregnancy can harm both you and your baby. If you eat too few calories or nutrients, fetal development can be less than ideal, and your baby may be underweight at birth. Low birth weight babies have an increased risk of short- and long-term health problems.

In the first weeks of your pregnancy — perhaps even before you know you're pregnant — most of your baby's major organs are forming. That's why it's so critical to make nutritious eating habits a part of your decision to begin a new life.

Weight gain

Pregnancy may be the one time in your life when you're encouraged to gain weight. But weight gain in pregnancy doesn't mean getting fat or eating whatever you want. Your size increases for various physical reasons, including the weight of the baby you'll deliver.

Over the years, the recommended amount of weight to gain during pregnancy has varied dramatically. Twenty or 30 years ago, minimal weight gain was thought to be best for mother and baby. Now research indicates that women who are normal weight at the time of conception have the healthiest pregnancies and babies if they gain approximately 25 to 35 pounds.

Your doctor will estimate the right amount of weight for you to gain. Individual recommendations vary based on factors such as your pre-pregnancy weight, your medical history, your health and the health of your developing baby.

How much weight you gain during your pregnancy partly determines your baby's weight, and a normal birth weight is important for good health. A desirable weight for a full-term newborn is between 6½ and 9 pounds. Babies born at these healthy weights have:

- A lower rate of infant death
- Fewer mental and physical handicaps
- Fewer serious childhood illnesses
- A head start, physically and mentally, over smaller babies

Strive for a slow and steady increase in your weight, but keep in mind that individual women gain at different rates. Here are some general guides to weight gain:

- First trimester: 1 to 1½ pounds a month
- Second trimester: ½ to ¾ pound a week
- Third trimester: ¾ to 1 pound a week

Calorie needs

Your developing fetus is exclusively dependent on the calories you provide through eating and drinking. This doesn't mean that you have to eat excessively, but you may need to eat more often than before your pregnancy. Some of the discomforts of early pregnancy — feelings of hunger or nausea and vomiting — are often relieved by intermittent snacking. If you feel more comfortable snacking, eat smaller meals to avoid excessive weight gain.

During your first trimester, an extra 200 calories a day over your normal intake will provide for the recommended 1 to 1½ pounds of weight that you should gain each month. It's important that these calories come from foods that offer the most nutrition for you and your

Where the Weight Goes

Your baby	6½-9 pounds
Placenta	1½ pounds
Amniotic fluid	2 pounds
Breast enlargement	1-3 pounds
Uterus enlargement	2 pounds
Fat stores and muscle development	4-8 pounds
Increased blood volume	3-4 pounds
Increased fluid volume	2-3 pounds
Total	22-32½ pounds

baby. You don't want a baby to grow on chips, sodas or fast foods. Your body will let you know that you need extra calories, but 200 extra calories isn't a big increase. For example, a slice of whole-grain bread, a glass of skim milk and 1 ounce of lean meat will add about 200 calories.

In your second and third trimesters, you'll need a total of 300 to 500 extra calories a day beyond your normal diet. The more active you are, the more calories you'll need. Even with this demand for more calories, you won't need to force yourself to eat more because your natural appetite almost always guides you to enough calories.

Food choices

While you're pregnant, you don't have to keep a food diary or analyze your meals and snacks, but do pay attention to some basic guidelines. Regularly eating a variety of foods is best for staying healthy. Try to eat the following types and amounts of food every day:

- *Grains: 6 to 11 servings.* Grains — cereals, breads, rice and pasta — are rich in energy-filled complex carbohydrates and provide important nutrients as well as fiber. Along with fruits and vegetables, grains should form the foundation of your diet.
- *Vegetables: At least 3 servings.* Vegetables are naturally low in calories and almost fat-free. They provide fiber, vitamins and minerals.
- *Fruits: At least 2 servings.* Fresh fruits generally have few calories and little or no fat, and they contain beneficial fiber, vitamins and minerals.
- *Dairy products: 2 to 3 servings.* Milk, yogurt and cheese are outstanding sources of calcium and vitamin D, which help your body absorb calcium. They also provide protein needed to build and maintain body tissues. Choose low-fat dairy products.

Vitamin and Mineral Supplements

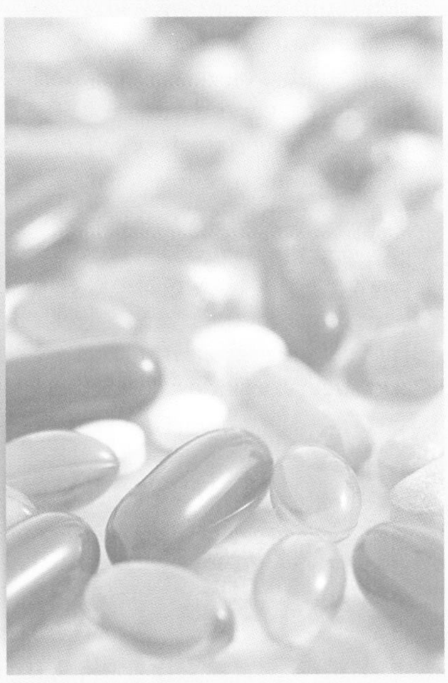

Pregnant women need more of almost every vitamin and mineral than do women who aren't pregnant. Guidelines from the National Research Council advise that pregnant women who eat a well-balanced diet don't need supplements. However, most pregnant women can't eat enough foods high enough in iron and folate to meet recommendations, and some women can't or won't eat enough high-calcium foods to meet the increased need for this mineral. Multivitamins that include folic acid taken early in pregnancy may help prevent birth defects and provide insurance that you get enough vitamins and minerals in your daily diet.

Folic Acid: A Pregnancy Must

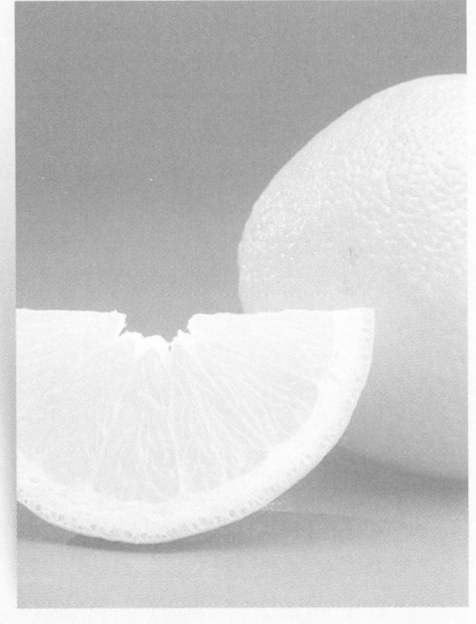

Folic acid is a synthetic form of folate, a vitamin found naturally in certain foods. It's an important nutrient, but never so much so as when you're considering becoming pregnant.

Some very important development takes place in the first several weeks of pregnancy. If you're planning on becoming pregnant, see your doctor to receive a prescription for folic acid supplements. Taking the supplements can help to avoid serious birth defects. In fact, the U.S. Public Health Service recommends that all women of childbearing age wanting to conceive children consume 400 micrograms (mcg) of folic acid daily as a means of reducing their risk of having a pregnancy with neural tube defects (NTDs), such as spina bifida. If you've had a pregnancy that resulted in a fetus with an NTD, you may decrease the risk of another NTD by 70 percent if before conceiving again you take 400 mcg of folic acid a day beginning 3 months before conception and continuing through the first trimester.

Folic acid is vital for cell growth and function and for the synthesis of DNA, the building blocks of your genetic code. You'll find folate in citrus fruits, beans, nuts, seeds, liver and dark green leafy vegetables such as spinach. But to get the recommended amount of folic acid, you'll need a supplement.

- *Poultry, seafood and meat: No more than 3 servings.* These foods are rich sources of protein with B vitamins, iron and zinc. Select lean varieties of meat and poultry to reduce fat and cholesterol.
- *Legumes: Frequently.* Low in fat and without any cholesterol, legumes — beans, dried peas and lentils — are the best source of plant protein. They're also excellent sources of fiber.
- *Fats and sweets: Sparingly.* Fats and sugars provide calories that can easily exceed your needs, leading to excessive weight gain.

Vegetarian diets

If you're a vegetarian, you can continue your vegetarian diet throughout your pregnancy and still have a healthy baby, but you'll need to pay additional attention to meal planning. Take time to review your food intake regularly. If you include fish, milk and eggs in your diet, it'll be easier to balance your nutritional intake. Eat a wide variety of foods each day and include one or two extra servings of plant foods high in iron.

Snacks

Healthy snacking is the perfect way to add the extra calories and nutrients essential during pregnancy. Well-planned snacks are also helpful for the times when you can't eat a full meal. In the early part of your pregnancy, frequent, small meals and snacks can help control nausea. In the last weeks, the pressure of

Key Nutrients in Pregnancy

More than 50 nutrients are essential for good health when you're pregnant. Here's a summary of those most critical for you and your baby:

Nutrient	Why you and your baby need it	Best sources
Protein	The main building block for your baby's cells. Provides reserves you'll need for labor and delivery.	Eggs, lean meats, poultry, fish, cheese, milk, dried peas, beans
Carbohydrate	Provides energy for you and your baby. Allows protein to be used for tissue growth.	Whole-grain and fortified breads and cereals, fruits, vegetables, rice, pasta, potatoes
Fat	Provides long-term energy for growth. Critical for the development of your baby's brain.	Lean meat, fish, poultry, eggs, nuts, seeds, peanut butter, oils, margarine, butter
Fluid	Helps increase fluid volume. Prevents constipation and dry skin. Needed for amniotic fluid.	Tap and bottled water, soup
Vitamin A	Promotes healthy skin, eyesight and bone growth.	Sweet potatoes, carrots, dark leafy greens, cantaloupe, apricots
Vitamin C	Forms healthy gums, teeth and bones for your baby. Keeps your tissues in top shape. Improves iron absorption.	Citrus fruits, broccoli, tomatoes, peppers, berries, melons, potatoes with skin
Folate	Helps blood cell and hemoglobin formation. Early in pregnancy, it may prevent birth defects in early fetal development (neural tube defects).	Dark leafy greens, dried peas and beans, whole-grain breads and cereals, citrus fruits, bananas, cantaloupe, tomatoes
Calcium	Helps form strong bones and teeth.	Milk, cheese, yogurt, collard greens, kale, sardines and canned salmon with the bones, broccoli, dried beans
Iron	A component of hemoglobin in red blood cells needed to deliver oxygen to your baby.	Lean red meat, spinach, tofu, dried fruits, whole-grain and fortified breads and cereals

your baby on your stomach may limit the amount of food you can comfortably eat at one time. Snacking may be more feasible.

Salt

Pregnant women were once encouraged to limit their sodium intake. New research suggests that it's better not to. During the last few weeks of pregnancy, almost all women have some swelling (edema) in their ankles, legs, fingers or face. Cutting back significantly on salt to reduce this swelling causes your body to conserve sodium and water, actually making the swelling worse.

If you have high blood pressure or develop complications later in your pregnancy, your doctor may suggest that you stay away from table salt and processed foods high in sodium.

Artificial sweeteners

More than 1,500 artificially sweetened foods line the shelves of your local grocery store. They include chewing gum, soft drinks, pudding, gelatin, drink mixes, yogurt and candy.

Although there's no conclusive evidence to support a recommendation either for or against the use of artificial sweeteners, pregnant women might want to consider limiting the amount in their diet. In all things, moderation.

Caffeine

Caffeine is a drug that has been part of the human diet for thousands of years. It's found naturally in coffee, tea, chocolate and cocoa. Caffeine is frequently added to soft drinks and over-the-counter medications, including many headache and cold tablets and allergy remedies.

An abundance of research indicates that moderate consumption of caffeine — 200 milligrams (mg) daily — has no negative effects during pregnancy. However, high amounts of caffeine — 500 mg or more daily — can increase the amount of time a fetus spends in an active, awake state and may cause a decrease in your baby's birth weight and head circumference.

Coffee is the most common source of caffeine. Drinking more than 3 cups of coffee a day isn't recommended. But don't assume switching to an herbal tea is safe. Because little is known about herbs and their effect on pregnancy, avoid herbal teas.

Pregnancy and Exercise

Today, an increasing number of health-conscious women are exercising throughout their pregnancies. This isn't to say that pregnancy is the time to embark on a vigorous fitness regimen, especially if you haven't been physically active

Smart Snacking

Here are some examples of healthy snacks:

Crunchy
- Raw vegetables
- Whole-grain crackers

Sweet
- Fresh fruit
- Dried fruit
- Low-fat yogurt
- A low-fat muffin

Thirst quenchers
- Ice water or sparkling bottled water
- Fruit juice fizz, which is made from juice and sparkling water
- A fruit shake made with skim milk
- Vegetable juice

Hearty
- A fruit muffin or bread
- Cereal with low-fat yogurt
- Vegetable soup
- A tuna sandwich

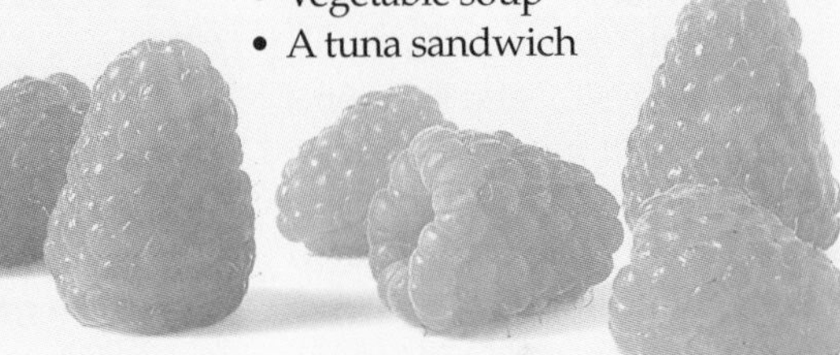

Caffeine Content

	Milligrams of caffeine	
	Average	**Range**
Coffee, 5 oz.		
Brewed, percolator	115	60-180
Brewed, drip method	80	40-170
Instant	65	30-120
Tea, 5 oz. hot or 12 oz. iced		
Brewed, imported	60	25-110
Brewed, U.S. brands	40	20-90
Instant	30	25-50
Iced	70	67-76
Soft drinks, 12 oz.	36	30-50
Cocoa, 5 oz.	4	2-20
Chocolate milk, 8 oz.	5	2-7
Semisweet chocolate, 1 oz.	20	5-35
Milk chocolate, 1 oz.	6	1-15
Chocolate syrup, 1 oz.	4	4-5

before. However, if you've been exercising regularly before pregnancy, you can continue to do so unless your doctor advises against it. Doctors even recommend that previously sedentary patients begin some form of mild exercise during pregnancy.

The long-term benefits of a regular exercise program for men and women are well-known. What impact, however, does exercising by an expectant mother have on the fetus? Studies indicate that exercise probably has no impact. However, it may increase maternal stamina.

The result of this increased stamina may be a successful vaginal delivery, possibly due to increased cardiorespiratory fitness and better endurance. Endurance is particularly valuable when a mother is pushing the baby out during delivery. Women who exercise regularly can often push for longer periods without fatigue.

Exercise, though, with caution. Because of physical and hormonal changes in your body, you're more vulnerable to injury. Your joints are less stable and more easily injured because your connective tissues now stretch more easily. Moreover, as you become larger, your center of gravity shifts, and you may find yourself losing your balance. Pay attention to your changing body.

Many sports and exercises are suitable for pregnant women. One of the best exercises during pregnancy is swimming. It provides a good cardiovascular workout with minimal risk of injury because of the water's buoyancy.

Low-impact aerobics also are fine, and in many communities low-impact aerobic classes for expectant mothers are available. Jogging and cycling also are good if you took part in these activities before conception. You may need to decrease your activity level if you find yourself becoming more fatigued than usual. Walking during pregnancy is often recommended, and it's usually the first exercise advised for previously inactive pregnant women who want to begin exercising.

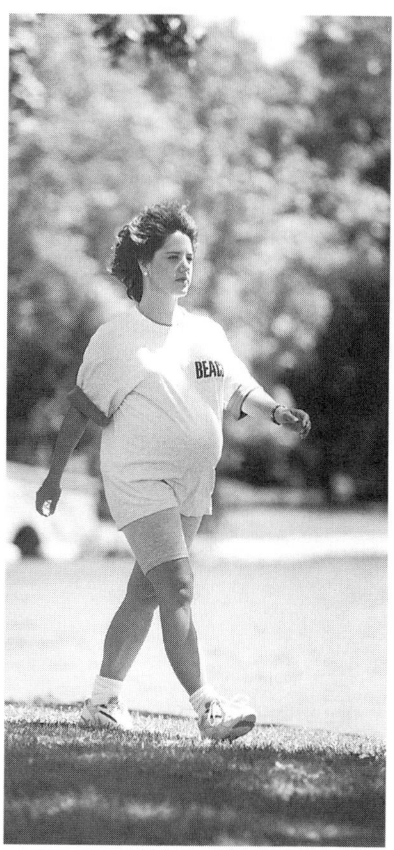

An invigorating walk is one of the safest, easiest forms of exercise during pregnancy. If you weren't physically active before pregnancy, walking is a good way to get started.

No matter what exercise you choose, check with your doctor before you begin. Although it's safe for most women to exercise during pregnancy, some pregnant women have medical problems that may make exertion inadvisable. In addition, never exercise to the point of exhaustion. Drink plenty of fluids to prevent dehydration during a workout.

Common Concerns

Most women come through pregnancy and childbirth healthy and with reason to celebrate. Still, few women escape without at least some discomfort. And along the way, they often have many concerns. Most doctors who deliver babies are accustomed to pregnant women asking questions — lots of them. Keep a notebook in which you can jot down questions as they come up and bring it with you to your checkups.

Morning sickness

Morning sickness is the term used to describe the queasiness, nausea or vomiting that about half of all pregnant women have during the first 12 weeks of pregnancy.

Although these conditions tend to be worse in the morning, they can occur at any point throughout the day. It's not understood why some women have nausea and vomiting. Hormonal changes may be responsible. Although morning sickness is certainly unpleasant, it's rarely dangerous.

If you experience morning sickness, you can do certain things to minimize your symptoms, although nothing is 100 percent effective. Many women find that the nausea is worse when their stomach is empty. By the time you feel hungry, it may be too late, and you may already feel the nausea creeping up on you. Make it a point to eat several small meals a day. Try keeping crackers at your bedside and eating a few before getting up in the morning. Keep stashes of nutritious foods that you can tolerate in strategic locations — your car, desk drawer or purse.

You may find the smell of certain foods nauseating. If this happens, avoid that particular food. Stick to a bland diet, avoiding spicy, rich and fried foods. On the other hand, eat whatever sounds good for your queasy stomach. If plain water upsets your stomach, try crushed ice, fruit juice or Popsicles.

Some medications may be effective for eliminating morning sickness. However, medications should generally be avoided except in severe circumstances. Most morning sickness goes away about 12 weeks into the pregnancy, although for some women it lasts longer.

Constipation

Constipation is marked by hard and occasionally painful bowel movements, a diminished frequency of bowel movements and difficulty in expelling stool. Constipation is a common problem during pregnancy. If you're normally constipated, you may find that the problem worsens during your pregnancy.

To alleviate the problem, drink plenty of fluids, exercise daily and make sure your diet contains several servings of fruits (prunes are particularly good), vegetables and grains, such as whole wheat and bran. Over-the-counter bulk-formers that contain psyllium also can be helpful. Don't take a laxative unless you check with your doctor.

Heartburn

Heartburn has nothing to do with your heart. Rather, the burning sensation in the middle of your chest and the bad taste in your mouth that sometimes accompanies it are the result of stomach acid refluxing up into your lower esophagus. It occurs when the muscle that closes off the stomach from the esophagus (esophageal sphincter) relaxes, allowing stomach juices to flow back up and irritate the esophagus.

About half of all pregnant women experience heartburn. It often worsens with advancing pregnancy because the stomach is displaced by the enlarging uterus, which delays the emptying of the stomach contents.

If you have heartburn, try eating smaller meals at more frequent intervals. Eat slowly and avoid greasy foods. Both regular and decaffeinated coffee may aggravate heartburn. Because heartburn is often worse when you lie flat, try sleeping with the head of your bed on 4- to 6-inch blocks. In addition, avoid eating for 2 to 3 hours before bedtime. If these practices don't help, talk to your doctor, who may recommend an antacid.

Backache

Low back pain is common during pregnancy. Often, it occurs when you're tired or have been bending, lifting or walking a lot.

When you're pregnant, your ligaments are more elastic, which allows your pelvis to expand during the birth of your baby. Although this is necessary, it makes your joints more prone to strain and injury. During pregnancy, as your center of balance changes, so does your posture, inflicting more strain than ever on your already vulnerable back.

Usually, the pain is in the lower back. Some women experience pain that starts at the lower back and radiates down one or both legs (sciatica).

Most women also have pain on the sides of the abdomen because of the stretching of the abdominal ligaments by the expanding uterus. Imagine your uterus being anchored by ligaments that extend down the sides of your abdomen. As your uterus grows, the ligaments stretch to accommodate it. Called round ligament pain, this pain is generally worse during the second trimester. Lying down on your left side may ease the strain.

Try not to gain more weight than is recommended because excess weight stresses your back. Backache can usually be relieved by eliminating as much strain as possible. Sometimes a maternity girdle can help. Your doctor may recommend exercises to relieve the pain. If the pain is severe, your doctor may recommend further evaluation to determine if an underlying problem is causing it.

Varicose veins

Varicose veins usually become worse in later pregnancy and are more pronounced in older mothers and in women who stand for long periods. Heredity also plays a role. As many as 20 percent of all pregnant women have varicose veins. The condition tends to appear earlier and is more pronounced with each pregnancy.

When you're pregnant, your blood vessels must accommodate an increased blood volume to supply the needs of your baby. Your uterus enlarges, and the flow of blood from your leg veins to your pelvis decreases. This combination can cause the veins in your legs to become swollen, creating leg discomfort.

If you have varicose veins, try to keep off your feet and elevate them when possible. Don't wear clothing that's tight around the thighs or waist. Support hose can help relieve the pain and swelling. Many doctors recommend that you put on support hose first thing in the morning and keep them on until just before you go to bed.

Surgery to treat varicose veins generally isn't recommended during pregnancy and rarely is the problem so severe that it becomes necessary.

Hemorrhoids

Hemorrhoids occur when the veins in the anal canal become enlarged due to pressure. When you strain during a bowel movement, the veins may protrude through the anus and cause pain and itching. Generally, they become worse during pregnancy and often occur in conjunction with constipation.

Prevention is the best treatment. Avoid becoming constipated to the point where you need to strain to expel stool. Eating food high in fiber, drinking plenty of water and exercising daily help prevent constipation.

If you feel pain during a bowel movement and feel a swollen mass near your rectum, you probably have a hemorrhoid. To ease the discomfort, take frequent warm-water baths. A cotton pad soaked with cold witch hazel cream and applied to the hemorrhoidal area also may help. Many women find relief with over-the-counter rectal suppositories that reduce the hemorrhoid and lubricate the anal canal.

Sleep difficulties

Sleep difficulties often occur during the later months of pregnancy. The frequent urge to urinate contributes to lack of sleep. The movement of your baby also may keep you awake. Some women simply have so much on their mind that sleep eludes them.

What should you do if you find yourself staring at the ceiling half the night? Avoid coffee, tea or cola drinks because they contain caffeine, which can keep you awake. In addition, don't eat a large meal just before bedtime.

Some doctors recommend exercising a little more so that you'll be more tired and more apt to fall asleep. But be sure to finish exercising several hours before bedtime.

For some pregnant women, a warm bath helps. If these ideas don't work, get up — read a book, pay some bills or catch up on household tasks. Try sleeping later.

If your lack of sleep becomes significant, talk to your doctor. Don't take any medications unless he or she recommends it.

Swelling

Swelling (edema) is common during pregnancy. Approximately one-quarter of your weight gain during pregnancy is fluid, which tends to congregate in various parts of your body, including the lower legs, feet and hands. You may notice swelling in your legs, ankles and feet after you've been standing for long periods.

The problem is usually worse at the end of the day and in warm weather. After a night of rest, the legs and feet return to their normal size in most women.

The fingers also are a common site for swelling. You may wake up in the morning with your fingers so stiff that you can't button your clothing. Your fingers may also be puffy.

Some women experience facial swelling. If your face becomes extremely swollen, especially around the eyes, you likely have preeclampsia (see page 274), a serious medical condition. Contact your doctor immediately.

Lying down and elevating your legs for an hour in midafternoon may reduce the swelling in your legs. Swimming and treading water also may temporarily relieve swelling in your legs and feet. Even standing in a pool can help.

Travel

There's no reason why you can't travel during your pregnancy unless your doctor advises against it.

Before you contemplate a cross-country car trip or a 2-week cruise, however, consider how you're going to feel. Many women, particularly during the first 3 months of pregnancy, have frequent bouts of nausea or morning sickness. Travel during this period may make the nausea worse.

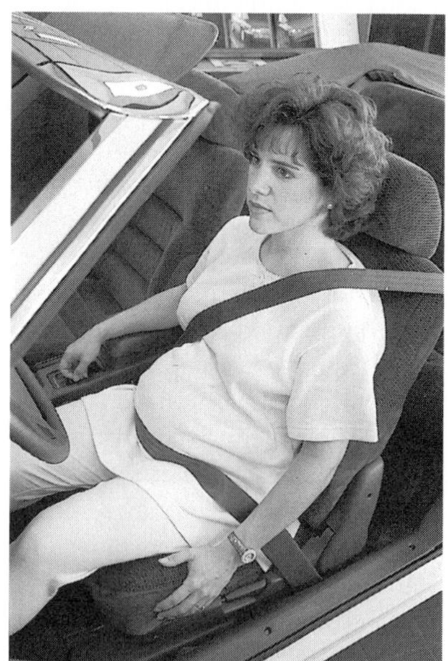

Place the lap portion of the seat belt blow your abdomen and across your upper thighs. Position the shoulder strap between your breasts and to the side of your abdomen.

A potential risk of traveling while pregnant is blood clots in your legs (thrombophlebitis), which can result from sitting for long periods of time. While traveling, get up and walk around for a few minutes every couple of hours to activate your leg muscles and increase blood flow.

Another consideration is the proximity to your due date. Most doctors advise against traveling during the last weeks of pregnancy, particularly if you have a history of any problems. Many airlines won't allow you to fly if you're close to your due date.

When traveling by car, remember to always wear your seat belt. Fasten a lap belt below your uterus, and place a shoulder harness between your breasts and to the side of your abdomen. You may find it helpful to put a pillow in the small of your back to prevent low back pain. Stop every couple of hours to get out and walk.

Medical Problems of Pregnancy

Most women go through pregnancy without any major complications. For a small percentage of women, however, this 9-month experience isn't without problems. This section explores some of the more common medical problems that can complicate pregnancy.

Anemia

Anemia occurs when a protein in blood that carries oxygen throughout the body (hemoglobin) falls below usual levels. A small decrease in hemoglobin is normal during pregnancy. Usually, anemia in pregnancy is due to an iron deficiency or an inadequate supply of folate.

If you have mild anemia, you may not have any signs or symptoms, and the condition may only be discovered during a routine blood test. With more severe anemia, signs and symptoms include fatigue, breathlessness, fainting, palpitations and pallor. Anemia can be risky for both mother and child. An anemic pregnant woman is less able to tolerate blood loss than is a woman with adequate hemoglobin.

Your doctor most likely will prescribe iron and folic acid supplements to prevent anemia. You can help prevent the condition by eating a diet rich in iron, which is found in foods such as liver, dried fruit, whole grains and beef. Dark leafy greens are a good source of folic acid. If you do develop anemia, your doctor will prescribe appropriate treatment.

Diabetes

Having diabetes doesn't preclude you from becoming pregnant. In fact, if you have diabetes, you have an excellent chance of having a healthy baby. However, before conception and during pregnancy, it's extremely important to keep your blood sugar (glucose) level under control through careful monitoring of your blood sugar. A satisfactory glucose level at the outset of pregnancy decreases your baby's risks of birth defects.

If you don't keep your blood sugar under good control, the excess blood sugar will travel through the placenta and cause an increase in your baby's blood sugar level. This activates the fetal pancreas to produce insulin, which acts as a growth hormone. Babies born to mothers whose diabetes is out of control often are extremely large, a characteristic that complicates labor and delivery. They also tend to have more congenital defects and are predisposed to diabetes.

For a pregnant mother with diabetes, the risks associated with the disease include infection, postpartum bleeding, heart and lung problems and a fourfold greater risk of preeclampsia than in mothers who don't have diabetes.

A woman with diabetes should seek the care of an obstetrician who specializes in high-risk pregnancies.

Gestational diabetes

Sometimes, women who don't have diabetes develop a condition called gestational diabetes during pregnancy. This form of diabetes also requires careful blood sugar control. Changes in your diet are the first step in treatment.

Your doctor may prescribe a medication called glyburide (DiaBeta, Micronase). It can prevent or forestall the need for insulin. Gestational diabetes usually goes away after the baby is born, but gestational diabetes increases your risk of developing diabetes later in life.

Your doctor may recommend a blood glucose screening test between 24 and 28 weeks into your pregnancy to check for gestational diabetes.

PREVENTION TIP

Be sure to make it to all of your scheduled prenatal checkups. Sometimes, it may seem like little happens at these appointments, but listening to the baby's heartbeat, measuring your weight gain and checking your blood pressure are vital to catching some problems before they become serious.

Asthma

Asthma is a chronic respiratory disease that afflicts about 3 percent of adults. The course of asthma during pregnancy is difficult to predict. In some women, the disease worsens with pregnancy. In others, it improves or remains the same.

If you have asthma, you may be more prone to respiratory infections during pregnancy. The emotional stress of pregnancy may make your attacks more intense. However, most asthmatic women can carry a baby to term safely. Many women with asthma require medication. Most asthma medication is safe to use during pregnancy.

High blood pressure

High blood pressure is a potentially dangerous problem during pregnancy. Pregnant women with high blood pressure tend to have small placentas, and their infants tend to be small at birth. The incidence of fetal death is higher in pregnant women with high blood pressure than it is in pregnant women without high blood pressure.

Some pregnant women have pre-existing high blood pressure, which means that they had it before they became pregnant. In others, pregnancy causes an elevation in blood pressure. You may have high blood pressure but no symptoms. The condition is easily detected during a routine blood pressure check, which is a part of every prenatal visit. Sometimes, bed rest is advised. If your blood pressure is extremely high, your doctor may prescribe medication.

Some women with mild pre-existing high blood pressure have no major problems during pregnancy. In others, their blood pressure continues to increase, and protein is detected in their urine, which is a sign of preeclampsia, a serious medical condition (see page 274). Preeclampsia typically occurs after the 20th week of pregnancy. Convulsions (eclampsia) can follow if preeclampsia isn't monitored and treated.

If you have high blood pressure, your doctor may request blood and urine tests to determine if your kidneys are functioning properly. He or she may also repeat ultrasound examinations to make sure your baby is growing properly.

Heart disorders

About 1 percent of all pregnant women have a pre-existing heart disorder. Although potentially serious, many women with heart disorders have successful pregnancies and healthy babies.

Pregnancy makes your heart and other organs work harder. Thus, if you already have a heart disorder, this extra load can cause complications. Make sure you discuss the risks of pregnancy with your doctor before you become pregnant.

Excessive weight gain, anemia and abnormal retention of fluid can be particularly dangerous for a woman with a heart disorder. Every effort should be made to avoid these problems. In some cases, bed rest for part of the pregnancy may be recommended.

Bleeding During Pregnancy

Bleeding from the vagina during pregnancy often is an indication that something is wrong. In the first 20 weeks of pregnancy, bleeding may be associated with miscarriage, ectopic pregnancy or other conditions.

Bleeding during a miscarriage may be slight or heavy. You may have no warning of vaginal bleeding or you may first notice some brownish discharge.

Approximately 20 percent of all pregnant women have some bleeding in early pregnancy that doesn't result in miscarriage. So don't necessarily assume the worst, but do check with your doctor.

After the 20th week of pregnancy, bleeding is much less common than in early pregnancy, affecting less than 2 percent of all pregnant women. Causes include placenta previa — a condition in which the placenta covers the cervical opening, the onset of premature labor, miscarriage and the separation of the placenta from the uterine wall (placental abruption).

Most often the bleeding (hemorrhaging) is mild. However, a severe hemorrhage can endanger your life and your baby's. If you begin bleeding after the first 12 weeks of pregnancy, see your doctor immediately. You may require hospitalization and diagnostic tests to determine the cause of your bleeding. If the bleeding is severe, blood transfusions may be necessary. Sometimes, labor is induced or a Caesarean delivery is performed.

Seizure disorders

If you take medication for a seizure disorder, such as epilepsy, you'll need special attention during pregnancy. Severe nausea and vomiting during early pregnancy may interfere with your ability to take your anticonvulsant medication. Expansion of your blood volume may change the levels of medication in your blood. These changes can increase the risk of seizures.

Medications used to control seizures may cause birth defects, some because they lower folate levels in your blood. Some medications are more apt to cause problems than others are. If you have a seizure disorder and you're contemplating pregnancy, make sure to discuss your condition and medication with your doctor.

Skin disorders

Skin pigmentation changes often occur during pregnancy. You may notice brownish spots on your face or on other parts of your body. This discoloration on your face is sometimes called the mask of pregnancy (chloasma). The pigmentary changes usually fade after the baby is born.

Other conditions that affect pregnant women are a type of hives (urticaria) and cholestasis. Hives are raised, red, often itchy welts of various sizes that appear and disappear on the skin. They may result from medications, allergic reactions or chemicals in foods, but often the cause is unknown.

Cholestasis is a condition that occurs when the flow of bile from the liver to the intestine is reduced or interrupted. Bile pigment (bilirubin) is deposited in skin tissues, causing itching. Itching without a rash generally occurs all over the body. In pregnant women, cholestasis is often due to hormonal changes.

Avoid scratching, which may cause infection. Wash with a mild soap. If your symptoms are severe, talk to your doctor, who may be able to provide some suggestions for relief.

Infectious diseases

Some common diseases that seem to do little more than make a pregnant woman miserable can, in fact, do irreparable damage to the fetus, depending on when in fetal development they strike.

German measles

German measles (rubella) is usually a mild viral disease that causes a mild, itchy rash and fever. If contracted during the first 10 weeks of pregnancy, however, the virus can cross the placenta and infect the fetus. More than half the infants born to women who have rubella during early pregnancy have congenital malformations such as cataracts, deafness, hernias, heart defects and defects of the central nervous system.

When contracted in later pregnancy, rubella doesn't cause congenital defects, but the infant is born with the virus, which can cause serious illness. Many of these babies later develop diabetes.

Your best defense against rubella is immunization. Most women in the United States have been vaccinated against German measles, but if you haven't and haven't had the illness, get vaccinated before you become pregnant.

Chickenpox

If you've never had chickenpox, consider getting the chickenpox vaccine before you become pregnant. Chickenpox (varicella) can be a serious disease in pregnant women, and it can be dangerous to the fetus. While in the uterus, the fetus may actually develop pocks. If these occur early in pregnancy, the pockmarks may cause some limb deformities.

The greatest risk to the baby seems to be exposure to the virus just before delivery. If the infant is delivered before receiving your antibodies against the virus, he or she may develop the disease. Immediate treatment may prevent serious complications or death in a newborn.

If you're exposed to the chickenpox virus during pregnancy and haven't had the virus, your doctor may recommend an injection of zoster immune globulin.

Fifth disease

Fifth disease is an infection most common among school-age children. Doctors call it parvovirus infection (erythema infectiosum). The most noticeable part of the infection is a bright red rash prominent on the cheeks, giving the impression of slapped cheeks. A lacy, red rash may also appear on the legs, trunk and neck.

Pregnant women are susceptible to developing fifth disease. Among those with the disease, about a third of their fetuses also show evidence of the infection. In the majority of cases, the mother delivers a normal, healthy baby. However, in some cases, fifth disease in a mother can lead to severe, even fatal, anemia in the fetus. This can result in congestive heart failure in the fetus.

Sometimes, it's possible to try to correct the anemia and heart failure with a fetal blood transfusion or administration of medication to the mother. The medication passes through the placenta to the fetus.

If you're pregnant and think you've been exposed to fifth disease, contact your doctor.

Toxoplasmosis

Toxoplasmosis is a disease that results from contact with the parasite *Toxoplasma gondii.* It's contracted by eating infected, undercooked meat or through contact with infected cat feces. The disease can be passed from an infected pregnant mother to her baby. If you're pregnant, be careful to not come in contact with cat feces. Wear gloves while gardening or cleaning the litter box and wash your hands thoroughly afterward.

As many as 25 percent to 45 percent of American women of reproductive age carry the organism, though they might not have symptoms. It's estimated that one fetus in every 800 to 1,400 pregnancies acquires toxoplasmosis. The disease is much more common in Europe, especially France.

Common symptoms are fatigue and muscle pain. You may feel like you have the flu. The disease is difficult to diagnose. If you have toxoplasmosis, your doctor will likely prescribe a medication to treat the infection.

Most infants born with toxoplasmosis don't immediately show evidence of having been infected, but many doctors advise treatment with antibiotics anyway. In addition, most infants are not infected despite maternal infection. Of those who are, most have only minor symptoms. A few, however, eventually develop neurologic problems and partial blindness. A small percentage of these infants die of the disease.

Group B streptococci

Group B streptococci are bacteria that can be transmitted to the fetus during childbirth. As many as 20 percent of pregnant women tested in the last trimester of pregnancy harbor these bacteria in their vagina but have no symptoms. If these bacteria are identified, you'll likely be treated with antibiotics during labor to prevent transmission of the bacteria to the baby as the baby travels through the vagina.

Although many infants are born with these bacteria, infection develops in only 2 or 3 per 1,000. An infant with group B streptococcal disease usually shows signs of infection within 48 hours after delivery, which include breathing problems and shock. Occasionally, an infant will be a week old before symptoms develop. Immediate treatment with antibiotics is necessary for infants with this infection.

Genital herpes

Genital herpes is a sexually transmitted disease (STD) that appears as painful blisters on the genitals. The cervix or upper vagina also may have blisters, which may not produce symptoms. In a newborn, herpes can cause serious damage to the eyes and central nervous system or, rarely, death.

There's no cure for genital herpes. After one attack, it may be a month or years before the next. Some women carry the virus but never have symptoms. If you have confirmed herpes or suspect that you have the virus, tell your doctor.

The danger to the baby is generally thought to result from exposure to the virus during an active (primary) infection in the mother as the baby travels down the birth canal. If an examination or test confirms that you have active herpes near your delivery time, your doctor may want to deliver the baby by Caesarean section. Women with herpes may be given preventive medications during the last 3 weeks of pregnancy to prevent a herpes outbreak during delivery.

Hepatitis B

Hepatitis B is a liver infection caused by the hepatitis B virus. This virus is transmitted through the exchange of bodily fluids. If you have the hepatitis B virus, it can be transmitted to your fetus through the placenta. Risk of premature birth is higher among women who have hepatitis B. In addition, a newborn baby can become infected by the virus.

A test for hepatitis B is generally done as part of prenatal care. If you have hepatitis B, your infant can be given an injection of antibodies against the virus following delivery.

Because the hepatitis virus also may be found in breast milk, a mother with hepatitis B shouldn't breast-feed.

Syphilis

Syphilis is a serious sexually transmitted disease that can be passed from a pregnant mother to her baby. If you have syphilis, you may see one or more lesions (chancres) on your genitals. Sometimes, they may go unnoticed. The lesions occur 10 to 90 days after exposure. About 6 weeks later, you may notice a rash.

During your first prenatal visit, you'll be tested for syphilis, as required by law. The disease can be treated with penicillin. At birth, your infant will be tested. If the baby has congenital syphilis, treatment is initiated immediately.

Gonorrhea

Gonorrhea is another sexually transmitted disease that can be effectively treated with antibiotics. However, if you have untreated gonorrhea, your baby will be exposed during the birth process.

Infection with gonorrhea may result in damage to your baby's eyes. For this reason, all newborns receive preventive treatment immediately after birth. This consists of an antibiotic ointment applied under the baby's eyelids.

A discharge of pus from the baby's eyes may be a sign that the infant has gonorrhea. If you have gonorrhea, your infant is treated with penicillin.

Chlamydia

Chlamydia, another sexually transmitted disease, can cause an eye infection (conjunctivitis) in a newborn. This usually appears during the second week of life. If treated with antibiotics, the infection doesn't have any long-term adverse effects. The antibiotic ointment used to treat gonorrhea usually prevents this eye infection as well.

Cytomegalovirus

Cytomegalovirus (CMV) is the most common virus affecting the fetus. Each year, about 1 percent of newborns — about 40,000 babies — are born infected with this virus.

Fortunately, most of these babies don't develop problems. But about 8,000 newborns do experience disabilities from the virus. It can cause death or numerous birth defects, such as blindness, deafness, seizures, anemia and neurologic disorders. There's no effective treatment.

CMV is acquired by contact with blood or other bodily fluids, often in a child-care setting. Careful attention to hygiene is important for protection in this setting. CMV infection brings the risk of hearing loss in otherwise healthy babies.

Human papillomavirus

Human papillomavirus (HPV) causes warts on the skin or cervix. Such warts found on the genitals are called venereal warts. They're highly infectious, sexually transmitted and occasionally painful. The warts tend to grow faster during pregnancy.

Often, treatment during pregnancy isn't effective. Sometimes, the warts are so large that they interfere with the baby's passage down the birth canal, necessitating a Caesarean section.

AIDS

A pregnant woman can be infected by the human immunodeficiency virus (HIV) that causes AIDS through sexual intercourse with an infected partner, by injecting drugs with contaminated needles, through artificial insemination with semen containing the virus or by a blood transfusion. Because of improved screening measures, acquiring HIV through a blood transfusion is now rare.

If you have HIV or AIDS and are pregnant, you can pass the disease to your baby. Transmission from mother to baby occurs 20 percent to 25 percent of the time, but risk of transmission may be reduced to as low as 8 percent if the mother receives appropriate medication during pregnancy.

Pregnancy Risk Factors

Most pregnant women deliver healthy, normal babies at or near term. Some factors, however, tend to increase the chances of complications such as miscarriage, stillbirth and premature birth. Some of these factors, such as age, are to a large extent beyond your control. Others, such as smoking and alcohol use, are dangerous practices you should avoid.

Age

Age is especially worthy of some attention because many women are delaying pregnancy until their 30s and even 40s. Most healthy women older than age 35 have uneventful pregnancies. Because many of these women have planned their pregnancies, they're often highly motivated and take especially good care of themselves. There remains, however, an increased risk for mother and child.

Pregnant women older than age 35 are at greater risk of developing gestational diabetes and high blood pressure. The rates of miscarriage and stillbirth also are slightly higher because there's an increased risk that the mother will pass on chromosomal abnormalities to the fetus. Placenta previa — a condition in which the placenta covers the opening of the cervix — is more common among older mothers. Labor also tends to be slightly longer in older first-time mothers.

Teenagers also are at higher risk of complications of pregnancy. The risk may not be so much age-related as the result of the youthful mother being less interested in taking care of herself. Too frequently, pregnant teens have inadequate diets, engage in illegal use of drugs and alcohol and get little or no prenatal care, which can result in a higher frequency of preeclampsia and eclampsia, a potentially fatal condition to both the mother and baby. In addition, they have higher rates of miscarriage, intrauterine growth restriction, stillbirths and premature births than do women a few years older.

Diet

An inadequate diet increases your risk of giving birth to an infant with a low birth weight, which makes the infant more vulnerable to infection, disease and death. Failure to gain an adequate amount of weight during pregnancy can adversely affect your baby. If you've been poorly nourished most of your life, the effects may be felt by your baby despite improved nutrition during pregnancy.

Smoking

Smoking is a difficult habit to break, but it's not impossible, as millions of Americans can attest. Studies show that mothers who smoke a pack or more of cigarettes a day consistently have smaller babies than do nonsmokers. A small baby is generally weaker and more vulnerable to illness than one of average size. Moreover, smokers are more apt to have their pregnancy end in miscarriage or stillbirth.

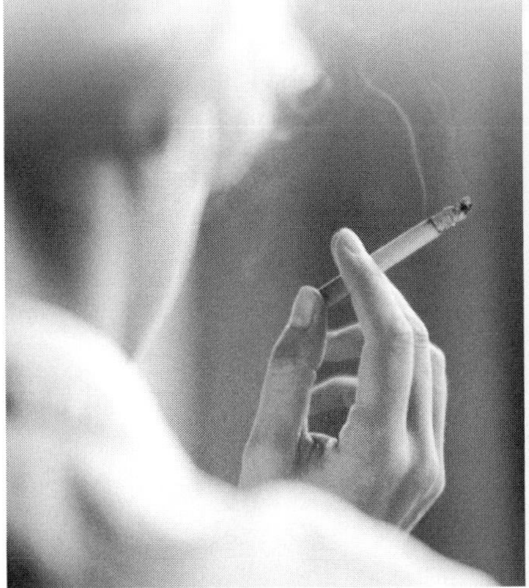

Alcohol

Alcohol use during pregnancy is the leading preventable cause of mental retardation in infants. There's no known safe level of alcohol use during pregnancy, so your doctor will probably advise you not to drink at all during your pregnancy.

If you drink excessive alcohol, your baby may be born with fetal alcohol syndrome. It's characterized by prenatal and postnatal growth retardation, facial abnormalities, heart defects, joint and limb problems and intellectual impairments. Results of studies using different methods and data sources suggest prevalence of the syndrome in the United States ranges from 3 to 22 cases per 10,000 births.

The more alcohol you drink, the greater the risk of having a child with fetal alcohol syndrome or other problems. Up to 33 percent of infants whose mothers are heavy

Intrauterine Growth Restriction

An infant who's born extremely small for its gestational age — below the 10th percentile — is considered to be growth restricted. Intrauterine growth restriction often occurs when the fetus doesn't get adequate nourishment from the mother through the placenta.

An infant born small for gestational age doesn't have the amount of body fat that a normal-sized newborn does. Thus, the infant has difficulty maintaining a normal body temperature and blood sugar level. Moreover, many growth-restricted infants grow slowly throughout at least early childhood. They may also have some delayed intellectual development.

Many conditions and lifestyle characteristics can produce intrauterine growth restriction. A woman who smokes, uses drugs illegally or drinks large amounts of alcohol is more likely to produce a small infant. A mother who's malnourished or fails to gain adequate weight also is in danger of giving birth to a small infant. Certain chronic diseases, such as cardiovascular disease, lupus or high blood pressure, also place you at risk.

Conditions related to pregnancy also can cause growth restriction. These include abnormalities of the placenta and cord, fetal infections or malformations and the presence of more than one fetus.

When a fetus isn't growing at a proper rate because of smoking, a poor diet or alcohol or illegal drug use, a change to a healthier lifestyle might help. If the fetus is still far from term, the risk of early delivery must be weighed against the risk of leaving it in the womb and allowing further malnutrition.

Congenital Defects

Birth defects, the leading cause of infant mortality in the United States, account for more than 20 percent of all infant deaths. In the United States, of approximately 120,000 babies born each year with a birth defect, 8,000 die during their first year of life.

Some defects correlate with the age of the mother. For example, if you're 30 years old, your chance of having a baby with Down syndrome is 1 in more than 900 births. If you're older than age 40, the incidence is about 1 in 100 births. Pregnant women who take certain medications or have diseases such as diabetes or alcoholism also are at increased risk of giving birth to a child with birth defects, as are women who have intrauterine infections.

drinkers have some congenital abnormality, whereas fewer than 5 percent whose mothers didn't drink during pregnancy have a congenital abnormality.

Illegal use of drugs

More infants are being born with both drug addiction and severe health problems. Pregnant women who use heroin or cocaine are two to six times more likely to have a baby who's born prematurely or at a low birth weight. The pregnancy also is apt to be complicated by high blood pressure or vaginal bleeding.

Approximately half the infants born to addicted mothers also are addicted to drugs. Generally, within the first day of life, the heroin-addicted infant becomes irritable and has convulsions, congestion, vomiting, diarrhea and fever. Frequently, sedatives are given to the baby and then slowly withdrawn. The withdrawal must be slow, or the infant may experience convulsions.

Medications

Almost any drug you take during pregnancy affects your baby too. Even a seemingly innocent over-the-counter drug travels through the placenta to your baby. Therefore, avoid taking medication unless it's approved by your doctor.

Sometimes, the effects of fetal exposure to a drug don't appear for many years. Such is the case with the female offspring of women who took diethylstilbestrol (DES). In the past, this medication commonly was prescribed for women who were thought to be in danger of miscarriage or who had a history of miscarriage. In the 1970s, many adolescent girls and young women were found to have unusual vaginal, cervical and uterine changes. The one thing they had in common was that their mothers had taken DES while pregnant.

Sometimes, medications can't be avoided during pregnancy. If you have a condition for which medication is necessary, your doctor can usually select one that will help your problem with minimal risk to your baby. Many pregnant women develop urinary infections that require antibiotics. And often doctors recommend that pregnant women with a high fever due to a viral illness take acetaminophen and stay well hydrated.

In general, the most dangerous time to take medication is during the first trimester of pregnancy, because that's when most fetal development occurs and when the fetus is most vulnerable to injury. However, some medications are more dangerous when taken later in pregnancy.

The medications listed below are known to cause or are suspected of causing birth defects. This is not a complete list. Check with your doctor before taking any medication.

- Isotretinoin (Accutane) is used for acne. It can cause heart disease and severe facial and ear abnormalities in a baby.
- The antibiotic streptomycin can cause infant deafness when it's used by a pregnant woman for a lengthy time. The antibiotic tetracycline can lead to retarded bone growth and damage to tooth pigmentation in a baby.
- Dicumarol is an anticoagulant sometimes taken by pregnant women with heart disease or excessive blood clotting. In their infants, it can cause abnormal facial features and mental retardation.
- Phenytoin (Dilantin, Phenytek), an anticonvulsant used for seizure disorders (epilepsy), can cause tumors, restricted growth or other abnormalities in a baby.
- If used in excess, diuretics, taken to relieve fluid retention, can interfere with fetal nutrition.
- Methyltestosterone, used to treat breast cancer, can cause masculinization of the female fetus.
- Tranquilizers may produce infant tremors that continue for months after birth.

PREVENTION TIP

While you're pregnant, avoid saunas, steam baths or immersion above your hips in a hot tub because of a possible association with fainting and resultant injury. Hot baths and showers are fine.

In some cases, a medication can be used to help the fetus. Some abnormalities in fetal heart rate can be treated with cardiac medications given to the mother, even though she doesn't have a heart abnormality. Similarly, if your doctor anticipates that labor will have to be induced before 32 weeks of gestation because of a medical problem, the infant can be given corticosteroid medications before labor that may enable the infant to breathe better after birth.

Radiation

Radiation from X-rays can damage the fetus, though the exposure level that may cause problems is fairly high. Nonetheless, avoid X-rays

? Question and Answer

Is it OK to go to the dentist while I'm pregnant?

You don't want to neglect your teeth during pregnancy. Some women notice that they're gums get more sensitive and bleed more easily during pregnancy. It's a good idea to visit your dentist right before you become pregnant and once during your pregnancy for a regular checkup and cleaning.

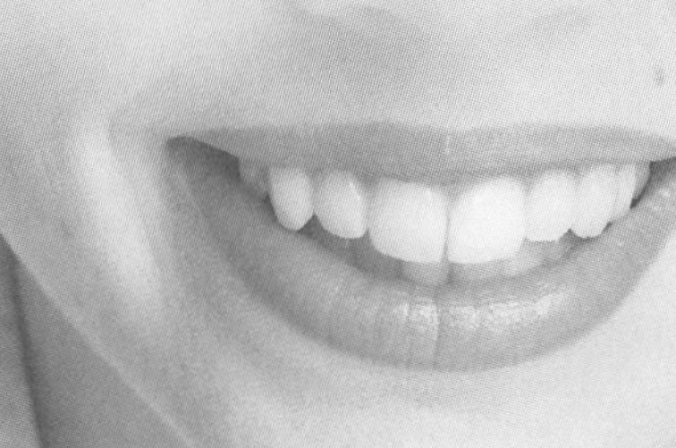

directed at the abdomen during pregnancy, if at all possible. Despite the risk, sparing use of X-rays may be necessary when a serious condition threatens the health of the mother.

Doctors are clearly aware of the potential risks of cumulative radiation to a fetus. Equipment also has improved so that less radiation is needed during diagnostic tests. These factors combine to make X-ray examinations relatively safe when a pregnant woman has a medical condition that requires them.

If you're pregnant, it's safe to have an X-ray of your teeth, head or extremities. Modern techniques protect your abdomen, and the only part of your body exposed to radiation is the area on which the X-ray is focused.

Prenatal Tests

Tests to determine if a fetus has a congenital defect are becoming increasingly common. In past years, women had to wait 9 months to know if their child had an abnormality. Now, women often can find out earlier in the pregnancy if the fetus they're carrying has a birth defect.

Life in the uterus isn't without risk. Sometimes, there's cause to suspect that your baby is in danger. Perhaps a previously active baby suddenly ceases to move, or blood tests reveal that an Rh-negative mother is developing antibodies against her Rh-positive fetus. Whatever the reason, if your doctor suspects something is wrong, several techniques can be used to evaluate fetal health, the goal being to find any sign of distress before irreparable damage is done.

One simple test is the Doppler ultrasound. It's used to detect the action of the fetal heart. It's a painless and noninvasive procedure in which a hand-held instrument is placed on your abdomen. This device can detect a heartbeat at 10 to 12 weeks and confirm a viable pregnancy.

Later in your pregnancy, you can document fetal movement each day by noting at least four movements in an hour during a time of day when the fetus is usually active. Fetal activity is generally felt more often after meals or at night when there are fewer external distractions. Keep in mind that the fetus has sleep cycles up to 1 hour throughout the day or night, during which time it won't move.

Ultrasound

The advent of ultrasound examination (ultrasonography) has made it possible to visualize the embryo as early as 6 to 7 weeks after your last menstrual period. This noninvasive and painless diagnostic tool uses high-frequency sound waves to produce an image of your baby. Safe for both mother and baby, it has proved invaluable in many instances.

In addition to its use in determining fetal age, ultrasound can show whether you're carrying more than one baby. It also allows your doctor to monitor your baby's rate of growth to determine if it's normal for gestational age.

With ultrasound, it may be possible to tell whether the fetus has kidney disease, an intestinal obstruction or is missing an arm or leg. The fetal brain can also be examined for some abnormalities using ultrasound. The position of the placenta and your baby's position in the womb can be determined. This diagnostic tool can also detect excessive amniotic fluid (hydramnios).

In many cases, ultrasound can also reveal the sex of your baby. An examination after 18 to 20 weeks of your pregnancy is an opportune time to obtain this information.

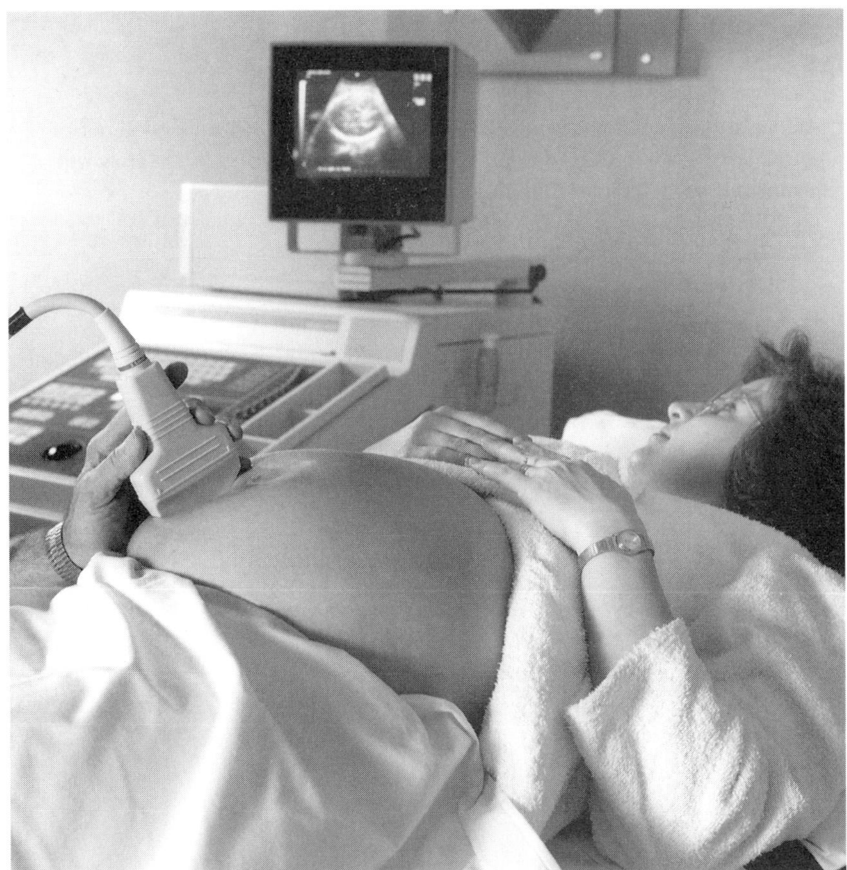

Ultrasound examination painlessly reveals the shape of the fetus within the uterus. Fetal age can be determined by measuring the width of the skull.

Triple test

The triple test is a set of biochemical tests that your doctor may offer between 15 and 18 weeks of your pregnancy. The triple test is a screening test, not a diagnostic test. Screening is done when no risk factors or symptoms are present. A screening test can only assess your risk of having a baby with a certain birth defect. A diagnostic test can usually show whether your baby has a birth defect.

The triple test looks at levels of three substances normally present in the bloodstream of a pregnant woman:

- Maternal serum alpha-fetoprotein (MSAFP), a protein produced by the fetus
- Human chorionic gonadotropin (HCG), a hormone produced by the placenta
- Estriol, an estrogen produced by both the fetus and the placenta

Blood is drawn from the mother and then tested in a laboratory. High levels of MSAFP may indicate that the fetus has a neural tube defect, most commonly spina bifida or anencephaly, which is a partially or completely missing brain. Low levels of MSAFP may indicate Down syndrome. Abnormal levels of HCG and estriol also may indicate chromosomal abnormalities. The timing of the tests is crucial, as the levels of these substances change throughout the pregnancy.

These tests aren't ideal. They're intended to screen rather than diagnose. This means that even among mothers who have a positive test result, their babies are only somewhat more likely to have one of the conditions. The opposite may be true as well — the tests don't catch all high-risk babies. There's a small chance that the results will be negative, indicating the baby is healthy, when in fact the child is born with a neural tube defect or Down syndrome.

Some women find the triple test reassuring. Some women find the inconclusiveness of the test to be more stressful than not having the information. If the results come back indicating a possible problem with the baby, often the next step is to have an ultrasound and amniocentesis.

Whether to have this set of tests is a personal choice. Talk to your doctor about the benefits and disadvantages and consider them carefully before making a decision.

Prenatal Tests: Factors to Consider

Asking questions and discussing concerns with your doctor or a genetics counselor before undergoing prenatal tests can be helpful. Here are some important points to consider and questions to ask:

1. What information can the test provide?
2. How accurate are the test results?
3. How often do you perform this procedure?
4. Is there a risk of miscarriage from the procedure?
5. If a problem is discovered, what are my options?
6. Can this information change the way I prepare for the baby?
7. Might this information change my mind about continuing the pregnancy?

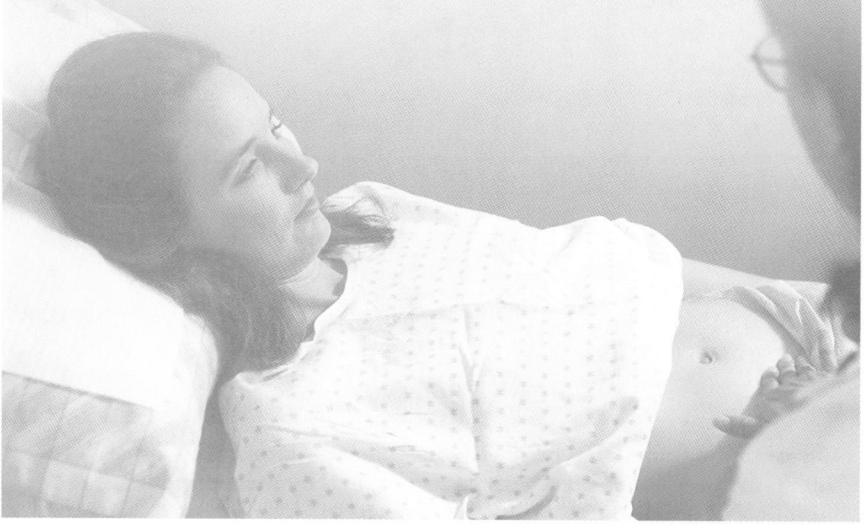

Amniocentesis

Amniocentesis is a test that you may choose to have performed early in the second trimester of pregnancy, usually between 14 and 16 weeks gestation. It may be offered to women 35 or older, women who have a family history of congenital abnormalities, such as Down syndrome or spina bifida, women who've previously given birth to a child with an abnormality, and women with an abnormal level of alpha-fetoprotein determined from a blood test.

Researchers are working on a more accurate blood test to identify Down syndrome. But currently the only way to be 100 percent certain if your child has Down syndrome or a variety of other defects is with an amniocentesis.

During amniocentesis, a doctor inserts a long, thin needle, guided by ultrasonography, into your uterus. The needle punctures the amniotic sac in which the fetus floats. A small amount of amniotic fluid is withdrawn, and the needle is then removed. The fluid is sent to the laboratory for tests. There's a 1 in 200 risk of losing the pregnancy as a result of the procedure.

Amniotic fluid contains valuable genetic information about your growing baby. After a few days in a culture medium, cells within the fluid can be studied for chromosome distribution.

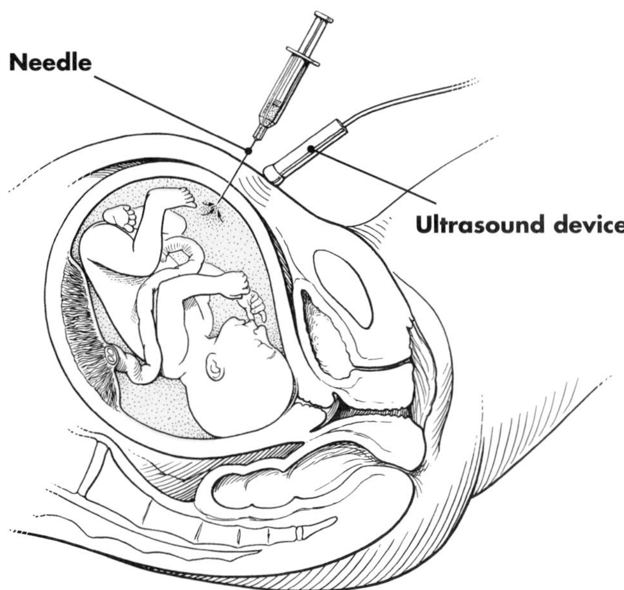

Amniocentesis involves removal of a small amount of amniotic fluid from the sac containing the fetus. Guided by an ultrasound image, a doctor inserts a long, thin needle into the uterus and withdraws fluid. Laboratory analysis of the fluid can reveal such things as your baby's sex, development and chromosome pattern.

The presence of Down syndrome, indicated by the presence of an extra chromosome 21, can be accurately diagnosed with amniocentesis. In addition, other defects such as neurologic problems, kidney diseases and metabolic disorders may be detected.

Amniocentesis can also be used later in pregnancy to monitor Rh incompatibility or to ascertain if the lungs are developed enough to withstand an early delivery.

Amniocentesis is usually safe for mother and child, but when it's done early in a pregnancy, it increases the risk of miscarriage after the procedure.

FISH

One of the difficulties of amniocentesis is the wait that's required for the results. If you undergo amniocentesis, you'll have to wait 7 to 14 days to find out if your baby has one of the detectable problems.

A test called FISH (fluorescence *in situ* hybridization) can identify the majority of chromosomal abnormalities in as little as 1 or 2 days. FISH can identify chromosome aberrations such as Down syndrome, trisomy 13 syndrome and trisomy 18 syndrome. The trisomies are rare genetic disorders usually involving severe mental retardation and severe physical defects. Most babies with trisomy 13 or trisomy 18 die before they're a year old.

The FISH test is used in conjunction with amniocentesis. The test uses some of the amniotic fluid collected from the amniocentesis, so you needn't go through an additional procedure.

FISH is highly accurate, but not perfect, in identifying chromosomal defects. If the test indicates that the baby doesn't have chromosomal irregularities, the amniotic cells are still cultured to verify that the fetus doesn't have an abnormality.

Chorionic villus sampling

Chorionic villus sampling (CVS) is similar to amniocentesis in that it's an invasive technique that can detect many genetic abnormalities, including Down syndrome. But rather than examining amniotic fluid, it examines tissue from the placenta. An advantage of this test is that it can be done between 9 and 11 weeks of gestation, earlier than other tests.

During CVS, your doctor uses ultrasonography to guide a small tube (catheter) into your cervix. He or she then uses a suction procedure to obtain a small piece of the placenta supporting the embryo. You might feel slight discomfort but little more than is normally felt during a pelvic examination.

The removed tissue contains the same chromosomes as your developing baby. Following analysis of the tissue, your doctor can determine whether your child has Down syndrome or other chromosome defects. The test also can determine the baby's sex.

CVS isn't as effective as amniocentesis for detecting some disorders, however. Sometimes, amniocentesis is used after chorionic villus sampling.

As with amniocentesis, CVS increases your risk of miscarriage. In addition, risk of intrauterine infection is greater than that associated with amniocentesis.

Percutaneous umbilical cord sampling

Percutaneous umbilical cord sampling is a technique that tests fetal blood from the umbilical cord for diagnosis of certain disorders. The procedure is done most easily in the third trimester.

Percutaneous umbilical cord sampling can also be used to determine oxygen and carbon dioxide levels in the blood, which may help diagnose growth restriction. In addition, the sampling can be used to check for infections such as cytomegalovirus.

Electronic fetal nonstress and stress tests

Electronic fetal nonstress and stress tests evaluate the fetal heart rate. The tests may be used when a woman notices a marked reduction

Rhesus (Rh) Factor Compatibility

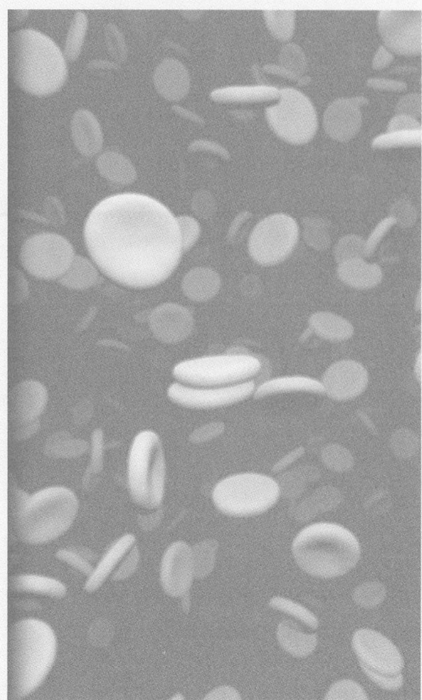

During pregnancy and especially at birth, some of your baby's blood can enter your bloodstream. If your blood and that of your child are compatible, no problem occurs. However, if they're incompatible, you can develop antibodies that could be a threat to subsequent pregnancies.

Blood groups are determined by the presence of certain protein molecules on the surface of blood cells. Rhesus (Rh) factor is one of these blood groups. Eighty-five percent of whites are Rh positive, which means they have the Rh component in their blood cells. Among black Americans, the percentage is slightly higher, and virtually all American Indians and Asians are Rh positive.

About 15 percent of whites and 7 percent of blacks are Rh negative. If you're Rh negative, you don't have a potential problem unless the father of your baby is Rh positive. If the baby inherits the father's Rh-positive blood, the blood of the baby is incompatible with your blood.

In most cases, the first child isn't at risk even if it's Rh positive because your Rh-negative blood hasn't had prior exposure to Rh-positive blood and so hasn't developed the antibodies that would attack the fetus. However, if you become pregnant again and the fetus is Rh positive, these antibodies can pass through the placenta and harm the developing baby. This risk increases with each Rh-incompatible pregnancy.

Rh disease isn't the problem it once was because of more thorough screening techniques, use of a serum that prevents the Rh-negative woman from developing antibodies and more effective therapy for infants who are affected.

If you're pregnant and your Rh factor isn't known, your doctor will order a blood test that can determine whether you're Rh negative or Rh positive. If you're Rh negative, periodic blood tests will be required throughout your pregnancy to check for development of antibodies. Although unlikely to occur during a first pregnancy, it isn't unheard of. If you've had a prior abortion or a miscarriage, it's possible that some of the fetus's blood cells entered your body and triggered the development of antibodies. There's also the possibility of small leaks of fetal blood during pregnancy.

Doctors often give pregnant women who are Rh negative a shot of RhoGAM at 28 to 30 weeks of gestation as a precaution should there be some early leakage of fetal blood. This serum masks any fetal red blood cells that have entered your circulation before your body has time to marshal its forces against them. There's almost no risk from the shot.

If antibodies have developed, the result may be mild or severe damage or death to the fetus, and an early delivery may be necessary. The infant may be given a blood transfusion while still in the womb. This is done to buy time until the baby's lungs are developed enough so that he or she can withstand an early delivery. After birth, additional blood transfusions will be needed.

in the amount of movement of the fetus, when she has a disease that threatens the fetus or when her baby's growth rate seems to be abnormally slow. They may also be used for women with symptoms of preeclampsia, a history of stillbirth or diabetes.

Nonstress test

The first step is often the nonstress test. During this test, you lie on your back and a recording device connected to an electronic monitor is attached to your abdomen. Fetal heart rate, uterine contractions and fetal movements are recorded.

Stress test

Contraction stress testing is usually done when the results of the nonstress test are abnormal. If your doctor recommends this test, you'll be given a medication that stimulates contractions. The effect of the contractions on the fetus is then monitored.

This test can help your doctor determine if your infant is at increased risk of dying in the womb (in utero). If so, a decision to induce labor may be made if the fetus is old enough to survive.

The test can also help your doctor determine if the infant is able to withstand a normal labor and vaginal delivery.

Biophysical profile scoring

A biophysical profile combines an ultrasound exam with a nonstress test. Most often, the following five factors of the fetus are monitored for a period of time, usually 30 minutes:

- Heart rate
- Breathing
- Body movement
- Muscle tone
- Amount of amniotic fluid

Each of these factors is given a score and added together for a final score. The results are on a scale of 1 to 10. A 10 is perfect. A score of 6 or less is cause for concern.

First Trimester

The first trimester of pregnancy can be difficult for an expectant mother and is the time when a developing embryo is most vulnerable. Virtually every organ in your baby's body is being formed during the first 3 months of pregnancy. Thus, the embryo is particularly sensitive.

If you take drugs, drink alcohol or are exposed to toxins or improper or excessive use of X-rays, the baby's development can go awry, and the result can be birth defects. Miscarriage also is more likely to occur during this critical first trimester.

The average time from fertilization to the birth of a baby is 266 days. Compared with the duration of gestation in most other species, that might seem an incredibly long time. Yet when you consider the magnitude of this creation, it's a wonder it doesn't take longer.

It's difficult to comprehend how something as complex as a human being can emerge from a single fertilized cell. Every aspect of this process, from the creation of the smallest fingernail to the brain itself, is set into an exquisitely scripted timetable that rarely falters. If it does, the result can be a miscarriage or birth defect.

Changes in you

For you, the first 3 months of your pregnancy can seem like riding a roller coaster. You're delighted yet have some fears. If the pregnancy was unplanned, you may be losing sleep figuring out how you'll cope with this enormous change in your life. Physically, you may feel drained and find yourself napping whenever you get the opportunity. Rest assured that these weeks will pass quickly and so will most of the symptoms.

The first sign of pregnancy for most women is a missed menstrual period. If your periods are usually regular and suddenly you're a week late and you've had intercourse during your cycle, take a pregnancy test. Sometimes, a woman will have what appears to be a period even though she is pregnant. However, the bleeding is usually scant.

Many pregnant women experience breast tenderness. Your breasts may seem fuller and tingle. The nipples are often extremely sensitive. Sometimes the breasts actually hurt. Many pregnant women experience morning sickness, which may range from a slightly upset stomach to incessant vomiting. This often begins a few days after the first missed period.

Fatigue is common during early pregnancy. If you're home during the day, you'll probably find yourself lying down for a nap. If you work outside the home, you may arrive home so tired you can't wait to go to bed.

Frequent urination is another sign of pregnancy. This occurs because the growing uterus exerts pressure on the bladder in the pelvis. As the size of your uterus begins to increase in your abdomen, this symptom will diminish. However, in the final weeks of pregnancy it returns, and many women find themselves unable to sleep through the night because of the need to urinate.

If you've missed a period and experienced some of these other signs and symptoms, give yourself a home pregnancy test or make an appointment to have a blood test at your doctor's office. Many women receive prenatal care from a doctor specially trained in the care of pregnant women and the delivery of babies (obstetrician). Some family doctors also offer this service to their patients. In some communities, licensed, certified nurse midwives also provide maternity care.

A certified nurse midwife has, at a minimum, a degree in nursing, specializing in obstetrics and gynecology, and has passed several examinations to receive certification. Nurse midwives provide complete obstetrical care for normal, healthy pregnancies and are trained to screen mothers for potential problems. In case of a problem, the mother is referred to a doctor.

In most states, nurse midwives are permitted to prescribe medications and vitamins, but they don't perform Caesarean deliveries or administer anesthetics. Most nurse midwives attend births in hospitals or birthing centers. Some with private, solo practices assist in births in the home. All nurse midwives are legally required to be associated with a backup doctor or group of doctors they can call on in case a problem develops.

Baby's development

So much happens to the fetus in the first 3 months. Still, the fetus is so small that for most women, no one can tell they're pregnant by just looking.

Fertilization

The process of fertilization begins with the penetration of the egg by a single sperm, one of the millions that traveled up the female reproductive system. Enzymes in the head of the sperm allow it to penetrate the firm capsule (zona pellucida) of the egg.

Swimming in an indirect path, the sperm swarm around the egg with the sides of their heads. Several sperm may begin to enter the outer egg capsule, but ultimately only one will enter the egg itself.

The egg and sperm each bring to the union 23 chromosomes containing thousands of genes. In these 46 chromosomes is the genetic material that determines sex, physical characteristics — such as eye, hair and skin color, body size and type, facial features — creativity and, to a large extent, intellectual capabilities and even personality. After the sperm penetrates to the center of the egg and the sperm and egg merge, fertilization is complete.

Multiple births result either from the fertilization of two or more eggs or from a single egg being fertilized

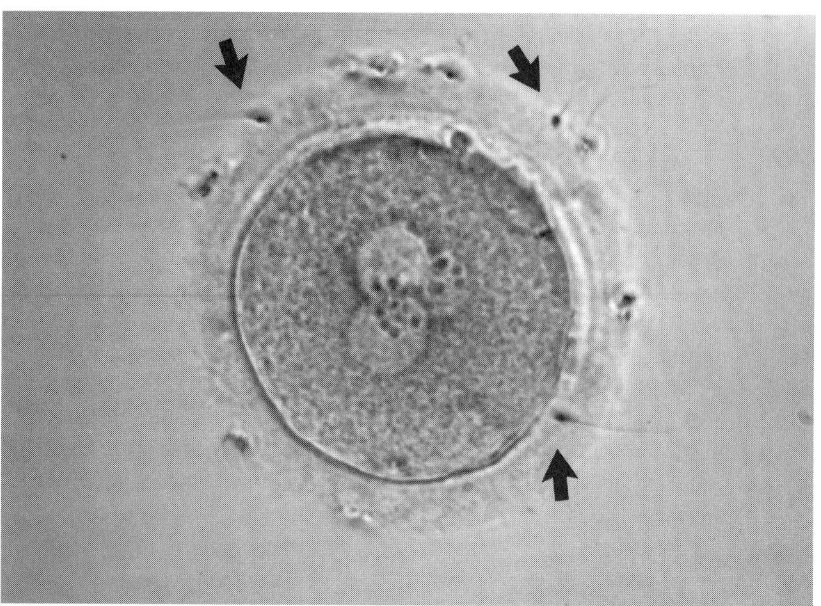

A recently fertilized ovum in an early stage of cell division. Some sperm entered the capsule but did not penetrate the egg (see arrows).

and then splitting to form two or more embryos.

Cell division

The next step in the process is cell division. Within 12 hours, the new cell has divided into two cells, each of which then becomes two cells, and so on, with the number of cells doubling every 12 hours. It's now called a zygote.

The new zygote continues to make its way slowly down the fallopian tube to the uterus, regularly doubling its cell numbers and becoming a bit larger and much more complex. Within 4 to 5 days after fertilization, the zygote — by this time made up of 500 cells — reaches its destination inside the uterus.

By the time the zygote reaches the uterus, it has changed considerably from a solid mass of cells to a group of cells arranged around a fluid-filled cavity called a blastocyst. One section of the blastocyst contains a compact mass of cells that will ultimately produce an embryo. The outer layer of cells (trophoblast) will produce the placenta, which provides nourishment.

While all this has been taking place, the rest of the female reproductive system hasn't been idle. The ovaries have been secreting the hormone progesterone into the bloodstream. The result of this hormonal surge is a uterine lining that's swollen with blood, the perfect environment for implantation to take place.

Initially, the blastocyst doesn't dig deeply into the uterus. It clings to the surface of the uterus for a few days. Then the blastocyst releases an enzyme that eats away at the lining of the uterus, allowing the mass to drop deeper into the lining, where it's surrounded by a pool of the mother's blood. Eight days have passed since fertilization took place. By the 12th day, the blastocyst will be firmly embedded in its new home.

At this point, you're pregnant, although it's too early for you to have missed a period or to have any other symptoms of pregnancy. In the initial days and weeks after fertilization, miscarriage is common, often before a woman knows she was pregnant. In fact, an estimated 50 percent of fertilizations end in miscarriage.

Organ formation

By the time the zygote burrows into the uterus, the placenta has begun to form. In another week, the rudiments of a spinal cord are evident and, within days, five to eight vertebrae are in place. In addition, the eyes and heart have begun to form.

It's during the third week after fertilization that the embryonic period begins. This is about the time that an expected period doesn't happen. If you take a pregnancy test, the results will probably be positive.

Over the next few weeks, the components of a human being develop, although at first the human baby is similar in appearance to the developing babies of some other mammals. The head begins to form, as does the intestinal tract.

At the end of the sixth week, the brain becomes more noticeable, and arm and leg buds begin to appear. Cells that will later become either ovaries or testicles have appeared. By the seventh week, the chest and abdomen are fully formed, and the lungs are beginning to develop. The embryo measures slightly more than a half inch and weighs a fraction of an ounce.

Your baby's face and features are forming in the eighth gestational week. Fingers and toes are beginning to develop, as are the ovaries or testicles. If the embryo is a male, his penis begins to appear at this time. At the end of the second

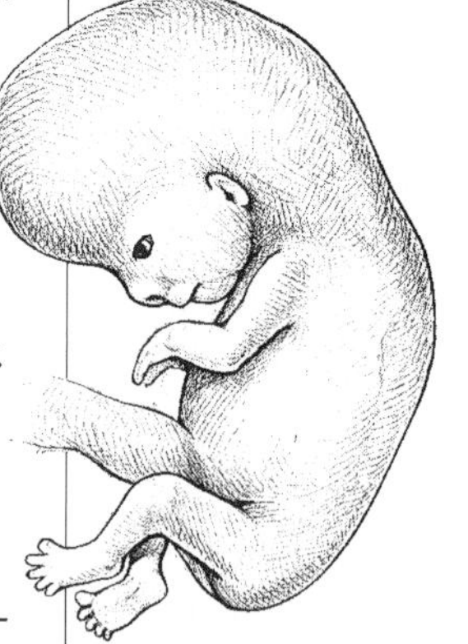

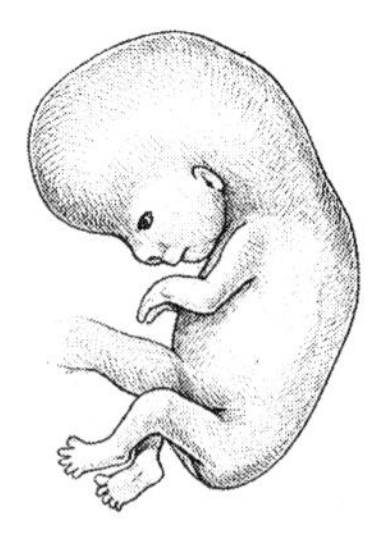

Actual size

At 8 weeks following conception, all of the major body organs are formed and growing. The embryo is about 1½ inches long from head to rump and weighs less than half an ounce.

Twins and Multiple Pregnancies

What are the chances that you're expecting twins? Without fertility assistance, a teenager has a 1 in 167 chance of having twins, but the rate for a 40-year-old woman is 1 in 55. In addition, having fraternal twins, or twins born of two separate eggs and sperm, may run in some families.

A multiple pregnancy occurs when more than one egg is fertilized or one egg splits after fertilization. Seven of 10 pairs of twins are fraternal, meaning they came from two eggs and two sperm. Abnormal weight gain or size, an excessive amount of movement and the detection of two heartbeats are common clues that you're carrying twins. If your doctor suspects twins, he or she will likely order an ultrasound examination.

With multiple births, try to increase the amount of rest you get, take in more calories and be diligent about your prenatal visits. Adherence to your prenatal checkup schedule is especially important because when you're carrying multiple fetuses, you have a higher risk of preeclampsia and eclampsia, placenta previa — a condition in which the placenta covers the cervix — and vaginal bleeding (hemorrhage).

Multiple pregnancies tend to be shorter, an average of 21 days shorter for women delivering twins. Unless there's a medical reason to indicate Caesarean delivery, twins can be delivered vaginally. And a woman with twins who wants to breast-feed can do so.

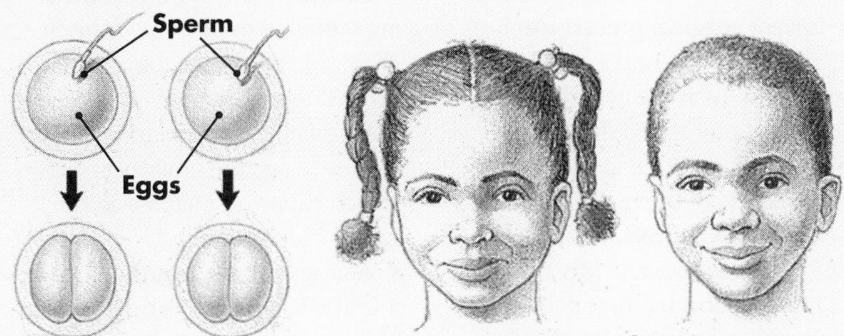

Fraternal twins, the most common kind, occur when two eggs are fertilized by two different sperm, leading to two individuals who are no more closely related than other brothers and sisters in a family.

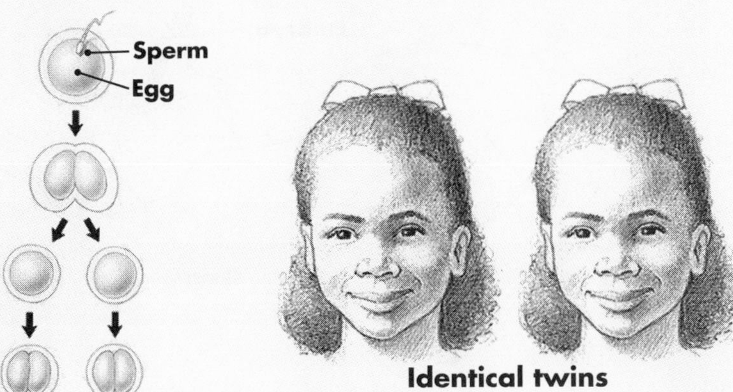

Identical twins occur when a single fertilized egg, for reasons that are unclear, splits and develops into two individuals who are genetically identical.

month of pregnancy, your baby looks much like a human infant, albeit in miniature.

By the tenth week, your baby's face is well developed. The heart has four chambers and beats 120 to 160 times a minute. Using a Doppler instrument, your doctor can hear the heartbeat somewhere between 10 and 12 weeks. At this point, the embryo is referred to as a fetus.

By the end of the first trimester, the fetus has a head that's disproportionately large compared with the rest of its body. Your baby is about 3 inches long and weighs little more than 1 ounce.

Possible problems

Having a baby today is safer than at any other time in history. We now know that a lot of problems can be prevented with good nutrition and regular prenatal care. But forming a new human being is still complex, and complications and problems do arise. Following are some of the troubles most common in the first trimester:

Miscarriage

Aside from the initial discomfort of pregnancy, the greatest threat in the first trimester is miscarriage (spontaneous abortion). Miscarriage and abortion refer to the termination of a pregnancy before the time the fetus can survive even for a few minutes outside the womb, which is generally before the 20th week after conception. A fetus born dead after the 20th week is termed stillborn.

About 50 percent of all fertilized eggs spontaneously abort, most of them before a woman is aware she's pregnant. The percentage of miscarriages in women who know they're pregnant is about 15 percent. Three-quarters of these miscarriages occur in the first trimester. Factors associated with miscarriage include older maternal age, difficulty in becoming pregnant and a history of miscarriage.

In the first trimester, miscarriage almost always occurs after the death of the embryo or fetus. Why does an embryo die in the uterus? The most common cause of miscarriage — an estimated 60 percent — is an abnormality in development, usually as a result of extra chromosomes. Other possible causes include infections, unrecognized diabetes in the mother and defects in the uterus.

Women who suffer a miscarriage tend to blame themselves. It's natural to seek an explanation when a miscarriage occurs, but try not to blame yourself. Almost never is miscarriage the result of stress or trauma.

The first symptom of a potential miscarriage is usually vaginal bleeding, with or without cramping. Approximately one in five women have some vaginal bleeding or bloody discharge during the first trimester, and less than half of these women lose their babies. However, if you have any bleeding, call your doctor immediately.

When the embryo or fetus dies, miscarriage is inevitable. An inevitable miscarriage is usually accompanied by pain in the lower abdomen or back. The pain may be dull and relentless or sharp and intermittent. Bleeding may be heavy. Tissue may emerge from your vagina. This is the embryo and placenta.

If possible, save it and give it to your doctor, who can examine it to be sure the pregnancy wasn't a tubal pregnancy, which is a type of ectopic pregnancy. Ectopic pregnancies can be dangerous and need immediate attention. With any kind of miscarriage, though, rarely can doctors determine the cause of death from such tissue.

Sometimes, only some of the products of conception are expelled. When this occurs, it is called an incomplete abortion, and the pain and bleeding can continue for several days. If there's no bleeding — neither the fetus nor the placenta is expelled — but the fetus has died, it's termed a missed abortion. You may feel pregnant and have no idea of a problem during a missed abortion, but the symptoms of pregnancy will eventually disappear. Your doctor may suspect miscarriage when your uterus fails to grow or when he or she can't detect a heartbeat during a visit. An ultrasound exam is often used to determine if you've experienced a missed abortion.

Once it starts, nothing can be done to prevent an inevitable, incomplete or missed abortion. With the use of vaginal ultrasound after spotting occurs, a doctor can usually tell if a miscarriage is inevitable.

When a miscarriage is inevitable, the mother has three options: She can wait for nature to take its course and the miscarriage to occur. This could take several weeks. She can have a surgical procedure called a dilatation and curettage (D and C), in which the embryo and placenta are removed. It carries a small risk of damage to the uterus. Or, she can take the medication misoprostal (Cytotec), which will provoke a miscarriage. Most doctors recommend waiting a few months after a miscarriage before trying to conceive again.

Ectopic pregnancy

Ectopic pregnancy occurs when the fertilized egg implants itself anywhere other than in the lining of the uterus. The fertilized egg may become implanted on the ovary or in the abdominal cavity, but in 95 percent of all ectopic pregnancies, the egg is implanted in the fallopian tube and is then called a tubal pregnancy.

You may have scanty, dark brown vaginal bleeding, abdominal pain, internal bleeding, severe cramping, a sudden urge to urinate or have a bowel movement or dizziness and fainting.

The interior of the fallopian tube is like a maze, with twists and turns and folds. Sometimes, for various reasons, the fertilized egg becomes stuck and implants in this unsuitable environment.

This growing zygote immediately begins to produce human chorionic gonadotropin (HCG), a hormone associated with pregnancy. The growing embryo then begins to secrete other hormones, which cause an increase in the tube's blood supply.

As the embryo continues to grow into the tube, vessels begin to bleed. Unlike the uterus, the tube wasn't made for pregnancy. As the embryo

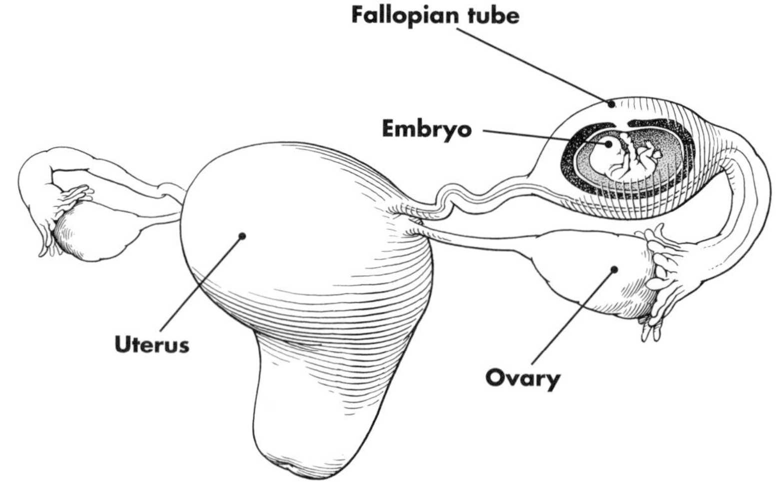

Potentially life-threatening, a tubal pregnancy occurs when a fertilized egg implants itself in the fallopian tube rather than the uterus. As the embryo develops, it causes the tube to expand beyond its capacity, causing bleeding (hemorrhaging) and potentially serious medical consequences.

grows, the tube becomes stretched beyond its capacity and significant bleeding (hemorrhage) often occurs. If the pregnancy continues long enough, the tube will rupture, a potentially life-threatening situation.

The frequency of ectopic pregnancy has increased in recent years. It now occurs in about 1 out of every 100 pregnancies. No one is certain why ectopic pregnancy has become more common. Some researchers speculate that an increase in the incidence of pelvic inflammatory disease may be at least partially responsible.

It's known, however, that some medical conditions tend to be associated with a higher risk of ectopic pregnancy. These include tubal adhesions caused by infection, appendicitis, endometriosis and the absence of one ovary.

If you have an ectopic pregnancy, initially you may not know that anything is wrong. Despite a missed menstrual period, results of a urine pregnancy test may be negative. If your doctor suspects an ectopic pregnancy, he or she will first do a pelvic examination to check for any abnormalities. An ultrasound examination or minimally invasive (laparoscopic) surgery may be done to confirm the presence of a mass.

If not detected early, an ectopic pregnancy is an extremely dangerous condition and is a leading cause of pregnancy-related death. There's no chance that the pregnancy can be carried to term or to a point at which the fetus has a good chance of surviving. Ectopic fetuses seldom develop beyond 3 months.

If you have an ectopic pregnancy, your doctor may want to operate immediately. If the embryo is still small and the fallopian tube hasn't been ruptured, the embryo may be squeezed out without further injury to the tube. Some doctors favor removing the injured part of the tube. If you've had massive hemorrhaging, a blood transfusion may be necessary. Removal of a tube and even of an ovary may be necessary.

Another option consists of using a powerful medication called methotrexate, which causes embryonic cells to stop growing and eventually disappear. In most cases, this replaces the need for surgery.

In women who've had one ectopic pregnancy, about 10 percent of subsequent pregnancies will be ectopic. If you've had two ectopic pregnancies, your chance of ever having a normal pregnancy is less than 50 percent. If the ectopic pregnancies have significantly injured both fallopian tubes but you still want to become pregnant, in vitro fertilization (see page 1069) may be the only option left.

Second Trimester

The middle part of the pregnancy is often the time when women feel their best. Usually, the morning sickness is gone, you have more energy and you start looking pregnant and feeling good. This is also the time when you'll start to feel those gentle flutters that will soon turn into strong kicks and elbowing from your growing baby.

Although the second trimester is the easiest part of pregnancy for most women, it's not without risks. Miscarriage isn't the risk that it was during the first 3 months, but some women begin premature labor during the second trimester. A fetus delivered this early isn't mature enough to survive. Although premature labor most often occurs during the third trimester, occasionally it may complicate the second trimester.

Changes in you

During the second trimester of pregnancy, your abdomen is enlarging slowly, and you'll probably need to start wearing maternity clothes. Your body is becoming rounder around the middle and probably at the hips, too, but it isn't yet unwieldy. For most women, the fourth, fifth and sixth months of pregnancy are uneventful and enjoyable.

At this stage, you're still seeing your doctor once a month, unless you have a medical condition that warrants more frequent visits. You're taking iron and folic acid supplements, and you're continuing to eat a balanced diet containing several servings each day of protein-rich foods including milk products, fruits, vegetables and grains.

If you've been contemplating travel, now is probably the best time during pregnancy to take a trip. As your due date approaches, your increased size will tax your energies, and you may be better off staying close to home.

Baby's development

During the second trimester, the fetus grows, and the organs that formed during the previous weeks mature.

At about 13 weeks, the fetus has tiny fingernails. The genitals are fully formed, and the sex can be determined with certain prenatal tests. The fetus can kick and move its toes. The mouth can open and close, and the fetus is capable of bending its arms and making a fist.

By the end of the fourth month, the heartbeat can be detected with a special stethoscope, though a Doppler instrument can detect a heartbeat much earlier. You're likely to feel the first signs of life in your abdomen. The fetus's skin is pink and less transparent than it was previously. Fine hair covers the entire body. The first eyelashes and eyebrows begin to appear.

At 20 weeks, the fetus may have hair on its head. Fat deposits begin to appear beneath the wrinkled skin. The fetus is now 12 inches long and weighs about 1 pound. If it's born at this time, it will attempt to breathe but will not survive.

Possible problems

As your pregnancy progresses, new dangers may emerge. While risks for miscarriage are greatly reduced, the concern now shifts to keeping the fetus growing and healthy in the uterus for the full term of the pregnancy.

Premature labor

Normally, labor occurs about 40 weeks (280 days) after the first day of your last period. If your baby is born between 37 and 42 weeks, delivery is considered to be at term. Sometimes, labor begins before term. You may have vaginal bleeding, mild to severe abdominal contractions or a gush or trickle of fluid from your vagina as your membranes rupture — or your water breaks, as it's often referred to.

Most often the precise cause of midpregnancy labor is never determined. However, the following conditions are associated with premature or preterm labor: spontaneous rupture of membranes, cervical infection, incompetent cervix, abnormal uterus, hydramnios, abnormal fetus or placenta, placenta previa — a condition in which the placenta covers the cervix — a retained intrauterine contraceptive device, preeclampsia and eclampsia, death of the fetus, history of premature delivery, multiple fetuses, cigarette smoking, bleeding (hemorrhaging), serious maternal disease and age. Teenagers and women older than age 40 are more likely to have premature labor.

Rupture of your membranes usually occurs after labor has begun, but occasionally it's the first step. If you have contractions that last for at least 30 seconds and occur every 10 minutes, and if your cervix is thinning and dilating, you're in labor.

Premature labor can be an ominous sign. The less time your infant has had in your womb, the less its chances of survival. In recent years, however, major advances have been made in the care of seriously ill or premature infants. Babies as small as 1 pound now have a chance of survival when cared for in specialized neonatal units.

A reasonable chance for survival of the baby is now being realized as early as 24 weeks gestation. Still, these babies often have serious, lifelong physical and intellectual developmental problems.

The treatment for premature labor varies and depends on the age of the fetus. Initially, many doctors prescribe bed rest and drinking plenty of fluid. This precaution alone is sometimes successful in stopping contractions. Cultures from the cervix and preventive antibiotics also may be considered because infection is believed to be one cause of premature labor.

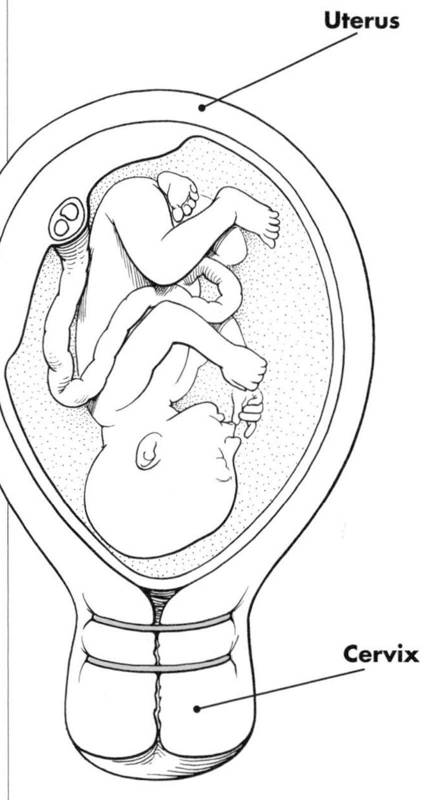

If the lower portion of your uterus (cervix) opens during pregnancy, a surgical procedure may be done to prevent premature delivery of your baby. Called cerclage, this procedure involves stitching the cervix closed to prevent expulsion of the fetus from the uterus.

There's no specific medication that's always successful in stopping premature labor. But several have had some degree of success. Under most circumstances, medications that can delay delivery are used only long enough to prepare for the delivery, such as getting the mother to a hospital equipped to care for premature babies. The drugs aren't used long term because they may pose risks and aren't effective over the long term.

If your premature labor is determined to be the result of a defect in your cervix, sometimes an operation can be done to forestall labor. A procedure called cerclage involves placing surgical stitches (sutures) around the cervix so that the infant can stay in the uterus until term.

Another cause of prematurity occurs when your doctor needs to induce labor early because the uterine environment appears to be increasingly harmful to your baby and its chances of survival are better outside the uterus. This usually doesn't occur until after 28 weeks of gestation.

Hydramnios

Hydramnios refers to a condition in which an excessive amount of amniotic fluid surrounds the baby. You may feel breathlessness, indigestion, nausea, abdominal distention and intense pain. You may also experience preterm labor.

Normally, the fetus begins to urinate and to swallow amniotic fluid in the second trimester of pregnancy. Later in the pregnancy, these functions may help control the amount of fluid in the uterus. Hydramnios often is associated with birth defects, particularly with malformations of the central nervous system and gastrointestinal tract. Some of these defects prevent the fetus from swallowing amniotic fluid, and others may cause it to excrete an excessive amount of urine.

If your doctor suspects hydramnios, he or she will probably want you to have an ultrasound examination. In most cases, the swelling of the uterus from the excess fluid is slight and harmless. In about 1 of 1,000 pregnancies, however, the condition is severe enough to cause premature labor. Women with diabetes and those carrying multiple fetuses have a higher incidence of hydramnios than other pregnant women.

If the condition isn't severe, no treatment other than additional rest may be prescribed. If the pain is severe, hospitalization and sedation may be necessary. You may be given medications to relax your uterus and reduce the chance of premature labor. Sometimes, amniocentesis is recommended to remove some of the excess fluid. Although this relieves pain, it must be repeated often.

Incompetent cervix
If you have an incompetent cervix, the lower portion of your uterus opens during the second trimester or early part of the third trimester. The result is a miscarriage or premature delivery.

A woman with an incompetent cervix usually has a history of miscarriage, typically in the second trimester of pregnancy. The cervix usually doesn't open before the fourth month of pregnancy because the fetus isn't sufficiently large to dilate it.

The cause of incompetent cervix is unknown, but the condition is often associated with trauma to the cervix after procedures such as dilatation and curettage (D and C) and with abnormal development of the cervix.

If your medical history indicates a possible incompetent cervix, surgery can be done to close your cervix during pregnancy. Called cerclage, the procedure is performed while you're under general anesthesia. Using strong thread, your doctor stitches around your cervix to close it to prevent you from expelling the fetus. After the procedure, you may be given medication to reduce the chance that the procedure could stimulate premature labor.

Cerclage is successful in 85 percent to 90 percent of cases. The thread is cut in later months of pregnancy.

Third Trimester

During the third trimester of pregnancy, what seemed so far off just a few months ago is now within reach — almost. If you haven't done so yet, it's a good time to start practicing relaxation techniques for labor. Toward the end of this stage, your baby has less room to move around and often settles down into position for labor.

The vast majority of women deliver near term and have no major complications. The problem of premature labor may occur in the third trimester as well as in the second, but the later in pregnancy it occurs, the better the outlook for the infant.

Some serious conditions are associated with late pregnancy. Preeclampsia and eclampsia are dangerous conditions that, when not detected early, can cause both fetal and maternal death. Other problems that your doctor will be watching for include bleeding (hemorrhaging), placenta previa — a condition in which the placenta covers the cervix — premature rupture of membranes, intrauterine death and intrauterine growth restriction.

Changes in you

No matter how well you've felt, this is probably the point when you ask, "When will it be over?" Your maternity clothes are getting tight. Your walk has given way to the pregnant waddle. You may notice stretch marks on your breasts and abdomen. Your feet and ankles may be so swollen that your shoes don't fit. You may be exhausted.

You can't seem to get comfortable at night, and when you do the baby starts kicking. Finally, the kicking stops and you sleep an hour or two, and then you wake up with a strong urge to urinate. You may awaken the next morning looking as though you've been up all night.

During the last trimester of pregnancy, many couples attend classes in preparation for childbirth. These classes teach you about the birth process, about exercises you can do to strengthen your pelvic muscles, enabling you to push more effectively, and about relaxation and breathing techniques that may help to relieve some of the pain during labor. Doctors recommend these classes even for women who know they want to use a pain relief medication during labor and delivery.

Many women, particularly those who've previously miscarried in early pregnancy, understandably are relieved to reach the late stage of pregnancy. With proper treatment in a specialized neonatal unit, babies born after 30 weeks have a good chance of survival. But there's no substitute for a full-term pregnancy. Therefore, one of your doctor's goals is to prevent premature labor whenever possible.

Your visits to the doctor will be more frequent during the final trimester. Up until now, you've probably been seeing the doctor every 4 to 6 weeks, unless you have a medical problem that warrants more frequent visits. After the 30th gestational week, your doctor may want to see you every 2 weeks until the 36th week, when you'll probably begin weekly visits. Toward the end of your pregnancy, your doctor may perform a pelvic examination to see if your cervix is beginning to dilate in preparation for labor.

Baby's development

The fetus takes on most of its weight after week 27 in the pregnancy. At the beginning of this last phase of development, the fetus weighs almost 2 pounds. The average baby is born 3 months later weighing $7\frac{1}{2}$ pounds.

When you're 28 weeks pregnant, your baby is covered with a thick, white protective coating called vernix. The infant's eyes are open, and a baby born at this time can cry weakly and move its limbs. Although infants born at this stage weigh about only 2 pounds and may experience significant medical problems, 85 percent to 90 percent of them survive because of recent advances in the care of premature and ill newborns.

One month later, the male infant's testicles descend into the scrotum. The infant now weighs about 3 pounds 12 ounces. With proper care, most of these infants are capable of surviving.

An infant born at term, 40 weeks after the mother's last menstrual period, has a more rounded body and is less wrinkled than babies born earlier. The skin may or may not still be covered with vernix. Most of the body hair is gone, although the shoulders and arms may still have a light covering. The fingernails and toenails may extend beyond the fingers and toes.

Possible problems

Chances are, especially if you've been healthy to this point, the third trimester will be medically uneventful for you and your baby. But some of the most serious problems of pregnancy do occur in the third trimester, and it's important to be aware of them.

Preeclampsia and eclampsia

Preeclampsia is one of the most dangerous complications of pregnancy. It's critical to address preeclampsia, or the result will be permanent harm to you or your baby. The signs and symptoms are:

Preeclampsia

- High blood pressure
- Excessive protein in the urine (proteinuria)
- Fluid retention that causes puffiness of the hands and face, particularly around the eyes
- Sudden and excessive weight gain
- Pain in the upper right side of the abdomen
- Severe headache
- Vision disturbances, including seeing flashing lights

Eclampsia

- Convulsions
- Unconsciousness

Preeclampsia can be a serious disease of late pregnancy that must be treated. Preeclampsia occurs in about 6 percent to 8 percent of all pregnancies, and the overall incidence of eclampsia is about 1 in 1,500 pregnancies.

Preeclampsia and eclampsia are often called toxemias of pregnancy, although no one has been able to identify a toxic substance in a pregnant woman's blood that can cause them. Hence, the cause remains unknown. The only known treatment is delivery of the baby. Doctors do know, though, how to diagnose the conditions and identify some women at higher risk.

If preeclampsia develops, you may not know it. Initially, you may feel normal because high blood pressure and protein in the urine do not cause symptoms. This is one reason it's so important to keep your prenatal appointments. As preeclampsia progresses, signs and symptoms may occur.

Preeclampsia can lead to bleeding in the brain, liver or kidneys, and it can be fatal for both mother and baby. Teenage mothers, women older than age 40, women in their first pregnancy, women with a history of high blood pressure and women who are carrying twins all are at higher risk of preeclampsia and eclampsia.

If you develop very mild preeclampsia, your doctor may instruct you to rest in bed, lying on your left side as much as possible to take the weight of the uterus off your major blood vessels. These precautions will help improve blood flow to your kidneys. Sometimes, this is all the treatment that's necessary.

If the condition is more serious, you may require hospitalization, during which you may be given medications to control your blood pressure and prevent seizures. The best treatment for severe preeclampsia is delivery of the baby. If you're near term, your doctor may induce labor or perform a Caesarean section. If the fetus isn't developed enough to have a good chance of survival, your doctor will try to forestall labor if the preeclampsia isn't too severe. You and your baby will be monitored continuously to make sure neither of you is in danger.

After delivery, symptoms of preeclampsia usually become less severe, although in some women eclampsia can still develop during the first 24 hours after delivery and rarely, later. Eclampsia isn't as frequent as it once was. If it does occur, your doctor will likely want you to deliver at once. Because of improved prenatal care, the vast majority of women with preeclampsia never progress to eclampsia.

Antepartum bleeding

If you have vaginal bleeding (hemorrhage) after the fifth month of pregnancy, you're experiencing antepartum (pre-birth) bleeding. Many conditions can cause antepartum bleeding in middle or late pregnancy, including placenta previa — a condition in which the placenta covers the cervix — cervical damage or separation of the placenta from the uterine wall.

Report any bleeding during pregnancy to your doctor immediately. He or she will want to determine the cause of the problem. You may need to be hospitalized for examination and tests.

Most often, antepartum bleeding is mild and no damage is done. However, if bleeding becomes heavy, it can be dangerous for both you and your baby. With a substantial amount of blood loss, a blood transfusion is often necessary. If the bleeding poses a threat, early delivery of the infant, either by inducing labor or by Caesarean section, is warranted.

Premature rupture of membranes

Normally, the membranes that surround the fetus rupture either just before or during labor. Occasionally, though, these membranes rupture weeks or months before the anticipated delivery date. If you feel a gush or a constant dribble of fluid from the vagina, your membranes may have ruptured, an event commonly referred to as your water breaking.

No one knows why membranes rupture prematurely, although growing data point to infection as a main cause. Call your doctor immediately. You'll likely be hospitalized. Amniocentesis or collection of vaginal fluid may be done to determine if your infant's lungs are mature enough for it to survive an early delivery.

When premature rupture of your membranes occurs, there's a high risk that your labor will begin within a few days — a dangerous prospect if you're in the middle of your pregnancy. In addition, there's a risk of infection once the membranes have ruptured.

If your baby's lungs are mature, your doctor may give you medications to induce labor. If your baby is too immature to have a good chance of survival outside the womb, your doctor may give you medication to help stimulate fetal lung maturity and to relax the uterine muscles to decrease the chance of early delivery. This can be successful, but risk of serious infection remains, so your condition must be monitored closely.

Placenta previa

In placenta previa, instead of being located high in the uterus, the placenta is partially or completely over the cervix. Late in pregnancy, as the uterus prepares for labor, the cervix expands and any placenta near it is torn loose. The result is a raw area that bleeds. You may have painless bleeding from the vagina, usually at the end of the second trimester or later. It often first occurs at night and usually stops on its own.

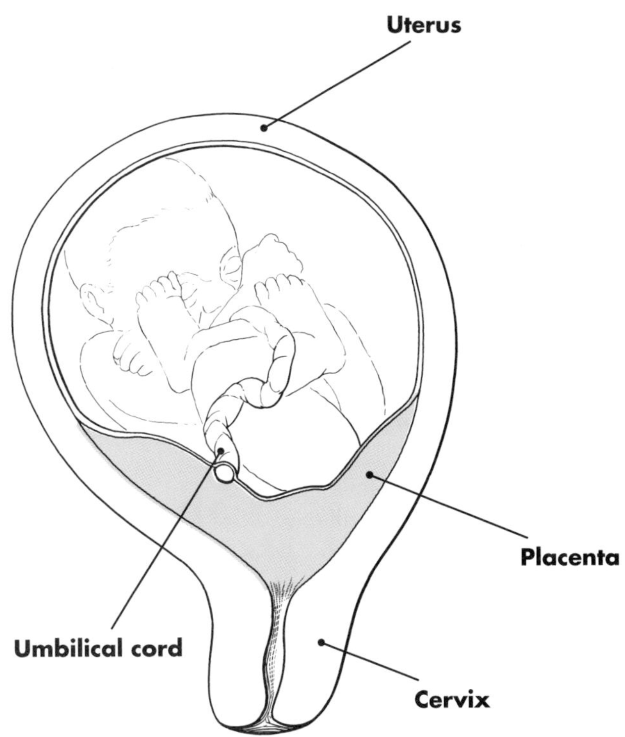

In a condition called placenta previa, the placenta is located over the cervix. Painless bleeding may occur. If this happens, see your doctor immediately.

Approximately 1 in 200 pregnancies that go beyond the seventh month have placenta previa. Uncommon in first pregnancies, placenta previa is more likely to occur with each subsequent pregnancy. Older mothers tend to be more at risk, as are women who've had Caesarean sections. If your doctor suspects placenta previa, he or she may request an ultrasound examination. Occasionally, magnetic resonance imaging (MRI) is necessary.

Bleeding with placenta previa can be severe and threaten the life of the mother and baby. If you're close to your delivery date, your doctor may want you to undergo a Caesarean section to prevent further bleeding. Blood transfusions may be necessary if the hemorrhaging is severe. You may be put on bed rest, and your doctor may have you forego intercourse and vaginal exams.

Placental abruption

Separation of the placenta from the uterine wall (placental abruption) before labor begins can decrease or interrupt the flow of oxygen-rich blood to the baby. Separation may be partial, involving only a part of the placenta, such as an edge, or the entire placenta may be separated from the uterine wall.

Women who have high blood pressure during their pregnancy — whether the condition first developed while they were pregnant or was present before — are more prone to placental abruption.

Placental abruption is one the leading causes of fetal death in the third trimester. It can also cause the mother to have severe circulatory problems or go into shock as a result of severe bleeding. Fortunately, with close monitoring of the mother and baby and prompt delivery at signs of trouble, the outlook for both is good.

Intrauterine death

Most fetal deaths occur as miscarriages in the first weeks of pregnancy. Occasionally, though, a fetus will die after the fifth month of gestation.

Several conditions are responsible for intrauterine death, including preeclampsia and eclampsia, maternal diabetes, antepartum bleeding, postmaturity, rhesus (Rh) disease and severe congenital abnormalities. The causes of many fetal deaths remain unknown.

Usually, the death of a fetus is silent. One day you may notice that you don't feel the baby move as you used to. When the doctor fails to detect a heartbeat, he or she will likely use ultrasound to determine if the fetus is still alive. Your doctor may want to do an amniocentesis to see if the cause of death can be determined.

Most often, labor begins within 2 weeks after fetal death, although it may be longer in middle pregnancy. If your labor doesn't begin on its own, you may be given medications to induce it. If your labor is too overdue, there's concern you may develop blood-clotting abnormalities that can set the stage for a life-threatening hemorrhage.

In most cases, the outlook for future pregnancies is the same as for first pregnancies. The biggest hurdle is the grief that every couple must work through after an intrauterine death.

Prolonged pregnancy

The average pregnancy lasts 40 weeks from the onset of the last menstrual period. Prolonged pregnancy (postmaturity) describes a pregnancy beyond 42 weeks.

As with prematurity, postmaturity can be dangerous. The overdue infant is dependent on an aging placenta that may fail to provide adequate oxygen. Moreover, the infant may continue growing, which may make delivery extremely difficult.

Occasionally, fetal growth may be halted altogether, and the infant may not be getting any nutrition. As a result, the stillbirth rate of these babies is twice that of those born after a pregnancy of normal length.

If your pregnancy continues to 42 weeks, your doctor will probably induce labor, provided he or she is sure that the baby is indeed overdue and there hasn't been a mistake in calculating the time of conception. If the baby is very large, assistance may be needed during the delivery or a Caesarean section may be performed.

Labor and Delivery

For many women, labor and delivery is the part of pregnancy that they look to with anticipation and, often, nervousness. Especially if you've never been through labor, you may wonder what it'll be like and how you'll make it through.

Try to relax. Most women make it through without any problem because women's bodies are made to accommodate labor and delivery. Although giving birth is difficult work, learning more about the process and practicing relaxation techniques can help to make your birthing experience go more smoothly.

First signs of labor

"How will I know when labor begins?" That's sometimes a difficult question to answer because each woman and each pregnancy are different. Maybe this is your first child, and you're confused by the advice of friends and relatives. Some people tell you that labor will be the toughest hours of your life, and others say that it won't be so bad. Perhaps you've already borne a child and you expect this labor to be similar to your previous one.

Whatever you expect, expect the unexpected. Every labor is different. But some good indicators can let you know that labor is beginning or about ready to begin:

1. A few days or hours before labor actually begins, you may have what's called bloody show. This is the discharge of a small amount of blood-tinged mucus. Actually, it's the mucus plug that formed the barrier between your uterus and vagina during your pregnancy.
2. The membranes that surround the amniotic fluid may rupture at the beginning of labor or as the labor progresses. When your membranes rupture (water breaks), you may feel a gush or slow trickle of fluid from your vagina.
3. Contractions may or may not be a sign that you're in labor. Throughout pregnancy, you may have noticed your uterus contracting. These are called Braxton Hicks contractions, and they usually don't cause discomfort until the last weeks of pregnancy. Many women then have these contractions and believe they're in labor. It's often difficult for pregnant women to distinguish between Braxton Hicks contractions and those of real labor. Sometimes, Braxton Hicks contractions stop if you lie down to rest or take a warm bath.

   As a rule, the contractions of real labor occur at regular intervals. The period between contractions slowly begins to get shorter, and the contractions become longer and more intense. The pain usually begins high in the uterus and radiates down the abdomen and to the lower back. Real labor contractions don't go away if you lie down and relax. If your contractions get longer, stronger and more frequent, chances are they're the real thing.

If you have any of these signs, notify your doctor or go to the hospital. Your doctor will likely want to examine you to see if your cervix is dilating and thinning (effacing), signs that the baby is getting ready to be born. If your membranes rupture, your doctor probably will

? Question and Answer

What's false labor?

Many women have one or more bouts of false labor before real labor begins. False labor is more likely to occur in the final weeks of pregnancy and in women who have already borne a child.

How can you distinguish false labor from true labor? With false labor you'll have contractions, but they'll usually be irregular and won't increase in frequency and intensity, as true contractions do. Moreover, the pain will be in the lower abdomen and groin, whereas true labor pains begin higher in the uterus and radiate down the abdomen and lower back.

When your labor is false, walking may stop the contractions, whereas with true labor, walking generally has no effect.

If you have doubts about your labor symptoms, seek medical advice. Many pregnant women have postponed going to the hospital, convinced it was only a false alarm, only to give birth before reaching the hospital.

want you to go to the hospital immediately.

Procedures

One of the reasons that labor is more safe today than ever before is that there are ways to monitor the mother's and the baby's health. It's important to understand common procedures before going into labor.

Labor is intense work, and it isn't the time to learn and make decisions about the procedures that your doctor recommends. Talk to your doctor beforehand about his or her preferences and usual practices. Ask questions so that you'll understand what's happening when it really matters.

Electronic fetal monitoring

Electronic fetal monitoring is commonly used to continuously record the unborn baby's heart rate during labor. Fetal monitoring may also be done before labor if the mother has a medical problem that may jeopardize the fetus.

As the uterus contracts during labor, the flow of blood through the placenta is temporarily reduced. Most fetuses tolerate this without problem, but if the fetus is otherwise compromised and in danger, changes in its heart rate occur. Many doctors recommend use of fetal monitoring during labor as a precaution to help ensure the safety of the unborn infant.

External monitoring

In external monitoring, two wide straps are placed around the mother's abdomen. One is placed high on the uterus and holds a gauge to measure and record the length and frequency of contractions. The other is placed lower on the abdomen. It holds a transducer that records the baby's heart rate. The gauge and transducer are connected to a monitor that displays and prints out both tracings simultaneously so that their interaction can be observed.

Internal monitoring

If during labor your doctor has a concern about the mother or fetus, he or she may recommend using an internal monitor. This is a more invasive procedure whereby an electrode is inserted through your vagina onto the baby's scalp. This is done after the membranes have ruptured (water has broken).

At the same time, a tube containing a gauge to measure your contractions (pressure catheter) is placed into the top portion of the uterus alongside the baby's head. Your contractions and the response of the baby's heart to these contractions are then recorded. If the baby's heart rate indicates possible distress, your doctor may decide it's safer to deliver the infant immediately by Caesarean section.

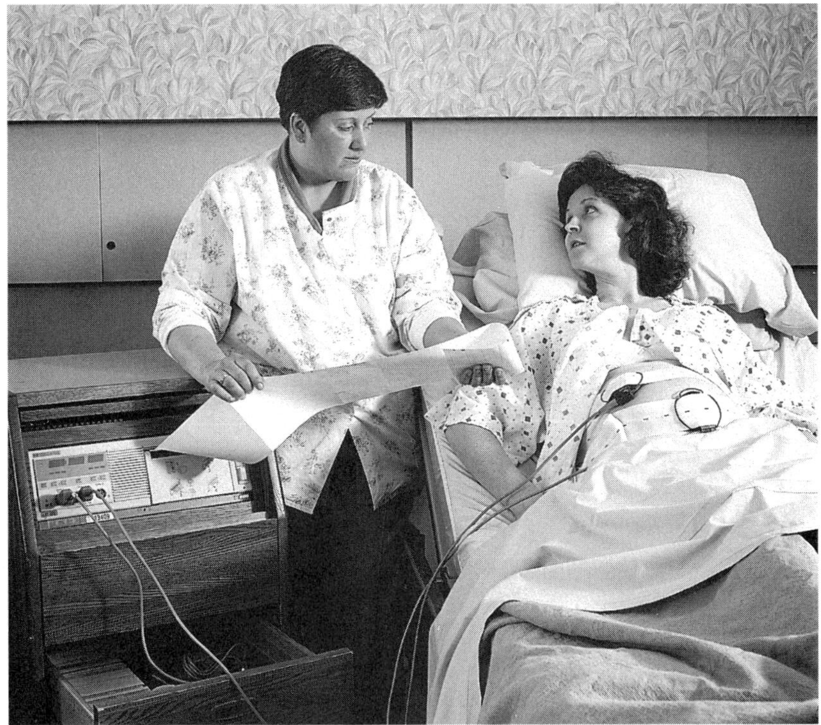

External fetal monitoring detects and records the baby's heart rate and the strength and frequency of contractions during labor.

Fetal pulse oximetry
Another type of fetal monitor measures the baby's blood oxygen level during labor and delivery.

The sensor is inserted into the mother's uterus and placed against the temple or cheek of the fetus, allowing your doctor to measure the level of oxygen in the baby's blood. This monitor can be used along with conventional electronic fetal monitoring when the fetal heart rate indicates that the baby may be in distress due to lack of adequate oxygen.

Fetal pulse oximetry is intended for use only on single, not multiple, fetuses of at least 36 weeks gestation, where the mother's water has broken and the baby's head is in the normal, head down, position for delivery. This procedure is new, and its effectiveness is still being evaluated.

Fetal blood sampling
Another method of helping to identify a fetus that's stressed during labor is by extracting a sample of fetal blood and measuring its acid (pH) content. If your doctor suspects your baby is getting an inadequate amount of oxygen, he or she may perform this test.

A funnel-shaped instrument called an endoscope is inserted through your dilated cervix to the baby's skin, usually the scalp. Two small incisions are then made in the skin, and a small amount of blood is drawn into a tube.

The pH of the blood is measured. If the pH is lower than normal, you may need an immediate Caesarean section.

Induction of labor
Sometimes, it's necessary to initiate (induce) labor. Although some mothers and doctors agree to induce labor because of convenience, this isn't recommended. Most labor inductions occur because the mother, baby or both are in danger if the pregnancy continues.

The most common medical reasons for inducing labor include preeclampsia and eclampsia and premature rupture of the membranes. In addition, labor may be induced when the doctor has a concern about the health of the fetus or the baby is overdue.

If your doctor recommends that labor be induced, he or she may first rupture your membranes. Sometimes this will bring on labor. At other times, medications such as oxytocin (Pitocin, Syntocinon) may be used after rupture of the membranes to bring on or enhance contractions.

Episiotomy
An episiotomy is an incision made just before delivery to widen the vulva so that the mother's tissues aren't torn. This surgical procedure is done to prevent severe damage to the mother's tissues that might otherwise occur with vaginal delivery of a very large baby.

If your doctor thinks that your vagina will be torn during delivery, he or she will inject a local anesthetic into the area between your vagina and rectum. An incision is then made just before the emergence of the baby's head.

After the delivery, the incision is sutured with stitches that dissolve. You may have some pain for a while. The pain may be relieved with hot baths or ice packs, pain medication and sprays that contain a local anesthetic.

Forceps
Forceps are two blunt blades that resemble a pair of tongs. They're used to pull the baby out of the vagina when the delivery isn't progressing as it should or when signs of fetal stress are evident.

Forceps may be used when labor stops progressing, when the baby is abnormally positioned or when there are signs that the baby isn't tolerating labor. Sometimes, use of forceps may be necessary when a woman doesn't have the strength to push the baby out. If a forceps delivery is necessary, often an episiotomy is too.

Complications from forceps deliveries are relatively rare. Occasionally, temporary bruises to an infant's face can occur. However, the skilled use of forceps has saved the lives of many babies.

Vacuum extraction
The vacuum extractor was designed as an alternative to forceps. A metal or silicone cup is fitted over the baby's scalp, and a pump is used to attach the vacuum extractor to the baby's head. Grasping the handle on the cup, the doctor can then move the baby's head to a better position and pull the baby out of the birth canal. Occasionally, some bruising occurs on the infant's scalp, which goes away in several days.

Stages of labor

As a rule, labor is usually longer with first babies. The cervix and birth canal of a first-time mother are less flexible, and therefore it takes longer for labor and birth. A first-time mother generally can expect about 13 hours to pass between the time she goes into active labor and the birth of her baby. Some women, however, are in labor much longer. For a woman who has previously given birth, the average time is between 4 and 8 hours.

Labor is divided into three stages:

First stage
The first stage of labor is the longest. During this stage, your cervix — the narrow passageway between your uterus and vagina — opens so that the baby can pass into the birth canal. Think of the uterus as a large, upside-down, elastic bottle. When labor begins, the cervix is about 3 centimeters ($1\frac{1}{2}$ inches) in length and almost closed.

Contractions cause the cervix to open (dilate) by creating pressure within the uterus. This force is tremendous and is directed through the uterus in two ways. During a contraction, the infant is subjected to an intense pressure that forces it against the cervix. The contractions cause the cervix to thin (efface) and pull up around the baby's head. Repeated contractions eventually stretch the cervix open. The cervix is fully dilated when it's open to a diameter of 10 centimeters (4 inches).

During the first stage of labor, your contractions become more frequent and last longer. You may be attached to a machine that monitors your infant's heart rate and charts the onset and cessation of each contraction. Your doctor or a nurse periodically does a pelvic examination to determine how you're progressing. If the contractions aren't forceful enough to open the cervix, you may be offered a medication to make your uterus contract.

Some women go through the entire labor process with no pain medication. These women usually have taken classes in prepared childbirth and learned a variety of techniques to control pain. They're also more likely to have a smooth and speedier delivery. Many women, however, choose pain relief. Every medication used to help relieve pain affects the baby in some way. Be sure you understand the benefits and risks of pain medication before you begin labor. Your doctor can help you decide what pain relief will be best for you and baby.

Sometimes, labor drags on without much progress. When this occurs, it can be because the contractions are poorly coordinated or not strong enough. If the cause is inadequate contractions, the uterus can be stimulated to contract by the intravenous infusion of a medication such as oxytocin (Pitocin, Syntocinon). In most cases, this is successful. If not, a Caesarean section may be necessary.

Conditions that can obstruct delivery include a head that's too large to pass down the birth canal or a fetal head position that makes delivery difficult. Sometimes, the cervix can be very resistant to stretching. In these cases, a Caesarean section may be necessary.

Second stage

The second stage of labor is when your baby is born. Your cervix is now fully dilated and effaced. This is the baby's signal to start the journey down the birth canal.

Once the cervix no longer offers resistance, each contraction serves to propel the infant downward. You may feel a tremendous urge to push, similar to that of a bowel movement. Sometimes, this urge to push comes before the cervix is fully dilated. However, you should wait for complete dilation before pushing.

Push only when you're having a contraction. In this way, two forces — that of the contraction and your pushing — combine to move the baby and conserve your energy.

Both the first and the second stages of labor are longer for first-time mothers. On average, it takes about 2 hours to push a first baby out, whereas women who have previously given birth usually complete the second stage in 15 to 40 minutes.

As you push and the baby begins to move, the vaginal opening becomes more and more dilated and begins to bulge. It takes several more minutes for the vulva to stretch to allow delivery.

After you've pushed the baby's head out, you're instructed to stop pushing for a moment while your doctor clears the baby's airway. You may find it difficult to stop pushing when told to, but try. It may help to blow air out of your mouth instead of pushing. Then, when you're encouraged to push again and with just a few more pushes, your baby is born.

The umbilical cord that connects the baby to the placenta is cut, and unless there's a problem, your baby is placed in your arms. Shortly after, the baby is weighed and examined.

Third stage

The third stage of labor is delivery of the placenta. Your uterus continues to contract to expel it, but you shouldn't feel much pain. It then continues to contract after expelling the placenta, but these too are generally mild contractions.

Pain relief

Most pregnant women — 80 percent to 90 percent — choose to use some type of pain medication during the birthing process. What you decide to use, if anything, depends on your preferences, your doctor's recommendations, what's available at the medical facility you've chosen and the specific character of your labor.

Learn about the different options ahead of time so that you can make knowledgeable choices regarding pain medication. Be sure to remain flexible, however, because you may need to change your mind if things don't go as you planned.

All medications involve some risk to the baby. These risks must be weighed against the desire to relieve pain.

Narcotics

Narcotics offer reasonable pain relief, don't interfere with your ability to push and can be given as an injection or intravenously. They do, however, have a sedative effect. They can also cause nausea and vomiting, dizziness, itching and, occasionally, respiratory problems.

Because narcotics can slow the baby's respirations at birth, they aren't given close to the time of delivery. Should the baby be affected by narcotics, medications to counter the effect can be given immediately to the newborn after birth.

Local anesthetics

A "local" is a medication that's injected directly into tissues, much as a dentist numbs your mouth before drilling. The simplest local used during the birthing process is one that numbs you before an episiotomy is made or a tear repaired.

A local anesthetic before an episiotomy has no effect on the baby, nor does it provide pain relief for labor. Injections at other sites have more widespread effects.

Paracervical block

A paracervical block is an injection into the tissues around the cervix that helps relieve the pain of uterine contractions and cervical stretching during early labor. Occasionally, a paracervical block slows the baby's heart rate. Today, because of the increased use of epidural or spinal anesthesia, paracervical blocks are less often used.

Pudendal block

A pudendal block is injected into the vaginal wall and the ligaments supporting the pelvic floor. Because it affects just the vagina and rectum, and gives no pain relief to the uterus or cervix, it's used only for the last part of labor and for an episiotomy.

Epidural and spinal blocks

Epidural and spinal blocks are increasingly popular pain relief options. Each of these procedures uses an anesthetic and narcotic mixture that's injected into the space surrounding the spinal nerves, temporarily blocking pain from the chest level down. These blocks can be used for labor as well as for an episiotomy and Caesarean birth. Their use, however, requires the services of an anesthesiologist.

Epidural and spinal anesthesia are the most effective forms of anesthesia for childbirth. You can receive good pain relief but still be awake and alert, able to push and able to enjoy your baby's birth.

Abnormal fetal positions

Most babies are born headfirst, with the face toward the mother's back. This position is called occiput anterior. It allows for the easiest passage through the birth canal. An estimated 4 percent of babies, however, enter the world in other positions, some of which are potentially dangerous and warrant special care during labor and delivery.

Breech

Breech presentation is the most common of the abnormal presentations. If your baby is breech, it's positioned with its buttocks near your cervix. Thus, either the buttocks or feet emerge first instead of the head.

Breech births are particularly common in premature infants because many babies don't assume the correct position until the last few weeks or even days of pregnancy. Other factors that predispose some women to breech birth include multiple fetuses, uterine abnormalities, tumors, hydramnios and placenta previa.

If your infant is in the breech position, in the last weeks of pregnancy, your doctor may attempt to turn the baby externally. If the baby doesn't turn before labor, most doctors perform a Caesarean section, which usually results in less risk to the infant but a slight increase in risk to the mother.

Transverse

Transverse presentation occurs when the infant lies crosswise in the uterus, usually with the shoulder over the birth canal. This presentation is more common in women who have had four or more children. Prematurity and placenta previa are other conditions associated with the transverse presentation.

Vaginal delivery is impossible when a live infant is in the trans-

Headfirst

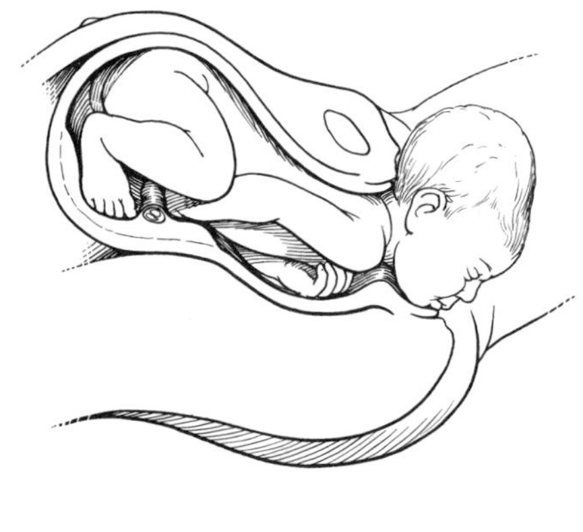

Transverse

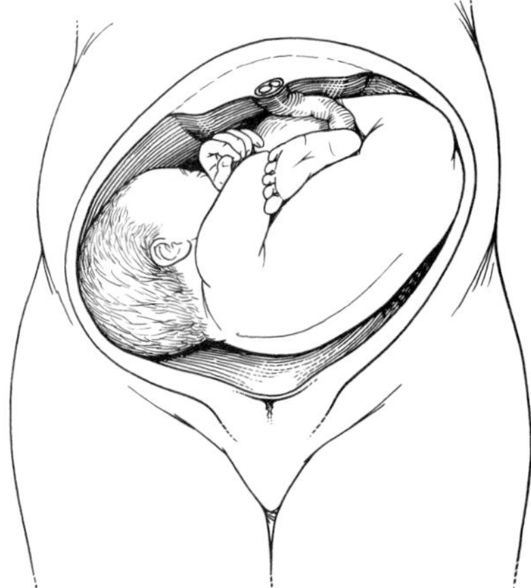

Breech

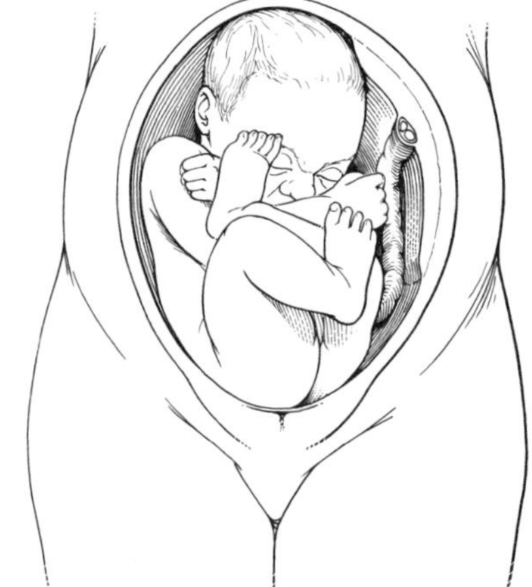

Occiput Posterior

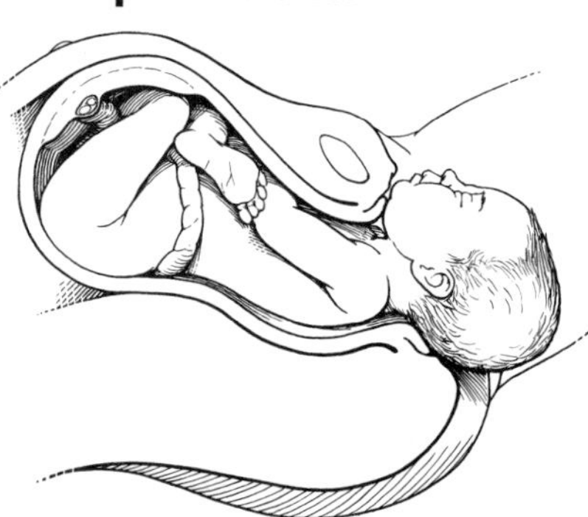

At the time of delivery, the normal position for the unborn baby is headfirst, with the face toward the mother's back. This position is called occiput anterior. Other presentations include breech, transverse and occiput posterior.

verse position. There's a real danger that the umbilical cord will become obstructed and cut off the infant's oxygen supply. An infant can't move through the birth canal in this position.

Caesarean section should be performed either before active labor begins or just after its onset. If a woman is allowed to labor too long, both she and her baby are at increased risk because of uterine rupture and the chance of cord damage.

Occiput posterior

Occiput posterior position is when the infant's head is positioned near the cervix but its face is toward the mother's front. This presentation can make it difficult for the infant to travel down the birth canal.

This position can delay delivery, especially if the infant is large. Forceps may be necessary for an occiput posterior presentation. Sometimes, a Caesarean section is necessary.

Caesarean delivery

A Caesarean delivery is birth by way of cuts (incisions) made through the abdominal wall and into the uterus.

Although recorded centuries ago as a method for attempting to save the baby after the mother's death, it wasn't until anesthesia and aseptic surgery were developed in the 19th century that Caesarean section became feasible as a means of saving both the baby and mother in a difficult delivery.

Childbirth by Caesarean delivery was once an operation of last resort, but it no longer is today. Ceasarean section presently accounts for more than 20 percent of all births in the United States. Even though many critics think the pendulum has swung too far toward the use of Caesarean sections, there's no doubt that many women and babies are alive today because of this alternative to vaginal childbirth.

When is Caesarean delivery necessary?

Many conditions call for a Caesarean delivery. Some premature infants have a better chance of survival when delivered in this way. Infants in breech or transverse positions more often than not are delivered by Caesarean delivery. When an infant is too large or a mother's birth canal is unusually small, a Caesarean delivery is the only safe way to deliver.

Sometimes, abnormalities of the uterus or vagina obstruct the birth canal and necessitate this operation. If a mother has preeclampsia, diabetes, genital herpes or high blood pressure and the fetus is having trouble, a Caesarean delivery may be indicated. Placental abnormalities such as placenta previa often make it necessary to do a Caesarean delivery.

In the event of multiple fetuses, many doctors advise this procedure. When labor is prolonged because of insufficient uterine contractions, a Caesarean delivery may be safer for both the mother and baby.

Some medical experts believe that the procedure is done too often and that doctors do a Caesarean delivery whenever they're faced with the possibility of a difficult birth, just to make sure that all precautions have been taken. Some of this so-called defensive medicine is practiced, but a potential lawsuit isn't the reason for most Caesarean births.

Improved fetal monitoring techniques now provide vital information about the status of the fetus and the ability to withstand labor and delivery. If it appears that the fetus may be jeopardized, most doctors proceed with a Caesarean delivery. In addition, improvements in the operation, in anesthesia and in antibiotics make the procedure safer for the mother than it once was.

As more women are postponing pregnancy until later in life, they and their infants are at higher risk of medical complications than are their younger counterparts. Hence, Caesarean births in this group are more common.

The need for a Caesarean section with subsequent pregnancies will depend on the type of uterine incision — how high the incision extends into the top of the uterus — and whether the circumstances that led to the first Caesarean section recur. Vaginal delivery after a Caesarean section always involves some risk.

The procedure

Women who have a Caesarean delivery are given an anesthetic. If the procedure is being done on an emergency basis, you may be put to sleep with a general anesthetic. Many hospitals now allow your partner to be in the operating room, unless you're having an emergency Caesarean.

It usually takes a little less than an hour to perform a normal Caesarean delivery. Two types of incisions into the abdomen can be used. One is the so-called bikini cut, which is a horizontal incision near

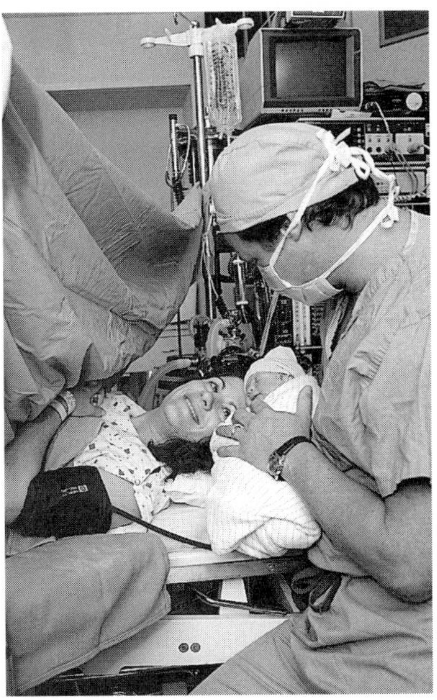

Often, the father can be present to witness a Caesarean birth. Within minutes of the birth, mom and dad can greet their baby while the surgeons finish the operation.

the pubic hair line. The other is a vertical cut from the navel to the pubis.

To open the uterus, one of two incisions can be made. The most common method is a horizontal incision in the lower part of the uterus, called a lower uterine transverse incision. This incision heals better and is associated with less chance of uterine rupture with a subsequent pregnancy.

On occasion, a doctor will use a vertical incision to open the uterus. This incision allows more access to your uterus and is used, for example, when an infant is very large or when an infant is premature and in an abnormal position.

After the uterus is opened, the baby is delivered, the umbilical cord is cut, the placenta is removed, and the uterine and abdominal incisions are stitched closed.

Complications

Although Caesarean delivery is safer than it used to be and most women recover well, it can result in complications. As with any operation, there's a risk of infection at the surgical site as well as bladder and kidney infections. Bleeding at the incision site is rare, but when it does occur, it can be severe.

The death rate for women who have a Caesarean delivery is two to four times higher than that for women who have a vaginal delivery. Many of the women who die, however, were ill before the operation, and most of these deaths have been associated with emergency conditions that led to the Caesarean section.

Recovery

Initially, you may feel groggy and uncomfortable and will need extra help caring for your baby. After the procedure, you'll be encouraged to try to move around your room on the same day. You can eat a regular diet when you have an appetite. You can hold your baby and begin breast-feeding just as you would if you had delivered your baby vaginally. Women who have a Caesarean delivery generally need to stay in the hospital one more day after the birth than women who have a vaginal delivery.

Future pregnancies

It used to be that once a woman had a Caesarean delivery, she would always have one for any subsequent births. This was done because of the risk of the uterine scar rupturing during labor, which often resulted in serious complications for both the mother and baby.

Now, many pregnant women who have had a previous Caesarean delivery may be able to have a vaginal delivery. This depends on the initial reason for the operation and if the condition is still present. For example, if the Caesarean section was done because of fetal distress, your next baby may be able to withstand labor and a vaginal delivery. Alternatively, if you had a Caesarean section because your pelvis is unusually small, your future deliveries may have to be Caesarean.

Other factors that determine if you can attempt a vaginal delivery are the type of uterine incision that was made and if the first Caesarean delivery was free of infection. If your uterine scar is the horizontal type (lower uterine transverse incision), you may be a candidate for vaginal delivery.

If you're attempting vaginal birth after a Caesarean, you'll want to take the following special precautions: Make sure to labor in a hospital. Don't labor at home and go to the hospital close to delivery. Make sure the hospital has a blood bank. And make sure the hospital has the ability to arrange for a Caesarean section within 15 minutes of recognizing a uterine rupture. Avoid having your labor induced.

Post-delivery problems

After the baby is born, the mother can sometimes experience health problems related to the delivery. Knowing what to expect in these situations may help ease some of the stress at a particularly emotional time.

Retained placenta

Normally, the placenta is delivered within 30 minutes after the baby. Your doctor may press on your abdomen to help expel the placenta. A retained placenta is one that's trapped in the uterus after delivery, often because it hasn't separated completely from the uterine wall.

Sometimes, the doctor has to peel the placenta from the uterine wall manually. You may need anesthesia during this procedure. If there's still a problem, a surgical procedure called a dilatation and curettage (D and C) may be necessary to remove the placenta.

Postpartum bleeding

Postpartum bleeding (hemorrhage) is the excessive loss of blood after delivery, as a result of heavy bleeding from the uterus. This is the most common type of serious obstetrical hemorrhage. It's often caused by an inability of the uterus to contract enough to control the bleeding that occurs when the placenta separates from the uterus. This inability can be the result of inadequate contractions of uterine muscles.

Other causes of postpartum bleeding include trauma to the vaginal wall from an episiotomy or lacerations, uterine rupture and retention of part of the placenta. The risk of postpartum bleeding increases with the delivery of an excessively large baby or more than one infant, a forceps delivery, vaginal delivery after a previous Caesarean section, several previous deliveries, hydramnios and labor that has been induced with medications.

If you have postpartum hemorrhage, the bleeding can vary from massive to just a steady seepage over a period of hours. Sometimes, the blood doesn't escape through the vagina but collects inside the uterus, causing the uterus to become distended.

Postpartum bleeding can usually be controlled with medications that make the uterus contract. If this treatment doesn't stop the bleeding, your doctor may do a pelvic examination to check for torn tissues.

An abdominal operation may be necessary if the bleeding can't be controlled. The first step is tying off the major blood vessels that supply your uterus. If this is successful, the bleeding will stop and your ability to have more children may not be hampered. If the hemorrhage continues, the uterus must be removed.

Following Pregnancy

If you've experienced an uncomplicated labor and delivery, no doubt you'll feel a great sense of relief after giving birth to a healthy baby. Accompanying that relief, however, is a whole new set of responsibilities and worries. There are decisions to make and more than a few problems and hurdles to deal with during the ensuing months.

In Chapter 12, "Infant and Toddler Years," many health matters concerning your baby are discussed in detail. However, you also may confront a few matters pertaining largely to your health.

Breast-feeding

The feeding of your newborn baby occupies a considerable portion of your time. Chapter 12 of this book discusses breast-feeding and bottle-feeding in detail. The discussion here is about what you'll experience when you breast-feed.

Most women are physically capable of breast-feeding. Some small-breasted women may think they won't be able to produce enough milk. This isn't true, because breast-feeding has nothing to do with breast size.

During pregnancy, your breasts are preparing to produce milk. The hormones estrogen and progesterone are produced by the placenta and promote the growth of special breast tissue designed to produce milk. Your breasts slowly increase in size, and the nipples change, becoming darker in color and more prominent.

After your baby is born, you'll probably be able to breast-feed immediately. The baby's suckling stimulates production of the pituitary hormone oxytocin, which helps contract the uterus. This helps your uterus return to normal size more quickly than if you don't breast-feed. In addition, breast-feeding can help prevent postpartum bleeding (hemorrhage) of the uterus.

Oxytocin also stimulates contraction of the muscles that surround the milk ducts, and this contraction, called the let-down reflex, releases colostrum, a thin, sticky fluid, into storage areas behind the nipples. Later on, colostrum is replaced by milk.

After the delivery of the placenta, release of the hormone prolactin is triggered, which in turn stimulates milk secretion. About 1 or 2 days after delivery, your breasts may feel engorged and uncomfortable. They'll be much larger than usual, tender and firm. You may notice prominent veins appearing.

These are normal changes caused by an increased blood flow and the production of milk. The best cure for this discomfort is a hungry baby.

The initial days and weeks of breast-feeding can be difficult under the best of circumstances. If you're having trouble, get help from someone with experience in breast-feeding. Many hospitals have lactation specialists who can help you get through the first couple of weeks as you and your baby learn to breast-feed.

Once you grow accustomed to the routine of breast-feeding, take advantage of its soothing effect on you and your baby. Learn to pay attention to your body's cues. If you're thirsty, get something to drink. If you're hungry, eat nutritious foods. If your baby cries, recognize that your first instinct is to feed your baby. Follow that instinct. If you feel sleepy, take a nap.

New mothers often wonder whether they're producing enough milk. If the baby is gaining weight and has at least six wet diapers and two or more stools during a 24-hour period, the amount is adequate.

Nutrition

During pregnancy, your body prepares for breast-feeding by storing additional nutrients and sources of energy. After your baby arrives, you may notice an increase in appetite and thirst and a change in dietary preferences.

The idea that you need to follow special dietary rules during breast-feeding is unfounded. Most important is that you eat a variety of foods at mealtime and nutritious snacks between meals and drink plenty of fluids to satisfy your thirst. You don't need to drink milk to make milk, but you do need to consume 1,200 milligrams of calcium daily from some source.

Your doctor may recommend that you continue taking your prenatal vitamins during lactation. Avoid crash diets to lose weight. Gradual weight loss of 1 to 4 pounds monthly is safe and healthy.

Breast problems

While breast-feeding, you may encounter the following problems:

Engorgement

Early, frequent and lengthy nursing helps prevent engorgement. Some engorgement is normal. However, increased fluid and accumulation of milk in the breasts can lead to severe engorgement. Hard, swollen, painful breasts can result. If your breasts are only moderately engorged, carefully position your baby and increase feedings. For severe engorgement, applying a warm washcloth compress and expressing milk by hand or with a breast pump may soften your breast and help to get your baby attached for feeding. Cold packs between feedings can help reduce swelling. For unmanageable engorgement, contact your doctor or a lactation consultant.

Cracked nipples

Cracked nipples most often occur because the baby is improperly positioned at the breast. Talk to a lactation consultant about the best way to hold your baby while breast-feeding. Correcting the position problem is the first step for healing.

Applying expressed breast milk to the damaged areas aids healing and provides antibacterial protection. It's not clear if creams aid in the healing process. Softening scabs with warm washcloth compresses also may help. For unmanageable nipple cracks or nipple pains, contact your doctor or a lactation specialist.

Blocked milk duct

A blocked milk duct leads to a small, hard lump in your breast. Sometimes, the lump will disappear on its own, or you can use hot water compresses, massage your breast and extend the length of breast-feeding sessions on the affected side. If it doesn't disappear, call your doctor.

Mastitis

Mastitis occurs when bacteria, most commonly *Staphylococcus aureus*, enters the breast. Part of the breast becomes red and is hard and hot. You may feel unusually tired and have chills and a fever. If you have these signs and symptoms, see your doctor.

Mastitis is treated with antibiotics. Continue breast-feeding and increase fluids and rest. You may be more comfortable breast-feeding your baby more often. You may notice a change in the color of your baby's stool because of the antibiotics.

With treatment, mastitis usually clears up within a few days. If it's untreated, an abscess may form, requiring surgical drainage.

Postpartum stress and depression

After having a baby, it's important to monitor your mental health and be aware if you may need help. Several mental health conditions can occur after delivery.

Contributing factors may include hormone changes, a perceived unsatisfactory birth experience, a sense of loss in no longer being pregnant, your level of marital satisfaction, a baby with a high level of needs, lack of social support, exhaustion or a family history of postpartum depression.

The transition from pregnancy to parenthood can be difficult. Experiencing depression, whether mild or severe, doesn't mean you've failed as a person or a parent. Expect to recover as you learn new ways to balance your daily life and responsibilities.

The blues

Having a baby is a powerful, exciting, frightening, joyous and awe-inspiring event. In the days that follow the delivery, you may be surprised and confused about the many and varied emotions you experience.

Having easily handled other responsibilities, as a new parent you may feel incompetent and overwhelmed with new responsibilities. Be patient with yourself as you make this transition and give yourself credit for how well you're doing.

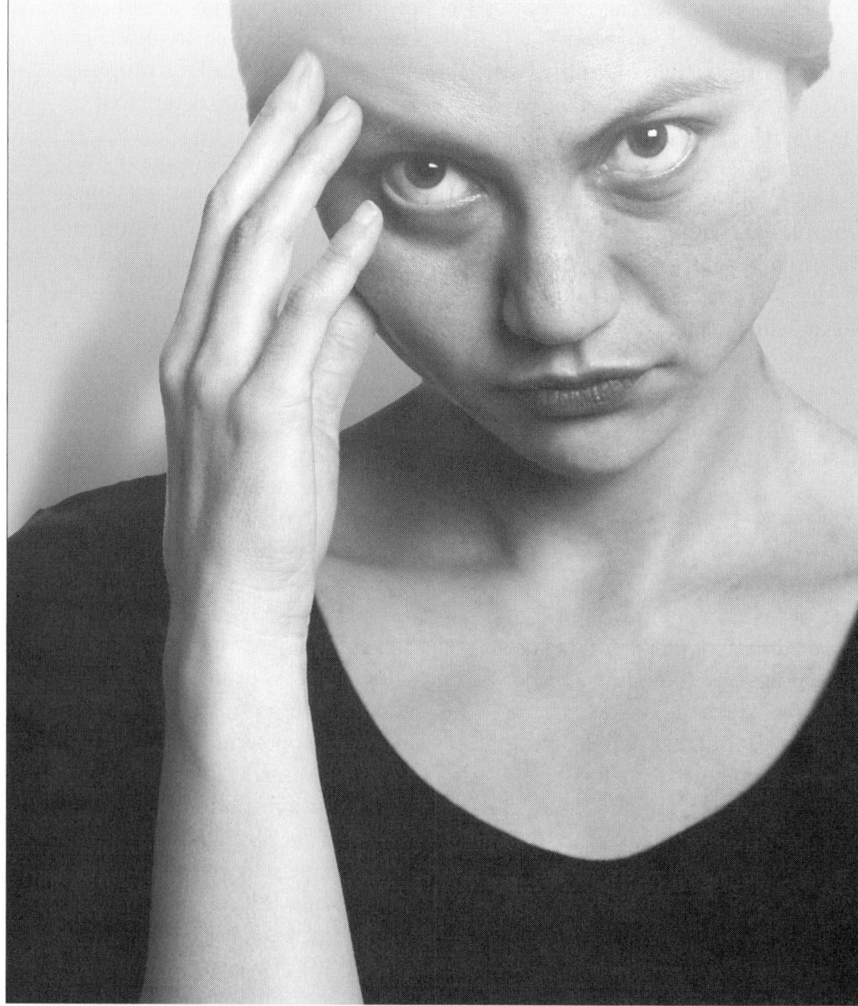

Common to 80 percent of new mothers is a mild depression called baby blues. This mild form of distress usually occurs a few days to weeks after birth. It's generally self-limiting, resolving spontaneously in a few weeks.

During this time, you may have feelings of sadness, anger, anxiety, irritability and incompetence. New mothers often experience uncontrollable crying for no identifiable reason.

Some mothers are surprised by occasional negative thoughts they may have about their baby and may interpret this as being a bad mother. It can be comforting to know that the baby blues are normal. In addition to accepting the blues as a normal part of birth, it's also important to take care of yourself.

Get adequate rest

Listen and respond to your body's cues for rest. Adequate rest has a significant effect on your emotional and physical well-being. Try sleeping during the day when your baby sleeps, to synchronize your rest periods.

You'll know you need more rest when things that didn't bother you before are now perceived as insurmountable events. Accepting assistance from others is sometimes difficult, but it may be just what you need for maintaining a positive and realistic emotional perspective.

Eat a nutritious diet

Good nutrition provides what your body needs during recovery from childbirth. A few small meals a day may be more comfortable for you than three large meals. Choose fruits and vegetables for snacking as healthy choices that also help with weight control.

Exercise

Light exercise can be helpful. Take a brisk, 30-minute walk as many days of the week as you can. You may enjoy your walk more if you take your baby with you in a baby carrier. Stretching and flexing as you play and talk to your baby will help tone your muscles. Your mind will be more at ease when your body feels good.

Socialize

Another normal part of the recovery process is to relive the birth process by sharing your childbirth experience with others. Having family and friends who truly listen and accept your feelings can greatly lessen depressive symptoms.

Postpartum depression

A more severe form of the blues, called postpartum depression, occurs in approximately 5 percent to 20 percent of new mothers. Symptoms are more intense and longer-lasting than those of the blues and can occur any time within the first year.

Additional symptoms may include constant fatigue, lack of joy in life, a sense of emotional numbness, withdrawal from family and friends, lack of concern for self or baby, severe insomnia, excessive concern for the baby, loss of sexual responsiveness, a strong sense of failure and inadequacy and severe mood swings. You may have high expectations and be overdemanding, have difficulty making sense of things or feel trapped.

Tell your doctor early on if your family or friends notice these symptoms. Early intervention may result in a more rapid recovery from postpartum depression. Treatment varies according to each individual's needs, but it may include behavioral therapy and antidepressant medication. You might also ask about a support group in your area.

Post-traumatic stress disorder

Post-traumatic stress disorder can occur following the birth of a child. It may be a response to a real or perceived traumatic childbirth, or it may arise from an unresolved past trauma — usually sexual in nature — that was triggered during childbirth.

Symptoms are similar to those of postpartum depression, but the cause is trauma related. When identified early, counseling, sometimes in combination with medication and stress reduction education, generally leads to recovery.

Sex Following Childbirth

Many couples want to know when they can resume sexual intercourse after the birth of a baby. The vagina of a woman who has just given birth has been through some trauma. Under the best of circumstances, it's bound to be tender. If you're breastfeeding, vaginal atrophy — thinning and drying of vaginal tissues — may occur as the result of less estrogen in your system.

Many doctors recommend waiting 4 weeks before having intercourse. Some ask couples to wait until after the new mother has a postnatal examination, which generally occurs 6 weeks after birth. During this time, you and your doctor can discuss contraceptive methods so that you're not faced with an untimely pregnancy.

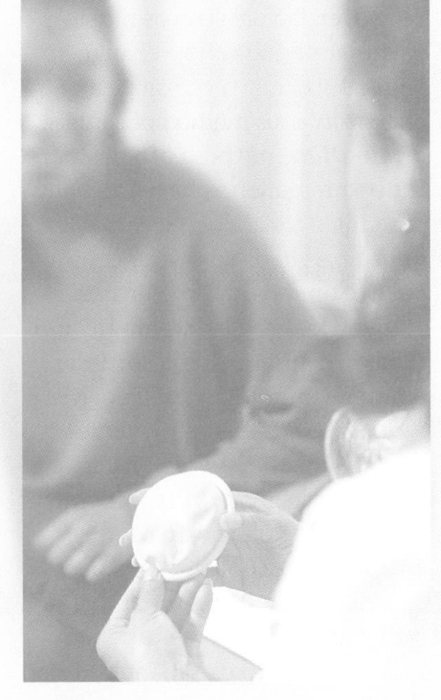

Postpartum psychosis

Another condition that can affect new mothers is postpartum psychosis. Fortunately, it is rare.

Symptoms, which may begin days or weeks after childbirth, may include severe depression, along with acute anxiety, racing thoughts, fear of harming yourself or your baby, hallucinations, irrational thoughts or statements, paranoia or hysteria.

The goal of treatment is to keep you and your baby safe and to preserve your sense of competence as a parent while you recover. This problem requires medical help.

Contraception

Some new mothers, particularly those who breast-feed, think they're protected from pregnancy. Don't make this mistake.

Breast-feeding does temporarily impair fertility to some degree, and many breast-feeding mothers don't menstruate for several months or even until the baby is weaned. Still, you can't rely on breast-feeding to prevent pregnancy. If you don't wish to become pregnant, use some form of contraception.

Your options for contraception are basically the same after delivery as they were before pregnancy. However, factors such as nursing, irregular periods and a change in vaginal size may necessitate a change in your method of contraception. One purpose of a postpartum examination, which is usually scheduled for about 6 weeks after delivery, is to discuss your contraceptive options and preferences.

If you've used a diaphragm and want to continue doing so, don't assume your old one will do. Many women require a slightly larger diaphragm after giving birth. Take your pre-pregnancy diaphragm with you to your postpartum examination. Your doctor can check whether it still fits and, if not, refit you.

If you want to use an intrauterine device, wait at least a month after the birth of your baby to have one inserted. If it's inserted before the uterus is firm, it may fall out.

Many women want to resume taking birth control pills but wonder if it's safe for a breast-feeding mother. There's no doubt that the use of some pills, most often the combination of estrogen and progestin pills, will somewhat reduce the milk supply in as many as one-third of women who use this method.

The reduction, however, is usually only temporary. Low-dose, progestin-only pills don't tend to reduce the milk supply, but they're not as effective a contraceptive as the combination pills. If you're nursing but want to take the pill, ask your doctor about the best option.

Several natural methods of contraception depend in part on a regular menstrual cycle. If you were using these methods before you became pregnant, it might be a good idea to use another method for the first few months after birth because your cycle may be irregular for a while.

Consult your doctor if your periods fail to return 3 to 4 months after delivery of your baby and you aren't breast-feeding. Women who are breast-feeding may not have a period for a year. ■

CHAPTER **16** PART II

Adult Years

Adulthood covers a longer span of time than ever before. The traditional marking of an adult — be it 18 or 21 years of age — can seem like just the beginning of life to someone who has lived to 96 years. More people than ever before are living well into their 80s, 90s and even 100s, and this trend is expected to continue as baby boomers age.

From raising families and building careers to perhaps retiring from work and planning how to spend your last years, adulthood encompasses many changes and adjustments. During this time, your body changes too.

This chapter outlines some of the changes associated with the various stages of adulthood and offers suggestions on managing the early and middle years and staying well in the later ones.

Family Life

In some respects, being an adult in the United States today is different than it was for adults at any other time in history. Not too many years ago, most 50-year-old parents were almost done with child rearing and were considering how to spend their time now that the house was emptied of children. Today, there are still parents readying for the empty nest at 50, but more and more, people are waiting even into their 40s to have children.

As a result, many 50-year-olds are still in the throes of child rearing. The family unit is also changing. Stepfamilies, rather than the traditional nuclear family, are becoming more common.

Adults in general, not just parents, are seeing changes too. Today, it's not unusual to see people in 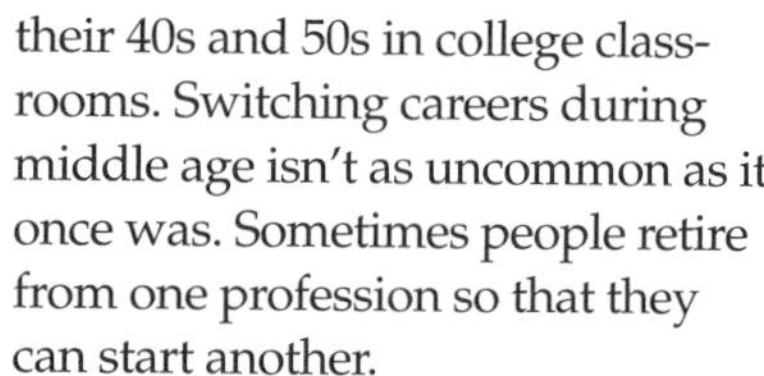their 40s and 50s in college classrooms. Switching careers during middle age isn't as uncommon as it once was. Sometimes people retire from one profession so that they can start another.

Even though the timing, configurations and pace of adult life may have changed, people still have high hopes for being part of a strong, loving family. Maintaining a strong family, though, takes work and commitment.

If you're raising children, caring for older parents and trying to find time for yourself, you may sometimes feel overwhelmed. But the payoffs of nurturing family ties are unparalleled. When adult siblings count each other as close friends, when teenagers open up to their parents, when family gatherings are warm events that everyone looks forward to, such love of family is well worth the effort.

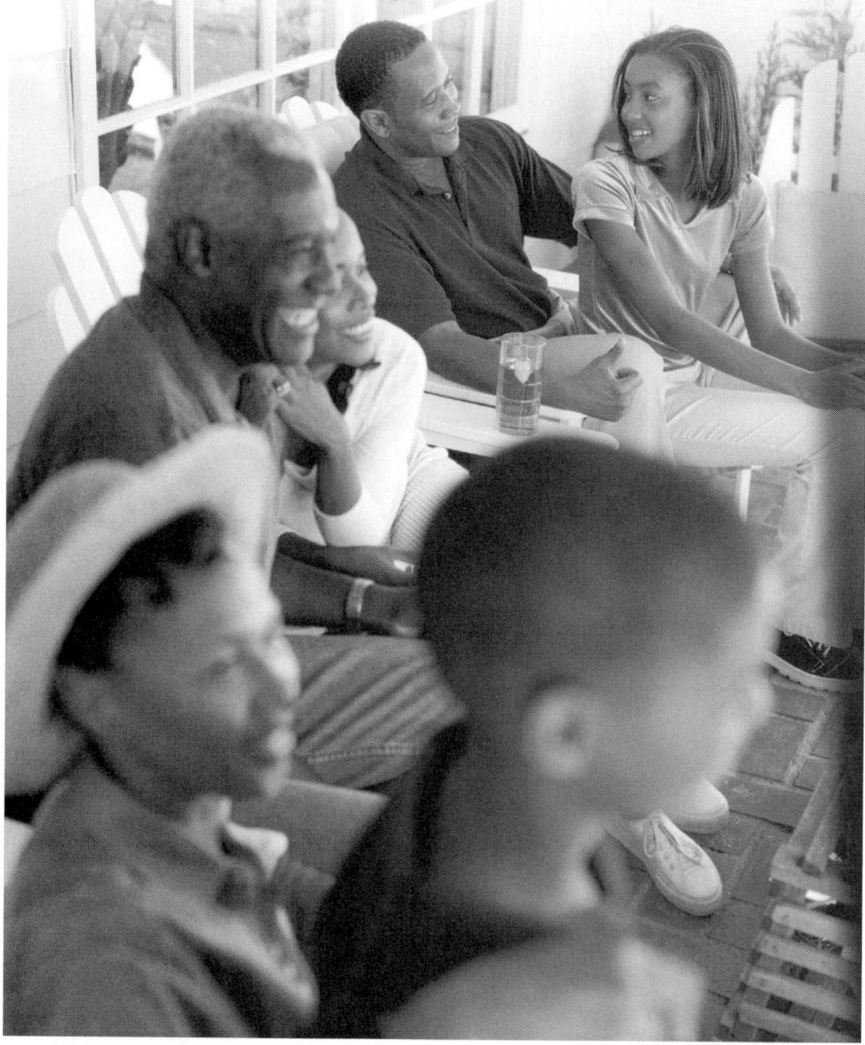

Building strong family ties

Building a strong family takes both consideration and communication. People in close families learn how to respect one another and how to disagree decently. Everyone needs to know that they're loved and will be cared for — no matter what happens. It's not always easy to deal with all of the changes that a family goes through, but a key to coping is knowing what to expect.

If you're raising toddlers, it's helpful to know that temper tantrums are inevitable so that you can plan your response. If your teenager spends all of his or her time in the bedroom with headphones on, it's comforting to know that eventually he or she will come out.

If you're widowed or divorced and remarry, understanding the unique demands on stepfamilies is crucial to success. And if you're caring for your older parents, it helps to know that many older adults forget things.

Sometimes, simply being aware of the typical stages of growth and aging can ease the stress. Another helpful tool is to think about the kind of family you have and the kind of family you'd like it to be.

Is your family one that likes to cook? Do you come from a family that devotes part of its time to helping others? Is dry wit part of your family's identity? Defining your family and nurturing such interests and strengths helps everyone feel a part of something solid.

Enjoying family activities

Close families often spend time together doing activities they enjoy, such as an annual camping trip or a sailing adventure. As everyone in the family gets older, the family campground may become a favorite summer gathering spot. Closer to home, some families set aside an evening each week as game night or movie night. Some families volunteer together.

The key is to get your family involved doing things together that are fun and meaningful. Grandparents can show pictures of their parents to their grandchildren and tell stories of their childhood. Computer-literate family members can teach the novices how to e-mail pictures and updates.

Activities are also a way to model good habits for your family. Kicking a soccer ball around in the park is a good way to get exercise. Making your daughter's track team competition a family outing shows her how important she is. Even cleaning the house can be more enjoyable when the whole family is involved.

Juggling family time

Maintaining a strong family isn't easy though, especially if both spouses work out of the home. You've worked a full week, attended two of your kids' games, made sure your father got to his eye appointment and taken the dog to the vet. It's Friday night, and you just want to collapse on the couch. But wait, there's still dinner to be made, laundry to be done, groceries to be bought — and the phone's ringing, probably your mother wondering if you could pick up a prescription for her.

Everyone has periods in life when there's so much to be done and never enough time. The stress can pile up right along with the list of unfinished projects. In times like these, it's critical to remember that it's unlikely you can do everything you want to do. The myth of needing to get it all done can be hard on both mental and physical health.

Cut yourself some slack. Sometimes, it makes more sense to live with some things undone and enjoy doing just those that are most essential. The following ideas can help you figure out how to fit in the things that matter most:

Prioritize
There will never be any shortage of things that it seems have to be done. Spend some time thinking about what needs to be done first and what's most important to you.

It might be helpful to have a long-term perspective. If you were looking back at your life as it neared the end, what would you hope to see? Is it more important to have had your closet organized or to have shared time with your daughter or son? If the closet is driving you crazy, maybe you can work on it 10 minutes a day until it's done.

Accommodate your priorities
If your priority is to spend a half-hour every night visiting with your spouse or going for a walk with your children, schedule other events around that time.

Delegate
Don't be afraid to ask for help when you need it. At home, try to arrange it so that everyone is working together to get the practical tasks done. If you're able, consider hiring help for some household work or lawn care.

Learn how to say no
Don't take on more than you can handle. Taking on nonessential responsibilities because you feel as if you should may leave less time and energy for the commitments you already have.

Working Life

For some people, work still means getting up and going to the same job every day until retirement. But the number of people spending their entire careers with the same employer is decreasing. More people switch companies, sometimes trading in one occupation for

Balancing Work and Family

One of life's biggest struggles is the pull between family and work. You want to give your best to both, and sometimes it feels as if they both suffer. Fight the guilt. Remember that having both a family and a job is normal today for both men and women. Also keep in mind that juggling the two is usually difficult for others too.

Do the best you can to accommodate both and expect that, at times, the needs of work will conflict with those of your family. Try not to resolve too many such conflicts, though, at the expense of your family.

If you have kids, don't be afraid to tell them how you're feeling. They may accept the situation more readily when they're assured that you're spending time away from them not because you don't love them but because sometimes you have to. In addition, ask your children about their feelings. Talking about the situation may help.

another. Others wait on careers until after their children are grown.

Starting new jobs and changing jobs can be exciting and challenging. Even retirement can be an eye-opener. Some people are surprised to find that retirement offers its own set of challenges.

Coping with workplace stress

If you dread going to work or often feel worn out or stressed after a day at work, you're facing a situation that could affect your professional and personal relationships, and even your livelihood and health. Overwhelming frustration or loss of interest in your job, persistent irritability, sarcasm and a quickness to argue are indicators of workplace stress.

Here are some strategies you can use to help overcome the challenges that work can pose:

- *Take care of yourself.* Eat regular, balanced meals, including breakfast. Get adequate sleep and exercise.
- *Develop friendships at work and off the job.* Sharing unsettling feelings with people you trust is the first step toward resolving them. Try to limit activities with people who reinforce bad feelings.
- *Take time off.* Go on a vacation or enjoy a long weekend. Plan private time each week when you don't answer calls or pages. During the workday, try to take short breaks.
- *Set limits.* When necessary, say no in a friendly but firm manner.
- *Choose battles wisely.* Don't argue whenever someone disagrees with you. Keep a cool head and save your arguments for things that really matter.
- *Set work goals.* Establish priorities and break big projects into smaller tasks. Being organized can help relieve stress.
- *Have an outlet.* Exercise, read, find a hobby or get involved in some other activity that you find relaxing and gets your mind off work.
- *Seek help.* If none of these steps relieves your feelings of stress or fatigue, ask a health care professional for advice.

Shift work

Some jobs entail working night shifts on a regular basis. Others require employees to rotate between day, evening and night shifts. Many different arrangements of shift work are used, but the one thing they all share is the toll they take on the body.

To remain healthy while working alternate hours, you need a healthy diet, adequate exercise and enough sleep. When you were younger, you could get away with temporarily shortchanging yourself on these healthy habits — subsisting on coffee and doughnuts for a meal and getting by with 4 to 5 hours of sleep. As you get older, your body becomes less forgiving.

Even if you get enough sleep, working shifts that change from week to week becomes increasingly difficult on your body. You get accustomed to a particular rhythm of waking and sleeping. Changing this rhythm requires a period of adjustment while your body experiences something akin to jet lag. This opens the way for health problems. Studies show serious consequences of shift work:

- Shift workers are usually sleepier when they're at work and more at risk of accidents.
- Family and social life are affected. Sometimes, children don't see a parent who works a night shift all week. Shift workers either miss out on events during the day or miss out on necessary sleep to attend them.
- Shift workers often switch to day hours on their days off, throwing their sleep patterns into further turmoil.
- Shift workers may experience more digestive problems than nonshift workers. Again, this is likely due to the interruption of

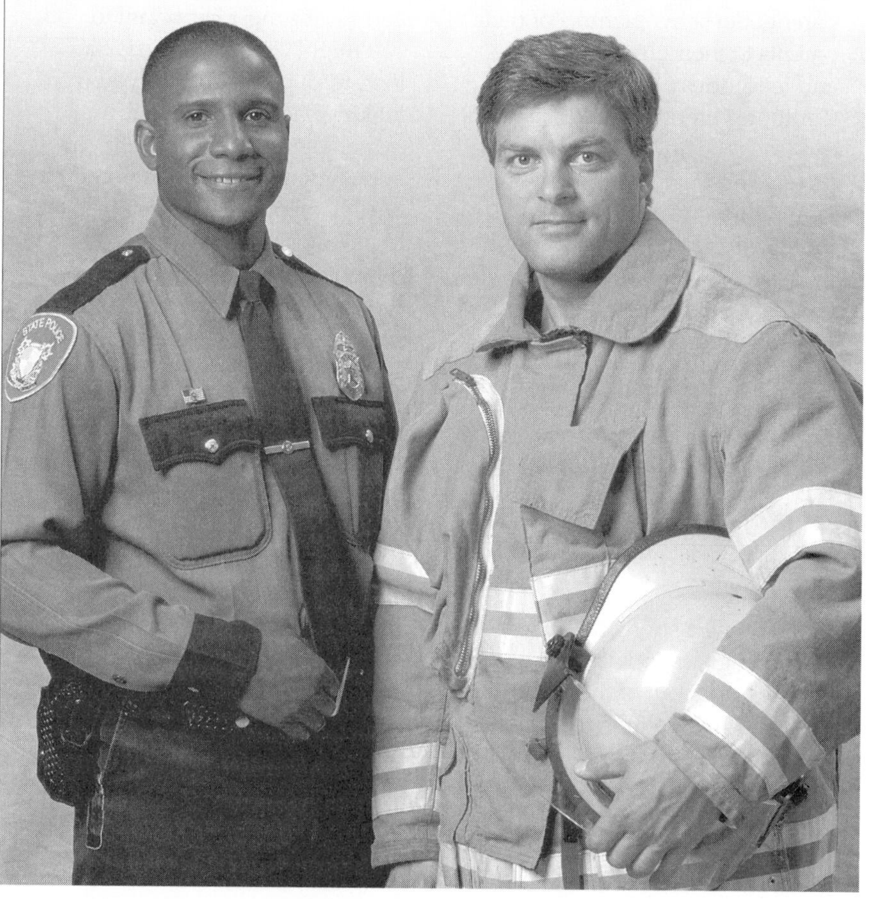

the body's natural sleep and rest patterns. Other practical matters, such as a lack of nutritious food on job sites in the middle of the night, may contribute to digestive troubles.

- Heart problems have been noted more frequently in shift workers. Again, it's difficult to separate lack of sleep and other factors — such as stress, diet, exercise and genetics — to determine what's behind the increase.

What you can do

Under such stressful working conditions, it's even more important that you give yourself the kind of care you need. Get enough sleep. Most people need a minimum of 6 hours' sleep each day. Many people need more than that. Experiment with different schedules to determine when you feel best rested after sleep. Some people sleep shortly after work and again before their shift, others sleep better in one longer block of time.

- Take naps. Be sure to nap long enough so that you're not more drowsy than before the nap — usually at least 20 to 30 minutes. Allow enough time between your nap and work to regain full alertness.
- Set the conditions for sleeping: make your bedroom dark, use earplugs, unplug the phone, ask family members to be quiet, find the quietest room in the house.
- Practice good sleep habits. Follow a routine for going to sleep that includes brushing your teeth and washing your face. Don't use your bed for lounging, reading or snacking. Go there to sleep.
- Establish a regular exercise routine. Exercise can promote improved sleep. Keep to a regular schedule — for example, after getting up or after work — but don't exercise close to bedtime.

Finding time for yourself

Are you the type of person who's so busy doing things for others that you don't have any time for yourself? Helping others is great, but you also need to take time for yourself, even if it's just 30 minutes a day.

Here are some ideas to help get you started:

- Tell the people closest to you — whether they be friends, a spouse, kids or parents — that you need a half-hour a day to yourself. Pick a time and stick to it. In the beginning, your family or friends may give you some resistance, but if you stick to your schedule, eventually everyone will know not to disturb you except in an emergency.
- Get away from the telephone, e-mails and the doorbell. Don't be tempted to get something done in your half-hour. Read a book or magazine, take a bath, meditate or exercise.
- Recast the frantic hour right after work as individual quiet time. This is the time that each person in the family can decompress in whatever way he or she likes.

Making It Through a Midlife Crisis

What constitutes a midlife crisis? Does everyone experience one? Is it possible to emerge from a midlife crisis unscathed or even better off?

Childhood is a period of growth and preparation for adulthood. As a young adult, you begin making your own way, exploring alternatives and striving to reach your goals. By your middle years, you likely have constructed a life of stability, comfort and familiarity. You may also have achieved adequate personal and financial resources. This can be a productive period, during which many people achieve their greatest accomplishments.

But a lot happens in these years. You may have to deal with difficulties in your work, marriage or parenting. You may have to deal with the loss of a parent or another loved one. Changes in your body make it clear that you're no longer as young as you once were. Suddenly, retirement and old age don't seem all that far away. If you haven't reached your goals, or what you anticipated for your level of success, you might consider yourself a failure.

It takes considerable personal stability to cope with the full array of changes and problems the middle years can bring. Individuals who feel unable to cope with the changes, who shift directions or who set new priorities and goals are often said to be experiencing a midlife crisis. During their middle years, some people also become mired in self-doubt, make sudden job changes, become obsessed with aging and mortality or have an extramarital affair. These actions also fall under the crisis heading.

Not everyone goes through a midlife crisis. If you do experience one, the outcome doesn't have to be detrimental. You can emerge from it better off — more aware of yourself as an individual and better able to direct your life under new and challenging circumstances. Taking stock of your priorities and where your life is headed is a positive thing, as long as you don't lose your way and take actions you may live to regret later.

If you find, though, that you're having trouble dealing with the difficulties of your middle years or in achieving a fresh perspective, don't be afraid to seek help. Talk with a family member or friend, a clergyperson, a counselor, your doctor or a mental health professional. Admitting that you're having difficulty and seeking help is not a sign of weakness but a sign of strength.

Changing Roles

Adulthood can present many life transitions. In fact, for some the changes can be so dramatic and intense that they make puberty seem like a breeze. Children grow up and leave home. Parents need extra help with day-to-day tasks. Friends or family members may go through midlife crises. Partners and close friends may die.

Caring for aging parents

Your parents once cared for you, but the time may now come when it's your turn to help care for them. Perhaps your parents are experiencing major health problems or are less able to get around to appointments and events.

It might be time for them to give up independent living, which poses a number of questions: Should they move in with your family? Choose a retirement community? Enter a nursing home?

It may be a stressful time for them, and they may seek your help in making these difficult decisions. Many resources are available to help you and your parents determine what the best living arrangement would be for them. For a list of resources, see page 1377.

The death of a parent is another situation you may have to deal with. It's a major loss and can trigger depression no matter what your age. Even at age 60, you can feel orphaned, unable to imagine life without a person who has been such a strong influence on you.

Grieving is the way to work through and accept such a loss. However, if grief becomes prolonged, or if you get stuck in one stage of grief and can't get out, seek help. Grief can lead to sustained depression.

Dealing with marriage difficulties

Changing goals and needs. Role reversals. Life stresses. Difficulties with children or parents. All of these affect a marriage.

Many people are reluctant to visit a marriage counselor when their marriage is in jeopardy, but sometimes a professional can help a couple communicate and, therefore, resolve conflicts and improve relationships. With something as important as a marriage at stake, counseling is certainly worth a try. Sometimes, though, even the best efforts at reconciliation fail.

Divorce is common among adults of all ages. Going through a divorce and adjusting to the new circumstances that follow the separation and legal proceedings can be among the most stressful events that take place during a person's lifetime. Divorce usually means fewer financial resources for both partners, requiring further adjustments in lifestyle.

If the divorcing couple have children, they'll have to make big adjustments as well — perhaps new homes, new schools and new people in their life. Some children adjust quickly and well, but others don't. If you're going through a divorce and have children, be sure to seek professional help if you or your children aren't coping well with the changes. One change almost always begets others. Too much change too fast can be extremely stressful.

Coping with the loss of a partner

In your younger years, accidents were the primary cause of death among people your age. As you get older, natural causes begin to take over. Heart disease, cancer and stroke are the primary killers of people older than 45. You attend more funerals. You no longer feel invincible, and increasingly, you sense your own mortality.

The loss of a spouse or a long-term partner can be devastating. You grieve on many levels: you've lost your best friend, you've lost the person around whom much of your daily life was structured, and your children, if you have any, have lost a parent.

Before you can regain order in your life, you must work through a period of grieving. However, if your grief seems prolonged or destructive and you have great difficulty coping, get professional help. Talk to your doctor, who may recommend that you see a psychiatrist or psychologist.

After losing a partner, you'll have to do things yourself that he or she used to do with you or for you. You'll have to develop new routines and fill the void in your life with new social bonds. In other words, you'll have to restructure some of your lifestyle.

More women than men go through loss of a spouse because three out of every four wives outlive their husbands. Surviving partners may experience economic hardship, particularly women who haven't been working outside the home. One solution is to re-enter

5 Things You Should Know

In case of an emergency, it would be helpful for you to know certain information about your parents. Know the answers to the following questions, or at least make sure the necessary information is readily accessible:

1. What are the names of your parents' doctors?
2. Who is your parents' health insurance provider? What type of coverage do they have?
3. Are your parents allergic to any medications?
4. What medications do they take?
5. Have your parents prepared an advance directive, such as a living will? Who has a copy of it?

the work force, intimidating as that may be. You can get counseling regarding job choices, and you can regain old skills or learn new ones by going back to school or taking community education courses.

If you're financially comfortable and don't need to work, think about volunteering. You'll fill up empty hours, add structure to your life and achieve a sense of accomplishment. Museums, schools, hospitals, libraries and social agencies are only some of the places where your experience and help will be welcome.

The Aging Process

If you're older than age 40, you've undoubtedly confronted some realities of growing older. You've probably peeked into a mirror at a face that has developed a few more wrinkles. You may have noticed that aches and pains linger a little longer after exercising or spending too many hours doing yardwork.

Until adults reach the fourth or fifth decade, aging rarely means much, even though it's a lifelong process that begins at birth. Childhood, adolescence and young adulthood are filled with feelings of immortality. It's only when certain physical changes begin to emerge that most individuals begin to accept that they may be getting older.

If you're older than age 60, you've not only encountered many realities of aging but also most likely realize that you've got a lot more life left. Whatever your life stage, aging sure beats the alternative. Understanding the changes that commonly come with age can help you accept the changes and possibly prevent certain diseases or disorders.

Flesh, bone and organs have a limited life span. Some parts tend to lose their shine and wear out sooner than others do. This section describes some of the ways that your organs and body systems change as you age. Not all of these changes are inevitable. Some of the decline typically blamed on aging is actually due to inactivity, an unhealthy diet and other lifestyle choices.

Vision changes

With age, the lenses of your eyes become less elastic. This change usually begins around age 40 and results in difficulty focusing on nearby objects. Around this age, many people find that they start needing the help of glasses for reading. If you don't need glasses at least some of the time by age 65, you're an exception.

Glaucoma, cataracts and macular degeneration can come with age. They're more serious and tend to develop in people in their 60s, 70s and 80s. However, these changes can occur in younger adults, especially in those with a family history of the disease.

These eye disorders can affect one or both eyes. Because they develop gradually and are usually

Warning Signs of Depression

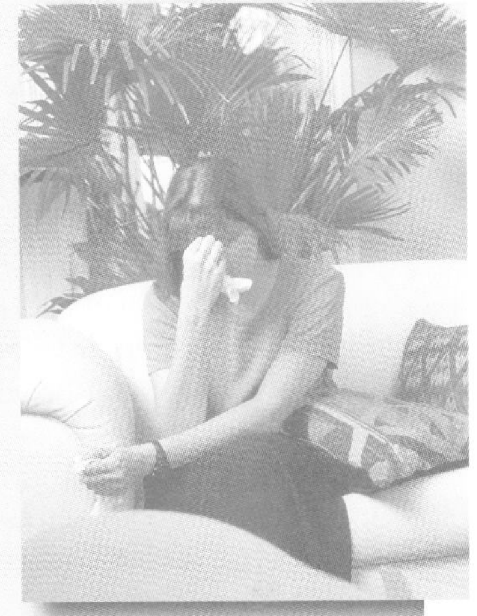

Everyone feels down from time to time. Generally, such sadness or despair passes on its own as the situation that caused it resolves or as you learn to cope with it.

Sometimes, though, the stresses of life can lead to depression. The sadness or despair doesn't go away and may get worse. Events that are common in the middle years — work difficulties, family struggles, caring for older parents — can trigger depression. In the later years, loss of a spouse, physical illness or retirement is commonly associated with depression.

Signs and symptoms of depression most often include several of the following:

- Persistent sadness
- Irritability
- Anxiety
- Loss of interest or pleasure in life
- Neglect of personal responsibilities or personal care
- Changes in eating habits
- Changes in sleep patterns, especially waking up in the middle of the night
- Fatigue or loss of energy
- Decreased concentration, attention and memory
- Extreme mood changes
- Feelings of helplessness, hopelessness, worthlessness or guilt
- Continuous negative thinking
- Physical symptoms that don't respond to treatment
- Increased alcohol or drug use
- Thoughts of death or suicide

Depression isn't a normal state of mind or something that you have to live with. Depression can often be successfully treated. Many individuals who have experienced an episode of depression are able to return to their normal life and live and work as they did before the depression occurred. If you feel that you or a loved one may be depressed, seek help. For more information on depression, see Chapter 37, "Mental Illness."

painless, they're often mistaken for the normal effects of aging.

It's important to visit an eye specialist regularly, especially as you begin to experience changes in your vision. Seek prompt medical attention if you develop a painful, red eye or if you lose some or all vision in an eye. Also seek attention if you experience flashes of light in your visual field. If left untreated, some eye disorders can cause permanent loss of eyesight.

Glaucoma

Glaucoma is a group of eye conditions resulting from abnormally high pressure in the eyeball. The result is a shrinking of the field of vision. About 3 percent of people older than age 65 have glaucoma.

Cataracts

A cataract is a clouding of the normally clear lens of the eye, resulting in blurred vision, double vision or seeing halos around lights. Cataracts are the leading cause of blindness in the world. Cataract surgery is one of the most common surgical procedures in the United States.

Cataracts affect nearly 20.5 million Americans age 40 or older, or about one in every six people in this age range. By 80 years of age, about half of all people develop cataracts.

Macular degeneration

Macular degeneration is a deterioration of the macula, the small, central part of the retina where images are focused. Macular degeneration affects reading acuity and visual sharpness. The disease is characterized by a black spot in the center of the visual field, affecting central vision. Peripheral vision is generally normal.

What helps

Even if you don't have vision problems, as you age you may need more light to see well. Try using a flexible light, such as a gooseneck lamp, to direct light onto your read-

Physical Changes that Occur with Age

Most adults generally experience common physical changes as they get older. The following list of some such changes comes from the Baltimore Longitudinal Study of Aging, published by the Department of Health and Human Services:

- Your heart grows slightly larger and maximum oxygen consumption decreases.
- Your systolic blood pressure increases and artery walls thicken.
- Your body redistributes fat.
- Your muscle mass and handgrip strength decline.
- Your ability to hear high-frequency sounds decreases, beginning around age 20, and low-frequency sounds become more difficult to hear during your 60s.
- Your maximum breathing capacity declines.
- Your brain sustains loss and damage of nerve cells.
- Your bladder loses capacity, leading to more frequent urination and, sometimes, incontinence.
- Your kidneys become less efficient in removing wastes from the bloodstream.

Remember, this information describes what happens on average to groups of people. It doesn't predict exactly how aging will affect you. If you take care of your health and stay active, you may be able to delay many of these occurrences.

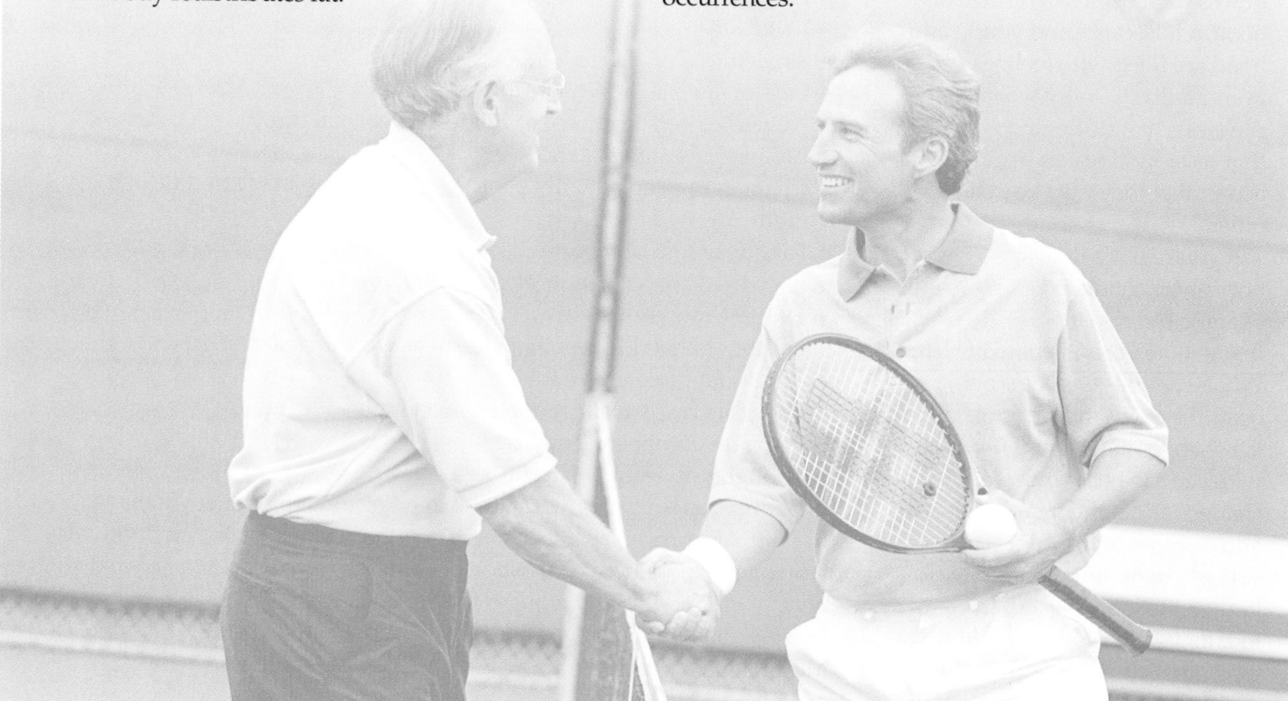

Problems with Night Vision

Night vision refers to how well you see in poor light or in the dark. With age, healthy eyes become a little less adept at seeing at night. One common and potentially dangerous consequence is difficulty driving. For example, your eyes may not be able to recover as rapidly from the momentary effect of looking at oncoming headlights.

Many eye disorders can result in reduced visual acuity at night. If you have trouble seeing well at night, consult your eye specialist. Don't just assume that it's a natural consequence of getting older.

ing or work. Higher-wattage light bulbs also may help. Use night lights to help you see better at night. This may also reduce the risk of falls.

If your only problem is trouble reading and you don't have any other vision disorder, you might wish to purchase nonprescription reading glasses, which are available in many drugstores and discount stores.

Hearing changes

Although some individuals retain excellent hearing throughout their life, most people gradually lose some hearing sensitivity, sometimes starting in their 20s. Hearing loss is one of the most common conditions affecting middle-aged and older adults. One in three people older than age 60 and half the people older than age 85 have significant hearing loss.

Age-related hearing loss usually first affects your ability to hear higher frequencies and later, lower frequencies. Some people find it difficult to follow conversations in a crowded room or restaurant.

Changes within the inner ear or in nerves attached to it, noise, earwax buildup and various diseases all can impair your hearing. If you or a family member suspects that you have hearing loss, see your doctor, who may refer you to a hearing specialist. Some hearing loss can be restored or improved with medical treatment or surgery.

Hearing aids can't help everyone, but they can improve hearing for many people. With the development of smaller hearing aids that are more effective and less noticeable, more people with hearing loss are turning to hearing aids to improve their hearing. For more information on hearing loss and hearing aids, see Chapter 24, "Ears, Nose and Throat."

Skin changes

With age, your body's largest organ, the skin, gradually loses some of its elasticity. The result: Your skin begins to wrinkle and sag. By keeping fit, you can keep many of your underlying muscles firm and taut, but in some locations, such as your face, your skin will sag a bit anyway.

Your skin also becomes a little thinner with age, allowing veins or discolorations beneath the surface to show through more readily. You may begin to lose your youthful color and glow. Decreased production of natural oils makes your skin drier. In addition, you perspire less.

How fast your skin ages depends on many factors. The most significant factor is sun exposure over the years. The more sun that your skin has been exposed to, the more damage. Smoking adds to skin damage, such as wrinkles.

Some changes are due in part to skin dryness, which can be minimized by good skin care throughout life. Nutrition and fitness also play a part. Your skin, like other organs, benefits from a good blood supply provided by a healthy diet and regular exercise.

Following are some common skin conditions that occur with age:

Wrinkles

Wrinkles are a natural consequence of aging. Taking care of your skin and keeping it healthy will help postpone wrinkles, but the effects of aging can't be stopped altogether.

Dry skin

Dry skin (asteatosis) is characterized by intense itching on your back, lower legs, hands or elsewhere. It results from loss of natural skin oils, producing scaly skin that, in some cases, can crack.

Restricting the frequency of baths or showers, not wearing wool next to your skin, increasing the humidity level in your house and applying lubricating cream or lotion can help combat the problem. However, see your doctor to make sure your itchy skin isn't the result of another condition.

Age spots

Age spots, also called liver spots, are flat, pigmented skin patches, from light brown to black. They can be anywhere from freckle sized to a few inches across. You may consider age spots to be cosmetically troublesome, but they're medically insignificant. Contrary to their name, they have nothing to do with the liver.

Purpura senilis

With age, tiny blood vessels just below the surface of the skin become fragile and bleed. This

Cosmetic Surgery

With the advent of wrinkles and sagging skin, some people consider cosmetic surgery a way to combat aging. Common questions about cosmetic surgery include:

What can it do?
The classic face-lift operation tightens and smoothes the skin, reducing coarser wrinkles and sags. Eyelid surgery removes puffiness and bags under the eyes and excess skin above the eyes. Eyelid surgery is also done for non-cosmetic reasons if sagging eyelids are impairing vision.

How is it done?
For a face-lift, a surgeon makes small incisions in the area of the sideburns, just in front of the ears, and behind the ears in the hairline. He or she then pulls the skin up and back and trims away the excess. Often, subcutaneous fat in the area of the chin is removed. Visible scarring is minimal.

Is it dangerous?
As with all operations, the procedure is subject to complications such as excessive swelling and bruising, infection and injury to nerves.

How long does recovery take?
Bruising and swelling from a face-lift largely disappear after 2 to 3 weeks.

How long do the results last?
Results can last from a few to many years.

causes superficial bruising called purpura senilis. The condition occurs mainly on the forearms. Certain medications taken to prevent blood from clotting, such as aspirin, can lead to or worsen purpura senilis. This condition is medically insignificant.

Hair changes

Hair changes with age, but the process varies greatly from person to person. On average, about 50 percent of adults are about 50 percent gray by age 50. Graying usually begins at the temples and slowly works its way up the scalp. The new hair is often different in texture.

Graying is considered attractive by some people and unattractive by others. How you view it is largely a matter of personal preference, your cultural background or current fashion.

Some thinning of hair also typically occurs in both men and women. About 60 percent of men experience hair loss or thinning by age 50. Male-pattern baldness typically involves a receding hairline and hair loss on the top of the head. Age, changing hormones and heredity cause some people to lose more hair than others.

A small number of women experience female-pattern baldness as they age. Instead of developing bald patches, women are more likely to notice a widening of their part and hair that looks and feels thinner. Hormone alterations that occur after menopause can cause facial hairs to coarsen and grow.

Dental changes

How your teeth and gums respond to age depends on how well you've cared for them over the years. But even if you're meticulous about brushing and flossing, you may notice that your mouth feels dry and your gums have pulled back (receded). Your teeth may darken slightly and become more brittle.

With less saliva to wash away bacteria, your teeth and gums become slightly more vulnerable to decay and infection. Smoking, illness and certain medications can aggravate these problems. Mild gum disease makes your gums red, puffy and sore. Left untreated, gum disease can progress until your teeth loosen and fall out.

Denture sores are usually due to improper fit. If you've worn your dentures for a while and begin developing sores, this irritation may indicate a change in the denture or in the alignment of your mouth. If your weight changes, your dentures may need to be refitted. Sores can also develop if food becomes trapped beneath the dentures. In rare cases, recurrent mouth sores can signal a health problem.

What you can do
Brush at least twice daily and floss daily. Be sure to clean both the outer and inner surfaces of your teeth and gums. If you have difficulty performing these tasks, try brushing with an electric toothbrush and using floss aids.

If you're having problems with denture sores, see your dentist to have your dentures adjusted. To avoid sores caused by trapped food, brush after every meal, take out your dentures at night and brush your gums, tongue and palate. Avoid using an over-the-counter ointment to numb denture-sore pain. In addition to daily oral care, visit your dentist at least annually for a routine cleaning and dental checkup.

Sleep changes

Your sleep needs change little throughout adulthood. If you need about 6 hours nightly, chances are you'll need about that amount — give or take 30 minutes — 10 years from now.

However, as you get older, you'll likely find that you sleep less soundly. Between ages 50 and 60, sleep often becomes less restful. After age 70, it's common to spend more time in bed but less time sleeping soundly. That's because delta sleep, the deepest, most restorative sleep, decreases with age. You may also get tired earlier in the evening and wake up earlier in the morning.

Insomnia tends to become more of a problem with age, for many reasons. Changes in your sleep patterns, activity level and health can disrupt your sleep schedule. Pain, depression, anxiety and stress also can interfere with sleep. Men who develop noncancerous (benign) enlargement of the prostate have their sleep interrupted by the need to urinate more frequently in the night.

Medications also can be at fault, as can a snoring bed partner. Lack of sleep due to insomnia isn't an inevitable part of aging. But with age, insomnia risk factors do increase.

Weight changes

For most people, maintaining a healthy weight or losing weight if they're overweight isn't easy. As you get older, these processes can become even more difficult. With age, your metabolism generally slows, meaning that your body functions by burning fewer calories than it once did. Calories that were once used to meet your daily energy needs instead are stored as fat. In addition, your level of activity may not be what it was. Often, the result is unwanted weight gain.

Cardiovascular changes

Your heart and blood vessels change with age, even in the absence of disease. Over time, the muscle of the heart becomes a less efficient pump, working harder to do the same job. You may also lose some pacemaker cells, which control the heart's rate and rhythm.

With age, your blood vessels naturally become less elastic. Hardened fatty deposits (atherosclerotic plaques) may accumulate in the walls of your arteries and narrow the passageway through the vessels. The natural loss of elasticity, in combination with atherosclerosis, makes the arteries narrower, causing your heart to work harder to pump blood through them. This can lead to high blood pressure (hypertension).

It's common for blood pressure to increase slightly with age. As long as your blood pressure remains within a satisfactory range, there's no cause for concern. But if the increase is significant enough to produce high blood pressure, the condition needs to be treated.

Cardiovascular changes typically occur gradually over a period of months or years. Between ages 40 and 65, the process already may be advanced, particularly in men, who have more cardiovascular problems than do women in this age group.

Despite age-related deterioration in your cardiovascular system, your heart is strong enough to meet the normal needs of your body, at rest or during exercise. However, it has less reserve capacity for overcoming injury or handling the sudden demands placed on it by increased physical activity, stress or illness. Atherosclerosis or high blood pressure can lead to heart attack or congestive heart failure.

> **? Question and Answer**
>
> **Is there a diet that can help me live a longer, healthier life?**
>
> No. There isn't one specific diet that can help all individuals live longer. The problems you accumulate as you age are unique to you. If you have high blood pressure, you may need to reduce your weight and avoid salt. If you have diabetes, you'll need to control sugar intake as well as your weight.
>
> The best advice is to follow a healthy diet that includes a variety of food groups. A balanced diet ensures proper intake of vitamins, minerals, proteins, carbohydrates and other food elements. In general, eat plenty of fruits and vegetables each day, while limiting fats and red meat. Eating moderate proportions is another important component of a healthy diet.

Digestive changes

Digestive changes often are so subtle that people don't begin to notice them until they reach their 60s.

In essence, with age, the digestive process slows. The swallowing action of the esophagus becomes somewhat slower. Similarly, the propulsion of digested food through the intestines slows down.

The amount of surface area within the intestines diminishes, reducing absorption. The flow of digestive secretions from the stomach, liver, pancreas and small intestine may decrease. These changes often are inconsequential or minimal and don't cause disruptive changes.

One of the common digestive conditions to occur with age is constipation. Constipation is marked by hard stool, less frequent bowel movements and difficulty having a bowel movement. Constipation may result from a diet low in fiber, changes in your diet, drinking too little fluids, use of medications, inactivity or natural changes, such as a slowing of digested food through the intestines.

Another condition more noticeable with age is heartburn.

Heartburn results when the valve between the esophagus and the stomach (lower esophageal sphincter) opens, allowing stomach contents to reflux into the esophagus.

Being overweight, smoking, overeating, consuming alcohol or caffeine or using certain medications can cause the sphincter muscle to relax and open.

In addition, with age this muscle loses tone and weakens. Frequent or constant heartburn is often associated with a common condition called gastroesophageal reflux disease (GERD).

Skeletal and muscular changes

Although you might think of bones as hard, rigid and unchanging, they're constantly undergoing renewal and responding to the demands placed on them. For example, a person who does a lot of heavy lifting not only develops larger and more powerful arm muscles than someone who doesn't do heavy lifting, but also develops stronger bones in the arms.

Your bones reach their maximal mass between ages 25 and 35. During subsequent years, they decline slightly in both size and density.

One consequence of this is that during the middle to later years of your life, your height may decrease. Another is that your bones become less resilient, making you more vulnerable to fractures.

In addition, muscles, tendons and joints generally lose a certain amount of their strength and flexibility. The result: You may not move as fast as you once did.

If you've had an active life, by age 60 your muscles will have lost little or none of the strength they had in your youth. However, you may notice that you're less flexible and your reflexes are slower.

Two of the more common skeletal and muscular disorders that come with age are osteoporosis and arthritis.

Osteoporosis

Osteoporosis is the term for loss of bone density, causing bone to become weak and susceptible to fracture. Although it typically results over time as people lose bone minerals during aging, long-term use of some medications, such as steroids, also can cause this condition.

Osteoporosis especially affects women after menopause. Men also lose bone density, but because they have more bone mass to start with and because they lose it at a slower rate, they're less likely to experience osteoporosis until advanced age.

The best treatment of osteoporosis is prevention, which should start well before you turn 40. Eating foods high in calcium, taking calcium supplements and getting plenty of weight-bearing exercise, such as walking, can help maximize bone mass before mineral depletion begins.

Smoking and excessive alcohol intake increase the risk of osteoporosis and should be avoided. After menopause, these preventive measures become even more important.

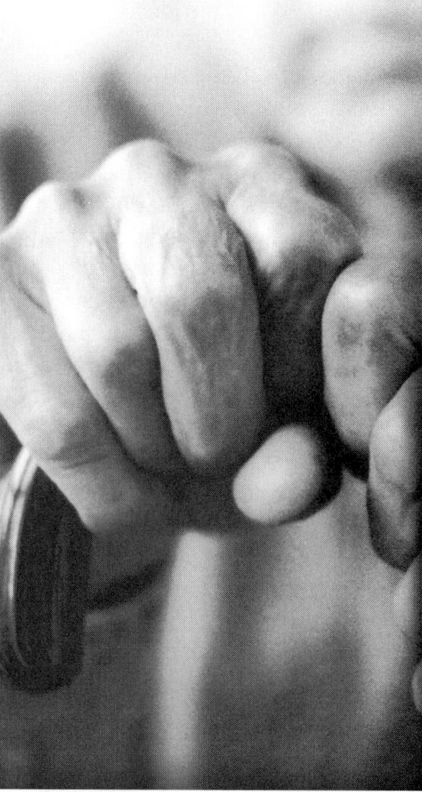

Arthritis

Most arthritis is simple deterioration of a joint. Heredity, diet and previous injuries and disease are causes of arthritis. Everyday wear and tear also can lead to the disease.

The two main forms of arthritis are osteoarthritis and rheumatoid arthritis.

Osteoarthritis

Osteoarthritis is the most common form of arthritis. During the middle years, most people have some arthritis in at least one joint. The symptoms are intermittent pain, stiffness and occasional swelling in the joint. Sometimes no symptoms are experienced. The disease is present to some degree in more than 80 percent of older adults.

Osteoarthritis typically causes pain and stiffness and starts in the spine or the large joints, such as your hips and knees. Because your natural response to a painful joint is to move it less, you use the muscles in the area less frequently, so they start to shrink and lose strength. This process produces a destructive cycle that increases the degree of disability.

Rheumatoid arthritis

Rheumatoid arthritis is less common and generally isn't closely associated with older age. Rheumatoid arthritis is an autoimmune disease in which your body's immune system attacks one or more joints. The disease generally affects your wrists, hands, feet and ankles. The disease most often develops in people between the ages of 20 and 50 and is twice as common in women as in men.

Sexual changes

Aging doesn't mean an end to sexual desire or function. In reality, sex can be more rewarding than it was during the frantic pace of your younger years. But with age, sexual needs, patterns and performance may change. For men, setting and mood often take on more importance. Touch and extended foreplay may become as enjoyable as release. Women may feel more relaxed, less inhibited and more confident in asserting their sexual desires.

The widespread misperception is that older adults aren't sexually active. The reality is that many older adults enjoy an active sex life that's often better than their sex life in early adulthood. The keys are caring, adapting and communicating.

Your brain is an important sex organ. Sexual arousal begins with stimulation of your senses — touch, sight, smell, taste and hearing. Because of this, orgasms are possible throughout life, although response may be diminished or delayed.

Changes in women

Menopause marks the end of menstruation in women. Common misconceptions about menopause are that it marks the end of interest in sex, triggers depression and brings on emotional instability. The fact is, if you were interested in and enjoyed sex as a younger woman, you'll probably feel the same way about it after menopause. Yet menopause does bring changes.

Desire

Although your sex drive is largely determined by emotional and social factors, hormones such as estrogen and testosterone do play a role. Estrogen is produced by your ovaries, and testosterone is made in your adrenal glands.

Surprisingly, sexual desire is affected mainly by testosterone, not estrogen. At menopause, your ovaries stop producing estrogen, but most women produce enough testosterone to preserve their interest in sex. Remember: The most important sex organ is the brain. Candlelight, music, food, conversation, books and thoughts can help create a mood for sex.

Vaginal changes

Estrogen deficiency following menopause may lead to changes in the appearance of your genitals and how you respond sexually. The folds of skin that cover your genital region (labia) shrink and become thinner, exposing more of the clitoris. This increased exposure sometimes reduces the clitoris' sensitivity or causes an unpleasant tingling or prickling sensation when it's touched. In addition, the opening to your vagina becomes narrower, particularly if you're not sexually active. And, the natural swelling and lubrication of your vagina occur more slowly during arousal. These factors can lead to difficult or painful intercourse (dyspareunia).

Sex and Illness

Changes in your body due to illness or surgery can affect your physical response to sex. They can also affect your self-image and ultimately limit your interest in sex. Here are tips to help you maintain confidence in your sexuality:

Know what to expect
Talk to your doctor about the usual effects of your treatment, including possible effects on sexual function.

Talk about sex
If you feel weak or tired and want your partner to take a more active role, say so. If some part of your body is sore, guide your mate's caresses to create pleasure and avoid pain.

Plan for sex
Try to have sex when you're rested and relaxed. Taking a warm bath first or having sex in the morning may help. If you take a pain reliever, such as for arthritis, time the dose so that its effect will occur during sexual activity.

Prepare with exercise
If you have arthritis or another disability, ask your doctor or therapist for range-of-motion exercises to help relax your joints before sex.

Find pleasure in touch
Touch is a good alternative to sexual intercourse. Touching can simply mean holding each other. Men and women can sometimes reach orgasm with the right kind of touching.

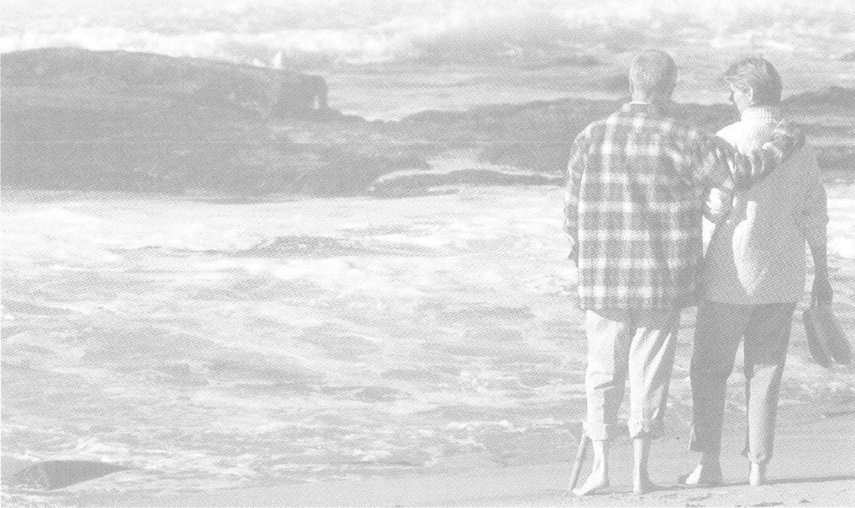

Longer foreplay sometimes helps stimulate your natural lubrication, or you can use a water-soluble lubricant such as K-Y jelly. Talk to your doctor about estrogen cream for your genital area or estrogen replacement therapy. Having intercourse regularly also helps. Women who are sexually active after menopause have better lubrication and elasticity of vaginal tissues.

Orgasm
Orgasms are possible throughout life. It may take longer as you age, but most people can still get there.

Emotional outlook
Study after study shows little connection between mood and menopause. Emotional reactions after menopause seem, instead, to be a result of whatever is going on in your life. Your expectations about menopause seem to influence how you experience the "change of life." If you think it will be difficult, it will. If you expect to breeze through it, you probably will.

Changes in men

With aging, the production of the hormone testosterone gradually declines but doesn't cease. However, physical changes in a middle-aged man's sexual response can parallel those in a postmenopausal woman.

Desire
You may experience a gradual lessening of sexual desire. Some men call this a focus on quality rather than quantity.

Excitement
You may require more stimulation to achieve and maintain an erection, and the erection may be less firm. You may need more partner involvement.

Orgasm
Ejaculation may expel less semen with less force than previously. After a climax, it may take longer before you can be stimulated to another.

Impotence
The inability to achieve and maintain an erection when desire and opportunity are present can affect men at any age, although it becomes more common as you get older. Nearly 20 percent of men are impotent at age 60.

Impotence is not an inevitable consequence of aging. Common causes are alcohol abuse, medications that affect sexual function and medical problems, such as diabetes and atherosclerosis. Stress, which can be plentiful during the middle years, also ranks high on the list of possible causes.

Don't interpret an episode or two of impotence as a signal that your sex life is about to end. If you regularly experience impotence, though, discuss the problem with your doctor. Chances are good that, regardless of the cause, it can be treated, especially if you seek therapy before the problem goes on too long.

Changes due to illness or disability

Illness or disability can interfere with how you respond sexually. In addition, certain medical conditions can affect sexual function:

Heart attack
If you or your partner has had a heart attack, fear of causing another one can affect your sexual behavior. But if you were sexually active before the heart attack, you can probably be so again. Even though pulse rates, respiratory rates and blood pressure increase during intercourse, after intercourse they return to normal within minutes. Sudden death during sex is rare.

If you have a type of heart disease with symptoms of angina, your doctor may recommend that you take nitroglycerin before intercourse.

Atherosclerosis
About half of all impotence in men older than age 50 is caused by damage to the nerves or blood vessels to the penis. Accumulation of plaques in your arteries (atherosclerosis) can damage small blood vessels and restrict blood flow to the genitals. This can interfere with erection in men and swelling of vaginal tissues in women.

Diabetes
Diabetes increases your risk of atherosclerosis. About half the men with diabetes become impotent. Men who've had diabetes for many years and who also have nerve damage (diabetic neuropathy) are more likely to become impotent.

If you're a woman with diabetes, you may suffer from decreased lubrication and painful intercourse. You may have more frequent vaginal and urinary tract infections.

Arthritis
Although arthritis doesn't affect your sex organs, the pain and stiffness of arthritis can make sex difficult to enjoy. If you have arthritis, discuss your capabilities and your desires openly with your partner.

Prostate surgery
In men, surgery for prostate cancer can cause impotence, but advances in surgery have reduced this risk in recent years. New treatments for impotence also are available.

Hysterectomy
A hysterectomy, by itself, doesn't interfere with a woman's physical ability to have intercourse or experience orgasm. Removing the ovaries, however, creates instant menopause and accelerates the physical and emotional aspects of this natural occurrence in a woman's life.

Medications
Some commonly used medications can interfere with sexual function. Drugs that control high blood pressure, such as thiazide diuretics and beta blockers, can reduce desire and impair erection in men and lubrication in women.

Other medications that may affect sexual function include some antihistamines, some antidepressants and medications that block secretion of stomach acid. If you take one of these and are experiencing side effects, talk with your doctor. Alcohol also may adversely affect sexual function.

Planning for Retirement

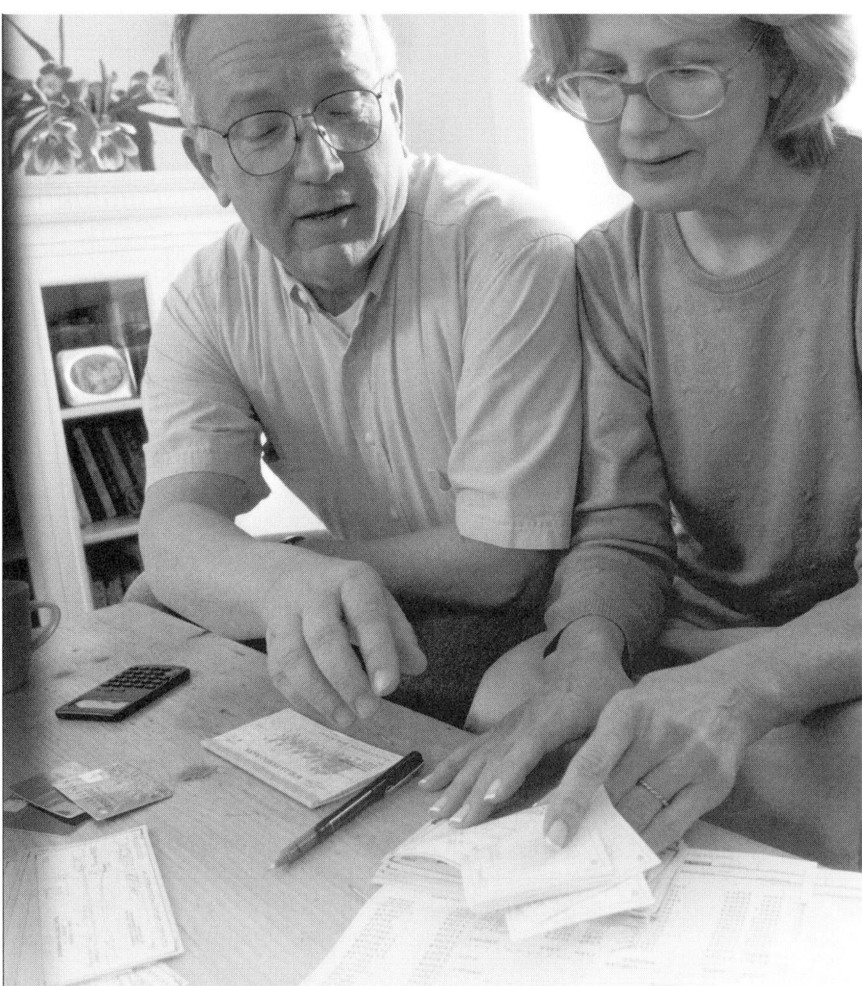

Retirement is a big adjustment. It can be a stressful time for which you're unprepared. Or it can be as rewarding and fulfilling as your early years. Which way it goes is, to a certain extent, up to you. Planning for your retirement will help ease the way for you to enjoy another phase of your life.

Financial security

"Money isn't everything," the old saying goes. And indeed it isn't. But money is one of the resources you need to make your way in the world. It helps you to live comfortably — whatever your definition of that is — and it helps you to be able to do many of the things you enjoy in your free time.

For some individuals, inadequate financial resources can make retirement difficult and be a major stress on their emotions that ultimately affects their health. People with sound finances generally tend to cope better with illness than do people who don't have the funds they need. In other words, along with a balanced diet, plenty of exercise and strong social ties, another component of well-being is adequate financial resources.

The means to achieving a financially secure retirement, however, have changed. For a growing number of individuals, the days of retired workers being taken care of entirely by company pensions and Social Security benefits are past. Increasingly, individuals are now largely responsible for planning their own retirement. Without good planning and discipline, there's no guarantee that your retirement income will cover your expenses, let alone allow you to fulfill your hopes for retirement.

If you haven't started planning for retirement already, a good way to begin is to look at how much money you think you'll need when you retire and compare it with how much money you're likely to have, based on your present saving and investment patterns. If you come up short, it may not be too late to take steps toward making up the difference.

Sources of retirement income

Your retirement income will probably come from a combination of sources. These are likely to include Social Security, savings and investments, retirement funds, pensions and earned income.

Don't forget about the effect of inflation — your money will buy less when you retire than it will today. And taxes will continue to take a portion of your money.

How much money will you need?

Retirement doesn't mean that bills stop arriving in your mailbox. It doesn't mean that you'll suddenly lose your desire to travel, eat in good restaurants or go to a ballgame. Nor does it mean that your roof won't leak and need replacement. Take all of these things into consideration when predicting how much money you'll need.

Estimate your life expectancy

In general, the average 65-year-old American man today can expect to live to age 81. An American woman the same age can expect to live to age 84. If you come from a family in which individuals tend to live much longer, you should adjust your estimated life expectancy accordingly.

Decide when you would like to retire
The age at which you retire can have a big impact on how much money you'll have for retirement. By working longer, you'll have more time to put money into your retirement accounts. In addition, you won't be drawing money out of them as soon, allowing them to continue to grow.

One thing to consider in determining when to retire is your Social Security benefits. See how your retirement age will affect your benefits. Each year the Social Security Administration is required to send you a Social Security statement. Under the benefits section, you'll find figures showing how much your monthly payment will be if you retire at age 62, age 66 or age 70.

You may have many good reasons to retire at a younger age. Just make sure that you're aware of the financial impact of working fewer years.

Calculate your expenses
Financial experts generally believe that the average retired couple should plan on their living expenses reaching 80 percent to 100 percent of their yearly gross preretirement income. Once again, take into consideration your specific plans.

If you plan to travel extensively or move to a more expensive area, you may need more money than you did before you retired. If your retirement goals are more modest, your annual living expenses may be less. Don't forget about important expenses such as health insurance and taxes.

Work it out
Once you've given thought to how and when you want to retire, do the math needed to clarify your financial picture. You may want to do this yourself or to seek the advice of a financial planner.

After you've determined when you'd like to retire, estimate approximately how many years from your retirement until your death. Calculate what you think your yearly living expenses will be and multiply that by the number of years that you expect to be retired. Compare your expected expenses with your retirement income to see if you'll have enough money.

Health insurance

The most expensive medical bills you'll ever have may be yet to come. A surprising number of middle-class people become impoverished when they reach their 70s and 80s because they had too many holes in their health insurance safety net. With age, health problems typically increase. It's important to make sure that you have adequate health insurance when you retire.

Medicare

Medicare is the federal health insurance program for Americans age 65 and older. If you're eligible for Social Security or have paid Medicare taxes for long enough, you're eligible for Medicare no matter how much money you have. Medicare offers several options.

Original Medicare
If you're eligible for Medicare, you'll be enrolled in Medicare Part A when you turn 65, unless you choose another option. Part A covers hospital bills and a few other services. There's no premium for Part A, but you pay a deductible, now around $800, if you're admitted to a hospital.

Another option is Medicare Part B. In order to be guaranteed coverage under this plan, you must sign up for it within 3 months of becoming eligible. Part B covers doctor visits, X-rays, laboratory tests and other diagnostic tests. You pay a monthly premium, an annual deductible and co-insurance — usually 20 percent of the Medicare-approved fee.

Under Medicare, you can use almost any doctor or hospital in the country. But some items — notably,

Deciding on Health Insurance

When choosing a health insurance plan, consider these points:

- *Coverage away from home.* If you travel often or live in another part of the country part of the year, make sure the plan covers you when you're away from home.
- *Access to specialists.* Medigap and fee-for-service plans let you see any specialist whenever you want to. Many HMOs require that you see only specialists who are part of the HMO network. If the specialists you want to see aren't part of your plan's network, you'll pay much more out-of-pocket if you see them.
- *Limited budget.* If you can't afford unexpected health care costs, original Medicare with a Medigap policy may be the right choice for you. Certain managed care plans also may be a good choice because their costs are usually fixed.
- *Prescription drugs.* If you take prescription drugs regularly and worry about being able to afford them, compare the drug benefits of a managed care plan with those of a Medigap plan. Original Medicare doesn't cover prescription drug costs.
- *Employer retiree coverage.* If you have good insurance through a former employer, original Medicare may be all you need. Don't give up good retiree coverage. It probably offers you more than original Medicare combined with a Medigap policy. However, many employers stop retiree coverage as soon as you enroll in original Medicare.

medications and some preventive services — aren't covered.

Original Medicare with a supplemental policy

Supplemental policies are often referred to as Medigap policies because they pay many of the things that original Medicare doesn't. Ten levels of supplemental policies, plans A through J, are sold by private insurance companies. The minimum benefits for each level are defined by the federal government. A Medigap policy may be a good way to add to your coverage.

If you want this additional coverage, you must buy a supplemental policy within a set amount of time after enrolling in Medicare. Some plans pay only for Medicare deductibles and coinsurance. More expensive plans or policies pay for prescription drugs and home care.

Medicare managed care

With Medicare managed care, you receive care from a managed care plan. It might be a health maintenance organization (HMO), a provider-sponsored organization (PSO) or a preferred provider organization (PPO). In all three, you receive care from a defined network of doctors and hospitals, often at lower cost to you than if you used original Medicare.

Choosing the managed care option means that you may be able to go only to hospitals and doctors that are affiliated with the managed care plan. For that reason, managed care plans may not be a good choice if you travel frequently or live in another part of the country for part of the year.

Private fee-for-service plans

With private fee-for-service plans, you choose a private insurance plan that accepts Medicare beneficiaries. The insurance company, not Medicare, decides how much it will pay and how much you'll pay.

With private fee-for-service plans, you can go to any doctor or hospital that deals with the plan. You get all of the services covered in Medicare Parts A and B. You may also receive benefits that original Medicare doesn't offer. Your premiums and out-of-pocket expenses may be higher than with original Medicare. You'll likely have a copayment for each visit or service provided.

The Aging of America

People are living longer than ever before. The number of people age 100 or older (centenarians) in the United States increased from 37,306 in 1990 to more than 50,000 in 2000. That's an increase of about 35 percent.

A large segment of the existing population is about to reach retirement years. In 2011, the postwar baby boomers — the generation born between 1946 and 1964 — will start turning 65. In that year, and for each of the 20 years that follow, the older adult population in the United States is expected to increase by about 1 million people.

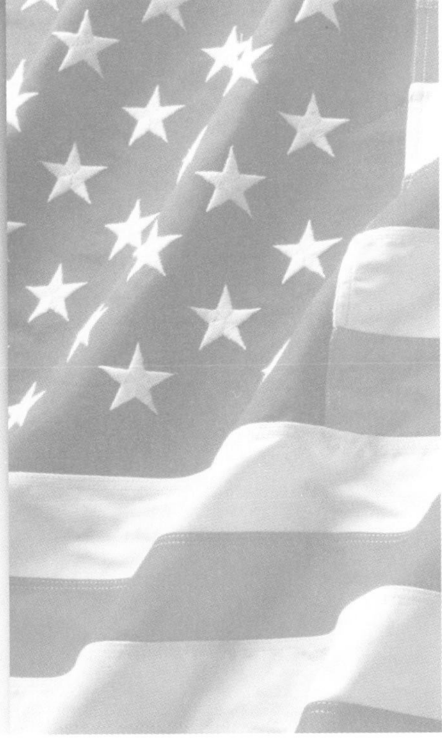

Emotional and psychological aspects

Changing your routine after years of working affects you emotionally and psychologically. For some people, the transition is difficult. A sudden, large increase in free time can take some getting used to.

Think of retirement as an opportunity for continued growth and enrichment. When you retire, it's important that you maintain social ties and address your emotional needs. Explore new ways to achieve a sense of accomplishment, structure and status. You might consider volunteering, spending more time with family, developing a hobby or working a part-time job that offers reduced hours and more flexibility.

Before you retire, think about what you'd like to do with your free time and try out that activity on weekends and vacations.

Retirement is often a good time to reassess marriage roles. If you're a homemaker, will having your spouse around more hinder or help your daily routine? If you've had a career, how can you become more comfortable at home during the day? If both you and your spouse work, how will your routines change if one of you retires and the other doesn't? Communication becomes even more important.

Even the best-planned retirement can have emotional bumps. Feelings of loss, restlessness, anxiety or depression are common during the first months. Acknowledge these feelings as normal. However, if the feelings seem overwhelming, or if you don't feel better at the end of the first year, get help.

Healthy Aging

No matter what your age, begin taking care of your health now to increase your chances of enjoying good health in your later years. If you're in your middle years, you've got plenty of time to gear up, whether it's initiating an exercise program, devising a more healthy diet or fine-tuning your social skills. If you're already retired, it's not too late to decide how — and how well — you want to live for the next 10, 20 or 30 years.

Aging isn't about retirement or even reaching a particular chronological age, such as 65. It's a lifelong process. The people who cope best are the ones who've successfully passed through each stage of life. Successful aging involves many factors within your control: your attitudes, your activities and your relationships.

Have a positive attitude

It's important to remember that attitude shapes reality. You're not suddenly old when you hit 65, become a grandparent or go through menopause. You're old only when you think you are. Although your body may age, your mind, for the most part, will stay as young as you feel.

If you expect to live a long life filled with physical vitality, humor and social connectedness, then that fundamental mind-set becomes an internal diagram that to a large degree will predict your future. But if you're convinced that old age will be a time of emptiness, depression and sickness, it more likely will be. In general, negative expectations can make you age faster than nature intended.

In all of life, stay focused on what's important and shrug off what isn't. A sense of humor and an ability to adapt to changes can help you cope.

Eat well

Numerous studies indicate that a healthy diet, when combined with regular physical and mental activity, can help you live longer and better. As you age, even if you've always maintained a healthy diet, your approach to food may have to be modified. With age your metabolism slows down, meaning that your calorie needs aren't as great. In addition to eating a nutritionally balanced diet, pay attention to serving sizes and calories. Eating too much food or a lot of high-calorie foods can more easily result in weight gain.

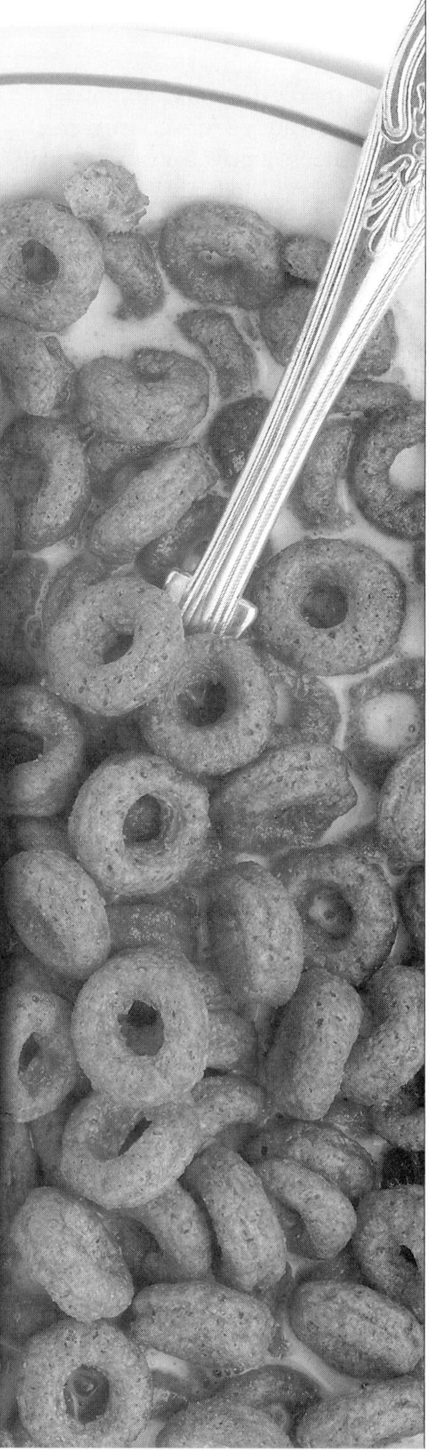

Increase fiber

A high-fiber diet can help prevent constipation and may decrease risk of some colon diseases, including colon cancer. Fiber may also help protect against diabetes, heart disease and high blood pressure.

Aim for 25 to 30 grams of fiber daily from a variety of foods. Eat whole-grain foods — like high-fiber cereals or whole-wheat breads — and fruits and vegetables. A couple of times a week, substitute legumes, such as beans or lentils, for meat. Read food labels to help find products with the maximum amount of fiber.

Choose nutrient-dense foods

Get the most out of every calorie you consume by eating foods that contain a lot of nutrients in relation to their calories. Richly colored fruits and vegetables offer lots of essential nutrients.

Whole-grain breads, rice, cereals and pastas contain more fiber than do enriched or refined products. They also contain more vitamins and minerals. You can't replace a balanced diet with liquid supplements.

Drink plenty of fluids

Water is important to your health. Try to drink plenty of nonalcoholic, caffeine-free liquids each day, preferably water. Inadequate fluid intake can contribute to problems such as chronic constipation, impaired kidney function and kidney stones.

Decrease fat, cholesterol and sodium consumption

There are several different kinds of fat. Saturated fat raises your blood cholesterol level more than anything else you eat does. Major sources of it are butter, cheese, whole milk, cream, meat, poultry, chocolate, coconut palm oil, lard and solid shortenings.

Trans fats, which can come from hydrogenated oils, can raise total cholesterol and low-density lipoprotein (LDL) cholesterol (the "bad" cholesterol). Trans fats can also lower high-density lipoprotein (HDL) cholesterol (the "good" cholesterol).

Polyunsaturated fats lower blood cholesterol but also seem to promote oxidation. Oxidation enables cells in your arteries to absorb fats and cholesterol. Over time, oxidation speeds up the buildup of the plaques that narrow arteries. Olive oil, canola oil and nuts contain mainly monounsaturated fat, which may help lower blood cholesterol. You'll find cholesterol in all animal foods, especially egg yolks, organ meat and whole milk.

Remember, too, that most people get plenty of salt in their regular diet. You need less than 1/4 teaspoon of salt daily to help regulate fluid balance. You can help avoid getting too much sodium by limiting processed foods. Canned foods and some frozen foods are often high in sodium. Read labels.

Limit alcohol

Alcoholism is a serious problem among older adults, many of whom didn't drink heavily until their 60s or 70s. Heavy drinking can be a way of responding to a major life change, such as the death of a spouse, divorce, retirement or loneliness. More women than men abuse alcohol later in life. Alcoholism may be undetected until major health consequences show up.

Too much alcohol — more than one drink a day for women or more than two a day for men — can harm almost every organ and system in your body. It increases your risk of cardiovascular disease, some cancers and liver and pancreatic diseases. Alcohol weakens your immune system, leaving you more vulnerable to infection. It clearly affects your cognitive abilities and your concentration, and it increases your risk of falling.

As you age, your body processes alcohol more slowly, so it takes fewer drinks to become intoxicated, and the effects last longer. Because alcohol's effects are magnified with age, the National Institute on Alcohol Abuse and Alcoholism recommends that people age 65 and older have no more than one drink a day.

If you enjoy a glass of wine with dinner, there's probably no reason to give it up. But if you find yourself drinking more than you used to, or if you turn to alcohol for comfort, then you may have a problem. Talk to your doctor.

Avoid nicotine

There's nothing good to say about nicotine. If you smoke or chew tobacco, then do your best to quit. It's never too late, even if you've used tobacco for years.

With one puff on a cigarette, you take in 4,000 chemicals. Nicotine is the one that hooks you. It can be harder to kick than heroine or cocaine. When you inhale, nicotine goes to your brain within 10 seconds. If you smoke a pipe or cigar or chew tobacco, the nicotine gets absorbed somewhat more slowly through the mucous membranes of your mouth.

Once nicotine reaches your brain, it increases production of the neurotransmitter dopamine, which regulates movement, motivation, emotion and pleasure. The acute effects of nicotine dissipate almost as quickly as they strike, which means you have to keep inhaling more to maintain the pleasurable feelings.

Because nicotine is so addictive, quitting smoking is hard. If you're a former smoker, quitting may be one of the hardest things you've ever done. If you want to quit, it may be the hardest thing you'll ever do. Withdrawal symptoms can last a month or more and can include irritability, craving, difficulty thinking and paying attention, sleep disturbances and increased appetite.

But there is help. Nicotine replacement products, such as gum, inhalers, nasal sprays and skin patches, as well as medication and behavioral therapy, have proved effective in helping people quit.

Think of the alternative. Smoking has been linked to gum disease, high blood pressure, heart disease, stroke, lung disease and a variety of cancers, particularly, but not exclusively, lung cancer. If you smoke and healthy aging is your goal, then you need to stop smoking.

Keep physically active

Physical activity is important throughout your life. And the earlier you begin and maintain an activity routine, the more benefit you'll see and feel as you age. The benefits of physical activity are seemingly endless and can include weight control, improved blood circulation, increased muscle mass, improved posture, greater flexibility, more endurance and improved balance.

Aging doesn't mean disability. Aches and pains are common, but your later years can be some of the most pleasant and productive years of your life. Strive to live life to the fullest by maintaining a reasonable level of fitness.

It's never too late to become more active. However, before you begin an exercise program that's more vigorous than walking, it might be a good idea to get a medical evaluation from your doctor. Then plan activities that you enjoy. If exercise is drudgery, you won't do it.

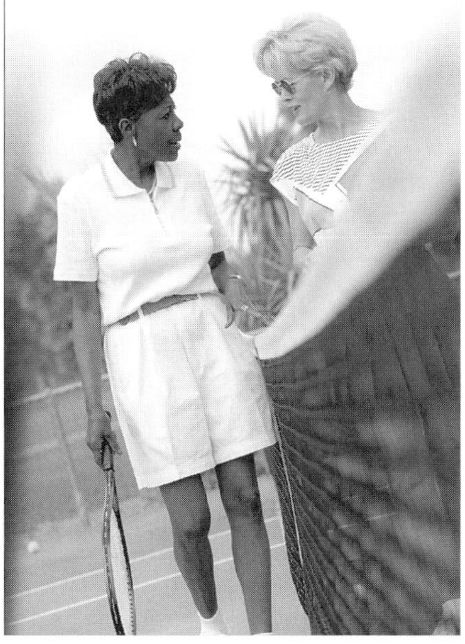

Control stress

When you're under stress, your body cranks out high levels of the stress hormone cortisol. If you're frequently under stress, excessive cortisol, over the long term, can be harmful to your health.

You can't always avoid stressful events, but you can control how you react to them. For more information on how to cope with stress, see Chapter 5, "Managing Stress."

Exercise your brain

Just when you're old enough to have acquired some wisdom, your mind starts to play tricks on you. You can't remember where you left your glasses or where you parked your car. You used to be able to do three things at once, but now you may be hard-pressed to focus on one.

Relax. Some memory slippage is normal as you age. Stress and anxiety also can interfere with your memory and your concentration. Aging doesn't generally affect immediate or long-term memory, but short-term memory often declines. To store and retrieve information, your brain performs a complex chain of chemical and electrical functions involving nerve cells. Over time, some of these cells may deteriorate and function less efficiently.

Your brain compensates in remarkable ways. Even though you might not have the same number of brain cells as a 19-year-old, consider how much more wisdom and judgment you have. These qualities are difficult to measure, but they reflect the ability to make sound decisions based on a lifetime of experience.

Keep in mind that your brain is like a muscle. You need to use it to keep it strong. Remember when you were in grade school and you had to memorize big chunks of information, such as the state capitals or the words to a lengthy poem? If you think that you were able to do that then only because of your youth, think again. You were able to do it because you worked hard at committing the information to memory. When was the last time you did that? Chances are, if you tried it now, you'd be as successful as you were then.

Just because you're older doesn't mean that you can't go back to college, learn new tasks, develop new hobbies or acquire new knowledge through reading. Lifelong learning is key to keeping your mind fit.

- Take classes. You can enroll in anything from a community education class to a college course.
- Keep a journal.
- Join a book club or other discussion group.
- Stay up-to-date on technology. Learn about computers and connect to the Internet. Use e-mail to stay in touch with friends and family.
- Explore the cultural life of your community. Attend concerts, lectures and plays.

Stay socially connected

Having strong ties with family and friends is always important. With age, those connections become even more crucial. Studies show that if you have few relationships or poor social ties, your risk of death is two to four times greater than that of individuals surrounded by many people they care about and who care about them. In fact, having a dependable group of friends and family is one of the most reliable predictors of longevity.

Balance your solitary activities with group activities. Instead of exercising by yourself, consider joining an exercise class. If you've always loved reading, consider joining a book discussion group. Take part in activities in your community, church, synagogue or mosque that maybe you declined in the past because you didn't have the time.

Many people stay socially connected by volunteering. You could volunteer at a local school or library or for a service organization such as Meals-On-Wheels.

According to researchers from the MacArthur Foundation Studies of Aging, strong social support can promote longevity by:

- Enabling you to get better or more prompt medical care
- Encouraging you to engage in healthful behaviors, such as regular walking
- Allowing you to receive direct expressions of affection, which in turn can improve your immune system
- Providing you with practical help when needed, such as assistance with household chores or transportation

Seek out spirituality

More studies are indicating that when you believe in something larger than yourself, you strengthen your ability to cope with whatever life hands you. People who attend religious services tend to enjoy better health, live longer and recover from illness faster and with fewer complications than those who don't. They also tend to cope better with illness and experience less depression.

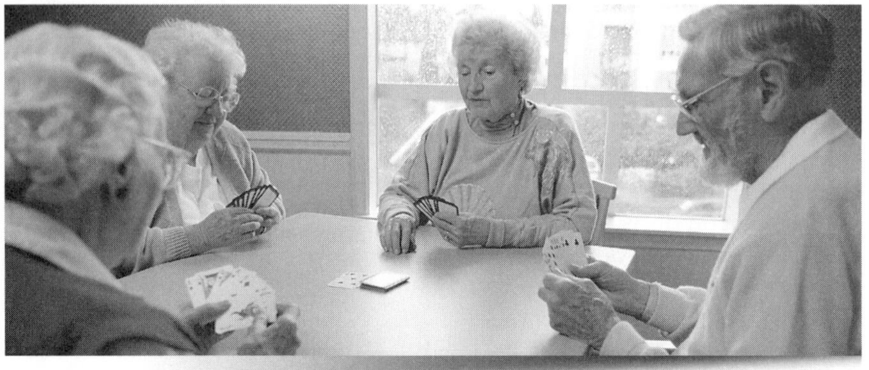

No one knows exactly how faith or spiritual belief and practice affect health. Some experts attribute the healing effect to hope, which has been shown to benefit your immune system. Others liken prayer to meditation, which decreases muscle tension and lowers heart rate. Still others point to the social connectedness, another healing factor that regular worship attendance fosters.

Everyone defines their spirituality differently. For some it's organized religion. For others it's feeling in tune with nature and the universe. For still others, spirituality is expressed through music, meditation or art.

A report from Mayo Clinic's Spirituality in Healthcare committee states that "spirituality as a dynamic process helps individuals discover meaning and purpose in their lives, even in the midst of personal tragedy, crisis, stress, illness, pain and suffering. This process is an inner quest. ... Spirituality empowers a person to be fully engaged in life experiences from birth to death."

Get regular medical exams

You need periodic health examinations for two main reasons. First, during a physical exam your doctor may be able to identify a medical problem early, sometimes even before you develop symptoms. That's generally when treatment is most successful.

Second, a medical evaluation can help to prevent a disease or disorder. For example, a blood test may reveal that your cholesterol level is rising. By changing your eating and exercise habits, you may be able to ward off high cholesterol levels, which can cause heart disease or a stroke.

Whether you need a checkup every year depends on your risk factors for specific diseases and your doctor's recommendations.

Vaccines Aren't Just for Kids

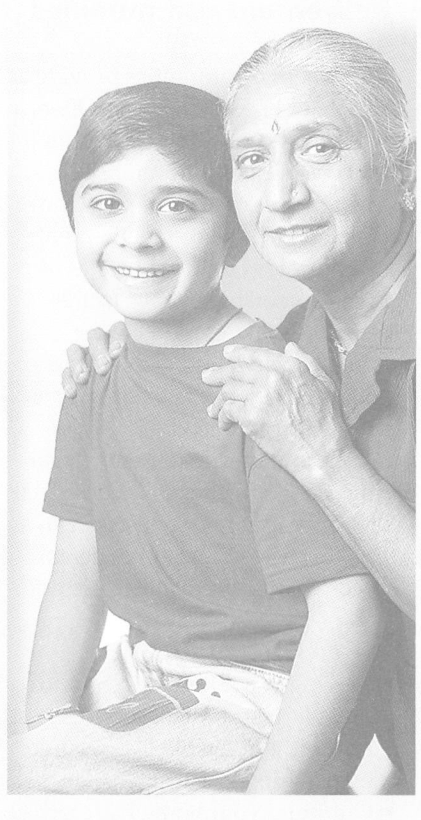

With age, you become more susceptible to certain infectious diseases, some of which are preventable with vaccines. In addition, the middle years frequently are a time when adults are more likely to travel internationally. To stay healthy, make sure you're up-to-date on vaccinations.

Flu shot

Older adults and people with underlying medical conditions are at increased risk of complicating illness, hospitalization and even death from flu (influenza) infection. All adults age 65 or older should receive this vaccine on an annual basis, as should younger adults with chronic lung disorders, cardiovascular disorders, diabetes, renal disease, liver disease, blood diseases, cancer or HIV infection and other diseases that suppress immunity.

In addition, get a flu shot if you're taking medications that suppress your immune system. Healthy adults living in a household with someone who has one of these disorders should get the vaccine to prevent transmission of the flu infection.

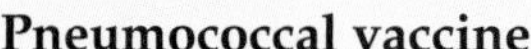

Pneumococcal vaccine

All adults age 65 or older should get the pneumococcal polysaccharide vaccine (PPV). It's also recommended for adults of any age who:

- Have a chronic, high-risk medical condition, such as diabetes or heart, lung or kidney disease
- Have an impaired immune system
- Have had their spleen removed
- Live in a nursing home or long-term-care facility
- Have received an organ transplant

People age 65 or older who are generally healthy may need only one shot. Those who received their first shot before age 65 may need a 5-year booster shot. You can get a pneumococcal vaccination any time of the year, but it's often convenient to get it when you receive your flu shot.

Tetanus and diphtheria vaccine

Because most children are vaccinated for tetanus and diphtheria (Td), in the United States these illnesses are now predominantly diseases of adults. Adults should get a booster dose every 10 years, or after 5 years if exposed.

Other vaccines

Certain lifestyles, occupations, hobbies and foreign travel plans may make other immunizations advisable. For more information on adult vaccines, see Chapter 1, "Getting Immunized." Ask your doctor for advice.

Residence Options in Your Later Years

Independence is a cherished ideal, especially in the United States. Most people would like to stay in their own home for as long as they live.

But sometimes, due to an accident or illness or other circumstances, you may find you need to look at alternative living arrangements. Here's an overview of some of those options.

Retirement communities

Retirement communities provide a variety of housing options. Often, a retirement community is a multiunit complex of condominiums, town houses or apartments. One of the major benefits of a retirement community is reduced hassles of home ownership. Such a facility also draws like-minded older adults together and delivers the community services that residents most want and need.

Continuing-care retirement communities go further still. These facilities offer multiple services on an a la carte basis so that as residents' needs change they can receive additional care within the same setting. A retirement community may provide the independent living setting that you want now and the assisted-living setting you may need in the future.

Loss of Independence

One of the toughest adjustments to make in the later years is the loss of independence. For one person, being independent means having time to read and a ready supply of good books. To another, it means a chance to golf several times a week. To another, it means not having to take orders from anyone.

To most people though, independence means the freedom to get up, move about, do things, have friends in, make telephone calls, go places and pursue activities they enjoy or that are important to them.

Before making changes in your living situation, think about what independence means to you. You may be able to adapt your current way of life, perhaps with only a few changes, to accommodate your needs.

If your current living arrangement doesn't seem to be working well, explore all options. Depending on your personal and physical needs and your financial situation, options may include:

- Moving to a smaller place with all rooms on one floor
- Moving to a retirement community with convenient services and without the hassles of home ownership
- Outfitting your home with special needs equipment to prevent falls or make daily tasks easier
- Hiring someone to help you with daily tasks
- Arranging for a companion to live with you and help you do things
- Seeking home health care services
- Moving to special housing for older adults, such as an assisted-living facility, which offers temporary or permanent nursing care
- Moving in with your family
- Moving in to a nursing home

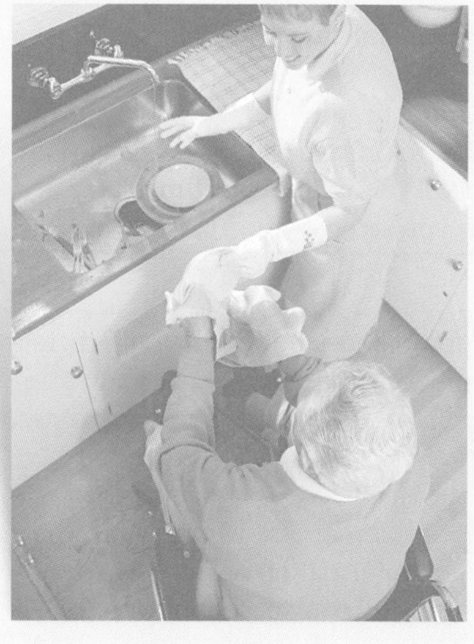

Assisted-living facilities

Assisted living is one of the fastest-growing living options for older adults. Many people want to maintain as much independence as possible but need or want some help with a few everyday activities.

Assisted-living centers can be ideal for individuals who need more help than they could receive in a simple retirement community but who don't require the kind of medical and nursing care provided by nursing homes. The goal of assisted living is to provide supervision, personal care assistance and health care services that emphasize an individual's right to control his or her life.

Types

Many different terms are used to describe assisted-living facilities. You may hear them referred to as board-and-care homes, retirement centers, congregate housing, senior residential housing or continuing-care retirement communities. Assisted-living services may be provided in free-standing facilities, on a campus with skilled nursing facilities or hospitals or at independent housing complexes. The kinds of services offered vary.

Residents

The typical assisted-living resident is a woman between 75 and 85 years old who's mobile but needs assistance with about two activities of daily living. Male residents make up only 31 percent of the assisted-living population.

Services offered by most facilities include help with bathing, dressing, eating and toileting. Eighty-one percent of residents need help with one or more of these activities. Residents may also receive help with other tasks, including telephoning, shopping, meal preparation, housework, taking medication and managing money.

Costs

Costs for assisted-living residences vary greatly and depend on the size of units, services provided and location. Assisted living is covered in a growing number of long-term-care insurance policies. The Health Insurance Association of America reported that all of the leading insurance companies that sell long-term-care insurance offer assisted-living coverage. However, the majority of people in assisted-living residences or their families pay for care themselves because many older Americans don't carry long-term-care insurance. For more information on long-term-care insurance, see page 310.

Assisted living isn't covered by Medicare, but certain services may be paid for through waivered grants. A number of states reimburse or plan to reimburse providers for assisted-living services as a waivered Medicaid service. Medicaid is the government's program of health insurance for low-income people. In addition, states have the option to pay for assisted living under Medicaid by including services in the state's Medicaid plan or petitioning the Department of Health and Human Services for a waiver. Grants are still only a small portion of the payments. Check with your county social services agency for information about what options are available in your area.

Finding the right facility

Because so many different assisted-living arrangements are available, it's important to research the options. Get a list of facilities in your area of interest. Call and ask each facility to send you some information. If after reviewing the costs, services and rules of each facility you're still interested in pursuing this option, narrow your choices to the places that you want to visit. While at the facility, ask questions and make notes. Equally important, trust your feelings about a place.

As you visit each facility, be observant and ask yourself questions about each of the following categories:

Setting

- Are the grounds clean?
- How does the facility smell?
- Do things appear to run well?
- Is the staff knowledgeable and helpful?
- Are bedrooms shared or private?
- Is there enough room for your personal belongings?
- Is there a private place for meeting guests?
- Will you be able to get around easily in the facility?
- Do residents seem happy?

Services and contract

- Is the facility licensed by the state and in good standing?
- What are the reasons for which you would be transferred or discharged?
- Is your doctor involved in your care plan?
- Is your family involved in your care?

Avoiding Falls

Falling is one of the biggest reasons people lose their independence. Half of all people older than age 65 who are hospitalized for a fall never regain their former level of independence. Here are some tips to help you avoid a fall:

Your health

- *Have your vision and hearing checked regularly.* If they're impaired, you lose important cues that help you maintain your balance.
- *Exercise regularly.* Exercise improves strength, muscle tone and coordination to help you prevent a fall.
- *Ask your doctor about your medications.* Some medications or combinations of medications used to treat conditions such as high blood pressure, angina, depression or insomnia can affect balance.
- *Avoid alcohol.* Even a little alcohol can cause a fall, especially if your balance and reflexes are already impaired.
- *Get up slowly.* A momentary decrease in blood pressure that accompanies a sudden change in position can cause dizziness.
- *Use supportive devices.* If you sometimes feel dizzy, use a cane or walker to help you keep your balance.
- *Select proper footwear.* Wear sturdy, low-heeled shoes with wide, nonslip soles.

Your home

- *All rooms.* Remove raised doorway thresholds. Rearrange furniture if necessary to keep electrical cords and furniture out of walking paths. Fasten carpets to the floor and don't use scatter rugs. Put night lights in electrical outlets in halls, bathrooms and bedrooms.
- *Stairways.* Be sure stairs are well-lighted and have sturdy handrails.
- *Bathrooms.* Install grab handles and nonstick mats inside and outside your shower or bathtub and near the toilet. Use a shower chair in your shower or a bath bench in your bathtub.
- *Kitchens.* Don't use difficult-to-reach shelves. Don't stand on a chair or stool to reach something. Use nonskid floor wax and wipe up spills immediately.
- *Bedrooms.* Put a light switch by the door and by your bed so that you don't have to walk across a dark room to turn on the light.

- What services does the facility offer?
- What is the ratio of staff to residents?

Food
- Are specialized diets available?
- Are cultural or ethnic preferences considered?
- Are residents involved in menu planning?
- Can you help with meal preparation and have access to the kitchen?
- Are snacks and beverages readily available between meals?
- Are extra helpings and substitutions available?

Socialization
- Are there activities that you're interested in?
- Are there places nearby for you to walk to?
- Is your family encouraged to visit?

Home health care

For most of people, a childhood illness meant staying home and being nursed back to health. As adults with a minor illness such as the flu or a cold, most people recover at home. Home care for a more serious or prolonged condition is essentially a variation on the same, familiar theme. For many people, the best place to get well is at home.

During illness or recuperation from an injury, sophisticated medical facilities are often unnecessary. As you recover from most illnesses or injuries, your own home is the most comfortable place to be. At home, most people sleep better, eat better and get well more quickly.

Home health care is also an option if you have a disabling illness. You may be well enough that you can still manage by yourself at home, but you can benefit from services provided by a home health care agency.

What's involved?

Many organizations in the United States provide home health services, including several private companies, hospitals, nursing homes, community social service agencies and city and county health departments. Services available to you depend on your needs and the particular program or programs that exist in your area.

Agencies that offer skilled nursing care may provide a nursing service to monitor your health status, give injections, change bandages and perform other nursing tasks. Sometimes, various forms of therapy are available in the home, including physical, occupational, speech, hearing and respiratory therapies. Meals and housekeeping services may be available.

Long-Term-Care Insurance

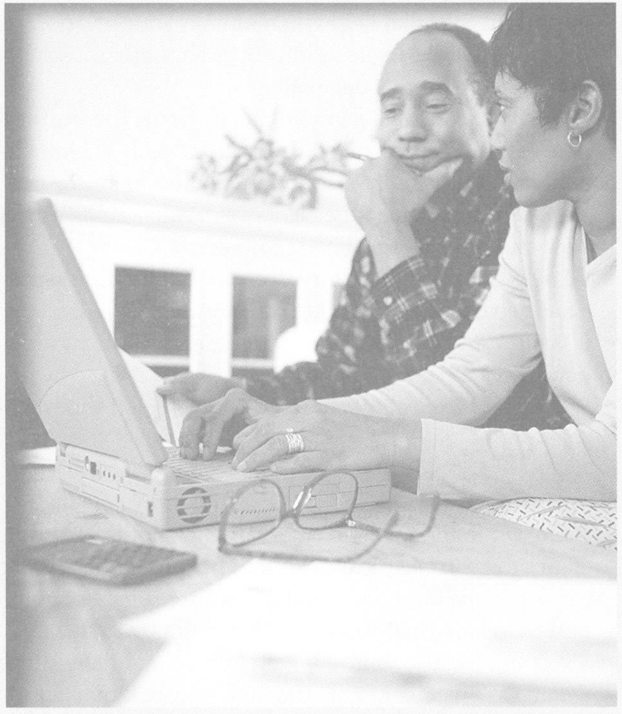

Chances are that during your lifetime you'll need some type of long-term care, which can be expensive and quickly eat up your savings. Medicare doesn't cover most types of long-term care. And many private insurance policies only pay a small portion of long-term-care services. Long-term-care insurance is designed to cover services such as nursing homes, assisted living, elder care and home health care.

An average nursing home stay costs $56,000 a year. Assisted-living facilities cost on average $26,000 a year. Elder care ranges from $30 to $130 a day, and home health care costs an average of $12,000 a year.

Not planning for the expense of long-term care is why many older adults become poor. Long-term-care insurance is expensive as well, although the younger you are when you enroll, the lower the premiums will be. But there's a trade-off. You may pay many years of unnecessary premiums. Some experts feel that a good time for many people to buy is when they're in their 60s.

Long-term-care insurance probably isn't the right choice if you have a limited income and few assets. Nor do you need it if you've saved enough to pay for long-term care, although you might still want to buy it to protect your assets.

Long-term-care insurance is complicated, and many different plans are offered. It's important to thoroughly research the various policies, including the services they'll pay for and how much the policies cost. It might also be helpful to talk with an individual who specializes in insurance or financial planning before you buy.

For more information on some agencies that provide information on long-term-care insurance, see page 1377.

Home care agencies that offer skilled nursing, therapeutic and supplemental services do so under the direction of your doctor. A medically trained caseworker or case manager may be responsible for coordinating the care provided to you or the individual in need of assistance.

Many organizations offer supportive rather than skilled services. In the case of supportive services, a home aide stops regularly at your home, perhaps every day or once a week. The aide may help with basic tasks such as bathing, shopping, cooking, eating and doing housekeeping chores.

A home aide can handle simple nursing tasks such as taking a temperature. For many people, help with some everyday activities can make it possible to continue living independently at home rather than in a nursing home.

Working to meet these varied needs, home health care agencies employ people with a wide range of skills. Another major advantage of home health care is that it's often less costly than a hospital stay.

Levels of care

Home health care is generally divided into three categories:

Skilled care

Skilled care is conducted under the direction of a doctor and consists of services provided by health care professionals, such as nurses and therapists. It may also include activities such as home dialysis, physical therapy or social services.

Home support services

Home support services include tasks such as cleaning the house, running errands and preparing meals. A home health care aide may perform many of these tasks under the direction of a case manager.

Combination care

Services might involve a home health care team made up of some combination of the following: a doctor, nurse, dietitian, therapist, social worker or home health care aide. This team carries out a plan to meet your needs.

Finding home health care

To find out which home health care services are available where you live, ask your doctor, a social worker, your local or county health department or your local senior citizens center. In addition, churches, synagogues, welfare departments and charitable organizations such as the United Way often can provide information on various services available.

If you live in an area that has multiple home care alternatives, compare the services offered. Important points to consider include:

- Will your insurance cover payment to the agency?
- Do the services match your present and future needs?
- How much medical or skilled supervision does the agency offer?
- Which hours of the day or week are covered?

Elder Abuse

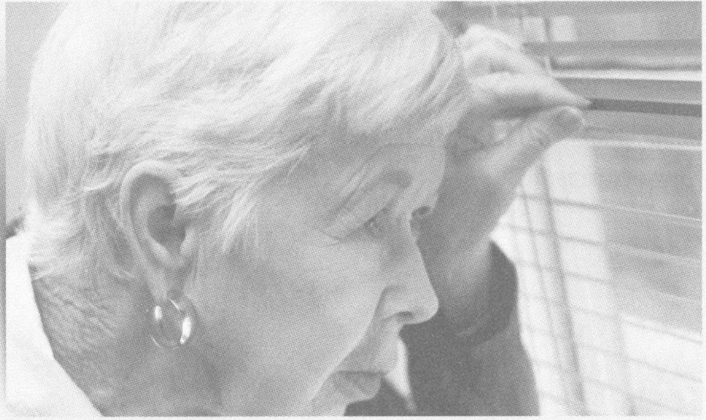

Abuse means anything from a consistent pattern of harsh words and marked unfriendliness to slapping, pushing, hitting and sexual molestation. One of the more common forms of abuse is neglect — when a caregiver fails to provide the goods or services an individual needs to function.

According to the American Medical Association, about 10 percent of people age 65 or older suffer some kind of chronic abuse. Frequently, the pattern emerges gradually, beginning with verbal abuse and progressing to physical abuse. Since 1981, there has been an increase in cases reported each year, to about 100,000 a year.

Who's most likely to be a victim?

Victims most often are individuals who are age 75 or older and who are dependent on others for basic care, such as bathing, dressing and eating. Abuse seems to occur in all economic and ethnic groups.

Who are the abusers?

In about half the cases, the abusers are the children or other younger relatives of the victim. About 40 percent of the time, the victim's spouse is the abuser. In institutions, professional caregivers also may be abusers.

What can be done?

Simply talking with the abuser about the problem isn't likely to help. If you're a victim of abuse or you suspect elder abuse, call the police or your county social services office, or ask a visiting nurse to contact the authorities. Doctors and social workers also can help. Most cities and counties, according to state law, protect a vulnerable adult from elder abuse through their welfare and social service agencies.

- Are replacement aides available to fill in when regularly assigned individuals can't come?

Also talk with people who've actually used the service and get their opinions.

In recent years, the number of home health care agencies has decreased. In many areas, there's a shortage of home health care workers. Medicare also has limited what it considers medical needs, and for how long it will pay. Sometimes, hospital discharges have to be delayed because no home help is available.

Reimbursement for services
Home health services are paid for in six main ways: by Medicare, Medicaid, private insurance providers, health maintenance organizations, the person being cared for and waivered service grants.

Make sure you understand what services Medicare or your insurance does and doesn't cover. In the case of home health services, limits usually are placed on the types of services, the length of visits and the number of visits.

Elder care

Elder care is a service that offers care in a supervised setting for older adults who can't be left alone during the day. Elder care is suitable for a person who is disabled, is recuperating or requires help performing everyday activities. The individual may live with family but need a place to spend the day when family members are at work.

Depending on the program, individuals can attend elder care daily or just a couple of days during the week. Transportation to and from the care center often can be arranged.

Elder care provides an opportunity to be with other individuals. Group activities are often part of the daily schedule, and some centers arrange formal activities. A midday meal is generally served.

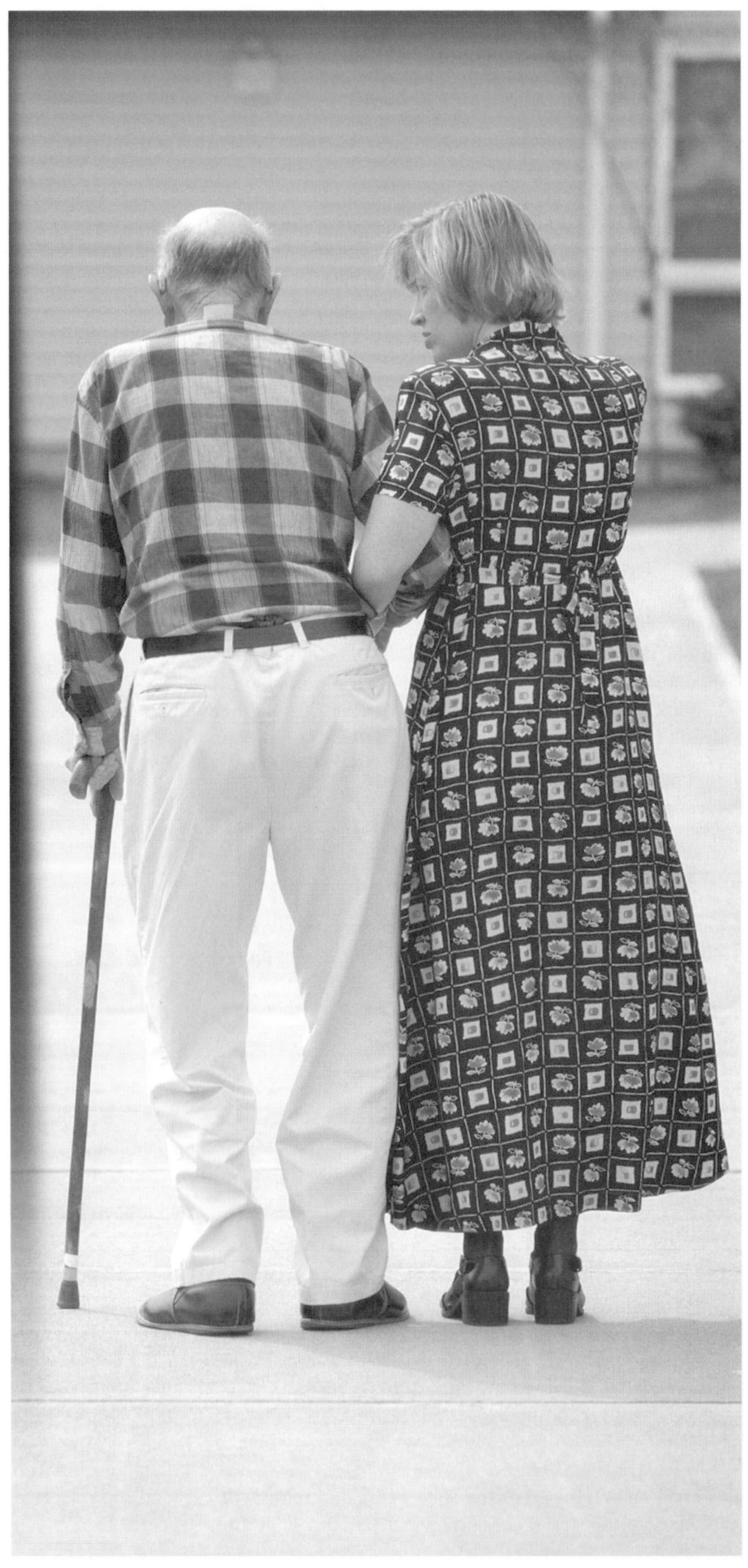

A variant of elder care is a medical elder care center. This type of service is sometimes referred to as day respite care. Here, medical and nursing attention is provided in addition to supervision, social activities and meals.

Individuals who qualify for this type of care can visit the facility on an as-needed basis for some particular medical procedure or therapy. Such a visit might be necessary once or twice a week or every day. Medical elder care is often located in a skilled nursing home.

Nursing homes

As more living options become available for older adults, nursing home use is declining. Still, 1.5 million Americans age 65 or older now reside in nursing homes. This is about 1 out of every 22 people age 65 or older. The percentage is small, but increases dramatically with age.

For people between the ages of 65 and 74, 1.1 percent live in nursing homes. For people between the ages of 75 and 84, 4.7 percent live in nursing homes. Among individuals 85 and older, it's 18.2 percent. Because women generally outlive men, the majority of nursing home residents are women.

Many older adults rank nursing homes as a last resort. People feel that such living arrangements signal not only a massive physical and mental decline but also a dramatic loss of independence. Despite such impressions, in the right circumstances, the fully supported care available in nursing homes can be the best option.

Many doctors recommend a stay in a nursing home to recover from a stroke, a hip fracture or some other mishap. Once rehabilitated, the individual is often able to return to independent living. This type of arrangement is often referred to as temporary rehabilitation or skilled nursing home care.

Other people enter a nursing home because they need full care for a condition that may not improve. Among the common problems that lead to nursing home admission are incontinence, memory disorders, stroke, walking disabilities, loss of a spouse or caregiver, and terminal illness.

When is a nursing home appropriate?

It's not inevitable that everyone who is old or who has a chronic illness has to enter a nursing home. Individual circumstances vary considerably. In addition, nursing home care is getting more expensive and difficult to arrange.

The single most important reason for entering a nursing home is the need for a level of nursing care that you can't receive at home or in an assisted-living environment.

Nursing home residents receive help with many of the routine activities of daily life. Eighty-five percent need help bathing, 70 percent need help dressing, more than 50 percent need help going to the bathroom and more than 30 percent need help eating. The average nursing home resident has several chronic illnesses that require medical attention. More than half have Alzheimer's disease or some other mental impairment.

When independent living, assisted living or care by family members isn't feasible or threatens to destroy the fabric of a family, a nursing home should be considered. If you're physically able to visit prospective nursing homes and psychologically fit enough to help make the decision, you should participate in the selection process.

Finding a good home

In selecting a nursing home, the first person to turn to for advice is a social worker, a hospital dismissal planner or your doctor. These people are often excellent sources of information on nursing homes and are familiar with entry criteria and options for different levels of care.

Service agencies funded by your county or the United Way are another source of help. Your state or county social services agency, health department or county medical society also can provide a list of nursing homes. These agencies may also have information on how best

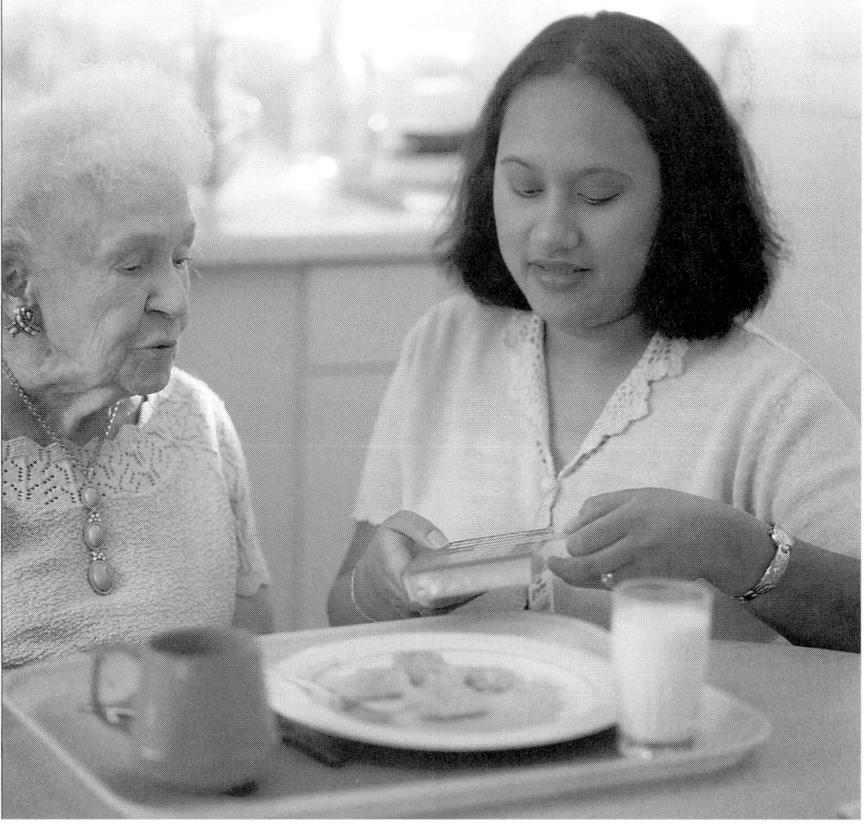

to evaluate and select a home. Some information from agencies or associations may be available via the Internet.

Most nursing homes now are termed skilled-care homes. So-called intermediate-care homes are being phased out in most areas. In a skilled-care home, you receive 24-hour nursing service as well as physical, occupational and other therapies. To select a nursing home, visit several. Before you go, write down the things that you want to find out. For example:

Atmosphere
- Are the staff members qualified?
- Is the staff friendly and caring?
- Do the residents seem happy?
- Is the facility clean?
- How does the facility smell?

Food
- Does the nursing home accommodate special dietary needs?
- What types of meals are served?
- Do residents get help in eating if they need it?

Activities
- What types of activities does the facility offer?
- Is there anything going on that interests you?
- Can you pursue your own hobbies and interests?
- Can you leave the home to go out and shop or just take a walk?
- Is it easy to get to a telephone?
- Can you have a say in choosing a roommate?
- Are private rooms available?

Medical care
- Will your doctor still be able to see you in the facility?
- Does the facility meet your medical needs?

Paying the bill

Nursing home care can be expensive. For some people, one helpful option is long-term-care insurance. Medicare may provide some initial financial assistance. Medicaid may provide long-term funding when patients have used up their own funds. Private health insurance policies, Veterans Affairs, trade unions and fraternal organizations also may pay for a portion of nursing home care.

In the United States, federal, state and local governments pay for more than half of the nursing home care. Individuals and their families generally fund a little under half. ■

CHAPTER 17 PART II

Death and Dying

It's never easy to think about your death or to face the reality of the death of loved ones. How you react to death depends on its circumstances and your personal beliefs and cultural influences. Because death challenges our understanding of the mystery of life, it will always be held in awe. The process of dying itself is also challenging. And scientific discoveries and medical advances have made death and dying even more complicated than in the past by often requiring people to make decisions about treatment options that were previously unavailable.

It's important to realize that death is quite different from the process of dying. Death is an endpoint when life ceases. But dying is the final part of the life process. Dying can be intense and shaped by the individual's history of illness, his or her response to stress, the nature of the illness and his or her interactions with others during the process. Cultural influences and belief systems also play a role.

For many dying people, life's experiences still have significant meaning and importance. Understanding the process of dying can often help terminally ill individuals and their families and friends cope during this difficult time.

Terminal Illness

The paths to death are as varied as the lives preceding it. Sometimes, death comes suddenly and without warning. Other times, people live with impending death as part of their life. With a terminal illness, the dying person, the attending doctor and a circle of family and friends are given time to prepare for death. They can discuss important issues, such as starting or stopping nutritional support, resuscitation and treatments such as medications, intravenous fluids or dialysis.

During a terminal illness, a dying person can often make clear his or her choices regarding an autopsy, organ donation, funeral arrangements — including burial or cremation — and legal matters. The reality of dying can be frightening to many people, but with support and encouragement, terminally ill individuals and their families can come to experience the remarkable possibilities that exist during this time in life.

Families, too, have to cope with complicated and painful emotional reactions when someone they love is terminally ill. Everyone copes in his or her own way. In some instances, the bereaved may choose to ignore or deny their loved one's inevitable death and avoid any talk of it, even with the dying person.

Although dying can be traumatic for everyone involved, it's also a time to come to terms with the ending of a life. Dying can be an occasion filled with moments of grateful remembrance and hope-filled meaning.

Discussing death

Most dying people can and should be told of their impending death. Unless a specific cultural tradition requires that the dying person not be told, people with a terminal illness generally want to be informed honestly of their situation. In most cases, a properly informed person is fortified, not undermined. In addition, this may give the dying person an opportunity to tell and see others, put affairs in order and leave memories, such as a journal.

That doesn't mean it's easy news to give or to digest. Dying people often fear abandonment, humiliation and loneliness at the end of their life. Some also fear dying in a hospital or on a machine. Others worry about becoming a burden to loved ones. And some believe that their personal relationships will suffer during this time and that they won't be treated as normal human beings. These concerns are often reinforced if the dying person is deprived of an opportunity to talk about feelings of fear and wonder when faced with death.

A person who's terminally ill may find it easier to talk to someone other than a relative. Most hospitals have a supportive-care program with trained staff members who can make it easier to get through this difficult time. In some instances, a social worker or a hospital chaplain can help a dying individual and family members talk about their attitudes toward death.

A dying person and his or her family members often need to discuss practical matters as well. It's helpful to understand the estimated length of the dying process, if it's known. Will it be days, weeks or months? This allows family members to adjust work schedules or consider taking time off. The 1993 Family and Medical Leave Act permits most employees up to 12 weeks unpaid leave for such a purpose.

The process of dying

Pain, both physical and emotional, is generally a dying person's principal fear. Fortunately, various methods of pain management make it possible to provide relief, with minimal side effects to compromise the comfort and dignity of dying. Many large hospitals operate pain clinics or offer hospice programs that include specialists trained in pain management. Pain-reducing drugs can successfully control most physical pain. Other therapies, such as biofeedback and relaxation therapy, also may be of benefit. These approaches alone may not relieve all of the pain, particularly the profound psychological pain that some people experience when dying.

Common reactions to impending death

When someone is told that he or she has a terminal illness, it's not uncommon for the person to feel a wide range of emotions — shock, anger, denial, depression. A dying individual may feel resentful toward anyone and everyone and robbed of the rest of his or her life. He or she may ask, "Why me?"

Some people attempt to negotiate or postpone the inevitable. There may be an element of bargaining with God or fate. Often the desired "deal" involves a period of time without pain and discomfort.

Others experience a peaceful acceptance of the importance and value of each day, for however long that may be. With this acceptance comes the ability to explore options and opportunities that present themselves at the end of life and to provide input into decisions that need to be made. This level of acceptance may come after having grappled with various and often-conflicting emotions and experiences. For some, this might come more easily and even automatically.

Role of a Chaplain

Hospital and hospice chaplains are often invaluable resources to individuals and families facing death. Chaplains can be from any faith tradition, but when they're ministering in a hospital setting, they're trained to be sensitive to an individual's personal religious beliefs. In most hospitals, chaplains are unit based, which means that they work with all of the patients and family members in a particular area of the hospital or hospice, regardless of a person's religious background.

Sometimes, a chaplain puts dying individuals in touch with members of their own faith. Other times a chaplain becomes integrally involved in an individual's care, working with doctors, nurses, therapists and social workers. A chaplain becomes familiar with medical procedures and recurring concerns and questions of people in a particular unit.

The hospital environment can create feelings of dependence and helplessness. A person in the hospital may feel alienated from family and friends. He or she may be unwilling to share feelings of guilt or anxiety. A chaplain can facilitate communication among family members and between the patient and the medical staff. In addition, a chaplain often helps terminally ill individuals and family and friends with coping mechanisms.

Chaplains are trained in dealing with important decisions such as maintaining or discontinuing life-sustaining measures and organ donation.

Perhaps the most important role of a chaplain is to provide comfort in the traditional role of offering individuals and their families a chance to share in the formal rituals of their faith community and to search for answers to difficult questions regarding suffering and dying. For people with specific cultural or religious convictions related to medical care, a chaplain can serve as a mediator between faith and scientific communities.

Hospice Care

Until the 20th century, most people spent their last days at home, comforted and cared for by family and loved ones. That tradition faded as hospitals became widespread. But recently, renewed interest in this time-honored philosophy has given rise to the field of hospice care.

Hospice care is a program focused on comfort. It's available to individuals with terminal illness. Hospices are based on the philosophy that people with no medical hope of recovery should be as comfortable as possible and in the setting they prefer. For many people, a hospital — with its busy atmosphere, numerous interruptions and focus on getting better — isn't where they prefer to spend their final days. By definition, hospice care is for people with 6 months or less to live.

Hospice addresses the two biggest fears that most dying people have — the fear of pain and other debilitating symptoms, and the fear of being alone. Although 80 percent of hospice care is provided at home or in

Creating a Memory Box

During a terminal illness, a dying person or family members may want to create a memory box. Gathering items with special meaning and writing down thoughts and wishes can be good ways to create special memories for family members. The box will be treasured for a lifetime, especially by young children of a dying parent.

Find a nice box and consider adding some of the following items:

- Favorite family pictures
- Special trinkets, books, knickknacks or medals
- A distinctive article of clothing, such as a favorite shirt, hat or scarf
- Beloved personal items, such as a pocket watch, reading glasses or a harmonica
- A journal in which everyone writes down his or her thoughts and memories
- An audiotape or videotape of the individual
- Letters written by the dying individual to family members

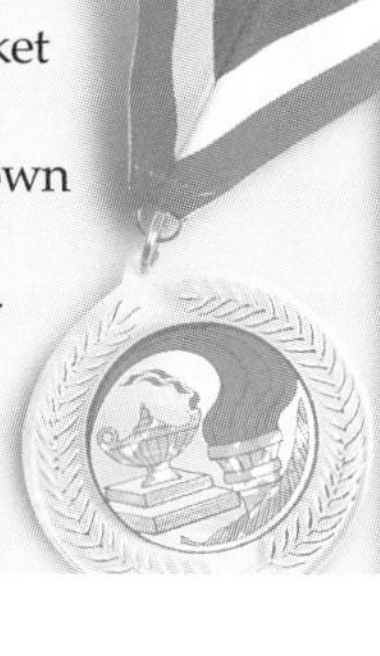

nursing homes, hospice is available wherever an individual may reside, including assisted-living facilities. Residential hospices, in which a dying individual can come to the hospice facility to spend his or her last days, also are available in some communities.

By choosing to receive hospice care, a terminally ill person accepts that death is near, and the treatment reflects that. Efforts to prolong life are cut back or stopped, and the emphasis shifts from finding a cure to maximizing the quality of life remaining. Although many people receiving hospice care have cancer, hospice is available to anyone of any age with any type of terminal illness.

Increasing popularity

In 1974, only one hospice program existed in the entire United States. Today, there are more than 3,000. The majority of hospice programs are run by nonprofit, independent organizations. Many are affiliated with hospitals, nursing homes or home health care agencies. Some programs are operated by for-profit organizations.

Hospice programs help individuals and family members meet the physical, emotional, social and spiritual challenges of a terminal illness. Hospice also offers bereavement services that tend to the needs of grieving family members. What distinguishes hospice is the nature of the care: The goal is to affirm life yet accept death as a normal part of the life process.

Cost

Cost is another factor in the growth of hospice care. Hospice care is often less expensive than traditional hospital-based care, especially when it's provided at home. The cost varies greatly depending on the length and type of care necessary and an individual's insurance coverage. Medicare — and in some states Medicaid — and most private insurance plans, including managed care organizations, cover hospice care. Coverage may be with benefits beyond standard plans. Medicare and Medicaid provide a package of services that includes professional services, medications related to the terminal illness, and supplies and equipment needed for management of symptoms at the end of life.

Family involvement

The core of hospice is an integrated and cooperative effort by family, friends and a team of professional and volunteer caregivers to meet a dying person's needs. In some situations, family members or friends are able to provide most or almost all of the care, with support and instruction from the hospice team. Other times, the hospice team plays a more active role.

A doctor leads the hospice team. A nurse typically coordinates the day-to-day care. Chaplains and social workers are available to counsel individuals and families and to make sure emotional, spiritual and social needs are being addressed. Trained volunteers perform a wide variety of tasks as needed, such as providing companionship, doing light housekeeping, preparing meals and running errands.

The National Hospice and Palliative Care Organization can provide information on hospice care available in your region (see page 1386).

Approaching Death

New technologies have forced a new definition of death. Today, doctors can keep people alive in circumstances that would have been impossible in the past. Most states recognize that a person is legally dead when he or she has experienced irreversible cessation of circulation and respiration or irreversible cessation and function of the entire brain, including the brainstem, which controls breathing.

Only a few years ago, anyone who had lost consciousness, was unable to breathe and had no heart-

Palliative Care

Modern-day palliative care grew out of the hospice movement, and it shares many of the same goals. The main difference between palliative care and hospice care is time. Hospice care is for people with 6 months or less to live. Palliative care is intended to span the period between acute medical care and hospice care. Palliative care generally covers the last year or so of life.

In practice, the two are quite similar. Both seek to include the active participation of family and friends in end-of-life care. The palliative care team encourages, and even may facilitate, open communication among family members and between the family and the medical team. This includes frank discussions of treatment options and disease progression. Emphasis is also placed on attending to the emotional, spiritual and psychological needs of family and friends. Like hospice care, palliative care involves not only doctors but also social workers and nurses.

Research shows that palliative care has a number of benefits:

- Less time in the hospital
- More time at home among friends and family
- Higher likelihood of dying at a place of one's own choosing
- Increased satisfaction with medical care
- Better control of symptoms, including acute and chronic pain
- Reduction in the cost of care

beat was considered dead. Now, in some instances, life-support systems can revive an individual not breathing and with no heartbeat and, in part, continue to support or replace some of these necessary functions. In addition, doctors often are able to maintain heart or lung function even when the brain ceases to function.

The remarkable ability to sustain life brings with it certain ethical, legal and medical concerns. Many of these issues are best dealt with before a person becomes unable to express his or her wishes (see Chapter 11, "Addressing End-of-Life Issues").

The moment of death

Caretakers' actions and attitudes, especially those of loved ones, can have a strong influence on the dying experience. For example, dying people frequently request that they not be left alone. They may fear not only the moment of death with its uncertainties but also abandonment. Offering consolation and reassurance at these moments is often difficult but necessary.

Many dying people are also comforted by their faith traditions and by having members of their faith community with them in their final moments.

Usually, there are signs that the moment of death is near. The dying person may become fidgety or restless and have irregular breathing. In such circumstances a doctor may provide medications or oxygen to make the person more comfortable. In some cases, the dying person's breathing can be eased if he or she is placed in a sitting position or allowed to lie on one side with a pillow under the head.

Even though the dying person may not be able to communicate, he or she often can hear much of what's being said. Despite any sense of powerlessness you may feel, your very presence can be all of the comfort a dying person seeks. Simply hold the person's hand or give him or her a hug. Physical contact is often soothing. If you don't know what to say, remember that silence can be golden.

The formalities of death

Death is a legal event that calls for several formalities.

The death certificate

Before a burial or cremation can take place, a medical death certificate must be obtained that shows the cause of death and formally registers the death. A death certificate is signed by a licensed physician. If a doctor has examined or treated a dying individual regularly or shortly before death, he or she generally isn't obliged to examine the body before signing the certificate. Sometimes, a medical examiner or coroner, rather than a family doctor or the physician in attendance, states the cause of death and signs the certificate.

In some instances, an autopsy may be ordered. An autopsy provides more information about a person's illness (see page 320). It may be required by law if the death resulted from an accident, is unexpected and unexplained or is a suspected homicide or suicide. After such matters are resolved, the family usually works with a funeral home on any final arrangements.

Funeral arrangements

If a loved one has died, a funeral director can be helpful in making virtually all of your decisions concerning funeral and burial arrangements. However, people who knew they were dying may have made these decisions with their family while they were still able to do so.

The funeral director will come to the deceased's home, hospital or nursing home to remove the body and take it to the funeral home. Later, members of the family meet with the funeral director to discuss funeral arrangements. Federal law requires that funeral homes provide consumers with itemized price lists of products and services to ensure that people pay for only what they want or need.

Family members should make it quite clear how elaborate or simple they want the funeral to be and how the details are to be handled. Because these are emotionally difficult times, you may want to seek help in making these decisions from someone who isn't personally involved, such as a member of the clergy, a close friend or an attorney.

Funeral decisions include the type and location of the funeral service and whether the remains are to be buried, cremated or both. If the body is to be donated to research, the funeral director will deliver the body to the designated institution.

Funeral ceremonies can be held at the funeral home or a place of

Organ Donation

As a family, discuss your wishes regarding organ donation so that if one of you ever becomes unable to communicate, others will know what to do in this regard after the death.

If you want to be an organ donor and have expressed that to your family, you may also want to indicate your intent on your driver's license, in a living will or by carrying a donor card. If you don't make your wishes clear, your family members may have to decide whether to donate your organs. Often this decision needs to be made when death is near or immediately following death, which can be an especially hard thing to do during an already difficult time. If they know your wishes ahead of time and understand the process, it can make this time much easier. For more information on organ donation, see page 144.

worship or both. If your family has a religious affiliation, the funeral director can contact your clergy member or recommend a member of the clergy or an appropriate authority. Fees and terms of payment are made with the funeral director at the time funeral arrangements are made. Usually, payment isn't required in advance, but these expenses become the first legal obligation of the estate of the deceased.

The estate

After the funeral, a probate judge may need to designate the executor or personal representative of the estate. This is often a member of the family, family attorney or close friend. The executor is responsible for the financial affairs of the deceased, which may include the funeral expenses.

After all payments are made, any remaining assets are distributed according to the deceased's will or the laws of the state in which the person lived. Procedures may vary from state to state. Some terminally ill people like to provide guidance to their family regarding estate and funeral matters to lessen the sense of burden that family members may feel.

The autopsy decision

Autopsy comes from Greek words meaning "to see with one's own eyes." An autopsy is a detailed examination of a deceased person's body to determine the cause of death. An autopsy is performed by a medical doctor who specializes in the nature of disease (pathologist). He or she then reports the findings to the attending doctor. On request, the doctor discusses the findings with the family.

In the 1940s, an autopsy was performed following about half the hospital deaths. Now only 10 percent to 15 percent of people who die are autopsied. One reason for this decline is that modern diagnostic measures performed on terminally ill patients make it clear what they are dying of.

Autopsies play an important role in medical science and can provide useful information for surviving family members and doctors.

Hereditary disorders

An autopsy may reveal conditions that could affect children and siblings. For example, if polycystic kidney disease is found, close relatives of childbearing age may want genetic counseling to determine if they're at risk of passing on the disease. An autopsy can also confirm some illnesses that have been diagnosed based on behavior alone, for example, Alzheimer's disease.

Emotional security

Family members often feel that they could have done something to prevent the death of a loved one. In the case of a fatal heart attack, they might berate themselves for not insisting that their loved one take it easier. An autopsy may reveal that the person had a preexisting heart condition that could have taken his or her life at any time — regardless of whether the person "took it easy."

Insurance settlements

Establishing the cause of death can help resolve disputes that may affect the benefits that survivors receive. For example, if a person with a heart problem dies from a fall, insurance benefits may vary depending on whether the death was accidental or the result of heart disease.

Benefits to medical science

Much of what researchers and doctors know about diseases, including statistical information, was discovered or confirmed through autopsies. Advances in medical knowledge depend in part on the study of

Bereavement

Humans experience many losses throughout life. The longer people live, the more losses they suffer. Bereavement is the natural response to a loss. Bereavement usually refers to feelings after the loss of a loved one — usually through death, but also after the dissolution of a relationship.

The death of a loved one is never easy to accept, and a sudden loss can be especially distressing. However, a long, terminal illness before a death can be emotionally, physically and financially draining.

To protect yourself from grief-related illness, take care of your own health. Monitor any medical problems you had before the loss, and seek professional help if new symptoms develop. Your ability to adapt to the stress of a death can influence your overall health. Severe or prolonged grief that disrupts daily routines or lifestyles can contribute to illnesses such as depression and alcoholism.

Although cultural norms for mourning determine behavior to some degree, there's no single right way to grieve. Nor is there a fixed timetable. Some people seem to return to normal emotions and activities within a month, but for others bereavement is measured in years rather than weeks or months.

People cope with their grief in different ways. Some people grieve openly, others privately. And it's not always evident that someone is grieving. During your bereavement, don't be afraid to seek help from clergy, friends and counselors. And remember that it's entirely appropriate — and essential for both your mental and physical health — to express your emotions. Healthy mourning is the process that helps you accept your loss so that you can go on with your life. Suppressing your emotions through excess activity, work, alcohol or drugs can prolong the mourning process.

human tissue removed at autopsy. Pathologic observations reveal a great deal about human disease. For example, such data helped to confirm the association between cigarette smoking and lung cancer. Autopsies also helped doctors discover the nature and character of conditions such as hyperparathyroidism and viral hepatitis. And they revealed the effects of toxic chemicals and other industrial hazards on body organs.

Quality assurance
Doctors use autopsy data to assess their accuracy in diagnosis and treatment. Autopsy findings also help assess the overall quality of care in a hospital and community.

Vital statistics
The causes of death keep changing. Deaths from infectious diseases are less common today, but degenerative illness takes a greater toll. Public health officials use information from autopsies to monitor such trends. Death statistics influence government spending for health care, the enactment of safety standards and the design of medical equipment.

Emerging illness
Early medical understanding of illness such as AIDS, Legionnaires' disease and toxic shock syndrome all came from autopsy studies.

Arranging for an autopsy

Autopsies are often required by state or local law when death results from an accident, is unexpected or unexplained or is a suspected homicide or suicide. Otherwise, autopsies require the permission of the next of kin.

When you sign an autopsy consent form, you can authorize a limited autopsy, which restricts the procedure to specific parts of the body, or a more thorough autopsy. A disadvantage of a limited autopsy is that it limits the amount of useful information the procedure provides and may leave some questions unanswered. Consent forms generally permit removal of internal organs and tissue.

There are many misconceptions about autopsy and tissue removal. In many cases, families are reluctant to permit an autopsy, believing that the procedure is degrading or that the deceased has "suffered enough." Another common misconception about autopsy is that it will disfigure the body. The truth is, an autopsy that's performed properly won't disfigure the body. At an open casket funeral service, observers won't be able to tell if an autopsy was performed. Autopsies don't interfere with embalming of the body, and the procedure doesn't need to delay the funeral. In addition, the majority of religious faiths allow autopsy.

In most instances, when you grant permission for an elective autopsy, the bill will be paid by the hospital. Medicare won't pay for the procedure. However, if the death occurs outside a hospital and family members request an autopsy, they usually must pay for it.

A dying individual who would like an autopsy performed after his or her death should make a provision for it in his or her advance directive (see page 141) and notify loved ones of the provision. This can help to spare loved ones the burden of having to make this decision during a time of grief.

Children and Death

Children are often overlooked in times of grief. But death is a crisis that should be shared by everyone in the family. Otherwise, children may experience silence and secrecy that isolates them from the rest of the family and denies them the opportunity to grieve with other family members.

Telling a child that a parent or sibling is going to die, or that he or she is dying, is difficult for everyone, including doctors and nurses. At the same time, children have a right to know about anything that affects them or their families. Not telling them is a breach of trust, and most children are aware that something is amiss in the family.

Why children need to know

Children can sense when something is wrong, but young children in particular usually can't interpret their suspicions. If left alone to wonder, small children may somehow feel responsible for the illness or death of a parent or sibling. They need help integrating their observations into day-to-day reality.

When informed in language that they can understand, most children have a remarkable capacity for dealing with death. Even the weight of very sad truths is preferable to the anxiety of too much uncertainty. If you talk with them, they won't feel cut off from that part of the family that "knows." In turn, you won't need to be secretive. You may even find your young children can be a comfort to you and others. Instead of burdening them with the darkness of unspoken fears, discussing death and loss with them permits them to live more freely.

Your local library and bookstores are good resources for books that explain death and dying in terms young children can understand.

When and from whom?

When should a child be told? Generally, as soon as possible. This information needs to be given in an age-appropriate way. Very young children, for example, won't understand that a parent is dying, but they may understand that the parent is sick or that people are sad because the parent is sick. Keep them informed as treatment progresses and tell them how it's affecting the person's health. Any change in appearance or disposition shouldn't go unexplained. Children of different stages of emotional development should probably be told individually. But after the initial disclosure, efforts should be made to make it a shared experience among all of the children.

It's generally best for a parent or both parents together to tell a child or children. And it's OK to cry. Tears give permission for your child to cry and to grieve with you. If you aren't available or are unable to tell your child, ask a friend or relative who's close to your child. Finally, the task can be left to a nurse or doctor. However, a young child may consider them strangers whose word is subject to disbelief.

How much information?

Children need to be told as much as they can understand. There's no single right way to tell children about death. They should be told what has happened and what will happen, although this isn't always clear early after the diagnosis. Parents should be guided by their own styles of communication and what they feel comfortable in discussing.

At all times, children should be told that no matter what the outcome, they will always be loved. They should be encouraged to ask questions, and these questions should be answered simply. Their fears may keep them from asking questions, so encourage them by asking them how they feel. At no time should you lie or make promises that you may not be able to keep. In addition, don't be afraid to say, "I don't know."

How will they respond?

Young children fear being separated from their parents. Being left in the care of strangers may suggest they've been abandoned.

When someone is sick, whether it's the parent or child, discipline can be difficult because children may need to seek extra attention by testing the limits of the rules. If you suspend the normal rules of conduct, it may be alarming to them. It's more appropriate to reassure children of your love while expecting the same cooperation and good behavior from them. As your child comes to learn what's happening, he or she should be assured that nothing he or she said or did, including any possible bad behavior, caused the illness or death.

Very young children — those younger than 3 years — believe everything is possible. There are no limits to their parents' powers. To preschoolers, death is still reversible. Nothing is final. School-age children younger than age 9 usually understand that death is a biological event rather than someone's appearing or disappearing in a supernatural form. But it's only at about age 9 that they're able to grasp death as the final, irreversible end of human life.

School-age children can become overly concerned about details and misjudge their significance. Guard against overwhelming them with specific data. Teachers and school counselors can be helpful in weighing the gravity and meaning of the information your child has learned from you.

It's important to try to maintain a sense of normalcy in view of a not-normal routine. Children need a sense of predictability to their day, and this can be challenging for parents dealing with their own emotions and needs in a difficult time.

The death of a parent

The death of a parent is a powerful and, at times, devastating event in the life of a child. Many children are able to resume a normal lifestyle in a matter of weeks. Others suffer the effects of an unhealed wound throughout their childhood and adult life. Why one child is able to deal with the death of a parent and another isn't depends in part on how the child is told about the death and how the rest of the family accepts the loss. Be aware of physical signs of grief, such as difficulty sleeping, a change in eating patterns or regressive behavior.

Children initially may deny the reality of the death, express anger or act out in rebellion. They may also repress any feelings associated with the loss. Caregivers should encourage children to share their feelings to whatever degree they can. Allow the child's friends to come into the home during the time of mourning. Friends can be a comfort, and the friends' knowing about the death can deepen the reality of the loss for the child.

Keep in mind that children have a remarkable capacity for adjustment. The changes they see in themselves, in the world around them and in those who surround them constitute an endless string of events to be absorbed. Whether the news is bad or good, children usually succeed in working their way through life's events — even those that seem unfair and unreasonable, like the death of a beloved parent. ■

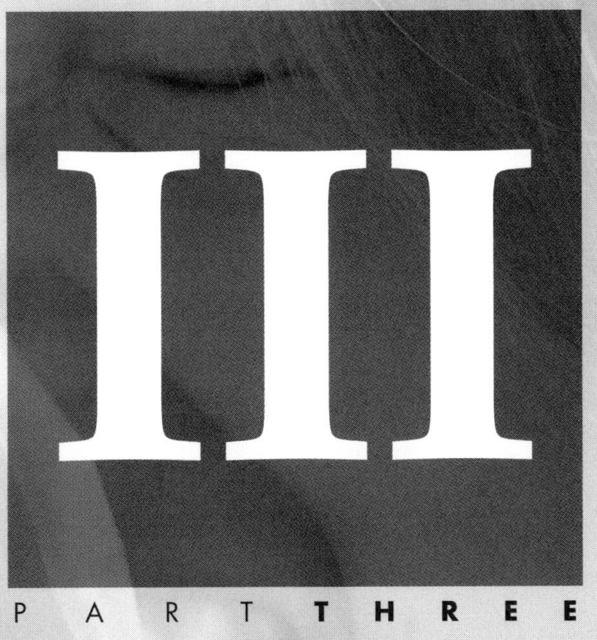

PART THREE

Making Sense of Your Symptoms

Making Sense of Your Symptoms

The human body usually operates effectively and reliably. At times, though, you may experience a breakdown in one of the body systems. Or an invader, such as a virus or bacterium, may affect normal functioning. When this happens your body usually gives off one or more signals to alert you that something is wrong. These are commonly referred to as signs and symptoms. A sign is an indication of illness that's noticeable to others, such as a cough or a red eye. A symptom is a sensation that only you can perceive, such as pain or stiffness.

Many times, it's easy to figure out what's triggering your signs and symptoms. Sneezing, a sore throat and a runny nose are usually indications of a common cold or an allergy. A deep, throbbing ache in a tooth is often associated with an abscess. Other times, it can be difficult to make sense of what your body is telling you. You may worry that a sign or symptom is a warning of one condition but later find out that it's really related to another. Or, you may be at a loss for what's causing it.

This section is intended to help you better understand what may be triggering a certain complaint. Following each sign or symptom is a list of diseases and disorders frequently associated with it. These are listed in alphabetical order, not by importance or frequency of occurrence.

By reading about each of the conditions listed, you may be able to better identify possible causes of the problem. Keep in mind, though, that the following information is only a guide. It may help you better understand the problem and assist you in communicating with your or your child's doctor so that he or she can more quickly get to the root of your ailment. Reading this section is *not* a replacement for seeing a doctor. In many cases, it's important that you get an expert opinion to be certain that what you think might be the cause of your sign or symptom is in fact the true culprit.

Warning!

If you or someone you know is experiencing signs and symptoms that might be a warning of a medical emergency, such as a heart attack or stroke, don't take time to read this section. Call for emergency medical help or have someone take you or the person in distress to the nearest hospital emergency department immediately. In a true emergency, time is of the essence. If you're not certain whether you're dealing with a medical emergency, call your doctor's office or the emergency department at your local hospital and describe the signs and symptoms being experienced by you or the person you're helping.

Signs and Symptoms Common in Adults

Listed here are 25 signs and symptoms commonly experienced by adults. These are some of the most frequent reasons that men and women see their doctors.

Abdominal pain

Abdominal pain can occur alone or with other signs and symptoms, such as nausea and vomiting. Occasional episodes of abdominal pain may be related to a bacterial or viral infection (gastroenteritis) or result from overeating or eating too much of the wrong foods — fatty or gas-producing foods or, for people with intolerance to milk sugar (lactose), dairy products. Abdominal pain that's recurrent, persistent or severe may signal a variety of other conditions. Abdominal pain is often associated with one of the following causes:

- **Abdominal wall pain (see page 995)**
  The pain is nagging and accompanied by tenderness in the abdominal muscles that increases when the muscles are tensed, such as when sitting up from a lying position. A specific spot (tender trigger point) can be located where the pain is worse with abdominal muscle tension.
- **Acute pancreatitis (see page 900)**
  Mild to severe pain in the upper abdomen or mid-abdomen may radiate through to the back. The pain may persist for hours or days without relief and be accompanied by nausea and vomiting. Alcohol and food may increase the pain. Bending forward or curling up in the fetal position may relieve it.
- **Appendicitis (see page 873)**
  Signs and symptoms often start with a loss of appetite, a low-grade fever and nausea with or without vomiting. The pain is initially located around the navel and later moves to the lower-right abdomen.
- **Diverticulitis (see page 879)**
  The pain typically comes on suddenly and is accompanied by a fever and nausea. The signs and symptoms are similar to those of appendicitis, except that the pain is usually located in the lower-left side of the abdomen instead of the lower-right.
- **Gallbladder attack (see "Gallstones," page 896)**
  The pain is usually in the upper-right abdomen or right midabdomen, and it may radiate to the back or right shoulder. It's unrelieved by changing positions or taking an antacid or pain medication. The pain often occurs 1 or 2 hours after eating, and it may be associated with nausea and vomiting.
- **Inflammatory bowel disease (see page 874)**
  The pain is caused by inflammation of the intestines.

It may be accompanied by cramping, diarrhea, weight loss, fatigue and intermittent fever.

- **Intestinal obstruction (see page 884)**
  The cramping, colicky abdominal pain comes and goes. It may be associated with visible bloating, bowel noise (rushes and gurgling), nausea and vomiting and, if the obstruction is complete or near complete, an inability to pass gas (flatus) or stool.
- **Irritable bowel syndrome (see page 879)**
  This chronic condition is associated with periods of diarrhea alternating with constipation and uncomfortable abdominal cramping and bloating. Irritable bowel syndrome isn't associated with a fever, weight loss or bleeding.
- **Malabsorption disorder (see page 871)**
  An intestinal sensitivity to a dietary protein, such as the gluten found in wheat and other grains, may result in abdominal pain, bloating, gas and diarrhea. A common malabsorption disorder is lactose intolerance, caused by an inability to digest the sugar in milk (lactose).
- **Peptic ulcer (see page 860)**
  The pain is gnawing and often located in the upper abdomen between the navel and breastbone. It's generally worse when the stomach is empty, so it tends to flare at night during sleep. Eating temporarily relieves the pain.
- **Shingles (see page 1192)**
  Symptoms may begin as itching or burning, tingling or knife-like pain on one side of your abdomen. The pain typically wraps around from the spine, following a nerve pathway. One to 5 days later, groupings of blisters appear in the same location.

Ankle and foot pain

Nearly everyone experiences an occasional episode of foot or ankle pain. Often, the pain is the result of a misstep that causes a sprain or fracture, or it's associated with a common problem such as a corn or callus. Many times, ankle and foot pain results from one of the following conditions:

- **Achilles tendinitis (see page 966)**
  The pain is located where the heel cord (Achilles tendon) meets the heel bone. The heel cord is tender to the touch.
- **Bone fracture (see page 949)**
  The pain is caused by a broken bone in a foot or ankle. Such injuries may occur during a misstep or accident.
- **Bunion (see page 971)**
  A bunion is a common deformity of the big toe joint. It causes painful swelling at the bump on the base of the big toe.
- **Gout (see page 1008)**
  Acute gout causes excruciating pain, often in the joint at the base of the big toe. The pain comes on rapidly and occurs with any movement of the affected joint. Even a bedsheet rubbing over an affected joint can be painful.
- **Metatarsalgia (see page 968)**
  The pain occurs on the bony prominences of the balls of the feet when you walk or stand.
- **Morton's neuroma (see page 969)**
  A burning or sharp pain is felt between the third and fourth toes. The pain is often worse when you wear tight shoes.
- **Osteoarthritis (see page 997)**
  The pain is chronic and slowly progressive. It may be worse with weight-bearing activity.
- **Plantar fasciitis (see "Heel pain," page 966)**
  The pain is located under the heel and is often most severe with the first steps out of bed in the morning or with the first steps after being seated for a while. Walking often improves the pain.
- **Sprain (see page 957)**
  A sprain occurs when a joint moves beyond its normal range of motion, stretching or tearing ligaments. The resulting pain is often accompanied by swelling.
- **Tendinitis (see page 992)**
  The pain is caused by an inflamed tendon in a foot or ankle.

Back pain

Low back pain not only is very common but also can result from injuries and diseases that range from minor to extremely serious. Back pain is often related to one of the following conditions:

- **Bone cancer (see "Bone tumors," page 987)**
  This is a rare cause of back pain. The pain is in the bone and is deep and aching. It's often worse with rest than during activity.
- **Bone infection (see "Osteomyelitis," page 987)**
  The pain is sudden and remains severe. It's often associated with a fever.
- **Herniated disk (see page 977)**
  The pain is typically in the lower back, and it may be accompanied by numbness or tingling that radiates into the buttocks and down a leg.
- **Muscle strain (see page 972)**
  Muscle stain is a common cause of sudden (acute) low back pain. Certain movements of the lower back worsen the pain.
- **Osteoarthritis (see page 997)**
  This common cause of back pain results from deterioration of bony joints. The pain is long term (chronic) and may worsen with weight-bearing activity and certain movements.
- **Osteoporotic compression fracture (see "Osteoporosis," page 981)**
  Sudden, severe back pain in a person with osteoporosis may be due to one or more small fractures in a spinal vertebra.

Chest pain

Chest pain may be a warning of a heart attack, but it can also occur for a number of other reasons. It may be caused by some other heart condition, or it may be associated with a chest wall or lung disorder. Chest pain can also stem from a gastrointestinal problem. Often, chest pain is related to one of the following conditions:

- **Angina (see page 754)**
  Discomfort, tightening or pressure occurs in the chest due to lack of blood flow to the heart muscle. Pain may also be felt in the jaw and inner-left arm or, occasionally, both arms. The pain or discomfort typically develops with physical exertion or high emotional stress. When you stop an activity or relax, symptoms often improve.
- **Chest wall pain (see page 995)**
  This is a common, harmless chest pain caused by muscle or cartilage tenderness in the chest wall. Pushing on a tender area in your chest with your finger reproduces the pain.
- **Esophageal spasm (see "Swallowing difficulties," page 854)**
  Tight, severe pressure develops under the breastbone, often after drinking a large gulp of cold or carbonated fluid. The pain usually improves in seconds. If prolonged, it can mimic a heart attack.
- **Gastroesophageal reflux disease (see page 850)**
  A warm, burning sensation (heartburn) develops in the upper part of the abdomen and the lower chest under the breastbone. You may get a sour taste in your mouth. Drinking a liquid antacid or chewing antacid pills usually relieves the discomfort.
- **Heart attack (see page 757)**
  Severe pain or pressure can be felt in the chest, neck, jaw or arms. It may be accompanied by shortness of breath, sweating, nausea and vomiting.
- **Pneumonia (see page 490)**
  Pneumonia is associated with a fever and a cough that may bring up colored sputum. You might experience shortness of breath and sharp chest pain when taking a deep breath.
- **Pulmonary embolism (see page 826)**
  Attempting to take a deep breath produces sharp chest pain. This may be accompanied by sudden shortness of breath and the coughing up of blood.
- **Rib fracture**
  A rib fracture can result from an injury or from severe coughing. Applying pressure to the fractured rib produces intense pain.
- **Shingles (see page 1192)**
  Symptoms may begin as itching or burning, tingling or knife-like pain on one side of the abdomen. The pain typically wraps around from the spine, following a nerve pathway. One to 5 days later, groupings of blisters appear in the same location.

Involuntary Weight Loss

For many people who struggle to shed pounds, unintentional weight loss might seem like a gift. However, significant loss of weight that occurs without trying can signify a serious medical disorder, and it should be investigated.

Involuntary weight loss is defined as a loss of more than 5 percent of your body weight over a 6-month span. For a 160-pound individual, a 5 percent loss would be about 8 pounds. If you're unsure about your original weight, other signs can help pinpoint if significant loss has occurred. Your clothes may fit more loosely, or you may be fastening your belt at a tighter notch. Friends and family members may comment that you've lost weight.

Questions

If you've lost weight without trying, ask yourself:

- Is the weight loss truly unintentional or have you modified your diet or activity level? Even small changes in either can cause weight loss if sustained over several months.
- How much weight have you lost and over how long of a period? This can help your doctor determine the potential seriousness of the problem.
- Is your appetite normal or has it decreased? Making this distinction can narrow the list of possible causes.
- Do you have other signs and symptoms? Other signs and symptoms also can help narrow the list of possible causes.

Causes of involuntary weight loss

The list of potential causes for involuntary weight loss is extensive. Although many people worry most

Cough

Occasional coughing is a normal part of everyday life. A cough that's severe or persists may be a sign of a variety of conditions, ranging from a medication side effect to lung cancer. A cough is often associated with one of the following conditions or medications:

- **Angiotensin-converting enzyme (ACE) inhibitors (see pages 747 and 1296)**
  These medications are used to treat high blood pressure or heart-related illnesses. In some people, they can cause a bothersome, dry cough.
- **Asthma (see page 532)**
  Shortness of breath, wheezing and tightness in the chest may accompany an asthma-related cough. Asthma may be triggered by allergies, a respiratory infection, cold air or exercise.

about cancer, the majority of people who experience unintentional weight loss don't have cancer. The largest studies of unintentional weight loss have shown that in nearly a quarter of the participants, no cause for the weight loss was found despite an extensive search.

Major causes of weight loss include:

- Cancer, most often of the gastrointestinal tract
- Depression
- Dementia
- Hyperthyroidism
- A gastrointestinal disorder, such as an ulcer, a malabsorption disorder or an inflammatory disorder
- Chronic lung disease
- Uncontrolled diabetes
- Some chronic infections, such as tuberculosis and human immunodeficiency virus (HIV)
- Alcoholism
- Certain medications, such as selective serotonin reuptake inhibitors (SSRIs) and nonsteroidal anti-inflammatory drugs (NSAIDs)

In addition, long-term (chronic) pain for almost any reason can cause weight loss. Pain and many of the medicines used to treat it decrease appetite.

When to see your doctor

If you've unintentionally lost more than 5 percent of your original body weight over a 6-month period, see your doctor. In preparing for the visit, list other signs or symptoms that you've been experiencing.

Your doctor will likely ask you a number of questions related to your weight loss and your overall health and conduct a physical examination. If you and your doctor think that the weight loss is significant, you may need to undergo diagnostic testing.

- **Bronchitis (see page 797)**
  The cough produces sputum, and it may be accompanied by wheezing.
- **Cold (see page 487)**
  The cough is usually accompanied by a stuffy nose, a sore and often scratchy throat, fatigue and a low-grade fever.
- **Foreign body (see page 857)**
  The cough follows inhalation of a foreign body, such as a piece of food, into the windpipe (trachea) or a bronchial tube.
- **Gastroesophageal reflux disease (see page 850)**
  The cough is typically accompanied by heartburn (acid reflux) and sometimes a sour taste in your mouth.
- **Pneumonia (see page 490)**
  The cough is associated with a lung infection and may produce colored sputum. Other signs and symptoms include shortness of breath, a fever and sharp pain when taking a deep breath.
- **Postnasal drip (see page 686)**
  Excess production of mucus that drains into the back of the throat causes the throat to feel full or "funny." The cough is an attempt to relieve the sensation.

Diarrhea

Everyone has loose, watery stools at one time or another. Often, diarrhea is a result of a viral or bacterial infection (gastroenteritis) or a side effect of medication. As the infection clears or your body becomes accustomed to the medication, the diarrhea usually stops. Persistent diarrhea generally indicates a gastrointestinal disorder. Diarrhea is often associated with one of the following conditions:

- **Antibiotic-associated diarrhea (see page 870)**
  Antibiotics can kill bacteria that normally live in the digestive tract, replacing them with diarrhea-causing bacteria. Up to 20 percent of people taking antibiotics experience this problem. Usually, the diarrhea is mild and of short duration. Occasionally, a serious colon infection can result, causing severe diarrhea.
- **Gastroenteritis (see "Gastrointestinal infections," page 866)**
  This condition is the most common cause of sudden, severe diarrhea. Other signs include nausea and vomiting.
- **Inflammatory bowel disease (see page 874)**
  Diarrhea may be accompanied by weight loss, fatigue, cramping, abdominal pain and intermittent fever. In some cases, the diarrhea may be bloody.
- **Intestinal obstruction (see page 884)**
  Diarrhea is accompanied by a cramping and colicky pain that comes and goes. Other signs and symptoms include visible bloating, bowel noise (rushes and gurgling), nausea and vomiting.
- **Malabsorption disorder (see page 871)**
  An intestinal sensitivity to a dietary protein, such as the gluten found in wheat and other grains, may result in abdominal pain, bloating, gas and diarrhea. A common malabsorption disorder is lactose intolerance, caused by an inability to digest sugar in milk (lactose).

Dizziness

Dizziness has many causes. Fortunately, most dizziness is mild, brief and harmless. The term *dizziness* is sometimes used by individuals to describe lightheadedness and a feeling of faintness. Other times, it's used to describe a feeling of imbalance — like walking in a rocking boat. More often it's used to describe the sensation that you or your surroundings are spinning (vertigo). To help your doctor understand your condition, it's important to clarify the type of dizziness you're experiencing.

A spinning sensation is often caused by one the following conditions:

- **Benign paroxysmal positional vertigo (see page 680)**
  Momentary dizziness occurs when turning your head from side to side, rolling over in bed or looking up suddenly. Intermittent episodes of these symptoms may occur over the years.
- **Labyrinthitis (see page 679)**
  Caused by an inner ear infection, this condition can produce vertigo with nausea and vomiting. Decreased hearing may result in the affected ear.
- **Meniere's disease (see page 677)**
  In addition to severe dizziness, signs and symptoms include ringing in the ear, pressure in the ear and hearing loss. The signs and symptoms come and go and might be recurrent every few months or years.
- **Middle ear infection (see page 668)**
  In addition to dizziness, pain and a plugged ear are other symptoms of middle ear infection (otitis media).
- **Stroke (see page 569)**
  Other signs and symptoms include numbness, tingling, weakness on one side of the body, difficulty speaking, double vision and facial droop. See a doctor immediately.
- **Transient ischemic attack (see page 568)**
  Often a precursor to a stroke, this condition can cause dizziness, numbness, tingling, weakness on one side of the body, difficulty speaking, double vision and facial droop. Unlike a stroke, the signs and symptoms of transient ischemic attack usually last a short time and then fully resolve.

Eye discomfort and redness

Many of the most common eye conditions don't pose a serious threat to vision, but they can be uncomfortable. Eye discomfort and redness is often associated with one of the following conditions:

- **Allergies (see "Respiratory allergies," page 527)**
  Airborne allergens, such as pollen, dust and smog, can produce itchy, pink-colored eyes.
- **Corneal abrasion (see page 634)**
  An injury to the cornea causes pain and a persistent feeling that you have something in your eye. Blinking makes it worse. Covering the eye improves the signs and symptoms.
- **Pinkeye (see "Conjunctivitis," page 642)**
  The white of the eye (sclera) has a pinkish discoloration. Other symptoms include itchiness and a gritty feeling in the eye when you blink. The eyelids may stick together while you sleep.
- **Subconjunctival hemorrhage (see "Blood in an eye," page 634)**
  A broken blood vessel causes a painless but alarming bright red area within the white of the eye. The condition is generally harmless.

Headache

Headaches are common and usually not due to a serious cause. Some headaches, though, can be a warning of a serious problem. Types of headaches and some conditions that can cause headaches include the following:

- **Brain tumor (see page 585)**
  A brain tumor is a rare cause of headache. Pressure from a tumor may cause chronic or persistent headaches in a person not prone to headache. Associated signs and symptoms may include weakness, clumsiness, vision changes, personality changes and vomiting.
- **Cranial (giant cell) arteritis (see page 660)**
  The headache may be mild or severe. The skin on one side of your face near the ear and temple is tender to the touch. Other signs and symptoms include a fever and aching of the shoulder and hip muscles.
- **Encephalitis (see page 577)**
  A headache associated with encephalitis is usually accompanied by a fever and sometimes pain behind the eyes. Signs and symptoms may be aggravated by light. You may feel lethargic, confused and experience an altered mental state.
- **Medication side effects (see "Medications Guide," page 1283)**
  Headaches are a side effect of a number of medications. Examples include nitrates, some antibiotics and oral contraceptives.
- **Meningitis (see page 576)**
  Meningitis is a life-threatening cause of headache. This type of headache is associated with a fever, a stiff neck and altered mental status. Attempting to bend the neck increases the pain.
- **Migraine (see page 557)**
  A migraine may be preceded by visual symptoms such as bright or colored light patterns or zigzags in the visual field (auras). Nausea and vomiting may accompany the headache.
- **Occipital neuralgia (see page 959)**
  With this condition, shooting pain in the back of the neck often travels up behind an ear to one side of the scalp. The discomfort can often be reproduced by firmly pressing on the bony bump in the back of the neck, where the occipital nerve is located.
- **Sinusitis (see page 687)**
  Sinusitis often follows an upper respiratory infection. In addition to a headache, signs and symptoms include nasal congestion, a runny nose, facial pain and pressure in the affected sinus. Head pain often increases when bending over or straining.
- **Subarachnoid hemorrhage (see "Hemorrhagic stroke," page 570)**
  Headache associated with this condition is often described as the "worst headache of my life." Severe pain comes on suddenly and lasts hours to days. It's often associated with nausea, vomiting and a stiff neck.

- **Temporomandibular joint disorder (see page 716)**
  This condition can cause facial pain, ear pain or a headache. Other symptoms may include clicking or catching of the jaw and soreness of the chewing muscles.
- **Tension-type headache (see page 556)**
  This is a common type of headache. The muscles of the back of the neck or scalp feel like they're tight and squeezing.
- **Tooth abscess (see page 701)**
  Throbbing around an abscessed tooth and gum may be mistaken for a headache.

Hip pain

Pain in the hip region is often related to one of the following conditions:

- **Bursitis or tendinitis (see pages 1008 and 992)**
  An aching pain is present in the outer hip region. Discomfort often worsens when you lie on the affected side or climb stairs. Sometimes, hip pain is referred, and the pain feels as if it's in the knee.
- **Claudication (see "Arteriosclerosis," page 785)**
  Pain develops in a hip or the buttocks or, more commonly, the thigh or calf muscles, when you walk. The pain goes away when you stop walking and stand still.
- **Hip fracture (see page 951)**
  The pain often occurs following trauma, such as a fall. Any movement of the hip produces severe pain.
- **Osteoarthritis (see page 997)**
  Aching or stiffness in the hip area may be felt in the groin. The pain worsens when you walk, climb stairs or stand for a prolonged period.

Knee pain

Knee pain can seriously impair walking and exercise. It's often related to one of the following conditions:

- **Cartilage tear (see "Knee injury," page 963)**
  The pain often develops after an injury in which the knee joint twists. The pain can be felt when pressing on the joint. It may be accompanied by swelling.
- **Gout (see page 1008)**
  The pain is sudden and severe and worsens when you move your knee. The knee is usually swollen and tender to the touch. Tests are necessary to differentiate gout from a knee infection.
- **Osteoarthritis (see page 997)**
  Slowly progressive discomfort occurs in the knee. The pain worsens when you walk, squat or stand for prolonged periods.
- **Patellar tendinitis (see "Runner's or jumper's knee," page 962)**
  The pain is accompanied by swelling and tenderness in the tendon below the kneecap.
- **Sprain (see "Knee injury," page 963)**
  A minor to severe tear of a knee ligament causes pain that may be associated with tenderness, swelling and loss of knee stability. A sprain is generally associated with trauma to the knee.

Lower gastrointestinal bleeding

Lower gastrointestinal bleeding, such as rectal bleeding, can be alarming. Frequently, the bleeding is due to a minor problem, such as hemorrhoids or an anal fissure. Other times, it may be a warning sign of a more serious condition, such as an ulcer or cancer. Lower gastrointestinal bleeding is often associated with one of the following conditions:

- **Anal fissure (see page 892)**
  The bleeding stems from a small tear in the anal tissue and may be accompanied by anal pain. The blood is typically bright red and is seen on toilet tissue or in the toilet bowl following a bowel movement.
- **Colon polyps (see page 886)**
  Small, precancerous growths in the colon may bleed occasionally. The blood may be bright red in the toilet or mixed in with stool.
- **Colorectal cancer (see page 887)**
  Blood, which may appear maroon-colored, may be mixed into the stool or show up in the toilet bowl. Other signs and symptoms include changes in bowel habits, cramping and weight loss.
- **Diverticular disease (see page 879)**
  Blood may be mixed in the stool or show up in the toilet bowl. The bleeding may be quite heavy.
- **Gastrointestinal infection (see page 866)**
  Some gastrointestinal infections cause cramping and bloody diarrhea.
- **Hemorrhoids (see page 890)**
  Hemorrhoids are the most frequent cause of rectal bleeding. Bright red blood usually shows up on toilet tissue or in the toilet bowl following a bowel movement. Bleeding may be accompanied by anal itching or discomfort.
- **Inflammatory bowel disease (see page 874)**
  Blood may be bright red or dark and mixed in with stool. Other signs and symptoms include a fever, cramps, diarrhea and weight loss.
- **Peptic ulcer (see page 860)**
  Bleeding from the upper gastrointestinal tract may cause stools to appear black or tarry. You may have gnawing pain in the upper abdomen between the navel and breastbone. The pain is worse when the stomach is empty. Eating may temporarily relieve the pain.

Nasal congestion

Nasal congestion is a common sign of a cold or an allergy, but it can also occur in other situations.

Nasal congestion is often associated with one of the following conditions:

- **Cold (see page 487)**
  A cold is a viral infection in the upper respiratory tract. In addition to nasal congestion, signs and symptoms include a runny nose, a sore or scratchy throat, fatigue, a cough and a low-grade fever.
- **Hay fever (see page 527)**
  Other signs and symptoms typically include sneezing and watery mucus from the nose. Itching of the nose, throat and eyes also is common.
- **Medication side effects (see "Medications Guide," page 1283)**
  Certain medications, such as the alpha-adrenergic blockers used to treat benign enlargement of the prostate gland, can cause mild nasal congestion as a side effect. Overuse of nonprescription nasal decongestant sprays also may result in a worsening of signs and symptoms, a condition referred to as a rebound effect.
- **Nasal polyps (see page 531)**
  Small growths in the nasal cavities can obstruct airways, leading to congestion. Polyps are most common in people with hay fever, aspirin-induced asthma and long-term (chronic) sinusitis.
- **Sinusitis (see page 687)**
  Inflammation of sinus membranes can cause nasal congestion. Sinusitis often follows an upper respiratory infection.
- **Vasomotor rhinitis (see page 686)**
  This condition mimics allergic rhinitis, with nasal congestion, sneezing and coughing due to phlegm in the throat. Other allergy symptoms — an itchy nose, eyes and throat — are absent. Triggers include cold air and strong smells.

Neck pain

Neck pain may be a short-term (acute) problem that improves on its own, or it may be long-term (chronic) and disabling. Neck pain is often associated with one of the following conditions:

- **Herniated disk (see page 977)**
  The pain begins in the neck and may radiate to a shoulder and down the arm. Other symptoms include numbness, tingling or weakness in the arm or hand.
- **Muscle strain (see page 972)**
  This is a common cause of sudden and sometimes severe neck pain. Moving your neck muscles produces pain.
- **Occipital neuralgia (see page 959)**
  Shooting pain in the back of the neck travels behind an ear to one side of the scalp. The discomfort can often be reproduced by firmly pressing on the bony bump in the back of the neck, where the occipital nerve is located.
- **Osteoarthritis (see page 997)**
  The pain is chronic and slowly progressive and may be accompanied by neck stiffness.

Numbness or tingling in a hand

Numbness or tingling in a hand is often associated with one of the following conditions:

- **Brachial plexus injury**
  Weakness, numbness and tingling develop in an arm and hand. This type of pain results from a shoulder or underarm injury that affects the network of nerves called the brachial plexus.
- **Carpal tunnel syndrome (see page 989)**
  Numbness and tingling may occur at night and radiate up an arm. The thumb, index finger and long finger are most often affected. Hand weakness also may occur.
- **Herniated disk (see page 977)**
  A compressed or damaged nerve in the neck can cause numbness and tingling that radiates down a shoulder into the arm, hand and fingers.
- **Peripheral neuropathy (see page 609)**
  Numbness and tingling or a crawling sensation are felt in both hands or both feet.
- **Stroke (see page 569)**
  Weakness or tingling occurs in an arm or hand and is usually accompanied by other symptoms, such as numbness and weakness in the face or a leg. Seek emergency medical care.
- **Ulnar nerve dysfunction (see page 991)**
  Trauma to the ulnar nerve at the elbow causes tingling and numbness from an elbow to the little finger and part of the ring finger. Bumping the area produces stinging pain. You may also have hand weakness.

Palpitations

Palpitations are an uncomfortable awareness of your heartbeat or a thumping sensation within your chest. They're often associated with one of the following conditions:

- **Anxiety and panic attacks (see "Anxiety disorders," page 1226)**
  Sudden episodes of intense fear prompt physical reactions, such as a racing heart, a flushed face, trouble breathing, dizziness, nausea and a sense of being out of control.
- **Atrial fibrillation (see page 766)**
  This condition is characterized by an irregular and often rapid heartbeat (arrhythmia).
- **Hyperthyroidism (see page 1039)**
  In addition to a rapid heartbeat, hyperthyroidism can cause weight loss, nervousness and tremor.
- **Premature contractions (see page 766)**
  Premature contractions (beats) are often described as

a skipped heart beat or a feeling that the heart turns over. They're usually harmless

- **Tachycardia (see pages 765 and 766)**
  Tachycardia is most often used to describe a racing, usually regular, heartbeat.

Shortness of breath

Shortness of breath is common after running hard, climbing a steep hill or exerting yourself in other ways. When you become short of breath without an obvious cause, you should seek medical attention. Shortness of breath is often associated with one of the following conditions:

- **Anxiety and panic attacks (see "Anxiety disorders," page 1226)**
  Sudden episodes of intense fear prompt physical reactions in your body such as trouble breathing, a racing heart, a flushed face, dizziness, nausea and a sense of being out of control.
- **Asthma (see page 532)**
  Breathing difficulty is often associated with a tight feeling in the chest, wheezing and coughing. It may be triggered by allergies, a respiratory infection, cold air or exercise.
- **Chronic obstructive pulmonary disease (see page 810)**
  In addition to shortness of breath, signs and symptoms of this condition include a barrel chest, minimal wheezing and, sometimes, pursing of the lips to help exhale.
- **Congestive heart failure (see page 761)**
  Shortness of breath may be worse when lying down. Other signs and symptoms include fatigue and swelling with accumulation of fluid (edema) in the feet, legs and trunk.
- **Pneumonia (see page 490)**
  Shortness of breath may be accompanied by a fever and sharp chest pain when you take a deep breath. Typically, pneumonia causes a cough that brings up colored sputum.
- **Pneumothorax (see page 817)**
  Abrupt chest pain and shortness of breath are the most common symptoms.
- **Pulmonary embolism (see page 826)**
  Along with sudden shortness of breath, you may cough up blood and have stabbing chest pain when you take a deep breath.

Shoulder pain

Pain that occurs when you move your shoulder is often due to a mechanical problem in the shoulder joint. Sometimes, illnesses in other parts of your body can cause shoulder pain (see "Referred shoulder pain," below). In such situations, moving the shoulder doesn't increase the pain. Shoulder pain is often associated with one of the following conditions:

- **Dislocation (see page 953)**
  The pain generally follows trauma to the shoulder. It improves with rest and worsens with movement. External rotation of the shoulder — such as when you swim the backstroke or cock your arm back to throw a football — can cause the head of the upper arm bone to slip out of the shoulder socket.
- **Frozen shoulder (see page 1009)**
  Symptoms include pain and tenderness with shoulder motion. Range of motion of the shoulder is severely limited.
- **Osteoarthritis (see page 997)**
  Osteoarthritis of the shoulder joint is relatively uncommon. Pain generally improves with rest and increases with activity. A grinding sensation or sound may occur with shoulder movement.
- **Rotator cuff injury (see page 1010)**
  This is the most common source of shoulder pain, especially in older adults. Pain occurs with shoulder movement, especially when reaching overhead, or with internal rotation of the shoulder. The pain may extend to the upper arm and be associated with weakness in the shoulder.

Referred Shoulder Pain

A number of conditions that occur in parts of the body other than the shoulder can cause pain that's felt in the shoulder. This is called referred shoulder pain. These conditions include:

- **Diaphragm irritation**
  The pain may be felt on the top of the shoulder and worsen with pushing on the abdomen or during a deep breath. The diaphragm is the thick, dome-shaped muscle that separates the chest and abdomen. When this muscle is irritated, such as with lower-lobe pneumonia, pain can result.
- **Gallbladder attack (see "Gallstones," page 896)**
  In addition to experiencing pain in the upper-right abdomen, you may feel it around the shoulder blade or top of the shoulder.
- **Heart attack (see page 757)**
  The pain may occur in the left shoulder, along with tight pressure in the chest, neck, jaw or arm.

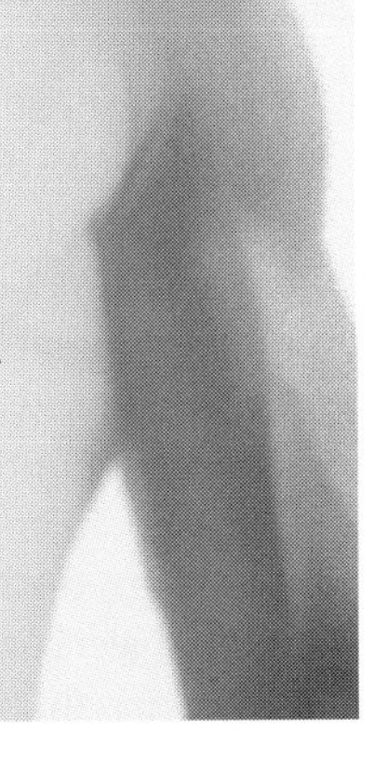

Sore throat

Everyone knows what a sore throat feels like. Often, it's not an indication of a serious problem, but sometimes a sore throat requires medical attention. A sore throat is commonly associated with one of the following conditions:

- **Cold (see page 487)**
  An upper respiratory infection, such as a cold, is the most common cause of a sore throat. Other signs include a cough, runny nose, scratchy throat and hoarse voice.
- **Epiglottitis (see page 691)**
  This condition generally causes a severe sore throat accompanied by a fever. You may drool or spit into a cup to avoid swallowing. See a doctor immediately.
- **Infectious mononucleosis (see page 494)**
  Signs and symptoms generally include a severe sore throat, fever, fatigue, headache and enlarged lymph glands in the front and back of the neck.
- **Strep throat (see page 491)**
  Other signs and symptoms include a fever, chills, fatigue and a headache. Lymph glands in the front of the neck may be painful.
- **Tonsillitis (see page 691)**
  Other signs and symptoms are a fever, chills, fatigue and painful glands in the neck. On examination, tonsils appear red and inflamed and may have a white covering.

Swallowing difficulties

Occasional difficulty in swallowing (dysphagia) isn't usually a serious problem and may simply stem from eating too fast or not chewing your food well enough. Difficulty swallowing may be associated with one of the following conditions:

- **Achalasia (see page 855)**
  The lower esophageal muscle (sphincter) doesn't relax properly to let food enter the stomach. This can cause regurgitation of retained "sweet tasting" food not mixed with stomach contents.
- **Aging (see "Swallowing difficulties," page 854)**
  With age the esophagus tends to lose some of the muscular coordination needed to push food to the stomach.
- **Esophageal stricture (see page 856)**
  Narrowing of the esophagus (stricture) causes large chunks of food to get hung up. Narrowing may result from formation of scar tissue or tumors.
- **Esophageal tumors (see page 858)**
  Difficulty swallowing gets progressively worse over several months. Other signs and symptoms include chest pain and weight loss.
- **Foreign body (see page 857)**
  An object becomes lodged in the esophagus, which causes pain and swallowing difficulty.
- **Gastroesophageal reflux disease (see page 850)**
  Damage to esophageal tissues from stomach acid backing up (refluxing) into the esophagus can lead to scarring and narrowing of the lower esophagus, making swallowing difficult.
- **Neuromuscular problems (see "Pharyngeal paralysis," page 856)**
  You may be unable to initiate swallowing despite repeated attempts. Food or fluid may enter the windpipe (trachea) or come out the nose.
- **Pharyngeal diverticulum (see page 855)**
  A small pouch forms in the throat. Food particles collect in this pouch, causing swallowing difficulty, gurgling sounds, bad breath and repeated throat clearing or coughing.

Swelling of the feet and legs

Swelling (edema) of the feet and legs is common after long periods of sitting, such as when you're on a long airplane flight. When the swelling occurs without an obvious cause, it may be a sign of a more serious problem. Swelling of the feet and legs is often associated with one of the following conditions:

- **Cellulitis (see page 1190)**
  This form of skin infection commonly causes redness, swelling, warmth and tenderness. It may be accompanied by a fever.
- **Congestive heart failure (see page 761)**
  Swelling occurs in both legs. It may be accompanied by abdominal swelling and shortness of breath with exertion and when lying down.
- **Deep vein thrombosis (see "Thrombophlebitis," page 789)**
  This condition typically causes sudden swelling of the lower leg accompanied by pain and tenderness behind the knee and calf. The leg may also appear dusky in color.
- **Lymphedema (see page 790)**
  Swelling occurs in one or both lower extremities and may extend to the toes and top of the feet.
- **Superficial thrombophlebitis (see page 789)**
  Pain, swelling, redness and tenderness occur near the surface of the skin in a leg vein — typically in a varicose vein.
- **Venous insufficiency (see "Varicose veins," page 790)**
  Swelling is typically worse when standing for a long time and better in the morning. You may also notice heaviness or aching in your lower legs, thickened, hardened skin and brownish skin pigmentation on an ankle.

Upper gastrointestinal bleeding

Upper gastrointestinal bleeding can manifest itself in several ways. Blood may be present in vomit and be either bright red or look like coffee grounds (digested blood). Upper gastrointestinal bleeding may also cause passage of black, tarry stools due to blood passing slowly from the stomach to the colon. If the bleeding is massive, stools may be maroon in color. Upper gastrointestinal bleeding is often caused by one of the following conditions:

- **Esophageal trauma (see page 859)**
  Bleeding may occur from a tear in the esophagus, often caused by trauma to the esophagus.
- **Esophageal tumor (see page 858)**
  Bleeding is accompanied by progressive difficulty in swallowing. You may experience chest pain and weight loss.
- **Esophagitis (see page 854)**
  An inflamed lining of the esophagus may bleed.
- **Gastritis (see page 864)**
  An inflamed lining of the stomach may bleed.
- **Peptic ulcer (see page 860)**
  Bright red blood may appear in vomit, or blood may appear in stool, causing it to be black and tarry. Gnawing pain in the upper abdomen between the navel and breastbone is common. The pain is generally worse with an empty stomach.

Urinary difficulties

Signs and symptoms associated with urinary difficulties vary from frequent, painless urination to the severe pain that accompanies passage of a kidney stone. Urinary difficulties are often associated with one of the following conditions:

- **Benign prostatic hyperplasia (see page 1123)**
  This condition affects men and is characterized by progressive slowing of the urinary stream, stopping and starting of the stream, an urgency to void and frequent urination during the night.
- **Kidney stones (see page 928)**
  Passage of a kidney stone or the lodging of a stone in the lower urinary tract may cause a constant feeling of the need to urinate. Kidney stone pain is felt in the lower abdomen. In men it may radiate to the tip of the penis or to the testicles. In women it may spread to the vaginal area.
- **Medication side effects (see "Medications Guide," page 1283)**
  Some medications interfere with the ability to urinate. For example, in some men with benign prostatic hyperplasia, pseudoephedrine, a drug found in some cold medications, can accentuate slowed urination or even cause an inability to void.
- **Overactive bladder (see page 945)**
  The bladder muscle becomes hyperactive, causing bladder spasm. You have an urgent, frequent need to urinate, even with an empty or near-empty bladder.
- **Prostatitis (see page 1122)**
  Urination is painful and may be accompanied by a fever and pain in the pubic area and pelvic floor muscles.
- **Urinary tract infection (see page 940)**
  This condition causes an urgent and frequent sensation that you need to urinate and a painful, burning sensation on urination. The urine may be cloudy or blood tinged.

Vomiting

Vomiting may stem from a gastrointestinal infection (gastroenteritis) or a more serious problem. It may be associated with one of the following conditions:

- **Appendicitis (see page 873)**
  Vomiting is generally accompanied by a loss of appetite, nausea and a low-grade fever. Pain begins around the navel and settles into the lower-right abdomen.
- **Gallbladder attack (see "Gallstones," page 896)**
  Pain often begins 1 or 2 hours after a meal and may be associated with nausea and vomiting. The pain is often directly below the breastbone and may radiate to the back or to the right shoulder.
- **Gastrointestinal infection (see page 866)**
  A viral infection of the gastrointestinal tract is a common cause of vomiting, which may be accompanied by diarrhea. Such infections usually improve in 1 to 3 days.
- **Intestinal obstruction (see page 884)**
  Nausea and vomiting are accompanied by cramping, colicky abdominal pain that comes and goes. Other signs and symptoms include visible bloating, bowel noise (rushes and gurgling) and, if obstruction is complete or near complete, passage of little or no gas or stool.
- **Medication side effects (see "Medications Guide," page 1283)**
  In some people, medications such as antibiotics, codeine and morphine can cause nausea and vomiting.

Wheezing

Wheezing is a musical-like sound heard when you breathe out (expire) through an obstructed airway. It's often associated with one of the following conditions:

- **Asthma (see page 532)**
  Wheezing may be accompanied by breathing difficulty, a tight feeling in the chest and coughing. It may be triggered by allergies, respiratory infection, cold air or exercise.
- **Bronchitis (see page 797)**
  Wheezing is generally accompanied by a cough that produces sputum.
- **Congestive heart failure (see page 761)**
  Fluid accumulation in the lungs resulting from heart failure can cause wheezing (cardiac asthma).

Signs and Symptoms Common in Children

Following are 15 signs and symptoms common to children and some of the most frequent reasons that children and adolescents see their doctors. Teenagers may also experience signs and symptoms that result from conditions similar to those that affect adults.

Abdominal pain

Occasional episodes of abdominal pain may be related to anxiety or a bacterial or viral infection (gastroenteritis). Abdominal pain that's recurrent, persistent or severe may signal a variety of other conditions. Abdominal pain is often associated with one of the following causes:

- **Antibiotic reaction (see "Antibiotic-associated diarrhea," page 870)**
  Some antibiotics cause abdominal pain. All antibiotics are capable of causing loose stools or diarrhea.
- **Anxiety (see "Fears and phobias," page 199, and "Anxiety disorders," page 1226)**
  Many children experience anxiety — often when they experience a new situation or encounter a frightening situation. Anxiety can lead to various physical symptoms, one of them being abdominal pain.
- **Appendicitis (see page 873)**
  Infection or obstruction of the appendix typically causes pain starting around the bellybutton (umbilicus) and settling in the lower-right abdomen.
- **Attention-seeking behavior**
  For whatever reason, a child may feel a need for more attention and may find that saying, "My stomach hurts," produces a quick response from parents.
- **Constipation (see pages 170 and 213)**
  Trouble passing stool can cause diffuse abdominal pain before a bowel movement and painful struggling during the bowel movement. This is one of the most frequent causes of abdominal pain in children.
- **Gas**
  Gas that's retained within the intestinal system is another common cause of abdominal pain in children from infancy through the elementary school years.
- **Gastroenteritis (see "Gastrointestinal infections," page 866)**
  Children often experience infection of the stomach or intestines due to a virus or, less commonly, a bacterium or parasite. In addition to abdominal pain, common signs and symptoms include nausea, vomiting and diarrhea. These typically improve in a day or two. See a doctor if they persist.
- **Malabsorption disorder (see page 871)**
  An intestinal sensitivity to a dietary protein, such as the gluten found in wheat and other grains, may result in abdominal pain, bloating, gas and diarrhea. A common malabsorption disorder is lactose intolerance, which is caused by an inability to digest the sugar in milk (lactose).
- **School phobia (see page 200)**
  A child who fears school or wants to avoid it may have poorly described abdominal pain that isn't associated with any other sign or symptom of illness and magically disappears if the child is allowed to stay home from school.

Constipation

Constipation in children is common and only rarely due to a serious problem. It may be related to one of the following conditions:

- **Congenital malformations (see "Congenital digestive and respiratory disorders," page 179)**
  Some babies are born with incomplete formation of part of the small intestine, which can cause intestinal obstruction. Constipation is one of the primary signs.
- **Functional stool holding**
  In some toilet-trained children, constipation may be a sign of a larger behavioral problem. The child may be reluctant to have bowel movements or to soil his or her underwear.
- **Hypothyroidism (see pages 156 and 1041)**
  Infrequently, constipation is associated with an underactive thyroid gland.
- **Intussusception (see page 873)**
  Intussusception is a telescoping of a segment of the intestines into itself that obstructs normal bowel flow. This generally causes sudden, severe abdominal pain, which may be accompanied by constipation.
- **Lack of dietary fiber and inadequate water consumption (see "Nutrition," page 205)**
  The most common causes of childhood constipation are inadequate water intake and lack of fiber in the diet. Eating too many fatty animal-based foods is another cause.

Other Important Concerns

Many times, parents make an appointment with their child's doctor not because their child is sick but because they're concerned about the child's behavior or eating or sleeping habits. Sometimes, the problem is a normal part of growth and development, and it improves on its own. Other times, it's more serious and requires treatment.

Because behavioral, eating and sleeping problems occur for various reasons and their characteristics vary considerably, it's difficult to include them in this brief overview of common childhood signs and symptoms. For more information on these conditions and how they affect children at different stages of life, see Chapters 12-14.

Cough

Cough is common and is often due to one of the following conditions:

- **Asthma (see page 532)**
  Asthma may cause coughing alone or coughing with other signs, such as wheezing.
- **Cold (see page 487)**
  The common cold often causes nasal mucus to drip into the throat, which can cause a cough.
- **Croup (see page 491)**
  Viral inflammation of the voice box (larynx) and windpipe (trachea) can cause a barky, harsh upper airway cough that's often accompanied by a high-pitched sound on inspiration (stridor).
- **Foreign body (see page 392)**
  Toddlers from 9 months to 3 years are at high risk of placing objects into their mouth, which then enter their airway, producing a cough and breathing difficulty. This requires immediate medical care.
- **Habitual cough**
  School-age or teenage children may cough out of habit. During sleep the cough isn't present. A habitual cough is diagnosed by excluding other possible causes.
- **Nasal allergies (see "Hay fever," page 527)**
  In addition to a cough, nasal allergies commonly cause nasal congestion and a runny nose. Nasal allergies are most common during warm weather during pollen season.
- **Pneumonia (see page 490)**
  Pneumonia typically causes a cough that brings up colored sputum. The cough is usually accompanied by a fever.
- **Secondhand smoke (see page 81)**
  When a child's airway is irritated from breathing in tobacco smoke, cough is common, especially if the child has asthma.
- **Sinusitis (see page 687)**
  Older children can get bacterial infections of the sinuses, although not as often as do adults. Cough that's accompanied by full or painful sinuses may be associated with sinusitis.

Decreased hearing

Decreased hearing may simply be due to a child's inattention, or it may be associated with one of the following conditions:

- **Fluid in the middle ear (see "Middle ear infections," page 668, and "Chronic ear infections," page 670)**
  The most common reason for poor hearing is a temporary collection of fluid behind the eardrum within the middle ear, leading to diminished hearing in that ear. Fluid buildup can lead to infection in the middle ear (otitis media).
- **Nerve damage or dysfunction (see "Hearing problems," pages 219 and 233)**
  Infectious diseases or a congenital deformity of the nerve that carries sound signals may cause hearing loss. Decreased hearing can also result from damage due to loud noise.
- **Selective hearing**
  This is a normal condition that occurs at several ages and stages of life. When a child is intently focused on something or isn't interested in the topic being discussed, he or she may tune out, creating the impression of hearing loss.

Diarrhea

Diarrhea is common in childhood and is often due to one of the following conditions:

- **Antibiotic reaction (see "Antibiotic-associated diarrhea," page 870)**
  Antibiotics can kill bacteria that normally live in the digestive tract, replacing them with diarrhea-causing bacteria. Up to 20 percent of people taking antibiotics experience this problem. Usually, the diarrhea is mild and of short duration. Occasionally, a serious colon infection can result, causing severe diarrhea.
- **Cystic fibrosis (see page 814)**
  Inadequate absorption of food due to this disease can result in fatty, malodorous, loose stools.
- **Eating disorders (see page 242)**
  Eating disorders are most common in teenagers. Anorexia nervosa and bulimia are associated with self-induced vomiting and use of laxatives as a means of losing weight. Laxatives cause diarrhea.
- **Gastroenteritis (see "Gastrointestinal infections," page 866, and "Diarrhea," page 212)**
  Children often experience intestinal infections due to a virus or, less commonly, a bacterium or parasite. The diarrhea usually stops in a day or two. Diarrhea associated with a fever and blood in the stool should receive prompt medical attention.
- **Inflammatory bowel disease (see page 874)**
  Teenagers are more likely than are younger children to develop inflammatory bowel disease. This chronic condition is often associated with bloody diarrhea, weight loss, abdominal cramping and other symptoms.
- **Intestinal obstruction (see page 884 and "Congenital digestive and respiratory disorders," page 179)**
  Blockages due to twisting or telescoping of the intestines can produce vomiting, diarrhea or constipation, as well as abdominal pain.
- **Malabsorption disorder (see page 871)**
  Chronic diarrhea can stem from an inability to digest milk sugar (lactose) or from an intestinal sensitivity to a dietary protein, such as the gluten found in wheat and other grains. Other signs and symptoms include

abdominal pain and bloating. Some children and teenagers can't tolerate sorbitol, a sugar substitute found in many diet foods.

Earache

Earache is very common in childhood and often occurs with head colds. Other causes of earache include the following conditions:

- **Ear infection (see pages 173 and 214)**
  Middle ear infection (otitis media) is common in children ages 4 months to 4 years. In addition to ear pain, common signs and symptoms include trouble sleeping, irritability and a fever. Older children will complain of ear pain and plugging of the ear.
- **Ear trauma (see "Ruptured eardrum," page 666)**
  Trauma to the ear that causes severe pain with bloody discharge from the ear canal requires immediate attention.
- **Swimmer's ear (see "Outer ear infections," page 664)**
  This condition is due to infection in the outer ear canal. Moving the ear or pressing on the entrance to the ear canal is painful. The condition is most common among children who spend considerable time swimming.

Eye discomfort and redness

Red- or pink-colored eyes are often associated with an eye infection, but they can also result from other causes:

- **Allergies (see "Respiratory allergies," page 527)**
  Airborne allergens, such as pollen, dust and smog, can produce itchy, pink-colored eyes.
- **Marijuana use (see page 93)**
  Chronically red eyes may be associated with marijuana smoking.
- **Pinkeye (see "Conjunctivitis," page 642)**
  The white of the eye (sclera) has a pinkish discoloration. Other symptoms include itchiness and a gritty feeling with blinking. The eyelids may stick together at night.
- **Secondhand smoke (see page 81)**
  Secondhand tobacco smoke can irritate a child's eyes as well as cause respiratory problems.

Headache

It's not uncommon for a child to experience a mild headache, especially during the adolescent and teenage years. However, head pain that's persistent or severe requires prompt attention. Head pain may be associated with one of the following conditions:

- **Attention-seeking behavior**
  If a parent has headaches, a younger child may complain of his or her own head aching as a way to get attention or support.
- **Headaches (see pages 217 and 233)**
  School-age and teenage children can experience tension-type headaches or migraines, although not as commonly as adults. A headache may be associated with an infection or other causes, such as stress or reaction to a medication.
- **Increased intracranial pressure (see "Structural disorders," page 582, "Subdural hematoma," page 572, and "Epidural hemorrhage," page 575)**
  Injury or certain conditions may lead to increased pressure on the brain and cause head pain, vomiting and other signs and symptoms.
- **Neck injury (see "Neck pain," page 959)**
  What presents as a pain in the head may actually originate from the neck.
- **School phobia (see pages 200 and 239)**
  A child who is fearful of or trying to avoid school may complain of poorly described head pain that magically disappears if he or she is allowed to stay home from school. The pain isn't associated with any other evidence of illness.
- **Sinusitis (see page 687)**
  Sinus congestion or a sinus infection can cause head pain that's typically accompanied by pain in the sinus cavities or facial pain or pressure when bending down.

Muscle and joint pain

Pain in a child's muscles and joints is often related to a child's active lifestyle or to one of the following causes:

- **Growing pains (see page 217)**
  Whether growth of long bones in the legs and arms actually produces pain isn't certain. During the years when children grow at a rapid pace, the most common reason for a child to complain of muscle or joint pain is simply that he or she is physically active, providing a challenging workout of his or her muscles and skeleton. This is sometimes called overuse syndrome.

Fever

Every child experiences a fever at some point. A fever may be associated with infection of any body organ. Low-grade fevers commonly occur with an upper respiratory infection, such as the common cold, and aren't to be feared.

A high fever — 103 F or higher — may suggest a more serious infection, especially if it persists. Seek prompt medical attention.

When a fever is long term (chronic) or recurrent without evidence of an infection, a doctor may look for other conditions that can cause a fever. These include rheumatic disorders, some vascular diseases and cancer.

- **Rheumatic disorders (see "Juvenile rheumatoid arthritis," page 1004)**
  Childhood rheumatoid arthritis and related disorders can produce painful, stiff, inflamed joints on a chronic or recurrent basis.
- **Sprain (see page 957)**
  Pain occurs when a joint moves beyond its normal range of motion, stretching or tearing ligaments. It's often accompanied by swelling.
- **Tendinitis (see page 992)**
  Repetitive motions such as those done while participating in athletics or playing a musical instrument can irritate and inflame one or more tendons. In addition to being painful, the joint may be stiff and tender to the touch.

Nasal congestion

A stuffy nose is a common part of childhood. Nasal congestion may stem from a variety of conditions:

- **Cold (see page 487)**
  Common signs and symptoms of a cold are nasal congestion, drainage of clear, gray mucus and a mild fever. Other signs and symptoms include irritability, lack of appetite and poor sleep.
- **Large adenoids (see "Adenoid and tonsil removal," page 691)**
  Snoring is the most common symptom of enlarged adenoids. In addition to a stuffy nose, swollen adenoids may give the voice a nasal quality.
- **Sinusitis (see page 687)**
  Prolonged nasal congestion with greenish or yellowish nasal discharge, facial pain, headache, bad breath, cough and a low-grade fever are common signs and symptoms of sinusitis.

Sore throat

An occasional sore throat is a normal part of growing up. But not all sore throats are trivial. A sore throat in children may be associated with one of the following conditions:

- **Cold (see page 487)**
  An upper respiratory infection, such as a cold, is the most common cause of sore throats. Other signs and symptoms may include a cough, runny nose, scratchy throat and hoarse voice.
- **Strep throat (see page 491)**
  Strep throat is the most common bacterial throat infection, generally occurring in children ages 5 to 15. In addition to a sore throat, signs and symptoms may include a fever, headache, abdominal pain and swollen lymph glands in the front of the neck.
- **Throat infection (see "Sore throat," page 690)**
  A bacterium or a virus can produce a painful throat infection. Even if a child's tonsils have been removed, the throat can become infected and produce signs and symptoms similar to those of tonsillitis.
- **Tonsillitis (see page 691)**
  Tonsillitis is an infection of the tonsils. Other common signs and symptoms are trouble swallowing, abdominal pain and a fever.

Urinary problems

Urinary problems may be associated with disorders and diseases that range from minor to serious. Urinary problems in children often are related to one of the following conditions:

- **Diabetes (see page 1018)**
  A child's first signs and symptoms of diabetes generally include increased thirst and frequent voiding of large volumes of urine.
- **Incontinence after toilet training (see "Bed-wetting," page 211)**
  If a toilet-trained child begins to wet the bed, either the passage of time or medical interventions may resolve the problem. Involuntary loss of urine during the day should be investigated by a doctor.
- **Urinary tract infection (see pages 218 and 234)**
  Frequent or painful urination may be associated with a urinary tract infection. Other signs and symptoms may include discolored urine, abdominal pain, a fever and chills.
- **Urine color change (see "Injury and inflammation," page 935, and "Urinary tract infections," page 940)**
  Certain kidney disorders, such as infection, inflammation and injury, may produce cloudy or dark urine. Swelling of the face and legs also may result.

Vision problems

Diagnosing vision problems in very young children can be difficult. As children get older, some of the following conditions may become more apparent:

- **Blurred vision (see "Common vision problems," page 622)**
  School-age children may develop visual disorders requiring corrective lenses. Typically, the child complains of trouble seeing and may squint to see better.
- **Color deficiency (see "Colorblindness," page 639)**
  This inherited condition usually occurs in males. People with this condition generally have trouble recognizing the colors red or green or both.
- **Double vision**
  Double vision can occur for a variety of reasons, some of them serious. See a doctor immediately.
- **Misaligned eyes (see page 640)**
  The eyes don't move in parallel motion. Instead, one eye turns inward or outward, either constantly or intermittently.

Vomiting

Vomiting in infants and young children is most often related to eating too much or to a mild intestinal infection. It may occur for the following reasons:

- **Congenital malformation (see "Congenital digestive and respiratory disorders," page 179)**
  Incomplete or incorrect formation of the small intestine can occur at the upper or lower ends of the intestinal tract, resulting in vomiting or constipation.
- **Eating disorders (see page 242)**
  Eating disorders are most common in teenagers. Anorexia nervosa and bulimia are associated with self-induced vomiting as a means of losing weight.
- **Excess consumption (see "Spitting up and vomiting," page 169)**
  Some infants eat more than their stomach can hold and spit up the excess.
- **Gastroenteritis (see "Gastrointestinal infections," page 866)**
  Children often experience infection of the stomach or small intestine due to a virus or, less commonly, a bacterium or parasite. Signs and symptoms commonly include nausea, vomiting, abdominal pain and diarrhea. They typically improve in a day or two. See a doctor if they don't.

Wheezing

Labored breathing with high-pitched sounds — usually during expiration — may represent asthma. But as an old saying goes, "All that wheezes is not asthma." A variety of airway or pulmonary problems may produce wheezing:

- **Asthma (see page 532)**
  Wheezing associated with asthma is often accompanied by breathing difficulty, a tight feeling in the chest and coughing. It may be triggered by an allergy, respiratory infection, cold air or exercise.
- **Bronchiolitis (see page 797)**
  The smallest airways in the lung can become infected with a virus, which may produce wheezing, cough and rapid breathing. This condition is different from bronchitis, which in children usually causes croup.
- **Hyperventilation (see page 353)**
  When some children become excited, anxious or fearful, they breathe too fast and produce a sound similar to wheezing.
- **Respiratory syncytial virus (see page 799)**
  This respiratory infection, commonly known as RSV, occurs mostly in children under age 4. In addition to wheezing, it causes a congested or runny nose, a cough and a low-grade fever. ■

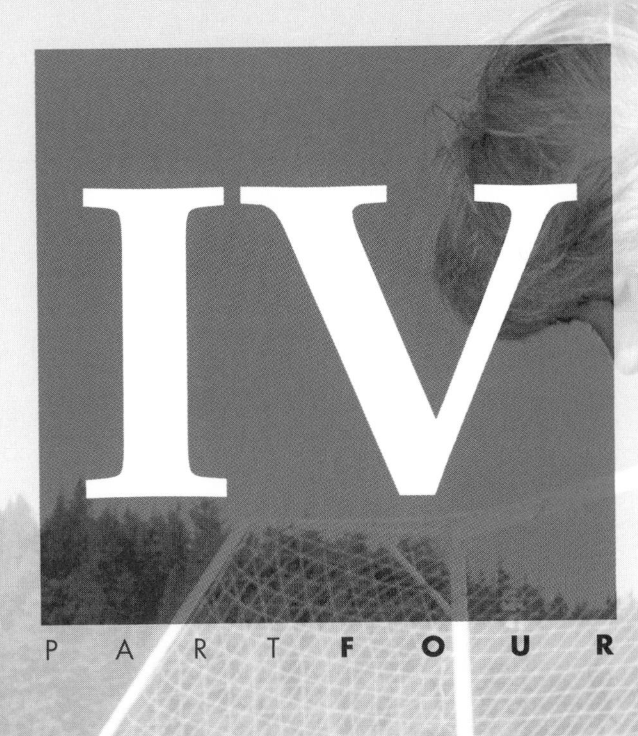

PART FOUR

First Aid and Emergency Care

First Aid and Emergency Care

Emergencies don't happen often, but when they do, you don't have much time to seek out first aid information. In order to react effectively, it's important to know what action to take when a person appears injured, seriously ill or in distress. Your skills could someday mean the difference between life and death for another human being.

This section provides valuable information on how to react in various emergency situations. You might, however, also consider taking a certified first aid course to learn lifesaving skills, such as the Heimlich maneuver, cardiopulmonary resuscitation (CPR) and how to respond to a heart attack or traumatic injury. To find out more about first aid courses offered in your community, check with a local hospital, Red Cross office, county emergency services office or American Heart Association chapter.

Emergency Warning Signs

If you're experiencing any of the following signs or symptoms, call for emergency medical help — 911 is the emergency phone number in most regions — or go immediately to the emergency department at the nearest hospital:

- Sudden or severe pain
- Pain or pressure in the upper abdominal area, which can signal a heart attack
- Difficulty breathing or shortness of breath
- Sudden dizziness, a sudden severe headache or a change in vision
- Sudden weakness or partial paralysis
- Severe or persistent vomiting or diarrhea
- Significant bleeding
- Suicidal or homicidal feelings

Choking and the Heimlich Maneuver

Choking is caused by a blockage of the respiratory passage in the throat (larynx) or windpipe (trachea). The flow of air to the lungs is blocked. This in turn cuts off the circulation of oxygen-rich blood to the brain and other organs. If the problem isn't corrected promptly, it can be fatal.

Choking is often due to a large piece of inadequately chewed food that becomes lodged in the throat or windpipe. Solid foods such as meat are usually the cause. Often, people who are choking had been talking while chewing a large piece of meat. False teeth also can increase the risk of choking because they interfere with how food feels in the mouth, making it harder to tell if the food is fully chewed. In addition, people with false

The Universal Choking Sign

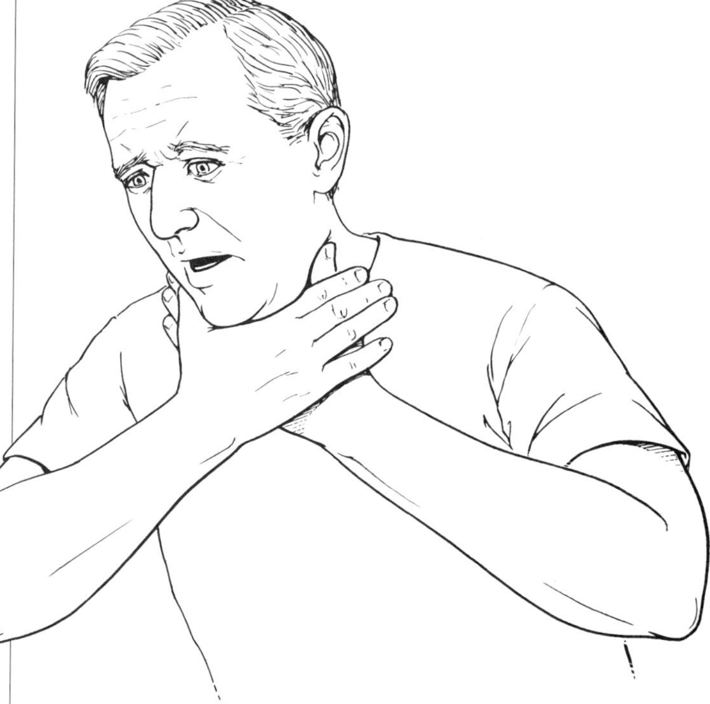

A person who's choking is unable to communicate except by hand motions. Often, the hand and arm motions are uncoordinated. It's important that both the person who is choking and the rescuer know the universal signal for choking: hands clutched to the throat, with thumbs and fingers extended.

The Heimlich Maneuver

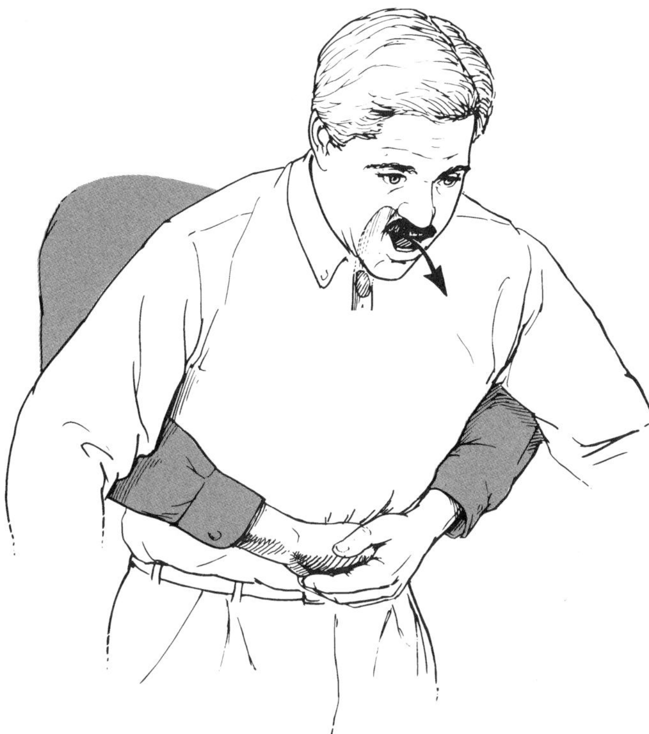

The Heimlich maneuver should be performed if there is complete or near-complete blockage of the airway.

The Finger Sweep

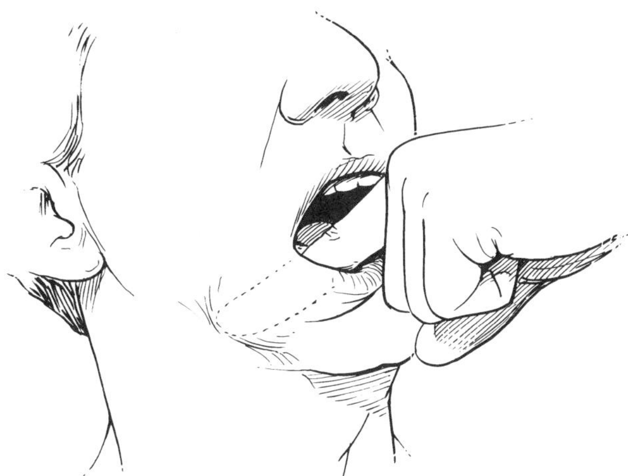

The simplest method for clearing an obstructed airway is to reach a finger into the back of the throat and sweep out the cause of the blockage, if it can be reached.

teeth can't chew food as thoroughly as they could with natural teeth because false teeth exert less pressure.

Other common causes of choking include:

- Drinking alcohol before or during a meal. Alcohol is a sedative — it dulls the nerves that help you sense how well your food has been chewed and that help you swallow.
- Eating too fast.
- Eating while laughing or talking hurriedly.
- Eating while walking, running or playing.

Panic is often one of the choking victim's first responses. The victim's face often assumes an expression of terror and then takes on a bluish or ashen color as he or she stops breathing. The person may wheeze or gasp.

Coughing vs. choking

If a morsel of food "goes down the wrong pipe," the coughing reflex will often quickly solve the problem. In fact, a person isn't choking if he or she is able to cough freely and has normal skin color. But if the cough is more like a gasp, he or she is probably choking and needs immediate help.

Ask the choking person to say something. If the person can talk, then the airway is not completely blocked, and oxygen is reaching the lungs.

Clearing an obstructed airway

You've seen it displayed on posters and performed on television, but do you know how to perform the Heimlich maneuver on someone who's choking?

The Heimlich maneuver is perhaps the best known technique for clearing an obstructed airway. It should be performed on someone only if there is complete or near-complete blockage of the airway. Indications of this would be that, in a choking situation, the person is unable to speak, has passed out or is making squeaky or gurgling sounds with great effort. The person's face may turn blue, gray or ashen.

To perform the Heimlich maneuver:

1. Stand behind the choking person and wrap your arms around his or her waist. Tip him or her forward slightly.
2. Make a fist with one hand and position it slightly above the person's navel.
3. Grasp the fist with the other hand and press hard into the abdomen with a quick, upward thrust — as if you were trying to lift the person off the ground. This action raises the diaphragm, putting pressure on the lungs and forcing air out of the lungs.
4. Repeat the Heimlich maneuver until the food or other blockage is dislodged.

Other techniques to clear a blocked airway may work in certain situations. But first determine that the individual is unable to breathe.

Clearing the airway using a finger sweep

The simplest method for clearing an obstructed airway is to reach a finger into the back of the throat and sweep out the cause of the blockage. Often, the blockage is too far down the throat to be seen. But if you can see it, sweep a finger into the back of the person's throat to clear the airway.

This method works only if the blockage is at the back of the throat or high in the throat. It should be attempted only if the blockage is visible. Be careful not to push the food or object deeper into the airway, which can happen easily in young children.

Clearing your own airway

If you begin to choke and no one is available to help you, use the following variation of the Heimlich maneuver on yourself:

1. Place a fist slightly above your navel.
2. Grasp your fist with the other hand and bend over a hard surface — a countertop or chair will do.
3. Shove your fist inward and upward.

Clearing the airway of a pregnant woman or an obese person

The abdomen of a pregnant woman or the large stomach of an obese person can prevent the effective use of the Heimlich maneuver abdominal thrust. Position your hands at the base of the breastbone, just above the joining of the lowest ribs. Proceed as with the Heimlich maneuver, pressing hard into the chest with a quick thrust. Repeat until the food or other blockage is dislodged or the person becomes unconscious.

Clearing the airway of an unconscious person

If the individual has collapsed, position the person on his or her back, look inside the mouth and do a finger sweep. To clear the airway of an unconscious person lying on his or her back, kneel over the individual and apply upward thrusts to the upper abdomen. When a person falls unconscious, relaxing muscles may loosen the object from the throat. If not, begin cardiopulmonary resuscitation (CPR). Chest compressions used in CPR also may dislodge the object. Each time you open the person's mouth to breathe into it, look first for any obstruction in the back of the throat. If you see an object, remove it.

Clearing the airway of a choking infant

If an infant is choking, assume a seated position and hold the infant facedown on your forearm, which is resting on your thigh. Thump the infant gently but firmly five times on the middle of the back using the heel of your hand. The combination of gravity and the back blows should release the object blocking the airway.

If the back blows are unsuccessful, hold the infant faceup on your forearm with the head lower than the trunk. Using two fingers placed at the center of the

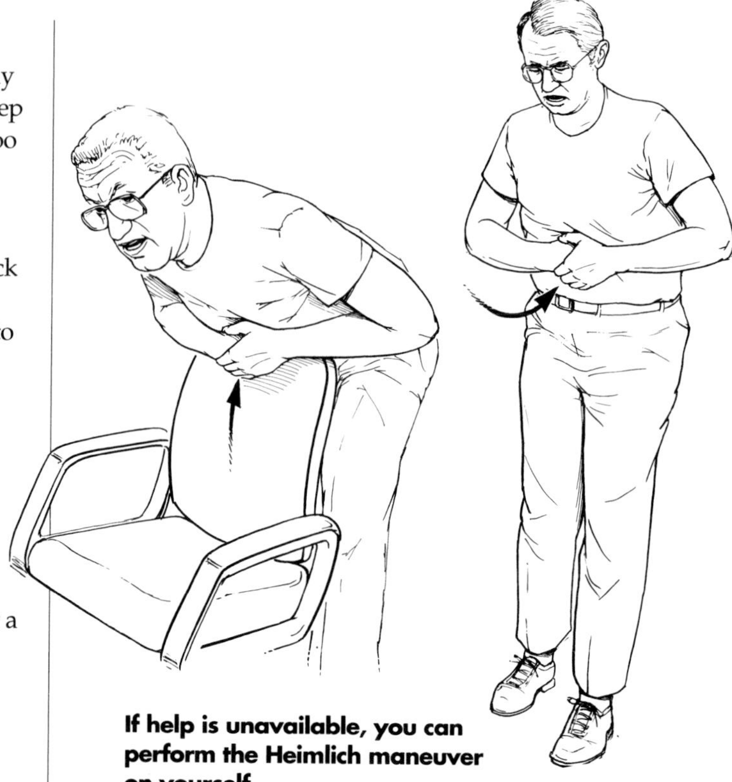

If help is unavailable, you can perform the Heimlich maneuver on yourself.

To clear the airway of an unconscious person lying on his or her back, kneel over the individual and apply upward thrusts to the abdomen.

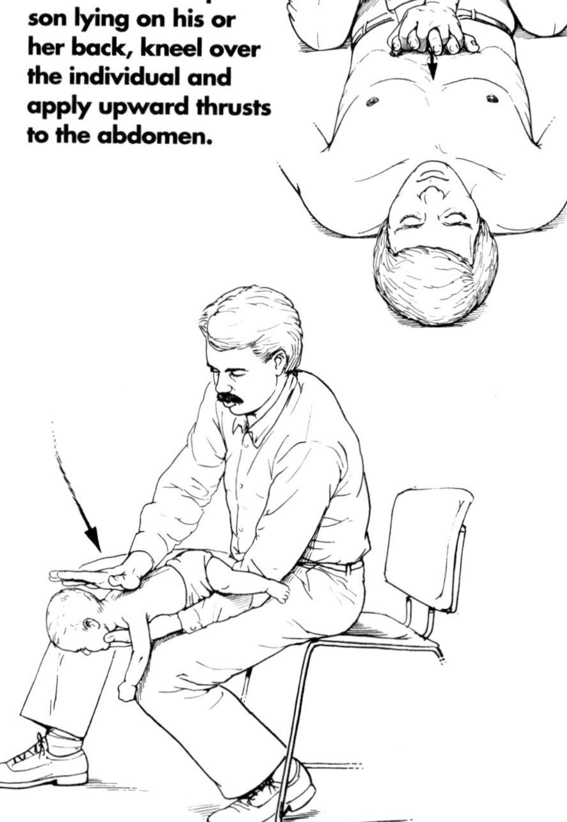

A gentle slap on the back can help clear the airway of a choking infant.

infant's breastbone, give five quick chest compressions. If breathing doesn't resume, repeat the back blows and chest thrusts. Call for emergency medical help.

If one of these techniques opens the airway, but the infant doesn't resume breathing, perform mouth-to-mouth resuscitation.

Cardiopulmonary Resuscitation

Cardiopulmonary resuscitation (CPR) is a lifesaving technique that's useful in a wide range of emergencies, such as a heart attack or near drowning, in which the person is unconscious and has stopped breathing.

Before you proceed with resuscitation, make sure that the person is actually unconscious and has stopped breathing. You can do harm by performing CPR on somebody who doesn't need it.

When the heart stops, the absence of oxygenated blood can cause irreparable brain damage in only a few minutes, and death can occur within 8 to 10 minutes. Time is critical when you're helping an unconscious person who isn't breathing.

If you're alone, the first priority is to call for emergency medical help. Generally, the number to call is 911. Then begin CPR. If you're not alone, have someone else call for help while you determine if the unconscious person is breathing. If he or she isn't, begin CPR.

Cardiopulmonary Resuscitation (CPR)

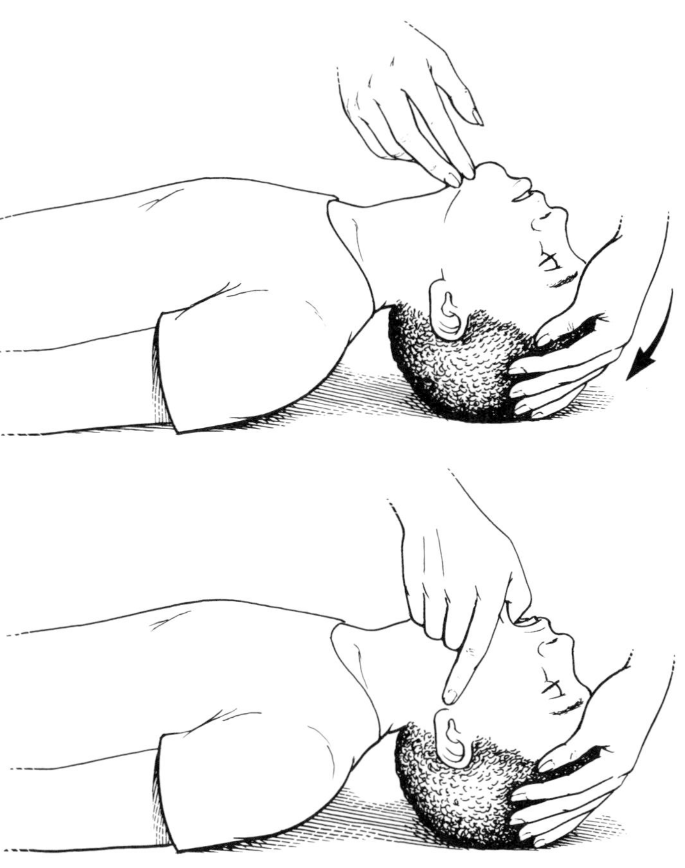

To perform CPR, first tilt the head and lift the chin to open the airway.

Performing CPR on an adult

The American Heart Association, which sets standards for cardiopulmonary resuscitation, distinguishes the three parts of the process with the letters *ABC*: *A* is for airway, *B* is for breathing, and *C* is for circulation. The three steps are described in order below:

A: Clear the airway

You can clear the victim's airway in several ways. But the first step is assessment.

1. Make sure that the unconscious person isn't simply resting or sleeping. Firmly shake or tap the person's shoulder and ask, "Are you OK?"
2. If you get no response, seek emergency help. If you're alone, find a phone and call for help before beginning CPR, unless the person is under age 8. Then begin CPR immediately. If you're not alone, have someone with you call for help while you begin CPR immediately
3. Lay the person on his or her back. If necessary, roll the person over so that he or she is faceup. Position yourself on your knees at a right angle to the person, by the person's neck and shoulders.
4. Tilt the head and lift the chin. This is the primary maneuver for opening an airway. Put your palm on

the person's forehead and gently push backward, then with your other hand lift the chin forward to open the airway. When a person is unconscious, muscle tone relaxes, and the tongue becomes a common cause of airway obstruction. Because the tongue is connected to the jaw, tilting the head and lifting the chin positions the tongue away from the airway.

If you suspect a neck injury, use a modified jaw thrust, without the head tilt. Place your hands on each side of the person's face, your thumbs on the cheekbones without pushing, and pull the jaw forward with your index fingers. Examine the mouth and throat to make sure no foreign material is present. If it is, sweep it out with a finger.

Check to see if the person is breathing by positioning your ear directly over the person's mouth. Look across the person's chest for the rise and fall of breathing. Listen for breath sounds. Feel for air on your face. If no breathing is evident, begin mouth-to-mouth resuscitation immediately.

B: Breathe for the person

If professional medical help or emergency equipment isn't available, mouth-to-mouth resuscitation is the best way to restore the flow of air to the lungs.

1. The basis of mouth-to-mouth resuscitation is simple: You breathe for the unresponsive person. Expel breath from your lungs into the victim's through that person's mouth. If the mouth is injured or can't be opened, breathe into the person's nose.
2. Position yourself at a right angle to the person's shoulder. Use the head tilt and chin lift maneuver and pinch the person's nose closed using your thumb and forefinger. This helps ensure that the air you breath into the person's mouth doesn't escape through the nose.
3. Take a deep breath. Open your mouth wide and place it tightly over the person's mouth. Exhale into the victim. Remove your mouth from the victim's, inhale and do it again. Deliver two big breaths. Observe the person's chest with each breath to note whether the air you're breathing into the person is actually causing his or her lungs to expand. Make sure you let the person exhale before delivering another breath. If the person's abdomen bulges excessively, the airway may be blocked, or your breaths may be too large.
4. Check for signs of circulation, such as breathing, coughing or movement. This should take no more than about 10 seconds. It was once recommended that you also check for a pulse. But studies indicate that doing so often takes too long and people aren't always able to correctly detect a pulse.
5. If there's no breathing, coughing or movement, begin cardiac compressions to circulate blood to the brain (see "C: Restore Blood Circulation"). If the person has signs of life but isn't breathing, continue

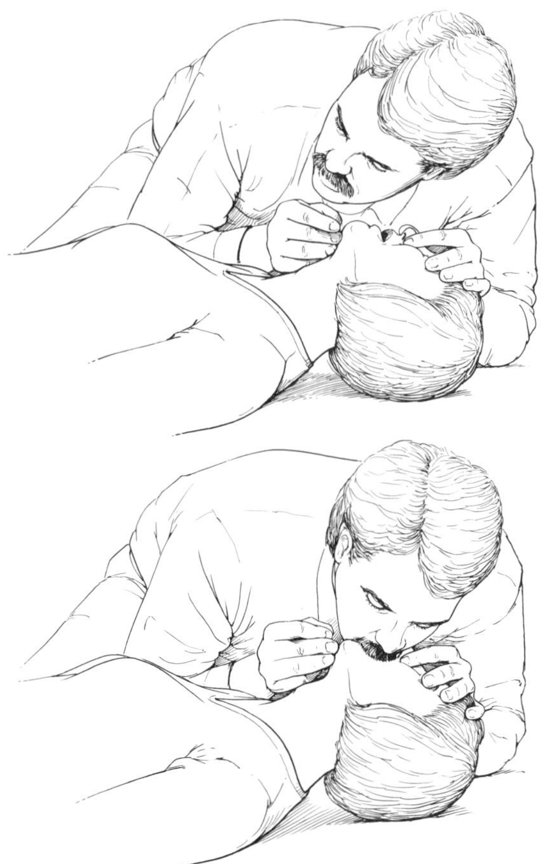

Look, listen and feel for air against your cheek to determine if someone is breathing (top). If you sense no indications of breathing, begin mouth-to-mouth resuscitation (bottom).

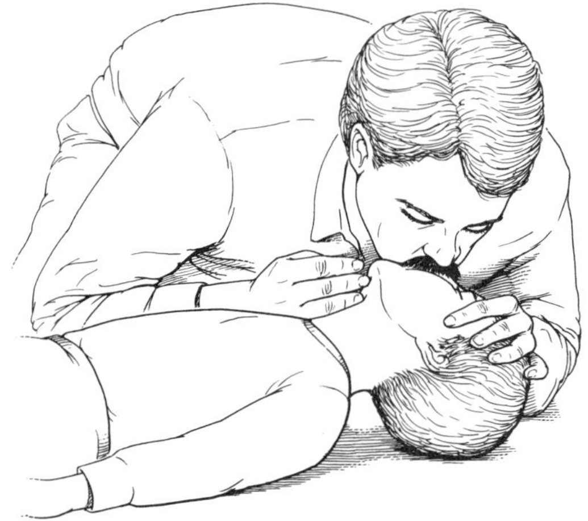

Use mouth-to-nose resuscitation if injury to the mouth or face makes mouth-to-mouth resuscitation difficult. Hold the person's mouth closed by lifting the chin. Then cover his or her entire nose with your mouth and blow into the nose. After exhaling, remove your mouth from the area to allow air to escape. Repeat these steps in a steady, rhythmic breathing pattern until the person resumes breathing or help arrives.

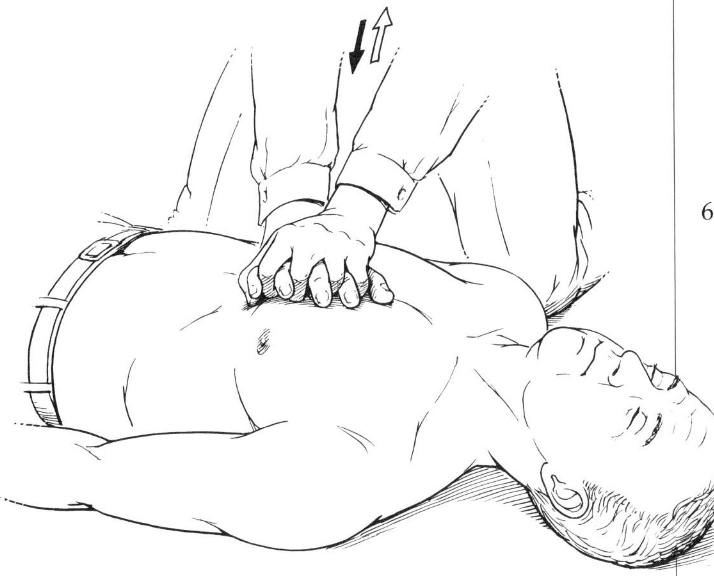

Heart compression (massage) must be coordinated with mouth-to-mouth resuscitation.

2-Person CPR

If someone else is available to help you perform cardiopulmonary resuscitation (CPR), assess the victim. Perform one-person CPR while the other rescuer calls for emergency assistance. When the other rescuer is available, begin two-person CPR.

Two-person CPR is similar to one-person CPR with the exception that one person provides breathing assistance while the other pumps the heart. Compress the heart at a rate of about 100 times a minute. After five compressions, pause to allow the second rescuer to give one breath to the victim.

mouth-to-mouth breathing. Using the same technique, blow a big breath into the individual every 5 seconds — 12 breaths a minute. Take your mouth away between breaths. Observe for signs of breathing and watch chest movement to make sure the air is expanding the lungs.

6. If the individual is breathing but the breaths are weak, shallow or labored, mouth-to-mouth resuscitation may still be helpful. However, coordinate your breathing assistance with the individual's breathing: Deliver a breath when he or she inhales and allow him or her to exhale before you breathe again.
7. Call for emergency medical assistance if you haven't already done so. Continue to breathe for the person until the individual breathes on his or her own or until emergency medical help arrives.

C: Restore blood circulation

In order to deliver oxygen to the brain, the person's blood flow must be restored. If you're unable to find signs of life in an unconscious person, heart compressions are necessary to restore circulation. Also referred to as closed heart massage, heart compressions must be coordinated with mouth-to-mouth resuscitation. The breathing delivers the air to the lungs, and the heart massage then pumps the oxygenated blood to the brain and other parts of the body. When you perform mouth-to-mouth resuscitation, you're acting as a breathing machine. When you perform heart massage, you're acting as a heart pump.

1. Work from a kneeling position at a right angle to the individual's chest. Put the heel of one hand in the center of the person's chest, between the nipples. With the other hand, grasp the first hand from above, intertwining the fingers. Or simply place the second hand on top of the first, with fingers extended. Be careful not to press on the rib cage. This could break ribs. It could also reduce the force of the compressions.
2. Shift your weight forward and upward so that your shoulders are over your hands. Straighten your arms and lock your elbows. This will assure that each chest compression is straight down on the sternum, so the person's torso doesn't roll. Rolling reduces the force of the compressions.
3. Shift your weight onto your hands to depress the victim's chest — it should fall about 1½ to 2 inches in an adult — then release the pressure to allow blood to flow into the heart. Each time you release, keep your hands in contact with the victim's chest, without changing the position of your hands. Count aloud as you do press, providing a total of 15 chest compressions in an even rhythm: one-thousand-one, one-thousand-two, and so on.
4. You must also give the person air. Use the same technique outlined for mouth-to-mouth resuscitation (see "B: Breathe for the Person," step 3): Use the

head tilt and chin lift maneuver to open the airway. Pinch the nose closed with the thumb and forefinger. Take a deep breath, then cover the person's mouth entirely with yours. Exhale into the unconscious person. Remove your mouth from the victim's, inhale and do it again.

5. Compress the chest 15 times, then give the person two breaths again. Establish a regular rhythm, counting aloud. Reassess breathing after four cycles of two breaths and 15 compressions. Call for emergency medical help if you haven't already done so. Continue until help arrives, if you're physically able to do so.

Performing CPR on a child

The procedure for giving CPR to a child age 1 through 8 is essentially the same as that for an adult. The differences are as follows:

- Use only one hand to perform heart compressions.
- Breathe more gently.
- Pump the child's chest five times and then breathe once for the child.

Begin CPR immediately, before calling for emergency medical help. If you're alone, the American Heart Association recommends that you do CPR for about 1 minute before taking time to call for help — generally 911.

As with adults, reassess the child's condition every few minutes.

Performing CPR on an infant

For infants — babies up to 12 months of age — CPR techniques are different. However, the goal is the same: restoring oxygen and blood flow to the brain.

Assess the baby

Be sure that the baby isn't simply resting or sleeping. Stroke the child and look for any response, such as movement. But don't shake the child. If breathing has stopped, start CPR immediately. If you're alone, perform CPR for about 1 minute before taking time to call for emergency medical help — you may be able to carry the child with you to a phone. If you aren't alone, direct someone to call for help. Making the call as soon as possible is important because most infants whose heart and breathing stop have an obstruction in their airway.

Position the baby

Place the baby on his or her back on a table. The floor or ground also will do. Gently tip the head back. This opens the airway. Examine the mouth to make sure no foreign material is inside. Check for breathing by positioning your ear directly over the baby's mouth and looking at the chest for the rise and fall of breathing. If no breathing is evident, begin mouth-to-mouth resuscitation immediately.

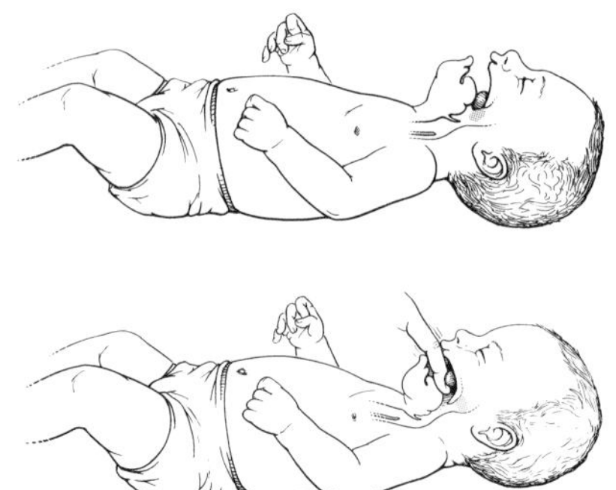

Before giving mouth-to-mouth resuscitation to an infant, tilt the child's head back to open the airway (top). If you see food or a foreign object in the infant's mouth, remove it with a sweep of your finger (bottom). Be careful not to push the food or object deeper into the child's airway.

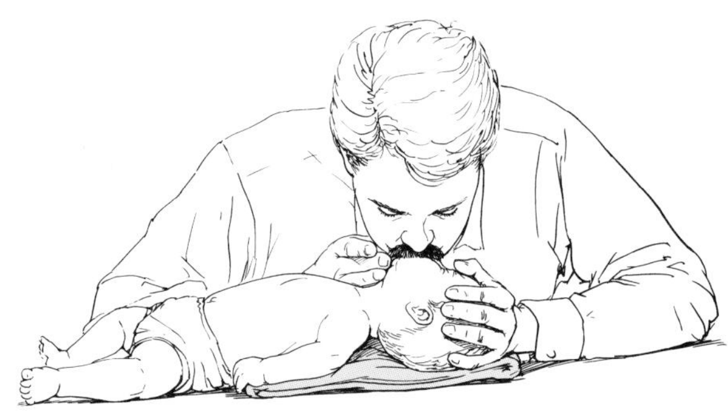

To perform mouth-to-mouth resuscitation on an infant, cover the baby's mouth and nose with your mouth. Using the strength of your cheeks, breath slowly two to five times.

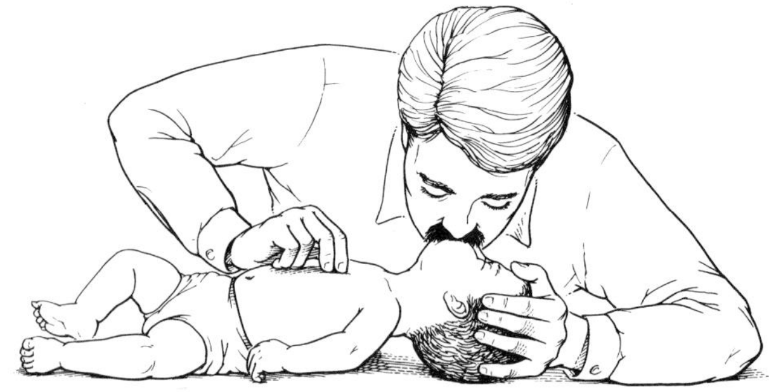

To perform cardiopulmonary resuscitation (CPR) on an infant, alternate compression of the baby's chest with gentle breaths from your mouth.

Deliver gentle breaths
Cover the baby's mouth and nose with your mouth. Using the strength of your cheeks rather than your lungs, breathe two to five times slowly — each breath taking 1 to $1\frac{1}{2}$ seconds to deliver. The breaths are more like puffs than deep exhalations. Too much air can result in a distended stomach and vomiting, a complication you want to avoid. But provide enough air to make the baby's chest rise.

Look for signs of breathing or movement
Check for signs of circulation: breathing, coughing or movement. This should take no more than about 10 seconds. The American Heart Association no longer recommends that you check for a pulse. Studies show that this wastes time and many people aren't always able to do so correctly.

Call for emergency medical help
If you're alone and haven't called for emergency help, call about 1 minute after beginning CPR. Continue to breathe for the baby until the child breathes on his or her own or professional medical help arrives.

Begin compressions
To pump the baby's heart, position your index and middle fingers on the baby's breastbone. Gently compress the chest no more than $\frac{1}{2}$ to 1 inch. Be gentle.

Count aloud as you pump in a fairly rapid rhythm. You should pump roughly $1\frac{1}{2}$ times a second, or about

Breathing Problems

Several disorders of the upper respiratory tract can produce difficulty breathing, especially in children. The most common include croup, epiglottitis and bronchitis.

Wheezing, the sound made by air passing through narrowed breathing passages, may be common to all three of these conditions and may sound similar to the wheezing of asthma. In fact, many individuals with asthma develop severe asthma attacks when they have an upper respiratory infection or bronchitis.

Croup
Croup is caused by a virus that infects the voice box (larynx), the windpipe (trachea) and the bronchial tubes. It's most likely to affect children between the ages of 3 months and 5 years. The signs and symptoms are fever, sore throat, hoarseness and cough. The cough often sounds like a bark (see page 491).

Epiglottitis
The epiglottis is the lid-like cartilage that covers the windpipe during swallowing. When it becomes inflamed, the condition is called epiglottitis. Signs and symptoms often include a very sore throat, fever, drooling, hoarseness and difficulty swallowing saliva due to pain (see page 691).

Bronchitis
Bronchitis is characterized by soreness and tightness in the chest. It's a common viral infection of the bronchi and trachea, the principal air passages in the chest. Accompanying signs and symptoms are cough, chills, overall discomfort and a slight fever (see page 797).

Treatment

If your child has any of these problems, carefully monitor his or her breathing because they each can lead to an obstructed airway caused by severe swelling of the tissues that line the airway. For croup and bronchitis, exposure to warm, humid air may provide relief. You could seat your child in the bathroom and quickly humidify the air by closing the door and filling the bathtub with hot water.

Seek emergency help if breathing becomes labored. Perform mouth-to-mouth resuscitation if breathing should stop.

100 times a minute. You can set this pace by counting: one-thousand-one, one-thousand-two, and so on. Breathe for the baby after every fifth compression.

CPR and specific emergencies

CPR can save lives in many kinds of emergencies. Some common situations in which it may be necessary to provide breathing assistance, as well as heart compressions, include heart attack, severe asthma attack, smoke inhalation, carbon monoxide poisoning, near drowning and electrical injury.

Heart attack

A heart attack occurs when one or more coronary arteries that supply oxygen-rich blood to the heart muscle become blocked. When deprived of blood, portions of the heart muscle gradually die. Sometimes, a heart attack is preceded by chest pain (angina) during or after exertion or even at rest. Other times, a heart attack occurs in the absence of any previous pain.

A heart attack is a medical emergency. If you think that you're having a heart attack:

1. Get immediate medical attention. Call for emergency medical help or have someone take you to the nearest medical emergency facility. Don't drive yourself. Delaying medical treatment is a mistake that costs thousands of lives every year.
2. While waiting for emergency help to arrive or while traveling to the emergency facility, chew and swallow an aspirin tablet. Aspirin helps prevent further blood clotting in the heart arteries. Chewing the tablet before swallowing it speeds its action.

If you're with an individual having a heart attack and the person stops breathing, perform CPR.

Severe asthma attack

People with asthma may experience occasional or even frequent attacks. Often, the individual's asthma medication is all that's needed to improve symptoms.

Occasionally, though, more serious or even life-threatening asthma attacks may occur. Signs and symptoms of a serious asthma attack may include extreme difficulty in breathing, a bluish cast to the face and lips, severe anxiety, a rapid pulse and excessive perspiration.

When a severe attack occurs:

1. Establish that the problem isn't a choking emergency. People with asthma, like the rest of us, can choke on food or other foreign objects that block the airway.
2. Keep calm.
3. Call for emergency medical help or take the person to the nearest emergency department.
4. If the person loses consciousness, begin CPR.

Smoke inhalation

Fire produces smoke that may contain poisons. When burned, plastics, synthetic fabrics, wood, chemicals and

Is It a Heart Attack?

A heart attack may cause one or more of the following signs and symptoms. If you experience any of these, call for emergency medical help.

- Intense, prolonged chest pain, often described as heavy pressure under the breastbone. The pain may extend beyond your chest, radiating to your left shoulder and arm, both arms, your back and even your teeth, jaw and neck. Sometimes, radiating pain may occur without chest pain. At times the pain may occur in the upper abdomen and feel much like severe indigestion. The pain may come on suddenly or gradually.
- Nausea and vomiting.
- Shortness of breath.
- Intense sweating.
- Weakness, restlessness and anxiety.

Occasionally, the only sign is loss of consciousness.

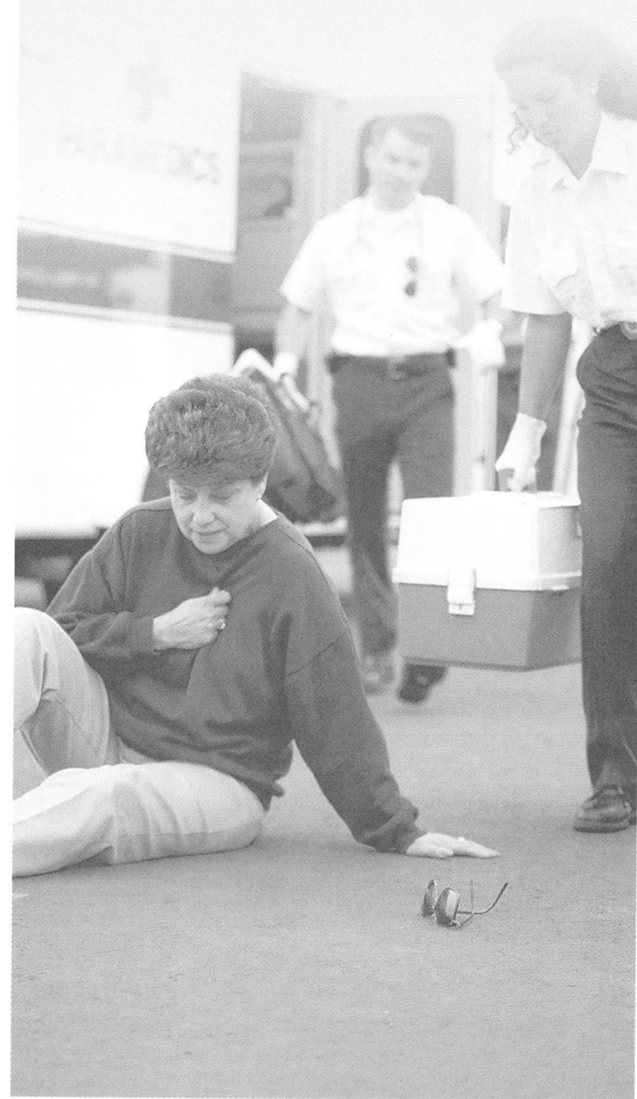

other flammable materials can generate carbon monoxide, cyanide and other toxic fumes. Inhaled smoke from these burning substances can cause breathing problems and damage your airway and lungs.

The key symptoms of smoke inhalation are irritated eyes and difficulty in breathing, such as gasping for breath. Any sign of breathing difficulty — even a cough — should be treated as an emergency because the problem will often get worse. To treat smoke inhalation:

1. Move the victim to a smoke-free area a safe distance from the fire or source of smoke.
2. Once the person is clear of the smoke, check for breathing. If the person isn't breathing, begin CPR.
3. If the person is breathing, loosen any tight clothing and make the individual as comfortable as possible. Summon emergency medical help — even if the person seems improved.
4. If necessary, treat for shock (see page 371).

Carbon monoxide poisoning

One byproduct of fire is carbon monoxide. When inhaled, carbon monoxide takes the place of oxygen in your bloodstream and reduces the supply of oxygen to your body's cells. Typical signs and symptoms of carbon monoxide poisoning are headache, nausea, vomiting and confusion. Seizures and death may occur when levels of carbon monoxide in the blood become high.

Inadequately vented furnaces and wood- or coal-burning stoves, among other things, can result in carbon monoxide accumulation in the home. To deal with carbon monoxide poisoning:

PREVENTION TIP

To prevent carbon monoxide poisoning, purchase carbon monoxide detectors for your home. The detectors sound a warning when carbon monoxide levels in a home or other building exceed an unsafe level. Look for the code UL 2034 on the box. This indicates the detector meets an industry standard that requires alarms to sound before a typical, healthy adult begins to experience symptoms.

Hyperventilation

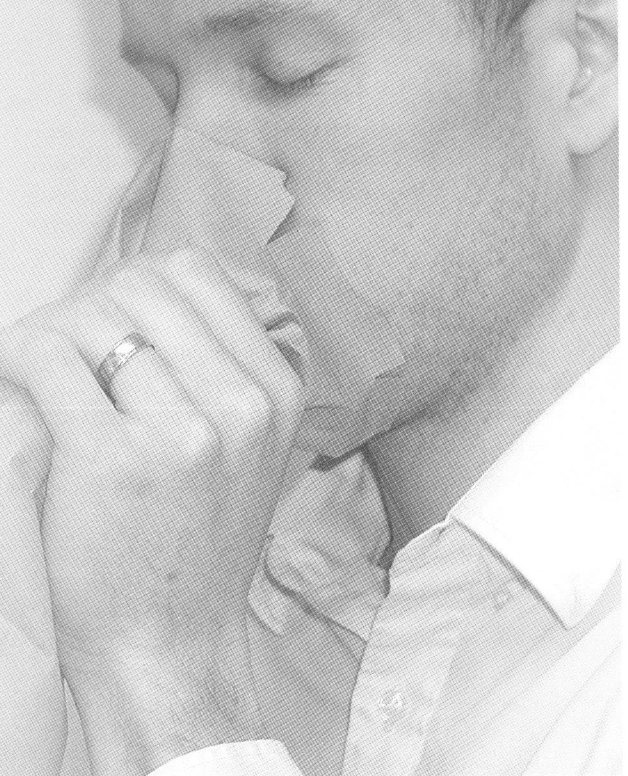

Fear or panic attacks can cause hyperventilation — overbreathing that results from taking too many breaths or breathing too deeply. Even though you're taking in extra air, you may feel as though you're not getting enough.

Hyperventilation can cause tingling and spasms of the hands, in which the fingers are extended while the thumb and fifth finger are drawn together. Your feet also have similar muscle spasms. Other symptoms include lightheadedness and tingling around the mouth. These symptoms are caused by emitting too much carbon dioxide through your lungs, creating a chemical imbalance in your body.

Treatment of hyperventilation consists of reassuring the individual that everything is OK and persuading the person to breathe more normally. Sometimes, breathing into a small paper bag helps because it restores the level of carbon dioxide in the body by requiring the person to rebreathe air from the lungs. The bag should expand and collapse when this is done properly.

If the person hasn't had such an incident before, he or she should see a doctor to be sure the episode isn't something dangerous that's mimicking a panic attack.

1. If you wake up at night with a headache — especially if another member of your family complains of headache or is hard to rouse — have everyone leave the house immediately. Go to a neighbor's home and call for emergency medical assistance.
2. If you're with someone who has been exposed to carbon monoxide, check to see if he or she is breathing. If not, begin CPR.
3. If the person is breathing, loosen any tight clothing on him or her and make the individual as comfortable as possible. Summon emergency medical help — even if the person seems recovered. He or she will benefit from high-flow oxygen as soon as it's available.
4. If necessary, treat for shock (see page 371).

Near drowning

If an individual is floundering or submerged in water and you believe that you're strong enough and sufficiently trained to rescue the person, do so immediately. If you're not a swimmer or are unsure that you can manage the person by yourself, get help.

To treat someone rescued from drowning:

1. Once the individual has been rescued, call for emergency medical help if you're alone. Then begin CPR. If you're not alone, send someone for help and begin mouth-to-mouth resuscitation as soon as it's safe to do so. This may mean starting the breathing process in shallow water even before the person has been positioned on shore.
2. Don't waste time trying to drain the person's lungs of water. Immediately begin to breathe for the person. Air should still be able to reach the lungs in spite of any residual water, and most of the time little or no water has actually entered the lungs.
3. Clear the airway and deliver two quick breaths. Continue to breathe for the person every few seconds while moving him or her to shore or a boat.
4. Near drowning can result in various medical complications, so seek emergency medical care for the victim even after successful CPR.

Electrical injury

Most people experience minor electrical shocks now and again. Such shocks are usually more surprising than dangerous because a reflex action almost instantly jerks you away from the source of electricity. Under certain circumstances, though, even small amounts of electricity can be life-threatening.

To treat someone with an electrical injury:

1. Move the person away from the source of the electricity. If you find a person who you think has been electrocuted, look but don't touch. This person may still be in contact with the electricity. Touching the victim could shock you as well. Turn off the appliance or the power when possible.
2. If that isn't possible, move the source of the electric-

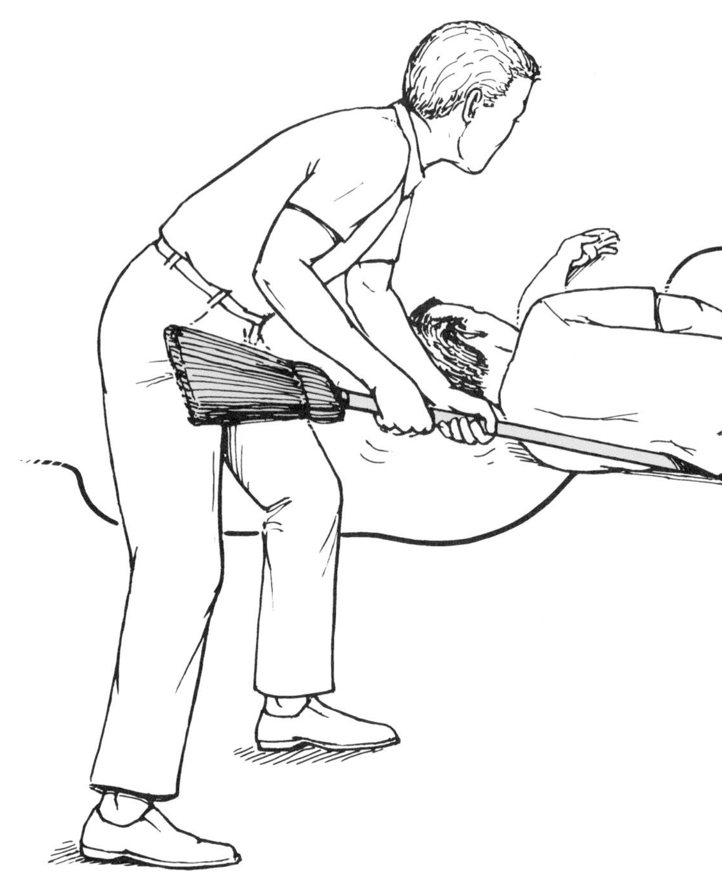

Use a nonconducting object — such as a dry, wooden or fiberglass broom handle — to pull or push a victim of electrical shock away from the live electrical source.

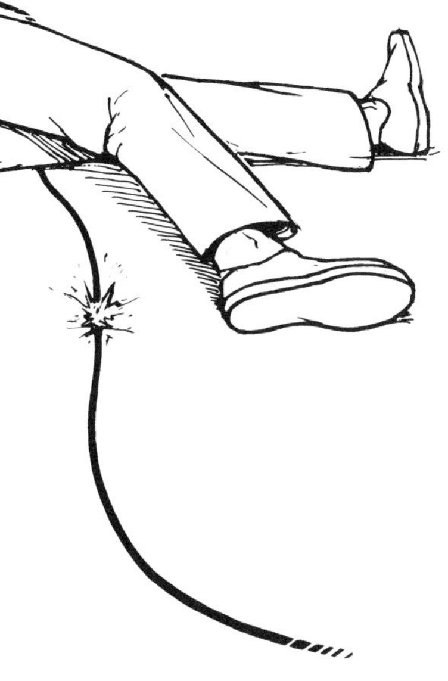

ity away from the victim. Use a dry, nonconducting object, such as plastic, rubber, fiberglass, wood (a broom handle, for example) or cardboard. Don't use a metal object.

3. Once the person is free of the electricity, check the individual's breathing. If it has stopped or seems dangerously slow or shallow, call for emergency medical help and then begin CPR.
4. If the person is faint or pale or shows other signs of shock, lay him or her down with the head slightly lower than the trunk of the body and the legs elevated.
5. Even if the person who received the electrical shock isn't unconscious or lethargic, make sure that he or she gets a medical evaluation to verify that no internal injuries resulted from the incident.

Severe Bleeding

When an injury results in bleeding, you need to take steps to stop the loss of blood. Most injuries don't cause life-threatening bleeding, but if substantial amounts of blood are lost, shock, unconsciousness and death can result. Appropriate care must be taken to stop the bleeding and also to avoid infection and other complications. The information that follows discusses appropriate emergency procedures to accomplish these goals.

Stopping severe bleeding

To stop a severely bleeding injury:

1. Lay down the bleeding person. If possible, position his or her head slightly lower than the trunk or elevate the legs. Either of these positions reduces the chances of fainting by increasing blood flow to the brain. If possible, elevate the site of bleeding. For example, hold an injured hand higher than the

Types of Bleeding

When you're assisting someone who's bleeding, it's often helpful to distinguish the type of bleeding that's occurring because treatment varies from one type to another. The three main classifications are:

Capillary bleeding

Capillaries are the most numerous and smallest blood vessels in the body. When a minor cut or skin scrape opens some capillaries, the bleeding is usually slow and small in content. The body's normal clotting action generally stops the bleeding in a matter of minutes.

Venous bleeding

Deeper cuts often open veins, releasing blood that's on its way back to the heart. Having delivered its load of oxygen to the cells, the blood is dark red. It flows steadily but relatively slowly. Placing direct pressure on the wound will usually stop the blood flow.

Arterial bleeding

The least common but most serious type of bleeding is caused by injury to an artery. The blood that's released is bright red and often spurts with each contraction of the heart. If a major artery is severed and not treated promptly, it's possible to bleed to death in as little as a few minutes. In most cases, though, direct, firm pressure on the wound will stop arterial bleeding.

heart. This reduces blood flow to the injury by forcing the heart to pump the blood upward, against the force of gravity.

2. Remove any obvious debris or dirt from the wound. Don't remove any objects impaled in the person. Don't probe the wound or attempt to clean it at this point. Your main concern is to stop the loss of blood.
3. Place pressure directly on the wound with a sterile bandage, a clean cloth or even a piece of clothing. If nothing else is available, use your hand.
4. Maintain pressure until the bleeding stops. When it does, bind the wound dressing tightly with adhesive tape. If none is available, use a piece of clean clothing.
5. If the bleeding continues and seeps through the gauze or other material that you're holding on the wound, don't remove the bandage. Rather, add more absorbent material on top of it.
6. If the bleeding doesn't stop with direct pressure, you may need to apply pressure to the major artery that delivers blood to the area of the wound. In the case of a wound on the hand or lower arm, for example, squeeze the main artery in the upper arm against the bone. Keep your fingers flat. With the other hand, continue to exert pressure on the wound.
7. Once the bleeding has been stopped, immobilize the injured area. Leave the bandages in place and call for emergency medical help or get the injured person to an emergency department as soon as possible.

Bleeding from an open wound

Bleeding from the surface of your body can range from very minor, such as a needle prick, to major, as with a deep gash in which an artery is severed. All wounds require appropriate care and treatment. Inadequate care can result in serious infection. One important precaution against infection is to make sure your tetanus immunization is always kept up-to-date.

Cuts

If you sustain a small cut that bleeds only slightly, wash the cut thoroughly with mild soap and water. Apply an antibiotic ointment to prevent an infection and a bandage to keep it clean.

If your cut is more serious — that is, the bleeding doesn't stop on its own in a few minutes or the cut is large, deep or rough on the edges — consult your doctor. But first stop the bleeding by applying pressure directly to the injury, using a sterile gauze pad or a clean cloth. Maintain pressure until the bleeding stops.

Bruises

Bruises (contusions) usually result from a blow or fall. Bleeding beneath the skin produces an accumulation of blood (hematoma). To reduce discomfort, elevate the injured area and periodically apply ice or cold packs for 20 minutes at a time several times a day for 1 or 2 days.

Arterial Pressure Points

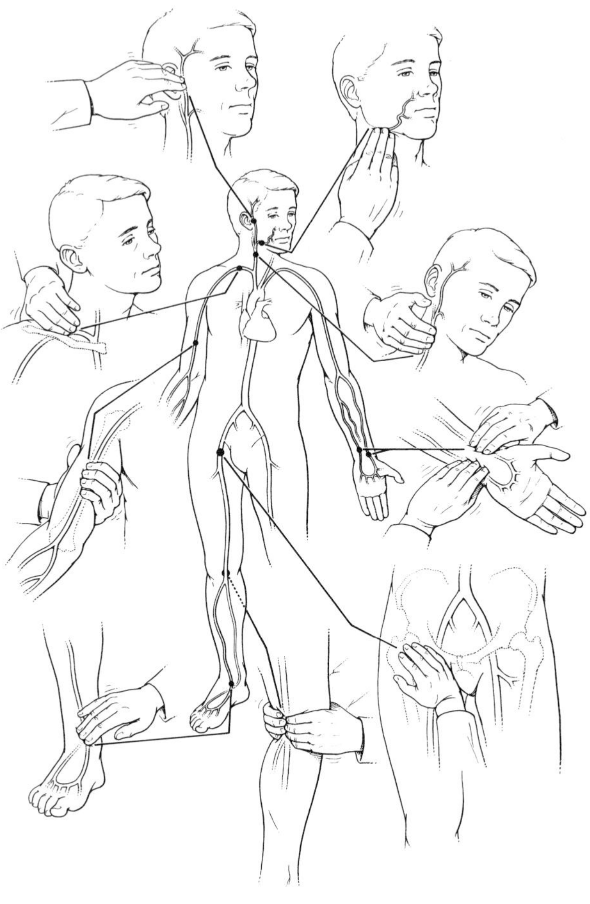

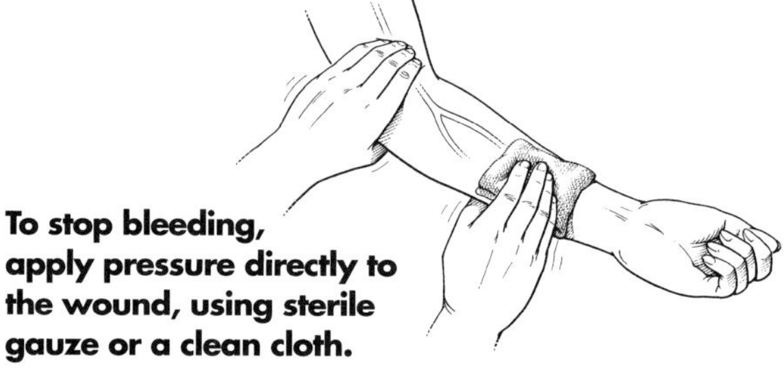

To stop bleeding, apply pressure directly to the wound, using sterile gauze or a clean cloth.

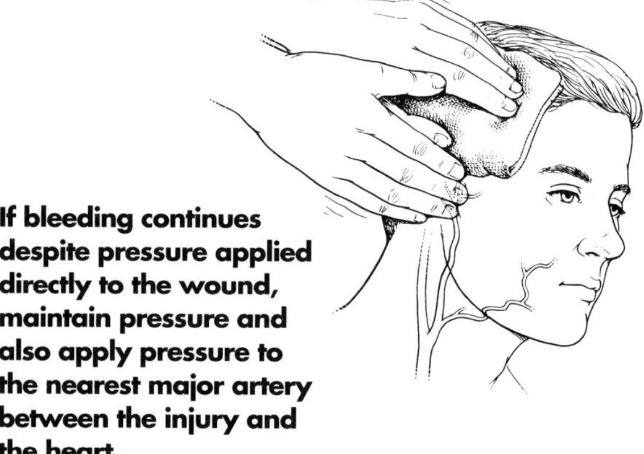

If bleeding continues despite pressure applied directly to the wound, maintain pressure and also apply pressure to the nearest major artery between the injury and the heart.

Tetanus Immunizations

A cut, laceration, bite or other wound, even if minor, can lead to tetanus that occurs days or even weeks later. Tetanus, also called lockjaw, causes stiffness of jaw muscles and other muscles. Other symptoms may include convulsions and breathing problems. The disease can be fatal.

Tetanus bacteria usually are found in the soil but can occur just about anywhere. If their spores enter a wound beyond the reach of oxygen, they germinate and produce a toxin that interferes with the nerves controlling your muscles. For more information on tetanus, see page 495.

Immunization for tetanus is important for everyone. The tetanus vaccine usually is given to children as a DTaP shot, in which diphtheria and whooping cough (pertussis) vaccines are included with the tetanus vaccine. Adults generally need a tetanus booster every 10 years. You may also get a booster shot if you suffer a deep or dirty wound and your most recent booster was more than 5 years ago. Boosters should be given as soon as possible after the injury.

If you haven't had a tetanus immunization previously, your doctor may administer tetanus immune globulin. It provides immediate protection that lasts only a few weeks. Several antibiotics can help eliminate the tetanus bacterium, but the best protection is proper care of the wound and a booster shot or tetanus immune globulin.

Punctures

Stepping on a nail is a common way to get a puncture wound. Such a wound usually doesn't result in excessive bleeding. Often, in fact, little blood flows and the wound seems to close almost instantly. This doesn't mean that treatment is unnecessary.

Puncture wounds are dangerous because of the risk of infection. The object that caused the wound, especially if it has been exposed to soil, may carry spores of tetanus bacteria or other bacteria. These can result in serious infections. A puncture wound through a shoe is particularly prone to serious infection.

If you sustain a puncture wound, stop the bleeding, if necessary, by applying pressure with a sterile gauze pad or clean cloth. Then seek emergency treatment to prevent infection. If the bleeding is minor, some doctors recommend allowing the wound to bleed for a short period of time to help flush it out. But it's unknown if this reduces the risk of infection.

Soft-tissue injuries

With a soft-tissue injury, the skin is damaged, as are underlying tissues such as muscle, supporting structures and blood vessels. These injuries can occur when an area is hit, when an area is badly cut, when skin is separated from the underlying tissues or when skin is forcefully torn away. Soft-tissue injuries require special emergency medical care. Apply pressure to the wound to stop bleeding and seek emergency care immediately.

Abdominal wounds

Because of the possibility of injury to internal organs, any wound that penetrates the abdominal wall is a potentially serious injury. If you or someone with you sustains such an abdominal wound, seek emergency care immediately.

Before moving someone with an abdominal wound, position the person on his or her back. If no internal organs protrude through the wound, use a gauze pad or sterile cloth and exert pressure on the injury to stop bleeding. When the blood flow has stopped, tape the bandage in place. If organs have been displaced, don't try to reposition them. Cover the injury with a dressing.

Bleeding from body openings

Bleeding from body openings can result from an internal injury or disease. Internal bleeding may accompany seemingly superficial injuries. For example, a blow to the head that produces minor bleeding from or under the skin may result in much more dangerous internal bleeding. In some cases, an internal injury may show no signs of external bleeding. In others, the person may vomit blood or bleed from the nose or mouth.

If the person has sustained an injury, such as during a fall, an automobile accident or an event involving violence, he or she may be bleeding internally.

Vomiting of blood

Vomiting of blood can occur as the result of injury to or disease of the throat, esophagus, stomach or the first portion of the small intestine (duodenum).

Call for emergency assistance. While waiting for medical help to arrive, have the person lie down with legs elevated, if possible. The person should not attempt to eat or drink — even if he or she complains of being thirsty. Food or liquids can worsen the problem.

Coughing up blood

When a person coughs up blood, the source of the blood is usually the lungs or windpipe. The blood that appears is usually frothy and bright red. Some possible causes include a bronchial or lung infection, a blood clot in the lung, a blunt injury to the chest or lung cancer.

Seek emergency help if the person coughs up large amounts of blood. While waiting for help to arrive, keep the individual's head elevated slightly and supported by pillows. Loosen clothing that's tight around the person's throat and chest. If the person complains of thirst, you may give small amounts of crushed ice.

Rectal bleeding

Bleeding from the anus can be the result of various problems. Hemorrhoids can cause bright red blood in the toilet bowl or on the toilet paper. Black, tarry stools, maroon stools or bright red blood in the stool may suggest bleeding higher in the gastrointestinal tract. If you observe rectal bleeding of an unknown cause, make an appointment to see your doctor. If rectal bleeding occurs in moderate to large amounts, seek emergency care.

Vaginal bleeding

Vaginal bleeding is a normal part of menstruation. However, bleeding from the vagina may also signal a wide range of gynecologic and other medical problems. See your doctor if you experience any unexpected vaginal bleeding. See your doctor immediately if you're pregnant and notice vaginal bleeding.

Blood in urine

Blood in urine can be frightening because it can appear as if you're bleeding more than you really are. A relatively small amount of bright red blood in the toilet may make the bowl appear to be full of blood. But chances are you've lost relatively little blood. See your doctor as soon as possible to determine the cause.

Nosebleeds

A nosebleed is a common condition that usually involves sudden bleeding from one nostril. It may result from trauma, breathing dry air, allergies or for no apparent reason. Most nosebleeds come from the septum, the cartilage that separates the nasal chambers and is lined with fragile blood vessels. This form of nose-

Detecting Internal Bleeding

In the event of a traumatic injury, internal bleeding may not be immediately apparent. Consider it a possibility if you observe any of the following signs or symptoms:

- Bleeding from the ears, nose, rectum or vagina
- Vomiting or coughing up blood
- Bruising on the neck, chest or abdomen
- Wounds that have penetrated the skull, chest or abdomen
- Abdominal tenderness, possibly accompanied by rigidity or spasm of abdominal muscles
- Fractures

Internal bleeding may produce shock. If the volume of blood in the body decreases, the person may feel weak, anxious and thirsty. In addition, the skin may feel cool. Other signs and symptoms of shock from internal bleeding include shallow and rapid breathing, a rapid and weak pulse, trembling and restlessness. The person may faint when standing or even while seated but soon recover when allowed to lie down. Elevating the person's legs may help.

If you suspect internal bleeding, request immediate emergency help. Try to keep the person still and loosen the person's clothing. In case of internal bleeding in an extremity, stop the bleeding by applying pressure directly to this area or manually compressing the major artery between the heart and the fracture or bruise.

Basic First Aid Supplies

Always keep your medicine cabinet or first aid kit well stocked. Include the following basic supplies:

- Adhesive or gauze wrappings or pads in several sizes
- Soap
- Absorbent cotton
- Tweezers
- Cotton-tipped swabs
- A thermometer
- Aspirin (especially for chest pain)
- Ibuprofen or acetaminophen (especially for pain and fever)
- Antiseptic solution (such as hydrogen peroxide, Betadine or Hibiclens)
- Antiseptic cream (such as Neosporin or Polysporin)
- Hydrocortisone cream (for bites and stings)
- Bandages or surgical tape
- Adhesive tape
- A sharp scissors
- Tissues
- A first aid manual
- Ipecac syrup (to induce vomiting)

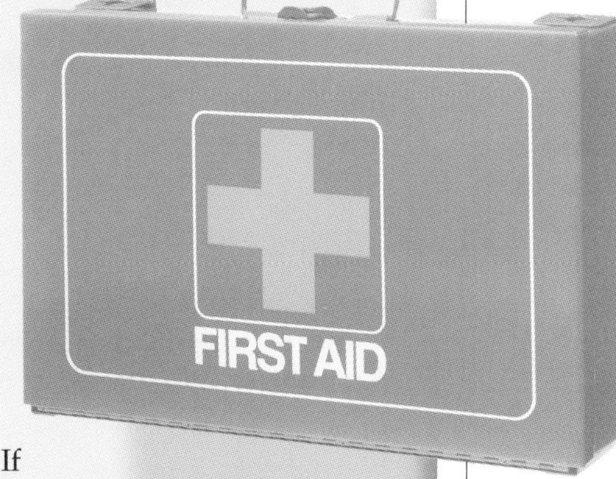

Other medications that you may want to have on hand include antihistamine tablets, antacids, an antidiarrheal medication and reserve supplies of medications taken by family members, such as insulin for diabetes. If you or a member of your family reacts severely to bee or insect stings, have a kit containing a syringe with adrenaline (epinephrine) readily available.

bleed isn't serious and is usually easy to stop. In some people, nosebleeds may begin farther back in the nose. These nosebleeds, which are less common, are often harder to stop. To stop the flow of blood:

1. Sit or stand upright. The upright position decreases the flow of blood into the veins of the nose. Don't tip your head back or insert anything in your nostril.
2. Pinch your nose with your thumb and index finger and breathe through your mouth. Do this for 5 to 10 minutes. This should stop the flow of blood.
3. If you succeed in stopping the flow of blood, there's no need to see a doctor. If the bleeding proves hard to stop, seek emergency care.

Burns

Burns come from many sources, including fire, the sun, steam, electricity, chemicals and hot liquids or objects. Burns may cause only minor injury that you can treat on your own or life-threatening emergencies that require intensive medical treatment.

Burn classifications

Distinguishing a minor burn from a more serious burn involves determining the degree of damage to body tissues. There are three classifications of burns:

First-degree burns

First-degree burns, the least serious burns, involve only the outer layer of skin (epidermis). The skin is usually reddened, and it may be swollen and painful. The outer layer of skin hasn't been burned through. Unless such a burn involves substantial portions of the entire body, it can generally be treated at home.

Treating Minor Burns at Home

To treat a minor burn:

1. Cool the burn by holding it under cold, running water for 15 minutes. If this isn't possible, immerse the burn in cold water or cover it with cold compresses. Don't put ice directly on the burn. Doing so can cause frostbite and further damage.
2. Once the burn is cooled, apply a lotion or moisturizer to soothe the area and prevent dryness. Don't apply butter to burned skin. Butter traps heat in the tissues and can cause more damage and increase the chance of infection.
3. Cover the burn with a sterile gauze bandage. Wrap it loosely to avoid putting pressure on the burn. Bandaging keeps air off the burn and reduces pain.
4. Fluid-filled blisters sometimes form to protect against infection. Don't break the blisters. If they break by themselves, wash the area with mild soap and water. Then apply an antibiotic ointment and gauze bandage. Dead skin from popped blisters may be trimmed away.
5. Acetaminophen (Tylenol, others) or ibuprofen (Advil, Motrin, others) may help relieve pain and swelling.

Second-degree burns

When the first layer of skin has been burned through and the second layer of skin (hypodermis) also is burned, the injury is a second-degree burn. Blisters develop, and the skin takes on an intensely reddened appearance and becomes mottled (spotted or blotchy). Severe pain and swelling are accompanying signs and symptoms. If a second degree burn is limited to an area no larger than 2 to 3 inches in diameter, you may be able to treat it at home. If the burned area of skin is larger or if the burn occurred on the hands, feet, face, groin, buttocks or a major joint, seek emergency medical care.

Third-degree burns

Third-degree burns are the most serious burns. They involve all of the layers of skin and sometimes deeper tissue. Third-degree burns usually have areas that are charred black. The person may experience severe pain or, if nerve damage is substantial, minimal or no pain at all. These burns need emergency care (see below).

Burns caused by fire

Burns caused by direct contact with fire — such as those that happen around campfires and to children playing with matches — should be treated according to the degree and extent of the burn. A first-degree burn on a small part of the body, such as a finger, can be treated as a minor burn. Burns that are extensive or that extend to deeper layers of tissue may require a visit to your doctor's office or to the emergency department of your local hospital.

Electrical burns

Any electrical burn should be examined by a doctor. An electrical burn may appear minor, but the damage can extend deep into the tissues beneath the skin. Electrical shocks can sometimes result in a heart rhythm disturbance, cardiac arrest or other internal damage from electrical current passing through the body. Sometimes, the jolt associated with the electrical injury can cause the person to be thrown or to fall, resulting in fractures or other injuries.

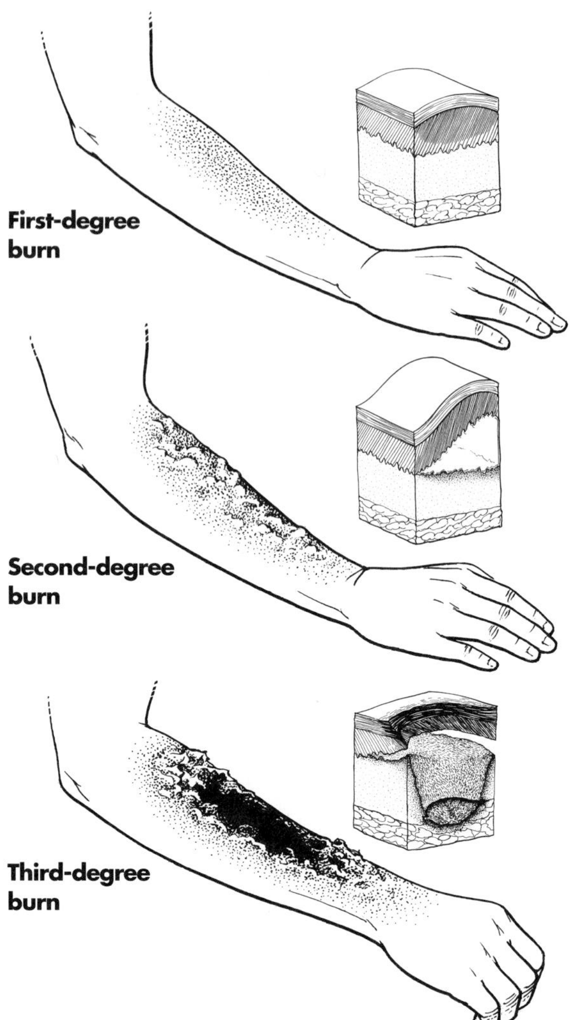

Burns are classified according to the degree of damage to skin and body tissue.

Treating Major Burns

Call emergency help immediately for all major burns. While waiting for medical help to arrive:

1. Make sure the cause of the burn has been extinguished or removed. Don't remove burned clothing that adheres to the skin, but make sure that the victim isn't in contact with smoldering materials.
2. Make certain the individual is breathing. If breathing has stopped, perform mouth-to-mouth resuscitation. If you suspect that the person's airway is blocked, attempt to clear it first.
3. If the individual appears to be in shock, take steps to treat the shock.
4. Cover the area of the burn with a dry, sterile bandage or clean cloth. Don't use a blanket or towel because of the fabric's tendency to stick to burns. A sheet will do if the burned area is large. Don't apply ointments and try not to break burn blisters.

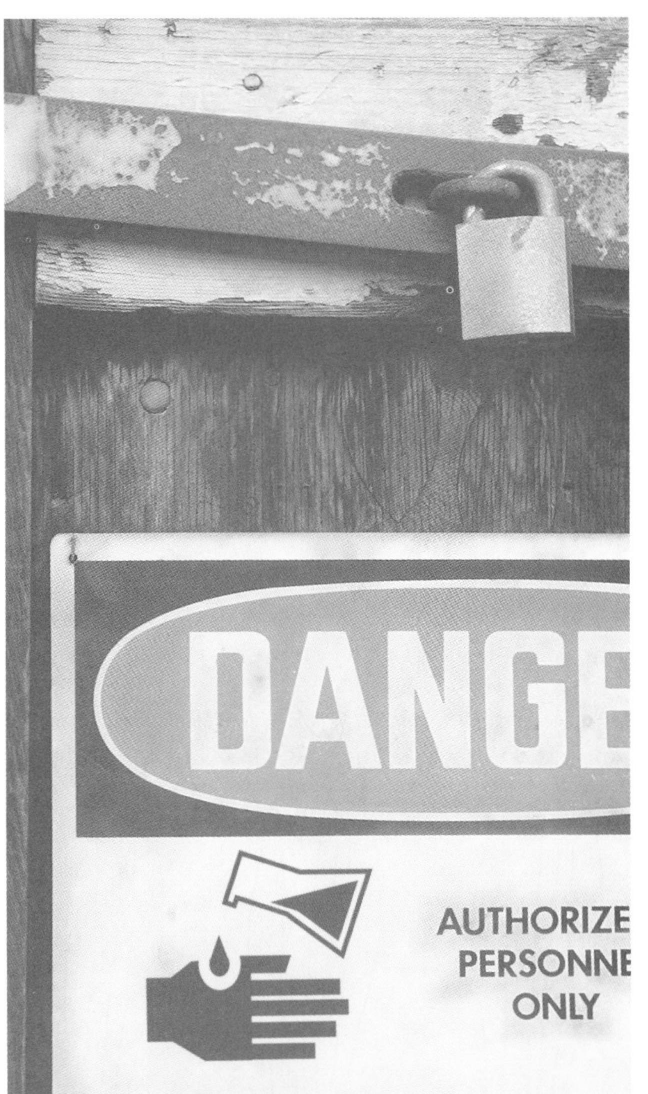

Chemical burns

To treat a chemical burn:

1. Make sure that the cause of the burn has been removed. Flush chemicals off the skin surface using cool, running water for 20 minutes or more. If the chemical is a powder-like substance, such as lime, brush it off the skin before flushing with water.
2. Treat the person for shock if he or she is faint, pale or breathing in a shallow, hurried fashion.
3. Remove any of the person's clothing or jewelry that has been contaminated by the chemical.
4. If the person complains of increased burning after you've washed the area, rewash the burn with water for several more minutes to further dissipate the chemical.
5. Wrap the burned area with a dry, sterile dressing or clean cloth.
6. If a chemical splashes into an eye, flush it with water immediately. Any source of clean drinking water will do. It's more important to begin the flushing than it is to find sterile water. Continue to flush the eyes with running water for at least 20 minutes. After washing the eyes thoroughly, close the eyelids and cover them with loose, moist dressings. Then seek medical attention for the injured person.
7. Minor chemical burns usually heal without further treatment. If the chemical caused a second-degree burn that's more than 2 to 3 inches in diameter, or the burn is on the hands, feet, face, groin, buttocks or a major joint, seek emergency medical help. Also seek emergency medical treatment if chemicals come in contract with one or both of your eyes.

Trauma

A traumatic wound is an injury caused by external force or violence. A broken bone, a severe blow to the head, a knocked-out tooth all are examples. Broken bones (fractures) are among the most common trauma injuries. The term *sprain* is frequently used to describe a wide range of injuries, but a sprain involves damage to the ligaments that connect the bones, not the bone itself.

Fractures, severe sprains, dislocations and other serious bone and joint injuries usually require professional medical care. You risk permanent disability, deformity and, in the case of skull, neck and spinal injuries, even death if you don't get prompt medical care. Likewise, head trauma, eye injuries and tooth loss should receive appropriate emergency treatment.

Fractures

A fracture usually occurs as a result of a fall, blow or other traumatic event. If you suspect a fracture, protect the injured area from further damage. Don't try to align the broken bone. Signs and symptoms of a fracture may include:

- Swelling or bruising over a bone
- Deformity of the affected limb
- Localized pain that's intensified when the injured area is moved or pressure is put on it
- Loss of function in the area of the injury
- A broken bone protruding from the skin

Treatment

To help protect against further injury from the fracture:

Check for a pulse

Check for a pulse below the fracture. Make sure that the wound is between the person's heart and the place

---

Types of Fractures

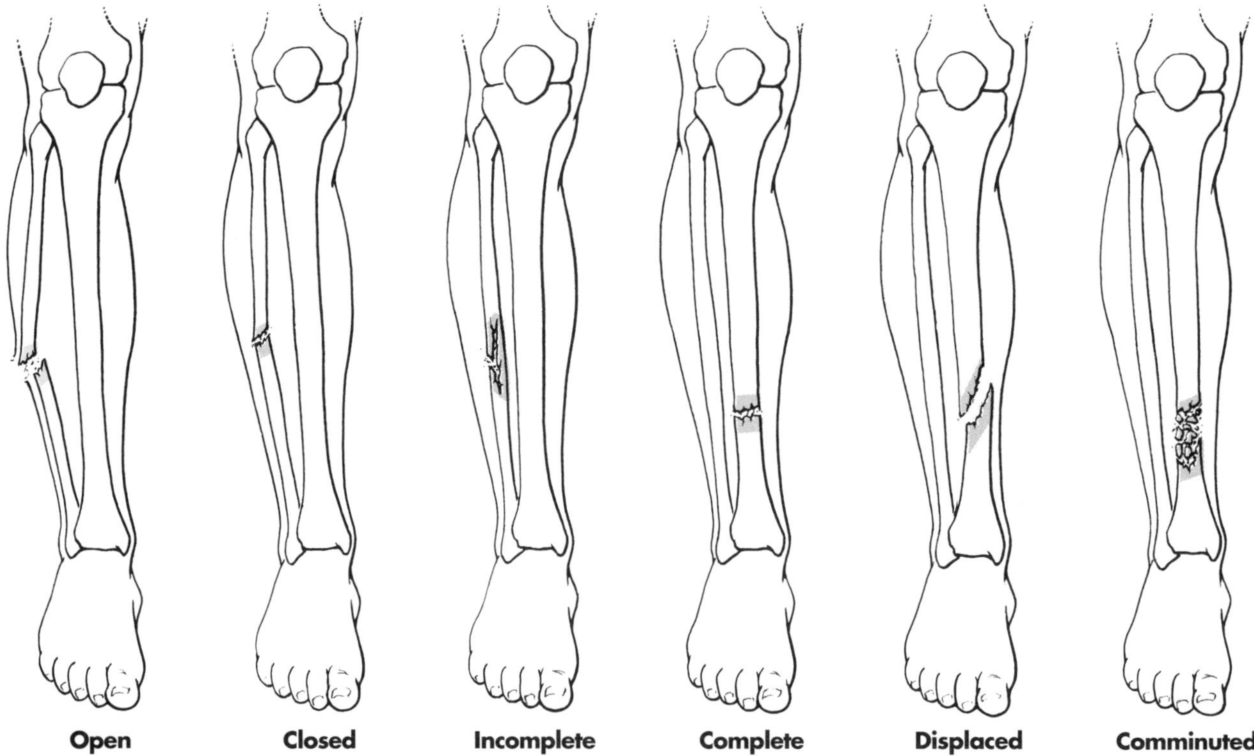

Open. The broken bone protrudes through the skin.

Closed. The broken bone doesn't protrude through the skin. This type of break is also called a simple fracture.

Incomplete. The bone is cracked but isn't separated into two parts.

Complete. The bone snaps into two or more parts.

Displaced. The two bone ends no longer line up.

Comminuted. The bone is splintered or crushed into several pieces.

Other types of fractures:

Impacted. One fragment of bone is embedded into another fragment of bone.

Pathologic. This type of fracture involves a bone break in a person whose bones are weakened by disease. Such a break may occur in an individual with bone cancer or decreased bone mass (osteoporosis). The break is called a pathologic fracture because an underlying disease is the main cause of the break.

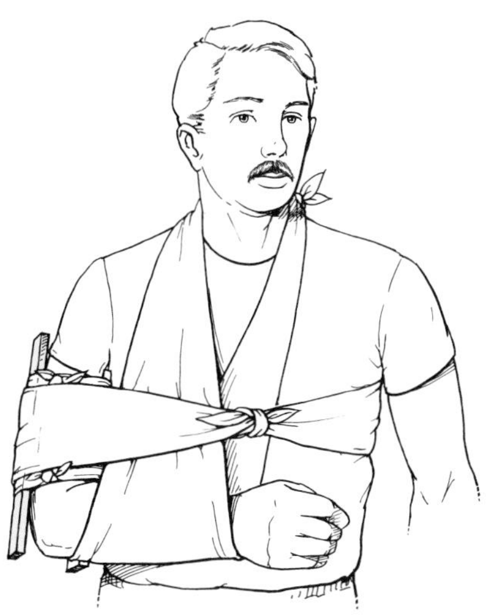

If professional help is unavailable, immobilize an upper arm fracture with a splint and a sling.

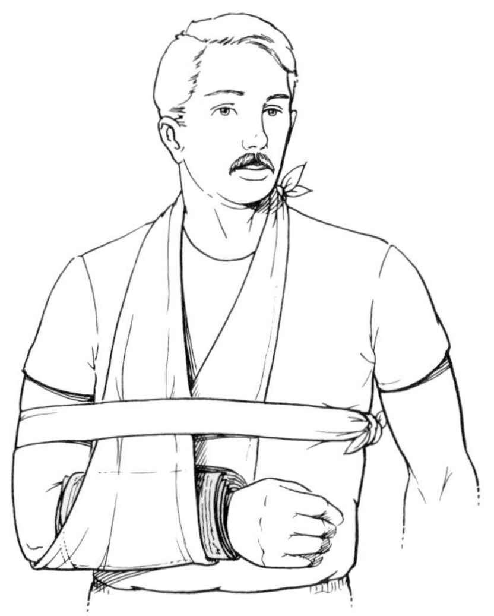

A rolled newspaper or magazine can serve as an effective temporary splint for a fracture of the lower arm.

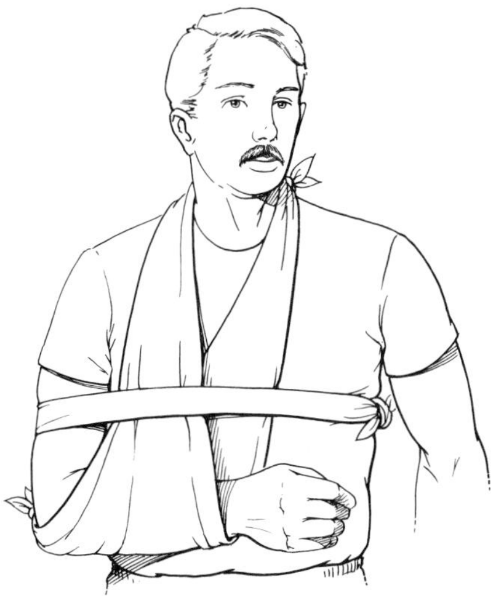

A simple sling can effectively immobilize an injured elbow.

where you're checking for the pulse. This will help you determine whether blood is still flowing past the break. If it's not — if there's no pulse — the person is at risk of losing the fractured extremity. Immediately transport the person to an emergency medical facility.

Stop the bleeding

If the break is an open fracture — the broken bone is protruding through the skin — or other bleeding is associated with the injury, apply pressure to stop the bleeding. Place pressure directly on the wound with a sterile bandage, a clean cloth or even a piece of clean clothing. If nothing else is available, use your hand. Maintain pressure until the bleeding stops. Elevate the site of the fracture to reduce blood flow.

Treat for shock

If the person is faint, pale or breathing in a notably shallow, hurried fashion, treat him or her for shock. Lay the person down with the head slightly lower than the trunk and legs.

Immobilize the bone

Before the person with the broken bone is transported, splint the bone to prevent its movement. Keep the joints above and below the fracture immobilized. A splint can stabilize the damaged area and prevent movement of broken bones that could aggravate tissue damage. Proper splinting may also reduce pain.

Splinting or immobilizing fractures

Splints can be made of wood, plastic, metal or another rigid material. Pad the splint with gauze or some other cloth, then apply it to the limb. The splint should be longer than the bone it's splinting and extend below and above the injury. Fasten the splint to the limb with gauze or strips of cloth, string or other material. Start wrapping from the extremity and work toward the body. Splint the limb firmly to prevent motions but not so tightly that blood flow is stopped.

How to splint the fracture depends on the location of the break. A spinal injury or a hip or pelvic fracture can't be splinted but must be immobilized in some other way.

Arm fractures

Rolled magazines or newspapers can be tied around a broken lower arm. A sling over the shoulder and a band around the sling can help immobilize an elbow.

Leg fractures

If a lower leg is broken, place the entire leg between two splints. If no splints are available, the healthy leg can be used as a splint to limit movement of the broken one. A broken thighbone requires that the hip joint also be immobilized.

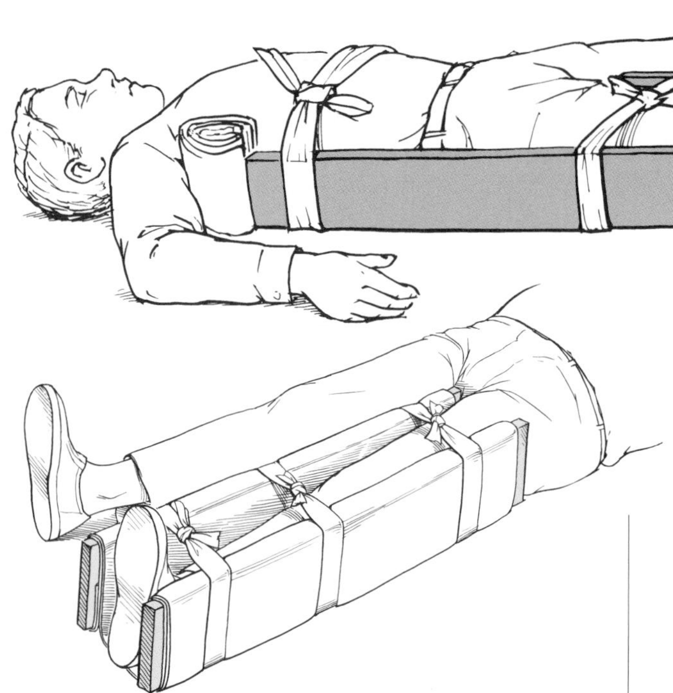

A leg splint can effectively immobilize a fracture of the lower leg (left). A fracture of a thighbone requires splinting of the trunk and lower leg (above).

Spinal injuries

If you suspect a neck or spinal injury, don't move the injured person. Permanent paralysis and other serious complications can result from moving a person with a spinal injury. The broken spine, if moved, could accidentally sever the spinal cord.

Assume the person has a spinal injury if:

- There's evidence of a head injury.
- The injury exerted substantial force on the back or neck.
- The person complains of severe pain in the neck or back.
- The person complains of weakness, numbness, paralysis or lack of control of the limbs, bladder or bowel.
- The neck or back is twisted or positioned oddly.
- The person is unconscious and can't describe the pain.

Call for emergency medical help. Keep the victim still and don't try to move him or her unless the person is choking or in immediate danger. If you need to move the person, gently reposition the individual on a board — a tabletop or a door will do. Get several people to help and make sure that the person's neck, head and spine are held firmly in alignment. Make sure the neck is stabilized. Use a heavy towel or scarf, a pocketbook or other soft, bulky material to prevent the head from rotating while the person is being moved.

Hip or pelvic fractures

Hip or pelvic fractures usually occur as a result of a fall or an accident. In some people whose bones are weakened from osteoporosis or bone cancer, such breaks can occur spontaneously. Suspect a broken pelvis or hip if the person complains of:

- Pain in the hip, lower back or groin area

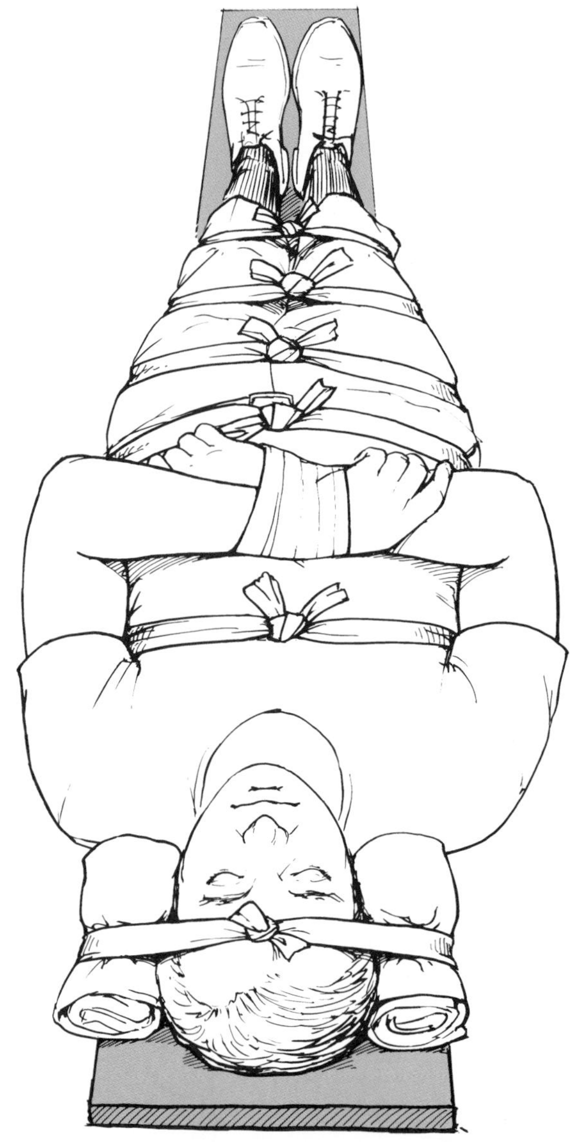

Neck and back injuries require special precautions. If medical help is unavailable and the injured person must be moved, recruit several people to help. Neck and back injuries can lead to permanent paralysis. Proper use of a backboard immobilizes the victim's head, neck and spine.

- Pain in these areas that worsens with movement of one or both legs

As with a spinal injury, call for emergency assistance and don't move the individual. If you need to move the person, gently reposition him or her on a board or a tabletop, just as you would a person with a spinal injury. Don't try to straighten an injured leg or hip that seems oddly positioned.

Other broken bones
When a fracture occurs in a bone in a finger, toe, rib or the face, splinting is usually unnecessary. Stop any bleeding and seek medical attention promptly.

Sprains

A sprain occurs when trauma such as a violent twist or stretch causes the joint to move beyond its normal

Amputation

When a finger, toe or larger body part is severed, life-threatening risks can include blood loss, shock and infection. Call for emergency medical help immediately. It's important that you quickly get the injured person and the severed part to a hospital, where the limb may possibly be reattached.

Until emergency help arrives:

Stop the bleeding
The first goal of emergency treatment is to stop blood loss. Whether the amputation involves an extremity as small as a toe or as large as a leg, apply pressure on the wound with a sterile bandage, clean cloth or piece of clothing. If possible, have the individual lie down. The limb with the injury should be slightly elevated. When the bleeding is under control, wrap the wound with additional layers.

If the bleeding continues
If a hand, foot, leg or an arm has been amputated, the bleeding may be hard to stop. First apply pressure to the artery that feeds the injured area. If that fails, a tourniquet may be necessary.

Use a tourniquet only as a last resort. Tourniquets are so effective at cutting off the flow of blood that they can cause tissue damage that makes it difficult or impossible to reattach the amputated part.

Wrap a necktie or other piece of cloth around the tissue immediately above — but not touching — the wound. The cloth must be long enough to wrap around the area twice with enough material left for a knot. Tie a half knot first, then place a screwdriver, stick, dowel rod or similar object on top of the knot and tie the second half knot. Twist the object to tighten the tourniquet. Tighten the cloth only as much as is required to stop the flow of blood. Note the time at which you applied the tourniquet. Tie the object in place with the cloth once bleeding has stopped.

Treat other injuries
When you have the bleeding at the site of the amputation under control, examine the person for other signs of injury, such as cuts or fractures.

Save the severed part
Once the person is stable and you're waiting for emergency medical help, carefully put the amputated body part in a clean plastic bag or wrap it in a clean cloth. If ice is available, place the bag with the severed body part in it inside a second bag containing ice. Don't put the ice in direct contact with the severed part and don't use dry ice. If ice isn't available, use very cold water.

Remarkable advances have been made in recent years in reattaching fingers, hands and even severed limbs. The results depend on many factors, but if you pay attention to caring for the severed body part and a qualified surgeon is readily available, reattachment may be possible.

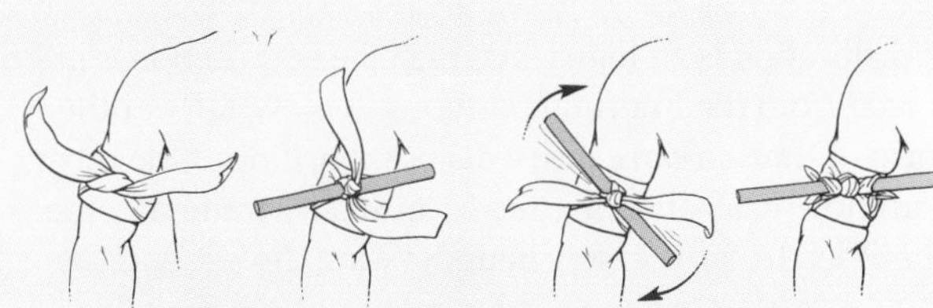

If all other methods to stop bleeding fail, apply and tighten a tourniquet.

range of motion, tearing ligaments attached to bone. Usual indications of a sprain include:

- Pain and tenderness in the affected area
- Rapid swelling, sometimes accompanied by discoloration of the skin
- Impaired joint function

Treatment

If a popping sound and immediate difficulty in using the joint accompany the injury, seek emergency medical care. If the symptoms are less serious, but you suspect bone or ligament damage in the joint, seek medical care as soon as possible. Also seek medical care if the pain or difficulty moving the joint doesn't improve within 2 or 3 days. Your doctor may order an X-ray to determine the extent and nature of the injury.

For most minor sprains, you can probably treat the injury yourself with an approach called PRICE (protection, rest, ice, compression and elevation):

Protection

Immobilize the affected area to encourage healing and to protect it from further injury. Use elastic wraps, slings, splints, crutches or canes as necessary.

Rest

Avoid activities that cause pain or swelling. Rest is essential to promote tissue healing.

Ice

Immediately apply ice to decrease swelling, pain and muscle spasm. Ice packs, ice massage or slush baths are all useful. Reapply ice periodically — for no longer than 20 minutes at a time — as long as the swelling lasts.

Compression

Swelling can cause loss of motion in an injured joint. To contain the swelling, compress the injured area until the swelling has stopped. Compressive wraps or sleeves made from elastic or neoprene are best.

Elevation

Raise the swollen arm or leg joint above the level of your heart to help reduce swelling. This is especially important at night.

Dislocations

A dislocation is an injury in which the ends of bones are forced from their normal positions. A blow, fall or other form of trauma can cause a dislocation. One of the most common dislocation injuries is caused by trauma to the shoulder. In some cases, an underlying disease such as rheumatoid arthritis, a congenital weakness or a joint weakened by previous dislocations may be responsible.

The usual signs of dislocation are:

- Swelling and intense pain

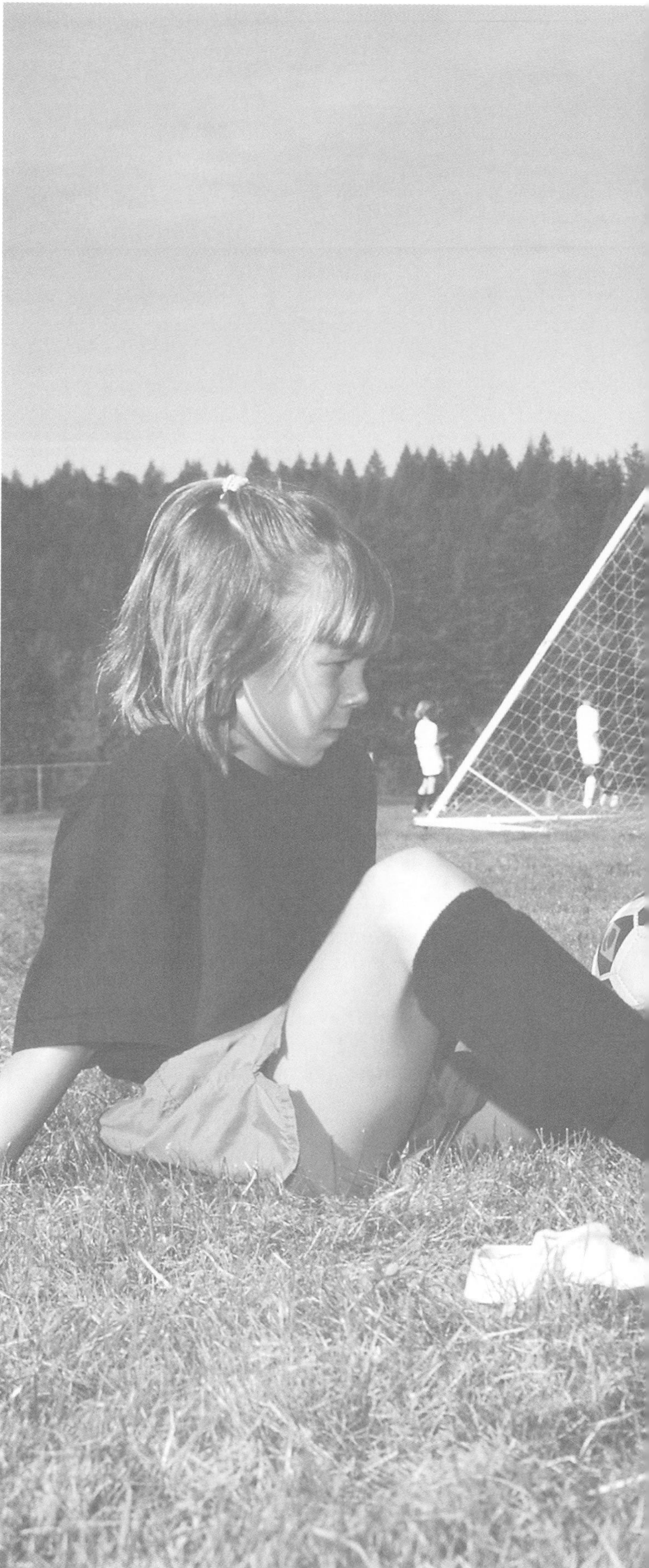

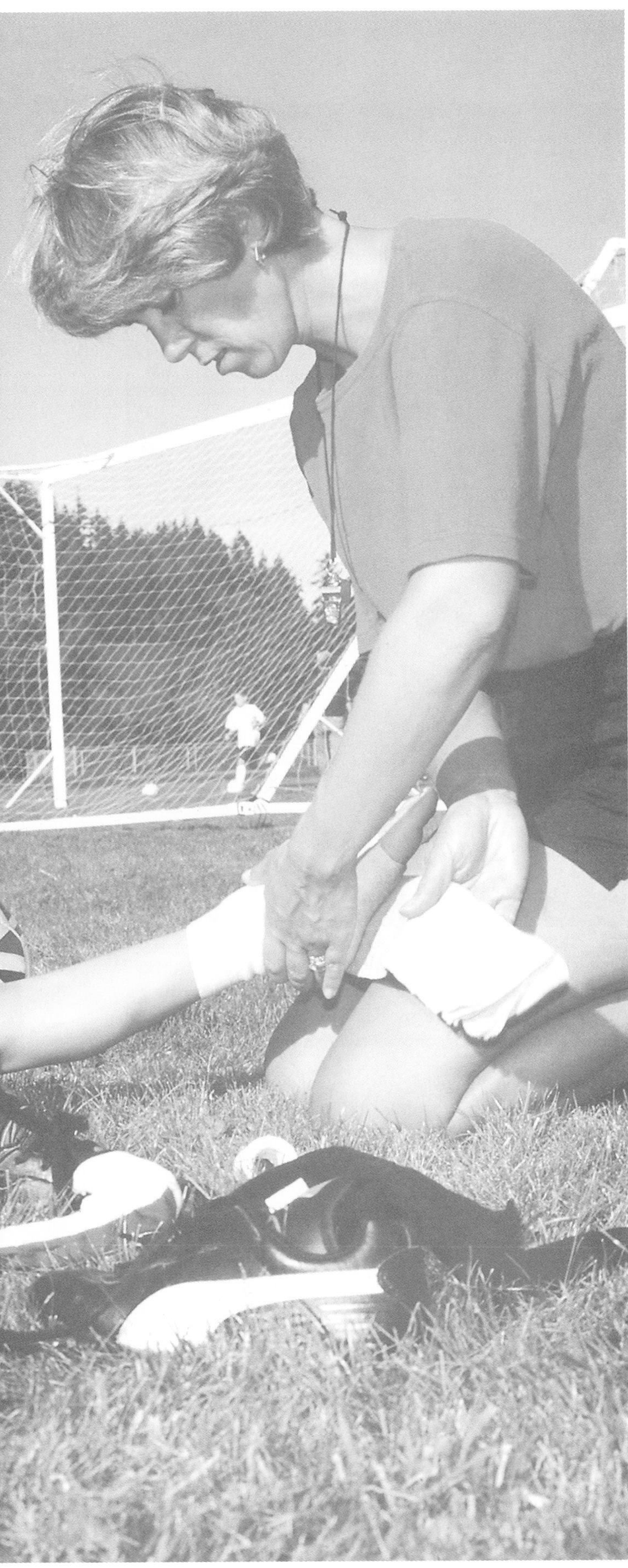

- A joint that's visibly out of position, misshapen and difficult to move

Treatment

Don't try to return the joint to its proper position unless you're trained to do so. Instead, splint the affected joint and seek medical care as soon as possible. If a dislocation isn't treated within 30 minutes, the swelling and pain can intensify and an anesthetic may be necessary before treatment. In the case of a suspected neck or spinal injury, don't move the injured person. Call for emergency medical help.

Head injuries

Most head injuries are minor because the skull provides considerable protection to the brain. Only about 10 percent of all head injuries require hospitalization, and simple cuts and bruises can often be treated with basic first aid techniques. Seek emergency medical care if any of the following signs or symptoms are apparent:

- Absence of breathing
- Severe head or facial bleeding
- Change in level of consciousness — confusion, lethargy or loss of consciousness, even if the person regains consciousness quickly
- Vomiting

Try not to move the neck because it may have been injured. If the person isn't breathing, begin cardiopulmonary resuscitation (CPR) right away, while trying to keep the neck as still as possible. If the person is bleeding, take steps to stop the bleeding.

Among the potential complications of head injuries are concussions, blood clots and skull fractures.

Concussions

When the head sustains a hard blow from being struck or from a fall, a concussion may result. The impact causes the brain to strike the inside of the skull.

Usually, a concussion, also called mild traumatic brain injury, doesn't cause loss of consciousness. It can, however, produce confusion, headache, loss of memory, dizziness or vomiting. More serious head injuries can cause a prolonged loss of consciousness, partial paralysis, shock or persistent symptoms of a concussion, such as confusion or a headache. A concussion requires emergency medical evaluation.

Intracranial hematoma

An intracranial hematoma results when a blood vessel — either an artery or a vein — ruptures between the skull and brain. Blood leaks between the brain and skull and forms an accumulation (hematoma), usually clotted, that presses on the brain tissue.

The most common cause of a hematoma is a blow to the head, such as from being hit by a baseball, falling off a stepladder or being in a car accident. Signs and symptoms may develop a few hours to several weeks after the head injury. They can include headache, nausea, vomiting, change in consciousness and pupils of unequal size. As more blood floods into the narrow space between the brain and skull, the person becomes progressively lethargic and possibly even unconscious. The condition can be fatal if not treated. Treatment often involves surgery to stop the bleeding and remove the excess blood.

Two kinds of hematomas can press on brain tissue: subdural and epidural. The difference between the two is their location. When an injury causes bleeding between the brain and the lining of the brain called the dura mater, blood accumulates within the brain, producing a mass called a subdural (below the dura) hematoma. When the bleeding occurs between the dura mater and the skull, the mass is known as an epidural (above the dura) hematoma.

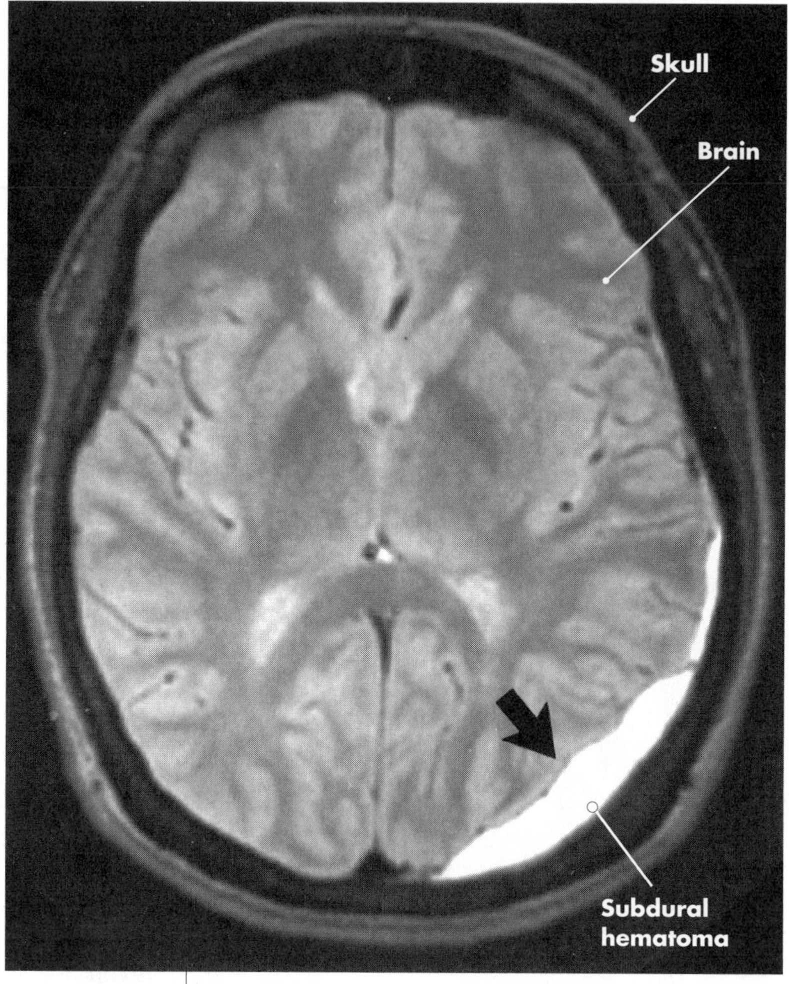

Hematomas are detected most often with the help of imaging a computerized tomography (CT) scan or magnetic resonance imaging (MRI). This MRI scan shows a subdural hematoma.

Skull fractures

Bleeding or visible bone fragments are obvious signs of a skull fracture. Other, less noticeable signs of a possible skull fracture include:

- Bruising or discoloration behind the ear or around the eyes
- Blood or clear, watery fluid leaking from the ears or nose
- Pupils of unequal size, accompanied by a change in mental status, such as confusion or unconsciousness
- Deformity of the skull, including swelling or depressions

A skull fracture is a medical emergency and must be treated promptly to avoid potential brain damage and even death.

Eye injuries

Traumatic injuries to the eye include corneal abrasions, blood in an eye and eyelid lacerations (see page 633 for additional eye injuries).

Corneal abrasion

The cornea is the clear structure at the center of your eye. It refracts light from the front of your eye to the retina at the rear of your eye. The cornea is easily injured — a speck of sand or even a contact lens that's worn for too long can scratch it.

Instantaneous pain at the moment of the injury followed by persistent pain and redness are the key signs and symptoms of a corneal abrasion. In some cases, the pain increases over a period of hours. If the pain persists after rinsing the eye to remove any foreign objects, close your eye, cover it with soft gauze or an eye patch and seek emergency medical care.

Blood in an eye

Blood visible through the pupil in the front chamber of the eye is called a hyphema. It can result from a blow to the eye or an injury that perforates the eye. Certain medical conditions also can cause the problem.

In most cases, the eye absorbs the blood within a few days. If it doesn't, a more serious eye injury may be apparent, and you may need to have the blood drained through a small opening in the eye. Seek the care of an ophthalmologist or see your personal doctor. This serious condition is different from the relatively harmless problem of bloodshot eyes, which are caused by broken surface blood vessels in the white part of the eyes, and subconjunctival hemorrhages, which are blotchy red spots that occur when small blood vessels break between the white of the eye and the membranes of the eyelid (conjunctiva).

Eyelid laceration

If an eyelid is cut or scraped, apply clean gauze to the eye without applying pressure and seek emergency medical care.

Tooth loss

When a permanent tooth is accidentally knocked out in one piece, it can sometimes be reimplanted, but only if you act quickly. A broken tooth, on the other hand, cannot be reimplanted.

Treatment

If a permanent tooth is knocked out, save the tooth and consult your dentist immediately. If the dentist is unavailable, go to the nearest emergency department.

Successful reimplantation depends on how soon the tooth is inserted. Within 30 minutes is ideal. Longer than 2 hours after the injury is often too long. Proper storage and transportation of the tooth also is essential. If a tooth is knocked out:

1. Handle the tooth by the top (crown) only. Don't touch the roots.
2. Don't rub or scrape the tooth to remove dirt.
3. Gently rinse the tooth in tap water but not under the faucet.
4. Try to replace the tooth in the socket and bite down gently on gauze or a moistened tea bag to help keep it in place.
5. If the tooth can't be replaced in the socket, immediately place it in milk, your own saliva or warm, mild salt water.

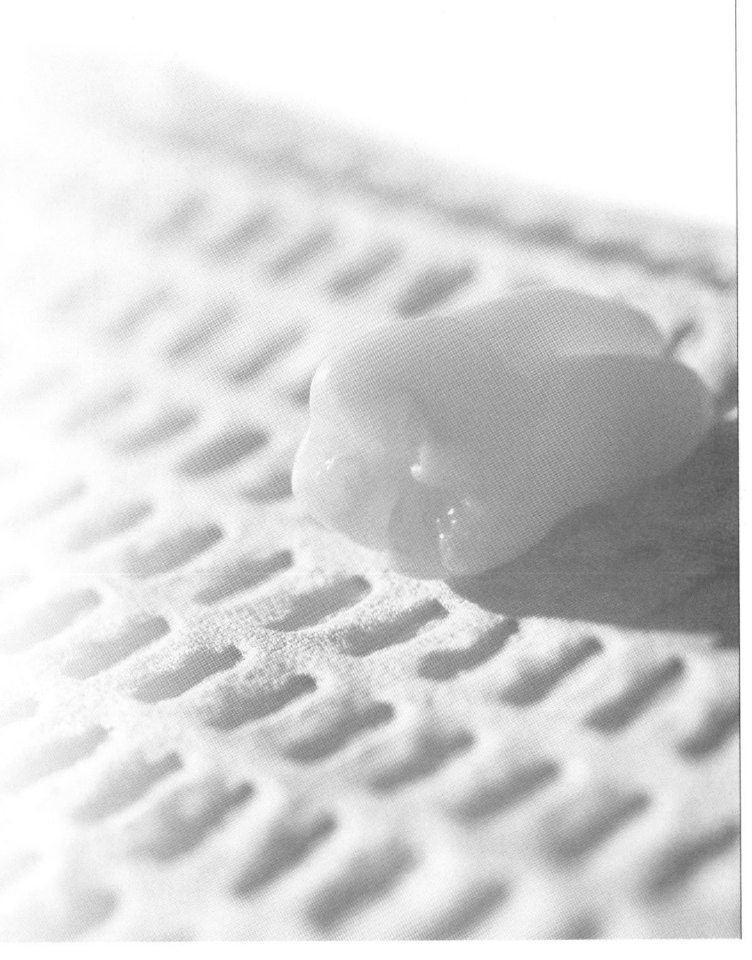

Shock

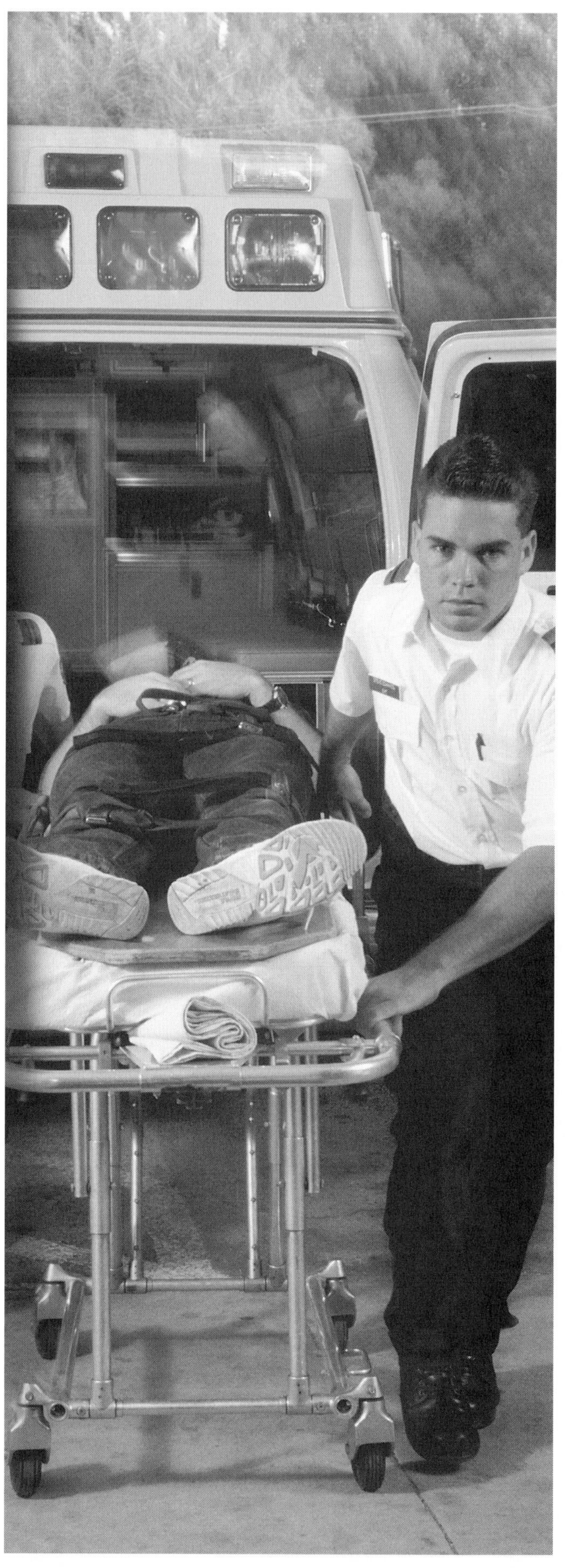

Shock is a common complication of blood loss, infection, a burn, a major fracture and other medical problems. It's a condition in which there's a reduction of blood flow throughout your body. This produces a decrease in your blood pressure and a reduction in the supply of oxygen to your tissues. This decrease may produce various signs and symptoms, including pale skin and a rapid, weak pulse. Shock can come on suddenly or be a delayed reaction to trauma. It can be life-threatening.

Types of shock

Shock is divided into three broad categories: hypovolemic, cardiogenic and vasogenic.

Hypovolemic shock

Hypovolemic shock results from serious bleeding, major trauma or dehydration resulting from loss of fluids due to vomiting or diarrhea. The term *hypovolemic* means there's too little blood volume. Severe hypovolemic shock may cause death in a matter of minutes if left untreated.

Cardiogenic shock

Cardiogenic shock is brought on by a heart that doesn't function properly. Causes of this type of shock include a heart attack, a very slow heart rate or an extremely rapid heart rate.

Vasogenic shock

Vasogenic shock is a direct result of blood vessel changes. This type of shock is caused by certain infections or severe allergic reactions to insect and bee stings (anaphylaxis).

Causes of shock

Shock may result for the following reasons:

Blood loss

Excessive loss of blood can produce hypovolemic shock, in which the volume of blood falls below a healthy amount. The bleeding may be external, as with a severe cut, or internal, as with a fractured pelvis or a rupture of an internal organ. Other sources of blood loss that can produce shock include ulcers and heavy vaginal bleeding.

Dehydration

A reduction in body fluids also can lead to hypovolemic shock. Usually, the fluid loss is obvious because the person experiences persistent vomiting, diarrhea or loss of fluid through urination. Conditions that can lead to fluid loss include stomach flu (gastroenteritis), excessive use of water pills (diuretics) and adrenal gland failure.

Recognizing and Treating Shock

Before you can effectively treat a person suffering from shock, you need to know how to recognize its signs and symptoms.

Recognizing shock

The following signs and symptoms may indicate the presence of shock in an ill or injured person:

Change in skin color

The skin may appear pale or gray and feel cool and clammy.

Rapid pulse and breathing

The heartbeat is weak and rapid and is accompanied by shallow, hurried breathing. Blood pressure drops and may not be measurable.

Staring eyes

The eyes appear dull, and the person appears to be staring. He or she may also have large (dilated) pupils, making the black center of each eye look large.

Unconsciousness, dizziness, agitation and thirst

The person may be unconscious. If not, he or she may feel faint, dizzy or weak or become confused or extremely anxious and agitated. Many people in shock complain of being thirsty.

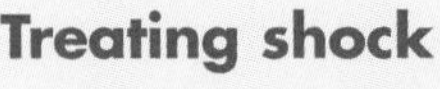

Treating shock

Seek emergency medical help if you observe the signs and symptoms of shock. While waiting for medical help to arrive:

Have the person lie down

Lay the person down on his or her back with the head lower than the feet. This position can help maintain blood flow to the brain and may relieve symptoms of faintness. Elevating the feet on a cushion or some other prop is usually the easiest way to establish this position. If the person has sustained an injury in which raising the legs will cause pain or further injury, leave the person flat on his or her back. Try to keep movement to a minimum.

Keep the person warm and comfortable

Loosen tight collars, belts or other constricting clothing. Cover the person with a blanket if the temperature is cold. If the floor or ground is cold, put a blanket beneath the victim. If it's hot, place the person in the shade or a cool area, if possible.

Take steps to prevent choking

If the person is vomiting or bleeding from the mouth, position the person on his or her side. This may help prevent choking or inhaling (aspirating) the vomit or blood.

Treat injuries

If an injury has occurred, treat it. Stop any bleeding, immobilize a fracture or take any other appropriate first aid steps. Pain from a fracture that isn't immobilized can worsen shock. Be especially careful when immobilizing someone who may have a spinal injury so that you don't further injure the spinal cord.

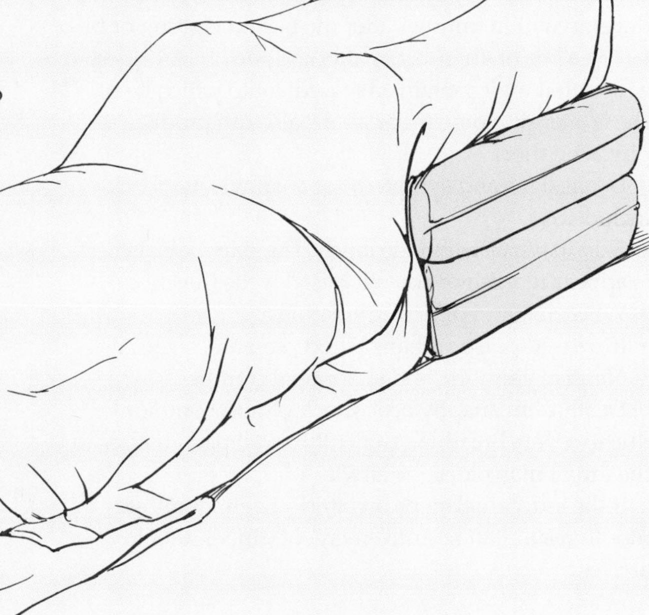

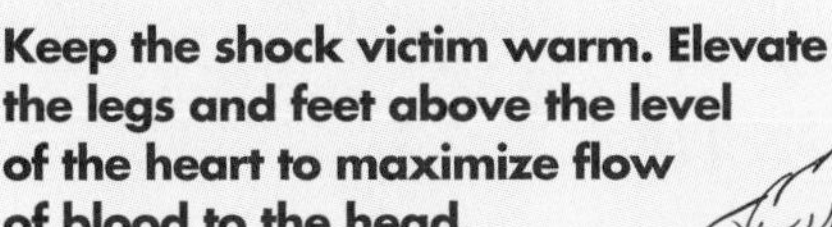

Keep the shock victim warm. Elevate the legs and feet above the level of the heart to maximize flow of blood to the head.

Heart conditions

Certain heart conditions, such as a heart attack, can cause a decrease in blood circulation, leading to cardiogenic shock. The supply of blood to the tissues falls below healthy levels due to inadequate pumping strength of the heart. Tissue cells don't have enough oxygen for normal functioning, resulting in shock.

Infection

If an infectious agent enters your bloodstream in an overwhelming manner and circulates throughout your body, it can produce what's called septic shock, a type of vasogenic shock. Your body fights back, destroying the unwanted bacteria. But in the process, the bacteria releases dangerous toxins that can cause tissue damage and interfere with normal blood circulation.

The presence of these toxins in your bloodstream can produce a variety of signs and symptoms, which may include reddened, flushed skin that's warm to the touch, chills and fever, rapid heartbeat and shallow breathing. Typically, these signs and symptoms last from 30 minutes to a few hours and then give way to cool, clammy skin, a drop in blood pressure, extreme thirst, shortness of breath and even respiratory failure.

Septic shock is more common among older individuals, the very young and people with certain lingering illnesses, such as diabetes, liver disease and blood-related cancers.

Severe allergic reaction

Some people react more strongly than others to certain allergens, and the introduction of the allergen into their systems can produce anaphylactic shock (anaphylaxis). This type of shock is a form of vasogenic shock, and it occurs most in people with a history of allergies.

You should suspect anaphylactic shock if symptoms develop within minutes after the person is stung or bitten by a bee or an insect or after the person has ingested a food that may contain an ingredient to which he or she is allergic. Some medications also can produce anaphylactic shock.

Usual signs and symptoms of anaphylactic shock include:

- Skin that's warm to the touch. The skin may also appear reddish or contain raised welts (hives).
- Wheezing and difficulty breathing.
- Increased pulse and low blood pressure.
- Nausea, vomiting and abdominal cramps.

Death from anaphylactic shock is most commonly due to severe breathing difficulty. Swelling of tissues in the throat may block the airway.

If the individual stops breathing, begin mouth-to-mouth resuscitation until emergency medical help arrives.

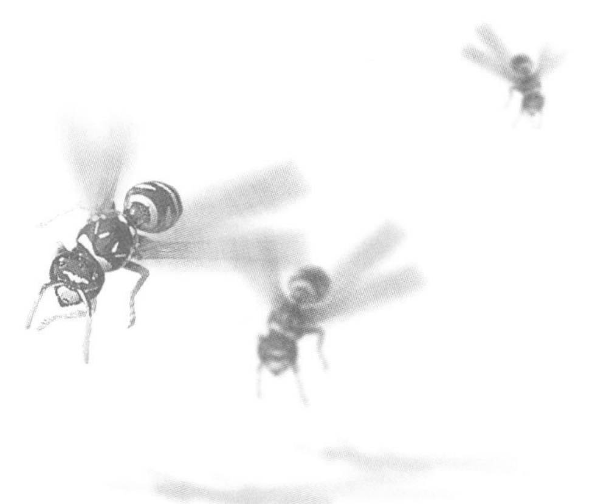

PREVENTION TIP

If you or a member of your family is severely allergic to bees, insects or certain foods, keep a properly equipped emergency kit available. The kit should include adrenaline (epinephrine) that can be administered with a hypodermic needle or a single-dose auto-injector in case of anaphylactic shock. Adrenaline quickly opens swollen airways, allowing you or your family member to breathe more easily. You can obtain this type of kit with a prescription from your doctor.

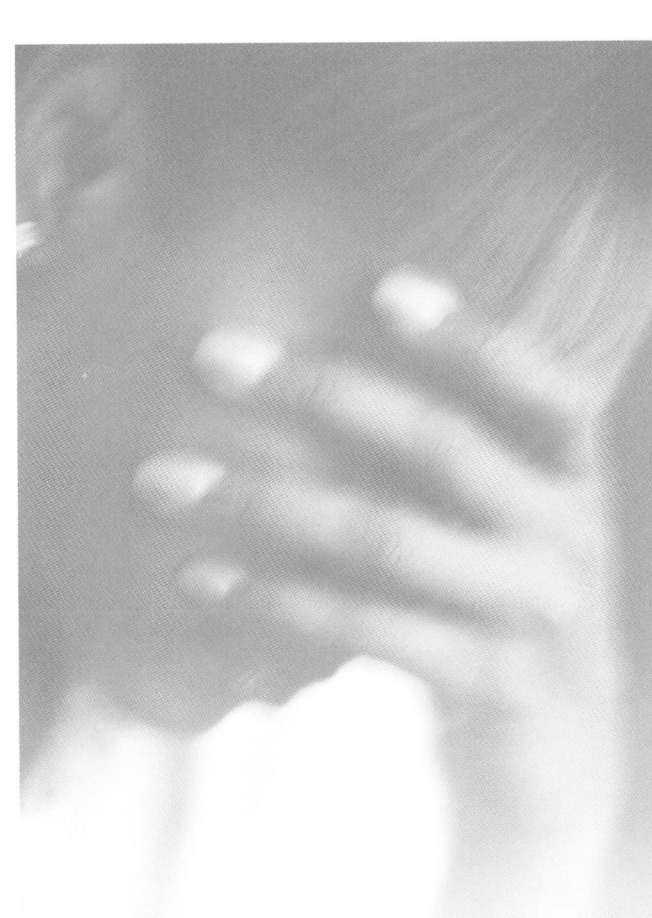

Fainting, Seizure and Stroke

Sudden loss of consciousness is one of the most alarming medical events. Fainting spells are generally the least serious of these events. For example, some perfectly healthy people faint at the sight of blood and recover completely in a matter of minutes. But all fainting, seizures and strokes must be treated as potentially serious medical emergencies. The unconscious individual should receive immediate care.

Fainting

People faint when the supply of blood to their brain drops too low. Someone who is fainting becomes pale because too little blood is reaching the skin, and then he or she temporarily loses consciousness. Usually within a minute of lying flat, the person's blood flow is restored, and he or she regains consciousness.

Fainting spells can have no medical significance, or they can be a sign of a serious disorder. Several medical disorders, including life-threatening heart rhythm disturbances and severe coughing spells, can produce fainting. Some people faint when they're extremely tired, when they receive news that's emotionally upsetting or when they see something disturbing. The heart slows and blood pressure falls. No matter how seemingly trivial, loss of consciousness should be treated as a medical emergency until the symptoms leave and the cause is known.

Treatment

You can do several things to help a person who has fainted or feels as if he or she is about to faint:

Have the person lie down

If someone complains of faintness or dizziness while sitting or standing, have the person lie down. If there isn't space to do so, have the individual lean forward while seated and put his or her head between the knees. This will help increase circulation to the brain. If a person faints, yet remains seated, quickly lay the individual on the floor.

Position the person on the back

If a fainting spell causes the person to slump to the floor, position the individual on his or her back. People who lose consciousness sometimes vomit, so you should carefully check the person's airway to make sure it's clear. Also check for vital signs. For example, is the person breathing? Can you feel a pulse? It may be weak and slow, so check carefully. If breathing has stopped, the problem is more serious than a fainting spell. Immediately begin cardiopulmonary resuscitation (CPR). Have someone call for emergency medical help.

If the person is breathing, rest the individual's legs on a chair or other elevated object so that the legs are higher than the head. This position allows gravity to increase blood flow to the brain. Loosen the person's belt, collar or other constrictive clothing. The person may revive quickly.

Check for other signs and symptoms
Does the person have chest pain or head pain? Is there apparent breathing difficulty? Does the person complain of numbness or continuing weakness? These may be signs of an underlying medical problem. If any of these signs and symptoms develop, seek emergency medical help.

Encourage the person to take it easy
After a fainting spell is over, the person's facial color should return to normal. Often, he or she will feel weak for a short time afterward, so lying quietly for a few minutes is a good idea.

Treat injuries
If the person was injured in a fall associated with the faint, treat any bumps, bruises or cuts. Seek emergency help if the injury appears serious.

Seizure

Normally, brain cells produce coordinated electrical discharges. When electrical discharges become disorgan-

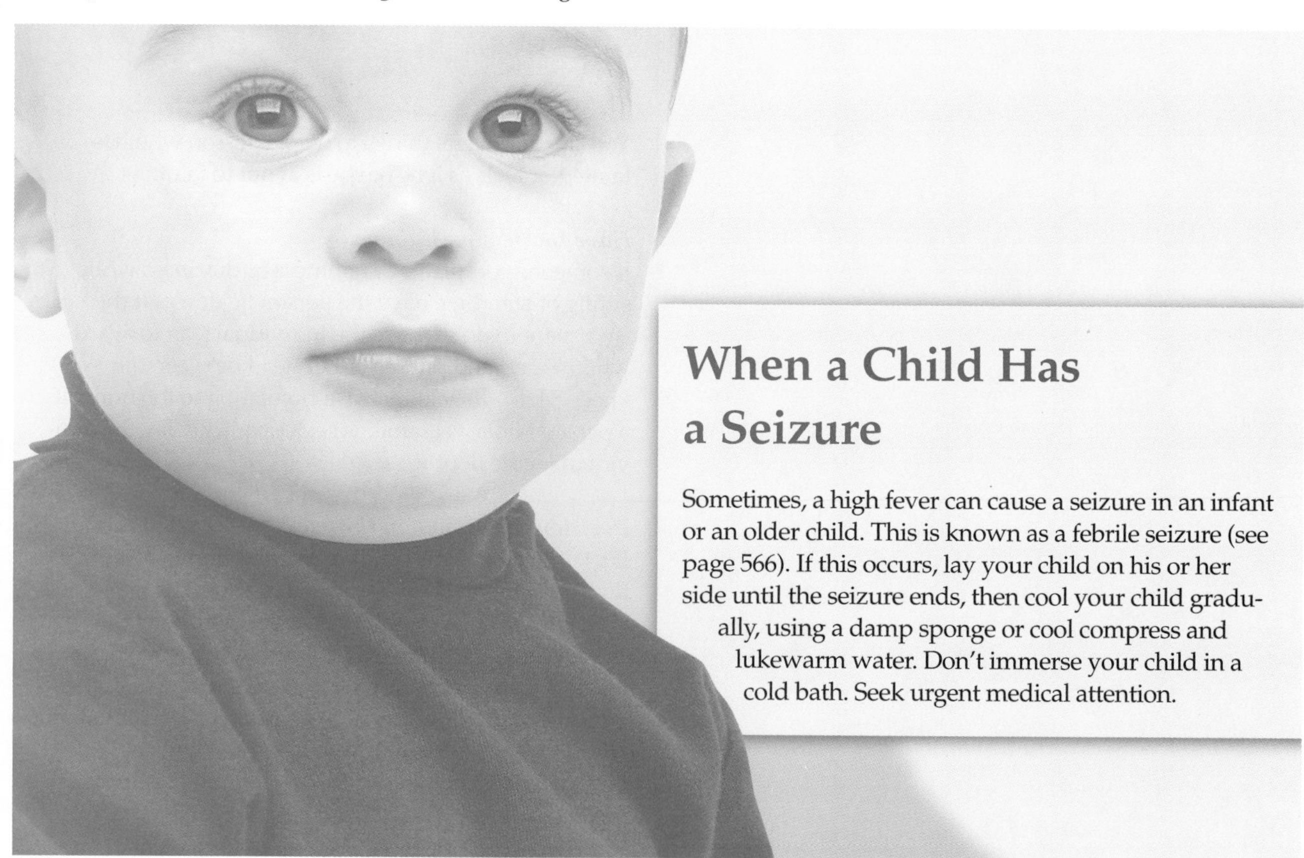

When a Child Has a Seizure

Sometimes, a high fever can cause a seizure in an infant or an older child. This is known as a febrile seizure (see page 566). If this occurs, lay your child on his or her side until the seizure ends, then cool your child gradually, using a damp sponge or cool compress and lukewarm water. Don't immerse your child in a cold bath. Seek urgent medical attention.

When a Fever Becomes an Emergency

Even when you're well, your body temperature varies, and that variation is normal. Doctors usually consider 98.6 F a healthy body temperature. But your normal temperature may differ by a degree or more. In the morning, your temperature is generally lower, and in the afternoon it's somewhat higher.

Fever itself isn't an illness, but it's often a sign of one. A fever tells you that something is happening inside your body. Most likely your body is fighting an infection caused by either bacteria or a virus.

Often, a fever isn't anything to worry about, but sometimes a fever should be evaluated, especially if it's accompanied by other severe symptoms. Contact your doctor in any of the following situations:

- Your temperature is more than 104 F.
- Your temperature has been more than 101 F for more than 3 days.
- A baby younger than 3 months has a temperature of 100.5 F or higher.

Seek emergency medical care if any of these signs or symptoms accompany a fever:

- Severe headache
- Persistent vomiting
- Mental confusion
- A seizure
- Severe swelling of the throat
- Unusual eye sensitivity to bright light
- A stiff neck and significant pain when you bend your head forward
- Difficulty breathing
- Extreme listlessness or irritability
- A bulging soft spot on a baby's head

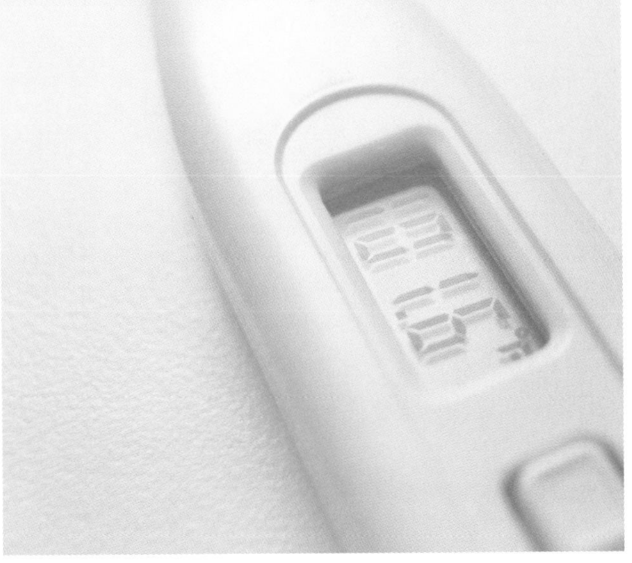

ized, a seizure can occur. A grand mal seizure, also called a convulsion, is an involuntary episode of alternating muscular contractions and relaxations accompanied by loss of consciousness.

Seizures caused by epilepsy are perhaps the most familiar kind, but several other disorders also can produce them. These conditions include kidney failure, meningitis, toxemia of pregnancy, head injury, sudden withdrawal from certain medications, such as benzodiazepines (Librium, Valium, others) and barbiturates (such as phenobarbital or amobarbital), and illegal use of some drugs. Rarely is a seizure the first sign of a brain tumor.

Treatment

When you're with a person having a seizure, take the following actions:

Keep the person from injuring himself or herself

If vomiting occurs, try to turn the person's head so that the vomit is expelled and isn't breathed in (aspirated) to the windpipe or lungs. Clear the area around the person of furniture or other objects to reduce his or her risk of injury during uncontrolled body movements. Don't try to limit the movements of a person who's having a seizure.

Although the person may briefly stop breathing — and a light-skinned person may turn bluish from lack of oxygen — breathing almost invariably returns without the need to assist breathing through cardiopulmonary resuscitation (CPR).

Position the individual on his or her side

Once the seizure is over, position the person on his or her side. This position allows for normal breathing and lets vomit or fluids drain from the mouth and airway. The person may have blood coming from the mouth if he or she bit the tongue or cheek. After the seizure, the person may be confused for a while. Watch the person until there's a complete return of mental function.

Seek emergency help, if necessary

Call for emergency medical help if someone is having a seizure and any one of these is true:

- The person has never had a seizure before.
- The episode lasts more than a few minutes.
- The seizure is a recurrence.

Try to keep at least mental notes about details of the seizure so that you can report them to the doctor. Important observations include the duration of the seizure, the extremities involved, possible factors that may have caused the seizure and any other details that you noticed.

Treat injuries

If the person is injured in a fall associated with the seizure, treat any bumps, bruises or cuts.

FIRST AID AND EMERGENCY CARE

Stroke

A stroke is a condition that results from bleeding into the brain or blockage of normal blood flow to the brain. Another term for stroke is *brain attack.* If you think that you or someone with you is having a stroke, seek immediate medical treatment. Just as with a heart attack, every minute may count. The longer a stroke goes untreated, the greater the potential damage.

Signs and symptoms of stroke include:

- Sudden numbness, weakness or paralysis of the face, arm or leg, usually on one side of the body
- Slurred speech or trouble talking or understanding speech
- Sudden blurred or decreased vision, usually in one eye
- Dizziness, loss of balance or loss of coordination
- Sudden, severe headache, with no apparent cause
- Difficulty swallowing due to lack of coordination

Signs and symptoms of a stroke may last only a few minutes, or they may persist for several hours. Even short-term warning signs should be taken seriously.

Treatment

While waiting for emergency medical help, pay attention to the person's breathing. If breathing ceases, begin assisting the breathing with cardiopulmonary resuscitation (CPR). Minor breathing difficulty may be alleviated by resting the person's head and shoulders on a pillow. Watch for vomiting. If vomiting occurs, turn the head to the side so that the vomit can drain out the mouth instead of being breathed into the lungs. Don't allow the person to eat or drink anything. If paralysis is present, protect the paralyzed limbs from injury that might occur when the person moves about or is transported.

High blood pressure crisis

High blood pressure is a common medical problem — about one-quarter of Americans have high blood pressure (hypertension). Unlike high blood pressure, which is very common, a high blood pressure crisis is extremely uncommon. The condition occurs when blood pressure in your arteries rises to a dangerously high level — when the second, or bottom, number in the blood pressure reading (diastolic pressure) spikes to more than 140 millimeters of mercury (mm Hg). A normal diastolic reading is 84 mm Hg or lower.

In addition to a very high blood pressure, the following signs and symptoms may indicate a high blood pressure crisis:

- Severe headache, accompanied by confusion and blurred vision
- Chest pain
- Nausea and vomiting
- A seizure

Possible causes of a high blood pressure emergency include a stroke, toxemia of pregnancy, kidney failure

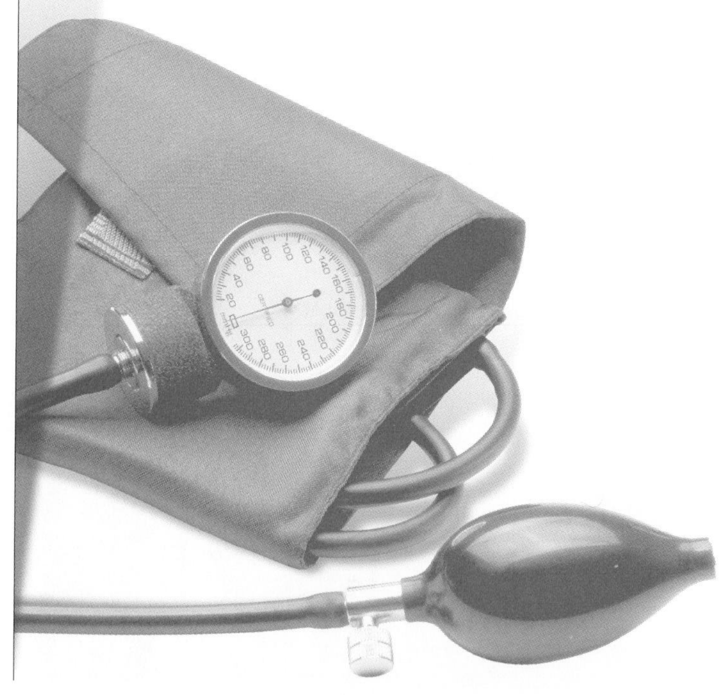

and severe drug interactions. The cause also can be simpler, such as not treating your high blood pressure or forgetting to take your medication, both of which can allow blood pressure to become dangerously high.

Treatment

When someone exhibits symptoms of a high blood pressure crisis, seek emergency medical help. While waiting for help to arrive, the person experiencing the symptoms should lie down and rest. Don't give him or her anything to eat or drink.

Diabetic emergency

People with diabetes may experience several types of emergencies. Among them are insulin shock, coma from increased blood acids and coma caused by high blood sugar.

Insulin shock

Insulin shock is also referred to as an insulin reaction or low blood sugar (hypoglycemia). This condition results from too much insulin and too little sugar (glucose) in your blood. Low blood sugar is most common among people with diabetes who take insulin. Rarely, an individual who isn't known to have diabetes may experience low blood sugar.

Signs and symptoms vary, but they may include nervousness, hunger, feelings of apprehension or confusion, cold and clammy skin, heavy sweating, loss of consciousness or a seizure. This progression of signs and symptoms may take place in less than an hour.

For people with diabetes who take insulin, blood sugar can decrease for many reasons. Some of the most common of them include:

- Skipping a meal
- Exercising longer or more strenuously than normal
- Not adjusting the medication to accommodate blood sugar changes

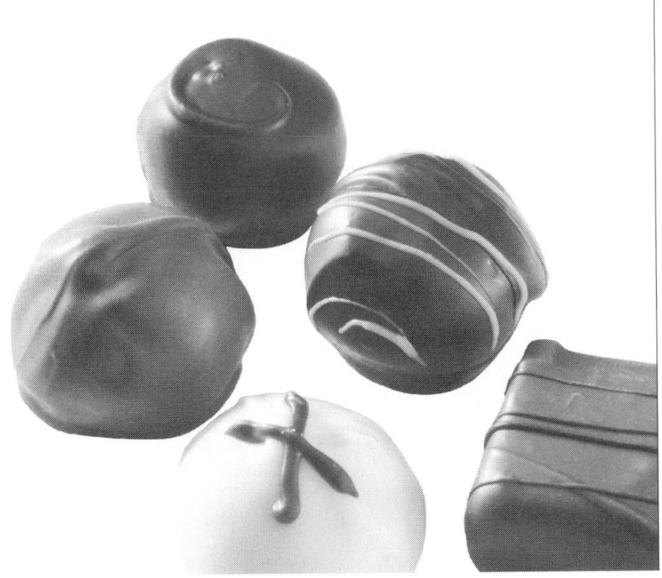

Treatment

Once you identify a person's problem as insulin shock, give him or her some kind of carbohydrate or sugar, if possible. Fruit juices, candy or sugar-containing soft drinks are effective. The person may stubbornly resist taking the food because low blood sugar has left him or her confused.

If the person vomits, wait a few minutes and then give small amounts of the carbohydrate cautiously. If the person is unable to cooperate in swallowing, you can try putting a teaspoonful of a syrup in his or her cheek at intervals of a few minutes. Often, 15 to 30 minutes will pass from the time the sugar is given until symptoms improve.

If the person is unconscious, he or she may need an injection of glucagon just under the skin to reverse the symptoms. Seek medical attention right away if recovery isn't prompt. Remain with the person for an hour or so after the apparent recovery because full mental function sometimes takes that long to return.

Increased blood acids

Increased blood acids, also called diabetic ketoacidosis (DKA), usually occurs when a person with type 1 diabetes (formerly called juvenile or insulin-dependent diabetes) skips an insulin dose, uses too small a dose or is stricken with a serious illness such as pneumonia. The muscle cells become so starved for energy that the body takes emergency measures and breaks down fat. As the fat is changed into energy, it produces blood acids known as ketones.

When a person's level of ketones rise, he or she may experience a variety of signs and symptoms. They begin more slowly than in an insulin reaction and usually progress over several hours or days before becoming severe. Among the signs and symptoms:

- Deep and rapid breathing
- Sweet, fruity smelling breath
- Loss of appetite
- Nausea and vomiting
- Fever
- Stomach pain
- Gradual change in consciousness, perhaps culminating in coma

Treatment

If you're not sure if a person's impaired condition is from an insulin reaction or from DKA, give sugar by mouth — just as you would for an insulin reaction. If there's no improvement within a few minutes, call for emergency medical help.

High blood sugar

Diabetic hyperosmolar syndrome (DHS) causes excessively high blood sugar levels, overwhelming the blood with sugar. The blood cells can't consume this much blood sugar, so the sugar passes from the blood into the urine. The filtering process to remove the excess sugar draws a large amount of fluid from the body and produces severe dehydration. If the person experiencing DHS doesn't consume enough water, the blood sugar progressively elevates and he or she gradually loses consciousness.

Signs and symptoms of DHS include:

- Excessive thirst
- Increased urination
- Weakness
- Leg cramps
- Confusion
- A rapid pulse
- Convulsions
- A coma

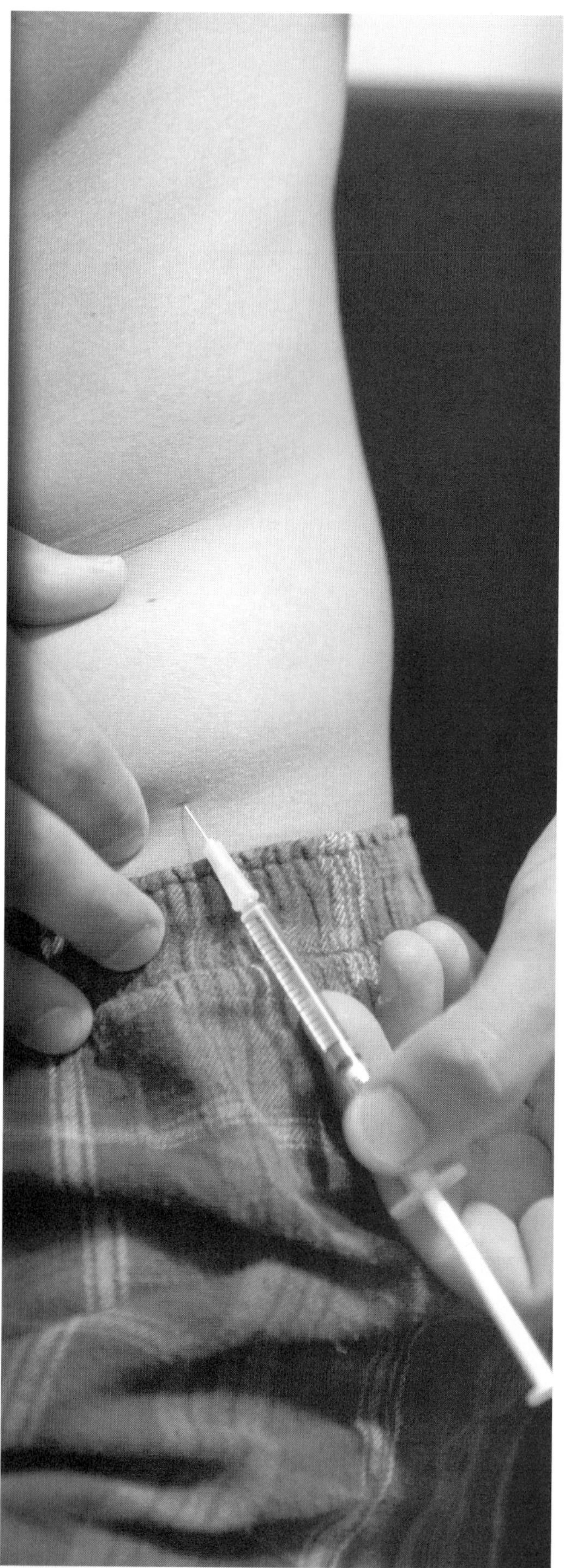

Treatment

If you think someone is experiencing a DHS coma, seek emergency medical help. A coma can be prevented by ensuring that people with diabetes drink generous amounts of water and by treating early signs of the illness promptly.

Poisoning

Any substance swallowed, inhaled, injected or absorbed by the body that interferes with the body's normal functioning is, by definition, a poison. Some poisons are well-known: pesticides, animal poisons and household chemicals bearing printed warnings. But there are many other less familiar poisons.

In fact, almost any nonfood substance is poisonous if taken in large enough doses. Aspirin is an excellent example of a nonfood substance that you might not think is poisonous. This useful medication is found in most homes and is safe when used properly. Yet each year more children die of aspirin overdoses than of overdoses of more familiar poisons, such as household cleaners or antifreeze.

When you suspect poisoning

Sometimes, poisoning is obvious. There's no denying it when a child is seated on the floor, surrounded by aspirin tablets, some half-chewed and others crammed like candy into the mouth. Many times, however, it's hard to tell whether someone has been poisoned. Look for these warning signs if you suspect poisoning:

- Burns or redness around the mouth and lips
- Breath that smells like chemicals, such as gasoline or paint thinner

PREVENTION TIP

Overdoses of seemingly harmless medications, such as the common painkillers aspirin and acetaminophen, take many lives each year. Numerous other over-the-counter (nonprescription) drugs also are dangerous if taken in large doses, especially by a child or an older adult. These include sedatives, antihistamines and iron and vitamin supplements.

Keep all of your prescription and nonprescription drugs and vitamins stored out of the reach of children. Don't put them out where they'll be available to a toddler, such as on a kitchen counter, on a bedside table or in a purse. Buy childproof packages. If you have medications that must be refrigerated, put them on a high shelf out of reach and sight of children. If medications are placed in drawers, lock them or install a latch that toddlers can't open.

Poison Control Centers

A poison control center isn't a hospital or treatment center. It's essentially a library staffed by experts familiar with poisoning. The information it can offer may be crucial to delivering fast and appropriate treatment in a poisoning emergency.

Poison control centers are often affiliated with large hospitals or emergency departments. Most states have at least one regional center required to meet reference material and personnel standards established by the American Association of Poison Control Centers. In most regions, the toll-free number to reach a poison control center is 800-222-1222. If that number isn't available in your area, check the emergency numbers in the front of your phone book for the poison control center nearest you.

- Burns, stains and odors on the person, his or her clothing or on the furniture, floor, rugs or other objects in the area in which he or she was playing or working
- Difficulty breathing
- Vomiting or other unexpected medical symptoms

Many conditions mimic the signs and symptoms of poisoning. These include seizures, intoxication, stroke and an insulin reaction. If you can't find any indication of poisoning, don't treat the victim for poisoning, but do call for emergency medical help.

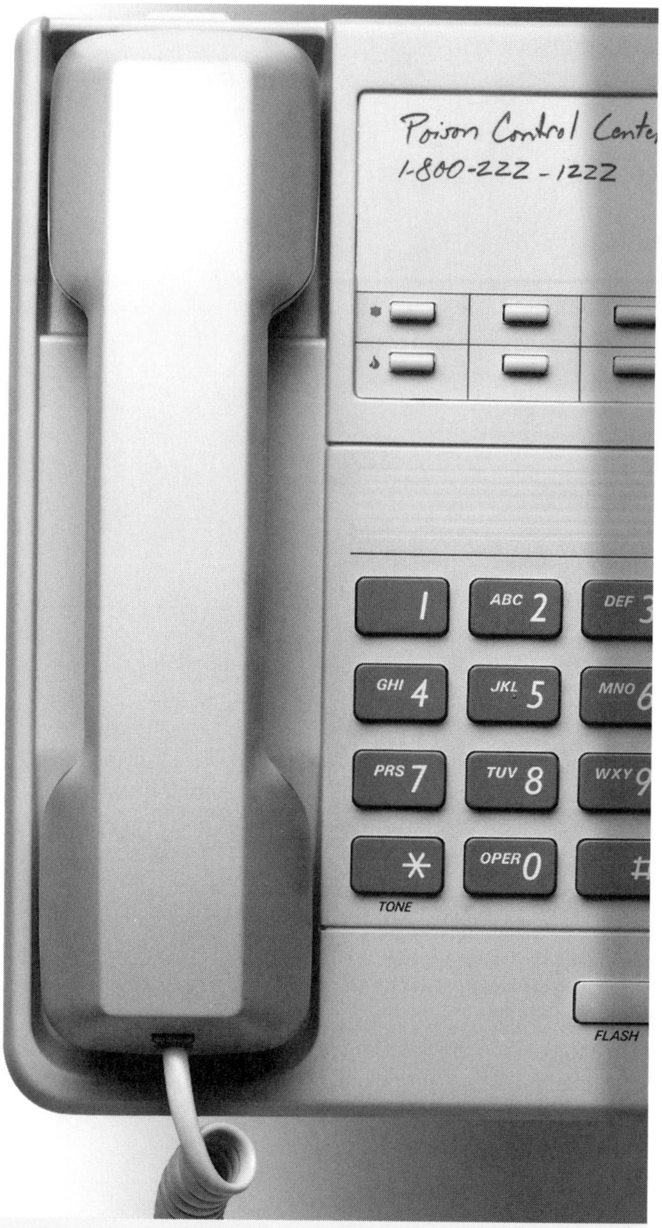

Treatment

If someone is unconscious and you think that he or she has ingested a poison, call for emergency medical help. If the person is awake and alert, take the following steps:

1. Call the poison control center. The toll-free number, which isn't available in all parts of the country, is 800-222-1222. In some communities, a local number is listed with other emergency numbers in the front of the telephone book. If you can't find one of the numbers quickly or if nobody answers immediately, call for emergency assistance or get the person to the nearest emergency department as quickly as possible.
2. When you call the poison control center or other emergency assistance, have the following information ready:
   - The poisoned person's condition, age and weight
   - The product container, for ingredients listed on the label
   - The time the poisoning took place
   - Your name, phone number and location
3. You will be asked other questions too, such as, "How much of the product do you think was consumed?" and "What have you done so far?"

When Not to Induce Vomiting

Some poisons, such as products that contain acids and alkalies, cause so much damage to body tissues they come into contact with that you shouldn't induce vomiting.

Acids you'll commonly find in the house include:

- Toilet bowl cleaners
- Shower cleaners
- Liquid rust remover
- Boric-acid-based laundry soap

Alkalies include:

- Oven cleaners
- Drain cleaners
- Window cleaners
- Liquid fabric softeners

Treatment

If the person who you suspect has ingested poison is unconscious, call for emergency medical assistance or take the individual to a hospital emergency department immediately. If the person is still conscious, call the nearest poison control center for instructions. Instead of inducing vomiting, you may need to dilute the poison or neutralize it with another substance.

To neutralize acids, you may be instructed to give milk of magnesia or another substance. To neutralize alkalies you may be told to give the victim lemon juice or diluted vinegar.

Common Plants That Can Be Poisonous

Name	Poisonous parts
Apricot	Pits
Cherry	Pits
Dieffenbachia	Leaves
English ivy	Entire plant
Foxglove (digitalis)	Entire plant
Holly	Leaves and berries
Jimson weed (thorn apple)	Entire plant
Lily of the valley	Entire plant
Mistletoe	Leaves and berries
Some mushrooms (especially amanita)	Entire plant
Philodendron	Entire plant
Plums	Pits
Poinsettia	Leaves, stem and sap
Potatoes	Sprouts, roots and vines
Rhododendron	Entire plant
Rhubarb	Leaves

4. Don't hang up. After quickly consulting reference materials, the person on the other end of the phone will tell you what to do.
5. Find out if you should induce vomiting. Certain poisons should be vomited; others, such as petroleum products, acids and alkalies, should not be. If you don't know what the poison is, don't induce vomiting.
6. If you're told to induce vomiting in the person who has swallowed the poison, use one of two methods:
   - Insert a finger into the person's mouth and touch the back of the throat. If the person is old enough, it may be easier for him or her to do it.
   - If you have ipecac syrup on hand — and every household with children should — give some to the poisoned person, along with a glass or two of warm water.
7. Whether vomiting is induced or occurs naturally, make sure that the person doesn't inhale (aspirate) vomit into the lungs. A small child can be held over your knees, facedown. A larger person should bend over or lie down on a bed with his or her head hanging over the side. The chin should be lower than the hips. After the person has vomited, give him or her milk or water.
8. Monitor vital signs. Be alert for changes in the person who has been poisoned. If breathing stops, immediately start breathing assistance with cardiopulmonary resuscitation (CPR). Watch for symptoms of shock.
9. If the poison has spilled on the person's clothing, skin or eyes, remove the clothing and flush the skin or eyes with water. You may need to hold the person's eyelids open while flushing the eyes.
10. Go to a hospital emergency department immediately. If you're unable to transport the poisoned person, call for emergency assistance. Take with you the container or packaging in which the poison was stored. If the identity of the poison is unknown, but the person has vomited, take a sample of the vomit for analysis.

Poisonous plants

Many plants — both cultivated and wild — are poisonous if swallowed. Be aware of plants in your home, garden and neighborhood and know which ones are poisonous. For example, apple seeds, potato vines and tomato leaves are poisonous. Lilies of the valley make lovely borders but are poisonous, as are daffodil bulbs, buttercups and the Christmastime favorites: holly and poinsettias.

Signs and symptoms that can result from eating a poisonous plant include:

- Burning pain in the mouth and throat
- Swelling in the throat that may lead to difficulty breathing

- Vomiting
- Abdominal pain or other gastrointestinal distress
- Hallucinations
- Seizures
- Unconsciousness

If you think that someone has ingested a poisonous plant, seek emergency medical help. If the victim is conscious, get a sample of the plant and call the nearest poison control center for instructions. If the person is unconscious, get the victim and the plant sample to a hospital emergency department immediately.

Food poisoning

Unwashed or improperly handled food of almost any sort — raw fish, undercooked meats, contaminated water — can lead to food poisoning. A good example is the potato salad left unrefrigerated for too long at a family picnic.

All foods naturally contain small amounts of bacteria. But when food is poorly handled or improperly cooked or stored, bacteria can multiply in great enough numbers to cause illness. If you eat contaminated food, whether you become ill depends on the organism in the food, the amount of exposure you've had to it, your age and your health. As you get older, your immune cells may not respond as quickly and effectively to infectious organisms. Young children also are at increased risk because their immune systems haven't fully developed.

Food poisoning can cause various types of sickness. If you become ill within 1 to 6 hours after consuming contaminated food or water, you probably have a common type of food poisoning. Signs and symptoms include nausea, vomiting, diarrhea and stomach pain.

Treatment

Rest and drink plenty of liquids. Don't use over-the-counter antidiarrheal medicines because they can slow elimination of the bacteria and toxins from your system. In most cases, the symptoms will go away within 12 hours. If they don't, contact your doctor if the symptoms are severe or if you have other health problems, such as diabetes, AIDS or cancer, that can magnify the effect of the food poisoning.

Prevention

To prevent food-borne illness, take the following steps when handling food:

- Plan ahead. Thaw meats and other frozen foods in the refrigerator, not on the countertop.
- When shopping, don't buy food in dented cans or in jars with bulging lids.
- Before preparing food, wash your hands with soap and water. Rinse produce thoroughly or peel off the skin or outer leaves. Wash knives and cutting surfaces frequently, especially after handling raw meat and before preparing other foods to be eaten raw.

Poison-Proofing Your Home

You can take several steps to protect your children from common household products that could poison them.

- Keep all medicine and poisonous household items, such as bathroom cleaners, in their original containers for easy identification.
- Lock medicine and poisons out of sight and reach of children.
- Keep purses and diaper bags containing medicine out of reach of children.
- Put child-resistant locks on cabinet doors.
- Don't tell your children that their medicine tastes like candy.
- Keep poisonous plants out of reach of children.
- Keep the number of your local poison control center on or near your phone.

Home Canning

Botulism is a potentially fatal food poisoning. You get it from eating foods containing a toxin formed by certain spores in food. Botulism toxin is most often found in home-canned foods, especially green beans and tomatoes.

Symptoms usually begin 12 to 36 hours after eating the contaminated food. They are headache, blurred vision, muscle weakness and eventually paralysis. Some people also report nausea, vomiting, constipation, urinary retention and reduced salivation. These signs and symptoms require immediate medical attention.

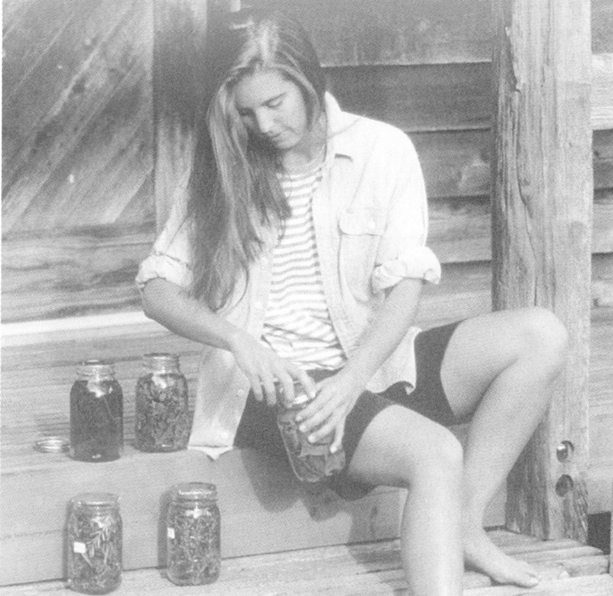

Troublesome Bacteria and How You Can Stop Them

Keep hot food hot. Keep cold food cold. And keep everything — especially your hands — clean. If you follow these three basic rules, you'll be less likely to get food poisoning.

Bacterium	How it's spread	Signs and symptoms	To prevent its spread
Campylobacter jejuni	Contaminates meat and poultry during processing if poultry feces contact meat surfaces. Other sources: unpasteurized milk, untreated water.	Severe diarrhea (sometimes bloody), abdominal cramps, chills and headache. Symptoms begin (onset) within 2 to 11 days. Lasts 1 to 2 weeks.	Cook meat and poultry thoroughly. Wash knives and cutting surfaces after contact with raw meat. Don't drink unpasteurized milk or untreated water.
Clostridium perfringens	Meats, stews and gravies. Commonly spreads when serving dishes don't keep food hot enough or when food is chilled too slowly.	Watery diarrhea, nausea and abdominal cramps. Fever is rare. Onset within 1 to 16 hours. Lasts 1 to 2 days.	Keep hot food hot. Hold cooked meats above 140 F. Reheat to at least 165 F. Chill foods quickly. Store foods in small containers.
Escherichia coli (*E. coli*) 0157:H7	Contaminates beef during slaughter. Spreads mainly by undercooked ground beef. Other sources: unpasteurized milk, unpasteurized apple cider, human stools and contaminated water.	Watery diarrhea may turn bloody within 24 hours. Severe abdominal cramps, nausea and vomiting. Usually no fever. Onset within 1 to 8 days. Lasts 5 to 8 days.	Cook beef to an internal temperature of 160 F. Don't drink unpasteurized milk or unpasteurized apple cider. Wash your hands after using the bathroom.
Salmonella	Raw or contaminated meat, poultry, milk and egg yolks. Spreads by knives, cutting surfaces or infected people who don't wash their hands before handling food.	Severe diarrhea, watery stools, nausea, vomiting and fever of 101 F or more. Onset within 6 to 72 hours. Lasts 1 to 14 days.	Cook meat and poultry thoroughly. Don't drink unpasteurized milk. Don't eat raw or undercooked eggs. Keep hands, cutting utensils and cutting surfaces clean. Wash hands after using the bathroom.
Staph (*Staphylococcus aureus*)	Spreads by hand contact, coughing and sneezing. Grows on meats and prepared salads, cream sauces and cream-filled pastries.	Explosive diarrhea, nausea, vomiting and abdominal cramps. Onset within 1 to 6 hours. Lasts 1 to 2 days.	Don't leave high-risk foods, such as potato salads and creamed sauces, at room temperature for more than 2 hours. Wash hands and utensils before preparing food.
Vibrio vulnificus	Raw oysters and raw or undercooked mussels, clams and whole scallops.	Chills, fever and skin lesions. Onset 1 hour to 1 week. May be fatal in individuals with a weakened immune system.	Don't eat raw oysters. Make sure all shellfish is thoroughly cooked.

- When cooking meat, use a meat thermometer. Cook red meat to an internal temperature of 160 F, poultry to 180 F. Cook fish until it flakes easily with a fork. Cook eggs until the yolks are firm and are no longer runny.
- When storing food, always check expiration dates. Use or freeze fresh red meats within 3 to 5 days after purchase. Use or freeze fresh poultry, fish and ground meat within 1 to 2 days. Refrigerate or freeze leftovers within 2 hours of serving.

Bites and Stings

A dog, spider, snake or even another person can deliver dangerous bites. And a bee, jellyfish or scorpion can pack a potent sting. Every one of these injuries should be treated promptly to minimize risks of infection, an allergic reaction or other complications.

Animal bites

Most animal bites are from household pets. But stray dogs and wild animals such as skunks, raccoons and bats also bite thousands of people each year. Animals living in the wild are especially dangerous because they're more likely to carry rabies than are household pets. Any animal — household, stray or wild — that bites a human should be impounded and checked for rabies.

Treatment

Any bite that penetrates the skin should be treated by a doctor for cleaning and possible antibiotic treatment. Your doctor will also want to make sure that you've had a tetanus shot within the past 10 years, or 5 years if the wound is very dirty or contaminated. You may need a booster shot (see page 16).

If the bite produces a deep puncture wound, if the skin in the bitten area is badly torn or if bleeding persists, apply pressure to stop the bleeding, then seek emergency medical help.

Watch for infection

No matter if the wound is superficial or deep, watch for any signs of infection in the hours and days after the bite. Swelling, redness, pus draining from the wound or increasing pain should be reported immediately to your doctor.

Certain diseases can be transmitted through bites and scratches, in which case in addition to swelling or soreness at the site of the wound, you may experience fever, headache and other flu-like symptoms. If these symptoms develop, consult your doctor.

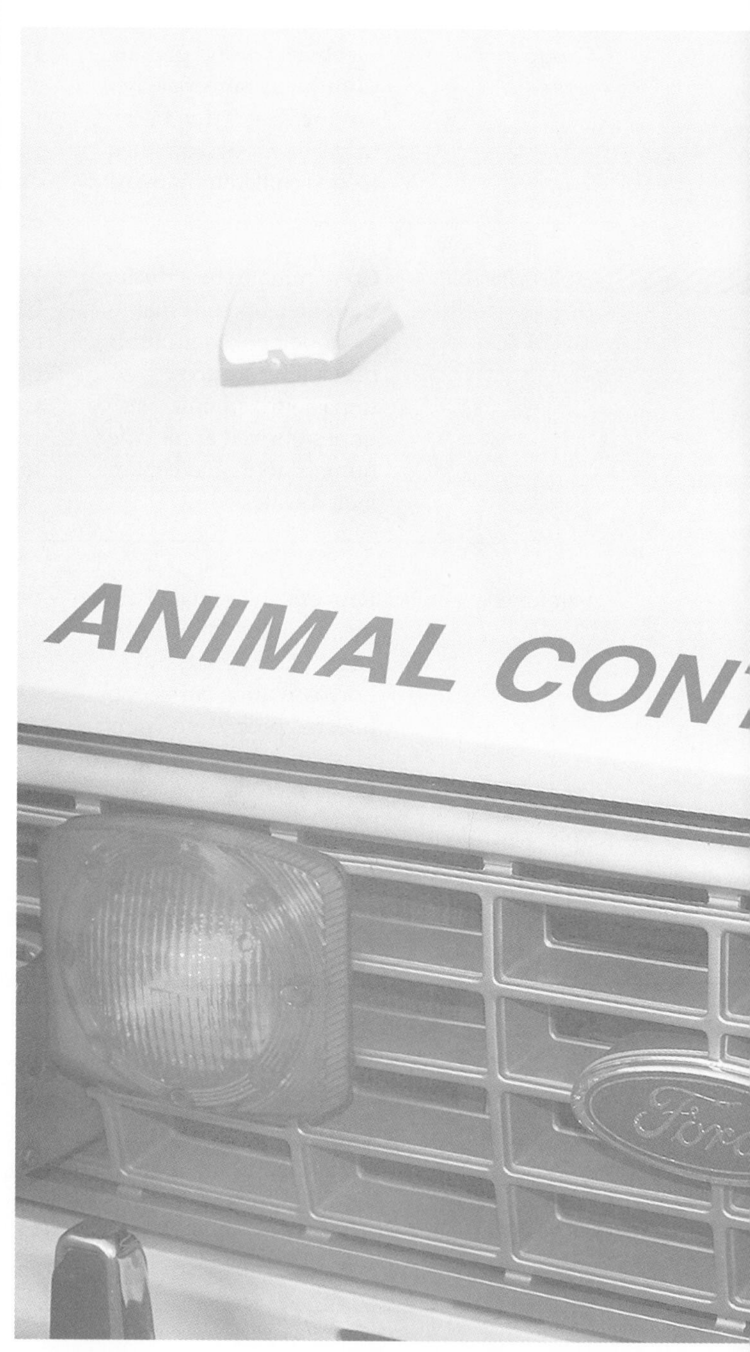

Human bites

There are two types of human bites. The first is what we usually think of as a bite: an injury that results from flesh being caught between the teeth of the upper and lower jaws. The second is an unintentional bite: a "fight bite" that occurs when, in the act of striking another person, an assailant accidentally cuts his or her knuckles on the opponent's teeth. In either kind of bite, the flesh can be torn open and infected with bacteria from saliva.

Human bites are among the most dangerous mammal bites — in part because people frequently delay seeking treatment out of embarrassment or fear of legal action. Human bites are also dangerous because of the considerable risk posed by the bacteria found in the

Risk of Rabies

Many wild animals carry rabies, but so can the usually friendly pooch next door, especially if it comes in contact with wild animals and hasn't been immunized for rabies.

Rabies is caused by a virus that affects the brain. It's most often transmitted to humans by saliva from an infected animal. However, a bite isn't necessary to transmit the virus. Even a licking from an infected animal can spread the disease if the animal's saliva comes in contact with a scratch or wound on your hand, arm or leg. Indirect contact can also produce rabies. If the animal comes into contact with your bedsheets, for example, the virus can linger there.

The rabies virus often takes 3 to 7 weeks to produce symptoms, and it can take much longer. If you think you may have been exposed to rabies, consult your doctor or health department right away. For more information on rabies, see page 498.

In the event of an unprovoked bite by an animal, the animal should be caught, confined and observed by a veterinarian for 7 to 10 days. If you can't catch the animal — as is often the case with wild animals — then contact your local health department, natural resources or law enforcement officials. The animal may have to be killed, and in such a way that its brain isn't damaged. Health or law enforcement officials will arrange testing of the animal for rabies. If the animal isn't caught, presume that it has rabies and act accordingly.

Symptoms

Often the first symptom of rabies is a tingling sensation that develops at the site of the animal bite. Skin at the site often becomes very sensitive. As the virus spreads, foaming at the mouth may occur — a consequence of excess saliva that can't be swallowed. Uncontrolled irritability and confusion may follow, alternating with periods of calm. Convulsions and paralysis leading almost inevitably to death will result if the rabies virus is untreated. In later stages, the virus may be present in the person's saliva and can infect others.

Treatment

Extensive cleaning of the wound with soap and water, followed by irrigation of the wound by a health care professional, should be carried out as soon as possible after the bite. Your doctor then must decide whether to treat you for rabies. Treatment consists of an antibody, about half of which is injected directly into the wound and the other half injected into a muscle, often at the hip. A vaccination then follows, which usually consists of five injections on five separate days over a 28-day period.

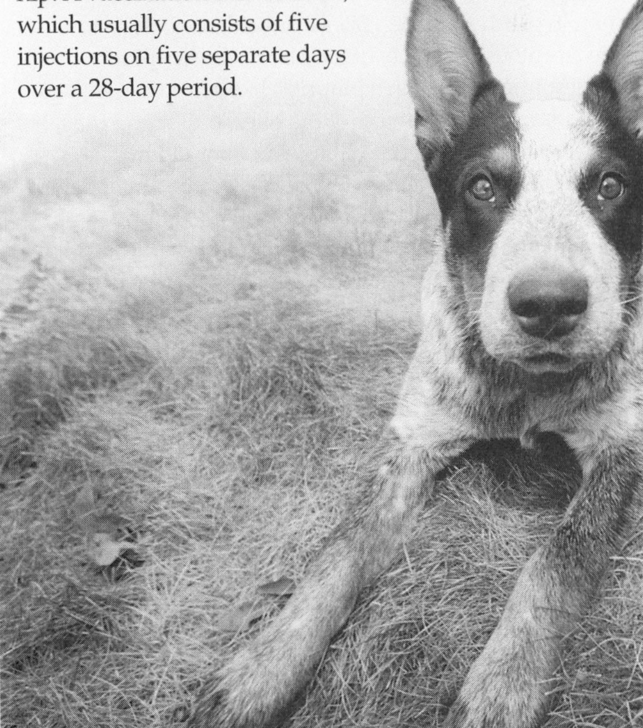

human mouth. Carried by the saliva, the bacteria enter the tissues at the site of the bite and can lead to serious infections. Bites also pose a risk of injury to tendons and joints when the cut extends below the skin.

Treatment

If you sustain a human bite that breaks the skin, see a doctor promptly. (A toddler's bite often leaves only a mark or a bruise.) Stop the bleeding by applying pressure, wash the wound thoroughly with soap and water, and bandage the wound. Then visit your doctor or an emergency department. Don't treat a human bite yourself. A serious infection could put you at risk of a prolonged hospital stay, permanent joint stiffness and even amputation.

Insect and spider bites and stings

Venom, saliva or other toxins injected into your skin are what cause the symptoms of an insect or spider bite or sting. With minor bites the reaction is temporary and limited to the area of the bite. A bump rises on your skin, the area may itch for a few hours, and then over a period of days the skin irritation and discomfort disappear. Typically, the bites of insects such as mosquitoes, fleas, flies, bedbugs, ants and chiggers follow this course.

However, your entire body can be affected if the venom is potent, as is the case with certain spiders and scorpions, or if you are hypersensitive to bee, wasp and yellow jacket stings.

Spider bites

Black widow and brown recluse spiders are present throughout the contiguous United States and are common in southern states. Bites from either can lead to serious illness. The bite of the black widow spider causes little more than a pinprick-like sensation — some victims aren't even aware of the bite. At first you may experience only slight swelling and faint red marks where you were bitten. Within a few hours, you'll begin to feel intense pain and stiffness. Other signs and symptoms include chills, fever, nausea and severe abdominal pain. The bite of a black widow spider is rarely lethal.

If you're bitten by a brown recluse spider, you'll experience mild stinging, followed by local redness and intense pain within 8 hours. A fluid-filled blister forms at the site and then develops into a deep, growing ulcer. Your body's reactions can vary from a mild fever and rash to nausea and listlessness. In rare cases death can result.

Tick bites

Ticks can be a threat to human health because some carry infections that can be transmitted to humans by a bite. Wood ticks can carry Rocky Mountain spotted fever, and deer ticks — which are much smaller than wood ticks — can carry Lyme disease. Rocky Mountain

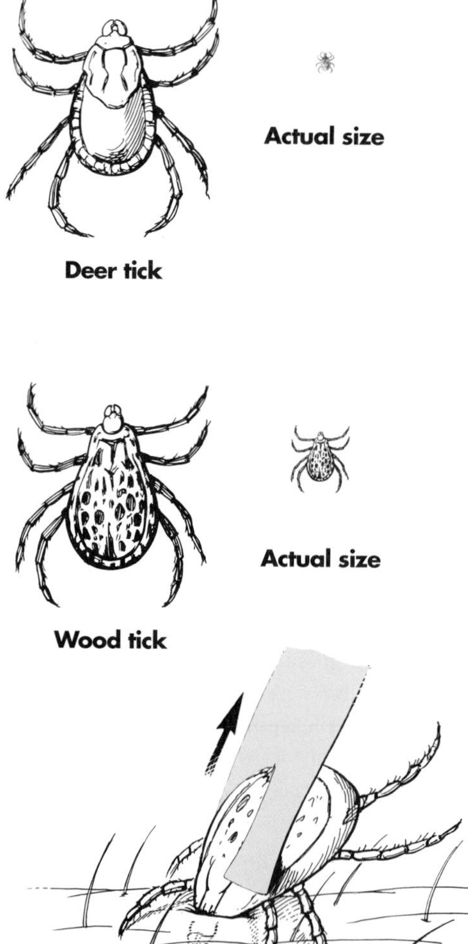

To remove a tick, use tweezers to slowly and steadily pull the tick away from the skin.

PREVENTION TIP

When walking in wooded or grassy areas, wear shoes, long pants tucked into socks and long-sleeved shirts. This can help prevent tick bites. In addition, stick to trails and avoid walking through bushes and tall grass. Insect repellents will often repel ticks. Among the longest lasting and most effective are products containing DEET. However, the American Academy of Pediatrics recommends that repellents used on children contain no more than 10 percent DEET. Tick-proof your yard by clearing brush and leaves and by keeping woodpiles in sunny areas.

spotted fever can produce chills and fever, severe headaches, widespread aches, restlessness and a red rash occurring between days 2 and 6 of the fever (see page 504). Lyme disease may produce symptoms similar to arthritis, but it may also cause a wide variety of other reactions (see page 504).

If you have a circular eruption on your skin after spending time in an area where ticks may live, it's possible that you've been bitten by a tick carrying an infectious agent. This can happen even though you didn't see the tick.

If you find a tick crawling on your skin, carefully remove it. Don't crush it between your fingers. Instead, burn it, bury it or flush it. Wash your hands afterward. If the tick has already bitten you and is holding on to your skin, remove it by gently grasping it near its head or mouth, preferably with a tweezers. Don't squeeze or crush the tick, but pull carefully and steadily. After the tick has been removed, wash the area thoroughly and apply antiseptic to the bite area. Watch carefully for the next week or two for a rash or other signs of illness.

Scorpion stings

Scorpions are found in the southwestern United States. Some scorpions have potentially lethal venom that's injected by a sting. Because it's difficult to distinguish the highly poisonous scorpions from nonpoisonous ones, all scorpion stings are treated as emergencies.

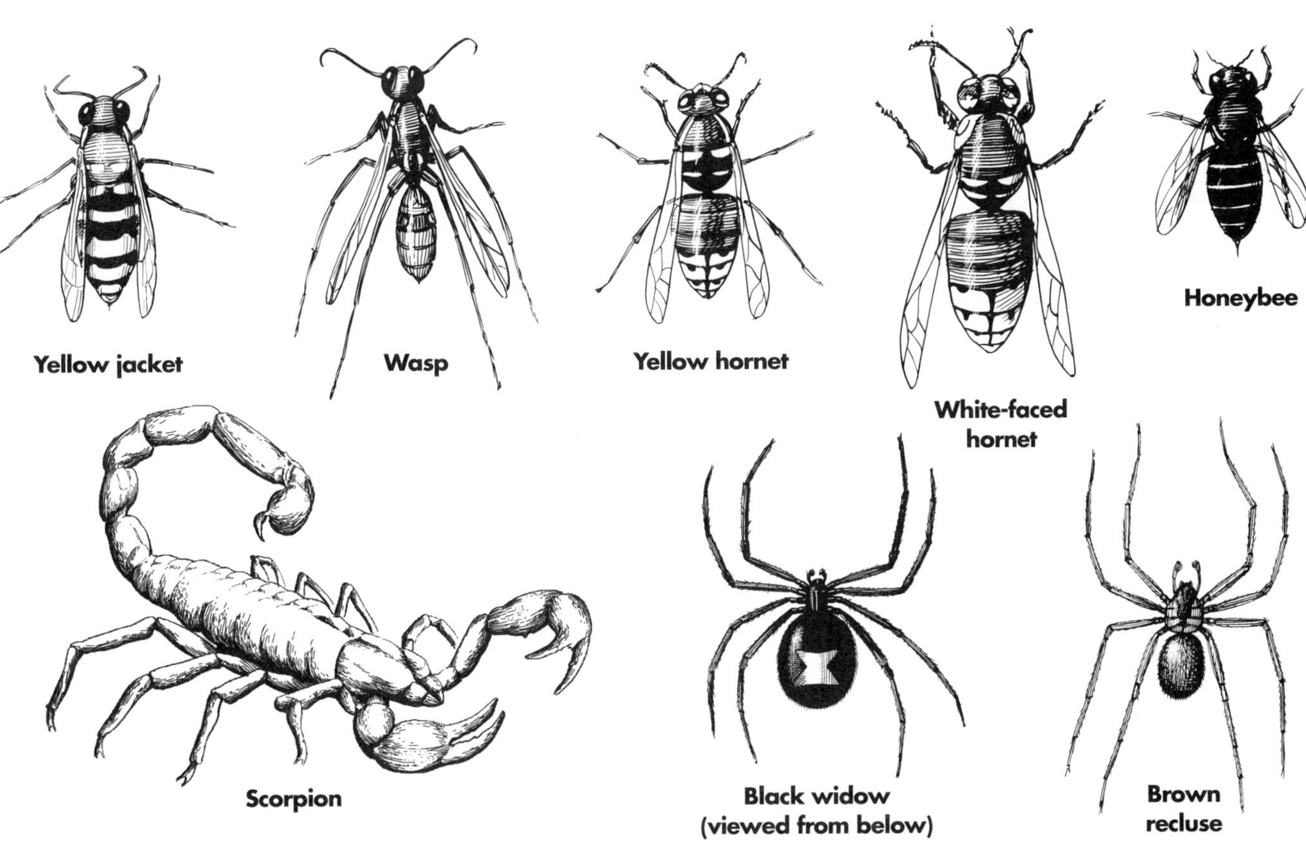

Distinctive marks of individual insects are emphasized to help identify them.

Other stings

Approximately 1 person in 50 is allergic to the venom of bees, wasps, hornets, yellow jackets or fire ants. For such sensitive individuals, getting stung can cause a life-threatening allergic response known as anaphylactic shock (see page 545).

Signs and symptoms include:

- Constriction of airways, including a swollen throat, resulting in breathing difficulty
- Shock associated with a severe decrease in blood pressure
- Rapid pulse
- Hives and welts below the skin surface (angioedema)
- Nausea, vomiting or diarrhea
- Dizziness, mental confusion, slurred speech or extreme anxiety
- Swelling of the lips and tongue
- Flushing of skin and intense itching

Treatment

Mild insect and spider bites and stings can often be treated with a baking soda paste, a cold washcloth or ice cubes to reduce the pain and swelling. You may also apply a hydrocortisone ointment or calamine lotion to reduce itching and inflammation. If you've been stung, check to see if a stinger is in the wound. If so, carefully remove it before treating the site. If you tend to react severely to bites or stings, consult your doctor.

If you're bitten or stung by a highly poisonous insect or spider — such as a black widow or brown recluse spider — or one that you're allergic to, seek emergency medical care.

While waiting for help to arrive:

1. Try to remain calm. Excessive excitement or activity increases the flow of venom through your bloodstream.
2. If you've been stung by an insect and you have an emergency kit containing antihistamine tablets and a syringe of adrenaline (epinephrine), prescribed by your doctor, use it.
3. Apply a clean cloth dampened with cold water or lined with ice to the bite or the sting. Remove it after 5 minutes.
4. If the sting or bite is on an arm or a leg, keep the limb dangling down so that gravity helps slow the circulation of the toxin.

Snakebites

Most snakes aren't poisonous, but a few are — such as rattlesnakes, coral snakes and water moccasins. So, unless you've been trained in identifying and handling snakes, avoid contact with any snake.

If you're bitten by a snake, it's important to determine whether the snake is poisonous. If it is, you'll need emergency treatment. Most poisonous snakes in North America have slit-like (elliptically shaped) eyes. Their

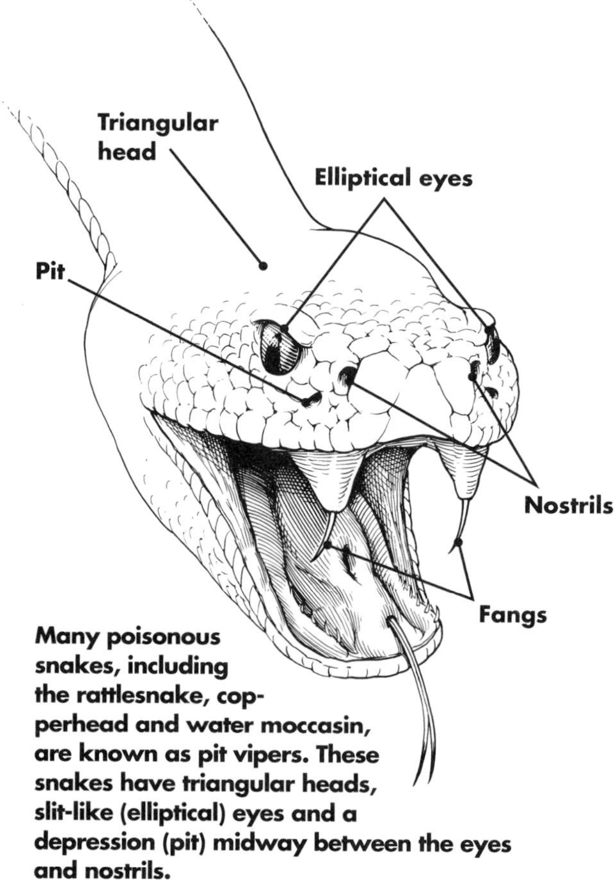

Many poisonous snakes, including the rattlesnake, copperhead and water moccasin, are known as pit vipers. These snakes have triangular heads, slit-like (elliptical) eyes and a depression (pit) midway between the eyes and nostrils.

heads are triangular with a depression, or pit, midway between the eyes and nostrils on both sides of the head, which is why they're also known as pit vipers. Other characteristics unique to certain poisonous snakes:

- Rattlesnakes make a rattling sound by shaking the rings at the end of their tail.
- Water moccasins have a whitish, cottony lining in their mouth.
- Coral snakes have red, yellow and black rings along their length.

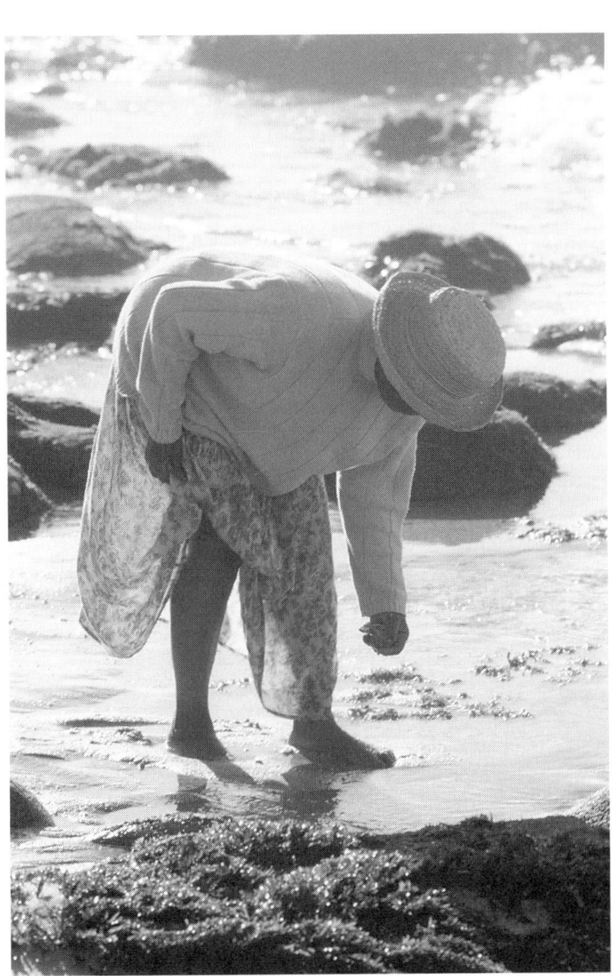

Treatment

If a nonpoisonous snake has bitten you, wash the bite thoroughly, cover it with an antibiotic ointment and bandage it. In general, this type of bite is more scary than dangerous. If you know or suspect the snake was poisonous, remain as quiet and still as possible after the bite. Lie down and, if possible, keep the bitten area lower than the level of your heart. This position uses gravity to help slow the circulation of the venom.

To treat someone with a snakebite from a poisonous snake:

1. If the area changes color, begins to swell or is painful, the snake was probably poisonous. Have the person lie down and, if possible, keep the bitten area lower than the level of the heart.
2. If the bite is on an arm or leg, immobilize the area with a splint, just as you would for a broken bone.
3. Don't cut the wound in an attempt to remove the venom. However, if you have a snakebite kit with a suction device, use that.
4. Call for emergency help or get to the nearest emergency department as quickly as possible.

Sea organism stings

Several sea organisms, including the jellyfish and Portuguese man-of-war, carry venom in their tentacles. This venom can be discharged on contact, in some cases even after the animals are dead. Stinging and pain are the key symptoms, along with a red, hive-like line of lesions. If a considerable amount of venom is injected, you may also experience shortness of breath, nausea and stomach cramps. Severe stings can lead to muscle cramps, fainting, coughing, vomiting, difficulty breathing and, in rare cases, death.

Portuguese man-of-wars are found in the waters of the Atlantic Ocean, ranging from Canada to the West Indies and Mediterranean Sea. They also live in the Pacific Ocean near Hawaii and southern Japan.

Treatment

If you're stung by a jellyfish or Portuguese man-of-war:

1. Get out of the water. Pain and cramps can be disabling, and you could drown.
2. Neutralize the poison. Sprinkle the area with meat tenderizer, vinegar, salt, sugar or even dry sand,

which contains some salt. Gently apply the material to the wound. This often offers quick relief.
3. Cleanse the wound. After 15 to 20 minutes, gently wash the area with seawater. Don't use fresh water and don't rub the skin because either action could trigger discharge of more venom.
4. Remove any stinging tentacles. Apply a paste made of seawater and sand (or baking soda, talcum powder or flour). Scrape the residue with a knife or other sharp object, such as a clamshell. It's best to wear gloves or use a towel when removing the Portuguese man-of-war debris.
5. Apply over-the-counter hydrocortisone ointment to reduce redness and swelling. A local anesthetic ointment, such as benzocaine or lidocaine, helps relieve pain, and a calamine-type lotion reduces itching.
6. For severe stings, seek emergency medical care.

Foreign Bodies

Children and adults alike occasionally get foreign objects in body openings — especially the eyes, ears and nose. Sometimes, you can get the objects out without the help of a doctor. Other cases require a doctor's expertise and equipment.

In the eyes

An eye often clears itself of foreign airborne objects, such as specks of dirt, by automatically tearing up and blinking. If you have something in your eye and tearing and blinking aren't enough to get rid of it, treat the condition promptly to avoid damage that can be caused by scratches, infection or exposure to chemicals.

Clearing your own eye

If an object is in your eye and no one is available to help you, try to remove the foreign matter yourself by flushing the eye with clear water as follows: Fill an eyecup or small juice glass with clean water. Position the eyecup or glass with its rim resting on the bone at the base of your eye socket and pour the water in, keeping the eye open. Even if you think the object has been removed, flush your eye if it still hurts and looks red. If you don't succeed in clearing the eye, seek emergency medical help.

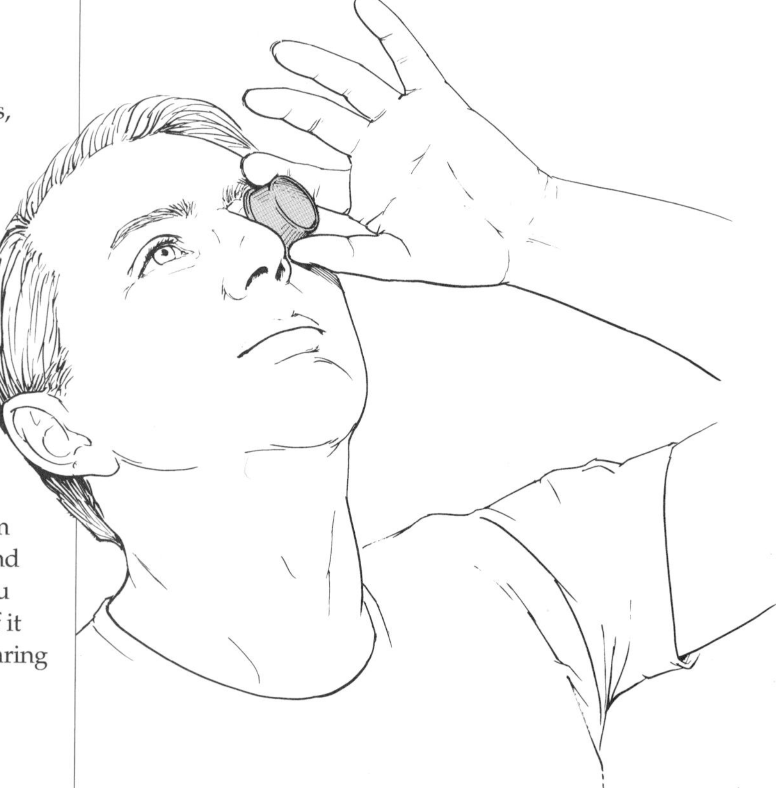

To remove a small object from your eye, flush it with a small amount of clean water.

Clearing someone else's eye

To clear someone else's eye:
1. Wash your hands before examining the eye. Seat the person in a well-lighted area.
2. Try to locate the object in the eye. Examine the eye by gently pulling the lower lid downward and instructing the person to look up. Reverse the proce-

PREVENTION TIP

A few simple steps can go a long way toward avoiding eye injuries:
- Wear goggles when working with tools.
- Wear safety glasses for sports.
- Pick up sticks and other loose objects on the lawn before mowing.
- Don't lean over a battery when attaching jumper cables.
- Store household chemicals out of reach of children.
- Supervise children at play, especially when they're playing with toys that can cause eye injuries, such as spring-loaded toy guns.

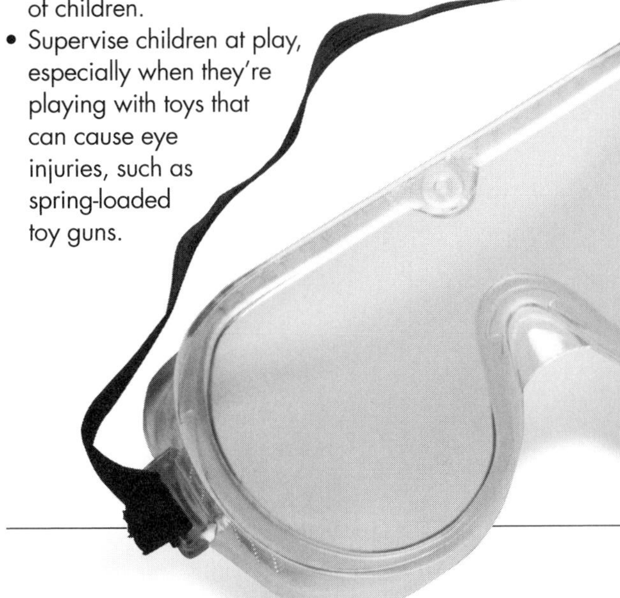

dure for the upper lid by holding the upper lid and telling the person to look down.
3. If it appears that the object is embedded in the eyeball, cover the eye with a sterile pad if available or a clean cloth. Don't try to remove the object. Go to the nearest emergency department for assistance.
4. If the object is large and makes closing the eye difficult, cover it with a paper cup and tape the cup to the face and forehead. Seek emergency medical assistance.
5. If the object is floating in the tear film or on the eye surface, try to flush it out or remove it manually. While holding the upper or lower lid open, use a moistened cotton swab or the corner of a clean cloth to remove the object. If you're unable to remove the object easily, cover both eyes with a soft cloth and seek emergency medical help.
6. If you do succeed in removing the object, flush the eye with an eye-irrigating solution or clean water.
7. If pain, redness or vision problems persist, seek emergency medical care.

In the ears

Children often insert objects into their ears, such as seeds, bits of plastic or tiny toys. Sometimes, an insect or an airborne object will accidentally enter the ear.

Treatment
If an object becomes lodged in an ear:
1. Don't try to remove the object by probing with a cotton swab, matchstick or any other tool. This risks pushing the object farther into the ear and damaging the fragile structures of the middle ear.
2. If the object is clearly visible, is pliable and can be easily grasped with a tweezers, gently remove it.
3. If the object isn't an insect, try using the pull of gravity: Tilt the head to the affected side. You may try shaking the person's head gently in the direction of the ground to try to dislodge the object.
4. If the object is an insect, tilt the person's head so that the ear with the insect is up. You can try to float the insect out by pouring a small amount of warm — not hot — mineral oil, olive oil or baby oil into the ear. As you pour the oil, you can ease the entry of the oil by straightening the ear canal: Pull the ear gently backward and upward. The insect should suffocate and may float out in the oil bath.
5. Don't use oil to remove any object other than an insect. And don't use this method if there's any indication of a perforation in the eardrum, such as pain or bleeding or discharge from the ear.
6. If these methods fail and the person continues to experience pain in the ear, reduced hearing or a sensation of something lodged in the ear, see a doctor as soon as possible.

In the nose

The nose is a favorite place for children and grown-up jokesters to insert things, such as a drinking straw, marble or piece of candy. Sometimes the object gets stuck.

Treatment
Try the following:

1. Direct the person with the object in the nose to breathe through the mouth until the object is removed. This helps avoid inhaling it.
2. Don't probe at the foreign object with a cotton swab, a matchstick or other tool. This risks pushing the object farther into the nose.
3. If the object is clearly visible, is pliable and can be easily grasped with tweezers, gently try to remove it.
4. Have the person gently blow his or her nose to try to free the object. Caution him or her to not blow the nose hard or repeatedly.
5. With a young child who can't blow his or her nose, you can try gently blowing once into the child's mouth, while at the same time pinching closed the unblocked nostril.
6. If these methods fail, seek emergency medical help.

In the windpipe and lungs

When an object is accidentally inhaled, sometimes it lodges in the windpipe (trachea) or the lungs. If an inhaled object causes choking, use the Heimlich maneuver to try to dislodge it. If that doesn't work, seek emergency medical help.

In some cases, a foreign body lodged in the windpipe or the bronchial tubes doesn't inhibit breathing, but it does constitute a health hazard. If you or someone with you inhales a foreign object, consult a doctor.

Swallowed

Occasionally, children swallow objects such as coins, pins, buttons, fruit pits and small toys. These foreign bodies usually pass through the digestive system without causing a problem, but sometimes they can become lodged.

Seek emergency help if the following signs or symptoms appear:

- Difficulty swallowing
- Spitting up saliva
- Abdominal pain or vomiting

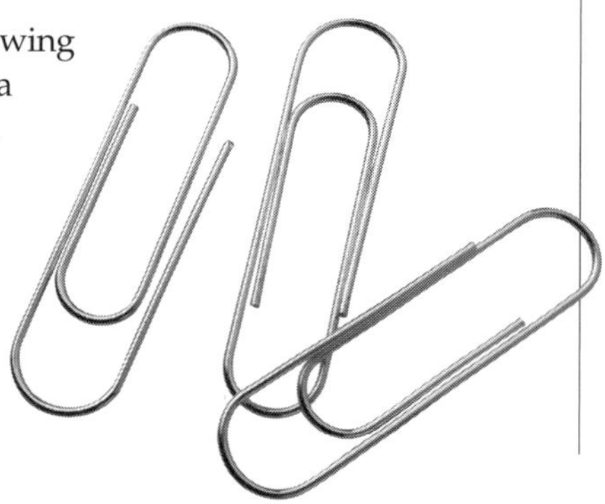

Children and Button Batteries

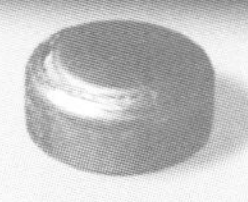

Button-sized batteries are common in portable electronic equipment, such as cameras, watches and hearing aids. To a curious child, these shiny objects can be intriguing. They're also dangerous when swallowed.

Button batteries contain dangerous alkali fluids. Some also contain potentially life-threatening amounts of mercury. If released into the stomach or intestine, the battery fluid may eat through the lining, producing signs and symptoms such as abdominal pain and tenderness, constipation, vomiting and fever.

If your child swallows a button battery, seek emergency medical care. Surgery may be necessary to remove the battery.

Store unused batteries out of reach of children. When disposing of used batteries, don't toss them into a wastebasket that a toddler can easily explore.

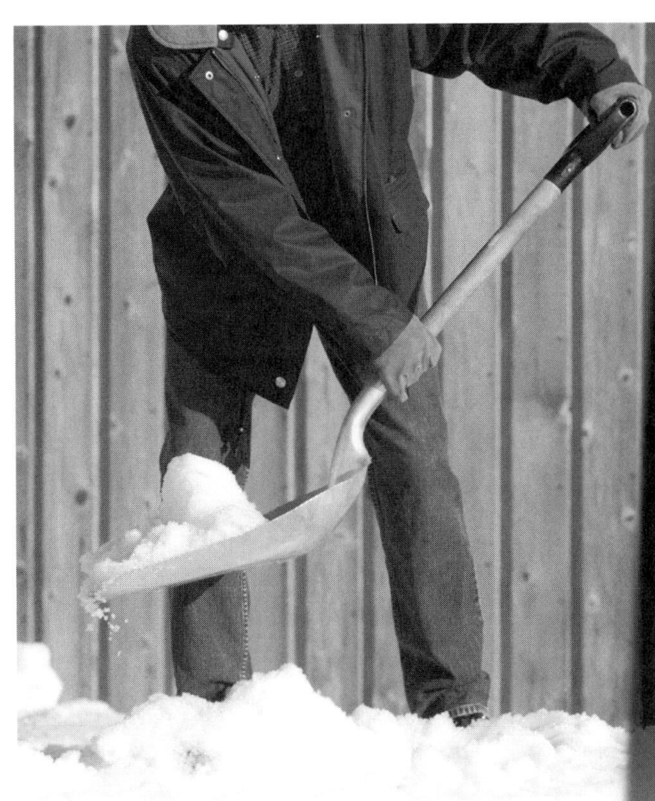

Cold-Related Emergencies

Overexposure to cold and damp weather can lead to frostbite or hypothermia.

Frostbite

When your skin is exposed to subfreezing temperatures, it and the underlying tissues may freeze. This condition is called frostbite. Wind and wet clothing can make the problem worse.

Frostbite can affect any part of your body, but your hands, feet, nose and ears are most susceptible because they're small and often exposed. Anyone can get frostbite, but people with circulatory problems are at greater risk. This includes people with atherosclerosis and those taking medication for a heart condition. Excessive consumption of alcohol or other drugs also puts you at increased risk.

The first sign of frostbite may be a slightly painful tingling sensation. This is often followed by numbness. Your skin may be hard, pale and cold. The area is likely to have a definite lack of sensitivity to touch. As the area thaws, the flesh becomes red and painful. In severe cases, the flow of blood to the affected area may stop. If this happens, seek immediate medical attention to try to reverse the damage.

Treatment

The first step in treating frostbite is to slowly warm the affected skin:

1. If possible, get out of the cold.
2. If you must remain outside and your hands are frostbitten, warm them by putting them on warmer areas of your body. You can tuck your hands into your armpits. If your nose, ears or face is frostbitten, warm the area by covering it with dry, gloved hands. If the skin tingles as it warms and has a burning sensation, circulation is returning. If numbness remains during warming, seek emergency medical care.

Altitude Sickness

If you live at a low altitude and make a trip to an altitude of more than 8,000 feet, you might experience altitude sickness. This condition is sometimes called acute mountain sickness. It can cause headache, nausea, fatigue, sleeplessness, shortness of breath and loss of appetite. It usually develops several hours after arriving at a high altitude, and it may last for several days. Skiers who travel to mountain slopes from lower elevations are commonly affected.

More serious forms of altitude sickness can produce severe breathing distress or severe brain illness that can become fatal if not treated.

Treatment

You can minimize the effects of mild altitude sickness by increasing your fluids and carbohydrates. In addition, your doctor may prescribe certain medications if you know that your travel plans will take you to high altitudes. For serious altitude sickness, you'll need to descend to a lower altitude. Oxygen and rest also are helpful.

3. Don't rub the affected area. Doing so can damage frozen tissues. Never rub snow on frozen skin.
4. If your feet are affected, don't walk.
5. Don't smoke. Nicotine shrinks your blood vessels and may reduce circulation.
6. If you aren't able to get emergency help, warm severely frostbitten hands or feet in warm — not hot — water.
7. Don't apply other heat sources, such as a heating pad, because you could burn the tissue.
8. Don't rewarm a frostbitten area if it's likely to refreeze. This can increase the damage.

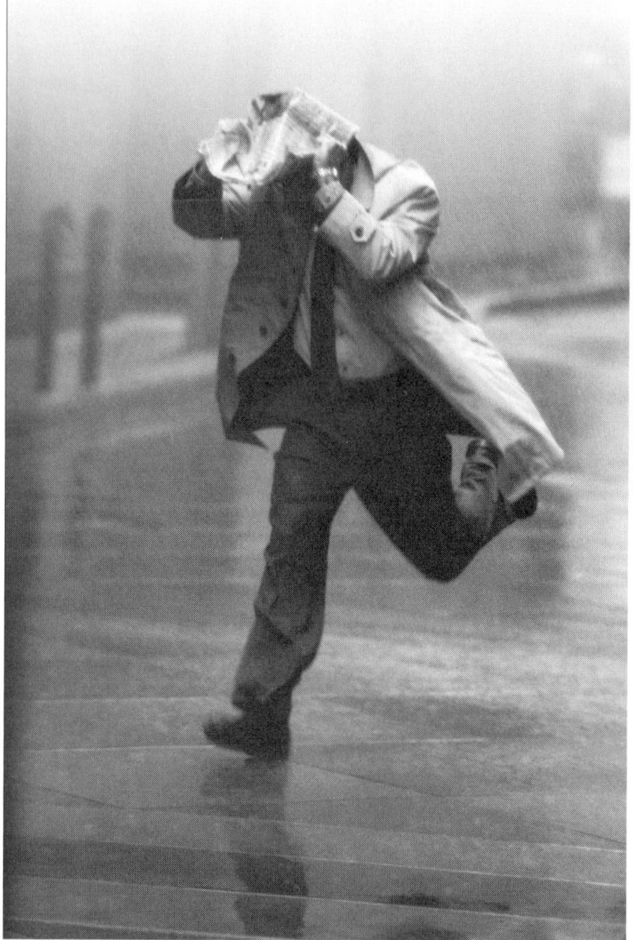

Hypothermia

Under most conditions your body is able to maintain a steady and healthy temperature. However, when you're exposed for prolonged periods to cold temperatures or a cool, damp environment — particularly if your clothing is wet or damp — the body's control mechanisms may fail to keep your body heat at a normal level. When you lose more heat than your body can generate, hypothermia begins. Common causes of hypothermia are falling into cold water and not wearing adequate warm clothing in winter weather.

The key sign of hypothermia is a body temperature that drops below 94 F. A normal body temperature is 98.6 F. Other signs and symptoms of hypothermia include:

- Shivering
- Slurred speech
- An abnormally slow rate of breathing

PREVENTION TIP

You can do several things to prevent injury from frostbite and hypothermia:

Stay dry
Your body loses heat faster when your skin is wet from rain, snow or sweat.

Protect yourself from the wind
Wind robs heat from your body by blowing it away from you. Exposed skin is especially vulnerable and can freeze in minutes when wind combines with subfreezing temperatures. Here's an example of what the wind can do. An outdoor temperature of -20 F combined with a 10 mph wind produces a wind chill factor of -46 F.

Wear warm clothing
Choose clothes that shield and breathe. Layers of light, loosefitting clothes trap air, which adds insulation. As an outer layer, wear something that's water-repellent and windproof.

Cover your head, neck and face
Much of your body heat is lost as it rises from the top of your body. Cap the heat in.

Wear warm socks and mittens
If you're going to be in subfreezing temperatures for more than a few minutes, wear two layers of socks. In addition, wear mittens, which protect your fingers more effectively than do gloves.

Stay alert to numbness
If part of your body gets so cold that it starts feeling numb, that's a clue your skin is beginning to freeze. Take time to rewarm yourself.

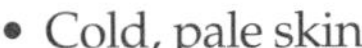

- Cold, pale skin
- Loss of coordination
- Tiredness, lethargy or apathy

Symptoms usually start with a gradual loss of mental sharpness and physical ability. If you're experiencing hypothermia, you may in fact be unaware that you need emergency medical treatment.

Older adults, young children and very thin people are at particular risk of hypothermia. Malnutrition, heart disease, diabetes and excessive consumption of alcohol or other drugs also put you at increased risk.

Treatment

To treat hypothermia:

1. If possible, get the person with hypothermia out of the cold.
2. If going indoors isn't possible, get the person out of the wind, cover his or her head and insulate him or her from the cold ground.
3. Remove the person's wet clothes and cover him or her with dry, warm clothes or blankets.
4. Call for emergency medical help.
5. While waiting for help to arrive, watch the person's breathing. If it stops, begin mouth-to-mouth resuscitation immediately.
6. If emergency help isn't available, warm the person with a bath of 100 F to 105 F. This water should be warm to the touch, but not hot. If this isn't possible, try to warm the person by sharing your body heat.
7. Don't give the person alcohol. Alcohol dilates blood vessels and gives only a temporary sensation of warmth. This dilation also increases the body's heat loss through the skin, further decreasing body temperature. Give the person warm nonalcoholic drinks, unless he or she is vomiting, in which case the individual should have nothing to drink.

Heat-Related Emergencies

Excessive sun exposure or heat can damage your skin and cause your body to overheat.

Sunburn

Prolonged exposure to the sun's ultraviolet rays produces red, tender or swollen skin. The skin may also develop water blisters. The swelling and redness of a sunburn are due to inflammation of the skin.

Treatment

Treatment for sunburn depends on the extent of the burn. You can treat most cases of sunburn without having to see your doctor.

PREVENTION TIP

To beat the heat:

Stay out of the sun
Avoid going outside during the hottest part of the day, from noon to 4 p.m.

Limit physical activity
Reserve vigorous exercise for early morning or the evening.

Dress for the heat
Wear clothes that are light-colored, lightweight and loosefitting.

Drink lots of liquids
Drink lots of liquids, but avoid alcohol and caffeine because they can cause dehydration.

Avoid hot and heavy meals
Smaller meals supplemented with healthy snacks are a good idea when the weather gets hot.

- Take a cool bath or shower. Adding a half cup of cornstarch, oatmeal or baking soda to your bath may offer some relief.
- Don't break water blisters because they help protect against infection and speed healing. If they burst, apply an antibacterial ointment on the open areas.
- Take ibuprofen to control the pain and to reduce swelling.

If sunburn is severe, contact your doctor. He or she may give you some medication to decrease your reaction and prevent some of the symptoms. You'll need to treat the sunburn as you would a minor burn.

Heat stress

Under normal conditions, your body's natural control mechanisms help you adjust to the heat: Porous skin allows excessive heat to escape, and perspiration generates a cooling evaporation. However, when you're exposed to high temperatures for long periods — especially when there's little breeze and high humidity — your body's normal control mechanisms may get overwhelmed. They simply can't handle the amount of intense heat bearing down on you. When that happens, problems develop. One of the most serious is heatstroke, which can be fatal.

Heatstroke

The two key signs of heatstroke are:

- A fever of 105 F or higher
- Hot, dry skin

Other signs include fainting, a rapid heartbeat, rapid and shallow breathing and elevated or lowered blood pressure. The person may also be confused or delirious. In extreme cases, seizures, coma and death may occur.

Heatstroke is predictable and preventable. Those most at risk are older adults and the very young. Others at high risk are people with previous heat-related illness and people who are dehydrated, who have heart disease and who drink excessive amounts of alcohol. Alcohol is dehydrating.

Certain medicines also can increase your chances of getting heatstroke. Some medications for motion sickness and depression can impair your ability to sweat. Drinking plenty of fluids, wearing cool clothing and having the ability to sweat are your main protections against heatstroke.

Treatment

The key to successful treatment of heatstroke is recognizing symptoms early. If you suspect that someone has heatstroke, get him or her out of the heat and into a cool spot. A cool, air-conditioned place is best. Call for emergency medical help. Extreme elevation of body temperature is a medical emergency requiring professional treatment to cool the victim, replace lost fluids and monitor heartbeat and breathing.

PREVENTION TIP

Damage to your skin from recurrent sunburns is cumulative, and continued overexposure to ultraviolet radiation can produce long-term problems. These may include skin discolorations, premature aging of your skin, increased wrinkling and skin cancer. To reduce your risk of these conditions, try to avoid being outside for long periods when the sun's ultraviolet radiation is at its peak — between 10 a.m. and 3 p.m. When you are outside for more than few a few minutes, cover exposed areas of skin, wear a broad-brimmed hat and use a sunscreen with a sun protection factor (SPF) of at least 15.

COMPLEMENTARY MEDICINE

Once a burn is completely cooled, a lotion, such as one containing aloe vera, or a moisturizer can make you feel more comfortable and prevent your skin from drying. Aloe vera comes from the aloe vera plant, also known as the burn plant. If you cut or break a leaf of this plant, soothing, healing sap oozes out. This sap has long served as a traditional treatment for burns, rashes and anything that inflames the skin. The sap seems to help reduce inflammation.

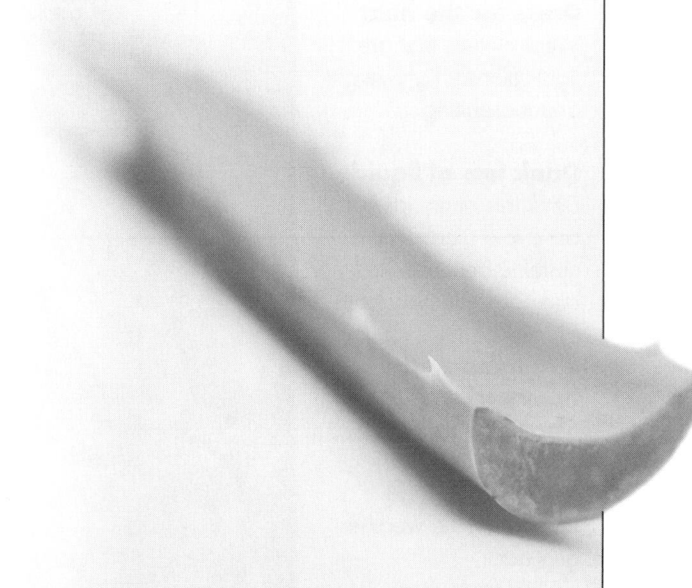

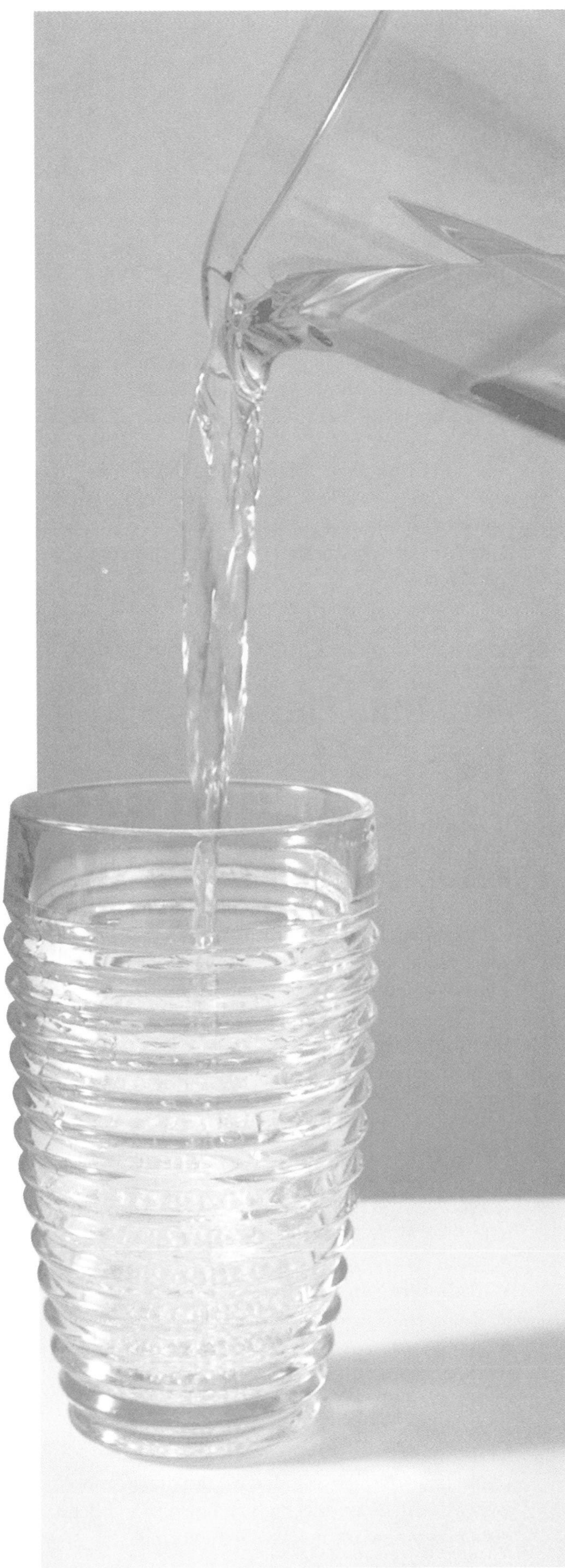

While you're waiting for the emergency help to arrive, cool the person by removing his or her clothing or spraying the person with water mist. Direct some air onto the person, either with an electric fan or by fanning with your hands or a newspaper. If possible, monitor his or her temperature with a thermometer. Stop cooling the person when his or her temperature returns to normal. If breathing stops, begin mouth-to-mouth resuscitation.

Heat exhaustion

Heat exhaustion isn't as dangerous as heatstroke, but it can quickly evolve into heatstroke. Think of heat exhaustion as a failure of your body's cooling mechanisms to respond properly to high temperatures bearing down on your body.

Heat exhaustion more often occurs in people taking water pills (diuretics) because they remove excess fluids from your body. Heat exhaustion can also occur following heavy sweating, when you've not had enough to drink to replace lost fluids.

Signs and symptoms often begin suddenly, which is why the condition is sometimes called heat collapse. They include:

- Faintness
- A rapid heartbeat
- Low blood pressure
- In light-skinned people, an ashen appearance
- Cold, clammy skin
- Nausea

Treatment

If you suspect that someone has heat exhaustion, get him or her out of the heat and into a cooler spot. A cool air-conditioned location is best. Have the person lie down and elevate his or her legs slightly. Loosen or remove most of the person's clothing. Give the person cold water to drink. Sports drinks also are good because they replenish electrolytes as well as fluids. If signs of heatstroke appear, seek emergency medical help.

Heat cramps

Heat cramps are painful muscle spasms that can occur after vigorous exercise and profuse sweating. Your abdominal muscles and other muscles that you use during exercise are most often affected. Heat cramps usually happen in warm environments, but they can also occur in cooler surroundings.

Treatment

If you experience heat cramps:

- Rest briefly and cool down.
- Drink water or a sports drink.
- Eat some salty food, such as salted nuts or salted pretzels. Sodium often helps relieve heat cramps.
- Massage the cramped muscles.

Mental Health Emergencies

Situations affecting an individual's mental health can also create medical emergencies. Similar to a physical injury, a mental illness may also require immediate, professional medical intervention.

Alcohol intoxication and withdrawal

Alcohol is a drug that depresses your central nervous system by acting as a sedative. In some people, the first reaction may be stimulation, but as drinking continues, sedating effects set in. At first, alcohol affects mainly your thoughts, emotions and judgment. But if you continue drinking, the alcohol impairs your speech and muscle coordination. Taken in large enough quantities, it can lead to a coma by depressing the vital centers of your brain.

The signs of alcohol intoxication range from slurred speech, uncoordinated movements and loud, unruly behavior to vomiting, lethargy and unconsciousness. The person may appear flushed and give off a noticeable odor of alcohol.

Serious symptoms can also occur when a habitual drinker suddenly stops drinking. Physical symptoms of withdrawal may occur within hours or several days later. The person may act strangely, hallucinate, become confused or restless and develop a noticeable trembling in the hands. These symptoms are sometimes called delirium tremens (DTs).

Treatment

If you're trying to help someone who you think is intoxicated or experiencing symptoms of alcohol withdrawal, if possible determine if his or her symptoms are caused by drinking alcohol or by withdrawal from it. Ask the person about this in a nonthreatening way. You're more likely to get an honest answer if you appear calm and nonjudgmental instead of angry and condemning. Also ask whether he or she has taken any medications while drinking. Mixing alcohol with certain drugs can cause the person's condition to quickly deteriorate and become life-threatening.

If the person vomits, try to prevent him or her from inhaling (aspirating) vomit into the lungs by bending the head between the knees or, if the person is lying down, by turning the head to one side. Most episodes of alcohol intoxication result in little more than a few hours of nausea and a morning-after headache. However, if you observe any of the following circumstances, seek emergency medical assistance:

- The person is withdrawing from habitual alcohol use.
- The person shows no evidence of alcohol consumption, but his or her behavior is unusual.
- The person is unconscious or has inhaled vomit.

Treating a Hangover

A lot of hangover remedies have been tried, but there isn't much evidence that they help. And some may hurt. Alcohol dehydrates you, as do caffeine drinks that are sometimes used to fight a hangover. If you have a hangover:

- Rest and drink plenty of bland liquids, such as water, soda, low-acid fruit juices and broth. Avoid drinks with lots of citric acid or caffeine.
- Take ibuprofen or another nonprescription pain medication.

Suicidal Thoughts and Behavior

It's commonly said that people who talk about committing suicide don't do it. That's an old cliche that simply isn't true. No two suicidal people are alike, but people thinking about suicide often express themselves with similar behavior. Here are some of those behaviors — common warning signs of potential suicide:

Suicidal threats

Sometimes, an individual will tell others outright that he or she is thinking of committing suicide. Or the person might try a less direct approach, such as saying that everyone would be better off if he or she had never been born or was dead. Take such words as a sign that he or she needs professional help.

Withdrawing from others

People at risk of suicide may be less willing to talk with others or may want to be left alone. Trouble at work or poor grades in school can be other signs of withdrawal.

Moodiness

We all have our ups and downs. But drastic mood swings — an emotional high on one day and deep discouragement the next — aren't normal.

Personality changes

Before someone commits suicide, you may notice marked changes in his or her personality and routines, such as eating or sleeping patterns. For example, an individual who's often shy becomes the life of the party, or an outgoing individual becomes withdrawn.

Risk taking

Uncharacteristically dangerous activities, such as high-speed driving, unsafe sex or drug abuse, may be a sign of an emerging desire to die.

Personal crisis

A major life setback, such as a divorce, a lost job or the death of a loved one, can be difficult for anyone to manage. Among people who are depressed, such a crisis can push them over the edge, triggering a suicide attempt.

Depression

Another warning sign is deep depression. Sometimes, the person is so depressed that he or she has difficulty functioning socially or in the workplace.

Gift giving

Sometimes before committing suicide, a depressed individual will give away his or her cherished possessions, believing that they won't be needed any longer.

- There's evidence that the person has taken alcohol along with other drugs.

Intoxication from other drugs

Many drugs — even prescription medications — can cause serious effects in people who are sensitive to the chemicals in the drug. Mixing drugs, such as alcohol and certain medications or illegally used drugs, can cause interactions that are particularly dangerous and potentially lethal.

Prescription medications

If you experience any of the following signs or symptoms after taking any medication, stop taking it and contact your doctor for advice. More serious signs and symptoms, such as loss of consciousness or seizures, indicate a need for emergency medical attention.

- Severe headache
- Confusion
- Emotional instability
- Anxiety
- Vision problems
- Rashes
- Seizures, a coma or a loss of consciousness

Illegally used drugs

Signs of illegal drug use vary according to the type of drug. With a drug such as marijuana, the effects may be subtle. You might notice dilated pupils or redness about the eyes of the user. You may also notice that the person's speech is faster than normal or is slow and confused.

Some street drugs produce profound changes in mood and thought processes, often resulting in hallucinations. Acute panic reactions may occur, as may a rapid heart rate, high blood pressure and tremors. Other street drugs may lead to a slower pulse, slower breathing and slurred speech, or they may cause depression, anxiety or impulsiveness. Still others produce excitement or euphoria and an absence of sensation, and in high doses they can cause drooling, vomiting, stupor or a coma. When there's a loss of contact with reality (acute psychosis), the person is at a high risk of suicide or violence toward others.

Treatment

Call for emergency medical help if you suspect a person has taken an overdose of drugs. Emergency signs and symptoms include:

- A loss of consciousness
- Breathing that has stopped or seems dangerously slow
- Behavior that's aggressive, fearful, panicky, hostile, delusional or violent

If you believe that the overdose occurred within the past hour, it may be appropriate to induce vomiting.

However, first check with a doctor or a poison control center (see page 379).

People who are long-term habitual drug users will probably experience withdrawal if they suddenly quit taking the drug. During withdrawal there's a danger of delirium tremens (DTs), seizures, or even death if the detoxification process isn't supervised by a trained person. Proper detoxification often takes a week or more of treatment, ideally in a hospital. Seek emergency medical help if you find someone experiencing signs of acute drug withdrawal.

Sudden personality changes

Sudden personality changes can result from drug use or from a severe form of mental illness. A quiet and thoughtful person can suddenly become disoriented, delirious or violent, and a previously outgoing person can become withdrawn, depressed or even suicidal.

If you find yourself dealing with a person who's acting or talking in a bizarre way, start by trying to talk calmly to that person. Try to reassure the individual that you're there to help. Listen and respond gently. With eye contact and a nonthreatening manner, try to establish some kind of interaction.

If the person has threatened suicide or harm to others, try to determine if the person is armed. Don't deal with someone who has a weapon and has threatened to use it. In addition, don't attempt to restrain a violent person unless you have proper training. A person in a disturbed state — especially if it's induced by drugs — can be more dangerous and stronger than you may imagine.

Call for emergency medical help or the police if the person is disoriented, agitated or poses a danger. Also seek help if you're unable to communicate with the person. A person reacting in this manner needs immediate medical attention.

Treatment

If a friend or a family member talks about committing suicide or behaves in a way that leads you to believe that suicide is a possibility, treat the person with respect and seriousness and seek professional help as soon as possible. Contact your family doctor, a mental health professional or a local suicide hot line. These sources will be able to suggest where you can get immediate help for the person. In the meantime, keep a close eye on him or her to prevent an opportunity for the suicide.

If you encounter a person who has just attempted suicide, seek emergency medical help. If the person has stopped breathing, begin assisting the breathing with mouth-to-mouth resuscitation. If the person is bleeding, try to stop the bleeding. If it appears the person has ingested a poison or taken an overdose of pills, try to find out what the person has taken and how much. Call a poison control center. ■

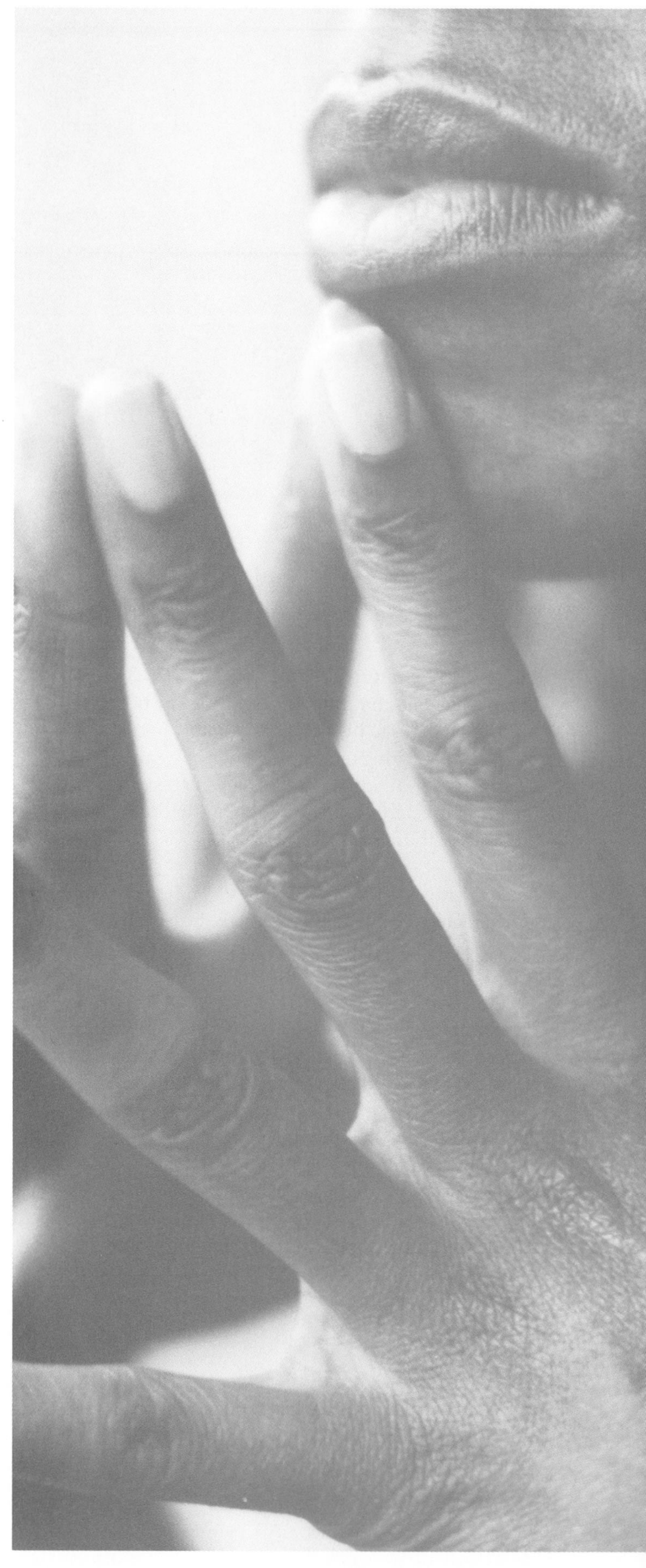

Visual Guide: Anatomy and Common Disorders

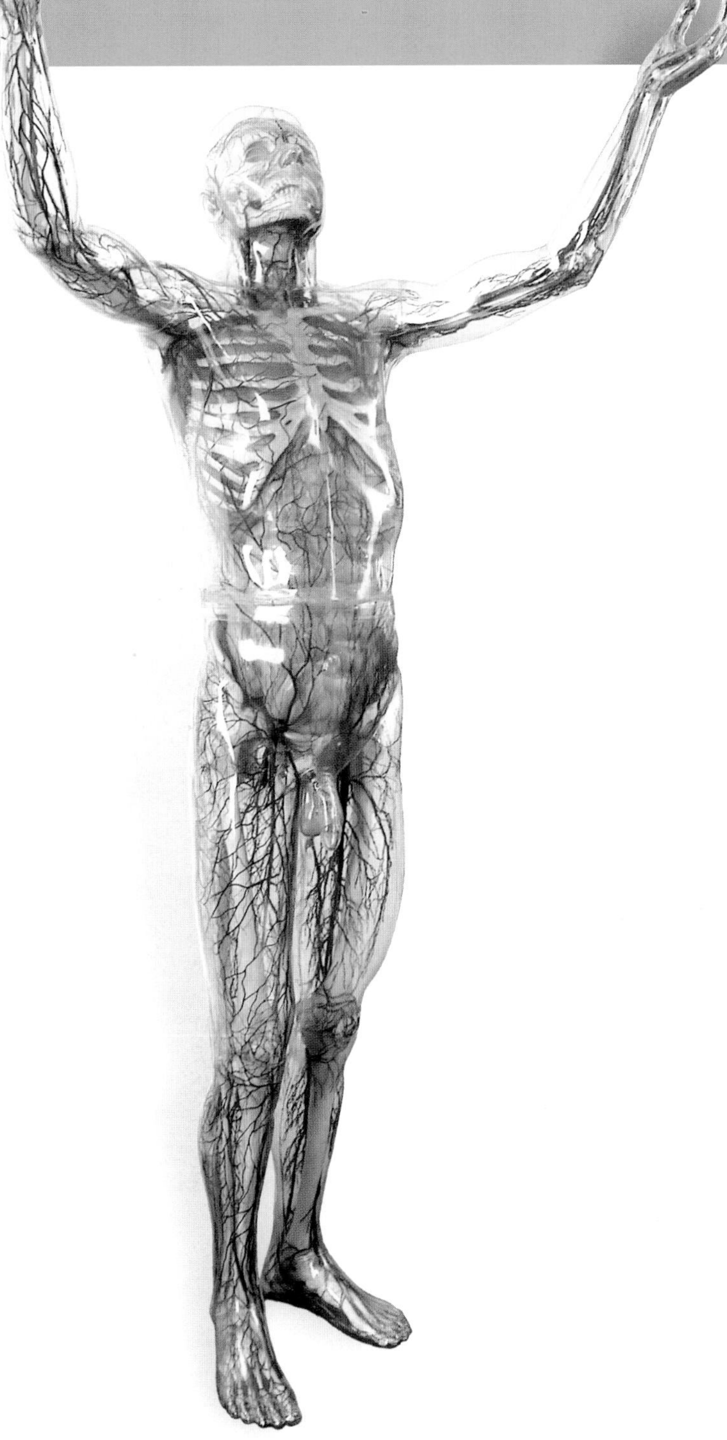

Bones and Joints

There are approximately 206 bones in your body. All of them are alive and continually changing, providing mobility, support and protection for your body. Some bones contain marrow, a soft core that manufactures blood cells. Ends of bone that meet at a joint are cushioned with a layer of cartilage, which absorbs shock or weight involved in movement. Ligaments bind the joint together, connecting bone to bone.

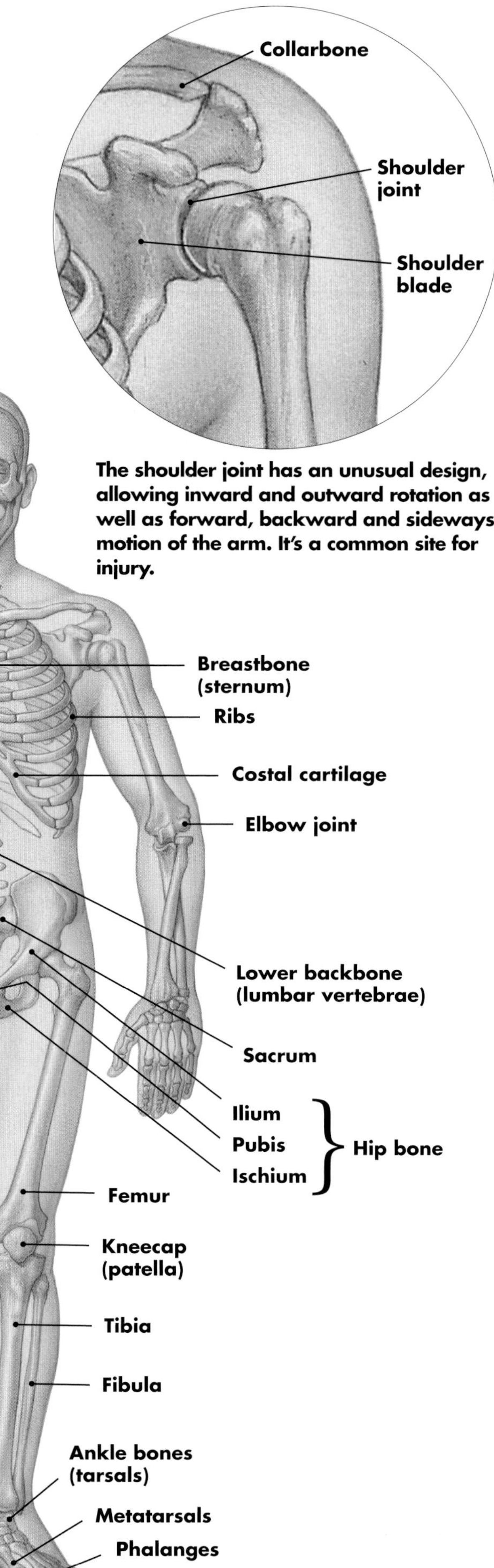

The shoulder joint has an unusual design, allowing inward and outward rotation as well as forward, backward and sideways motion of the arm. It's a common site for injury.

The knee joint has a hinge design, allowing bending (flexion) and straightening (extension) of the leg. It is also a common location for injury.

Your skull and vertebrae protect your brain and spinal cord. A column of bones called vertebrae makes up the spine. In between the vertebrae are spongy structures called disks. The vertebrae and disks are held together by a network of ligaments.

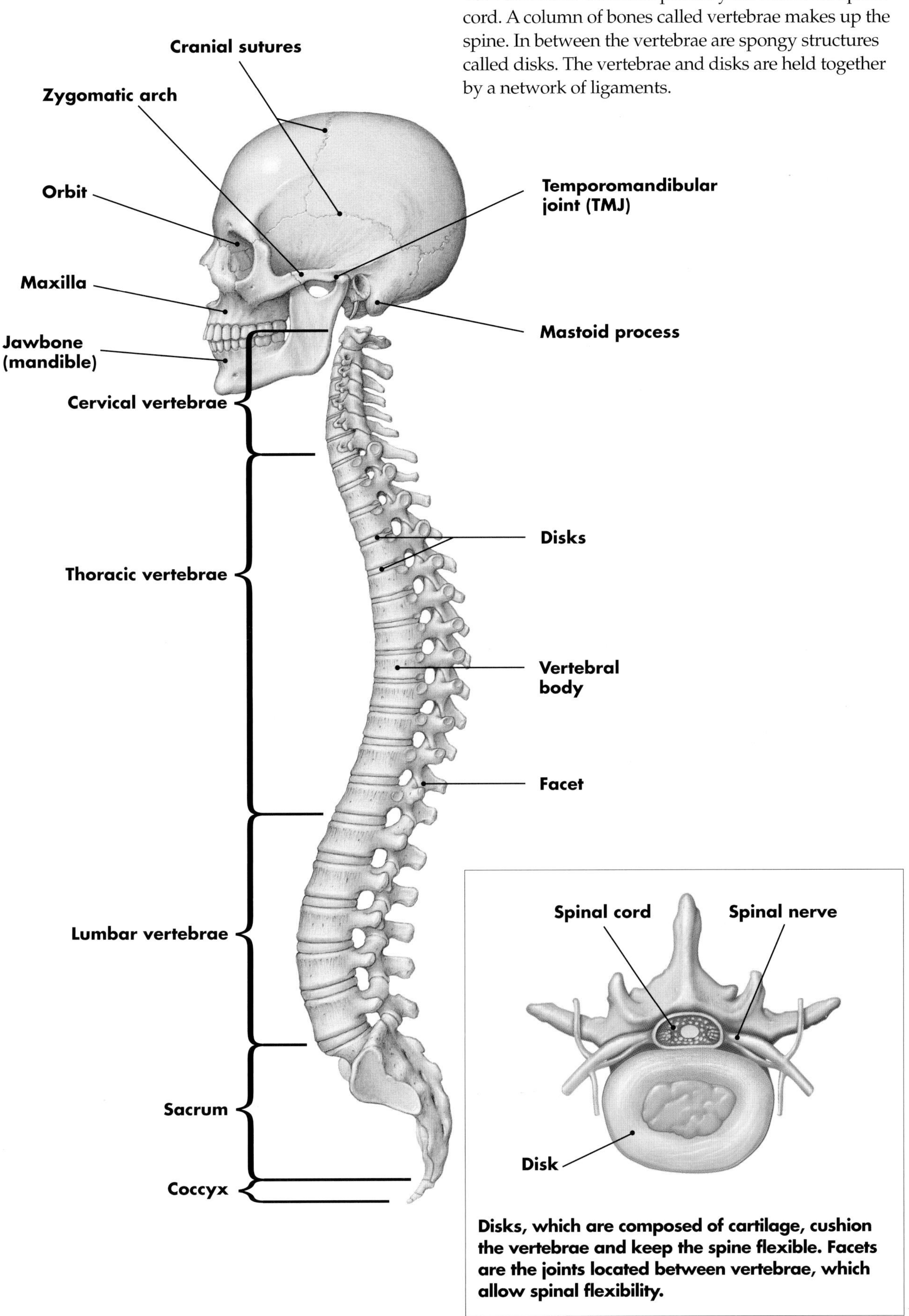

Disks, which are composed of cartilage, cushion the vertebrae and keep the spine flexible. Facets are the joints located between vertebrae, which allow spinal flexibility.

Muscles

The superficial and deep muscles of the musculoskeletal system contract to produce movement at the joints. Virtually all of these muscles are paired. For example, contraction of the biceps muscles causes the forearm to flex, whereas contraction of the opposing triceps muscles causes the forearm to extend. Many muscles are connected to bones by tendons.

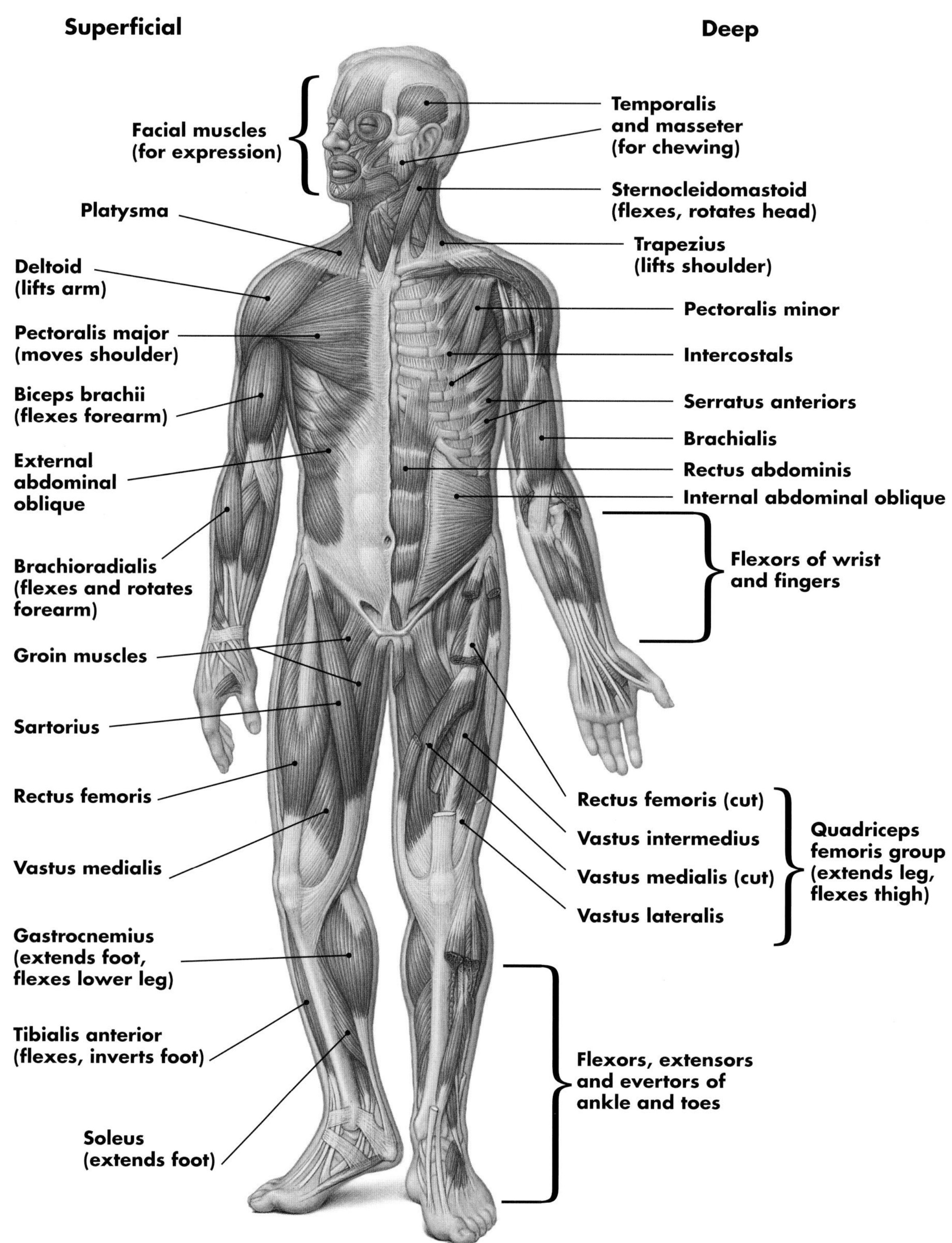

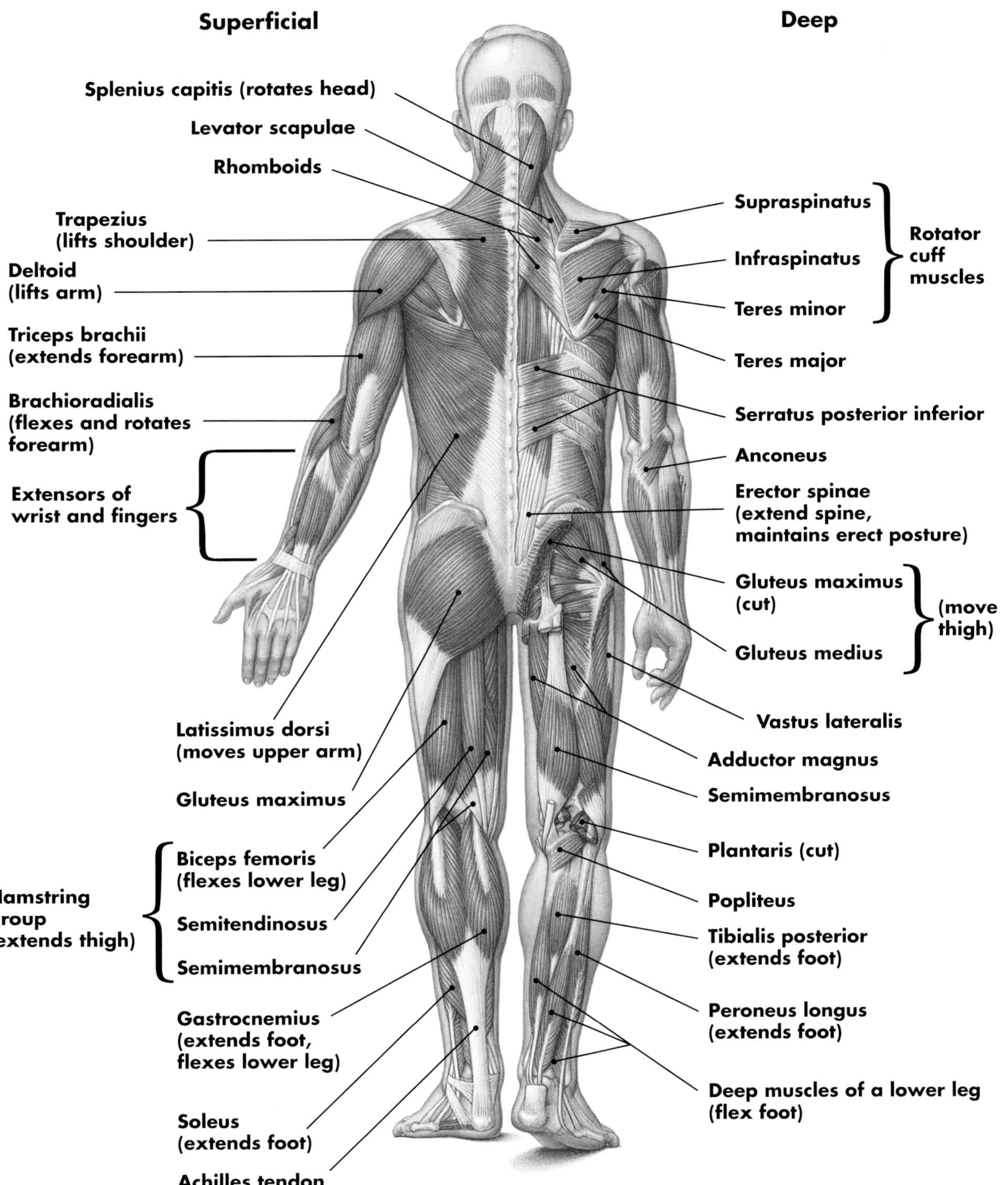
Superficial
Deep
Splenius capitis (rotates head)
Levator scapulae
Rhomboids
Trapezius (lifts shoulder)
Deltoid (lifts arm)
Triceps brachii (extends forearm)
Brachioradialis (flexes and rotates forearm)
Extensors of wrist and fingers
Latissimus dorsi (moves upper arm)
Gluteus maximus
Hamstring group (extends thigh)
Biceps femoris (flexes lower leg)
Semitendinosus
Semimembranosus
Gastrocnemius (extends foot, flexes lower leg)
Soleus (extends foot)
Achilles tendon
Supraspinatus
Infraspinatus
Teres minor
Rotator cuff muscles
Teres major
Serratus posterior inferior
Anconeus
Erector spinae (extend spine, maintains erect posture)
Gluteus maximus (cut)
Gluteus medius
(move thigh)
Vastus lateralis
Adductor magnus
Semimembranosus
Plantaris (cut)
Popliteus
Tibialis posterior (extends foot)
Peroneus longus (extends foot)
Deep muscles of a lower leg (flex foot)

Organs

Protected by skin and bones, the body's internal organs function day and night, serving the body's needs. The insets on the right show how the body's internal organs appear on computerized tomography (CT) scans.

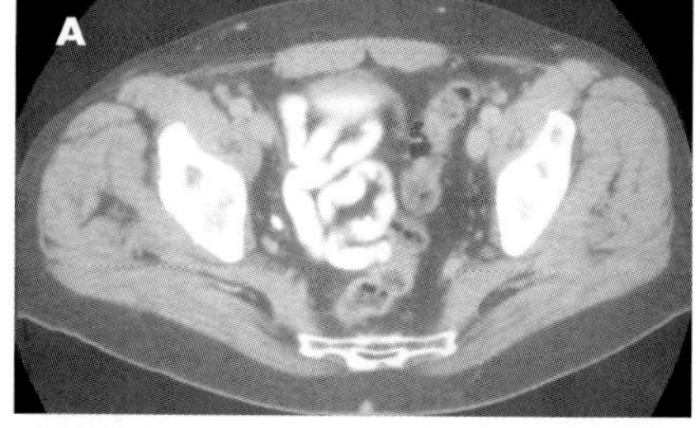

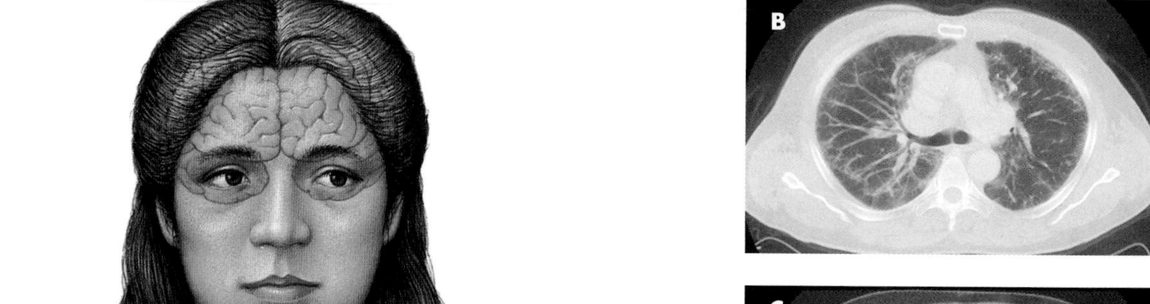

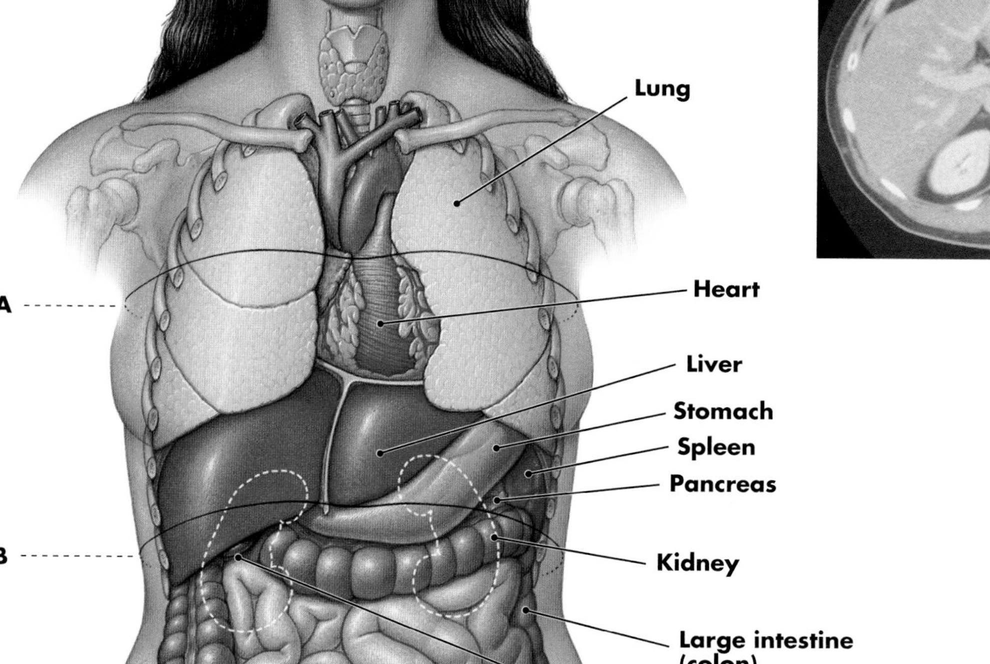

Cystic duct
Common bile duct
Gallbladder
Pancreas
Duodenum (cut)
Pancreatic duct

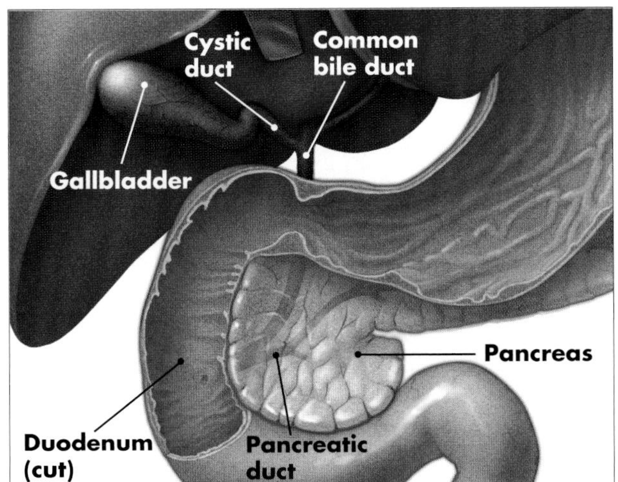

Digestive System

Digestion begins when food enters the mouth. Food is broken down by chewing and salivary gland enzymes. Once swallowed, wave-like muscular contractions (peristalsis) move the food through the digestive tract. Food nutrients are absorbed and waste products eliminated.

The small intestine is the body's main digestive organ. Digestive juices are released into the upper portion of the small intestine (duodenum) from the pancreas, liver and gallbladder by way of a system of tiny ducts.

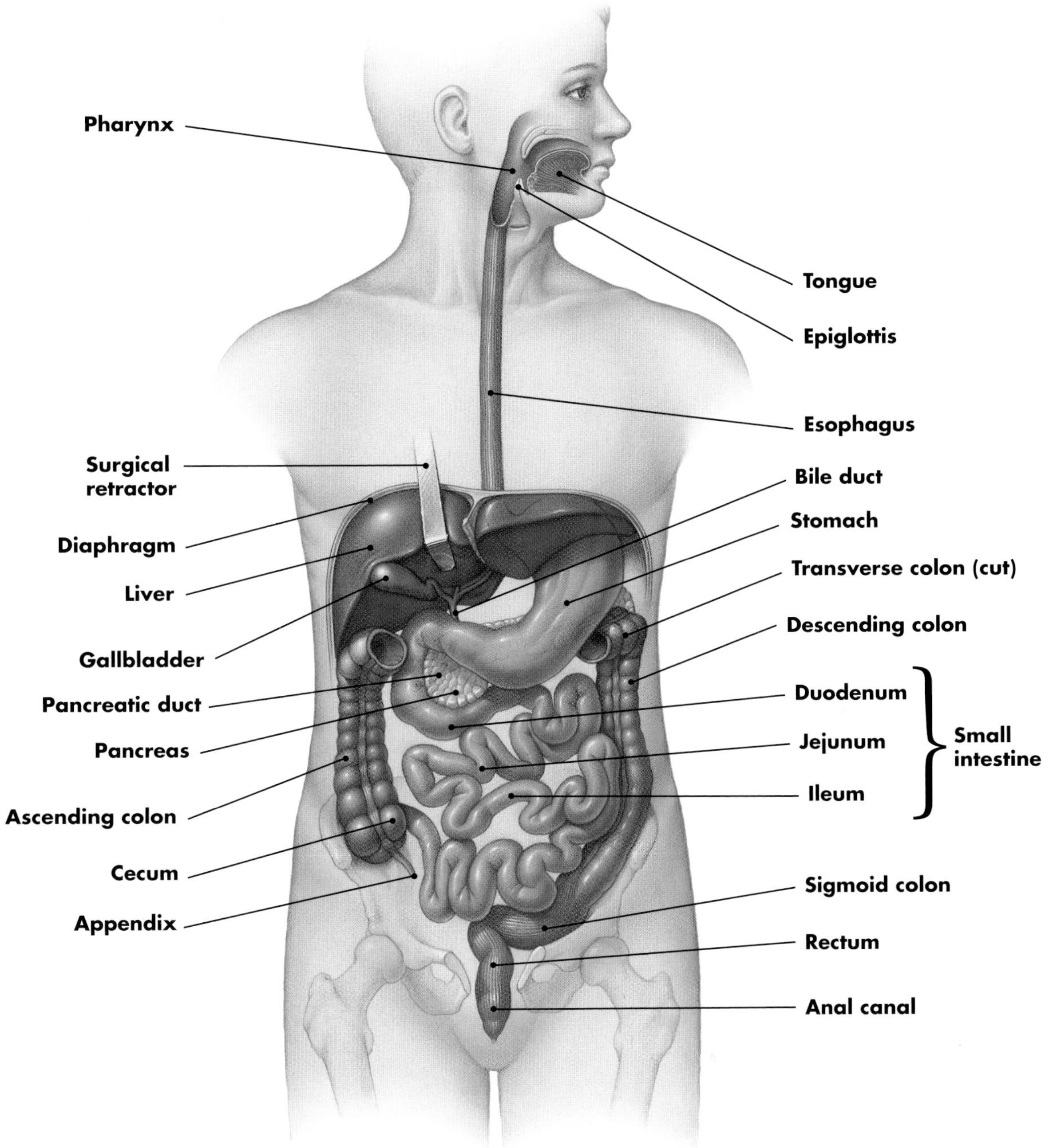

Pharynx
Tongue
Epiglottis
Esophagus
Surgical retractor
Bile duct
Stomach
Diaphragm
Transverse colon (cut)
Liver
Descending colon
Gallbladder
Duodenum
Pancreatic duct
Pancreas
Jejunum
Small intestine
Ileum
Ascending colon
Cecum
Sigmoid colon
Appendix
Rectum
Anal canal

VISUAL GUIDE

Heart and Blood Vessels

The heart and blood vessels supply body tissues with life-sustaining oxygen and nutrients. The heart pumps blood into the arteries (red). The major arteries that emerge from the heart are the aorta and pulmonary arteries. Veins (blue) return blood to the heart. The large veins that enter the heart are the superior vena cava, inferior vena cava and the pulmonary veins.

The coronary arteries supply nourishing blood to the heart muscle itself. Coronary arteries emerge from the aorta and extend over the surface of the heart. Blood returns from the heart muscle through coronary veins.

Adventitia (outer layer)
Tunica media vasorum (muscle layer)
Endothelium (inner lining)

The artery wall consists of three layers: the smooth inner lining (endothelium), the middle layer of muscle (tunica media vasorum) that controls the width of the artery to regulate blood flow through it, and the outer layer (adventitia).

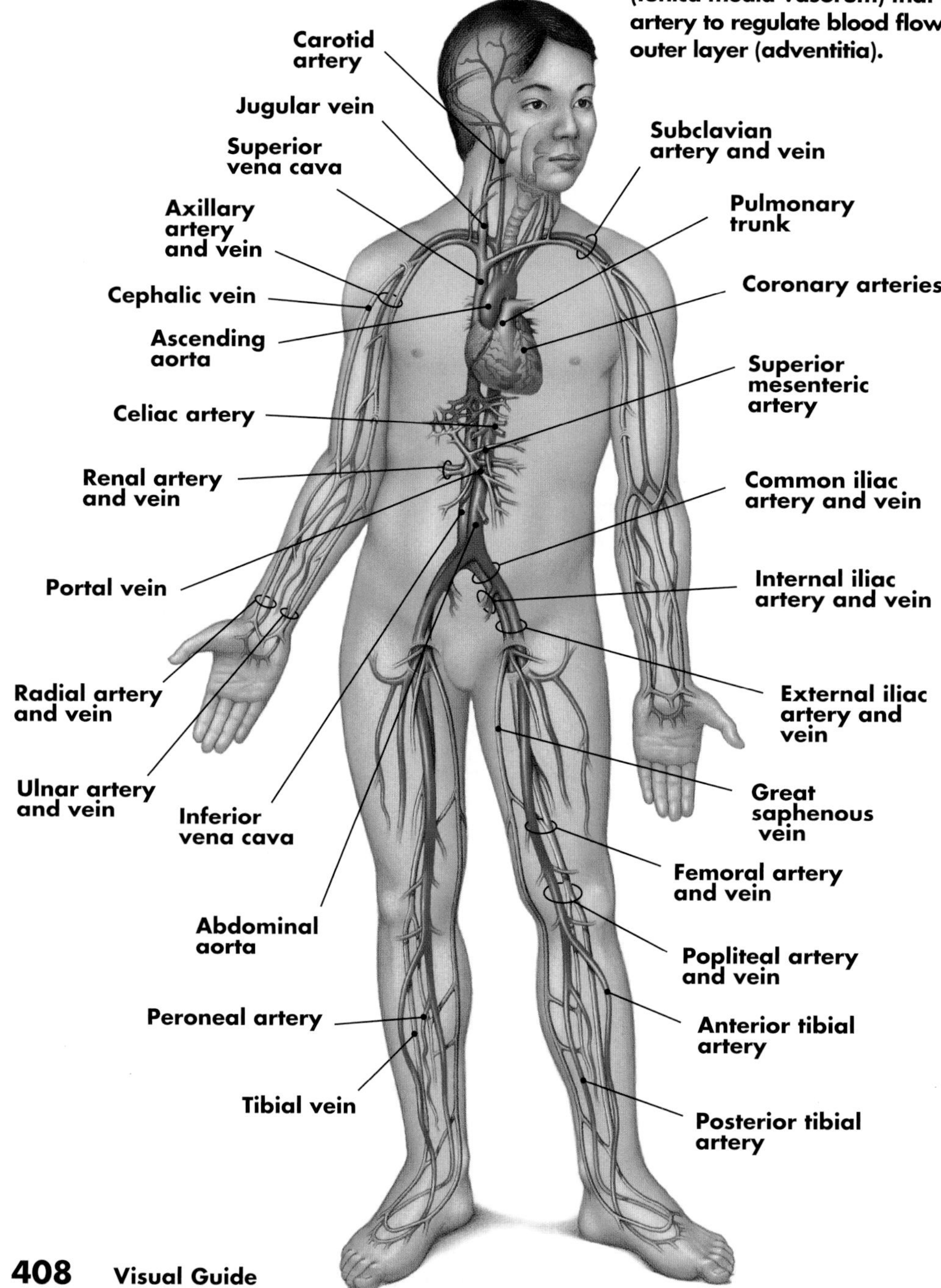

Contraction (systole)

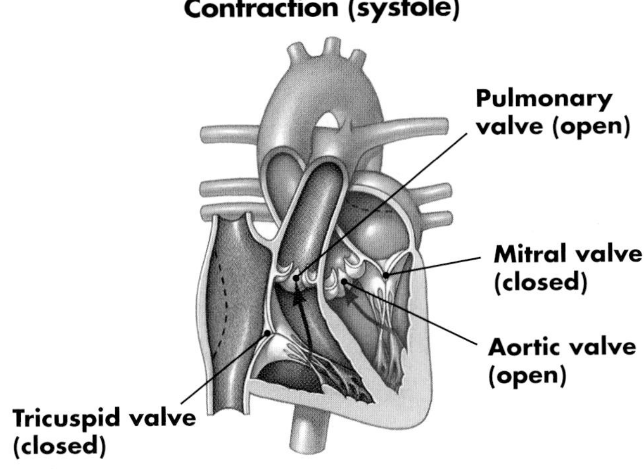

The heart has four chambers connected by valves. Blood from the veins flows through the superior and inferior vena cava into the right atrium, and then through the tricuspid valve into the right ventricle. The right ventricle pumps blood through the pulmonary valve and into the lungs via the pulmonary arteries. Reoxygenated blood from the lungs enters the left atrium via the pulmonary veins and flows through the mitral valve into the left ventricle. The left ventricle pumps the blood through the aorta for delivery to body tissues.

Valves keep blood flowing through the heart in one direction. As the ventricles relax (diastole), pressure within them decreases. The mitral and tricuspid valves are forced open, allowing blood to flow from the atria into the ventricles. The aortic and pulmonary valves are closed to prevent the return of blood pumped out on the previous beat. During contraction (systole), pressure pushes the aortic and pulmonary valves open, and the mitral and tricuspid valves are forced shut.

Relaxation (diastole)

Pulmonary valve (closed)
Aortic valve (closed)
Mitral valve (open)
Tricuspid valve (open)

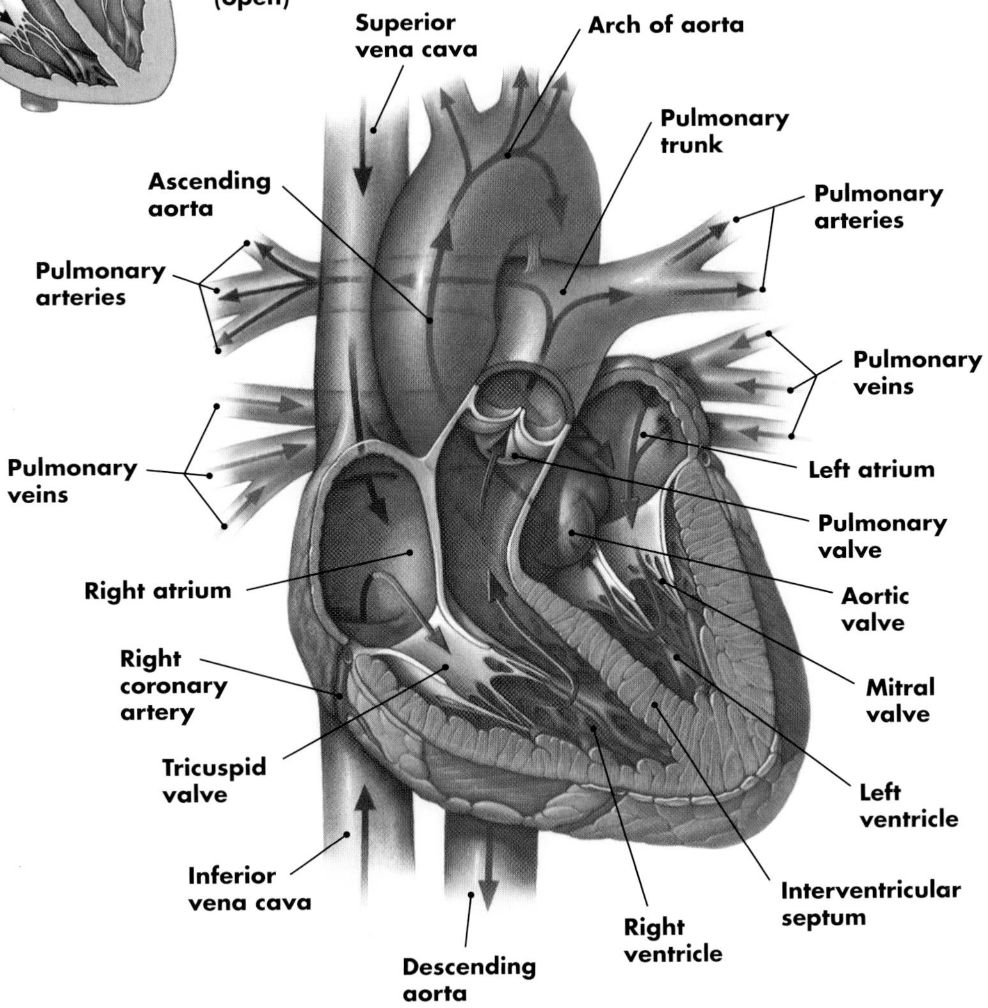

Superior vena cava
Arch of aorta
Pulmonary trunk
Ascending aorta
Pulmonary arteries
Pulmonary arteries
Pulmonary veins
Pulmonary veins
Left atrium
Pulmonary valve
Right atrium
Aortic valve
Right coronary artery
Mitral valve
Tricuspid valve
Left ventricle
Inferior vena cava
Interventricular septum
Right ventricle
Descending aorta

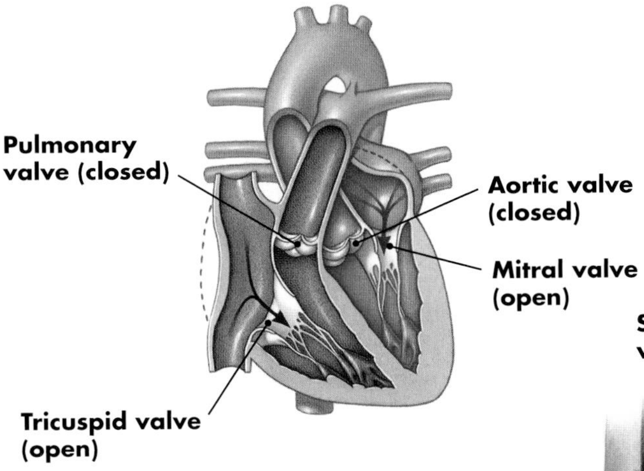

Lungs

The lungs supply oxygen to blood and remove carbon dioxide from it. This exchange takes place in tiny air sacs called alveoli. Oxygen passes from the air in the alveoli into the blood. The oxygenated blood flows through tiny capillaries surrounding the alveoli into the pulmonary veins. The pulmonary arteries carry the blood to the lungs. Pulmonary veins return the blood to the heart.

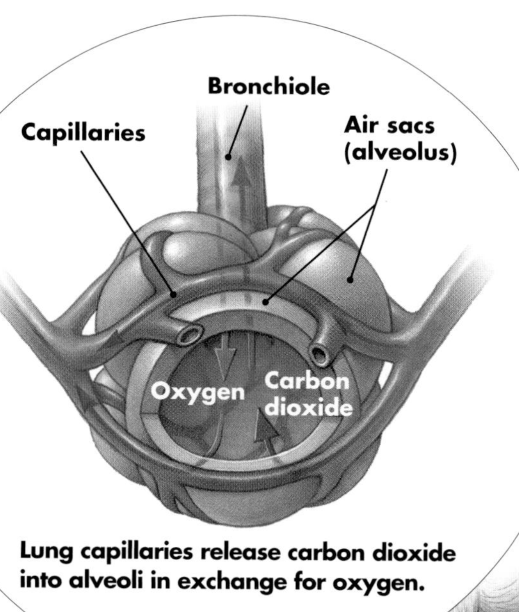

Lung capillaries release carbon dioxide into alveoli in exchange for oxygen.

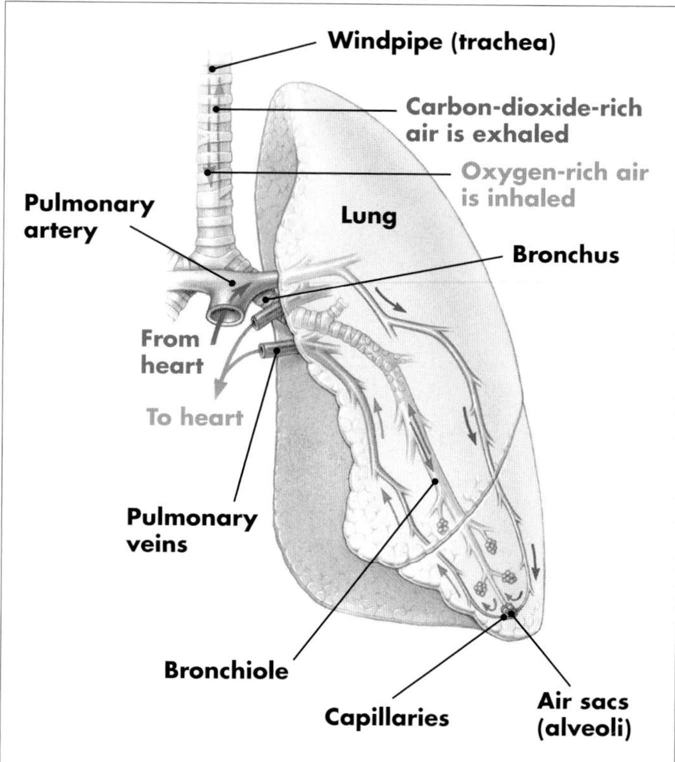

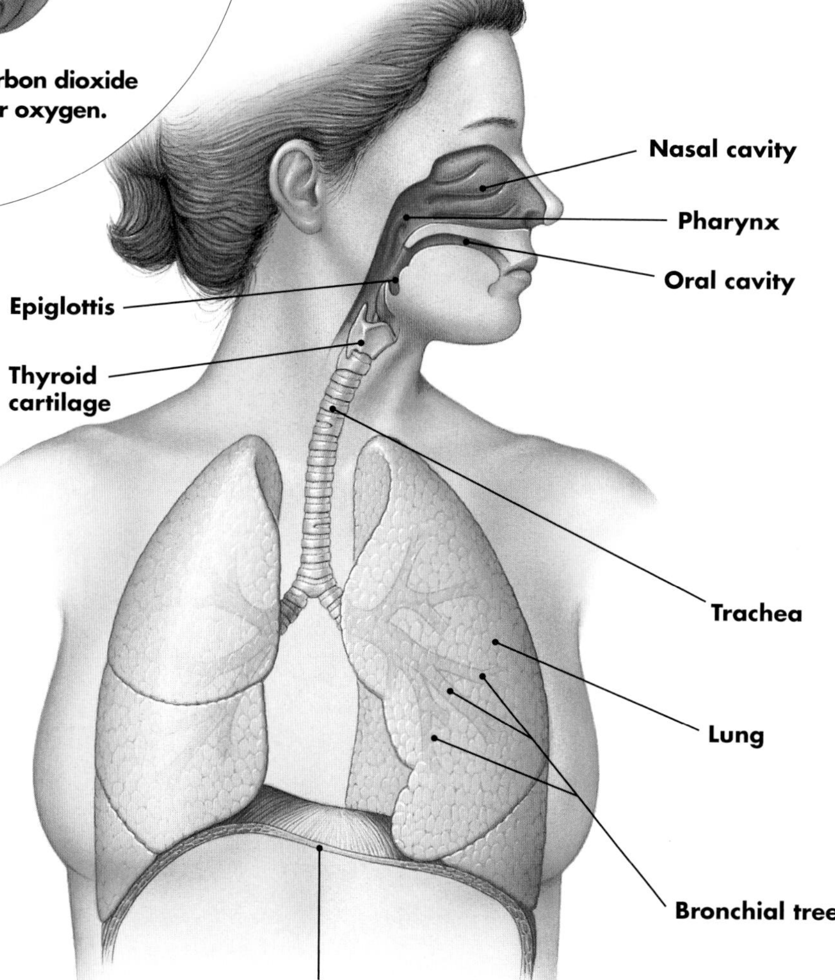

Endocrine Glands

The endocrine glands control many body activities as well as the response of body systems to usual and stressful events. The glands secrete hormones into the bloodstream. These chemical messengers deliver instructions to organs and tissues.

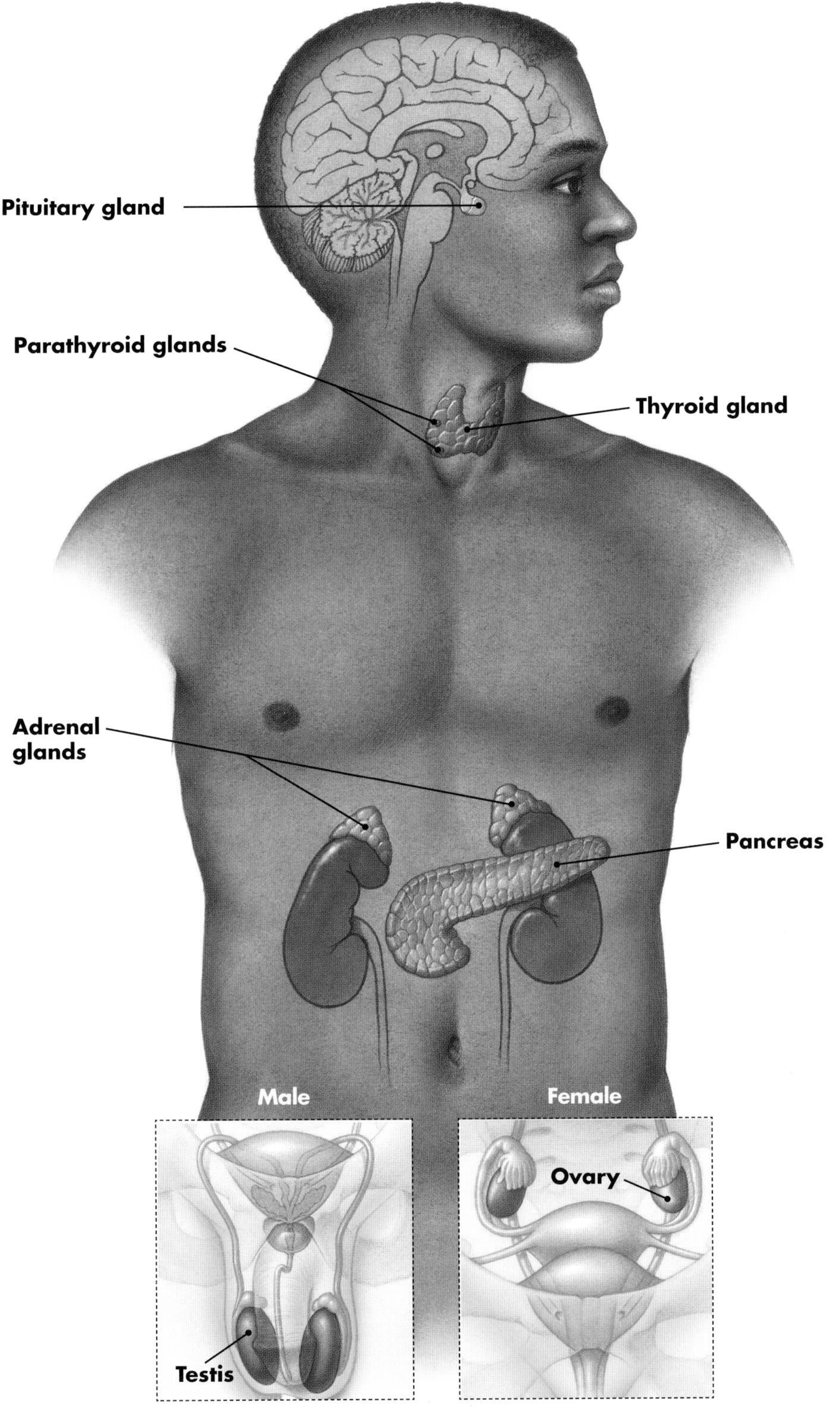

VISUAL GUIDE

Breast and Female Reproductive Organs

The female breast produces milk to feed infants. Each breast has between 15 and 20 sections (lobes). Each lobe is made up of many smaller structures (lobules) that end in tiny bulbs that can produce milk. The lobes, lobules and bulbs are linked by a network of thin tubes (ducts). Ducts carry milk from the bulbs to the dark area of skin in the center of the breast (areola), where it's expressed from the nipple.

Female reproductive organs include the ovaries, which release an egg at ovulation, the fallopian tubes, where an egg may meet with the sperm, and the uterus, where the fertilized egg implants itself and grows into a fetus. The reproductive organs are located near the bladder and the urethra.

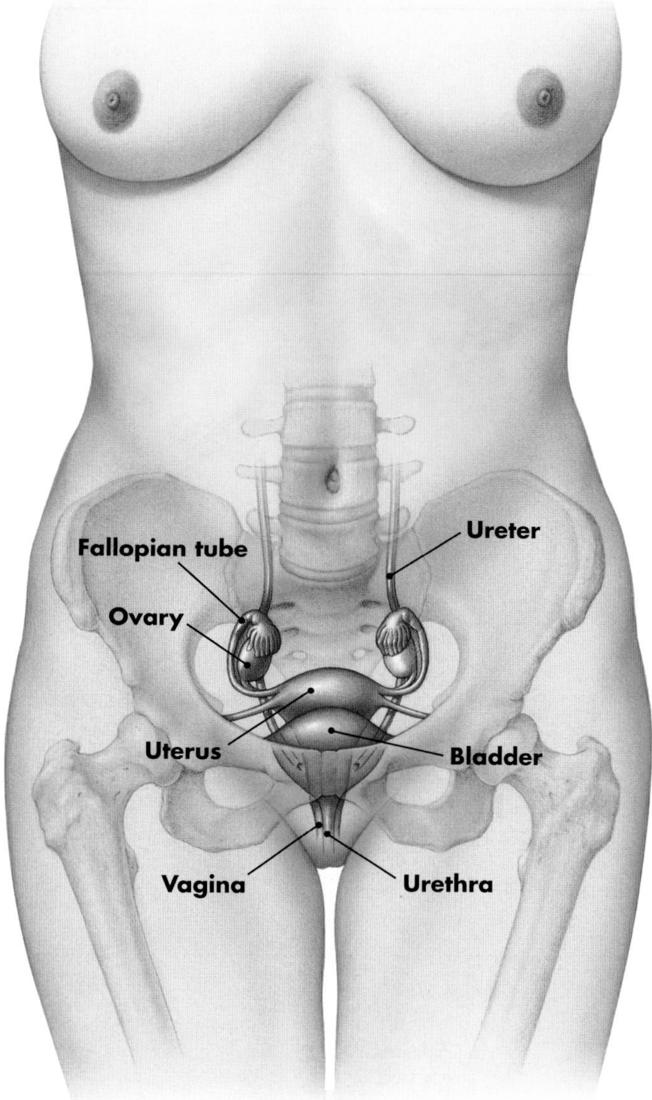

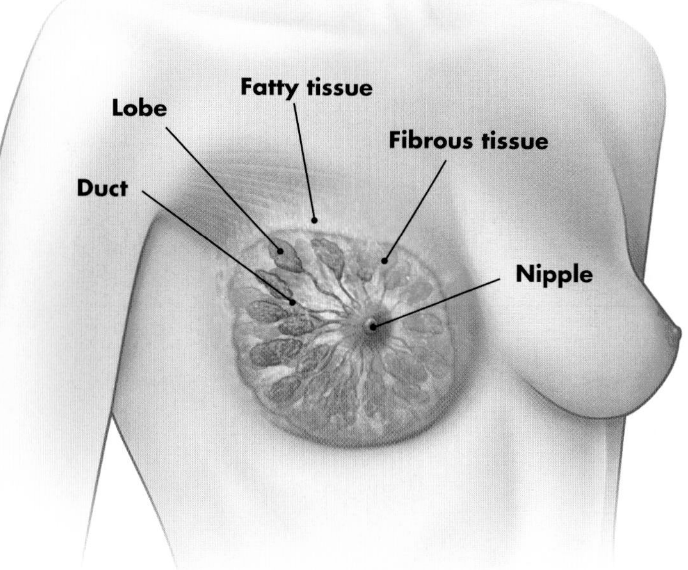

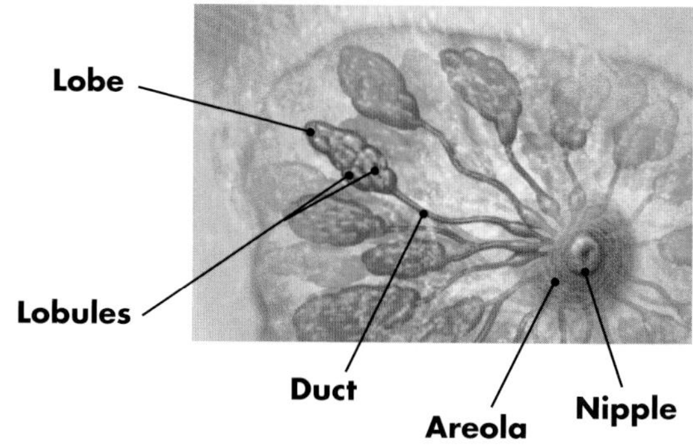

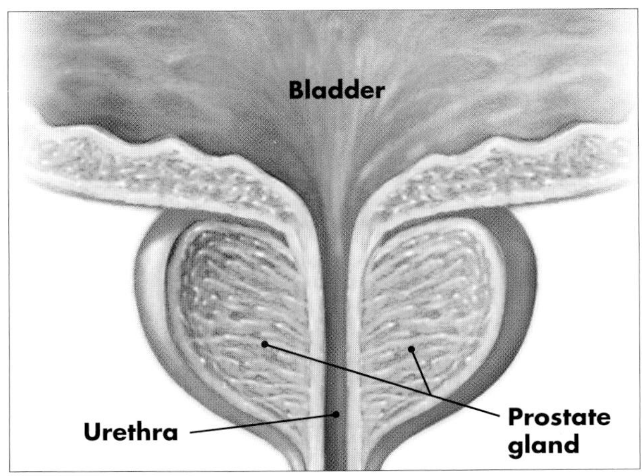

The primary function of the prostate gland is to produce most of the fluid in semen. Tiny ducts within the prostate convey the fluid to the urethra, where it mixes with sperm. About the size of a walnut, the prostate gland is located just below the bladder, and it surrounds the top portion of the urethra.

Male Reproductive Organs and Urinary Tract

Male reproductive organs include the testicles, where sperm are produced, the epididymides and vasa deferentia, which transport sperm into the seminal vesicles and prostate gland. Fluids from the seminal vesicles and prostate gland are mixed with the sperm and ejaculated as semen through the urethra.

In men, the urethra serves both the reproductive and urinary systems — transporting both semen and urine. The urinary tract includes the kidneys, ureters, bladder and urethra. In both men and women, the kidneys cleanse blood of excess fluid and waste products as they manufacture urine, which is passed to the bladder by way of the ureters. The bladder stores urine and expels it through the urethra.

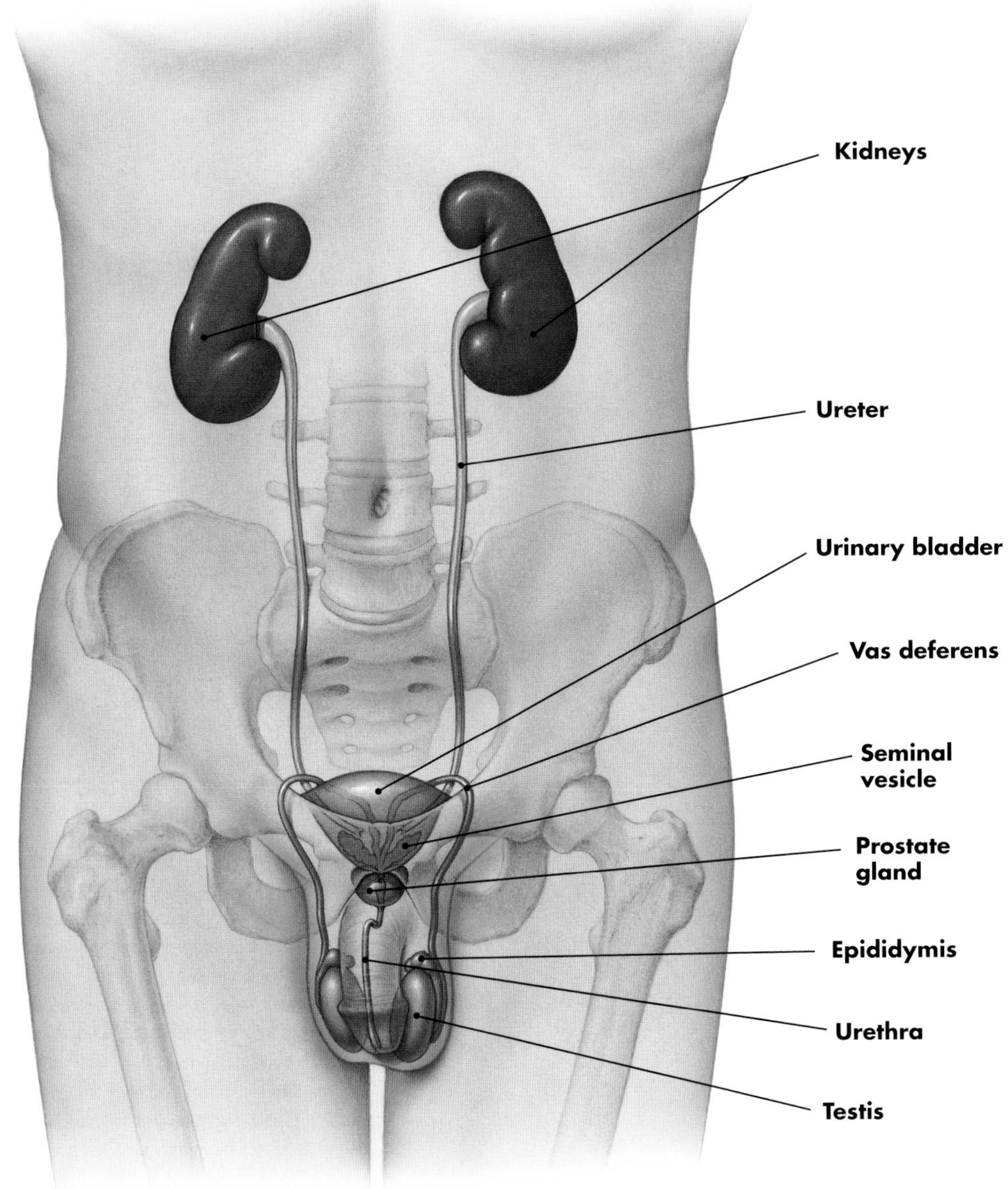

Brain

The brain controls virtually all of the body's activities, from basic instincts of survival to intellectual analysis and creative thought. It organizes and shapes emotions and monitors and directs body functions and physical actions. The basic structures of the brain include the brainstem, the cerebellum, responsible for balance and movement, and the cerebrum, the largest structure of the human brain and perhaps the most recognizable, due to its heavily folded appearance. The cerebrum (see opposite page) is divided into two hemispheres. Each hemisphere is composed of four lobes — frontal, parietal, temporal and occipital — each of which directs different activities.

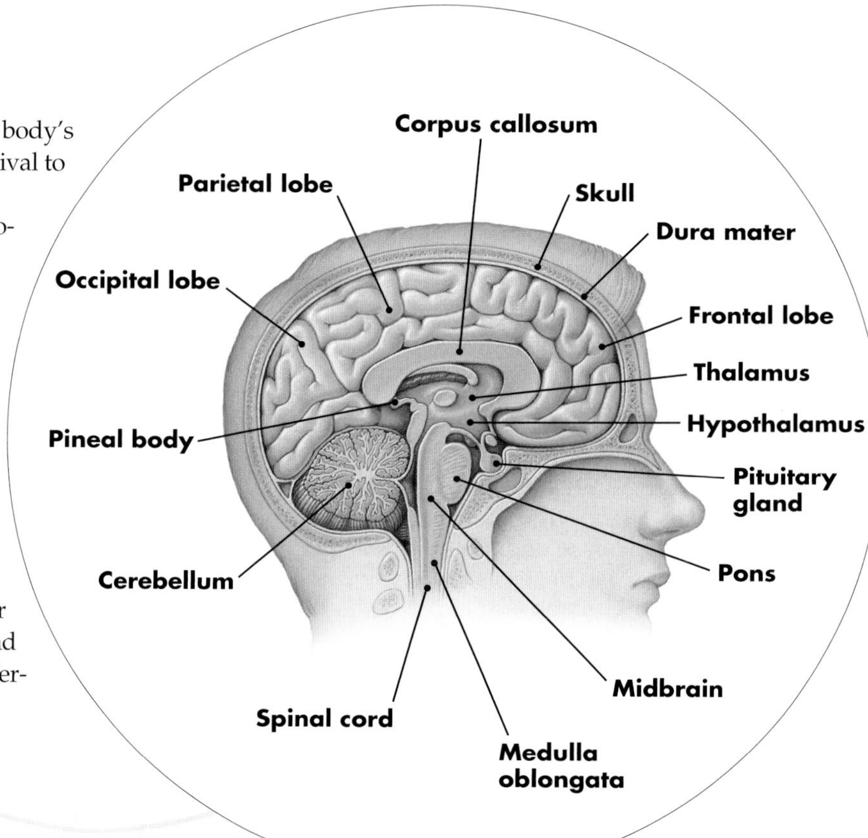

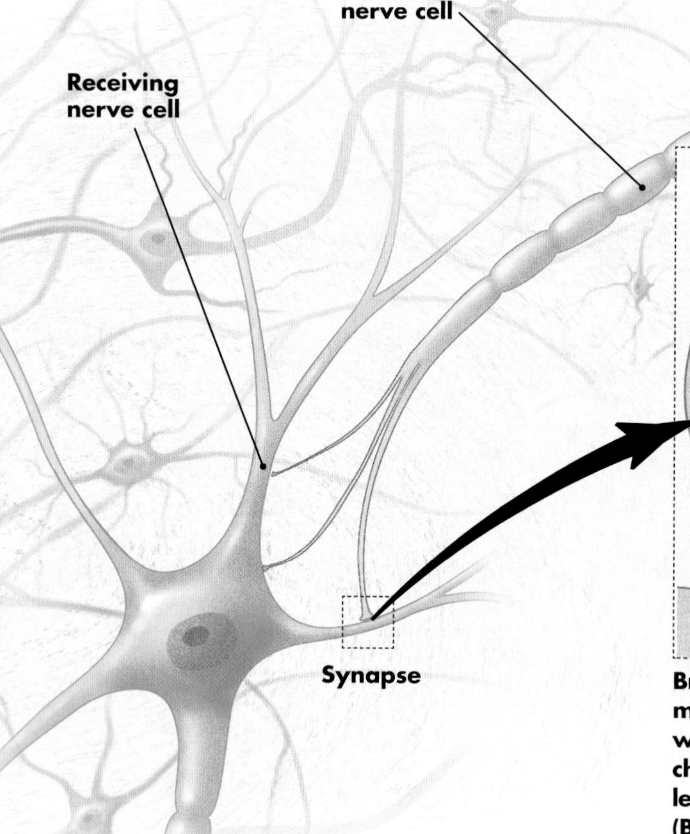

Brain cells communicate by exchanging chemical messages. When a sending nerve cell communicates with a receiving nerve cell: (A) Packages containing chemical messengers (neurotransmitters) are released into a gap (synapse) between the two cells. (B) The neurotransmitters bind with receptors on receiving nerve cells. (C) Once communication is complete, the neurotransmitters return to the synapse. (D) The neurotransmitters re-enter the sending nerve cell. (E) The neurotransmitters are repackaged for future use or broken down by enzymes.

Nervous System

The human body communicates by its nervous system, which is composed of the brain, spinal cord and peripheral nerves. Peripheral nerves receive messages from various body parts and the outside world. These messages are transmitted to the spinal cord and passed on to the brain, which interprets and responds to the messages. The spinal cord continuously transmits messages back and forth between the brain and the outermost regions of the body.

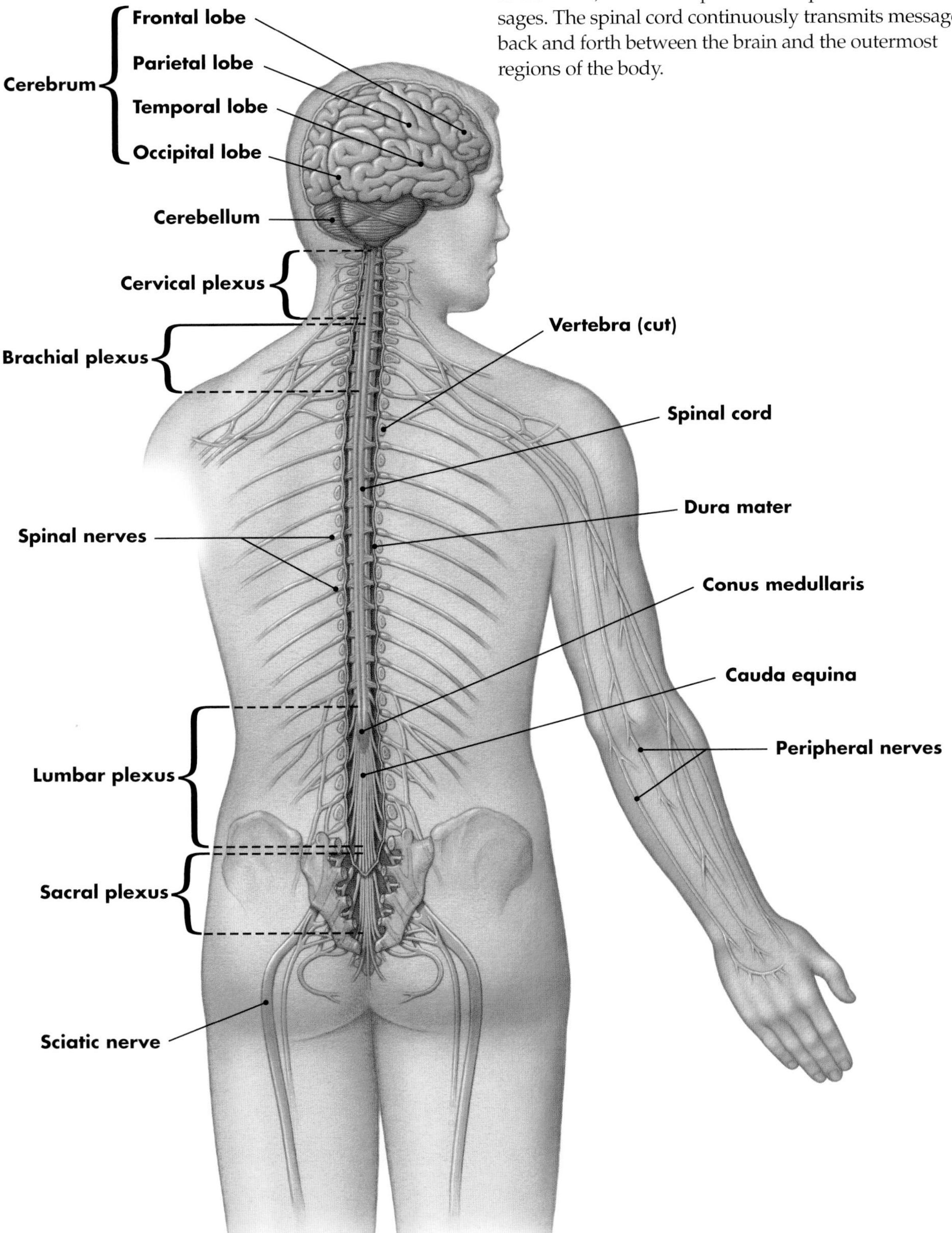

VISUAL GUIDE

Eyes and Ears

An image passes through the pupil at the front of the eye and onto the lens, located behind the pupil. The lens projects the inverted image onto the retina, located at the back of the eye. The retina, which is composed of light-sensitive cells, converts the image into electrical impulses that are delivered to the brain by way of the optic nerve.

The two main functions of the ears are hearing and balance. The eardrum transmits sound by means of tiny connective bones (hammer, anvil, stirrup) to the inner ear. There, sound is transmitted as electrical impulses to the brain via the auditory nerve. The inner ear also contains the semicircular canals of the vestibular labyrinth, structures essential to balance.

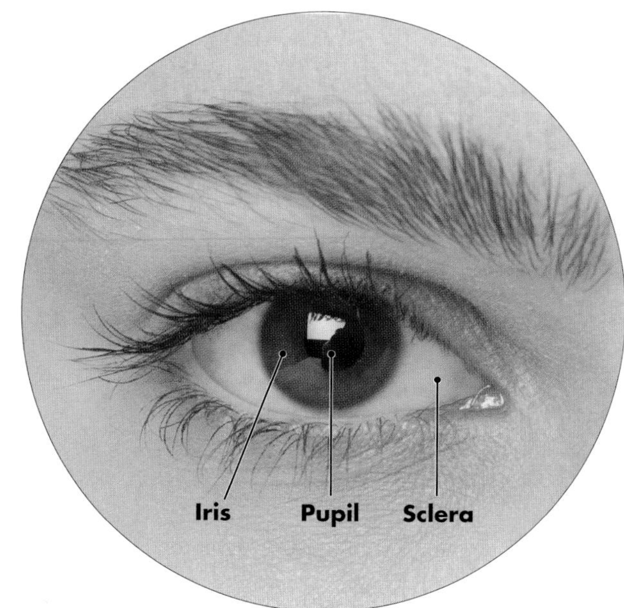

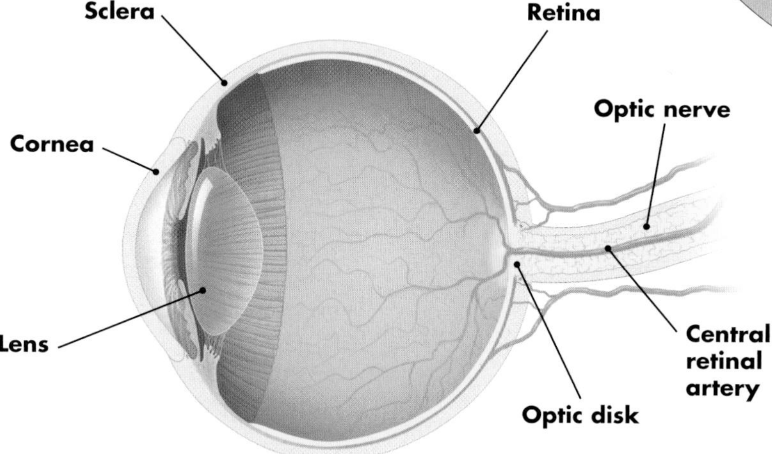

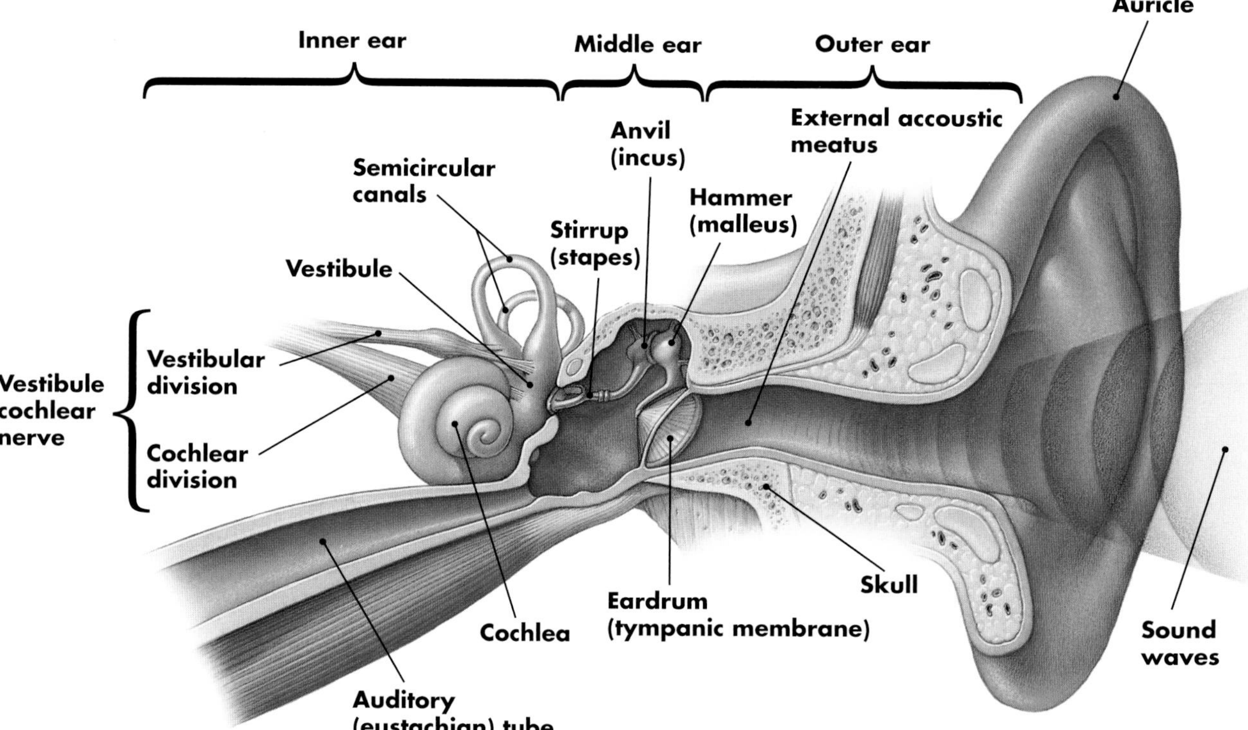

Nasal and Oral Cavities

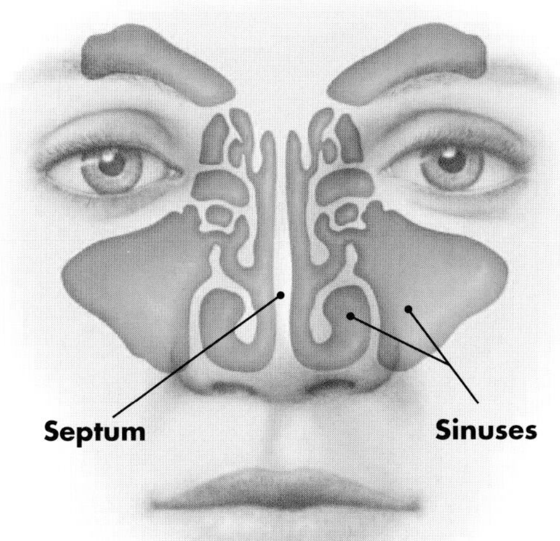

The nose is divided into two identical passages called nostrils, which are separated by a partition (septum) of cartilage and bone. The nasal passages also open into the sinuses, tiny air-filled cavities in the skull. The adenoids are an aggregation of lymphatic tissue located behind the nasal passages.

The oral cavity is composed of the mouth and teeth. Many important acts, such as speaking and singing, use the teeth and mouth to shape sounds. The teeth and mouth are also responsible for the first phase of digestion.

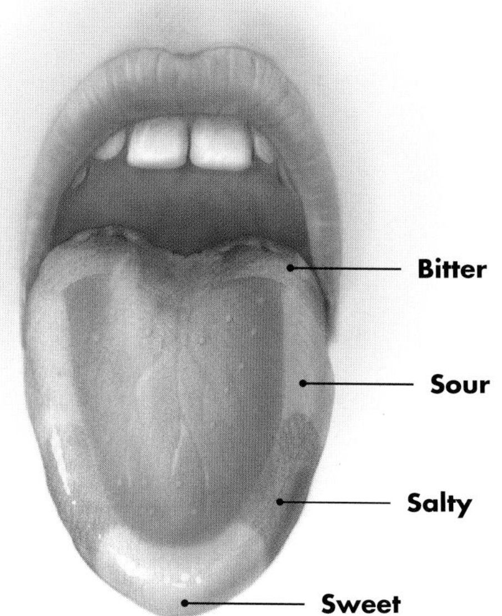

Working in conjunction with your sense of smell, your taste buds can distinguish sweet, salty, sour and bitter flavors.

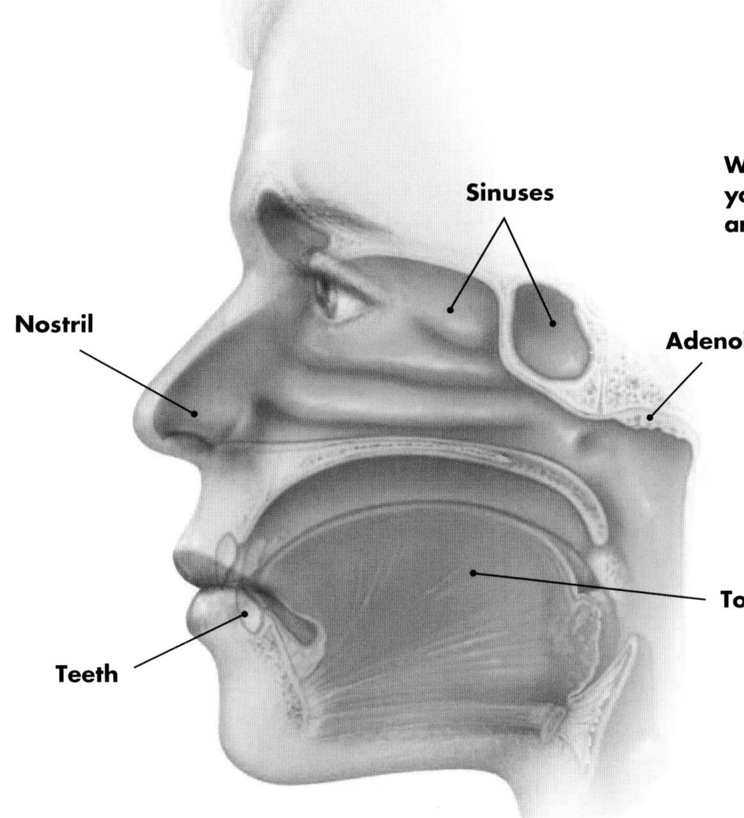

Skin

Skin keeps out invaders, helps control body temperature and protects vital internal organs. The adult human body has 2 square yards of skin. One square inch of skin contains millions of cells and includes structures such as oil glands, hair roots (follicles) and sweat glands. Specialized nerve endings in skin sense heat, cold and pain.

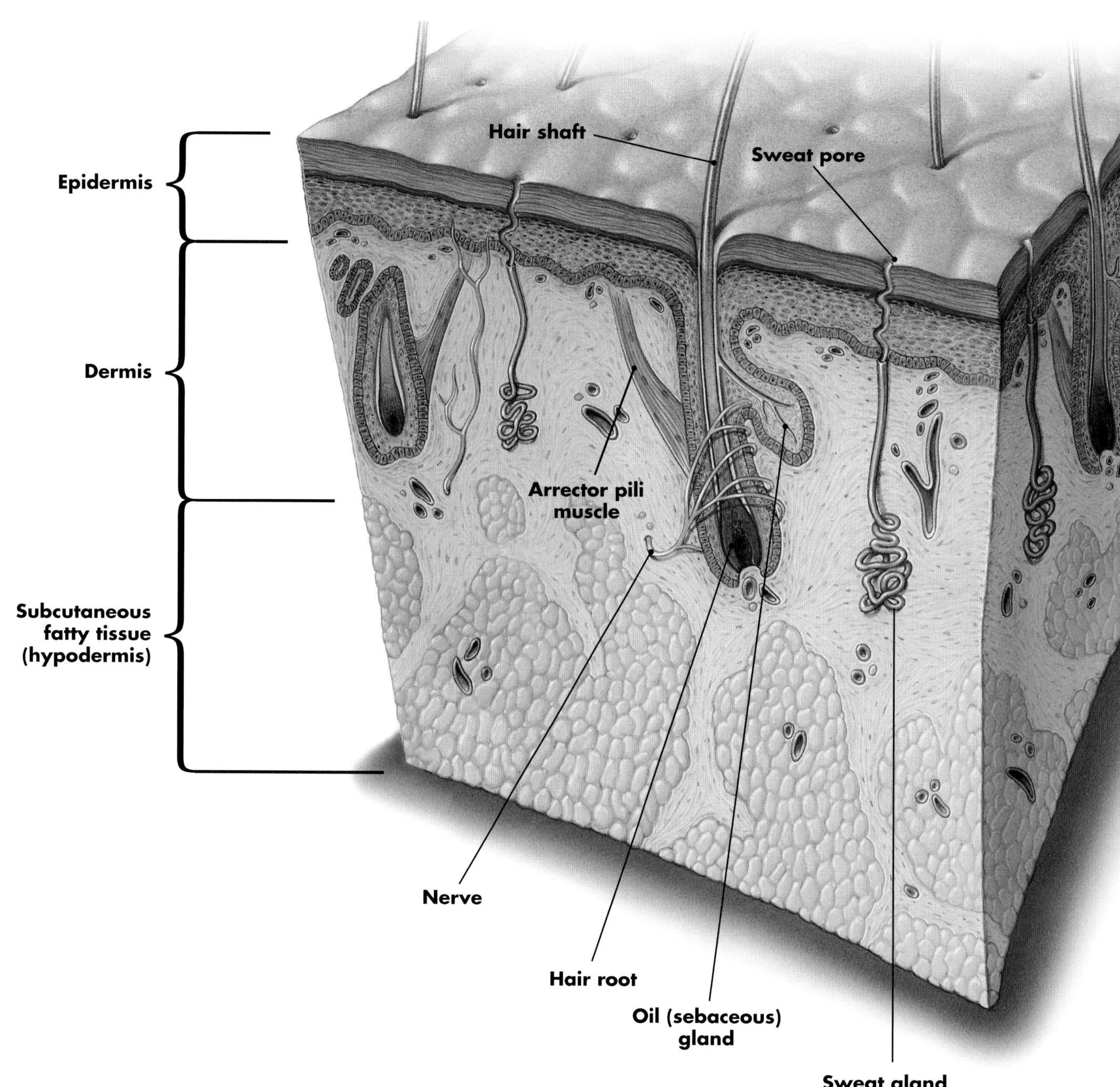

Immune System

The immune system is a complex array of organs, cells and molecules distributed throughout the body, responsible for protecting the body from harmful invaders (antigens), such as germs, viruses and other foreign substances. Each part of the immune system contributes to the growth, development or activation of lymphocytes, specialized white blood cells that play a major role in the body's immune response. White blood cells originate in bone marrow. Some migrate to the thymus gland and develop into specialized types of immune cells. Some white blood cells from bone marrow and the thymus gland gather in lymph nodes and other immune organs, including the spleen, tonsils, adenoids and appendix. Other cells circulate throughout blood and lymphatic vessels.

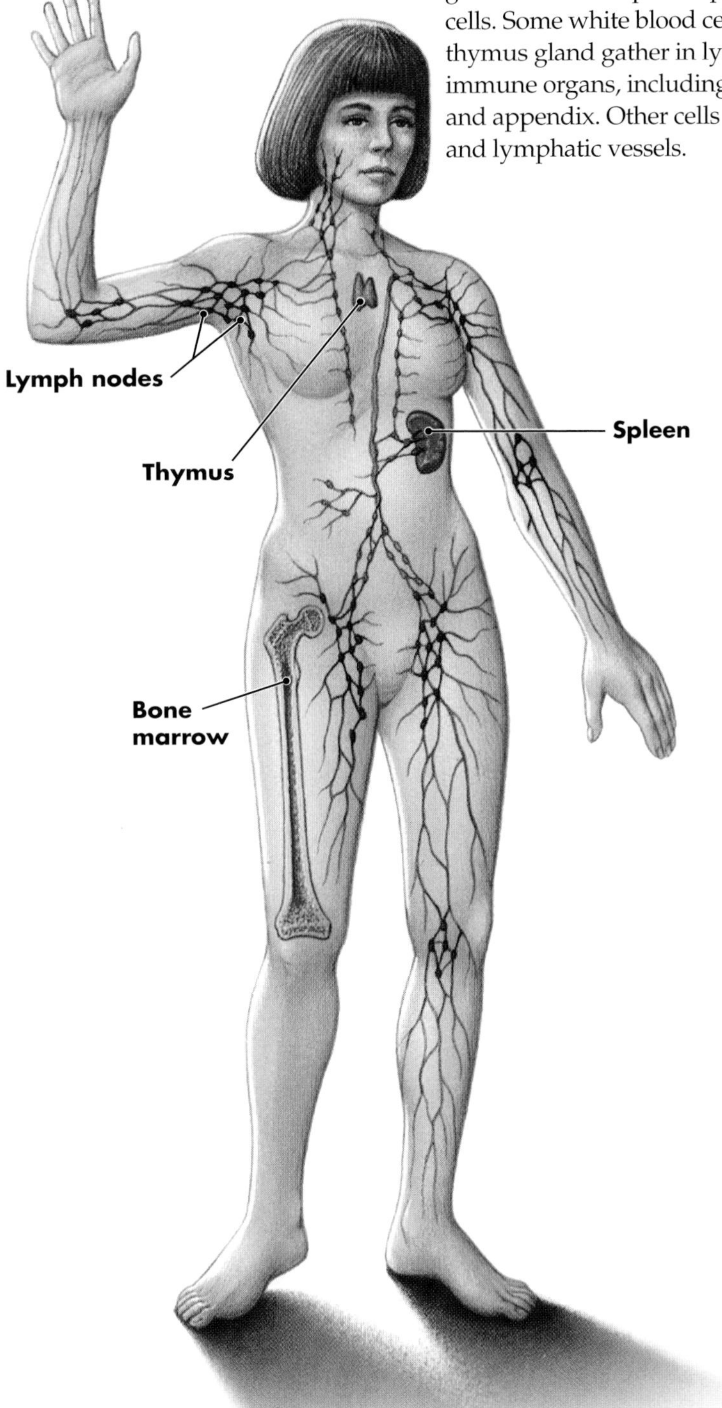

Genes

1. Your body is made up of cells — about 100 trillion of them. Different kinds of cells — for example, skin, muscle, bone and blood — perform different functions. Each cell has a control center called the nucleus.

2. Within the nucleus of each cell are 23 pairs of structures called chromosomes. Half of a person's chromosomes are inherited from the mother and the other half, from the father.

3. Each chromosome contains strands that resemble a twisted ladder. The strands, called deoxyribonucleic acid (DNA), are held together by chemical "rungs."

4. Chromosomes are made up of genes. Each gene is composed of sequences of thousands of pairs of the chemicals adenine (A) and thymine (T), and the chemicals cytosine (C) and guanine (G). The precise sequence of these chemical pairs in the gene directs the cell to produce another chemical, usually a protein, which has a specific task to do. This is how each gene tells each cell in your body precisely how to act — controlling your features and growth, and influencing or directly affecting the function of your organs.

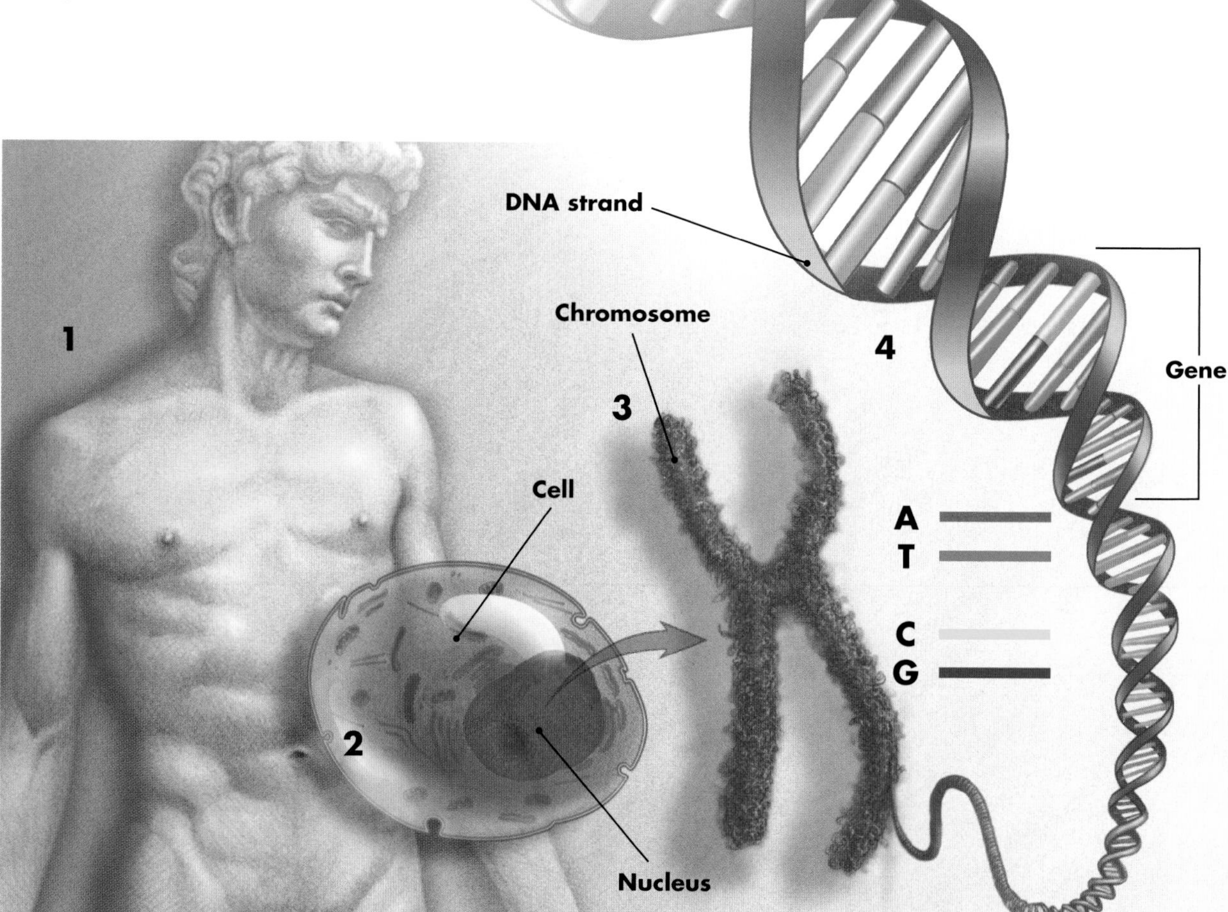

Spinal Disorders

Many types of spinal disorders cause back pain. Back pain generally isn't life-threatening, but the pain can make you miserable.

Pain radiating from your back down your buttock to your lower leg, called sciatica (see left), may be associated with inflammation or compression of the roots of the sciatic nerve.

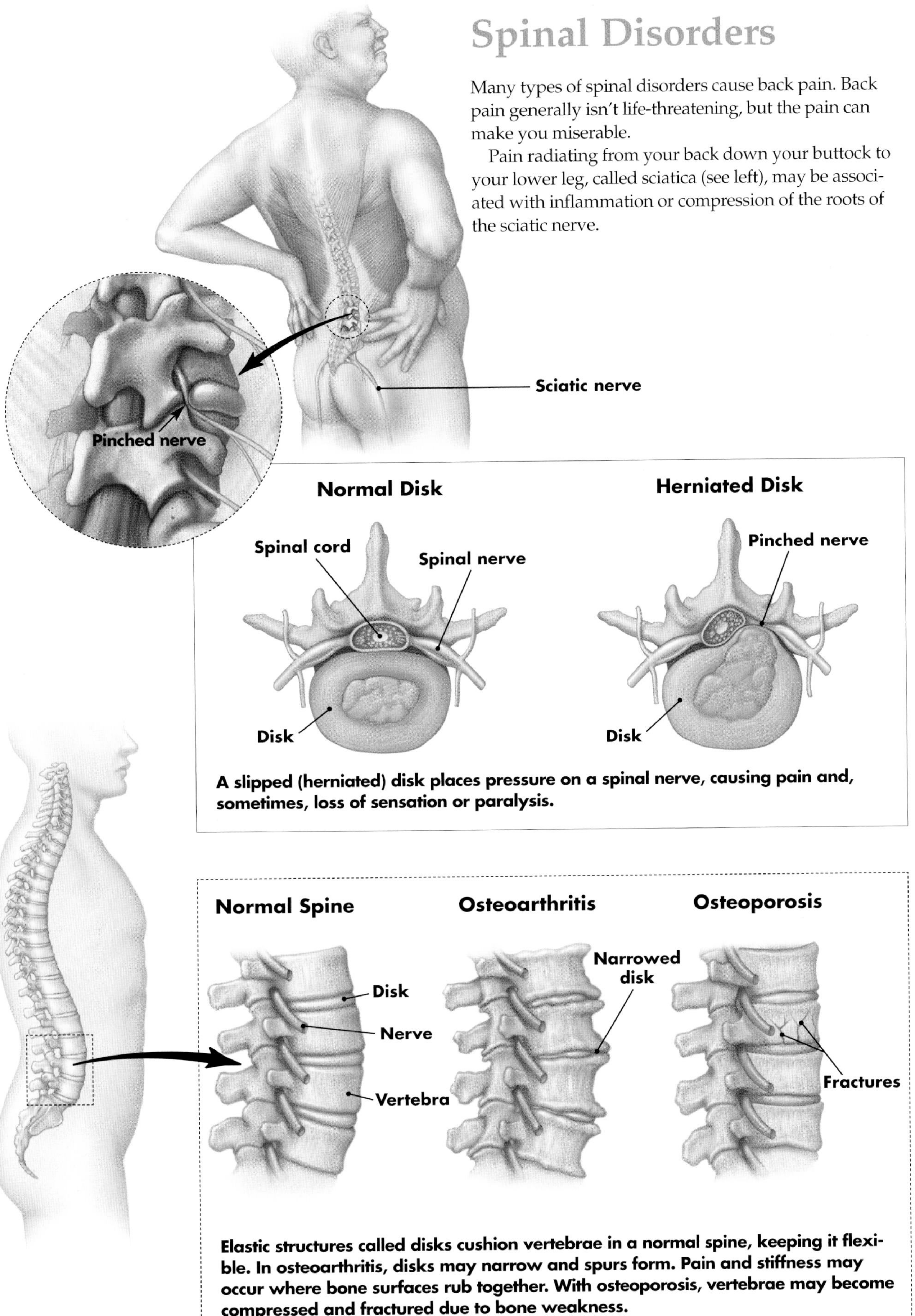

A slipped (herniated) disk places pressure on a spinal nerve, causing pain and, sometimes, loss of sensation or paralysis.

Elastic structures called disks cushion vertebrae in a normal spine, keeping it flexible. In osteoarthritis, disks may narrow and spurs form. Pain and stiffness may occur where bone surfaces rub together. With osteoporosis, vertebrae may become compressed and fractured due to bone weakness.

Joint Disorders

Pain and stiffness in a joint often results from osteoarthritis. This common form of arthritis affects nearly all adults older than age 60. Joint replacement surgery can help restore near-normal, pain-free joint movement. Many joints, including the hip, knee, shoulder, elbow, wrist and even finger joints, can be replaced.

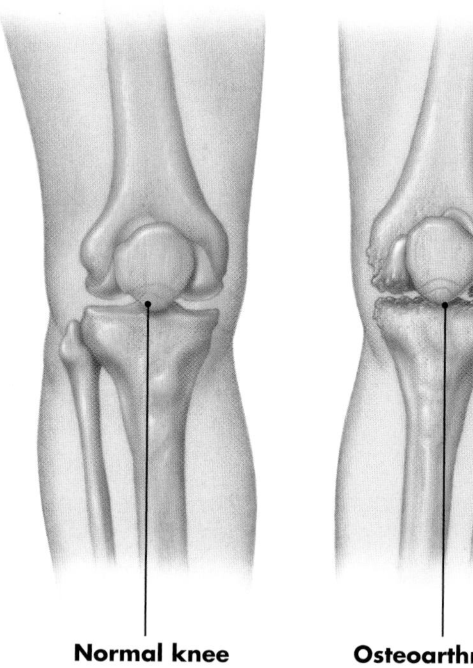

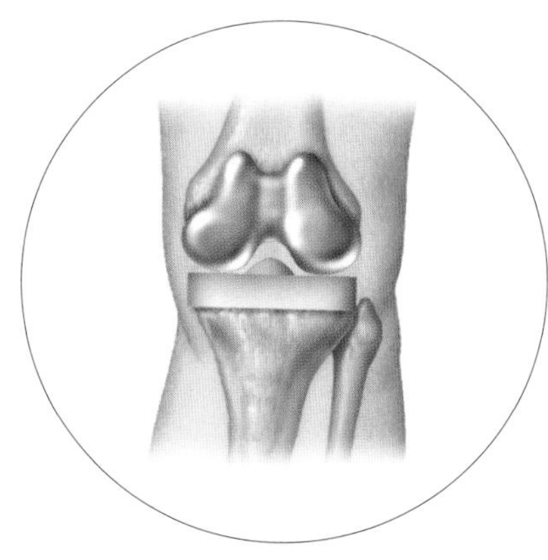

At right, a normal knee joint and a knee damaged by osteoarthritis. The inset above shows a knee repaired by total knee replacement.

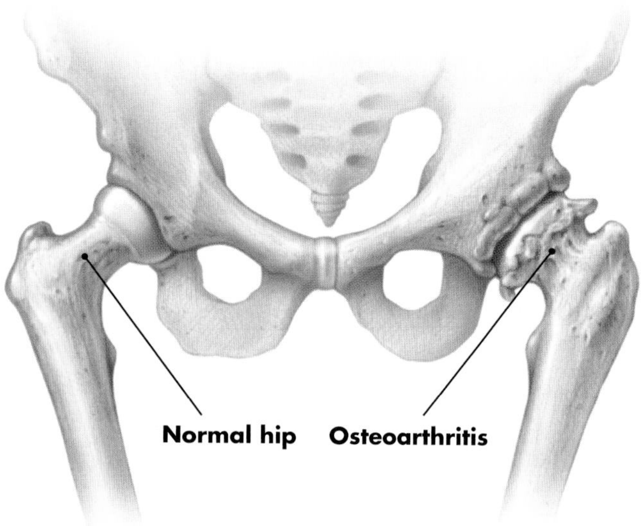

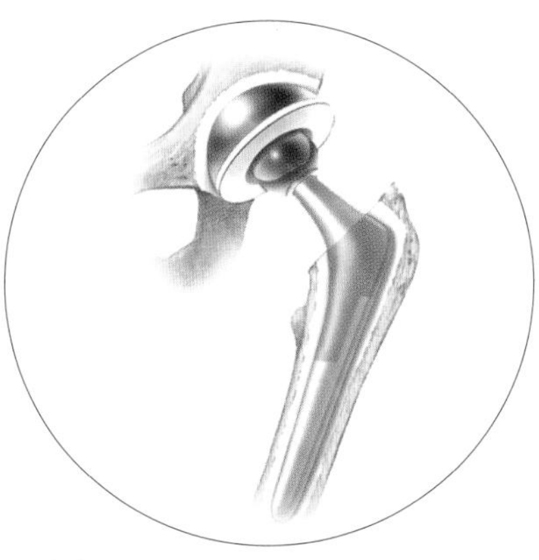

At left, a hip showing a normal joint and a joint that has been damaged by osteoarthritis. The inset above shows how an implant can replace a damaged joint.

Joint Disorders

The meniscus is the crescent-shaped cartilage in the knee situated between the ends of the bones of the thigh and lower leg. A meniscus tear is a common knee injury. If the tear is severe, surgical repair may be necessary. The photos below show a normal meniscus (left), a partial tear of the meniscus (right) and a meniscus tear (bottom).

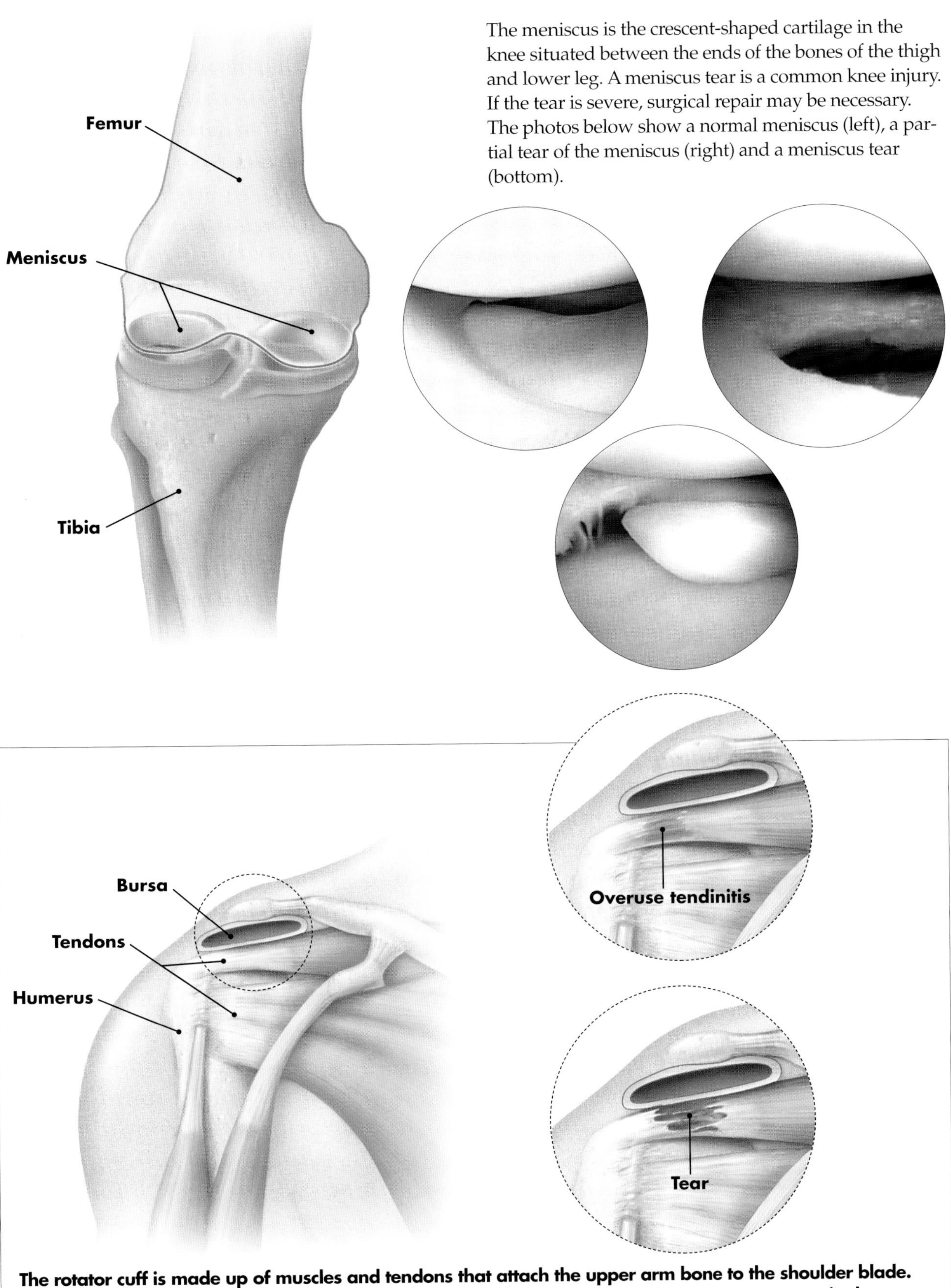

The rotator cuff is made up of muscles and tendons that attach the upper arm bone to the shoulder blade. Typical rotator cuff injuries involve inflammation of the tendons (tendinitis) or one or more tears in the tendons.

Breast Disorders

All breast lumps need to be taken seriously and investigated promptly. However, the vast majority of lumps are noncancerous (benign) and may be associated with a woman's monthly menstrual cycle.

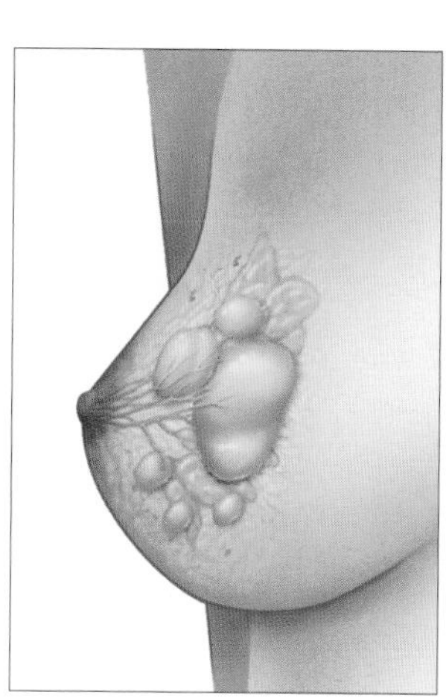

A breast cyst (see above) is a fluid-filled sac that tends to enlarge near the end of a woman's menstrual cycle, when the body is retaining more fluid. Some cysts are tiny, but others can be as large as an egg.

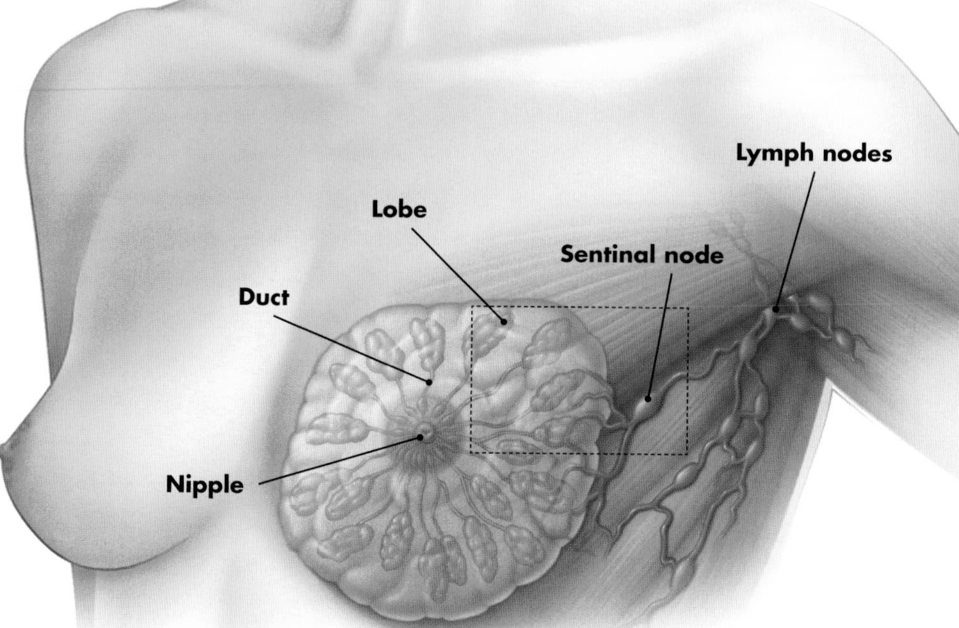

The sentinel node is the first lymph node into which a tumor drains. By finding the sentinel node before surgery, doctors can remove the node for study during surgery. If the sentinel node is free of cancer, it's unlikely the cancer has spread.

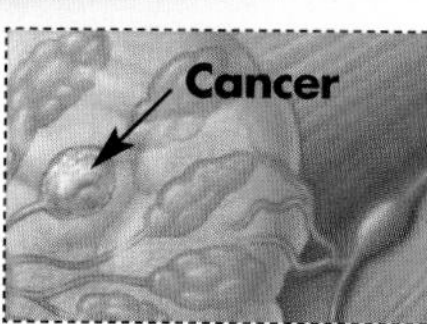

Early breast cancer is confined to the duct

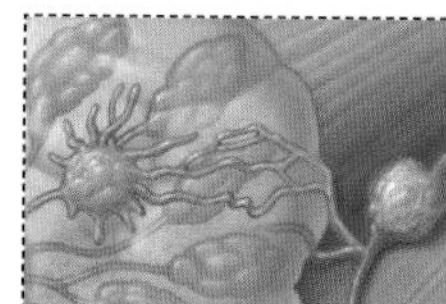

Invasive breast cancer has spread from a duct into adjacent breast tissue and the nearby sentinal node

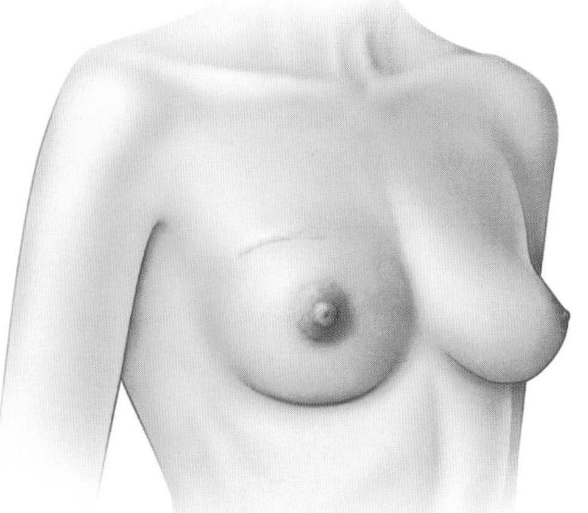

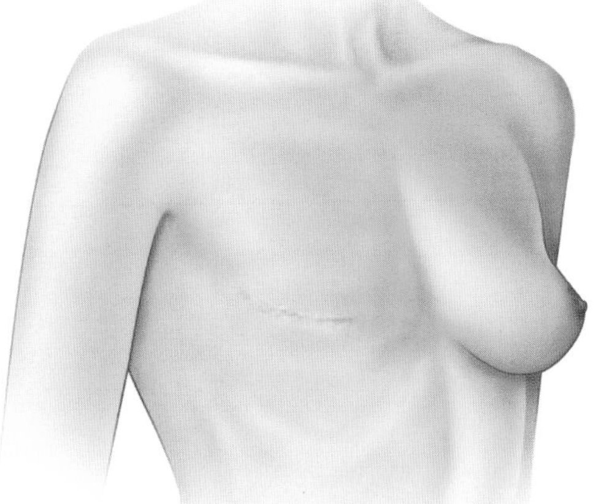

During a lumpectomy, the tumor is removed along with some of the lymph nodes. During a modified radical mastectomy, the breast is removed, and possibly some underarm lymph nodes. Chest muscles are left intact.

Prostate Disorders

Benign prostatic hyperplasia (BPH) is a noncancerous enlargement of the prostate gland that's common in older men. Your prostate gland may enlarge and gradually compress your urethra, slowing the flow of urine.

A more serious disorder is prostate cancer. Prostate cancers grow within the gland. The tumor may not produce any signs and symptoms.

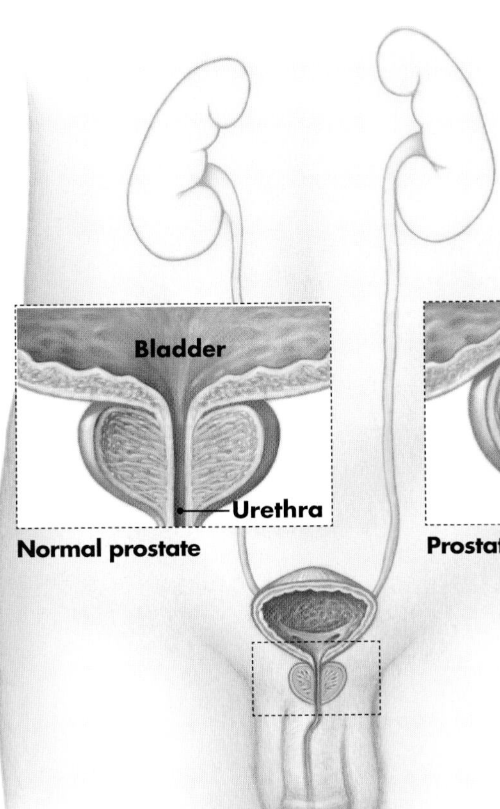

Normal prostate

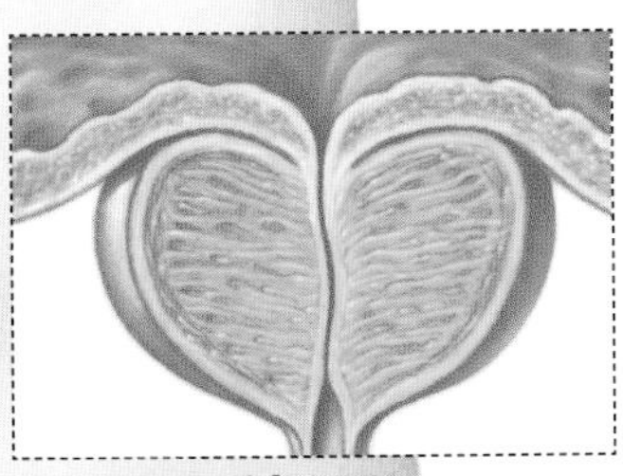

Prostate with BPH

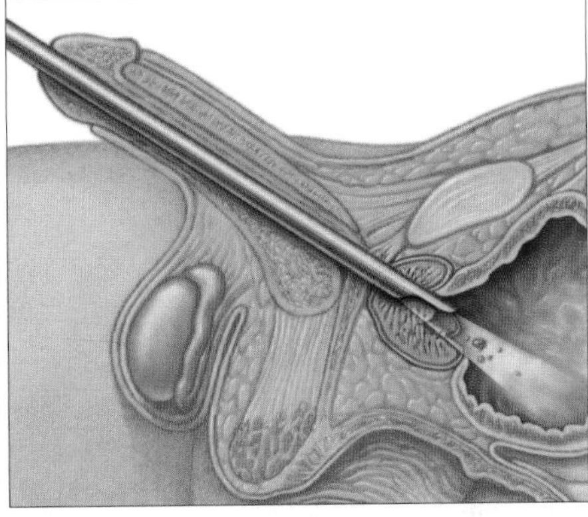

For BPH, a surgeon can reduce the size of the prostate gland with a procedure called transurethral resection of the prostate (TURP). Other procedures also may be used.

Staging and grading prostate cancer. When a biopsy confirms the presence of cancer, the cancer is staged to determine how far it has spread, with stage I being the most confined and stage IV the most widespread. The cancer is also graded to determine whether it's a slow- or fast-growing form. The most common scale runs from I to V, with I being the least aggressive form of cancer.

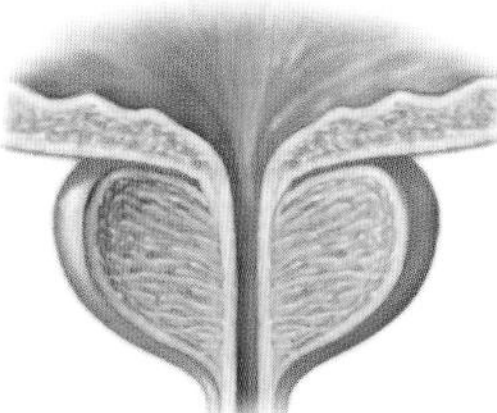

Stage I. Very early cancer that's confined to microscopic particles that can't be felt on examination.

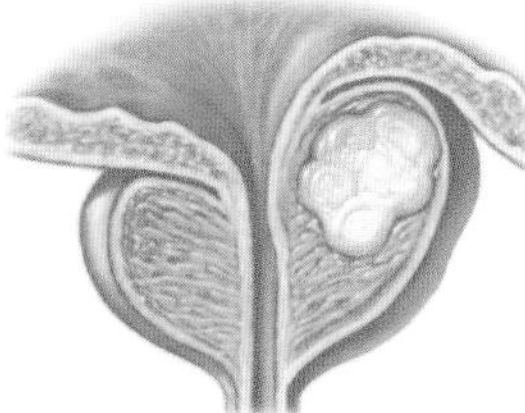

Stage II. Cancer that can be felt but is confined to the prostate.

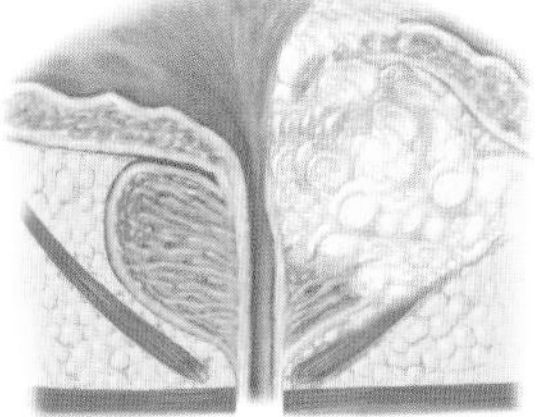

Stage III. Cancer that has spread beyond the prostate to seminal vesicles or adjacent bladder tissue.

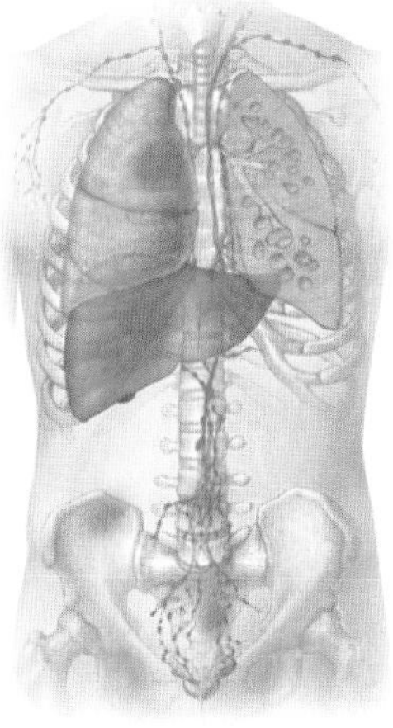

Stage IV. Advanced cancer that has spread to lymph nodes, bones, lungs or other organs.

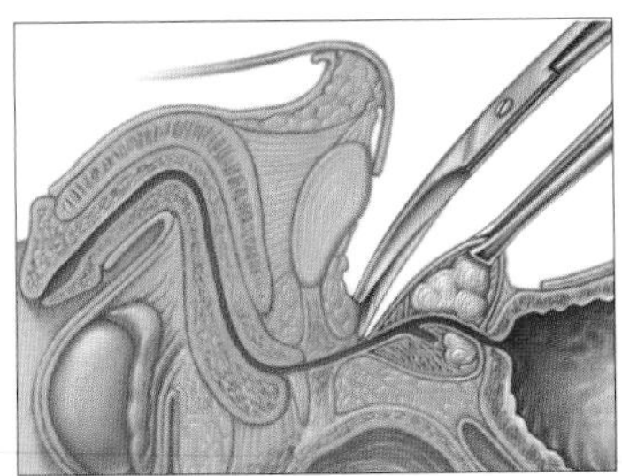

For prostate cancer, removal of the prostate gland (radical prostatectomy) is a common treatment option. Other procedures also may be used.

Heart Disorders

Coronary artery disease is a common cause of heart disease. In this condition, fatty deposits (plaques) accumulate on the interior walls of the arteries in your heart. This narrowing reduces blood flow and can cause chest pain (angina) or lead to a heart attack. A common procedure to widen arteries and restore circulation is balloon angioplasty followed by placement of a stent (see below).

An alternative to opening blocked arteries is coronary bypass surgery (see right). Bypass surgery involves rerouting blood around blockage sites. Bypasses can be surgically constructed out of veins taken from a leg or from arteries arising near the collarbone. A double bypass operation (see right) routes blood around blockages in two vessels.

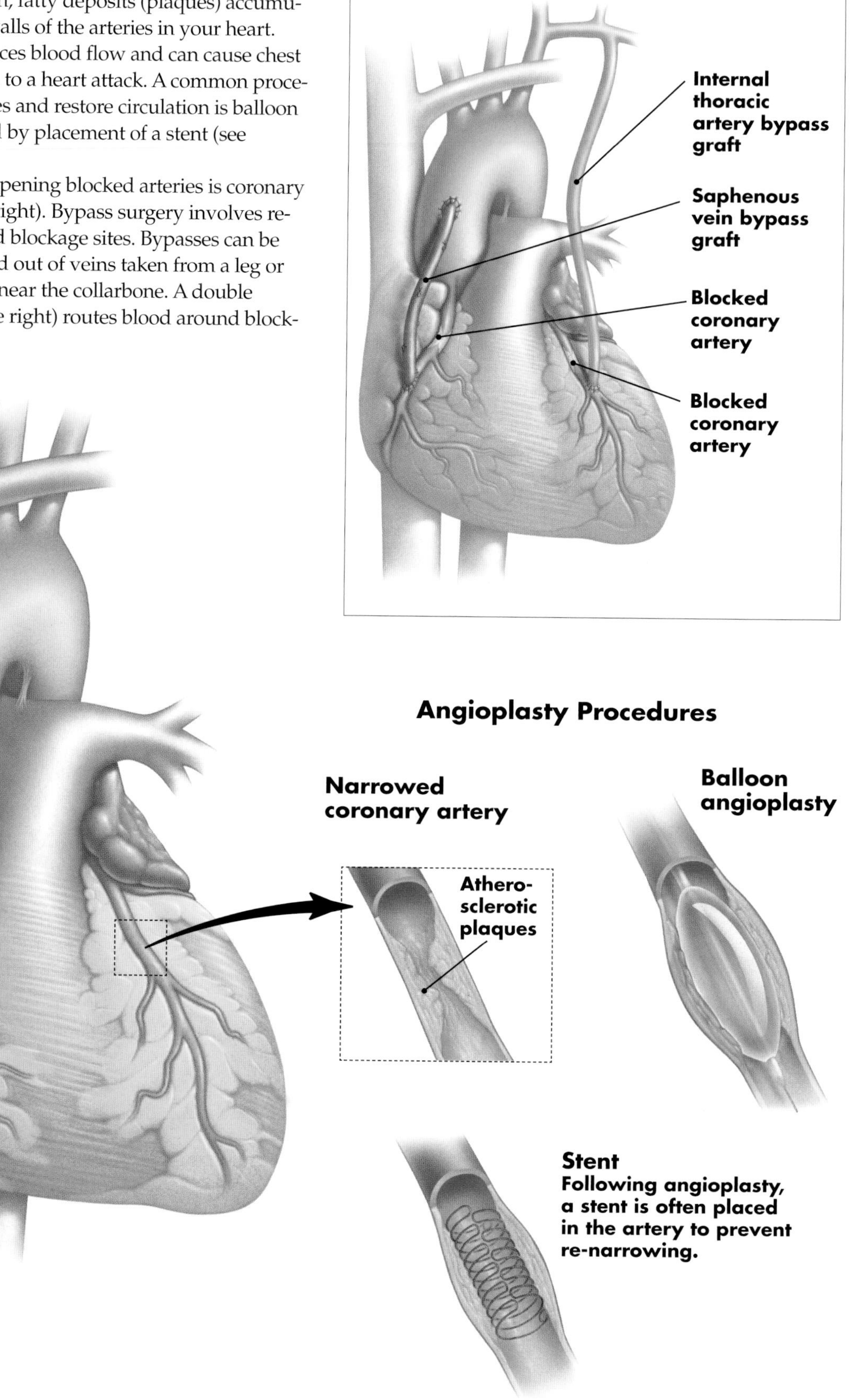

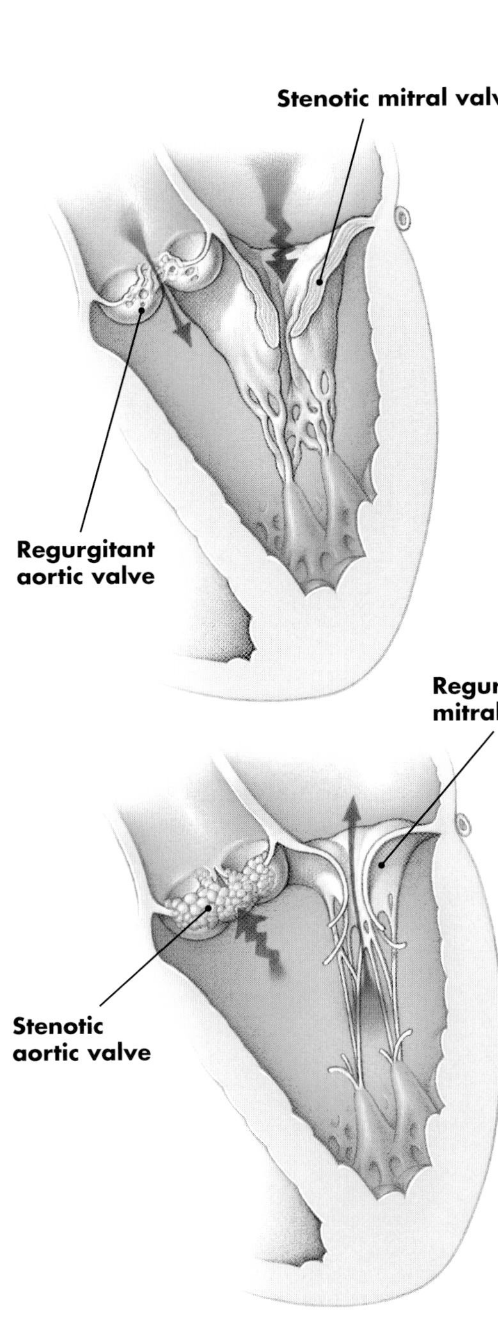

Heart valve disease can cause the valves to narrow, restricting blood flow through them (valve stenosis). Valves may also not close properly, allowing blood to flow backward (valve regurgitation).

Top-left illustration
A narrowed (stenotic) mitral valve impedes blood flow from the left atrium to the left ventricle. A leaky (regurgitant) aortic valve allows blood to flow from the aorta back into the left ventricle when the ventricle relaxes.

Middle-left illustration
A narrowed (stenotic) aortic valve reduces blood flow from the left ventricle into the aorta. A leaky (regurgitant) mitral valve allows blood to flow back from the left ventricle to the left atrium when the ventricle contracts.

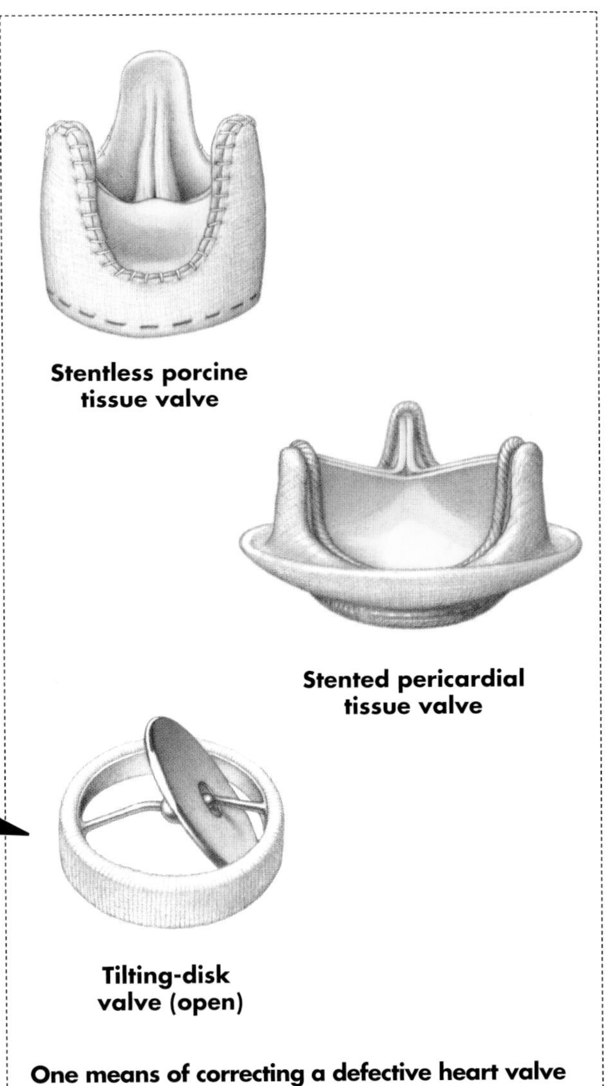

One means of correcting a defective heart valve is for a surgeon to remove it and replace it with an artificial valve. Various types of artificial (prosthetic) valves are availabe, each with its own advantages.

Lung Disorders

Three common chronic lung disorders restrict the flow of air out of the bronchial passages: chronic bronchitis, emphysema and asthma. Another lung disorder, lung cancer, is the leading cause of cancer deaths in the United States.

In asthma (see right), lung airways become inflamed and swollen. Muscles surrounding the airways tighten and constrict, and membranes in airway linings secrete excess mucus.

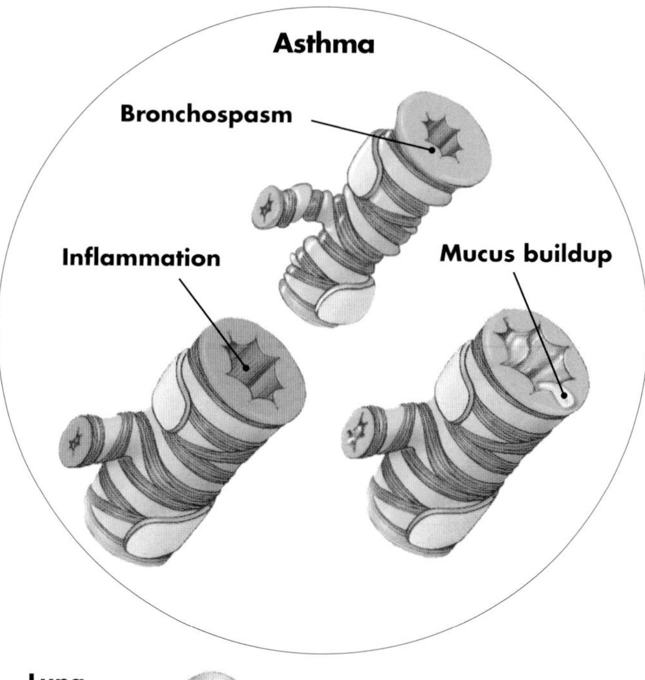

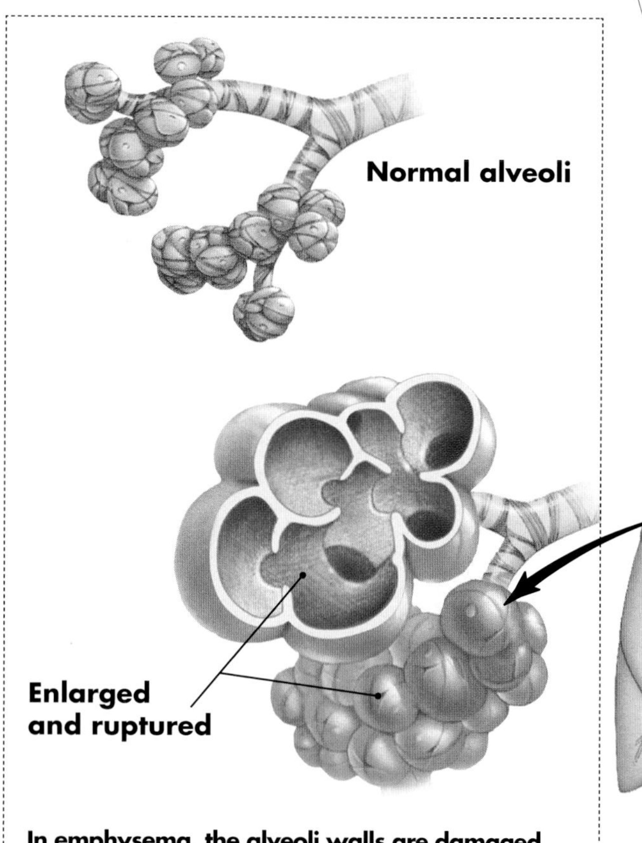

In emphysema, the alveoli walls are damaged by inflammation. Alveoli can lose their natural elasticity, become overstretched and rupture.

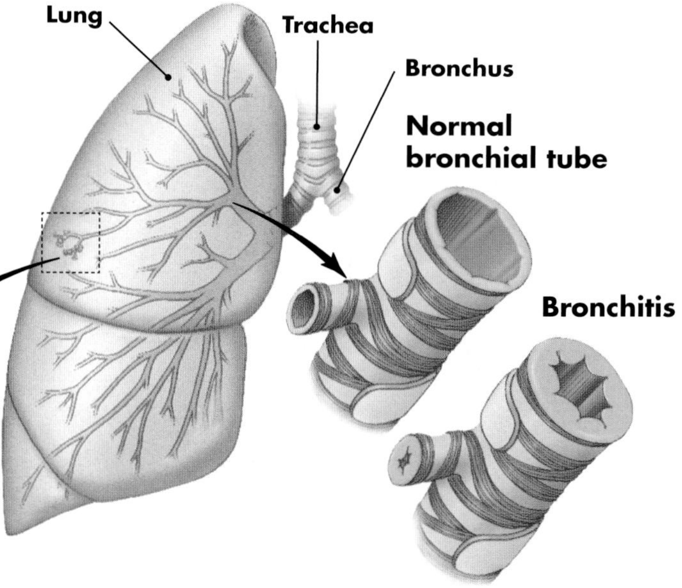

Chronic bronchitis is a chronic inflammation and thickening of the walls of the bronchial tubes, which narrows them.

Lung Cancer

Surgery to treat lung cancer involves removing the cancer and a portion of surrounding lung tissue. The most common surgery is lobectomy.

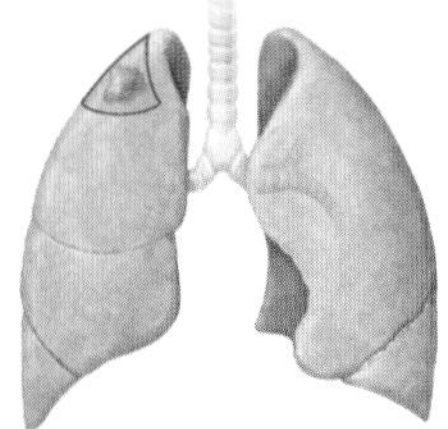

Wedge resection is removal of a small portion of a lobe.

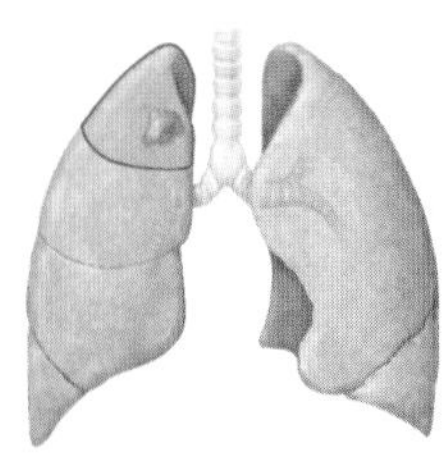

Segment resection is removal of a larger portion of a lobe.

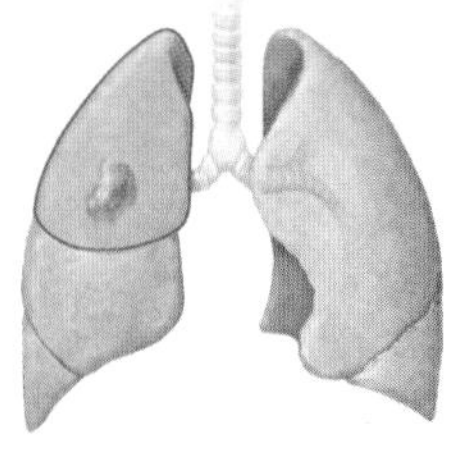

Lobectomy is removal of an entire lobe.

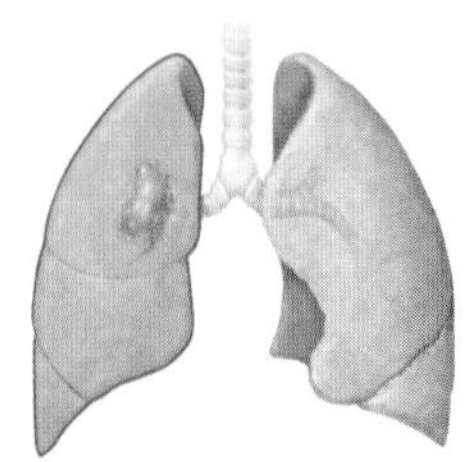

Pneumonectomy is removal of an entire lung.

Blood Disorders

There are many blood disorders, each caused by a malfunction of a certain blood component. Anemias are caused by too few red blood cells and leukemias by too many white blood cells. Bleeding disorders are often caused by defects in platelets or clotting factors.

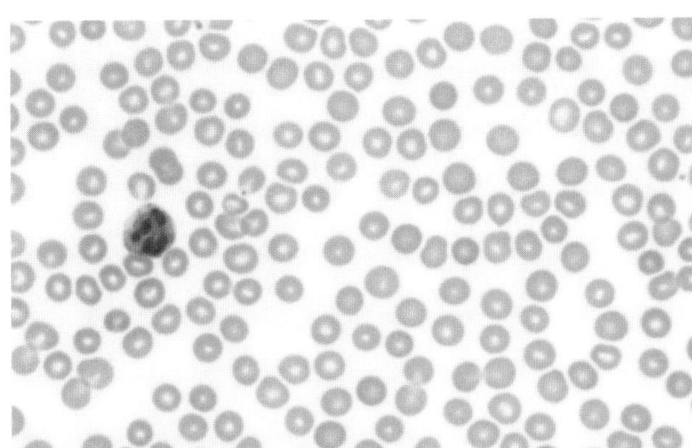

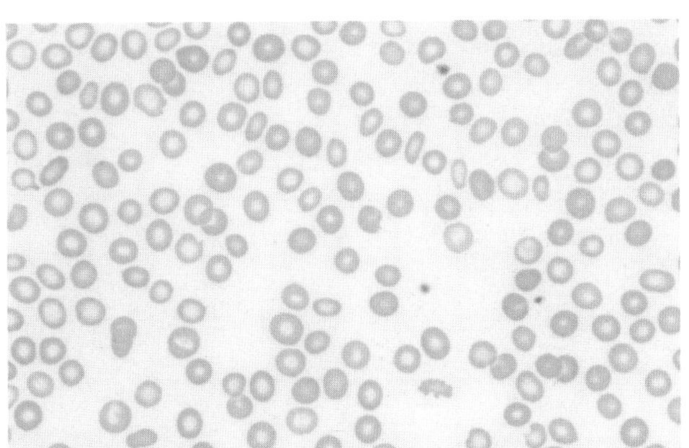

On the left is a normal blood smear. On the right is a blood smear showing iron deficiency anemia. The cells are smaller, and the white area in the middle of the cells is larger (increased central pallor).

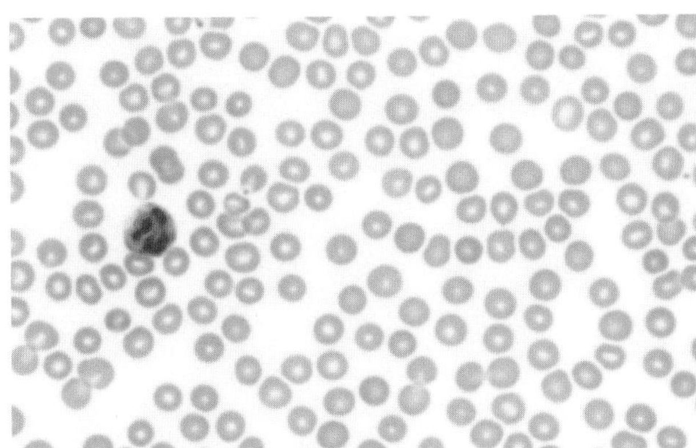

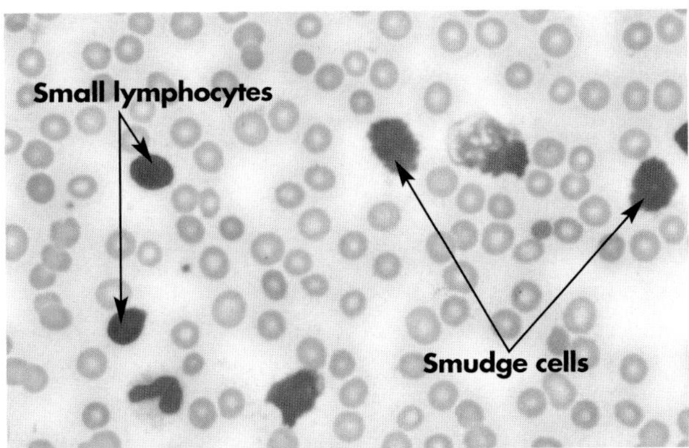

On the left is a normal blood smear. On the right is a blood smear showing chronic lymphocytic leukemia. There's an increased number of small lymphocytes and some smudge cells.

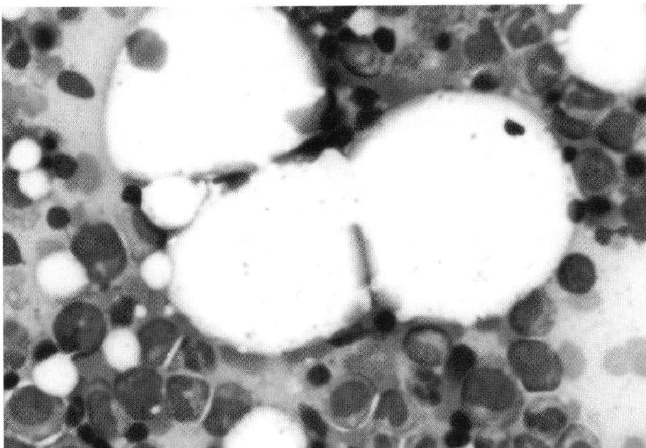

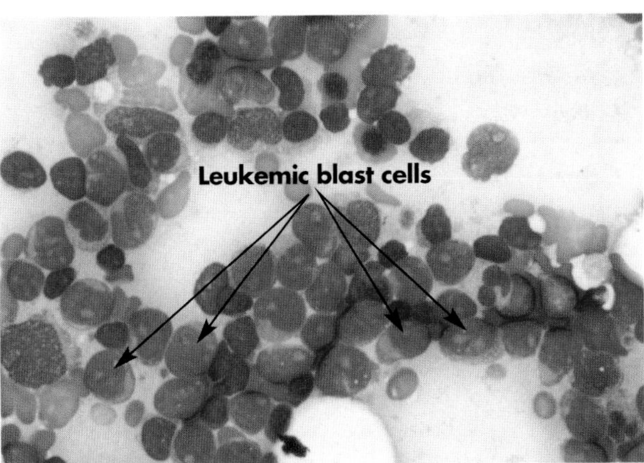

On the left is a slide of normal bone marrow showing a variety of cells. On the right is a slide showing acute leukemia, a primary cancer of bone marrow. Most of the cells on the slide to the right are leukemic blast cells.

Gastrointestinal Disorders

The digestive system is composed of a complex network of organs that convey and convert food into energy the body needs. There are many disorders that can affect this intricate system.

Gallstones (shown below) are made up of various components of bile and form in the gallbladder. If the stones leave the gallbladder, they can become lodged in ducts and cause problems.

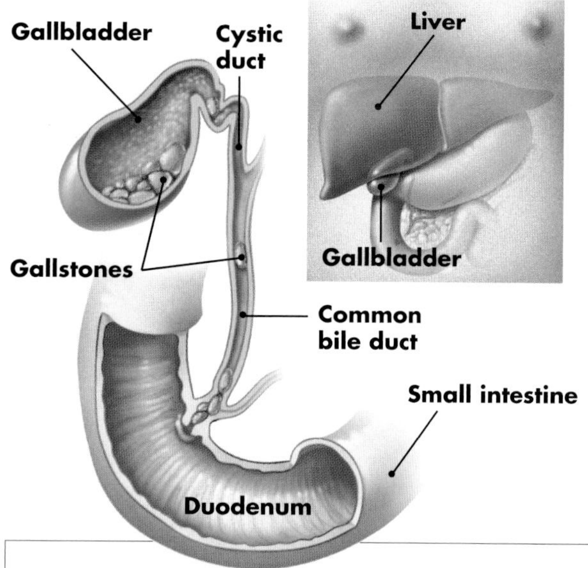

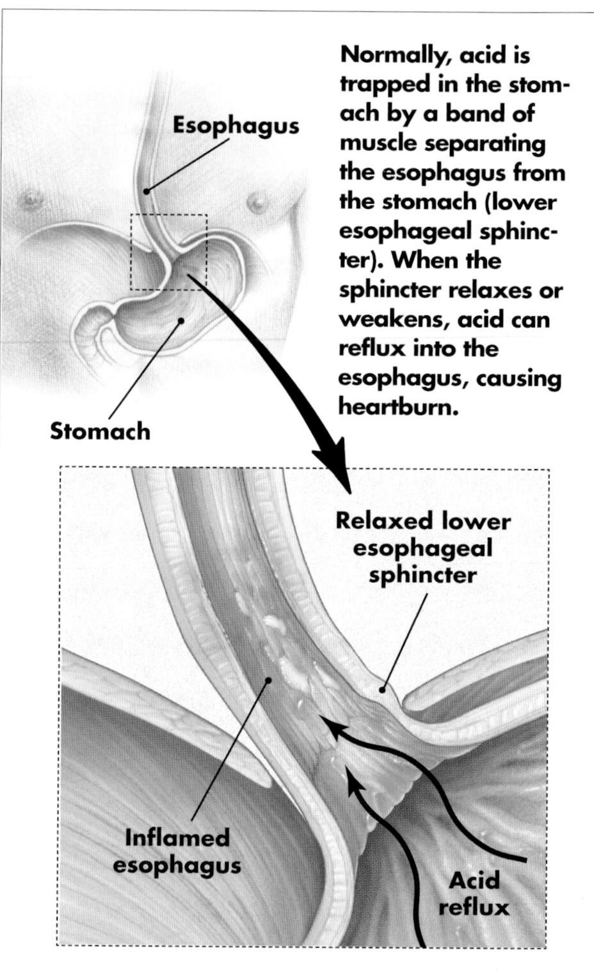

Stage 0. The cancer is in its earliest stage. It hasn't grown beyond the inner layer (mucosa) of the colon or rectum.

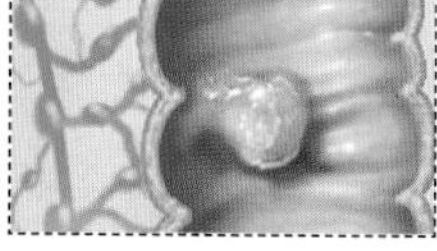

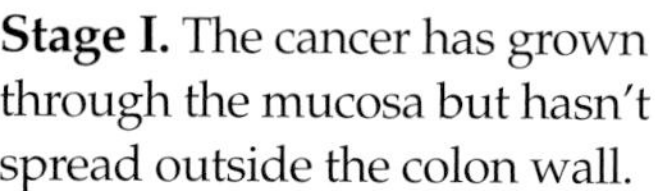

Stage I. The cancer has grown through the mucosa but hasn't spread outside the colon wall.

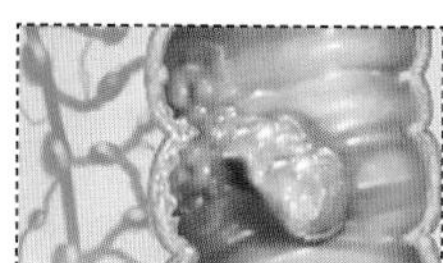

Stage II. The cancer has grown through the wall of the colon or rectum but hasn't spread to nearby lymph nodes.

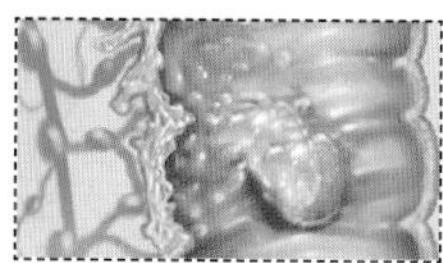

Stage III. The cancer has spread to nearby lymph nodes but hasn't spread to other parts of the body.

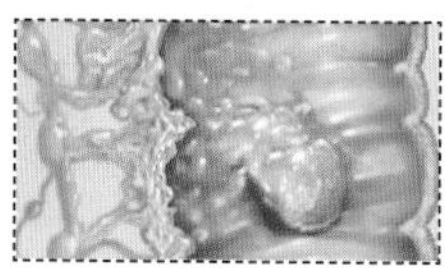

Stage IV. The cancer is advanced and has spread to distant organs, such as the liver or lungs, or the lining of the abdominal cavity.

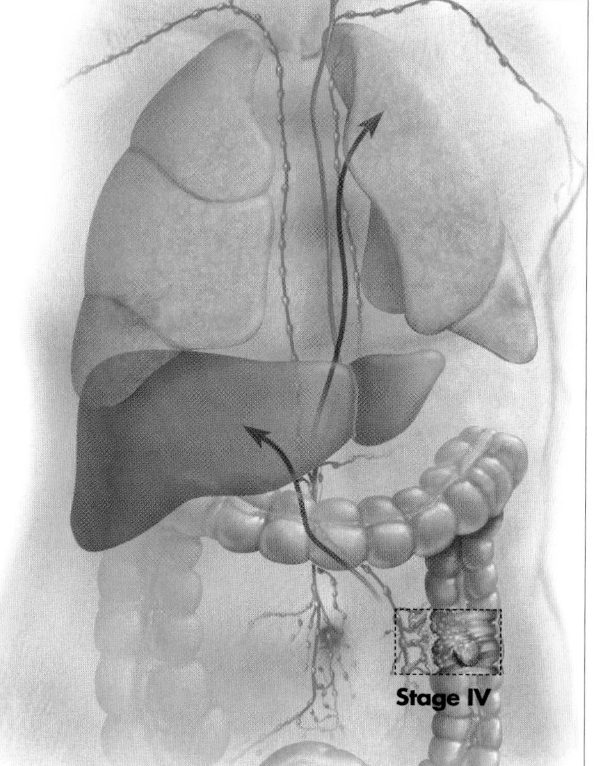

Unlike some other cancers, the size of the cancerous tumor isn't a major factor in determining the outcome of colorectal cancer. Of greater importance is how far the cancer has spread.

Eye Disorders

The delicate structures of the eye often change with age, making it more difficult to see. Aging also increases the risk of serious eye disorders.

Although certain vision problems may be an unavoidable, natural part of aging. Others can be prevented. Even those that are unavoidable can often be slowed or stopped through early detection and treatment.

Some of the most common eye disorders include cataracts, glaucoma, macular degeneration and diabetic retinopathy.

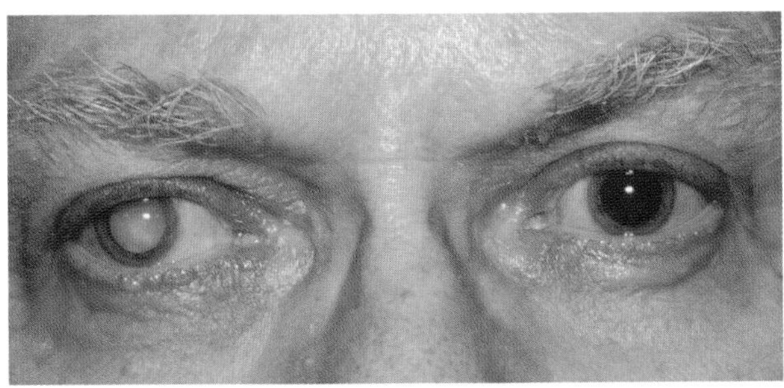

A cataract occurs when the lens of the eye becomes cloudy (left eye), giving the pupil a white appearance.

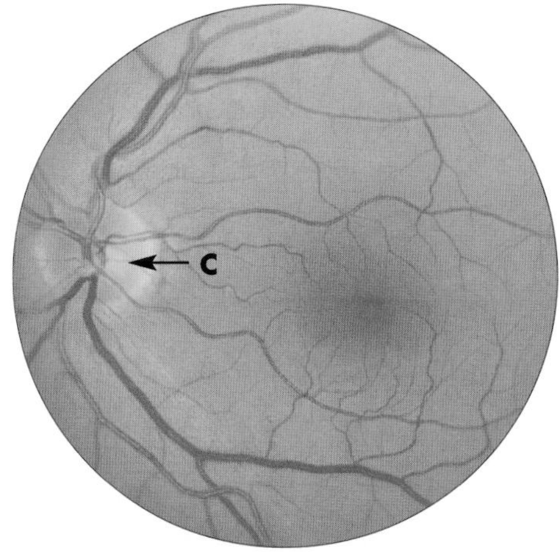

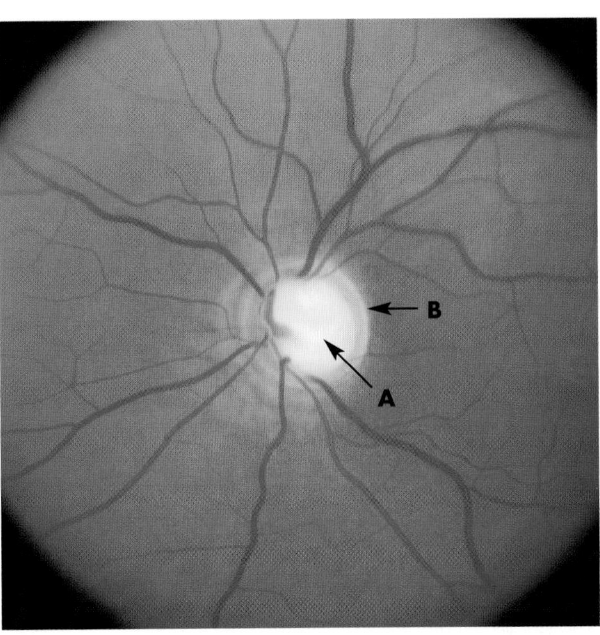

The photo on the right shows an optic nerve that's damaged by advanced glaucoma. This is evident from the evacuation (cupping) at the center of the optic disk (A). Only a narrow rim of optic nerve tissue remains (B). In comparison, the optic disk of a healthy eye (above) has more even and reddish coloration (C).

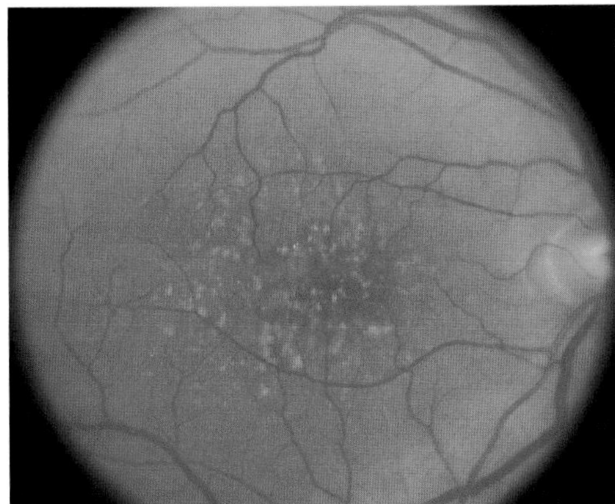

The hallmark of early-stage dry macular degeneration is the appearance of waste deposits (drusen) in and around the macula. Drusen have the appearance of yellow spots.

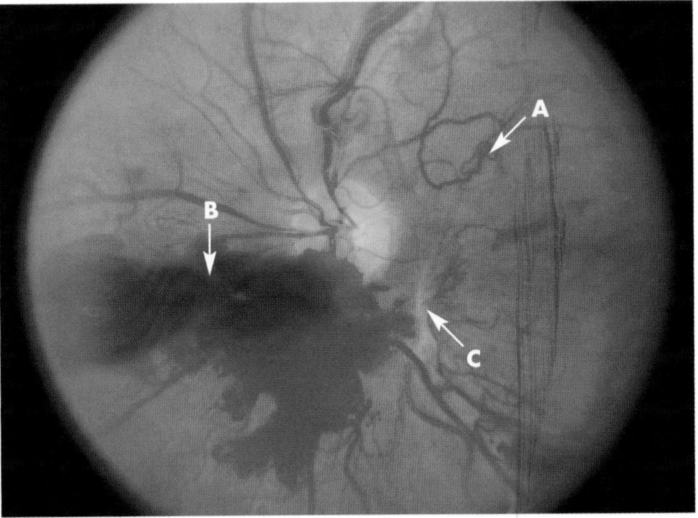

In late-stage proliferative diabetic retinopathy, abnormal blood vessels grow on the optic nerve and the retina and into the vitreous cavity (A). These blood vessels break, causing bleeding (B) and the formation of scar tissue (C).

Skin Disorders

The color and texture of your skin can reveal a great deal about the health of your skin and your health in general. Sometimes the first clue to illness is revealed by a rash or welts. At other times, the skin disorder itself is the only abnormality.

Psoriasis and Dermatitis

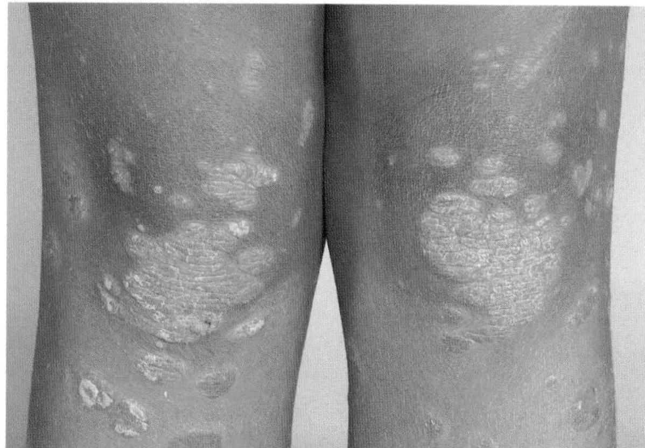

Psoriasis. Areas of skin are covered with dry, red patches with silvery scales. Lesions may itch.

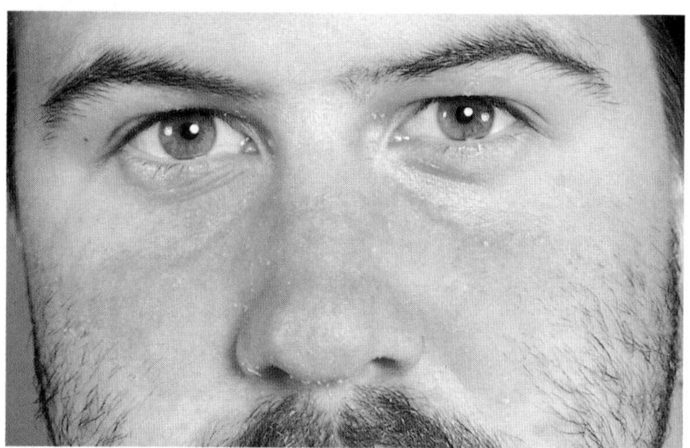

Seborrheic dermatitis. Greasy-appearing, scaly, itchy areas on the sides of the nose, between the eyebrows, behind the ears or on the scalp.

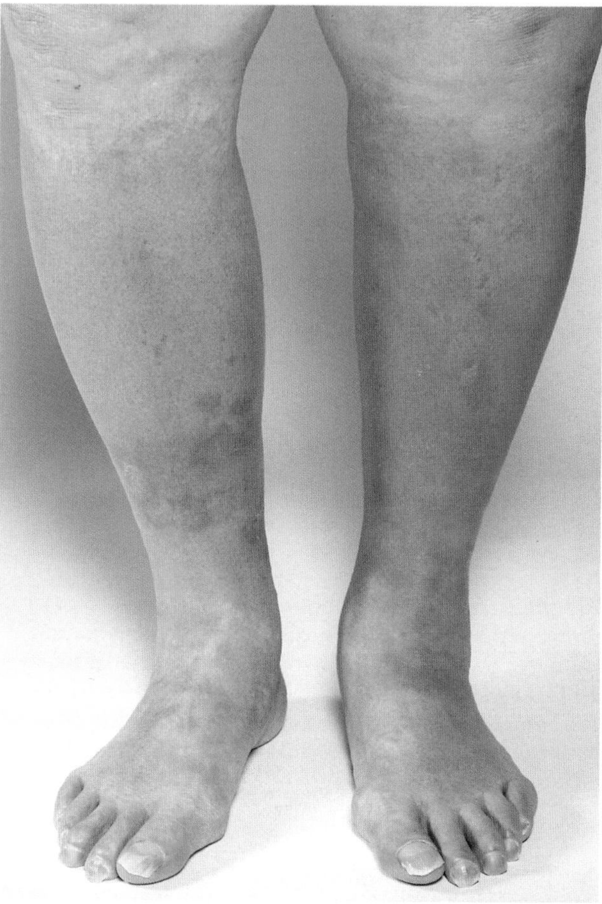

Stasis dermatitis. Thickening, redness and itching of the skin of the lower legs and ankles, often associated with varicose veins.

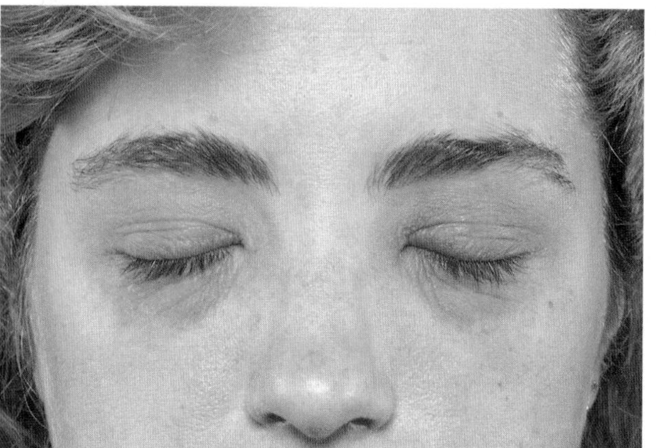

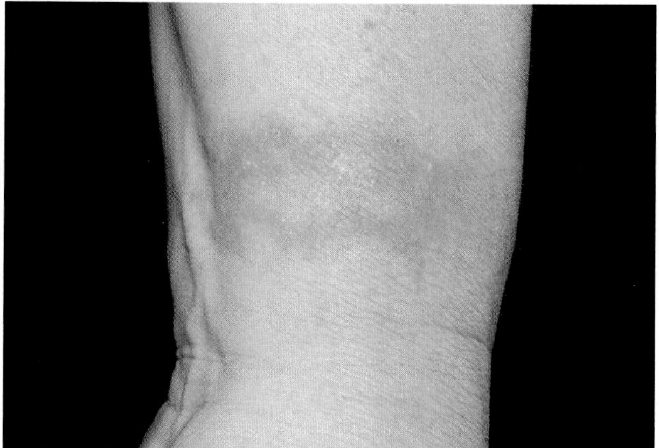

Contact dermatitis. Skin redness and itching resulting from direct contact with a plant, chemical or other substance, such as makeup (left) or a bracelet made from nickel (right).

VISUAL GUIDE

Pigmentary Disorders

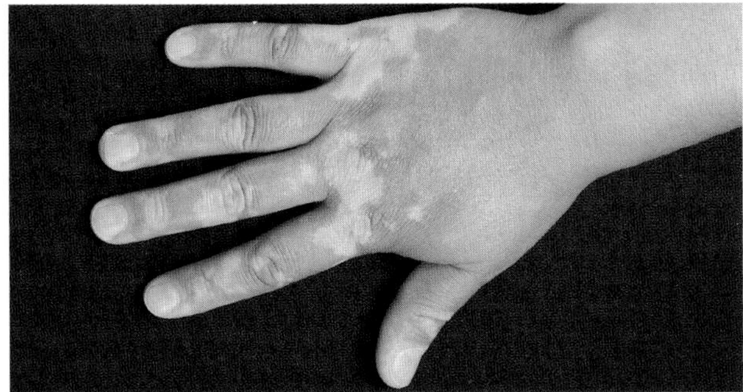

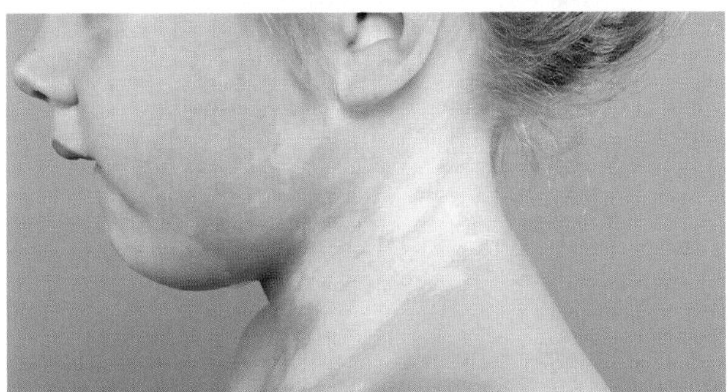

Vitiligo. The development of patches of white or depigmented skin.

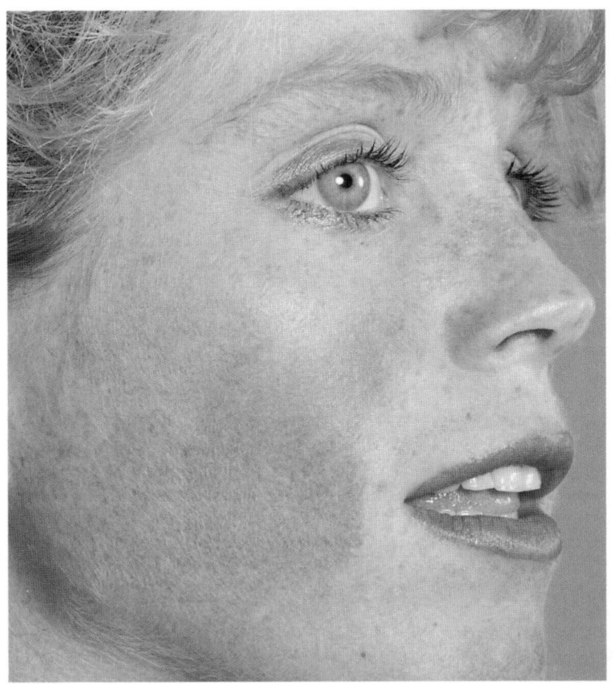

Chloasma. Patches of darker skin, most commonly found on the face. Results from excessive melanin in the skin. Condition is common during pregnancy.

Aging Skin

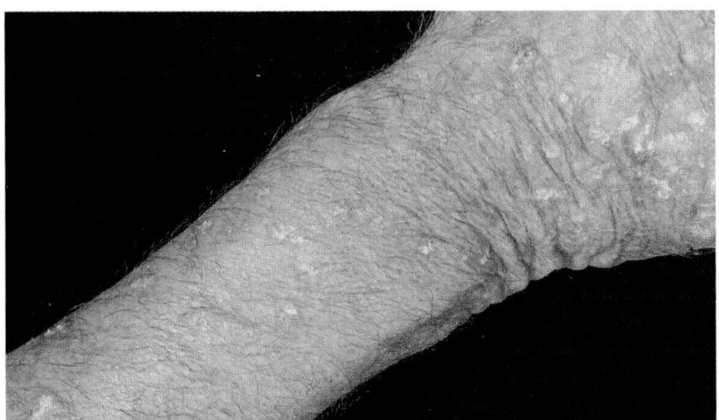

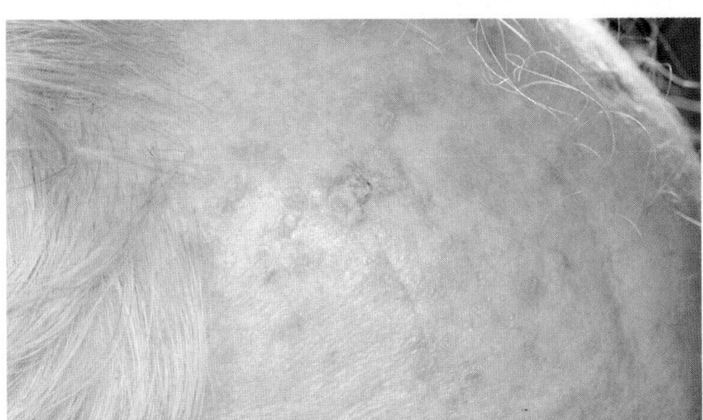

Actinic (solar) keratoses. Gritty, scaly, gray to dark pink patches on face, scalp and back of hands. The patches have a sandpaper surface. They may be precancerous.

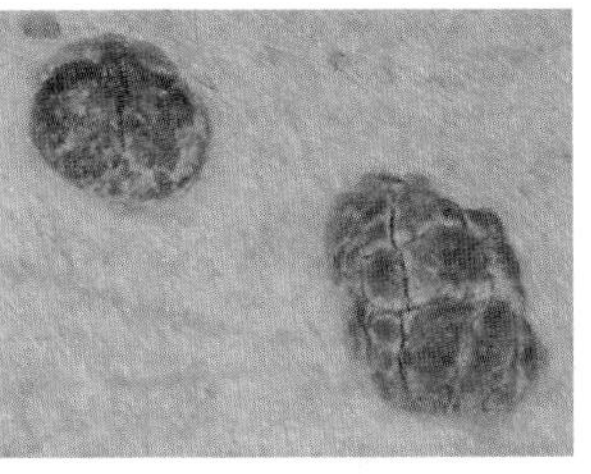

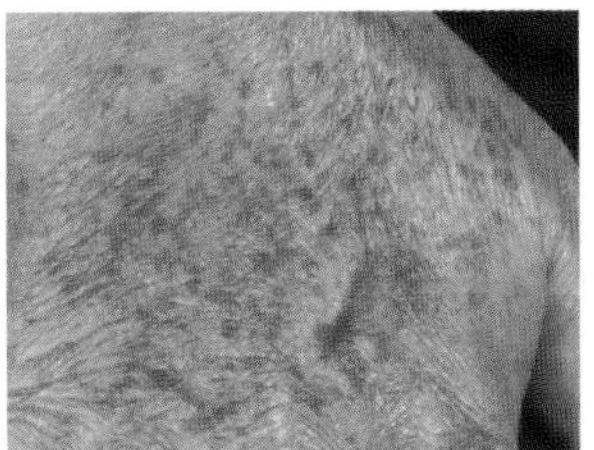

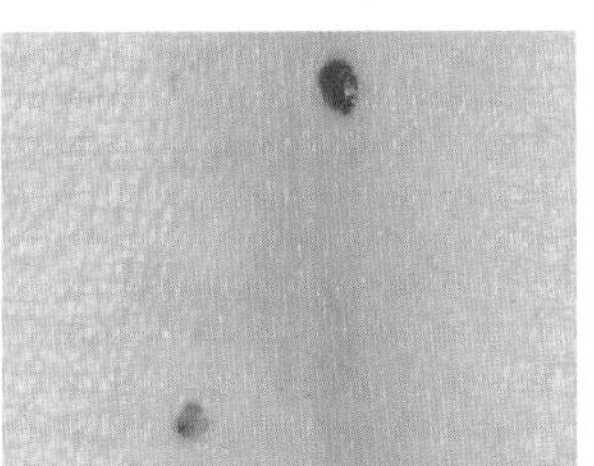

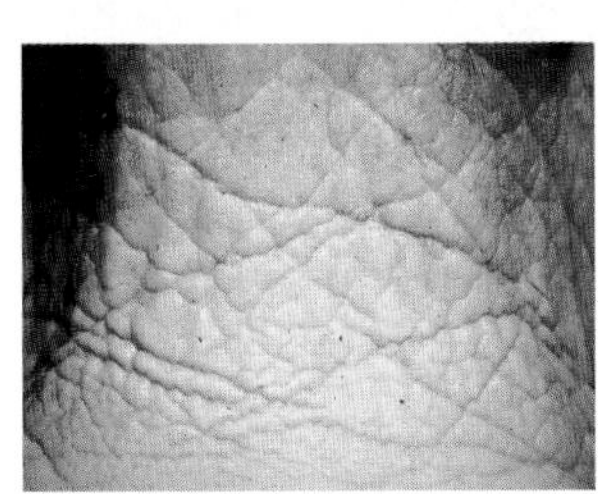

Seborrheic keratoses (upper left). Oval lesions with a waxy, scaly, slightly elevated appearance.

Solar lentigines (upper right). Flat patches of increased pigmentation that range from freckle sized to a few inches across. Also called liver spots.

Cherry angiomas (bottom left). Characterized by small, smooth, cherry-red bumps on skin. Range in size from a pinhead to ¼-inch across.

Sun-damaged skin (bottom right). Coarse wrinkles, sagging folds, dryness or leathery toughness.

Skin Cancer

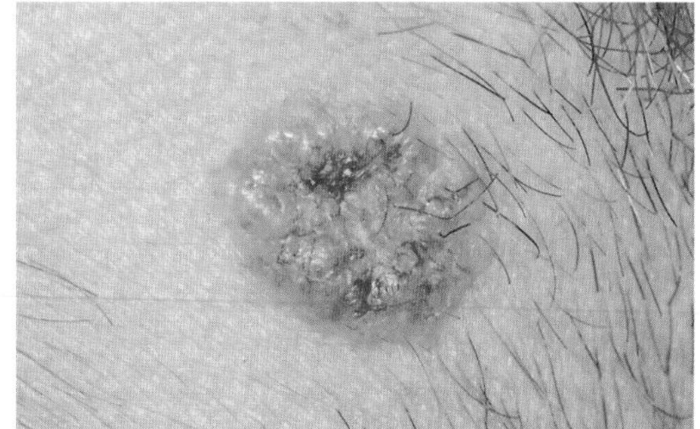

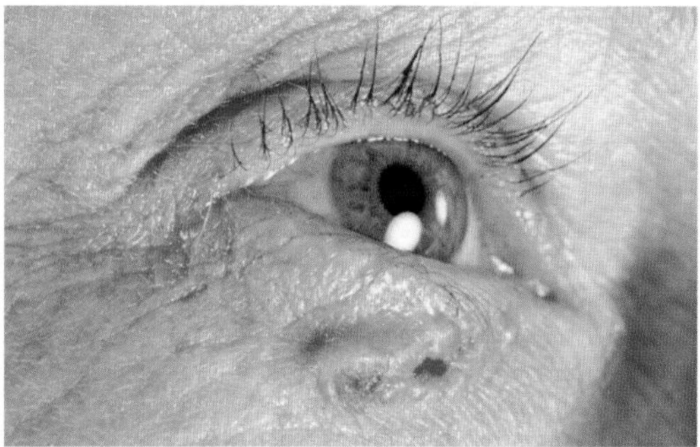

Basal cell cancer. The most common malignant skin tumor. Characterized by a pearly or waxy bump commonly found on the face, ears or neck. Or it may be a flat, flesh-colored or brown scar-like lesion.

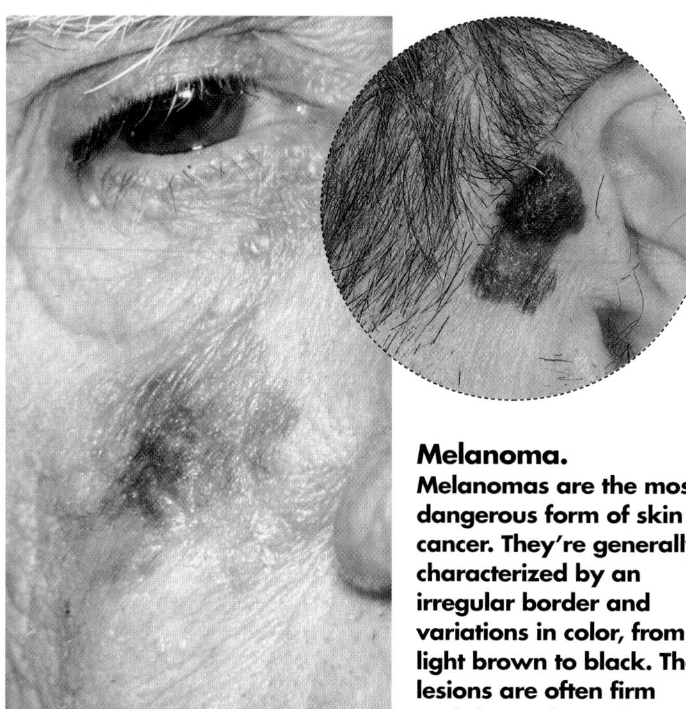

Melanoma. Melanomas are the most dangerous form of skin cancer. They're generally characterized by an irregular border and variations in color, from light brown to black. The lesions are often firm and dome shaped.

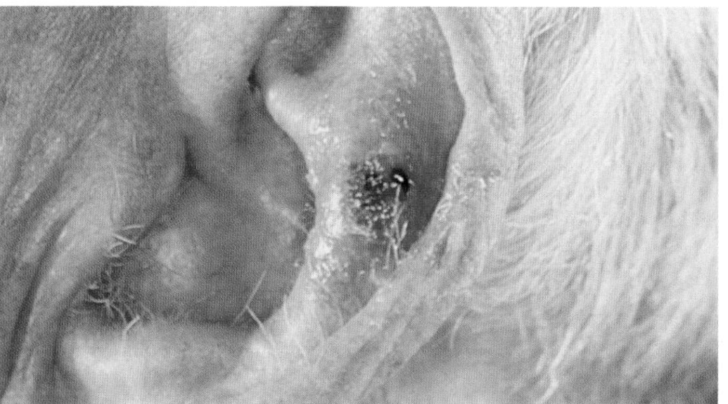

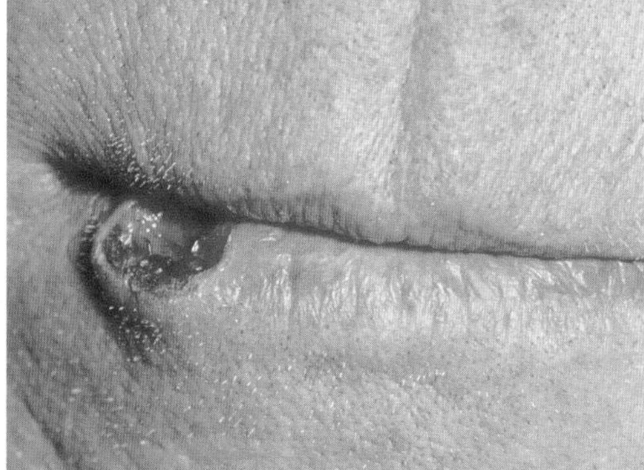

Squamous cell cancer. This skin cancer typically appears in areas exposed to sun. The lesion is generally firm, red, nodular or flat and has a scaly, crusted or ulcerated surface.

Noncancerous (Benign) Growths

Skin tag. Tiny, soft growth attached to a narrow stalk. Often skin colored but may be darker.

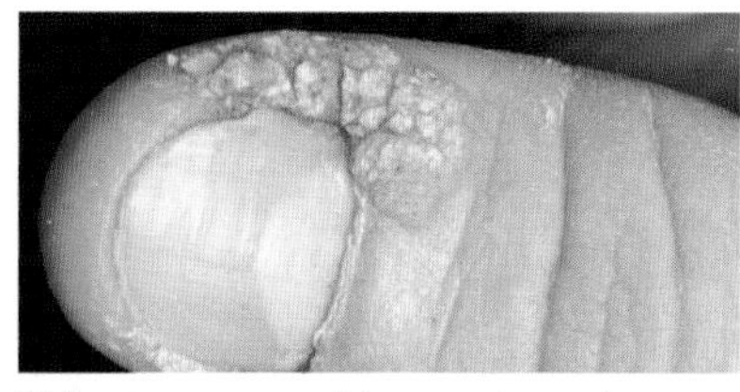

Warts. Caused by a virus that stimulates rapid reproduction of skin cells. Most commonly occur on hands or feet.

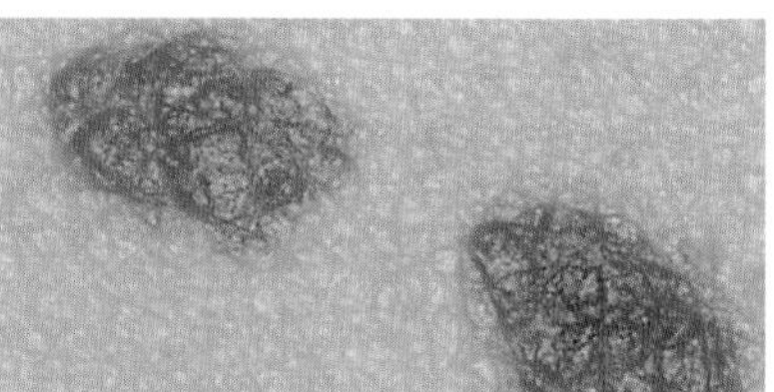

Moles. Accumulations of pigment cells. May stay smooth or become raised or wrinkled, and may contain hair.

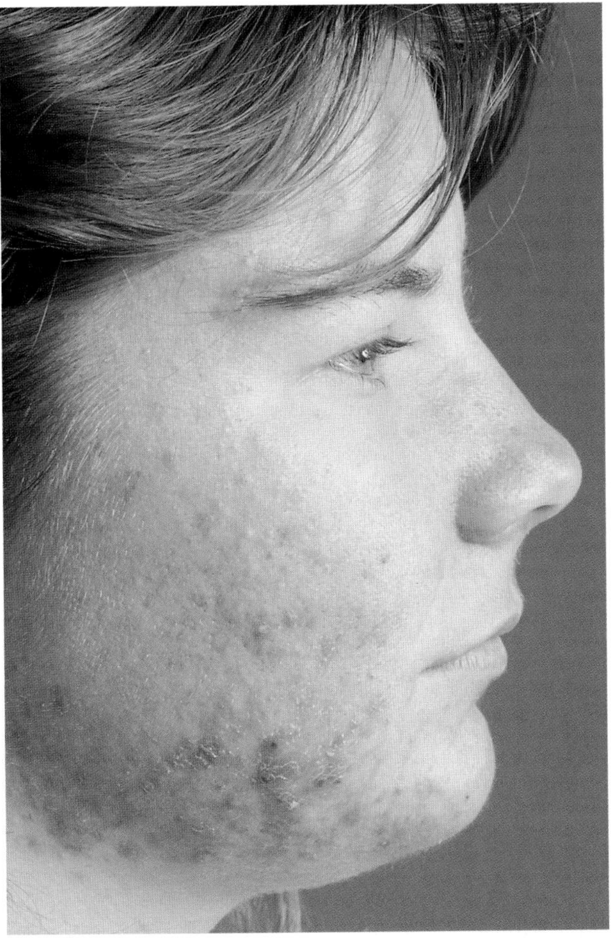

Common acne. Clogging of hair pores (follicles) in skin, causing the development of whiteheads or blackheads on the face, neck, shoulders or back.

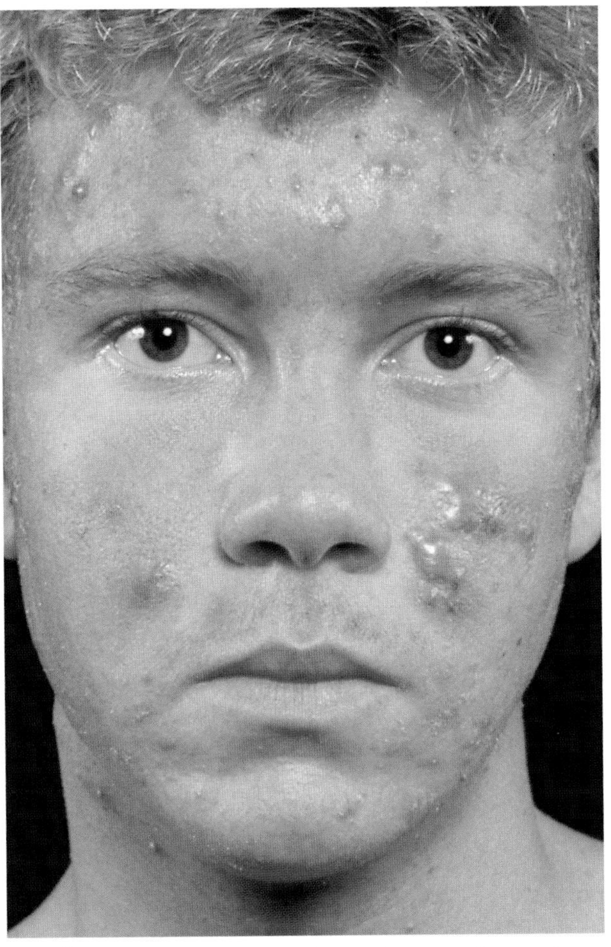

Cystic acne. Most severe form of acne. Clogged pores cause boil-like infections (cysts) in the skin.

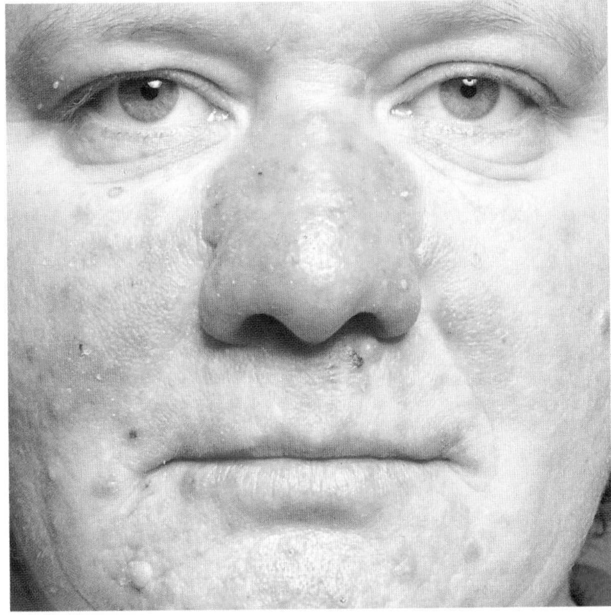

Acne rosacea. Chronic inflammation of the central face with pustules in the reddened area. Occurs most often in adults.

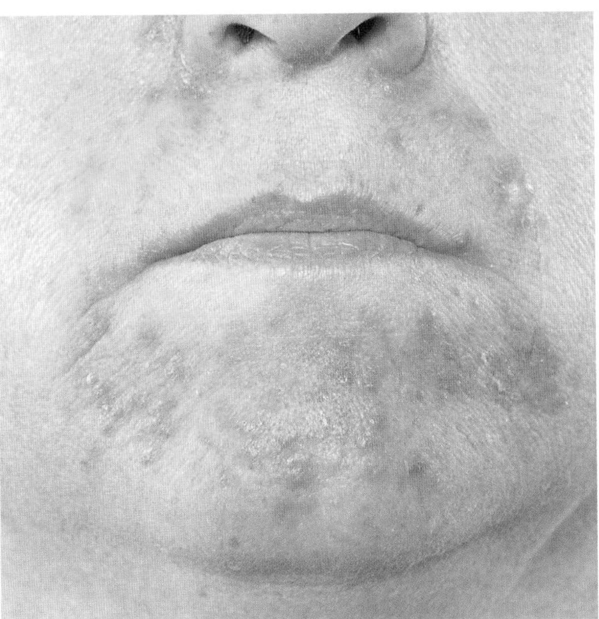

Perioral dermatitis. Red, often bumpy, rash around the mouth and chin. An area of normal skin usually separates the edge of the lips from the rash.

Childhood Diseases

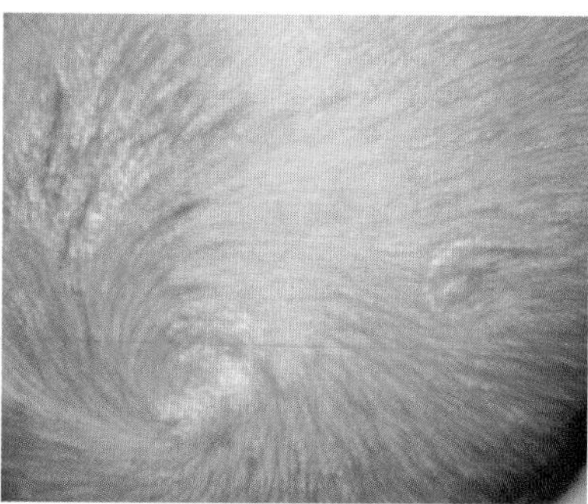

Cradle cap (infantile seborrheic dermatitis). Dry, scaly patches. Yellow crust may form over the patches.

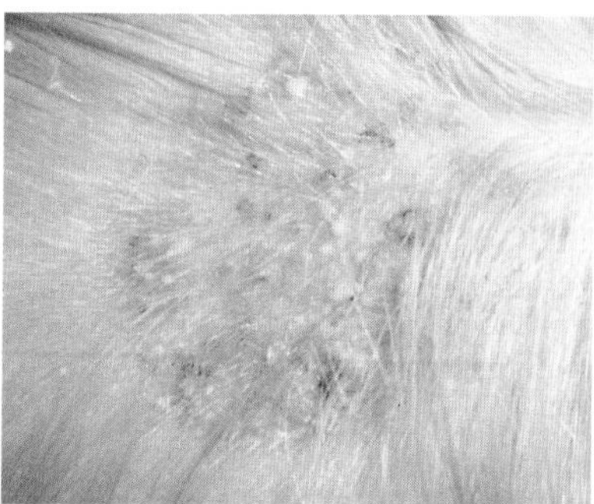

Scalp ringworm (tinea capitis). A fungal infection that causes an itchy, red, circular patch on the scalp.

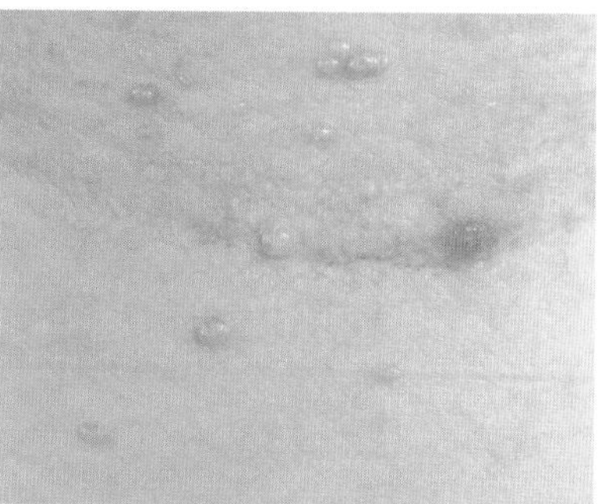

Molluscum contagiosum. Tiny pearl-like projections with a white, cheesy core.

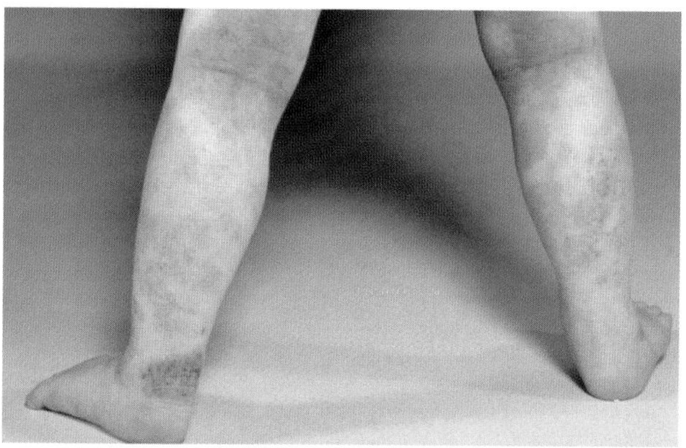

Infantile eczema. Rough, red, patchy rash usually associated with extremely dry skin.

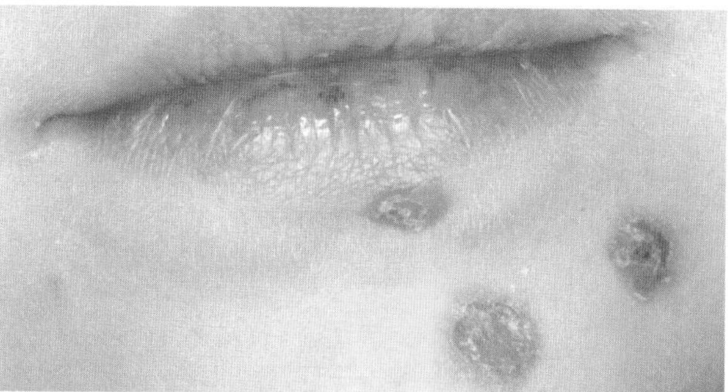

Impetigo. Bacterial infection that starts with a red sore, blisters briefly, oozes and forms a thick crust.

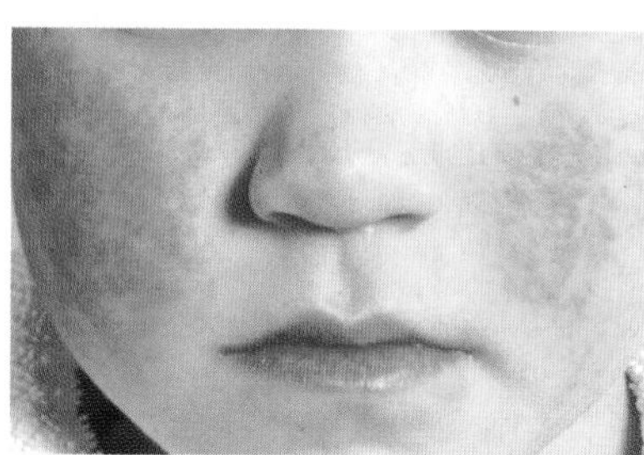

Fifth disease. A viral infection that causes a red rash on the cheeks, appearing as if the cheeks have been slapped.

Keratoses pilaris. Dead skin cells plug hair follicle openings, causing small, pointed pimples.

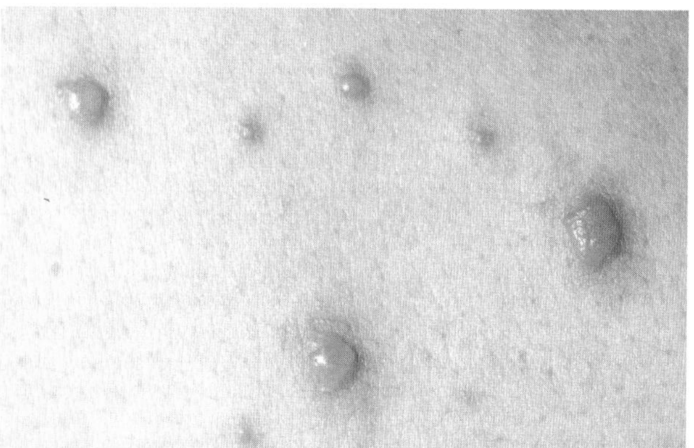

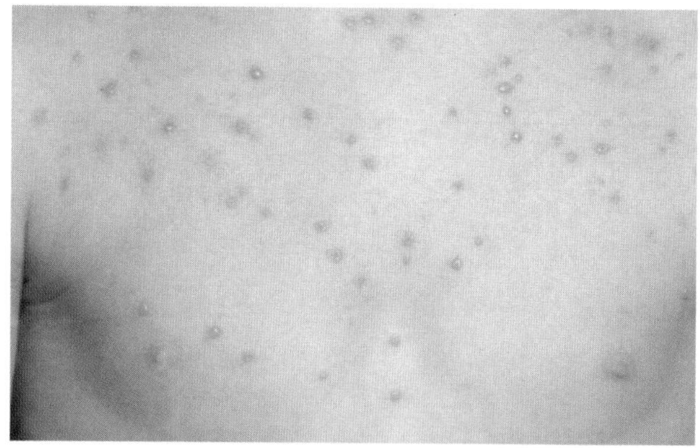

Chickenpox (varicella). Itchy, red rash that breaks out (erupts) on the face, scalp, chest, back, and arms and legs. Spots fill with clear fluid, rupture and then crust over.

Infestations and Bites

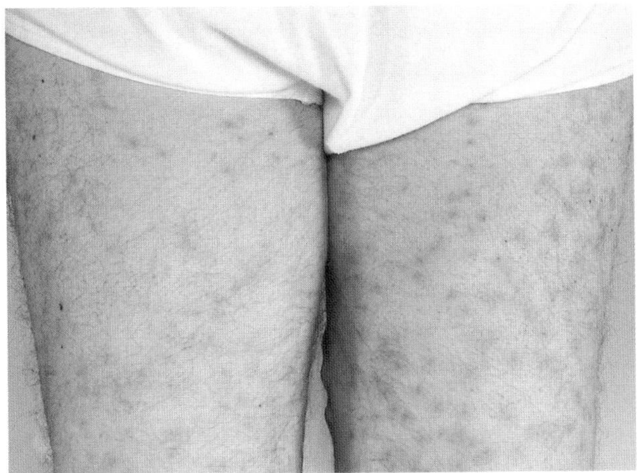

Swimmer's itch. Sandpaper-like rash caused by parasitic infestation. Develops after swimming in fresh water. Most noticeable beneath swimsuit.

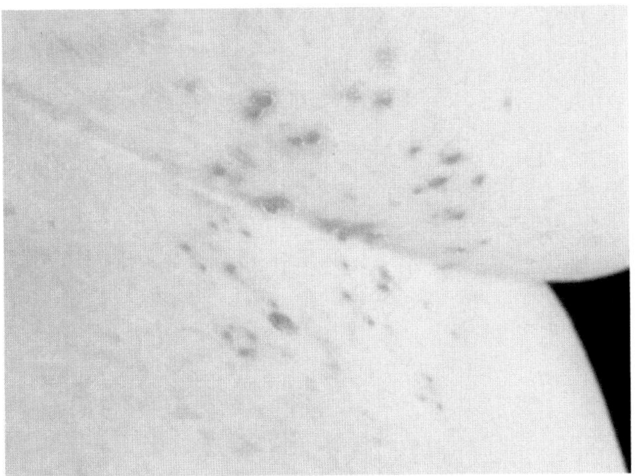

Scabies. Lesions where tiny mites burrow in the skin. Itching is often severe.

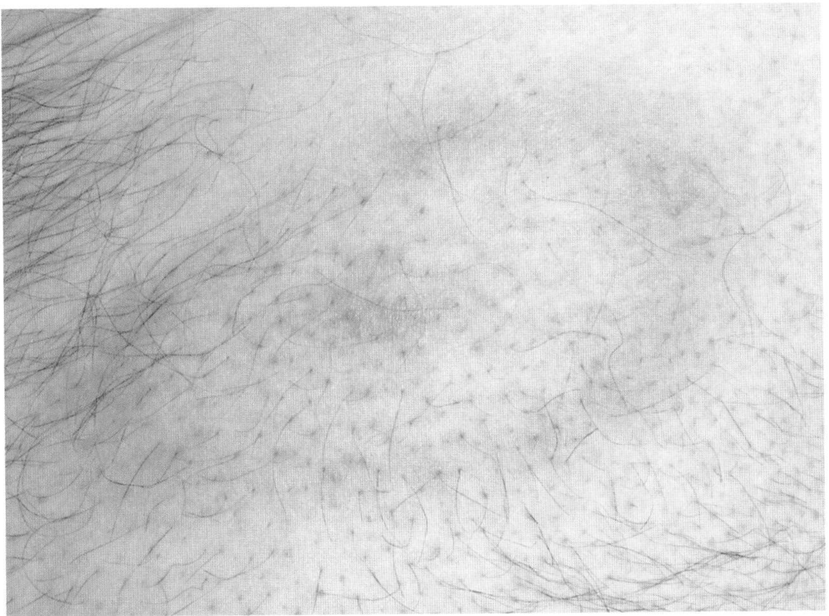

Lyme disease. Red rash that usually occurs at the site of a tick bite. Central portion clears as the rash spreads outward.

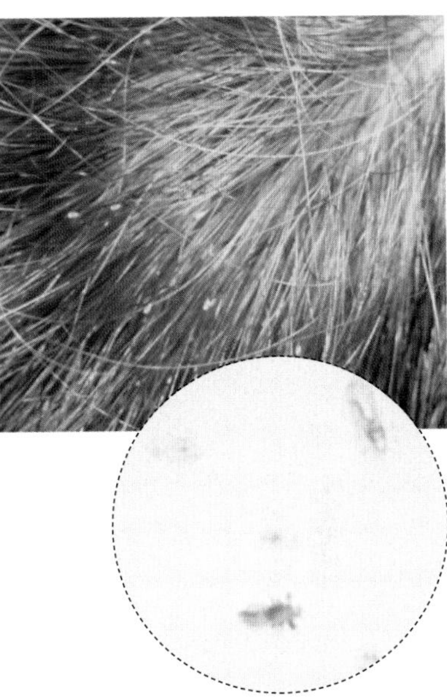

Head lice. Tiny insects found on the scalp. Small nits (eggs) resembling tiny pussy-willow buds are found on hair shafts.

Hives

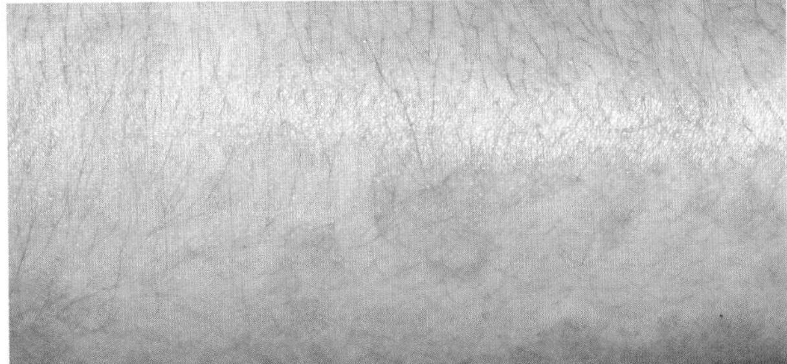

Hives (uticaria). Characterized by raised, red, itchy welts of various sizes on the surface of the skin.

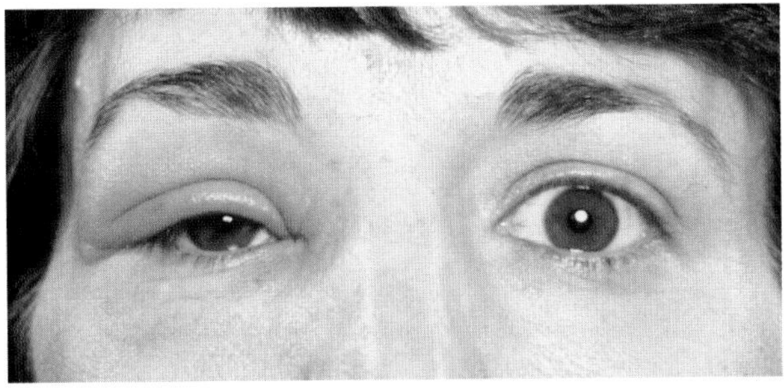

Angioedema. Large welts develop below the surface of the skin, particularly on the eyes and lips, but also on the hands, on the feet and in the throat.

Fungal Infections

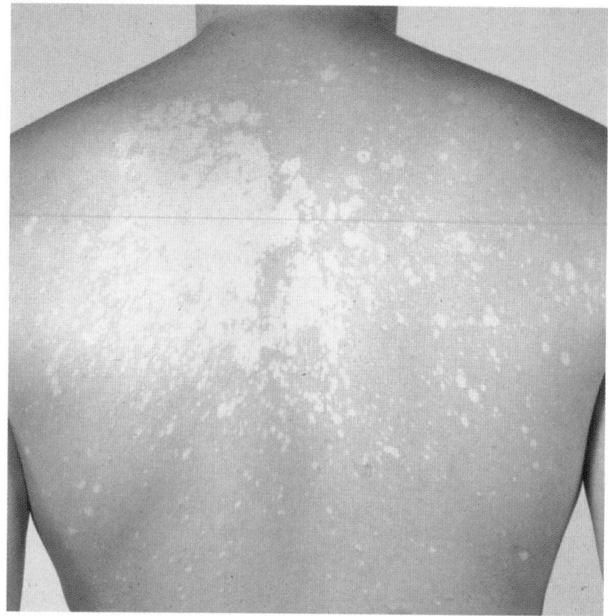

Tinea versicolor. Characterized by small, scaly, pale patches on the upper body and neck or face.

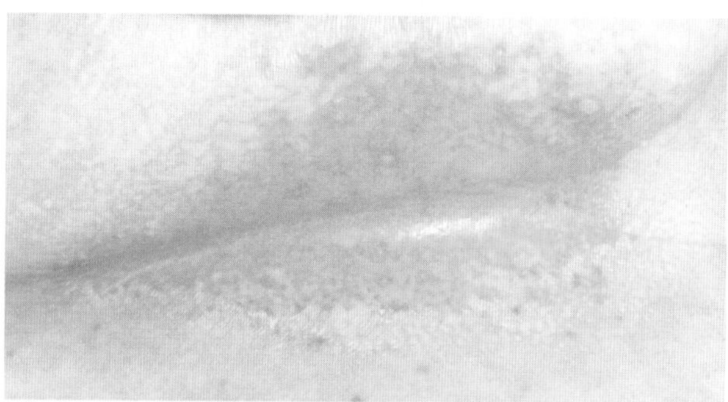

Intertrigo. Red, moist patches rimmed with small, red bumps found under the breasts, in armpits, in groin or buttock folds or between fingers or toes.

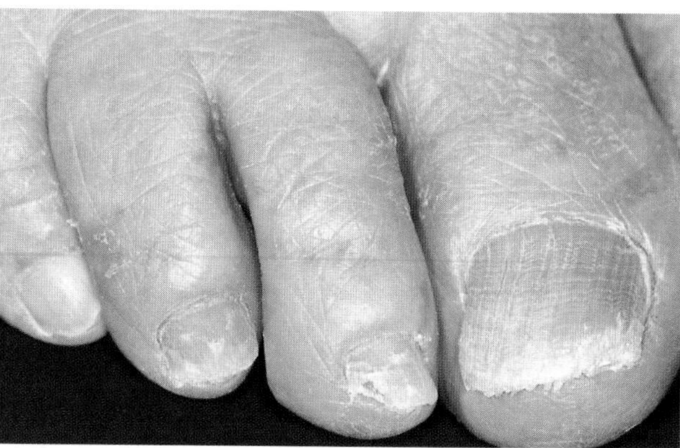

Onychomycosis. Fungal infection in the toenails or fingernails. Nails become discolored, pitted and may thicken.

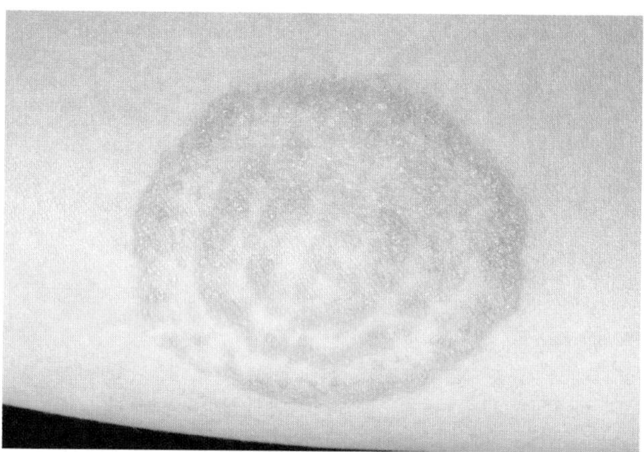

Ringworm (tinea corporis). Itchy, red, scaly, slightly raised expanding rings on the trunk, face, groin or thigh.

Other Infections

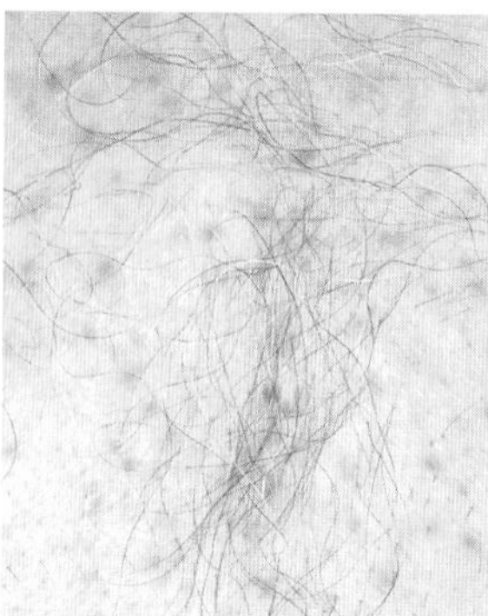

Folliculitis. Infection of hair follicles caused by bacteria or fungi.

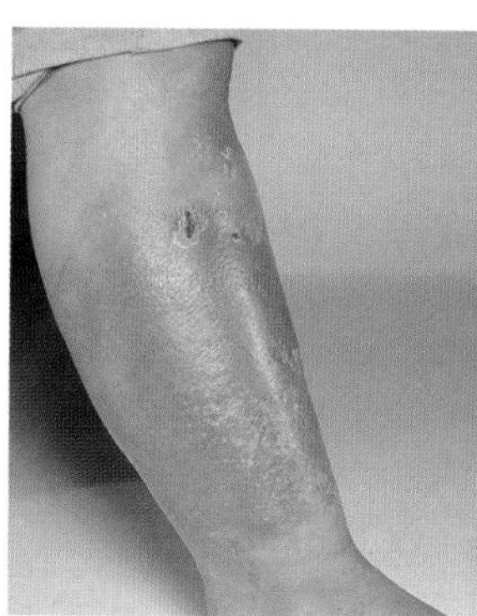

Cellulitis. Generally caused by bacterial infection. Characterized by hot, red, swollen and painful skin.

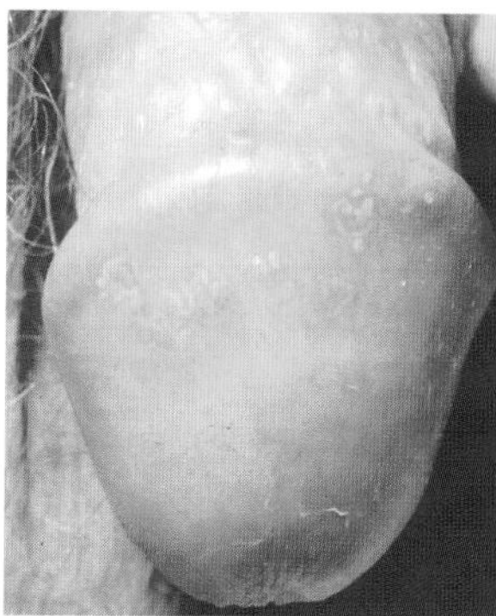

Genital herpes. Lesions characterized by blisters or open sores (ulcers). Often accompanied by burning or tingling sensation or pain.

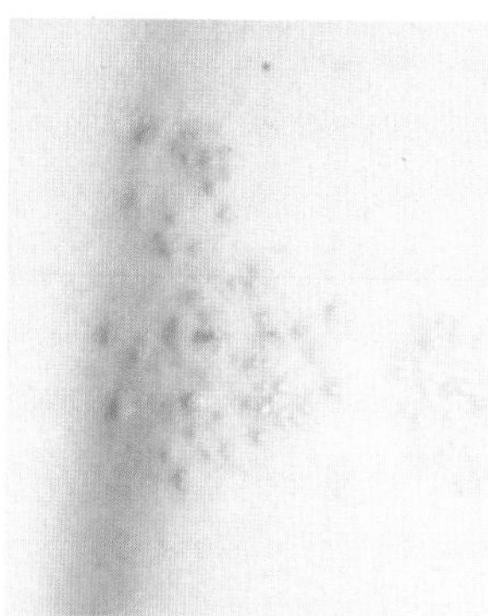

Shingles (herpes zoster). A red rash with small fluid-filled blisters, often extending out from the spine along a nerve pathway.

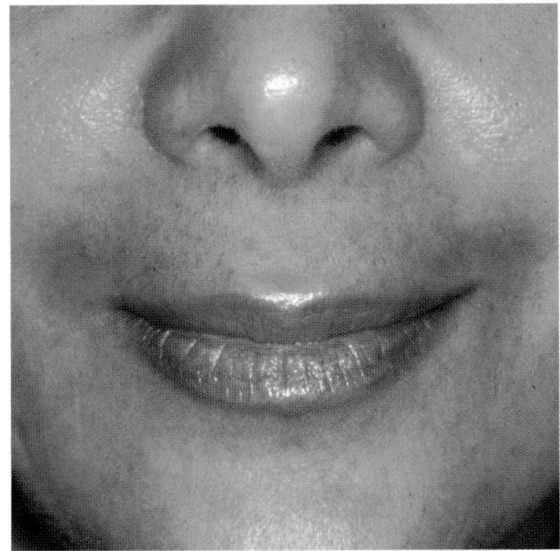

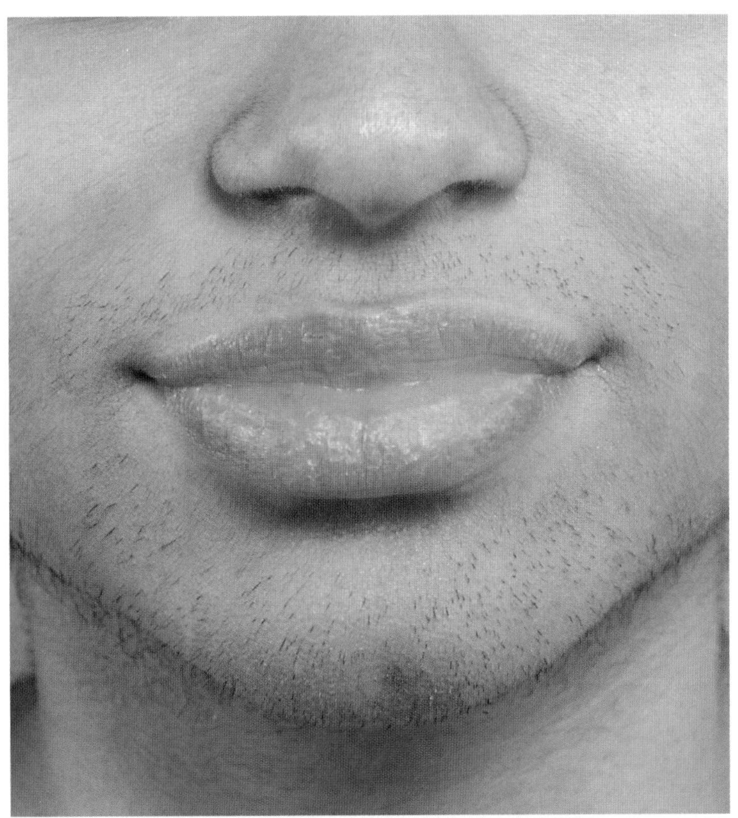

Hirsutism. Excess hair. Most often noticeable around the mouth and on the chin and neck of women.

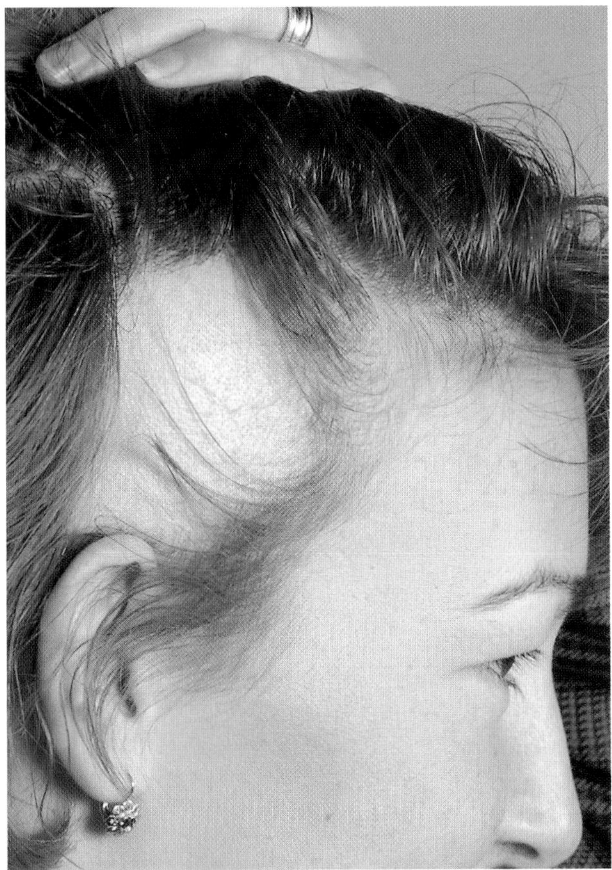

Alopecia areata. Hair loss that often starts with circular bald patches, which may overlap.

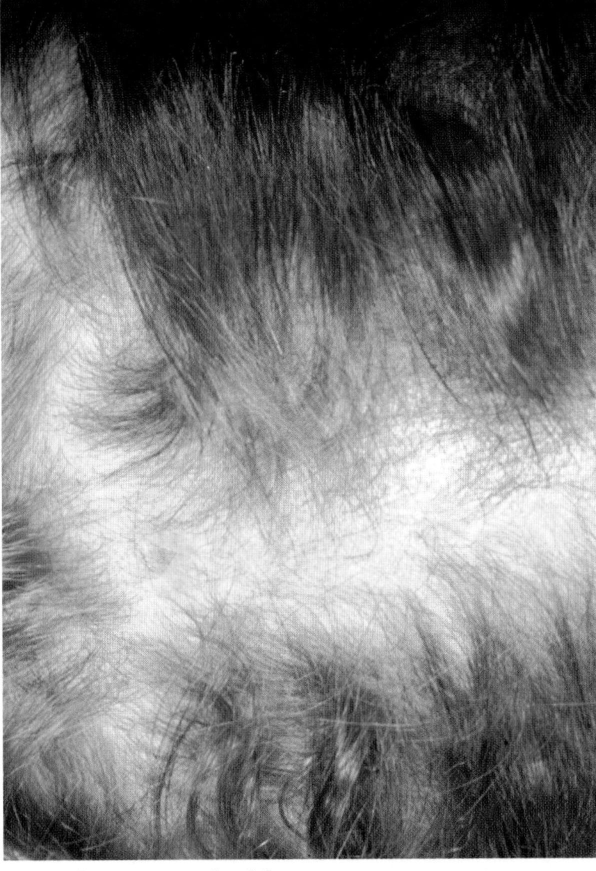

Female-pattern baldness. Generally, thinning of the hair all over the head, especially on the crown.

Oral Disorders

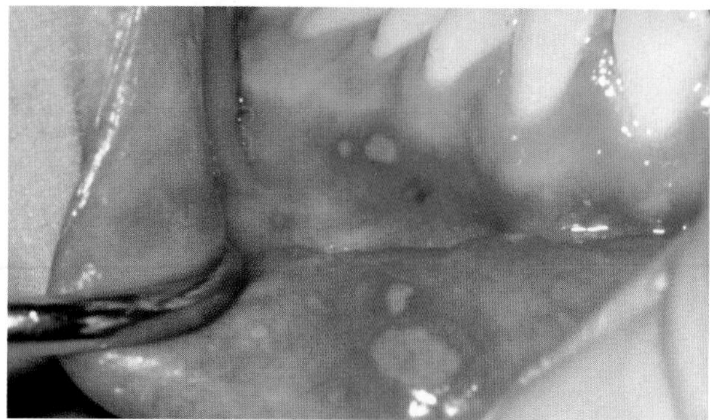

Canker sore. Occurs inside the oral cavity. A painful sore with a white or yellow center and a red border.

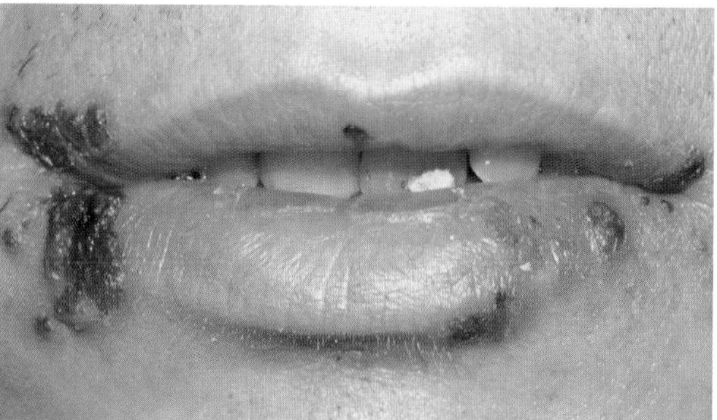

Cold sore (herpes simplex). Small, fluid-filled blisters on a raised, red, painful area. Blisters break and ooze. Yellow crust forms that sloughs off.

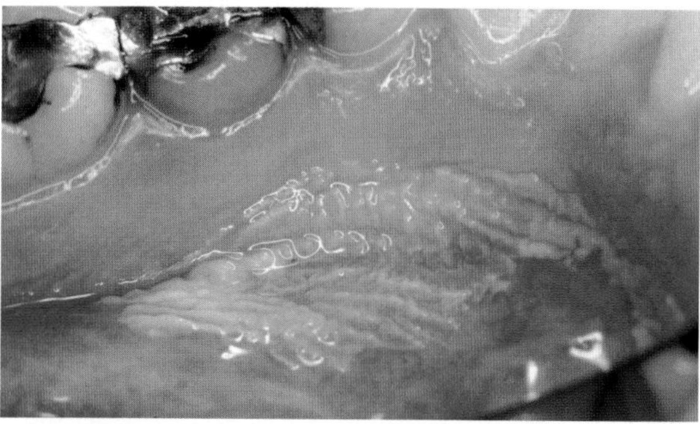

Leukoplakia. Thickened, hardened white patch on the cheek or tongue. May be a precancerous lesion.

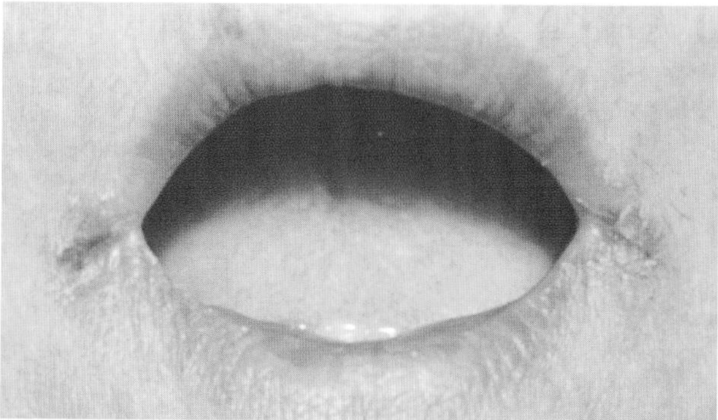

Cheilitis. Corners of the mouth become irritated, red and cracked. Fungus can grow in the corners of the mouth, keeping them inflamed and sore.

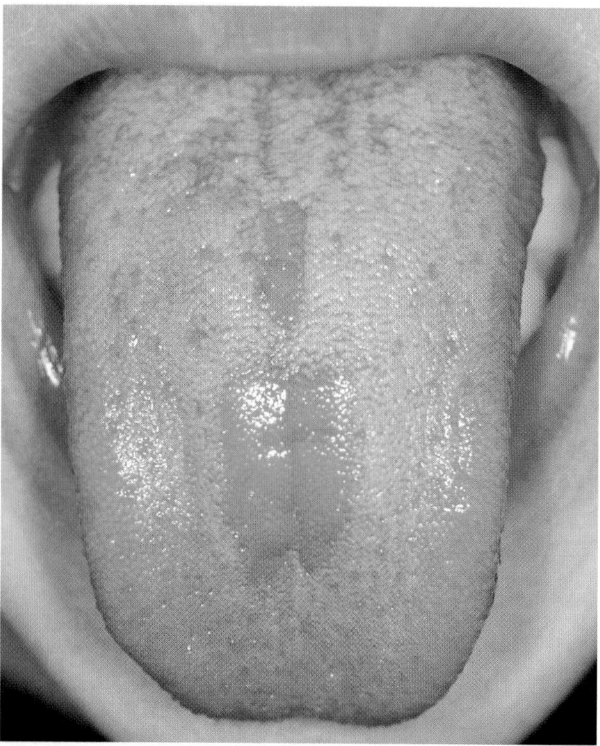

Geographic tongue. Patches with an absence of papillae, making the tongue appear smooth and bright red in the patches.

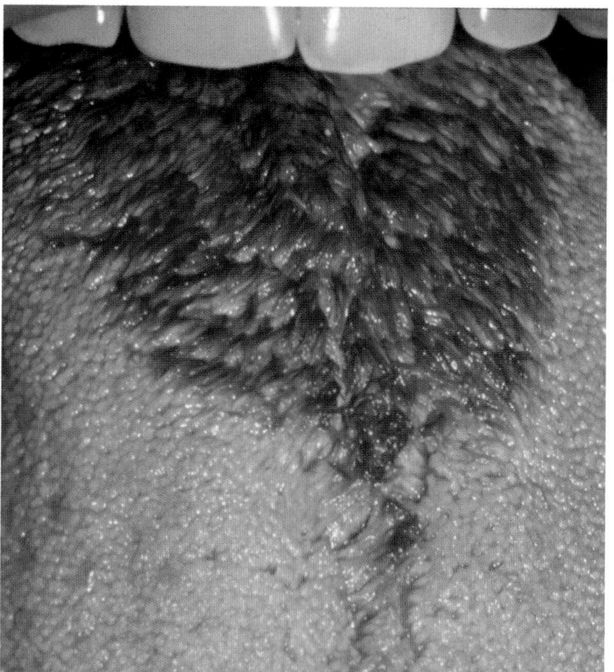

Black, hairy tongue. Hair-like projections that grow on the tongue, giving it a hairy appearance.

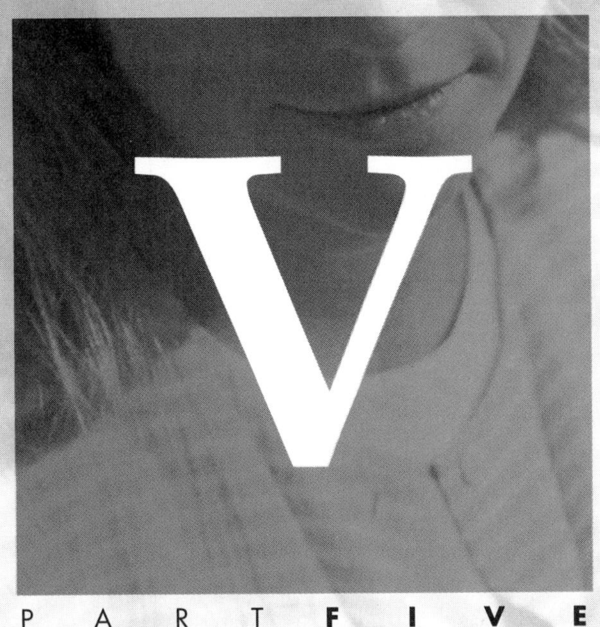

PART FIVE

Diseases and Disorders

CHAPTER **18** PART V

Genetics and Disease

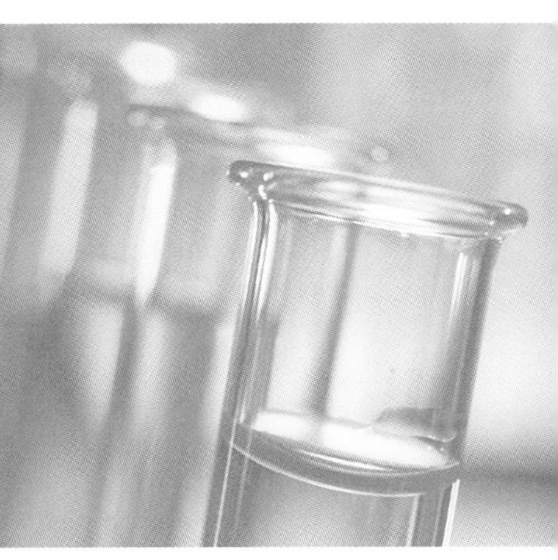

Let's say you want to make a cake. If you don't know the ingredients and instructions by heart, you'll probably start off by finding a recipe. It should contain a detailed list of the ingredients that you'll need and directions on how to put them together so that the end result is a cake that's good to eat.

In much the same way, there's a recipe that makes you a living, breathing human being, entirely different from any other person on the planet. A complete version of this recipe is contained in virtually every cell in your body. Passed along to you from your parents, the recipe is coded into a long, twisted molecule of a chemical called deoxyribonucleic acid (DNA).

DNA is tightly packed into a set of structures — called chromosomes — within the nucleus of your cells. Within your chromosomes, DNA is arranged into segments called genes. Each one of your genes contains specific instructions for making a particular protein — a molecular structure that can do any number of jobs, from making up your skin and hair to acting as a hormone or enzyme and controlling chemical reactions in your cells. Just as ingredients such as flour, water and eggs come together to produce a cake, when these proteins are put together, they result in a human body.

When a cell divides, each gene must be copied so that the two resulting cells each has a complete set of genes. Mistakes in this copying process can and do occur. Quite often these mistakes are harmless and easily repaired, but sometimes they can cause disease and premature death. Genetics — the study of genes and diseases that genetic anomalies may cause — is a rapidly advancing medical field that's receiving a lot of attention.

Scientists recently mapped out a rough draft of the specific components that make up the human genome — a complete set of the 30,000 to 40,000 genes typically present in a human being. The hope is that by studying and understanding the role of each of these genes, doctors and scientists will gain a better understanding of why and how things go wrong that cause illness.

In order to gain better insights into how genetics and disease are intertwined, it's helpful to understand some basic information about genes and chromosomes, inheritance patterns and how living beings progress from a single cell to a fully formed adult. It's also useful to learn how some diseases may be passed on from one generation to the next, how genes and environment can work together to produce illnesses and how the study of genes may lead to better treatment and, perhaps, even the cure or prevention of some diseases.

The Basics of Genetics

Your body is made up of trillions of microscopic cells. A typical human cell is about one-tenth the diameter of a human hair. Your cells are categorized into approximately 200 different types. For example, skin, muscle, bone and blood cells all perform different functions: making your skin soft, your muscles flexible, your bones solid and your blood fluid. Each cell's function is largely determined by which of its

The Human Genome Project

The Human Genome Project is an international research effort begun in 1990 to create a literal map of all of the genes contained in the human genome. A rough draft of this map, which currently shows 30,000 to 40,000 genes, was finished in June 2000. The map details the sequence of the 3 billion base pairs (nucleotides) that make up the 6 feet of DNA contained in the human genome of each cell. The genome map also shows genetic landmarks along each of the 23 chromosomes, including the locations of genes that are known to mutate and cause disease and other genes that are known to repair DNA.

The human genome is not the only type of DNA being sequenced. Genetic maps have been completed for other organisms, including the fruit fly and the *Escherichia coli (E. coli)* bacterium. Efforts are under way to map the genomes of the mouse, rat and zebra fish as well. These genomes can provide a source of comparison for the human genome.

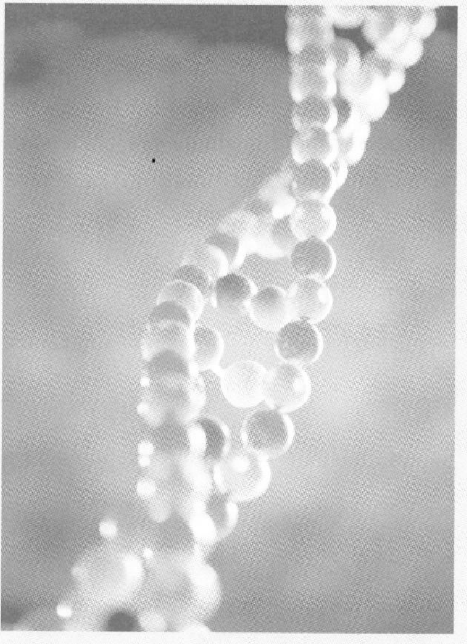

The next step in the Human Genome Project is to refine the current rough draft. Scientists are seeking to understand the function of each gene as well as its location on a particular chromosome. Researchers are also investigating variations within a particular gene between different individuals and how these variations may cause susceptibility to disease or varied responses to medications. Another goal of the genome project is to determine the role of the proteins that are coded by various genes.

approximately 40,000 genes are activated.

Chromosomes, genes and DNA

Each cell, except for mature red blood cells, has a control center called the nucleus. The nucleus houses your DNA, contained in two sets of 23 chromosomes, for a total of 46 chromosomes. One set comes from your mother, the other from your father. Two of these 46 chromosomes — called X and Y — are the sex chromosomes, which determine whether you are male or female. Females have a pair of X chromosomes. Males have an X chromosome and a Y chromosome. All other chromosomes are called autosomes.

The only cells that don't contain two sets of chromosomes are the egg and sperm. Known as your sex cells, each contains only one set of chromosomes. When an egg cell and sperm cell join together to form a zygote, the zygote contains the complete 46 chromosomes. This is how you get one set of 23 chromosomes from each parent.

The DNA contained in your chromosomes is a double-stranded structure composed of sugar and phosphate molecules that are joined together by paired chemicals called nucleotide bases. Four types of nucleotide bases are found in DNA: adenine (A), thymine (T), cytosine (C) and guanine (G). Adenine always pairs up with thymine, and cytosine always pairs up with guanine. The end result, known as the double helix, resembles a long, twisted ladder.

Cell proteins

One of the most important functions of genes is to produce proteins. Just as many kinds of genes control your traits, many kinds of proteins play various roles in your body. Some function as structural components, others as enzymes that control chemical reactions within your body. Other proteins help convert food from your diet into energy. Proteins are vital to the development and maintenance of your body. In fact, the two main components of your body are water and protein.

Amino acids are the basic building blocks of proteins. There are 20 kinds of amino acids in total, and they come together in various combinations to form different proteins. Proteins can be simple structures, made up of only a few amino acids, or complex, made of several chains of amino acids.

Some genes continuously produce proteins for basic cell metabolism, and other genes are activated ("switched on") only when their protein-coding information is needed. In fact, some genes in a particular cell may be permanently "switched off." In other words, not all genes are activated in a cell at any given time.

When a cell needs a specific protein, it initiates a process called transcription. Transcription uses the blueprint provided by DNA to produce a protein. First, an enzyme called ribonucleic acid (RNA) polymerase makes an exact copy of a gene's DNA. This copy, called messenger RNA (mRNA), then

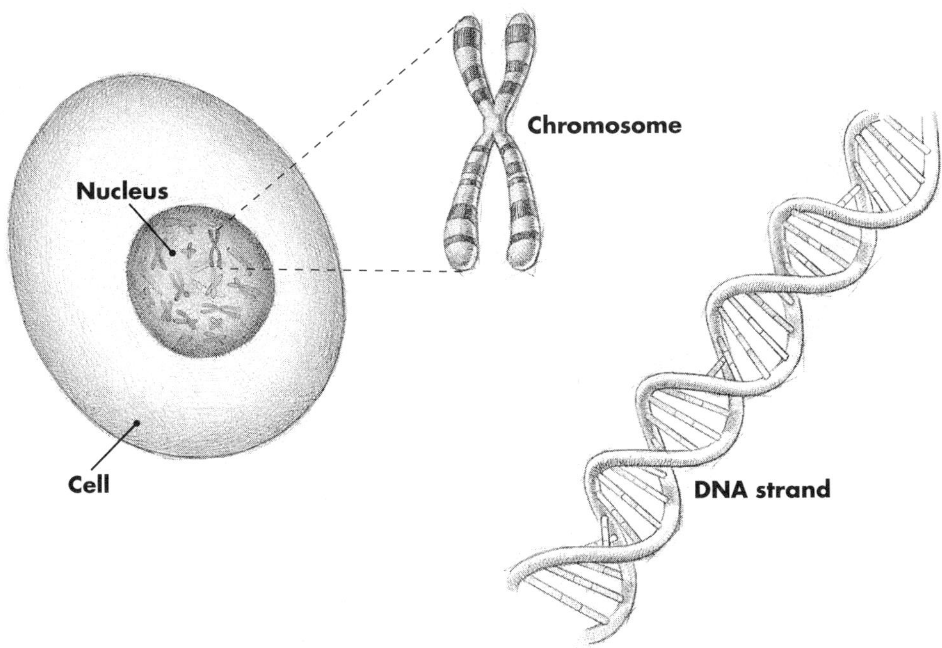

Virtually every cell in your body has a nucleus that contains 46 chromosomes (23 pairs) — half coming from each parent. Each chromosome consists of spirals of deoxyribonucleic acid (DNA), divided into units called genes. Your genes control the traits you inherit from your parents and can pass on to your children.

travels outside of the nucleus to the outer part of the cell, where it links up with an enzyme called a ribosome. The ribosome creates a corresponding chain of amino acids based on the genetic sequence carried by the mRNA. This chain of amino acids then folds into a unique shape and forms a protein, ready to perform its function.

Controlling cell function

Throughout your lifetime, your body is in the business of generating new cells. During growth and development before adulthood, your cells are particularly busy dividing and specializing — developing your brain, increasing your height and creating a fully functional immune system, among myriad other things.

The exact way in which your cells are able to selectively activate or deactivate parts of the genome remains a mystery, but your health depends on it. For example, it's believed that cancer results in part from the failure of a growth-control gene to switch off properly or failure of a tumor-suppressing gene to turn on, resulting in uncontrolled growth of cells.

In order to know what to do and when to do it, each new cell requires a complete set of your genetic material (genome). When a cell divides, its DNA is replicated so that the newly formed cells have a complete copy of the genome. Sperm and egg cells undergo yet another division process, resulting in four cells with half the original amount of genetic material. This prepares the sperm and egg cells for a potential union. When a sperm and egg unite, the new structure (zygote) has 46 chromosomes in 23 pairs. This is how the number of chromosomes and genes remains the same from one generation to the next.

Genes and inheritance

The genes you inherit from your parents are expressed in a variety of ways, but are perhaps most discernible in your physical characteristics, such as the shape of your ears, your eye color and your body build. Genes can also influence certain mental and personality traits, such as a talent for music or organization.

Genes can be either dominant or recessive. In a gene pair, the effects of a dominant gene will take precedence over the effects of a recessive gene. For example, if you inherit a gene for brown eyes, which is dominant, from your mother and a gene for blue eyes, which is recessive, from your father, your eye color will be brown because the dominant gene takes precedence. This is called autosomal dominant inheritance.

Logically, if you inherit two dominant genes for brown eyes, your eye color will be brown as well. On the other hand, if you inherit two recessive genes for blue eyes, your eye color will be blue. This is called autosomal recessive inheritance. In general, for a recessive gene to express itself, it must be paired with a similar recessive gene.

Variations in genes (polymorphisms) occur on a regular basis and can influence the way genes are expressed. And rarely does a single gene pair control one specific trait. Most of the time, traits are governed by the interplay of a variety of genes.

Genetic Disorders

Understanding how DNA normally functions can help you understand how genetic information might go awry. The topic of genetics and disease is frequently reported in the news, with many reports speculating on how a particular disease may be related to your genetic makeup. Understandably, some of the most frequent questions people now ask of their doctors relate to whether a disease can be inherited.

Genetic disorders can be caused by an abnormality (mutation) in your DNA that's significant enough to alter the function of a specific protein. This abnormality can involve an entire chromosome or a single gene or gene pair.

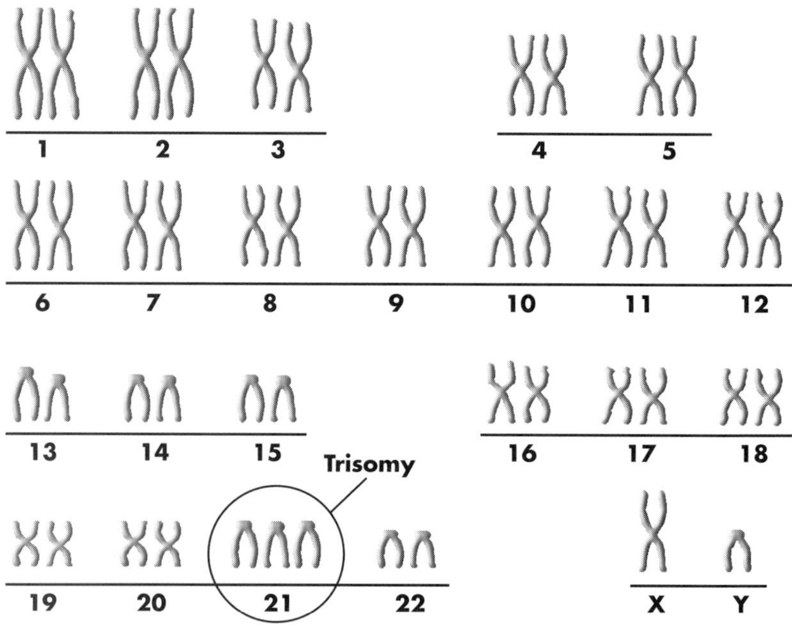

Down syndrome occurs when one of the reproductive cells from the parents that combine at fertilization contains extra material from chromosome 21. Individuals with Down syndrome usually have three copies of chromosome 21 (Trisomy 21) instead of two copies.

Chromosome abnormalities

Chromosome abnormalities typically consist of an extra, missing or incomplete chromosome. An example is Down syndrome, a condition caused by the presence of extra genetic material from chromosome 21 — most of the time an entire extra copy of chromosome 21 is present (trisomy 21). Chromosome anomalies such as trisomy 21 may cause mental retardation and other birth defects.

Gene abnormalities

Diseases may also be caused by abnormalities within a single gene or gene pair, often referred to as a gene mutation. A common example of a single gene disorder is cystic fibrosis. About 30,000 people in the United States have this disorder. It results from abnormalities in the gene known as the cystic fibrosis transmembrane regulator. Cystic fibrosis is a recessive disorder, so an affected person must have two mutated copies of the gene.

Some diseases, called multifactorial conditions, are thought to require the presence of one or more genetic mutations and specific environmental factors. Scientists have discovered that some people who develop cancer have both a genetic predisposition to the disease as well as a history of exposure to environmental toxins.

Breast cancer is a much-publicized example. Defects in one of several genes — especially BRCA1 or BRCA2 — put you at greater risk of developing breast cancer. Usually, these genes help prevent cancer by making proteins that keep cells from growing abnormally. If these genes have a mutation, they're not as effective at blocking unwanted cell growth.

On the environmental side, factors such as excess body weight and long-term exposure to estrogen may increase your risk of breast cancer. Similarly, a combination of a genetic defect and smoking may increase your risk of the disease.

Genes mutate in several ways:

- *Substitution.* When DNA is copied, one nucleotide base may be substituted for another (such as C for T), resulting in a different sequence than the original. When a ribosome reads the DNA in order to gather the appropriate amino acids for the desired protein, one of the amino acids will be the wrong one.
- *Deletion or insertion.* Sometimes a nucleotide base is dropped or ignored as the DNA is being read. Other times an extra base is added to the sequence. The result

Genes and Alzheimer's Disease

Alzheimer's disease is a progressive degeneration of the brain that affects millions of Americans. The exact cause of Alzheimer's remains a question, but researchers have located four specific genes associated with the disease and suspect that there may be more. One of the interesting results of the genetic research on Alzheimer's is that it's sometimes classified as a single-gene disorder and sometimes as a multifactorial condition.

Only rarely has Alzheimer's been identified as a single-gene disorder. More commonly, several factors are thought to play a role in its development.

Single-gene disorder

Some forms of Alzheimer's disease, called familial Alzheimer's disease (FAD), appear to be inherited. Other forms are sporadic, with no clear hereditary pattern. Familial Alzheimer's disease, which generally begins before the age of 65, constitutes less than 5 percent of all Alzheimer's cases. Scientists have isolated mutations in three genes that relate specifically to different forms of FAD. All three gene mutations have an autosomal dominant pattern of genetic transmission. This means that if one parent has the mutation, each child has a 50 percent chance of inheriting it.

Multifactorial condition

Because most people with Alzheimer's disease have no family history of the disease and none of the genetic mutations associated with FAD, researchers continue to search for and identify other factors that may be associated with the disease or that increase risk. Scientists believe that a number of factors contribute to sporadic Alzheimer's, including age and environmental exposures.

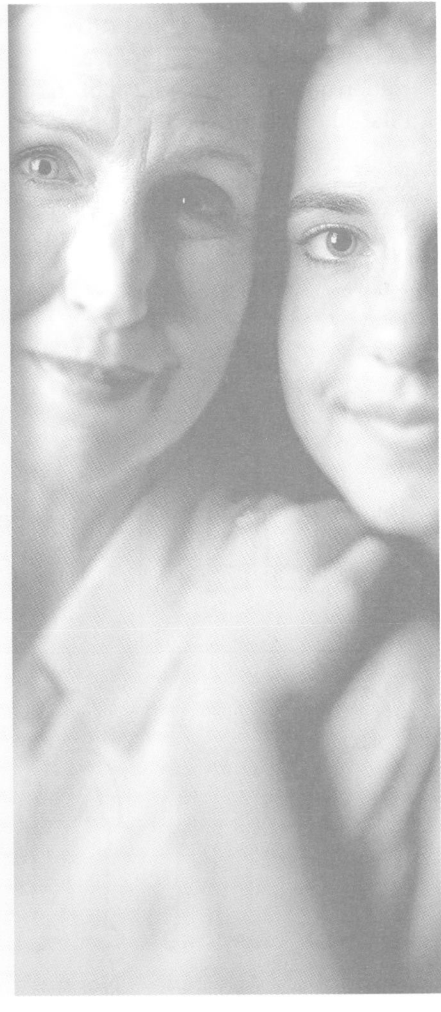

is a different amino acid chain.

- *Repetition.* A portion of the DNA strand may be accidentally repeated more times than it should, resulting in an extra-long protein.

Each of these gene alterations results in a change in protein shape and function, which may in turn alter your body's chemistry and result in disease.

Acquired and inherited mutations

If a genetic mutation occurs during a person's lifetime, it's called an *acquired* mutation. For example, skin cancer is most often caused by damage to skin cell DNA from ultraviolet B (UVB) radiation given off by the sun or by special lights used for tanning. An acquired mutation is typically present in just one or a few cells.

A gene mutation is termed inherited if it's present in reproductive cells or occurs at the time of fertilization and is thus present at birth. Like other inherited traits, the mutation may reside in a dominant or recessive gene, or it may be located on a sex chromosome. An inherited gene mutation is present in every cell of the body.

Dominant gene mutations

If you inherit a dominant gene mutation for a disorder, you'll eventually develop that condition because the dominant gene takes precedence over the recessive gene it's paired with. In addition, each of your children will have a 50 percent chance of inheriting your dominant gene mutation and developing the disease.

Disorders caused by dominant gene mutations are called autosomal dominant disorders. An example is familial hypercholesterolemia, a condition marked by very high levels of blood cholesterol.

Recessive gene mutations

A recessive genetic disorder requires inheritance of a recessive gene from each parent in order for the disease to develop. If you inherit only one such recessive gene, the dominant normal gene it's paired with takes over, and you won't develop the disorder. But you still are a carrier of the gene mutation and can pass it on to your children. If you have children with someone who's also a carrier, each child has a 25 percent chance of inheriting both recessive gene mutations and developing the associated disease. It's relatively rare for two people to be carriers for the same mutated recessive gene.

When both genes of a pair are required to cause a particular condition, this is called autosomal recessive disorder. Cystic fibrosis is an autosomal recessive disorder that results from an abnormality in the copy of the cystic fibrosis gene inherited from each parent. Another example is the blood disorder sickle cell anemia.

Sex chromosome mutations

Some mutations that cause disease are found only on the female sex (X) chromosome. These are called X-linked disorders. Men are more likely to develop these disorders

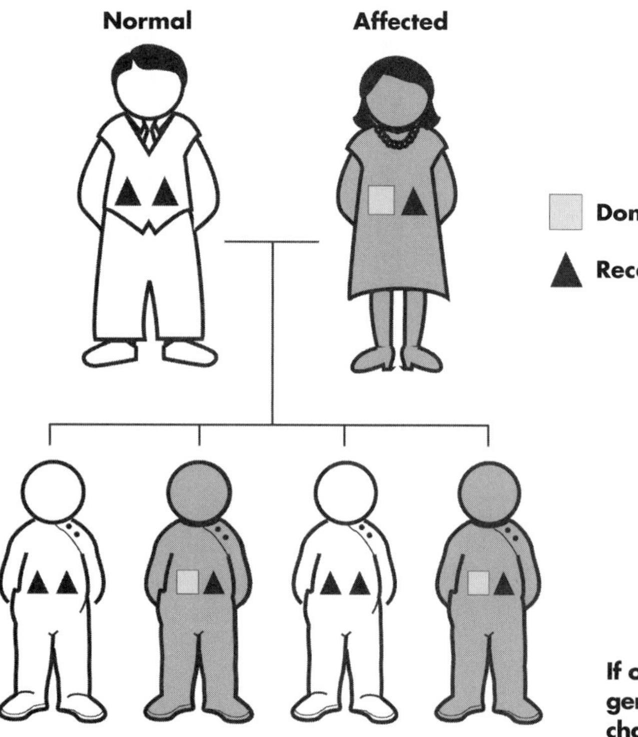

If one parent carries an altered (mutated) dominant gene, such as the gene for Huntington's disease, the chance is 50 percent the couple's baby, regardless of sex, will be born with the disease.

Recessive Gene Mutations

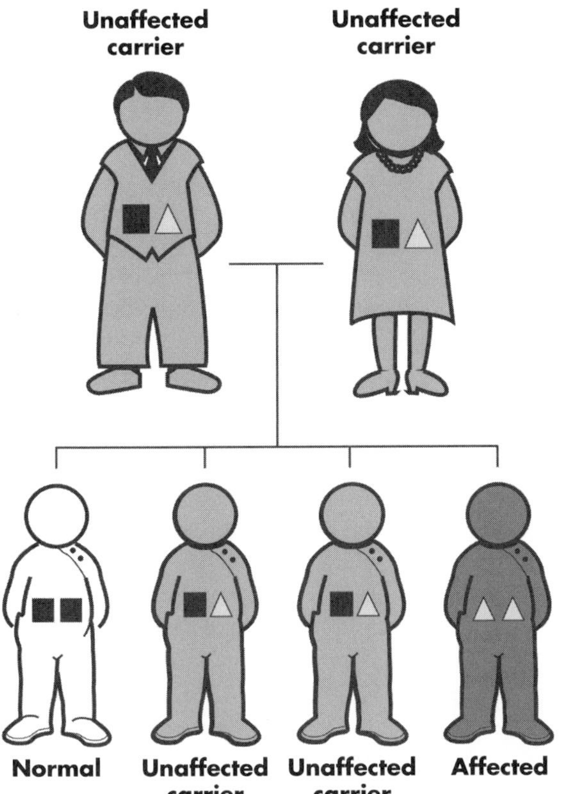

Dominant gene (normal)

Recessive gene (altered)

Recessive disorders, such as cystic fibrosis, can occur even if neither parent has the disorder. If both parents are carriers of an altered (mutated) recessive gene their offspring may be affected. The chance is one in four that their child, regardless of its sex, may be born with cystic fibrosis, two in four that it will be a healthy, unaffected carrier and one in four that it will neither carry the gene nor have the disease.

Sex Chromosome Mutations

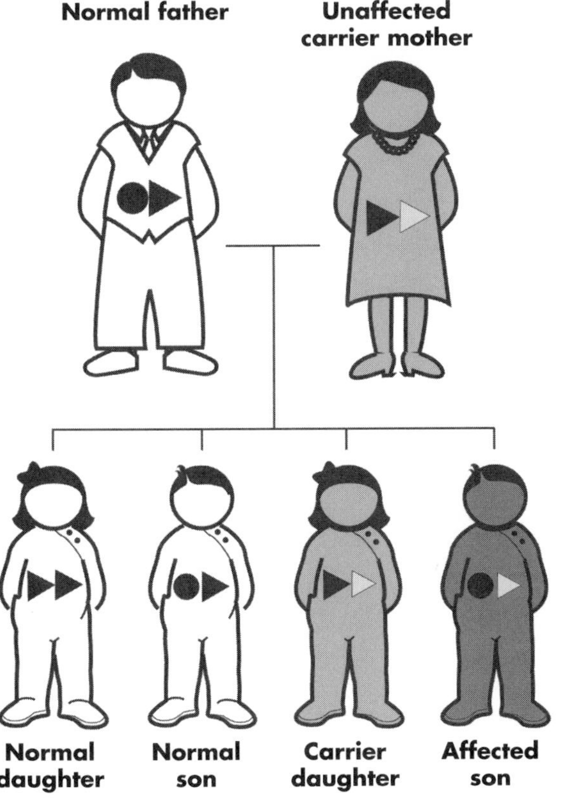

Some genetic conditions affect only males. Females may be carriers of the disorder but remain healthy. For example, when a couple has a son with hemophilia, the mother is the carrier of the altered (mutated) gene and the father is normal. A son of this couple has a 50 percent chance of inheriting the condition. A daughter of this couple has a 50 percent chance of being a carrier of the gene, like her mother.

X chromosome

X chromosome (recessive)

Y chromosome

Normal male

Normal female

Unaffected carrier female

Affected carrier male

because they have only one X chromosome. (The other male sex chromosome is the Y chromosome.) Women, on the other hand, have two X chromosomes, and the normal X chromosome generally takes over for the mutated one. Thus, women are more likely to carry the mutation than to develop the related disorder. A father with the disease will pass the mutation on to his daughters, who will almost always be unaffected because they'll have one normal X chromosome from their mother that will counteract the mutated X they received from their father. Hemophilia is a fairly common example of an X-linked disorder.

These patterns of disease inheritance may seem fairly straightforward, but in real life things are much more complicated. Remember how some people have green or hazel eyes? Diseases are the same way. People express genes in a number of ways, and thus may express a disease differently as well.

This is why two people who both have cystic fibrosis may not have the same symptoms or experience the same degree of severity in their disease. With multifactorial conditions, the influence of a person's individual genome and personal life experience can be even more pronounced. Thus, multifactorial disorders can vary significantly from one person to the next. So even though scientists are coming to a better understanding of genetic disorders and inheritance patterns, many more contributing factors have yet to be explored.

Cancer Family Syndromes

Cancer family syndromes are often inherited in an autosomal dominant fashion. This means that if a parent has the condition, each child has a 50 percent chance of inheriting the mutated gene.

The hereditary nonpolyposis colon cancer (HNPCC) syndrome is a relatively common example. This condition is thought to be responsible for about 2 percent to 10 percent of all colon cancers. Other cancers that occur with increased frequency in HNPCC families include endometrial, ureteral, pancreatic and ovarian cancers. When an individual inherits a gene responsible for HNPCC, the lifetime risk that he or she will develop colon cancer is about 80 percent. This is much higher than the risk for individuals who don't carry this gene. Thus the genes that cause many familial cancers act in a dominant fashion but don't express themselves 100 percent of the time.

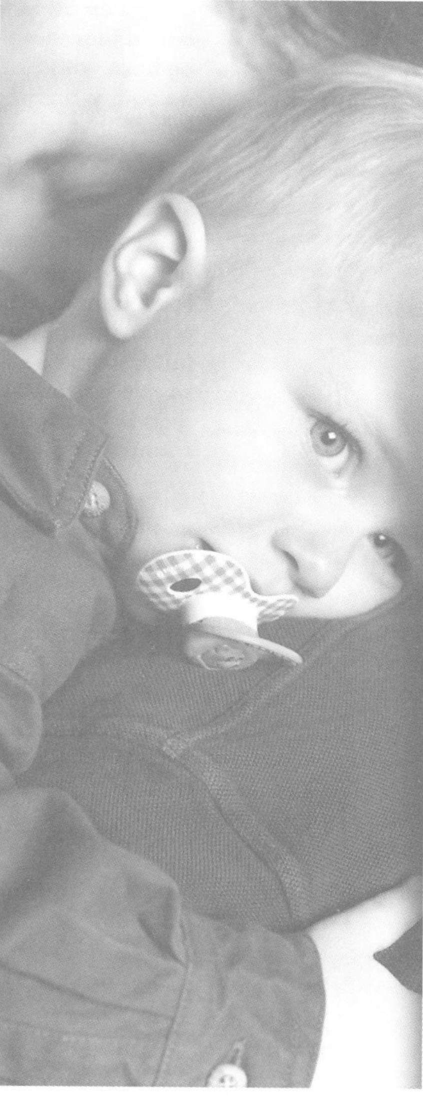

Gene Testing

More than ever before, laboratory tests can detect genetic disorders. The rate at which new DNA tests have been developed in the last 10 years has been staggering. Several dozen genetic conditions can be diagnosed using DNA testing.

Obtaining DNA tests often requires the assistance of a medical geneticist or genetic counselor to coordinate the genetic testing. The number of tests available and the locations of the laboratories doing the tests change frequently. In addition, the sample requirements may differ from laboratory to laboratory and even within one lab over time. Providing such specific information is one of the ways a medical geneticist can be of assistance.

Types of tests

For genetic testing to be performed, DNA must first be isolated from one of your cells. DNA is fairly stable and can be obtained from any living cell with a nucleus. The most commonly used cell type is the white blood cell because it's easy to obtain from a blood sample. In

? Question and Answer

How accurate is genetic testing?

Genetic testing isn't always 100 percent predictive. Even when a genetic test reveals that a person has the gene for a particular disorder, the following may remain uncertain:

- Whether the disorder will actually appear
- When the symptoms may begin
- Which symptoms will occur first
- How severe the condition will be
- How the condition will progress over time

other cases, fetal or bone marrow cells are used. There are several ways to test DNA.

Chromosome analysis

Chromosome analysis (karyotyping) looks for defects in a chromosome rather than a particular gene. It's often performed to evaluate DNA from couples with a history of miscarriages or to check for fetal abnormalities, such as Down syndrome. Cells are grown in a laboratory and then stained to highlight the chromosomes under a microscope. The chromosomes are photographed to provide a picture of their arrangement and structure, and any possible abnormalities.

Most often cells are obtained from a blood sample. In some cases, a bone marrow sample may be taken to test for a specific chromosome abnormality related to a certain type of leukemia. To check for abnormalities in a fetus, samples may be taken from the fluid that surrounds the fetus (amniotic fluid) by a procedure called amniocentesis. A thin, hollow needle is inserted into the uterus and into the amniotic sac, which surrounds the baby. A small amount of amniotic fluid, which contains fetal cells, is withdrawn for examination in the laboratory.

A piece of tissue from the placenta also can be used for fetal genetic testing. Samples of the cells that line the placenta (chorionic villi cells) are removed during a procedure called chorionic villus sampling and analyzed in the laboratory. To obtain the sample, your doctor may either withdraw the cells through a needle inserted into your abdomen or suction a few cells through a catheter threaded into your cervix.

Typically, chromosomes from a number of cells are analyzed to avoid possible error due to abnormal growth of the cells after they've been removed from the body.

DNA analysis

DNA analysis is often used to test for a single-gene disorder such as cystic fibrosis or hemophilia. After DNA is isolated from a cell sample, it's cut into usable pieces by a restriction enzyme that works like a molecular scissors to cut DNA into 4- to 8-base fragments.

The DNA is then sorted according to size by placing it within a gel medium and using electricity to separate the fragments. The smaller fragments move away from the larger fragments, distinguishing the DNA fragments so that they can be looked at separately. A small piece of radioactive single-stranded DNA called a probe is then added to the solution. The probe is designed to be the same sequence as the known gene or a nearby "landmark," called a genetic marker. When the probe finds the gene or marker, it binds to the fragment like a key in a lock. Researchers can tell where the gene or genetic marker is by radioactive signals from the probe, which can be seen on an X-ray.

One laboratory technique that has proved useful to scientists in finding different genes or genetic mutations is polymerase chain reaction (PCR). This technique allows very small amounts of DNA to be reproduced in a test tube, eliminating the need to obtain large numbers of living cells from the person being tested. In some cases, PCR is used to multiply the DNA from a single cell. The technique also speeds up testing in the laboratory by providing researchers with multiple copies of the DNA sample.

One drawback is that PCR DNA testing is vulnerable to contamination. For instance, skin cells from a laboratory worker could contaminate the test. If this occurred, the DNA from the lab worker as well as from the patient would be multiplied. Avoiding contamination requires strict laboratory techniques.

Protein analysis

In some cases, DNA alterations are detected indirectly through the presence or absence of the gene's product (protein or enzyme) in a bodily sample, usually of blood, urine or amniotic fluid or cells.

Phenylketonuria (PKU) is a rare autosomal recessive disorder caused by a missing enzyme (phenylalanine hydroxylase). Deficiency of this enzyme prevents the amino acid phenylalanine, present in foods such as milk and eggs, from being metabolized properly. This leads to elevated levels of phenylalanine in people with PKU. A buildup of this amino acid in the brain can lead to severe mental retardation.

Because PKU can be treated with a diet low in or free of phenylalanine, newborn screening for the disease is mandatory throughout most of the United States. A small heel prick is usually sufficient to obtain a blood sample. The phenylalanine test may also be done for prospective parents with a history of the disease or for a prenatal diagnosis. Tay-Sachs disease, which causes

Finding Diseases that Run in Families

With some genetic disorders, the exact mutation isn't known, but the general location of the mutated gene on the chromosome is known. In such cases, scientists begin by studying families in which multiple members across several generations have developed the condition. By comparing DNA samples of relatives who have the disease with samples from relatives without the disease, researchers can identify genetic markers that are consistently inherited by people with the disease. These markers are usually located in the vicinity of the mutated gene or genes. This process of DNA comparison is called linkage analysis.

deterioration of the nervous system, is another condition caused by the lack of an enzyme (hexosaminidase) due to genetic mutation. In this case, the enzyme itself is tested. Tay-Sachs is more common among people of Ashkenazi Jewish descent.

How are genetic tests used?

Genetic tests are used to determine if a person may have a genetic mutation that causes a disease or increases susceptibility to a disease. The tests also may be used to identify carriers of a genetic mutation or to confirm a suspected genetic disorder.

Newborn screening

Screening newborns for treatable genetic disorders is the most common form of genetic testing in the United States. Examples of diseases in which newborn screening is used include phenylketonuria (PKU), an enzyme deficiency, and the blood disorder sickle cell disease. By identifying these conditions at a very early age in life, many of the adverse effects can be prevented through appropriate therapy.

Carrier testing

Couples with a family history of genetic disorders such as cystic fibrosis, Tay-Sachs disease and sickle cell disease may use DNA testing to see if either partner carries the altered recessive gene associated with the disease. If both carry the recessive gene, there's a 25 percent risk that their children will develop the disease and a 50 percent risk that their children will be carriers. If only one parent carries the recessive gene alteration, the children won't develop the disease, but there's still a 50 percent chance that each child will be a carrier.

Knowing the results of the test may assist couples with family planning. A medical geneticist or genetic counselor can help couples better understand potential risks (see page 453).

Prenatal diagnostic testing

Prenatal testing can offer information about the sex of a fetus, as well as potential genetic problems and physical deformities. The four most common prenatal tests include ultrasound, amniocentesis, chorionic villi sampling and the maternal serum alpha-fetoprotein blood panel screen (see page 263).

Testing is usually offered to parents with specific risk factors:

- The mother is age 35 or older.
- The father is age 45 or older.
- The family has a history of congenital malformation, mental retardation, chromosome abnormality or neural tube defects.
- The parents are known carriers of a genetic condition that can be determined via prenatal testing.
- The mother was exposed to a harmful chemical agent during pregnancy.
- Prenatal screening tests produced abnormal results.

Prenatal diagnostic tests aren't mandatory. Indeed, for many parents, the decision to undergo testing is difficult because of the psychological consequences of knowing this genetic information. Moral, ethical and religious beliefs can all affect a family's choice. In addition, the potential risks of the test procedures themselves must be considered. For example, the risk of miscarriage due to amniocentesis is between 1 in 200 and 1 in 400.

If you're faced with these choices, it's important to discuss them with your doctor, a medical geneticist or a genetic counselor to help determine the best course of action. Perhaps most important of all is to take the time to consider all possible scenarios and work through your responses to each.

Some questions to ask yourself and your doctor before undergoing prenatal testing include:

- How accurate are the test results?
- How often does my doctor perform the procedure?
- How concerned am I about the risk of miscarriage?
- How much do I want to know about the future health of my baby?
- What might change my mind about continuing the pregnancy?
- Will this information change the way my doctor and I prepare for the birth of my baby?
- If a problem is discovered, what are my options? Is termination of pregnancy an option for me?
- Will knowing this information cause me to make decisions I might not otherwise make?

Predictive testing

Predictive gene tests focus on identifying disease-causing gene alterations before evidence of the disease appears. These tests are generally aimed at people at high risk of a disease because of a strong family history of it. Some testing, such as that for a known single-gene disorder, indicates whether a person will develop the disease. If you have the faulty gene, you'll eventually develop the disease. Tests that are currently available include those for some forms of amyotrophic lateral sclerosis (ALS or Lou Gehrig's disease), some forms of ataxia and most forms of cystic fibrosis, hemophilia, Huntington's disease, sickle cell disease, thalassemias and Tay-Sachs disease.

Other predictive tests can only estimate your susceptibility to a particular disorder. In other words, having the faulty gene may increase your risk but it doesn't guarantee that you'll develop the disorder. Susceptibility to certain forms of inherited breast, ovarian and colon cancer can be genetically tested. There's also a test for a gene variation that may increase your risk of Alzheimer's disease.

The benefit of these tests — particularly in the case of single-gene disorders — is that they can help you prepare for what may come. In addition, if you know that you have a genetic predisposition to a certain cancer, you can pursue more aggressive screening options for prevention or early detection.

If test results show that you don't have a faulty gene, this knowledge may relieve unnecessary worry and anxiety. On the other hand, knowing that you've inherited an altered gene, may impose an emotional burden. With some diseases, positive results of a susceptibility test are especially difficult to interpret because they don't predict with absolute certainty whether you'll develop the disease.

Confirming a diagnosis

Sometimes, a doctor may use gene testing to confirm a diagnosis in a person with signs and symptoms suggestive of a genetic disorder. In the case of cystic fibrosis, genetic testing is able to detect about 88 percent of gene mutations. Thus the DNA test can confirm the diagnosis of cystic fibrosis in a person with clinical symptoms. For many genetic disorders, though, gene alterations responsible for the disease haven't yet been identified, and no specific gene test can confirm the diagnosis.

Genetic Counseling

Medical geneticists and genetic counselors are often called upon to help individuals understand inherited diseases and disorders. A medical geneticist is a doctor who has completed 2 to 3 years of additional training in medical genetics. Genetic counselors have 2 years of specialized training in medical genetics beyond a college degree. Look for individuals who are board certified.

In the past, people were most often sent to a medical geneticist for evaluation of a relatively rare disorder caused by a single-gene abnormality. Now doctors and scientists realize that many complex and common disorders are due in part to genetic factors. For instance, a congenital abnormality of one of the major organ systems, such as a congenital heart defect, is often due in part to genetic factors and may prompt genetic evaluation. If a person has multiple congenital anomalies, a genetic component is almost always involved. Sometimes, a person has a family history of a known inheritable disorder, such as cystic fibrosis, sickle cell anemia or hemophilia.

Benefits of counseling

If you're considering genetic testing for yourself or your child, there are many issues to think about. Speaking with a geneticist or a genetic counselor can help you sort them out.

These health care professionals are specially trained to deal with the complex issues surrounding genetic testing. They won't tell you what to do, but they can offer valuable information before you make your decision. Should you choose to go ahead with the testing, they can help you interpret the results and provide support in the weeks and months ahead. Some issues to think about include:

- What treatments are available for the genetic disorder under consideration?
- What impact might test results have on your relationships with your spouse, family, children and friends? For some people, family relationships improve after genetic testing. For others, they become more complicated.
- Will genetic testing cause fears of having "good" or "bad" genes or cause others to think less of you?
- Results of a genetic test sometimes can give unexpected information. For example, revealing nonpaternity — that a child's father isn't the biological father.
- Who will give you emotional support through the process?
- How will you react if your test results are uncertain?
- What are your plans and hopes for having children?
- What are your career interests, and how might the testing affect your choices?
- What is the cost of the test, and who will pay?
- Do you want your insurance company to know the results? Can these results be used to discriminate against you, or will they be regarded as a pre-existing condition?
- Will the results become a part of your medical record?
- Would you like to be tested at this time, or would postponing the testing be better?

Family health history

If you're referred to a medical geneticist for evaluation, it's helpful to put together your family health history, also called a family pedigree or family health tree, before the appointment. For instance, in the case of a family history of cancer, it's helpful to know the type of cancer in each affected family member and the person's age at diagnosis. It's also important to know about unaffected family members because this information can be helpful in interpreting the family pedigree and in creating a risk assessment.

The more information you provide about the health conditions in your family, the better a geneticist can help you. He or she analyzes the family pedigree in order to determine the inheritance pattern of a disorder in the family. This pedigree analysis often helps the geneticist to develop a screening or treatment plan for those who may be at risk or have the disorder.

Creating a family pedigree

You can create a family health history by asking about the health of relevant family members, which typically involves first- and second-degree relatives. First-degree relatives are your parents, sisters, brothers and children. Second-degree relatives include aunts, uncles, grandparents and grandchildren.

On the family health tree, for each family member record relationship, sex, year of birth, illnesses and age at diagnosis, and significant lifestyle factors (when known), such as tobacco and alcohol use or obesity. If anyone on your health tree has died, note the age at death and cause of death. Other things you might want to include are:

Race or ethnicity
The race or ethnic background of the family is important. For instance, if the family is of Northern European background, the risk of family members being carriers for a cystic fibrosis gene mutation is increased. Likewise, if the family is black, the risk of family members being carriers for sickle cell anemia is increased. Remember that a carrier of a genetic disorder doesn't have the condition.

Intermarriage
When taking a family history, pay attention to the possibility that a couple may have been blood relatives. This increases the risk of certain disorders in their children.

History of birthing difficulty
A history of previous miscarriages or stillborn or neonatal deaths also may be relevant. For example, it's estimated that 12 percent of neonatal deaths are due to a disorder in a single-gene pair.

Environmental exposures
Illnesses can also be influenced by exposure to factors such as illicit drugs, prescription medications, radiation and toxic chemicals.

Gene Therapy

One of the biggest hopes behind genetic studies is that understanding the human genome will enable treatment to cure or even prevent genetic diseases. Now that a map of all human genes exists, the next goal of researchers is to better understand the individual function of each gene and how a breakdown in its function may cause disease. This understanding may allow scientists to replace or supplement flawed or missing genes with healthy ones, addressing the problem at its root, rather than treating its consequences. This is known as gene therapy.

Applications

Although many researchers already have begun experimenting with gene therapy, this area is still in its early stages. Most gene therapy currently takes place within carefully controlled clinical trials. Nonetheless, almost every common disease is being studied from a genetic point of view as well as from a more conventional standpoint. Some of the major potential applications of gene therapy include:

Replacing a damaged or defective gene
Replacing a damaged or defective gene is a method that targets diseases caused by a single-gene defect. For example, cystic fibrosis, hemophilia, Huntington's disease and Tay-Sach's disease all have been traced to mutations in one or both copies of a particular gene pair. Replacing or supplementing the flawed genes with healthy ones could potentially halt or reverse progression of the disease. This might also work for certain cancers where a specific gene has failed to suppress the abnormal growth of cells. Injecting healthy genes into cells may also be useful for supplementing protein deficiencies, as in certain types of anemia.

Killing harmful cells
Killing harmful cells involves inserting a gene into these cells so that they produce a protein that causes cell suicide (apoptosis) or that makes the cells susceptible to drugs that can destroy them. Studies show potential for the use of this application in combination with currently available medications and radiation to more effectively kill harmful cells. This type of therapy could be helpful in treating cancerous (malignant) tumors.

Methods of delivery

A basic challenge of gene therapy lies in delivering healthy genes efficiently, accurately and safely to the appropriate cells targeted for alteration or destruction. Researchers are investigating the following methods:

Stem cell transplantation
Stem cells are nonspecialized cells that have the ability to replicate themselves and then divide into more specialized cells. Currently, the biggest use for stem cells is in bone marrow transplants to treat people with conditions such as leukemia, lymphoma, aplastic anemia and some inherited immune disorders. Bone marrow contains blood stem cells that produce red and white blood cells and platelets.

One way to introduce new copies of genes into body cells is through transplantation of stem cells into bone marrow. This can be done in two ways. One method involves using chemotherapy to destroy unhealthy bone marrow of an affected person and then transplanting healthy stem cells from a compatible donor, such as a brother or sister, into the destroyed bone marrow to produce healthy new blood cells.

White blood cells are often the cells of interest because they're capable of producing enzymes that may be deficient in the affected person. For example, early clinical trials in children with the degenerative condition Maroteaux-Lamy found that when newly generated white blood cells produced even as little as 10 percent of the normal amount of the missing enzyme, the child's condition improved. Unfortunately, stem cell transplantation is expensive. The procedure also carries risks, such as infection and death, and sometimes works for only a short period of time.

Stem Cell Research

Stem cells and their potential for curing disease are growing and popular topics. But what exactly are stem cells and why are they so important?

What are stem cells?

Stem cells are primitive, undifferentiated cells that have the ability to self-replicate and produce any number of increasingly specialized cells. They're most important during the fetal stage, where they engineer the growth and development of a single cell into a fully formed human being. Embryonic human stem cells have the potential to divide and specialize into any type of cell in the human body. Following birth, stem cells still exist in your body (adult stem cells) but are limited to reproducing cells as needed for the specific tissues and organs in which they reside, such as your skin or bones.

Using stem cells as treatment

Stem cells have captured scientific and public interest because of their potential ability to replace damaged or diseased cells. Currently, the biggest use for stem cells is in bone marrow transplants used to treat people with conditions such as leukemia, lymphoma, aplastic anemia and some inherited immune disorders. Bone marrow, and even the bloodstream, contains blood stem cells capable of producing healthy, new red and white blood cells and platelets.

In 1998, researchers made a scientific advance by isolating embryonic stem cells and growing them in a laboratory. Researchers also discovered how to stop these cells from specializing and how to keep them at a state of maximum potential for differentiating. This set the stage for researching how to direct these cells to treat disease — for instance, how to stimulate them to form new brain cells or a new kidney. Such cells possibly could be used to treat conditions like Parkinson's, Alzheimer's or kidney failure that currently have no effective treatment.

Another important discovery in recent years was finding that adult stem cells exist in a number of tissues previously thought not to contain them, such as the brain, skeletal muscles, liver, pancreas and the cornea of the eye. If these cells were to be properly isolated and grown in culture, they might be used to form healthy tissue where needed. In addition, some evidence suggests that adult stem cells might even be stimulated to form one of several different tissues, not just the one of their origin.

Stem cell cultures may also be used to test the effects of certain medications on various cell types. If cell testing proves the drugs to be safe and beneficial, they might be tested on animals and humans.

Obstacles

Major challenges in the field of stem cell research are yet to be faced. Scientists need to better understand how stem cells specialize in order to stimulate them into forming different tissues. There's also a concern that the transplanted cells could be rejected because cells derived from embryos or fetal tissue would be genetically different from those of the person receiving them.

One way to avoid rejection involves taking a cell including its nucleus from the potential recipient (other than an egg or sperm cell) and fusing it with a donor egg cell that has had its nucleus removed (somatic cell nuclear transfer). The fused cell would contain the recipient's own DNA and, therefore, wouldn't provoke immune system rejection. This process of DNA transfer is referred to as therapeutic cloning.

Another way to avoid rejection is to use the person's own adult stem cells for transplantation. The problem with this is that adult stem cells are present in small numbers within the body, so it can be difficult to isolate and remove them. In addition, they don't multiply and remain viable in the laboratory as well as embryonic stem cells do. And they may contain DNA mutations that have occured over the person's lifetime.

Stem cell research is ongoing and treatment applications, for the most part, are still years away. But if progress with blood and bone marrow transplants is any indication, stem cells will someday help many people.

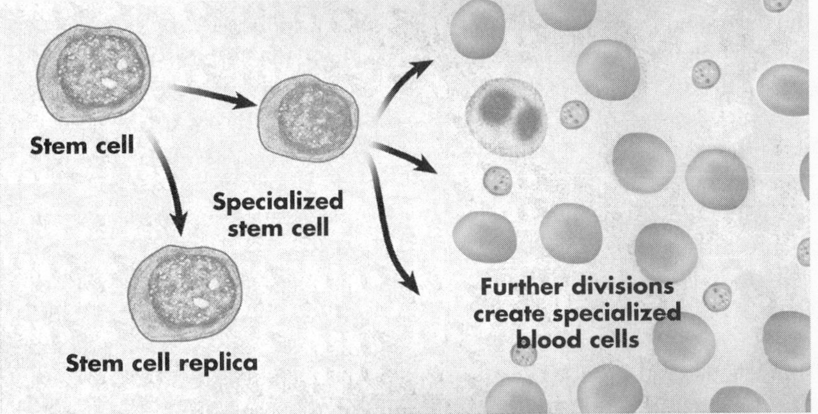

When a stem cell divides, it creates a stem cell that's specialized — a cell that can create cells that perform specific functions, such as blood cells. It also creates an exact replica of itself.

A second way to treat people with an enzyme disorder is to take immature white blood cells (stem cells) out of the bone marrow and insert in them appropriate enzyme-generating genes before transplanting the cells back into the individual. This method is less hazardous because there's no need to destroy the person's own bone marrow with radiation and chemotherapy. New cells in the marrow can exist with the old cells. It doesn't matter if the old cells produce deficient or abnormal enzyme as long as the new cells produce even a relatively small amount of normal enzyme. One of the challenges to this type of treatment has been delivering the replacement gene into the nucleus of the cell where it can be activated.

Viral carriers

Another form of gene therapy uses viruses as carriers (vectors) of healthy DNA. The virus most commonly used in gene therapy experiments is the adenovirus, which causes the common cold. Other viruses used include retroviruses, poxviruses and the herpes virus. Viral vector therapy takes advantage of what viruses do naturally — spread throughout the body and deliver their own genes into human cells.

To perform this procedure, a sample of cells, usually stem cells from bone marrow, is taken from the person who's to receive the genetic therapy. The cells are then grown in a laboratory. Doctors remove disease-causing genes from the vector virus and insert therapeutic genes into the viral particles. The virus is then allowed to infect the bone marrow stem cells and, it's hoped, incorporate the corrective genes into the cells' DNA. These infected cells are then transplanted back to the person through an intravenous solution. Once in the body, they migrate to the person's bone marrow and begin producing the corrective protein.

Unfortunately, the therapeutic viral genes don't always infect enough bone marrow cells in the laboratory to be effective once transplanted into the body. Most diseases occur when there's less than 1 percent to 10 percent of the normal enzyme or protein produced from a particular gene. Treating a disorder requires that the individual produce at least this amount of normal enzyme, but achieving even these small amounts has been difficult.

Another problem with viral-based gene therapy is that the replacement gene may be lost in transfer and not attach to a cell's DNA. Even if bone marrow cells are infected in sufficient numbers, if DNA is lost during subsequent cell division, the therapy won't be successful.

In addition, the virus itself may multiply when it's injected into the person's body, and this may cause problems. Viral vectors may also generate an immune system response or infection when they're injected. If the person has generated an immune response to the virus, the virus can no longer get into the person's cells to allow for transfer of the corrective DNA. If this happens, the vector gradually becomes ineffective in leading to production of the normal protein.

Nonviral carriers

Researchers have tried other ways to place corrective DNA into the cells of an individual with a particular genetic disease. One method is to use tiny fat globules as carriers (vectors) of the corrective gene. When the fat globules join with fat in cell membranes, the DNA inside the globules is released into the cells.

This method relies on the corrective DNA being able to join with the person's own DNA inside the cell. This means that the corrective DNA must not only get into cells but also get into the nuclei of the cells. The procedure is most effective in cells capable of dividing. Thus, white blood cells are good candidates for this type of therapy because they divide. Most brain cells, which don't divide, aren't good candidates. Researchers are still working on ways to enhance the efficiency with which the corrective DNA attaches to the person's DNA.

Systemic delivery

The hope is that one day doctors simply will be able to inject gene-carrying vectors directly into the bloodstream, and the vectors will transfer their therapeutic genetic material into specific targeted areas. To achieve that, though, the vectors must be protected from destruction by the body for long periods of time so that they can reach the target cells. They must also be able to enter the target cells from the bloodstream.

Antisense therapy

Instead of trying to incorporate corrective genes into cells, another technique is to curtail the activity of known harmful genes. For a gene to produce a protein, the gene's sequence must be copied and sent outside of the cell's nucleus to be translated into amino acids. The copy of the gene's sequence is known as a "sense" sequence. One way to stop mutated genes from producing harmful proteins is to jam up the sense sequence with antisense molecules. This stops the harmful protein from being made.

Like corrective gene therapy, delivery of antisense molecules to cells poses a significant challenge, as does protection of the molecules until they reach their target.

Obstacles

Although the promise of gene therapy is exciting, many issues need to be resolved before gene therapy becomes a standard form of medical practice. In addition to developing effective methods of delivery, other major hurdles facing scientists include:

Unknown genetic effects

Little is known about the activity of specific genes at different times in different cells. If new genes are introduced, will they express themselves long enough and at high enough levels to accomplish their mission? In addition, could the new genes alter more than the intended cells, or could they overexpress themselves, producing so much of the new protein that it becomes harmful? There's also the question of whether inhibiting some activities of a gene will lead to unintended effects on as-yet-undiscovered functions of that same gene.

Multifactorial conditions

Only a small percentage of diseases are caused by a single-gene disorder. Most diseases are due to abnormalities of several genes, as well as environmental factors. Understanding the root causes of each disorder and how to address them effectively is a tremendous challenge.

Ethical issues

Gene therapy has attracted much public attention regarding concerns about short- and long-term consequences of manipulating the human genome. Currently, gene therapy focuses on delivering corrective genes to diseased cells. It doesn't involve altering the genome in reproductive cells, which would permanently change the genetic characteristics of future generations.

Manipulating genetic information in reproductive (germ) cells is called germline therapy. Presumably germline therapy could be used to correct defective genes so that a family could be free of a disease, such as hemophilia. But might it also be used in an attempt to enhance genetics traits, such as intelligence or athletic ability? If this were done, would a short stature or an average IQ eventually be considered defects?

Germline therapy isn't approved by the National Institutes of Health,

What's Cloning?

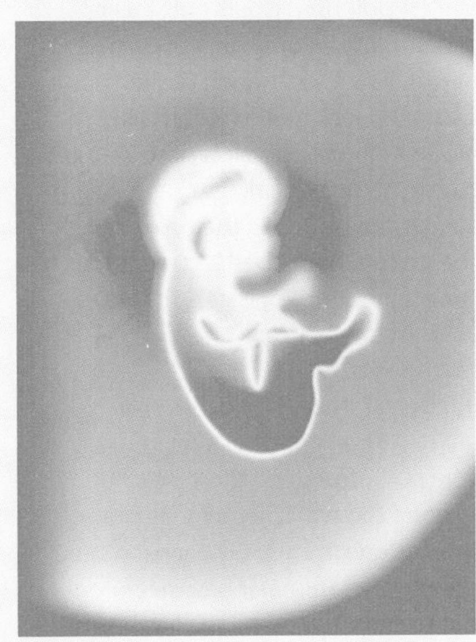

Cloning involves taking a single organism's genetic material and using it to create a genetically identical organism, without the use of sexual reproduction. This process basically has three steps:

1. First, an egg cell is obtained from a donor, and its nucleus (genetic material) is removed.
2. Next, any cell other than an egg or sperm cell (somatic cell) is taken from the organism that's to be cloned.
3. The somatic cell is fused with the DNA-less egg cell and stimulated to start dividing into an embryo that could develop into a fully formed organism.

When most people think of cloning, they think of creating a whole new child or animal. Animal cloning has been done successfully, with Dolly the sheep the most famous example. After Dolly was cloned in Scotland in 1997, other animals have also been successfully cloned. But the subject of most debate is human cloning. There are actually two types of human cloning: reproductive cloning and therapeutic cloning.

Human reproductive cloning is the attempt to create a new person genetically identical to the person who donated his or her DNA. After an embryo is cloned in a laboratory, it would be implanted in the uterus of the surrogate mother who donated the egg cell. A host of ethical and legal issues surround this topic. To date, no human has been successfully cloned. In fact, cloned human embryos have yet to reach a stage beyond a few cells.

Many scientists are opposed to reproductive cloning because of the dangers involved, as illustrated by animal cloning. For every 100 animal cloning attempts, only three, at the most, produce actual offspring, and even then survival beyond birth is improbable. If cloned human babies survive birth, it's likely that many of them would have severe birth defects, malfunction of various body systems and premature death. Not many people want to pay this sort of price for the ability to create a human clone, regardless of how they feel about its moral aspects.

Another form of human cloning that particularly interests scientists is therapeutic cloning. The goal of therapeutic cloning is to provide a source of genetically compatible embryonic stem cells to a person with a severe disorder. Embryonic stem cells are nonspecialized cells produced in very early embryonic stages. These cells have the potential to become any cell type in the body. When transplanted into a person with a disease, they could potentially replace damaged tissues or organs with healthy new cells. This type of cloning hasn't been successful yet either.

Human cloning is a hotly debated topic. On one side, many people see it as a major technological and medical advance toward the treatment of incurable diseases. On the other side are those who regard it as irresponsible use of human life. Some countries, such as Britain, have authorized human therapeutic cloning. In other countries, such as Japan, it's a punishable crime to create any type of human clone. Currently the U.S. government is debating legislation to address human cloning in America.

but its potential exists and this is what many people are concerned about. The U.S. branch of the Human Genome Project has set aside a specific portion of its budget to study the ethical, legal and social issues surrounding the project with the goal of being better prepared for other complex issues that may arise in the future.

The future

The power of gene therapy to change the way medicine is practiced is enormous. Like most other great innovations, it has the potential for great good as well as harm. It's possible that diseases that are now common could some day be merely the subjects of history books. However, discussion is needed on how to maintain respect for the cycle of life and avoid situations that begin to resemble selective breeding.

In the meantime, there's still much to learn and understand about genes and the role they play in our lives. ■

CHAPTER 19 PART V

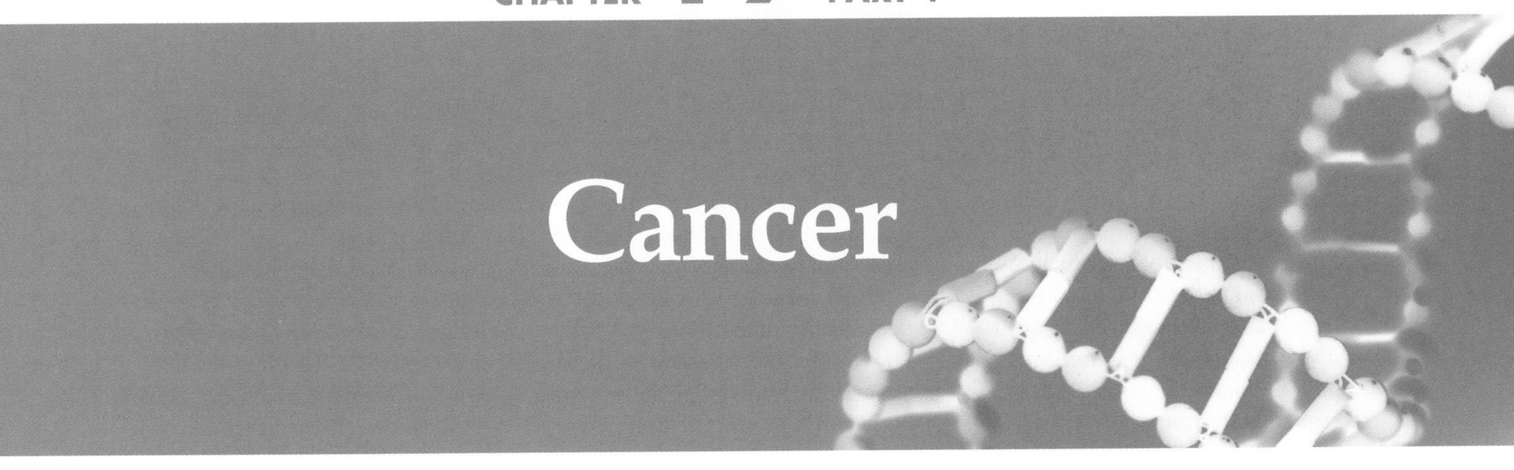

Cancer

Many people have a fear of cancer, perhaps because they view it as an incurable disease. But the truth is that although cancer remains a serious illness, it's no longer the inevitable death sentence it once was. Instead, it's increasingly becoming a tale of survivorship.

It's estimated that approximately 22 million people in the world today have survived cancer. Well over 8 million living Americans have a history of cancer. In the United States, 2 million women are breast cancer survivors, and 1 million men are prostate cancer survivors. In fact, the cancer death rate is declining, as is the rate of new cancer cases.

But the battle against this disease isn't over. Annually, cancer (excluding nonmelanoma skin cancer) is diagnosed in almost 1.3 million Americans. In the United States, cancer causes more than 500,000 deaths each year — nearly one of every four deaths.

There are at least 200 different kinds of cancer. Some cancers affect just one organ, and others are more generalized. But the basic characteristic of all cancers is the same — uncontrolled growth and spread of abnormal (malignant) cells.

Why cancer develops in some people but not in others isn't fully known. But medical professionals are gaining knowledge about what factors may contribute to the development of cancer. These factors include those that may be controlled or eliminated, such as certain dietary habits and use of tobacco.

Researchers know also that most cancers develop slowly. You may not detect evidence of the disease for 5 to 40 years after you've been exposed to a cancer-causing agent. Cancer of the lung, for example, may not appear until 25 years or more after sustained exposure to tobacco smoke. This long delay between exposure and development of the disease may partly explain why so many people ignore the warnings associated with smoking.

This chapter provides an overview of cancer: what it is, how it develops and how it's detected and treated. It also offers some guidelines on potential ways to prevent cancer, as well as what to do when you have cancer. Other chapters in this book offer more detailed information on specific types of cancer. Cancers are generally named according to the primary body system or organ affected.

The following list shows you where to find more specific information on some of the more common cancer types:

New Cases of Cancer and Cancer Deaths by Site and Sex — 2001

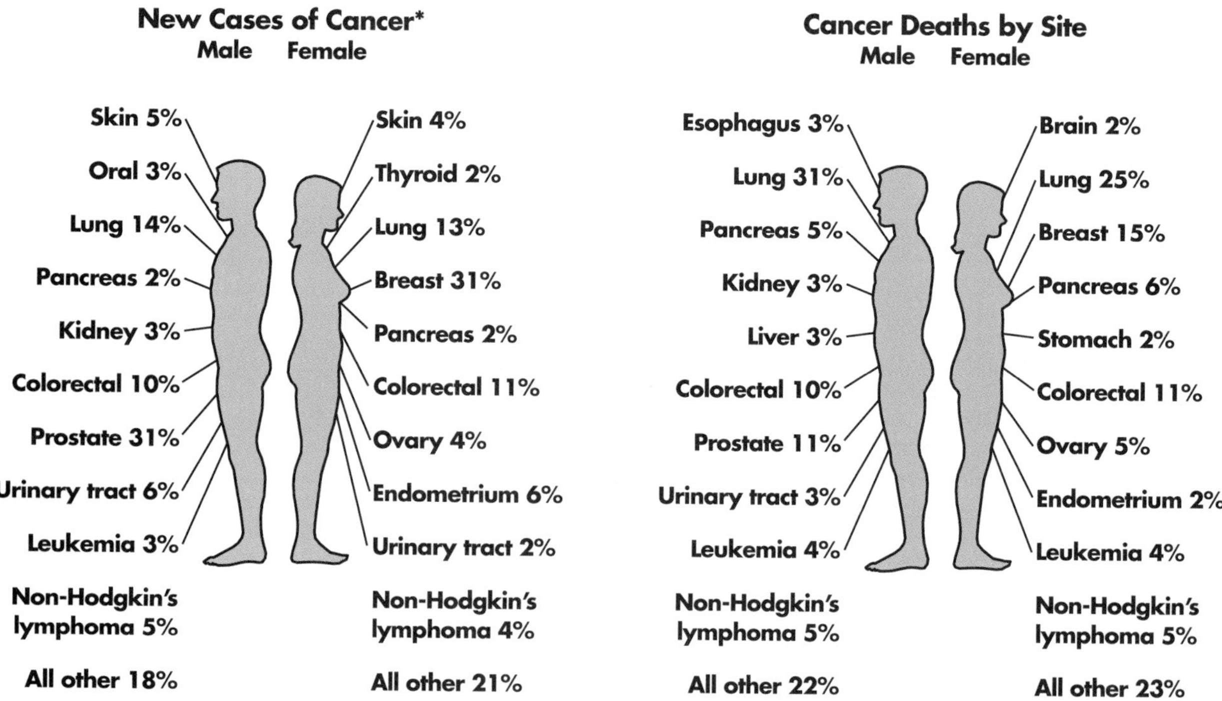

*Excluding basal and squamous cell skin cancers and *in situ* carcinomas, except bladder cancer.
Source: American Cancer Society

Bladder cancer, see page 933.
Breast cancer, see page 838.
Cervical cancer, see page 1098.
Colorectal cancer, see page 887.
Endometrial cancer, see page 1097.
Kidney cancer, see page 932.
Lung cancer, see page 817.
Oral cancer, see page 721.
Prostate cancer, see page 1124.
Skin cancer, see page 1200.
Testicular cancer, see page 1119.
Throat cancer, see page 695.

What Is Cancer?

Your body is made up of trillions of individual cells. It grows and develops as a result of increases in the numbers of new cells that become different types of tissue.

New cells are created through a process of cell division called mitosis. Cells acquire various specialized functions through an accompanying process called cell differentiation.

In the early developmental years of your life, cells divide rapidly in order to bring your body and all of its organs to full growth and maturity. Once you reach adulthood, most of your cells switch into maintenance mode, dividing only to replace cells that are injured or dead. Normal cellular function and, in turn, the overall health of your body depend largely on the delicate balance between cell growth and a process of programmed cell death called apoptosis.

Unlike normal cells, cancer cells either lack the controls that switch off growth or lose their ability to undergo apoptosis or both. They divide without restraint, crowding out neighboring normal cells. In addition, they affect the function and growth of normal cells by competing with them for available essential nutrients.

Uncontrolled cells can grow into a mass called a tumor that can invade and destroy nearby normal tissue. Cancer cells can also spread to other parts of the body via the bloodstream or lymphatic system in a process called metastasis.

Not all cells that exhibit rapid or uncontrolled growth patterns are cancer cells. Cells may accumulate as benign tumors, which often don't damage surrounding tissues. Benign tumors grow only locally and typically aren't life-threatening unless they're in a confined space, such as the skull.

Cancer cells, on the other hand, generally spread beyond their place of origin and, if not detected early, are often life-threatening. Cancer can develop in several forms.

Carcinomas

Cancers that originate on external or internal body surfaces, such as skin and colon cancers, are called carcinomas. These are the most common types in the United States.

Sarcomas

Sarcomas develop in the body's supportive tissues, such as bones and muscles.

Lymphomas

Lymphomas originate in the lymph nodes and immune system.

Leukemias

Leukemias originate in the bone marrow and are evident in the bloodstream.

Damaged DNA

What goes awry to produce cancer cells? This is a basic question scientists are still attempting to answer. Although they have yet to understand the exact processes by which all cells grow, divide, communicate and differentiate, they have learned much about what goes on within a cell to activate or alter normal cells to become cancerous.

Your body contains approximately 100 trillion cells. In the core (nucleus) of each cell reside 23 pairs (46 total) of structures called chromosomes — half of them inherited from each parent. Each chromosome is composed of long, double-stranded sequences of a material called deoxyribonucleic acid (DNA), arranged as a double helix.

Normal Cells

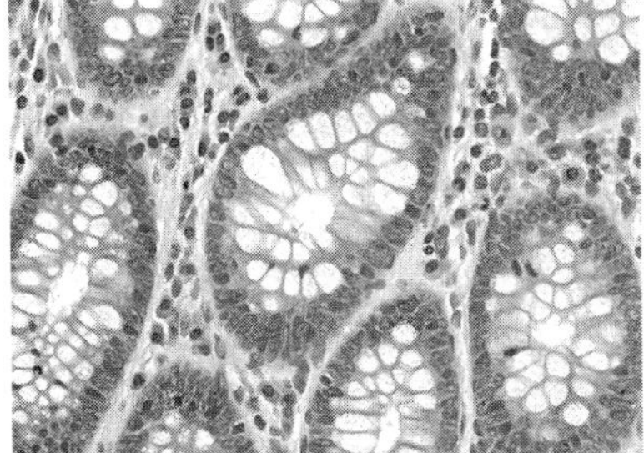

This slide shows normal tissue cells. The cells are oval shaped, with all of the cells looking similar. They're very well organized into a single layer of cells.

Cancer Cells

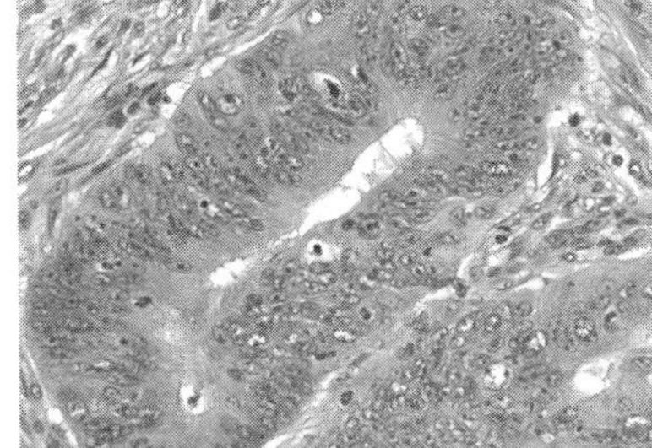

This slide shows cancer cells. Cancer cells are stacked up and highly disorganized. They also look very different from each other.

Benign Tumor Cells

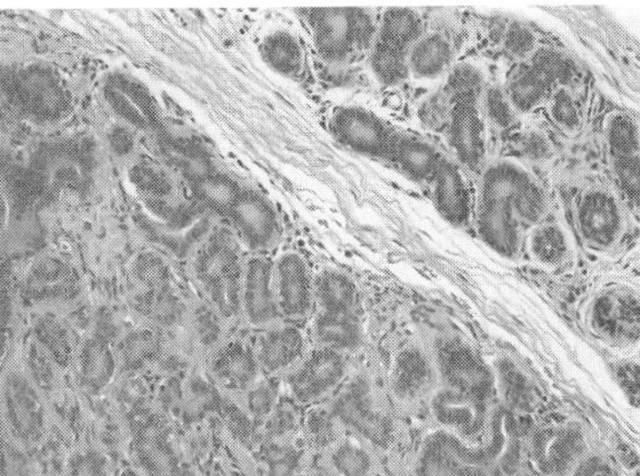

This slide shows a benign tumor (fibroadenoma). Unlike cancer, the cells remain well-formed. Benign tumors also don't invade normal surrounding tissue.

Each chromosome is made up of smaller units called genes. Each gene consists of a specific section of DNA. Encoded within the DNA is a set of instructions that determines almost everything about you, from the color of your eyes to your susceptibility to different diseases.

The code used in these instructions is composed of four chemical components: adenine (A), thymine (T), guanine (G) and cytosine (C). Different sequences of these molecules within a gene are translated or expressed as different proteins, substances that make up practically every part of your body and play a role in most of your body's activities (see Chapter 18, "Genetics and Disease"). Each cell contains between 30,000 and 40,000 genes, forming a complete recipe for a human being.

Not all genes are active all of the time. Cells selectively switch on certain genes in response to stress, injury, infections, hormones, growth factors and many other external stimuli. Some genes act as control (regulatory) genes. Some control genes can cause other genes to manufacture their protein continuously, such as an enzyme required for cells to transform nutrients into energy. Others can adjust genes' production in response to a particular need of the body, such as for insulin, which is a hormone necessary to control blood sugar levels. Still others can regulate cell division and differentiation.

When the genetic programming of a normal cell is disrupted or mutated, serious harm may result, many times in the form of disease.

Advances in Cancer Research

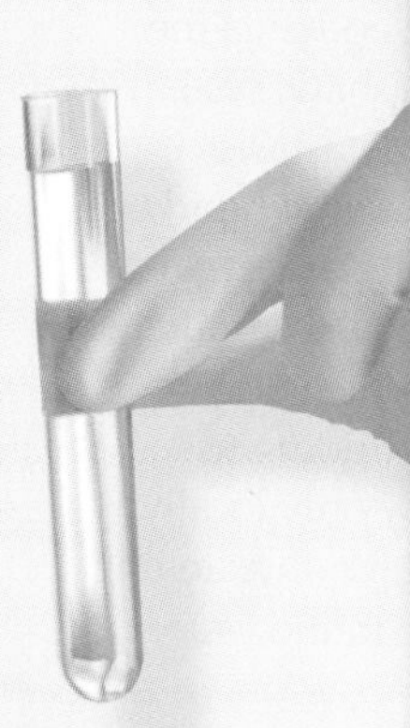

During the past three decades, great strides have been made in understanding how genes are activated and inactivated. This progress is due in great part to the development of recombinant DNA technology, a laboratory procedure that allows the genetic information contained in the DNA of a particular organism to be spliced (manipulated).

This technology allows scientists to isolate and observe the actions of individual genes. For example, a gene suspected of causing a particular disease in humans is inserted into a mouse's DNA. As the mouse's DNA is reproduced, so is the inserted gene. Scientists then observe what happens in the mouse as a result of its recombined DNA.

Recombinant DNA technology has made it possible for scientists to show that multiple mechanisms (agents) may be involved in activating cancer-causing genes (oncogenes). Altered chromosomes have long been suspected of playing a role in the origin of tumors. Research on a family of tumor-producing viruses (retroviruses) led investigators to specific genes associated with cancer in humans and to the exploration of whether chromosome rearrangement may be one way that proto-oncogenes, the precursors to oncogenes, are activated.

Such discoveries were possible partly because of the development of polymerase chain reaction (PCR), a laboratory procedure by which a small fragment of DNA can be quickly reproduced millions of times, making it easier to study. PCR led to the identification of the first genetic marker for cystic fibrosis and is now aiding scientists in the search for specific cancer genes.

Investigators have also discovered a set of genes that actually plays a protective role against cancer development, particularly in inherited cancers. Known as tumor-suppressing genes, these genes act to prevent the unregulated growth of cancer cells and the cancer-inducing effect of activated oncogenes. If one of these tumor-suppressing genes is absent or its protein product is unable to work properly, the cancer-producing action of an oncogene may not be completely suppressed and a tumor may develop.

Researchers continue to investigate how transformed or mutated cells are able to bypass the body's immune response to avoid being recognized as a foreign substance and attacked. One theory suggests that proteins made under the direction of oncogenes cause these abnormal cells to send messages that alter and evade the body's immune response.

Through the use of genetic engineering — a process whereby individual genes can be isolated and altered — scientists have produced biologic response modifiers (BRMs), natural substances that mesh with the body's own immune defenses in response to cancer. BRMs offer hope that new treatments for cancer may work by enhancing the body's own system to control cancer.

A major roadblock remains in finding a way to safely deliver immune system antibodies or anticancer drugs to the site of the cancer. One approach is monoclonal antibodies, artificial agents designed to attach themselves to cancer cells and deliver antibodies or drugs with great precision. The potential of these immunologic "bullets" in locating and treating cancer is an exciting prospect (see page 468).

Strategies to conquer cancers are progressing. The oncogene hypothesis, the discovery of tumor suppressors and the application of recombinant DNA techniques are a few of the advances now revolutionizing our understanding and treatment of cancer. The future holds the promise of applying such new information to the diagnosis, treatment and, ultimately, prevention of this complex disease.

Genes that have the potential for initiating cancer are known as proto-oncogenes. Normally, these genes perform useful functions, such as regulating cell division and tissue repair. But when a gene's DNA is disrupted or damaged, these functions may be altered. Proto-oncogenes can become cancer-causing genes called oncogenes (the root word *oncos* comes from the Greek word for "mass" or "tumor"). Oncogenes convert normal cells into cancer cells.

Damage to DNA can result from a variety of environmental factors, including chemicals, radiation, tobacco use and viruses. Damage can also occur because of factors inside your body, such as abnormal functioning of hormones, immune and metabolic disorders, and inherited genetic mutations. Some factors are avoidable; others are not.

Very few cancers are directly inherited. Eighty percent to 90 percent of people who develop cancer have no family history of the disease. Scientists have, however, identified many of the controllable factors that increase a person's chances of getting cancer (see page 479). Most researchers believe that a complex mix of such factors, acting together or in a sequence of events, promotes cancer cell growth.

Diagnosing Cancer

Along with prevention, one of the best approaches to fighting cancer is an early diagnosis. In most cases the earlier a cancer is detected, the greater are the chances it can be treated before it spreads to other tissues or organs. With the cancer-screening procedures available today, many cancers can be detected early enough to be cured.

Every diagnosis of cancer attempts to identify the type and location of the cancer. Each type has its own characteristic rate of growth, tendency to spread and particular set of tissues or organs to which it's likely to spread. Identifying the type of cancer you have enables your doctor to anticipate how it's likely to behave. This allows you and your doctor to plan appropriate treatment procedures.

If your doctor suspects that cancer may be present, because of signs or symptoms or the results of a cancer-screening procedure, a biopsy may be done. A biopsy involves taking a sample of the affected tissue for microscopic examination. Tissue samples may be removed surgically or with a needle. A biopsy can help determine if a tumor is benign or malignant. Biopsies are also used as screening tools to check for cellular abnormalities (precancerous changes) that often occur before cancer development.

Grading

The microscopic examination of a tissue sample may also provide clues about the way the tumor will behave or respond to treatment. The more normal the cells appear and the fewer the number of dividing cells, the more likely the cancer is to be slow growing and responsive to treatment. Based on the sample's cellular appearance, a grade is assigned to the tumor, usually ranging from I to IV. A lower grade generally indicates fewer cellular abnormalities. Higher grades indicate more abnormalities.

Staging

If a tumor is benign, your doctor may advise its removal to avoid the possibility of it becoming cancerous. If the tumor is cancerous, your doctor will want to determine if or how far the cancer has spread, a process called staging.

Staging is accomplished through a number of steps. It begins with a thorough history and physical examination and is followed by diagnostic tests, which might include a computerized tomography (CT) scan or magnetic resonance imaging (MRI), bone scans, X-rays, blood tests or other laboratory procedures. Staging is different for each type of cancer.

Information obtained from these tests is used to help classify the stage of the cancer. There are different ways of assigning malignant tumor classifications. The most common method is the TNM system. This system evaluates three components — the primary tumor (T), the nodes (N) and metastasis (M) — by answering the following key questions:

- T – How big is the tumor, and has the cancer spread locally?
- N – Have cancer cells spread to nearby lymph nodes?
- M – Has the cancer spread (metastasized) to other, distant areas of the body?

Numbers are assigned to each of these categories, indicating the degree to which the tumor has grown or spread. Once the TNM classifications have been determined, your doctor can determine the stage of your cancer. Like cancer grades, a lower number indicates that the cancer is still in its early stages, and a higher number means it's a more advanced cancer.

If cancer cells are present in a particular location but haven't begun to invade nearby tissues, the stage can also be described as *in situ* — a Latin term meaning "in place." This is a very early stage of cancer development and generally carries a very good prognosis. If the cancer has invaded nearby tissues, then it's called invasive. If the cancer has traveled to a different part of the body, it's known as metastatic.

Estimating a survival rate

Doctors often use statistics to help them estimate a prognosis, which is a prediction of the course and outcome of the disease and the likelihood of recovery. A common statistic used in the study of cancer is the 5-year survival rate. This rate is based on people who have survived the cancer for a period of 5 years, whether the cancer is receding (in remission), cured or under treatment. This statistic provides only a rough estimate of how the average person may do with a specific type of cancer. Your situation may be different.

Evaluating the results

All of these diagnostic tools — laboratory tests, imaging scans, grading and staging classifications, and statistical averages — can help guide you and your doctor toward the type of treatment best suited to your cancer. The diagnosis and staging of your cancer may require several days or weeks. Your therapy depends on a thorough and accurate evaluation.

Screening for Cancer

A number of tests are helpful in screening for cancer. They vary in complexity and cost. Most of the widely used tests are designed to discover the more common forms of cancer in people at high risk and for whom an early diagnosis may allow more effective treatment and better chances of survival.

Because everyone is different, the screening methods you and your doctor choose should address your specific circumstances and the type of cancer for which you may be at increased risk. Ideally, a test should detect the cancer early enough that chances for a full recovery are high.

Safety is important also. The test shouldn't pose a significant health threat. Twenty years ago the procedure used to detect breast cancer (mammography) had a relatively high radiation exposure that may have been a factor in later cancer development. Today, mammography exposes women to only small amounts of radiation, so the examination is much safer.

Screening tests for cancer don't have the same preventive value in all cases and for all types of cancer. With lung cancer, for example, sputum analysis or frequent chest X-rays typically don't identify the disease in its early stages. Only 15 percent of lung cancers are detected early enough to make a significant difference in survival rates. Other cancers are more easily detectable in their early stages, such as the detection of cervical cancer through a routine Pap test.

The cancer-screening tests and procedures described here are part of a cancer prevention program recommended by the American Cancer Society (ACS).

Breast cancer

Warning signs: An abnormality on a mammogram, any lump or thickening in the breast, bleeding or discharge from the nipple
Risk factors: Breast cancer occurs most often in women who:
- Are older than age 50
- Have never given birth
- Had their first child after age 30
- Have never breast-fed
- Are more than 40 percent over their ideal weight
- Reached sexual maturity early or had a late menopause
- Have a family history of premenopausal breast cancer, cancer in both breasts or ovarian cancer

Checkup guidelines: It's recommended that every woman examine her breasts carefully once a month (see page 836) and that women ages 20 to 39 have their breasts examined by a doctor every 3 years.

Not all doctors agree on how often women should have mammograms, and there are conflicting studies as to the benefits of an annual mammogram. The ACS recommends that women age 40 and older have a breast examination by a doctor and a mammogram every year. Some doctors and other organizations think an annual mammogram after age 50 is more appropriate. You and your doctor will make the final decision, based on your individual situation.

Cervical cancer

Warning signs: Abnormal vaginal bleeding
Risk factors: Cervical cancer is associated with:
- Genital herpes or genital wart infections
- Onset of sexual activity shortly after reaching puberty
- Many sexual partners
- Tobacco use

Checkup guidelines: If you're a female who's sexually active or older than age 18, it's recommended that you have a Pap test (see page 1100) and a pelvic examination annually. After you've had three or more consecutive normal annual examinations, your doctor may decide that the Pap test can be performed less frequently.

Colorectal cancer

Warning signs: Rectal bleeding or a long-term change in bowel habits
Risk factors: Colorectal cancer is associated with:
- A history of colorectal polyps
- A family history of colorectal cancer or inflammatory bowel disease
- Tobacco use
- Physical inactivity
- A high-fat diet
- A low-fiber diet
- A diet low in fruits and vegetables
- Alcohol consumption

Checkup guidelines: If you're an adult age 50 or older who's at average risk of colorectal cancer, it's recommended that you have one or more of the following screening procedures:
- A fecal occult blood test annually
- A flexible sigmoidoscopy every 5 years
- A fecal occult test blood annually *and* flexible sigmoidoscopy every 5 years

- A barium enema every 5 years
- A colonoscopy every 10 years

A digital rectal exam should be done at the same time as a sigmoidoscopy, colonoscopy or barium enema.

Of the first three options listed, the American Cancer Society prefers the third option. Mayo Clinic cancer specialists recommend periodic evaluations of the entire colon by either barium enema or colonoscopy. If you're at an increased risk of this type of cancer, your doctor may request more frequent screening.

Endometrial cancer

Warning signs: Abnormal vaginal bleeding
Risk factors: Endometrial cancer is associated with:

- A history of infertility or failure to ovulate
- Late onset of menopause or prolonged estrogen therapy or tamoxifen use after menopause
- Obesity
- Diabetes
- Gallbladder disease
- High blood pressure
- Hereditary nonpolyposis colorectal cancer (HNPCC)

Checkup guidelines: Most endometrial cancer is detected early due to postmenopausal bleeding. If you're a woman with a personal or family history of HNPCC, consider an annual endometrial biopsy beginning at age 35.

Lung cancer

Warning signs: A persistent cough, coughing up blood, bronchitis, chest pain, and recurrent pneumonia in the same location
Risk factors: Lung cancer is associated with:

- Tobacco use
- Exposure to secondhand smoke
- Exposure to environmental pollutants such as asbestos and arsenic
- Exposure to radon and radiation
- Tuberculosis

Checkup guidelines: If you're older than age 40, consider having a baseline chest X-ray. Subsequent chest X-rays may be done at the discretion of your doctor. Low-dose helical (spiral) computerized tomography (CT) scans and molecular markers in sputum are being studied for possible use in early lung cancer detection.

Oral cancer

Warning signs: A change of color inside your mouth, a lump or thickening in your mouth or a sore inside your mouth that fails to heal
Risk factors: Oral cancer is associated with:

- Being male and age 40 or older
- Use of chewing tobacco
- Heavy use of smoking tobacco
- Excessive alcohol consumption

Checkup guidelines: See a doctor or dentist if you have a sore in your mouth that fails to heal or if you notice a lump inside your mouth.

Prostate cancer

Warning signs: Often none. Some men experience difficulty urinating. Blood in the urine or persistent pain in the lower back, pelvis or upper thighs.
Risk factors: Prostate cancer occurs most often in men who:

- Are over 65
- Are black
- Have a family history of the disease

Checkup guidelines: If you're older than age 40, it's recommended that you have a digital rectal examination at the time of your annual physical. At age 50 — or at an earlier age if you're black or have a family history of prostate cancer — discuss with your doctor the benefits of having a regular prostate-specific antigen (PSA) blood test.

The accuracy of the PSA test is frequently debated, and some health experts think that it can be a needless and expensive procedure. Mayo Clinic urologists agree that the test isn't ideal, but they support its use because it's the best screening tool available for identifying prostate cancer. Along with the ACS and the American Urological Association (AUA), Mayo Clinic urologists recommend a yearly PSA test beginning at age 50. After age 75, Mayo urologists believe a yearly digital exam to be sufficient, although the ACS and AUA recommend lifelong screening. For more on the PSA test, see page 1125.

Skin cancer

Warning signs: Skin cancer can present itself in many ways:

- A small lesion with an irregular border
- A firm bump, nodule or lesion — from pearl colored to black — anywhere on the skin
- Dark lesions on the palms, the soles of your feet or the tips of your fingers or toes
- A shiny, waxy, pearl-colored bump on your face, ear or neck
- A firm, red nodule or a flat lesion with a scaly or crusted surface
- A change in a mole
- A sore that fails to heal

Risk factors: Skin cancer is associated with:

- Fair skin
- Blue eyes
- Red hair
- Severe sunburns in childhood
- A family history of birthmarks or moles
- Exposure to coal, tar, pitch, creosote, arsenic compounds or radium

Checkup guidelines: If you have a skin lesion that exemplifies the warning signs listed above, see your doctor.

Testicular cancer

Warning signs: Any lump on the testicle, a change in its size or a sensation of fullness
Risk factors: Testicular cancer strikes younger men and is uncommon after age 40. A known risk factor for this cancer is undescended testicles — one or both — at birth.

Checkup guidelines: Beginning in their late teens, it's recommended that men examine their testicles monthly (see page 1119).

Throat cancer

Warning signs: Hoarseness
Risk factors: Heavy smoking, particularly when coupled with excessive alcohol use
Checkup guidelines: Have a throat examination annually if you're a heavy smoker or in the event of unexplained hoarseness or a change in the character of your voice lasting more than a few weeks.

Urinary tract and bladder cancer

Warning signs: Blood in urine, back pain, loss of weight and appetite, a persistent fever and anemia
Risk factors: Urinary tract and bladder cancer is associated with:

- Being male and age 50 or older
- Tobacco use
- A history of chronic urinary tract infections

Checkup guidelines: A routine urinalysis during an annual physical examination may reveal blood in your urine (hematuria), the most common warning sign.

Treating Cancer

More than ever before, many cancers can be successfully treated. The probability of a complete cure or extended survival is continuously improving because of growing knowledge and understanding of cancer. As a result, new therapies that selectively kill cancer cells are steadily being developed. Such therapies are not only more effective but also safer. In addition, management of cancer pain has improved to the point that most people with cancer can live and work comfortably while undergoing cancer treatment.

Treatment regimens for cancer are based on the needs of the individual being treated and the type of cancer he or she has. But the basic therapeutic options available to most people with cancer are similar. Why one form of treatment is more appropriate than another for a given person depends on a variety of factors, including the diagnosis, the stage of the disease, the individual's age, sex and general health, and his or her individual choice. In women, menopausal status also can be a factor in treatment decisions.

During the diagnostic phase, your doctor is usually able to determine if a localized form of treatment, such as surgery or radiation therapy, can treat your cancer, or if a total body (systemic) form of treatment, such as chemotherapy, is necessary because cancer cells have spread to other body parts.

Surgery

Surgery has long been the foundation of cancer treatment. The goal of any operation can vary — it may be to determine whether a growth is malignant, to remove a cancerous growth from the body or to learn if malignant cells have spread to other body parts. Sometimes, surgery is directed primarily toward relief of an obstruction, for example, removing a growth that's obstructing the bile ducts. At other times, when it's not possible to remove all of the cancerous growth, a surgeon may remove as much as possible (a debulking procedure) in order to make chemotherapy or radiation more effective.

Surgery is most successful if the cancer is contained in one location (localized). Sometimes, however, cancer cells spread from the site where the cancer first appeared (the primary tumor) and travel by way of the bloodstream or the lymphatic system to other sites in the body to form secondary tumors (metastases). If cells spread before the primary growth is taken out, cancer may recur at other locations, even after the primary tumor has been fully removed.

Metastatic tumors are still named based on the primary location of the cancer. For example, breast cancer that has spread to the lungs is called breast cancer metastasis, not lung cancer.

Cancer Clusters in Populations

Data collected by public health officials sometimes show an increase in the frequency of occurrence of a certain type of cancer or group of cancers in a region or community. This increase is often referred to as a cancer cluster.

Further study usually finds that such clusters are explained by the laws of chance or by changes in medical referral patterns. Sometimes, though, the increase is traced to an environmental factor.

The laws of chance tell us that most communities or groups of people of similar age and background will have about the same frequency of various diseases. They also suggest that from time to time there will be an unusual concentration of one disease or another within certain groups of people.

This statistical phenomenon might be compared to dealing a hand of cards. Usually, the cards in a hand will be fairly evenly distributed among the four suits, but you can also expect that now and then you'll be dealt a hand composed almost entirely of one suit. Mathematicians can even calculate the odds of such an event occurring.

It's important to separate cancer clusters that are merely random from those related to environmental factors. Scientific proof that a cancer cluster is a consequence of exposure to potentially toxic substances depends on careful evaluation.

If the cancer is widespread, an operation is rarely able to cure it. Occasionally, a single metastatic tumor appears after removal of the primary cancer and, in some cases, the surgical removal of this single lesion can result in a complete recovery. This situation may be experienced by people with cancer of the colon or testicles, among others. Metastatic tumors, in most of these circumstances, are located in the lung, liver or brain.

Radiation therapy

Radiation is another option for destroying cancer cells. Radiation therapy — also referred to as radiotherapy, X-ray therapy, cobalt treatment or irradiation — may be one part of a treatment regimen or the only form of treatment. Radiation affects only the cancer cells located within the area of the body (field) receiving the radiation.

Radiation is sometimes used before surgery to shrink a cancerous tumor, after surgery to destroy any remaining cancer cells, in combination with anticancer drugs or alone. Radiation is particularly effective on certain types of localized cancers, such as malignant tumors of the lymph nodes or vocal cords.

Like surgery, radiation isn't usually curative if the cancer cells have spread throughout the body or outside the field of radiation. It may still be used even if a complete recovery isn't probable because it can shrink tumors to decrease signs and symptoms the cancer is producing, such as pressure, pain or bleeding.

Generally, radiation produces less physical disfigurement than radical surgery, but it may produce some troublesome side effects, such as irritated or thickened skin, difficulty swallowing, dry mouth, nausea, diarrhea, hair loss and loss of energy. How serious and extensive these side effects become depends on where and how much radiation is used.

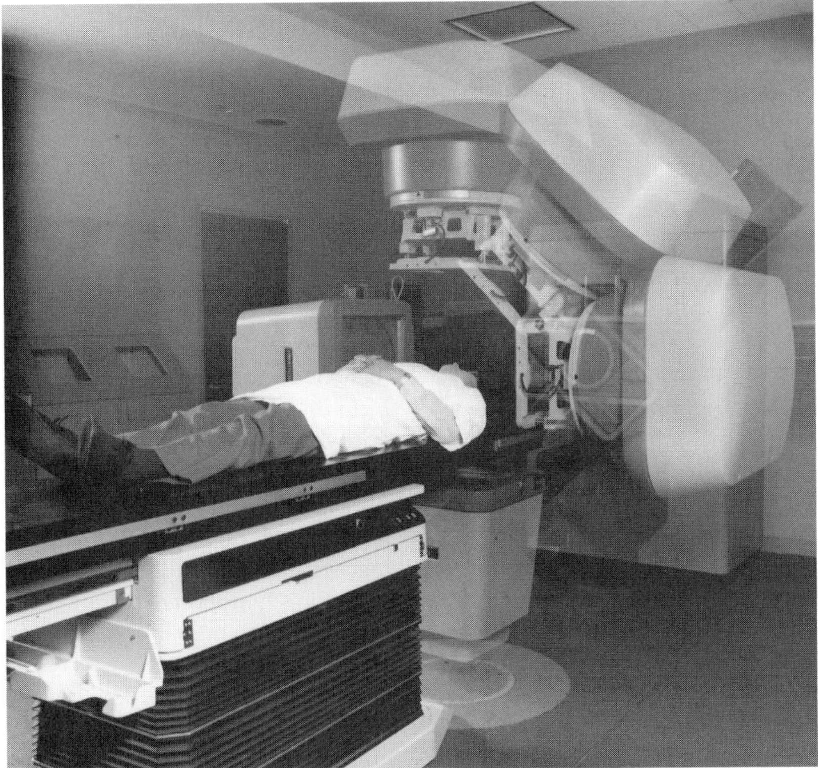

Radiation therapy can effectively destroy cancer cells. During treatment this radiation source slowly rotates to deliver radiation more effectively.

Chemotherapy

Chemotherapy is the systemic use of medication to treat cancer. The medication is generally administered by injection or intravenously. For some types of malignancy, such as Hodgkin's disease, leukemia and testicular cancer, chemotherapy may produce a full recovery even when the cancer is widespread.

Chemotherapy is more frequently being given following an operation to remove the cancer even when there's no clear sign of the cancer having spread. This is referred to as adjuvant chemotherapy. For some cancers, especially breast and colorectal, adjuvant chemotherapy has been shown to decrease the chance the cancer will return. And people with cancer who receive this therapy generally live longer than those who don't have the treatment.

Chemotherapy may also be given before an operation to shrink the cancer and make the operation easier or more successful. This is called neoadjuvant chemotherapy and is used in cancers of the head, neck and breast. In instances in which the cancer isn't curable, chemotherapy can relieve symptoms and enhance quality of life. This is called palliative treatment.

Chemotherapy may involve the use of more than one medication. Combination chemotherapy consists of giving a group of drugs that work together to kill cancer cells. The downside of anticancer medications is that they often affect normal tissue cells as well as cancer cells.

Normal cells most likely to be affected are those that divide rapidly, such as those found in bone marrow, the lining of the gastrointestinal tract, the reproductive system and hair follicles. After treatment is complete, these cells usually recover.

Depending on the specific medications used, chemotherapy can produce various side effects. They include hair loss, mouth sores, difficulty swallowing, dry mouth, nausea, vomiting, diarrhea, bleeding and infection.

Less common problems include damage to the heart, liver, lungs, kidneys or nerves. Nerve damage typically results in numbness or tingling of the hands or feet. In most instances, the side effects disappear once the treatment is complete. Health care experts are working to reduce and even eliminate these side effects.

Immunotherapy

Your body's immune system acts as a surveillance system to guard against the presence of what it interprets to be foreign substances. For example, when your immune system detects harmful bacteria or a virus in your body, it responds by producing specific proteins (antibodies) that attack and destroy the invaders.

Your immune system also views cancer cells as foreign invaders. But due to a failure in the system, it often doesn't recognize cancer cells. For years, researchers have been trying to find ways to enhance the body's natural immune reaction to cancer cells.

Using the immune system to attack and destroy cancer cells is called immunotherapy. Other names for the technique include biological therapy, biotherapy or biologic response modifier therapy. Immunotherapy may be prescribed alone or in combination with other cancer treatments.

One variation of immunotherapy is to administer substances that stimulate the immune system — nonspecific immunomodulating agents. Two such agents are used in conjunction with surgery for bladder cancer and surgery for advanced colon cancer.

Another variation is to produce specific immune system proteins (cytokines) in the laboratory and then use them in treatment. These proteins — called biologic response modifiers (BRMs) — account for the majority of immunotherapeutic agents currently being used or studied. BRMs include:

Interferons

Interferons are cytokines that occur naturally in your body. There are several types of interferons. The type most commonly used in cancer treatment is called interferon-alpha. Interferons may directly inhibit cancer cells, or they may stimulate other immune system cells to help in the battle.

Interferons are used in the treatment of a number of conditions, including hairy cell leukemia, melanoma, chronic myeloid leukemia and AIDS-related Kaposi's sarcoma. They're also being studied for potential use in the treatment of metastatic kidney cancer and non-Hodgkin's lymphoma.

Interleukins

Like interferons, interleukins are a type of cytokine. Interleukin-2, the most widely studied interleukin, works by stimulating other immune system cells that can destroy cancer cells. It has been approved for the treatment of metastatic kidney cancer and metastatic melanoma and is being studied as a treatment for several other cancers.

Colony-stimulating factors

Rather than interacting directly with cancer cells, colony-stimulating factors (CSFs) encourage production of white blood cells. Chemotherapy tends to impair the functions of your bone marrow, including production of white blood cells, platelets and red blood cells. Reduced numbers of these cells make you more vulnerable to infection. CSFs may allow you to tolerate chemotherapy with a lower chance of developing an infection or with less fatigue caused by chemotherapy-induced anemia.

Monoclonal antibodies

Monoclonal antibodies are designed and produced in a laboratory to target specific types of cancer. By attaching themselves to tumor cells, they can either react with that cancer cell or be used to deliver anticancer medications or radiation.

The Food and Drug Administration has approved two monoclonal antibodies — rituximab (Rituxan), for the treatment of recurring B cell non-Hodgkin's lymphoma, and trastuzumab (Herceptin), for use against metastatic breast cancer that produces too much of a protein called HER-2. Additional monoclonal antibodies are being developed and studied for use in other types of cancer. These include other lymphomas, leukemias, brain tumors, as well as cancers of the lung, colon, rectum and prostate.

Vaccines

Researchers are working on vaccines that can help your immune system recognize cancer cells. Unlike infectious disease vaccines, which are given to prevent a disease, cancer vaccines are given only after a tumor develops. The vaccine is intended to help your body reject the tumor and prevent the cancer from recurring.

Side effects

Side effects of BRMs may include a rash or swelling at the site of injection, flu-like symptoms and fatigue. CSFs may cause bone pain, fatigue, fever and appetite loss. Muscle aches and fever may occur after a cancer vaccine.

Some BRMs may cause allergic reactions. Side effects can be severe at times, so it's always important to talk with your doctor about possible side effects of your particular cancer treatment.

As researchers learn more about how the immune system recognizes and attacks malignant cells, their studies may lead to effective immunotherapy techniques against many types of cancer.

Hyperthermia therapy

Hyperthermia therapy involves exposing body tissue to high temperatures — up to 106 F — harming some tumors by damaging the cells or depriving them of nutrients. This therapy can be performed in a small area, for example, on a limb or an organ, or on the whole body in cases of metastatic cancer. The treatment can be uncomfortable and may cause blisters if applied directly to the skin, although the blisters generally heal quickly.

Researchers have evaluated hyperthermia in conjunction with radiation and chemotherapy to treat cancer of the breast, lymph nodes, skin, eye and cervix. Its role is still being investigated.

Cryotherapy

Cryotherapy is the opposite of hyperthermia therapy. It uses extreme cold to destroy cancer cells. Cryotherapy consists of the application of liquid nitrogen to a tumor. It's used most often to treat early-stage skin cancers and precancerous skin conditions, as well as cancer of the retina (retinoblastoma). Researchers are studying cryotherapy as a possible treatment for some internal cancers, such as those affecting the prostate and the liver. For these cancers, liquid nitrogen reaches the tumor through a device called a cryoprobe.

Stem cell transplantation

Stem cell transplantation is used to replace cells within bone marrow that have been destroyed by radiation or chemotherapy. During the procedure, you receive a supply of stem cells — immature cells that haven't yet differentiated into the various types of blood cells. You may receive your own stem cells (an autologous transplant), stem cells from an identical twin if you have one (a syngeneic transplant) or stem cells from a sibling or a parent or even an unrelated donor (an allogeneic transplant). Knowing that you'll have a supply of healthy stem cells available to you allows your doctor to use higher doses of chemotherapy or radiation therapy. Stem cell transplantation is used most often as a treatment for leukemia and lymphoma.

Angiogenesis inhibitors

All tumors require new blood vessel development to supply oxygen and nutrients to their cells so that they can grow. The formation of new blood vessels is called angiogenesis. Scientists are studying the use of both natural and synthetic inhibitors of angiogenesis to shrink tumors or prevent them from growing by blocking the formation of new blood vessels.

Coping with Side Effects

Sometimes the side effects of cancer treatment are temporarily more distressing than the cancer itself. Both

Emerging Therapies

Cancer treatment is constantly evolving. Some of the methods described here are now accepted therapy, and others are under investigation and remain experimental. Doctors often combine these approaches with chemotherapy and radiation.

Gene therapy
Tumors grow because normal genes become damaged, causing healthy cells to turn cancerous. Genes that suppress cancer can also fail to work properly. The intent of gene therapy is to repair or replace defective genes and increase the production of healthy ones.

Molecularly directed therapy
The Food and Drug Administration has approved the use of imatinib mesylate (Gleevec, STI-571) to treat chronic myeloid leukemia, a rare form of cancer. This leukemia is caused by a genetic mutation that allows a blood cell enzyme to be switched on permanently. The drug works by inhibiting the enzyme and thus the abnormal growth of white blood cells.

Trastuzumab (Herceptin) is another treatment aimed at a specific protein, called HER-2-neu, that's made by a defective gene. The protein is found in about one in four people with breast cancer. Herceptin is a monoclonal antibody that binds to the defective protein, resulting in a decrease in cell growth and even death of the cancer cells. Unlike most monoclonal antibodies, it doesn't depend on the immune system to be effective against cancer cells.

Laser surgery
Laser beams are powerful tools for accomplishing precise surgical procedures. Laser surgery is frequently used in treating cancers of the skin, lungs, vocal cords, vagina, vulva, cervix and penis. The heat emitted by a laser can also shrink tumors, relieving cancer-related symptoms.

Photodynamic therapy
During photodynamic therapy, cancer cells are treated with photosensitizing agents and then exposed to laser light. Light absorbed into tumor cells from the laser causes a chemical reaction, destroying the tumor cells. The advantage of this therapy is that it's highly selective, affecting only cancer cells while leaving normal cells alone. This procedure uses laser light that's able to pass through only a thin layer of tissue, so it's useful for surface cancer but not as effective against cancer located deep inside an organ. Researchers are working to improve this aspect of photodynamic therapy.

radiation therapy and chemotherapy have common side effects that include fatigue, nausea, hair loss, skin problems, mouth and throat difficulties, diarrhea, and constipation. Immunotherapy also can cause fatigue.

Although scientists have made strides in modifying the severity of such problems, including effective nausea medications, you'll likely experience some side effects during your treatment.

Many people continue to work or go to school — though perhaps on a less demanding schedule — and carry on daily activities while receiving cancer treatment. You can do things to reduce side effects and improve your quality of life during this period.

Fatigue

People frequently feel more tired during cancer treatment. The level of fatigue can vary — you may feel a mild lack of energy, or you may feel completely wiped out. Your fatigue also may last for several months after completion of your treatment.

Regardless of your level of fatigue, pay attention to it. Try to get a good night's sleep and rest as needed throughout the day. Light activity is usually beneficial to help you maintain energy, but let others help you do things too. It's also important that you eat well and drink plenty of fluids. For more on managing fatigue, see page 476.

Nausea

Antinausea medications help prevent or decrease nausea and vomiting in many people undergoing cancer treatment.

To prevent nausea, also try these measures:

- Eat bland foods such as toast, crackers and Popsicles.
- Drink small amounts of clear liquids frequently.
- Avoid dry foods if you have a dry mouth or mouth sores.
- Eat cold foods because hot foods tend to have a stronger smell.
- Eat foods that you like.
- Wear loose clothing.
- While you're eating, distract yourself with conversation, a movie or a favorite hobby.

Hair loss

Certain chemotherapy drugs and radiation therapy to the head can cause hair loss (alopecia). The hair tends to come out in clumps, most often during washing or brushing.

Your doctor can tell you in advance if hair loss is a likely side effect of your treatment. If you know hair loss is likely, you may wish to purchase a wig or hair piece before the treatment begins so that you can match hair color and texture. Some people choose to wear turbans or scarves. Others have their hair cut short before it begins to fall out so that the process of losing their hair isn't quite as overwhelming.

Treat your hair gently with mild shampoos and soft brushes and avoid high heat when drying your hair. Use sunscreen to protect your scalp from the sun.

Skin problems

Dry skin can be another side effect of radiation therapy or chemotherapy. The following practices can help to reduce the effects of dry skin:

Cancer Centers

Choosing doctors and a hospital to treat your cancer can be stressful. Sometimes the process seems automatic. Your family doctor may refer you to a cancer specialist (oncologist) within the same practice or at an associated medical facility. Sometimes you're faced with many options. Before making a decision, ask for advice from your personal physician or another doctor with whom you feel comfortable and have confidence. This person can help you locate and evaluate an appropriate cancer facility.

Most large medical centers are equipped to treat cancer cases that don't require a high degree of specialization. However, if you need complicated or experimental treatment or if the doctors at your local hospital are inexperienced in treating your specific type of cancer, you might want to consider seeking care at a specialized cancer center.

Usually, a hospital directly connected to or affiliated with a medical school offers a broader range of treatment options because these types of institutions often draw prominent clinicians, researchers and educators to their medical facilities and teaching staff. Teaching hospitals — those that train doctors but don't necessarily have a direct medical school affiliation — also often are good facilities.

Teaching hospitals and hospitals associated with medical schools often conduct clinical trials in which they investigate potential new cancer treatments. If you're offered a chance to enter one of these trials, make sure that you fully understand the possible risks and benefits. Although clinical trials are clearly experimental, the therapies under investigation often include some of the most promising treatments.

The National Cancer Institute has designated more than 40 medical centers throughout the United States as comprehensive cancer centers. These centers provide leadership in cancer research and education and develop programs involving scientists and physicians from many fields. Comprehensive cancer centers generally offer the most extensive range of cancer treatment found in the United States. To find out more about these centers, see the National Cancer Institute on page 1385.

- Avoid hot baths.
- When you do take a bath, add bath oil to the water.
- Don't bathe more than once a day.
- Apply moisturizers and lotions while your skin is still moist.
- Avoid skin products that contain alcohol.

Mouth and throat disorders

It's important to maintain good oral hygiene during cancer treatment because gum disease, mouth sores and mouth dryness can result from chemotherapy. Radiation therapy to the chest or throat area also can cause gagging, coughing or swallowing problems. Remember to take the following measures:

- Brush your teeth and gums after every meal.
- Use a soft toothbrush and don't brush too hard.
- Rinse your mouth often with warm salt water.
- Avoid mouthwashes with alcohol.
- Eat soft foods, such as ice cream, mashed potatoes, yogurt or macaroni and cheese.
- Keep your lips moist with lip balm or petroleum jelly.
- Avoid spicy or acidic foods, such as tomato and citrus.
- Carry a water bottle with you and sip throughout the day.

Diarrhea

Treatment can affect the cells that line your intestines, causing diarrhea. The following habits can help to control your bowel movements:

- Drink plenty of mild, clear liquids, such as water, ginger ale, clear broth, weak tea or sports drinks. Diarrhea can cause dehydration.
- Eat several small meals throughout the day rather than three larger meals.
- Eat low-fiber foods, such as white rice, noodles or chicken.
- Eat foods rich in potassium, a vital nutrient that's lost through diarrhea. Foods with plenty of potassium include bananas, oranges, potatoes and apricots.
- Avoid beverages containing alcohol or caffeine, sweets, dairy products and extremely hot or cold foods because these can make diarrhea worse.

If you have diarrhea for more than 24 hours, or if it's associated

Complementary and Alternative Therapies

When cancer is diagnosed, many people look beyond standard medical practices to help fight the cancer or cope with its side effects. Although some nontraditional therapies may be helpful, others may be harmful, especially if they're used in place of proven treatments.

Complementing standard care

Complementary and alternative therapies for cancer are most often used in conjunction with standard medical treatments. These therapies won't cure your cancer, but they may enhance your quality of life by reducing stress, lessening side effects of treatment and improving your general sense of well-being. In addition, because most complementary and alternative methods are self-managed, they can give you a sense of control over your situation.

The types of complementary therapies that may accompany cancer treatment are many and varied:

- Meditation
- Acupuncture or acupressure
- Therapeutic massage
- Music, movement and art therapy
- Prayer and other spiritual practices
- Yoga
- Tai chi
- Hypnosis

To improve your sense of well-being, you don't necessarily have to enroll in an organized program. Taking the time to relax and enjoy the small things in life is a complementary therapy in and of itself.

In place of standard care

Some people explore complementary and alternative therapies in an effort to replace more standard treatment. But the safety and effectiveness of these alternative therapies is often not tested, and some may even be harmful. The National Cancer Institute has established a section devoted to studying the effectiveness of alternative treatments. Some popular alternative therapies have included high doses of vitamin C, laetrile, coffee enemas and ozone therapy. Herbal supplements, which many people think of as "all natural," are not regulated in the same manner as foods and drugs and may contain a host of contaminants.

A good rule of thumb in terms of complementary and alternative therapies is to first discuss them with your doctor and avoid any treatment that promises a cure, encourages you to give up conventional therapies or requires you to travel to another country. See Chapter 43, "Complementary and Alternative Medicine," for more information.

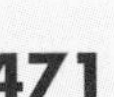

with abdominal pain or cramping, contact your doctor.

Constipation

Certain medications, physical weakness, lack of activity or a diet low in fiber and liquids can cause constipation. If you experience constipation for more than 1 or 2 days, your doctor may prescribe a stool softener or laxative. Try taking these steps too:

- Increase the amount of high-fiber foods in your diet, such as whole-grain breads, raw fruits and vegetables, fruit juices or dried fruits.
- Drink plenty of liquids.
- Exercise lightly every day.
- Avoid foods that commonly cause constipation, such as chocolate, cheese and eggs.

Appetite and weight changes

If you eat a balanced diet, you'll most likely be better able to tolerate the side effects of chemotherapy, radiation and surgery. Good nutrition also enhances your immune function and sense of well-being.

Common and difficult problems often associated with cancer are weight loss and malnutrition. Many factors can contribute to weight loss. Cancer or its treatment can decrease appetite and food intake or interfere with your body's consumption, digestion and absorption of food. In addition, many people experience appetite and weight changes even before a diagnosis of cancer is made.

Often a person with cancer who experiences severe weight loss simply can't eat in spite of his or her understanding that nourishment is important. Some people are unable to taste their food, and it's not uncommon to feel full after eating only a few bites.

Radiation therapy, chemotherapy or surgery also may cause signs and symptoms — such as nausea, alterations in sense of taste or smell, a sore mouth, diarrhea, anorexia or difficulty swallowing — that increase chances of nutritional problems.

If you're one of these people, you can take many simple, constructive steps to improve your appetite during cancer treatment and prevent weight loss (see page 476). Various feeding techniques, such as tube feedings, intravenous feedings or oral supplements, also can help people with cancer — even those with complicated nutritional problems — get adequate nutrition. A medication called megestrol (Megace), taken as a pill or syrup several times each day, has been shown in clinical trials to increase weight in individuals with cancer.

Clinical studies also indicate that a good nutritional state can improve a person's chance of undergoing successful treatment and withstanding the effects of cancer. But no conclusive evidence indicates that decreased or excessive amounts of any nutrient have a beneficial role in the treatment of cancer. Your doctor or a registered dietitian can provide advice on how to maintain adequate nutrition.

Pain

Cancer doesn't always cause pain. More than half the people with cancer don't experience significant pain. Some people, though, have severe pain. In general, the more advanced the cancer, the greater likelihood of periods of severe pain.

Causes

Cancer pain may be dull, aching, sharp, constant, intermittent, mild, moderate or severe. The pain may stem from the destruction of healthy tissues around the primary tumor or other areas in the body where the cancer has spread. Or, it may result from pressure on nerves, bones or other organs as the cancer continues to grow.

Cancer treatments are another source of pain. Surgery can be painful. Radiation therapy may lead to skin reactions or scars that are painful. And chemotherapy can cause potentially painful side effects due to mouth sores, diarrhea or damaged nerves. Emotional responses to the cancer, such as anxiety, depression or feelings of hopelessness, can make the pain seem worse.

Treatments

Pain relief can be obtained in many ways. Through a combination of pain-relieving medications and other forms of treatment, most people with cancer don't have to deal with severe pain. One of the components of cancer treatment is to decrease pain with as few side effects as possible.

Cancer treatments

The ideal way to treat cancer pain, when possible, is to remove the source of pain through surgery, chemotherapy or radiation therapy.

Medications

Pain medications (analgesics) are another option. Many drugs are used to treat cancer pain, but most fall into two categories: non-narcotics and narcotics.

- *Non-narcotics.* Non-narcotics include acetaminophen and nonsteroidal anti-inflammatory drugs (NSAIDs). NSAIDs are also helpful if inflammation is responsible for some of the pain. Antidepressants and antiseizure medications and steroids are other non-narcotic agents that may help control cancer pain.
- *Narcotics.* Narcotics, such as morphine and codeine and its derivatives, are more powerful painkillers most often prescribed for moderate to severe pain. People with cancer often worry that using narcotics will lead to addiction. It's true that people who use narcotics for purposes other than pain control, such as to achieve an altered state of mind, may become addicted to them. But when taken for pain and under proper direction, narcotics rarely cause addiction. If a

narcotic is needed to relieve severe pain for a long time, the comfort it provides often outweighs the risk of addiction.

A common side effect of narcotics is constipation. It can be treated with appropriate measures prescribed by your doctor. Other side effects can include confusion, lethargy and sleepiness. These usually occur when the pain medication is initiated, but once a steady amount of the medicine stays in your body, the side effects generally go away.

Occasionally, tranquilizers (sedatives) are used in combination with analgesics. Tranquilizers provide no pain relief, but they may help you tolerate the discomfort and can be an integral part of treatment. Tranquilizers or large doses of narcotics can cause confusion or delirium. This may limit their usefulness in some cases, but such side effects usually go away with appropriate, steady dosing.

Most pain medications can be taken orally, so they're easy to use. Others are given by injection or intravenously, which introduces the medications into the bloodstream in a controlled flow through a needle inserted into a vein in an arm. Some pain medications are available in patch form. For some people with cancer, this is a convenient and effective way of providing durable pain relief.

Other therapies

Beyond medications, other options for treating pain include:

- *Nerve blocks.* In this procedure, nerve pathways that carry pain impulses to the brain are blocked either by injection of substances into or around nerve fibers or by surgery. Nerve blocks carry some risks, but for people who can't tolerate the side effects of pain medications, they can be helpful. Nerve blocks are frequently used for pancreatic cancer and some other types of cancer.
- *Behavior modification therapies.* These therapies are used most often in combination with other pain relief treatments. They help decrease anxiety and can build confidence in your ability to cope with pain. Behavior modification therapies include hypnosis, biofeedback, relaxation exercises and massage. For more information on some of these procedures, see Chapter 43, "Complementary and Alternative Medicine."

Childhood Cancer

Approximately 8,600 new cases of childhood cancer are diagnosed each year in the United States, making cancer a rare condition among children. In addition, modern treatment now makes prolonged survival and recovery not only possible but likely with many childhood cancers — more than 70 percent of all children with cancer in America now survive.

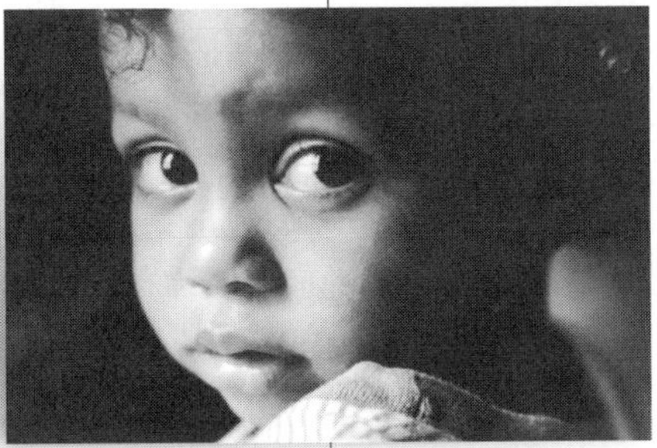

Still, cancer remains responsible for more deaths than any other disease in school-age and preschool children. Only accidents claim more lives in these age groups.

The most common childhood cancer is leukemia. It accounts for about one-third of childhood cancers. With new treatments the outlook for children with this disease has brightened considerably. The other major cancer, responsible for approximately 20 percent of childhood cancers, is a malignant brain tumor. Less common cancers that occur in children include a tumor of the kidney (Wilms' tumor), a nervous system cancer (neuroblastoma), cancer of the eye (retinoblastoma) and bone cancer (osteosarcoma). The causes of these cancers remain largely unknown.

It's important to choose carefully when deciding where to have your child treated for cancer. A team of specialists in childhood cancer is usually able to deliver the best treatment. This team includes pediatricians, pediatric surgeons and pediatric nurses.

With the help of your child's doctor, seek out a medical center where the staff is experienced in providing the latest advances in treatment. The center and its staff should also offer emotional support for the entire family.

Dealing with your child's cancer

Having a child with cancer is very stressful for even the strongest of families. The best approach is to be honest with your child about his or her disease and to be supportive. Both you and your child's health care team should prepare your child thoroughly for the experiences involved in his or her treatment. Reassure your child that everybody is trying to make him or her better. Ask doctors and nurses to help answer your child's questions.

The goal of pediatric cancer treatment is not only to get rid of the cancer but also to help your child continue to function at an age-appropriate level — developmentally, psychologically and emotionally.

Although it's important to support and console your child, it's also critical to maintain as much normalcy as possible in his or her life. Keeping schedules, rules, family activities and previous expectations in place conveys a message that you trust your child's ability to cope with this difficulty. It also suggests that, as a parent, you'll help him or her prepare for a long future.

While your child is receiving cancer treatment, communicate closely with school personnel to establish behavioral and academic expectations that are as realistic as possible. Most schools are able to provide individualized instruction if required during periods of intense treatment. In addition, they often have school re-entry programs for children who have been out for a period of time.

In addition to caring for your sick child, it's also important to take care of yourself and one another. Siblings can be very supportive of their ill brother or sister but must know that their own special place in the family is secure.

Economic stress isn't unusual for families with a seriously ill child. Financial burdens not only include the cost of treatment but also may involve the costs of travel, lodging and child care. Incomes also may be affected by disrupted work schedules.

Many pediatric cancer centers are staffed with child life specialists, mental health professionals, social workers and clergy who are trained to help families with difficult emotions and situations. In spite of the difficulties, many families develop closer, more supportive and trusting relationships as a result.

Living with Cancer

A diagnosis of cancer can change your life. The disease can dominate your thoughts and actions and produce long-lasting effects on your daily routine, your relationships with others and your view of life.

But these effects don't have to be negative. Armed with the advice of health professionals and the insights of others who have dealt with cancer, you can learn to cope with cancer's impact. Life with and after cancer not only is possible but also can be lived fully.

Pursuing rehabilitation

Rehabilitation is an important component of cancer treatment. Whatever form your rehabilitation happens to take, the goal is always the same — to restore your life to as normal as possible.

This might mean developing an exercise program, learning to use a prosthesis after an amputation or even retraining for a job. Such wide-ranging tasks and goals usually call for a team approach.

Depending on your needs, you may work with a number of health care professionals, including physical therapists, occupational therapists and social workers. The initial stage of the rehabilitation may begin in a hospital, or all of the rehabilitation may be offered in your home or in an outpatient center.

Don't be discouraged if at first you find the process difficult and the results disappointing. Progress may come slowly, and the effort may be intense. If you have problems, don't hesitate to discuss them with your therapist, physiatrist — a physician whose specialization includes rehabilitation — or another doctor.

Preparing for follow-up visits

Going in for checkups is one thing that many people with cancer fear. Several days before each visit, you may start worrying, afraid that your doctor will find something terribly wrong. And once you get to the doctor's office, the sights, sounds and smells may bring back memories you'd prefer to forget.

This is natural. But try to balance these negative associations with positive ones. Keep in mind that the medical treatment you have received, and continue to receive, is good. It's helping you stay alive.

Asking plenty of questions during your first few visits also can help to make later visits less worrisome. Before a follow-up checkup, write down any questions that have come up and bring them with you so that you can ask your doctor for answers and advice.

The National Cancer Institute has made a list of some questions you may want to ask your doctor:

- How often will I need a checkup?
- What will my checkups consist of, and will they always be the same?
- What are some signs or symptoms that the cancer has returned or progressed?
- How likely are these signs or symptoms to occur?
- What changes might I notice that are OK, that aren't danger signs?
- Should I change my diet?
- Do I need to alter my daily routine?
- If I experience pain, what should I do?
- What's the best way for me to get in touch with you if I have questions or concerns?
- Is there someone else I can talk to if you aren't available?

Dealing with cancer's emotional toll

There is no right way to act or feel if you have cancer. The disease generally produces a roller coaster of emotions in each individual. What's important is that you recognize and accept your actions and emotions and find healthful ways to deal with them.

Here are some common emotions that accompany cancer:

Disbelief

When you learn that you have cancer, shock may be one of the first feelings you experience. You can't believe this is happening. You might find yourself walking around in a dream-like state for a period of time, unable to concentrate or make decisions.

Fear

Next may come the consuming fear that often accompanies acute distress. All you can think about is the cancer. You start to imagine all of the terrible things cancer might do to you. It could kill you. It could force you to live the rest of your life in pain, with no dignity and no ability to take care of yourself. It could prevent you from doing things you enjoy.

Anger
Once the reality begins to sink in that you have cancer, you may find yourself suddenly engulfed with anger over the unfairness of it all. You might even take out some of that anger on people who are trying to help you — your family, your doctor, your friends, your co-workers — because they're the most available.

It's certainly understandable for you to be angry. But if you allow your anger to control you, it can become as disruptive to your life as the cancer itself.

Anxiety
If you experience side effects from your treatment, such as hair loss or skin reactions, you may feel embarrassed, worry what others will think and lose your self-confidence. This can make you anxious. You might also withdraw from others and from social and business gatherings. These feelings can be especially difficult if you've always been a self-confident person.

Cancer Coping Strategies

You may not be able to get rid of distressing feelings, but you can find positive ways to deal with them so that they don't take over your life. The following strategies can help you cope with the difficulties of cancer:

Be prepared
Ask your doctor questions and read about your specific type of cancer and its potential side effects. The fewer the surprises, the more quickly you'll adapt.

Maintain a routine
Don't let the cancer or side effects of treatment dominate your day. Try to follow at least some of the routine and lifestyle you had before learning of your cancer. Go back to work, take a trip, visit your children or grandchildren. You need activities that give you a sense of purpose, fulfillment and meaning. But realize that initially you may have some limitations. Start slowly and gradually build up your level of endurance.

Set reasonable goals
Having goals helps you feel in control and can give you a sense of purpose. But don't choose goals you can't possibly reach. You may not be able to work a 40-hour week, for example, but you may be able to work at least half time. In fact, many people find that continuing to work can be helpful.

Get plenty of exercise
Exercise helps fight depression and is a good way to relieve tension and aggression.

Try not to wallow in sad feelings
Seek diversions and plan at least two or three enjoyable experiences a week. These might include a new hobby, playing golf or going to a movie. Make it something you enjoy and look forward to.

Enjoy some humor and laughter
Find ways to help lighten your day with laughter, whether by spending time with someone who makes you laugh or watching a funny movie. Laughter helps distract your attention from your health problems. It's also a kind of analgesic — that is, it promotes the release of chemicals that help fight pain and reduce depression.

Take time for yourself
Eating well, relaxing and getting enough rest can help combat the stress and fatigue of cancer. Plan ahead for the down times, when you may need to rest more or limit what you do.

Look for ways to compensate
If you have trouble eating, for example, reserve mealtimes for when you're at home and plan outings that don't revolve around food. If you frequently need to use the bathroom, sit in the back of the movie theater or the meeting room so that you'll feel less conspicuous if you need to leave.

Open up to a friend, family member or counselor
Sometimes it helps to talk with someone about your feelings and fears. Your mind and body aren't separate. The better you feel emotionally, the better able you are to physically cope with your illness.

Don't avoid sexual contact
People with cancer sometimes feel as if they're no longer adequate as sexual beings. Don't fall for this feeling. You can express your sexuality in many ways. Touching, holding, hugging and caressing may become far more important to you and your partner. In fact, the closeness you develop through these actions can produce greater sexual intimacy than you've ever had before.

Look for the positive
Cancer doesn't have to be all negative. Good can come out of it. Confrontation with cancer may lead you to grow emotionally and spiritually, to identify what really matters to you, to settle long-standing disputes and to spend more time with people who are important to you.

Emptiness
If you've had surgery to remove part of your body, you may feel a void that's hard to describe. Women may feel less feminine after a hysterectomy or breast removal. Men may feel like less of a man following prostate removal.

Depression
Depression is common among people with cancer. You may grow deeply sad and discouraged over what has happened. You may become pessimistic about your future. Such feelings may last only a short time, or they may linger for weeks or months.

Depression that lingers can interfere with your ability to manage your life. It can precipitate a downward spiral that makes you more and more miserable. Because you're depressed you don't feel motivated to cope with your daily problems. When the problems become worse, so does your depression. To find out the common warning signs of depression, see page 1221.

If you think you may be depressed, talk to your doctor or a therapist. With treatment, which may involve counseling or taking antidepressant medications or both, the majority of people affected by depression show significant signs of improvement.

Regaining your strength

Fatigue is a common side effect of cancer and treatment. Your body is dealing with a number of physical challenges, and the effort involved in coping with them is often exhausting and stressful. Fatigue can be a frustrating obstacle when you're struggling to keep a normal schedule and maintain a good quality of life.

To help reduce fatigue, consider taking the following steps:

Tell your doctor
Don't hide or ignore your fatigue. Tell your doctor about it because it may have a treatable physical cause, such as anemia.

Rest
Don't fight fatigue. If you need short naps during the day, take them.

Go easy on yourself
Take one day at a time and try not to overdo it. But don't sit back and do nothing, either. Inactivity also produces fatigue.

Delegate
You may need to ask others to do tasks that traditionally you've done, such as cutting the grass or shoveling snow.

Practice relaxation techniques
Wrestling with heavy emotions, such as anxiety and fear, can contribute to your fatigue. Talk with your doctor, nurse or counselor about stress reduction techniques and which ones might work best for you.

Try to get a good night's sleep
Establishing a nightly relaxation routine, such as reading a book or taking a warm bath, may make it easier to fall asleep. Avoiding caffeine, getting some exercise during the day and keeping your bedroom at a comfortable temperature also can be helpful sleep inducers.

Eating better to feel better

A nutritious diet provides the fuel that lets your body maintain its strength and operate at its best. That's why a nutritious diet is especially important if you have cancer. If you don't eat enough food or the right kinds of food, your body resorts to using stored nutrients. This weakens your natural defenses against infection, a major threat for people with cancer. In addition, the better you eat, the more able you may be to handle treatment, such as radiation therapy, which in turn improves your chances of destroying the cancer.

When you have cancer, what you should eat and how often you should eat may be different from when you're healthy. Normally, nutrition recommendations stress eating plenty of fruits, vegetables and grains and cutting back on fat, sugar and salt. But if you're having difficulty maintaining your weight because of your cancer or your cancer treatment, proper nutrition involves eating more high-calorie foods to promote strength and energy, and eating more foods that are high in protein. Protein helps repair body tissues.

The following steps can help to add more calories and protein to your diet:

- *Emphasize dairy products.* Milk, cream, cheese and cooked eggs are good sources of calories and protein.
- *Eat plenty of peanut butter.* Spread it on toast, fruit slices, crackers or celery. Peanut butter is high in calories and protein.
- *Choose breaded or fried meat.* Beef, poultry and fish prepared this way contain more calories. Meat is also a good source of protein.
- *Add high-calorie toppings.* Top your hot cereal with brown sugar, honey or cream. Top your pie, cake, pudding and gelatin with ice cream or whipping cream. Top fruit with sugar or cream.
- *Drink high-calorie beverages.* Good choices include milk, fruit juice, lemonade, fruit-flavored drinks, malts, floats, soft drinks, cocoa and eggnog. Water, black coffee and tea have no calories.
- *Stock up on nutritional drinks.* These products, available as a liquid or powder, are sold under brand names such as Ensure, Sustacal, Boost and Carnation Instant Breakfast. The drinks are high in both calories and protein, and they contain extra vitamins and minerals.

If you don't feel like eating, nutritional drinks can be used as snacks or as meal substitutes. Some people find nutritional products difficult to drink because they don't care for their flavor or texture. If this is true for you, you may want to try this recipe: Combine one can of a liquid drink with a piece of fruit or scoop of ice cream or both. Blend the mixture in a blender and serve it over ice. If you're not certain whether you could benefit from a nutritional drink, talk with your doctor or a registered dietitian.

Stimulating your appetite

Loss of appetite is common when you're ill or recovering from an illness. The nausea, vomiting, depression and fatigue that often accompany cancer can make food unappealing. Try the following suggestions to improve your diet and stimulate your appetite:

- *Eat whenever you're hungry.* If your appetite and taste buds seem in disarray, eating smaller meals throughout the day may work better for you than trying to eat three big meals. Taking just a few bites of the right food or a few sips of a nutritious drink every hour or so can help a lot.
- *Prepare and freeze meals ahead of time.* This way you won't have to cook when you don't feel like it.
- *Choose foods that look and smell good.* Cancer treatment can alter your sense of taste and smell. If red meat is unappetizing, try other sources of protein: chicken, fish or dairy products. Most people with cancer find that soups and soft foods, such as pasta or mashed potatoes, are the easiest to eat and digest. If your favorite foods suddenly don't look appetizing anymore, don't force yourself to eat them.
- *Enhance the flavor.* Food may taste bland to you. Try small amounts of seasoning or marinate meat and vegetables with a flavorful preparation.
- *Drink less with meals.* Although you should aim to drink 6 to 8 cups of fluids daily, limit beverages at mealtimes because they can make you feel full and keep you from eating adequate amounts of food. Drink beverages after your meal.
- *Change the atmosphere.* Eating in a different setting may stimulate your appetite. Invite a friend to join you, play music, light some candles or watch a video or TV program.

If you're still having trouble eating a few weeks after your treatment, contact your doctor. He or she may want you to talk with a registered dietitian. Some dietitians specialize in assisting people with cancer and can help devise a customized eating plan that meets your individual needs.

Getting back to work

Work is an important part of life, providing personal fulfillment, income or enjoyment. If you have cancer, work can also be rehabilitative and uplifting, especially if you're treated as a valuable team member. Many people with cancer find getting back to work helps them regain a sense of normality and control over their lives.

If you're an employee, having cancer doesn't mean that your career is ruined or that you'll never again pull your weight at work. In

Telling Your Children You Have Cancer

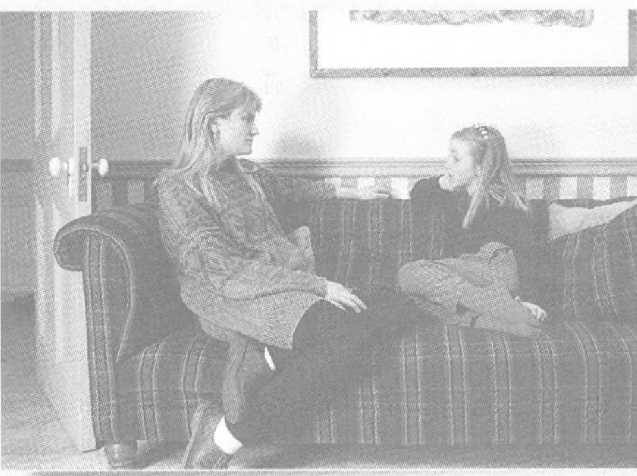

If you've received a diagnosis of cancer and have children, the prospect of telling them about your cancer can be overwhelming. It helps to come to grips with the diagnosis yourself before communicating it to them. But at some point, your children must be told. Remember too, that children, particularly younger children, don't understand cancer in the same way that adults do, so often they don't experience the shock, anxiety or fear that parents expect them to. Here are some suggestions as to how you might explain your cancer:

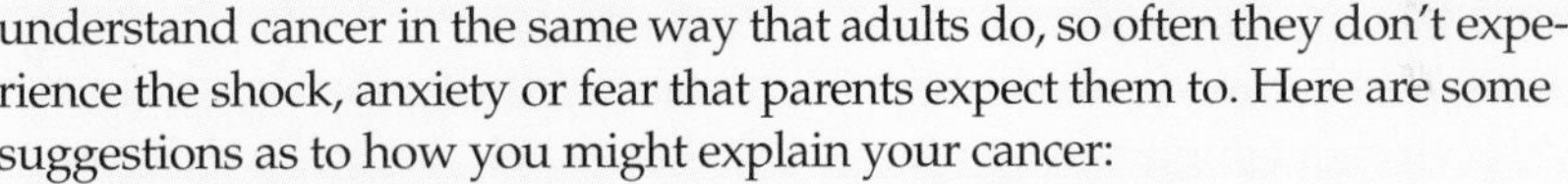

- Be honest with your children about your diagnosis, what you're going through and what they can expect at each of the various stages of your disease and treatment.
- Encourage your children to ask questions, share their feelings and help out around the home or with your care.
- Reassure your children that nothing they did or thought caused your cancer, that it's not contagious and that they'll continue to be loved and cared for no matter what happens to you.
- Enable your children to carry on as normal a schedule as possible — and assure them that it's OK to do so.
- Alert your children's teachers, counselors and child-care providers of your situation.
- If you need it, ask for help from doctors, nurses, social workers, counselors, support groups, psychologists and psychiatrists.
- Continue to discipline your children as you normally would.
- Give answers that are truthful yet hopeful. Children can sense when something is wrong and might imagine the worst.
- Don't put too much responsibility on your children. It's reasonable for them to help, but they shouldn't become another adult in the home.
- If possible, avoid sending your children away to a friend or relative. Being sent away increases children's feelings of abandonment.

fact, 8 of 10 employees with cancer return to their jobs. And surveys show that employees who have had cancer are just as productive as other workers, and no more likely to take sick days.

At first, you may need to make a few adjustments, such as working fewer hours. But eventually you should be able to resume your regular schedule and activities. Before you return to work:

- Talk with your doctor about how much you should work. It's often best to ease back into your work schedule.
- Talk with your supervisor about adjusting your hours or duties when you first return.
- Consider how you'll respond to co-workers who may have questions about your cancer and how you're doing. Practicing what you're going to say ahead of time can make the interchange more comfortable.

Communicating with family and friends

Cancer has a way of stifling communication when you need it the most. Family members may find it difficult to come to grips with your illness, so they aren't able to talk with you about important issues. And well-meaning friends — not knowing what to say or do, and not wanting to upset you — may steer clear of conversations about your health.

Here are some ways you can make it easier for family and friends to give you needed support:

Give it time
You may want to talk about important issues related to your illness before some of your family and friends are ready. Interpret their body language, such as whether they make eye contact. If they aren't ready to talk, give them a little more time to adjust.

In the same way, if some of your loved ones are ready to talk before you are, acknowledge their feelings but say that you're not ready to talk yet.

Not all families are open and sharing. Sometimes it's easier to open up to someone outside your immediate circle of family and friends, such as a counselor or someone else who has experienced cancer.

Reach out to family and friends
Reach out to the people you care about. You may think it should be the other way around. And with some of your closest family and friends, it will be. They'll come to you. But try to remember people you knew who were ill and how hard it was for you to think of what to say or do to help them.

Think of ways to put family and friends at ease. Ask a busy friend what projects he or she has going. Invite a friend who's not a great talker to help you with a chore, such as cleaning out the garage. For friends who have plenty of their own problems, ask how things are going.

Accept help
Don't be afraid to ask for help either. Many times your family and friends are waiting for clues as to how they can help. When they say, "Let me know how I can help," go ahead and tell them. Most family and friends are grateful to have a chance to show you, in tangible ways, that they care.

Joining a support group

Not everyone with cancer needs a support group. Having family and friends may be all of the support you need. But some people find it helpful to have people they can turn to outside of their immediate circles.

In general, support groups fall into two main categories: those led by health care professionals, such as a psychologist or nurse, and those led by group members. Some are more educational and structured and may include discussions on new treatments. Others emphasize emotional support and shared experiences.

In addition, the Internet now offers online virtual support groups in which you can converse with others by way of your computer. But be careful about the reliability of information on therapy or treatment you may find online. Talk with your doctor to make sure it's accurate and, more importantly, not harmful.

If you think that you would like to join a support group, check with your doctor, hospital or community health services. A variety of volunteer support groups exist that can help you during this transition in your life.

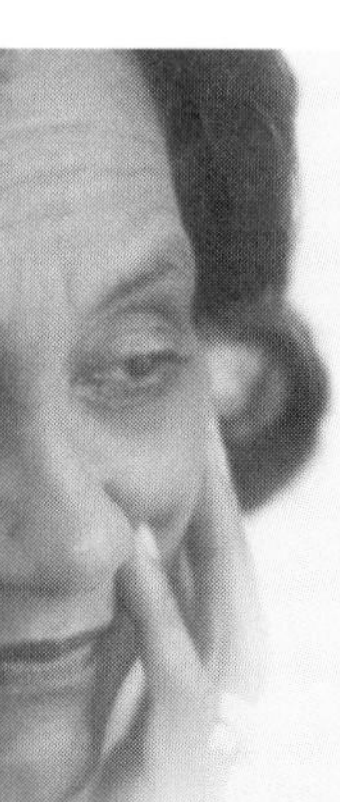

Hospice Care

The word *hospice* comes from the Latin word for "guest." It's the root that forms the words *hospital*, *hospitality* and *hostel*.

In the Middle Ages, a hospice was a way station for travelers. Today *hospice* has another meaning. Hospice is a program that offers a coordinated, interdisciplinary program of care and services for terminally ill people and their families. The program may be in a medical center, the ill person's home or in a separate facility dedicated to hospice care.

Hospice care neither hastens nor postpones death. Rather, hospice programs emphasize quality of life, with the focus on the management of side effects and psychosocial counseling instead of on treatment of the disease.

The goals of hospice programs are to allow people to adequately prepare for death and to live their last days in as much comfort as possible.

For more information on hospice care, see page 317.

Preventing Cancer

Scientists and doctors don't understand many of the reasons why people develop cancer, but there's still a lot that you can do to help decrease your risk of getting it. Smoking causes approximately 30 percent of cancer deaths. Evidence suggests that another third of cancer deaths may be due to dietary factors. If Americans applied to their lives everything known about cancer prevention, cancer rates might be reduced significantly.

Cancer prevention can take the form of a few simple decisions in your everyday life. No matter what your age, it's never too late to set a course that could help you avoid cancer down the road. Here are some strategies to get you started on a healthier lifestyle.

Tobacco use

If you smoke, you likely find it to be an enjoyable habit. Perhaps you smoke to calm your nerves or to curb your appetite. People smoke for a number of reasons. Combine that with the addictive nature of nicotine, and the prospect of quitting becomes fairly unappealing and frequently difficult.

But there's no two ways around it. Not using tobacco, or deciding to stop using it — whether it's cigarettes, chewing tobacco, pipes or cigars — is one of the most important health decisions you can make.

You may have heard it a hundred times, but it's true. Tobacco use can be fatal in the long run. If you smoke cigarettes, you're inhaling air that contains about 43 substances that can cause cells to become cancerous (carcinogens). Tar in cigarette smoke also forms a sticky brown layer on the lining of your lungs and air passageways. This layer traps the carcinogens you inhale when you smoke, enhancing the development of cancerous cells.

Smoking is responsible for 85 percent to 90 percent of all lung cancer cases. Smoking also increases your risk of cancer of the esophagus, larynx, mouth, bladder and kidneys. In addition, tobacco use is linked to emphysema, bronchitis, cardiovascular disease and stroke. Chewing (spit) tobacco isn't harmless, either. Evidence indicates that chewing tobacco increases your risk of oral cancer.

Healthy diet

Your diet is another important risk factor for cancer — second only to smoking — that you can control.

Quitters Do Win

Tobacco users who quit, regardless of their age, live longer than those who continue to use tobacco. By quitting, you can reduce your chances of getting lung cancer by more than half, as well as reduce your risk of other types of cancers and diseases.

A number of aids are available to help you break nicotine's grip. They include the following products and medications:

Nicotine patch
Now available over-the-counter, the nicotine patch is placed on your skin, where it gradually releases nicotine into your body. This helps battle nicotine addiction by reducing nicotine cravings when you cut back or stop smoking. Eventually you taper off using the patch.

Nicotine gum
You can also buy nicotine gum over-the-counter. When you chew the gum, it releases nicotine into your body. The lining of your mouth absorbs the nicotine. After you get the initial burst of effect from the nicotine, you can "park" the gum alongside your cheek until you have another nicotine craving.

Nicotine nasal spray
Your nose is yet another way to get nicotine into your body. A nicotine nasal spray, available by prescription, may get nicotine into your body faster than nicotine gum or patches because it's absorbed by the lining of your nose.

Nicotine inhaler
A nicotine inhaler, available by prescription, looks like a plastic cigarette. One end has a plastic tip like that used on some cigars. When you put this tip in your mouth and inhale as if you were puffing on a cigarette, the inhaler releases nicotine vapor into your mouth, where it's absorbed.

Non-nicotine medication
Bupropion (Zyban) is an antidepressant medication that has been proved to help people combat nicotine addiction. It's the first non-nicotine medication approved by the Food and Drug Administration as a smoking cessation aid. It's available only by prescription.

You can try to quit on your own, or you can join a stop smoking program or support group. Your doctor can advise you on the effective use of nicotine replacement products or a smoking cessation program. Programs are often available through hospitals and clinics or your local public health department. National health organizations such as the American Cancer Society and the American Lung Association are excellent sources of information and can offer tips and strategies to help you stop.

Reducing Your Risks

Here's how your health improves after stopping smoking:

Immediately	The air around you is no longer dangerous to children and other adults.
20 minutes	Your blood pressure drops to normal. Your pulse rate drops to normal. The temperature in your hands and feet increases to normal.
8 hours	The carbon monoxide level in your blood drops to normal. The oxygen level in your blood increases to normal.
24 hours	Your chance of having a heart attack decreases.
48 hours	Your senses of smell and taste improve.
2 to 12 weeks	Your circulation improves. Your breathing improves. Your walking becomes easier.
1 to 9 months	Your coughing and sinus congestion decrease. Your shortness of breath decreases. Your overall energy increases. The ability of your lungs to self-clean and reduce infection increases.
1 year	If you're a man, your risk of premature heart disease is half that of a male smoker.
5 years	Your risk of stroke is comparable to that of a nonsmoker.
10 years	Your life expectancy is comparable to that of a nonsmoker. Your risk of dying of lung cancer is about half that of a smoker. Your risk of cancers of the mouth, throat, esophagus, bladder, kidney and pancreas decreases.
15 years	All other factors being equal, your risk of heart disease is comparable to that of a nonsmoker.
Before age 50	Your risk of dying in the next 15 years has decreased by 50 percent compared with that of continuing smokers.

Although making healthy food selections can't guarantee you won't get cancer, it can help reduce your risk. The American Cancer Society recommends the following nutritional guidelines:

Eat foods from plant sources
Whether it's cauliflower or cranberries, eating more fruits and vegetables may play a role in preventing a variety of cancers. The same is true of foods made from whole grains, such as breads and cereals.

Plant foods contain more than 100 vitamins, minerals, fibers and other beneficial substances. Fruits, vegetables and whole grains are excellent sources of fiber, which may help reduce your risk of colorectal cancer. Green and dark yellow vegetables, soybean products and vegetables such as broccoli and cauliflower may play a role in reducing your risk of cancer of the colon, rectum and stomach.

Most Americans get far less plant foods than they should. To help reduce your risk of cancer, try to eat five or more servings of fruits and vegetables and 6 to 11 servings of grains each day.

PREVENTION TIP

There are no miracle foods for cancer prevention. Eat as though your diet were an investment. Just as you would diversify your portfolio, diversify your diet. Eating a variety of foods provides a variety of nutrients that promote health.

Question and Answer

Can eating more soy foods reduce my risk of cancer?

Some studies suggest that substances in soy may cause changes at the cellular level that hinder cancer cell development and growth. In addition, some kinds of cancer occur far less often in cultures where soy is a food staple, such as many of those in Asia. Although soy hasn't been proved to help prevent cancer, it's an excellent source of protein and a good alternative to meat in your diet.

Choose fewer high-fat foods
Studies suggest that people with high-fat diets that include a lot of high-fat meats are at increased risk of cancer of the prostate, colon, rectum, uterus and breast. Less than 30 percent of the calories you consume each day should come from fat. Pay attention to food labels. They typically list how many fat grams you're getting in a serving. Based on an average 2,000-calories-a-day diet, you want to limit fat to 65 grams or less a day.

Physical activity and weight

Regular physical activity plays a key role in helping you stay healthy and control your weight. When you're at a healthy weight, you lower your risk of many kinds of cancer.

Studies suggest that obesity is a risk factor for cancer of the prostate, colon, rectum, uterus and, in postmenopausal women, the breast. What is a healthy weight for you? See Chapter 3, "Controlling Your Weight."

Despite the benefits of exercise, many people avoid it. About 70 percent of older adults — the age group with the highest risk of cancer — are inactive.

One reason may be that many people believe that exercise must be strenuous, even painful, to be beneficial. The truth is, the frequency and duration of physical activity are more important than the activity's intensity.

Experts recommend that you get 30 minutes or more of physical activity most days of the week. That may sound daunting, but those 30 minutes can include activities such as a brisk walk, raking the yard and ballroom dancing.

Alcohol use

Your risk of cancer increases with the amount of alcohol you consume and the length of time you've been consuming alcohol on a regular basis. Even a moderate amount of alcohol — two drinks a day if you're a man, one drink a day if you're a woman — may increase your cancer risk.

This is particularly true if you smoke. Using both alcohol and tobacco significantly increases your risk of cancer of the mouth, esophagus and larynx. Some studies also suggest that alcohol use may put you at greater risk of developing breast cancer.

Skin protection

Skin cancer is one of the most common forms of cancer, and one of the most preventable. Although repeated exposure to X-rays or contact with certain chemicals can play a role in this disease, sun exposure is by far the most common cause of skin cancer.

Approximately 90 percent of skin cancer occurs on parts of the body that usually aren't covered with clothing — your face, hands, forearms and ears.

Cancer Warning Signs

The American Cancer Society recommends that you see a doctor as soon as possible if you have any of these seven warning signs:

- Unexplained changes in bowel or bladder habits
- A sore that doesn't heal
- Unusual bleeding or discharge
- Thickening or a lump in a breast or elsewhere in your body
- Indigestion or difficulty swallowing
- An obvious change in a wart or mole
- A nagging cough or hoarseness

PREVENTION TIP

Many skin cancers are curable if detected early. But your best bet is to prevent it in the first place. That means adopting sun-sensible habits:

- Avoid peak radiation hours. The sun's ultraviolet (UV) radiation is at its peak between the hours of 10 a.m. and 3 p.m. Try to minimize or avoid being outside during that time.
- Stay in the shade. If you must go outside, minimize your sun exposure by staying in the shade.
- Wear clothing that protects you from the sun's rays. A broad-brimmed hat can protect your face and neck.
- Choose the right sun protection. Make sure your sunscreen has a sun protection factor (SPF) of at least 15 and that it's a broad-spectrum sunscreen, which means it blocks both UVA and UVB radiation — two types of ultraviolet light that can damage your skin. If you'll be swimming, make sure your sunscreen is waterproof. To have the best effect, sunscreens need to be applied 30 minutes before you go outside. Use generous amounts and reapply it every 90 minutes.
- Protect your children from sunburns. Repeated sunburns in childhood is the biggest risk factor in the development of melanoma later in life.
- Avoid reflective surfaces. Snow and water can reflect up to 85 percent of the sun's damaging rays.
- Don't use indoor tanning beds or sunlamps. They can be just as damaging as the sun.

Cancer signals

Knowing your risk of cancer and being aware of changes in your body can help you prevent cancer or help your doctor detect it early, increasing your chances of a full recovery.

One way to assess your cancer risk is to find out if your family has a history of cancer. If so, find out what type of cancer and at what age the person who had it received a diagnosis. In general, the more frequent and earlier that cancer occurs in your relatives, the more likely you're at risk. But just because someone in your family had cancer doesn't mean you'll get it.

If you see a pattern of cancer that occurred at an early age, you may wish to schedule a visit with your doctor. He or she can help you decide your next step, which may include seeing a medical geneticist. Genetic testing can help determine if you may have inherited an increased risk of some types of cancer. For more information on genetic testing, see Chapter 18, "Genetics and Disease."

You also need to stay alert to changes in your body that could signal cancer. If you notice warning signs, talk to your doctor.

Regular checkups

You and your doctor can discuss which cancer screening tests are best for you, based on your age, occupation, lifestyle, family history and personal preferences.

Between doctor visits, examine yourself at home for changes that may signal some kinds of cancer, including cancers of the breast, skin and testicles. If you aren't familiar with when and how to do such self-exams, ask your doctor during your next visit. If you already perform self-exams, your doctor can help you determine if you're doing them correctly. ■

CHAPTER 20 PART V

Infectious Diseases

Keeping infectious microorganisms out of your body and destroying any that get in are the missions of your immune system.

Less than 30 years ago, scientists had only fragments of information about how the variety of cells that make up your immune system interact to help protect you against disease. But through research advances, scientists now believe that more than 100 million types of immune cells exist. For each virus or bacterium, there seems to be an immune cell that's specifically designed to hunt it down and destroy it.

However, viruses and bacteria are cunning adversaries, constantly seeking new ways to breach your immune system's defenses. In addition, some antibiotics long used to treat infections are becoming less effective.

Understanding Your Immune System

Your immune system is a complex array of organs, cells and molecules distributed throughout your body. Each part of the system contributes to the growth, development or activation of lymphocytes, sophisticated white blood cells that play a major role in your body's immune response.

White blood cells originate in bone marrow. Some then migrate to your thymus gland, where they develop into specialized types of immune cells. Some of these cells from bone marrow and the thymus gather in lymph nodes and other organs involved in immunity, including your spleen, tonsils, adenoids, appendix and small intestine. Other white blood cells circulate throughout your blood and lymphatic vessels. Lymphatic vessels transport lymph, a colorless fluid that can carry microorganisms and dead cells from distant infections into lymph nodes, where they're eliminated. Lymph vessels also transport white blood cells to sites of infection.

Immune army 'soldier' cells

The key to your immune response is a remarkable arsenal of white blood cells. The main "soldiers" include B cells, T cells, phagocytes and chemical killers.

B cells and T cells

B cells and T cells are white blood cells that recognize and then coordinate the attack against foreign invaders, also known as antigens.

Your Immune Armament

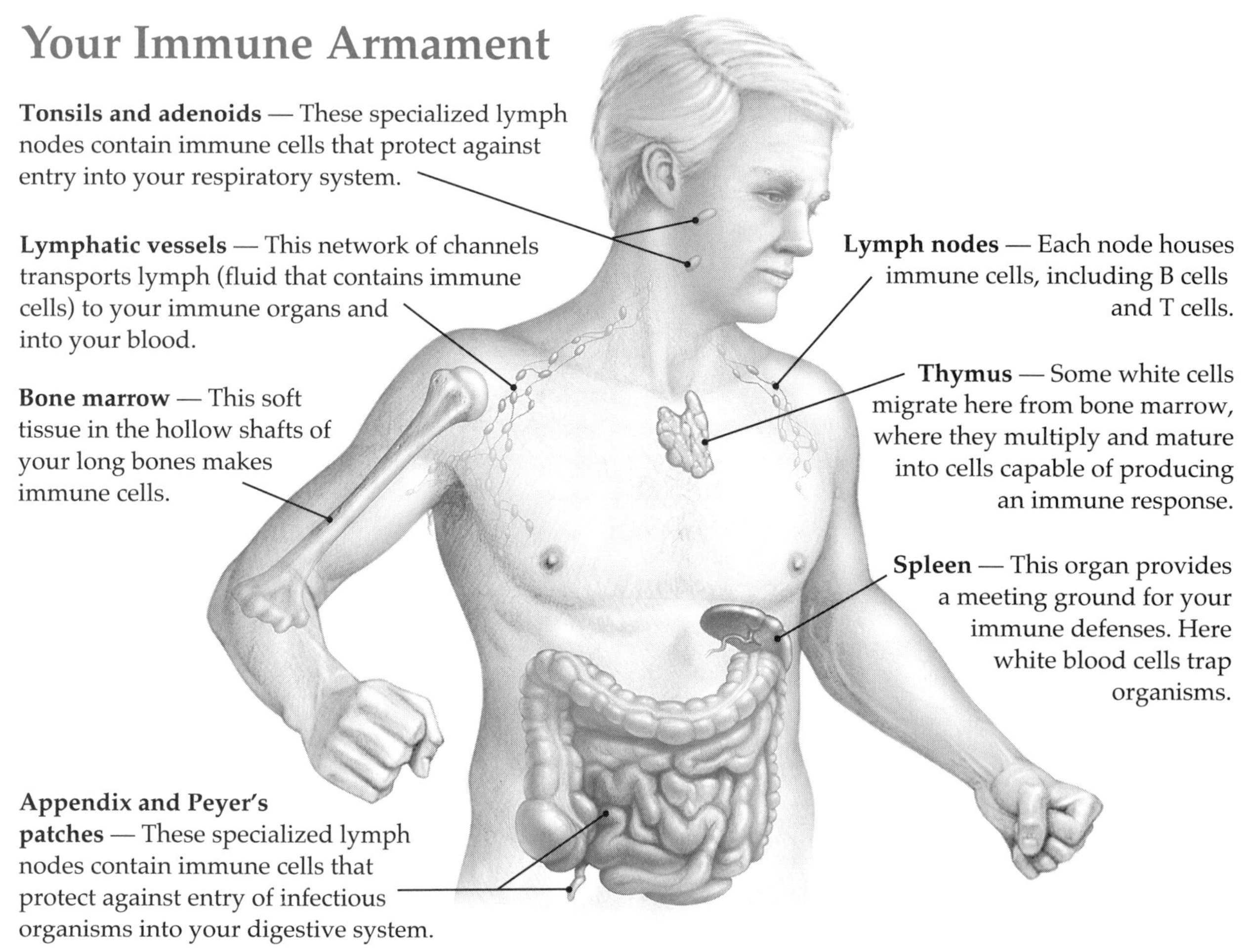

B cells work chiefly by producing antibodies, substances that attach themselves to and destroy antigens. Each antibody is designed to attack a specific antigen. T cells coordinate immune defenses and kill organisms in cells on contact. And they secrete potent chemicals, called lymphokines, which are particularly good at attacking cancerous cells or cells infected by viruses.

Phagocytes

Phagocytes are another type of white blood cell. The main function of these "eater" cells is to gobble up anything unwanted, from a speck of dust or pollen to a virus. The macrophage is a specific type of phagocyte that helps initiate the immune response.

Chemical killers

Some white blood cells are chemical killers called neutrophils, eosinophils and basophils. These cells also ingest unwanted microorganisms and release powerful chemicals that help destroy such microorganisms.

Lines of defense

As antigens attempt to invade your body, they're confronted by increasingly sophisticated layers of protective defenses.

Physical barriers

Your skin effectively shields your body from invaders, whether they're harmful or not. Your respiratory system also helps keep out microorganisms. Defenses include trapping irritants in nasal hairs and mucus, carrying the mucus upward and outward on tiny hair-like projections lining the respiratory tract (cilia), coughing and sneezing.

Your skin and the mucous membranes lining your respiratory and gastrointestinal tracts also contain macrophages and antibodies. Fluids such as saliva, sweat and tears contain destructive enzymes. Stomach acids also play a role, killing most microorganisms ingested in food or water.

General defenses

Invaders that slip through physical barriers are met by scavenger cells circulating in your blood and lymphatic vessels. One general defense mechanism is the inflammatory response. It halts disease-causing microorganisms early in their invasion and confines them to a localized area. Immune cells cause small blood vessels near the invasion site to widen (dilate), causing redness and warmth. Swelling occurs when immune cells cause blood vessels to leak fluid into surrounding tissue. Nearby lymph nodes then trap the microorganisms and trigger production of more immune cells that kill the organisms and limit the infection.

Complement defenses

Complement defenses involve a complex series of circulating proteins that complement the work of antibodies. When a complement protein comes in contact with an invading organism, each component of the complement system is activated. The result is a protein complex that attaches to the organism's surface and destroys it by puncturing its cell membrane.

Antibody defenses

Unwanted microorganisms that pass through the front-line defenses confront even more sophisticated defenses. As soon as they identify an antigen, B cells produce antibodies that attach themselves to the antigen, neutralizing it or rendering it harmless. Antibodies are specific: Each is effective against only the antigen that led to its creation.

Cellular defenses

T cells concentrate on trickier assignments, such as finding microorganisms hidden within cells. For help in finding the foe, macrophages act as undercover agents, moving among cells, checking for foreign substances.

Building resistance

When you're born, your immune system is relatively weak. It becomes stronger as you mature and are exposed to infectious agents and receive vaccinations. This is known as post-exposure immunity.

Each time you're exposed to a foreign invader, your immune system creates T and B memory cells specific to the invading organism. After you recover, your immune system stores a few of the memory cells. The next time you come into contact with that same type of organism, the memory cells rapidly multiply to stop the infection.

Vaccines work in a similar manner. When you're vaccinated, a killed or weakened virus or bacterium is injected into your body. Although the injected organism isn't strong enough to make you sick, it still stimulates an immune response. Memory cells are formed, providing immunity against the disease for years or even a lifetime.

The Enemy

Substances that can invade your body live everywhere — in the air, on food and plants, on and in animals, in the soil and water and on virtually every other surface. They range from microscopic organisms to larger parasites. The vast majority of these organisms don't produce disease because they're kept under control by your immune system. But if that system becomes weakened or you encounter an organism to which you haven't built up resistance, illness results. Many types of organisms cause infectious disease.

Bacteria

Bacteria are one-cell organisms that are visible only under a microscope. They appear as short rods (bacilli) or round cells (cocci), are self-sufficient and multiply by subdivision.

When infectious bacteria gain entry to your body, they increase in number and potentially produce powerful chemicals, called toxins, that damage specific cells in the tissue they've invaded, causing you to become ill.

A few of the more common groups of disease-causing bacteria include staphylococcus, escherichia (the principal species of which is the well-known *E. coli*), streptococcus, chlamydia, haemophilus, gonococcus and rickettsia.

Not all bacteria are harmful. Some bacteria that reside in the body — such as in the mouth and intestinal tract — are actually of benefit.

Infectious Agents

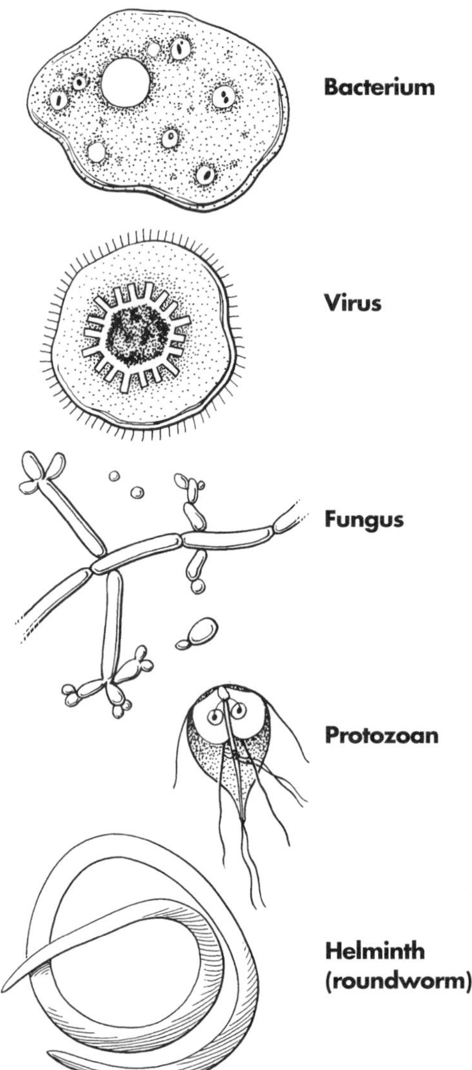

Viruses

In its simplest form, a virus is a capsule that contains genetic material. But it isn't able to reproduce on its own. When a virus invades your body, it enters some of your cells and takes them over, instructing these host cells to manufacture the parts it needs to multiply. In the process, the host cells are eventually destroyed. Polio, AIDS and the common cold are viral illnesses.

Fungi

Molds, yeasts and mushrooms all are types of fungi. Obviously, mushrooms aren't infectious, but certain yeasts and molds can be. These single-cell organisms are slightly larger than bacteria. Candida is one example of a yeast that causes infection. It can produce thrush — an infection of the mouth and throat — in infants, in people taking antibiotics and in people with impaired immunity. It's also responsible for most types of infection-induced diaper rash.

Protozoa

Protozoa are single-cell organisms that can live within you as a parasite. Many protozoa reside in the intestinal tract and are harmless. Others may cause disease. Often, these organisms spend part of their life cycle outside of humans or other hosts, living in food, soil, water or insects. The diseases malaria and giardiasis are caused by protozoan parasites.

Helminths

Helminths are among the larger parasites. The word *helminth* comes from the Greek for "worm." If this parasite or its eggs enter your body, they take up residence in your intestinal tract, lungs, liver, skin or brain, where they live off the nutrients in your body. The most common helminths are tapeworms and roundworms.

Treating Infections

Medication is available to fight many of the infections that your immune system may not be equipped to handle. Most bacterial infections can be treated with antibiotics, substances produced by microorganisms that destroy other bacteria. Some antibiotics are produced from synthetic antibacterial agents.

Unfortunately, antibiotics have no effect on viruses. A few medications have been developed that help to control viral infections, but these drugs usually don't cure the infections. However, the development of vaccines that can prevent certain viral infections has led to the eradication of a number of deadly diseases, including smallpox and polio. Some vaccines are also effective against bacterial infections, such as tetanus and diphtheria.

Parasitic infestations caused by protozoa and helminths often can be successfully treated with appropriate medications. Malaria, a protozoan infestation, may be prevented through regular intake of certain drugs. Antifungal medications exist to treat infections such as athlete's foot, jock itch and ringworm.

Antibiotics

Before penicillin was discovered, very few medications were available to combat bacterial infections. Now antibiotics are common, and new drugs are continuously being developed.

Specificity
Each antibiotic works against specific types of bacteria. Some destroy only one or two kinds of bacteria. Others affect many. When your doctor first suspects that you have an infectious disease, he or she may take samples of your blood, pus, urine, stool or sputum to grow (culture) the offending organism in a

Antibiotic Resistance

When bacteria are exposed to an antibiotic, they can develop a resistance or tolerance to that antibiotic. This may happen quickly or slowly.

Because of this, some antibiotics have become less useful today than they were in the past. Newer antibiotics are constantly being developed. However, it's likely that they too will become less effective in future years.

To help prevent antibiotic resistance, it's important to take antibiotics only when they're needed. If you take an antibiotic unnecessarily — such as for the common cold, which is caused by a virus and not bacteria — you increase your chances of developing drug-resistant bacteria. Such resistance makes future treatment more difficult.

laboratory. This is done to try to identify the organism and determine how resistant or susceptible that particular strain is to a variety of antibiotics. It usually takes at least 24 hours to get the results of these tests. Therefore, depending on the diagnosis, your doctor may first prescribe an antibiotic that attacks a broad array of bacteria (a broad-spectrum antibiotic) and then, depending on the organism identified by the culture results, change your prescription to a more specific antibiotic.

Topical vs. oral

For certain localized infections, such as of the eye or skin, antibiotics may be applied on the surface (topically) as a solution or ointment. In most cases, though, antibiotics are taken orally or administered intravenously or as an injection into muscle. Antibiotics are given intravenously or intramuscularly if the infection is serious or if the drug isn't properly absorbed when taken orally.

Types

Once absorbed into your bloodstream, the antibiotic circulates rapidly throughout your whole body. It takes only about 1 minute for your heart to circulate all of the blood in your body. However, the antibiotic acts only where it encounters particular bacteria. Depending on the type of antibiotic and the dosage, the medication works either by killing the bacteria or preventing it from multiplying.

Antibiotics such as penicillins and cephalosporins kill bacteria by interfering with their ability to form cell walls. This ultimately causes their death. Most other antibacterial agents, including tetracyclines, sulfonamides, aminoglycosides (gentamicin, streptomycin) and macrolides (erythromycin), interfere with the proteins and chemicals the bacteria need to multiply and survive. This allows your body's immune system to take control of and eliminate the bacteria.

Common Infectious Diseases

A wide range of diseases can challenge your immune system. Some seem to occur rather frequently, others once in a lifetime, if at all.

In the following pages, we discuss several of the most common infectious diseases. Some are also discussed in other chapters, especially those that affect predominantly only one organ or body system. The following list shows you where to find more information on such diseases:

Gastrointestinal infections, see page 866.
Heart infections, see pages 778-785.
Respiratory infections, see page 797.
Skin infections, see page 1188.
Urinary tract infections, see page 940.

Colds

Signs and symptoms

- A watery, runny nose, progressing to nasal congestion
- Sneezing
- Watery eyes
- A sore throat and hoarseness
- Coughing
- Slight fever that may be accompanied by muscle aches and chills
- Headache
- An overall feeling of being unwell

Everyone experiences a cold now and then. In fact, perhaps as many as half of all short-term illnesses are colds or another type of viral respiratory illness, such as croup, pharyngitis, laryngitis or bronchitis.

Colds are most common during childhood. Children usually experience their first cold during their first year of life and are especially susceptible to them until about age 6, when their immunity seems to be established. Adults tend to be less vulnerable to colds, but statistics suggest that on average each person gets three or four colds a year.

Colds are caused by viruses. More than 200 different types or viral strains can produce respiratory illness. These include the rhinoviruses, the group most often associated with the so-called common cold, which primarily affects the nose and throat.

Colds are spread primarily by two routes. The first and most effective route is direct contact with infected secretions. Shaking hands with a person who has been blowing his or her nose or has coughed into his or her hand is a common way of coming in contact with that person's virus. The second route is open sneezing and coughing. These actions spread the virus into the air to be inhaled by others. However, this is a less efficient method of transmission.

Myths and popular wisdom about catching colds abound: If you get wet in a rainstorm or go out with wet hair, you'll surely catch one. If you're exposed to cold air, you'll come down with a cold. Fatigue and lack of sleep can cause colds. However, none of these has been proved in clinical studies to increase your risk of getting a cold.

Colds, though, do have a seasonal pattern. More people have colds during fall, winter and spring than during summer.

Diagnosis

General signs and symptoms of a cold include nasal and head congestion, coughing, sneezing, hoarseness and watery eyes. Because many different viruses cause colds, the symptoms can vary.

Symptoms usually develop within 1 to 2 days after exposure and may be signaled at first by an itching or sore throat, increasing nasal congestion and mild body aches or headache. A watery, runny nose is often the first major sign. After a while the discharge becomes thick and turns yellowish green.

A normally healthy person has no need to see a doctor for a cold. However, if it lasts more than 2 weeks, see your doctor to make sure that a secondary bacterial infection of the lungs, larynx, trachea, sinuses or ear hasn't set in. If you have a history of any such infections, consult your doctor without delay.

How serious is a cold?

Colds are general nuisances that for the most part must just be waited out. Occasionally, a more serious secondary bacterial respiratory infection can follow a cold and require medical treatment.

Treatment

Because a cold is a viral infection, antibiotics aren't beneficial. Antibiotics work primarily on bacterial infections. A cold usually lasts 3 to 4 days, but it may last up to 10 to 14 days. Therefore, treating a cold is largely a matter of patience.

Certain actions may help you feel better if you have a cold. Get plenty of rest. Staying at home helps prevent infecting others. Remain in a warm — not hot — room in which the air is moistened by a humidifier or vaporizer. Drink lots of fluids to loosen the mucus. Adults can take aspirin for aches and pains. Children should use acetaminophen (Tylenol, others) instead.

Zinc lozenges are frequently mentioned as a treatment for colds, but as of yet no conclusive evidence shows that zinc is effective. If you do use zinc, take it within 24 hours of the onset of symptoms for it to be of possible benefit.

Children, women who are pregnant and people with chronic illnesses should avoid zinc until its safety has been proved for them. Zinc lozenges cause nausea in some people.

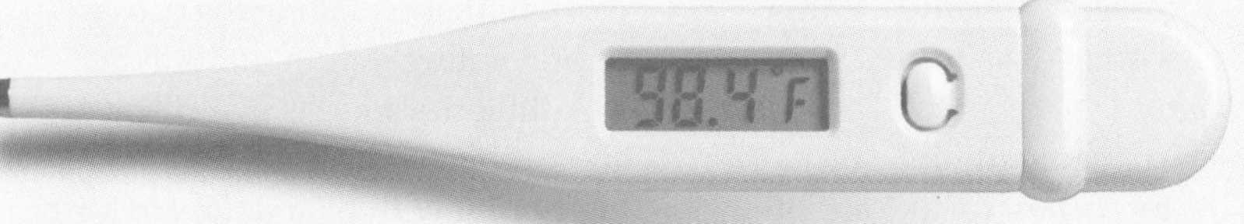

Temperature and Thermometers

Normally, your body temperature shows a definite pattern: low in the morning, gradually increasing during the day and reaching its maximum during late afternoon or evening. Ordinarily, body temperature varies by 1 to 2 degrees Fahrenheit over the course of the day but usually doesn't exceed 99.9 F.

Thus, the mark at 98.6 F on your thermometer is only a general guide. A reading slightly above 98.6 F isn't abnormal and doesn't automatically signal illness. An increased body temperature usually isn't considered dangerous until it goes above 105 F.

What's a fever?

Ordinarily, your body controls its temperature to be within a range of 97 F in the morning to 99 F in the evening. When fever is present, the mechanisms that control body temperature are set a few degrees higher. This increase in temperature is usually triggered by an immune system response to a foreign invader. When the cause of the fever disappears, or if you take medication to reduce the fever, the set-point returns to the normal range.

Taking your temperature

There are several ways to take your temperature. Older oral and rectal thermometers were essentially glass tubes containing a column of mercury. As the mercury expands, in response to the heat from your body, it moves up the column. These types of thermometers, however, pose a risk of mercury contamination and are being replaced by nonmercury thermometers.

Other types of thermometers include electronic thermometers and temperature strip thermometers. These are generally safer, although they may be slightly less accurate than the older, mercury-containing thermometers.

When taking someone's temperature, follow the instructions that came with the thermometer. In adults and children 7 years old or older, you usually take the temperature orally by inserting the bulb end of the thermometer under the tongue and having the person close his or her mouth. After about a minute, you can remove the thermometer and read it. Some newer thermometers may be even faster and generally work by gently inserting the end of the device into the ear canal.

Nonprescription cold remedies, decongestants and cough syrups may help to relieve some of the symptoms, but these products won't cure your cold or make it go away more quickly. Be careful not to use nasal sprays or drops — except for saline drops — in young children.

Gargling with warm, salty water several times a day can help relieve a sore throat. A nonprescription topical anesthetic also may help relieve throat discomfort. Sucking on hard candy helps keep your throat lubricated.

Flu (influenza)

Signs and symptoms

- Fever and chills
- A sore throat
- Coughing
- Muscular aches and pains
- Fatigue and weakness
- Nasal congestion
- A flushed face

Like the common cold, the flu (influenza) is primarily spread among people who are indoors, especially at schools, nursing homes and other places where large numbers of people gather. Outbreaks of influenza usually occur in the winter and early spring.

PREVENTION TIP

The primary way to prevent the flu (influenza) is with a flu shot (influenza vaccine), given each fall. Because influenza can lead to complications, the flu shot is strongly recommended for people at increased risk of acquiring the disease. For more information on the flu shot, see page 13.

The medications amantadine and rimantadine are 75 percent to 90 percent effective in preventing influenza A and may be used in conjunction with a vaccine. Although zanamivir and oseltamivir aren't yet approved for flu prevention, studies suggest that they're effective in this capacity as well.

Unfortunately, many viral diseases that aren't influenza are called flu, which causes considerable confusion. There are three types of true influenza viruses: A, B and C. All of them are spread from person to person by direct contact, such as by shaking hands with someone who has sneezed or coughed into his or her hands, or by inhaling infected droplets from the air.

Type A usually is responsible for the large flu outbreaks. Types B and C generally aren't as widespread. Type B causes smaller, more localized outbreaks. Type C is the least common and usually causes only a mild illness.

Types B and C are fairly stable viruses. However, the type A virus changes (mutates) frequently, with new strains appearing regularly. This generally results in a new epidemic every few years. Every 10 to 40 years, influenza breaks out as a pandemic, affecting people all over the world.

Diagnosis

The flu usually has a sudden onset with fever, chills, muscular aches and pains, weakness, malaise, nasal congestion, a flushed face, a dry cough and a sore throat. All of the signs and symptoms are similar to those of the common cold but tend to be much more severe.

Influenza typically develops 1 to 4 days after coming into contact with the virus. The fever may last 3 to 5 days, although it can last as little as 1 day or as long as 1 week.

Diagnosing the flu with complete certainty requires a lab culture. What makes the diagnosis difficult is influenza's similarity to many other illnesses.

If your doctor suspects the flu, he or she may be able to isolate the virus from throat washings or may do a blood test to look for antibodies to the virus. These tests are mainly of value to public health officials, who can better advise the public if they know the character and extent of the disease circulating in a community.

How serious is the flu?

Isolated cases of the flu generally last several days and resolve without complications. However, flu epidemics still are responsible for an average of approximately 20,000 deaths each year in the United States.

The illness can result in complications such as bronchitis, pneumonia and worsening of existing chronic diseases, such as heart disease or asthma.

Complications of influenza are more common in older adults and in individuals with weakened immune systems or chronic medical disorders.

Treatment

Rest is the primary treatment for the flu. In some cases, medication is effective at shortening the course of the illness.

In the United States, four antiviral drugs have been approved for treating influenza: amantadine (Symmetrel), rimantadine (Flumadine), zanamivir (Relenza) and oseltamivir (Tamiflu).

Amantadine and rimantadine, both of which are taken orally, are effective against the influenza A virus only. They can relieve symptoms and shorten the illness. Side effects of the medications may include insomnia, dizziness or difficulty in concentrating, especially in older adults.

Zanamivir and oseltamivir are used to treat both influenza A and B and can shorten the duration of your illness by a day or two. The medications are members of a new class of antiviral agents called neuraminidase inhibitors. These drugs work by inhibiting the activities of an enzyme, called neuraminidase, which plays an important role in the spread and growth of the viruses from infected cells.

Zanamivir, which is inhaled, is available to people age 13 and older. Oseltamivir, an oral medication, is only recommended for people older than age 18.

Pneumonia

Signs and symptoms

- Coughing
- Shortness of breath
- Pain in the chest (pleurisy)
- Chills
- Fever

Pneumonia is an inflammation of the tissues of your lungs. Rather than being one specific infection, however, what your doctor calls pneumonia may actually have more than 50 different causes. The results range from a mild condition that accompanies a cold to a life-threatening illness.

Pneumonia can result from bacteria, such as pneumococci or streptococci, a virus, such as influenza, or a chemical irritant. To make pneumonia more easily understood, the many varieties can be classified into various subtypes.

Community-acquired pneumonia

Community-acquired pneumonia gets its name from the way it's transmitted — in the community at large rather than in a hospital. Common causes include pneumococci and mycoplasma. The influenza virus also can cause pneumonia.

Hospital-acquired pneumonia

This type of pneumonia is acquired in the hospital. The number of potential infecting agents is generally much greater with hospital-acquired pneumonia than with community-acquired pneumonia. These agents also tend to cause more severe illness.

Aspiration pneumonia

Aspiration pneumonia results from bacteria being breathed into the lungs. Usually, this occurs when the contents of your stomach enter your lungs after you've vomited. It can also occur with diseases that interfere with swallowing.

Pneumonia caused by opportunistic organisms

Pneumonia is more likely to strike people with impaired immune systems. Organisms that aren't harmful in healthy people can be extremely dangerous in people with diseases such as AIDS, sickle cell anemia and other conditions that impair the immune system. Medications that suppress your immune system, such as corticosteroids or certain types of chemotherapy for cancer, also increase your risk of opportunistic infections.

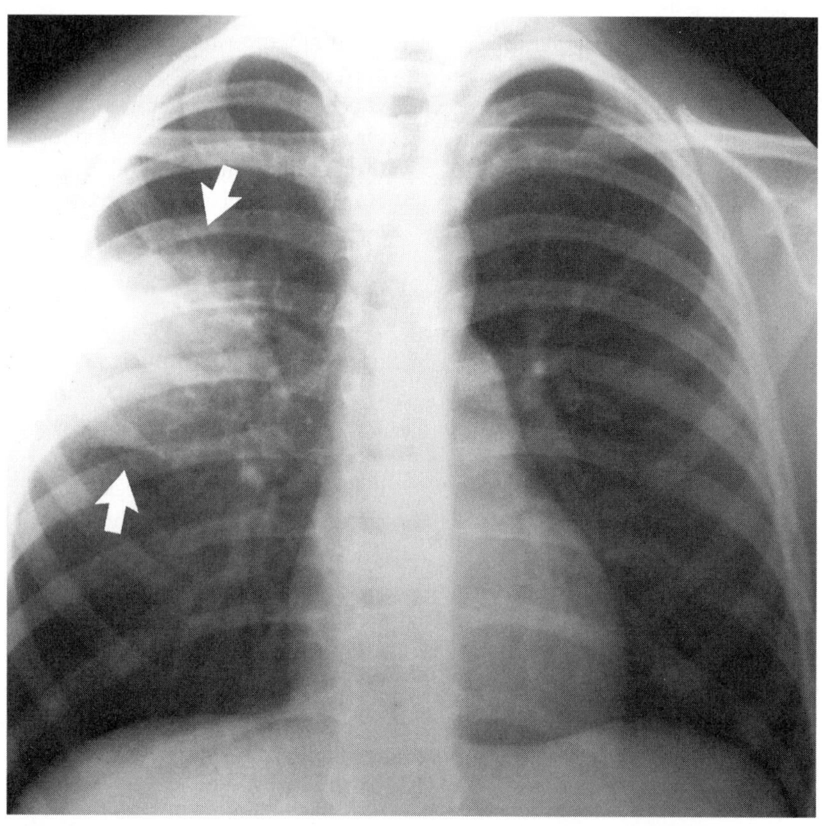

This chest X-ray reveals pneumonia in the upper lobe of the lung (see arrows).

Diagnosis

Signs and symptoms of pneumonia vary depending on the type and extent of infection. At first, pneumonia may appear to be a cold or it may develop as a complication of a cold. A fever typically accompanies most types, as does a cough. The cough may be dry or it may produce colored or bloody sputum. If the inflammation spreads to the surface of your lungs (pleura), you may experience sharp pain that's aggravated when you breathe (pleurisy).

Using a stethoscope, your doctor may detect distortions in the sounds of your breathing that suggest the presence of infection. Chest X-rays also may help identify the location and extent of the infection. A sample of your sputum may be tested (cultured) to identify the infecting agent.

PREVENTION TIP

You can reduce your risk of one type of pneumonia with the pneumococcal vaccine. The vaccine protects against a common form of the disease that results from the pneumococcus bacteria. It's recommended for healthy adults age 65 or older and for people with a weakened immune system due to a chronic illness, such as cardiovascular disease, lung disease or alcoholism. The vaccine is also recommended for people who've had their spleen removed. For more on the pneumococcal vaccine, see page 15.

How serious is pneumonia?

Pneumonia is common, occurring in more than 1 in every 100 people annually. The seriousness of this disorder depends largely on the cause of the illness and your overall health.

A healthy person generally has sufficient defense mechanisms to be able to resist or control the invading organism. In young people, pneumonia is often a passing discomfort that remains undiagnosed and is regarded as simply a cold.

Susceptibility of pneumonia is increased among individuals whose defense mechanisms are impaired by aging, a chronic illness, alcoholism or the use of immunosuppressant drugs. In older adults and people weakened by another disease, pneumonia can be fatal. Proper medical care, adequate rest and careful monitoring are essential.

Treatment

The treatment your doctor recommends depends on the cause of the pneumonia — whether it's a bacterium, virus or other agent — and the severity of your symptoms. If the cause is bacterial, you'll likely receive an antibiotic.

The choice of antibiotic is determined by several factors, including the specific bacteria causing the infection. Hospitalization may be necessary in severe cases.

Strep throat

Signs and symptoms

- A sore throat
- Red, swollen tonsils
- Swollen lymph glands in the front of the neck
- Fever
- Headache
- Muscle aches
- Abdominal pain and possibly vomiting

Strep throat occurs most commonly between the ages of 6 and 12 years. It's caused by the bacterium *Streptococcus pyogenes* (group A beta-hemolytic streptococcus). The bacteria spread through airborne droplets or direct contact, such as touching a contaminated doorknob or other surface.

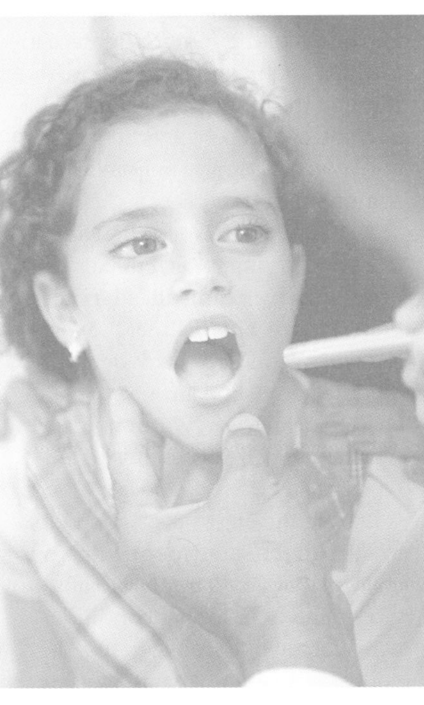

Diagnosis

Because the symptoms of strep throat are similar to those of several other illnesses, including colds, your doctor will likely do a throat culture test for strep infection. For this test a cotton swab is rubbed against the back of your throat, and secretions on the swab are taken to a laboratory for analysis.

For some time, a rapid test has been available that gives an initial diagnostic result within 1 hour. However, it misses up to 30 percent of strep cases, requiring the need for a traditional throat culture. More recently, Mayo Clinic developed a new diagnostic test that provides a final, confirmed result in about 8 hours, compared to 1 to 2 days for a throat culture.

How serious is strep throat?

Although strep throat usually isn't dangerous, it may lead to complications if left untreated. These can include scarlet fever, sinus infection and ear infections, as well as more serious delayed complications, including kidney disease (nephritis) and rheumatic fever.

Treatment

Because strep throat is a bacterial infection, it's usually treated with antibiotics. Once treatment is started, symptoms often improve within 1 or 2 days. Although you'll feel better, it's important to finish the entire prescription. Stopping the medication early can create strains of bacteria that are resistant to antibiotics. It may also lead to more cases of strep throat and other complications, such as rheumatic fever.

Prevention

If your child has strep throat, make sure no one else uses his or her drinking glasses and eating utensils. Wash those items carefully in hot, soapy water or a dishwasher. In addition, you might want to give the sick child a new toothbrush.

Croup

Signs and symptoms

- Loud, brassy coughing
- Difficulty breathing

Emergency signs and symptoms

- Drooling or great difficulty swallowing
- An inability to bend the neck forward
- Blue or dusky lips
- High-pitched noises when inhaling
- Coughing that worsens
- Increased difficulty breathing
- A heart rate exceeding 160 beats a minute
- Unconsciousness

Croup is an infection of the voice box (larynx), windpipe (trachea) and bronchial tubes that's caused by a virus. It occurs most often between the ages of 3 months and 5 years. Boys are more likely to get it than are girls. An upper respiratory illness of several days' duration usually precedes symptoms of croup.

A narrowing of the airway that occurs with croup causes a tight, brassy cough that may resemble the barking of a seal. If your child has croup, his or her voice will probably be hoarse, and he or she will

Aspirin and Children

Aspirin is an effective drug for treating a wide range of symptoms and disorders in adults. It's generally thought of as mild and harmless, but in certain cases, it can be very dangerous, particularly when given to children. Aspirin use is related to a serious childhood condition called Reye's syndrome (see page 579). You shouldn't give aspirin to your child for any reason unless it's prescribed by a doctor.

Instead, try acetaminophen, which can help relieve minor aches and pains and is available over-the-counter with different names, such as Tylenol, Panadol, Liquiprin and Tempra. Acetaminophen also comes in several forms, including drop, liquid and tablet. Each form has a different strength, so read labels and follow directions carefully, paying particular attention to dosage instructions for age or weight.

have difficulty inhaling. Your child will probably be more comfortable sitting up than lying down.

Croup typically lasts 3 to 4 days. During that time, it may go from mild to severe several times. Usually, the condition worsens at night and improves in the morning.

Treatment

Because croup is caused by a virus, antibiotics aren't helpful. Antibiotics work against bacteria, not viruses.

If your child has croup, warm, moist air may relieve some of the airway swelling and ease the cough. Run hot water in your shower for 10 minutes with the bathroom door closed. Once the room looks like a steam bath, take your child into the bathroom for at least 10 minutes. Another method of creating increased humidity is to use a vaporizer in the child's room. Have the child put his or her face in the mist and breathe deeply through the mouth. A wet washcloth placed loosely over the nose and mouth also may help relieve symptoms.

A child with croup is often agitated and crying, which makes breathing more difficult, so try to both reassure and distract him or her with a cuddle, a book or a favorite game. Encourage your child to drink clear, warm fluids, which may help loosen thickened secretions.

During the illness it's a good idea to sleep in the same room with your child so that you'll be alert to any worsening of his or her condition. Don't let anyone smoke in the house because smoke will worsen the symptoms.

If the symptoms persist for more than a few days or become severe, contact your child's doctor. Occasionally, croup may cause complete obstruction of the airway. This is an extreme emergency situation that usually develops over the course of several hours. To guard against this dangerous complication, be alert for emergency signs and symptoms and seek urgent medical attention if they occur.

Chickenpox (varicella)

Signs and symptoms

- Fever
- Weakness
- A red, itchy rash

Chickenpox, also known as varicella, occurs primarily in children, although adults also can contract the disease if they haven't had it already or been immunized.

Chickenpox is spread by inhaling infected respiratory droplets or by direct contact with the fluid from a blister when it ruptures. In people who've had chickenpox, the virus can reactivate later in life and cause shingles (see page 1192).

Diagnosis

The most recognized symptom of chickenpox is the itchy, red rash and small blisters that break out on the face, scalp, chest, back and, to a lesser extent, arms and legs (see the color illustration on page 436). The rash usually appears about 2 weeks after exposure to the virus and begins as superficial spots.

The blisters quickly fill with a clear fluid, rupture and turn crusty. They then slough off in 1 to 2 weeks. The rash continues to break out for 1 to 5 days, so blisters at various stages of development may be present at the same time. Fever and malaise, often mild in children and more severe in adults, also develop.

How serious is chickenpox?

In children, chickenpox is often a mild disease, but in adults it can be more serious. In adults, pneumonia may develop. In people with suppressed immune systems, the disease can be very serious. Although uncommon, inflammation of the brain (encephalitis) may occur, but recovery usually is complete.

If a pregnant woman contracts chickenpox during the first or second trimester, there's a small risk the child will be born with a congenital deformity. When a pregnant woman contracts the disease within 5 days before delivery, there's a high risk of the newborn having serious disease. The newborn generally should be immunized immediately with varicella-zoster immune globulin (VZIG).

Chickenpox seldom lasts for more than 2 weeks, from the appearance of the first blisters to the disappearance of the last one. A secondary bacterial infection of the ruptured blisters may cause fever and skin scarring.

Treatment

To prevent spreading the disease, isolate the person with chickenpox until the rash crusts over. Keep the skin moist with frequent baths or, once the fever has subsided, showers. Cool, wet compresses or tepid water baths may help to relieve itching.

Escherichia Coli O157:H7

In 1982, 47 people in two states became sick with bloody, watery diarrhea, severe cramps and abdominal pain. Public health officials were stumped. Although it appeared obvious it was a gastrointestinal infection of some sort, how could so many people, across two states, become sick at the same time with similar signs and symptoms? What was the cause of such an outbreak?

After 3 months of investigation, medical experts found the answer. All of the individuals affected had eaten hamburger from the same stock at a national fast-food restaurant. The infectious culprit in the meat was a strain of bacteria we now know as *Escherichia coli* O157:H7. *E. coli* O157:H7 adheres to the intestine wall after being ingested. Once established, it produces a toxin that can cause bloody diarrhea.

Since that initial outbreak, many similar outbreaks have occurred. According to the Centers for Disease Control and Prevention (CDC), approximately 73,000 cases of *E. coli* O157:H7 infection and 61 deaths occur each year in the United States. The CDC reports that outbreaks have occurred in more than 30 countries on six continents.

As a result, the Department of Agriculture has changed its regulations on meat handling. It now requires safe handling labels on raw meat and poultry products and has instituted monitoring programs to test random beef samples. Meat processing plants are required to take steps to prevent contamination from pathogens and other hazards.

Transmission

The bacterium can live in the intestines of healthy cows and is found on some cattle farms. Eating meat that hasn't been cooked enough, particularly ground beef, is the most common way of acquiring an *E. coli* O157:H7 infection. The bacterium has also been found in unpasteurized milk and juice, and in produce such as lettuce and alfalfa sprouts.

In addition, you can become infected through contact with contaminated stool. This is particularly apt to occur with young children who are still being toilet trained or still learning how to properly wash their hands. Families and people at child care centers with infected children are at increased risk of developing the illness.

Treatment

Within a day to 2 weeks of exposure to the bacteria, you may experience watery diarrhea and abdominal cramps. In most people, this eventually progresses to bloody diarrhea. Generally, the symptoms resolve within 1 to 9 days.

For mild diarrhea, drink plenty of fluids to avoid dehydration. This is especially important for children. As you begin to feel better, you might try eating semisolid foods and low-fat fibers, such as soda crackers and toast. Diarrhea is your body's way of attempting to get rid of the offending organism. For this reason, health experts generally don't recommend antidiarrheal medications, as they may contribute to keeping the bacteria from being eliminated.

In a small percentage of people infected with *E. coli* O157:H7, particularly the very young and the very old, a serious complication called hemolytic uremic syndrome (HUS) may occur. HUS destroys red blood cells and causes kidney failure (see page 923). It requires intensive care and may lead to further kidney complications and possibly the need for kidney dialysis later in life. In a few cases, it may be fatal. Antibiotics may increase the risk of developing HUS.

Prevention

According to food safety experts, the best way to prevent such an infection is to use common sense. Avoid having raw meat come into contact with other foods. Cook your meat until it's done. For hamburger, meat should reach at least 160 F, and for steaks and roasts, between 145 F and 170 F.

In addition, properly wash hands, foods and cooking utensils that have come in contact with raw meat. Keep meat and produce separate while in the refrigerator and while cooking. Wash vegetables and fruits thoroughly, especially if they'll be eaten raw. Don't drink unpasteurized milk or fruit juices.

Practicing proper hand-washing techniques along with your children can go a long way toward preventing a host of infectious diseases.

Antihistamines may help relieve severe itching that can accompany chickenpox. The medication acyclovir may be used to treat severe complications, such as pneumonia or encephalitis. Routine use of acyclovir in all people with chickenpox isn't considered necessary.

People with suppressed immune systems who aren't immune to chickenpox generally should receive varicella-zoster immune globulin (VZIG) after known exposure to chickenpox.

Prevention

A chickenpox vaccine is available and might be useful for the following people:

- Children ages 12 to 18 months
- Healthy children who are older than age 13
- Adults who haven't had chickenpox and have never been immunized against the disease

If you or your child is in one of these categories, consider asking your doctor about this vaccine. It's given in two doses 4 to 8 weeks apart.

Infectious mononucleosis

Signs and symptoms
- Fever
- A sore throat
- Loss of appetite
- Fatigue and weakness
- Sore muscles
- Swollen lymph glands
- Pain in the upper-left side of the abdomen

Infectious mononucleosis (mono) is caused by the Epstein-Barr virus. This infection most often occurs in people between the ages of 16 and 25. It's thought to be spread through saliva. The incubation period for the disease is usually 7 to 14 days in children and teenagers. The incubation period is longer for adults, sometimes as long as 30 to 50 days.

Diagnosis
Infectious mononucleosis causes a wide variety of signs and symptoms, including fever, sore throat, swollen lymph glands and enlargement of the spleen. Nausea, jaundice, headache, stiffness, chest pain, coughing and a rapid or irregular heartbeat also may result. Loss of appetite, muscle pain, fatigue and weakness are often present, and a red rash appears on some individuals. This wide variety of signs and symptoms can make diagnosis difficult. If your doctor suspects mononucleosis, he or she may advise a blood test called a Monospot test, which checks for evidence of the Epstein-Barr virus in your bloodstream.

How serious is infectious mononucleosis?
Mononucleosis isn't a serious disease, except in rare cases in which the spleen becomes severely enlarged and ruptures or when other vital organs, such as your liver or heart, are infected. Seek urgent medical care if you experience sudden sharp pains in the upper-left side of your abdomen. This could mean a rapidly enlarging or ruptured spleen. If a ruptured spleen should occur, emergency surgery may be required to control the bleeding.

In most cases, the fever, swollen lymph nodes and enlargement of the spleen improve after 10 days. However, it may take 2 to 3 months before you feel completely normal. Even though most of the symptoms aren't severely debilitating, the disease may cause prolonged fatigue and weakness.

Treatment
Treatment for mononucleosis generally depends on its symptoms and severity.

Medication
There's no specific drug treatment for viral infectious mononucleosis, but the sore throat that accompanies the disease occasionally is aggravated by a strep infection. Strep requires treatment with an antibiotic. Sometimes, your doctor may prescribe a course of corticosteroids to help relieve symptoms.

Self-care
Rest is an important part of treatment. Don't expect to return to your normal routine for at least 2 to 3 weeks. Your doctor may ask you to avoid contact sports for several months if your spleen is enlarged. Drinking plenty of fluids helps to relieve the fever and sore throat and keeps you from becoming dehydrated. For a sore throat, try gargling warm, salty water several times a day.

PREVENTION TIP

Proper hand washing is the best way to prevent many infections. That's why it's important to wash your own hands regularly and to show your children how to wash their hands properly.

The Centers for Disease Control and Prevention recommends taking the following steps:
- Use soap and running water.
- Rub your hands vigorously as you wash them.
- Wash all surfaces, including backs of hands, wrists, between fingers and under fingernails.
- Rinse well and leave the water running until after drying hands.
- Dry hands with a single-use towel.
- Turn off the faucet using a paper towel.

Gastrointestinal infections

Signs and symptoms
- Watery diarrhea
- Nausea and vomiting
- Fever
- Abdominal cramps
- Occasional muscle aches and headache

Emergency signs and symptoms
- Profuse diarrhea, to the point of causing lightheadedness
- Bloody diarrhea

Bacteria, viruses, fungi and parasites can cause gastrointestinal infections. These infections are most commonly contracted by drinking contaminated water, eating unwashed raw fruits or vegetables or eating meat or fish that hasn't been cooked properly.

One of the most common viral infections of the gastrointestinal tract is rotavirus. This infection occurs mainly in infants between the ages of 6 and 24 months. Other types of gastrointestinal infections include *Campylobacter jejuni, Escherichia coli (E. coli), Staphylococcus aureus* and salmonella.

Diagnosis
Most gastrointestinal infections take a day or two to cause any signs or symptoms, depending on the incubation period of the infectious agent. Diarrhea is the most common symptom of a gastrointestinal infection. If the lining of the intestine is damaged, stool may be bloody.

Vomiting also is common. In some cases, fever, loss of appetite, abdominal cramps, nausea and weight loss occur.

Diarrhea and vomiting that begins within several hours of ingesting a food generally suggests food poisoning due to a preformed toxin, rather than a toxin that's released after the bacteria have lodged in your intestine. To determine the cause, your doctor may take blood or stool samples to be grown (cultured) and analyzed in a laboratory.

How serious are gastrointestinal infections?
In the United States, gastrointestinal infections generally aren't serious, although they can be fatal in small children, the very old and people with impaired immune systems. In developing countries, where sanitation levels are often poor and health care is often less than adequate, diarrheal diseases are among the top causes of sickness and death.

The loss of fluids brought on by diarrhea can cause dehydration, a serious problem in older adults and young children. For this reason, it's important to drink plenty of safe liquids throughout the course of the illness. Avoid alcohol, caffeine and milk products.

If your child exhibits signs of dehydration — dry mouth, pale skin, sunken eyes, decreased urination — talk to your doctor. Other reasons to call your doctor include severe or prolonged diarrhea or vomiting, either high fever or a sudden drop in body temperature, changed levels of consciousness, severe abdominal pain or bloody stools.

Treatment
For the most part, gastrointestinal infections get better within a few days and complete recovery occurs without treatment. During your illness stay hydrated with nonalcoholic, noncaffeinated fluids. Water and sports drinks, which contain sodium, potassium and other nutrients, are generally best. If you're severely dehydrated, you may need an intravenous electrolyte solution.

If the intestinal infection is caused by bacteria, antibiotics may shorten the illness. Or in some instances — such as diarrhea caused by *E. coli* 0157:H7 — they may lead to serious complications. Signs and symptoms such as nausea, vomiting, abdominal pain and diarrhea are some of the possible side effects of antibiotics.

Prevention
Good hygiene is a key element in the prevention of gastrointestinal infections. Frequent hand washing is one of the most effective ways of getting rid of germs. In addition, wash any areas that have been in contact with raw meat — especially poultry — with hot, soapy water.

Make sure all meat is thoroughly cooked before you eat it. If you're traveling in a foreign country, avoid local drinking water and ice cubes, unsanitary eating establishments and raw fruits and vegetables, unless you peel them yourself.

Other Infections

Many other infectious diseases occur less often than the illnesses described so far, but they can cause very serious illness. Immunizations now make it possible to avoid many — but not all — of these.

Tetanus

Signs and symptoms
- Stiffness of the jaw, neck and other muscles
- Irritability
- Spasms of the jaw and neck muscles
- Painful convulsions

Tetanus, also known as lockjaw, is caused by the bacterium *Clostridium tetani,* whose spores are found in soil. If the spores enter a deep wound with low oxygen content, they germinate and produce a toxin (tetanospasmin) that interferes with nerves that control your muscles. The incubation period from the time of the injury until symptoms appear is 5 days to 3 weeks (usually 8 to 12 days).

Diagnosis
Although some people with tetanus experience only pain and tingling at the wound site and some spasms in nearby muscles, most of them have a stiff jaw and neck, difficulty swallowing and irritability. Spasms of the jaw or facial muscles often follow, progressing to spasms and rigidity of the neck, abdominal and back muscles. Finally, painful convulsions caused by minor stimuli affect the respiratory muscles so that the individual is unable to breathe.

How serious is tetanus?
If muscle spasms develop early, chances of recovery are poor. Tetanus is serious and often fatal, especially in small children and older adults. Prevention is the best treatment.

Treatment
Consult your doctor immediately if you incur a wound that may be contaminated with soil, particularly if the wound is deep. If you've received the initial series of tetanus vaccinations and more than 5 years have passed since your last booster shot, your doctor may give you another booster shot. Your body will quickly manufacture the needed antibodies to protect you against tetanus.

The doctor might also prescribe antibiotics and open the wound so that he or she can clean it. If you acquire tetanus, immediate hospitalization is necessary.

Prevention
Immunization is vital for everyone. The tetanus vaccine is usually initially given to children as part of the diphtheria-tetanus-pertussis (DTaP) vaccine, with tetanus booster shots every 10 years, or at the time of a major injury if it has

been more than 5 years since your last booster. For more information on the vaccine, see page 12.

Measles (rubeola)

Signs and symptoms

- Fever
- Coughing
- Sneezing
- Inflamed eyes
- A sore throat
- Tiny white spots on the lining of the cheek
- A rash

Measles (rubeola) was a common childhood illness before widespread use of the measles vaccine. The virus that causes the disorder is transmitted by inhalation of infected droplets in the air, such as from a sneeze. Measles is most contagious before its rash appears, making it difficult to avoid the disease. Once you've had measles, you're permanently immune to the disease.

Diagnosis

Measles begins with fever, accompanied by a persistent cough, sneezing, inflamed eyes (conjunctivitis) and a sore throat. After about 4 days, a red, blotchy rash appears on the face and behind the ears. The rash spreads to the chest and back and, finally, to the arms and legs. By the time it reaches the arms and legs, it usually has begun to fade from the face.

The symptoms usually appear 10 to 14 days after exposure to the virus. The diagnosis is typically made on the basis of the characteristic rash and the small, white spots on the lining of the cheek.

How serious is measles?

Typically, a measles infection lasts 10 days to 2 weeks and you recover completely. In a small number of cases, pneumonia or other bacterial infections develop in the course of the illness, or complications such as encephalitis arise immediately after appearance of the rash. Encephalitis can cause vomiting, convulsions, coma and brain damage.

Treatment

Acetaminophen (Tylenol, others) can help relieve fever, and a sedative cough medicine may help relieve coughing. A person with measles should remain isolated until a week after the rash disappears, and he or she should stay in bed until the fever disappears. Severe symptoms may require additional treatment.

Prevention

The measles vaccine is effective and is usually given as a combined measles-mumps-rubella (MMR) inoculation. Doctors recommend that the MMR vaccine be given to children between 12 and 15 months of age, and again between 3 and 6 years of age.

German measles (rubella)

Signs and symptoms

- A rash
- Mild fever

German measles (rubella) is only moderately infectious. It's transmitted by inhalation of droplets of moisture carrying the virus. The incubation period is 2 to 3 weeks, and the affected person is contagious for 1 week before the rash appears.

Diagnosis

The symptoms of this disease are usually mild and sometimes hardly noticeable. They may include mild

Making Vaccines Safer

In the past, the diphtheria-tetanus-pertussis (DTP) vaccine used whole cells of the pertussis bacterium. Common DTP side effects included fever and inflammation at the site of the injection. More serious side effects, such as seizures, were far more rare, but they still raised concern among public health officials. The newer DTaP vaccine uses only the parts of the bacterium cell needed for immunity. This is called an acellular vaccine, thus the *a* preceding the *P*. The DTaP vaccine has fewer side effects than the DTP vaccine. The DTP vaccine is no longer used in the United States.

In 2001, the Food and Drug Administration (FDA) approved a new formulation of the vaccine that contains no preservatives other than thimerosal and contains 95 percent less thimerosal than before. Thimerosal is a mercury-containing preservative used in small amounts in some vaccines to keep microorganisms from contaminating the vaccine. Although there's no evidence that any child has been harmed by thimerosal found in vaccines, health officials are working to reduce levels of the preservative in vaccines to minimize possible exposure to mercury.

Given the FDA approval of the reformulated DTaP vaccine, all routine pediatric vaccinations are now being reformulated to contain trace amounts, if any, of thimerosal.

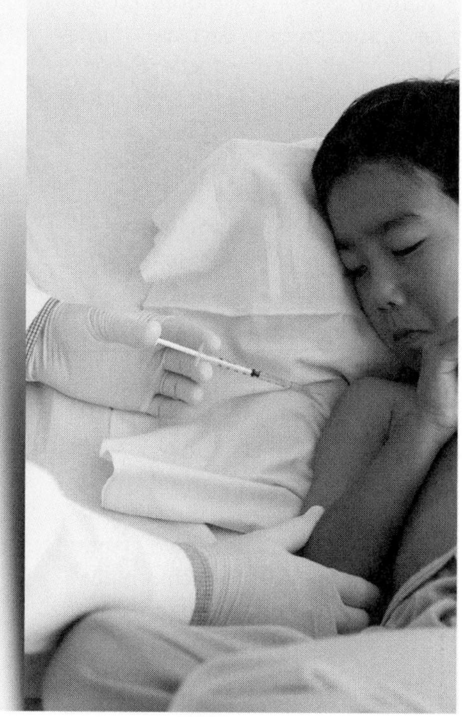

fever, enlarged lymph nodes and a fine, pink rash that appears on the face and trunk and then the arms and legs. The rash usually disappears in 3 to 5 days, lasting no more than 1 day on each portion of the body. In many cases, a rash doesn't occur. Your doctor may take a blood sample to check for antibodies to the virus.

How serious is German measles?

In itself, German measles is a mild infection. Once you've had the disease, you are usually permanently immune. However, if a woman has rubella when she's pregnant, the consequences for her unborn child may be severe. The child may have one or more problems, including growth retardation, cataracts, rashes, deafness, congenital heart defects and defects of other organs. The highest risk to the fetus is during the first trimester, but rubella during the second trimester also is dangerous.

Treatment

The standard treatment for rubella is to let the infection run its course. Taking acetaminophen (Tylenol, others) may help to relieve symptoms. If you're exposed to rubella while you're pregnant, contact your doctor promptly.

Prevention

A vaccine is available to protect against the disease. It's usually part of the combined measles-mumps-rubella (MMR) vaccination schedule (see page 8). If a woman is given the vaccine, she should be cautioned to not get pregnant for at least 3 months after vaccination.

Roseola

Signs and symptoms

- High fever
- Swollen lymph nodes in the neck
- A rash on the trunk and neck

Roseola is caused by the human herpes virus 6. The route of transmission is thought to be through the respiratory system. This viral infection usually affects children ages 6 months to 3 years, but it can at times affect adults. The infection typically isn't serious, but sometimes complications occur.

Diagnosis

The primary sign of roseola is a sudden, high fever that typically occurs in a child 6 months to 3 years old. The child may be irritable, and his or her lymph nodes may become swollen. As the fever goes down, a rash appears on the trunk and neck and lasts a few hours to a few days. Roseola is usually diagnosed by its signs and symptoms and can be confirmed by an antibody blood test.

Treatment

Treatment consists of acetaminophen (Tylenol, others) and applying cool sponges or washcloths to lower the fever. In some cases, a high fever can cause convulsions (a febrile seizure). Contact your doctor if this occurs.

Whooping cough (pertussis)

Signs and symptoms

- A hacking cough, often followed by explosive coughs that end in a high-pitched whoop
- Sneezing
- Nasal congestion
- Tearing
- Loss of appetite
- A general feeling of unease and discomfort (malaise)

Emergency signs and symptoms

- Difficulty breathing
- Blue lips

Pertussis gets its name from the Latin word for "intensive cough." The condition is also known as whooping cough because of the high-pitched whooping sound characteristic of the disease. The condition is caused by the *Bordetella pertussis* bacterium.

Whooping cough primarily occurs in infants younger than 2 years and is contracted by inhaling infected airborne droplets, often from an adult with a mild case of the disease. The disease is most contagious early on, but it can be transmitted until the infection is completely cleared.

Diagnosis

Diagnosing whooping cough in its early stages can be difficult because symptoms resemble those of a cold. After 10 days to 2 weeks, the characteristic whooping may develop when the person has spasms of rapid, consecutive coughs followed by a strained, hurried, deep inhalation with a high-pitched sound.

Coughing attacks can be set off by sneezing, crying, anger or fright. The person may cough up large amounts of thick phlegm. Vomiting is common. About 4 weeks after the coughing attacks begin, symptoms gradually disappear.

Whooping cough is less common in the United States than it was decades ago because of the widespread vaccination of children. However, it's becoming slightly more common in adults and adolescents. About 25 percent of whooping cough now occurs among teenagers and adults. In countries in which immunization against pertussis has lagged, the consequences have been disastrous, with deaths occurring from the reemergence of the disease.

How serious is whooping cough?

With proper care, most people recover from the illness without incident. However, it can lead to pneumonia with subsequent damage to the lungs. In very severe cases, lack of oxygen (asphyxia) may lead to brain damage. If a person's lips turn blue, this means that he or she is having severe difficulty breathing and needs emergency medical care.

Treatment

Your doctor will likely prescribe an antibiotic. In more severe cases, corticosteroids also may be used.

Drink plenty of fluids and eat smaller, more frequent meals rather than large ones. Cough medicines provide little benefit.

Prevention

Vaccination for whooping cough is generally given as part of the diphtheria-tetanus-pertussis combination vaccine (DTaP) administered during childhood.

Mumps

Signs and symptoms

- Swollen, painful salivary glands
- Fever
- Weakness and fatigue
- Inflammation of the pancreas, testicles, ovaries or brain

Mumps is mainly a childhood disease but can occur in adults. The medical term for the illness is *epidemic parotitis*.

It's caused by a virus spread by inhalation of infected droplets in the air. The affected person becomes contagious a day before the symptoms appear, is highly contagious for another 3 days and then less contagious as the swelling goes down.

Diagnosis

Mumps signs and symptoms usually appear 2 to 3 weeks after the infection begins. The primary — and best known — sign is swollen, painful parotid salivary glands (located at the back of the jaw), causing the cheeks to puff out. In small children, fever is usually slight.

Occasionally, the illness can lead to more serious signs and symptoms. If the person experiences headaches and becomes lethargic, inflammation of the brain and its lining (meningoencephalitis) may be present.

Pain in the upper abdomen, nausea and vomiting may indicate inflammation of the pancreas. Lower abdominal pain in women may mean inflammation of the ovaries. This is often difficult to diagnose.

About a quarter of teenage boys and adult men who contract mumps experience inflammation of the testicles (orchitis).

Your doctor can confirm a diagnosis of mumps by identifying the mumps virus in your saliva or by finding an increase in mumps antibodies in your blood. However, this testing is rarely necessary.

How serious is mumps?

Mumps makes you uncomfortable, but it's usually not a serious disease and rarely lasts more than 2 weeks. Encephalitis, an uncommon but serious complication of the illness, can cause neurologic symptoms and, rarely, is fatal. Orchitis is uncomfortable and occasionally causes male infertility.

Treatment

There's no specific treatment for mumps. Your doctor may advise bed rest until the fever disappears. Isolation to prevent the spread of the disease is sometimes appropriate. For most of the complications that may arise, treatment depends on the symptoms.

Prevention

The vaccine against mumps is safe and effective and should be given to all children more than 1 year old. It may be given by itself or combined with other vaccines. Use of this vaccine has greatly decreased the incidence of mumps in the United States.

Fever of Unknown Origin

Fever is the most common reaction to an infection. But a fever doesn't always signify that you have an infection. Fever can also be a sign of a noninfectious disease or result from a medication. Sometimes, the cause is unapparent. If you have recurrent temperatures greater than 100.5 F for more than 3 weeks and there's no obvious cause, even after extensive evaluation, the diagnosis may be "fever of unknown origin." However, with persistence, a cause can usually be identified.

Some of the tests that your doctor may use to try to identify the cause of unknown fever include blood tests, X-ray examinations, computerized tomography (CT) scans and biopsies of the arteries, lymph nodes, bone marrow, liver or muscles.

Rabies

Signs and symptoms

- Pain, and then tingling, at the site of an animal bite
- Skin sensitivity
- Excessive drooling of saliva
- An inability to swallow liquids
- Rage alternating with calm
- Convulsions and paralysis leading to death

Rabies results from a virus (belonging to the rhabdoviridae family) that affects the brain. It's transmitted to humans through saliva when they're bitten or licked by an infected animal. Dogs and cats may be infected, and many bats, skunks and foxes are infected. Rodents are unlikely to be. The incubation period from the time of exposure until symptoms appear is usually 3 to 7 weeks, but this can range from 10 days to 2 years.

Diagnosis

Untreated rabies begins with pain followed by tingling at the site of the animal bite. You become extremely sensitive to temperature changes and air currents and tend to choke whenever you try to swallow liquids. Restlessness, muscle spasms, rage, extreme excitability and excessive drooling also are present. Finally, convulsions and paralysis ensue.

How serious is rabies?

Rabies is almost always fatal. Death, due to heart or respiratory failure and paralysis, usually occurs 7 to 25 days after symptoms appear.

Treatment
If you're bitten by a dog, cat or farm animal, it should be caught, confined and observed by a veterinarian. If you're bitten by a wild animal, the animal should be killed, if possible, and the brain tested for rabies. Wild raccoons, skunks, bats, coyotes, wolves and foxes are generally presumed to have rabies.

If you waken and find a bat in your room or in your child's room and you can't be positive there was no contact, kill the bat and talk to your doctor about having it tested for rabies. If the bat has escaped, it's best to assume there has been contact and proceed with treatment.

Treatment consists of administering an antibody, half of which is injected directly into the wound and the other half into surrounding muscle. You'll also receive a vaccine, given as five injections. The first injection is given along with the antibody, and the others are given 3, 7, 14 and 28 days after the first shot.

Scarlet fever

Signs and symptoms
- A sore throat
- Fever
- Chills
- A rash on the neck and chest

Scarlet fever was once a common, serious childhood illness but is now rare. Caused by the toxin from a specific type of streptococcal bacteria, scarlet fever usually begins suddenly with a sore throat, fever and chills. The bacteria produce erythrogenic toxin that causes a rash. Within 12 to 36 hours, the rash appears on the neck and chest but not on the face. Then it spreads over the body. The rash has a sandpaper consistency. Often the area of greatest involvement is above the armpits and the groin. The tongue may become swollen and bright red. The rash usually disappears after 3 days. The tongue may remain swollen for somewhat longer, but recovery usually is complete.

Treatment
Penicillin or another antibiotic is usually given for a minimum of 10 days. Bed rest and drinking plenty of liquids also are important.

Typhoid fever

Signs and symptoms
- Fever
- Headache
- Weakness and fatigue
- A sore throat
- Coughing
- Diarrhea

Emergency signs and symptoms
- A sudden drop in body temperature
- Shock, characterized by decrease in urination, a lightheaded feeling particularly on standing up, lethargy and a change in level of consciousness

Typhoid fever is caused by the bacteria *Salmonella typhi* and *S. paratyphi*. It's acquired by consuming contaminated food or fluids. It's rare in industrialized countries but more common in developing countries. The bacteria penetrate the wall of the small intestine and cause inflammation of the lymph nodes and spleen. Chronic carriers are possible sources of the disease.

A chronic carrier is someone who carries typhoid bacteria in his or her intestinal tract for years but has no symptoms. In developing countries with poor sanitary conditions and unsafe water supplies, epidemics of typhoid fever still occur.

Diagnosis
Although it may come on suddenly with chills and fever, especially in children, typhoid fever usually develops slowly. It begins with headache, coughing, weakness and fatigue, generalized aches and a sore throat. Vomiting, constipation or diarrhea, and abdominal pain are often present as well. Fever usually is highest in the evening.

If the disease isn't treated, a second stage follows in which the individual often becomes extremely ill. Fever becomes continuous, and the person either develops severe constipation or diarrhea with the consistency and color of pea soup. In severe cases, the person may develop the "typhoid state," lying motionless with eyes half-closed and appearing wasted and exhausted. After about the second week, a rash may appear on the chest and back. It typically disappears in 3 to 4 days. Improvement often comes slowly. Abdominal

Smallpox

The eradication of smallpox is a success story of modern medicine. Smallpox was once a highly infectious viral disease that would spread in epidemics, causing death in up to 40 percent of its victims. The disease caused severe headache, fever and a red, blistering rash that often left scars. At the end of the 18th century, Edward Jenner, an English physician, discovered that inoculation with cowpox virus, which is usually harmless, prevented smallpox. Campaigns were launched in the United States and Europe to inoculate people against smallpox. However, as late as 1967, when the World Health Organization launched a global campaign to eliminate this disease, outbreaks still occurred regularly in many countries.

After 10 years of effort, this international campaign was successful and the disease was eradicated. Smallpox vaccination is no longer necessary, and in 1972 routine vaccination in the United States stopped.

The potential use of smallpox as a biological weapon has renewed interest in the disease, spurring the manufacture of the vaccine. Vaccination would only be reinstituted as a defense against biological warfare.

symptoms disappear gradually, and the fever decreases, becoming normal after another week to 10 days. However, symptoms can recur at any time up to 2 weeks after the fever has subsided.

About one-third of people with typhoid develop complications. Intestinal bleeding, usually during the third week, is manifested by a sudden decrease in blood pressure, increase in pulse and signs of shock followed by blood in the stool. Perforation of the intestine also may occur in the third week. This development causes abdominal pain with rigidity and soreness and an increase in body temperature and pulse. Other, more rare, complications include pneumonia, psychosis, meningitis and infection of the bladder, kidney or spine (osteomyelitis).

To diagnose typhoid fever, your doctor may take samples of your blood, urine and stool so that they can be cultured for *S. typhi*.

How serious is typhoid fever?

Untreated, typhoid fever is very serious. Even when treated, a few people don't survive the disease's complications. Older adults and people with chronic illnesses are especially vulnerable. In children, the disease usually is milder. A few people become chronic carriers.

Treatment

Antibiotics are available to treat typhoid fever. The choice depends on the strain of the bacteria. Other treatment steps include drinking fluids to avoid dehydration and eating a high-calorie, nonbulky diet to supply your body with the nutrients it may lose during the illness. At times, administration of fluids through a vein (intravenously) is necessary. Because the bacteria are present in the stool and urine, proper hand washing is important. Also avoid contact with contaminated clothing and bedding.

Prevention

Currently, two types of typhoid vaccines are available — an oral form and an injected form. The oral vaccine is given as four capsules, taken one a day every other day. The injectable vaccine is given in a single dose. Both vaccines are less than 100 percent effective. People who plan to live or to travel in an area where the disease is prevalent or who may have been exposed during an epidemic outbreak should be immunized. Carriers should not work as food handlers or in child care centers.

Diphtheria

Signs and symptoms

- A sore throat and hoarseness
- Nasal discharge
- Malaise
- Fever
- A thick gray membrane covering the throat and tonsils
- A rapid pulse

Diphtheria is an acute infection caused by the bacterium *Corynebacterium diphtheriae*. It usually attacks the respiratory tract. Infection occurs by inhalation of airborne droplets exhaled by a person with the disease or by a carrier who has no symptoms. The organism can also infect skin wounds or any mucous membrane. The disease is now rare in the United States.

Diagnosis

After an incubation period of 2 days to a week, a mild sore throat, fever and general unease (malaise) develop. Your doctor looks for a gray membrane covering your throat and tonsils.

How serious is diphtheria?

With proper treatment and no complications, the prognosis is good. However, the gray diphtheria membrane in the upper airway can be dangerous because it may obstruct breathing. In addition, the disease may cause a serious heart infection called myocarditis. Sometimes, the bacteria affect the cranial nerves, causing nasal-sounding speech, regurgitation of food and an inability to swallow. This is seldom fatal, unless paralysis of respiratory muscles develops. If the person survives these complications, recovery is slow but complete.

Treatment

If you have diphtheria, it's essential that you receive diphtheria antitoxin. You'll also be given antibiotics for the infection and to prevent you from becoming a carrier of the bacterium. You'll also need bed rest and 10 to 14 days of isolation.

Prevention

The diphtheria vaccine can prevent the disease. It's ordinarily given in infancy, often in combination with the whooping cough (pertussis) and tetanus vaccines, the combination of which is called the DTaP vaccine. The vaccine is very effective. A booster shot every 10 years is appropriate, especially if you travel to an area where diphtheria is common.

Wound infections

Signs and symptoms

- Swelling, discoloration and death of the surrounding tissue
- Hot, inflamed skin around a wound
- Elevated temperature
- Decrease in blood pressure
- Rapid heartbeat

After an injury causes a break in the skin or after an operation, various wound infections may occur. The infection can range from minor to severe, depending on the cause of the infection and how quickly it's identified and treated.

Some severe wound infections include:

Necrotizing subcutaneous infection

This infection is caused by bacteria that infect tissue through wounds. Primary symptoms are swelling, discoloration and death of the surrounding tissue. The skin around the wound becomes hot, inflamed, tender and red. If the infection worsens, the skin becomes discolored and gangrene may develop. Occasionally, a necrotizing subcutaneous infection is referred to as "flesh-eating bacteria" infection.

To determine the correct antibiotic to treat the infection, your doctor will take a sample of pus from the wound for culture to identify the bacteria present.

Your doctor also may have to thoroughly open the wound so that all infected tissue can be removed. One operation usually isn't sufficient to remove all the dead tissue. A second operation frequently is necessary. If the infection involves an arm or leg, amputation may even be necessary.

Gas gangrene

Gangrene is defined as death of infected tissue. Gas gangrene results when a wound becomes infected by a certain type of bacteria, usually clostridium bacteria.

The infection causes sudden pain and swelling around the wound, a moderate increase in temperature, a decrease in blood pressure and a rapid heartbeat.

Skin around the wound becomes pale due to fluid that builds up under it. A watery, foul-smelling, brownish-red fluid is released later. The tissue changes from pale to dusky to highly discolored as the infection worsens. Left untreated, stupor, delirium, coma and death can result.

Treatment of gas gangrene consists of penicillin given intravenously. Surgical removal of infected tissue is essential, and removal of surrounding tissue usually is necessary.

Cutaneous abscess

A cutaneous abscess resulting from a bacterial infection causes a pus-filled sore on the skin. Sometimes the lymph glands in the area become swollen, and you may have a fever.

Treatment consists of opening the infected area, thoroughly cleaning and irrigating the wound with saline, and packing it with gauze for 24 to 48 hours to absorb the pus and discharge. Application of heat and, if possible, elevating the affected area, may help relieve the inflammation. Your doctor may recommend antibiotics, sometimes administered initially via injection.

Insect and Mite Infestations

Small insects can sometimes attach themselves to your skin and feed on your blood. In the United States, these infestations are annoying but rarely dangerous. However, some insects do transmit viruses or bacteria that can cause serious illness in humans.

Lice

Signs and symptoms

- Intense itching
- Lice on the scalp, body, clothing, pubic hair or other body hair
- Nits (eggs) on hair shafts

Lice are tiny parasitic insects. Head lice (*Pediculus humanus capiti*) are often spread among schoolchildren by contact, clothing, combs or hairbrushes. Body lice (*P. h. corporis*) are generally spread through clothing or bedding. Pubic lice (*Phthirus pubis*), also known as crabs, can be spread by sexual contact, clothing, bedding or even toilet seats.

Diagnosis

The first sign of lice is intense itching of the affected area. People with body lice may develop hives or abrasions from scratching. Head

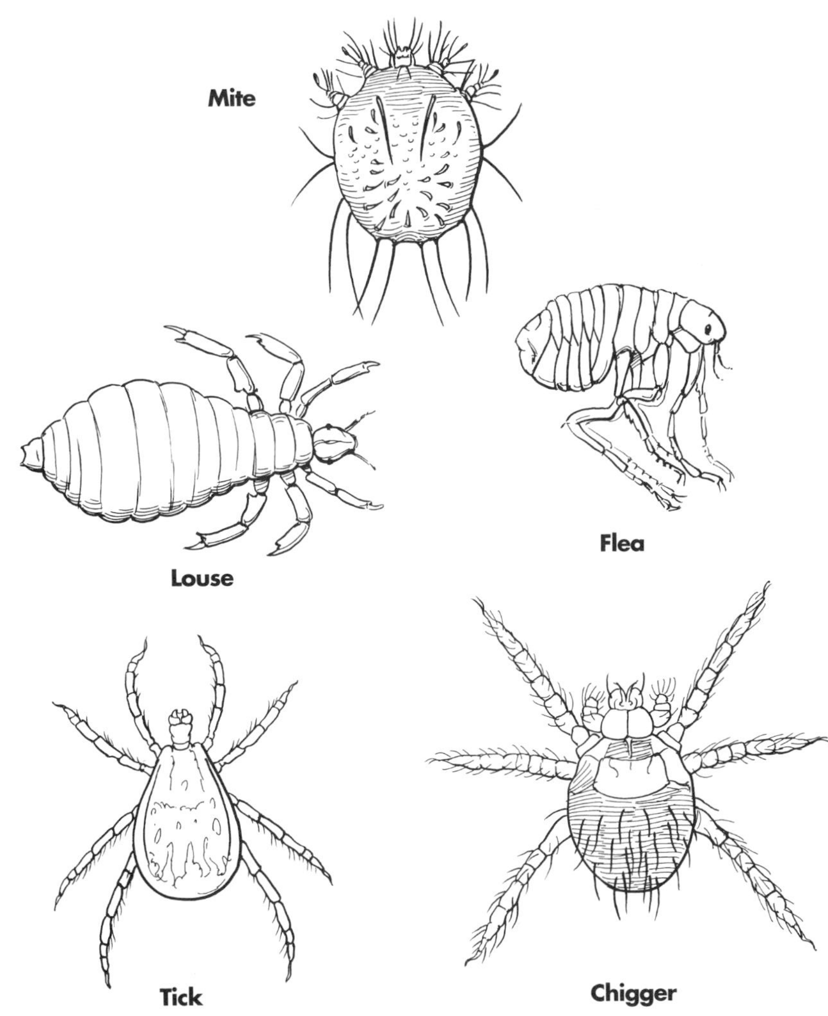

lice are found on the scalp and are easiest to detect at the nape of the neck and over the ears. Small nits that resemble tiny brown buds can be found on the hair shafts (see the color illustration on page 437). Body lice are difficult to find on the body because they burrow into the skin, but they usually can be detected in the seams of underwear. Pubic lice are found on the skin and hair of the pubic area. They can be annoying and are easily spread.

Treatment

Several lice-treating lotions and shampoos, both prescription and over-the-counter, are available. Examples include lindane (Bio-Well, Kwell, others) and permethrin (Acticin, Elimite) solution. Apply the product to all infected and hairy parts of the body.

After shampooing your hair, treat it with vinegar. Grasp a lock of hair with a cloth soaked in vinegar and strip the hair downward to remove any remaining nits. Repeat until you have treated all of your hair this way.

You can also remove the nits with a tweezers or fine comb. Your sexual partner should be examined and treated if infected. Children should be kept at home until at least one treatment has been applied. Sheets, combs, brushes and hats should be washed in hot, soapy water.

Scabies

Signs and symptoms

- Itching at night
- Thin, irregular marks on your skin

A scabies infection involves mites that are almost impossible to see without a magnifying glass. They cause severe itching, which is usually worse at night. Found worldwide among all groups of people and of all ages, scabies often infest an entire family. Scabies are spread by close physical contact and, less often, by sharing clothing or bedsheets with an infested person. Canine scabies can be transmitted from dogs to humans.

Diagnosis

The mites prefer to burrow into certain areas of the skin, such as between your fingers, in your armpits, around your waist, along the insides of your wrists, on the backs of your elbows, on your ankles and the soles of your feet, around the breasts and genitals and on your buttocks. They make a characteristic burrow that looks like a thin, irregular pencil mark (see the color illustration on page 437).

Your doctor may look for such a burrow and remove the mite located at the end of one to confirm the diagnosis. Although not serious, scabies are very annoying.

Treatment

Treatment involves eliminating the infestation. Several creams and lotions are available and are usually applied all over the body, from the neck down, and left on for 8 to 10 hours.

Two medications commonly used are 5 percent permethrin (Acticin, Elimite) cream or lindane (Bio-Well, Kwell, others). Your doctor will recommend the appropriate medication. Because of the high rate of infestation, it may be appropriate for all family members and sexual partners to be treated, even if no infestation is apparent.

Fleas

Signs and symptoms

- A localized rash
- Severe itching

Fleas are small insects that suck blood from dogs, cats, humans and other animals. By using their tremendous jumping ability, they often spread from family pets to their owners. Eggs laid in bedding hatch and remain there to feed off animals or humans.

Diagnosis

Fleabites cause intense itching. Clusters of bites can be seen around the waist, along the ankles, in the armpits and in the crooks of elbows and knees. Hives may develop in people who are especially sensitive to flea saliva. The surest way to diagnose flea infestation is by identifying the tiny insects themselves. In the United States, having fleas isn't serious, and you normally don't need to see your doctor if you have them. Nonetheless, they're annoying and should be eliminated to relieve symptoms.

Treatment

Calamine lotion may help to relieve the itching, but the problem will continue until the fleas are eliminated. Persistent treatment of animals and their living areas is necessary. Once fleas are established, getting rid of them is difficult, and just putting a flea collar on your pet isn't sufficient.

Various flea insecticides are available. Spray one of these on your pet's bedding, as well as on your own, if you suspect that fleas have established there. Furniture and carpeting also should be sprayed. Home foggers help eliminate the insects. However, be careful to remove other pets, such as birds and fish, because they're very sensitive to these insecticides. If you have a heavy infestation of fleas, or other treatments aren't effective, you may have to call a professional exterminator.

Chiggers

Signs and symptoms

- Intense itching
- Pimple-like bumps or hives

Chiggers, also known as redbugs or harvest mites, are the larvae of a type of mite. In North America, they're found primarily in the South but can be found as far north as Canada.

Chiggers live in areas of tall grass or brush and on the edges of woods. Farmers, hunters, hikers, and others who spend a lot of time in the woods are most likely to become infested.

Diagnosis

The larvae prefer warm, moist places and usually take up residence around your waist, on your ankles, in the crooks of your elbows and armpits, in the groin area and wherever clothing is tight. These small, red insects attach themselves to the skin and insert a feeding tube to reach a source of blood. This causes small, red pimples and sometimes hives. Several hours after they've inserted their feeding tube, you'll experience intense itching at the site.

Chiggers feed in the same spot for 1 to 4 days and then drop off. The best way to diagnose an infestation of chiggers is by identifying the mites. They can be found in the center of pimples that have not yet been scratched.

In the United States, chiggers don't cause any diseases but are annoying because of the intense itching.

Treatment

The aim of treatment is to relieve the itching. Your doctor may prescribe an antihistamine. Corticosteroid creams or lotions also can be applied directly to the pimples.

Ticks

Signs and symptoms

- Itching
- A tick embedded in your skin
- A small, hard lump surrounded by a red circle

Ticks are small, flat insects that feed on blood. They live in tall grasses, brush and wooded areas and attach to animals or people passing by.

Diagnosis

After walking through areas that might contain ticks, check to see if any have attached themselves to your skin or clothing. They can lodge anywhere but are often found in hair, around ankles and in the genital area. Once embedded, they can cause a small, hard, itchy lump surrounded by a red halo.

How serious is a tick bite?

A tick bite can be serious because ticks may be carriers of Lyme disease or Rocky Mountain spotted fever. A condition called tick paralysis may occur after a tick has fed on a person for several days. The condition can resemble poliomyelitis, a viral disease that affects your spinal cord. Tick paralysis can be very serious, but if the tick is removed, the symptoms usually disappear.

Treatment

Don't detach a tick from a pet with your bare hands because infection may result. Don't scratch a tick bite. If you do, the body of the insect may break off, leaving the head embedded in your skin. Treatment

Deer tick

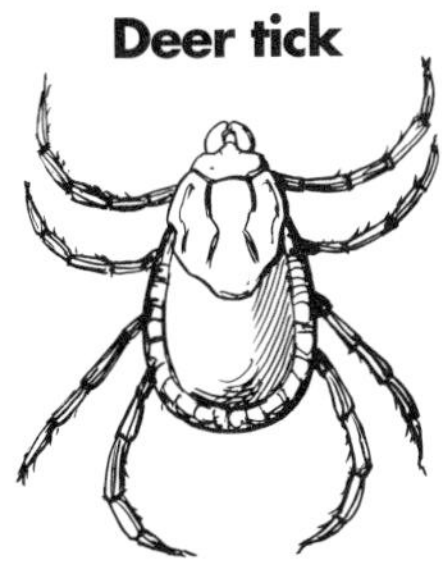

Actual size

Wood tick

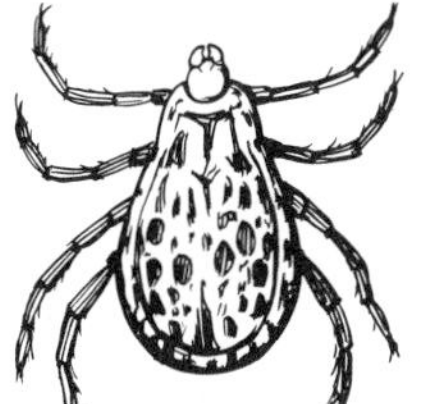

Actual size

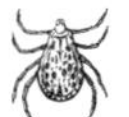

The deer tick and wood tick are two common ticks.

Tick-Transmitted Diseases

Although tick bites are usually harmless, they can at times pass on infectious organisms that cause serious illness. In addition to Lyme disease and Rocky Mountain spotted fever, ticks can transmit other less familiar diseases. The following diseases have a number of signs and symptoms in common, including chills, headache, fever, profuse sweating, muscle aches, nausea and weight loss. Antibiotics are generally the recommended treatment.

Human granulocytic ehrlichiosis

Signs and symptoms of human granulocytic ehrlichiosis generally develop about a week after the bite. In addition to the common tick-bite symptoms, diarrhea, altered mental state, rash and other problems also may develop later. In some cases, the condition can be fatal.

Human babesiosis

Human babesiosis is a rare disease that's most likely to occur in people who are beyond age 40 or who have a damaged spleen or no spleen. The infectious agent's incubation period can last weeks to months. It may be treated with antimalarial medications, such as quinine. Severe cases may require a blood transfusion.

Q fever

Q fever can be acquired by inhaling contaminated dust particles and drinking unpasteurized milk from infected farm animals. A vaccine is available for people who may be frequently exposed to the harmful organism causing the disease.

Tularemia

Tularemia can be acquired from tick bites or from eating improperly cooked meat or drinking contaminated water. Among reported cases in the United States, the death rate is less than 2 percent. It can be treated with intravenous (IV) antibiotics.

consists of gently — slowly and steadily — removing the tick using a tweezers. Place the tweezers as close to the head of the insect as possible (see page 386).

Lyme disease

Signs and symptoms

- A characteristic red rash at the site of a tick bite
- Headache
- Chills and fever
- Body aches
- Joint inflammation and arthritis

Named after a large outbreak among children in Lyme, Conn., this disease is caused by an organism (spirochete) that's transmitted by a species of very small ticks, called the deer tick. From May to October, this tick is found throughout the United States, especially on the East and West Coasts and in Wisconsin and Minnesota.

Diagnosis

Lyme disease is difficult to diagnose because it mimics several other diseases. A characteristic target-shaped red rash usually occurs at the site of the tick bite (see the color illustration on page 437), followed by headache, chills, fever, body aches and stiffness.

Sometimes, the bite may go entirely unnoticed. A few weeks to months later, the person who was bitten may experience facial paralysis, joint inflammation, various neurologic symptoms and sometimes heart palpitations and heart block, a condition where impulses are improperly conducted within the heart.

Your doctor may perform a blood test to check for antibodies to the organism. However, the test isn't always conclusive.

How serious is Lyme disease?

If detected in its early stages, the disease can be treated with medication. If not treated early, complications involving the joints, heart and central and peripheral nervous system can occur.

Treatment

Treatment consists of antibiotics, such as doxycycline or amoxicillin. Aspirin and other anti-inflammatory drugs may help to relieve joint inflammation.

Prevention

When walking in wooded or grassy areas, wear shoes, light-colored clothing, long pants tucked into your socks and long-sleeved shirts. Apply tick repellents to skin or clothing.

Check yourself and your pets often for ticks. If you find any, remove them by using a tweezers. Grasp the tick close to the head and pull directly outward. Don't yank or crush the tick. Pull carefully and steadily. If the tick has been attached for less than 24 hours, infection usually doesn't follow, but it's still a good idea to see your doctor.

Rocky Mountain spotted fever

Signs and symptoms

- Chills and fever
- Severe headache
- Widespread aches and pains
- Restlessness
- A red rash occurring between days 2 and 6 of fever

Rocky Mountain spotted fever, caused by the organism *Rickettsia rickettsii,* is transmitted to humans in the western United States by wood ticks and in the eastern United States by dog ticks. In the southern United States and Central and South America, the disease is transmitted by other types of ticks. In the United States, Rocky Mountain spotted fever occurs primarily during the late spring and early summer and is most common in the eastern part of the country.

Diagnosis

Three to 10 days after being bitten by an infected tick, you develop nausea, headache, loss of appetite and a sore throat. As the disease develops, fever, chills, tenderness and soreness in the bones and muscles, restlessness, insomnia, abdominal pain and vomiting occur. You may have a cough and, possibly, delirium, lethargy and stupor.

Between the second and sixth days of the fever, a red rash appears on your wrists and ankles. The rash spreads up your arms and legs to your chest. Your doctor may attempt to establish a diagnosis of the condition by doing a blood test or examining a specimen of the rash to search for the presence of the organism.

How serious is Rocky Mountain spotted fever?

A mild case of Rocky Mountain spotted fever that's treated promptly is fairly benign. Even without treatment, mild cases may disappear after 2 weeks. In a small percentage of infected people, the disease can be serious or even fatal, especially in older adults.

Treatment

The infection is treated with antibiotics. Prompt treatment is important because the disease can progress rapidly.

Parasitic Infestations

Parasites range from microscopic, single-celled organisms called protozoa to larger parasites called helminths. Protozoa often spend part of their life cycle outside of humans, living in food, soil, water or insects. The protozoan that causes malaria is a well-known example. Some types of protozoa are commonly present in your body but are kept under control by your immune system.

Tapeworms and roundworms are the most common types of helminths. If they enter your body, they may take up residence in your intestinal tract, lungs, liver, skin or brain, where they live off nutrients available at those sites.

Malaria

Signs and symptoms

- Sequential chills, fever and sweating
- Headache
- Muscle pains
- Anemia

Malaria is spread primarily by the female anopheles mosquito. It may also be transmitted through contaminated blood transfusions and by the sharing of contaminated needles. The disease is found primarily in the rural areas of tropical and subtropical countries. It's one of the leading infectious killers in the world, particularly of children.

Approximately 300 to 500 million cases of malaria occur worldwide each year, and more than 1 million people die of this disease annually. In the United States, about 1,200 cases are reported each year, primarily among people returning from areas where this genus of mosquito thrives.

The female mosquito becomes infected with the malarial parasite when it bites a human who has malaria and ingests blood containing the protozoa. After developing in the mosquito, the parasite is then transmitted to other humans by subsequent bites of the mosquito. In humans, the parasite migrates to the liver. Later it enters the bloodstream and infects red blood cells. The parasites multiply in the cells and, 48 to 72 hours later, depending on the species, cause the red blood cells to rupture, releasing a new generation of parasites.

Diagnosis

The symptoms of malaria relate closely to the parasite's life cycle. After an incubation period of anywhere from 8 days to 8 months, chills and fever begin, lasting 15 minutes to an hour, which correspond to the rupture of the red blood cells. Headache, vomiting and nausea also may occur. Fever remains high for several hours, and then sweating begins as body temperature falls. The cycle may recur every 48 to 72 hours, depending on the species of protozoan.

If you experience any of these signs and symptoms within a year of traveling to an area where malaria is present, see your doctor promptly. A blood smear can often identify the parasite. Because malaria infection is often initially thought to be a flu-like illness or some other viral disease, be wary if you develop an illness with fever within 12 months after traveling to a malaria area. Tell your doctor about your trip. A blood test can determine if you have the disease.

How serious is malaria?

Left untreated, some forms of malaria can be fatal. The disease may resolve after 6 to 8 months, but it can persist for up to 3 years or even longer with certain species. Malaria may cause miscarriage or stillbirth in pregnant women. Falciparum malaria, one of four types, can lead to death in a matter of hours after the first symptoms appear.

Treatment

Acute malaria is a serious illness that requires hospitalization. Antimalarial medications such as chloroquine (Aralen), quinine (Formula Q, Legatrim), primaquine and mefloquine (Lariam) are used to treat the infection. Resistance to the drugs is growing, however, and worldwide health programs are being initiated to develop more effective ways to treat the illness.

Prevention

There is no vaccine for malaria. However, many of the same drugs used to treat it are also effective preventive medications. In most countries of the world where malaria exists, resistance has developed to chloroquine. If you'll be traveling in malaria prone areas, your doctor may instead prescribe mefloquine, the antibiotic doxycycline or a newer combination antimalarial called Malarone. Start taking either of these medications 1 week before you leave home. Continue to take the medication while you're traveling and for 4 weeks after leaving the malaria prone area.

Discuss with your doctor possible reactions to mefloquine, such as nausea, dizziness, insomnia and vivid dreams. Also be sure to review with your doctor your past and current medical history for any indications that you shouldn't take this type of medicine. People with epilepsy or other seizure disorders shouldn't take mefloquine. Children under age 8 should avoid doxycycline, as it can permanently stain their teeth. Malarone shouldn't be taken by people with severe kidney impairment. The drugs that prevent malaria may cause miscarriage or stillbirth in pregnant women.

Take precautions in a malaria prone area to avoid being bitten by mosquitoes. Sleep under mosquito netting, stay in buildings with screens on doors and windows, stay indoors between dusk and dawn — times when the mosquitoes feed — and wear mosquito repellent.

Tapeworms

Signs and symptoms

- The presence of eggs in stool or worm segments in clothing, bedding or stool
- Hunger
- Dizziness
- Fatigue
- Loss of appetite and weight
- Vomiting
- Irritability

The tapeworms usually found in humans represent only six species. The beef tapeworm (the largest, can grow to 75 feet long), fish tapeworm and pork tapeworm are usually acquired by eating infected raw or undercooked beef, fish or pork, respectively.

The dwarf tapeworm is transmitted directly from one person to another. The rodent tapeworm, which is common in rats, is transmitted by accidentally swallowing infected rat fleas, beetles or

Tapeworm

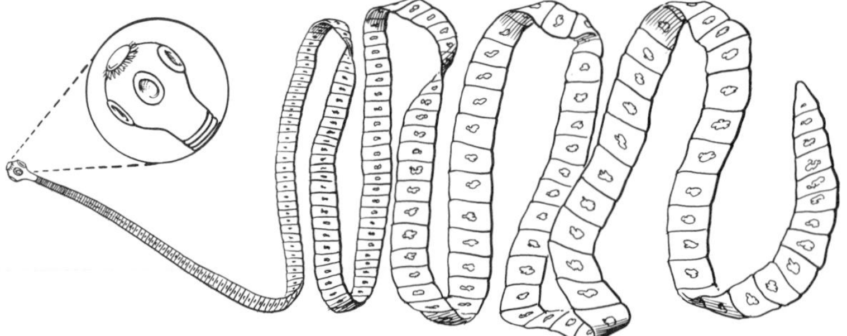

The largest species of tapeworm can grow up to 75 feet long.

cockroaches, usually after they've gotten into cereals or other stored foods.

The dog tapeworm is typically found in children who come into close contact with infested dogs or cats and have swallowed infected fleas or lice.

Diagnosis

Tapeworms usually cause few symptoms. The beef, pork and fish tapeworms may cause hunger, dizziness and fatigue. The three smaller tapeworms may cause loss of appetite, weight loss, vomiting and irritability — especially in children. In severe cases, nausea, diarrhea and abdominal pain may be present.

Tapeworms are usually discovered when eggs are found in the stool or worm segments are found in the stool, bedding or clothing. A doctor generally makes the diagnosis by obtaining eggs or segments and examining them under a microscope.

How serious is a tapeworm infestation?

Usually, the presence of tapeworms in the intestines isn't a serious situation. But some types of tapeworms can penetrate the intestinal wall and spread to various internal organs. The resulting condition may become very serious.

Treatment

Many prescription medications are available to treat tapeworm. A worm in the intestines usually begins to disintegrate after treatment and is passed out of the body within 24 to 48 hours.

It's generally assumed that the entire worm has been eliminated if no segments reappear after 3 to 5 months.

Trichinosis

Signs and symptoms

- Diarrhea and cramps
- Malaise
- Fever
- Muscle pain and tenderness
- Facial swelling

Trichinella spiralis lives in the intestines of most carnivores, including marine animals. The female worm releases larvae that enter muscles and form cysts. When the infected muscle is eaten, the cysts develop into a new generation of worms.

Humans usually get trichinosis from eating infected raw or undercooked pork or pork products or from eating beef that has been ground in a contaminated meat grinder or mixed with infected pork. The incidence of infection has been greatly decreased by public health measures, but meat from wild animals, especially bear, is still a source of infection.

Diagnosis

Two to 12 days after eating infected meat, you may experience diarrhea, abdominal cramps, and malaise lasting 1 to 7 days, although some people have no symptoms. When muscles are invaded by the larvae, muscle pain and tenderness, fever, swelling of the face, weakness, sensitivity to light and conjunctivitis may develop and last about 6 weeks. Your doctor may use a blood test and a muscle biopsy to diagnose trichinosis.

How serious is trichinosis?

Except in severe cases, trichinosis usually isn't serious and often gets better on its own.

Treatment

In most cases, treatment isn't necessary. Pain relievers may be given for muscle aches. An anthelmintic medication called albendazole (Albenza, Eskazole, Zentel) may be prescribed for intestinal infestation, but it's not effective if the worm has established itself in the muscle.

Prevention

Trichinosis is easily prevented by thoroughly cooking meat or freezing it at 5 F for 3 weeks.

Pinworms

Signs and symptoms

- Severe itching of the anal area at night
- Insomnia, irritability and restlessness
- Vague gastrointestinal symptoms

Humans are the only host of the pinworm, which lives in the large intestine of an infected person. At night, the female worm migrates out through the anus, lays large numbers of eggs and dies. After a few hours, the eggs can be spread to other individuals or can reinfect the host if they're transferred to the mouth by contaminated food, drinks or hands. After the eggs are swallowed, they hatch in the small intestine and migrate to the large intestine. The entire cycle takes 3 to 4 weeks, and the eggs are contagious for up to 2 to 3 weeks. Pinworms occur more frequently in children than in adults.

Diagnosis

The primary symptom is severe itching around the anus, particularly at night, although some peo-

Pinworm

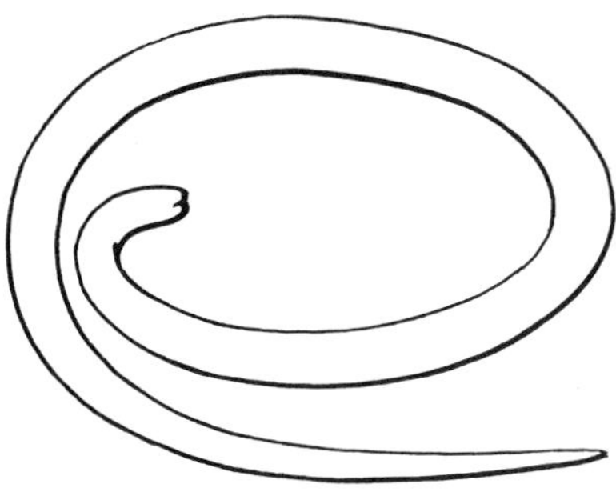

ple experience no noticeable symptoms. Pinworms are diagnosed by identifying eggs taken from the skin around the anal area. The most reliable method is to apply a short piece of cellophane tape to the area and take the tape to your doctor, who will put it on a slide for microscopic examination. Gather the tape sample in the morning before your child has defecated or bathed.

How serious is pinworm infestation?

A pinworm infestation is annoying, but it isn't serious. It's easily treated, but reinfection is common.

Treatment

People with pinworm symptoms — and often other members of the household — should be treated. Medications such as mebendazole (Vermox) are very effective. Try to avoid scratching the anal area and take special care to keep fingernails clean.

Make sure everyone in your family washes his or her hands after defecating, and wash bedding to help prevent spread of pinworms or recurrence of the infection.

Strongyloidosis

Signs and symptoms

- Small, sometimes itchy skin lesions
- Diarrhea, sometimes alternating with constipation
- Abdominal pain
- Gas (flatulence)

Strongyloidosis is caused by the small worm *Strongyloides stercoralis*. Also known as threadworm, it's found in many tropical and subtropical areas. Strongyloidosis sometimes occurs in temperate areas, including the United States. It's common in overcrowded, unsanitary conditions.

Diagnosis

The first sign of a strongyloidosis infestation is the appearance of small, red and sometimes itchy lesions caused by the larvae entering the skin. The larvae travel through the bloodstream to the lungs, from which they rise to the throat and are swallowed. They then inhabit the intestine and cause abdominal pain, flatulence and diarrhea, which sometimes alternates with constipation.

The abdominal pain is similar to the dull burning caused by an ulcer. Nausea, vomiting and loss of appetite also may occur. In severe cases, diarrhea is accompanied by blood and mucus. While they're in the lungs, the larvae may cause a dry cough, irritation of the throat, a low-grade fever and difficulty breathing. Determining the cause of the disease is difficult because of the wide variety of symptoms. Finding the larvae in stool or fluid from the small intestine confirms the diagnosis.

How serious is strongyloidosis?

Unless the infection is overwhelming, most people recover completely once the worms are eliminated.

Treatment

A strongyloidosis infection is treated with anthelmintics, medications used to treat worm infections.

Ascariasis

Signs and symptoms

- Vomiting, accompanied by stomach pain and bloating
- Wheezing, coughing and difficulty breathing

Ascaris lumbricoides is the largest of the roundworms and the most common intestinal worm. It's found wherever human feces are used as fertilizer or in places of poor hygiene. The worm affects only humans, and infestation is most severe in children. The eggs are found in the soil and enter humans who consume contaminated food or drink. After migrating to the lungs, the larvae rise to the mouth and are swallowed. Eventually, they take up residence in the small intestine, where they develop into an adult form that lives for a year or more.

Diagnosis

Examination of a stool sample for eggs or segments of the worm can confirm a diagnosis.

How serious is ascariasis?

Ascariasis generally isn't a serious condition and sometimes may get better without treatment. While in the lungs, however, the larvae cause wheezing, cough and difficulty breathing and can cause permanent damage. In the intestines, the adult worms cause vomiting, upper abdominal discomfort, distention and occasionally a bowel obstruction.

Treatment

Treatment consists of anthelmintics, medications that kill parasites.

Ascaris lumbricoides

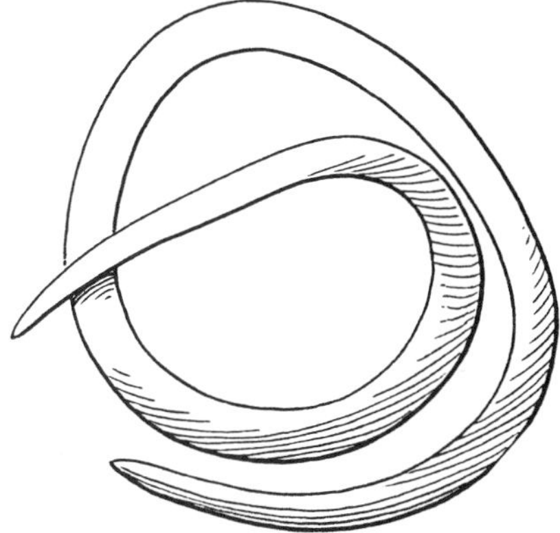

Ascaris lumbricoides is the largest of the roundworms, ranging in length from 6 to 14 inches.

Hookworms

Signs and symptoms

- A dry cough
- Difficulty breathing
- A low-grade fever
- Weakness and fatigue
- Loss of appetite
- Diarrhea
- Ulcer-like abdominal pain
- Pallor
- Blood-tinged sputum

Hookworm infections are widespread in tropical and subtropical areas. The larvae live in damp soil and can penetrate the skin between the toes, enter the bloodstream and proceed to the lungs.

From the lungs, the larvae go to the throat, are swallowed and attach to the lining of the small intestine, where they develop into half-inch-long adult worms. The disease may affect anyone, but children are particularly susceptible to severe infestations.

Diagnosis

At the spot where the hookworms enter the skin, the larvae cause an itchy rash called ground itch. When in the lungs, they provoke a dry cough, wheezing, difficulty breathing, a low-grade fever and sputum tinged with blood. Two weeks after entering the skin, they reach the intestines.

You may experience no symptoms, but in people with serious infestations or without adequate iron intake, the worms can cause a loss of appetite, bloody diarrhea, abdominal pain, weakness and fatigue, pallor and anemia. Finding microscopic hookworm eggs in the feces confirms the diagnosis.

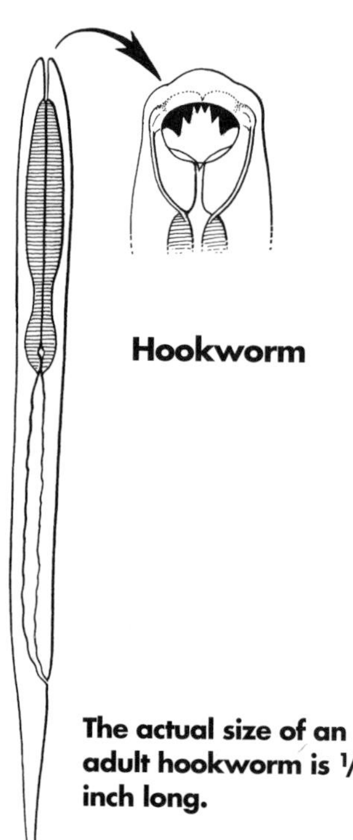

Hookworm

The actual size of an adult hookworm is ½ inch long.

How serious is hookworm infestation?

Because hookworms don't reproduce in humans, they die and disappear in 1 to 5 years, depending on the species. People with mild or severe cases usually recover completely if they're treated adequately and aren't reinfected.

Treatment

If you have no intestinal symptoms, treatment for hookworms is unnecessary. The worms eventually will be passed out of your system. If you have a heavy infestation, an antiparasitic medication is necessary. Several types of prescription medications are available. However, certain drugs shouldn't be used by pregnant women. If you're pregnant, be sure to tell your doctor. A diet high in protein, vitamins and iron supplements will prevent malnutrition and anemia until the infestation is eradicated.

Prevention

Toilet facilities that prevent fecal contamination of the soil will break the cycle of infection. In addition, always wear shoes when in contaminated areas.

Sexually Transmitted Diseases

Several bacterial and viral infections are sexually transmitted diseases (STDs), that is, they can be transmitted by sexual contact. Gonorrhea, chlamydia and syphilis are bacterial infections. Herpes and venereal warts are viral infections. Many other diseases also can be sexually transmitted, such as hepatitis (see page 903). In addition, the presence of STDs may facilitate the transmission of human immunodeficiency virus (HIV) infection.

Gonorrhea

Signs and symptoms

- Thick, pus-like discharge from the urethra
- Burning, frequent urination

Gonorrhea, caused by the bacterium *Neisseria gonorrhoeae,* is a common sexually transmitted disease (STD). In the United States, almost 500,000 cases of gonorrhea are reported each year. It's most common in people 15 to 29 years

The Importance of Safe Sex

The Centers for Disease Control and Prevention reports that approximately 15 million new cases of sexually transmitted diseases (STDs) occur each year in the United States. About half of these are lifelong infections. Although some sexually transmitted diseases, such as syphilis, are less common, epidemics of others, such as genital herpes, gonorrhea and chlamydia, continue to occur.

Many STDs are treatable, but some aren't and they can be fatal. AIDS, in particular, has no cure, and death will eventually occur in most cases.

For information on how to reduce your risk of acquiring a sexually transmitted disease, see Chapter 6, "Addressing Risky Behaviors."

old. It occurs in both men and women.

About half of infected women don't experience symptoms at all, which increases the risk of their spreading the disease. Homosexual men also may not have symptoms, especially when the infection affects the pharynx or rectum.

Diagnosis

In men, the first symptoms of gonorrhea generally appear between 2 days and 2 weeks after exposure to the bacteria. First you may experience a tingling sensation in the tube that carries urine from the bladder (urethra). A few hours later, urination becomes painful and a milky discharge is noted. As the infection progresses, urethral pain becomes more pronounced and large amounts of creamy, pus-like discharge are produced.

In women, symptoms may not appear for 1 to 3 weeks, if at all. The infection usually affects the cervix and other reproductive organs as well as the urethra. You may develop frequent, urgent and painful urination, and a pus-like discharge from the vagina or urethra.

In about 50 percent of women, the only symptoms are a slight increase in vaginal discharge and some inflammation, which may be evident only on pelvic examination. The symptoms are often so mild that many women don't realize they have the infection. In many cases, the only suggestion that a woman may have gonorrhea is the knowledge that someone with whom she has had sexual contact has the disease.

In both sexes, rectal gonorrhea may result from anal intercourse with an infected person or from the infection spreading to the rectum from the genital area. It may cause discomfort in the anal area and rectal discharge, but in many cases no symptoms are present. Oral sex can produce pharyngeal gonorrhea, resulting in a sore throat and painful swallowing. Again, many people have no symptoms. If the infection spreads to the eyes, it can cause a red, inflamed eye (conjunctivitis).

To confirm a diagnosis of gonorrhea, your doctor takes specimens of the discharge or infected tissue for laboratory examination. This must be done before antibiotics are taken. The symptoms of gonorrhea are similar to those of a number of other STDs, so it's important to know exactly what's causing them. Sometimes, more than one STD may be present, so if you have gonorrhea, a doctor usually does a blood test for syphilis too.

How serious is gonorrhea?

Gonorrhea is an acute infection that can become chronic if not treated. In men, gonorrhea may lead to epididymitis (see page 1117). In women, it can spread to the uterus and fallopian tubes, causing pelvic inflammatory disease. PID can result in scarring of the tubes and infertility.

Gonorrhea can also spread through the bloodstream to cause infection in other parts of the body. Fever, rash, joint pain and stiffness are possible. These complications can cause permanent joint damage. If treated appropriately, gonorrheal infections usually can be cured. However, several strains of gonococci are already resistant to many antibiotics.

Treatment

If you have gonorrhea, it's important that you abstain from sexual contact until your infection is completely eliminated. Your doctor will prescribe antibiotics to treat the infection. He or she may also recommend over-the-counter pain relievers.

General therapy for complications in men consists of hot sitz baths and, if epididymitis is present, bed rest, cold packs and immobilization. In women, infection of the fallopian tubes requires bed rest and possible surgical treatment if the infection doesn't clear. Your doctor will probably recommend follow-up testing to assure eradication of the infection.

Chlamydia

Signs and symptoms

- Painful urination
- In women, vaginal discharge
- In men, urethral discharge

Chlamydia is a genital infection in men and women that's caused by the bacterium *Chlamydia trachomatis,* which is transmitted by either vaginal or anal sex. Touching the eye with a hand that's moistened with infected secretions can cause a serious eye infection. *C. trachomatis* is the most common cause of blindness worldwide. It causes serious eye infections in children in many developing areas, including India, Africa and the Middle East. A mother can pass the infection to her newborn during delivery, causing pneumonia.

Diagnosis

Diagnosing genital chlamydial infection can be difficult because symptoms may be slight or nonexistent. When symptoms are present, they're similar to those of gonorrhea. In men, chlamydial infection may cause a burning sensation during urination and a discharge from the urethra. The symptoms are milder than those caused by gonorrhea and may appear 1 to 3 weeks after exposure. Women may have no symptoms, or they may experience burning urination, a thin vaginal discharge or lower abdominal pain. But many must rely on having their sexual partners inform them that they have the disease.

Tests for chlamydial infection involve identifying the bacteria in secretions from the cervix (in women) or from urethral or seminal fluid (in men).

How serious is chlamydia?

In men, chlamydial infections can cause epididymitis and inflammation of the urethra. In women, they cause urethral infection and inflammation of the cervix and other pelvic organs. If you engage in anal sex with an infected partner, the organism may cause inflammation of the rectum. In a newborn, conjunctivitis or pneumonia may occur during the first 2 weeks after birth.

Treatment

All of the sexual partners of an infected person must be treated, even if they have no symptoms. Otherwise they may pass the disease back and forth. With antibiotic treatment the infection should disappear within 1 to 2 weeks. If it doesn't, check again with your doctor. He or she may order additional laboratory tests to determine another treatment.

Syphilis

Signs and symptoms

Primary

- Painless sores on the genitals, rectum, tongue or lips
- Enlarged lymph nodes in the groin

Secondary

- A rash over any area of the body, but especially on the palms of the hands and soles of the feet
- Mouth sores
- Fever
- Headache
- Soreness and aching in the bones and joints

Tertiary

- Widespread infection affecting internal organs, including bones, heart, brain and spinal cord

Syphilis is a complex disease caused by the bacterium *Treponema pallidum.* Although once very prevalent, this disease has become less common among heterosexual people, compared with gonorrhea and chlamydia. But recently, the incidence of syphilis has increased in poor, urban areas of the United States and in people with AIDS. Usually transmitted by sexual contact, the organism gains entrance to the body through minor cuts or abrasions in the skin or mucous membranes. The disease can also be transmitted by infected blood and from a mother to her unborn child during pregnancy (congenital syphilis).

Diagnosis

Syphilis has three active stages. In the primary stage, sores appear on the genitals, the genital area, the rectum or the tongue and lips, 10 days to 6 weeks after exposure. Generally, these lesions are painless but are extremely infectious. Pain does occur if the sore becomes infected with other bacteria.

Your doctor also looks for swollen lymph nodes in the groin area. Sometimes, a rapid diagnosis can be made by microscopic examination of discharge from open sores. Your doctor can also use a blood test to check for the presence of the infection.

The second stage begins anywhere from a week to 6 months after the first stage. A red rash may appear on any surface of the body, including the palms of the hands and soles of the feet. You may also have flu-like symptoms — headache and aching in the bones and joints.

An intermediate period is called latent syphilis, during which no symptoms are present. During this time, syphilis can be detected by special blood tests. If the disease hasn't been treated adequately, the bacteria continue to spread and you may experience a relapse.

The last stage, known as tertiary syphilis, includes widespread infection, which is often serious. By this time, the bacteria have spread throughout the body and may affect any of the internal organs, including your bones, heart, brain and spinal cord. Examination of your spinal fluid may be necessary to determine whether the nervous system is involved.

How serious is syphilis?

Syphilis can be cured if the diagnosis is made early and the infection is treated appropriately. However, if it's not treated, the disease can be fatal. If a woman contracts the disease while she's pregnant, it can be transmitted to her unborn child, causing deformities or death of the child.

Treatment

Antibiotics are often successful in treating the primary and secondary stages of syphilis. Penicillin is highly effective in treating syphilis. If you're sensitive to penicillin, your doctor will prescribe another type of antibiotic.

The disease is very contagious during both of these stages, especially the secondary. If you have syphilis, don't engage in sexual contact until at least two blood tests after your antibiotic treatment indicate that the infection has been eliminated. There's no vaccine against syphilis. Follow-up blood tests are required at regular intervals for at least 1 year to monitor response to treatment.

Genital herpes

Signs and symptoms

- Pain or itching in the genital area
- Water blisters or open sores

Herpes is caused by the herpes simplex virus (HSV). There are two types — oral (see page 1191) and genital. That which affects the mouth and lips, causing a cold sore, generally stems from herpes simplex virus type 1 (HSV-1). That which affects the genital area is typically caused by herpes simplex virus type 2 (HSV-2). Genital herpes may be transmitted by vaginal or anal sex. The virus enters the body through tiny cuts in the skin or mucous membranes. It can infect the eyes by contact with a contaminated finger. It affects both men and women.

Diagnosis

The initial symptom of HSV-2 is pain or itching of the skin covering the genital area. This stage is known as the prodromal period and begins 2 to 7 days after exposure to the virus. Anywhere from a few hours to several days after this prodromal stage, sores begin to appear.

In women, they may erupt in the vaginal area, external genitals, buttocks and anus. In men, they're generally on the penis, scrotum, buttocks, anus and thighs (see the color illustration on page 438). Sores may be present but invisible inside the cervix, for women, and the urethra of men.

While the sores are present, it may be painful to urinate. They generally begin as small, tender, red bumps and become watery blisters within a few days. Then they rupture, becoming ulcers that ooze or bleed. After 3 to 4 days, scabs form and the ulcers heal. You may experience pain and tenderness in the genital area until the infection clears. During the very first outbreak, you may experience flu-like signs and symptoms, such as headache and fever, as well as swollen lymph nodes in the groin.

Your doctor can confirm a diagnosis of herpes by growing (culturing) swab samples of the water blisters or early ulcers. A thorough examination for other sexually related diseases is important. Often, at least one other sexually transmitted disease is present in addition to herpes.

How serious is genital herpes?

Herpes has no cure or vaccine. The virus remains dormant in the infected areas and periodically reactivates, causing symptoms. The disease is very contagious whenever sores are present.

Besides the sores, herpes generally doesn't cause any other serious permanent complications in adults. However, infants can become infected as they pass through the birth canal of mothers with open sores, which may result in brain damage, blindness and death. This infection is more common in infants of mothers who are having their first outbreak of active herpes infection at the time of delivery. The rate of herpes infection in newborns is increasing as the rate of genital herpes in women increases.

Treatment

Because herpes can't be cured, treatment consists of controlling symptoms and trying to keep the infection from reactivating. During the initial outbreak, antiviral drugs such as acyclovir (Alti-Acyclovir, Zovirax) and famciclovir (Famvir) in oral form help speed healing. This initial treatment doesn't prevent recurrences. If recurrences are frequent, acyclovir can be taken daily to suppress the herpes virus. Topical treatment consists of keeping the sores clean and dry.

Prevention

Herpes is very contagious when sores are present. If you have herpes and sores are present, abstain from sexual contact until they're completely healed. If you don't have herpes, using a condom during sexual intercourse may reduce the risk of acquiring the infection. If you're sexually active, a monogamous sexual relationship with an uninfected partner is the surest way of avoiding the disease.

Venereal warts

Signs and symptoms

- Wart-like growths on the genitals

Venereal warts, also called genital warts, are caused by the human papillomavirus (HPV). Venereal warts affect both men and women and are easily transmitted through sexual contact. People with an impaired immune system and pregnant women are even more susceptible.

Diagnosis

Venereal warts may be similar to common skin warts in appearance. They may develop from 3 weeks to 3 months after exposure to the virus. In men, they usually appear near the tip or on the shaft of the penis and sometimes on the scrotum. In women, they may appear on the vaginal lips, inside the vagina, on the cervix or around the anus. HPV can also cause lesions on the cervix.

Often, a doctor can diagnose venereal warts simply by physical examination.

How serious are venereal warts?

Venereal warts generally aren't life-threatening, although they are contagious. Women with cervical lesions caused by HPV have a higher risk of cervical cancer. Women with such lesions should have a Pap test each year.

Treatment

All of the sexual partners of an infected person must be treated, and all of the warts must be removed. Medications applied directly to the warts may be helpful. A procedure involving freezing of wart tissues (cryosurgery) may be used. Other options for removal of large venereal warts include use of a laser or a procedure called electrodesiccation, in which electrical current is used to destroy wart tissue, followed by removal of the wart at its base. These treatments may require local or general anesthesia. Regardless of the treatment, venereal warts tend to recur frequently.

HIV and AIDS

Acquired immunodeficiency syndrome (AIDS) is a chronic condition affecting the immune system caused by human immunodeficiency virus (HIV). The virus causes a progressive weakening of the immune system.

By damaging or destroying the cells of your immune system, HIV interferes with your body's ability to effectively fight off viruses, bacteria and fungi that cause disease. This weakening also makes you more susceptible to infections that your body would normally resist, such as some types of pneumonia, meningitis and cancer.

Infection with the virus is known as an HIV infection. The term *AIDS* denotes the late stages of HIV infection. In everyday language, though, both terms are used to refer to the same disease.

HIV and the immune system

When your immune system is healthy, specialized white blood cells (lymphocytes) and antibodies help to resist germs to keep you free from disease. When most unwanted organisms enter your body, they're attacked and destroyed. This response is coordinated by a type of lymphocyte known as helper T cell.

When HIV enters your body, it can't live on its own. It must take over another living (host) cell to survive. HIV enters helper T cells by attaching to a protein on the surface of the cells called CD4 — thus the name CD4 cells for helper T cells. Once inside the CD4 cells, the virus inserts its own genetic material into the cells and uses them to make copies of itself.

When the newly formed viruses burst out of the host cells, they find other cells to attack. In the meantime, the old host cells die. The cycle repeats itself again and again. In the process, more than 10 billion new HIV particles can be produced every day. Your immune system tries to overcome this massive infection by producing antibodies and forming more helper T cells, turning out as many as 2 billion new CD4 cells daily.

Ultimately, the virus wins the race. The number of CD4 cells your body can produce progressively decreases, and you develop a severe immune deficiency. Your body is no longer able to effectively fight off infection.

A global problem

In nearly two decades — since the first reports of the disease — HIV infection has become a global epidemic, affecting more than 36 million people in more than 190 countries. Since the epidemic began, 21.8 million people have died of AIDS, including 4.3 million children. According to the United Nations Program on HIV/AIDS (UNAIDS) and the World Health Organization (WHO), 5.3 million new HIV infections occurred during the year 2000, and AIDS-related deaths reached a high of 3 million.

Sub-Saharan Africa continues to be the world's most affected region, accounting for approximately 70 percent of all AIDS cases reported worldwide. According to UNAIDS 2000 estimates, the total number of people currently living with HIV in this region is over 25 million. At the same time, almost 2.5 million people died of AIDS in Africa, up from 2.2 million in 1999. A new epidemic is taking place in Eastern Europe, where 700,000 people are now living with HIV, compared with 420,000 in 1999.

In Asia, an estimated 6.4 million people have HIV and AIDS, with 700,000 new cases in south and southeast Asia in 2000. In Latin America and the Caribbean, approximately 210,000 adults and children became infected during this same year, leading to a total of 1.8 million people with the disease in that area.

In the United States, approximately 900,000 people are living with HIV and AIDS. More than 438,000 AIDS-related deaths have been reported to the Centers for Disease Control and Prevention since the beginning of the epidemic.

In the past few years, the AIDS epidemic in the United States has changed — it now affects mainly minority communities, particularly blacks and Hispanics.

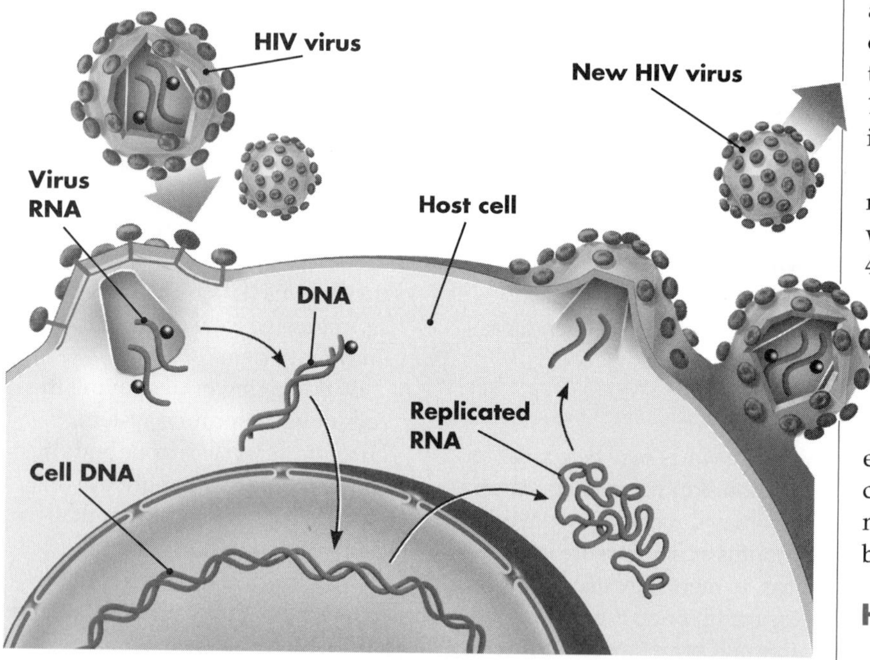

Human immunodeficiency virus (HIV) belongs to a family of viruses called retroviruses. These viruses carry their genetic information on single-stranded ribonucleic acid (RNA). Once inside a host cell, HIV uses an enzyme called reverse transcriptase to convert its RNA into double-stranded deoxyribonucleic acid (DNA). The viral DNA enters the nucleus and is inserted into the host cell's DNA. After this, HIV is able to reproduce (replicate) itself. When the cell bursts, the replicated viruses are released.

How do you get HIV?

You can be infected with HIV in the following ways:

Sexual activity

You may become infected if you have vaginal, anal or oral sex with an infected partner and his or her blood, semen or vaginal secretions enter your body. You can also become infected from shared sexual devices if they're not washed or covered with a condom. The virus is present in the semen or vaginal secretions of someone who's infected. It enters your body through small tears that can develop in your rectum or vagina during sexual activity.

If you already have another sexually transmitted disease, you're at much greater risk of contracting HIV. Contrary to what researchers once believed, women who use the spermicide nonoxynol-9 also may be at higher risk of acquiring HIV infection. This spermicide irritates the lining of your vagina and may cause tears that allow the virus into your body.

Infected blood

In some instances, the virus may be transmitted through blood and blood products — including whole blood, packed red cells, fresh-frozen plasma and platelets — that you receive in blood or blood-product transfusions.

In 1985, American hospitals and blood banks began screening the blood supply for HIV antibodies. This testing, along with improvements in donor screening and recruitment practices, has substantially reduced the risk of acquiring HIV through transfusions.

Currently, the chance of transfusion-associated HIV transmission in the United States is about 1 in every 450,000 to 1 in every 600,000 transfusions.

Needle sharing

HIV is easily transmitted through needles and syringes contaminated with infected blood. That's why sharing intravenous drug paraphernalia puts you at high risk of HIV, as well as infectious diseases such as hepatitis. Your risk is increased if you inject illicit drugs frequently or also engage in high-risk sexual behavior.

Avoiding the use of injected illegal drugs is the most reliable way to prevent infection. If this isn't an option for you, one way to reduce your risk is to use household bleach to sterilize injection paraphernalia. Another option is to participate in a needle exchange program in your community. Such programs allow you to exchange used needles and syringes for sterile equipment. Finally — and most importantly — consider seeking counseling or other treatment for your drug abuse problem.

Accidental needle sticks

Transmission of the virus between HIV-infected patients and health care workers through needle sticks and cuts is low. Over 99 percent of needle sticks or cut exposures don't lead to infection.

Transmission from mother to child

Between one-quarter and one-third of untreated pregnant women infected with HIV pass the infection to their babies. Among women who receive treatment for their HIV infection during pregnancy, the risk to their babies decreases by as much as two-thirds.

Other routes

In very rare cases, the virus may be transmitted through organ or tissue transplants or unsterilized dental or surgical equipment.

How HIV Is *Not* Transmitted

There are many myths regarding human immunodeficiency virus (HIV) transmission. You *can't* become infected through ordinary contact, such as hugging, dancing or shaking hands, with someone who has HIV or AIDS. And you *can't* be infected in any of the following ways:

- Coming into contact with the sweat or tears of someone with HIV or AIDS.
- Sharing food, utensils, towels, bedding, a swimming pool, a telephone or a toilet seat with someone who has the virus.
- Being bitten by bedbugs or mosquitoes.
- Kissing someone who's HIV-positive or who has AIDS. There's no evidence that the virus is transmitted through kissing. Although HIV is sometimes found in the saliva of people with the virus, it occurs in low concentrations. In addition, natural inhibitory substances in saliva help prevent the virus from being transmitted.
- Donating blood. Donation centers use new, sterilized needles for each person donating blood. They also employ screening methods to test donated blood for disease-causing agents.

Signs and symptoms

The signs and symptoms of HIV and AIDS vary, depending on the phase of the infection.

Early infection

When first infected with HIV, you may have no symptoms. It's common to develop a brief flu-like illness 2 to 6 weeks after being infected. But because the symptoms of an initial infection are similar to those of other diseases, you might not suspect you have HIV.

Even if you don't have symptoms, you can transmit the virus to others. Once the virus enters your body, your own immune system also comes under attack. The virus multiplies in your lymph nodes and slowly begins to destroy your helper T (CD4) cells.

You may stay symptom-free for as long as 8 or 9 years. But the virus continues to multiply and destroy immune cells. Tests are likely to show a sharp decline in the number of these cells in your blood. Eventually, you may develop mild infections or these chronic signs and symptoms:

- Swollen lymph nodes
- Diarrhea
- Weight loss
- Fever
- Cough
- Shortness of breath

Late infection

During the last phase of HIV, which occurs approximately 10 to 11 years after the initial infection, these more serious signs and symptoms may appear:

- Soaking night sweats
- Shaking chills or fever higher than 100 F for several weeks
- Dry cough
- Shortness of breath
- Chronic diarrhea
- Persistent white spots or unusual lesions on your tongue or in your mouth
- Headache
- Blurred and distorted vision
- Weight loss
- Persistent, unexplained fatigue
- Swelling of lymph nodes for more than 3 months

At its late stage, the infection may meet the official definition of AIDS — a positive HIV-antibody test plus at least one of the following:

- Development of an opportunistic infection, such as *Pneumocystis carinii* pneumonia (PCP). Healthy people normally can resist this lung infection. But in people with weakened immune systems, the organism can multiply in the lungs and cause difficulty breathing. Children are susceptible to the same opportunistic infections as adults and may have severe forms of common childhood illnesses, such as ear infections (otitis media), pneumonia and tonsillitis.
- A CD4 cell count of 200 per microliter of blood or less. A normal CD4 count ranges from 600 to 1,000 cells. Some people with a count of less than 200 still don't look sick. However, the low count is an indication that the individual's immune system is failing. The disease AIDS doesn't occur immediately after an individual becomes infected with HIV. In fact, the average time between exposure to HIV and development of AIDS is typically 10 to 12 years.

Are You at Risk?

The human immunodeficiency virus (HIV) crosses all cultures, national borders and religions. Anyone, of any age, race, sex or sexual orientation, can become infected. But you're at greatest risk of HIV and AIDS if you:

- Have unprotected sex with multiple partners. Unprotected sex means having sex without using a new, latex or polyurethane condom every time.
- Have unprotected sex with someone who's HIV-positive.
- Have another sexually transmitted disease, such as syphilis, herpes, chlamydia or gonorrhea.
- Share needles during intravenous drug use.
- Have hemophilia and received blood products between 1977 and April 1985, before standard testing of blood products for HIV began.
- Received a blood transfusion or blood products before 1985.

Newborns or nursing infants whose mothers have tested positive for HIV also are at high risk.

Testing and diagnosis

Diagnosis of HIV generally begins with a blood test to check for the presence of antibodies to the virus. This test is most accurate 3 to 6 months after a person suspects he or she was exposed to HIV. An HIV test isn't accurate soon after exposure because it takes time for your body to produce the antibodies. The time between exposure to HIV and a positive HIV-antibody test is called the window period. Most often it's 6 to 12 weeks.

HIV-antibody testing may involve a combination of procedures. Most blood is first tested with an antibody screening test. If this detects HIV antibodies, the test is repeated. If the second test also shows antibodies, a confirming test, known as the Western blot, is done. The combination of these testing methods makes identification of HIV antibodies nearly 100 percent accurate.

Testing for HIV and AIDS can be done on an anonymous or confidential basis. Confidential testing means that your results will be recorded, but no one can give them out without your permission, except where required by law. Anonymous testing means that your name is not recorded and only you can learn the results of your test.

If you test positive for HIV, it's vital that you tell your sexual partner or partners promptly so that they can be screened and take steps to protect themselves. If you're pregnant, use of specific medications during your pregnancy can greatly reduce the chances that you'll pass the infection to your baby.

Complications

HIV infection weakens your immune system, making you highly susceptible to a large number of bacteria, viruses, fungi and parasites. You may also be more vulnerable to certain types of cancers. Treatment with antiretroviral drugs can markedly decrease risk of these conditions.

Bacterial infections

A number of bacterial infections may occur:

Bacillary angiomatosis

Bacillary angiomatosis is rarely seen in people who don't have HIV. This bacterial infection first appears as purplish to bright red patches on your skin. Often, it resembles the rash that occurs with a type of cancer called Kaposi's sarcoma. It can also cause disease in other parts of your body, including your liver and spleen.

Mycobacterium avium complex

Mycobacterium avium complex (MAC) is an infection caused by a group of bacteria. Normally, these bacteria cause an infection of the respiratory tract. But if you have advanced HIV infection and your CD4 lymphocyte count is extremely low, you're more likely to develop a systemic infection that can affect almost any internal organ, including your bone marrow, liver and spleen.

Salmonellosis

Salmonellosis is a bacterial infection that's transmitted through contaminated food or water. Although anyone exposed to salmonella bacteria can become sick, salmonellosis is 20 times more common in HIV-positive people. Proper hand washing and careful food handling can reduce risk of this illness.

Tuberculosis

Worldwide, tuberculosis (TB) is the most common opportunistic infection that affects individuals with HIV. It can strike people with HIV no matter what their CD4 cell level is. If you find out that you're HIV-positive, you'll need a skin test for TB early on. If the test is positive, you'll need a chest X-ray and other tests to make sure that you don't have an active infection. If you have inactive TB, your doctor will give you treatments to help prevent it from becoming active in the future.

Viral infections

Infections that may stem from other viruses include:

Cytomegalovirus

Cytomegalovirus is a common virus transmitted in body fluids such as saliva, blood, urine, semen and breast milk. A healthy immune system inactivates the virus, and it remains dormant in your body. If your immune system is impaired, the virus may resurface and cause damage to your eyes, digestive tract, lungs and other organs.

Herpes simplex virus

The herpes simplex virus that usually causes genital herpes (HSV-2) may be transmitted during unprotected anal or vaginal sex. If you have HIV, your skin infection resulting from the disease is likely to be more severe than in people who don't have HIV, and the sores may take longer to heal.

Human papillomavirus

Individuals with HIV are particularly susceptible to human papillomavirus (HPV) infection and more prone to recurrent infections. HPV puts women at risk of cervical cancer and both men and women at risk of anal cancer. About half of all women with HPV have no symptoms. Most doctors recommend that you have an annual pelvic exam and Pap test to check for cervical cancer, HPV and other sexually transmitted diseases.

Progressive multifocal leukoencephalopathy

Progressive multifocal leukoencephalopathy (PML) is an extremely serious brain infection. Signs and symptoms vary and may include speech problems, weakness on one side of the body, partial loss of vision or numbness in one arm or leg. PML usually occurs only when your immune system has been severely damaged.

Viral hepatitis

Viral hepatitis causes inflammation of the liver. There are several types of viral hepatitis. Among individuals with HIV who develop hepatitis, HIV may progress more rapidly. These individuals are also more likely to develop liver toxicity from their medications.

Fungal infections

Fungal infections include:

Candidiasis

Candidiasis is a common HIV-related infection. It causes inflammation and a thick, white coating on the mucous membranes of your mouth, tongue (thrush), esophagus (Candida esophagitis) or vagina.

Cryptococcal meningitis

Meningitis is an inflammation of the membranes surrounding your brain and spinal cord (meninges). Cryptococcal meningitis, the most common central nervous system infection associated with HIV, is caused by a fungus present in soil. With early treatment, cryptococcal meningitis can be successfully treated with medication.

Pneumocystis carinii pneumonia

Pneumocystis carinii pneumonia (PCP) is a common infection among individuals with AIDS. It's caused by a microorganism that occurs naturally in the lungs of people and animals.

In healthy people, it doesn't cause disease, but it can lead to illness in someone with an impaired immune system. PCP is the leading cause of death in children with HIV. Fortunately, in recent years antiretroviral medications that boost the immune system have helped reduce the number of people who get this serious disease.

Parasitic infections

Parasitic infections are common complications of an HIV infection. They include:

Cryptosporidiosis

Cryptosporidiosis is an infection caused by an intestinal parasite commonly found in animals. It's generally acquired by ingesting contaminated food or water. The parasite grows in the intestines and bile ducts and causes severe, chronic diarrhea.

Toxoplasmosis

Toxoplasmosis is the most common cause of brain lesions in people with advanced HIV. It's caused by a parasite found primarily in cat feces or raw or undercooked meat, especially pork, lamb and venison. Once you're infected with these parasites, they can spread throughout your body, including to your heart, eyes and lungs.

Cancers

HIV increases the risk of the following cancers:

Kaposi's sarcoma

Kaposi's sarcoma is a tumor of the blood vessel walls. It's the most common cancer in people with HIV infection and is rare in people not infected with HIV.

This cancer usually appears as pink, red or purple lesions on your skin and in your mouth. In people with darker skin, the lesions may look dark brown or black. Kaposi's sarcoma can also affect your internal organs, including your digestive tract and lungs.

Non-Hodgkin's lymphoma

Non-Hodgkin's lymphoma is a cancer that originates in a type of white blood cell (lymphocyte). Although lymphomas can start in other organs, they usually begin in your lymph nodes. The most common early sign is painless swelling of the lymph nodes in your neck, armpit or groin.

Treatment

A panel of leading AIDS specialists has developed a set of guidelines for treatment of individuals with HIV. These guidelines are regularly refined and updated. Treatment generally focuses on achieving the maximum suppression of viral replication for as long as possible while maintaining an acceptable quality of life.

This aggressive approach is known as highly active antiretroviral therapy (HAART). Its aim is to reduce the amount of the HIV virus in blood to very low, or even nondetectable, levels. However, the virus never disappears entirely. This is usually accomplished with a combination of three or more drugs.

If you have HIV, it's important to choose a doctor who's both supportive and experienced in the management of HIV infection. Your doctor monitors your immune system and assesses your general health at regular intervals to evaluate the status of your disease and to determine whether additional action is required.

It's also important that you take an active role in treatment decisions. If you and your doctor discuss the risks and benefits associated with various therapies, you can make informed choices.

Medication

Since 1995, the number of medications available to treat HIV and AIDS has more than tripled. Powerful combinations of newer antiretroviral drugs have helped reduce serious complications of the disease and prolong life.

Antiretroviral drugs

The most effective medications for HIV and AIDS are antiretroviral drugs. These drugs attack the virus itself. They're designed to interfere with the growth and replication of HIV at various stages of its life cycle, prolonging survival of people with HIV infection.

If you're receiving antiretroviral drugs, your response to the treatment is measured by the levels of HIV in your blood (viral load). These levels should be tested at the start of treatment and then every 3 to 4 months while you're on therapy. Some people are tested more often.

- *NRTIs.* The earliest antiretroviral drugs are known as nucleoside analogue reverse transcriptase inhibitors (NRTIs). They act by incorporating themselves into the DNA of the virus and blocking an enzyme called reverse transcriptase, which HIV needs to replicate.

  NRTIs include zidovudine (Novo-AZT, Retrovir), lamivudine (Epivir, 3TC), didanosine (ddI, Videx), zalcitabine (ddC, Hivid), stavudine (d4T, Zerit) and abacavir (Ziagen).
- *NNRTIs.* Non-nucleoside reverse transcriptase inhibitors (NNRTIs) inhibit the reverse transcriptase enzyme as well, but they do so by binding directly to the enzyme. NNRTIs include nevirapine (Viramune), delavirdine (Rescriptor) and efavirenz (Sustiva).
- *Protease inhibitors.* Another class of medications is called protease inhibitors because they inhibit replication of HIV protease, a different enzyme needed for formation and assembly of HIV proteins. Inhibition of this enzyme causes HIV particles to become structurally disorganized and

noninfectious. Examples include saquinavir (Fortovase, Invirase), ritonavir (Norvir), indinavir (Crixivan), nelfinavir (Viracept), amprenavir (Agenerase) and lopinavir (Kaletra).

Medications for opportunistic infections

If you have an accompanying infection, your doctor may recommend other medications, such as antibiotics, to treat the infection. Some opportunistic infections may also be prevented with medication.

Self-care

To reduce your risk of additional infections and to keep your immune system as healthy as possible, practice good hygiene, eat well and exercise as able. One of the most crucial aspects of HIV and AIDS treatment is emotional support. Seek support from health professionals, family and friends in dealing with your illness and its treatment.

Prevention

A vaccine for HIV and AIDS is being pursued. Unfortunately, certain characteristics of HIV make a vaccine difficult to develop. HIV lives in cells, multiplies in great numbers and mutates rapidly — it creates slightly different versions of itself. For now, the best way to fight HIV is through education, awareness and avoidance of behaviors that may transmit HIV.

Emerging Diseases

Infectious agents can be powerful organisms. Even as we conquer one infectious disease, a new one emerges or an old one resurfaces. This is not new. Germs have traveled for centuries, carried around the globe by rodents, fleas, insects, birds and humans. Sadly, as they spread from one area to another, they can wreak havoc within human lives, causing epidemics of diseases such as bubonic plague, smallpox and now AIDS.

Environmental factors also can influence emergence of disease. Floods may carry disease-causing organisms. Weather changes may create an environment that promotes the increase of disease carriers, such as rodents. Suburbs in wooded areas provide more exposure to infected ticks and other insects.

Germs also have the capability of changing themselves. Bacteria and viruses frequently mutate into new variants. They can become not only more virulent but also resistant to drugs and medications used to combat them.

The following section discusses a few of the infectious diseases that have recently emerged or re-emerged. The diseases aren't necessarily new or common. Rather, they've reminded us that — in spite of all our knowledge of medicine and technology — the fight against disease is never really over.

Anthrax

Signs and symptoms

The signs and symptoms of anthrax vary according to type:

- A raised, itchy bump that develops into an open sore with a black center
- Nausea and vomiting
- Loss of appetite
- Fever
- Abdominal pain
- Bloody diarrhea
- A sore throat
- Muscle aches
- Chest discomfort and difficulty breathing

Anthrax infection is caused by the bacterium *Bacillus anthracis*. The disease usually affects livestock, but it can also occur in humans. Anthrax was once common in areas where livestock was raised, but animal vaccination programs have greatly reduced the natural occurrence of the disease among animals and humans.

Anthrax has renewed importance because of its use as a biological weapon. The anthrax bacillus is commonly used in research, and it generally isn't difficult to obtain and grow. It's also highly lethal. However, making enough anthrax spores in a form that can cause widespread damage (aerosolized) is much more difficult than growing a lab culture and is dangerous to those working with it.

In addition, the release of anthrax spores could be difficult to control once deployed because of the wind, making anthrax a less effective weapon of mass destruction. Refined anthrax spores form a fine, white dust. Crude preparations have a brownish sand-colored tint and are clumpier.

There are three forms of the infection — skin (cutaneous) anthrax, intestinal anthrax, which is contracted from eating infected meat, and inhalation anthrax, the deadliest form.

Skin anthrax

Skin anthrax occurs when a cut, blister or other skin wound comes into contact with anthrax spores. The infection usually becomes apparent within 7 to 12 days of the exposure. It begins as a raised, sometimes itchy bump. Within 1 or 2 days, it develops into an open sore with a black center.

Intestinal anthrax

Intestinal anthrax results when a person eats undercooked meat from an infected animal. It causes sores (ulcers) within the intestines.

The first signs and symptoms generally show up a day to a week after eating contaminated meat. They may include nausea and vomiting, fever and loss of appetite, followed by abdominal pain and bloody diarrhea.

Inhalation anthrax

Inhalation anthrax occurs if enough anthrax spores are inhaled. Once inhaled, the spores can take anywhere from a day to 2 months to become active.

Initial signs and symptoms are similar to those of the flu or a cold and may include a sore throat, fever, fatigue, muscle aches and chest discomfort. These may last a few hours or a few days. Within 3 days of onset, the disease progresses, producing high fever and breathing problems. This type of anthrax destroys lung tissue and may spread to the brain, causing meningitis.

Diagnosis

Tests to detect the presence of anthrax bacteria include skin biopsy, sputum tests and blood tests. A rapid anthrax test allows doctors to diagnose anthrax in blood samples in less than an hour. To confirm evidence of inhalation anthrax, a chest X-ray may be taken. Endoscopy and stool samples can be used for diagnosing intestinal anthrax, and a spinal tap may be done to check for anthrax meningitis.

How serious is anthrax?

Cutaneous and intestinal anthrax are rarely fatal when treated adequately. Inhalation anthrax is dangerous because its early symptoms are often difficult to distinguish from the flu or a common cold. Once the disease has spread, inhalation anthrax is often lethal.

If you believe that you're at risk of anthrax exposure — for example, you work in an environment where anthrax was detected — see your doctor. If you develop signs and symptoms of the disorder following exposure to animals or animal products in parts of the world where anthrax is more common, seek prompt medical attention.

Treatment

All three forms of anthrax are treated with antibiotics.

Prevention

An anthrax vaccine for humans was approved by the Food and Drug Administration in 1970, but it's currently unavailable to the public, and the supply is limited. The vaccine is presently recommended for military personnel and people who work with anthrax or who live or travel in areas of high exposure. Two new vaccines are being tested.

Hantavirus

Signs and symptoms

Early

- Fatigue
- Fever
- Muscle aches, especially the thighs, hips and back
- Headache
- Dizziness
- Abdominal problems

Late

- Coughing
- Severe shortness of breath

The first prominent outbreak of hantavirus pulmonary syndrome (HPS) in the United States occurred in 1993, in the Four Corners area — where the borders of Utah, Colorado, New Mexico and Arizona meet. Other cases of hantavirus infection likely occurred before then but weren't recognized as such.

The hantavirus is a distant cousin of the Ebola virus and can cause respiratory failure in infected people. The virus has been known to cause disease in China for many years.

Since the 1993 outbreak in the United States, additional cases involving several types of hantaviruses have been reported in the Western states and many Eastern states. Cases have also been reported in Canada and several countries in South America.

The virus is transmitted by certain types of rodents. So far, the deer mouse, cotton rat and rice rat have been identified as carriers in the United States. Other types of animals, such as cats, dogs and farm animals, are not known to carry the virus. Neither are mosquitoes. In addition, a person can't transmit the virus to another individual.

Experts believe the sudden outbreak in the Four Corners area was caused by a rapid increase in the rodent population due to a period of heavy snowfall and rain following an extended drought.

The virus, which doesn't cause disease in the animal, is shed in the rodent's saliva, urine and feces. Humans are thought to become infected when they breathe air contaminated by rodent droppings or nests. This may happen when a person is cleaning out sheds, barns, attics or other areas that have been infested by infected rodents, and contaminated dust is kicked up into the air.

Diagnosis

Like many infections, the early signs and symptoms of HPS are similar to those of the flu (influenza). Virtually everyone with HPS initially experiences fever, fatigue and muscle aches, especially around the thighs, hips, back and sometimes shoulders. About half the infected individuals also have headaches, dizziness, chills and abdominal problems, such as nausea, vomiting, diarrhea and abdominal pain.

Symptoms may appear to improve, but within 1 or 2 days coughing and shortness of breath occur as the lungs fill with fluid. Breathing difficulty may be subtle at first but rapidly gets worse. Internal bleeding develops followed by respiratory failure. Besides blood tests, chest X-rays are sometimes used to check for abnormalities in the lungs. Tests using serums (serologic tests) may be used to identify the virus.

How serious is hantavirus?

HPS is a serious infection that usually requires hospitalization and intensive therapy. Among diagnosed cases, the death rate has been over 50 percent. If you have a history of contact with rodents and subsequently experience abrupt, flu-like symptoms or have difficulty breathing, see your doctor immediately. Tell your doctor of your contact with rodents so that he or she may know to look for the hantavirus as a possible cause of your illness. When treated early in the disease process, chances of recovery may be better.

Treatment

There's currently no effective treatment for HPS. Oxygen therapy is given to help with severe breathing distress. People who are severely ill may be given a breathing tube and ventilator to provide respiratory support.

Prevention

The best way to prevent HPS infection is to avoid contact with rodent feces, urine and nests. In your home, try to maintain a rodent-free area by setting mousetraps and patching up potential entry holes. If you're hiking or camping, avoid pitching your tent in areas that have mice droppings or mice dens. If you're sleeping on the ground, use a tarp or pad to avoid direct contact with possibly contaminated dust. Air out and disinfect cabins and shelters before using them. Stand upwind when cleaning out birdhouses.

If you're cleaning out a barn or shed or other area that may contain rodents, follow these guidelines from the Centers for Disease Control and Prevention:

- Wear latex gloves. Surgical masks also may be protective.
- Don't vacuum or sweep up droppings, urine or nesting materials, as this will stir up dust.
- Air out the space for 30 minutes before cleaning. Leave the area while it's airing.
- Spray the building or area with a disinfectant — a household detergent will do. Then leave the area for another 30 minutes.
- Thoroughly wet rodent droppings and nests with a 10 percent chlorine solution or similar disinfectant and let the wet materials sit for 30 minutes. Using rubber gloves, move the materials to a plastic bag, seal it and place it in the trash or an incinerator. Dispose of the gloves in the same way.
- Wash all potentially contaminated surfaces with a disinfectant. Avoid vacuuming the area until it has been thoroughly decontaminated. Then, do so only with adequate ventilation.

New variant Creutzfeldt-Jakob disease

Signs and symptoms

- Behavior changes
- Unusual sensations
- Progressive impairment of memory, judgment and thinking (dementia)
- Loss of coordination
- Loss of vision, partial or complete
- Involuntary muscle movements
- A coma

Bovine spongiform encephalopathy (BSE) is a brain disorder in cattle, more popularly known as mad cow disease. So far, BSE has been found only in Europe with the majority of cases occurring in the United Kingdom. An epidemic of BSE in the United Kingdom peaked in 1993 at about 1,000 new cases a week.

BSE gained wide public attention when it was linked to a form of Creutzfeldt-Jakob disease (CJD), a human brain disorder that usually occurs in people around age 60. The new variant of Creutzfeldt-Jakob disease — known as nvCJD — is similar to the classic form in that it causes a rapidly progressive loss of memory, thinking and reasoning skills (dementia), as well as personality changes and problems with muscular coordination. However, nvCJD affects people as young as 12 years old, begins primarily with psychiatric symptoms and has a longer duration than CJD, which usually lasts about a year from onset of symptoms to death.

Some evidence suggests that eating meat contaminated with BSE may be the cause of nvCJD, although this hasn't been proved. The fact that no cases of nvCJD have been confirmed in places where BSE is absent may indicate a causal relationship between the two disorders. In addition, the time period between likely exposure to contaminated beef and onset of new nvCJD cases (around 10 years) is similar to incubation periods for CJD. Preliminary animal studies also have linked the two disorders.

Diagnosis

CJD can be diagnosed with 100 percent accuracy only with a brain biopsy or autopsy, when examination of the brain reveals characteristics of the disease, such as prion protein buildup.

So far, no cases of BSE or nvCJD have been confirmed in the United States. Public health officials and regulators began monitoring the food industry in the United States after BSE first appeared in the United Kingdom in 1986. British authorities eventually traced the outbreak to meat-and-bone meal, a type of feed made from remnants of slaughtered animals. In 1997, the Food and Drug Administration banned the use of this type of feed to protect the food supply from contamination by imported feeds. Regular inspection of cattle in the United States hasn't found any cases of BSE.

According to the Centers for Disease Control and Prevention, the risk of nvCJD to travelers in Europe is almost nonexistent. One preventive measure that may be taken, however, is to avoid eating beef and beef products while in Europe.

Treatment

Currently, there's no cure for the disease and treatment is aimed at relieving symptoms.

West Nile virus

Signs and symptoms

- Fever
- Headache

- Body aches
- Skin rash
- Swollen lymph glands

Emergency signs and symptoms

- A stiff neck
- Stupor
- Disorientation
- Tremors or convulsions
- Paralysis
- A coma

West Nile virus made its first appearance among Americans in August 1999, when an outbreak occurred in and around New York City. An epidemic of the virus resulted in severe illness in 59 people and seven deaths.

The virus was first identified in Uganda in 1937. It has since been found throughout Africa and the Middle East and in parts of Europe, Russia, India, Indonesia and the United States. Health officials aren't sure how the virus arrived in the United States, but some suspect it may have been brought in by an imported bird or a newly infected human arriving from a place where the virus is present.

Mosquitoes transmit the virus to humans. The main reservoirs for the virus are birds. It's of particular concern that the migratory patterns of birds have led to the spread of the virus to new locations. Since the outbreak in New York, the virus has been detected in several states.

Infection with the virus occurs primarily when the weather is mild and mosquito populations are active. It takes 5 to 15 days from the time of infection before symptoms of the illness appear.

Diagnosis

West Nile virus can be confirmed by rising levels of antibodies to the virus in your blood, or from a positive culture of West Nile virus drawn from a blood sample. Finding West Nile virus genetic material in body fluids also confirms an infection.

How serious is West Nile virus?

Anyone bitten by an infected mosquito is at risk of acquiring the virus, although the chance of developing a West Nile virus-related illness after being bitten is lower than 1 percent, and even less in some areas.

In most cases, people who become infected recover fully. Risk of severe infection is greater for people who are over age 50 or who have weakened immune systems.

Treatment

There's no specific treatment for West Nile virus and no vaccine is currently available, although steps are being taken in this direction. Severe cases may require hospitalization.

Prevention

The best way to prevent a West Nile virus infection is to take the normal precautions against exposure to mosquitoes. This includes wearing pants and long-sleeved shirts and using insect repellent. Mosquitoes are most active between dusk and dawn. Avoid having standing water around the home, where mosquitoes can breed and multiply. ■

CHAPTER 21 PART V

Allergies and Asthma

Allergic reactions serve no useful purpose. They're simply misguided immune system reactions to a normally harmless substance that you happen to eat, inhale or touch. But allergies and asthma, a respiratory condition that often accompanies allergies, are nothing to sneeze at. The two are common and often annoying. Without proper treatment they can sometimes be fatal.

The job of your immune system is to protect your body from harmful invaders (antigens), such as germs, viruses and other foreign substances. Your immune system is continuously searching for and destroying unwanted organisms.

Fortunately, your immune system doesn't attack everything foreign that enters your body. Most of the foods, drinks and drugs that you ingest don't trigger an immune response. Occasionally, though, the immune system goes astray and reacts — or rather overreacts — to an innocent invader such as pollen or cat dander, causing allergies. Your immune system perceives the substance as harmful and launches an attack against it.

Allergic Reactions

To fully understand allergies and asthma, it's important to know how your body's immune system works. The main players in an allergic reaction are white blood cells known as lymphocytes.

Lymphocytes are manufactured in enormous quantities in bone marrow. Some migrate to your thymus, where they develop into specialized types of immune cells. Some lymphocytes migrate from bone marrow and the thymus to your lymph nodes and other organs, including your spleen, tonsils, adenoids, appendix and small intestine. Other lymphocytes circulate throughout your body in blood and lymphatic vessels.

The role of lymphocytes is to seek out and destroy harmful foreign invaders that enter your body. In people with allergies, lymphocytes perceive innocent substances such as pollen, dust mites and dander as harmful and launch an attack against them. These innocent substances are known as allergens.

When allergens enter your body, lymphocytes called basophils and mast cells combat them by releasing a variety of chemicals. One of these is called histamine, which acts as an

An Allergic Response

When an allergen, such as pollen, enters your body, the following processes occur:

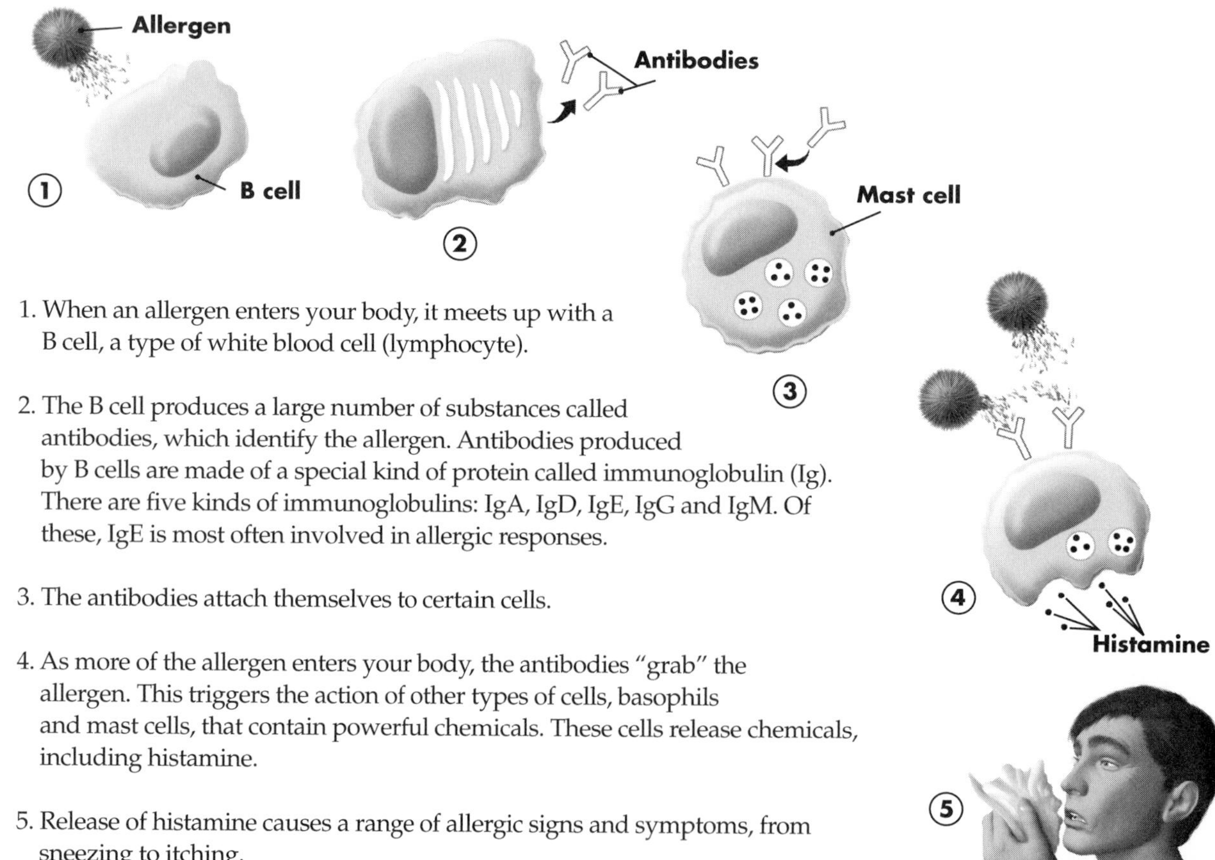

1. When an allergen enters your body, it meets up with a B cell, a type of white blood cell (lymphocyte).

2. The B cell produces a large number of substances called antibodies, which identify the allergen. Antibodies produced by B cells are made of a special kind of protein called immunoglobulin (Ig). There are five kinds of immunoglobulins: IgA, IgD, IgE, IgG and IgM. Of these, IgE is most often involved in allergic responses.

3. The antibodies attach themselves to certain cells.

4. As more of the allergen enters your body, the antibodies "grab" the allergen. This triggers the action of other types of cells, basophils and mast cells, that contain powerful chemicals. These cells release chemicals, including histamine.

5. Release of histamine causes a range of allergic signs and symptoms, from sneezing to itching.

irritating stimulant. Often other white blood cells, called eosinophils, also respond to allergens by releasing powerful chemicals intended to destroy them. When they detect an invader, eosinophils can also increase in number in your blood and in your nasal and bronchial secretions.

These immune responses result in a host of signs and symptoms that vary in severity. Some people have only mild sniffles during ragweed season, and others react with a severe asthma attack.

When histamine and other chemicals are released in the lungs, lung tissues become inflamed, causing the secretion of mucus and the swelling and narrowing of air passages. This leads to wheezing, coughing and, sometimes, shortness of breath.

When these chemicals are released in nasal cavities, they cause a runny nose, teary eyes and itching in the nose, throat, roof of the mouth and eyes. Histamine in the skin produces hives and other rashes. When the chemicals are activated in the digestive system, abdominal cramps and diarrhea may result.

Occasionally, your entire body is affected in a serious allergic response known as anaphylactic shock (anaphylaxis). Blood vessels dilate and air passageways narrow, causing a drop in blood pressure, difficulty breathing and other symptoms. Unconsciousness or death may result (see page 545).

Each allergen stimulates its own specific set of antibodies. For this reason, a person may be sensitive to ragweed but not to mold allergens. It is, however, fairly common for a person who's allergic to one substance to be allergic to others.

Allergic reaction triggers

A surprising number of substances found outdoors, indoors or in foods can trigger an allergic reaction. You may be allergic to substances present in certain medications, parts of plants (such as pollen), dust mites in household dust, animal dander, molds, fungi or insect venom. Some people are also sensitive to chemical changes in response to exercise or exposure to heat or cold.

Paths of exposure

Different allergens have different routes of entry into the body.

Contact

Exposure to plant allergens such as the resins of poison ivy, poison oak and poison sumac occurs when you come into contact with the resin. For instance, you can get poison ivy by accidentally brushing against the plant's leaves while walking in a wooded area, by handling the plant — leaves, stems or roots — while gardening or even by touching clothing that has had resin deposited on it. The allergic reaction usually occurs on your skin wherever contact was made.

Other contact reactions can occur from prolonged exposure to certain metals, such as nickel and chromium. People who are sensitive to components in cosmetics can develop rashes after exposure to nail polish, hair dyes, eye makeup or lipstick. Health care workers may become allergic to latex after repeated exposure to gloves and other latex-containing products.

Inhalation

Inhalation is the most common way of being exposed to allergens. Millions of people have hay fever (allergic rhinitis) due to sensitivity to certain plant pollens. Spring, summer and fall are the pollen producing seasons.

Because pollen is easily airborne, during these seasons exposure is inevitable. As part of their reproductive cycle, molds also release particles that travel in the air. When inhaled, these particles can trigger an allergic reaction.

A similar reaction can occur when a sensitive person inhales animal dander or dust mites, which are common in household dust. In northern regions, exposure to these allergens tends to increase during the winter months because people tend to spend more time indoors. Substances in the air such as smoke, fumes, mists and baby powder also may cause an allergic reaction.

The reaction to an inhaled allergen typically is characterized by signs and symptoms such as a drippy nose, a cough, and itchy, teary eyes. An inhaled allergen can also trigger asthma symptoms.

Wheezing associated with asthma can occur when airways in the lungs become inflamed and swollen. Other asthma symptoms include a feeling of tightness in the chest, a cough and the production of thick mucus.

PREVENTION TIP

The best way to prevent allergies is to avoid the allergen, which can be fairly easy in the case of something like poison ivy or penicillin. It's more difficult to avoid pollens, molds and dust because they're airborne and present even in the best-kept homes.

When you're indoors, you can minimize exposure to pollens and outdoor molds by keeping your doors and windows closed and, when needed, using an air-conditioning system equipped with good filters. Discard any moldy or mildewed items from your home.

If you're allergic to dust, keep your house and work environment as dust-free as possible. This means vacuuming, dusting and damp-mopping frequently. Avoid decorating with items that trap dust, such as bed ruffles and curtains.

Common Myths

Allergies often appear to be mysterious in origin and unpredictable in response. At times they can also be difficult to treat. So it's not surprising that misconceptions and myths regarding allergies abound.

Myth: Allergies are all in your head
Fact: For most people, allergies are a real medical condition. However, allergy symptoms may be aggravated by stress or emotions. Although stress and emotions don't cause allergies, they can exaggerate your body's response to the allergens. Scientists don't fully understand the relationship between allergic responses and emotions.

Myth: Moving to Arizona will cure allergies
Fact: For years people bothered by seasonal allergies to pollens and molds thought that if they moved to the desert Southwest, where the foliage and climate are different from other regions, their allergies would disappear. Although the desert is lacking in maple trees and ragweed, it does have other pollen-producing plants, such as sagebrush and cottonwood, ash and olive trees. People who are sensitive to some pollens and molds often find that in a new environment they eventually develop sensitivities to new allergens. For example, people sensitive to ragweed may become sensitive to sagebrush pollen.

Myth: Short-haired pets don't cause allergies
Fact: The length of an animal's fur doesn't determine its allergic potential. In fact, the fur itself isn't the culprit. The cause is the dander, the scales of skin that are constantly shed by all animals with hair or feathers. In addition, saliva and urine may trigger a sensitivity. If you have allergies to furry pets, the only really safe pets are fish and reptiles.

Myth: You won't get poison ivy unless you touch the plant
Fact: It's true that the plant resin responsible for a sensitivity to poison ivy, poison oak and poison sumac must actually touch your skin to cause a reaction. But that resin may first touch your clothing and then later be transferred to your skin quite easily while you're handling that clothing. This may explain why people who haven't touched the plants do have reactions. These resins can even be carried in smoke if the plants are burned.

Myth: Most people outgrow hay fever
Fact: Many people believe that hay fever is a childhood disorder that you outgrow by the time you reach adulthood. On the contrary, hay fever can develop at any life stage, and you can recover from it at any point in your life.

Myth: No one ever dies of allergies
Fact: Although it's true that many allergies are merely an inconvenience, some allergic reactions can be serious. People who are highly sensitive to allergens can experience life-threatening shock (anaphylaxis) after being stung by a certain insect, being injected with a certain drug or eating a certain food. Asthma attacks also can be fatal. Severe reactions must be taken seriously and treated promptly and properly.

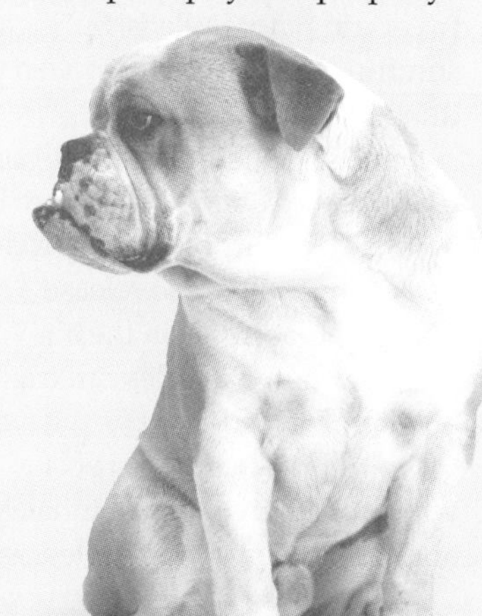

Absorption
Certain foods and medications that are absorbed into the body by way of digestion or injection can cause an allergic response in some people. The foods most likely to produce reactions include milk, eggs, soy, peanuts and other legumes, tree nuts, wheat, shellfish, fish and corn.

Almost any medicine has the potential to cause an allergic reaction. The most common offenders by far are penicillin and its relatives, followed by other antibiotics, insulin, local anesthetics and the intravenous contrast agents used in certain X-ray tests. Some people are sensitive to aspirin and react to it by having a rash, hives or aggravation of asthma.

Stings
Some allergens find their way into people by way of stings. For most people, venom from the sting of a bee, wasp or yellow jacket causes an allergic reaction that's locally uncomfortable for a couple of hours. But in people who are highly sensitive to these allergens, such a sting can trigger a whole-body (systemic) reaction that can be fatal without immediate treatment.

Other sensitivities
In rare cases, people are sensitive to heat, cold, pressure, light, sun rays or exercise. They may experience responses such as rashes or hives. These responses generally don't involve the antibodies responsible for most allergic reactions.

Diagnosing Allergies

To determine if you have an allergy, your doctor may ask you a series of questions about your symptoms, your family's medical history, any past medical problems, past or current emotional or relationship problems and your lifestyle, including work, eating and recreation habits.

You can also expect questions about possible exposure to allergens. This interview is one of the most important sources of information in making a diagnosis.

For example, because the tendency to develop allergies is inherited, it's important for your doctor to know whether your parents have or had allergies. People who have allergies frequently have a close relative with allergies — although the types of allergies may not be the same. You're less likely to inherit a sensitivity to a specific agent than the general tendency to develop sensitivities.

Testing for allergens

When being evaluated for allergies, you may undergo one or more tests to see if your body responds when exposed to certain allergens.

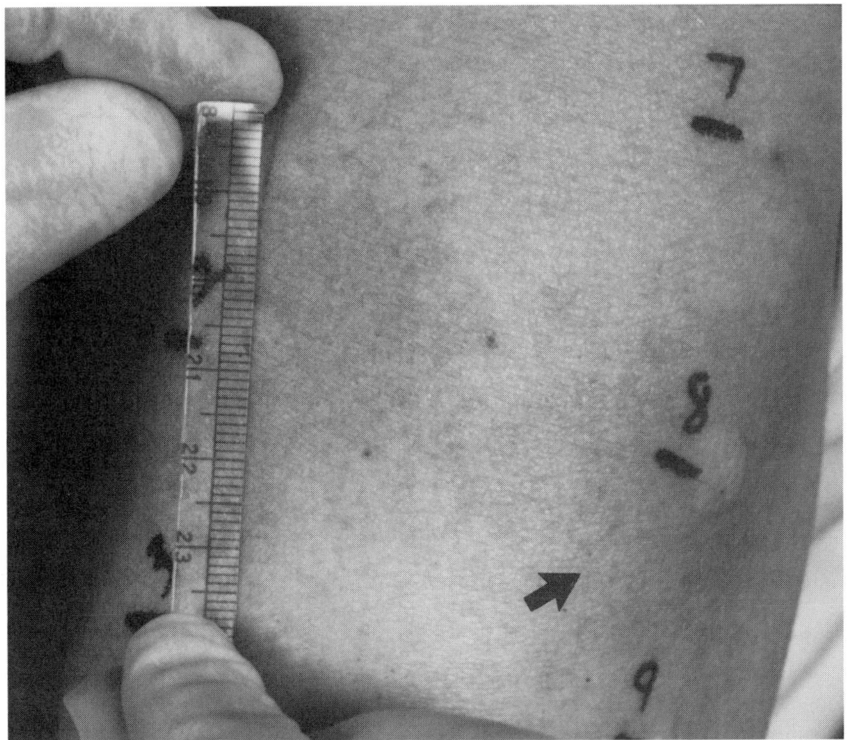

An area of red and swollen skin (see arrow) resulting from a skin test indicates that this person is allergic to the allergen introduced beneath the skin surface.

Skin test

The skin test is the most commonly used test, and it can be administered in several ways. Generally, a small amount of a suspected allergen is placed on your forearm, upper arm or back. The area is then pricked or scratched to introduce the allergen just beneath the skin.

Another method involves injecting a tiny amount of an allergen directly into the skin. With either method, the results are checked after 15 minutes. If the skin at the test site is swollen and red, the test is considered to be positive for that allergen. Several allergens are generally tested at the same time to eliminate possible allergens and because people are often sensitive to several substances.

Skin tests aren't foolproof. You may test positive and yet not respond to the allergen in daily life, and a negative result doesn't rule out sensitivity to that allergen. Or, if too much allergen is placed on the skin, you may get a positive reaction even if you aren't allergic to the substance. In rare instances, someone with an extreme sensitivity to an allergen can have an anaphylactic reaction requiring immediate treatment with an injection of adrenaline (see page 545). Therefore, skin tests must be conducted carefully and interpreted cautiously.

Positive results in skin tests involving food allergens tend to have the widest margin of error; negative tests mean a food allergy is unlikely. Skin tests are particularly useful for respiratory allergies, insect sting allergies, latex allergy and penicillin allergy. Other than for penicillin and closely related drugs, skin tests generally aren't useful in diagnosing a drug allergy.

In vitro allergen-specific IgE antibody test

The in vitro allergen-specific immunoglobulin E (IgE) antibody test, formerly known as a radioallergosorbent test (RAST), is a blood test that's useful for diagnosing sensitivity to inhaled allergens, such as pollen. It measures the amounts of specific IgE antibodies in your blood. In contrast to skin tests, this test may be more convenient, and it doesn't pose any risks because all of the testing is done on a blood sample in a test tube (in vitro). In addition, any antihistamine drugs you're taking won't affect the test.

The downside to the in vitro allergen-specific IgE antibody test is that it may not be as sensitive as skin tests. The blood sample also must be analyzed in a specialized laboratory, a process that takes a day or longer. The test may also be more expensive than skin tests.

Treating Allergies

Several strategies are effective for treating allergies. The best approach is simply to avoid exposure to the allergic substance, but that may not always be possible. Medications and allergy shots are other options.

Avoidance

Avoiding a known allergen is fairly simple in the case of an allergy to

Inappropriate Tests and Treatments

If you think that you may have food allergies, be wary of certain tests and treatments that haven't proved valid. Avoid procedures such as cytotoxic testing, provocation and neutralization testing, and systemic yeast hypersensitivity treatment.

Cytotoxic testing involves mixing extracts of foods with samples of a person's white blood cells. Some people believe that if the cells change shape in any way, the individual is allergic to that food. However, no proven correlation exists between such a change and a food allergy.

With provocation and neutralization testing, an individual is injected with a small amount of food extract to provoke symptoms. When symptoms occur, he or she is given "neutralizing" injections of the food, on the theory that this will neutralize the effects of the first dose. This also is an unproven diagnostic test.

Systemic yeast hypersensitivity treatment is based on the theory that a yeast-like fungus called *Candida* is the cause of all food allergies. This treatment is given to people who think they have food allergies.

They're told to remove from their diet all foods containing yeast and mold — including fruits, milk, refined carbohydrates, such as breads, and processed foods. Supposedly, this enables the body to correct the condition. No evidence supports the notion that *Candida* has any relation to food allergies.

penicillin or poison ivy. Avoidance isn't so simple for people allergic to such things as pollen and dust mites. Pollen is constantly in the air during certain months of the year, and even the best-kept homes contain dust. For tips on reducing exposure to these and other inhalant allergens, see page 527 for information on pollen and page 529 for information on animal dander, mold and dust allergies.

Medications

Several medications are available to relieve the effects of allergies, with antihistamines being the most common. All of these medications may cause side effects — some more serious than others — that you may want to discuss with your doctor.

Antihistamines

The most common medication for many allergies, particularly hay fever (allergic rhinitis), is an antihistamine. It blocks the action of histamine, the substance that's largely responsible for the signs and symptoms that accompany allergies, such as congestion, a runny nose, watery eyes and an itchy throat.

Antihistamines are available both over-the-counter and in prescription form. Over-the-counter antihistamines include products such as diphenhydramine (Benadryl, Sominex, others) and clemastine (Contac, Tavist). Prescription antihistamines include products such as fexofenadine (Allegra), loratadine (Claritin) and cetirizine hydrochloride (Zyrtec). For many people with allergies to pollen, mold or dust mites, these drugs can provide relief.

Corticosteroids

Corticosteroid medications, such as cortisone and prednisone, are generally prescribed for more severe symptoms. These powerful anti-inflammatory drugs come in various forms and may be administered by injection, metered-dose inhaler, nasal spray, pill or topical cream. Except for the mild topical creams, these drugs are available only by prescription and can be very useful in treating allergies. However, they may have side effects that need to be weighed against the seriousness of the symptoms.

Corticosteroids are typically taken by way of metered-dose inhalers or nasal sprays, both of which reduce the dosage compared with oral or injected forms of the drug. Still, side effects can be a risk if you use corticosteroids on a long-term basis. They include bruising, glaucoma, cataracts, osteoporosis and suppressed growth in children. Corticosteroid-containing creams may cause skin problems in people with sensitive skin, so they too should be used with care.

Cromolyn

Cromolyn is a nonsteroidal drug that's used to treat seasonal or chronic hay fever. The drug is available as a nasal spray (Nasalcrom) or as eyedrops (Crolom, Opticrom). You begin taking cromolyn before allergy season because it must be used for several weeks before its benefits start to become apparent.

Adrenaline

The most severe allergic reaction is anaphylaxis, which can cause blood vessels to dilate and air passages in the lungs to constrict. This reaction can cause severe wheezing, low blood pressure, unconsciousness and, in some instances, death. Treatment for anaphylaxis involves an injection of adrenaline (epinephrine). Adrenaline quickly opens narrowed airways and constricts blood vessels.

Allergy shots

Certain allergies may be treated with what's commonly referred to as allergy shots. Another term for this type of treatment is *immunotherapy*. It involves injecting very small amounts of known offending allergens under the skin in the upper arm. The intent is to decrease your immune system's reaction to the allergens by helping your body learn to accept them as the harmless substances they are.

Medication Side Effects

Antihistamines can be very useful in treating allergy symptoms, but side effects need to be considered. Antihistamines can cause drowsiness, dryness of the nose and mouth and blurred vision. One study reported that diphenhydramine, an antihistamine in some over-the-counter allergy and cold remedies (Benadryl, Sominex, others), can cause more driving impairment than being legally drunk. Nonsedating prescription antihistamines such as fexofenadine (Allegra) and loratadine (Claritin) tend to cause much less drowsiness. Cetirizine hydrochloride (Zyrtec) is less sedating than older antihistamines such as diphenhydramine.

You may want to avoid driving a car or operating heavy machinery when you're taking an over-the-counter antihistamine. Even if you don't feel drowsy, your driving may be impaired as long as the drug is in your system. Also avoid alcohol, which speeds the absorption of some antihistamines and intensifies the drowsiness.

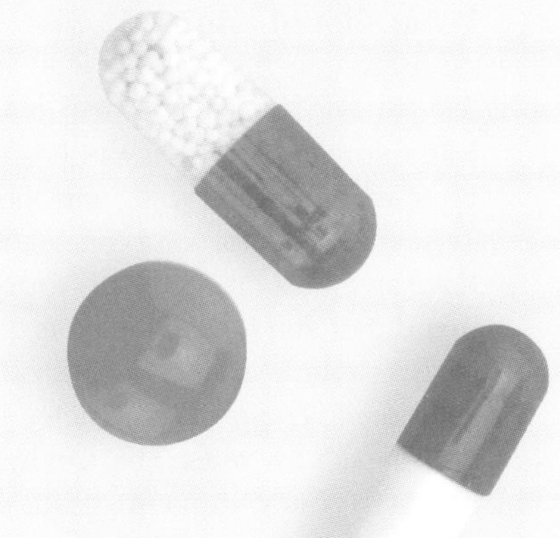

Question and Answer

Do HEPA filters relieve symptoms of allergy and asthma?

Although high-efficiency particulate air (HEPA) filters may help a select group of people, there aren't many good studies to confirm this. The filters only take out airborne allergens, such as mold spores and pollen. They can remove animal dander, too, but if the source of the dander is in your home, you won't benefit from the filter. A HEPA filter won't remove the microscopic mites that live in house dust because they're dense and tend to accumulate on surfaces rather than remain suspended in the air.

Simply keeping your home closed up and using an air conditioner will get rid of about 75 percent of outdoor airborne allergens. If you're still considering a HEPA filter, make sure the type of allergy you're dealing with is one that this system could help, for example, a pollen or mold-spore allergy. Then choose one of an appropriate size for the space you need to filter.

The treatment requires regular injections, often weekly, of increasing doses of the allergens until a maintenance dose is established. Then, injections of the maintenance dose are given monthly for up to several years.

Severe reactions to immunotherapy are rare but can occur. As a precaution, your doctor will likely recommend that you stay in a waiting room for a period after you receive the injections. An adverse reaction, if it happens at all, typically occurs within 30 minutes after an injection.

Allergy shots may provide hay fever relief that continues even after the shots are discontinued. A British study found that immunotherapy given for 3 years to treat grass-pollen allergy can provide symptom relief that continues for 3 years or more after the shots are stopped.

Respiratory Allergies

Allergies of the respiratory tract often produce signs and symptoms that are similar to those of a cold: a congested head and chest, stuffy or runny nose, coughing, sneezing and wheezing. In fact, allergies and colds are often confused. Some allergy symptoms typically last far longer than those of a cold. Others may appear and disappear briefly, which is also uncharacteristic of the common cold.

For some people, allergy symptoms appear during a pollen season. For others, the symptoms manifest primarily when their homes are closed to ventilation and dust mites and mold allergy exposure is common. Still others experience symptoms only during certain events, such as when visiting a home occupied by a cat or dog.

Hay fever (allergic rhinitis)

Signs and symptoms

- Stuffy or runny nose
- Frequent sneezing
- Itchy eyes, nose, roof of mouth or throat
- Coughing

It's springtime. The air is sweet with the smell of fresh, new flowers, but you can't enjoy it because your head is stuffed up, your nose is sore and your throat itches. Or, it's fall and ragweed and other plants are spreading their wind-blown pollen everywhere, including into your respiratory system — making your eyes teary, your head and nose congested, and the roof of your mouth itchy.

These signs and symptoms are characteristic of allergic rhinitis, commonly referred to as hay

Question and Answer

I have respiratory allergies and asthma. I'll be traveling to an area with many plants and trees. What should I do?

See your doctor for a pre-trip evaluation and advice. Make sure your allergies and asthma — particularly your asthma — are well controlled before you leave.

Ask your doctor for a contingency plan in case you have an attack on your trip. Your doctor may recommend that you take along emergency medications such as antihistamines, bronchodilators or corticosteroids. Take a peak flowmeter with you to monitor your peak flow rates. This can help guide adjustments to your asthma medication.

In addition:

- Pack all of your medications in your carry-on luggage so that you have them in case you need them en route or if your luggage doesn't arrive on time. Be sure to pack more medication than the minimum you'll need. Store medications in their original containers. The containers provide instructions on dosages and refills and identify the drugs for customs officials when needed.
- Smoke can irritate asthma, so if you're traveling abroad, you may want to book a nonsmoking flight. If this isn't possible, ask for seats far away from the smoking section. Commercial flights within the United States are smoke-free.
- If you cross several time zones, allow for time differences so that you maintain your medication dosage schedule.
- Find out ahead of time if and how your health insurance plan handles medical care abroad, in case you should need medical treatment.

fever — although allergens other than hay usually cause the condition, and no fever is present. An estimated 35 million Americans have hay fever.

No one knows why some people are more susceptible than others are to the tiny airborne pollens of certain plants. In all likelihood, the sensitivity is partly an inherited trait that affects the ability of the immune system to deal with potential invaders.

Many people believe that hay fever is a childhood disorder that you outgrow by the time you reach adulthood. On the contrary, hay fever can develop at any life stage, and you can recover from it at any time. A person who has conditions such as eczema or asthma or who has relatives with allergies is more likely to have hay fever.

Some people with hay fever are sensitive to only one or two substances. Others are sensitive to many substances.

When you inhale pollen to which you're allergic, your immune system antibodies react with the pollen. This triggers the release of histamine, which comes in contact with the lining of your nose, sinuses, eyelids and eyes. Your sinuses may become congested, your nose may run, and your eyes, nose, throat and roof of your mouth may itch. You may sneeze, sometimes violently and repeatedly. A hay fever attack generally lasts about 15 to 20 minutes and recurs several times a day. For people with severe hay fever, the condition can disrupt their lives. For those with minor symptoms, the illness is only an annoyance.

Diagnosis

To help in identifying the cause of your hay fever, your doctor may ask you a series of questions as to the severity of your symptoms, when you first noticed them and if they seem to get worse at any particular time. You may be asked to keep a diary to determine accurately when your allergic reactions occur most frequently.

If your symptoms occur only in the spring, then you're probably allergic to pollens found only in the spring. If you have allergy attacks throughout the growing season, you may be allergic to several different pollens.

Your doctor may recommend tests such as skin prick tests or an in vitro allergen specific IgE antibody test, formerly known as a radioallergosorbent test (RAST), to determine which pollens you're most sensitive to.

Treatment

For mild hay fever, nonprescription oral antihistamines and decongestants are often effective. However, over-the-counter antihistamines can produce drowsiness and dryness of the throat and mouth, causing as much discomfort as that of the hay fever. Nonsedating prescription antihistamines such as fexofenadine (Allegra) and loratadine (Claritin) have less tendency to cause drowsiness (see page 526).

Avoid regular use of over-the-counter decongestant nasal sprays. These sprays should only be used twice a day for a maximum of 3 to 4 days. Although they relieve symptoms at first, they can make the problem worse. If used too often or for too long, they cause your nose to become increasingly congested, and more frequent doses are needed to clear it. The only way to resolve the problem is to stop using the spray and wait for the congestion to subside. This may take a month or two. Inhaled corticosteroids often help relieve the symptoms while you're waiting for the problem to resolve.

For moderate to severe hay fever, treatment may include a prescription antihistamine. Your doctor may also prescribe a corticosteroid

That Pesky Pollen

Wherever plants grow, pollen is in the air at some time of the year. Trees, both deciduous and evergreen, produce pollen in spring. Grasses and most flowers produce their pollen during summer months. Late-blooming plants such as ragweed produce pollen in early fall. In warm climates with long growing seasons, pollen may be present in the air for 10 months of the year. In climates with shorter growing seasons, the pollen is present for less time.

Ragweed, a roadside plant, heads the list of hay-fever-causing plants east of the Rocky Mountains. Other plant pollens that produce allergy symptoms include sagebrush, tumbleweed, redroot pigweed, spiny amaranth, burning bush and English plantain.

Grasses that cause troublesome pollens include rye, timothy, redtop, Bermuda, orchard, sweet vernal and bluegrass. Most trees, including maple, oak, ash, birch, poplar, elm, pecan, juniper and cottonwood, produce pollens that can trigger hay fever.

Pollens that are carried by insects from one plant to another tend to be larger grains that are relatively harmless. Those carried by the wind are lighter and smaller and can cause hay fever. The amount of pollen in the air depends on the weather. Hot, dry breezes stir up pollen, whereas dampness washes the pollen to the ground.

Most pollen particles are so small that they can be carried by the air into a house through doors and screens. It doesn't take much pollen to produce an allergic reaction — as little as 20 particles per cubic yard. Many plants can produce up to a million such particles.

The most effective way to avoid pollen is to stay indoors, especially when pollen counts are high. Keep doors and windows closed. Air conditioning also is helpful.

nasal spray or the medication cromolyn in nasal spray form (Apo-Cromolyn, Nasalcrom). These products help reduce nasal congestion. You may need to use the products for several weeks before you experience benefits. If you're bothered by watery or itchy eyes, your doctor may recommend a prescription eyedrop such as levocabastine (Livostin), ketorolac (Acular) or olopatadine (Patanol).

The closest thing to a cure for hay fever is immunotherapy to desensitize your immune system to allergens. Increasing amounts of the offending allergen are injected under your skin over a period of months. Many people who undergo this therapy lose their sensitivity to a particular allergen, usually within 2 years. But this therapy isn't appropriate for all individuals.

Animal dander, mold and dust allergies

Signs and symptoms

- Stuffy, runny nose
- Frequent sneezing
- Itchy eyes, nose, roof of mouth or throat
- Coughing
- Wheezing

Not all respiratory allergies are caused by pollen. Identical allergic reactions can occur because of sensitivity to molds, animal dander and the microscopic mites that live in house dust. For some people, mold, dust or animal allergies are an inconvenience, producing mild symptoms that last only a few weeks each year. Others experience more severe, and sometimes year-round, symptoms.

Animal dander

Some people are allergic to the dander of animals and birds. The fur and feathers themselves are not the cause of year-round irritation. It's the scales shed from the skin that cause the allergy, along with the pet's saliva and urine. People allergic to pollens or molds may be allergic to animal dander as well.

The only way to eliminate the problem is to avoid the source. This means not keeping pets. If you're sensitive to the tiny amounts of dander found in wool, avoid products made mostly of wool. Don't buy furniture or rugs that contain animal hair.

Molds

People with many allergies are sensitive to the spores of common molds carried in the air. Outdoor molds produce spores mostly in the summer and early fall, although in warm climates they can be present all year. Indoor molds shed spores all year long, producing constant problems for people who are sensitive to them.

Molds thrive indoors in damp locations, such as basements and bathrooms, and in upholstered furniture and beds, rugs, stuffed animals, wood, books and wallpaper. Outdoors they live in the soil and on compost or damp vegetation. People who are susceptible to mold spores react most noticeably when they're mowing grass, harvesting crops or walking through tall grass and plants. Common offending molds include the indoor molds *Penicillium*, *Aspergillus*, *Mucor* and *Rhizopus* and the outdoor molds *Alternaria* and *Hormodendrum*.

Keep doors and windows closed as much as possible and, when needed, use air conditioning in your home, car or office. Dry out a damp basement by using a dehumidifier. Be sure to clean the dehumidifier regularly so that molds and other growths don't develop inside it. Clean bathroom and basement walls with disinfectants. Instead of using wallpaper, paint walls with mold-proof paint.

Dust

House dust harbors all kinds of substances, including pollen, mold spores and animal dander. However, the primary cause of an allergic reaction to dust is microscopic mites. Mites thrive in damp, warm environments.

The best way to deal with dust is to keep your home as dust-free as possible and the humidity low. This means not only vacuuming visible dust but also damp-mopping and dusting often. Wash throw rugs and furniture covers weekly. If you're the one with the allergy, if possible, have someone else do the cleaning or wear a dust mask.

Avoid using overstuffed furniture and dust trappers such as bed ruffles, canopy beds, bunk beds, carpeting, curtains, Venetian blinds and upholstered furniture. Enclose pillows, mattresses and box springs in allergen-proof coverings.

A central heating and air-conditioning system that filters the air is a big help. You may also want to use a dehumidifier.

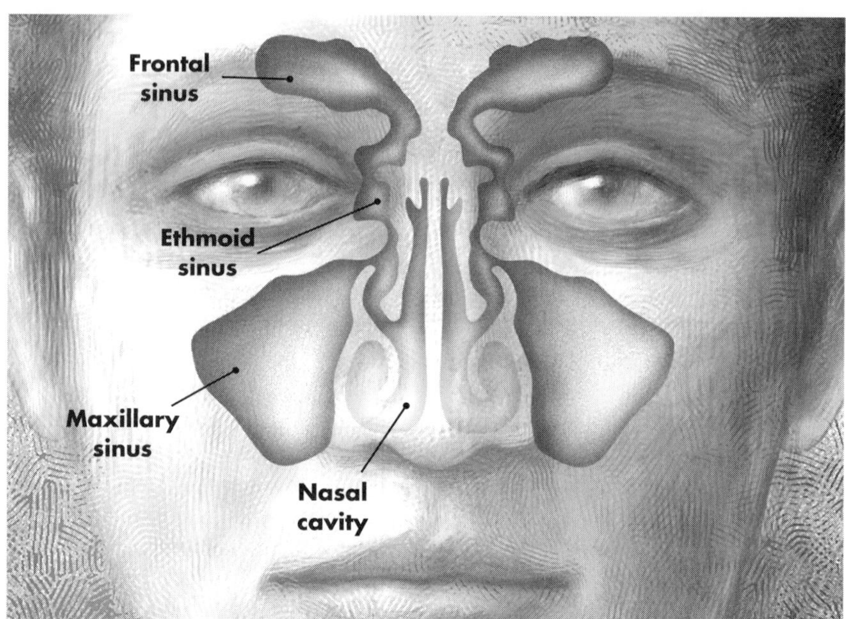

Sinuses are hollow spaces within the bones of your face. They produce mucus, which normally drains through sinus openings into your nose. If drainage is blocked, a sinus infection can result.

Miscellaneous irritants

Dozens of other inhaled substances can cause reactions among a small percentage of people. These include:

- Industrial smoke and fumes
- Tobacco smoke
- Face and baby powder
- Powdered soaps and detergents

People who are sensitive to respiratory allergens are more likely to be sensitive to such irritants. If you seem to be bothered by these substances, try to avoid them as much as possible.

Diagnosis

To determine the cause of your allergy symptoms, your doctor may ask you questions to determine how severe the reaction is, how often it occurs, whether it's year-round or seasonal, and the situations in which it occurs most frequently. A series of skin tests may help identify the allergens to which you're most sensitive.

The in vitro allergen-specific IgE antibody test, formerly known as a radioallergosorbent test (RAST), may be used to check for specific

Reducing Cat Allergy Symptoms

Despite the ability of cats to make more people scratch and sneeze more than any other pet, feline fancy often wins over practicality. Of the 6 million Americans who are allergic to cats, about one-third still keep a cat in their home.

If you have a cat allergy but can't bear to get rid of your cat, follow these suggestions to help you live in your home more comfortably:

- *Wash your cat once a week.* This can reduce the amount of your cat's airborne allergen by close to 90 percent.
- *Avoid carpets and upholstered furniture.* Mop floors frequently and vacuum using a high-efficiency filter attachment.
- *Use a high-efficiency particulate air (HEPA) filter to decrease cat allergens in dust.* This type of air cleaner appears to remove the majority of dust particles that pass through the filter.
- *Keep the cat out.* If you have an outdoor cat, let it stay outside as much as possible and make off-limits your bedroom and other rooms in which you spend a lot of time.
- *Increase ventilation.* This will help decrease allergen levels.

If you or someone in your home has asthma triggered by cat allergy, it's best to find your cat a new home. Continued exposure to cat allergens may lead to narrowing of the airways even after the exposure stops. After you find a new home for your cat, thoroughly clean your house. But remember that it can take weeks, even months, for cat allergens to disappear from carpeting and upholstered furniture.

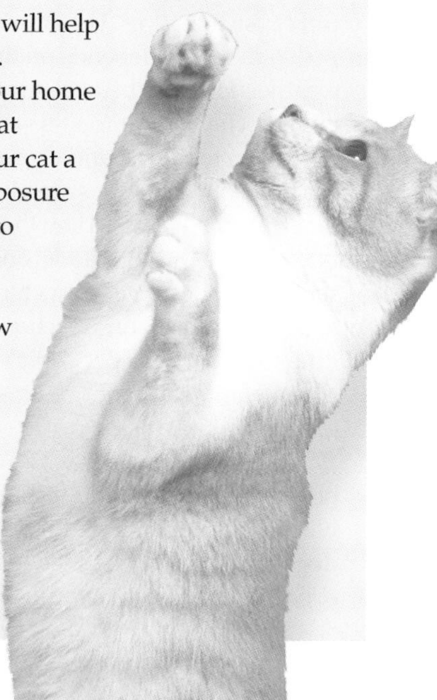

antibodies in blood. Because some people are sensitive to more than one allergen, it can be difficult to pinpoint which allergens cause the most trouble.

How serious are these allergies?

The cold-like symptoms of this type of allergy are inconvenient and annoying, but they're generally not a serious health threat.

Treatment

The most effective treatment for allergy to molds, dust and animal dander is avoidance. This may be easier said than done because some allergens, particularly mold spores, are windborne just like pollen. With pollen, staying indoors in an air-conditioned atmosphere is often the most useful preventive measure.

When the allergen is house dust or animal dander, you can take steps to decrease your exposure. In addition, medications such as antihistamines and corticosteroids can help alleviate symptoms, and allergy shots (see page 526) may help desensitize your immune system to the allergens.

Chronic sinusitis and nasal polyps

Signs and symptoms

- Pain around your eyes or cheeks
- Tenderness of your sinuses to pressure or touch
- Headache
- Fever
- Difficulty breathing through your nose

Your sinuses are hollow spaces within the bones of your face, behind and above your eyes and nose. They help humidify and warm the air you breathe, aid your sense of smell and improve the sound of your voice. They also secrete mucus, which cleans and moisturizes your nasal passages.

Inside your sinuses, tiny hair-like projections called cilia constantly sweep mucus out of your sinuses and into your nose and throat. Your sinuses drain into your nose through small openings called ostia. When ostia become blocked, mucus accumulates in sinus cavities. Microorganisms such as viruses and bacteria can multiply and cause infection. Infection produces swelling, which can decrease sinus drainage.

Sometimes, respiratory allergies can lead to infection or inflammation of your sinus cavities, causing pain and difficulty breathing through your nose. If you've had sinusitis for 3 weeks or longer and it doesn't respond to antibiotics, you may have chronic sinusitis caused by allergies.

Chronic sinusitis is different from acute sinusitis caused by a bacterial infection, which typically responds to treatment within a few weeks. Chronic sinusitis is also associated with nasal polyps, small, benign tissue growths within nasal passages that hinder breathing.

Causes

Allergies to such elements as pollen, animal dander and dust mites can cause a stuffy nose, leading to chronic sinusitis. With seasonal allergies, symptoms tend to occur during distinct seasons. With nonseasonal allergies, symptoms may appear and reappear at random times. Fungi can cause a specific type of chronic sinusitis called allergic fungal sinusitis.

Nasal polyps also can obstruct sinus drainage. Nasal polyps occur when the mucous membrane that lines the inside of the nose swells and protrudes into the nasal passage. Nasal polyps are caused by an overproduction of fluid in the mucous membrane, sometimes as a result of hay fever or some other nasal allergy.

Often, no specific cause can be identified. Polyps may appear singly or in clusters, making breathing difficult and interfering with your sense of taste and smell.

Diagnosis

People often have several episodes of severe but temporary (acute) sinusitis before developing long-lasting (chronic) sinusitis. If you've had sinusitis a number of times and the condition doesn't respond to treatments such as nasal sprays, decongestants and antibiotics, you might have chronic sinusitis.

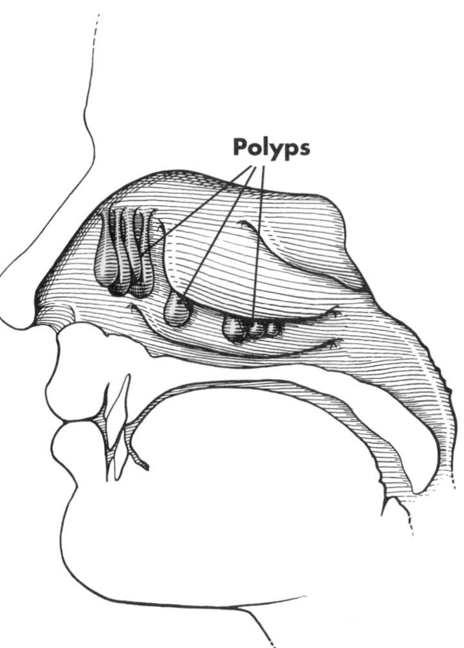

Pearl-like lumps in the lining of the nasal passage are called nasal polyps. If they cause breathing difficulty or recurrent sinus infections, these polyps can be removed surgically.

Your doctor may be able to tell whether allergies are the reason for your sinusitis. Allergy testing may yield important information about your allergic sensitivities.

The following procedures help in diagnosing chronic sinusitis:

Nasal endoscopy

During a nasal endoscopy, a thin, flexible tube with a fiber-optic light attached to it (endoscope) is inserted into your nose. This allows your doctor to visually inspect the inside of your sinuses.

Imaging

Computerized tomography (CT) images show details of your sinuses and nasal area and can reveal a deep inflammation or infection that may be difficult to detect using an endoscope.

Nasal speculum
If your doctor thinks that you may have nasal polyps, he or she can look for them using a device called a nasal speculum, which looks like a pair of sugar tongs. If you have polyps, you may be able to see them yourself by shining a light up your nostril and examining the nasal passage with a mirror. Polyps are pearl-like lumps, but if they're at the back of the nasal passage, they won't be easy for you to see.

Treatment
Treatments for chronic sinusitis include:

Antibiotics
The condition may require a long period — about 3 or 4 weeks — of antibiotic treatment, often using medications that are effective for a wider variety of bacteria than those used for acute sinusitis.

Corticosteroids
If you have intense inflammation of your sinuses, your doctor may prescribe a corticosteroid nasal spray. If you have severe sinusitis, your doctor may recommend oral corticosteroids or a corticosteroid shot to shrink the inflamed sinus membranes, followed by a corticosteroid nasal spray to prevent them from swelling again.

Antifungal medications
To treat allergic fungal sinusitis, doctors will sometimes prescribe a nasal solution containing an antifungal agent to wash out (irrigate) and then drain sinus cavities.

Surgery
Surgery is most often performed when chronic sinusitis doesn't respond to medications or when polyps are blocking nasal passageways. Surgically enlarging a narrow sinus passage or removing a bone or polyp that's blocking a passage will allow better drainage. This type of surgery is most often performed using an endoscope with attached cutting tools.

Allergy shots
If your sinusitis is allergy related, allergy shots may prevent future bouts of the condition.

Asthma

People don't often think of asthma as a killer disease, yet more than 5,000 Americans die of asthma each year. Asthma also accounts for more than 400,000 hospitalizations annually. An estimated 17 million Americans have asthma — about 6.4 percent of the U.S. population. Of these about 4.8 million are children. Asthma is the leading cause of chronic illness in children.

Asthma is a chronic condition that occurs when your lungs' main airways (bronchial tubes) become inflamed. The muscles of the bronchial tube walls tighten, and mucous membranes that line the tubes produce extra mucus, causing the airways to narrow. This can lead to everything from minor wheezing to severe difficulty breathing. Attacks can last minutes to days.

Some people with asthma have persistent symptoms. For others, symptoms are intermittent. With professional help, asthma attacks can be controlled and are seldom disabling or life-threatening.

Fortunately, asthma is a treatable disease, and most flare-ups and deaths can be prevented. In recent years scientists have gained a better understanding of asthma's causes. New drugs have been developed to replace older medications, and greater emphasis is now being given to managing the condition, much as people manage diabetes.

Together, you and your doctor can gain control over your symptoms, reduce your risk of severe attacks and help you maintain a normal life.

Signs and symptoms
- Wheezing
- Difficulty breathing
- Tightness in the chest
- Coughing

Emergency signs and symptoms
- Extreme difficulty breathing
- Bluish lips and nails
- Severe breathlessness
- Increased pulse rate
- Sweating
- Severe coughing

Risk factors

You're more likely to develop asthma if others in your family also have the disease or if you have allergies. About half the children who develop asthma do so before age 10. Adults can develop asthma at any age — even into their 70s and beyond.

For people under age 30, asthma is typically triggered by allergies. Forty percent to 70 percent of people age 30 and older with asthma also have respiratory allergies.

For individuals in whom allergies aren't a factor, asthma may be related to an irritant or a medical condition. In most cases, asthma is the result of a combination of allergic and nonallergic responses.

Airway
Mucous membrane
Smooth muscle

Normal airways in your lungs

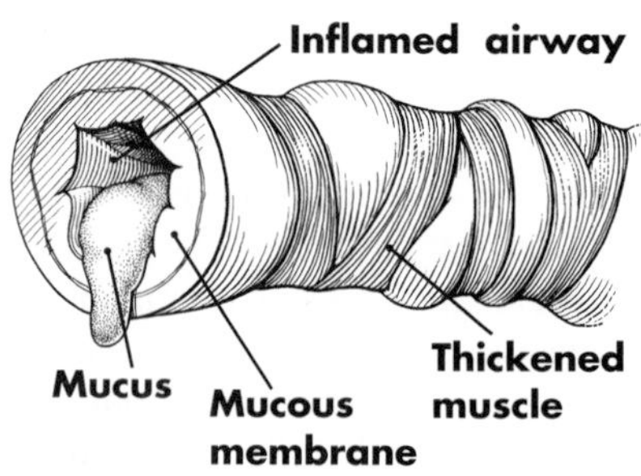

In asthma, airways in your lungs are inflamed and swollen.

Occupational Asthma

Some people regularly experience wheezing, coughing or shortness of breath at work that may be accompanied by itchy eyes or a runny nose. When they leave work, their signs and symptoms improve.

This is commonly referred to as occupational asthma. It's caused by inhaling dust, vapors, gases or fumes particular to the workplace. These substances can irritate your respiratory system.

Occupational asthma generally develops in one of two ways:

Direct response to an irritant
Asthmatic symptoms occur immediately following exposure to substances like ammonia, hydrochloric acid, sulfur dioxide or environmental smoke. This is especially common in people who already have asthma.

Long-term sensitization
Continued exposure — sometimes over months or years — causes an allergic response. Symptoms develop more gradually. An example is a veterinarian who after regular exposure to animals develops an allergy to one or more of them.

Common irritants

It's estimated that occupational asthma may account for up to 15 percent of all asthma cases in the United States. About 11 million workers are exposed to substances known to cause occupational asthma, and as many as 1.5 million workers are directly affected by the disease.

More than 240 substances are currently known to cause occupational asthma when inhaled, and the list keeps growing. These substances generally fall into one of these categories:

- Chemicals such as anhydrides, diisocyanates and acids that are used in the manufacture of paints, varnishes, adhesives, laminates and soldering fluxes (resin used in soldering)
- Enzymes used in detergents, flour conditioners, some pharmaceuticals and meat tenderizers
- Proteins found in animal dander, hair, scales, fur, saliva and body wastes
- Flour and grain dust
- Proteins found in rye, barley, oats, rice and soy
- Products used during seafood and egg processing
- Chlorine gas, sulfur dioxide, hydrochloric acid and smoke

If your asthma is severe and there's a strong connection between your illness and your job, your doctor might recommend that you eliminate any exposure to irritants or other substances that can cause asthma. This might mean that you can't work in the same location, at the same job or in the same industry.

Changing jobs is a difficult decision with many potential consequences, and such a recommendation is never made without careful consideration. Working with your doctor, you can arrive at the best decision for your overall health.

Researchers have identified a number of factors that may increase your chances of developing asthma:

- Exposure to secondhand smoke
- Living in a large urban area, especially an inner city, where your exposure to many environmental pollutants may be increased
- Exposure to occupational triggers
- A family history of asthma
- Low birth weight
- Obesity
- Gastroesophageal reflux disease (GERD)

PREVENTION TIP

If you have asthma, you're more likely to be bothered by stomach acid backing up (refluxing) into your esophagus, a condition called gastroesophageal reflux disease (GERD). In some cases, GERD may actually cause asthma symptoms. To help prevent GERD, don't eat or drink for several hours before going to bed. You may also find it helpful to elevate the head of your bed. See page 850 for more information about GERD.

Diagnosis

Episodes of wheezing, coughing or difficulty breathing are the primary signs and symptoms of asthma. Airflow obstruction results from an inflammation of the bronchial tube walls, tightening of the bronchial smooth muscle fibers and increased production of mucus. Inhaling and exhaling through narrowed bronchial tubes is what produces a wheezing sound.

Doctors use various tests to help diagnose asthma and its causes. A complete physical examination, breathing tests and allergy tests may be needed.

Your doctor may also ask you to perform a peak flowmeter breathing test at home to determine if there's a pattern to the attacks, helping to narrow the list of possible causes (see page 539).

Asthma Medications

Most people with asthma can effectively manage their disease with medications. Asthma medications fall into two main categories: those you take continuously to prevent attacks and those you use to relieve symptoms during an attack.

Preventive medications

Preventive medications are generally taken once or twice daily to prevent asthma attacks. They work by reducing inflammation in lung airways and thus preventing spontaneous spasm of airway muscles.

If one drug doesn't keep your asthma under control, you may need to take a combination of medications. Preventive medications include:

Inhaled corticosteroids

Inhaled corticosteroids are commonly used to treat asthma, unless the symptoms are only mild or intermittent. They include medications such as fluticasone (Flovent), budesonide (Pulmicort), triamcinolone (Azmacort), beclomethasone (Beclovent, Vanceril) and flunisolide (Aerobid).

The medications act locally on lung tissues to reduce inflamed mucous membranes, mucus production and airway hyperresponsiveness ("twitchiness"). Common side effects of inhaled corticosteroids include hoarseness, an oral yeast infection (thrush) and skin bruising.

Oral corticosteroids

Oral corticosteroids are most often prescribed to adults or children for poorly controlled or severe asthma. The most commonly used oral corticosteroid is prednisone. It's effective at controlling airway inflammation, but it can cause many side effects, especially when taken for an extended time. Side effects include bruising, glaucoma, cataracts, osteoporosis and growth suppression in children.

Cromolyn and nedocromil

Inhaled cromolyn (Intal) and nedocromil (Tilade) are anti-inflammatory drugs that can help prevent attacks in people with mild to moderate asthma. They're also effective at preventing exercise-induced asthma. These drugs are often prescribed for children or young adults with asthma.

Leukotriene blockers

Leukotriene blockers, introduced in 1996, are the first new class of asthma medication in 20 years. These drugs prevent the actions of a group of powerful asthma mediators called leukotrienes.

Leukotriene blockers include the medications zileuton (Zyflo), zafirlukast (Accolate), montelukast (Singulair) and others. The medications are safe and effective in controlling symptoms of persistent asthma in many people. Because they're taken orally, leukotriene blockers are preferred by some people who dislike or have difficulty using inhalers.

Long-acting beta agonists

Long-acting beta agonist inhalers include the medications salmeterol (Serevent) and formoterol (Foradil). They relieve airway constriction for up to 12 hours and are often used to prevent signs and symptoms of asthma, including nighttime attacks.

Because they take longer to act, these medications aren't recommended for immediate relief during an attack. Beta agonists are also available as tablets, but tablets aren't as speedy as inhalants and can cause more side effects.

Theophylline

Theophylline (Elixophyllin, Uniphyl) is often used when other medications aren't effective. Taken in pill form, it's both a short- and long-acting medication. Theophylline isn't as effective as a beta agonist, but it lasts longer than the short-acting beta agonists.

Theophylline can be difficult to use because it interacts poorly with some other medications and commonly causes side effects. However, it's an effective treatment for some people.

The Cockroach Connection

For reasons no one quite understands, the number of asthma cases has risen dramatically in the past decade, especially among children living in the inner city. Asthma is the most common chronic illness of childhood. One potential reason for the increase in asthma in children is the lowly cockroach. Many allergists and asthma researchers have long suspected a strong connection between cockroaches and inner-city asthma.

The focus on cockroaches as an asthma trigger comes as investigators are trying to explain a worldwide increase in asthma. Other hypotheses include increased air pollution, changes in ozone levels and the increased time people spend indoors, where allergens may exist in greater amounts and for longer periods.

Researchers can now test some of these possibilities using sample-gathering techniques developed in recent years. These techniques can measure the amount of allergens — including cockroach body parts and droppings — in indoor air and dust.

Unfortunately combating cockroaches isn't as simple as just doing a better job of housekeeping. Cockroaches are very mobile and may be found throughout an apartment building or a single-family dwelling and will quickly return to an area from which they have been exterminated. There's no perfect solution, but preventive measures include cleaning up food, keeping it stored in tight containers, and using roach traps and safe pesticides.

Relief medications

Medications that relieve asthma symptoms include short-acting beta agonists, a type of bronchodilator. They open constricted airways and improve symptoms during an asthma attack. They don't correct inflammation and should be used only as needed for occasional symptoms. Sometimes, however, a doctor will recommend regular use of a bronchodilator in conjunction with a preventive medication for people having difficulty controlling their asthma.

Short-acting beta agonists include the inhaled medications albuterol (Proventil, Ventolin) and pirbuterol (Maxair). They act quickly to open airways during an asthma attack. The medications may also be taken before exercise or exposure to cold air. They often relieve symptoms for up to 6 hours.

Combination therapy

If one drug isn't keeping your asthma in check, your options generally are to increase the strength (dose) of that medication or to take an additional medication of a different type.

A number of studies indicate that adding another medication is often the most effective therapy. Combining two different medications may reduce the risk of potential side effects from taking a high dose of one drug, such as an inhaled corticosteroid. In addition, the different drugs treat asthma in different ways. For example, one drug may control inflammation to prevent attacks, while another may help keep airways open.

Some combination drug products are now available on the market, such as Advair Diskus, an inhaler that combines the corticosteroid fluticasone and the bronchodilator salmeterol. Asthma medications can be prescribed in a number of combinations. An inhaled corticosteroid often is one component. Some combinations include:

- *An inhaled corticosteroid and inhaled, long-acting bronchodilator.* In this combination the inhaled corticosteroid helps control inflammation, while the long-acting bronchodilator salmeterol, also taken by inhaler, helps open narrowed airways. Many studies show this combination to provide better asthma control than increasing the dose of an inhaled corticosteroid alone, particularly at night.
- *An inhaled corticosteroid and a leukotriene blocker.* Although not as well studied as the previous combination, studies show this duo to be more effective at controlling asthma than an inhaled corticosteroid alone.
- *An inhaled corticosteroid and oral theophylline.* Theophylline can be difficult to use because it interacts poorly with some drugs and commonly causes side effects, but it has proved effective for some people.

If your asthma isn't well controlled with two medications, you may benefit from a three-pronged approach: an inhaled corticosteroid, a leukotriene blocker and a long-acting bronchodilator.

The right combination depends on the severity of your asthma and your treatment goals. For instance, you may prefer a pill instead of an inhaler. Perhaps you experience greater problems at night or during a favorite activity. Maybe you've experienced certain side effects with one drug but not with another. By discussing these issues with your doctor, the two of you can select the treatment program that controls your symptoms and works best for you.

Future Therapies

Asthma is likely the result of a combination of genetic and environmental factors. Researchers have discovered several genes associated with airway inflammation and constriction. These discoveries may lead to new therapeutic approaches to the prevention and treatment of asthma. As their understanding of asthma evolves, scientists are developing many new classes of drugs that interrupt the asthma process at key points.

Asthma Inhalers

Inhalers have transformed asthma treatment. They enable people with asthma to deliver medication directly to their lungs almost anytime, anyplace. During the past several decades, a variety of inhalers have been developed to relieve or prevent asthma symptoms. The most common device used to deliver inhaled medication is a metered-dose inhaler.

There's one catch, however. Metered-dose inhalers help only when you know how to use them. It takes a certain amount of coordination and skill to use a metered-dose inhaler properly. Many surveys have shown that most people who use a metered-dose inhaler — maybe up to two-thirds — use it improperly. But studies also show that with careful and repeated instruction, more than 90 percent of people who use inhalers can learn to do so correctly.

Types of inhalers

Inhalers are hand-held, portable devices that deliver medication directly to the lungs. A variety of inhalers are available, but basically they fall into two categories — metered-dose and dry powder.

Metered-dose inhalers
Metered-dose inhalers use a chemical propellant to push the medication out of the inhaler. The inhaler includes a pressurized canister with measured doses of medication inside. To use a metered-dose inhaler, you must perform two actions —

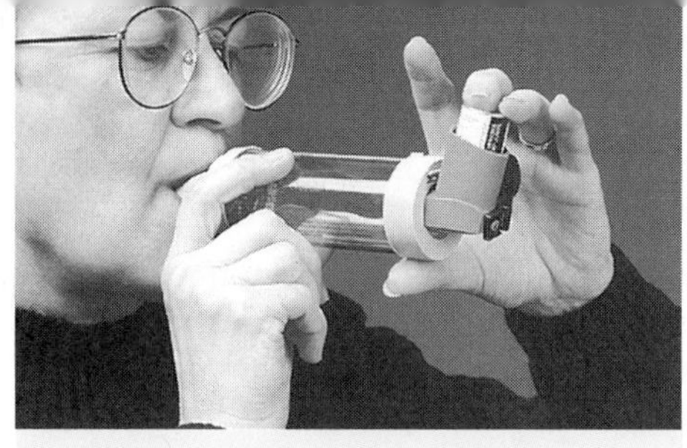

To use a metered-dose inhaler, follow these steps:

1. Shake the inhaler well, perhaps five or six times.
2. Attach a spacer to the nozzle end of the inhaler. A spacer is a 4- to 8-inch-long plastic tube that helps to distribute the medication evenly in the bronchial tubes. It also acts as a holding chamber that keeps your medication from escaping into the air. Releasing your medication into the chamber gives you time to inhale more slowly. It decreases the amount of medication that's deposited on the back of the throat and increases the amount that reaches the lungs. You can buy a spacer or make your own.
3. Hold your head erect and sit up straight. Breathe in and out normally once, then stop for a moment. Don't try to push all of the air from your lungs.
4. Close your mouth around the end of the spacer.
5. Squeeze the inhaler once as you breathe in slowly, like you're sipping hot soup. Keep inhaling even after finishing the squeeze. Continue inhaling for a total of 5 to 7 seconds.
6. After inhaling, remove the spacer from your mouth and hold your breath for 10 seconds. Then exhale through your nose.
7. If you've been directed to take two doses at a time, breathe normally four or five times and repeat steps 1 through 6.
8. Gargle with water or brush your teeth after using an inhaled corticosteroid. Spit out the water. This reduces the amount of drug that's swallowed and absorbed into the body by way of the stomach. It also reduces side effects such as mouth and throat irritation and oral yeast infections (thrush).

push down on the canister and inhale the medication through a tube called a spacer. The idea is to inject the medication into the incoming air and slowly breathe this mixture into your lungs.

Dry powder inhalers

Dry powder inhalers are breath-activated. The medication is released when you suddenly inhale from the device. A dry powder inhaler requires you to place your lips on the mouthpiece and inhale more rapidly than with a traditional metered-dose inhaler. Some people find dry powder inhalers easier to use than the conventional pressurized metered-dose inhalers because hand-lung coordination isn't required. Spacers shouldn't be used with dry powder inhalers.

Carefully follow the instructions that come with your inhaler and ask your doctor, nurse or pharmacist for a demonstration. Try using the inhaler in front of this person and ask for feedback. Then practice at home in front of a mirror.

Who should use an inhaler?

Both children and adults can use inhalers. Generally children age 6 and older can be trained to use an inhaler properly, and some children as young as age 4 may be able to use the device. Parents should supervise their children's use of all medications.

For people who are unable to use an inhaler, a nebulizer is generally recommended. Nebulizers are most commonly used by infants, young children and people who are seriously ill. The device includes a compressor-driven pump that converts the medication into a mist that's inhaled.

Inhaler pros and cons

The benefits of inhalers are that they're convenient to carry and use and they can provide immediate relief. But they need to be used properly to be effective. Noncompliance is a problem for many people with asthma who use metered-dose inhalers to manage their disease — either they forget to take the prescribed medication, or they use the inhaler incorrectly.

This can lead to the second problem: People with asthma can rely too much on short-acting bronchodilator inhalers.

These fast-acting medications can relieve symptoms quickly. But they're no substitute for the long-term medications that keep asthma under control. Maximum daily use of a bronchodilator is two puffs every 4 to 6 hours. If you're using one more frequently to control symptoms, you need a more effective program of preventive medications. Overuse of a bronchodilator can also put you at risk of toxic drug levels, which can cause an irregular heartbeat, especially if you have a heart condition.

Managing Asthma

In addition to medication, self-care is of paramount importance in controlling asthma. The best way to overcome anxiety and the feeling of helplessness that can accompany asthma is to take steps to reduce your risk of an attack. Try to take breaks between tasks and allow yourself some time to rest. Also avoid or limit activities that seem to make your asthma worse.

Take precautions when exercising

For many people with asthma, exercise can induce airway spasms. This doesn't mean you should eliminate exercise from your life. In fact, regular exercise is good for you. It helps keep your muscles in tone, which is important to your overall health. But do take precautions. Exercise only under the following conditions:

- You're feeling well and aren't bothered by a cold or another type of viral illness.
- You're properly warmed up. Five to 10 minutes of stretching or light exercise can help relax and open your airways.
- You've taken precautions for cold weather, if you plan to exercise outdoors and the weather is accommodating. Cold air and dry air are more likely to provoke a bronchospasm. Simple cold-weather protection includes breathing through your nose — to warm and humidify the air before it enters your lungs — and using a scarf or cold-air mask. Recent evidence suggests that repeated cold-air exercise can make asthma worse over the long term. Exercising in cold weather should be approached with caution, and preventive treatment should be considered to avoid loss of asthma control. You may want to choose an exercise that can be done in a warmer, more humid environment, such as an indoor pool.
- You've taken your medications as recommended. Your doctor may recommend that you take your medication immediately before exercising to help prevent asthma symptoms.

If you start to feel asthma symptoms coming on during a workout, you may be able to continue if the symptoms remain mild. Otherwise pause and take two puffs of your bronchodilator inhaler. If your asthma symptoms persist or get worse, it's probably a good idea to stop exercising for the time being.

If you have asthma, be sure to talk to your doctor about how to incorporate exercise into your lifestyle. Studies of athletes with asthma show that it's possible for many people with asthma to participate in any sport and at any level of performance — including the Olympic level.

Know and avoid triggers

Identify the things that trigger your symptoms. This can be one of the most important ways to take control of your life. More than 2,000 indoor irritants can trigger an attack. Common triggers include tobacco smoke, house dust and pets. Frequent outdoor triggers include pollen, mold and cold air.

Take the following precautions to reduce your exposure to asthma triggers and lessen the possibility of attacks:

- Avoid all types of smoke, even smoke from a fireplace or burning leaves. Smoke irritates the eyes, nose and bronchial tubes. If you have asthma, you shouldn't smoke, and people should never smoke in your presence.
- Because influenza can set off a serious asthma attack, get an annual flu shot, unless you've had an allergic reaction to chicken eggs, which are used in the preparation of the vaccine. The shot won't protect you against common colds, which also can trigger an attack. To help avoid a cold, wash your hands frequently and thoroughly.
- If you're allergic to pollen, use an air conditioner and keep windows and doors closed during the pollen season. This helps reduce your risk of an attack due to exposure to airborne pollen from trees, grasses and weeds.
- Limit use of contact lenses. Try substituting eyeglasses for your contacts when the pollen count is high. Pollen grains can become trapped under the lenses.
- Attach a two-ply microfiltration bag or electrostatic filter to your vacuum cleaner if you're allergic to house dust. You may also want to consider adding a high-efficiency dust filter to your ventilation system, although they're expensive and they haven't been proved to be beneficial.
- Maintain optimal humidity in your home and office — 40 percent to 50 percent — to reduce your exposure to dust mites, which thrive in warm, damp conditions. If you live in a damp climate, consider talking to your doctor about using a dehumidifier.
- Decontaminate your decor. To minimize dust that may aggravate nighttime symptoms, encase

COMPLEMENTARY MEDICINE

Although more research is needed, some evidence suggests that vitamin C may improve lung function and help prevent exercise-induced bronchospasms. The elements manganese and magnesium also may be beneficial in helping to control asthma.

Evidence also points to acupuncture as a complementary therapy that may help prevent asthma attacks. Researchers have yet to determine why acupuncture may be beneficial. One theory is that it stimulates the release of certain body chemicals. These might include vasoactive intestinal peptide, a chemical that works as a bronchodilator. Some studies suggest that inserting acupuncture needles at certain points on the chest wall leads to decreased airway resistance, as well as decreased sputum stickiness (viscosity) and improved sleep patterns.

Adverse side effects from acupuncture are rare, but they do occur. Infectious diseases, including hepatitis B, can be transmitted from needles that aren't properly sterilized.

It's always a good idea to check with your doctor before trying a new therapy. And never replace a proven treatment, such as medication, with a treatment that isn't proved.

Allergy Shots and Asthma

For some people with both asthma and allergies, avoiding triggers and taking medication isn't enough to control their symptoms. Allergy shots (immunotherapy) may be an option. With this treatment, tiny amounts of the substance to which you're allergic are injected underneath your skin. The substance is injected in progressively larger doses over several months to gradually increase your tolerance to it. In some cases, immunotherapy can help prevent airway inflammation and other symptoms that result when you come in contact with the allergen. Immunotherapy seems to work best for allergies to dust mites, pollen and cat dander.

Severe reactions to immunotherapy are rare but can occur. As a precaution, your doctor will recommend that you stay in a waiting room for a period after you receive the injections. An adverse reaction, if it happens at all, typically occurs within about 30 minutes after the injection.

mattresses, pillows and box springs in dustproof covers that can be removed and cleaned frequently. Avoid using dust attractors such as dust ruffles and curtains. Replace bedding made of down, kapok or foam rubber with synthetic materials such as Dacron. Wash sheets, pillowcases and mattress pads weekly in hot water. Replace synthetic pillows every 2 to 3 years.

- Keep the air in your home clean. Have a utility company check your air conditioner and furnace once a year. Change the filters in your furnace and air conditioner according to the manufacturer's instructions. If you use a humidifier, change the water daily.
- Avoid projects that raise dust. If you can't do that, wear a dust mask, available at drugstores and hardware stores. Also avoid projects that might expose you to asthma triggers such as paint vapors or wood dust.
- Reduce pet dander. If you're allergic to dander, avoid pets with fur or feathers. Having pets regularly bathed or groomed may reduce the amount of dander in your surroundings.
- Clean regularly. Clean your home at least once a week. Because cleaning stirs up dust, wear a mask or have someone else do it.
- Reduce stress and fatigue.
- Some adults with asthma experience severe attacks after taking nonsteroidal anti-inflammatory drugs (NSAIDs), including aspirin or ibuprofen (Advil, Motrin, others). You may need to avoid over-the-counter cold remedies and pain medications containing aspirin or ibuprofen.
- In some people, sulfites can trigger an asthma attack. Sulfites are found in various foods and beverages, including wine, beer, fresh and dehydrated fruits, seafood, maraschino cherries and some soft drinks. If you react to sulfites, ask the server when you're eating away from home if sulfites have been added to the food. At home check food labels for the terms *sodium bisulfite, potassium bisulfite, sulfur dioxide* and *potassium metabisulfite.*

Monitor your breathing

You may recognize signs of an impending attack, such as coughing, wheezing or shortness of breath. But lung function may decrease well before you begin to notice symptoms. So it's important to measure peak airflow with a home peak flowmeter.

If you have severe asthma, your doctor may recommend that you take a peak flow measurement at least once a day. Like a thermometer or blood pressure device, a peak flowmeter gives an objective measure of your condition. This device can be your asthma early warning system. A peak flowmeter measures the rate at which you can expel air. It's exhaling, not inhaling, that's most affected by inflamed airways associated with asthma. A reading that's lower than usual may be a warning of an impending flare-up.

Your doctor may give you specific instructions on how to deal with a decrease in your readings. If you have more severe asthma, you may need to use a peak flowmeter several times a day.

Develop an action plan

Consider your doctor as your partner in managing your asthma. With your doctor and other members of your health care team, write a detailed plan for taking maintenance medications and for managing an acute attack. Then be sure to follow your plan.

Asthma is an ongoing condition that needs to be regularly monitored and treated. Taking control of your treatment can also make you feel more in control of your life in general. Follow the plan as long as it's effective. If you experience difficulty, contact your doctor for additional instructions.

Pay attention to your symptoms

Be aware of symptoms that generally precede an asthma attack and respond to them when they occur. Don't wait for wheezing. It may disappear when airflow is severely restricted. Seek emergency care in the following situations:

- Breathing becomes difficult and your neck, chest or ribs pull in with each breath.
- Your nostrils flare.
- Walking or talking becomes difficult.
- Your fingernails or lips turn blue.
- Peak airflow, as measured with a peak flowmeter, decreases to half of your normal level or doesn't improve after you take your medication.

Treat attacks early

If you act quickly, you're less likely to have a severe attack. And you won't need as much medication to control your symptoms. When your peak flow measurements alert you to an impending attack, take your medication as instructed and immediately stop any activity that may have triggered the attack. If your symptoms don't improve, be sure to get medical help as directed in your action plan.

Children and Asthma

Nearly 5 million people under age 18 in the United States have asthma. Many more probably have hidden (undiagnosed) asthma.

With effective treatment, many children with asthma can enjoy a full range of activities, including exercise and sports. In many cases, their symptoms decrease in their adult years.

Follow a treatment plan

Work with your child's doctor to develop a treatment plan. The two overall objectives are to:

- Minimize the frequency and severity of asthmatic episodes
- Control the condition to allow for a normal quality of life

Your child's treatment plan may include several strategies:

- Medications
- Avoidance of asthma triggers
- Daily use of a peak flowmeter
- Allergy shots

Be supportive

Attitudes can be especially important. Children with asthma may emphasize what they can't do. Help them focus on what they can do — and how they can help keep their asthma under control. Be encouraging and supportive.

Be prepared for an attack

An asthma attack can be an anxious time for you and your child. That's exactly why you need to prepare for how to handle the situation. Your doctor can help you put together a written contingency plan that outlines what to do in an asthma attack. This plan will help you avoid panic when an attack does occur.

Copies of the plan should be kept in places where they're accessible at a moment's notice. Be sure that your child and everyone who cares for him or her — such as grandparents, a baby sitter and schoolteachers — know where the plan is kept. Also keep copies of the plan in your wallet or purse, the car and your child's backpack in case an asthma attack occurs away from home.

Although every child's plan will be different, it should contain the phone number of your child's doctor and this basic information:

- *Warning signs.* Symptoms and peak flowmeter readings that often are a precursor to an attack.
- *How to manage an attack at home.* Medications that should be used during an asthma attack — also where they're located and how to use them.
- *Indications of a serious attack.* Information needed to evaluate if your child needs medical care. List criteria for determining how much difficulty your child is having breathing. Note what level of medication use indicates a serious attack. List instructions for using medications that are designed specifically for treating a serious asthma attack.
- *What to do in an emergency.* Warning signs of a life-threatening asthma attack, emergency phone numbers and the location of the nearest hospital.

If you're in doubt about the seriousness of your child's symptoms, it's better to be safe than sorry. Call your child's doctor. There's no such thing as an inappropriate call about asthma. Successful treatment of asthma attacks depends on recognizing symptoms and acting early.

Work with school personnel

Every parent of a child with asthma faces the dilemma of how to help the child control his or her asthma at school. According to the American Lung Association, asthma leads to 10 million missed school days every year. That makes asthma the No. 1 cause of school absenteeism due to chronic illness. You can help keep your child from adding to that statistic. Create a feedback system to detect how well your child is managing asthma during the school day.

Share your child's treatment plan

Share your child's treatment plan with all of the adults who regularly interact with him or her:

- Homeroom teacher
- School nurse

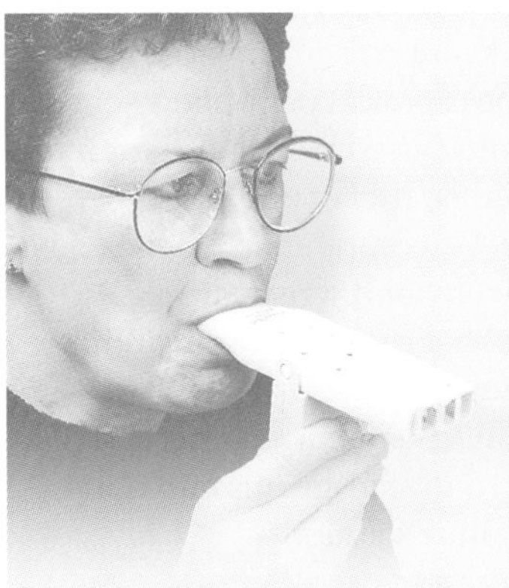

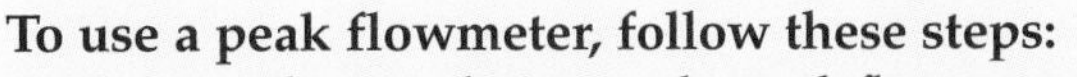

To use a peak flowmeter, follow these steps:

1. Connect the mouthpiece to the peak flowmeter.
2. Push the indicator to the bottom of the scale.
3. Take a deep breath and blow as hard and fast as possible — like you're blowing out a candle 6 feet away — with your lips tight around the mouthpiece.
4. Note the reading of the indicator. This is your peak flow rate.
5. Slide the indicator back to the bottom of the scale and repeat the test two more times.
6. Record the highest reading of the three tests.

Children and Corticosteroids

For several years, the Food and Drug Administration has required drug manufacturers to add language on the labels of corticosteroids stating that they may reduce the rate of growth in some children. Does this mean that it's not safe for a child to take inhaled or intranasal corticosteroids?

Inhaled and intranasal corticosteroids are, by expert consensus, still the best and most effective medications for asthma. Most doctors appropriately continue to recommend these products for many, if not most, people with asthma.

Corticosteroid use may reduce growth rates in some children. It's not possible to predict accurately which children will be affected. Studies don't reveal conclusively whether the slowed growth rate is permanent or whether affected children "catch up" later.

Asthma is a chronic disease that can be debilitating and even life-threatening. For children with asthma, the benefits of inhaled corticosteroids largely outweigh the risk of a potential reduction in growth.

To reduce possible side effects, it's important to use inhaled or intranasal corticosteroids with care. Here are some important things to remember if your child is taking these medications:

- Carefully follow the instructions.
- Together with your child's doctor, determine over time the lowest dose of inhaled or intranasal corticosteroids that will manage your child's allergies or asthma.
- Discuss other options with your child's doctor. Other medications for allergies and asthma do exist. But they also have possible side effects and may not offer the same benefits as inhaled or intranasal corticosteroids.
- Talk to your child's doctor before discontinuing inhaled or intranasal corticosteroids. Stopping the medication suddenly without careful follow-up could seriously impair your child's health.
- Be sure your doctor monitors your child's growth.

- Specialists, such as music, art and physical education teachers
- Classroom aides
- Counselors
- Coaches

Meet with your child's teachers and other school personnel early in the school year. Describe any medications that your child takes, how those medications are administered and possible side effects. Explain how your child can manage an asthma episode. Finally, provide a phone number where you can be reached during the school day.

Set up a medication location
Your child might feel self-conscious about taking medication at school. Make arrangements for your child to take his or her daily medication with minimal disruption.

Meet with the physical education teacher
Flexibility is key in physical education. Ask your doctor to write a letter to your child's physical education teacher. This letter may include guidelines for appropriate levels of exercise and explain your child's symptoms and asthma management plan.

Evaluate the school environment
Check that your child's classrooms are as free as possible of dust, mold and odors from chemicals such as glues and paints. Hamsters, guinea pigs and other animals in a classroom also might pose a problem. You may want to request a change in your child's homeroom.

Monitor your child's learning
Ask your child's teachers to contact you if he or she has difficulty paying attention or following instructions, and follow up promptly on any decline in grades. Asthma symptoms or medications might be playing a role.

Assess the results
Observe your child's symptoms. If you notice any change, consult your doctor.

Skin Allergies

Most Americans experience skin reactions at some time during their lives. The most common sensitivity is to plants such as poison ivy, poison oak or poison sumac. In people who are susceptible to these plants, contact with the irritants of these plants produces an itchy rash that may blister. Many other substances also can produce skin allergies.

Contact dermatitis

Signs and symptoms

- Itchy rash consisting of small bumps, blisters or swelling
- Burning sensation of the eyes and mucous membranes

Each year millions of people experience contact dermatitis, an irritation of the skin caused by direct contact with certain plants, cosmetics, chemicals, metals, drugs and adhesives. Contact dermatitis is a hypersensitivity reaction produced by immune cells in the skin.

The most common skin irritants include:

- The resins of poison ivy, poison oak and poison sumac
- The chemical para-phenylenediamine, used in hair and fur dyes, leather, rubber and printing
- Nickel compounds, often used in jewelry and wristwatches
- Rubber compounds, including latex
- Ethylenediamine, a preservative used in skin creams and ophthalmic solutions

- Dichromates, used in textile ink, paints and leather processing
- Formaldehyde, found in products ranging from permanent-press clothing to dyes, polishes, plaster, paper, rugs, foam insulation and particleboard used in home construction and furniture

Diagnosis

With contact dermatitis a rash generally develops within 2 days of exposure to the allergen. In people with a high sensitivity to the allergen, it can develop within just a few hours.

The affected area reddens and swells, and small, itchy blisters form. The blisters first fill with clear fluid and then burst, revealing raw skin susceptible to bacterial infection. The itching ranges from minor to severe. The rash usually reaches its peak after about 5 days and is usually gone in 1 to 2 weeks. In the case of formaldehyde, a burning sensation of the eyes and linings of the nose, mouth, throat or eyes may develop.

How serious is contact dermatitis?

Contact dermatitis is irritating. It causes pain and discomfort, and the blisters can become infected. It may be temporarily debilitating, but it has no lasting effects.

Treatment

The itching often can be relieved by applying a paste made of water and baking soda or Epsom salts, or applying calamine lotion or nonprescription hydrocortisone cream to the rash. Some people are sensitive to the agents in certain creams and lotions, which can aggravate the condition. Don't apply alcohol to the rash because this tends to make the itching worse. Cover open blisters with sterile gauze to prevent infection. Creams and lotions don't help much when the blisters open, but they can be used again when the blisters heal. Try not to scratch.

For severe contact dermatitis in sensitive areas, such as your face, eyes and genitals, see your doctor. He or she may prescribe an antihistamine or a stronger cortisone ointment or oral cortisone medication.

Prevention

Avoidance is the best way to prevent contact dermatitis. Allergens in household agents aren't always easy to detect, but harmful plants are. Learn to recognize offending plants and avoid them or wear protective clothing.

If you're allergic to a chemical such as formaldehyde, take steps to avoid exposure to it. For example, wash all new permanent-press clothing several times before wearing it and avoid insulating your home with formaldehyde foam. In the case of nickel sensitivity, wear solid (not plated) gold and sterling silver jewelry.

> **? Question and Answer**
>
> **I've heard conflicting reports on home humidifiers. Should someone with asthma use a humidifier?**
>
> It's a good question with a complicated answer. On one hand, high indoor humidity can promote mold and dust mites — both of which can trigger asthma and allergy symptoms. In addition, humidifiers can be a source of airborne bacteria and fungi. On the other hand, low indoor humidity also can aggravate nasal dryness and coughing — especially in people who have a cold, the flu or croup.
>
> The best advice is to use humidifiers cautiously. Keep indoor humidity no higher than 50 percent. Clean the humidifier regularly according to instructions. Consider limiting humidifier use to those times when someone in the house has a cold, the flu or croup.

Eczema

Signs and symptoms

- Extreme, persistent itching
- Thickening of the skin in patches

Eczema, also known as atopic dermatitis, usually occurs in babies and children, although it can occur later in life. About 70 percent of people with eczema have a family history of the condition. In addition, approximately 40 percent to 60 percent of individuals with eczema have respiratory allergies such as hay fever and asthma.

Diagnosis

Eczema consists of patches of dry, extremely itchy, thickened skin. Characteristically it affects the skin behind the knees and in the folds of the elbows. The itching is persistent and often drives people to frantic scratching. Babies and children who have the condition sweat more than normal, and they have dry skin that has a greater-than-normal tendency to itch. Most infants with eczema come from families in which other members have allergy-related diseases, such as hay fever or asthma.

Children usually outgrow their eczema by about age 6, although among some individuals, improvement doesn't occur until puberty or adulthood.

How serious is eczema?

Eczema is irritating, but for most people it's a passing problem. Some people have severe eczema.

Treatment

Treatment for eczema primarily involves use of creams, lotions and antihistamines. The objective is to stop the intense itching because it leads to scratching and thus more itching.

Give children short baths no more than three times a week, using a mild, neutral soap. Use of bath oil sometimes keeps the skin from drying too much. Keep their fingernails short to decrease the damage caused by scratching.

Latex Allergy

Allergic reactions to latex — a substance found in many health care and consumer products — have become increasingly common. Latex is a natural rubber product derived from the milky sap of the rubber tree. It may be found in examination and surgical gloves, intravenous and respiratory supplies and many other medical and dental products. Consumer products containing latex include condoms, diaphragms, rubber gloves, balloons and tires.

Reactions to latex allergy can take two forms. One is a skin rash (contact dermatitis). It's often seen in people who wear latex gloves, and it resembles the skin rash of poison ivy. This type of allergic response generally isn't a reaction to the latex but to the chemical additives used in the manufacture of latex products. The second type of reaction is a classic allergy reaction, and it can be more serious. In this case, the allergens are proteins in the latex itself. Signs and symptoms include hives, hay fever, a runny nose and those associated with occupational asthma (see page 533).

The best way to avoid latex allergy reactions is to avoid latex or reduce your exposure to it as much as possible. If you think that you may have a latex allergy, visit an allergist to find out. A medical history and allergy tests can determine your sensitivity to latex.

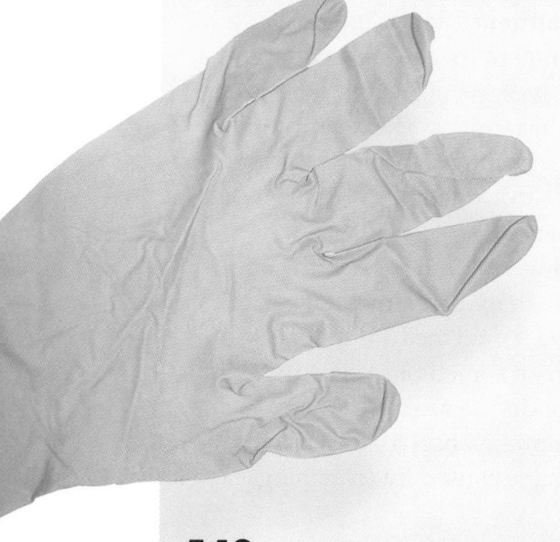

Use creams and lotions to keep the skin moist. To reduce inflammation and itching, apply a corticosteroid cream or ointment. If that doesn't help, tell your doctor; he or she may prescribe an antihistamine.

When the condition has been present for months or years, it causes the skin to become thickened and leather-like — a process called lichenification. In such cases, doctors will sometimes recommend ointments that contain coal tar, a thick liquid obtained from distilling coal. Coal tar contains chemicals that may have a therapeutic effect, but the ointments can be messy and have a strong odor.

Prevention

Avoid sweating and overheating, which are the most common triggers of itching associated with eczema. Although allergens don't directly cause eczema, they can trigger a flare-up.

Inhalant allergens such as pollen, dust mites and animal dander are of particular concern. Dry air also can irritate eczema, so consider using a home humidifier during dry seasons.

Hives and angioedema

Signs and symptoms

Hives

- Raised, red, often itchy welts of various sizes that appear and disappear at random on the surface of the skin
- The development of welts where the skin is scratched (dermatographism)

Angioedema

- Large welts below the surface of the skin, particularly around the eyes and lips but also on the hands and feet and in the throat

About 20 percent of people experience hives at one time or another. The medical name for hives is *urticaria*, from the Latin word *urtica*, for "nettle." Hives usually occur in batches rather than singly, and they may last a few minutes or several days. Hives occur on the surface of the skin. Angioedema is a similar swelling that occurs deeper in the skin.

Hives and angioedema are thought to result from the release of histamine and other chemicals into the bloodstream. The cause of the release is unknown, although a range of substances have been found to cause hives, including foods, pollen, animal dander, drugs, latex, insect venom, infections, illness, cold, heat, light and emotional distress. As with many allergies, heredity may play a role in the development of hives and angioedema.

Foods that may cause hives in sensitive people include shellfish, fish, nuts, eggs and milk. Penicillin and aspirin also are known culprits. Some people experience hives from coming in contact with pollen and animal dander.

Diagnosis

The primary sign of hives and angioedema is a swelling of the skin in the form of red welts. With hives, the welts are on the surface of the skin. They're often intensely itchy.

In the case of angioedema, the welts are deeper and appear primarily around the eyes and mouth, making them appear swollen. Welts may occur on the hands and feet, although less frequently.

To help determine the cause of your condition, your doctor may ask you to create a detailed diary of exposure to possible allergens over a period of 2 weeks to a month and a record of when hives occur.

Because hives and angioedema can be triggered by many different things and because they can also be exacerbated by stress and other emotions, it's sometimes impossible to determine the cause.

How serious are hives and angioedema?

Hives and angiodema are generally harmless. They leave no lasting marks and sometimes cause few symptoms. But when angioedema

Leaves of Three, Let It Be

The phrase, "Leaves of three, let it be," is familiar to many people, and with good reason. Certain three-leaved plants, especially poison ivy and poison oak, are the most common cause of contact dermatitis.

Poison sumac, which has many leaves, is a common offender as well. Four of every five Americans become sensitive to these plants to some degree. The problem-causing substance is the same for each plant, an oily resin called urushiol.

A reaction to urushiol occurs when a sensitive person comes in contact with the resin by brushing against the plant or something, such as clothing or pet fur, that has brushed against it.

It takes only a tiny amount of urushiol to cause a reaction, but direct contact is essential. The resin can be spread by accidentally rubbing it onto other areas of the skin before all of the resin is washed off.

If you come in contact with a poisonous plant, washing off the harmful resin with soap within 5 to 10 minutes after exposure can help avert an episode of contact dermatitis. Don't try to remove the resin by taking a bath, because this can spread the resin to other parts of your body.

Carefully remove and wash clothing, jewelry, shoes and shoelaces that may have come in contact with the resin.

Poison Ivy

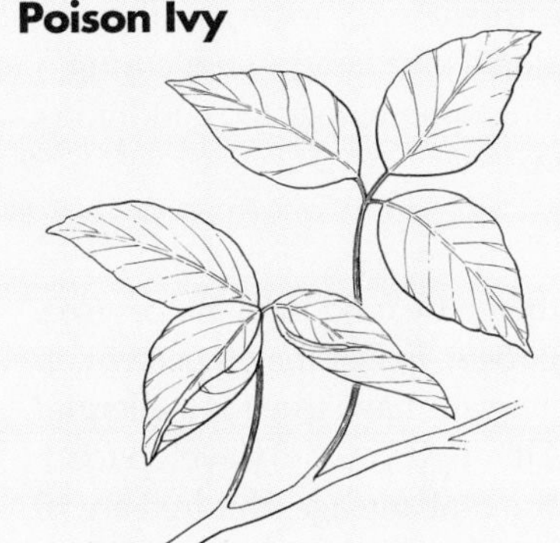

Poison Oak

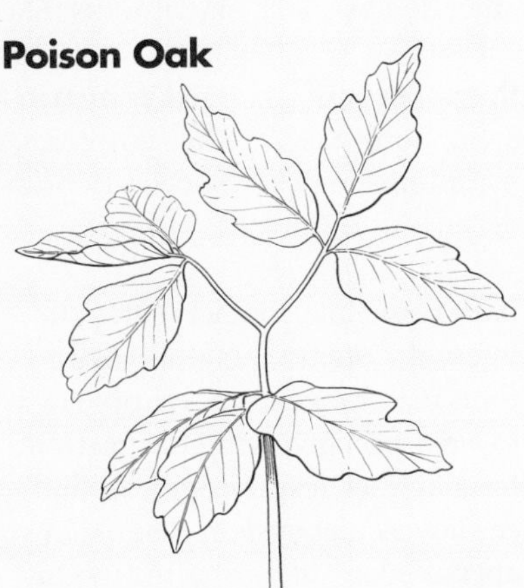

Poison Sumac

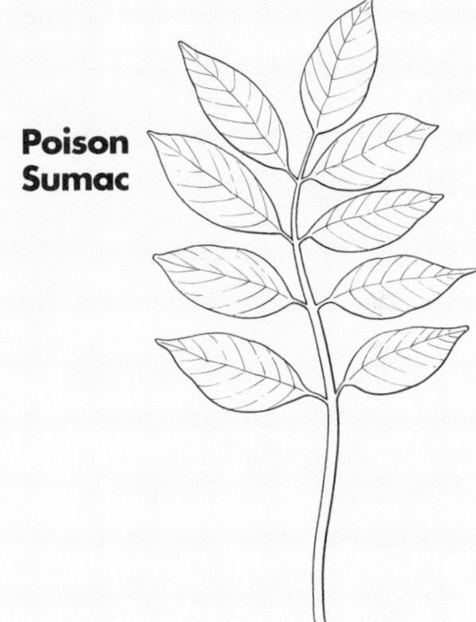

Poison ivy can be a low-growing plant, bush or vine. Its elliptical leaves grow in groups of three on a stem. Poison oak can grow as a low plant or bush. Its leaves, which resemble oak leaves, also grow three to a stem. Poison sumac may be a bush or tree. It has two rows of leaflets on each stem and a leaflet at the tip. The smooth edges of its leaves distinguish it from its harmless sumac relatives.

affects the throat or tongue, it can obstruct the air passage and be life-threatening.

In addition, hereditary angioedema, a rare form of the condition, is more troublesome and can be especially dangerous. It results from a blood protein disorder involving your immune system response. The symptoms of this disorder include nonitchy swelling, possibly with painful abdominal cramping and diarrhea.

Treatment

The standard treatment for hives and angioedema is an antihistamine. For more severe cases, other drugs may be used, such as an injection of adrenaline (epinephrine). Occasionally, doctors prescribe a corticosteroid medication. To prevent hives and angioedema, avoid substances known to trigger an allergic response.

Reactions to heat, cold or light

Signs and symptoms

- Rash
- Welts such as hives that appear as a result of exposure to heat, cold, sun or rubbing

Emergency signs and symptoms

Emergency signs and symptoms can occur as a result of immersion in cold water. They include:

- Muscle cramping
- Vomiting
- Fainting

One of the most puzzling allergy-like reactions is that to physical stimuli, such as pressure, heat, cold, light and sunlight. People who have this type of response often have very sensitive skin. Sometimes, just rubbing a blunt object on the skin produces swelling within a few minutes.

Diagnosis

Signs and symptoms include tiny hives that may result in response to vigorous exercise, a hot shower, emotional stress or a rewarming of body parts that have been exposed

Feel Like You're Allergic to Almost Everything?

For most people allergic reactions stem from sensitivities to specific agents, such as pollen or mold. Some people, though, feel as if they're allergic to almost everything around them. Strong fragrances, exhaust fumes, new carpet, cigarette smoke, solvents, plastics, formaldehyde and pesticides are among the irritants people cite as causing an array of symptoms.

These individuals may experience dizziness, impaired concentration, headache, joint pain, fatigue, memory loss and heat intolerance. The condition is known by several names, including multiple chemical sensitivity, total allergy syndrome and idiopathic environmental intolerances — the term recommended by the World Health Organization.

Allergies aren't the cause of such symptoms. Several theories as to a cause have been proposed, but none has been proved. Some scientists believe the symptoms may be related to an immune deficiency. Others believe they may be due to immunologic hypersensitivity, overstimulation of the olfactory (smell) area of the brain, damaged tissues, stress, depression or an anxiety disorder. About half the people with idiopathic environmental intolerances also have depression or anxiety. It's uncertain whether these cause the condition or are merely associated with it.

People with idiopathic environmental intolerances sometimes become frustrated when doctors can't find a physical cause for their symptoms, and they often consult other health care providers in search of an explanation for their illness. Some take drastic measures that are expensive and disruptive to their lives. These may include quitting a job to move to the mountains, living in a home free of synthetic materials or eating only organic foods. Despite such measures, rarely are the symptoms relieved permanently.

The most effective treatment tends to be a multifaceted approach that includes controlling — not curing — the symptoms and treating other associated conditions, such as depression or anxiety.

to cold air. Swelling of the hands and feet may occur in response to pressure. In testing for heat and cold reactions, your doctor may apply cold and hot objects to your skin to see if a reaction occurs.

Treatment

The best method for treating hypersensitivity to heat and cold is to avoid temperature extremes whenever possible.

You can prevent sun-induced hives by avoiding sun exposure or using sunscreens, especially if you're taking antibiotics, antihistamines, diuretics, antifungal agents, tranquilizers or hypoglycemics, which may make your skin more sun sensitive. Some perfumes also may cause sun reactions.

Food, Drug and Insect Sting Allergies

Allergies to foods, drugs and insect stings are thought to result from an antibody response to allergens that have come into contact with your internal systems. Signs and symptoms may range from a simple rash to a reaction involving the gastrointestinal tract, respiratory tract and cardiovascular system. They may appear soon after a specific food is eaten, a drug is administered or an insect sting occurs.

Food allergies

Signs and symptoms

- Abdominal pain, diarrhea, nausea or vomiting
- Fainting
- Hives, eczema or swelling beneath the skin
- Swelling of the lips, eyes, face, tongue and throat
- Nasal congestion
- Asthma

Emergency signs and symptoms

- Severe symptoms of the reactions listed above
- Anaphylactic shock

Few things are more distressing than a reaction to food because food represents something that nourishes and comforts. An estimated 40 percent of Americans believe they're allergic to specific foods, but in actuality most are bothered by food intolerances (see page 546). Fewer than 1 percent of Americans have true food allergies.

Although you can develop food allergies at any age, children are 10 times more likely to have a food allergy than are adults. Ninety percent of food allergies are caused by milk, eggs, soy, peanuts, wheat, fish, shellfish and tree nuts, such as cashews, almonds and Brazil nuts. Other foods that can cause problems include corn and legumes. Chocolate, long thought to be allergenic, seldom causes allergy.

Fortunately, many children outgrow allergies to milk, eggs and wheat by about age 6. Allergies to nuts and shellfish are more likely to be lifelong.

Diagnosis

Most food allergies provoke an almost immediate reaction. If you eat something and within a few minutes your tongue and lips are swollen, it's fairly easy to suspect the cause. It's unusual for a food to cause a reaction that begins more than 2 hours after eating.

Your doctor may take several steps to determine if you have a true food allergy. You'll need to review your symptoms and when they occurred, and you may be asked to keep a detailed diary of everything you eat and drink for several weeks, as well as any medications you take. Various tests may help determine specific allergens.

Skin test
A skin test is used to see if you develop allergic symptoms when a small amount of food extract is pricked into your skin. Negative skin tests are usually reliable in excluding a food allergy, but positive skin tests are less accurate.

One approach is the double-blind challenge test. In this test, you're given skin pricks of extracts of suspected foods in disguised form so that neither you nor your doctor knows what food is being administered. These results are more conclusive, but this test can be difficult to conduct and is time-consuming.

Immunoassays
These tests involve examining a blood sample for immunoglobulin E (IgE) antibodies specific to certain foods. A negative test essentially excludes a food allergy.

How serious are food allergies?

For most people, food allergies are merely a nuisance, but for a few they can be life-threatening. Responses vary from minor sniffles and a cough to life-threatening anaphylactic shock.

Treatment

The only completely effective treatment for a food allergy is to avoid the food that causes the problem. For some people this is no problem. For people allergic to foods or food ingredients that are common in the average diet, it means living on a severely restricted diet.

Emergency treatment, including an immediate injection of adrenaline (epinephrine) is necessary when anaphylaxis develops. If you have a food allergy, talk to your doctor about carrying such medication for emergency use.

Drug allergies

Signs and symptoms

- Rash
- Hives
- Generalized itching
- Wheezing and difficulty breathing

Anaphylactic Shock

Anaphylactic shock, also called anaphylaxis, is the most severe and frightening allergic response. Luckily, it's also the most infrequent, although each year several hundred Americans die of this reaction.

Anaphylaxis is an immunoglobulin antibody response to a large number of different antigens. The response is sudden, beginning seconds or minutes after an offending allergen is encountered.

Signs and symptoms

- Constriction of airways, including swollen throat, resulting in breathing difficulty
- Shock associated with severe decrease in blood pressure
- Rapid pulse
- Hives and welts below the skin surface (angioedema)
- Nausea, vomiting or diarrhea
- Dizziness, mental confusion, slurred speech or extreme anxiety
- Swelling of the lips and tongue
- Flushing of skin and intense itching

The anaphylactic reaction is systemic, meaning that it's not limited to the site of the irritation. Its most characteristic symptom is constriction of air passageways in the bronchial tract or throat or both.

The constriction is often accompanied by shock — a situation in which there can be a sudden decrease in blood pressure that causes a rapid pulse as well as weakness, paleness, mental confusion and unconsciousness. Anaphylaxis requires immediate treatment and can cause death if it's not treated quickly.

A person who experiences only a mild reaction may have a severe reaction with a subsequent exposure. A person may also become hypersensitive at any time, whether previously sensitized or not.

Causes

Almost any allergen can cause the response. Anaphylaxis occurs more commonly after certain insect stings or intravenous injection of certain drugs. Certain foods such as peanuts, tree nuts and shellfish also can cause fatal reactions. Only rarely do pollens cause the anaphylactic response. Some people have anaphylactic reactions for which no cause can be found.

Treatment

The standard treatment for anaphylaxis is injection of adrenaline (epinephrine) as soon as possible. It opens airways and improves blood circulation.

Cardiopulmonary resuscitation (CPR) and an emergency tracheotomy — an incision creating an opening in the windpipe through the neck — sometimes have to be performed as lifesaving measures.

If you observe someone experiencing an allergic reaction with signs of anaphylaxis, summon emergency medical personnel immediately. Check to see if the person is carrying special medication — to inhale, swallow or inject — to counter the effects of an allergic attack. If you're trained in CPR, perform the procedure if the person isn't breathing or has no pulse.

Emergency signs and symptoms

- Obstruction of the throat due to swelling
- Severe asthma
- Anaphylactic shock

Almost any drug can cause an adverse reaction that may range from irritating to life-threatening. Some reactions are true allergic responses — antibodies are mobilized against the offending drug and histamine is released. Nonallergic reactions also can occur.

Penicillin and its relatives are responsible for many drug allergy reactions, including mild rashes, hives or even anaphylactic shock. Most reactions are minor rashes.

Other drugs that cause allergic reactions include sulfas, barbiturates, anticonvulsants, insulin and local anesthetics. In addition, contrast dyes injected into blood vessels to outline major organs in X-ray studies contain iodine, which may cause an allergic reaction.

Diagnosis

A rash is the most common allergic reaction to drugs. Penicillin and its relatives can cause a rash, similar to hives, and another reaction known as serum sickness. This reaction, which can take up to 3 weeks to develop, is characterized by fever, aching joints, swelling of the lymph glands and a rash. In some cases, these medications, as well as streptomycin, insulin and tetracycline, can cause anaphylactic shock.

Sensitivity to penicillin drugs can be diagnosed with a skin test, but sensitivities to other drugs aren't as easy to detect because skin testing for most other drugs is either ineffective or dangerous. This means that the doctor must rely on a patient's memory about when and how certain drugs were taken.

How serious is a drug allergy?

Severe reactions such as anaphylaxis or acute asthma can be life-threatening. But such reactions are rare. Most reactions are limited to rashes and hives, but this doesn't mean that they can be ignored.

Allergy vs. Intolerance

Food allergies and food intolerance are often thought to be the same thing, but they're not. In a true allergic reaction, the body releases histamine and other substances that produce the gastrointestinal, respiratory and skin symptoms associated with food allergies. Only about 1 percent of the population has true food allergies.

Food intolerance can produce allergy-like symptoms, but the chemistry is quite different, as no histamine is released. In addition, if you have a food intolerance, you can usually eat a small amount of the problem food without a reaction. By contrast, if you have a true food allergy, even a tiny amount of the food may trigger an immediate allergic reaction.

One of the tricky aspects of diagnosing a food intolerance is that some people are sensitive not to the food but to a substance or ingredient used in the preparation of it. This is particularly true of foods containing lactose, wheat, monosodium glutamate (MSG), sulfites, salicylates and possibly tartrazine.

Causes of food intolerance include emotional and physical stress, irritable bowel syndrome and the absence of an enzyme needed to digest a specific food, causing incomplete digestion (malabsorption). Malabsorption disorders include:

Lactose intolerance

As most people grow older, they're less able to tolerate lactose, a sugar found in milk and some other dairy products. Even in infancy 1 percent to 3 percent of all babies are lactose intolerant. For more information on this condition, see page 872.

Wheat and vegetable intolerance

Intolerance to gluten, found primarily in wheat products, most commonly occurs in young children, who may or may not outgrow their sensitivity. Vegetables to which some people are intolerant include broccoli and peas, which produce intestinal gas, and mushrooms and wines, which produce indigestion and diarrhea.

MSG intolerance

MSG, a commonly used flavor enhancer, may cause flushing, headache and numbness around the mouth in people who are sensitive to it. Because many Chinese restaurants use MSG, this type of intolerance is sometimes called Chinese restaurant syndrome. MSG is also found in some seasoning mixtures and prepared foods.

Sulfite intolerance

Sulfites are present in various foods and beverages, particularly wine, beer, fresh and dehydrated fruits, seafood, dehydrated soups, maraschino cherries and some soft drinks. The sulfites help sanitize and preserve foods. Although few people are sensitive to sulfites, this type of intolerance occurs in up to 8 percent of people with asthma.

Treatment

The most common drug allergy reactions — rash, itching and hives — are treated with antihistamines or, occasionally, steroid drugs. Asthma reactions are treated with bronchodilators and steroids. Anaphylaxis is treated with adrenaline (epinephrine) injections.

In some cases, sensitivity to penicillin can be reduced with treatment so that the person can tolerate the drug. Small amounts of the drug are given in slowly increasing amounts. Sometimes, antihistamines and steroids are given before and with the penicillin doses to lessen the allergic reaction.

Prevention

If you know that you're allergic to certain drugs, avoid them. This means alerting your doctor of your drug sensitivities.

People sensitive to aspirin should avoid all aspirin-containing drugs. Wearing a medical alert necklace or bracelet at all times can alert medical personnel to your allergy in case of an emergency.

Nonallergic Drug Reactions

Many drugs can cause adverse reactions that mimic the symptoms of an allergy, but the reactions aren't the result of an immune system response, as are true allergies. Almost 1 million Americans, primarily adults, have reactions to the common drug aspirin. The reaction can include hives, welts (angioedema) and anaphylaxis. About 10 percent of people with asthma are sensitive to aspirin. In these individuals, aspirin can cause asthma to worsen. Reactions can also occur with other nonsteroidal anti-inflammatory drugs, such as ibuprofen (Advil, Motrin, others).

Angiotensin-converting enzyme (ACE) inhibitors, a class of drugs that relax blood vessels and are used to reduce blood pressure or treat congestive heart failure, sometimes cause cough and angioedema that aren't allergy related. Opiates such as morphine and codeine can cause reactions that mimic allergic anaphylaxis.

Some antibiotics, such as erythromycin, can cause stomach upset or diarrhea, and the antibiotic ampicillin may cause a rash that isn't allergy related.

Insect sting allergies

Signs and symptoms

- Hives
- Itchy eyes
- Constricted feeling of the throat and chest

Emergency signs and symptoms

- Swelling of the throat that causes difficulty breathing
- Coughing or wheezing
- Severe hives
- Mental confusion
- Slurred speech
- Abdominal cramps, nausea and vomiting
- Decrease in blood pressure that may result in unconsciousness

For most people, the sting of a bee or wasp is a temporary irritation. The area may swell and itch or sting for several hours, but then it returns to normal.

For 1 percent to 2 percent of people, however, such stings cause serious symptoms. These people are extremely sensitive to some insect venoms, particularly that of bees, wasps, hornets, yellow jackets and fire ants. An immunoglobulin antibody response occurs, releasing histamine into the body. Spiders, ticks, mosquitoes and biting flies are just a few of the creatures that can cause a nonallergic reaction.

Diagnosis

Symptoms of an insect sting allergy usually appear within a few minutes after the sting occurs. In addition to pain and an intense itch around the site of the sting, a mild reaction might include hives and itchy eyes. Extremely sensitive people may have more serious signs and symptoms such as severe hives and anaphylactic shock (see page 545).

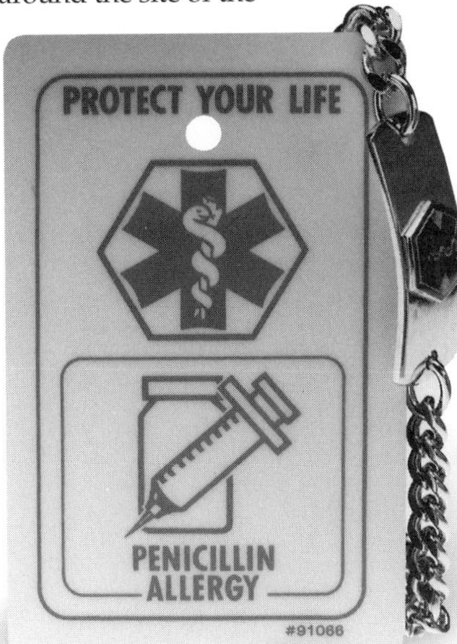

If you have a drug allergy, carry appropriate identification, such as a drug alert necklace or bracelet, at all times.

Severe reactions to insect stings can happen within 2 or 3 minutes. Generally, the sooner the reaction begins, the more severe it will be. To confirm an allergic response to a certain insect, your doctor may perform skin tests several weeks after the incident.

How serious are insect sting allergies?

Reactions to insect stings range from mild to life-threatening. If you know that you're sensitive to stings, seek medical attention for any sting. Many people don't know they're highly sensitive, and their past experience isn't always dependable because sensitivity can develop at any time.

Treatment

In the case of severe reactions, an injection of adrenaline (epinephrine) to open constricted airways will be administered. Corticosteroids, which act over a longer period of time than adrenaline, are often prescribed to reduce hives and other swelling. If the person stops breathing, cardiopulmonary resuscitation (CPR) may be needed.

Occasionally, if the throat is constricted enough to block an air passage, a tracheotomy will be performed, and a tube will be inserted into the throat.

When the reaction is less severe, you can minimize the effects by keeping the venom as localized as possible. Remove the stinger if it's present and place a cold pack on the wound to limit swelling and reduce itching.

Prevention

Once an insect sting allergy is confirmed by testing, immunotherapy may be used to increase your tolerance to the offending venom. Injections of small amounts of the venom will be administered every week until you can tolerate the amount of venom in a sting. From then on, you receive maintenance injections every 4 to 6 weeks for a 3- to 5-year period.

It's also important to avoid exposure to the insect as much as possible. For example, when you're outside, avoid wearing clothing with flowery prints or bright colors, which are attractive to certain insects. Don't use sweet perfumes, scented soaps, suntan lotions and cosmetics. Wear shoes and long-sleeved shirts as much as possible. And try to stay away from places where stinging insects are found, such as orchards, flower gardens and fields or lawns containing clover. If you feel in danger of being stung, stay calm. Move away from the insect slowly and without sudden movement. Panicky flailing only agitates insects, increasing risk of a sting.

People who are extremely sensitive to insect stings can safeguard themselves by carrying an emergency kit containing antihistamine tablets and a syringe of adrenaline (epinephrine). Your doctor can prescribe such a kit. Wearing a medical alert bracelet or necklace or carrying a medical identification card will provide helpful information in case of an emergency. ■

CHAPTER **22** PART V

Brain and Nerves

You might think of your brain as the chief executive organ in your body. It shapes and controls all of your thoughts and emotions and virtually all of your bodily functions and physical actions. Together with your spinal cord, it makes up your central nervous system.

The peripheral nervous system extends from your spinal cord and branches out to the tips of your fingers and toes. Sensory nerves are continuously gathering information from both inside and outside your body, busily sending messages to your brain.

Your brain receives hundreds of impulses from this network of nerves. While it interprets the messages, it sends information to different parts of the brain for memory storage. It then shoots back instructions that determine the appropriate response of your fingers, legs, mouth or other body part. By processing, sorting, filing and responding to incoming information, your brain gives meaning to the world around you. The individual manner in which your brain does this makes you the unique person you are.

Structures of the Brain

Your brain is made up of many structures that have specific functions. In a healthy brain, these parts work together in an efficient yet incredibly complex fashion. Although scientists are still discovering basic information about the workings of the brain, they know much more about it now than they did even 10 years ago. Advances in science and technology have provided so many new insights into this vital part of the human body that the U.S. Congress labeled the 1990s as the Decade of the Brain.

Some of the brain's basic structures include the brain stem, cerebellum, cerebrum and limbic system. The brain stem, located at the base of the brain, is responsible for regulating some of your most basic survival functions, such as breathing and heart rate. The cerebellum, which sits at the back of the brain stem, controls movements such as brushing your teeth and riding a bike. The cerebrum, resting on top of the brain stem, is the largest part of the human brain and the most easily recognized. It's responsible for all of your intellectual activities — your ability to think, reason, remember, imagine and plan for the future.

The limbic system, located in the deeper regions of the brain and responsible for emotions, is composed of the following structures:

- *Hypothalamus.* It controls body functions and urges — such as eating, sleeping and sexual behavior — and regulates body temperature.
- *Thalamus.* It acts as an information relay center, sorting and sending messages to and from various parts of the brain.
- *Amygdala.* It governs such emotions as anger and fear and triggers your response to danger, whether it be confronting the situation or fleeing it, a reaction commonly called the fight-or-flight response.
- *Hippocampus.* It plays an important role in forming and retrieving your memories, sending them to be stored in appropriate sections of the cerebrum or cerebellum and recalling them when necessary.

The cerebrum is divided into left and right hemispheres. Putting your two fists together in front of you can give you a rough picture of what your cerebrum looks like. Each hemisphere is subdivided into four lobes that control different activities. The frontal lobes in each hemisphere, located directly behind your forehead, govern such activities as speech production, abstract thought and voluntary movement. Behind the frontal lobes are the parietal lobes, which receive sensory information such as pain, taste and touch. Situated under the frontal and parietal lobes are the temporal lobes, areas that help you hear and interpret sounds and that are responsible for memory. The temporal lobe of the dominant half of your brain — usually the left — plays a major role in language func-

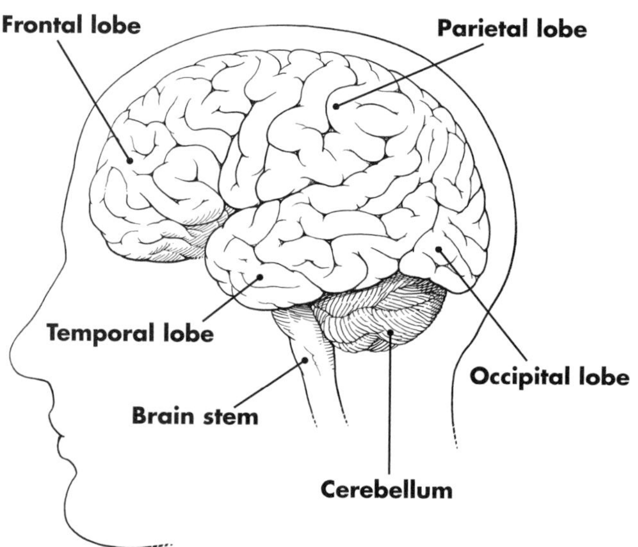

The outer cerebrum is composed of the frontal, parietal, occipital and temporal lobes. Other major areas of your brain include the brain stem and cerebellum.

tion. At the back of the brain are the occipital lobes, responsible for your vision.

Covering your cerebrum is a layer of tissue less than a quarter-inch thick. Grayish-brown and wrinkled in appearance, this layer is the cerebral cortex — commonly called the gray matter. The cerebral cortex is where most information processing in your brain takes place. All of the grooves, bulges and folds in the cortex allow a greater surface area to fit inside the skull, thus increasing the amount of information that can be processed. The human brain has more wrinkles than any other animal brain.

In addition, there are structures under the cortex called the basal ganglia. They play a critical role in relaying messages between different areas of the brain. Some disorders, such as Parkinson's disease, involve abnormalities in the basal ganglia.

Your brain and spinal cord are encased in bone. The brain is protected by the skull, and the spinal cord is protected by the vertebrae. The brain and spinal cord are sheathed in three layers of membranes (meninges): the outermost layer is called the dura mater, the middle layer the arachnoid and the innermost layer the pia mater. These layers provide cushioning for the brain and spinal cord. In addition, a liquid called cerebrospinal fluid, located between the arachnoid and pia mater, further protects your brain and spinal cord from injury.

Structures of the Nervous System

Peripheral nerves run from the spinal cord to all other parts of your body. Parts of the peripheral nervous system are named for the four spinal regions from which they branch: neck (cervical), chest (thoracic), lower back (lumbar) and pelvis (sacral). The spinal cord acts as a central communication network to transmit signals back and forth between your brain and the farthest reaches of your peripheral nervous system.

Your autonomic nervous system distributes nerves to smooth muscles in blood vessels (vascular) and internal organs (visceral), to exocrine and endocrine glands and to function-controlling cells of internal organs. This intricate system controls unconscious but vital activities such as distribution of blood flow, regulation of blood pressure, heartbeat, sweating and body temperature. Connections between autonomic and other brain functions occur in the brain stem and hypothalamus.

Cranial nerves are those nerves connected directly to your brain. They exit from the brain to control muscles in your face, eyes, tongue, ears and throat. They also convey sensations from these parts back to the brain.

Your arteries, which carry oxygen and nutrients from your lungs and heart, are critical to the functioning of your brain. Despite its small size and weight, your brain uses 20 percent of the heart's output of blood and 20 percent of the oxygen consumed by your body at rest. Blood is brought to the brain by the paired vertebral and carotid arteries, which extend up through your neck from your aorta. These large

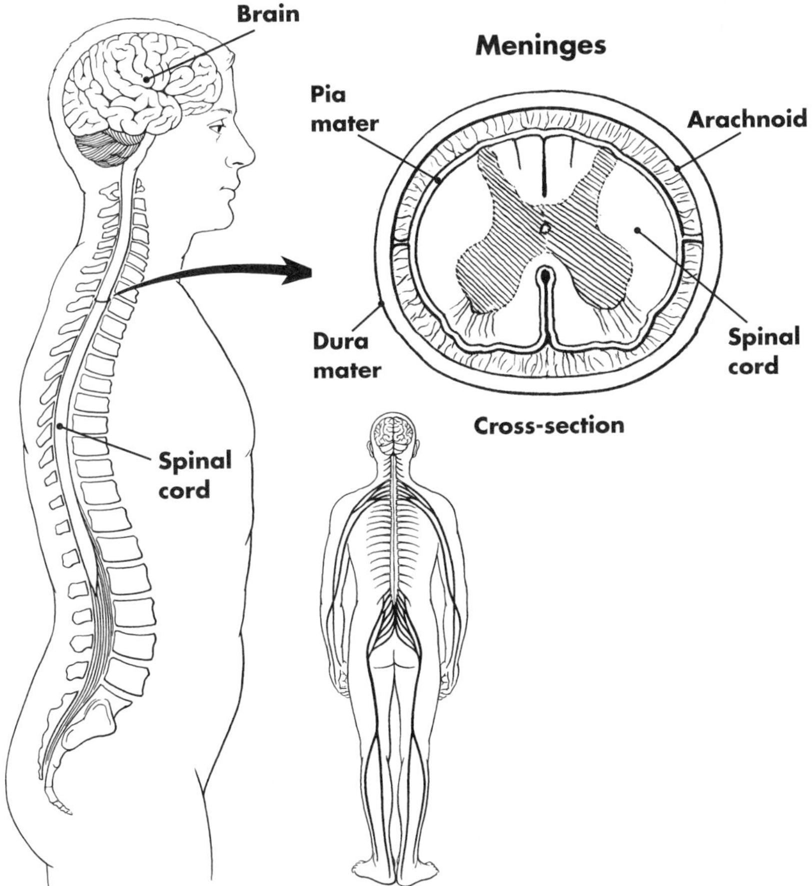

Your central nervous system, composed of your brain and spinal cord, is protected by your skull and vertebrae and by three layers of membranes: dura mater, arachnoid and pia mater — collectively known as meninges. Your peripheral nervous system (lower right) extends from your spinal cord to all other parts of your body.

arteries then divide into smaller ones to distribute blood to various regions of your brain.

A Healthy Brain at Work

The basic unit of your brain and nervous system is a nerve cell called a neuron. Neurons allow different parts of your body to communicate. They do so by generating electric impulses — messages — and relaying them near and far, to and from your brain and the rest of your body. Surrounding the neurons are glial cells that act as bodyguards — protecting, nourishing and supporting neurons. The human brain contains about 12 billion neurons and 50 billion glial cells.

Each neuron is made up of a cell body, which contains a nucleus and several other structures essential to the neuron's functioning. Extending from the cell body are branches called dendrites, which receive incoming messages from other nerve cells. Also extending from the cell body is a larger branch called an axon. Axons carry outgoing signals from the cell body to other cells, such as a nearby neuron or a muscle cell. Interconnected with each other, neurons are able to provide efficient, lightning-fast communication.

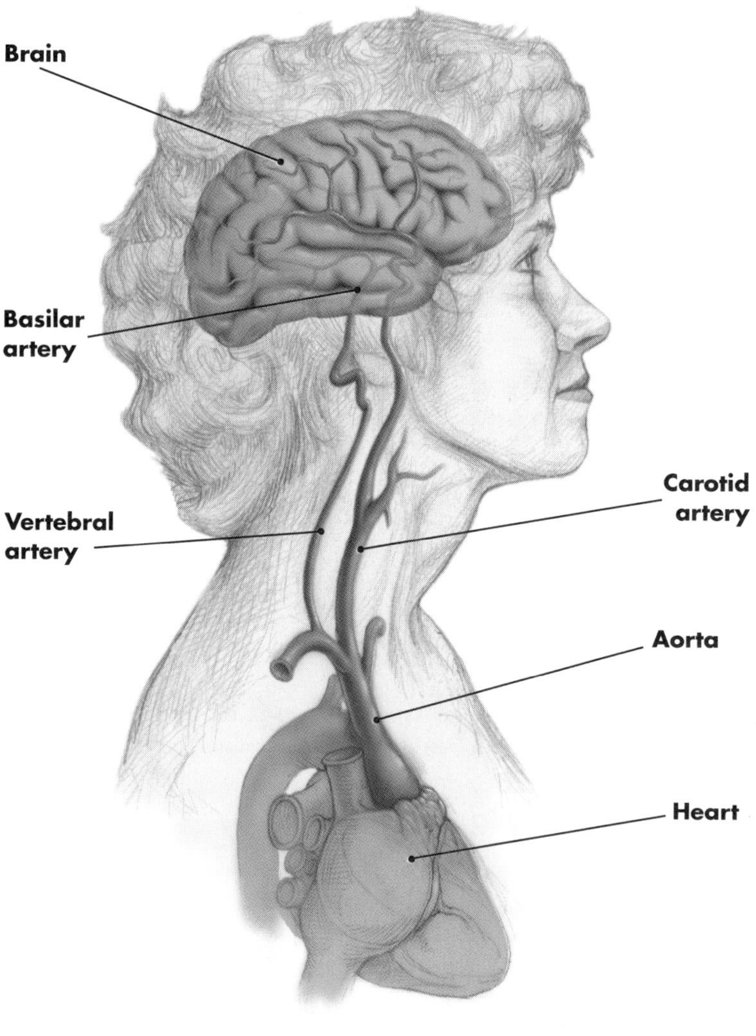

Your brain needs a constant supply of oxygen and nutrients from blood delivered through several key arteries.

Covering some axons is a white fatty substance called myelin. Myelin helps insulate the axons and speeds the transmission of impulses.

A neuron communicates with other nerve cells or body cells through electric impulses. In order to send an impulse, the neuron must be stimulated by something, which can range from a prick on your finger to a funny scene in a movie to an incoming impulse from an adjoining neuron. The message is then passed from one neuron to the next.

Within a neuron, the impulse travels through the cell body to the tip of the axon where there are tiny sacs containing neurotransmitters, chemicals that act as data messengers. The arrival of an electric impulse signals the release of the neurotransmitters into the synapse, the tiny gap between two nerve cells. In the synapse, the neurotransmitters bind to receptors on a receiving cell. This allows the impulse to enter the receiving cell and pass on to that cell's axon. Once the neurotransmitters have done their job, they're released back into the synapse and return to their cell of origin, where some of them may be reused (see the color illustration on page 414). This process is repeated from neuron to neuron as the impulse travels to its destination.

Neurons maintain their health by converting nutrients found in circulating blood, such as glucose and oxygen, into energy by a process called metabolism. Neurons are constantly renovating and repairing themselves so that they can continue to function properly. These processes are key to a healthy brain.

When things go wrong

Like a finely tuned machine, your brain and nervous system depend on a harmonious balance among all of their parts for efficient operation. Your brain and nervous system are vulnerable to a wide variety of injuries.

Interruption of the blood supply to the brain causes strokes. Degeneration of nerve cells causes illnesses such as Alzheimer's disease, amyotrophic lateral sclerosis and Parkinson's disease. An inflammatory reaction of the brain to an infection can cause meningitis and encephalitis. A head injury or brain tumor may cause structural damage. Problems in mental processing and learning are called cognitive disorders and can result from a variety of conditions affecting special brain functions. Seizures are caused by abnormal firing of nerve cells.

Neurologists and neurosurgeons are the medical specialists who treat brain and nervous system disorders. Diagnosis can be difficult

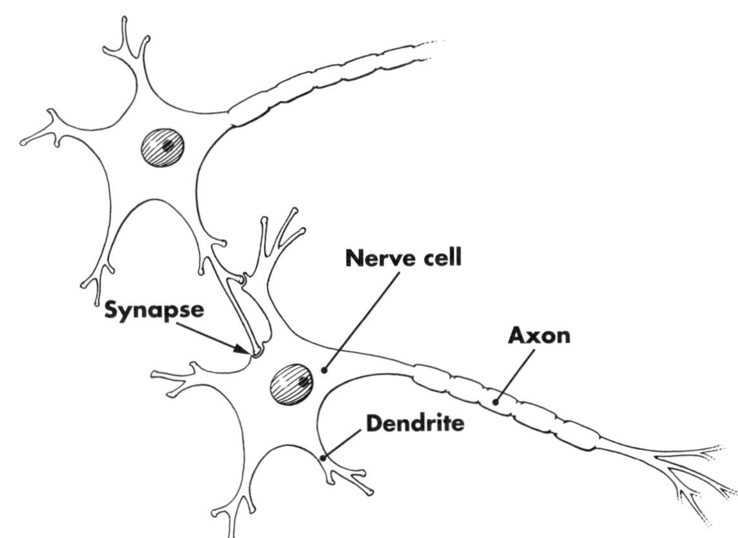

The nerve cell (neuron) is the basic unit of the brain and nervous system. It consists of the cell body, a major branching fiber (axon), and numerous smaller branching fibers (dendrites). Every nerve cell is linked to adjacent nerve cells at contact points called synapses.

A Neurologic Examination

The most important element in the diagnosis of a nervous system disorder is a description of your signs and symptoms and how they developed. Headaches, blurred vision or tingling sensations, for example, can be caused by many disorders. To determine what condition you might have, your doctor will likely ask detailed questions about your signs and symptoms and then conduct a neurologic examination.

A neurologic examination systematically tests how well the various parts of your nervous system are functioning. Many abnormalities that you may not notice can be detected with simple tests done in your doctor's office. The tests aren't painful, and no surgical procedure or injections are required.

Some of the routine tests for nervous system functions are described here:

Tendon reflexes

Your tendon reflexes are tested to evaluate motor and sensory nerve functions, spinal cord connections and peripheral nerve conditions. For example, your doctor may stimulate your reflexes by tapping your knee or ankle lightly with a special rubber-tipped hammer.

Babinski's reflex

Light stroking of the underside of your foot may produce a certain type of involuntary movement of your big toe, which can suggest an abnormality in the nerve tracts that originate in the brain or spinal cord.

Muscle strength

Weakness of a muscle or group of muscles can be a manifestation of a neurologic disorder. Therefore, your doctor may test the strength of various muscles as part of your examination.

Muscle tone

To test your muscle tone, a doctor moves your arm or leg to assess the ease and range of movement. For example, both legs may be tested to check for differences between the two sides of your body. Increased tone (spasticity or rigidity) or decreased tone (flaccidity) can indicate particular problems in the nerves that control different muscle groups.

Sensory function

Sensory tests are important in a neurologic examination because sensations such as pain, heat, touch and vibration travel through your peripheral nerves to your central nervous system. Your doctor evaluates these functions by asking what you feel when your skin is touched lightly by a pinprick, a hot or cold object, a cotton ball or a tuning fork.

Nervous system disorders can also affect your eyes and senses of taste, smell and hearing. Eye testing is particularly useful. The size of your pupils, a difference between the sizes of the pupils, range of eye movement, gaze and field of vision are often useful for diagnosing disturbances that may include the nerves that control your vision.

Gait, posture, coordination and balance

To evaluate these abilities, your doctor may ask you to stand, walk or move your body in a particular way to reveal possible abnormalities.

Mental status

Your doctor may also ask you questions that help determine whether your thinking, judgment or memory is impaired.

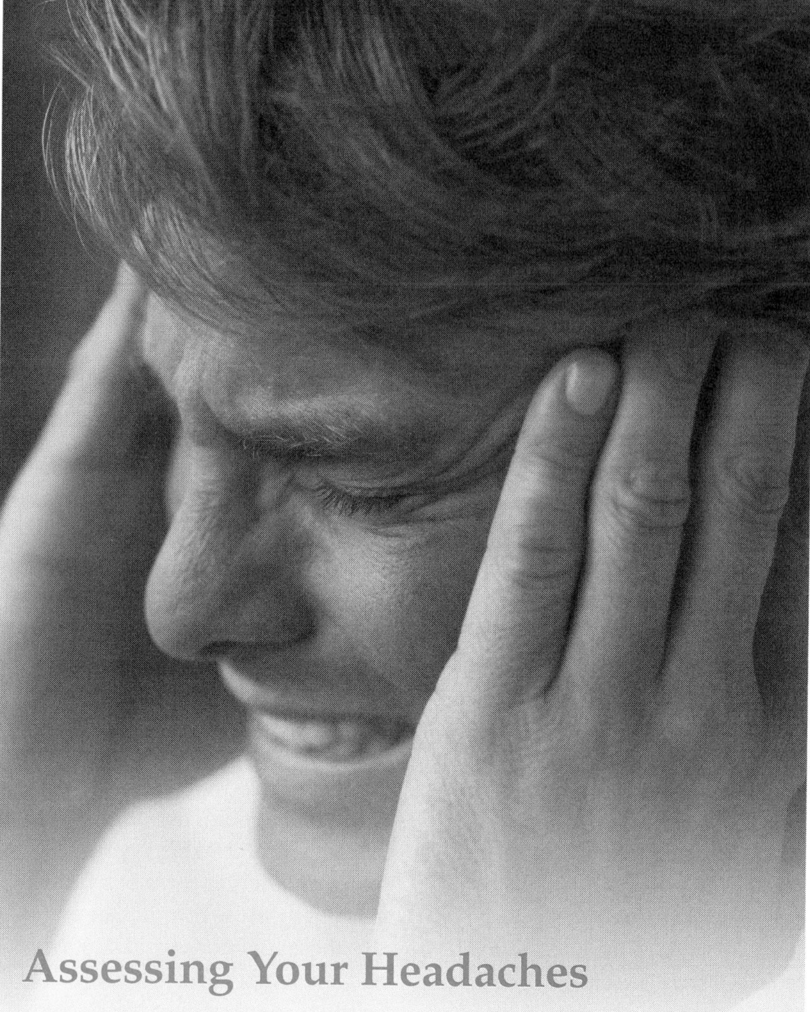

Assessing Your Headaches

To help assess your pain, your doctor may ask several questions about your headaches, such as:

- Do certain things trigger your headaches?
- How frequently do your headaches occur?
- Do they occur at regular intervals, and if so, at what time of day or night?
- Where do you experience the first pain?
- What does the pain feel like? Is it intense?
- Do your headaches begin slowly or rapidly? How soon does the pain peak?
- How long do your headaches typically last?
- Do other signs and symptoms precede your headache?
- Do other signs and symptoms accompany your headache?
- What relieves your headaches?
- Is there a history of headaches in your family?
- How do you respond to headache medication?
- Do your headaches affect your ability to work or participate in other activities?
- What thoughts do you have about your headaches?
- Why are you seeking help now?

If you have frequent headaches, it may be useful to keep a headache diary, including answers to the questions listed above. Such a journal may help you and your doctor identify headache triggers to avoid in the future.

because signs and symptoms can be numerous and diverse. Difficulties may also be encountered in distinguishing between neurologic and psychiatric disease. A careful assessment of the character and pattern of signs and symptoms over time, in addition to laboratory tests, are sometimes necessary to reach an accurate diagnosis.

Headaches

Almost everyone experiences a headache at one time or another. Headaches are among the most common medical complaints. Headaches have many causes, and the site, severity and frequency with which they occur vary greatly. About 95 percent of all headaches are primary headaches, meaning that they aren't caused by an underlying disease or tumor. Sometimes, a headache may result from a serious medical problem, but this is uncommon.

What causes head pain?

Although your brain tissue can't ache, there's evidence that certain pathways within the brain stem and other portions of the brain may contribute to the production of various types of headaches. In fact, pain can't occur in most of your skull and a large portion of your brain membranes. Observations made during surgery indicate that only certain structures in your head are pain sensitive. These structures include skin and tissues lying just beneath it on the outside of your skull — muscles, arteries, the skull coating, eyes, ears and nasal and sinus cavities. Pain sensitive structures inside your skull include arteries, venous sinuses and their tributary veins, parts of the outer membrane at the base of the brain and certain cranial and cervical nerves.

Cranial or cervical nerves send pain sensations from these parts of your head to your central nervous system. Dental and jaw pain, for example, are conveyed by the cranial nerves. Your cervical nerves also convey messages about pain in your neck and at the base of your head.

Outside of your skull, pain may result from inflammation or tension in muscles, inflammation of scalp arteries or inflammation in your sinuses, ears or gums. Inside your skull, enlargement or contraction of arteries, inflammation of brain membranes or pressure from a tumor or hemorrhage can produce a headache.

Although the exact nature of headache pain is unclear, research suggests that headaches may occur as a result of changes in the levels of brain chemicals (neurotransmitters), such as serotonin and noradrenaline. An imbalance in the levels of these neurotransmitters may lead to inflammation of scalp arteries and subsequent irritation of pain sensitive structures. This causes pain impulses to travel along the trigeminal nerve, a major pathway for pain, into the brain. The level of endorphins, natural painkillers produced by your brain and spinal cord, also may be disrupted, causing pain.

Your headache might feel dull, throbbing (pulsatile) or sharp. Precise description of your pain can be helpful in diagnosing what type of headache you have. Primary headaches are generally classified into three categories: tension-type, migraine and cluster.

Tension-type headaches usually produce a dull pain, knot or pressure in your forehead, scalp or the back of the neck. Migraines are associated with severe pain on only one side of your head and are often accompanied by nausea or transient visual disturbances. Cluster headaches are characterized by a steady pain in and around one eye or on one side of the head and tend to occur in episodes.

An unrelieved headache that's disabling and continues for 6 months or more is considered chronic. Approximately 42 million Americans have chronic headaches, of which migraines and tension-type headaches are some of the most common forms.

Although the exact cause of headaches is uncertain, they can be triggered by any number of things. Headaches, especially migraines, occur in some women just before or during a menstrual period. Such headaches are likely related to hormonal fluctuations. Headaches from high blood pressure tend to occur on awakening in the morning, but this type is uncommon and occurs only with severe high blood pressure.

A headache that results from an infection in your nasal cavity can

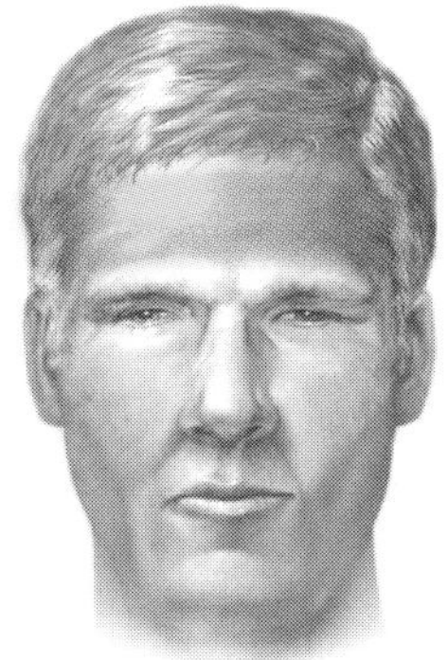
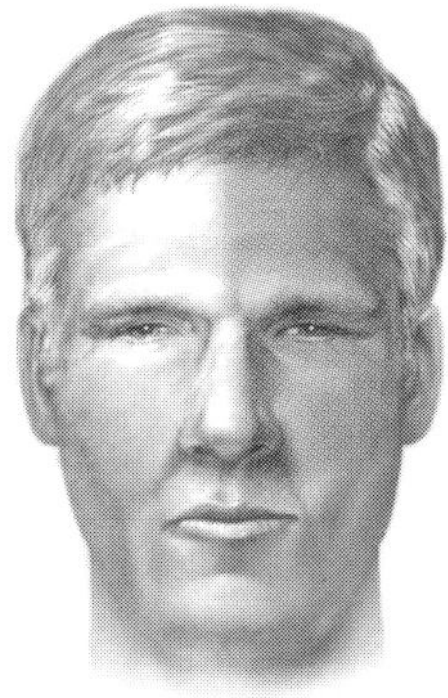
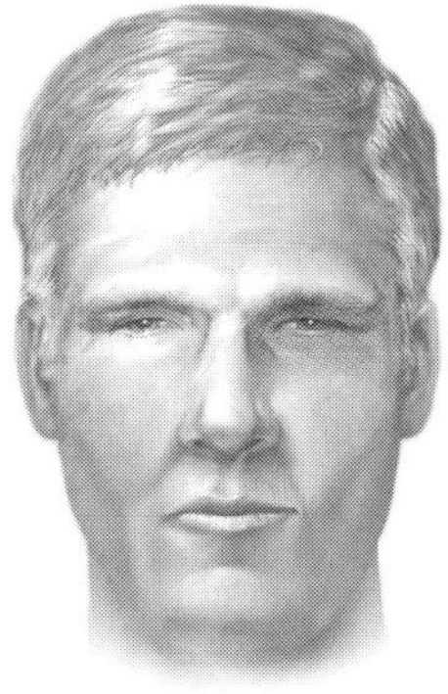

The three most common types of headaches cause different types of pain. The pain of a tension-type headache is usually a dull, squeezing pain that may involve the forehead, scalp, temples or back of the neck. A migraine commonly occurs on only one side of the head. Cluster headaches usually occur on one side of the head or as a stabbing sensation in an eye.

When a Headache Spells Trouble

Headaches that signal a serious medical condition are uncommon, but a headache can accompany conditions such as a cerebral hemorrhage, brain tumor and weakened blood vessel (aneurysm).

If you have one or more of the following headache warning signs, seek urgent care:

- Abrupt, severe headache, often like a thunderclap
- Headache with fever, stiff neck, rash, mental confusion, seizures, double vision, weakness, numbness or speaking difficulties
- Headache after a head injury, even if it's a minor fall or bump, and especially if it gets worse
- Chronic, progressive headache that worsens after coughing, exertion, straining or a sudden movement
- New headache pattern after age 55

A rare headache-related condition that almost always begins after age 55 is temporal arteritis, an inflammation of arteries in your scalp, brain and eyes. It's treatable, but if ignored, it can lead to blindness or, rarely, stroke.

You generally need not be concerned by an occasional headache. Most everyone experiences them, and they're usually related to common conditions such as stress, allergies or overuse of alcohol. If, however, your headache appears with other signs and symptoms or you have one that you might call the worst ever, seek medical help.

Rebound Headaches

If you find yourself taking pain relievers for headaches three or more times a week on a regular basis, you may be experiencing a rebound effect. In other words, your medication may actually be contributing to your head pain.

Although scientists aren't sure why this happens, they think that overuse of pain medications may short-circuit your brain's pain control system. When your pain reliever wears off, your headache returns, at times even stronger than before.

Signs and symptoms

Rebound headaches are typically continuous throughout the day but not necessarily severe. You may notice increasing pain at certain times, especially when your pain reliever begins to wear off. Often, the headaches can be triggered by just minor mental or physical stress.

Nausea, anxiety, restlessness, irritability, difficulty concentrating and depression may accompany rebound headaches.

Breaking the cycle

To break the rebound cycle, you'll need to wean yourself off your pain medications. Start by making an appointment with your doctor or a headache specialist.

Depending on what you've been taking, you may be advised to temporarily stop all pain medication. Doing so will likely mean increased headaches for the next week to 10 days. But most people who successfully stop pain relievers experience significant pain relief within 2 months.

Once you've broken the cycle, you can work with your doctor to set up an appropriate headache management plan. Often, daily preventive therapy is available for different types of headaches, such as avoiding or minimizing certain headache triggers — caffeine, stress or irregular eating patterns. In addition, your doctor may prescribe a specific medication to treat your headaches, matching it with the type of headache to which you're prone.

Alternative pain management

Instead of pain medication, try some of the following techniques. They may be just as effective as medication, without the side effects:

- *Rest in a quiet, dark room.* Place a cold towel on your forehead and compress your temples. Ice also may help.
- *Take a hot shower or warm bath to relax.* Massage your scalp, face, neck and shoulder muscles.
- *Learn stress relief techniques.* These include relaxed breathing, yoga and meditation.

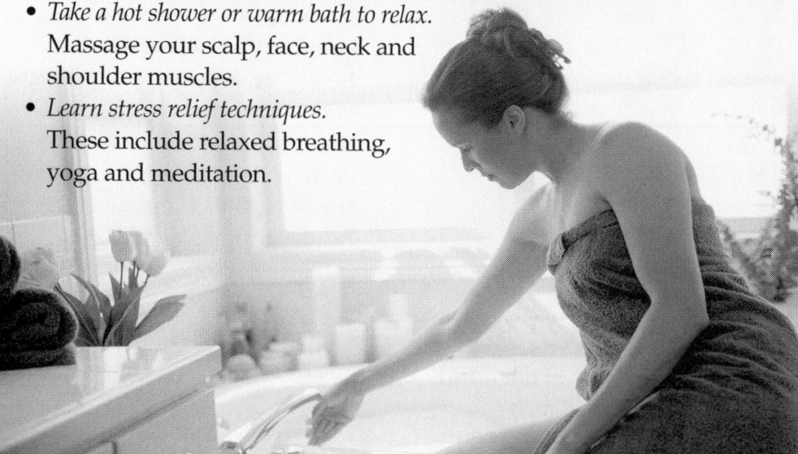

be particularly painful when you bend over. It's is usually accompanied by other signs and symptoms of infection. Eyestrain headaches may occur after long periods of reading or driving a car at night. Headaches also result from overexertion.

Making a diagnosis

Diagnosis of a headache is generally based on a medical history and examination. If your headache is of recent onset, occurs in abrupt attacks, is triggered by exertion, is typically present in the morning and accompanied by vomiting or is associated with other signs and symptoms, further testing may be required.

Testing may include a computerized tomography (CT) scan or magnetic resonance imaging (MRI) of your head to look for any structural abnormalities and to examine your sinuses, facial bones and neck tissue and bones. X-rays of the upper spine may be needed if your headaches began after a head or neck injury.

Your doctor may need other tests, such as a spinal tap, or lumbar puncture (see page 578), or cerebral arteriography, to establish the diagnosis.

Tension-type headaches

Signs and symptoms

- A dull or pressure-like pain in the forehead, scalp, temples or back of the neck

A tension-type headache is often diffuse and intense pain over the top of your head or the back of your neck. It may feel like fullness or pressure, as if your head were surrounded by a constricting band or vise. You may find it difficult to sleep. Many people complain of tight muscles in the neck and shoulders.

Tension-type headaches that occur two or more times a week for a period of months or longer are considered chronic. Some people experience such headaches over a period of years or even decades. The headache pain usually has a waxing and waning quality.

Tension-type headaches are probably the most common head pain. Stress, depression and anxiety are the most common triggers. Some tension-type headaches may be triggered by poor posture, working in awkward positions or a sudden strain. Because they respond well to over-the-counter pain medications, people with tension-type headaches usually don't consult their doctors.

These headaches may strike people of any age or sex. The chronic form most frequently develops during middle age, and it can last for several years after onset.

Diagnosis

To establish a diagnosis, your doctor will likely ask questions or have you undergo tests to exclude other possible sources of your pain. Tests may include a urinalysis, vision tests, a sinus X-ray and a magnetic resonance imaging (MRI) or computerized tomography (CT) scan.

Your doctor may look for evidence of anxiety or depression. You may be asked if any particular stress in your job or family situation might be associated with worsening of the headache.

How serious are tension-type headaches?

These headaches don't lead to more serious disorders. They may, however, be a sign that you're stressed, anxious or depressed.

Treatment

Tension-type headaches usually respond well to relaxation techniques, such as massage, hot showers, warm baths, biofeedback and meditation. Adequate exercise and rest also can be helpful. Sometimes, physical therapy is recommended. Keeping a headache diary may help you identify and avoid what triggers your headaches.

Medication

Pain relievers such as acetaminophen, aspirin or ibuprofen are usually effective. Antidepressant medications may be prescribed for a chronic problem. Avoid tranquilizers.

Medication is not a cure, however. Overuse of pain relievers can even lead to headaches, known as rebound headaches. In addition, the effectiveness of your pain medication may eventually wear off. If tension-type headaches persist, your body may be telling you that serious changes are needed in your lifestyle.

Migraines

Signs and symptoms

- Moderate to severe head pain
- Nausea and vomiting
- Sensitivity to light and sound
- Fatigue
- Sparkling, rainbow-like colors or blank spots in your field of vision (aura)

A migraine usually begins in the early morning or during the day with intense, gripping pain on one side of your head that may gradually spread. It typically reaches the peak of severity in minutes to an hour or two and lasts for hours to up to 2 days, unless treated. Sleep generally improves signs and symptoms, but you may be listless after waking up. The frequency of attacks can range from daily to occasional. Migraine attacks can be associated with nausea and, at times, vomiting.

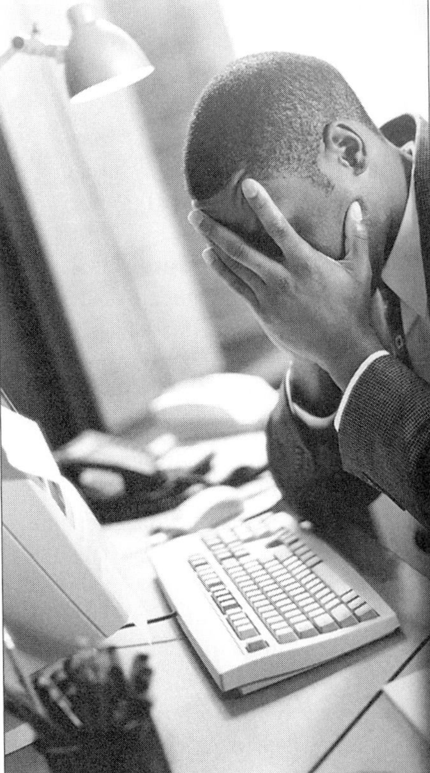

The exact cause of migraines is unknown. Scientists suspect they're related to an imbalance of serotonin and possibly other brain chemicals (neurotransmitters). Serotonin regulates pain messages moving through the trigeminal nerve pathway, a major pathway for pain. Changes in noradrenaline activity may be responsible for an aura many experience just before the headache.

During a headache, the brain's serotonin levels drop. Researchers believe this causes the trigeminal nerve to release substances called neuropeptides, which travel to your brain's outer covering. There they cause blood vessels to become dilated and inflamed. The result is headache pain.

Much is still unknown about migraines, but experts believe this type of headache starts in the brainstem of the cerebral cortex. It then follows a trail to the trigeminal nerve system — a major pain pathway in your brain. From there it moves to the blood vessels in the outer covering of the brain. The blood vessels become dilated and inflamed, causing pain. Because levels of magnesium drop right before or during a migraine, it's possible that low amounts of this mineral, which is involved in nerve cell function, may cause nerves in the brain to misfire.

Types

Migraines have several clinical patterns:

Migraines with aura

With a classic migraine, some people get a neurologic warning 5 to 20 minutes before their headache begins. The warning, called an aura, may include sparkling flashes of colored light, dazzling zigzag lines, slowly spreading blind spots and dizziness. You may also have a feeling of numbness on one side of your body. Less commonly, the symptoms include a slowly spreading weakness or numbness of your face or a hand or leg, tingling and numbness in your lips or difficulty talking or writing. Rarely, these symptoms may persist, presumably because of a stroke.

Migraines without aura

A common migraine begins gradually with no characteristic warning symptoms. Hours before the headache, you may be elated, full of energy, thirsty, hungry for sweets, drowsy, irritable or depressed. These are sometimes referred to as premonitory symptoms. The headache usually builds to full intensity over several minutes or longer.

Others

Less common types of migraines include:

- *Migraine with aura and paralysis.* Called familial hemiplegic migraine, this type of migraine results in paralysis of one side of the body. The affected person has at least one immediate relative who has identical attacks.
- *Migraine aura without headache.* This form occurs mostly in older adults.
- *Status migrainosus.* This is a migraine that persists longer than 72 hours.
- *Migrainous infarction.* In this condition one or more aura symptoms persist for longer than 21 days.

Migraines may begin in childhood, adolescence or early adulthood and taper in number and intensity as you grow older. In more than half of all cases, there's a family history of migraines. Women are three times more likely to have migraines than men are. Attacks tend to decrease during pregnancy, generally during the second trimester.

The biologic causes of migraines are unknown, but many triggers have been identified. A period of hard work followed by relaxation may lead to a weekend migraine. Stress, hormonal fluctuations during menstruation, alcohol consumption, hunger or use of oral contraceptives can cause migraines in some people.

Certain foods may produce attacks, including red wine, chocolate, aged cheese, milk, chicken livers, meats preserved in nitrates or anything prepared with monosodium glutamate. Some people report that exposure to sunlight or exercise triggers their attacks. Many migraine attacks have no apparent trigger.

Diagnosis

If you have migraines with characteristic warning symptoms or a family history of this type of headache, your doctor may have little difficulty diagnosing the condition. If you don't have these traits or if the headaches are severe and of recent onset, you may need testing to look for other causes, such as a tumor, aneurysm or other structural disorder. In some cases, a doctor will request tests such as a spinal tap to analyze cerebrospinal fluid (see page 578), a sinus X-ray, vision tests and a computerized tomography (CT) scan or magnetic resonance imaging (MRI).

How serious are migraines?

Migraines are a chronic disorder without a cure. The headaches aren't life-threatening, and there's no proof that they lead to other disorders. With treatment you should be able to reduce the number and severity of attacks.

Sometimes, complications result from efforts to control your pain. If you take over-the-counter or prescription headache medications more than three times a week, you may be setting yourself up for a complication known as rebound headaches (see page 556). Although these drugs can give you temporary relief, your body gets used to them over time. The result is that your headaches may become worse or more frequent. You then use more pain medication, which traps you in a vicious cycle.

In addition, nonsteroidal anti-inflammatory drugs (NSAIDs), such as ibuprofen (Advil, Motrin, others) and aspirin, may cause side effects such as stomach pain, bleeding and ulcers, especially if taken in large doses or for a long period of time.

Treatment

Medications that may help treat migraines fall into two classes — those that stop or decrease pain once it has started and those that reduce or prevent migraines.

Acute medications

Acute (abortive) medications stop or decrease pain after a migraine starts. You may have better results from these medications if you rest or sleep in a dark room after taking them:

- *Pain relievers.* Analgesics such as acetaminophen (Tylenol, others) or NSAIDs may ease mild to moderate migraines in as many as 50 percent of the people who experience them. If over-the-counter medications don't help, your doctor may suggest a prescription-strength version of the same drug. Be aware that new over-the-counter medications marketed specifically for migraines, such as Excedrin Migraine, Advil Migraine and Motrin Migraine Pain, contain the same amount of pain reliever as the original versions of these drugs and usually aren't effective for people seriously disabled by their headaches. Taken too often or for long periods of time, NSAIDs can lead to ulcers, gastrointestinal bleeding and rebound headaches.
- *Triptans.* Sumatriptan (Imitrex) was the first drug specifically developed to treat migraines. It mimics the action of the brain

chemical serotonin by binding to serotonin receptors and causing blood vessels to constrict. Sumatriptan is available in oral, nasal and injection form. With tablets, relief occurs in about 2 hours. Injections may bring relief in as little as 15 minutes. The nasal form acts more quickly than the tablets but slower than an injection. Injections may be inconvenient, however, and you may develop irritation at the injection site. Sumatriptan is expensive, and its effectiveness is limited. It relieves pain for about 5 hours.

Since the introduction of sumatriptan, a number of similar drugs have become available, including rizatriptan (Maxalt), naratriptan (Amerge), zolmitriptan (Zomig), almotriptan (Axert) and frovatriptan (Frova). Rizatriptan and zolmitriptan are effective in 60 percent to 80 percent of people with migraines.

Side effects of triptans include nausea, dizziness and muscle weakness. Although rare, stroke and heart attack also are possible complications of these drugs. In rare cases, people taking Imitrex have developed severe abdominal pain, cramping and bloody diarrhea due to decreased blood flow to the intestine (mesenteric ischemia). This may require hospitalization or even surgery.

If you're taking the class of antidepressants known as monoamine oxidase inhibitors (MAOIs), don't use triptans. Be sure your doctor knows all of the medications you're taking.

- *Ergot derivatives.* Medications such as ergotamine and dihydroergotamine (D.H.E. 45) are thought to help relieve pain by binding to serotonin receptors, just as the triptans do.
- *Metoclopramide.* Metoclopramide (Reglan) is useful in relieving nausea and vomiting associated with migraines.

If your migraine is prolonged and associated with continued

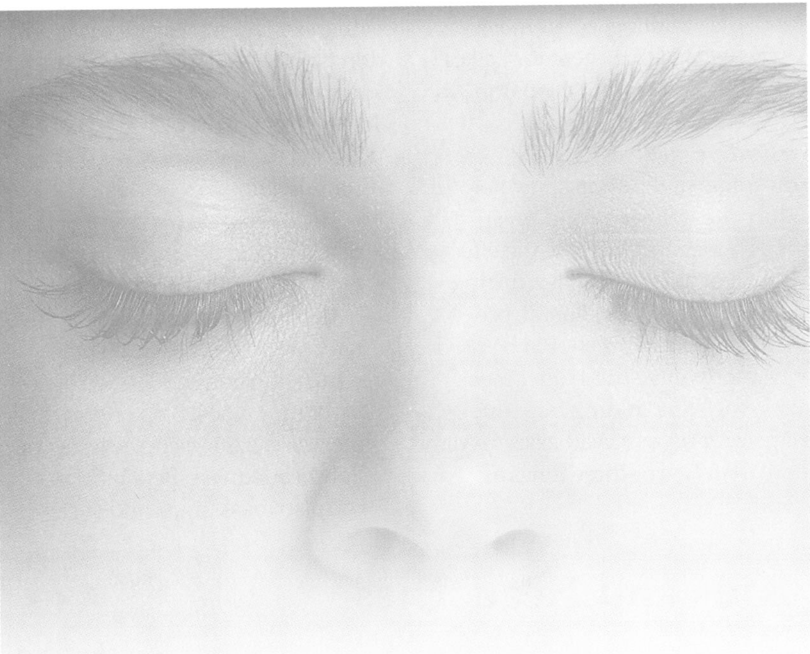

Muscle Relaxation

People sometimes develop habitual muscle responses to stress — a tension habit. Muscle relaxation techniques can reduce pain from muscle tension. These techniques have been useful in disorders such as tension headaches, temporomandibular joint (TMJ) syndrome and backaches.

Practiced relaxation techniques are successful stress relievers for many individuals. If you feel anxious, try the following relaxation strategy:

1. Sit in a comfortable chair or lie down. Close your eyes. Begin to breathe slowly and deeply. Keep breathing deeply and rhythmically for a number of minutes. As you breathe in, let your abdomen and chest expand with air. Contract them as you breathe out. In between, hold your breath for a few seconds. After some practice, a few breaths taken this way can calm you down during stressful situations.
2. Tense the muscles of your toes and press down your feet. Hold them taut. Feel the tension in your toes and feet. Notice where the tightness is. Keep the muscles tight and concentrate on the tension for about 20 seconds. Then relax your toes and feet. Feel the tension leave your muscles. Feel them become more and more relaxed, more and more heavy. Feel the warmth circulate through them as the tension drains away. Say the words *calm* and *relax* silently to yourself. When your feet and toes feel limp, go through the same procedure with another set of nearby muscles, moving very slowly up your body with one group of muscles at a time: your ankles and lower legs, your thighs, your pelvis and buttocks, your abdomen, your fists, your arms and your shoulders.
3. Press your head into the cushion or pillow and tense the muscles in your neck. Clench your jaws. Frown and squint your eyes. Then relax. As you relax each section of your neck and head, keep saying *calm* and *relax.* Breathe deeply and fully.

For more information on reducing stress, see Chapter 5, "Managing Stress."

attacks of vomiting, seek emergency medical treatment to replace lost fluids and control the pain.

Preventive medications

Preventive medications may help reduce the frequency and severity of migraines and increase the effectiveness of relief medicines during migraine attacks. In general, preventive medications should be used only after you've tried other measures, such as avoiding migraine triggers, or if your headaches occur more than two or three times a month.

In most cases, these medications don't prevent all migraines, and some can have serious side effects. To be effective, they need to be taken every day or as your doctor recommends.

- *Cardiovascular medications.* Beta blockers and calcium channel blockers, commonly used to treat high blood pressure and coronary artery disease, may help reduce the frequency and severity of migraines. Side effects can include dizziness, drowsiness or lightheadedness. Beta blockers can also mask signs and symptoms of low blood sugar in people with diabetes and worsen asthma.
- *Antidepressants.* Certain antidepressants are effective in preventing all types of headaches, including migraines. Most effective are tricyclic antidepressants, such as nortriptyline (Aventyl, Pamelor) and amitriptyline (Elavil). These medications may reduce migraines by affecting the levels of serotonin and other brain chemicals.
- *Antiseizure medications.* Some antiseizure medications, such as val-

Kids and Headaches

Headaches are one of the top reasons older children miss school. Recurrent headaches are common during late childhood and adolescence, although they're rarely due to a serious problem. Headaches are associated with many viral illnesses. However, if your child frequently complains of a headache, even during times when he or she is otherwise well, consult your doctor.

A headache may indicate stress related to school, friends or family. It may be a reaction to a medication, particularly a decongestant.

If you think it's a tension-type headache, help your child find ways to relax and avoid unnecessary stress. If headaches occur frequently, help your child keep a headache diary. Use acetaminophen (Tylenol, others) or ibuprofen (Advil, Motrin, others) sparingly and briefly to avoid missing serious problems that the pain reliever may be masking.

Don't give aspirin to children under age 16 unless instructed to do so by a doctor. Aspirin use in children is associated with Reye's syndrome, a rare and potentially life-threatening condition.

Migraines also may occur in children and are often accompanied by vomiting, light sensitivity and sleepiness. Recovery typically follows within a few hours.

If your child's headache persists, comes on suddenly without explanation or gets steadily worse, call your doctor. Also seek medical help with a headache that follows a recent ear infection, a toothache, strep throat or other infections.

Be sure to tell your doctor if there's any family history of migraines. That information could help lead to a diagnosis.

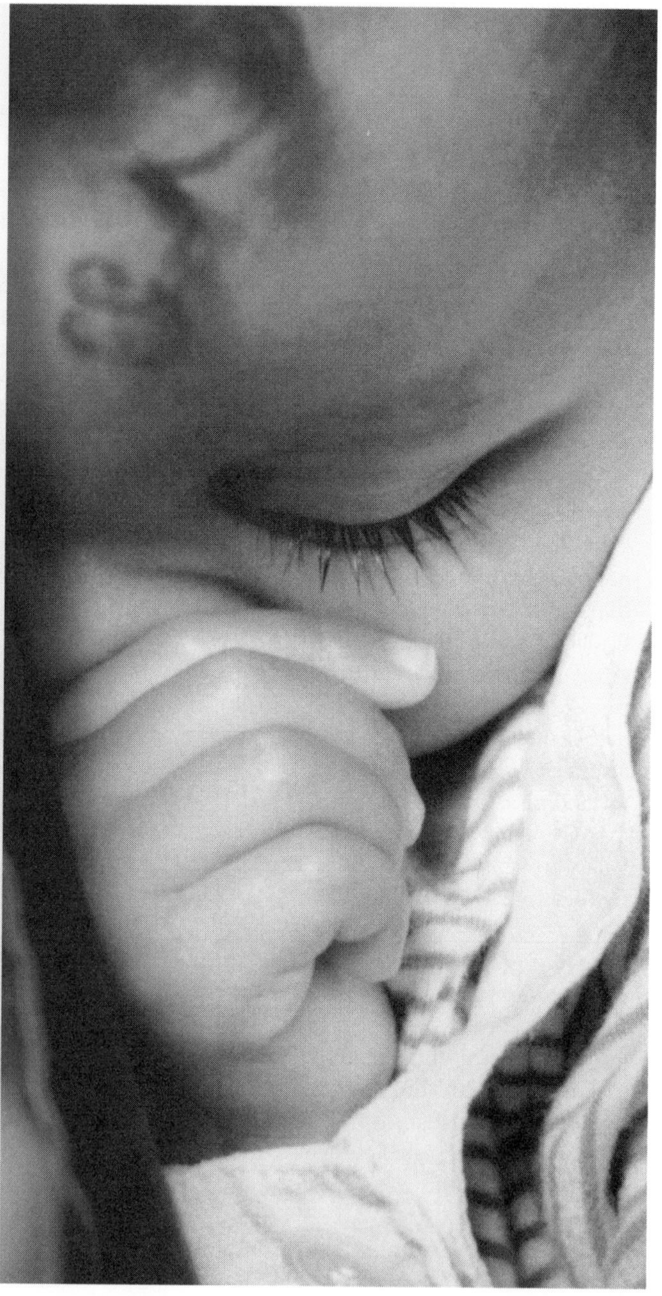

proic acid (Depakene) and gabapentin (Neurontin), primarily used to treat epilepsy and bipolar disease, may prevent migraines. Valproic acid can cause side effects such as nausea and vomiting, heartburn, diarrhea, cramps, hair loss and confusion. Side effects of gabapentin may include fatigue, dizziness, blurred or altered vision, unsteadiness and nausea or vomiting. If you're pregnant, don't use these medications.
- *Cyproheptadine.* The antihistamine cyproheptadine (Periactin) affects serotonin activity. It's sometimes used as a preventive measure in children with migraines.
- *Riboflavin.* A high dose of riboflavin — about 400 milligrams daily — may prevent migraines. Riboflavin (vitamin B-2) may correct brain cell deficiencies possibly associated with migraines in some people. Large doses of this vitamin should be taken only with medical supervision.

Self-care

If you know that certain foods trigger a migraine, avoid them. For some people, maintaining a regular sleep schedule, including on weekends, helps reduce or prevent migraines.

Aerobic exercise — about 30 minutes on most days — reduces tension and can prevent migraines in some people. Be sure to warm up slowly because sudden, intense exercise can actually trigger a headache. Relaxation techniques also can be helpful.

If you think your migraines may be related to medications, such as birth control pills or hormone replacement therapy, consider discontinuing their use. These medications contain the hormone estrogen, which can trigger or contribute to headaches. Talk to your doctor about other options or dosages for you.

If you have frequent headaches, keep a diary to see what triggers your attacks. Note the time a headache began, what you ate during the preceding 24 hours, how you felt and what you were doing when the headache started, any unusual stress, how long the headache lasted and what made it stop. You can also use this diary to help review your signs and symptoms with your doctor.

Cluster headaches

Signs and symptoms

- Steady pain in and around one eye, occurring in episodes that often begin at the same time of day or night
- Watering and redness of an eye, with nasal stuffiness on the same side of the face

Cluster headaches are characterized by intense burning, boring pain usually located in or around one eye and temple and occasionally in one cheek or jaw. Your affected eye is bloodshot and teary. The nostril on that side often becomes blocked and may run profusely. Other possible signs are reduced pupil size and a drooping eyelid.

The pain swiftly intensifies within 5 to 10 minutes to a peak that typically persists for 30 minutes to 2 hours. Affected people usually don't lie down during an attack because this position increases the pain.

Cluster headaches have a rapid onset and can occur at any time, but they often occur 2 to 3 hours after you fall asleep, usually during the phase of deep sleep known as rapid eye movement (REM). Headaches can occur daily for days, weeks or months before a remission period that may last weeks or years (episodic attacks), or they can occur for a year or more without remission (chronic attacks). A chronic phase may follow a period of episodic attacks.

Unlike migraines, which more often affect women, cluster headaches predominantly affect men. The first attack most frequently strikes men during adolescence or their early 20s. Almost all affected people are heavy smokers. There's usually no family history of similar headaches.

No specific cause has been found for cluster headaches. Some researchers believe these headaches are related to a chemical present in the brain and certain cranial nerves. The chemical causes blood vessels to enlarge and become painful.

Recent studies suggest abnormal activity in the hypothalamus may cause cluster headaches. The hypothalamus has many functions, including control of the sleep-wake cycle and other biological clocks. Abnormal activity in the hypothalamus could explain the nighttime and seasonal nature of the attacks.

Consumption of alcohol can trigger cluster attacks if you're predisposed to them. Rarely, some foods may trigger a cluster headache.

Diagnosis

If your signs and symptoms are typical of cluster headaches, your doctor may have little difficulty in diagnosing the condition. Nevertheless, you may need tests to exclude other problems that can cause similar pain, such as an aneurysm of an artery in your head, a tumor made up of newly formed blood vessels, sinusitis or glaucoma.

How serious are cluster headaches?

Cluster headaches are a chronic problem. There's no known cure and little understanding of the periodic pattern of attacks. The headaches can be a lifelong disorder. The pain during an attack can be debilitating, but there's no permanent physical harm, and the condition doesn't lead to other disorders.

Treatment

Cluster headaches are often resistant to pain relievers because these drugs take effect too slowly. Some prescription medications can help ease or prevent headache pain.

Acute medications
Acute (abortive) medications stop or decrease pain after a cluster headache starts:

- *Sumatriptan.* Sumatriptan (Imitrex) in injectable form is used to relieve cluster headaches. The medication may work in as little as 15 minutes. Sumatriptan mimics the action of the brain chemical serotonin by binding to serotonin receptors and causing blood vessels to constrict.
- *Ergot derivatives.* Medications such as ergotamine (Ergomar) and dihydroergotamine (D.H.E. 45) constrict swollen blood vessels in your brain and scalp. This is effective for some people, but the dosage must be limited to avoid side effects, especially nausea. Ergot derivatives come in tablet or aerosol form. The medication may also be prescribed to prevent attacks.
- *Oxygen.* Inhalation of 100 percent oxygen often provides relief. This may be the most effective treatment for frequent cluster headaches that occur primarily at night.

Preventive medications
Preventive medications may help reduce the frequency and severity of cluster headaches and increase the effectiveness of relief medicines during cluster attacks.

- *Methysergide maleate.* This drug may be used to relieve and prevent attacks. About 60 percent of people with cluster headaches respond to this medication. It inhibits serotonin action and prevents the release of histamine from cells. It's used during periods of pain and is tapered off slowly during remission.
- *Lithium carbonate.* One of the effects of this compound is to block the action of serotonin in the brain. It can be effective during a chronic phase of cluster headaches. During remission its dosage is tapered to avoid side effects.
- *Calcium channel blockers.* Medications such as verapamil (Calan, Isoptin) relax blood vessel muscles and are effective for the prevention of cluster headaches in many people. The medication may be continued for 3 to 4 weeks after the last headache and then is gradually tapered and discontinued under the direction of your doctor. Occasionally, if the headaches are chronic, long-term use is required.
- *Corticosteroids.* Medications such as prednisone may help stop a cluster headache. They may be prescribed if your cluster headaches are of recent onset or if you have a pattern of brief attacks and long remissions.

Surgery
Rarely, surgery on certain groups of nerve cells near the brain may be recommended if drug management doesn't work. Surgery provides relief for approximately 60 percent of people with chronic cluster headaches. The operation carries a risk of permanent residual muscle weakness or sensory loss in certain areas of the face and head.

Seizures

Brain cells communicate with each other through electric signals. Seizures occur when there's a sudden change in these signals, causing them to become disorganized. During a seizure, some brain cells send abnormal signals, which stop other cells from working properly. Abnormal signals may cause temporary changes in sensation, behavior, movement or consciousness.

Seizures can occur as a result of a disease or accident that affects the brain or for no clear reason. If you have a single episode, it doesn't necessarily indicate that you have

When to See a Doctor

Seek medical evaluation as soon as possible after your first grand mal seizure. If your medical evaluation shows that you have epilepsy, you don't need to seek medical help each time you have a seizure. But do seek prompt medical advice if any of the following conditions are present:

- The seizure lasts longer than 5 minutes.
- Recovery from the seizure is slow.
- A second seizure follows immediately.
- You're pregnant.
- Signs of injury or illness are present.
- Your seizures become more frequent.
- There's a change in the way you feel during and after the seizures occur.
- You have changed your seizure medication or started taking other medicines.

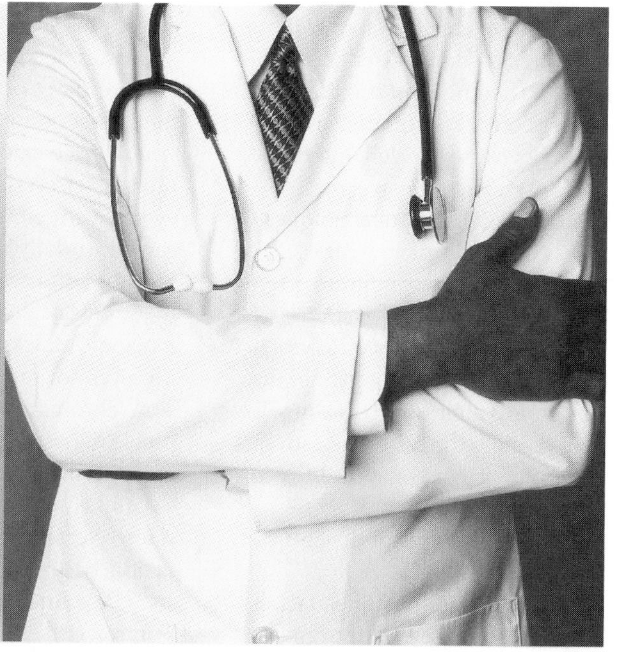

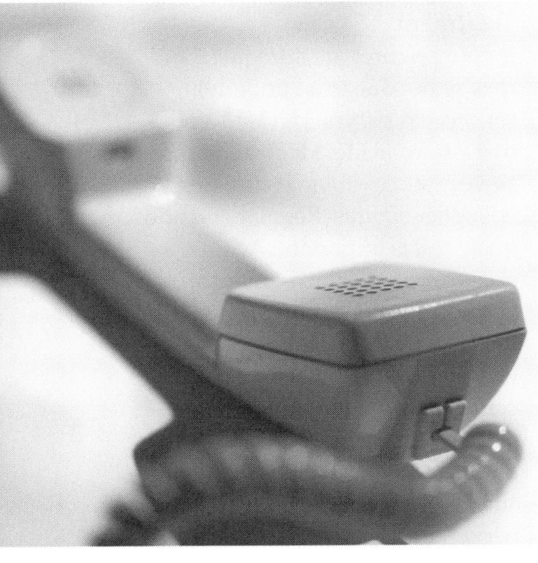

What to Do When Someone Has a Seizure

If you come across someone having a seizure, promptly call for medical help and follow these instructions:

- Gently roll the person onto one side and put something soft under his or her head.
- Loosen tight neckwear on the person.
- Don't try to put your fingers or anything else in the person's mouth. The tongue can't be swallowed.
- Don't try to restrain the person.
- Look for a medical alert bracelet on the person. It should state who to contact in an emergency and what medications he or she uses. Allergies to medications may be noted.

epilepsy. When seizures recur spontaneously, the condition is called epilepsy. Seizure disorder is a broader term that includes both a single seizure and epilepsy.

Seizure disorders aren't mental disorders, although mental health can influence control of seizures. They also don't cause psychiatric problems or mental retardation, even though people with epilepsy may also have those conditions. In some people, hereditary or environmental factors may contribute to repeated seizures.

Grand mal seizure

Signs and symptoms

- An episode of loss of consciousness with convulsions

A grand mal seizure (generalized tonic-clonic seizure) starts with a 15- to 20-second period of muscle rigidity (tonic phase) and then a 30- to 60-second period of rhythmic jerking (clonic phase). Loss of consciousness occurs, which may be accompanied by falling. The seizure ends with a few minutes to a few hours of deep, relaxed sleep before consciousness returns with no memory of the seizure. Headache and drowsiness or confusion may follow a grand mal seizure.

Grand mal seizures are due to abnormal electric activity that rapidly spreads throughout the brain. In most cases, the seizures seem to occur randomly in time, but for some people, they're associated with menstruation, sleep deprivation, low blood sugar, increased stress or, rarely, reactions to a specific stimulation by light, sound, touch or reading. Sometimes, the seizures involve only a few muscles (focal seizure), such as an extremity or one side of the face.

Sometimes, seizures run in families. In fact, a number of genes have been linked to certain seizure syndromes. Other identified causes of recurring seizures include scar tissue from prior brain disease or injury, a brain infection, tumor, abscess or hemorrhage, alcohol or drug withdrawal and metabolic disturbances from diabetes, kidney or liver disease. When the disorder begins before age 25, the cause is frequently unknown. Seizures that start after age 25 are more likely to be due to a slowly growing brain tumor.

Approximately 2 million Americans have epilepsy, and up to 5 percent of the population has had a single seizure episode. Most of the people in this single-seizure group have a grand mal seizure, sometimes in combination with another type of seizure.

Diagnosis

A grand mal seizure is easily recognized, but the cause may be difficult to diagnose. Your doctor will want a detailed medical history. After a physical examination, you may need a test called electroencephalography (EEG), which records the electric activity of your brain cells.

Other diagnostic tests may include a computerized tomography (CT) scan or magnetic resonance imaging (MRI) and blood tests. Focal seizures are sometimes caused by scarring or by a tumor in a specific part of the brain. A CT scan or MRI may help reveal such a cause.

How serious is a grand mal seizure?

The seriousness of a grand mal seizure depends on what caused it. Therefore, it's important to see a doctor when a grand mal seizure has occurred.

When a seizure results from a condition such as low blood sugar and the condition is corrected, seizure disorder isn't serious. In some cases, though, a seizure may be due to a serious medical disorder such as a brain tumor or brain infection.

A seizure that produces loss of awareness or loss of control can be dangerous if you're driving a vehicle or operating certain types of equipment. Therefore, many states have driving restrictions that are related to how well your seizures are controlled. Seizures can also result in injuries due to falling.

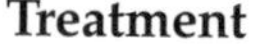

Antiseizure Medications

Medication can control or greatly reduce the number of seizures for many people with a seizure disorder. Drug selection and dosage require close medical supervision and testing. You may have side effects such as drowsiness, upset stomach and a rash.

In some cases, the medication can be discontinued after several years without seizures, but this must be done by a gradual decrease in dosage and under the supervision of your doctor. If your seizures are due to an underlying condition, such as an infection or stroke, your doctor may decide that your antiseizure medication can be eliminated after the underlying cause has been treated and is under control.

Commonly prescribed antiseizure (anticonvulsant) medications include:

- Carbamazepine (Carbatrol, Tegretol)
- Clonazepam (Klonopin)
- Ethosuximide (Zarontin)
- Phenobarbital (Luminal, Solfoton)
- Phenytoin (Dilantin)
- Primidone (Mysoline)
- Valproic acid (Depakene)
- Divalproex (Depakote)

In the past decade, newer antiseizure medications have been developed, including the following:

- Gabapentin (Neurontin)
- Felbamate (Felbatol)
- Lamotrigine (Lamictal)
- Topiramate (Topamax)
- Tiagabine (Gabitril)
- Oxcarbazepine (Trileptal)
- Levetiracetam (Keppra)
- Zonisamide (Zonagran)

For prolonged or cluster seizures, your doctor may prescribe a sedative, such as diazepam (Diastat, Valium) or lorazepam (Ativan). For a child who has a type of epilepsy called infantile spasms, or severe seizures that don't respond to more commonly used medications, a steroid drug called adrenocorticotropic hormone (ACTH) is sometimes prescribed and given as an injection.

Many seizure medications can increase the risk of birth defects. If you're considering becoming pregnant, talk to your doctor about your seizure disorder and your medications.

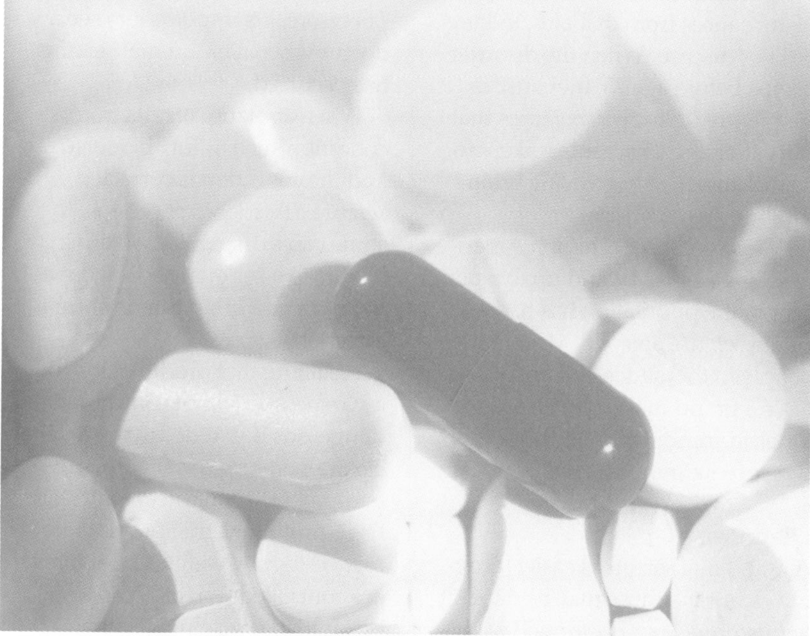

Treatment

If your seizures are infrequent and they're not due to an underlying serious illness, you can lead a relatively normal life. Medication can be very successful in controlling epileptic seizures. Regular and adequate rest is important. Avoid excess alcohol, which can increase your chances of having a seizure. Wear a medical alert bracelet or necklace stating who should be contacted if a seizure occurs.

If medication doesn't work, other options may be available, such as surgery or a treatment called vagal nerve stimulation.

Medication

Medication is the first line of treatment for seizure disorders, and for many it's an effective way of controlling the condition. Discuss the side effects of your specific medication with your doctor. Most antiseizure medications are taken orally. It's important to take them according to the instructions on the prescription or as otherwise directed by your doctor. Taking the medication on time helps to keep a steady level of the drug in your body.

Pregnancy may alter your need for medication, so promptly inform your doctor if you're contemplating becoming pregnant or when you have become pregnant while taking antiseizure medications.

Surgery

Seizures caused by a brain tumor, abscess or hemorrhage may not recur after surgical removal of the abnormality. Occasionally, if the seizures are limited to a particular part of the brain and that part can be removed without serious consequences, surgery may be an option. The location of seizure activity can be identified using EEG and magnetic resonance imaging (MRI).

In children who don't seem to have a brain region where seizures begin and who regularly fall to the ground with their seizures, surgery to split the fibers that connect the two brain hemispheres (corpus callosum) may dramatically reduce seizures without tremendously affecting other brain functions. This type of surgery is considered when medications fail to control seizures.

Ketogenic diet
If your child doesn't benefit from medication or if the side effects are intolerable, your doctor may suggest a specialized diet that's high in fat and low in protein and carbohydrates. The goal of the diet is to get the body to produce ketones, which cause the body to use fat instead of glucose for energy. This process has an effect against seizures, although the exact way in which it works is unclear.

The ketogenic diet is a complex treatment and requires careful involvement by a doctor, a dietitian and family members. The diet, which prescribes exact amounts of specific foods and beverages for each meal, must be strictly followed in order to be effective. Even a tiny intake of sugar can significantly alter the effectiveness of the diet. Nonetheless, it has proved helpful in two out of three children placed on the diet. It's usually implemented for a limited period of time. It's not as effective in adults as it is in children.

Vagal nerve stimulation
A device called a vagal nerve stimulator may be an option if medications are ineffective or if they cause serious side effects. The stimulator is implanted under the collarbone. Wires from the stimulator are wrapped around the vagus nerve in your neck. This nerve connects the lower part of your brain to your heart, lungs and gastrointestinal tract.

The device stimulates your brain and turns on and off according to an adjustable program. The stimulation has the effect of inhibiting seizures in some patients, although the exact mechanism by which this occurs is unclear.

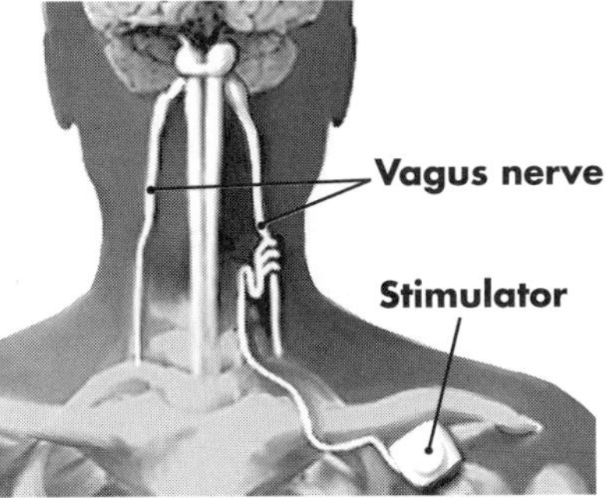

A vagal nerve stimulator delivers tiny, intermittent electric pulses to the vagus nerve. In some people, the pulses inhibit seizures.

Absence seizure

Signs and symptoms
- Brief staring spells with loss of awareness
- Eyelid fluttering during the spells
- Prompt recovery of awareness when the spells end

Absence seizure epilepsy (petit mal seizure epilepsy) is another type of epilepsy. Each absence seizure lasts only seconds, but tens to hundreds of such seizures may occur each day.

During an absence seizure, there's a brief lapse of awareness, often with fluttering of eyelids or twitching of hands. Full recovery occurs immediately at the end of the seizure, and no confusion follows. Usually, the person who had the seizure has no memory of it.

Absence seizures typically begin in children ages 6 to 12 and rarely start after age 20. After onset, they may occur for weeks or months before an adult notices them because they're usually very brief, with little abnormal movement. Your child may exhibit learning problems before you or a teacher discovers the seizures.

Less than 10 percent of all people with seizure disorders have absence seizures. Sometimes, they occur in combination with other types of seizures. Usually, no identifiable cause is found for the seizures, and your child probably has no other neurologic problems.

Atypical absence seizures, however, are often associated with neurologic disorders such as congenital malformations in the brain, chemical disturbances from kidney or liver disease or brain tissue scarring from head trauma or birth injuries. Compared with an absence seizure attack, an atypical absence seizure attack is usually longer and has more abnormal movements.

Diagnosis
Electroencephalography (EEG), which measures brain wave activity, is generally used to look for signs of the distinctive brain electric pattern associated with absence seizures. In some instances, a doctor may also order blood tests or a computerized tomography (CT) scan or magnetic resonance imaging (MRI) to check for other possible causes of the seizures.

How serious are absence seizures?
Most children with absence seizures have significantly fewer or no seizures when they take medication. Up to 70 percent of children with petit mal seizures stop having them by late adolescence. At this age, most teens may be able to discontinue their medication under their doctor's supervision.

Treatment
Most children with typical petit mal seizures can live fairly normal lives and should be encouraged to do so. Your doctor will probably advise you that your child can participate in physical activities and schoolwork with few restrictions. Restrictions on driving or operating certain types of equipment when your child gets older will depend on the degree of seizure control.

Medication
Petit mal seizures are usually very responsive to antiseizure medications. Medical evaluation is required to determine the best drug and dosage for your child. Possible side effects of the medications include dizziness, upset stomach and lethargy.

Febrile seizure

Signs and symptoms

- A brief episode of loss of consciousness and convulsions during fever

A febrile seizure is a convulsion triggered by a high fever that occurs in young children. The seizure typically lasts 5 minutes or less. After the seizure, your child may cry or be quite sleepy. Most children who experience a febrile seizure are between the ages of 6 months and 5 years.

Febrile seizures are the most common type of seizure in children. They occur in about 4 percent of children before the age of 4 years. Some children inherit a tendency to have a seizure along with a fever. Febrile seizures usually stop by the time a child is 5 or 6 years old.

A febrile seizure may be triggered by a rapid onset of fever, which is commonly caused by an infection, such as a middle ear infection.

Diagnosis

If your child has a convulsion while a fever is present, seek medical attention immediately. Often, these seizures occur when body temperature is rising rapidly. Diseases such as meningitis may first become apparent with this combination of signs and symptoms, and emergency treatment may be required.

Your child's doctor will likely ask about your family medical history and perform a physical examination on your child. If the fever is clearly due to a common childhood illness, an electroencephalography (EEG) test to check brain wave activity may be the only test needed. If there's no sign of an abnormality, the diagnosis is usually febrile seizure.

How serious is a febrile seizure?

Although a febrile seizure may be alarming to you as a parent, it's usually harmless to your child and generally doesn't lead to a long-term or ongoing problem. Approximately 90 percent of febrile seizures stop on their own within 5 minutes, and the risk of future mental impairment is minimal. Still, a febrile seizure always warrants medical attention to determine the cause of the fever.

Risk of epilepsy increases if your child has a complex febrile seizure. A complex febrile seizure lasts longer than 15 minutes, occurs more than once within 24 hours or affects one side of the body more than the other. With use of medication, future seizures can usually be controlled or their frequency or severity reduced significantly.

Treatment

Place your child on the ground lying flat and remove any nearby objects that could be a source of injury. Gently roll your child onto his or her side. Don't put anything into his or her mouth during a seizure. Keep attentive to your child's needs during the entire seizure.

Following the episode, report the seizure to your doctor. Rapidly cooling the child doesn't prevent further seizures. If the seizure lasts longer than 5 minutes — or if your child has two or more seizures — seek emergency medical attention.

Medication

After your child has a single episode of seizure during a fever, his or her doctor may or may not prescribe antiseizure medication to prevent recurrence.

When susceptibility to a febrile seizure is demonstrated by at least two episodes, your child's doctor may recommend quick and vigorous control of fever during childhood illness as a way to prevent febrile seizures. This might include giving your child acetaminophen (Tylenol, others) or ibuprofen (Advil, Motrin, others) at the first indication of fever.

Avoid giving aspirin for fever because it may trigger a rare but potentially fatal disorder known as Reye's syndrome.

A small number of children require continuing treatment with antiseizure medication (see page 564) until age 3 or 4. Antiseizure medications are effective in preventing febrile seizures, but they often cause significant side effects.

Children who have frequent or prolonged febrile seizures may

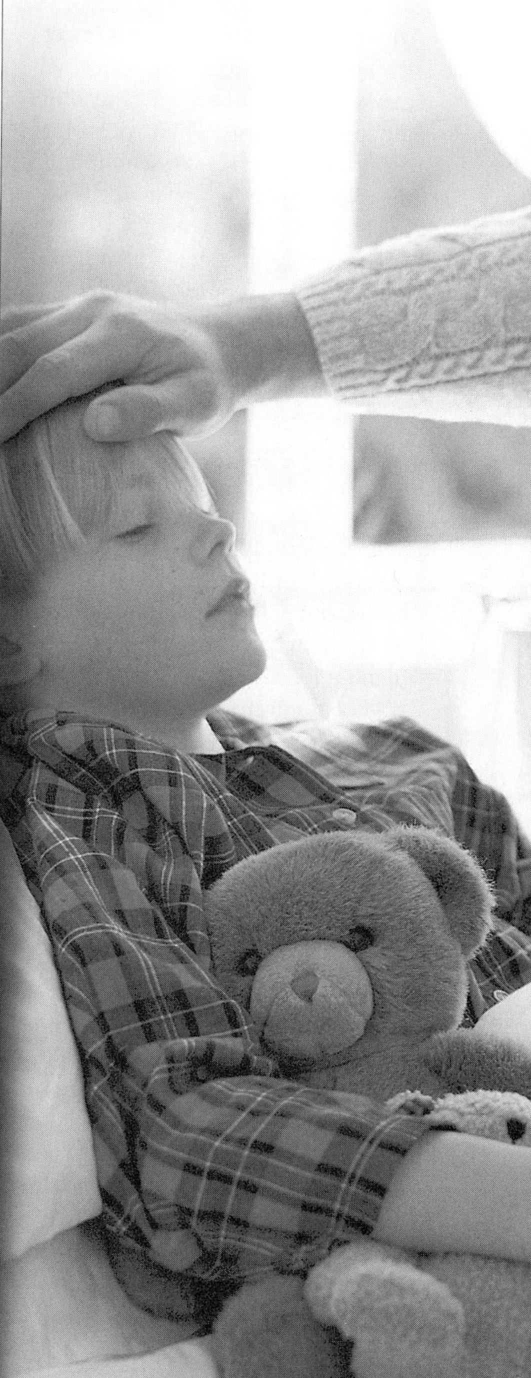

benefit from preventive treatment with oral or rectal diazepam (Diastat, Valium) when a fever occurs.

If no seizures occur after a few years and results of EEG and neurologic examinations are normal, your doctor may recommend reducing your child's medication dosage. Many children eventually can stop taking all medication and remain free of seizures.

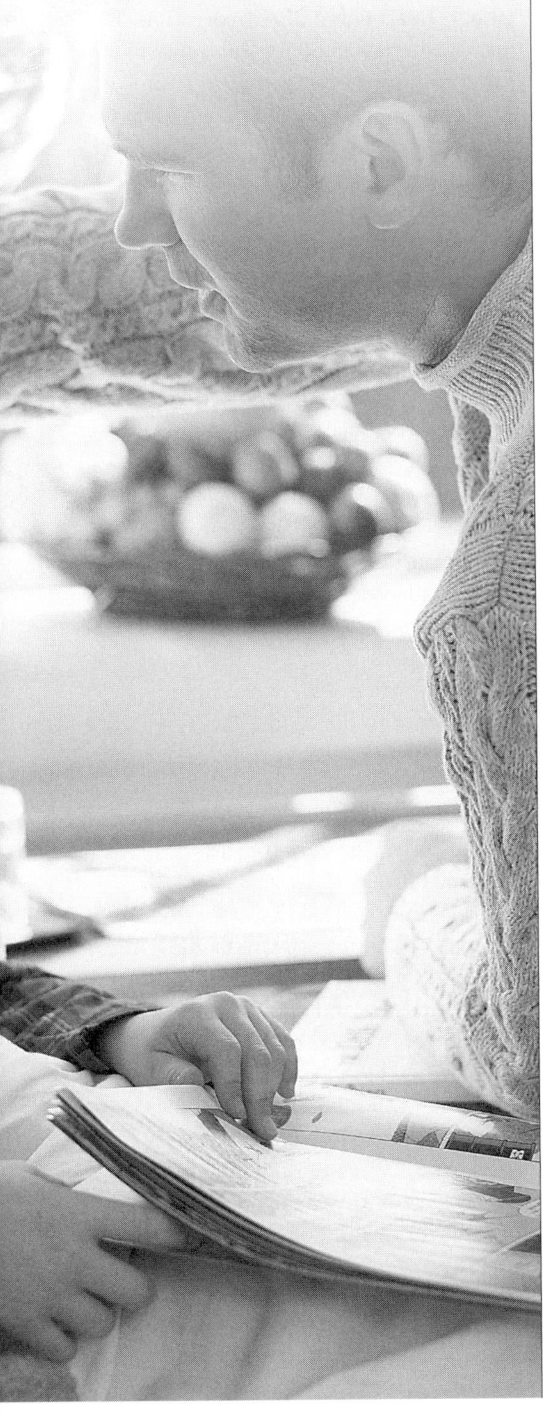

Temporal lobe seizure

Signs and symptoms

- Preceding the seizure, sparkling colors or blank spots in your field of vision (aura)
- A transient loss of awareness
- A simple, repetitive act, such as lip smacking

These seizures most often originate in the temporal lobe, the part of your brain that extends from your temple to just behind your ear. If the seizure is associated with altered consciousness, it's called a complex partial seizure.

Temporal lobe seizures are frequently preceded by a peculiar sensation (aura) that's followed by 1 to 2 minutes of loss of awareness or contact with surroundings. The physical component can be a simple repetitive act such as lip smacking, repeated swallowing or picking at clothes. These movements are called automatisms. After the seizure has ended, it may take minutes to hours to recover normal mental activity, and you may not remember the seizure.

The aura, which usually precedes the seizure by seconds or a few minutes, is variously described as hallucinations of smell, sight or sound. Aura is also experienced as altered perceptions such as deja vu or recurrent memory, or sudden emotion of anxiety or fear.

Seizures are sometimes caused by a specific disorder in the temporal lobe, such as scar tissue or tumor, but often there's no identifiable cause. Long-term (chronic) temporal lobe seizures are known as temporal lobe epilepsy. About half of all people with complex partial seizures also have grand mal seizures.

Diagnosis

Your doctor will want to know your medical history and that of your family. Diagnostic tests usually include electroencephalography (EEG) to check for abnormal electric activity in the brain, blood tests to detect chemical imbalance and computerized tomography (CT) or magnetic resonance imaging (MRI) to check for structural abnormalities of the brain that may be the cause of seizures.

How serious are temporal lobe seizures?

The seizures themselves aren't generally life-threatening, but they can cause injuries associated with falling. A seizure that produces either loss of awareness or control can be dangerous if you're driving a car, swimming, working at heights or operating certain types of equipment. In some cases, seizure disorders may require restrictions of physical activities. Still, limitations are often temporary, and many people with a seizure disorder are able to live an active life.

A medical alert bracelet can be helpful. These bracelets state who should be contacted if a seizure occurs and what medications are to be administered.

Treatment

The goal of seizure treatment is to eliminate or reduce seizures, minimize side effects of treatment and allow you to live a normal, healthy life. This may involve the use of medications, surgery or, in some cases, a treatment called vagal nerve stimulation.

Medication

To minimize seizures, you may need to take medications regularly (see page 564). Selection of the drug and its dosage requires medical evaluation and testing. These medications may sometimes produce side effects, such as dizziness and sedation.

Surgery

In some cases of temporal lobe seizures — such as when the cause of the seizures can be localized to an area within one temporal lobe — an operation may be recommended if medications fail to satisfactorily control the seizures. Surgery is generally more effective early in the treatment process — when the first two medications fail to control seizures.

An evaluation at a comprehensive epilepsy center is needed to see if you're a good candidate for surgical treatment. The evaluation typically involves identifying the site where your seizures originate. The evaluation generally requires an MRI, as well as an EEG and hospitalization so that your seizures can be recorded with a video camera.

Improved surgical techniques have led to success rates as high as 95 percent in properly selected cases. The success rate depends on the type of seizures, their cause and whether other brain disorders are present. In some people, the success rate may be more modest and in the range of 60 percent to 70 percent. Success is defined as being free of seizures or having only auras that don't interfere substantially with daily activities.

Like all surgical procedures, surgery to treat seizures carries certain risks. Although rare, it's possible that new neurologic problems may result from surgery.

Vagal nerve stimulation

A device called a vagal nerve stimulator may be an option if medications are ineffective or cause serious side effects and surgery isn't an option (see page 565). The chance of dramatic control of temporal lobe seizures with vagal nerve stimulation is only 4 percent to 5 percent, but 50 percent of individuals experience reduction of seizures by at least one-half.

Stroke and Vascular Disorders

Two major artery systems extend through your neck to carry blood to your brain. An interruption of blood flow in one of these systems — even for a few seconds — usually produces a dramatic effect on your brain's functions. Depending on what areas of your brain are affected, you can have vision or speech difficulties, paralysis in part of your body or loss of consciousness. If this interruption continues for more than a few minutes, brain cells in the affected area may die, causing permanent impairment or death. Two conditions that can affect blood supply to brain cells are reduced blood flow (ischemia) and bleeding (hemorrhage).

Transient ischemic attack

Signs and symptoms

- Sudden onset of weakness or numbness of the face, arm or leg, often on one side of the body
- Sudden lack of coordination of the limbs
- Sudden vision loss or double vision
- Sudden difficulty speaking or understanding others
- Sudden severe dizziness, loss of balance or difficulty walking

A transient ischemic attack (TIA) is caused by a temporary deficiency in blood supply to the brain. Most episodes last only a few minutes, but some last up to 24 hours. A TIA has the same origins as ischemic stroke.

Most TIAs are due to atherosclerosis, a condition where cholesterol-containing fatty deposits (plaques) form inside arteries. Plaques narrow the pathway of blood through the artery and decrease flow. A blood clot (thrombus) can form on an injured plaque. A plaque fragment or a small piece of clot forming in the heart can break off and lodge in a smaller artery. When the clot or fragment temporarily blocks blood flow at a distant site in the brain, the result is a TIA.

The signs and symptoms of a TIA are similar to those of ischemic stroke, with an important difference — the signs and symptoms disappear completely within 24 hours. A TIA may be repeated in the same day or some time later, and each episode typically lasts only a few minutes.

Various factors can increase your risk of a TIA. Risk factors that you can change or control include high blood pressure, tobacco use, diabetes and abnormal blood cholesterol levels. Certain cardiovascular diseases also can make you more prone to a TIA, including congestive heart failure, a previous heart attack, heart valve disease or valve replacement and an irregular heart rhythm (atrial fibrillation).

Blacks are at greater risk of a TIA than are whites, partly because of their higher prevalence of high blood pressure and diabetes. Risk is also greater if one of your parents or siblings has had a TIA or stroke.

Diagnosis

The most significant feature of a TIA is the speed with which it comes and goes. Rapid onset, brief duration and then a return to normal is the usual sequence. Recurrent episodes of similar signs and symptoms also are significant.

A detailed description of your signs and symptoms can help in the diagnosis of a TIA. Weakness in only one arm or leg, for example, may point to a disturbance in a branch of the internal carotid artery, whereas weakness in both arms or legs suggests disturbances in blood flow through the vertebral arteries or basilar artery.

Other information that your doctor may obtain to assist in diagnosis includes your eye pressure and arm blood pressure and noise (bruit) heard over the neck with a stethoscope when blood flow in various arteries is impaired.

You may also need to undergo tests to gather additional information and provide images of brain arteries for evaluation. These may include a computerized tomography (CT) scan or magnetic resonance imaging (MRI), cerebral arteriography, magnetic resonance angiography (MRA), carotid ultrasonography or transesophageal echocardiography to check for blood clots in a chamber of your heart.

How serious is a transient ischemic attack?

You should regard a TIA as a warning that a stroke may follow. Approximately one-third of people with TIAs later have a stroke, a third have more TIAs, and a third have no further brain-related signs or symptoms.

Treatment

The purpose of treatment for a TIA is to prevent future episodes or a subsequent stroke.

Medication

If you have high blood pressure and TIAs, medication will likely be prescribed to lower your blood pressure. In the absence of high blood pressure, antiplatelet medications may be prescribed to reduce the tendency of your blood to clot.

The most common antiplatelet medication is aspirin. In addition to its pain-relieving ability, aspirin inhibits clumping of blood platelets. The presence of such clumps of platelets at a narrowed site in an artery further compromises blood flow to the brain.

A combination drug including aspirin and dipyridamole (Aggrenox) may also be used to reduce blood clotting. If aspirin isn't effective or you can't take aspirin, your doctor may prescribe similar-acting drugs such as clopidogrel (Plavix) or ticlopidine (Ticlid). Both require monitoring by your doctor.

Anticoagulant medications such as heparin or warfarin (Coumadin) may be recommended in some situations. Anticoagulants reduce the tendency of the blood to clot as well, but they affect clotting factors (proteins) instead of platelet function. These medications are sometimes referred to as blood thinners, although they don't actually thin blood.

Surgery

If you have a moderately or severely narrowed carotid artery in your neck, your doctor may suggest a surgical procedure called carotid endarterectomy (see page 573). This preventive surgery can remove plaques to prevent another TIA or a stroke.

If you're not a good candidate for this surgery, a procedure called carotid angioplasty with stent placement may be used instead. It involves threading a balloon-tipped catheter into the obstructed area of an artery. The balloon is inflated, compressing the plaques against the artery walls. A metallic mesh tube (stent) may be placed in the artery to keep it from narrowing again.

Stroke

Signs and symptoms

- Sudden onset of weakness or numbness of the face, arm or leg, often on one side of the body
- Sudden lack of coordination of the limbs
- Sudden vision loss or double vision
- Sudden difficulty speaking or understanding others
- Sudden severe dizziness, loss of balance or difficulty walking
- Sudden severe headache

Stroke is the common name for several disorders that occur within seconds or minutes after the blood supply to the brain is disturbed. When blood flow to the brain is blocked, nerve cells are deprived of oxygen and nutrients. As a result, the function of brain cells may be altered or permanently damaged. Brain tissue may die.

Prompt medical assistance is required. Just as for a heart attack, every minute counts. The longer a stroke goes untreated, the greater the damage. Success of treatment depends in part on how soon care is given.

Stroke is the third leading cause of death in industrialized countries. Approximately 750,000 Americans suffer a stroke each year. One-fourth of them die, and half of the survivors have long-term disabilities. Stroke is more likely to occur as you get older, and your risk doubles each decade after age 35. Five percent of the population older than age 65 has had a stroke.

Warning signs may be temporary, such as a transient ischemic attack (TIA), lasting from a few minutes to 24 hours. Even symptoms lasting only a short time may indicate an impending stroke. It's important to take them seriously.

Symptoms may progress or fluctuate during the first day or two after they begin. This is called stroke in evolution. When no further deterioration occurs, the condition is considered to be a completed stroke. The only warning signal that suggests you may be prone to a stroke is a transient ischemic attack. A TIA is a temporary condition that usually lasts less than an hour and leaves no permanent physical or cognitive effects.

Types

Strokes are characterized by the location and type of disturbance. The two basic types are ischemic stroke and hemorrhagic stroke.

Ischemic stroke

The most common blood flow disturbance is an inadequate supply of blood through an artery (ischemia). When this happens, nerve tissue served by that artery rapidly loses its ability to function and may die. The dead tissue is called an infarct.

Many factors that contribute to your risk of ischemic stroke are cumulative. Perhaps that's why the majority of ischemic strokes occur in people beyond age 65.

Atherosclerosis is the condition that often leads to ischemic stroke. It's where cholesterol-containing fatty deposits (plaques) gradually accumulate on the inside of your artery walls. The accumulation narrows, hardens and roughens the inside surface of your arteries. A blood clot (thrombus) may then develop and block the flow of

Emergency Treatment

While waiting for emergency help to arrive, carefully watch the person suspected of having a stroke. If breathing ceases, cardiopulmonary resuscitation (CPR) is necessary.

If the person is having difficulty breathing, position the person's head and shoulders on a pillow. If vomiting occurs, turn the person's head to the side so that he or she doesn't choke on the vomit.

Don't let the person eat or drink anything.

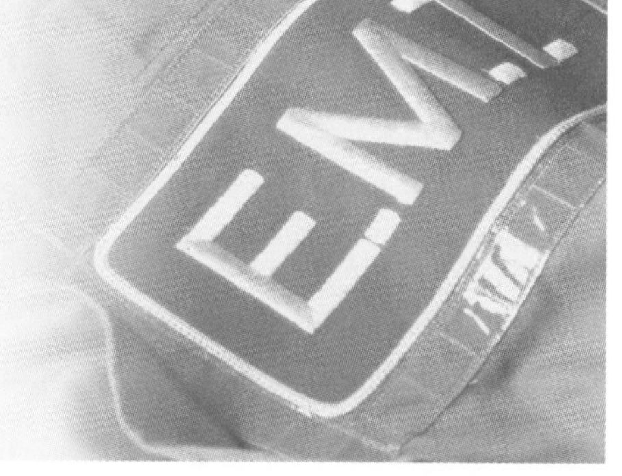

blood. This type of ischemic stroke is called a cerebral thrombosis.

Another type of ischemic stroke, called a cerebral embolism, is caused by an embolus lodging in a cerebral artery and blocking blood flow. An embolus is a fragment of plaque or a blood clot that has broken loose from a heart valve or an artery.

Hemorrhagic stroke

A hemorrhagic stroke occurs when an artery in the brain leaks or ruptures. When an artery leaks blood into the brain, causing compression, displacement and death of nerve tissue, it's called an intracerebral hemorrhage. The initial effect of an intracerebral hemorrhage is often more severe than that of an ischemic stroke. The long-term effects, however, are similar in both cases.

Another type of hemorrhagic stroke, accounting for 5 percent to 10 percent of all strokes, is a subarachnoid hemorrhage. This occurs when there's bleeding within the space between the surface of the brain and the skull. Spontaneous subarachnoid hemorrhage most commonly occurs after the rupture of an aneurysm — a balloon-like bulge that develops in an artery wall.

A subarachnoid hemorrhage is often signaled by a sudden thunderclap headache that's more severe than any you've ever felt. About half of all cases are fatal, and many people who survive are left permanently disabled. Bleeding from an aneurysm also may produce an intracerebral hemorrhage.

Less frequently, hemorrhage can occur as a result of rupture of an arteriovenous malformation. This congenitally malformed tangle of thin-walled blood vessels can cause headaches, seizures and, when ruptured, an intracerebral or subarachnoid hemorrhage.

A severe headache followed by other signs and symptoms is more typical of a hemorrhagic stroke than an ischemic stroke. Many cerebral hemorrhages are due to the long-term effects of high blood pressure. Uncontrolled high blood pressure can cause small arteries inside the brain to become susceptible to rupture.

Diagnosis

A diagnosis of stroke doesn't depend on any single symptom, but on a rapid development of symptoms. The presence of specific symptoms that correspond to specific arterial areas within the brain is further evidence of stroke. However, even with a completed stroke, early care may decrease the amount of damage.

Other possible causes of your signs and symptoms, such as a tumor, need to be excluded. One or more of the following diagnostic tests may be used to evaluate your blood vessels: carotid ultrasonography, cerebral arteriography, computerized tomography (CT), magnetic resonance imaging (MRI) and magnetic resonance angiography (MRA).

How serious is stroke?

Stroke is potentially a very serious illness that warrants prompt medical attention. After any kind of stroke, an area of dead brain tissue (cerebral infarct) may remain. Recovery depends on whether other nerve tissue can assume the function of that area. A series of strokes can lead to a long-term (chronic) brain disorder called vascular dementia.

Stroke most frequently results from chronic conditions such as high blood pressure, atherosclerosis and heart disease. If you have one or more of these chronic disorders, see a doctor regularly.

Treatment

Intensive care for a comatose stroke victim includes life-support equipment to supply oxygen, nutrients and medication, and catheterization for bladder function. Ability to

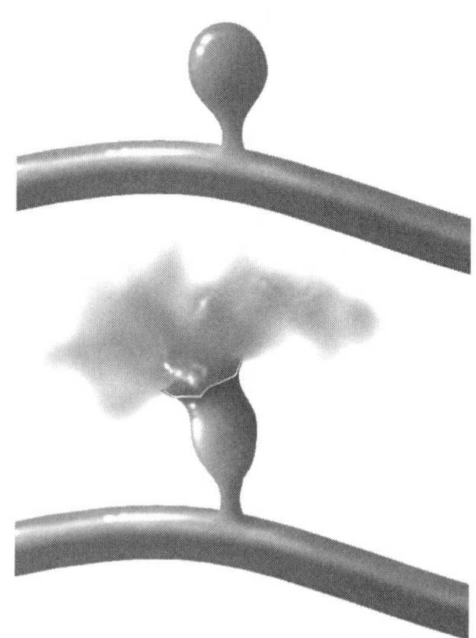

An aneurysm is a ballooning of an artery from a weak area in its wall. Over time, the wall stretches and becomes thin enough to rupture.

Are You at Risk?

Many risk factors for stroke are the same as those for a heart attack. These include:

- *Family history.* Your risk of stroke is greater if one of your parents or a brother or sister has had a stroke or TIA.
- *Age.* Your risk of stroke increases as you get older. It doubles each decade past age 35.
- *Sex.* Men are at greater risk of ischemic stroke than are premenopausal women. Men and women have similar risks of intracerebral hemorrhage, but women are more likely to have subarachnoid hemorrhage.
- *Race.* Blacks are more likely to have strokes than are whites. The increase is partly due to greater risk of high blood pressure and diabetes.
- *High blood pressure.* High blood pressure increases your risk of both ischemic and hemorrhagic stroke. It can weaken and damage blood vessels in and around the brain, leaving them vulnerable to hemorrhage and atherosclerosis. Excessive dietary salt, lack of exercise and excess weight contribute to high blood pressure.
- *Cardiovascular disease.* Several other heart and blood vessel conditions can increase your risk of a stroke: congestive heart failure, a heart attack, aortic heart valve disease or valve replacement and an irregular heart rhythm (atrial fibrillation). With these conditions, your heart doesn't pump blood efficiently or it beats irregularly. This can lead to formation of blood clots (thrombosis) in a chamber of the heart or on a diseased valve. About 15 percent to 20 percent of all ischemic strokes occur in people with atrial fibrillation.
- *Tobacco use.* If you smoke, your risk of a stroke may be two or three times greater than if you don't. Smoking contributes to the formation of fatty deposits (plaques) in your arteries. Nicotine makes your heart work harder, increasing your heart rate and blood pressure. The carbon monoxide in cigarette smoke replaces oxygen in your blood, decreasing the amount of oxygen delivered to the walls of your arteries and tissues, including tissues in your brain. The combination of smoking and using oral contraceptives greatly increases your risk of stroke.
- *Diabetes.* Diabetes doubles your risk of a stroke. It increases the severity of atherosclerosis and interferes with normal breakdown of fibrin, a protein in your blood that binds clots together.
- *Undesirable blood cholesterol levels.* High levels of low-density lipoprotein (LDL, "bad") cholesterol and low levels of high-density lipoprotein (HDL, "good") cholesterol increase your risk of narrowed or blocked arteries, including those leading from your heart to your brain (carotid and vertebral arteries).
- *Previous transient ischemic attack (TIA) or stroke.* If you've had a TIA, your risk of a stroke increases significantly. The more frequent the TIAs, the greater your risk. If you've already had a stroke and you're over age 45, your risk of having another increases by about 10 to 20 times.
- *Elevated homocysteine level.* This amino acid occurs naturally in your blood. Studies indicate that people with elevated levels of homocysteine may have a higher risk of heart and blood vessel damage.
- *Sedentary lifestyle.* Lack of physical activity on a regular basis increases the risk of stroke.

Decreasing your risk of stroke involves many of the same lifestyle changes as those for decreasing your risk of cardiovascular disease, such as quitting smoking, limiting fat and cholesterol in your diet, exercising regularly, controlling blood pressure and diabetes and managing stress.

It may not be easy to change an old habit, or to start a new one such as daily exercise. But doing so may help protect you from the most common cause of serious, long-term disability and the third most common cause of death in the United States — stroke.

Talk to your doctor about your stroke risk factors and the treatments, medications and resources that may be available to help you reduce your risk.

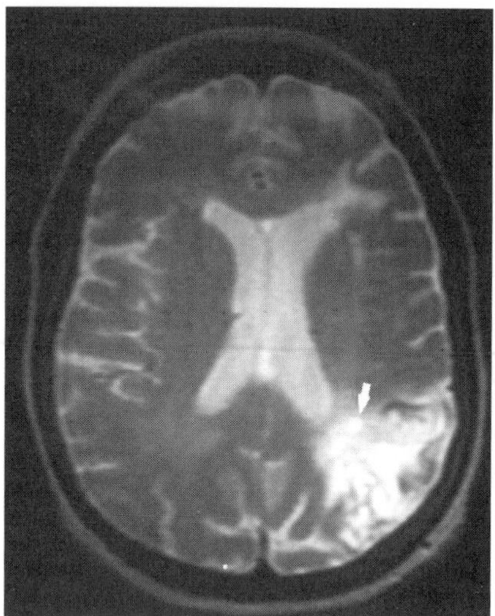

The arrow reveals an area of brain tissue affected by a stroke as shown on a magnetic resonance image (MRI).

swallow may be lost. It may return within 1 to 2 weeks, or it may never return. In the interim, food and water can be supplied intravenously or directly to the stomach following a procedure called a gastrostomy. Some strokes result in much less damage and require less care.

Medication

In case of an ischemic stroke, immediate treatment aims to improve blood flow. Several drugs can help:

- *Aspirin, dipyridamole and aspirin (Aggrenox) and clopidogrel (Plavix).* These are examples of platelet-inhibiting medications. They reduce the tendency of blood to clot by preventing blood platelets from sticking together as they pass through narrowed arteries.
- *Warfarin (Coumadin).* This drug is an anticoagulant medication. It also helps prevent blood clots, but it takes several days for this drug to become fully effective.
- *Heparin.* This drug works immediately and may be injected intravenously or under the skin to reduce clotting while waiting for warfarin to take effect.
- *Tissue plasminogen activator.* Thrombolytic therapy using tissue plasminogen activator (TPA) may prevent or minimize damage to your brain by dissolving a blood clot and restoring blood flow. However, this type of clot-busting medication is of benefit only within 3 hours of stroke onset. It also increases the risk of bleeding in your brain. Before receiving TPA, you may undergo a computerized tomography (CT) scan to detect any existing bleeding. It's also important before you take this medication that your blood pressure be under control.

Anticoagulant medications are potentially dangerous in people with high blood pressure or extensive brain tissue damage because they increase the possibility of bleeding (hemorrhaging). Thus, they aren't used as treatment for hemorrhagic stroke.

Treatment for a hemorrhagic stroke is complex. Therapy typically involves controlling blood pressure and limiting fluids, and it may involve giving medications to minimize swelling of brain tissue. Pain relievers may be prescribed to relieve headache. If nausea and vomiting are present, intravenous administration of nutrients and fluid may be necessary for a few days.

Surgery

Following an ischemic stroke, you may need a carotid endarterectomy in addition to medication. This procedure may be used if you've previously experienced symptoms of stroke and you have a neck (carotid) artery that's moderately or severely narrowed. The intent is to clear the carotid artery of plaques before another stroke can occur. Typically, a surgeon makes an incision to open the artery, removes the plaques and then closes the artery.

In some cases, angioplasty may be used instead of carotid endarterectomy. In this procedure, a doctor places a small wire tube into a narrowed artery. The tube contains a balloon that inflates to widen the artery. A small metallic mesh tube (stent) may be placed in the widened artery to keep it from narrowing again.

In cases of subarachnoid hemorrhage, cerebral aneurysm repair may be necessary. A surgeon may clamp the aneurysm at its base or use a procedure known as coiling. In this procedure, a catheter is passed through a blood vessel in your groin to reach the aneurysm. A tiny platinum coil is pushed through the catheter and positioned inside the aneurysm. The coil fills the aneurysm, causes it to clot and seals it off. Eventually the clot becomes harmless scar tissue.

Rarely, surgery is needed to remove blood that has leaked into the tissues from a cerebral hemorrhage. If an arteriovenous malformation is small and located in an easily accessible portion of the brain, it may be removed surgically to eliminate the risk of rupture.

PREVENTION TIP

Alcohol can be both a risk factor and a preventive measure for stroke. Binge drinking and heavy alcohol consumption increase your risk of hemorrhagic stroke. However, light to moderate alcohol use — no more than one drink daily for women and one to two drinks daily for men — can increase your high-density lipoprotein (HDL or "good") cholesterol and decrease your blood's tendency to clot. Both factors may contribute to a reduced risk of ischemic stroke.

Subdural hematoma

Signs and symptoms

- Steady or fluctuating headache, drowsiness, seizures or confusion after a head injury
- Partial paralysis on one side of the body
- Slowed thinking, changes in personality

Emergency signs and symptoms
- Convulsions, stupor or loss of consciousness after a head injury
- Enlarged pupils

Subdural hematoma (subdural hemorrhage) is caused by an injury to the head. It may be the result of a car accident or a seemingly trivial bumping of your head. Bleeding occurs when blood vessels — usually veins — rupture between the brain and the outermost of three membrane layers that cover the brain (dura mater). The leaking blood forms a mass (hematoma) that compresses brain tissue. If the hematoma keeps enlarging, you may experience a progressive decline in consciousness that can culminate in death.

The interval between injury and the onset of significant signs and symptoms, such as headache, confusion, paralysis and loss of consciousness, can vary. A hematoma is considered acute if the interval is less than 48 hours, subacute if it's between 48 hours and 2 weeks and chronic if it's more than 2 weeks. Infants and older adults are at higher risk of this condition. The injury that caused it may not be apparent or remembered.

Carotid Endarterectomy

Endarterectomy is a surgical procedure that removes cholesterol-containing fatty deposits (plaques) from inside a blood vessel. Plaques can reduce the flow of blood through an artery or break off and travel to, and lodge in, the brain. Plaque formation (atherosclerosis) is common. It frequently occurs in the neck arteries to the brain, particularly in the carotid artery where it branches.

Plaque formation at this junction is a common cause of transient ischemic attack (TIA) or ischemic stroke. Carotid endarterectomy is usually done after one or more TIAs to prevent their recurrence or a subsequent stroke. Occasionally, carotid endarterectomy is performed during the first few hours of an evolving ischemic stroke.

Carotid endarterectomy is also effective in reducing the risk of stroke in people who have severe narrowing of the carotid artery but haven't yet experienced symptoms.

Benefits vs. risks

Although it has a high success rate, the procedure has risks. Your doctor will discuss them with you and determine whether to recommend the procedure for you. In addition to the severity and location of the narrowing, your doctor will consider other factors before recommending this operation, such as whether you have high blood pressure or other forms of cardiovascular disease. Unstable coronary artery disease may make the risk of this operation too great.

In individuals for whom the risks of the surgery may be too high, nonsurgical therapy is considered. This generally includes medication to prevent blood clotting.

The procedure

The procedure begins with an incision in the neck to expose the carotid branching site (bifurcation). Clamps are inserted to stop blood flow. The artery is opened to remove the plaques. Closure of the artery may require a patch of synthetic material. Restoring blood flow through the artery must be done carefully to prevent clots from entering the blood flow.

Complications, including stroke, can arise during this operation. To minimize the risk of stroke during surgery, brain activity is monitored by a test called electroencephalography. It allows the surgeon to determine if circulation to the brain is adequate while the carotid artery is clamped for repair. If not, steps can be taken to improve blood flow. Sometimes, the person undergoing surgery is kept awake to allow cooperation with surgical staff.

As with any surgical procedure, the success rate of carotid endarterectomy depends on the expertise of the doctor and surgical team. Blockage may recur, but that's uncommon. In properly selected individuals, the operation usually eliminates risk of further transient ischemic attacks (TIAs) and reduces the chance of a stroke.

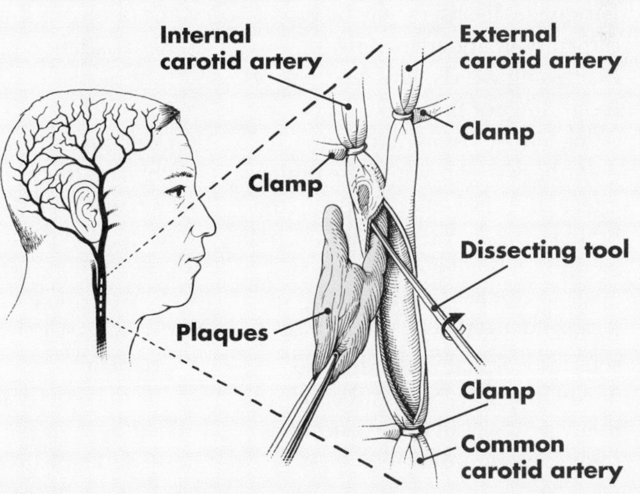

If blood flow to the brain is blocked by an obstruction in the carotid artery, a surgical procedure called an endarterectomy may be done. Clamps are placed on the artery to stop blood flow while fatty deposits (plaques) inside the artery are removed with a dissecting tool.

Stroke Rehabilitation

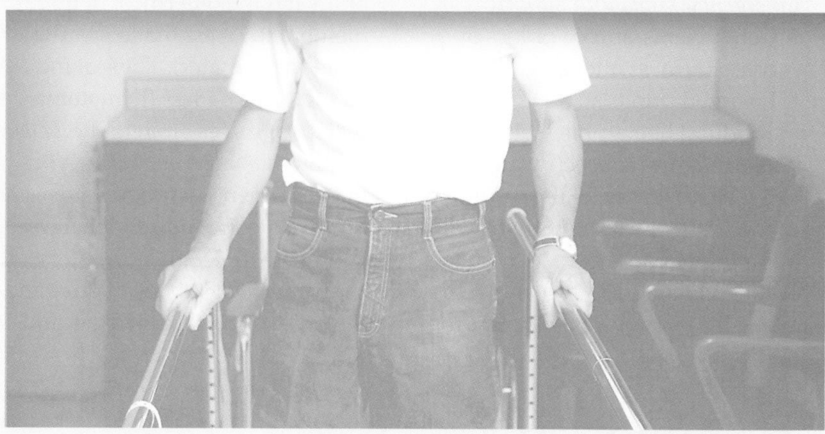

There are approximately 4.5 million stroke survivors in the United States today. Some have only minor disabilities, and well over half of all stroke survivors regain their independence. But 2 out of 10 stroke survivors require extended care, some because of permanent mental or physical disabilities and others because they lack home care.

Following a stroke, rehabilitation is crucial for morale and a return to maximal function. Recovery and rehabilitation depend on the area of the brain involved and the amount of tissue damaged. Stroke may affect you physically, psychologically and cognitively.

Physically
Harm to the right side of the brain may impair sensation and movement on the left side of the body. Damage to brain tissue on the left side may affect movement on the right side and may also cause speech and language disorders. Language disorders may include difficulty in understanding or expressing words. This can be very frustrating for the stroke survivor. Some loss of vision may occur regardless which side of the brain is affected. A stroke that occurs in the brain stem can cause disturbances in breathing, swallowing, balance, hearing and eye and tongue movements. You may also have a loss of sensation. Initially, bladder and bowel function are disturbed in many people, but these conditions frequently improve.

Psychologically
In addition to the various physical effects, depression is a common response to stroke. Affected individuals may feel helpless, frustrated and uninterested in activities they once enjoyed. Diminished sex drive, mood changes and thoughts of suicide aren't unusual.

Cognitively
The way in which a person learns, remembers, interacts with others or interprets everyday events may be affected. These side effects may be due in part to changes in the production of brain chemicals. Antidepressant medications may be prescribed.

Stroke rehab team

A stroke rehabilitation team can help you get started on your way to recovery. The team may include some or all of the following people:

- Rehabilitation physician (physiatrist)
- Nurse
- Dietitian
- Physical therapist
- Occupational therapist
- Recreational therapist
- Speech therapist
- Social worker
- Psychologist
- Chaplain

The makeup of the team is determined by your particular needs. Early and repeated tests to determine the status of your improvement are used to design your rehab program. Therapy is focused on maximizing your capabilities, such as getting you back to work or improving mobility at home and in the community. Many stroke survivors regain partial use of affected limbs, especially with the help of rehabilitation professionals.

Recovery

Some individuals recover satisfactorily without specific rehabilitation therapy. Others require it. In some, the damage is so severe that intensive rehabilitation is impractical. Among individuals in whom rehabilitation may not be possible, the goal of treatment and care is to prevent complicating muscle contractures, skin ulcers, pneumonia, malnutrition, bowel and bladder dysfunction, social isolation and depression. The most important and effective help over the long term may come from family and friends, and it requires patience and persistence.

A supportive home environment has a beneficial effect on rehabilitation. Regardless of age, stroke survivors who can go home to a healthy spouse or other companion are more likely to become independent and productive. In case of severe damage, the home environment can reduce risk of further complications. Encouragement is important.

Various adaptive devices and architectural modifications such as ramps, hand bars on the tub and toilet, and bath benches or shower chairs facilitate independence and safety. Contact your doctor, local rehabilitation professionals or independent living center for information and assistance.

Diagnosis

Chronic subdural hemorrhage can be difficult to diagnose. Progressive loss of consciousness following a head injury, however, generally should be presumed to be caused by a hemorrhage inside the head until proved otherwise. The best method to define the position and size of the hematoma is a computerized tomography (CT) scan, if there's time to perform it. In some cases, magnetic resonance imaging (MRI) may be used instead. Sometimes, immediate surgery is necessary, leaving no time to perform tests.

How serious is a subdural hematoma?

Acute subdural bleeding (hemorrhaging) is often fatal with or without immediate surgery, and death may occur despite prompt medical attention.

Subacute and chronic forms have less risk, but require medical attention as soon as signs and symptoms are apparent, or permanent brain damage may result. Risk of serious complications is greater for people who use aspirin and anticoagulant medications on a daily basis.

Treatment

Treatment of a hematoma usually requires surgery. If the blood is localized and liquid, the only procedure necessary may be the creation of a hole through the skull to drain the blood. Large hematomas or clotted blood may require that a section of skull be opened (in a procedure called craniotomy) to remove the blood. Some subdural hematomas are small and don't cause symptoms or need to be removed.

Intensive care includes various procedures and medications to control brain swelling (edema) caused by other fluids accumulating following a head injury. After surgery, antiseizure medications, such as phenytoin (Dilantin), may be prescribed to control or prevent posttraumatic seizures. Seizures can begin as late as 2 years after the trauma.

Amnesia, giddiness, attention difficulties, anxiety and headache may occur and continue for some time. In adults, most recovery occurs within the first 6 months, and smaller improvements occur over 2 years. Incomplete recovery is a result of brain damage. Children usually fare better than adults. They have better immediate recovery, and small improvements spread over a longer period.

Epidural hemorrhage

Signs and symptoms

- Headache, drowsiness or confusion after a head injury
- Paralysis on one side of the body
- Nausea, vomiting or dizziness

Emergency signs and symptoms

- Enlarged pupils

Epidural (extradural) hemorrhage occurs when a blood vessel, usually an artery, ruptures between the outer surface of the dura mater — the outermost of three membrane layers that cover the brain — and the skull. The blood vessel is usually damaged by a skull fracture. Blood then leaks between the dura mater and the skull to form a mass (hematoma) that compresses the brain tissue.

Epidural hemorrhage is usually caused by a head injury resulting from an automobile or motorcycle accident. There may be no visible signs, such as an open head wound or bruise.

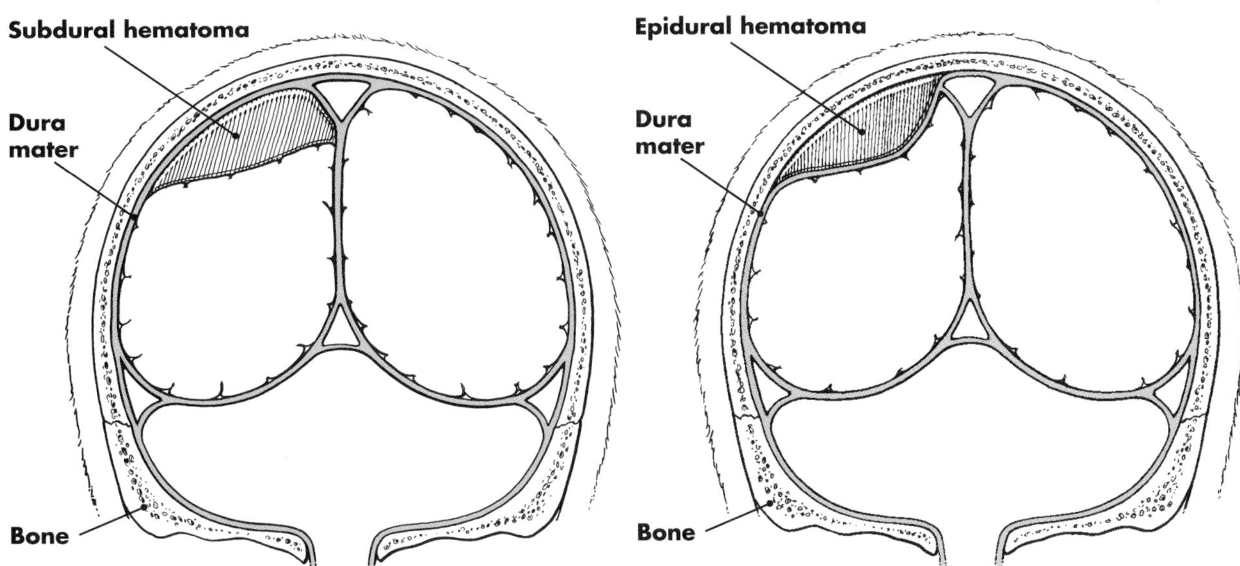

When an injury results in bleeding between the brain and the outer membrane of the brain (dura mater), blood may accumulate, producing a mass called a subdural hematoma (left). When bleeding occurs between the dura mater and the skull, the accumulation is termed epidural hematoma (right). Both can put pressure on the brain.

In epidural hemorrhage, pressure on the brain increases as more blood flows into the narrow space between the brain and skull. The pressure may rapidly lead to unconsciousness, permanent brain damage and even death. Prompt diagnosis and treatment are important.

Diagnosis

Signs and symptoms are likely to occur within minutes to hours after the injury. Several tests, such as computerized tomography (CT) or magnetic resonance imaging (MRI), may be required to locate and assess epidural hemorrhaging. Sometimes, there's no time to perform such tests, and an immediate operation is required.

How serious is epidural hemorrhage?

Although the percentage of head injuries that result in acute epidural hemorrhage is small, the risk of death is substantial unless prompt treatment is available. Up to a third of victims may remain conscious, but most are drowsy or comatose from the moment of trauma.

Treatment

If diagnostic tests indicate the presence of epidural hemorrhage, an operation will be necessary to stop the bleeding. Surgery involves excising a portion of the skull (craniotomy) to remove the blood clot and stop the bleeding. Prompt surgery usually results in complete recovery.

A significant period of recovery is often required following an epidural hemorrhage. Headache may occur and continue for some time, along with anxiety, amnesia and difficulty concentrating. Speech disorders and paralysis usually resolve. In adults, most recovery occurs within the first 6 months, but smaller adjustments may be made over 2 years. Incomplete recovery is due to permanent brain damage. Children fare better than adults — they have better immediate recovery and improvements continue over a longer period.

Infections

Infections can attack your central nervous system in several ways. They may result from a direct invasion by a virus, bacterium or fungus. A minor condition, such as an ear infection or the measles, can lead to central nervous system involvement. You can also be infected from tick bites or mosquito-borne agents.

Infections vary in seriousness. They may result in several days in bed, months of sickness with residual mental and physical impairment, or even death.

Meningitis

Signs and symptoms

- Fever
- Severe headache
- Vomiting
- Confusion
- Seizures
- Progressive lethargy
- Drowsiness
- In infants, bulging in the soft spot of the skull
- Stiff neck

Emergency signs and symptoms

- Stupor
- Coma
- Convulsions

Meningitis is an infection and inflammation of the membranes (meninges) and fluid surrounding your brain and spinal cord (cerebrospinal fluid). It's most often caused by a bacterial or viral infection. Of the two, bacterial meningitis is usually much more serious.

Meningitis usually strikes suddenly, with a high fever, severe headache and vomiting. Seventy percent of cases of meningitis occur in children under age 5, but the disease is increasing in frequency among people between ages 15 and 24. Older adults also tend to have increased incidence of meningitis.

Some types of meningitis are contagious. You may be exposed to the bacteria when someone with the infection coughs or sneezes. The bacteria can spread through kissing or sharing eating utensils, a toothbrush or a cigarette. You're also at increased risk if you live or work with someone with the disease.

The infection often starts as a respiratory illness. An infection of the heart valves, bones or some other organ can spread to the meninges via the bloodstream. Infection can also occur by direct invasion of bacteria already localized near your central nervous system, for example, from an infected ear, sinus, nose or tooth.

The *Streptococcus pneumoniae* (pneumococcus) bacterium is the most common cause of meningitis in adults and children. It most often occurs when the bacterium enters your bloodstream and migrates to your brain and spinal cord. You may also have this type of bacterium in your lungs, where it can cause pneumonia. Pneumococcal meningitis can also follow an ear infection or head injury.

The bacterial strain meningococcus may cause local epidemics within relatively confined environments, such as universities, boarding schools or military bases. It produces a purplish rash in 50 percent of cases. Other bacterial strains that cause sporadic cases of meningitis include *Haemophilus influenzae* type b and staphylococcus.

Less frequent causes for acute bacterial meningitis include an epidural abscess and medical procedures such as a spinal tap (lumbar puncture). Alcoholism, diabetes, AIDS and immunosuppressant medications taken following organ transplantation may make you more vulnerable to meningitis.

Other, normally less life-threatening, forms of the disease include aseptic (viral), chronic and recurrent meningitis. Aseptic meningitis is most commonly caused by certain viruses but also can be a reaction to certain medications or chemicals that aren't normally present in cerebrospinal fluid. This form of meningitis causes many of the same signs and symptoms as does a bacterial infection.

Human immunodeficiency virus (HIV), tuberculosis, fungal infections, malignant cancer cells or syphilis may cause chronic meningitis. Signs and symptoms often evolve over a period of weeks.

Recurrent meningitis may be the result of a channel of communication between the nose and the linings of the brain (subarachnoid space). This channel, usually the result of a head injury, permits loss of cerebrospinal fluid through the nose. It also may allow bacteria to travel from the nose or sinuses into the subarachnoid space.

Recently, the herpes simplex virus has been recognized as another cause of recurrent meningitis. The virus can lie dormant in the body but be reactivated from time to time, causing meningitis.

Diagnosis

Signs and symptoms of meningitis may not develop early in the course of the infection. If you experience signs and symptoms consistent with meningitis, your doctor will likely examine your head, ears and skin — especially along the spine — for evidence of infection. You may have X-rays taken of your chest, skull and sinuses. A computerized tomography (CT) scan may be done to determine if there's an abscess. A definitive diagnosis, however, will likely require analysis of your cerebrospinal fluid, obtained by a spinal tap. One of the main laboratory signs of meningitis is an increased white blood cell count in the fluid. Some of the fluid can be cultured to determine the type of organisms present.

How serious is meningitis?

Acute bacterial meningitis is a medical emergency. The longer you have the disease without treatment, the greater your risk of permanent neurologic damage, such as hearing loss, brain damage, loss of memory or death. Meningitis is most dangerous to infants and older adults. In infants, a bulging in the soft spot of the skull (fontanel) and a stiff neck are key signs.

Meningococcal meningitis may be rapidly fatal if not treated promptly with an appropriate antibiotic. Viral meningitis is usually mild and often resolves on its own in 1 to 2 weeks.

Treatment

For acute bacterial meningitis, antibiotic drug therapy is generally instituted immediately. The choice of antibiotic depends on the type of bacteria causing the infection. In some cases, treatment for brain swelling, shock, convulsions or dehydration may be necessary, as well.

Drainage of infected sinuses or mastoids is sometimes required. If fluid has accumulated between layers of the meninges, the fluid may need to be drained or surgically removed.

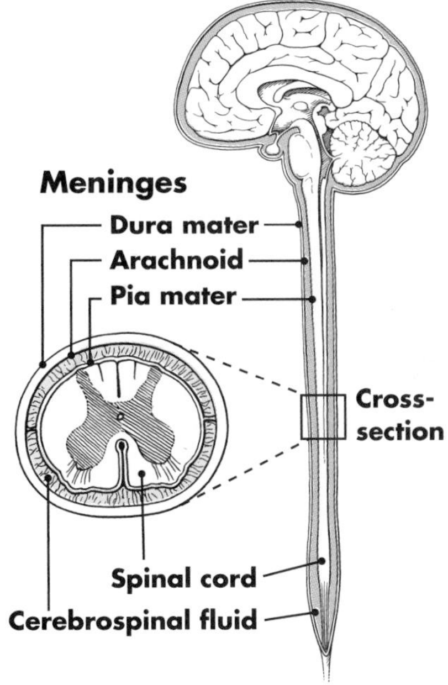

Like the brain, the spinal cord is protected by several layers of membranes (meninges): dura mater, arachnoid and pia mater. Cerebrospinal fluid (shown in blue) surrounds the brain and spinal cord. Meningitis affects the meninges and cerebrospinal fluid.

Prevention

Many children now routinely receive vaccines against *Streptococcus pneumoniae* (pneumococcal conjugate vaccine) and *Haemophilus influenzae* type b (Hib vaccine), starting at about 2 months of age. If your child hasn't been vaccinated for these diseases, talk to your doctor.

A vaccine also is available that offers some protection against four of the five strains of bacteria responsible for meningococcal meningitis. Both the Centers for Disease Control and Prevention and the American College Health Association recommend this vaccine for college students, especially those living in campus dormitories. The vaccine is also recommended for people traveling to countries where meningitis is common. It's important to receive the vaccine at least 1 week before your departure.

If you've been exposed to someone with meningitis, talk to your doctor about medication that may help protect you from the disease.

Encephalitis

Signs and symptoms

- Drowsiness
- Confusion and disorientation
- Seizures
- Sudden fever
- Severe headache
- Nausea and vomiting
- Tremor
- Occasionally, a stiff neck

Emergency signs and symptoms

- Altered levels of consciousness

Encephalitis is a rare but severe inflammatory disease of the brain that's usually caused by a viral infection. Encephalitis sometimes occurs due to a direct viral invasion of your central nervous system.

Another form is secondary (postinfectious) encephalitis, which follows or accompanies a viral illness such as measles, chickenpox, German measles (rubella) or mumps. The cause of secondary encephalitis is believed to be an overreaction of the immune system to a foreign substance.

Secondary encephalitis arises from within your body, but the primary viral form results from the environment around you. Viral encephalitis can occur sporadically at any time of the year or as an epidemic. The most common sporadic form is herpes simplex encephalitis. It can start as a minor illness with headache and fever. This is followed by neurologic signs and symptoms, which may include difficulty in talking, weakness, confusion, unconsciousness or repeated seizures.

Epidemic varieties are commonly caused by mosquito-borne viruses and occur during the summer months. The major types of mosquito-borne encephalitis in the United States are eastern equine encephalitis, western equine encephalitis, St. Louis encephalitis, La Crosse encephalitis and, more recently, West Nile encephalitis, caused by the West Nile virus (see page 519).

Diagnosis

In children, seizures, severe headache and sensitivity to light may be early signs and symptoms.

A Spinal Tap

A spinal tap (lumbar puncture) is used to measure pressure in your cerebrospinal fluid and to remove some of the fluid for laboratory analysis. This procedure is also used to inject spinal anesthetics, some medications and substances for diagnostic imaging.

The procedure

A local anesthetic is used at the puncture site. A thin, hollow needle is then inserted between two vertebrae in your lower back (lumbar region), through the spinal membrane (dura) and into the spinal canal. The vertebrae must be spread apart slightly to provide access, so you'll be asked to lie on your side with your knees drawn up to your chest and both arms clasped around your knees. This position flexes the back and spreads the vertebrae. Some conditions require the puncture to be made between two cervical vertebrae in your neck rather than the lower back.

Once the needle is in place, fluid pressure is measured, a small amount of fluid is withdrawn, and the pressure is measured again. If a drug or substance is being injected, its volume will equal the volume of the fluid that's withdrawn. The procedure usually takes about 30 minutes if only cerebrospinal fluid is being extracted, but more time may be required for an injection. After the procedure, the puncture site is covered with a bandage.

You may have a feeling of pressure during the procedure. Afterward, you may have a headache due to a decrease in cerebrospinal fluid pressure, especially if there is a persistent leak of fluid into tissues. Lying down usually alleviates the headache, and it usually goes away as the pressure returns to normal in a few days.

Uses

A sample of cerebrospinal fluid can aid in the diagnosis of various diseases. These include multiple sclerosis, Reye's syndrome, Guillain-Barre syndrome, infections of the central nervous system, certain kinds of tumors and subarachnoid hemorrhage. A cerebrospinal fluid sample can be tested for protein, sugar, red and white blood cells and cancerous (malignant) cells. The fluid can also be cultured to identify bacterial and viral organisms.

A spinal tap may also be used for injecting dye (contrast material) or radioactive substances into cerebrospinal fluid when needed to make diagnostic images of the fluid's flow, a procedure called myelography (see page 610). Occasionally, a spinal tap is used to inject medications such as antibiotics and chemotherapy drugs.

Risks

Some risks accompany lumbar puncture, although they're fewer now than they once were. Greater care is used to prevent infection, and the procedure is used more selectively. The availability of improved imaging procedures has reduced the need for a spinal tap in many conditions.

You're at increased risk of complications from a spinal tap if you have a blood-clotting disorder or increased spinal fluid pressure, which can lead to compression of the brain stem after a sample of cerebrospinal fluid is removed.

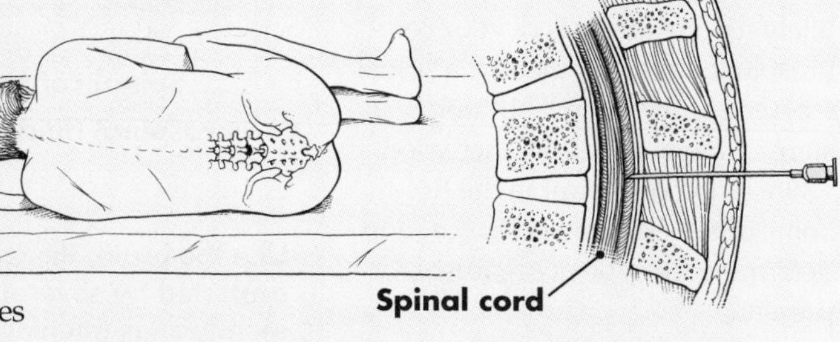

In a spinal tap (lumbar puncture), you lie on your side, knees pulled to your chest, while a needle is inserted into an anesthetized site between two vertebrae and a small amount of cerebrospinal fluid is extracted for laboratory testing.

In adults, mental disturbances, from severe disorientation to coma, may be the predominant initial symptom.

The onset of neurologic signs and symptoms can be variable. You may be severely ill within 24 hours after initial signs and symptoms, or a week may pass before neurologic involvement is apparent. In the case of secondary viral encephalitis, the disease may develop 7 to 30 days after onset of the initiating viral infection.

Encephalitis usually is diagnosed by analyzing your cerebrospinal fluid, removed by a spinal tap (lumbar puncture). Analysis of the fluid reveals an increased white blood cell count, which signals that your body is fighting infection, and absence of bacteria, which helps to rule out acute bacterial meningitis. When hemorrhages are part of the illness, your cerebrospinal fluid may be slightly bloody. Electroencephalography, magnetic resonance imaging (MRI) or a computerized tomography scan (CT) can help establish the diagnosis of encephalitis.

Diagnosis of herpes simplex encephalitis is sometimes difficult. Recent advances using sensitive DNA methods have allowed detection of the virus in spinal fluid, confirming the diagnosis. If results are negative, and if signs and symptoms warrant, a brain biopsy may be necessary. Because this biopsy involves some risk, treatment with an antiviral agent is initiated early. If no response occurs with antiviral treatment, a brain biopsy may be advised.

How serious is encephalitis?

The course of viral encephalitis is variable. It may be of short duration and leave no lasting effects, or it may strike with great severity and leave significant neurologic impairment. This can include loss of memory, the inability to speak coherently, lack of muscle coordination, paralysis or hearing or vision defects.

The most severe (acute) phase of the illness may last from a few days to a week. The duration of the fever may be 4 to 14 days. Resolution is sometimes gradual, other times abrupt. Resultant neurologic defects may continue to resolve over weeks or months. Even severely ill individuals can have a complete recovery.

Treatment

Because viruses that cause encephalitis don't respond to antibiotics, basic treatment generally consists of rest, nourishment and sufficient fluid intake to let your natural defenses fight the virus. Early on, irritability is common. For those who experience mental impairment, physical and speech therapies may be necessary.

In the case of herpes simplex encephalitis, antiviral agents such as acyclovir (Zovirax) have been used with success in early stages. For some people, antiseizure medication may be needed.

Prevention

Even though viral encephalitis is rare, a good way to prevent secondary encephalitis is to make sure that you and your children are immunized against viral infections that may lead to encephalitis — chickenpox, measles, mumps and German measles (rubella).

To protect yourself and your family against mosquito-borne encephalitis during an outbreak of the disease:

- Wear long sleeves and pants if you're outside between dusk and dawn.
- Apply mosquito repellent that contains DEET to your skin and clothing. However, exercise caution when using repellents on children.

  The American Academy of Pediatrics recommends using a repellent made for children — containing no more than 10 percent DEET — and applying it to their clothing rather than skin when possible.
- Repair all holes in screens on doors and windows.
- Eliminate standing water by emptying buckets, discarded tires, birdbaths, drains, wheelbarrows, flowerpots and similar containers. Be sure to change your pet's water dish daily.
- Fill ornamental pools with mosquito-eating fish.
- Clean your gutters, and drain flat roofs regularly.
- Drain puddles when possible.
- Fill holes in trees and stumps with mortar.
- Put screens on rain barrels and openings to water tanks.

Reye's syndrome

Signs and symptoms

- Persistent nausea and vomiting after a viral infection

Emergency signs and symptoms

- Drowsiness
- Stupor
- Loss of consciousness or coma
- Delirium, seizures or convulsions

Reye's syndrome is a relatively rare but serious illness that can follow a viral infection in children. It affects the blood, liver and brain. Characteristics of the syndrome include high levels of ammonia and acidity and low levels of sugar in blood, fat deposits and swelling in the liver, and brain swelling that may cause loss of consciousness, delirium or seizures.

Reye's syndrome was first identified as a distinct disease in 1963, and the number of recognized cases began to increase in the 1970s. The number of cases in the United States peaked at 555 in 1980, after which they began to decrease sharply. Presently, only a few cases are reported each year. Many people assume the decline is the result of the warnings against children taking aspirin, which has been associated with the syndrome, but that may be only part of the reason.

Although the use of aspirin may trigger it in children, the specific cause for Reye's syndrome is unknown. The condition occurs almost exclusively in children between ages 2 and 16, following a viral infection such as chickenpox or influenza or even an ordinary upper respiratory infection. Some researchers believe Reye's syndrome may be an underlying metabolic condition unmasked by a viral illness.

Diagnosis

Signs and symptoms typically start a week after the viral infection. At first your child experiences persistent nausea and vomiting for 1 to 3 days, followed by a progressive decline in mental alertness as brain swelling increases. This progresses from lethargy and drowsiness to stupor and deepening stages of coma. Episodes of agitation, seizures or convulsions may occur. These signs and symptoms develop rapidly over a few days, and immediate medical attention is required.

To diagnosis the condition, your doctor may request blood tests, but a liver biopsy — in which a tissue sample is removed for laboratory study — is the definitive test.

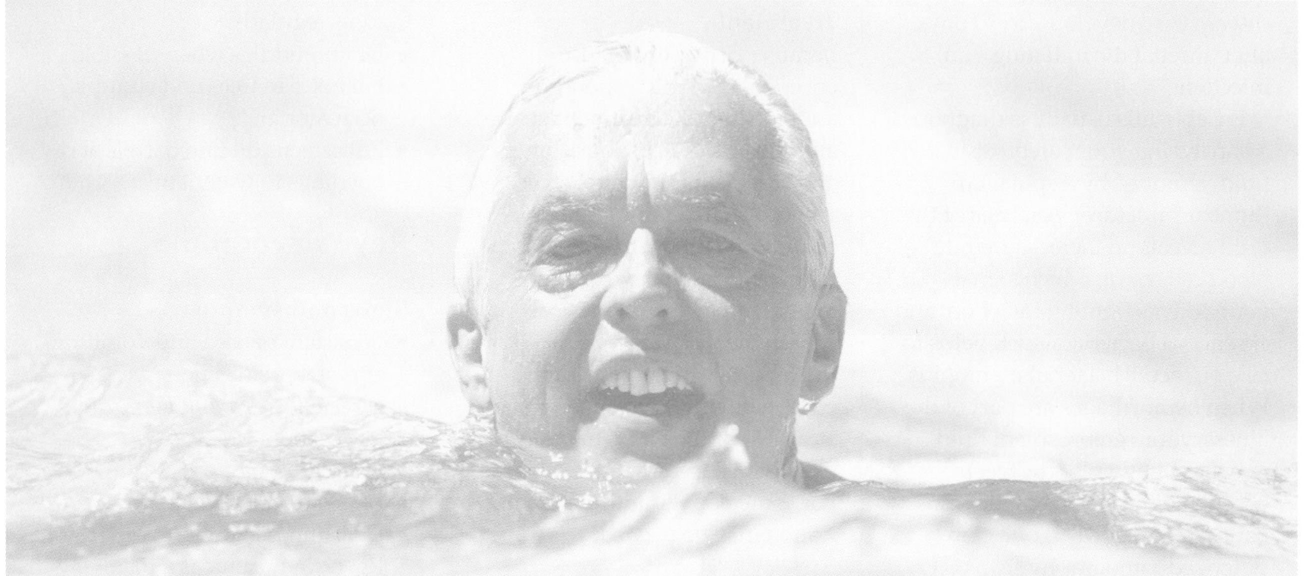

Post-Polio Syndrome

Late effects of polio, which some doctors call post-polio syndrome, can resemble arthritis, tendinitis or amyotrophic lateral sclerosis (ALS). Weakness can develop in any muscle, whether or not it was involved during the earlier polio attack. Joint pain and flu-like aching of the muscles are common. The syndrome affects about 25 percent of polio survivors.

Scientists aren't sure of the exact cause of post-polio syndrome. It appears to not be a reactivation of a long-dormant virus or a new infection. Because most individuals with post-polio syndrome are in their 30s or 40s, it can't be attributed to aging either.

Current research focuses on nerve cells in the spinal cord. Normally, these cells deteriorate over time, but other cells compensate for their loss. Polio survivors, however, lost some of their nerve cells during their initial illness. People who recovered and then led physically active lives may have unknowingly overworked their remaining spinal nerve cells. Overuse of undamaged muscles in an effort to compensate for those that have been damaged can lead to pain and weakness after many years.

To confirm the diagnosis of post-polio syndrome, doctors generally look for these criteria:

- *Previous exposure to polio.* The syndrome usually occurs in people who were age 10 or older during the initial attack of polio and whose symptoms were often severe.
- *Long interval period.* The onset of late effects varies widely but typically begins about 30 years after the initial infection.
- *Gradual onset.* Weakness can develop quickly over a few months but may be imperceptible until it interferes with daily activities. You may awaken refreshed but feel exhausted by midday, tiring after activities that once were no problem.

It's difficult to forecast the course of symptoms. Fortunately, the progressive weakness in post-polio syndrome commonly is mild.

Although there's no specific treatment for the syndrome, see your doctor if you're a polio survivor experiencing new muscle weakness or pain. Medications, including aspirin and other nonsteroidal anti-inflammatory drugs (NSAIDs), may relieve some of the signs and symptoms. An occupational or physical therapist can analyze the ways that you move during work or leisure and suggest ways to reduce muscle fatigue. Try swimming or water aerobics and avoid overuse of your muscles.

Your attitude also plays an important part in your adjustment. Many communities are developing support groups for polio survivors that offer counseling, self-help tips and practical advice.

Cerebrospinal fluid may be obtained by a spinal tap (lumbar puncture) to exclude other diseases with similar signs and symptoms, such as meningitis or encephalitis.

Your doctor may also evaluate the possibility that your child has one of the rare, inherited metabolic disorders that can mimic the signs and symptoms of Reye's syndrome. The key to diagnosing or excluding these unusual conditions is obtaining blood and urine samples during the acute phase of the illness and having them analyzed in a qualified biochemical genetics laboratory. Many of these metabolic conditions are termed mitochondrial diseases because the problems arise from the part of body cells called the mitochondria.

If a child dies of a Reye's-like illness, it may be important to obtain blood and urine to check for such metabolic conditions, which might affect other family members.

How serious is Reye's syndrome?

Although its severity varies greatly, Reye's syndrome is usually a severe, life-threatening disorder. Emergency treatment is required. The chances for your child's survival depend on how far the disease has progressed, how soon treatment is started and how quickly body chemistry is stabilized.

Previously, the fatality rate was more than 40 percent. With earlier diagnosis and better treatment, this rate has decreased to about 10 percent. Most children recover completely in 2 to 3 months, but in a few cases brain damage persists.

Treatment

Medications are given, usually intravenously, and vital signs are monitored. Your child's low blood sugar level is treated by giving glucose, blood chemistry values are corrected with electrolyte solutions containing sodium, potassium and chloride, and acidity is treated with counteracting basic solutions. Small amounts of insulin may be given to increase glucose metabolism.

Brain swelling is generally controlled with a corticosteroid (dexamethasone) that reduces inflammation, and a diuretic (mannitol) may be given to increase fluid loss through urination. Other medications may include purgatives, vitamin K-1 and an oral nonabsorbable antibiotic (neomycin).

Monitoring of the pressure inside your child's skull may be used to guide the effectiveness of therapy. Other common procedures include the insertion of a tube into your child's airway to aid breathing.

Prevention

The occurrence of Reye's syndrome is reduced by avoiding the use of aspirin (acetylsalicylic acid) in children younger than age 16 during a viral illness. Aspirin isn't recommended for children younger than age 12 with any illness.

Keep in mind that other common medications, including Alka-Seltzer and Pepto-Bismol, contain salicylates and should be avoided by children.

Epidural abscess

Signs and symptoms

- Ear or nose pain with pus
- Unrelenting headache
- Fever
- Nausea and vomiting
- Back pain and tenderness

Emergency signs and symptoms

- Reduced consciousness
- Increasing loss of sensation, weakness or paralysis in one side of the body or both legs
- Seizures or convulsions
- Speech disturbance

Epidural abscess is usually due to a bacterial infection that causes pus to form between the outermost brain membrane (dura mater) and the bones of the spine or skull. Sometimes, it invades the bone surface inside the skull or vertebrae. It can also penetrate membrane layers to become a subdural abscess, a brain abscess or meningitis.

Epidural abscesses in your head may develop from infections in your sinuses, ears or the mastoid bones behind your ears. Occasionally, bacteria are carried by the blood to the epidural space from an infection elsewhere in the body. Abscesses in the spine can start from a boil on your skin, an infection in your lung or abdomen or an infection following surgery.

Progressive headache or back pain with fever and tenderness around the infection site may develop. As the abscess enlarges, it can cause direct pressure on the spinal cord or brain, resulting in pain and the loss of neurologic function.

Epidural and similar abscesses are now relatively rare because antibiotics can control many infections in their early stages. The greatest risk is from chronic sinus or ear infections.

Diagnosis

The diagnosis of an epidural abscess is suggested by the presence of an infection and the subsequent development of signs and symptoms. Your doctor will probably order an X-ray or magnetic resonance image (MRI) or computerized tomography (CT) scan of your head or spine to establish the diagnosis.

How serious is an epidural abscess?

An epidural abscess can cause serious neurologic damage or even death if it's not treated promptly. Prompt treatment generally results in a complete recovery.

Treatment

Intravenous antibiotic therapy is generally initiated immediately to control the infection. However, the abscess sometimes isn't cured by antibiotics alone, and an operation may be necessary to drain the infected area. A section of your skull or spine is opened to provide access to the abscess and to facilitate drainage. If the abscess has penetrated any area of your skull or vertebrae, some of the affected tissue may be removed. Sometimes, it's difficult to find and remove all traces of the infection, and your recovery may be complicated by reinfection. After such an operation, antibiotics are usually given for 1 to 2 months.

Botulism

Signs and symptoms

- Weak, limp muscles within 12 to 36 hours after consuming contaminated food
- Double vision
- Dry mouth
- Speech disturbance
- Difficulty swallowing
- Vomiting and cramps

Emergency signs and symptoms

- Rapidly progressive weakness or paralysis
- Breathing difficulty

Botulism is a form of poisoning caused by the toxin produced by the microorganism *Clostridium botulinum,* commonly found in soil. The organism is similar in many ways to the one that causes tetanus. The toxin blocks nerve signals to the salivary glands and to muscles. This effect begins 3 hours to 14 days after consuming the poison.

Botulism poisoning can result from eating canned or home-preserved foods that weren't cooked enough to destroy the organism's spores. Usually, but not always, the lids or sides of containers contaminated by this organism will bulge.

Diagnosis

A diagnosis of botulism is generally based on signs and symptoms and is confirmed by identifying the toxin in blood, food or feces.

How serious is botulism?

Respiratory failure due to weakness of the muscles that control breathing causes death in 10 percent of botulism cases and in 2 percent of botulism cases in infants. The disorder is now very rare because of careful food preparation. Heating foods to boiling temperatures for 10 minutes destroys the toxin.

Treatment

Treatment consists of administering antitoxins. In most individuals treatment is effective and recovery is usually complete.

Avoid food containers that appear to be bulging, as they may be contaminated.

AIDS and the Nervous System

AIDS is caused by the human immunodeficiency virus (HIV) and may lead to various nervous system diseases. HIV may directly infect your central nervous system and cause progressive degeneration of nerve cells. The virus also suppresses your immune system. HIV can infect any component of the nervous system, including the outer covering of the brain (meninges), the brain, spinal cord or peripheral nerves.

Approximately one-third of individuals with AIDS develop nervous system diseases, including viral, fungal or bacterial infections that cause meningitis, encephalitis or myelitis. Other diseases of the nervous system that occur in association with AIDS include parasitic cysts in the brain, abnormal growth of lymphoid tumors in the nervous system and a progressive form of dementia. Peripheral nerve disease also can be associated with AIDS.

Some AIDS-related diseases of the nervous system are treatable, but the effectiveness of standard treatments, such as antibiotic therapy for bacterial infections, is limited by the immunodeficiency. Treatment often requires lifelong therapy.

Triple-drug treatment of the HIV infection has lessened the frequency of opportunistic infections in the brain. Research on treatment is very active, and new medications are being tested.

Structural Disorders

The nerve tissue in your brain is delicate and easily torn, bruised or damaged by pressure. Under ordinary circumstances, your skull and spinal membranes (meninges) provide protection. But upon sudden or severe impact, such as in a motor vehicle or industrial accident, the skull and membranes may prove inadequate. Structural damage to your brain from an accident can range from a mild concussion to permanent disability or death.

Other structural problems described in this section include a disruption in the balance of cerebrospinal fluid in your brain (hydrocephalus) and tumors inside your head.

Concussion

Signs and symptoms

- Brief loss of consciousness or memory after a head injury
- Headache
- Faintness
- Nausea or vomiting
- Slightly blurred vision
- Difficulty concentrating

Emergency signs and symptoms

- Persistent confusion or delirium
- Persistent drowsiness
- Progressive lethargy
- Dilation of a pupil
- Speech disturbance
- Partial paralysis
- Stupor
- Coma

A concussion is the result of brain injury from a violent jar or shock to the head, causing at least a temporary loss in brain function.

Normally, the brain floats within the skull surrounded by cerebrospinal fluid, which cushions it from the light bumps of everyday activity.

But the fluid may not be able to absorb the force of a sudden blow or a quick stop. The impact of a blow to the head creates a sudden movement of the brain within the skull, causing it to become bruised. Such traumatic movement can produce a wide range of injuries. Concussion is the mildest form of these.

Although losing consciousness is a common symptom of a concussion, it's possible to suffer a concussion without being completely "knocked out."

Head injuries are usually caused by motor vehicle or industrial accidents, falls or physical assaults. Accidents are the leading cause of death in people younger than 44 years, and head injuries occur in many of these accidents.

The fatality rate due to head injury has been reduced in recent years through the use of motorcycle and sports helmets, hard hats and seat belts and because of better emergency services. Nevertheless, head injuries remain a serious problem.

Diagnosis

Get prompt medical attention for any impairment of consciousness or dazed feeling following a head injury. Diagnostic considerations include serious bleeding within the skull, which could require emergency surgery.

Symptoms of serious brain damage may be immediately obvious, or they may not appear until hours or days after the injury. Your state of alertness and attentiveness provides key information about the extent of damage.

A doctor will examine you for evidence of skull fracture and brain damage. A computerized tomography (CT) scan or magnetic resonance imaging (MRI) may be required to determine if potentially serious damage has occurred or whether your injuries are limited to a concussion. An observation period of 24 to 48 hours is generally recommended in a hospital or at home with your family or friends checking to see if further symptoms develop.

How serious is a concussion?

A concussion is a minor, temporary injury without permanent brain damage. Accidental head injuries, however, can cause death or brain damage in some cases, and any head injury is potentially serious. Thus, any traumatic injury to your head should be medically evaluated.

The loss of memory (amnesia) associated with concussion usually involves only your memories just before and during the accident that caused the concussion. It may, however, encompass a few weeks (or rarely months) before the accident. Your recovery of memory is likely to progress from the more distant past to the recent experience.

Some people with concussion have a combination of signs and symptoms, called postconcussion syndrome or post-traumatic syndrome, for some time after a head injury.

In addition to headache and dizziness, these signs and symptoms may include insomnia, irritability, restlessness, inability to concentrate, depression or personality changes, such as moodiness. Precisely why these signs and symptoms occur in some people isn't known.

Treatment

If there are no complications, a concussion generally requires little or no treatment. Your doctor may prescribe acetaminophen or a stronger pain medication to relieve your headache. Aspirin should be avoided because it can contribute to bleeding. Rest and relaxation with limitation of activities requiring concentration or vigorous movement will usually facilitate recovery within a few days.

Athletes, such as football players or boxers, who've had a concussion should have a medical evaluation before returning to their sport.

Other traumatic brain injury

Signs and symptoms

- Headache

Emergency signs and symptoms

- Persistent confusion, drowsiness or delirium
- Speech disturbance
- Difficulty breathing
- Difference in size of eye pupils
- Partial paralysis
- Seizures or convulsions
- Stupor
- Coma

Traumatic brain injury may result from a blow to the head or from an object that penetrates the skull, such as a bullet or piece of industrial equipment. Traffic accidents, falls, industrial accidents and physical assaults are the major causes of such injuries.

About 1.5 million cases of traumatic brain injury are reported each year in the United States. These injuries range from mild concussions to severe brain damage. About 3 percent of these injuries end in death. Most head injuries are mild.

Moderate to severe brain injuries can be associated with a skull fracture, torn covering membranes or nerve tissue, and bruises or hemorrhaging within your brain. You may experience brain swelling or leaking of cerebrospinal fluid. Subdural or epidural (extradural) hemorrhage also is possible. Symptoms may not appear for several days after an accident.

Diagnosis

Get prompt medical evaluation for any head injury that causes even a brief loss of consciousness or persistent symptoms.

Your doctor may recommend hospitalization for observation, testing and treatment if you show any indications of possible brain injury. Diagnostic tests such as a computerized tomography (CT) scan or magnetic resonance imaging (MRI) may be necessary to observe the structure of your brain.

How serious is a traumatic brain injury?

The severity and effects of a head injury depend on the extent of damage and which area of the brain was most affected. Previous injuries and diseases as well as your overall state of health can play a role in potential complications. Most people with moderate head injuries recover in weeks to months, although some disability may persist. Severe injuries can be fatal or permanently disabling despite the best medical and surgical treatment.

Treatment

Emergency treatment is required for people who have entered a coma. A comatose state usually is indicative of severe brain injury. Brain swelling, which can cause death, may require treatment with medications such as corticosteroids and, possibly, surgery. Surgery may also be done to remove bone fragments, blood clots or damaged tissue, or to insert a shunt to control the pressure inside the brain.

Hydrocephalus

Signs and symptoms

- In newborns, abnormal enlargement of the head
- Mental decline
- Slow and restricted body and eye movements
- Urinary incontinence

Hydrocephalus — *hydro* meaning "water" and *cephalus* meaning "head" — is a condition in which excess fluid accumulates in the brain. Although hydrocephalus is often referred to as water on the brain, the "water" is actually cerebrospinal fluid — a clear fluid surrounding the brain and spinal cord.

Normally, this fluid is produced in the brain, flows through the four ventricles of the brain, exits into closed spaces (cisterns) that serve as reservoirs at the base of the brain, cleanses the surfaces of the brain and spinal cord and is then absorbed into the bloodstream. The balance between production and absorption of cerebrospinal fluid is critical.

Usually, the fluid is almost completely absorbed into the bloodstream as it circulates. However, some circumstances prevent or disturb the production or absorption of cerebrospinal fluid or inhibit its normal flow. When this balance is disturbed, hydrocephalus results.

Hydrocephalus may be present at birth (congenital) or acquired. Congenital hydrocephalus can be due to a blockage in the brain's cerebrospinal fluid circulation system or to an inability to reabsorb the fluid. The resulting pressure expands the loosely connected sutures in the skull so that in a newborn or young child, the head is enlarged abnormally in all directions, especially in the frontal area.

Your infant's symptoms may be mild and the progression might stop but then reappear in later childhood. The skull becomes firmly closed by age 5 years, so subsequent symptoms don't include further appreciable head enlargement.

Congenital or childhood hydrocephalus due to a blockage in the circulation of cerebrospinal fluid in the brain may be caused by various congenital malformations of the brain, a fetal infection, birth injury or tumor. Hydrocephalus due to problems of reabsorption can result from brain malformation, an infection such as bacterial meningitis, subarachnoid hemorrhage or spinal cord defects such as syringomyelia or myelomeningocele.

In adults, a variation of hydrocephalus may occur in which cerebrospinal fluid pressure is normal but reabsorption of cerebrospinal fluid is defective. Symptoms arise slowly after meningitis, head injury or subarachnoid hemorrhage or they may develop for no known reason.

Hydrocephalus is relatively uncommon, occurring in approximately 1 in 1,000 children. In adults, normal-pressure hydrocephalus is also uncommon and occurs most frequently among older adults.

Diagnosis

Your child's head may be measured at birth. If the circumference of the head exceeds a certain size, your doctor may measure the head frequently during the first weeks of life. If the soft spot (fontanel) on your infant's head is still open, an ultrasound of the head can distinguish between a normal large head (macrocephaly) and hydrocephalus. If the results of the ultrasound are abnormal, your infant will need further evaluation.

In later childhood and adulthood, signs and symptoms such as mental decline and slowed body movements may lead to further testing. In all cases, a diagnosis generally requires a computerized tomography (CT) scan or magnetic resonance imaging (MRI) and an examination and culture of cerebrospinal fluid obtained by a spinal tap (see page 578).

How serious is hydrocephalus?

The severity of this condition depends on the child's age at onset and whether the disease is progressive. If the condition is well advanced at birth, major brain damage and physical handicaps are often inevitable. Death usually occurs early from an underlying infection. In less severe cases, with proper treatment, 40 percent of affected individuals have a nearly normal life span and intelligence.

Treatment

The goal of treatment is to re-establish the balance between cerebrospinal fluid production and reabsorption. In young children with a slowly progressive condition, the drug acetazolamide (Dazamide, Diamox) sometimes diminishes cerebrospinal fluid production. When the imbalance is due to a reabsorption problem, treatment may consist of repeated spinal taps to relieve pressure.

An operation to implant a flexible tube (shunt) is effective in many children and adults. A shunt is placed to circumvent the blockage or to divert excess cerebrospinal fluid into the bloodstream or abdominal cavity, where it's reabsorbed. A successful shunt procedure will allow an infant's head size to become normal and will relieve signs and symptoms in older children and adults. Shunt tubes may require replacement as a child grows. Successful shunts usually are maintained for life, but shunt infections are a serious complication.

Brain tumor

Signs and symptoms

- Headache of recent onset
- Vomiting
- Weakness and lethargy
- Personality change
- Double vision
- Recent incoordination or clumsiness of an extremity
- Intellectual deterioration

Emergency signs and symptoms

- Vision, sight or speech difficulty
- Seizures
- Stupor

A tumor is caused by abnormal growth of cells. Tumors can be noncancerous (benign) or cancerous (malignant). The two major categories of brain tumors are primary and secondary.

A primary brain tumor originates and develops within brain tissue. The cause is generally unknown. Occasionally, a benign or malignant brain tumor is present at birth (congenital), and some are hereditary. About 17,000 Americans a year receive a diagnosis of a primary brain tumor.

A secondary (metastatic) brain tumor spreads to the brain from a malignant tumor elsewhere in your body, such as the lung or breast. Metastatic brain tumors are more common than primary brain tumors. They occur in approximately 90,000 Americans a year.

Both primary and secondary tumors may be located within your brain or in proximity to it, such as in the skull, brain membranes, supportive tissue, cranial nerves, or pituitary or pineal gland. Tumors can also originate in these locations, and each type may have its own signs and symptoms, treatment and prognosis.

Although brain tumors can occur at any age, they're most common in children ages 3 to 12 and adults ages 40 to 70. Most brain tumors in children are primary.

A brain tumor, primary or secondary, can directly compress or invade brain tissue, damaging or destroying areas responsible for sight, movement, balance, speech, hearing, memory or behavior. Pressure from a brain tumor can also cause surrounding brain tissue to swell, leading to an increase in pressure and symptoms.

Diagnosis

Initially, signs and symptoms of a brain tumor may be vague and intermittent, making it difficult to diagnose. In addition, other diseases can cause similar signs and symptoms.

Most headaches don't signal a serious medical condition. But headaches that progressively worsen or that are worse in the morning than in the afternoon, accompanied by nausea or vomiting or by blurred or double vision should be brought to the attention of your doctor. Early diagnosis of a brain tumor can lead to earlier, and perhaps more effective, treatment.

If you have emergency signs and symptoms, seek prompt medical attention because they may indicate the onset of serious neurologic disorders.

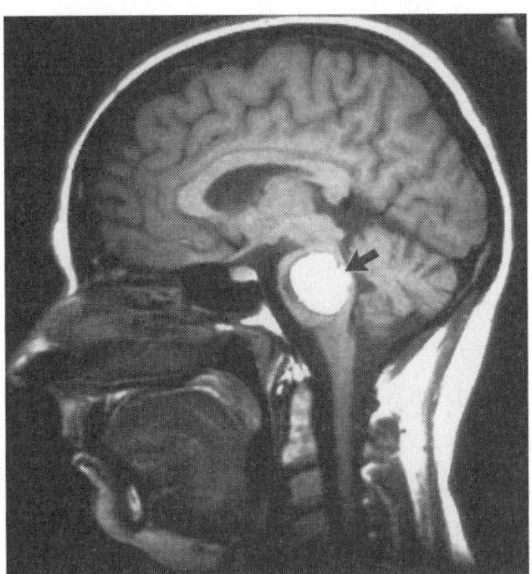

A magnetic resonance image (MRI) shows a tumor in the brain stem (see arrow).

Diagnosis of brain tumor usually involves several steps. A thorough physical and neurologic examination might lead to suspicion of a brain tumor. Depending on the results of that exam, your doctor may request a computerized tomography (CT) scan or magnetic resonance imaging (MRI) of the head to obtain detailed images of the brain. Cerebral arteriography may be needed to show the location of blood vessels in and around a brain tumor.

Tests that evaluate other areas of the body may be needed to search for a tumor that may spread to the brain. Other tests, such as magnetic resonance spectroscopy (MRS), single-photon emission computerized tomography (SPECT) or positron emission tomography (PET) scanning, can help doctors gauge brain activity by observing brain chemistry and blood flow.

A biopsy, which involves removing a piece of the tumor so that it can be examined under a microscope, may be needed to identify the type of brain tumor.

How serious is a brain tumor?

When a brain tumor causes neurologic signs and symptoms, it's extremely important to proceed quickly with appropriate treatment. Benign tumors are frequently curable, although sometimes their location makes total removal impossible. If a tumor infiltrates the brain so that tumor tissue can't be totally removed, recurrence following surgery is likely. Both benign and malignant tumors can produce profound and irreversible neurologic impairment. Most malignant brain tumors — primary or secondary — are not curable.

Brain tumors may block the flow of cerebrospinal fluid in the brain, leading to the buildup of fluid in and around the brain and increased pressure on the structure of the brain. This is a serious complication known as hydrocephalus. The fluid may require drainage to relieve pressure and reduce the risk of further brain injury.

Treatment

Treatment of a brain tumor may include surgery, irradiation to kill tumor cells or chemotherapy to halt progression of the disease. Hormone therapy may be used for certain tumors, such as those located in the pituitary gland. Corticosteroids to diminish brain swelling, antiseizure medications to control seizures and painkillers for headaches also may be prescribed.

Some benign and malignant tumors can be removed surgically. Many can be removed only partially and some not at all.

Advances in computer-assisted (stereotactic) surgery make it possible to remove some tumors deep within the brain. A treatment that precisely focuses radiation beams to the tumor is called stereotactic radiosurgery. No scalpels are involved. So-called Gamma Knife radiosurgery delivers radiation beams in the exact size and shape of the tumor, with the aid of tumor imaging techniques.

If widespread cancer is present, the primary consideration is to provide comfort and preserve neurologic function, when possible.

Neuroblastoma

Signs and symptoms

- An abdominal mass, perhaps accompanied by liver enlargement
- Bone pain, if a tumor has spread to bone
- Respiratory distress, if a tumor has spread to the chest
- Pallor
- High blood pressure
- Diarrhea

A neuroblastoma is a cancerous tumor made up of neuroblasts, embryonic cells from which nerve tissue is formed. Neuroblastomas can originate in nerve tissue in the neck, chest or pelvis, but occur most often in the abdomen, generally near the adrenal gland. The disease then may spread to the liver, bone marrow and bones.

Unlike most tumors, a neuroblastoma has a high rate of decreasing in size without treatment (spontaneous regression). Neuroblastomas occur mostly in children, and 75 percent of cases are diagnosed by the time a child is age 5. The disease may be present at birth but usually isn't detected until later.

Diagnosis

The site and extent of a suspected tumor determine what diagnostic tests will be needed. If there's an abdominal mass, a computerized tomography (CT) scan or magnetic resonance imaging (MRI) may be done. A bone scan or bone marrow biopsy — in which a tissue sample is removed for laboratory study — may indicate whether the cancer has spread to bone.

How serious is a neuroblastoma?

The prognosis of this disease depends on the age of the child and how advanced the disease is. Spontaneous regression is more common in very young infants. The older the child and the more widespread the disease, the more likely it is that the cancer won't respond to treatment.

Treatment

If the tumor is small and localized, surgery alone or with local radiation therapy may offer a cure. In more advanced disease, chemotherapy may be successful. In children with the most advanced disease, intensive treatment followed by bone marrow transplantation may be an option. The chances of long-term survival decrease significantly at this most advanced stage of the cancer.

Bell's palsy

Signs and symptoms

- Sagging muscles and weakness on one side of the face
- An inability to close one eye

Bell's palsy (facial palsy) causes a weakness or paralysis of the muscles that control expression on one side of your face. The condition results from damage to the facial nerve, which runs beneath the ear to the facial muscles of the same side.

The cause of the disorder is unknown, and its development isn't well understood. The prevalent theory is that the facial nerve becomes swollen, perhaps by a viral infection, such as shingles (herpes zoster). The nerve has no room to expand within the bony channel it runs through. Bell's palsy results from nerve injury due to restriction or compression.

Complete paralysis on one side of your face leaves you looking expressionless because you have no movement of the muscles from the forehead to below the mouth on the paralyzed side. The corner of your mouth may droop, and you may have difficulty retaining saliva on that side of your mouth. When you move the muscles of the unaffected

? Question and Answer

What's a meningioma?

A meningioma is a noncancerous brain tumor that originates in the cells of the outer covering of the brain (meninges). The site and location of the meningioma determine its seriousness. Treatment is usually by surgical removal of the tumor. If the tumor is located in an area that isn't very accessible, complete removal may be difficult or impossible. Sometimes, functions of the brain already affected by pressure from the meningioma may be permanently damaged.

side, the face is distorted. The eye on your affected side may close only partially if at all, so tears may leak from that eye.

Some people complain of pain behind the ear, in the jaw or on the entire side of the face. You may feel that the unaffected side seems twisted or contracted, and you may experience changes in salivation and sense of taste, heightened sensitivity to sound or difficulty in speaking or eating.

Bell's palsy can occur at any age, but it's most common between ages 30 and 60. Sometimes, it's associated with an infection of the middle ear. Each year, about 40,000 Americans get the disorder. If both sides of the face are simultaneously involved, a disorder such as Lyme disease or sarcoidosis may be the cause.

Diagnosis

The onset of Bell's palsy tends to be fairly abrupt. You may notice it when you wake up. Pain behind your ear can precede the palsy by a day or two. Maximal weakness or paralysis may be apparent within 48 hours after onset.

Your doctor may be able to make a preliminary diagnosis by looking at your face and asking you to try to move your facial muscles. Other conditions, such as a stroke, can cause one-sided facial paralysis, and careful evaluation is needed to exclude these disorders. Bell's palsy usually affects all of the muscles on one side of the face equally, including the forehead muscles. Strokes usually don't cause paralysis of the forehead muscles on the affected side of the face.

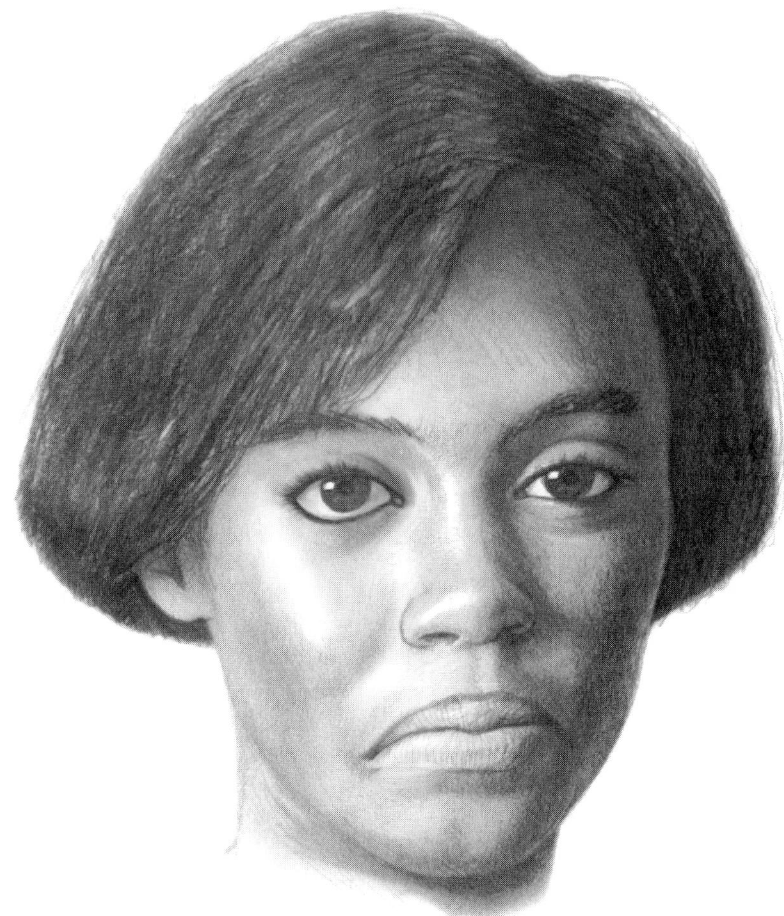

Bell's palsy may cause the corner of your mouth to droop, and you may have trouble retaining saliva on that side of your mouth. The condition may also make it difficult to close the eye on the affected side of your face.

Your doctor may also arrange for you to be tested by electromyography. This test measures a muscle's electrical activity in response to stimulation, to determine the severity of nerve damage.

How serious is Bell's palsy?

Bell's palsy is usually a temporary problem. In 80 percent of cases, recovery begins within 2 to 3 weeks and is complete within a few months. A mild case may be noticeable only when you smile. Improvement of the paralysis by the end of the first week suggests a favorable outcome.

Recovery is variable, and electromyography may be helpful in determining the prognosis. If the damage to the facial nerve is unusually severe, the fibers may be irreversibly damaged. A complication can arise from misdirected regrowth of nerve fibers. The misdirected fibers can cause unintended contraction of some muscles during facial movement.

Treatment

Most people recover fully without treatment. Doctors aren't sure that any treatment changes the ultimate outcome of Bell's palsy.

If you can't completely close your eye, however, you'll need to take steps to protect it from excessive dryness, which can lead to a corneal ulcer.

Use of a temporary eye patch or shield or an ointment may help during sleeping. Use of moisturizing eyedrops, such as methylcellulose drops, help guard your eye from dust and dryness.

Doctors sometimes prescribe a corticosteroid medication, such as prednisone, to reduce possible swelling of your facial nerve. Antiviral medication, such as acyclovir (Zovirax) or famciclovir (Famvir), may help limit or reduce damage to the nerve from viral causes.

Your doctor may also recommend physical therapy and facial massage to preserve muscle tone.

Degenerative Disorders

Your brain, spinal cord and peripheral nerves form an intricate system consisting of billions of nerve cells. These cells are complex transmitters that carry electric and chemical signals to make your muscles move and to relay information throughout your nervous system.

If a few scattered cells die or malfunction, you likely won't notice any change because surrounding cells will carry the transmissions. When there's progressive deterioration in any part of your nervous system, you eventually lose some ability to function. This loss can be related to mental ability, muscular movement and muscular control and coordination.

Degenerative disorders may be disabling and, in most cases, there's no known cure. Nonetheless, research is progressing rapidly. Scientists have discovered and learned more about the brain and its disorders in the last decade than in the previous 50 years. The hope is that increased understanding will lead to new methods of treatment and prevention.

Alzheimer's disease

Signs and symptoms

- A gradual loss of memory for recent events and an inability to learn new information
- A progressive tendency to repeat oneself, misplace objects, become confused and get lost
- A gradual disintegration of personality and judgment
- Increasing irritability, anxiety, depression, confusion and restlessness

Alzheimer's disease is the most common cause of dementia, accounting for approximately 50 percent to 60 percent of all cases. About 4 million people in the United States have Alzheimer's disease.

The chance of developing Alzheimer's increases with age, and the number of people with the disorder is expected to triple in the next 20 years as more people live into their 80s and 90s. Alzheimer's disease is rare in young people and uncommon in middle age.

Everyone has occasional lapses in memory. Alzheimer's disease — a progressive, degenerative brain disease — goes beyond simple forgetfulness. It may start with slight

Dementia

A number of disorders that cause progressive deterioration in any part of your nervous system (neurodegenerative disorders) produce a collection of signs and symptoms (syndrome) called dementia.

Dementia is characterized by a progressive decline in intellectual and social abilities to a degree that interferes with daily functioning. Signs and symptoms vary from individual to individual, depending on a person's genetic makeup, lifestyle, cultural background and personal life experiences. Some of the more general characteristics of dementia include a reduction in or loss of memory, reasoning, judgment and language. Personality changes and abnormal behavior also may occur as dementia progresses. Eventually, people with dementia may lose the ability to perform even the most basic of tasks, such as speaking or eating.

Such signs and symptoms can be evidence of Alzheimer's disease, vascular dementia or other brain disorders known to cause dementia. In the past, people referred to dementia as senility and considered it to be an inevitable part of aging. Today, we know that dementia isn't a normal part of the aging process but is caused by an underlying condition affecting the brain.

If you notice such manifestations in yourself or a loved one, it's important not to brush it off as simply "getting old." An early diagnosis is important because prompt treatment may affect the course of the disease.

Brain disorders that cause dementia

Diseases of the brain that can cause dementia include:

Alzheimer's disease

Alzheimer's disease is the most common cause of dementia. Changes in the brain of people with Alzheimer's disease include a loss of nerve cells in the areas vital to memory and other mental functions. Individuals with Alzheimer's disease also have lowered levels of brain chemicals that carry messages back and forth between nerve cells. The first sign of Alzheimer's disease may be worsening forgetfulness. As the disease progresses, it affects your language, reasoning, understanding, reading and writing. Eventually, you may become anxious or aggressive.

Vascular dementia

Vascular dementia results either from narrowing and blockage of the arteries that supply blood to the brain or from strokes that result from an interruption of blood flow within the brain. The onset of symptoms is often abrupt, but sometimes the disease progresses slowly, making it difficult to distinguish it from Alzheimer's disease. It's common to experience problems with thinking, language, walking, bladder control and vision.

Parkinson's disease

As many as 30 percent to 40 percent of people with Parkinson's disease develop dementia late in the disease. Conversely, some people with Alzheimer's develop physical signs and symptoms similar to those in

memory loss and confusion, but it gradually worsens and leads to severe, irreversible mental impairment that destroys a person's ability to remember, reason, learn and plan for the future.

The course of the disease and how rapidly changes occur varies from person to person. For some, the progression from simple forgetfulness to severe dementia takes 5 to 8 years. For others, it can take a decade or longer.

Alzheimer's generally progresses from mild to moderate to severe. People with mild Alzheimer's can usually live alone and function fairly well. People with moderate Alzheimer's have greater difficulty coping without supervision. People with advanced Alzheimer's disease generally can no longer care for themselves.

Alzheimer's disease affects the brain by destroying its basic component, the nerve cell (neuron). A healthy brain has close to a billion neurons. Neurons generate electric and chemical signals that are relayed from neuron to neuron to help your body perform a host of functions, including thinking, learning and remembering. Chemicals called neurotransmitters help these signals flow seamlessly between neurons.

In people with Alzheimer's disease, neurons in the brain slowly die. As they die, lower levels of neurotransmitters are produced, creating signaling problems in the brain.

Alzheimer's disease is named after German neurologist Alois Alzheimer. In 1906, he examined the brain of a woman who had died after years of progressive dementia. Her brain tissue contained abnormal clumps and irregular knots of brain cells. Today, these clumps (now called plaques) and knots (now called tangles) are considered hallmarks of Alzheimer's disease.

Researchers continue to study plaques and tangles to better understand why brain cells slowly die. In the meantime, scientists have theories that may explain how these structures are involved in Alzheimer's disease:

- *Plaques.* Plaques are made up of a normally harmless protein called amyloid-beta. Scientists believe that plaque deposits form between neurons early in the disease process, before neurons begin to die and signs and symptoms develop. Although the ultimate cause of neuron death in Alzheimer's isn't known, mount-

Parkinson's disease, such as stiffness of the limbs, shaking at rest (tremor), speech impairment and a shuffling gait.

Lewy body dementia

Lewy bodies are protein deposits found in deteriorating nerve cells. They often appear in damaged regions deep within the brain of people with Parkinson's disease. When widespread throughout the brain, Lewy bodies cause signs and symptoms similar to those of Alzheimer's disease.

Lewy body dementia can affect your dreams, speed of thinking, memory, language, judgment and reasoning. It can also cause you to hallucinate and lose your sense of direction, which may result in a tendency to get lost.

Huntington's disease

Huntington's disease stems from an inherited disorder within the brain that causes certain nerve cells in the brain to waste away. As the disorder progresses, you experience personality changes and a decline in intellect, memory, speech and judgment. Dementia may develop in the later stages of the disease.

Creutzfeldt-Jakob disease

Dementia that sometimes occurs in young or middle-aged people may be caused by Creutzfeldt-Jakob disease. This rare and fatal brain disorder is thought to be caused by prions, infectious agents that can transform normal protein molecules into transmissible, deadly ones.

The earliest signs and symptoms of the disease may be memory impairment and behavior changes. The disease progresses rapidly with mental deterioration, muscle jerks (involuntary movements), weakness in the limbs, blindness and eventually coma. Bovine spongiform encephalopathy, commonly known as mad cow disease, is believed to be a prion disorder.

Frontotemporal dementia

Frontotemporal dementia is an uncommon brain disorder characterized by disturbances in behavior, personality and eventually memory. The disease is relentless in its progression and may ultimately include language impairment, erratic behavior and dementia. Pick's disease is a form of frontotemporal dementia.

Disorders that mimic dementia

Some conditions produce signs and symptoms similar to those of dementia, particularly in older adults. Two conditions sometimes mistaken for dementia are depression and delirium.

Depression can cause difficulty in remembering, thinking clearly and concentrating. Sometimes, depression occurs in conjunction with dementia. In these cases, the deterioration of emotions and intellect can be more extreme.

Delirium is an acute state of temporary mental confusion. It tends to be most common in older adults who have lung or heart disease, infections, poor nutrition, medication interactions or hormone disorders. A person who exhibits sudden disorientation, loss in mental skills, or loss of consciousness is likely to have delirium rather than dementia.

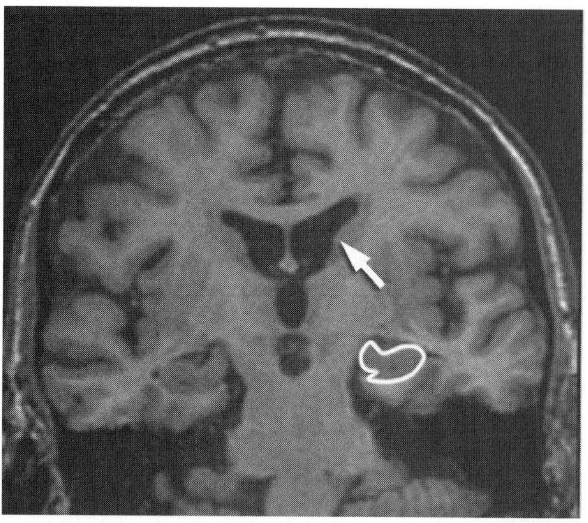

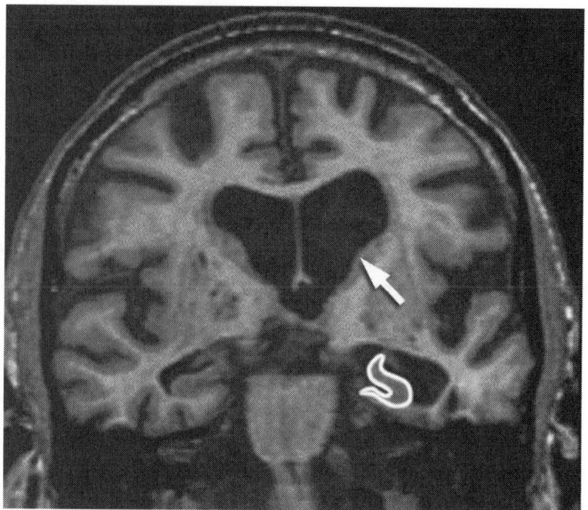

These magnetic resonance images (MRIs) of the brain show a person without Alzheimer's disease (left) and a person in the moderate stage of the disease (right). Signs of Alzheimer's disease include noticeable shrinkage of the hippocampus (circled in white) and enlarged interior cavities of the brain that have filled with cerebrospinal fluid (see arrows).

Mild Cognitive Impairment

Mayo Clinic researchers have recently identified a state of memory loss called mild cognitive impairment that may one day come to be known as pre-Alzheimer's.

This memory loss falls somewhere between that associated with normal aging and that common in early Alzheimer's disease. People with mild cognitive impairment may experience forgetfulness beyond what's typical for their age, but not have full symptoms of Alzheimer's.

Identification of this category of memory loss could help doctors more accurately diagnose and advise patients. It could also alert individuals to an increased risk of developing Alzheimer's disease.

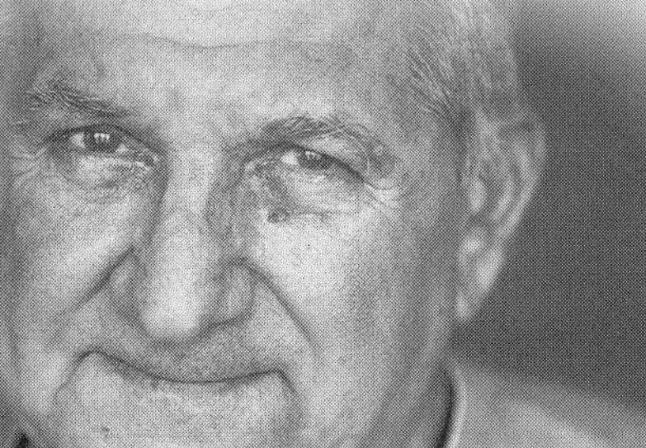

ing evidence suggests that a form of amyloid-beta protein may be the culprit.

- *Tangles.* The internal support structure for brain neurons depends on normal functioning of a protein called tau. In people with Alzheimer's, threads of tau protein undergo alterations that cause them to become twisted. Many researchers believe this may seriously damage neurons and even destroy them.

Researchers are also studying the role genetics play in Alzheimer's disease. Certain rare forms of early-onset Alzheimer's that occur before age 65 are caused by specific genetic mutations. But the number of people with these mutations is extremely low — about 200 families worldwide. The sporadic form of Alzheimer's, which has no known cause, accounts for the vast majority of cases. The presence of a gene known as apolipoprotein E (APOE 4) also may increase a person's risk of developing Alzheimer's, but it doesn't guarantee that the disease will actually occur.

Diagnosis

The only test that can confirm a diagnosis of Alzheimer's disease is examination of brain tissue obtained by a biopsy or an autopsy. Nonetheless, increased understanding of Alzheimer's in recent years allows doctors to recognize some of the disease's earliest manifestations through a variety of tests and examinations, resulting in a diagnosis that can be quite accurate.

Some of the signs and symptoms of the disorder, such as disorientation and confusion, may also occur with conditions such as vitamin B-12 deficiency, hypothyroidism, depression, an adverse reaction to medications or a chronic subdural hematoma. Because many of these disorders can be treated, it's important for an individual with mental status abnormalities to have a careful medical evaluation.

An early clinical diagnosis of Alzheimer's is important because it may allow medications to have more of an effect on the disease's signs and symptoms.

In addition, an early diagnosis can help both the person with Alzheimer's and his or her family make financial, legal and health care decisions for the future. The sooner these decisions are made, the less stressful the disease may be in the long run.

A person with dementia may lack insight into his or her disability. Consequently, if you know someone who shows signs of changes in mental ability, strongly suggest a medical evaluation. The assistance of family and friends is essential in helping diagnose dementia or Alzheimer's disease and is also needed for ongoing support.

To help differentiate Alzheimer's disease from other causes of memory loss, doctors typically rely on a thorough medical history and description of symptoms as well as a variety of tests, including physical and neurologic examinations, neuropsychological testing and a number of laboratory tests, such as brain scans and blood and urine tests.

Alzheimer's Warning Signs

When people forget something, they often joke that they're developing Alzheimer's disease. But having Alzheimer's isn't the same as having an occasional memory lapse. Alzheimer's is a condition that becomes progressively worse. Most people with Alzheimer's share certain characteristics. These may include:

Increasing and persistent forgetfulness
At its onset, Alzheimer's disease is marked by periods of forgetfulness, especially of recent events or simple directions. But what begins as mild forgetfulness persists and increases. People with Alzheimer's may repeat things and forget conversations or appointments. They routinely misplace things, often putting them in illogical locations. They frequently forget names, and eventually they may forget the names of family members and everyday objects such as a comb or watch.

Difficulties with abstract thinking
People with Alzheimer's disease may initially have trouble balancing their checkbook, a problem that progresses to trouble understanding and recognizing numbers.

Difficulty finding the right word
It may be a challenge for individuals with Alzheimer's to find the right words to express their thoughts or even to follow conversations. Eventually, reading and writing also are affected.

Disorientation
People with Alzheimer's disease may lose track of time and dates. They may find themselves lost in familiar surroundings. Eventually, they may even wander from home and get lost.

Loss of judgment
Solving everyday problems, such as knowing what to do if food on the stove is burning, becomes increasingly difficult. Alzheimer's is characterized by difficulty doing things that require planning, decision making and judgment.

Difficulty performing familiar tasks
Once-routine tasks that require sequential steps, such as cooking, become a struggle as the disease progresses. People with Alzheimer's may forget how to do the most basic things, such as brushing their teeth.

Personality changes
Individuals with Alzheimer's may exhibit mood swings. They may express distrust in others, show increased stubbornness and withdraw socially. Early on, this may be a response to the frustration they feel as they notice uncontrollable changes in their memory. Depression often coexists with Alzheimer's disease. Restlessness also is a common sign. As the disease progresses, individuals may become anxious or aggressive and behave inappropriately.

How serious is Alzheimer's disease?

Alzheimer's disease isn't an acute condition, and it rarely requires emergency treatment. Abrupt changes in mental status are usually due to other diseases, which may require an immediate evaluation. Alzheimer's disease, however, is ultimately fatal. Individuals with the disease may become bedridden and unable to care for themselves. They often die of pneumonia or other infections because of the disability. People with Alzheimer's may become disoriented, increasing their risk of falls, which can cause serious fractures or head injuries.

Treatment

Currently, there's no cure for Alzheimer's disease. Medications and caregiving are the primary treatments. During the early stages of the disorder, care can often be provided at home under the direction of a doctor. Providing care for an individual with Alzheimer's disease can be very challenging and stressful to the spouse and family members. Often, those providing care need assistance from support organizations and a network of family and friends. Eventually, the individual's condition deteriorates so that full-time nursing care is required, and it's often necessary to place the person in a long-term-care facility.

Medication

Current medications for Alzheimer's disease can't stop or reverse the underlying disease process, but they may decrease symptoms.

All of the medications currently approved by the Food and Drug Administration for treating the cognitive impairment of mild to moderate Alzheimer's belong to a family of drugs called cholinesterase inhibitors. These drugs work by improving levels of acetylcholine in the brain, a neurotransmitter that plays an important role in memory skills. They include:

- *Donepezil (Aricept).* Donepezil is the most commonly prescribed medication for Alzheimer's. Its side effects, which include nausea, diarrhea and fatigue, are usually mild and of short duration.
- *Rivastigamine (Exelon).* Rivastigamine also reduces symptoms of mild to moderate Alzheimer's. Side effects include nausea and vomiting.
- *Galantamine (Reminyl).* Galantamine is the newest drug on the market for mild to moderate Alzheimer's. It also improves cognition, function and behavior. Its long-term effects have not yet been observed, but it was well tolerated during clinical trials.
- *Tacrine (Cognex).* Tacrine was the first drug approved for Alzheimer's disease, but now it's rarely used. It requires monitoring of liver function and must be given four times a day.

Occasionally, mild sedatives, antidepressants or antipsychotic medications may be necessary to improve behavioral problems that often accompany Alzheimer's, including sleeplessness, wandering, anxiety, agitation and depression. These drugs, often used in low doses, can improve a person's quality of life and assist the family in caring for their loved one.

Caregiving

Education is very important for caregivers. Learning more about the disease process and techniques for dealing with problems can be beneficial to family and friends of the person with Alzheimer's disease.

An individual with Alzheimer's disease should be encouraged to continue his or her daily routines, physical activities and social interactions as much as possible. Proper nutrition and fluid intake are critical, but special diets and supplements are usually unnecessary. Exercise is important, and your doctor may recommend physical therapy. Travel with a supportive companion may be possible if arrangements aren't overly complicated.

Whenever possible, avoid dramatic changes, such as moving to a new location, arranging furniture and disrupting established routines. Also avoid dangerous equipment or materials in the living environment, and monitor carefully the person's ability to drive.

You can use notes as reminders of activities and a calendar listing routine tasks and directions for daily activities. A medical alert bracelet may be helpful in case the person becomes disoriented and wanders into an unfamiliar setting.

Alzheimer's disease can be a difficult disorder to deal with, but concern and compassion on the part of the individuals providing care can make a major difference.

Future therapy

Research on Alzheimer's disease continues to move forward. Understanding how development and progression of Alzheimer's disease unfolds in the human brain is one of the main concentrations of researchers. This information can help experts find better methods of prevention, diagnosis, treatment and care.

Strategies being studied include:

- *Anti-amyloid treatment.* Better understanding of the mechanisms underlying the formation of amyloid plaques and their potentially toxic accumulation in the brain of people with Alzheimer's disease has led many scientists to pursue ways of removing the protein aggregations or preventing them from forming. Whether a decrease in amyloid plaque formation is effective in preventing Alzheimer's is an issue that investigators hope to resolve in the near future.
- *Anti-inflammatory agents.* A number of anti-inflammatory agents are being investigated in an attempt to prevent further degen-

Use It or Lose It?

Studies suggest that maintaining mental fitness may delay the onset of dementia.

One study focused on a large group of nuns reported to have low rates of Alzheimer's disease, even though their average age was 85 and many were in their 90s. Many of the nuns had advanced academic degrees and led intellectually challenging lives into old age.

Some researchers believe that lifelong mental exercise and learning may promote the growth of additional connections between neurons (synapses) and delay the onset of dementia. Other researchers argue that advanced education gives a person more experience with the types of memory and thinking skills used in tests to measure dementia. This advanced level of education simply may help some people "cover" their condition longer.

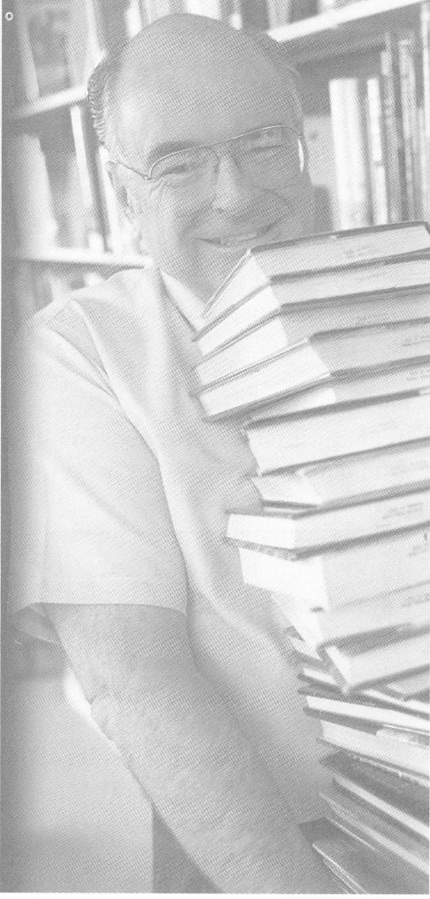

eration of neurons by reducing the inflammatory response triggered in the brain of individuals with Alzheimer's. Some of the medications being studied are prednisone, nonsteroidal anti-inflammatory drugs (NSAIDs) and COX-2 inhibitors.
- *Estrogen.* Some research indicates that hormone replacement therapy after menopause may reduce a woman's risk of developing Alzheimer's disease by 40 percent to 50 percent. But when estrogen was given in trials as a form of treatment to women with Alzheimer's, the results were negative. Because the effects of estrogen still aren't proved, women shouldn't begin hormone replacement therapy solely to prevent Alzheimer's disease.
- *Antioxidants.* Vitamin E, selegiline and ginkgo biloba are antioxidants that may help prevent brain cell damage by destroying toxic free radicals. Free radicals are byproducts of normal cell function. An excess of them may disrupt brain cell function.
- *Neurotrophic agents.* Neurotrophic factors are proteins that assist in the development and survival of neurons. One theory in the treatment of Alzheimer's disease is that introducing these factors into the brain may help damaged neurons.

Vascular dementia

Signs and symptoms

- A relatively abrupt loss of memory or other cognitive functions
- Cognitive loss, usually accompanied by the signs and symptoms of a stroke
- Walking disturbances
- Loss of bowel or bladder control
- Sudden, involuntary laughing and crying

Emergency signs and symptoms

- An abrupt change in mental state

Vascular dementia is caused by a series of strokes or loss of blood supply to parts of the brain, resulting in areas of dead brain tissue (infarcts).

The disorder produces a step-by-step or gradual decrease in mental ability. Strokes and resulting vascular dementia are typically the consequences of one or more underlying disorders, including high blood pressure and atherosclerosis. Approximately 10 percent to 15 percent of all cases of dementia are classified as vascular.

Memory — particularly of recent events — may be affected first. Depending on the location of the damage, other functions may be involved. In the early stages, before too much damage has occurred, the affected person often is aware of impaired ability, and frustration tends to increase the characteristic depression.

Diagnosis

Diagnosing vascular dementia requires fulfilling certain criteria and eliminating other possible causes of dementia that might be treatable, such as normal-pressure hydrocephalus, vitamin deficiencies or hypothyroidism.

This is generally accomplished through a series of tests, including physical and neurologic examinations, neuropsychological testing and various laboratory tests. A history of high blood pressure, transient ischemic attacks (TIAs) or stroke may be an indication that the dementia is vascular in origin.

How serious is vascular dementia?

Vascular dementia is a disorder that becomes progressively worse. There may be periods where signs and symptoms improve, followed by further decline. Death may result

Dementia and Communication

People with dementia often have problems using language and understanding others. Common changes in the ability to communicate include repetition and the use of inaccurate and socially inappropriate words that may reflect jealousy, paranoia or impulsiveness. Here are some tips to help communicate with someone who has dementia:

- Approach the person from the front, identify yourself and address the person by name.
- Speak slowly and clearly in a gentle, relaxed tone.
- Use short, simple and familiar words. Repeat when necessary, using the same words.
- Use one-step commands and requests.
- Ask one question at a time, preferably those that can be answered with a yes or no. Give the person extra time to respond.
- Offer encouragement when the person has difficulty expressing thoughts and feelings.
- Don't interrupt, criticize, correct or argue. Be patient and flexible.
- Avoid pronouns. Identify people by name.
- Avoid negative statements and quizzing, such as, "You know who that is, don't you?"
- Let the person know you're listening and trying to understand.
- Maintain eye contact to show interest.
- Don't talk to others about the person as if he or she weren't there.
- Use nonverbal communication, such as pointing and touching, when appropriate.
- Provide appropriate touch. This is perhaps the greatest form of communication in the later stages of dementia. Offering hugs, applying hand lotion and giving back rubs can be wonderful ways of communicating care and acceptance.

Question and Answer

What's cognition?

Cognition comes from the Latin word *cognoscere*, meaning "to know." Thus, your cognitive skills are the ones that enable you to know things. This includes your powers of awareness, intuition and memory, combined with your ability to perceive, reason and make judgments. Cognitive impairment is the loss of these powers.

from a stroke or complications such as pneumonia or infection.

Treatment

Prevention of further strokes is the best treatment for this dementia. If you have high blood pressure or TIAs or if you've had a stroke, see your doctor regularly to minimize your signs and symptoms, to lessen the chance of recurrence of a stroke or TIA and to avoid vascular dementia. Drugs prescribed for Alzheimer's disease are being evaluated as treatments. People with this disorder generally require care similar to that for Alzheimer's disease.

Parkinson's disease

Signs and symptoms

- Shaking (tremor) at rest
- Masking (reduction) of facial expression and blinking
- Slowness of movements
- A shuffling gait with short steps
- Stiffness or rigidity of limbs
- A slow, soft, monotone voice
- Difficulty in maintaining balance
- A stooped posture
- Small, illegible handwriting
- Dementia

Parkinson's disease was first described by James Parkinson in England in 1817. It's a progressive degeneration of nerve cells (neu-

Tests for Dementia

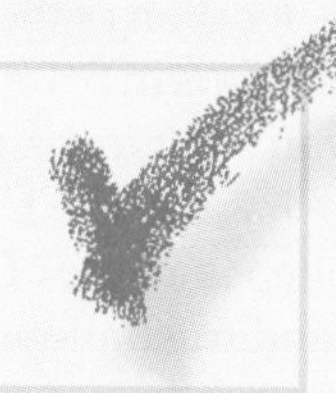

One of the purposes of testing for dementia is to help identify a possible treatable cause. Therefore, an accurate diagnosis is important.

Evaluation of a person with dementia typically begins with a detailed history, followed by physical and neurologic evaluations. Depending on the results, laboratory tests are selected. Neuropsychological testing can provide additional information about a person's cognitive abilities, including memory, judgment, reasoning and planning skills. Some of the things a doctor typically evaluates include:

Mental status

A mental status assessment is often included in the neurologic exam. This test assesses various mental functions, such as memory, attention, language and perception skills. A doctor or clinical psychologist may ask questions to assess several mental processes. These questions may include an evaluation of:

- *Insight into symptoms.* What do you think your problem is?
- *Orientation.* What's the date, month and year? Where are you now?
- *Memory.* Memorize a list of words and repeat them later.
- *Recall.* Remember information learned at a previous time.
- *Abstract reasoning.* Explain a proverb.
- *Attention.* Recite the months of the year forward and backward.
- *Thought content.* What are your fears and concerns?
- *Language.* Name objects and demonstrate an ability to read, write and comprehend the spoken word.
- *General knowledge.* Who's the president? How many weeks are there in a year?

Memory

Memory tests may be used to evaluate a person's ability to learn verbal and nonverbal information and to recall items from the remote past. The ability to construct objects by drawing also may be assessed, and the person may be asked to recall these drawings at a later time.

Cognitive skills

Cognitive function may be assessed by formal neuropsychological testing. This examination uses standardized tests of intelligence, memory, language and prior academic achievements. Typically, an individual's performance score is compared with scores obtained from other people of the same age and education level. These tests help determine if changes in mental status performance are within the normal range of aging or if an underlying disease may be involved. For example, depression may interfere with some attention and memory tasks in a manner somewhat similar to that found in Alzheimer's disease.

Several laboratory tests may be performed to identify a disease that may be causing the signs and symptoms. These tests include a computerized tomography (CT) scan or magnetic resonance imaging (MRI), electrocardiography, a chest X-ray, blood chemistry and urine tests and drug screening. Additional neurologic tests that may help in the diagnosis include electroencephalography, spinal tap (lumbar puncture) and radioisotope studies.

rons) in parts of the brain that control muscle movements.

This particular group of neurons, called the substantia nigra, releases a chemical called dopamine. Dopamine is important for transmitting signals from the substantia nigra to another part of the brain called the corpus striatum. These signals help your muscles make smooth, controlled movements. In Parkinson's disease, the substantia nigra is damaged or destroyed, resulting in impairment of walking, arm movement and facial expression.

Parkinson's disease manifests itself in various ways. It may be evident only on one side or both sides of the body. Blinking, smiling and swinging your arms when you walk all are unconscious acts that are part of human behavior. In Parkinson's disease, these acts tend to be lost. Many develop a fixed staring, expression and unblinking eyes — the so-called masked face of the disease. And instead of gesturing while talking, some people lack animation when they speak.

People with Parkinson's disease may gradually develop a slow, shuffling walk with an unsteady gait, stooped posture and a tendency to fall. In the later stages of the disease, their muscles may freeze up, making it hard to initiate normal movement. This is especially distressing because it can make performing the simplest tasks difficult and time consuming. Even the functioning of the digestive tract may slow down, causing problems with swallowing, digestion and elimination. In fact, constipation is often a major problem for people with Parkinson's disease.

Tremors often start with a slight shaking in one finger that later may spread to the whole arm. Sometimes, tremors in the hand cause a back-and-forth rubbing of the thumb and forefinger known as pill rolling. A person with Parkinson's may also develop tremors in the head, lips or feet. These signs and symptoms may occur on one or both sides of the body and may be more noticeable under stress. Although tremors can be very distressing, they're usually not disabling and often disappear during sleep.

Muscle stiffness (rigidity) often occurs in the limbs and neck. When stiffness is severe, it limits the size of movements. For example, the handwriting of people with Parkinson's disease often becomes extremely small. In addition, many people with Parkinson's disease have trouble speaking, and their voice may become a soft monotone.

During the later stages of the disease, as many as 30 percent to 40 percent of people with Parkinson's disease develop dementia, with the loss of intellectual and social abilities.

Although much research has been done on Parkinson's disease, its cause remains unknown. Scientists suspect that Parkinson's may result from a combination of genetic and environmental factors. Studies indicate that people who have a first-degree relative, such as a parent or sibling, with Parkinson's are at greater risk of developing the condition themselves, suggesting a genetic connection.

Other studies have linked the disease to exposure to herbicides and pesticides. Certain drugs prescribed for psychiatric disorders, nausea and epilepsy may cause Parkinson's-like signs and symptoms (parkinsonism). Alzheimer's disease, as well as other neurologic diseases, can sometimes cause tremors. Exposure to toxins such as manganese or the chemical MPTP, a byproduct of heroin production, can lead to parkinsonism.

In about 5 percent to 10 percent of cases, Parkinson's begins before age 50. More commonly, signs and symptoms start later in life and develop very slowly. More than 1 million Americans have the disorder.

Diagnosis

A diagnosis of Parkinson's disease is made primarily on the basis of a medical history and a comprehensive neurologic examination. Similar signs and symptoms can result from certain medications, especially some drugs used to treat nausea or severe psychiatric disorders. In addition, your doctor will consider a variety of other degenerative brain conditions that share some of the features of Parkinson's disease but differ in other respects.

Tremors may result from other causes, such as essential tremor (see page 598). Many people with Parkinson's disease have little or no tremor.

The precise time of onset of Parkinson's often isn't known. You may not recognize the early signs and symptoms as a medical problem. One of the first signs or symptoms you experience may be a slight dragging of a foot while walking, a sense of stiffness in a limb or a mild tremor in the fingers of one hand. Signs and symptoms beyond these early indicators, however, typically become so clear-cut that your doctor may suspect the disorder by simple observation.

How serious is Parkinson's disease?

Parkinson's disease tends to be progressive — its signs and symptoms gradually worsen. The time involved in this process varies greatly. You may have years of active living after developing this disease. For others, the progression is more rapid. During the later stages of the disease, many individuals need assistance. In its most severe form, the disease can leave you incapacitated by rigidity and tremor, although this occurs in only a small minority of cases.

Many people with Parkinson's disease experience depression. In addition, some degree of mental deterioration occurs in about one-third of individuals with the disease. In the later stages, auditory and visual hallucinations may develop. These signs and symptoms may be caused by medication prescribed to improve other manifestations of the disease.

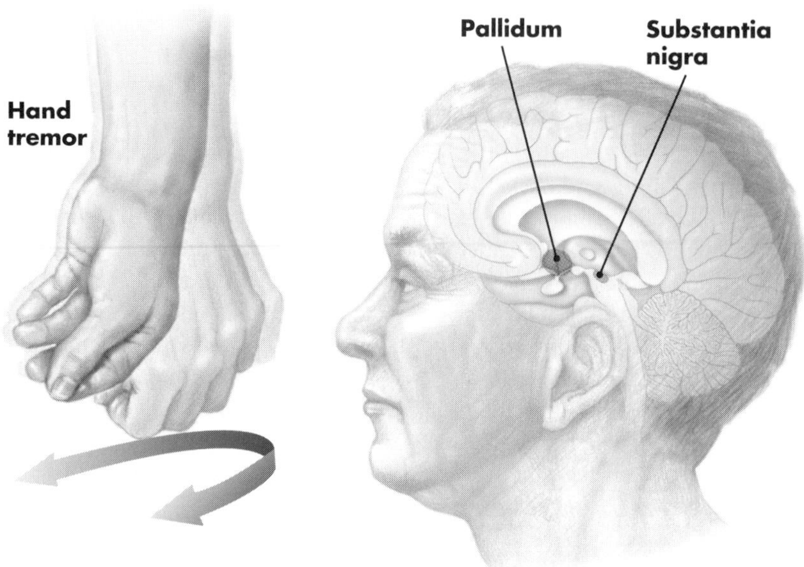

Movement problems associated with Parkinson's disease, such as tremor, are caused primarily by inadequate levels of the brain chemical dopamine, which transmits messages from the substantia nigra to other parts of the brain. One treatment involves surgically destroying tissue in the part of the brain called the pallidum.

Treatment

In the early stages of the illness, you may not need treatment. When the disease reaches the point at which it interferes with daily activities, medication is frequently prescribed.

It's important to maintain your general health and continue to exercise. Your energy level may vary, and you'll need to adjust your activities accordingly. Rest periods during the day are often needed. Fatigue, anxiety and unhappiness may aggravate your signs and symptoms considerably.

Emotional support and encouragement from family, friends or members of a support group help many people deal with the illness. Getting involved in a physical or occupational therapy program also can be both physically and emotionally stimulating. This can help individuals with Parkinson's disease maintain a positive mental attitude and avoid depression.

Medication

The main goal of treatment is to reverse the problems with tremors, walking and other movement by restoring your brain's supply of dopamine.

- *Levodopa.* Since its introduction in the 1960s, levodopa has become the standard drug therapy for Parkinson's disease. Levodopa is the synthesis of a chemical found in plants and animals that's converted into dopamine by nerve cells in the brain. The increase in dopamine may reverse many of the disabling signs and symptoms of Parkinson's disease, but as time passes, side effects may increase and require adjustments of the dosage.

  Treatment with dopamine itself isn't possible because dopamine doesn't cross the body's blood-brain barrier. This is a meshwork of tightly packed cells in the walls of the brain's capillaries that screen out certain substances. Levodopa, on the other hand, does cross this barrier, but only a small amount actually reaches the brain. Combining levodopa with carbidopa (Sinemet), allows more levodopa to get to the brain and reduces some of the side effects of this therapy. Sinemet CR is a prolonged-release version of this combination drug.

  During early treatment, side effects from levodopa usually aren't a major problem. But as the disease progresses, the drug works less uniformly. As a result, some people experience involuntary movements (dyskinesias), especially when the medication is at peak effect. Over time, waxing and waning of the drug's effects is also common. The period of time that each dose is effective decreases, requiring more frequent doses.

  Other side effects may include hallucinations, a drop in blood pressure — especially in the standing position — and nausea. Still, levodopa often allows people with Parkinson's disease to extend the time they're able to lead relatively normal lives, in many cases, for a number of years.
- *Dopamine agonists.* Unlike levodopa, these medications aren't changed into dopamine. Instead, they mimic the effects of dopamine in the brain and cause neurons to react as though sufficient amounts of dopamine were present. This class of drugs includes the older dopamine agonists bromocriptine (Parlodel) and pergolide (Permax), and the newer medications pramipexole (Mirapex) and ropinirole (Requip).

  Dopamine agonists are primarily used in addition to levodopa therapy. Occasionally, they're used alone early in the treatment of Parkinson's disease, especially in younger adults. Some researchers have suggested that early use of dopamine agonists may forestall some of the complications of levodopa, but this is controversial. The side effects of dopamine agonists are similar to those of levodopa. These medications aren't recommended for individuals with hallucinations or confusion.

- *Selegiline.* Selegiline (Eldepryl) is used as an adjunct to levodopa therapy. It prevents the breakdown of both naturally occurring dopamine and dopamine formed from levodopa. It does this by inhibiting the activity of monoamine oxidase B (MAO-B) — the enzyme that metabolizes dopamine in the brain. It was once thought that this drug might slow the progression of Parkinson's disease, but this doesn't appear to be true. Toxic reactions have occurred in some patients who took selegiline with the narcotic drug meperidine (Demerol).
- *COMT inhibitors.* A newer class of medications, COMT inhibitors prolong the effect of levodopa therapy by blocking an enzyme that breaks down dopamine. Tolcapone (Tasmar) is a potent COMT inhibitor that easily crosses the blood-brain barrier and, in clinical trials, reduced the amount of levodopa needed by 25 percent. But because tolcapone has been linked to liver damage and failure, the drug is normally used in people who don't respond to other therapies. Entacapone (Comtan) is a milder COMT inhibitor that may help manage fluctuations in the response to levodopa in people with Parkinson's disease.
- *Anticholinergics.* Before the introduction of levodopa, these drugs were the main treatment for Parkinson's disease. In general, they help control tremors in the early stages of the disease. They're only mildly beneficial, and sometimes the benefits are offset by side effects such as dry mouth, nausea, urine retention and severe constipation. Anticholinergics can also cause mental problems, including memory loss, confusion and hallucinations. Anticholinergic drugs used to treat Parkinson's disease include trihexyphenidyl (Artane) and benztropine (Cogentin). The antihistamine diphenhydramine (Benadryl) and antidepressants such as amitryptiline (Elavil) work much like anticholinergics and may be used in older adults who can't tolerate anticholinergics therapy.
- *Amantadine.* This antiviral drug may be of benefit for people in the latter stages of Parkinson's disease, especially if they have problems with levodopa-induced dyskinesias. Side effects of amantadine (Symmetrel) include swollen ankles and a purple mottling of the skin.

Most people respond in some degree to drug therapy. Some people are almost completely relieved of signs and symptoms. However, over a period of years, control of signs and symptoms may decrease and the response to medication may vary.

Surgery

The following procedures may be options when signs and symptoms can't be controlled with medications:

- *Thalamotomy.* This procedure has been used for years to reduce tremors in people with Parkinson's disease. Thalamotomy involves the destruction of small amounts of tissue in the thalamus — a major brain center for relaying messages and transmitting sensations. But because the surgery can cause extreme weakness and slurred speech if it's performed on both sides of the brain, thalamotomy is usually performed on only one side of the brain. Thus, tremor relief is confined to one side of the body.
- *Pallidotomy.* Improved imaging techniques that allow surgeons to pinpoint troubled areas with greater precision have renewed interest in pallidotomy. In this procedure, an electric current is used to destroy a small amount of tissue in the pallidum, a part of the brain responsible for many features of Parkinson's disease. Pallidotomy may improve tremors, rigidity and slowed movement (bradykinesia) by interrupting the neural pathway between the pallidum and thalamus. It may also decrease the involuntary movements caused by drug therapy.

  Although pallidotomy may help certain people, it's not a cure and, in many cases, its benefits don't last. In addition, the surgery carries a number of risks, including slurred speech, disabling weakness and vision problems, especially when performed on both sides of the brain.
- *Deep brain stimulation.* This procedure involves implanting a stimulating device into the brain to control the shaking and trembling caused by Parkinson's disease. A deep brain stimulator consists of a pacemaker-like unit implanted in the chest that transmits electric pulses through an electrode implanted in the thalamus. The pulses appear to interrupt signals from the thalamus that may play a role in tremors. Potential risks exist with this form of treatment, including infection caused by the wire connecting the electrode to the stimulator and the need to perform minor surgery to change the unit's battery.

  More recently, deep brain stimulation has been extended to other brain areas, particularly the subthalamic nucleus. Stimulation within this brain center may markedly improve many aspects of parkinsonism.

Experimental therapy

Researchers continue to work on the development of new medications for Parkinson's disease. Great interest also exists in finding a way to replace the dopamine-producing cells in the substantia nigra. One approach has been fetal cell transplantation, a procedure in which fetal cells are implanted into the brain of people with Parkinson's disease.

Unfortunately, a large study published in 2001 suggested that fetal cell implants only benefit people under age 60, and about 15 percent of study participants later developed severe involuntary movements as a result of too much dopamine. In addition, the use of fetal cells raises a number of moral and ethical issues.

The answer, many researchers believe, lies in the use of embryonic stem cells. Stem cells are the parent cells of all tissues in the body. Researchers have been able to isolate and culture undifferentiated human stem cells in the laboratory. The hope is that they may one day be able to direct these cells to become specific types of cells — such as dopamine-producing neurons — that can be used to treat Parkinson's.

Stem cells used in research are derived from embryos that were produced in a laboratory to treat infertility, and they're used only with the informed consent of the donors. The use of embryonic stem cells is a controversial topic, and has been very limited.

Researchers are also investigating genes that code proteins responsible for producing dopamine, drugs that block the action of glutamate, an amino acid that destroys nerve cells, and the role of the antioxidant coenzyme Q-10 in stopping the progression of Parkinson's disease.

Essential tremor

Signs and symptoms

- Rhythmic, alternating movement of your hands, head, tongue or voice box (larynx)
- Hand tremor that worsens with use

Essential tremor is a common movement disorder. Almost half of all cases run in families, appearing from adolescence to later in life. It most commonly begins in middle to late life and progresses slowly. Over time, the tremor may affect your hands, head or voice. Voluntary movements, such as holding a coffee cup or a fork, usually make the tremor worse. This is in contrast to Parkinson's disease, in which the tremor tends to decrease with such movement.

The tremor usually stops when you're at rest. Jerky movements begin when you start a voluntary action, such as eating or writing. Essential tremor can make coordinated movements, such as touching your nose, difficult. Signs and symptoms may increase the more active you are. Fatigue or stress can make the tremor worse. The tremor disappears when you're asleep.

Diagnosis

Diagnosing essential tremor generally involves ruling out other conditions that can result in hand, head or voice tremors. Your doctor will likely ask about your medical history and perform a physical and neurologic exam. You may be asked to write, drink from a glass or hold a piece of paper.

You may also undergo blood, urine and neurologic tests to check for other causes, including thyroid disease, drug side effects and other neurologic disorders, such as Parkinson's disease.

How serious is essential tremor?

Essential tremor isn't life-threatening and usually is only a mild nuisance. But if it becomes disruptive, treatment is available to keep it under control.

Treatment

Lifestyle changes, for example avoiding stressful situations and stimulants such as caffeine, may ease the signs and symptoms.

Medications

The first line of treatment for essential tremor is often a prescription medication that affects your central nervous system. Medication can reduce tremor severity by about 50 percent to 60 percent. These medications include:

- *Beta blockers.* Often used to treat high blood pressure, beta blockers may also help control tremors. The most effective beta blocker for treating essential tremor is propranolol (Inderal).
- *Antiseizure medications.* These include the medication primidone (Mysoline).
- *Tranquilizers.* Tranquilizers include the medications diazepam (Valium) or alprazolam (Xanax).
- *Carbonic anhydrase inhibitors.* These include the medication methazolamide (Neptazane).
- *Botulinum toxin.* This chemical is produced by a bacterium that causes food poisoning (botulism). When injected into affected muscles, the toxin helps relax them.

Surgery

If medications aren't effective and signs and symptoms are disabling,

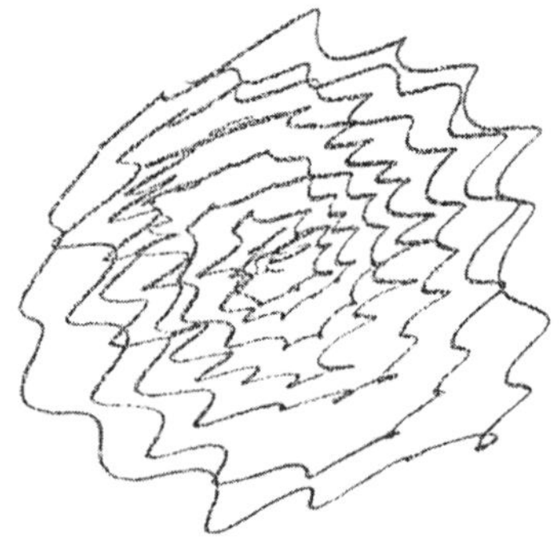

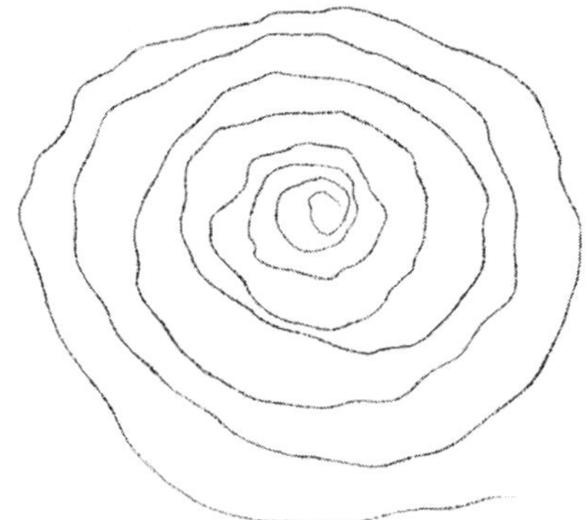

One test used to evaluate essential tremor involves having you draw a spiral. The spiral on the left was drawn by a hand affected by essential tremor. The spiral on the right was drawn by an unaffected hand.

the following types of surgery may be of benefit:

- *Thalamotomy.* This procedure may help the small number of people whose essential tremor is disabling.

  Thalamotomy involves destroying a tiny part of your thalamus, a message relay center deep within your brain. Destruction of a small region of the thalamus on one side of your brain typically relieves a tremor on the opposite side of your body. Between 70 percent and 80 percent of people who undergo the operation experience substantial relief from essential tremor. However, the operation generally relieves tremors only on one side of your body. Surgeons usually don't operate on both sides of the thalamus because doing so poses risks of speech impairment and other complications.
- *Deep brain stimulation.* This treatment involves use of a brain implant device called a thalamic or deep brain stimulator. It may be appropriate if you have severe tremors and medications aren't effective.

  A pacemaker-like unit implanted in the chest transmits electric pulses through a wire to an electrode in your thalamus. The pulses, which are painless, interrupt signals from the thalamus that help cause tremors. You turn the pulse generator on and off by passing a magnet over it. This procedure doesn't pose the risks of thalamotomy, and it can be performed on both sides of your brain.

Tic disorders

Signs and symptoms

- Habitual, repetitive movements or twitches of the face and body

Tics are semivoluntary mannerisms that usually develop in childhood. Grimaces, eye or mouth twitches, head turning, and shoulder shrugging are examples of common tics. Adolescents sometimes have such tics, which resolve as they get older.

A condition called Tourette's syndrome is characterized by multiple, more prominent tics that develop in youth and include vocalizations, such as sniffing, grunting and compulsive swearing. This syndrome is four times more frequent in boys than in girls and sometimes runs in families.

The tics of Tourette's syndrome aren't exactly involuntary, but compulsive or urgent, like the urge to scratch an itch. Sometimes, they can be suppressed, but ultimately the tics are expressed. The cause of this condition is not known but may be associated with abnormal metabolism of certain brain chemicals.

Diagnosis

A history and physical examination can help your doctor determine if you have a tic disorder, as well as its type and severity. Tests to exclude other disorders also may be necessary.

How serious are tic disorders?

Tic disorders typically are more frustrating than serious. Emotional stress can aggravate signs and symptoms and focus inordinate attention on the disorder.

Some conditions that may accompany Tourette's syndrome include obsessive-compulsive disorder, autism, anger control problems and poor social skills. People with Tourette's may experience periods free of signs and symptoms. Signs and symptoms often decrease with age and, in some cases, may eventually disappear.

Treatment

Often, no treatment is needed. In some cases, small dosages of dopamine agonists may be helpful. Examples of dopamine agonists include bromocriptine (Parlodel) and pramipexole (Mirapex). For mild tics, your doctor may also suggest small dosages of the blood pressure medication clonidine (Catapres) or the antiseizure medication clonazepam (Klonopin).

Low doses of antipsychotic drugs (neuroleptics), such as haloperidol (Haldol), pimozide (Orap) and fluphenazine (Prolixin), may control multiple tics more effectively, but they have significant side effects and are generally reserved for more severe disorders.

Multiple sclerosis

Signs and symptoms

- Numbness, weakness or paralysis in one or more limbs
- Brief pain, tingling or electric shock sensations
- Impaired vision with pain during movement in one eye
- Tremor, lack of coordination or unsteady gait
- Double vision or rapid, involuntary eye movement
- Fatigue
- Dizziness
- Exacerbations and remissions of signs and symptoms

Multiple sclerosis (MS) is a chronic, potentially debilitating disease that affects your brain, optic nerves and spinal cord (central nervous system). Strong evidence suggests that the illness is an autoimmune disease, one in which your immune system turns against your own body.

Normally, nerve fibers are coated with a protective sheath of a fatty substance called myelin. This sheath functions in a way that's similar to the way insulation shields electrical wires.

With MS, immune cells mistakenly destroy the cells that produce the myelin sheath. Myelin becomes inflamed, damaged and detached from the fibers. Eventually, the detached myelin is destroyed. Firm or hardened (sclerosed) patches of scar tissue form over the fibers. These damaged areas block or delay nerve impulses traveling to or from your brain, often disturbing muscle strength and coordination, as well as vision.

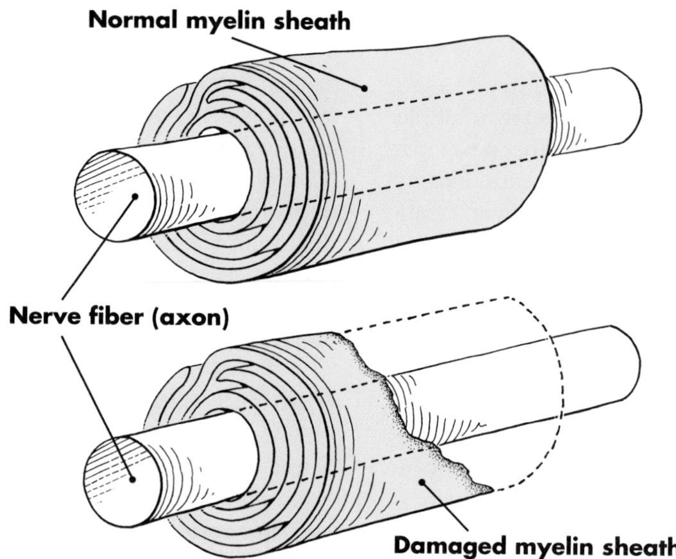

Your nerve fibers are protected by an insulating sheath (myelin). In multiple sclerosis, the sheath is damaged.

Ultimately, this process leads to degeneration of the nerves themselves, which likely accounts for permanent disabilities that develop in MS. No one knows what triggers this process, but some researchers suspect a virus or other infectious agent in an individual who is genetically susceptible to the disease.

MS generally occurs in episodes (attacks) that last weeks or months and are separated by periods in which signs and symptoms improve or disappear (remission). Disability may persist and the signs and symptoms may increase in severity. Apart from traumatic injury, MS is the leading cause of major disability in adults of working age.

MS occurs in five main forms:

- *Benign.* In 10 percent to 15 percent of people with MS, signs and symptoms are mild to moderate. They don't worsen or lead to permanent disability.
- *Relapsing-remitting.* In this type, one or two flare-ups of MS occur every 1 to 3 years, followed by periods of remission. The flare-ups typically appear over a number of hours, last a few weeks or months and gradually disappear. Signs and symptoms may increase with each recurrence. About 85 percent of people with MS begin with this form.
- *Primary progressive.* After signs and symptoms first appear, they progress without acute attacks or periods of remission. About 15 percent of people with MS have this pattern of disease.
- *Secondary progressive.* After years of relapsing-remitting MS, at least half of all affected individuals experience slow but continuous deterioration. Occasional relapses may be superimposed upon the continuous deterioration.
- *Progressive relapsing.* This is primary progressive MS with the addition of sudden episodes of new signs and symptoms or worsened existing ones. This form occurs in less than 5 percent of people with MS.

Attacks are most frequent during the first 5 to 10 years of the disease. The first attack most commonly occurs between the ages of 18 and 55 years. However, the range of onset of MS spans from early childhood to older adulthood.

More than 300,000 Americans have MS. Women are at higher risk of this disease than are men. Your risk of MS is greater if a relative has the disease. The disease is not, however, passed on reliably from one generation to the next like other genetic diseases. First-degree relatives have approximately a 3 percent to 5 percent chance of developing MS. Whites of Northern European descent, especially those of Scandinavian heritage, are more susceptible to MS.

Diagnosis

The signs and symptoms of MS are variable, so the disease can be difficult to diagnose in its initial stages. However, the sequence of an attack, remission and recurrent attack limited to the central nervous system strongly suggests MS. An accurate diagnosis is important as other conditions may mimic MS. Many people with fatigue, pain and nonspecific tingling don't have MS. If MS is suspected, your doctor will probably refer you to a neurologist for a detailed examination.

Criteria for diagnosing MS are evolving but currently include a reliable history of attacks or sustained neurologic deterioration and an observable abnormality of the central nervous system, such as weakness and altered reflexes or sensation. Because lesions of MS are distributed randomly in the brain and spinal cord, signs and symptoms can vary considerably. A neurologic examination systematically tests various parts of your nervous system.

Laboratory tests may be used to help establish the diagnosis. You may be given a standard visual stimulus test to determine how fast your optic nerve conducts electric signals. A magnetic resonance imaging (MRI) scan of the brain and spinal cord is usually of help in diagnosis. A spinal tap (lumbar puncture) also may be used to check the concentration of immune cells, antibodies and proteins in your cerebrospinal fluid (see page 578).

How serious is multiple sclerosis?

As noted, the course of MS varies widely. The average life expectancy of more than 35 years after onset of the disease has increased 10 to 15 years in the past few decades as a result of better medical care, particularly in dealing with complications of the disease. Most people with MS are ambulatory, and many are employed even after having MS for 20 years. It's very uncommon to be permanently disabled within weeks or months of initial signs and symptoms of MS.

Treatment

If your attacks are mild or infrequent, your doctor may advise a wait-and-see approach, with counseling and observation. However, if you have a relapsing form of the disease, your doctor may recommend medications to reduce new attacks, slow the disease process and alleviate symptoms.

Medications

Medications prescribed to slow the course of MS include:

- *Beta interferons.* Interferon beta-1b (Betaseron) and interferon beta-1a (Avonex) are genetically engineered copies of proteins that occur naturally in your body. They help fight viral infection and regulate your immune system. With Betaseron, you inject yourself with the medication approximately every other day. You need to inject Avonex once weekly. These medications have reduced flares of MS by up to 30 percent. It's unclear which of their many actions leads to a reduction in disease activity and what may be their long-term benefits.

  The Food and Drug Administration has approved beta interferons only for people with relapsing forms of MS who can still walk. The medications don't reverse nerve damage, and it hasn't been conclusively proved that they prevent long-term permanent disability. A small percentage of people develop antibodies to beta interferons, which may make them less effective. Other people can't tolerate the side effects, which may include inflammation and pain at the injection site, flu-like signs and symptoms and abnormalities of liver function.

  Mayo Clinic neurologists generally recommend beta interferons for people who have significant attacks of MS, particularly those who don't recover fully after flare-ups. This treatment may also be used for people who have a significant increase of new lesions as seen on an MRI scan, even when there aren't major new signs and symptoms of disease activity.
- *Glatiramer acetate.* This medication is an alternative to beta interferons if you have relapsing-remitting MS. Doctors believe that glatiramer acetate (Copaxone) works by blocking your immune system's attack on myelin. Glatiramer acetate is as effective as beta interferons in curbing MS attacks, but it doesn't reduce new lesions to the same degree. You need to inject glatiramer once daily. Side effects may include flushing and tightness in your chest following injection.
- *Mitoxantrone.* This chemotherapy agent is administered by intravenous infusion once every 3 months. It works by suppressing immune cells believed to attack myelin. It's typically prescribed only when interferons or glatiramer acetate haven't been effective. Its use may be associated with a risk of bladder infections and pneumonia as well as hair loss and menstrual irregularities. At higher doses, it may be toxic to the heart muscle, so regular monitoring with electrocardiograms and heart ultrasounds (echocardiograms) is important.

Medications taken to relieve signs and symptoms in MS include:

- *Corticosteroids.* Doctors most often prescribe brief courses of oral or intravenous (IV) corticosteroids to reduce inflammation in nerve tissue and shorten the duration of flare-ups. Prolonged use of these medications isn't recommended because it isn't helpful and may lead to side effects such as osteoporosis and high blood pressure.
- *Muscle relaxants.* If you have MS, you may experience muscle stiffening or spasms, particularly in your legs, which can be painful. Tizanidine (Zanaflex) and baclofen (Lioresal) are used to reduce this muscle spasticity. Baclofen may increase weakness in the legs. Tizanidine appears to control muscle spasms without leaving your legs feeling weak, but it can be associated with drowsiness and a dry mouth.
- *Medications to reduce fatigue.* These may include the antiviral drug amantadine (Symmetrel) or a medication used for narcolepsy called modafinil (Provigil). The benefit of these medications appears to be due to their stimulant properties.

Many different medications may be used for muscle stiffness, depression, pain and bladder control problems often associated with MS. Some arthritis drugs, such as azathioprine (Imuran) and methotrexate (Rheumatrex), that suppress the immune system also may slow progression of MS in some cases.

Other therapies

In addition to medications, physical and occupational therapy can help you preserve independence through the use of strengthening exercises and assistive devices to ease daily tasks. Individual or group counseling may help you and your family cope with MS and reduce emotional stress.

Experimental treatments

Researchers are evaluating various experimental approaches to treating MS:

- *Plasma exchange.* This procedure involves removing blood and mechanically separating the blood cells from the fluid (plasma). Your

blood cells then are mixed with a replacement solution, typically albumin, or a synthetic fluid with properties similar to plasma. The new solution is returned to your body. Replacing your plasma may dilute the activity of the destructive factors in your immune system and help you to recover. The treatment is only an option for people with sudden, extremely severe attacks of MS who don't respond to high doses of steroid treatment. It's most helpful for people with a relatively mild preexisting disability before the attack.
- *Intravenous immunoglobulin.* Intravenous immunoglobulin (IVIg) therapy involves receiving injections of antibodies from a group of donors. Studies in Europe have reported that IVIg can reduce the number of attacks in relapsing forms of MS. IVIg has been studied at Mayo Clinic for the potential to stimulate growth of myelin. Current commercial preparations of IVIg seem to be ineffective in doing so. More specific antibodies that appear to promote myelin growth in animals with diseases that mimic MS may be evaluated in humans in the future.
- *Antiviral medications and antibiotics.* Presently, no infectious agent has been identified that conclusively causes MS. For this reason, these medications aren't currently recommended outside of controlled experiments evaluating their safety and effectiveness.

Amyotrophic lateral sclerosis

Signs and symptoms

- Slow loss of strength and coordination in one or more limbs
- Muscle twitches or cramps
- An increasingly stiff, clumsy gait
- Difficulty swallowing, speaking or breathing

Amyotrophic lateral sclerosis (ALS) is a progressive degeneration of the nerve cells in the brain and spinal cord that control your voluntary muscles. It's commonly called Lou Gehrig's disease after the New York Yankees baseball player who died of ALS in 1939.

The affected nerve cells shrink and disappear with no other signs of abnormality. Muscles then waste away because the nerves that stimulated them are gone.

About 30,000 Americans have ALS. It occurs worldwide and appears to affect men and women equally. A defective gene has been identified in some cases of inherited ALS. The disease isn't contagious.

The onset of the disease is often gradual. Generally, there's increasing weakness in one limb, especially a hand. Later, other limbs may be affected. This may be accompanied by muscle twitching and cramping. Additional muscles become affected as ALS progresses, and complete paralysis may result. The disease eventually affects semivoluntary muscles, such as the ones used for chewing, swallowing, speaking and breathing.

Diagnosis

The disease is often well advanced before people seek medical attention. In these instances, a doctor may be able to make a diagnosis based on signs and symptoms. Electromyography to test for nerve damage may be required.

How serious is amyotrophic lateral sclerosis?

ALS is a chronic degenerative disorder that becomes progressively worse. Most people with ALS die of respiratory failure due to paralysis of the muscles used in breathing. Sometimes, people with ALS stop breathing because they inhale (aspirate) food and oral secretions into the lungs. Generally, death occurs within 2 to 10 years after diagnosis and only one in five people with the disease live longer than 5 years.

Treatment

There's no cure for ALS. Individualized therapy is useful for maintaining muscle function and general health during the disease's early stages. ALS doesn't affect your mind, and several years of productive and enjoyable life may be possible. The complications of aspiration of food and saliva inhaled into the windpipe (trachea) can be avoided by insertion of a tube through the wall of the abdomen and into the stomach through which liquid feedings can be given.

The Food and Drug Administration has approved the medication riluzole (Rilutek) for the treatment of ALS. It may slow the progression of the disease slightly in some people. Emotional support from family and friends is important.

Huntington's disease

Signs and symptoms

- A wide, swinging gait
- Hesitant or slurred speech
- Involuntary, jerky movements in arms, neck, trunk and face
- Clumsiness or problems with balance
- Personality changes, such as moodiness and paranoia
- Intellectual deterioration, including memory loss and inattention

Emergency signs and symptoms

- An abrupt change in mental state

Huntington's disease, also known as Huntington's chorea, is a progressive degenerative brain disease that causes certain nerve cells to waste away. As a result, emotions, motor skills and mental skills are typically affected.

Huntington's disease is an inherited condition resulting from a single abnormal gene. If one parent has the faulty gene, the chance of inheriting the defect is 50 percent in each offspring. Because the onset is typically in middle age, many parents are unaware that they carry the gene until they've already had children.

The disorder was first identified in 1872 by American physician George Huntington. *Chorea* comes from the Greek word for "dance" and refers to the incessant, quick, jerky and involuntary movements of people with the disease.

Signs and symptoms usually appear between the ages of 35 and 50. Individuals who develop the disease at a younger age often have a more severe condition, but the disease is rare in children. About 1 in 10,000 Americans have the disease, with about 30,000 known cases in the United States.

Progression of the disease is slow. Personality changes, from moodiness to paranoia, may occur first. Involuntary facial movements such as grimacing may be mild initially. Other signs and symptoms, including severe chorea and mental impairment (dementia), appear as the disease progresses.

Diagnosis

The diagnosis of Huntington's disease is generally based on a medical and family history and a physical examination. Your doctor may also recommend neurologic studies including a computerized tomography (CT) scan or magnetic resonance imaging (MRI) of the brain.

How serious is Huntington's disease?

After onset of the disease, signs and symptoms will progress in severity until death occurs. Although signs and symptoms vary from person to person, vital functions such as swallowing, eating, speaking and walking usually deteriorate over time. Death generally occurs as a result of complications of the disease, such as an infection or a fall.

Treatment

Most people who have Huntington's disease eventually become physically and mentally disabled. In earlier stages of the disease, they may require short-term hospitalization. As the disease progresses, long-term nursing home care may be necessary.

No treatment is available to stop or reverse Huntington's disease, but some approaches can decrease its signs and symptoms.

Medications

Tranquilizers such as clonazepam (Klonopin) and antipsychotic drugs such as haloperidol (Haldol) and clozapine (Clozaril) may help control involuntary movements, violent outbursts and hallucinations.

Various medications including fluoxetine (Prozac), sertraline (Zoloft) and nortriptyline (Aventyl, Pamelor) may be used to control depression and the obsessive-compulsive rituals that some people with Huntington's disease develop. Medications such as lithium (Eskalith, Lithobid) can help control extreme emotional fluctuations and mood swings.

Side effects from many of the medications used to treat signs and symptoms of Huntington's disease can include hyperexcitability, fatigue and restlessness.

Speech therapy

Huntington's disease can impair speech, affecting the ability to express complex thoughts. Speech therapy may help. Remind friends, family members and caregivers that if a person with Huntington's doesn't speak, it doesn't necessarily mean that the person doesn't understand what's going on. Ask people to continue talking to the person, and keep his or her environment as normal as possible.

Friedreich's ataxia

Signs and symptoms

- Difficulty in maintaining balance while walking or standing
- Abnormal speech rhythm or articulation
- Weakness in limbs
- A tremor of the hands or arms
- Deformed spine or feet
- Paralysis, particularly of the legs

Friedreich's ataxia was named in 1863 for German physician Nikolaus Friedreich, who first described the condition. *Ataxia* is the medical term for coordination problems, such as clumsiness or difficulty maintaining balance. Ataxia can be caused by many different conditions.

Friedreich's ataxia, a rare, inherited disease, is due to nerve fiber degeneration in areas of the spinal cord, peripheral nerves or cerebellum caused by a faulty gene. Normally, nerve fibers are encased in a sheath of a fatty substance called myelin, which enables smooth conduction of electric impulses between cells. In Friedreich's ataxia, nerve fibers lose some of their myelin sheath, and the spinal cord becomes thinner.

Signs and symptoms of the disease typically begin between the ages of 5 and 15. The condition affects about 1 in 50,000 people in the United States. In addition to problems with coordination and speech, many people develop curvature of the spine (scoliosis) and deformities in their feet. This often occurs as muscles weaken.

Friedreich's ataxia is an autosomal recessive disorder. You must inherit the abnormal gene from both parents in order to develop the condition. You may also be a carrier of the gene, without ever developing signs and symptoms, if you inherit it from only one parent. If there's a history of the disorder in your family, you may wish to speak with a genetic counselor before beginning a family.

Mutation of the gene responsible for the disease causes reduced production of a protein called frataxin. Research suggests that a lack of frataxin leaves nerve cells vulnerable to oxidative stress, a harmful condition caused by molecules called free radicals. Free radicals normally assist in your body's processing of fuel for energy, but too many of them can be damaging.

Diagnosis

Diagnosis of this disorder is based on family history and neurologic findings including tests such as an electromyogram, which measures electrical activity in muscle cells, or an electrocardiogram (ECG). Tests to exclude other disorders may include a computerized tomography (CT) scan or magnetic resonance imaging (MRI) of the brain and spinal cord, and a spinal tap (lumbar puncture) with analysis of cerebrospinal fluid. Genetic testing can confirm the diagnosis.

How serious is Friedreich's ataxia?
Although signs and symptoms vary from person to person, most people with this disease eventually need a wheelchair to get around. Complications include various forms of cardiovascular disease, such as enlargement of the heart, heart failure, impairment of the conduction of electric impulses within the heart (heart block) and abnormal heart rhythms (tachycardia). Diabetes also may develop. Survival beyond early adulthood is rare. Death is frequently caused by a heart condition.

Treatment
No specific treatment is available for Friedreich's ataxia. Continued physical activity is recommended for general health and physical therapy is often helpful.

Treatment of heart problems and diabetes can help maintain quality of life for a longer time. Orthopedic problems may be improved through surgery or the use of a brace.

Investigators hope that identifying the genetic cause of the disorder will lead to effective methods for a prevention or cure.

Myasthenia gravis

Signs and symptoms
- Facial muscle weakness, including drooping eyelids
- Difficulty breathing, talking, chewing or swallowing
- Double vision
- Muscle weakness in the arms or legs

Emergency signs and symptoms
- Increasing difficulty breathing or swallowing

Myasthenia gravis is a chronic disorder characterized by weakness and rapid fatigue of your voluntary muscles. Muscle weakness develops gradually and may affect any of the muscles that you control voluntarily. It commonly affects muscles of the face, eyes, arms and legs, and those involved in chewing, swallowing and breathing.

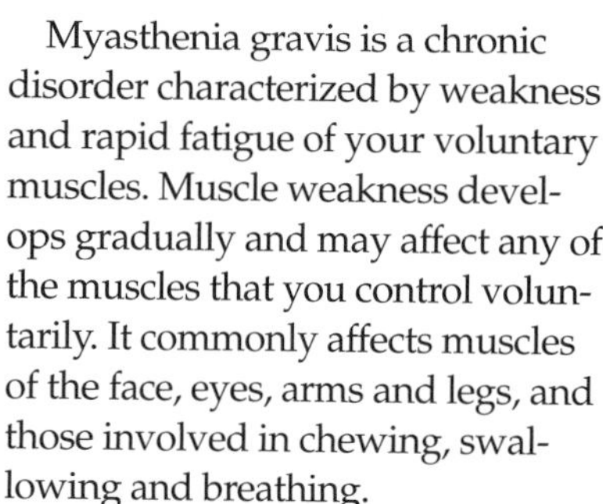

The more a muscle action is repeated, the worse the weakness becomes. In myasthenia gravis, good days alternate with bad. Remissions may occur, however, and can last for months. In rare cases, breathing or swallowing problems worsen, requiring emergency medical care.

Myasthenia gravis is an autoimmune disease, which means that antibodies normally formed to fight infection instead attack normal tissue. When your nervous system is functioning normally, the chemical acetylcholine transmits nerve impulses to muscles. At specialized areas of your muscles, called neuromuscular junctions, receptor sites receive these impulses and signal your muscles to contract, allowing you to, for example, raise a spoon to your mouth.

In myasthenia gravis, there's a breakdown in communication between your nerves and muscles. For unknown reasons, myasthenia gravis causes your immune system to produce antibodies that block or destroy many of your receptor sites — up to 80 percent of them. With fewer receptor sites, your muscles receive fewer nerve signals, causing weakness.

The thymus gland, a part of your immune system located in the upper chest beneath the breastbone, may trigger or maintain the production of these antibodies. Large in infancy, the thymus gradually shrinks in healthy adults. However, some people with myasthenia gravis have an abnormally large thymus gland. About 10 percent to

Torticollis

Torticollis, sometimes called wryneck, is an intermittent or continuous spasm of the large muscles of the neck. It's a form of dystonia — sudden, involuntary contractions of a muscle or group of muscles. The condition may be inherited or acquired after damage to the neck muscle, or it may develop for no apparent reason.

The spasm is usually more prominent on one side than the other. This may cause permanent turning or tilting of the head. Stress or anxiety may make signs and symptoms worse.

Application of heat and massage may ease head and neck pain. Stretching exercises and a neck brace may improve spasms. Injections of botulinum toxin (botox) to relax the muscles may provide relief, although repeat injections are usually required. In severe cases, surgery may be an option.

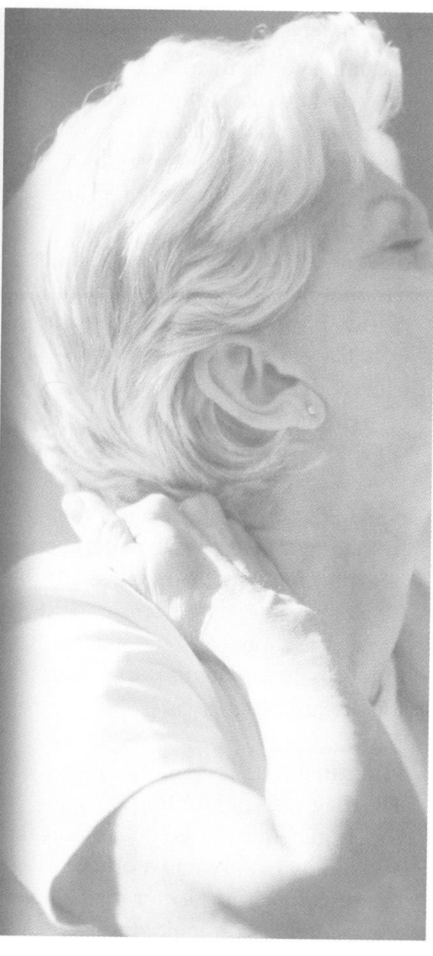

Physical Therapy for Neurologic Problems

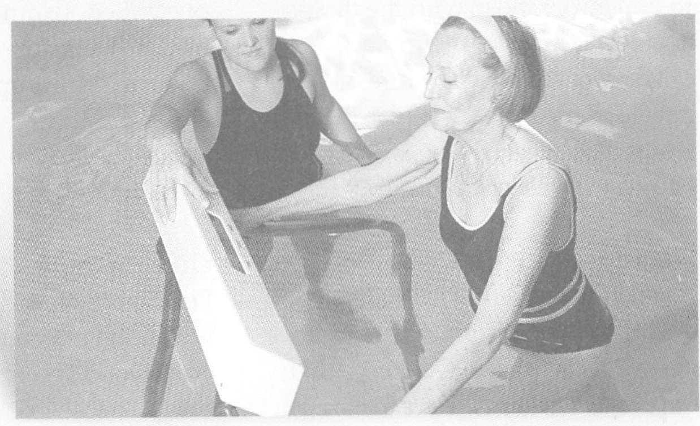

Physical therapy is used to achieve maximal potential in people with disabilities, including those resulting from neurologic diseases and disorders. Physical therapy treatments can be valuable in helping to relieve pain, improve strength and mobility and perform essential tasks to maintain independence.

Before you begin a program of physical therapy, have a complete medical examination with diagnostic, functional and psychological testing, as determined by your doctor. A physical therapist generally consults closely with your doctor to plan a program that will work for you. The therapist and your doctor will also re-evaluate the therapy frequently as you make progress.

Your physical therapy program may address problems related to joint mobility, muscle strength, coordination, heart and lung capacity, posture and ability to change position, walk, communicate, follow directions and perform other daily activities.

Physical therapists are trained and licensed in the use of a variety of therapies that may help relieve signs and symptoms of disease. Some of the therapies they may use include:

Exercise

Exercise is the most varied and widely used of all physical therapy techniques. Your exercise routine will be designed to overcome the manifestations of your disorder as much as possible, whether it be to increase the degree of joint mobility or to retrain your muscles to contract and relax in useful coordination with other muscles.

Exercises may be simple or complex. They may be performed actively by you alone or with the help of your therapist or passively as your physical therapist moves your arm or leg through a range of motions. Active exercises are necessary to improve your muscle function, but passive exercises are helpful when you have muscle contractures or need to relearn certain movements. Resistance exercises can improve muscle strength.

Various types of equipment may be used, including an exercise table or mat, a stationary bicycle, walking aids, a wheelchair, practice stairs, curbs, ramps, parallel bars and pulleys and weights.

Hot and cold treatment

Heat can stimulate circulation, relax tense muscles and relieve pain. It can be applied with warm-water compresses, infrared lamps, short-wave radiation, ultrasound, hot paraffin wax or warm baths. In some cases, cold treatment with ice packs or cold-water soaking may be necessary. Alternating hot-and-cold water immersion of the hands or feet is used in certain circumstances.

Whirlpool baths

Whirlpool baths can ease pain from muscle spasms and help guide or strengthen your movements because the water partially supports you but provides resistance to your motion.

Massage

Massage therapy can improve circulation, help you relax, relieve local pain or muscle spasms and reduce swelling. It can be done by trained therapists with special equipment or by family members trained in proper techniques.

Electricity

Electric currents of very low strength applied through your skin can stimulate superficial muscles and make them contract. This helps to produce response in paralyzed or weakened muscles. Certain medications can even be administered through your skin by means of a low-voltage electrical apparatus. Portable electric current devices called transcutaneous electronic nerve stimulation, or TENS, units are sometimes used to control chronic pain (see page 1333).

Assistive devices

Your therapy may include learning how to use assistive devices for walking, such as a cane, brace or walker, or a mobility aid such as a wheelchair or motorized scooter. You may also receive training in use of devices that can make it easier to fasten buttons, hold a fork, dial a telephone or drive a car.

Other therapies

In addition to your doctor and physical therapist, you may meet with an occupational therapist to help you regain the ability to perform routine daily tasks such as grooming and dressing or develop alternative methods of compensating for lost function.

15 percent of those with the disease develop tumors of the thymus.

Myasthenia gravis is rare. It develops most frequently in women between the ages of 20 and 40 and men older than age 60.

Diagnosis

A key symptom that may alert your doctor to the possibility of myasthenia gravis is muscle weakness that improves with rest. Tests to confirm the diagnosis may include a neurologic examination, electromyography and a blood analysis for the presence of certain antibodies. After the strength of various muscles is tested, you may be given a drug called edrophonium (Tensilon). Improved muscle strength after taking this drug is suggestive of myasthenia gravis.

How serious is myasthenia gravis?

There's no cure for myasthenia gravis, but treatment can often lead to a remission. In a crisis phase of the illness, affected individuals become so weak that they need help breathing or swallowing, but this rarely persists beyond a few weeks. With proper treatment, most people can lead productive lives.

Treatment

Plan activities to take advantage of your energy peaks, and schedule daily rest periods. To relieve double vision, wear an eye patch. Because stress can worsen your condition, try to avoid situations that may provoke unnecessary anxiety. Enlist family and friends to help you minimize your level of stress.

Medication

A drug called pyridostigmine (Mestinon, Regonol) is often prescribed to improve signal transmission between your nerves and muscles. Arrange to eat meals about 30 minutes after taking the medication to minimize chewing and swallowing difficulty. Medications that suppress or alter your immune system may also be prescribed. Examples include prednisone (Deltasone, Sterapred), azathioprine (Imuran), cyclosporine (Neoral, Sandimmune), mycophenolate (CellCept) and intravenous immunoglobulin.

Other therapies

Plasmapheresis is a treatment in which the plasma component in your blood is removed and discarded because it contains antibodies that may contribute to your disease. Other fluids to replace your plasma are mixed with your blood cells and returned to your body. This treatment may reduce the immune response and improve muscle strength temporarily.

Surgery

In some cases, removal of the thymus gland may be recommended. This can lead to permanent improvement in signs and symptoms. This procedure is used mainly in young individuals because the thymus gland shrinks with advancing age. As with any type of surgery, there are associated risks.

Spinal Cord and Peripheral Nerve Disorders

Your peripheral nervous system runs from your spinal cord to all other parts of your body. It's the network of nerves that you use to initiate movements and perceive sensations. Damage to your spine or peripheral nerves can interfere with communication between your brain and other areas of your body.

Damage to your peripheral nerves or spine can result in numbness or abnormal sensations and an inability to move your muscles. The seriousness of these disorders may range from temporary numbness to permanent paralysis.

Spinal cord injury

Emergency signs and symptoms

- Weakness, incoordination or paralysis in a part of the body after an accident
- Numbness or loss of sensation
- Loss of bladder or bowel control

Most spinal cord injuries are the result of traffic or industrial accidents, falls, gunshot wounds and recreational or athletic injuries. Sometimes, a relatively minor injury can produce severe damage if you have a predisposing condition, such as rheumatoid arthritis.

Your spinal cord is composed of long nerve fibers leading to and from your brain. The nerve fibers of the spinal cord feed into nerve roots that emerge between the vertebrae and organize into peripheral nerves that extend to your skin and muscles.

If the spinal cord is injured, the nerve fibers passing through the injured area can be affected. Part or all of your corresponding muscles and nerves below that injury site may be impaired.

Spinal injuries occur most frequently in the lower back (lumbar) and neck (cervical) areas. A lumbar injury can affect leg, bowel and bladder control and sexual function. A neck injury may affect breathing as well as movements of your upper and lower limbs. Injury to one side of the spinal cord typically impairs the muscles on the same side and some sensations on the same and opposite sides of your body.

Injury may result from your spinal cord being stretched, compressed, pushed sideways or cut. It could also result from bleeding or the accidental insertion of a fragment of bone or metal into your spinal cord. Striking your chin on the steering wheel during a traffic accident, for example, may stretch your spinal cord and cause injury. A bullet or knife wound can sever the cord.

Often, injury to the spinal cord in the neck area results from a sharp bending of the neck during contact

PREVENTION TIP

To reduce the risk of spinal cord injuries:

- Wear a seat belt whenever you're in an automobile. Make sure your children are safely buckled in too. A seat belt is one of the most effective devices in reducing spinal cord injuries resulting from car accidents.
- Wear a helmet when in-line skating, riding a bicycle or operating a motorized vehicle such as a motorcycle.
- Always wear appropriate equipment and safety gear when engaging in sports.
- If you own a firearm, take a firearm or hunting safety course and keep the firearm locked away when not in use.
- Prevent falls by using a step stool to reach things and installing safety devices such as handrails, window guards and safety gates at the top and bottom of stairs.

while playing football, from a shallow-water dive or from a motor vehicle accident. Injury to the lower spine, another common result of car and motorcycle accidents, may result in a crushing injury of the spinal cord.

Bleeding within the spinal cord can cause some permanent loss of sensation and muscle weakness. Bleeding around the spinal cord may compress it and result in weakness or loss of sensation in your limbs and trunk.

Compression may also occur from fluid accumulations and swelling in your spinal cord. The resulting paralysis may continue for several days and then improve dramatically when the swelling subsides or the accumulated fluid is removed surgically, although some impairment may persist.

Most cuts and other severe forms of trauma to the spinal cord cause permanent disability or paralysis because nerve fibers seldom regenerate. Paralysis below the neck can involve all four extremities, a condition called quadriplegia, or only the legs and lower body, resulting in paraplegia.

Approximately 10,000 to 15,000 people — mostly young and otherwise healthy — become paraplegic or quadriplegic each year in the United States because of spinal cord trauma. Trauma is most common among men between the ages of 15 and 35.

Diagnosis

Numbness or paralysis may occur immediately after a spinal cord injury or develop gradually as bleeding or swelling occurs in or around the spinal cord. Urgent medical attention is required to minimize long-term effects of such trauma.

After a physical and neurologic examination, other diagnostic tests may be needed. These usually include X-rays, a computerized tomography (CT) scan or magnetic resonance imaging (MRI) or myelography (see page 610). Occasionally, spinal tap (lumbar puncture) is necessary.

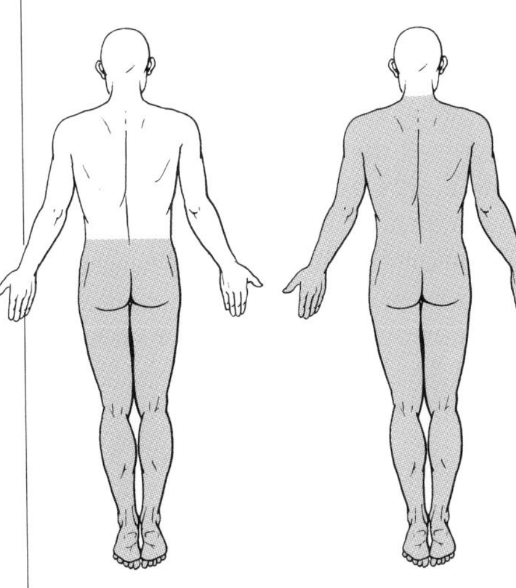

Paralysis of the lower body is called paraplegia. Paralysis below the neck is called quadriplegia.

How serious is spinal cord injury?

The immediate effect of a spinal cord injury is often paralysis or loss of sensation in part of your body. This can be fatal if a neck injury has paralyzed breathing. The time between injury and treatment is a critical factor that can determine the extent of your recovery.

Recovery of movement or sensation within the first week is usually followed by eventual recovery of most or all functions. Any impairment remaining after 6 months probably will be permanent. If your bladder control is lost, your risk of recurring urinary tract infections increases. You also become susceptible to injury of any part of your body that has impaired sensation.

Treatment

Treatment consists of emergency care, hospitalization while the injuries heal and rehabilitation.

Medication

Corticosteroid medications can help reduce swelling that may be compressing your spinal cord. Antibiotics may be required for urinary tract infections.

Surgery

Surgical procedures may be necessary to remove fragments of bone or foreign objects, to fix fractured vertebrae by fusing the bone or inserting metal pins, or to decompress the spinal cord.

Other therapies

Traction may reduce some dislocations of your spine and immobilize the back during healing. Sometimes, traction is accomplished by placing metal braces, attached to weights or a body harness, into the skull to hold it in place.

Bed rest is the primary treatment. Further neurologic assessment is used to check for signs that reflexes and sensations are returning. Injuries usually heal in 2 to 4 months, and then a doctor can estimate how much disability will remain.

Your doctor may recommend physical therapy to obtain the most benefit from remaining muscle function and strength or to learn how to move with mechanical assistance.

Spinal tumor

Signs and symptoms

- Steadily increasing back pain
- Muscle weakness in the limbs
- Numbness or cold sensations

Emergency signs and symptoms

- Loss of bowel or bladder control
- Progressive loss of lower limb strength or sensation

Spinal tumors are abnormal growths that can occur within your spinal cord, between its covering membranes or outside of the membranes in the spinal canal. These growths are cancerous (malignant) in 40 percent of cases. Spinal cord tumors are similar to brain tumors but are much less common.

Sometimes, tumors of the spine start elsewhere in your body, usually a lung or breast, and move through your bloodstream (metastasize) to the spinal area. More commonly, they originate in the bony spine itself. The cause is often unknown, although nonmalignant tumors can be present from birth (congenital) or hereditary.

Signs and symptoms generally appear when the growing tumor presses against the spinal cord.

Rehabilitation in Paraplegia and Quadriplegia

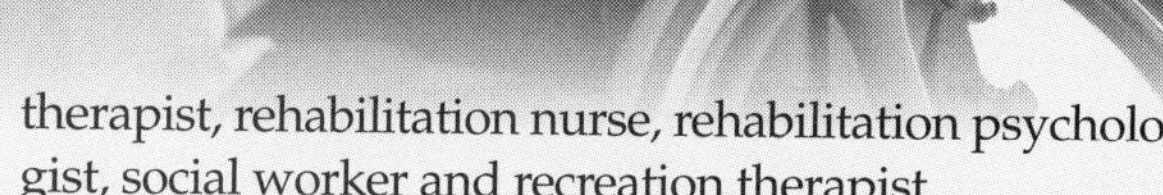

An accident that results in paralysis is a life-changing event, whether you've lost movement in your legs and lower body (paraplegia) or all four extremities (quadriplegia). Recovery from such an event takes time, but many people who are paralyzed move on to lead productive and fulfilling lives. The will to live is amazingly strong in humans, and the creativity with which many affected people lead their lives is infinite.

Initial recovery

In the early stages of paraplegia or quadriplegia, your doctor will treat the injury or disease that caused the loss of function. He or she will also watch for possible dangers such as stool or urine retention, respiratory or cardiovascular difficulty, stomach or intestinal ulcers, skin problems, muscle contractures and formation of deep vein blood clots (thrombosis) in the extremities.

After the initial injury or disease stabilizes, attention will be given to problems that may arise from immobilization, such as deconditioning, muscle contractures, bedsores, urinary infection and blood clots. Early care will likely include changing your position frequently, range-of-motion exercises for paralyzed limbs, help with your bladder and bowel functions, applications of skin lotion and use of soft bed coverings or flotation mattresses. Hospitalization can last from several days to several weeks, depending on the cause and extent of the paralysis and the progress of your therapy.

Rehabilitation team

During this time, a rehabilitation team will work with you to improve your remaining muscle strength and to give you the greatest possible mobility and independence for living a full and active life. Your team may include a physiatrist, physical therapist, occupational therapist, rehabilitation nurse, rehabilitation psychologist, social worker and recreation therapist.

Rehabilitation therapy

Rehabilitation therapy may include exercise and various therapeutic methods, such as whirlpool baths and massage, to relieve pain and relax your muscles. You may receive training on day-to-day tasks and on the devices you'll need to assist you, such as a wheelchair or equipment that can make it easier to fasten buttons or dial a telephone. This therapy may require several months in a rehabilitation facility.

Transitioning home

The rehabilitation team may smooth your transition to living at home by means of short-term leaves from the hospital. Such visits can acquaint you with support services in your community. Your doctor will continue to monitor your health and help you, with the assistance of your family or friends, to adapt to a lifestyle that's healthful and as independent as possible.

Rehabilitation professionals can help you select needed equipment and modifications in your home. The goal is optimal independence and efficiency at minimal cost. Your rehab team can also help you address transportation needs.

Your part

Your mental state is extremely important. Sudden disability can be followed by depression. Many people with a disability learn to counter their depression by vigorous rehabilitative activity. It's essential for you to find or rediscover interesting things to do for yourself as well as with others. Don't hesitate to seek out support groups and peer counselors to help you.

Back pain and muscle weakness become progressively worse, and cold sensations may be felt in the legs, fingers or hands. Loss of bowel and bladder control and muscle spasms sometimes occur. Early treatment of a spinal tumor is important, so have your signs and symptoms evaluated by a doctor as soon as possible.

Diagnosis

Similar signs and symptoms can result from other spinal disorders, so an accurate diagnosis is important. If a spinal cord tumor is suspected after a physical and neurologic examination, your doctor may request diagnostic tests, which may include X-rays, a computerized tomography (CT) scan, magnetic resonance imaging (MRI) or myelography (see page 610).

How serious is a spinal tumor?

If you're diagnosed with a spinal tumor, proceed with treatment as quickly as possible to minimize risk of permanent impairment. Early diagnosis and treatment provide a higher success rate, although neurologic signs and symptoms may continue after initial treatments.

Treatment

Corticosteroids, such as dexamethasone, are used to reduce spinal cord swelling. Surgical removal is usually successful for isolated tumors outside the spinal cord. Other tumors may not be completely removable, and radiation therapy may be necessary. Physical therapy programs are often needed to help with rehabilitation after completion of surgical or radiation therapy.

Cervical spondylosis

Signs and symptoms

- Pain or stiffness in the neck
- Pain, numbness, or pins-and-needles sensation in the shoulder or arm
- A burning sensation or clumsiness in fingers
- Bladder control problems
- Numbness or weakness in the legs or arms
- Imbalance or stiffness of the legs

Cervical spondylosis (cervical osteoarthritis) is due to growth of bone spurs on the vertebrae in your neck.

Although a neck injury can lead to spondylosis many years later, bone spurs generally result from normal aging as the bone-cushioning cartilage within joints deteriorates and roughens. Eventually, if the cartilage wears down completely, you may be left with bone rubbing on bone — causing the ends of your bones to become damaged and your neck joints to become painful.

Your body attempts to fix the damage, but repairs may result in growth of new bone along the sides of the existing bone, which produces prominent lumps or bone spurs.

This happens slowly, and your neck gradually becomes stiff. The bone spurs eventually may press against nerve roots leading to your shoulders and arms. This compression causes pain or other sensations in these areas. If the spurs also press against your spinal cord, your leg muscles and bladder and bowel control may be affected.

The signs and symptoms are similar to those due to a herniated disk, but spondylosis is usually much less acute.

Diagnosis

A stiff neck is the key symptom, and it may not be very painful. If your signs and symptoms become troublesome, your doctor may request a neck X-ray or a computerized tomography (CT) scan or magnetic resonance imaging (MRI) to assess how much the spurs interfere with your nerve roots and spinal cord and if there's a need for surgery.

If you have pressure on the spinal cord or nerve roots, your doctor may recommend a myelogram (see page 610) to obtain additional diagnostic information.

How serious is cervical spondylosis?

The signs and symptoms of cervical spondylosis are often mild and may not require medical treatment. Your discomfort may be long term or occur only under certain circumstances, such as sleeping in the wrong position or turning your head suddenly. In a few cases when there's pressure on the spinal cord or nerve roots, cervical spondylosis can cause permanent disability.

Treatment

For mild cervical spondylosis, your doctor may recommend exercises, the use of a neck collar or traction therapy. Traction involves using a head halter, carefully selected weights and a pulley arrangement to stretch your neck for 15 to 30 minutes at a time. For a more severe case, hospitalization may be required.

Medication

To relieve pain, your doctor may prescribe pain medication or a muscle relaxant.

Surgery

Surgery may be required to remove the bone growths and to fuse your vertebrae. Fusion of two or more vertebrae stiffens that part of the neck or back. This helps prevent painful movement or neurologic problems related to compression of the spinal cord or nerve roots by the unstable spine.

Peripheral neuropathies

Signs and symptoms

- A tingling sensation in the hands or feet
- Numbness in the same areas
- Unsteadiness or lack of coordination
- Weakness and pain of the feet and hands

Your peripheral nervous system is the network of nerves necessary to initiate all bodily movement (motor nerves) and allow sensation (sensory nerves). This network reaches all parts of the body and is connected to your central nervous system at the brain stem and at many points along the spinal cord.

Your peripheral nerves allow communication between the brain and organs, blood vessels, muscles and skin. Your brain's commands are conveyed to muscles by motor nerves and information is delivered to your brain via sensory nerves.

Damage to a peripheral nerve can interrupt communication between the area it serves and your brain. This can impair your ability to move muscles or feel normal sensations, or both, in an affected area. A damaged nerve can also produce tingling, burning and other painful sensations in the affected area.

Peripheral neuropathy is the term used to describe damage to your peripheral nerves. With minor damage, you may have acute burning pain, whereas major damage can result in imbalance or muscle weakness. You may have damage to a single nerve, as in carpal tunnel syndrome, or damage to many nerves, as in Guillain-Barre syndrome.

The causes of peripheral neuropathy are numerous. A partial list includes traumatic injury, pressure on a nerve and nerve damage from autoimmune diseases such as lupus and rheumatoid arthritis. Some liver, kidney and thyroid diseases also can damage peripheral nerves.

Myelography

Myelography is a diagnostic examination that produces detailed X-ray images of your spine after injection of a dye into the spinal canal. It can be helpful in determining if undue pressure is being placed on your nerves or spinal cord.

Generally, hospitalization is required for the test, and no food or drink is allowed for several hours before it. You may be given a sedative.

The procedure

The test is performed while you're lying facedown on an X-ray table that can be tilted. A local anesthetic is injected into the skin over the small of the back. You're given a spinal tap, a procedure in which a needle is inserted between two of your lower vertebrae and a small amount of your cerebrospinal fluid is withdrawn.

A contrast medium is injected slowly through the needle used in the spinal tap. A series of X-rays is made to show the configuration of the space around the spinal cord and determine if it's distorted by the presence of a protruded disk, bony spur or tumor. The diagnostic team can see the contrast medium in your spinal area on the X-rays. The table can be tilted up and down to move the medium to the location of the suspected disorder in your spine.

Once the contrast medium is in the appropriate location, X-rays are taken from different angles until the problem area can be seen clearly. While the contrast is still in, a computerized tomography (CT) scan may be done to further evaluate the area of concern. Most contrast agents are absorbed by the bloodstream and excreted in the urine. They generally don't have to be removed when the procedure has been completed.

You may feel some pressure or nausea during the injection, although preparation beforehand should minimize these effects. The procedure generally takes 45 to 90 minutes. After the procedure, you may have a headache because of changes in the pressure of your cerebrospinal fluid. Lying down will help alleviate your headache, which is usually short-lived.

Risks and benefits

Some risks are associated with myelography. Certain conditions, such as pressure on your spinal cord from a tumor or herniated disk, can be worsened by the change in cerebrospinal fluid pressure. A prompt operation may be necessary, but significant complications are rare.

Noninvasive diagnostic tests, such as a computerized tomography (CT) scan or magnetic resonance imaging (MRI), provide good resolution and are often used for general diagnosis of spinal disorders. In many cases, though, myelography combined with CT continues to be the preferred test because its resolution is generally sharper. In addition, cerebrospinal fluid obtained from the spinal tap can be used to check for evidence of infection, inflammation and cancer.

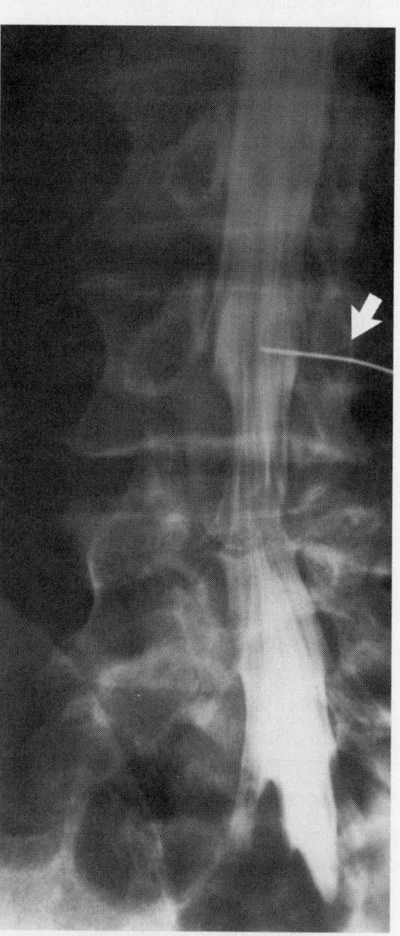

In myelography, a liquid dye (contrast medium) is injected through a needle (see arrow) into the space around your spinal cord.

Microorganisms can attack your nerves directly and result in peripheral nerve damage. Toxic substances, including heavy metals (lead, mercury, arsenic), carbon monoxide, organic solvents and even some medications, especially those used to treat cancer, can damage peripheral nerves.

The most common causes of peripheral neuropathy, though, are diabetes, alcoholism associated with poor nutrition and vitamin deficiency. With diabetes, signs and symptoms of a peripheral neuropathy may first appear after you've had the disease for many years. If your diabetes is poorly controlled, signs and symptoms may occur much earlier.

Among individuals with alcoholism, an inadequate diet — especially one deficient in the vitamin thiamine — can contribute to neuropathy. Pernicious anemia also may occur and increase the chances for peripheral neuropathy. Pernicious anemia occurs when your body is deficient in vitamin B-12.

Signs and symptoms of peripheral neuropathy usually progress over many months, but in certain cases, such as arsenic poisoning, the onset may be abrupt.

A tingling sensation (paresthesia) usually begins in your toes or the balls of your feet and spreads upward. Occasionally, it begins in your hands and extends up your arms. Numbness may proceed in the same way. Your skin may become sensitive, and even the lightest touch can be painful. In some peripheral neuropathies, weakness may come before or may be more noticeable than the sensory signs and symptoms.

A common peripheral neuropathy called meralgia paresthetica is characterized by burning sensations, numbness and sensitivity on the outside of your thigh.

Diagnosis

Because peripheral neuropathies can result from a wide range of diseases and conditions, the cause for your particular disorder may be difficult or impossible to diagnose. Your doctor may begin by asking you several questions about your signs and symptoms, medications you're taking, recent viral illnesses, alcohol consumption, possible toxic exposure and whether your family or co-workers have similar signs and symptoms.

A physical and neurologic examination may follow. Possible diagnostic tests will depend on your answers to the questions and the results of the examinations. They may include blood tests, urinalysis, a chest X-ray, metabolic tests, thyroid function studies, electromyography, a spinal tap or, possibly, a nerve biopsy, in which sample nerve tissue is removed and examined under a microscope.

How serious are peripheral neuropathies?

In contrast to the nerves in your central nervous system, peripheral nerves may regenerate with proper care. In some disorders, recovery occurs, but signs and symptoms may recur if the cause isn't eliminated.

Diabetic neuropathy can affect many parts of your body and may cause a number of complications. For instance, if the nerves related to digestion are damaged, your stomach may empty slowly resulting in nausea, vomiting and bloating. Or you may have frequent constipation or diarrhea. Damage to the nerves in your feet increase the risk of pressure-related injuries and, along with poor circulation, can lead to skin ulcers and even gangrene.

Treatment

Therapy is directed at the cause of the neuropathy. This may mean better control of the underlying cause, such as getting regular injections of vitamin B-12 for pernicious anemia, keeping your blood sugar (glucose) level close to normal if you have diabetes or avoiding alcohol.

Physical therapy may help you to maintain muscle strength and avoid muscle cramping or spasms. Mechanical devices may also be needed for mobility.

Medications

Medications can ease pain symptoms, but most have side effects, especially if taken for long periods of time. If you take pain medication regularly, including over-the-counter products, discuss the benefits and side effects with your doctor. Medications that may help relieve neuropathic pain include:

- *Pain relievers.* Nonprescription medications such as acetaminophen (Tylenol, others), aspirin, and ibuprofen (Advil, Motrin, others) usually help mild symptoms. For more severe symptoms, your doctor may recommend prescription nonsteroidal anti-inflammatory drugs (NSAIDs).

  If you take aspirin or other NSAIDs for long periods of time or in large doses, you can develop nausea, stomach pain or bleeding, ulcers and kidney problems. Risk of these conditions increases as you grow older, especially for a woman.
- *Tricyclic antidepressants.* Antidepressant medications, such as amitriptyline (Elavil), nortriptyline (Aventyl, Pamelor), desipramine (Norpramin) and imipramine (Tofranil), may relieve mild to moderate pain by interfering with chemical processes in your brain that cause you to feel pain.

  Common side effects of these medications include dizziness, dry mouth, nausea, tiredness or weakness, constipation and weight gain. To help reduce these symptoms, your doctor may start you off at a low dose and slowly increase the amount of the drug you take.
- *Antiseizure medications.* Drugs developed for seizure disorders, such as gabapentin (Neurontin), carbamazepine (Carbatrol,

Tegretol), phenytoin (Dilantin), along with other, newer anti-seizure medications, are often prescribed to treat jabbing or burning pain. Side effects of these medications may include drowsiness and confusion.
- *Other drugs.* Mexiletine (Mexitil), a drug used to treat irregular heart rhythms, sometimes helps relieve burning pain. Side effects of mexiletine range from dizziness and lightheadedness to nausea, vomiting, shaking hands and difficulty walking. The topical ointment capsaicin (Capzasin, Zostrix) may help ease the pain of small-fiber neuropathies typically associated with diabetes. It may take 1 to 2 weeks before you see results with capsaicin, but aside from a mild tingling, burning or slight skin irritation where you apply the ointment, there are few side effects.

Guillain-Barre syndrome

Signs and symptoms
- Numbness and tingling beginning in the fingers or toes
- Muscle weakness

Emergency signs and symptoms
- Widespread tingling and numbness
- Difficulty breathing

Guillain-Barre syndrome is a collection of signs and symptoms resulting from inflammation and destruction of the protective covering (myelin sheath) surrounding the peripheral nerves, those outside the brain and spinal cord. The syndrome is acute and frequently causes severe damage to part or all of your peripheral nervous system.

The cause of Guillain-Barre syndrome is unknown, but many doctors and scientists now believe that it's a disorder of the immune system. Research indicates that the immune system may attack the myelin sheath that covers the peripheral nerves, preventing the nerves from transmitting signals to the muscles. If muscles are unable to receive nerve commands, weakness or paralysis may occur. The brain also receives fewer sensory signals, resulting in the inability to feel heat, cold, pain and other sensations.

In two-thirds of the cases, the syndrome follows an infectious illness, such as flu, a cold, Epstein-Barr virus or campylobacteriosis, a gastrointestinal syndrome caused by the bacteria *Campylobacter jejuni.* Hodgkin's disease also may precede the syndrome. Guillain-Barre syndrome sometimes follows a medical procedure. Five percent to 10 percent of all cases occur following an operation.

For a brief period, a vaccine was thought to be a potential cause. Initial concern was raised when many cases of Guillain-Barre syndrome were reported after a major flu (influenza) vaccination program in 1976 and 1977. Further study revealed that the number of cases was no greater than would've occurred without the vaccination. People who receive influenza vaccine aren't at increased risk of developing Guillain-Barre syndrome.

Signs and symptoms can appear within 1 to 4 weeks after an infection or operation. Tingling sensations in your fingers and toes may be followed by general muscle weakness. A sensation of weakness usually spreads from your legs to

COMPLEMENTARY MEDICINE

Several drug-free therapies and techniques may help relieve pain associated with peripheral neuropathy. These therapies are frequently used in conjunction with medications, but some may be effective on their own. Complementary therapies used in the treatment of peripheral neuropathy include:
- Biofeedback
- Acupuncture
- Hypnosis
- Relaxation techniques

For information on these therapies, see Chapter 42, "Pain Management," and Chapter 43, "Complementary and Alternative Medicine."

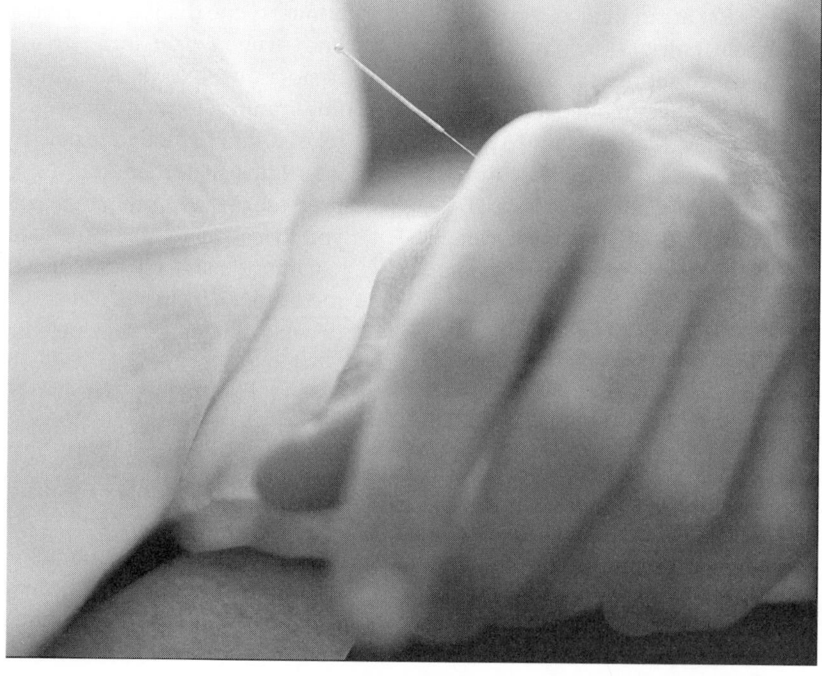

your arms and face. In some cases, the weakness may be severe enough to produce paralysis, and your respiratory muscles may be affected. The muscles responsible for eye movement, facial movements, speaking, chewing and swallowing may become weak or paralyzed.

The syndrome can strike at any age and occurs at a rate of 3,500 cases annually in the United States and Canada.

Diagnosis

A diagnosis of Guillain-Barre syndrome is generally based on signs and symptoms, a physical examination and diagnostic tests, including an analysis of cerebrospinal fluid obtained by a spinal tap, or lumbar puncture (see page 578).

How serious is Guillain-Barre syndrome?

In its most severe form, Guillain-Barre syndrome is a medical emergency that requires hospitalization. Some people with Guillain-Barre syndrome need respiratory assistance at some point during the illness. Fifty percent to 90 percent of individuals affected recover completely over a period of months. If you're severely affected, you'll likely need long-term rehabilitation to regain your independence. Some permanent impairment remains in about 15 percent to 20 percent of cases. The mortality rate is 5 percent or less.

Treatment

Guillain-Barre syndrome generally is treated by supportive care. A procedure called plasmapheresis, which removes plasma and damaging antibodies from your blood, may be used during the first few weeks of a severe attack. Intravenous infusions of immunoglobulin, which contains healthy antibodies from blood donors, also may be beneficial, especially if given early. These treatments may improve your chance of a full recovery.

Once your condition is stabilized, rehabilitation therapy will likely be initiated. Whirlpool hydrotherapy may be used to relieve pain and facilitate movement retraining. Physical therapy that includes passive exercise can be done safely during the acute phase of the illness. After your signs and symptoms subside, your rehabilitation team will prescribe an active exercise routine to help you regain muscle strength and independence. For some individuals, training with adaptive devices, such as a wheelchair or a brace, may be necessary.

Charcot-Marie-Tooth disease

Signs and symptoms

- Weakness in the legs and, to a lesser degree, the arms
- Absence of muscle-stretch reflex
- Foot deformity

Charcot-Marie-Tooth disease is a broad term for a group of hereditary disorders caused by degeneration of peripheral nerve fibers or the insulating covering (myelin sheath) over the fibers. The disease is named after the three doctors who simultaneously described it over a century ago — Jean Martin Charcot and Pierre Marie in France and Howard Henry Tooth.

The disorder most often affects the legs, feet and hands. It generally results in muscle weakness and loss of muscle bulk. In some cases, it may cause a mild loss of sensation. Initial signs include foot abnormalities, such as an excessively high arch or flexed toes. It may be difficult to lift your foot.

Signs and symptoms frequently become obvious between mid-childhood and age 30, but they may also appear late in life. They tend to develop slowly and sometimes appear to stabilize spontaneously. The disorder affects about 100,000 to 125,000 people in the United States.

Diagnosis

A diagnosis of Charcot-Marie-Tooth disease generally includes a physical and neurologic examination, electromyography and, rarely, a biopsy of a nerve in the leg. Genetic tests are now available that may help diagnose some of these neuropathies.

How serious is Charcot-Marie-Tooth disease?

The disorder isn't life-threatening. The severity of signs and symptoms varies from person to person, but foot abnormalities and difficulty walking are generally the most serious problems. Only rarely is a wheelchair necessary. Most people with this disorder can lead active, vigorous lives.

Treatment

Vocational counseling or leg braces may be needed, as may an orthopedic operation or corrective shoes to improve walking. Future treatment could possibly include use of gene replacement therapy.

Syringomyelia

Signs and symptoms

- Gradual loss of sensation in the nape of the neck, shoulders and upper arms
- Weakness of the arms or legs

In syringomyelia, a fluid-filled cavity forms on the spinal cord, usually in the neck area. The cavity may expand gradually along the spinal cord. Pressure from the cavity may damage the cord, producing a number of signs and symptoms. Initially, the sense of heat or touch may be reduced, followed by the wasting of muscles.

Syringomyelia may result from spinal cord trauma, a tumor or a congenital defect that triggers the disease in adolescence or early adulthood.

Diagnosis

A neurologic examination can reveal loss of sensation or movement. Tests to determine the severity and location of the cavity may include computerized tomography (CT), myelography (see page 610) or magnetic resonance imaging (MRI).

How serious is syringomyelia?
Often, the progression of signs and symptoms is slow, but if untreated, severe disability can develop.

Treatment
Surgical therapy to drain the cavity and decompress the spinal cord frequently stops progression of the disorder. About half the individuals with syringomyelia improve significantly after the operation.

Myelomeningocele

Signs and symptoms
- A sac protruding from the spinal cord on a newborn's back
- Weakness of the lower limbs

Myelomeningocele (open spina bifida) is a congenital defect that leaves a baby's spinal canal open along several vertebrae in the lower or middle back. It's a severe form of spina bifida, a condition where a baby's neural tube — the embryonic structure that develops into the spinal cord — fails to develop or close properly.

In myelomeningocele, the spinal cord and membranes protrude at birth because of the opening, forming a sac on the baby's back. In some cases, skin covers the sac. In other cases, tissues and nerves are directly exposed, making the baby prone to life-threatening infections. Either partial or complete paralysis is common.

The cause of the disorder is unknown, although factors that may increase risk of myelomenigocele include a neural tube defect in a previous child, lack of folic acid during pregnancy, certain antiseizure medications and diabetes.

Diagnosis
The condition is apparent at birth. In some cases, prenatal testing to check for spina bifida may be warranted.

How serious is myelomeningocele?
Most babies survive, although they may experience physical and neurologic problems, including lack of normal bowel and bladder control, and partial or complete paralysis of the legs. Between 70 percent and 90 percent of babies born with myelomeningocele also have excess fluid in the brain (hydrocephalus).

Children with both myelomeningocele and hydrocephalus may have learning disabilities. Other congenital malformations are often associated with myelomeningocele, such as syringomyelia, clubfoot or hip dislocation. Meningitis can occur with a leaking sac, so this defect should be promptly treated with surgery.

Treatment
Myelomeningocele usually requires surgery within hours to days after birth. Early surgery can help minimize the risk of infection associated with exposed nerves. It may also help protect the spinal cord from additional trauma.

During the procedure, a neurosurgeon places the spinal cord and exposed tissue inside the body and covers them with muscle and skin. Sometimes, a ventriculoperitoneal shunt, a tube that allows fluid in the brain to drain into the abdomen, is placed during the operation on the spinal cord. At times, the shunt placement isn't needed until weeks to months later.

Paralysis and bladder and bowel problems usually occur with the disorder, and treatment for those conditions typically begins soon after birth.

In case of partial paralysis, special exercises that work the baby's legs and feet may be prescribed. They help prepare the child for walking with braces or crutches when he or she is older.

Many babies with myelomeningocele have spinal cords that are less able to properly grow in length as the they grow. This progressive tethering can cause loss of muscle function to the legs, bowel or bladder. Spinal cord surgery may allow the child to regain a normal level of functioning.

Neuralgias

Signs and symptoms
- Attacks of extremely sharp, stabbing pain or constant burning pain

Neuralgias are severe jabs of pain that extend along the path of one of your nerves. They may be due to injury or irritation of the nerve but, in many cases, the cause is unknown.

Your pain may include a background sensation of burning and aching with sharp, stabbing jabs superimposed on it. The pain comes in episodic attacks that might last for seconds or minutes, and the episodes may recur for days or weeks.

During an acute phase of the disorder, you may be hypersensitive to touch and to any slightly painful sensation. You may even find that sensations that normally aren't painful cause you pain.

Some neuralgias can occur as a result of the herpes zoster virus that causes shingles (postherpetic neuralgia) or a herpes simplex virus infection. Postherpetic neuralgia can be debilitating. It typically produces constant burning pain that's more prominent than the brief shooting or jabbing component. Contact or movement — even a movement such as sneezing — may provoke a new pain attack. Nerve pain can continue for weeks, months or sometimes years after all other signs of herpes virus infection have disappeared.

Trigeminal neuralgia, the most common of all neuralgias, is characterized by severe, sharp, electric shock-like pain on one side of your face, often triggered by talking, chewing or brushing your teeth (see page 616). A type of neuralgia called glossopharyngeal neuralgia is characterized by recurrent attacks of severe pain in the back of the pharynx, tonsils, middle ear and base of the tongue. The attacks may be precipitated by movements such as talking or swallowing, and the pain can be intense. Occipital

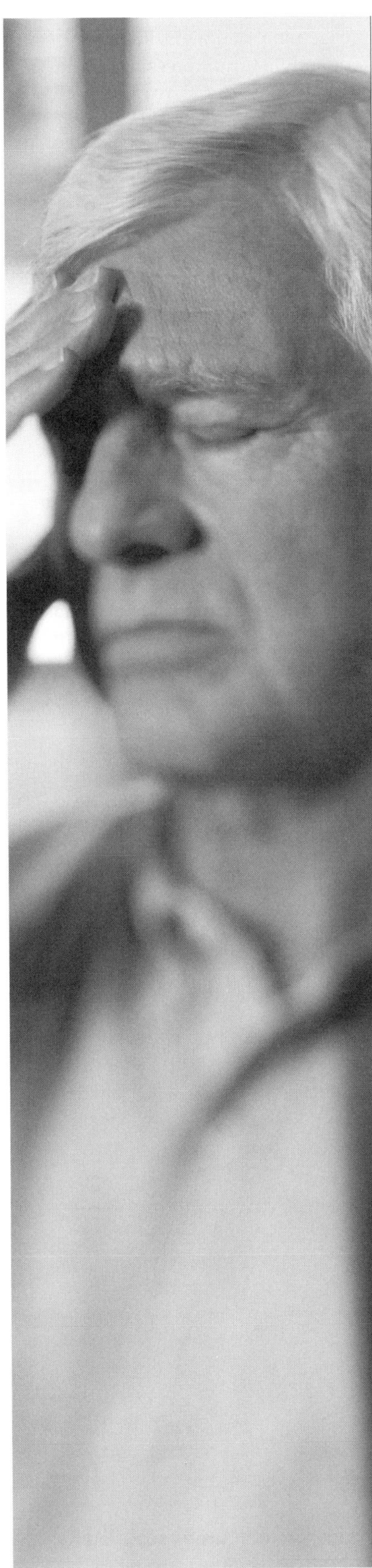

neuralgia causes pain in the back of your head that usually shoots into the scalp from behind the ears. Intercostal neuralgia occurs between your ribs.

Neuralgias usually strike after age 40 and occur most commonly in older adults.

Diagnosis

A diagnosis is generally determined by your signs and symptoms and by the exclusion of other disorders that may cause similar signs and symptoms.

How serious are neuralgias?

Although your pain may be incapacitating, the condition isn't life-threatening. Your attacks may come and go variably, but the time between them may grow shorter as you get older.

Treatment

The first line of treatment usually consists of medications to ease signs and symptoms. The type of medication your doctor prescribes will depend on the type of neuralgia you have and the severity of your signs and symptoms. If medications aren't effective, other procedures, including surgery, may be considered.

Medications

Medications that may help provide pain relief for neuropathy include:

- *Pain relievers.* Nonprescription pain relievers, such as acetaminophen (Tylenol, others), and nonsteroidal anti-inflammatory drugs (NSAIDs), such as aspirin and ibuprofen (Advil, Motrin, others), may help mild symptoms. For more severe symptoms, your doctor may recommend a prescription NSAID.

  If you take NSAIDs for long periods of time or in large doses, you may develop nausea, stomach pain or bleeding and ulcers. Large doses of NSAIDs can also lead to kidney problems and heart failure. Risk of these conditions increases as you grow older.
- *Topical analgesics and anesthetics.* Aspirin mixed into an absorbing cream or a nonprescription-strength lidocaine cream may reduce skin hypersensitivity.
- *Capsaicin.* This nonprescription cream, made from the seeds of hot chili peppers, may relieve skin hypersensitivity. Capsaicin (Capzasin, Zostrix) depletes your nerve cells of a chemical called substance P, which is involved in sending pain messages to your brain. You periodically rub the cream on the involved area of skin, usually three times a day.
- *Lidocaine skin patches.* These are small, bandage-like patches that contain the local anesthetic lidocaine. The patches, which must be prescribed by a doctor, are designed to be applied directly to painful skin and deliver relief for 4 to 12 hours.
- *Antidepressants.* Tricyclic antidepressant medications, such as amitriptyline (Elavil) and nortriptyline (Aventyl, Pamelor), may provide relief for mild to moderate symptoms by interfering with chemical processes in your brain that cause you to feel pain. They don't eliminate the pain, but they may make it easier to deal with. Other antidepressants that may be used to treat symptoms include venlafaxine (Effexor), bupropion (Wellbutrin), sertraline (Zoloft) and fluoxetine (Prozac).

  Common side effects of these medications include dizziness, dry mouth, nausea, weakness, constipation and weight gain. To help reduce these symptoms, your doctor will likely start off at a low dose and slowly increase the amount of drug you take.
- *Antiseizure medications.* Medications developed to treat seizures, such as gabapentin (Neurontin), carbamazepine (Carbatrol, Tegretol) and phenytoin (Dilantin), are often prescribed for jabbing pain. Side effects may include drowsiness and confusion.

- *Nerve block.* Doctors may use medications to block affected nerves. A local anesthetic can be injected to numb the area, relieving pain for a limited time. A long-term approach may involve blocking the nerves with oral drugs called neurolytics. These drugs destroy nerve tissue in a limited area, helping to relieve pain.
- *Other drugs.* Mexiletine (Mexitil), a drug ordinarily used to treat irregular heart rhythms, sometimes helps relieve burning pain. Side effects range from dizziness and lightheadedness to nausea, vomiting, shaking of the hands or difficulty walking.

Other procedures

Physical therapy may ease some neuralgias through the use of desensitization techniques. The following procedures are sometimes used for postherpetic neuralgia:

- *Transcutaneous electrical nerve stimulation.* Transcutaneous electrical nerve stimulation (TENS) involves placement of electrodes over the painful area. The electrodes are attached to a small, portable stimulator that you wear. The stimulator delivers tiny painless electric impulses that pass through the electrodes to nearby nerve pathways. You turn the TENS unit on and off as needed to control pain. Exactly how the impulses relieve pain is uncertain. One theory is that the impulses stimulate production of endorphins, your body's natural painkillers.
- *Nerve surgery.* A surgical procedure called dorsal root entry zone (DREZ) is considered a last resort by many doctors. The surgery involves destroying the point where damaged nerves join your central nervous system. This prevents the nerves from passing inappropriate pain messages to your brain. The surgery is risky because it involves disrupting several vertebrae in your spine.

Trigeminal neuralgia

Signs and symptoms

- Brief flashes of excruciating pain in the lips, gums, cheek, chin or, rarely, forehead

Trigeminal neuralgia, also called tic douloureux, is a condition of recurring pain on one side of your face. The pain — which emanates from one or more of the three branches of the fifth cranial (trigeminal) nerve — may be described as a ripping, darting or sharp cutting sensation that occurs in a portion of the face. An attack may last for seconds or a few minutes. Its intensity may cause facial muscle contraction, hence the term tic. Episodes may recur for days or weeks or months.

The pain associated with trigeminal neuralgia is caused by a disturbance in the function of the trigeminal nerve, which carries sensation from your face to your brain. However, there's no clearly identifiable cause for the disorder.

In many cases, a blood vessel that compresses or kinks part of the trigeminal nerve has been linked to trigeminal neuralgia. Less frequently, a tumor pressing on the nerve's covering may cause pain.

These painful attacks can be spontaneous. They may also be provoked by mild stimulation of the facial region that occurs when brushing your teeth, shaving or putting on makeup. The pain may be confined to a fairly small area of the face, or it may spread rapidly over a wider area. But it's always confined to areas where sensation is carried by the trigeminal nerve.

The disorder is seen most often in individuals over age 50 and frequently in those older than 70 years. Women are three times more likely to have trigeminal neuralgia than are men. For unknown reasons, the condition occurs more frequently on the right side of the face than on the left and doesn't occur simultaneously on both sides.

Diagnosis

The disorder is often diagnosed after excluding other conditions that may cause pain in your head, jaw, teeth or sinuses. Frequently, a person may undergo ineffective

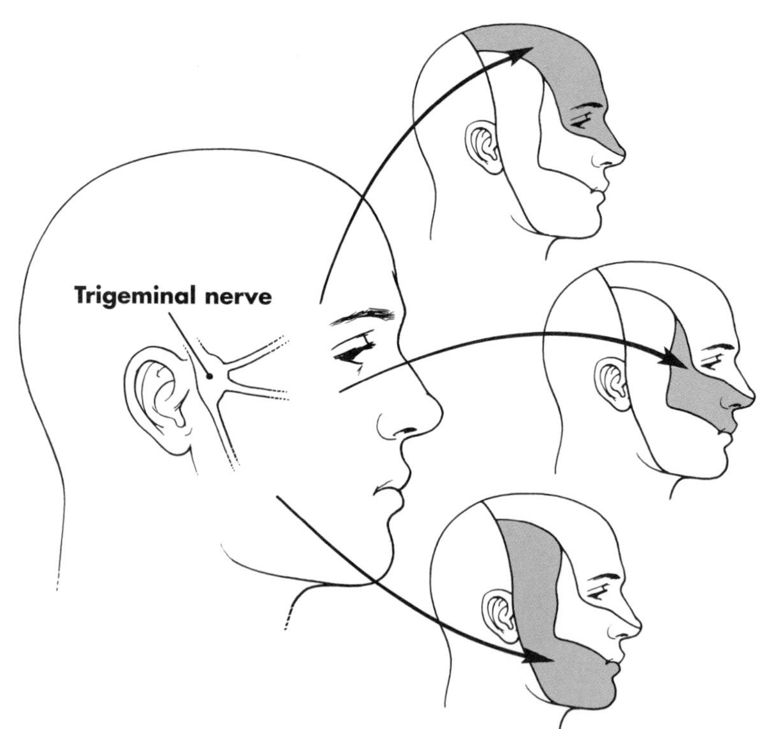

If you have trigeminal neuralgia, pain may occur in areas supplied by one of the three branches of the fifth cranial (trigeminal) nerve.

dental procedures to correct the pain before a diagnosis is made.

How serious is trigeminal neuralgia?

Although the pain may be incapacitating, it's not life-threatening. Attacks come and go variably, but periods of remission may grow shorter as you age. The condition can usually be effectively managed through the use of medication and other treatments.

Treatment

The main treatment options for people living with trigeminal neuralgia include medication to manage the pain and procedures that interfere with nerve function or that relieve the pressure on the trigeminal nerve.

Medications

Some of the more commonly used drugs include:

- *Carbamazepine.* Carbamazepine (Carbatrol, Tegretol) is the medication most commonly used to treat trigeminal neuralgia. In the early stages of the disease, carbamazepine controls pain 70 percent to 80 percent of the time. Over time, the effectiveness of the drug tends to decrease. Side effects of this medication include dizziness, double vision, sleepiness and nausea.
- *Phenytoin.* Phenytoin (Dilantin) was the first medication used to treat trigeminal neuralgia. Its effectiveness may increase if used in combination with carbamazepine or baclofen. Side effects of this medication include severe drowsiness.
- *Baclofen.* Baclofen (Lioresal) is a muscle relaxant often useful in treating trigeminal neuralgia. Its effectiveness may increase if used in combination with carbamazepine or phenytoin. Side effects of this medication include confusion, depression and severe drowsiness.
- *Oxcarbazepine.* Oxcarbazepine (Trileptal), an antiseizure medication, may be useful in treating trigeminal neuralgia. Side effects of this medication include dizziness and double vision.

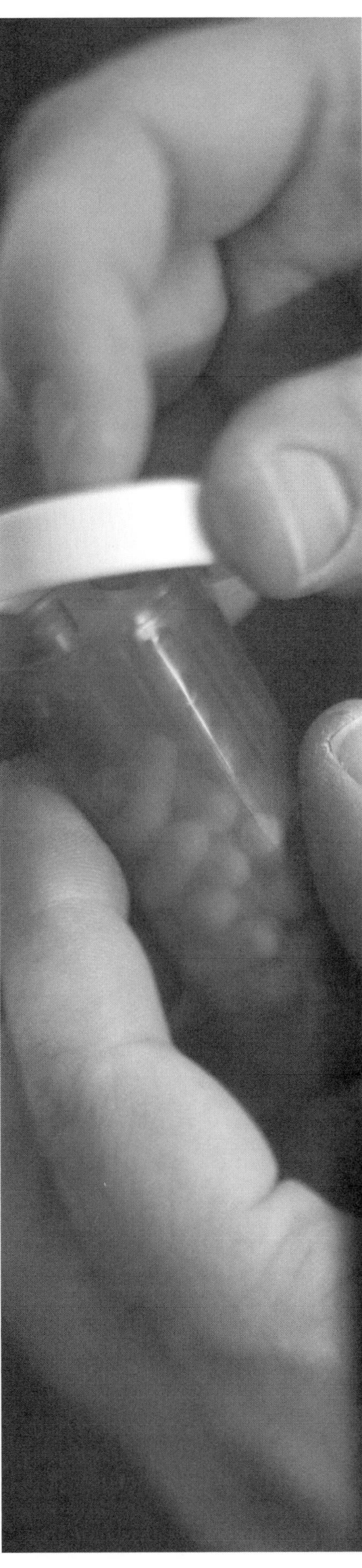

Percutaneous procedures

These procedures are intended either to interfere with nerve function or to numb the area where the pain occurs. Alcohol injections given under the skin of the face can offer temporary relief by numbing painful areas for days or months. Repeated injections are often required.

Several more invasive — albeit longer-lasting — procedures focus on damaging the nerve root (ganglion) to reduce or eliminate the sensation of pain. In each of these procedures, a hollow needle is inserted through the face into one of the openings in the skull. The tip of the needle is positioned near the ganglion. The needle is used as a pathway to damage the nerve.

- *Percutaneous balloon compression of the trigeminal nerve.* Pressure is applied to the root of the trigeminal nerve to reduce or eliminate pain. A balloon at the end of the catheter is inflated with enough pressure to damage the nerve so that pain signals are blocked. This treatment is successful in about 80 percent to 90 percent of people who undergo it.
- *Percutaneous glycerol rhizotomy.* A substance called glycerol is injected through the needle to damage the trigeminal nerve and block pain signals. Initially, the procedure works in about 80 percent to 90 percent of people who undergo it, but the pain recurs in about 60 percent of people, and as many experience mild facial numbness or tingling.
- *Percutaneous stereotactic radiofrequency thermal rhizotomy.* An electrode is threaded through the needle and advanced until it rests against the nerve root. An electric current is passed through the electrode, creating a lesion on nerve fibers to block pain. The procedure is successful in about

80 percent to 90 percent of cases. A common side effect is mild to severe facial numbness.

Surgery

Surgical procedures to manipulate nerve pathways also are available, but they often carry the greatest risk:

- *Microvascular decompression.* This neurosurgical procedure works to remove or relocate blood vessels that may be putting pressure on the trigeminal nerve. Although microvascular decompression has the highest success rate, it also carries a risk of significantly decreased hearing, facial weakness, and, in rare cases, major stroke or death.
- *Gamma Knife radiosurgery.* This is a noninvasive treatment that delivers single high doses of radiation to the root of the trigeminal nerve in an effort to damage the nerve ending and eliminate the pain. Because it's relatively new, long-term effects of the procedure aren't known. ■

CHAPTER 23 PART V

Eyes

Your eyes are a small part of your body, but they play a large role in your life. They're exceptional and unique instruments, able to receive in an instant millions of unrelated pieces of information about the world around you. With your eyes you experience the shape, color and motion of your surroundings.

The eye is often compared to a camera, and there are some similarities. Like a camera, the eye lets light enter through a small opening. An adjustable lens focuses the light onto a layer of light-sensitive cells at the back of the eyeball, comparable to the light-sensitive film in a camera.

This comparison, however, doesn't do justice to your eyes. They're far more complex and sophisticated than any technology developed. Thousands of times a day, your eyes move and focus on images near and far, picking out objects for inspection and interpretation from a vast available field.

Parts of the Eye

The eye is composed of many intricate parts. Each one plays an essential role in the healthy functioning of the eye.

Orbit

Your eyes are cradled in sockets formed by a protective structure of bone known as orbits. The orbits include portions of the bones of the cheek, forehead, temple and nose. Unlike many other bones in your body, these eye protectors usually don't weaken or thin with age. Small deposits of fat cushion the eyeball within the orbit.

The upper and lower eyelids help protect the front of your eyeball by blocking dirt and bright light that can damage your eyes. The eyelids also lubricate your eyeball during each blink. Blinking washes away dust, pollen and other foreign bodies. The lubricant, familiar to us as tears, comes from lacrimal glands above each eye. Tears drain from each eye into your nose through a tiny opening close to where the eyelids join your nose. From this opening, tears are channeled to your nose by the nasolacrimal ducts.

Sclera

When you look in the mirror and see the white of your eye, you're looking at the sclera. This tough, white, leathery coating forms the circular eyeball shape and protects the eye's delicate internal structures. The sclera has an opening at the front that allows light to enter the eyeball.

A thin, moist, clear membrane called the conjunctiva covers the exposed front portion of the sclera. This tissue layer also lines the inside of your eyelids. The conjunctiva helps lubricate your eye.

Cornea

At the front of your eye, covering the opening in the sclera, is a domed layer of clear tissue called the cornea. The cornea juts out from the eyeball as a tiny bulge. Its convex surface bends the light as it enters the eye, helping to focus the images you see. The cornea, in fact, provides about two-thirds of the focusing power of the eye.

The cornea also protects your eye. It's packed with sensitive nerve endings. If even a tiny speck of dust hits the cornea, you get the message instantly. If tears can't wash away the foreign material, continuing pain prods you to locate and remove the material.

Pupil

The pupil lies behind the cornea. The pupil is the dark spot in the center of your eye. It's through the pupil that light passes into your eye.

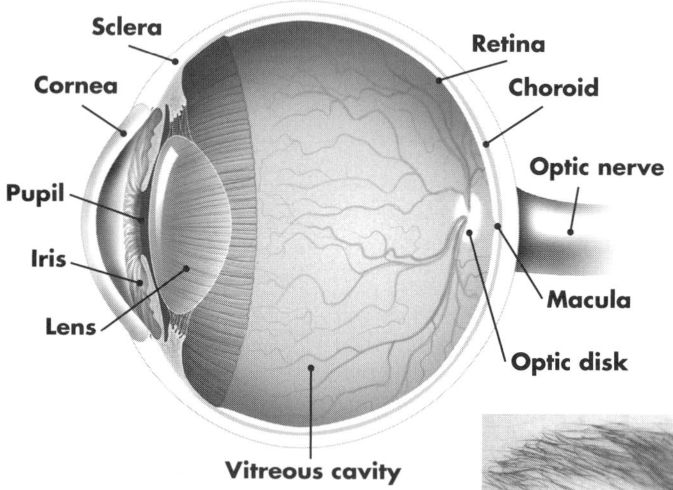

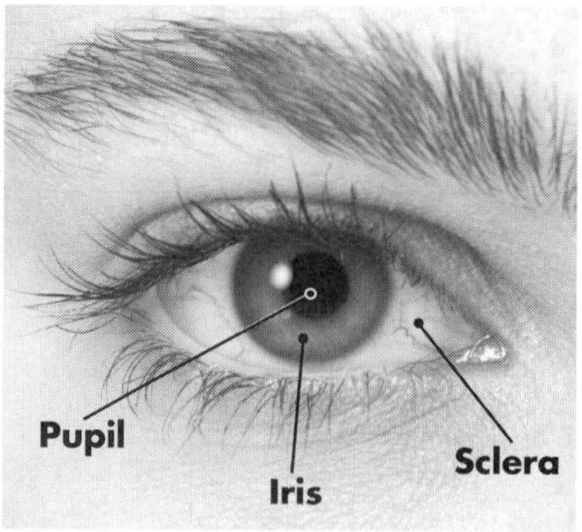

The eye is a complex and compact structure measuring about 1 inch in diameter. Yet in an instant, the eye can receive millions of pieces of information about the outside world, which are quickly processed by the brain.

Iris

Surrounding the pupil is the iris, the colored part of the eye. Its color comes from a pigment called melanin in the iris tissue. The more pigment, the darker the color. Brown eyes have a lot of pigment. Blue or green eyes have less.

The iris does more than add color to your eye. It contains a ring of muscle fibers that can expand or contract the size of the pupil to control the amount of light that enters the eyeball. In bright light, the iris reduces the size of the pupil. When the light is dim, the iris enlarges the pupil to let in more light.

The space between your cornea and iris is called the anterior chamber. It's filled with a clear fluid called the aqueous humor, which nourishes the cornea and lens, removes waste products and plays an important role in maintaining normal pressure in the eye. Fluid is continuously produced and circulated through the anterior chamber before draining out of the eye.

Lens

Behind the iris and anterior chamber is the lens, a clear elliptical structure. A circular muscle surrounds the lens. By relaxing or contracting, this muscle changes the lens' curvature to sharpen the focus of whatever you're looking at. When an object is nearby, the muscle contracts and the lens thickens. When an object is farther away, the muscle relaxes and the lens becomes thin. These adjustments allow the lens to change its focusing power. With age, the lens loses its elasticity, making it more difficult for you to focus on close objects.

Vitreous cavity

The vitreous cavity extends from the back of the lens to the retina, which covers the back of the eyeball. The cavity is filled with a colorless, gelatinous substance called vitreous humor. Both the aqueous humor in the anterior chamber and the vitreous humor maintain the pressure and shape of the eyeball.

You may occasionally notice what looks like tiny bits of string or lint moving through your vision. These "floaters" are tiny bits of material suspended in the otherwise clear vitreous humor. Usually, floaters are a result of aging, but they can be a sign of a more serious eye disorder.

Retina

Lining the interior back wall of the eyeball is a thin layer of tissue called the retina. The retina consists of millions of light-sensitive cells and nerve connections that capture the images focused by the cornea and lens.

The light-sensitive cells are shaped like either rods or cones. There are about 20 rod cells for every cone cell. Rod cells allow you to see in dim light, and they assist with your ability to see to the side while looking ahead (peripheral vision), but they can't distinguish colors. Cone cells distinguish color but require more light to function. This is why it can be hard to detect color in dim light. Cone cells are concentrated in the center of the retina and allow you to see sharp detail when looking straight ahead at a well-lit object.

Light striking the rods and cones triggers a chemical reaction. This in turn generates electric impulses that are relayed through the optic nerve and beyond to the visual cortex, the seeing portion of your brain.

The outer portion of the retina is nourished mainly by a layer of arteries and veins called the choroid, which is sandwiched between the retina and sclera. The inner part of the retina receives its nutrition from retinal blood vessels.

Macula and fovea

At the center of the retina is the macula, a small area that's densely packed with cone cells. The macula provides your central vision and allows you to see fine detail. A small depression in the center of the macula, called the fovea, contains only cone cells and provides the sharpest vision.

PREVENTION TIP

To help protect your eyes and vision:

- Have your vision checked regularly.
- Protect your eyes against sun damage. Buy sunglasses with ultraviolet-blocking lenses.
- Eat foods containing vitamin A and beta carotene, such as carrots, yams and cantaloupe.
- Optimize your vision with the right glasses when necessary.
- Use good lighting.
- Control chronic health conditions such as diabetes and high blood pressure.
- Recognize warning signs, such as sudden onset of hazy or blurred vision, flashes of light, black spots, halos or rainbows around lights or sudden loss of vision in one or both eyes.

Optic nerve

Visual information gathered by the retina is transmitted along nerve fibers to the optic nerve, a bundle of more than 1 million nerve fibers that connects the rear of the retina to the brain. The optic nerve serves as a communication cable between the eyes and brain.

Muscles of the eyeball

Each eye has six muscles attached to the sclera, allowing you to move both eyes and track an object without necessarily turning your head. These eye muscles, working independently or together, allow you to shift your visual field left, right, up, down, around and diagonally. Your brain coordinates these muscles so that both eyes move in unison.

How you see

A listing of all of the eye's parts may make the organ seem complicated. Yet the basic mechanism of sight is relatively simple.

Rays of light project through the cornea, the pupil and then the lens. Internal eye muscles help adjust the shape of the lens to focus the light rays on the retina. There, rods and cones turn the light into electric impulses that are carried by the optic nerve to the brain.

A special part of the brain — the visual cortex — interprets the electrical impulses. The image that the retina receives is upside-down and reversed — just like it is in a camera — because of the optical properties of the cornea and lens. The brain reinterprets the information so that you see the images in their correct orientation. The brain also processes the separate images from each eye and produces a three-dimensional image.

Common Vision Problems

You can see an object clearly only when it's properly focused. That means the cornea and lens have adjusted the point of focus by bending (refracting) the light rays so that the image falling onto the retina is sharply focused. If the focusing powers of the cornea and lens aren't coordinated with the length or shape of the eyeball, the image is blurry.

The most common eye problems — nearsightedness, farsightedness, astigmatism and presbyopia — are due either to errors of refraction of the lens and cornea or to an abnormal eye shape. Most of these conditions can be corrected with eyeglasses, contact lenses or surgery that changes the curvature of the cornea (refractive surgery).

Nearsightedness

Signs and symptoms

- Distant objects appear blurry

Nearsightedness (myopia) affects about 30 percent of the population. With this condition you can see clearly objects that are near to you, but objects farther away are blurry. If you're nearsighted, your eye is probably too long from front to back, causing the light rays refracted by the cornea and lens to meet in front of — rather than on — the retina.

The degree of your nearsightedness determines your focusing ability. People who are severely nearsighted are able to see clearly only objects that are a few inches from their eyes. Individuals who are mildly nearsighted may see clearly objects that are several yards away.

Occasionally, nearsightedness results not from an elongated eyeball but from too much focusing power in the lens and cornea. The result is the same — the light rays focus in front of the retina.

Nearsightedness often is first detected during childhood, from early school years through the later teens. A child may persistently squint, sit close to the television, movie screen or class chalkboard, hold books very close while reading and seem to be unaware of distant objects. The condition affects boys and girls equally and tends to run in families. Changes in vision may develop rapidly or slowly and gradually worsen during childhood and adolescence. The condition tends to stabilize during young adulthood.

Treatment

Nearsightedness is easily corrected. An eye specialist will perform a series of tests to determine the extent of the condition and the level of correction needed. Nearsightedness may be treated with eyeglasses or contact lenses. Another option is refractive surgery (see page 631).

Normal Vision

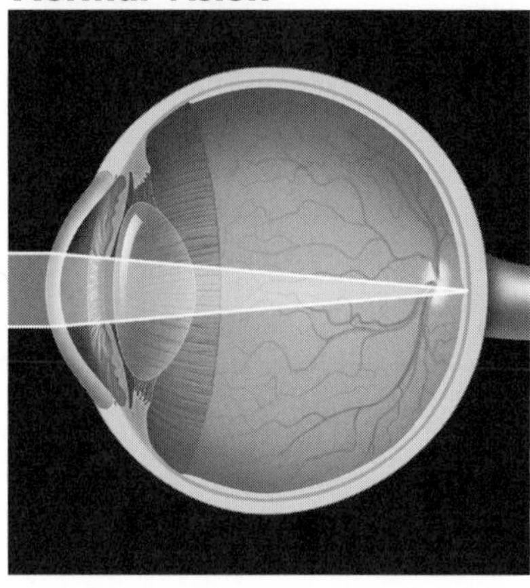

Nearsightedness

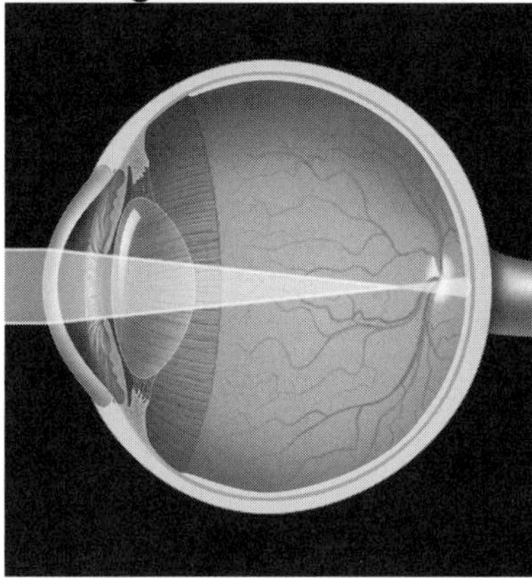

Farsightedness

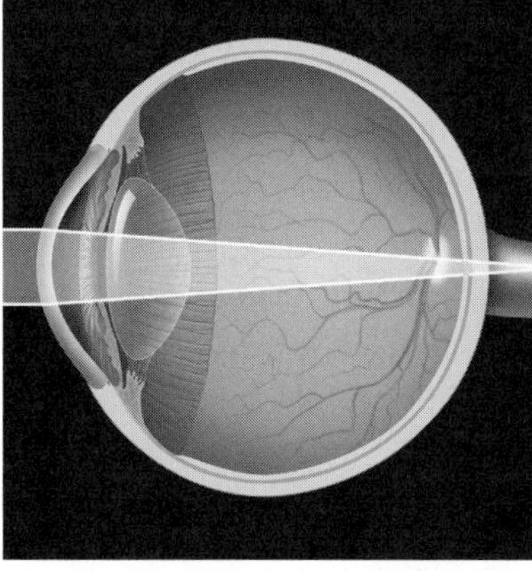

With normal vision, the image is sharply focused onto the retina. In nearsightedness (myopia), the point of focus is in front of the retina, making distant objects appear blurry. In farsightedness (hyperopia), the point of focus falls behind the retina, making close-up objects appear blurry.

Farsightedness

Signs and symptoms

- Nearby objects appear blurry
- Eyestrain, including aching eyes and headache

Farsightedness (hyperopia) is another common condition. You're able to see objects at a distance clearly but have difficulty focusing on objects that are near.

This condition usually results from the eyeball being too short from front to back. The rays of light coming into your eye aren't focused when they reach the retina, located at the back of the eye. Instead, the point of focus falls behind the retina. Farsightedness may also result from a weakness in the ability of the lens and cornea to focus because one or the other doesn't have a steep enough curvature.

Farsightedness usually is present at birth and tends to run in families. Most young people don't know they have the condition because their lens is flexible enough to compensate for the condition. So most young people with farsightedness don't need corrective lenses. But as they age, the lens becomes less elastic and unable to make the necessary adjustment. By middle age, most farsighted people need corrective lenses to improve their near vision.

Common symptoms of farsightedness include difficulty focusing on objects close at hand and sometimes headaches or general eye discomfort after doing close tasks such as reading, writing or drawing.

Treatment

If you're experiencing symptoms of farsightedness, see an eye specialist. He or she will conduct a series of tests to determine the nature and extent of the problem and the level of correction required to improve your vision.

Farsightedness is treated easily with eyeglasses or contact lenses. Surgery to treat farsightedness is available but the surgery isn't widely used.

Astigmatism

Signs and symptoms

- Portions of your visual field are distorted
- Vertical, horizontal or diagonal lines appear blurry

Astigmatism is a refractive error caused by an uneven curvature of the cornea. In a normal eye, the dome of your cornea is curved evenly and smoothly in all directions. In an astigmatic eye, the cornea typically has areas that are steeper or flatter than normal, blurring only some of what you see. In some instances, astigmatism results from abnormalities of the lens inside the eye, and the cornea is normal.

Astigmatism is usually present at birth and may occur in combination with nearsightedness (myopia) or farsightedness (hyperopia). The condition tends to remain constant, neither improving nor deteriorating significantly with age. Sometimes, astigmatism develops after an eye injury, disease or surgery.

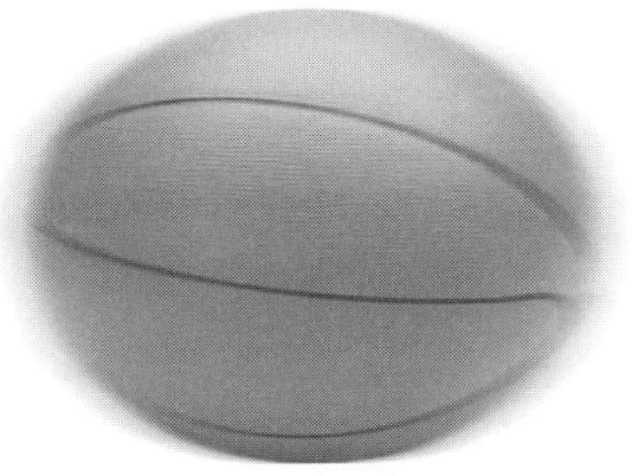

Astigmatism is caused by the uneven curvature of your cornea, which is unable to focus the light entering your eye evenly and creates distorted, blurry vision.

Eye Specialists

There are three main types of eye care professionals. They differ in their level of training and the tasks they perform.

Ophthalmologists

An ophthalmologist is a medical doctor (M.D.) who has, in addition to medical school training and a hospital-based general internship, at least 4 years of specialized training in caring for the eyes and diagnosing and treating eye ailments. In addition to providing complete eye examinations and eye care, an ophthalmologist also treats eye injuries and performs various surgical procedures.

An ophthalmologist is well trained in the use of specialized instruments to make a correct diagnosis, even if eye problems aren't obvious or are obscure. This can be crucial if the problem is serious and a delay of a few hours may make the difference between good vision and blindness.

Optometrists

An optometrist is trained to diagnose common eye conditions, such as refractive errors, and to prescribe corrective lenses. An optometrist graduates from a school of optometry and earns a doctor of optometry (O.D.) degree.

Optometrists can conduct certain tests, and often they can detect signs of eye disease from examination of the retina. Optometrists may be licensed to prescribe medications to treat eye diseases.

Opticians

An optician is a technician who fills eyeglass and contact lens prescriptions written by ophthalmologists and optometrists. An optician grinds and fits lenses but doesn't examine eyes for refraction problems or disease.

Vision Changes with Age

As you get older, your vision changes. If it doesn't, you're a rare exception. Many of these changes are primarily an annoyance, and most people learn to adjust.

- Often, the retina loses some of its sensitivity to light. To compensate, add brighter lighting to your workstation or favorite reading chair.
- Lenses in the eye may become less elastic and lose their ability to adjust their focus. You may need reading glasses or a magnifying glass for reading small print.
- Lenses in the eye may become cloudy and cause your visual acuity to decrease, colors to appear dim and glare to form when light shines directly at you. In this case, you may want to avoid night driving.
- Sometimes, the vitreous humor shrinks, which can produce bothersome floaters in your visual field. With time, most people get used to them. However, if you notice a sudden increase in the number of floaters, you should contact an eye doctor.

Older individuals are also at higher risk of other eye diseases and disorders. Although some vision problems are unavoidable, others can be prevented. And even those that are unavoidable often can be slowed or stopped through early detection and treatment. That's why it's important to have your eyes examined frequently.

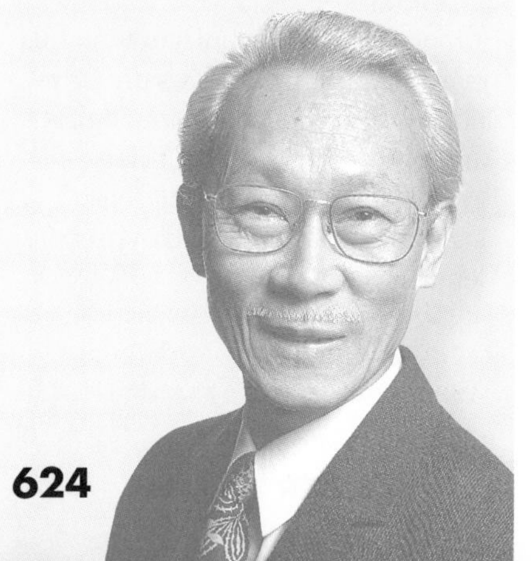

Treatment

Minor astigmatism may not cause signs or symptoms. The condition is generally first identified during an eye examination. Astigmatism is treated with a cylindrical corrective lens that corrects for the uneven curvature of the cornea. Hard contact lenses used to correct nearsightedness or farsightedness also correct astigmatism. Another option is surgery to reshape the curvature of the cornea. The procedure is similar to the surgery used to correct nearsightedness and farsightedness.

Presbyopia

Signs and symptoms

- Nearby objects appear blurry
- Eyestrain, including tired eyes and headache

The name *presbyopia* may be unfamiliar to you, but the condition probably isn't. With age, the lens becomes harder and less elastic, making it more difficult for you to see nearby objects clearly. This hardening process is a normal part of life, and it happens to everyone to some degree.

Many people begin to notice a change in their vision around age 40. If you're farsighted, you may encounter this problem even earlier in life. If you're nearsighted, you'll eventually experience presbyopia, although later in life than a normal-sighted person will.

Close-up objects that were once easy to see become blurred. The print in newspapers, books and restaurant menus seems smaller, and you instinctively hold them farther away from your eyes to be able to read them.

Treatment

An eye specialist can easily test your eyes for presbyopia. The condition is usually treated with glasses and only occasionally with contact lenses. As your lenses lose the ability to adjust, you may need a change in prescription every few years until about age 65. At that point, the lenses generally have lost most of their ability to accommodate, so changes in your prescription become less frequent.

If you're nearsighted or have astigmatism, you may need new lenses to counteract the effects of presbyopia. Fortunately, you don't have to constantly shuffle glasses because they can be made with lenses that have two or even three corrections. In a double (bifocal) lens, first introduced by Benjamin Franklin, the upper segment of the lens corrects your distance vision, and the lower segment corrects your near vision (see page 628).

Hereditary Disorders of the Eyes

Some conditions and diseases affecting the eyes can be passed from one generation to the next. These conditions range from simple nearsightedness (myopia) and farsightedness (hyperopia) to more serious eye diseases.

Heredity seems to play a role in the incidence of misaligned and weak eyes (strabismus and amblyopia). Defects of color vision (colorblindness) usually are present from birth. These defects are often passed down through the mother, usually to her sons. Eye diseases with a genetic factor include glaucoma, cataracts, retinitis pigmentosa and retinoblastoma.

Retinoblastoma, a cancerous tumor of the eye that affects young children, has a genetic component in 30 percent to 40 percent of cases. Other general disorders that can affect vision and have a hereditary component include diabetes and high blood pressure.

An Eye Examination

It's recommended that everyone have an eye examination from time to time. Individuals who wear glasses or contact lenses should have their eyes checked every year. People who don't wear glasses or contacts don't need an examination as often, unless they have a vision disorder or experience eye symptoms.

Infants usually get an eye exam from their pediatrician between birth and age 3 months and again between ages 6 months and 1 year. It's also recommended that children have their eyes examined at about ages 3 and 5. Children and adolescents should have an eye examination whenever they experience any problems with vision or symptoms of eye trouble.

If you don't wear glasses or contact lenses and don't have an eye disorder, consider having comprehensive eye examinations on the following schedule:

- At least once between ages 20 and 39
- Every 2 to 4 years between ages 40 and 64
- Every 1 or 2 years beginning at age 65

An eye examination involves a series of tests to evaluate different aspects of your vision, check for signs of disease and assess whether damage has occurred.

Visual acuity test

Acuity refers to the sharpness of your vision — how clearly you see an object. Using a Snellen chart, your eye doctor will check how well you read letters of decreasing size from across the room. Having 20/20 vision means that you can read letters that individuals with normal vision can read from 20 feet away.

Refraction assessment

Refraction refers to how lightwaves are bent as they pass through your cornea and lens. A refraction assessment helps your eye doctor determine a corrective lens prescription that will give you the sharpest vision.

Your eye doctor may use a computerized refractor to measure your eyes and estimate the prescription you need to correct a refractive error. Or he or she may use a technique called retinoscopy. In this procedure, your doctor shines a light into your eye and measures the refractive error by evaluating the movement of light that's reflected by your retina.

An eye doctor fine-tunes the refraction assessment by asking you to look through a Phoroptor, a device that contains wheels of different lenses. You look at the Snellen chart through various lenses and judge which combination of lenses gives you the sharpest vision.

Visual field test

Your visual field is the area in front of you that you can see without moving your eyes. Visual field testing (perimetry) is done in several ways. In one test, you look at a screen on which a computerized machine flashes spots of light in different locations and of varying brightness. You press a button each time you see a flash. The machine records your responses and maps the area you see. Gaps in your field of vision may indicate a serious eye disorder.

Another test uses the Amsler grid, named after the Swiss ophthalmologist who developed it. In the center of a square grid is a black dot. With one eye covered, you focus on the dot and tell your eye doctor whether you can see the entire grid clearly.

Glaucoma test

By measuring the internal pressure of your eye, your eye doctor can determine whether you're developing glaucoma. Two common techniques are used to measure eye pressure — air-puff tonometry and applanation tonometry. Both measure the amount of force needed to momentarily flatten (applanate) your cornea.

Visual Acuity Test

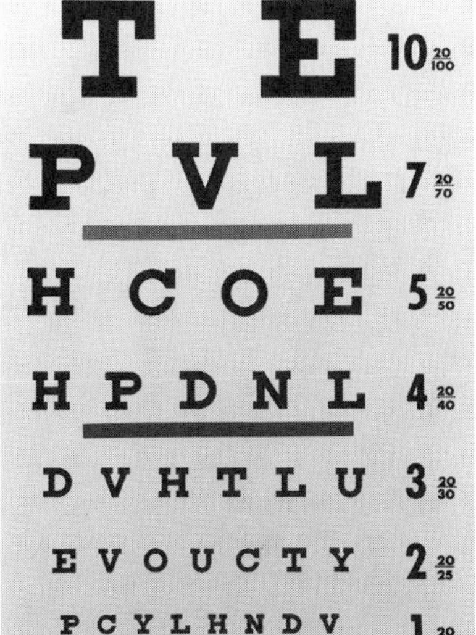

During a visual acuity test, you're asked to read letters of decreasing size on a chart at a fixed distance from you, usually 20 feet.

Refraction Assessment

A Phoroptor is a device that allows you to view a Snellen chart through different lenses. The lenses are changed until a combination is found that you feel gives you the sharpest vision.

External eye exam

An external eye exam is a quick check of your eyes with no special instruments other than a light. The eye doctor checks your pupils to see if they respond normally, your cornea and iris for clarity and shininess, and your eyes and eyelids for position and movement.

Slit-lamp examination

A slit lamp allows an eye specialist to see the structures at the front of your eye under magnification. The microscope is called a slit lamp because it uses an intense line of light — a slit — to provide a cross-sectional (oblique) view of the cornea, anterior chamber and lens. The illumination allows a doctor to detect and precisely locate any abnormalities.

When examining problems involving the cornea, your doctor may use fluorescein dye. The dye spreads across your eyes and appears bright yellow when hit with blue light. This causes tiny cuts, scrapes, tears, foreign material or infections on your cornea to stand out.

Retinal examination

In a retinal exam, your eye doctor puts dilating drops in your eyes to open your pupils wide and provide a better view of the back of your eye. Using a slit lamp or ophthalmoscope — an instrument that shines a bright light into your eye — an eye doctor can see abnormalities in the structures in the back of the eye, including the retina. This type of exam can help the doctor detect important clues about the presence of disease, such as diabetes and high blood pressure, elsewhere in the body.

Fluorescein angiography

Fluorescein angiography is a diagnostic test used to evaluate diseases of the retina and choroid. Fluorescein

Glaucoma Test

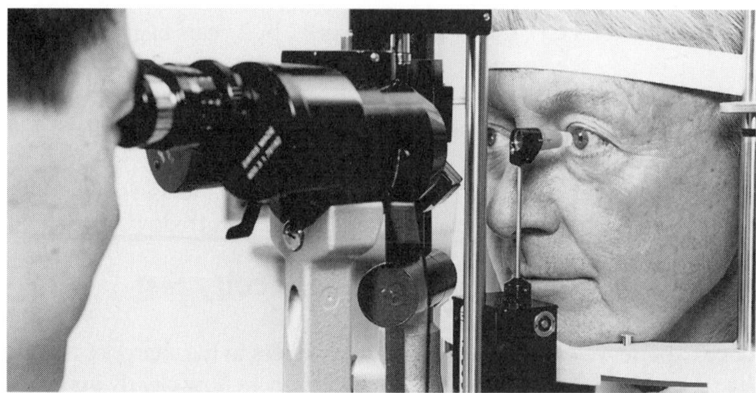

A tiny, flat-tipped cone is mounted on a slit lamp and positioned in front of your eye. By lightly touching the surface of the eye, the doctor measures internal eye pressure. High internal pressure may indicate glaucoma.

Slit-Lamp Examination

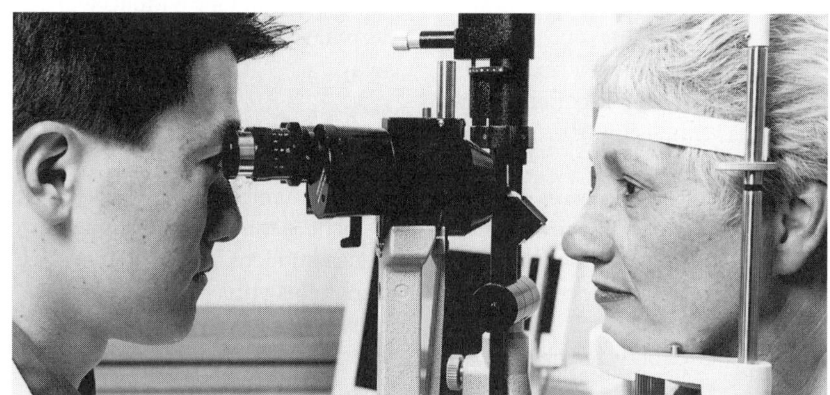

A slit of light is focused to provide an oblique view of the cornea. An eye specialist can also focus this light for a detailed view of the lens.

Retinal Examination

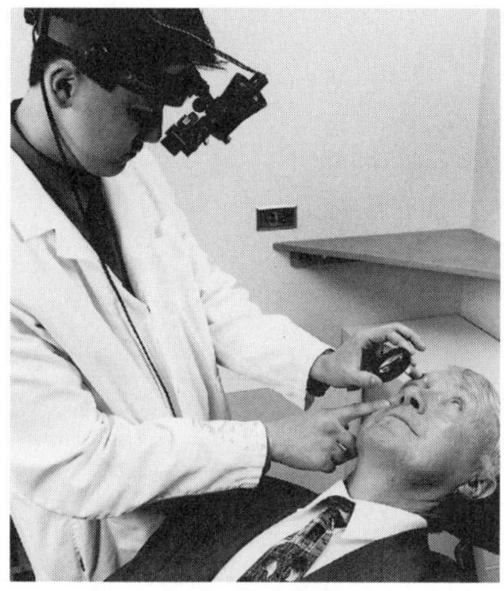

With the ophthalmoscope mounted on his head and a powerful lens held in front of the eye, an eye specialist shines a bright light into the eye to examine the entire retina.

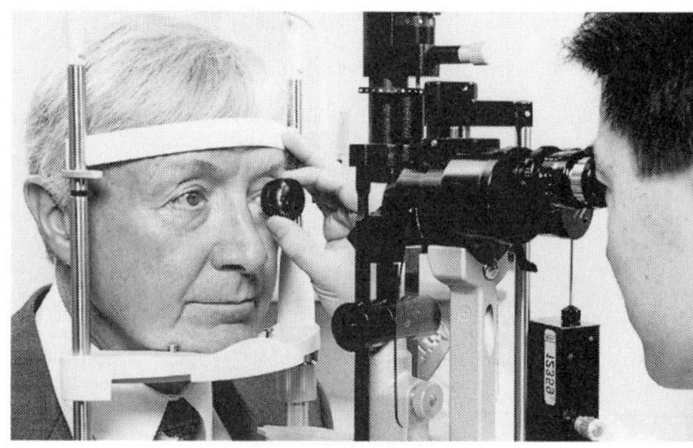

A slit lamp, assisted by a magnifying lens in front of the eye, gives an eye specialist a clear view of the central retina.

dye is injected into an arm vein. As the dye circulates through your eye, the blood vessels in your retina and choroid stand out as bright yellow, and pictures of your retina are taken. The images allow your doctor to assess blood vessel damage and to note the formation of any abnormal blood vessels. This is helpful in diagnosing conditions such as macular degeneration and diabetic retinopathy.

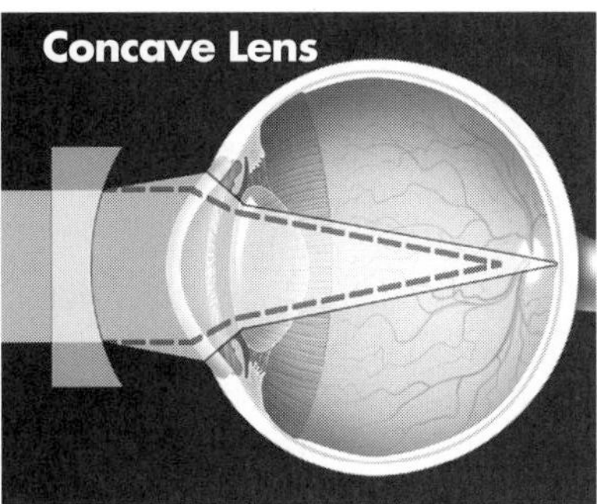

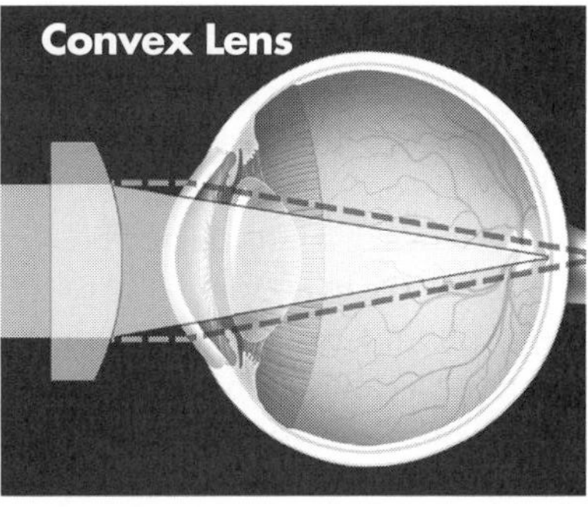

A concave lens (left) corrects for nearsightedness (myopia). The dashed line indicates where the point of focus would be without the corrective lens. A convex lens (right) corrects for farsightedness (hyperopia) and is commonly used in reading glasses. The dashed line indicates where the point of focus would be without the corrective lens.

Correcting Imperfect Vision

If you need to sharpen your vision, whether to see clearly at a distance or to read fine print, you have many options to choose from. These include a variety of eyeglasses and contact lenses and, in some cases, surgery to change your cornea's curvature.

You and your eye doctor can decide which option may work best for you. You'll want to take your individual needs into consideration. If you play sports, are very active or hate the look and feel of glasses, you may prefer contacts or the more permanent solution of surgery.

How corrective lenses work

Many vision problems are treated with lenses that compensate for abnormalities in the shape of your eye or the curvature of your cornea or lens. There are three basic shapes for corrective lenses:

- *Concave lenses* are thinner in the middle than on the edges. They correct for nearsightedness (myopia).
- *Convex lenses* are thicker in the middle than on the edges, as in a magnifying glass. These lenses correct for farsightedness (hyperopia) and are commonly used in reading glasses.
- *Cylindrical lenses* are curved more in one direction than the other to compensate for astigmatism.

If after a routine eye exam your doctor determines that you need corrective lenses, he or she will give you a prescription. It indicates the refractive power that each lens needs in order to correct your specific vision problem. The prescription numbers determine the shape and thickness of your lens. The higher the prescription numbers, the stronger the prescription — meaning the more that light must be refracted, the thicker the lens needs to be.

Eyeglasses

About 6 out of 10 Americans wear some kind of corrective lenses. About 8 out of 10 of those needing vision correction choose eyeglasses. Eyeglasses are available in many frame styles and lens designs. You can also purchase them in a variety of locations, including eye doctors' offices, eyeglass shops and discount stores.

Lens materials

Eyeglass lenses can be made of glass or plastic. Most eyeglass wearers choose plastic. Although glass lenses are usually more scratch resistant than plastic, they can be about twice as heavy. Another drawback of glass lenses is that they're more prone to break or chip, though the lens material must pass a breakage standard set by the Food and Drug Administration.

There are several types of plastic lenses:

- *High-resin plastic.* These plastic lenses are a bit thicker than glass but about half the weight. They're also easy to scratch, and for that reason some manufacturers routinely put a scratch-resistant coating on them.
- *High-index plastic.* This material is lighter and thinner than high-resin plastic lenses. That makes these featherweight lenses ideal for strong corrections. Unfortunately, they cost considerably more than high-resin plastic. They generally include a scratch-resistant coating and ultraviolet (UV) protection.
- *Polycarbonate plastic.* These are the strongest lenses available, which makes them a good choice for active kids and for use in safety glasses and sports glasses. Although they aren't as lightweight as the high-index lenses, they're lighter than high-resin. They generally come with scratch-resistant coating and UV protection.

Lens coatings

Lenses may be coated to offer:

- *Scratch protection.* A clear, hard coating is applied to lenses to make them more resistant to scratching. If you buy high-resin plastic lenses, you may want to pay the extra money for this treatment. Other plastic lenses have already been treated. Have both sides of a lens treated because you can accidentally scratch the inside when cleaning them. Be careful where you store your glasses because scratch-protection coating can crack and peel in extreme temperatures.

- *UV protection.* UV rays may contribute to several age-related eye diseases, such as cataracts and macular degeneration. When you're outside it's a good idea to wear glasses that filter out 100 percent of both UVA and UVB light. High-index plastic and polycarbonate plastic lenses have UV protection.
- *Anti-reflection coating.* Reflection and glare can make driving difficult, particularly at night. Anti-reflection (AR) coating helps block the light reflected off surfaces such as pavement, water, snow and glass. This is a big help if you have a strong prescription, which increases glare.

  AR coating has a few disadvantages. The chemical makeup makes it harder to keep your lenses clean. And frequent, hard cleaning can rub the coating off. Try to wipe them carefully with a lint-free cloth moistened with water or a lens cleaning solution. In addition, the scratch-resistant coating is generally applied before the anti-reflection coating, leaving the AR coating vulnerable to scratches.

Lens treatments

A final consideration in choosing lenses is whether you want any special treatment:

- *Photochromic lenses.* Photochromic lenses are chemically treated so that they automatically become dark in direct sunlight and clear in lower light. However, they won't get dark while you're driving unless the sun is shining directly on your face. So you may need sunglasses or clip-on sunglasses for driving. In addition, this treatment doesn't work as well on plastic lenses as it does on glass.
- *Tints.* Unlike photochromic lenses, which respond to various levels of brightness, tinted lenses remain a constant shade in all lighting conditions. Adding color to your glasses can help if you're especially sensitive to light and wish to use your lenses as sunglasses. Almost any color can be chosen for a tint. Sunglasses are often gray or brown. A yellow tint helps keep blue light from entering the lens and can make objects appear sharper.
- *Edge treatment.* If you're very nearsighted, the edges of your lens will be thick and can look unattractive. They also add unnecessary weight to your glasses, especially if you choose large frames. A skilled optician can grind the edges so that they blend into the frame.

Bifocal and trifocal lenses

Many people need only single-vision lenses to correct for nearsightedness (myopia), farsightedness (hyperopia) or astigmatism. Some need multifocal lenses, which are two or more lenses combined into one.

If you're nearsighted, farsighted or have major astigmatism, chances are that by the time you're in your 40s, you'll also need bifocals and eventually trifocals.

In bifocal lenses, the top portion is used for seeing at a distance and the bottom for reading. Trifocals add a third power, to help you see objects at an intermediate distance, such as a computer monitor, items on the grocery store shelf or books on a library shelf.

There are several common designs for multifocal lenses:

- *Flattop semicircle.* The reading, or up-close, section in bifocals and trifocals appears as a clearly defined semicircle at the bottom of each lens. The line separating the up-close correction from the rest of the lens can be polished out so that people don't know you have multifocal glasses. But your vision will be distorted in the small area where one corrective power merges into the other.
- *Executive style.* Instead of a semicircle, the line dividing the corrective powers runs all the way across the lens. This type of lens gives you the widest possible field of vision for close work and is often used with trifocals.
- *Progressive.* A progressive lens has no division lines. Trifocal correction is built into the lens, and the prescriptions change smoothly as

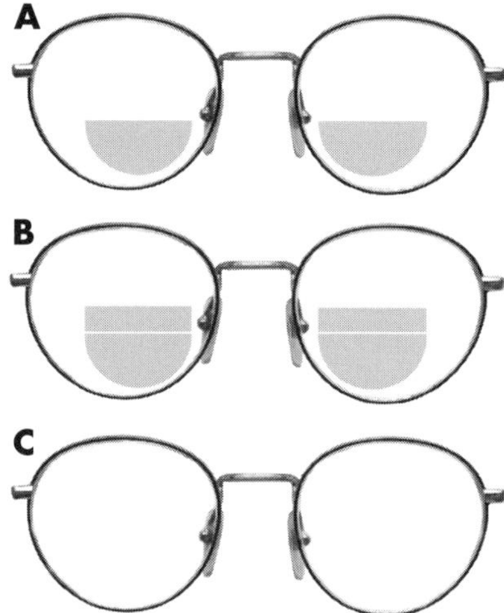

Bifocals (A). As the name implies, the bifocal style combines two focal powers in one lens. The top part of the lens corrects your distance vision, while the lower part (shaded) allows you to read and see objects clearly from a foot or so away.

Trifocals (B). The trifocal lens adds a third power for an intermediate focus between the other two. The added power helps you focus clearly on objects approximately 2 to 4 feet away, such as a computer monitor on a desk, packages on grocery store shelf or books on a library shelf.

Progressive (C). A progressive lens has no division lines in it. Instead the focal powers change smoothly as your eyes move from top to bottom. This means a trifocal, or intermediate, correction is built into the lens.

your eyes move from top to bottom. If you require a bifocal correction for the first time, many eye doctors suggest you try progressive lenses to avoid the occasionally bothersome lines separating the segments. One disadvantage of a progressive lens is that there may be some distortion along the bottom edge, near the reading section.

It takes practice getting used to bifocals and trifocals. Be sure your frames are properly adjusted to fit your head. As you tilt your head up and down, your line of vision should move smoothly from one segment of the lens to the other segment in both eyes at precisely the same time.

Nonprescription reading glasses

As you enter your 40s, you may find that you need glasses for reading only. You might be able to save some money by purchasing these glasses at a pharmacy or discount store.

Nonprescription reading glasses with lenses of various strengths are often on display alongside the sunglasses. Reading glasses can also be worn over your contact lenses that correct distance vision.

If your eye doctor has told you the correction that you'll need, look for lenses of that power. Otherwise try the trial-and-error method. The weakest reading lenses are labeled +1.00 diopters, and the strongest are +3.00. Test a few different powers by holding printed material about 14 to 16 inches from your eyes.

When you find a pair that allows you to read comfortably at that distance, that's probably the power you need. To give you an idea of the power you might need, here's a general guide that shows which power is commonly associated with each of several age ranges:

Eyeglass Frames

When you're looking for new glasses, you may be tempted to start with frames on the display rack. If you want to save time, start by considering your prescription. Your lens may be best suited to a frame that's a certain shape or size. For example, if your prescription calls for a thick lens, a thin wire frame might not be able to support its weight. A skilled optician can tell by your prescription what kinds of frames will work best for you.

When shopping for a pair of frames, keep these tips in mind:

- The size of your frame is important for your vision as well as your appearance. Very large frames can pick up too much glare from overhead lights and distort your vision. If the frame is too small, your field of vision may be limited.
- If you need strong — and therefore, thick — lenses, choose smaller frames. This will reduce the weight of your glasses and may eliminate distortion created when the size of your lens extends beyond your field of vision.
- Thin metal frames are usually the lightest. But plastic frames tend to be more durable and better able to support thick lenses.
- Both metal and plastic frames come in different grades, or levels of quality. Generally, you'll get what you pay for. Metal frames made of titanium, carbon graphite and flexon — a titanium-based alloy — are more expensive but are especially durable. Propionate plastic is used in cheaper frames, and Kevlar and Optyl (a resin) are more durable.
- If your glasses fit correctly, they'll feel snug and secure, yet they won't rub behind your ears or irritate the bridge of your nose. If the frames do bother you, they can be adjusted at the hinges, bridge or temples, the side arms that rest on your ears.
- New glasses require a short adjustment period. You may experience some eye ache, but it shouldn't be unbearable or persistent. If your eyes bother you so much that you can't wear the glasses, or the discomfort lasts more than a couple of weeks, check back with the optician. Your frames or prescription may need to be adjusted. It's a good idea to have the fit of your glasses checked every year or so because they become easily misaligned.

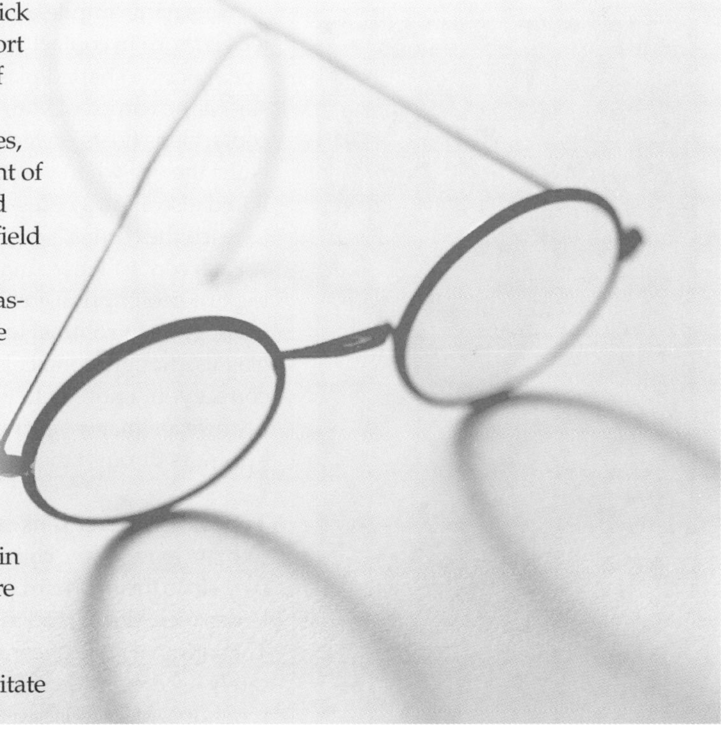

Ages	*Power (in diopters)*
40 to 45	+1.25
45 to 50	+1.50
50 to 55	+1.75
55 to 60	+2.00
60 to 65	+2.25
Over 65	+2.50

You'll need prescription glasses if each of your eyes requires a different lens power. If you do a lot of reading, you may prefer prescription glasses, which can be more accurate and made of higher-quality material. But inexpensive glasses made of lower-quality materials won't damage your eyes. Whether you decide on prescription or nonprescription reading glasses, it's a good idea to see your eye doctor whenever you notice vision changes.

Contact lenses

For many people, contact lenses are a good alternative to glasses. Unlike glasses, they don't slide around, fog up or attract dirt. Contact lenses can also correct vision problems that before could only be corrected with eyeglasses. You can even get bifocal contacts.

Contacts are most useful for people with refractive errors such as nearsightedness (myopia), farsightedness (hyperopia) and astigmatism. In addition, some unusual conditions such as keratoconus (cone-shaped cornea) are better treated with contact lenses than with glasses.

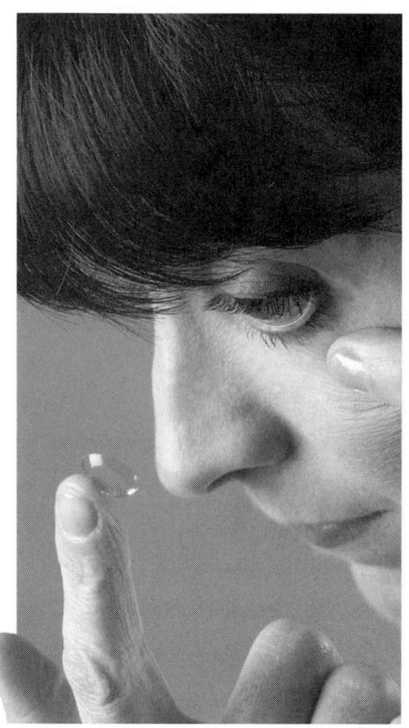

As its name implies, a contact lens is worn in contact with the eye. The specially shaped plastic disc sits on the cornea of your eye. The contact lens floats on tears that bathe the eye when you blink. This liquid also allows necessary oxygen to reach the cornea.

Each contact lens is made according to a prescription, just as eyeglasses are. In contrast to eyeglasses, though, contact lenses correct your entire field of vision because all images reaching the eyes pass through the lenses.

Types of contact lenses

Contact lenses have come a long way since the first hard plastic lenses were developed in the 1940s. That original style of contacts is rarely used anymore. The two basic types of contact lenses used today are rigid gas-permeable lenses and soft lenses.

Rigid gas-permeable lenses

Rigid gas-permeable lenses are slightly flexible hard contacts that are more porous to oxygen. They're comfortable and offer excellent correction for a wide range of vision problems. They're more durable than soft contacts and may provide sharper vision. But they have several drawbacks. You have to wear them regularly to keep your eyes used to them. They can slip off the cornea and even pop out of your eye more easily than soft contacts. And it's easier for dust to get under gas-permeable lenses and irritate your eyes.

Soft lenses

Soft contact lenses hold water, which is what makes them soft and comfortable. Soft contacts allow oxygen to pass through the plastic and nourish your cornea. These contacts are more comfortable and easier to adjust to than are rigid gas-permeable lenses. But they

Contact Lens Options

To improve or fine-tune your vision, your eye doctor may recommend one of the following types of contact lenses:

Bifocal

Bifocal soft lenses, like bifocal glasses, have a reading correction and a distance correction on each lens. The lower section of the lens is weighted, so that it stays at the bottom of your cornea and is there when you look down to read. Sometimes, however, when you blink, the lens can momentarily twist around and blur your vision.

Monovision

With monovision lenses, you wear a lens with reading correction in only one eye and a lens with just distance correction in your other eye. Your brain may adjust to this unequal correction, but your vision will be a bit more blurry than normal. Generally, you'll have sharper vision with a bifocal contact lens in each eye.

Toric

Toric lenses are designed to correct astigmatism, as well as nearsightedness or farsightedness. The lenses are weighted to keep them in place. It's important to have toric lenses fitted properly because if the lens moves as you blink or move your eye, your vision won't be sharp.

PREVENTION TIP

One of the more common problems with contact lenses is overuse. If you wear them for too long at a time, your corneas may not get enough oxygen. This causes blurry vision, pain, tearing, redness and sensitivity to light.

If you experience such signs and symptoms, remove your lenses immediately. Always keep your lens case readily available so that you can remove and safely store your lenses if your vision becomes blurry or your eyes start to hurt. It also helps to carry a pair of glasses as a backup in case such problems develop.

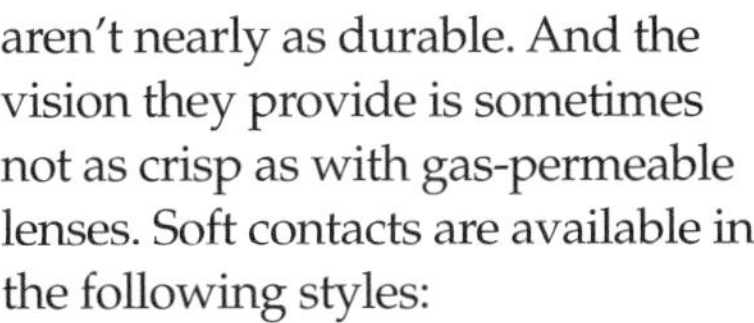

aren't nearly as durable. And the vision they provide is sometimes not as crisp as with gas-permeable lenses. Soft contacts are available in the following styles:

- *Daily wear, or conventional.* These plastic lenses conform to the shape of your eye. As the name implies, they're designed to be worn when you're awake and taken out before you go to sleep. You shouldn't wear them overnight. It's important to clean them every day after you wear them and to replace them each year.
- *Disposables, or frequent-replacement.* These lenses are thinner and more porous to oxygen than daily wear lenses, which makes them even more comfortable. As the name suggests, disposables are intended to be replaced at regular intervals. Some are designed to be worn only 1 day, others 2 weeks and others 1 to 3 months. The length of time you can wear them depends on the design and material and how well you take care of them.

  Like other soft lenses, disposables can be torn if you handle them roughly. They generally require less care than conventional soft lenses.
- *Extended wear.* These contacts are usually disposable and are designed for more than 24 hours of wear without being removed. The lenses are approved for up to 7 days of continual wear. However, most doctors don't recommend extended-wear contact lenses because, regardless of the material they're made of, your eyes receive less oxygen when you wear contact lenses while sleeping. The lenses also put you at increased risk of an eye infection because bacterial growth increases dramatically on them if you wear them overnight.

Buying and fitting contact lenses

Whichever form of lenses you choose, make sure that you have the services of a professional who can determine your exact needs. Good vision, comfort and the health of your eyes require that contact lenses be fitted properly.

Prescribing contact lenses is more complex than it is for eyeglasses. Contacts require measurements for power, curvature, diameter and thickness as well as a selection of design and material. A contact lens prescription is determined after an initial evaluation and a follow-up visit or two.

Caring for contact lenses

Proper care of your contact lenses is vital to your comfort and the overall health of your eyes. Each kind of lens has its own requirements, but no matter what type you wear, the first rule is to keep them clean.

1. Before handling your contacts, wash your hands with a mild soap. Rinse and then dry your hands with a lint-free towel.
2. Never use tap water or saliva to clean your lenses. These fluids may contain microorganisms that can cause infection. Use only sterile cleaning and disinfecting solutions.
3. For daily wear and rigid gas-permeable lenses, use an additional protein-removing enzyme cleaner.
4. Some bacteria can penetrate soft contact lenses. After cleaning each lens by gently rubbing it in cleaning solution in the palm of your hand for a few seconds, soak the lenses in cleaning solution for at least 4 hours before wearing them again. This kills most of the remaining bacteria.
5. Replace your lens case every 3 months.

Refractive surgery

An increasingly popular alternative to wearing glasses or contact lenses is laser surgery to correct the curvature of the cornea. Refractive surgery can correct farsightedness (hyperopia), nearsightedness (myopia) and astigmatism, though it can't help with presbyopia, the waning of your near vision that starts around age 40.

The burst in popularity of refractive surgery is due partly to intensive marketing and partly to the treatment's effectiveness. It allows many people to get rid of their glasses or contacts. Yet this type of surgery does have risks. If you're content with your glasses or contacts, you may not want to take any risks.

Typical candidates for refractive surgery are healthy adults ages 18 to 55 whose vision hasn't changed in the past year and who have mild to moderate nearsightedness, farsightedness or astigmatism. You may not qualify if you have dry eyes, cataracts or other eye problems, or if you're pregnant, because your vision can change during pregnancy.

LASIK surgery

The most common type of refractive surgery is LASIK, short for laser-assisted *in-situ* keratomileusis. This procedure is currently the gold

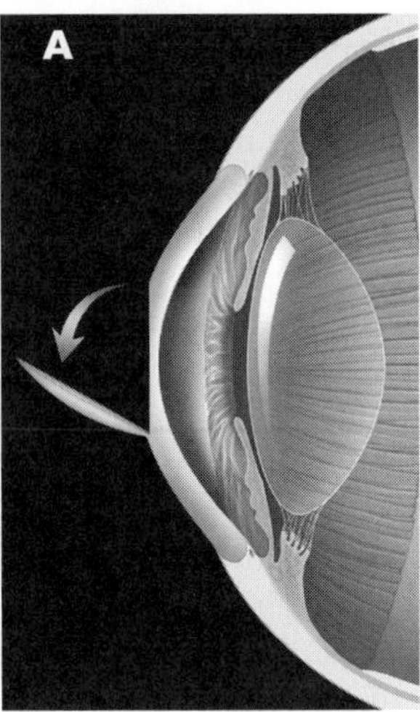

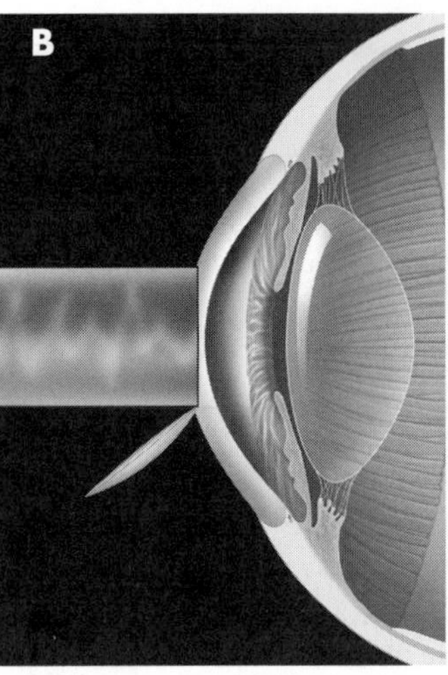

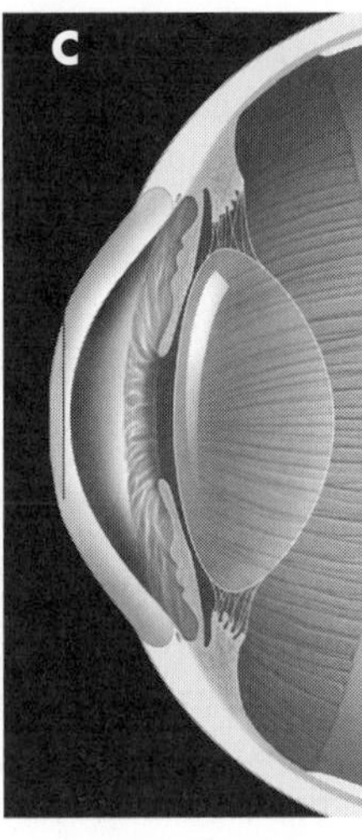

During LASIK surgery: (A) A circular flap of tissue is cut from the cornea and folded back. (B) A cool laser (excimer laser) reshapes the underlying layer of the cornea. (C) When the reshaping is complete, the corneal flap is returned to its position over the treated area.

standard for surgical correction of nearsightedness. The entire procedure takes only 10 to 20 minutes, and the laser beam is generally used for less than 1 minute.

Anesthetic drops are put in your eye. Then a delicate cutting instrument (microkeratome) is used to cut a circular flap of tissue from the center of your cornea. This flap, still hinged to your cornea, is about the size and shape of a contact lens. The surgeon folds the flap out of the way and uses a special laser to reshape the layers of your cornea, removing one microscopic layer at a time.

A computer, reading a topographical map of your cornea, tells the surgeon exactly which bits of tissue to remove. The laser is known as a cool laser (excimer laser) because it vaporizes tissue without causing heat damage.

If you're nearsighted, layers are removed from the center of your cornea to flatten its dome shape. If you're farsighted, the surgeon trims away a doughnut-shaped ring to produce a steeper curve. And if you have astigmatism, the surgeon can smooth out the distortion in your cornea's curvature.

After this sculpting, the surgeon returns the corneal flap to its position over the treated area, then places a clear shield over your eye. You wear this shield overnight. The flap quickly reattaches to your cornea without stitches.

Photorefractive keratectomy

Another surgery used with similar success is photorefractive keratectomy (PRK). Instead of sculpting the inner layers of your cornea, the surgeon uses the excimer laser to reshape the outer corneal surface. After removing the thin, protective epithelial layer of the cornea, the surgeon flattens the cornea's curvature. The epithelium grows back and conforms to the new shape of the cornea.

Expect to be at the doctor's office about 1 to 2 hours. Follow-up appointments are routinely at 1 day, 1 week, 1 month and 1 year.

Benefits and disadvantages of surgery

Refractive surgery allows about 70 percent of nearsighted people to achieve 20/20 vision without corrective lenses. More than 90 percent achieve at least 20/40 vision, the level usually required to pass an eye exam for a driver's license. These percentages continue to rise as a result of improved technology and surgical skill.

Functional vision — the ability to do most daily activities without corrective lenses — returns about 1 day after LASIK and in 7 to 10 days after PRK. When the anesthetic drops wear off after LASIK, you may feel a scratchy sensation in your eyes for a day or so. Yet LASIK is the less painful of the two procedures because the exposed nerve endings of your cornea are covered by the corneal flap. With PRK the pain may be much more intense for several days and may require strong painkillers.

After LASIK surgery about 2 percent of people don't see as clearly as they did before, compared with about 1 percent following PRK surgery. Between 5 percent and 15 percent of recipients undergo a second surgery to further sharpen their vision. Other possible problems that may arise after refractive surgery include:

- Increased sensitivity to light
- Problems with glare
- Clouded vision, which typically resolves over time
- Decreased night vision and halos around lights
- Intolerance of contact lenses

Selecting the right surgeon

For your surgery, choose an ophthalmologist with special training in the procedure, experience in the procedure you're having done and a high rate of success. Start by asking your primary care doctor for recommendations.

Once you identify a possible surgeon, ask the following questions. You have only one pair of eyes, so choose carefully whom to trust them with.

- How long have you been doing this kind of surgery? (Look for someone with years of experience, not months.)
- About how many of these surgeries have you performed, and how many do you do in an average week or month? (Choose someone who does some of these surgeries every week and who has performed the surgery hundreds of times.)
- What percentage of the people you've treated achieve 20/20 vision without corrective lenses?

What percentage achieve 20/40 vision? (Look for someone whose numbers are at or above the national average of 70 percent for 20/20 vision and 90 percent for 20/40 vision or better.)

- What percentage of your clients return for an additional surgery? (The average is 5 percent to 15 percent.)
- What are the risks and possible complications? (If the doctor guarantees the surgery will eliminate your need for glasses or contacts, or that the risks are almost nonexistent, look for another surgeon.)

Eye Trauma

From time to time, eye injuries of one kind or another happen — from a stray foul ball, a grain of sand or a splash of a household chemical, for example.

Foreign objects

Signs and symptoms

- Sudden pain in the eye
- Sudden decrease in vision
- A red eye

Everyone occasionally gets a speck of dust in the eye, and often just blinking can help wash the particle away. But if you find that this doesn't work or know that something more serious has entered your eye, seek medical attention promptly. A foreign object in the eye can be a serious threat to sight, particularly if the object enters the eye itself or damages the cornea or lens.

Diagnosis

If you go to a doctor for help with a foreign object in your eye, he or she will likely examine your eye with a slit lamp — an instrument with a light source and high magnification. If the object has entered the eye itself, an X-ray or a computerized tomography (CT) scan may be needed.

Treatment

If the object can be seen on the eye surface, the doctor may be able to remove it with surgical tweezers. If the object is no longer present but has scratched the cornea, you may need a topical antibiotic to protect against infection. Your doctor may also suggest that you wear a patch over the eye to protect it until the cornea heals. If an object has entered the eye, surgical removal will likely be necessary.

Chemical burns

Signs and symptoms

- Pain in the eye
- Decreased vision
- Increased sensitivity to light

Chemical burns of the eye can endanger your vision. If your job

Protecting Your Eyes

Myths about eye care are common. For example, the warnings that reading in dim light or sitting too close to the television screen will damage your eyes aren't true. Reading by flashlight is also harmless, as is sitting in the front row of a movie theater. These activities may make your eyes feel tired or strained, but they don't harm them.

However, many other situations can seriously damage your eyes. Some of the most common injuries are the result of accidents while doing everyday tasks such as cooking, cleaning or working in the yard. To help protect your sight:

Wear safety goggles or glasses

Wear safety goggles or glasses while working with industrial chemicals, power tools and hand tools. Make sure that your children also get in the habit of wearing protective eyeglasses when helping with hazardous housework, cooking, gardening or mowing lawn. Teach children early to wear goggles when using tools.

It's also a good idea to wear safety glasses or shields for sports such as racquetball, basketball, squash and tennis. Use appropriate headgear, such as a batter's helmet for baseball and a face mask for hockey. If a hockey puck or racquetball hits your eye, it can cause serious internal damage. Basketball players frequently suffer corneal abrasions from finger pokes.

Be careful when applying makeup

Take care when using anything near your eyes, from brushes to hair spray. You can injure your cornea by hastily applying mascara or accidentally squirting hair spray in the eyes.

Follow instructions

Read the instructions on detergents, ammonia, cleaning fluids and other household chemicals. When using fluids that come in spray containers, point nozzles away from your eyes at all times. Store household chemicals safely and out of children's reach.

Remove dangerous toys

Keep children away from toys that could lead to eye injury. Examples are BB guns, plastic swords or spring-loaded toys that shoot darts. Don't allow children to have fireworks.

Be careful around car batteries

When you're attaching jumper cables, a battery can explode and acid can get into your eyes.

Question and Answer

Will wearing sunglasses protect my eyes from disease?

Long-term exposure to ultraviolet (UV) radiation from the sun can contribute to eye disease, particularly cataracts and age-related macular degeneration. The easiest way to protect your eyes from such damage is to wear sunglasses. Generally speaking, you don't need to wear them every time you step outside. But if you spend much time in the sun, wear sunglasses that screen out UV radiation.

Choose sunglasses that provide maximum protection from both ultraviolet A (UVA) and ultraviolet B (UVB) light. The greater the blockage of UV light, the lower your risk of damage. To minimize UV light that can enter from the sides, choose sunglasses that fit close to your face or wraparound glasses. Wear your sunglasses on cloudy days as well as sunny days because clouds don't block all UV radiation.

For activities on water, sand or snow, gray-tinted, polarized lenses can reduce glare. Gray- or green-tinted lenses offer the least color distortion.

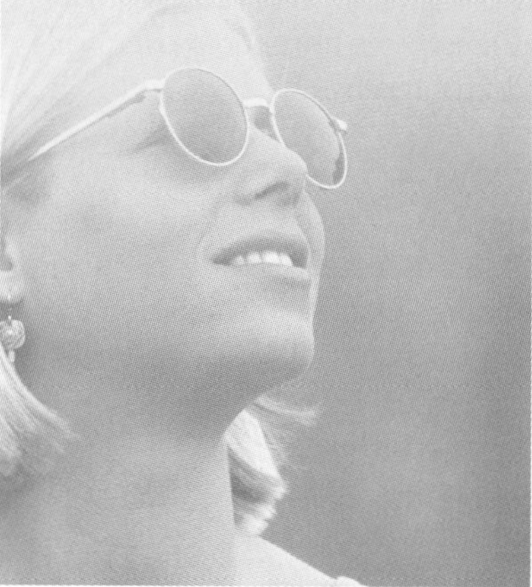

entails the use of hazardous chemicals, be aware of the dangers, protect your eyes with goggles or protective glasses, and know where the closest source of clean water is in case you need to flush your eyes. Remember that household cleaning products, particularly those that contain ammonia or bleach, and garden chemicals also can cause serious harm.

Direct contact — a chemical splashed in your eyes — is most hazardous, but concentrated fumes and aerosols also can cause injury. You'll know if a chemical has burned one or both of your eyes. They may hurt, be sensitive to light, and your vision may be blurred.

Treatment

Immediately flush the eye with clean water and continue doing so for 15 to 30 minutes. To flush your eye, hold your head under a water faucet or pour water into your eye from a clean container. Keep your eye open as wide as possible during flushing.

Chemical burns to the eyes are a medical emergency and should be treated promptly. Go to the emergency department at your local hospital or contact your ophthalmologist. The doctor examining and treating the eye may use a local anesthetic to lessen the pain. Depending on the extent of injury, the eye may be bandaged or treated with an antibiotic and allowed to heal. Serious damage to the conjunctiva, cornea or eyelid may require surgical repair later on.

Black eye

Signs and symptoms

- Bruising around the eye
- Swelling of the lid and tissue around the eye

A bruise around the eye — a so-called black eye — results from bleeding under the skin. The injury may be limited to a small amount of bleeding that provides the characteristic black-and-blue bruising. Sometimes a black eye indicates a more extensive injury, even a skull fracture, particularly if the area around both eyes is bruised or you have a head trauma.

Treatment

Using gentle pressure, apply ice to the soft tissue around the injured eye for 10 to 15 minutes. Take care not to press on the eye itself.

Seek medical care promptly if you experience vision problems such as double vision or blurring or if you have severe pain or bleeding in the eye or from the nose. A doctor can determine whether more serious damage has occurred.

Blood in an eye

Signs and symptoms

- Bleeding within the front portion of the eye

Bleeding into the front portion of the eye (hyphema) may follow direct trauma to the eye. It can result from a blunt injury or a sharp injury that perforates the eye's coating. At times, hyphema may result from severe inflammation of the iris (iritis), a blood vessel abnormality or cancer within the eye. When the bleeding is caused by trauma, the blood is usually absorbed completely within a few days. Recurrent bleeding in the eye can reduce vision and damage the cornea. In some cases, glaucoma can result.

Treatment

A doctor may recommend hospitalization, especially if repeat bleeding occurs. Medication may decrease the risk of repeat bleeding. For severe bleeding, a doctor may choose to drain the blood through a small opening in the eye. This drain can be reopened later if further bleeding occurs.

Corneal abrasion and injury

Signs and symptoms

- Severe eye pain
- A red eye
- Swollen eyelids

The cornea is the curved, transparent covering at the front of the eye. Along with the cornea, the lens focuses images on the retina. As the most exposed part of the eye, the cornea is susceptible to various injuries, ulcers and infections. The most common corneal injury is an abrasion — irritation caused by scratching or rubbing. This can happen when a speck of sand or sawdust scratches the cornea or you wear contact lenses for too long. Your cornea can also be burned from exposure to ultraviolet radiation after you've been sitting in the sun or under a sunlamp for too long or looking into a welding arc without proper eye protection.

Following corneal injury, the tissue around your eye may swell, and the eye itself may redden and hurt intensely. You may blink more than usual. Some people don't feel any symptoms for several hours after the injury, then suddenly find themselves in extreme discomfort for no apparent reason.

Treatment

Eyedrops containing a dye can help a doctor identify damage to the cornea. Simple corneal abrasions and injuries are treated by removing any foreign material, covering the eye with a patch and letting the eye heal itself. The cornea usually heals quickly, in as little as a day or two. Your doctor may also apply an antibiotic ointment to prevent infection and prescribe a pain reliever for the first day or two to relieve the discomfort. More serious injury to the cornea may require surgical treatment.

Eyelid Disorders

The eyelids, though thin and delicate, are extremely important in protecting the eyes. Quick and powerful reflexes make the eyelids close when an object nears or when irritating particles are in the air. The eyelids also lubricate the eyes and wash foreign particles from them.

Lacrimal glands located above each eyeball produce tears, which are spread by the eyelids as a thin film. The tears drain from the eyes through nasolacrimal ducts, which have openings at the inner corner of each eyelid. The nasolacrimal ducts carry the tears to the nose — which explains why crying causes your nose to run. The eyelids are lined with the conjunctiva, the transparent mucous membrane that also covers the white surface of the eye.

Sties and lumps

Signs and symptoms

- Painful swelling on the edge of the eyelid
- Slightly blurred vision

A sty (hordeolum) is an infection around the root (follicle) of an eyelash. A sty resembles a pimple or boil. You may get more than one sty at a time or several in succession because bacteria that initially infect one hair follicle can spread and infect others.

A sty usually develops gradually, forming a painful red lump. Eventually, the lump fills with pus and bursts. The release of pus relieves the pain, and after a few more days the sty usually disappears.

Another form of swelling on the lid is called a chalazion. Unlike a sty, a chalazion is relatively painless. It results from a blockage of one of the small glands (meibomian glands) that produce part of the tear layer. Bacteria may grow within the blocked gland. A chalazion develops a little farther up on and within the eyelid. Most chalazions are only mildly uncomfortable, but they may be unsightly.

Treatment

Sties and lumps are almost always harmless to the eye and sight. However, if a sty interferes with your vision or doesn't disappear on its own, or if you have recurrent infections, see a doctor.

To treat a sty, apply a warm compress to it for about 10 minutes four times a day. To make a compress, soak a clean cloth in warm water and wring it out before applying it to your eye. Warm compresses can help relieve the pain. Don't squeeze the sty in an effort to remove the pus. Let the sty burst on its own, then wash your eyelid thoroughly. If the sty is stubborn or you have recurring infections, your doctor may prescribe an oral antibiotic or an antibiotic cream to apply to the

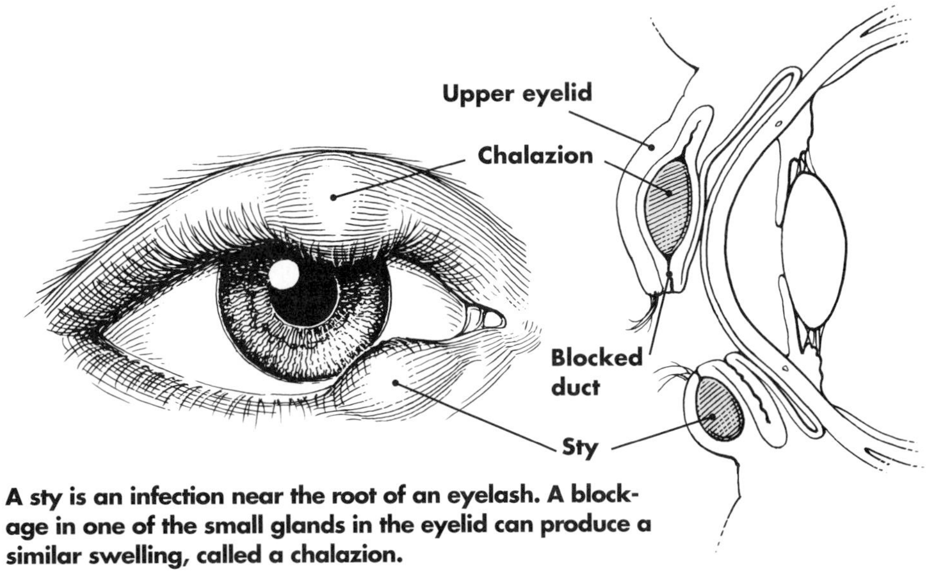

A sty is an infection near the root of an eyelash. A blockage in one of the small glands in the eyelid can produce a similar swelling, called a chalazion.

Eyedrops

Many brands of eyedrops can be purchased without a prescription. They fall into two general categories: artificial tears and vasoconstrictors.

Artificial tears

Artificial tears contain substances, such as methylcellulose, that hold water and resemble your own tears. One or two drops in each eye usually provide lubrication and comfort for several hours. You can use artificial tears as often as needed.

Vasoconstrictors

Vasoconstrictors (Murine, Visine) contain a medication that causes the tiny blood vessels in the conjunctiva to constrict. If you have bloodshot eyes — redness and visible blood vessels — one or two drops in each eye will usually relieve the redness for several hours and often provide comfort as well. Some vasoconstrictors also contain an antihistamine to provide added relief for allergies.

Vasoconstrictors shouldn't be used more than two or three times a day for more than 3 days, unless otherwise directed by your doctor. Overuse leads to a rebound effect of increased swelling and redness that persist even after you stop using the drops.

Follow the directions carefully for whatever eyedrops you use. A pharmacist can help you select the type of eyedrops you need and inform you how to use them. After placing an eyedrop in your eye, follow these simple steps:

1. Keep the eye closed for 30 to 60 seconds. This encourages absorption and minimizes drainage through your tear duct into your nose.
2. Don't blink. Blinking tends to move the liquid from your eye into your tear duct.
3. Use your index finger to apply firm pressure for a minute or two over the junction of your lower eyelid and nose to block the opening of your tear duct.

eyelid. A particularly persistent sty may need to be lanced and drained.

A chalazion usually disappears without treatment in a month or two. Applying warm compresses may help speed the healing. Your doctor may prescribe an antibiotic ointment. If these methods prove unsuccessful or if the chalazion continues to enlarge, it can be removed surgically. After the procedure the eye usually is covered with a patch for several hours.

Tearing problems

Every time you blink — every few seconds — tears lubricate your eyes. The fluid is essential for your eyes to function properly. Problems may develop with the tear glands that result in continuously watering eyes or dry eyes.

Dry eyes

Dry eyes, caused by an inadequate amount or quality of tears, can lead to an uncomfortable sensation. Your eyes may feel hot and gritty and appear swollen and red. The condition usually affects both eyes.

Dry eyes may result from an allergy to eyedrops used for another condition or from Sjogren's syndrome, a connective tissue disorder often associated with rheumatoid arthritis, or they may occur for no apparent reason. Dry eyes are most common among women following menopause, probably due to hormonal changes.

Problems unrelated to tear production also may cause your eyes to feel dry and scratchy. These may include:

- Eyelid inflammation (blepharitis)
- Entropion or ectropion (see page 639)
- Environmental irritants, such as smoke, sun, wind and indoor heating
- Disruption of the blink reflex
- Eyestrain

In addition, a variety of common medications, both prescription and over-the-counter, can cause dry eyes. These include diuretics, antihistamines and decongestants, sleeping pills, tricyclic antidepressants, some drugs for treating acne and opiate-based pain relievers, such as morphine.

Treatment

Although the condition generally isn't a threat to sight, the discomfort of dry eyes may require medical treatment. Your doctor will likely prescribe artificial tears that you can use to bathe your eyes whenever needed. If your condition is caused by an allergic reaction to eyedrops, discontinuing them should help.

Watering eyes

Too much tearing can result from either excessive tear production or inadequate drainage by the nasolacrimal ducts, the tubes that drain tears from the eyes to the nose. This occurs mostly among adults.

PREVENTION TIP

Like any liquid, tears evaporate when exposed to air. These are simple steps you can take to help slow evaporation and minimize problems of dry eyes:

1. Don't direct hair dryers, car heaters, air conditioners or fans toward your eyes.
2. Wear glasses when outside on windy days and goggles while swimming.
3. Keep your home humidity between 30 percent and 50 percent. In winter a humidifier can add moisture to dry indoor air.
4. Remember to blink. Consciously blinking repeatedly helps spread your own tears more evenly.

However, about 5 percent of babies are born with a tear duct that has failed to open. In most of these infants, the tear ducts open spontaneously within a few weeks. Usually, only one eye is affected by continuous tearing. Other causes include irritation of the eye due to an abrasion, infection of the eyelid, inward-growing eyelashes, allergies or nasal problems.

Treatment
Your doctor will examine the eye carefully for signs of blockage of a nasolacrimal duct or of excessive tear production. He or she may also ask you questions to identify other possible causes. These might include scarring of the nasolacrimal duct caused by chronic sinusitis, chronic allergies or injury to the nose. Treatment for a blocked duct generally includes probing and irrigating (flushing) the tear drainage system. In some cases, an operation may be needed.

Infection of the tear duct
Occasionally, the nasolacrimal duct can become infected (dacryocystitis). When this happens, the tissues between the inner angle of the eye and the bridge of the nose become swollen, red and tender. Tears can no longer make their way into the nose, causing excessive tearing.

Treatment
Your doctor may prescribe an antibiotic for the infection. To relieve discomfort apply a warm compress to your eye several times a day. Soak a clean, lint-free cloth in warm water, wring it out and place it over the affected eye for about 10 minutes.

Once the infection has cleared, a new tear drainage opening may need to be created surgically. In this operation, called dacryocystorhinostomy, the doctor may use thin silicone tubing to keep the new tear duct open while healing occurs. In rare cases, it may be necessary to surgically implant an artificial tear duct. The artificial duct is made of unbreakable glass and is placed in the inner corner of the eyelid.

Twitchy Eyelid

From time to time, you may experience a twitch in an eyelid. This involuntary quivering usually lasts only a few seconds, but it can be recurrent and irritating and make you wonder if something is wrong with your eyes.

A twitch is almost always harmless. Eye twitches are similar to the common experience of an occasional muscle twitch in a hand, forearm, leg or foot. These muscle flutters (fasciculations) last only a few seconds, although they may happen often.

No one knows exactly what causes most twitches, although they're often associated with fatigue and stress. Very rarely, a twitching eyelid is a symptom of a muscle or nerve disease, but symptoms of these diseases tend to be distinct from an ordinary eye twitch.

You may be able to relieve the twitching by gently massaging the affected eyelid.

Itchy Eyelid

Itchiness around the eyes often accompanies seasonal allergies, but itchy eyelids may be a manifestation of contact dermatitis, a skin inflammation that results when your fingers come in contact with some irritating or allergy-causing substance and then touch your eyes. Cosmetics also can cause allergic reactions on the sensitive skin of the eyelids.

If your eyelids itch, don't rub or scratch them excessively. Rubbing ultimately can result in eczema, with thickening patches of skin and persistent itching. If your eyelids are sensitive to certain cosmetics or other materials, avoid using them.

Blepharitis

Signs and symptoms
- Sticky, crusty and reddened eyelids
- Itchy, burning, swollen eyelids
- Pinkeye (conjunctivitis)
- A grainy feeling with blinking
- Loss of lashes

Blepharitis is an inflammation of the eyelid edges that's due to a bacterial infection. When the glands near the eyelashes produce excess oil, it creates an environment favorable for bacterial growth. The result is a crusty inflammation that's uncomfortable and unsightly but rarely a threat to sight.

You may find that you have to pry your eyes open in the morning, because the sticky secretions seal the eyelids shut overnight. In severe cases, small ulcers may develop on the edges of the lids, and the cornea can become scarred. People with blepharitis often have a history of recurrent sties and chalazions.

Treatment
Cleaning your eyelids carefully is important for treating blepharitis. In the morning, soak a clean, lint-free cloth in warm water, wring it out and place it over the eyes as a compress. This will loosen the crusty scales. Then gently scrub your eyelashes and eyelid edges with a cotton-tipped swab soaked in diluted baby shampoo. This will help remove the crust.

If self-help measures don't clear up the problem, your doctor may prescribe — in addition to eyelid scrubs — an ointment or eyedrops containing antibiotic and corticosteroid medications to clear the

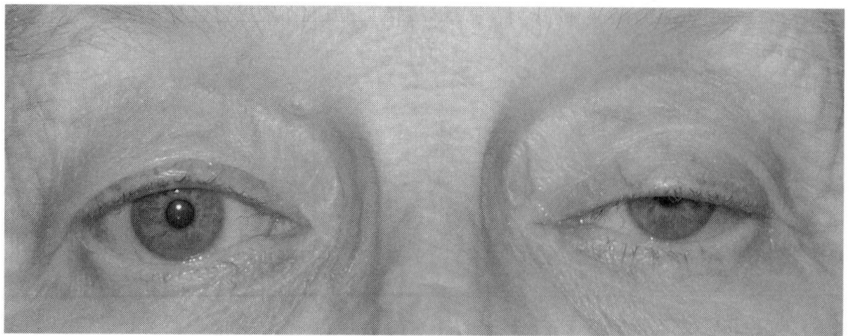

Drooping of the upper eyelid (right) is known as ptosis.

infection and reduce the swelling. If topical treatment is unsuccessful, oral antibiotics may be prescribed.

Drooping eyelid

Signs and symptoms

- Drooping of one or both upper eyelids

Drooping eyelid (ptosis) is caused by a weakness of the muscle that raises the upper eyelid and keeps it open. Some children are born with the condition. When present from birth, it usually affects only one eye. Ptosis often runs in families.

In adults, some drooping of the eyelids can occur as a normal effect of aging, as the eyelid muscles lose tone. Less often, a drooping eyelid may be the result of an injury or a disease, such as diabetes, myasthenia gravis, stroke, a brain tumor or cancer, all of which can affect nerve and muscle function. A drooping eyelid that develops suddenly requires immediate attention. It may be a sign of stroke or another acute problem within your nervous system. If the problem develops over several years, it may be due to the effects of aging.

Diagnosis

If your child's eyelids are noticeably uneven, especially to the degree that vision is obscured, have her or him evaluated by a doctor. If you notice that one or both of your own eyelids have gradually become droopy, ask your doctor about it the next time you have an appointment. If the drooping came on suddenly, see your doctor right away. A thorough examination may be needed to determine whether a more general health problem could be the cause.

Treatment

For children born with ptosis, surgical correction may be necessary to prevent poor vision in the affected eye. Among adults, if the drooping is the result of aging or injury, your doctor may recommend that you have an operation to shorten the muscle, lifting (elevating) the lid. If the cause is a more general health problem, such as myasthenia gravis, stroke or diabetes, treatment

Eyelid Surgery

With age, eyelid tissue loses elasticity, strength and tone. Fat accumulates around the eyes. Your eyelids may droop, and you may have bags beneath your eyes. Heredity also can lead to droopy eyelids. Whatever the cause, you may appear to always look tired. Perhaps the sagging skin even interferes with your sight.

Surgery

Blepharoplasty is a surgical procedure to remove excess skin and fat from the upper and lower eyelids. The procedure usually is done using a local anesthetic. The surgeon makes an incision in the fold of the eyelid near the lashes. Excess skin, muscle and fat are removed, and the incision is closed. Mild cases are sometimes treated with laser surgery. In this procedure, the laser shrinks and tightens the skin and muscles without removing them.

Recovery

Blepharoplasty shouldn't interfere with your vision, and you may wear your eyeglasses the day after the procedure. Wearing glasses can also help protect your eyelids from injury. Any swelling, tenderness and pain should subside within 2 to 4 weeks.

You may experience some temporary problems. Because many tiny blood vessels are disturbed during the procedure, you may experience areas of blood under the skin (hematomas). These usually subside after a few days and leave no permanent sign. Some people have temporary double vision the first few hours after the operation. Many people report excessive tearing for a few days, but this usually disappears.

An infection following surgery is uncommon but can occur. See your doctor if you experience:

- Excessive swelling that doesn't improve gradually
- Redness that increases over several days
- Tenderness or pain in the eyelid that doesn't resolve gradually
- Problems with vision

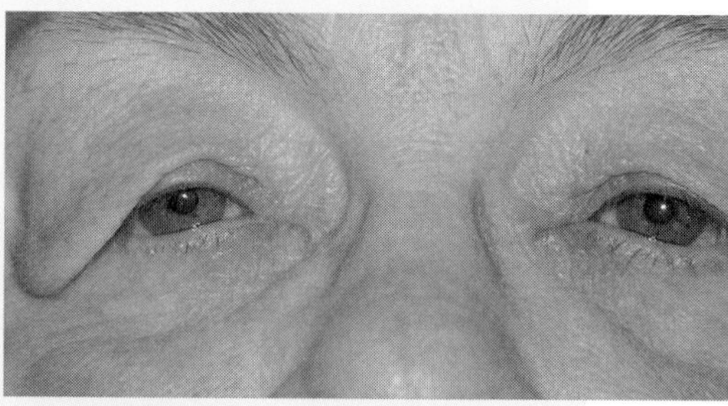

Relaxation of the tissues of the upper eyelid may cause it to droop over the eyelashes and interfere with vision. This is known as blepharochalasis.

of the underlying disorder may help relieve the eyelid problem.

Entropion and ectropion

Signs and symptoms

- Eyelashes scratching the eye
- Excessive tearing
- Eye irritation and matter in the eye when you wake up

Entropion and ectropion generally are due to aging. In entropion, the upper or lower lid turns inward, causing the lashes to scratch the eye. In severe cases, this can cause an ulcer or scarring of the cornea. One of the first signs of entropion is irritation and excess matter in the eyes in the morning. This usually improves later in the day. As the disorder advances, the irritation may persist longer or become constant. You may also notice your lashes turning in toward the eyes.

Ectropion, the reverse problem, is often the result of muscle weakness. It also may be related to an underlying condition such as allergic dermatitis or lupus erythematosus.

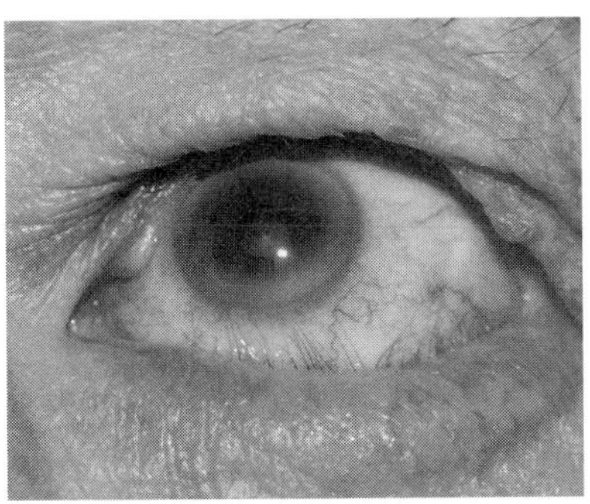

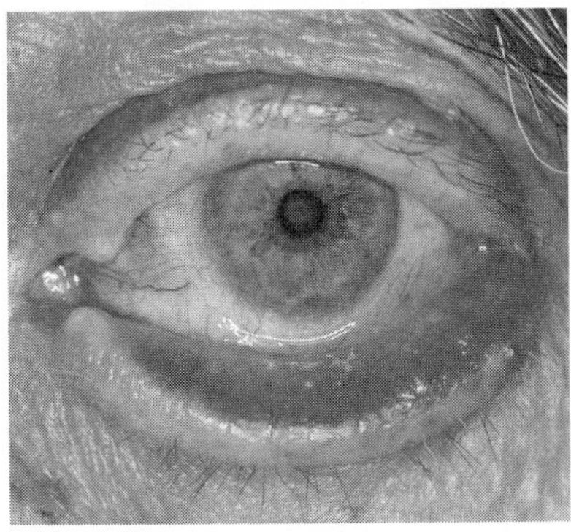

With entropion (top) the eyelid turns inward so that the lashes rub against and irritate the eye. With ectropion (bottom) the eyelid turns outward and sags away from the eyeball.

The lower lid turns outward, sometimes causing tears to flow over the lower lid edge and down your cheek rather than into the tear drainage system.

Treatment

Both entropion and ectropion can be corrected by surgery that repositions the muscles holding the lids in place. The procedures are usually performed on an outpatient basis with a local anesthetic. When an underlying condition is the cause of ectropion, the first step is to treat the underlying cause.

Eye Disorders and Diseases

The eyes are susceptible to various disorders and diseases. Many eye conditions don't seriously affect your ability to see, but they can be annoying or over time may present more serious risks to your vision. Among the most serious disorders are those related to the functioning of the eye. These include glaucoma, cataracts and problems involving the retina, including retinal detachment and macular degeneration.

Colorblindness

Signs and symptoms

- Certain colors are muted and difficult or impossible to see
- An inability to distinguish between certain shades of color
- Seeing everything in shades of gray (extremely rare)

Although most people call it colorblindness, life for a person with poor color vision is usually not black and white. Only rarely is everything seen in shades of gray. Most people with poor color vision are unable to distinguish between certain shades of color.

Your ability to view the world in hundreds of hues begins with just three colors — red, blue and green. As light rays pass through the lens and the transparent, jelly-like substance (vitreous humor) that makes up much of your eye, they interact with light-sensitive chemicals in cone cells in the retina. As long as the cones can accurately distinguish red, blue and green, these colors can be further blended to produce a continuous band (spectrum) of colors. If the cones lack one or more light-sensitive chemicals, you may see only two colors, such as either red and green or blue and yellow. The most common color deficiency is an inability to see red and green.

Defects can be mild, moderate or severe, depending on the amount of light-sensitive substances missing from the cones. In addition, a reduced sensitivity to red is seldom as severe as a reduced sensitivity to green. So more people struggle to see green than red. Interestingly, most people with a red-green deficiency aren't aware of their problem. To them, leaves are green and roses are red, but their "green" may be what normal-sighted people call yellow.

Causes

The causes of color vision deficiencies are as follows:

Genetic

The genetic defect responsible for color vision deficiencies is passed from mother to son. Because women usually have genes that compensate for the deficiency, the condition seldom affects them. The gene that carries this defect also determines whether the condition will be mild, moderate or severe. The degree of color deficiency you inherit remains the same throughout your life. Most people who have an inherited color deficiency can see normally in all other respects.

Acquired

Color deficiencies can accompany various forms of eye disease. People may develop problems seeing blue and yellow when the retina is affected by disease. Disorders of the optic nerve also can affect your color vision. Cataracts also impair color perception.

Age

Aging can bring on color deficiency. During childhood and adolescence, your ability to see colors steadily improves and peaks in your 30s. Color vision then gradually deteriorates as a normal part of aging.

Diagnosis

An ophthalmologist can test for a color deficiency. Many ophthalmologists use a book containing multicolored dot patterns as a simple and accurate screening test for color vision deficiencies. An ophthalmologist can help you find out what type of color deficiency you may have and determine if you have any associated eye disease.

Treatment

No treatment can correct inherited color perception deficiencies. Wearing a colored filter over eyeglasses or a colored contact lens may enhance your perception of contrasts. But such lenses won't improve your ability to discern colors. And because they're usually worn over only one eye, they can distort depth perception.

If you have an acquired color deficiency, it may worsen as the disease that causes it progresses. Treatments that slow or reverse the course of the underlying disease often improve color vision.

Misaligned eyes

Strabismus and amblyopia, conditions that affect eye alignment, are usually first observed during early childhood. *Strabismus* is the general term for crossed eyes or those that are misaligned in some other way. Amblyopia, often called lazy eye, can be a consequence of strabismus.

Babies are born with the ability to see, but, at first, they can't focus. The nerve connections between the eyes and brain haven't yet become fully organized. During the first few weeks of life, your baby's eyes may appear to wander. At times, they may seem to work independently, sometimes crossing and at other times roving outward. This is normal. By the end of the second or third month, however, your baby's eyes should appear to be working in parallel and able to focus on small objects. No one knows why some children's eyes are misaligned, although it tends to run in families.

Strabismus

Normal vision depends on the eyes focusing together, producing binocular vision. When the eyes don't function in tandem, double vision results. In a young child with strabismus, however, the brain will ignore the images from one eye, and the nerve connections between that eye and the brain fail to develop normally.

About 4 percent of children have strabismus. It seems to affect boys and girls equally. If not treated before age 5 or 6, they risk permanent loss of visual acuity in the nondominant eye.

The most common forms of strabismus in children are cross-eye (esotropia) and walleye (exotropia). Esotropia is characterized by one eye turning inward. Exotropia occurs when an eye turns outward. Sometimes the eye will turn down

Normal Pattern

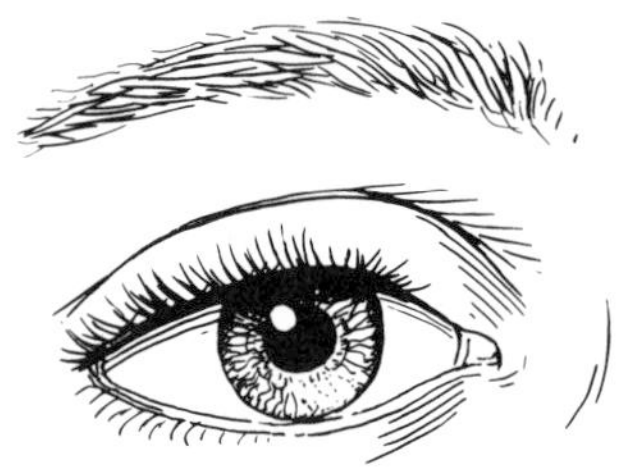
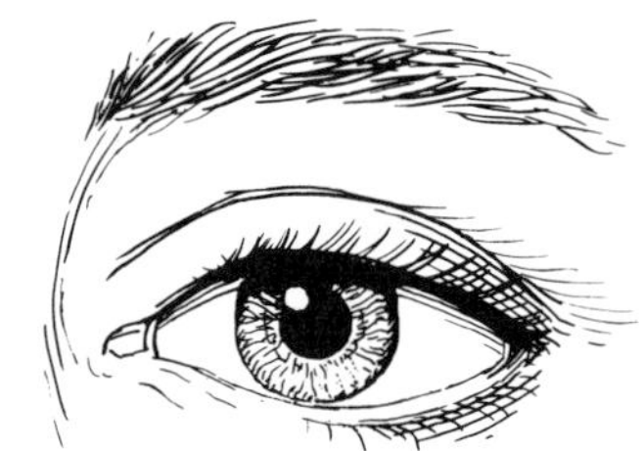

Cross-Eye (esotropia)

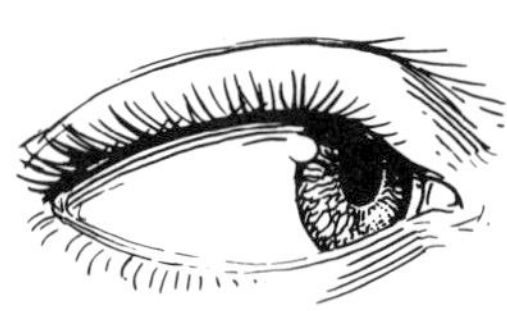
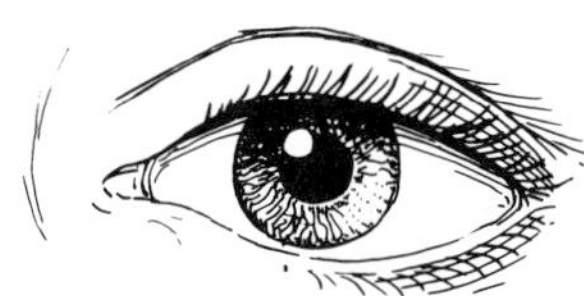

Walleye (exotropia)

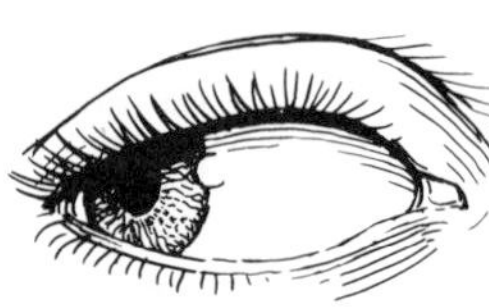
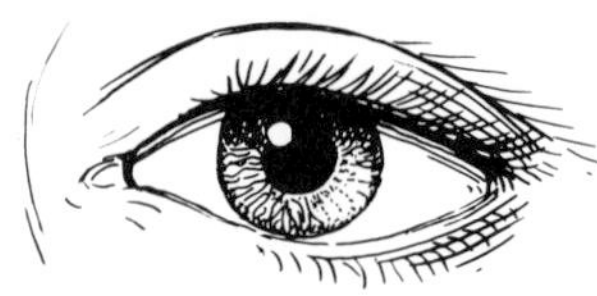

Some children have eyes that are misaligned, a condition called strabismus. Two common forms of strabismus are esotropia, in which an eye turns inward, and exotropia, in which an eye turns outward.

or up. The deviations may be constant or occasional, such as when the child is tired and the eye muscles weaken.

The resulting poor vision prevents a child from having normal depth perception, which good binocular vision produces. The affected eye probably won't develop good vision unless it's used. This can be accomplished by surgery to bring the eyes into alignment or perhaps by wearing a patch over the unaffected (dominant) eye, forcing the affected eye to focus and see.

Amblyopia

Amblyopia is a condition in which vision in the nondominant eye is poor, usually as a result of strabismus. Amblyopia can also result from a greater degree of farsightedness (hyperopia), nearsightedness (myopia) or astigmatism in one eye or from the rare occurrence of a childhood cataract. The brain then "turns off" the more affected eye, and the stronger eye becomes dominant and retains good vision.

Diagnosis

The key to treating strabismus and amblyopia is early detection. Strabismus is usually easy to recognize, but amblyopia in a child may not be evident because he or she often doesn't realize that vision is poor in one eye. Testing of visual acuity may be needed to discover amblyopia. Following is a list of things to look for:

1. Do your child's eyes work together? Have your child follow your hand moving back and forth. Notice if the eyes seem to move and follow as one.
2. Cover one of your child's eyes and move your hand or a toy back and forth. Does the uncovered eye follow the object? Cover the other eye and repeat.
3. Can your toddler gauge depth when playing with objects?
4. Does your child seem cross-eyed when playing with toys or other close objects but normal when looking into the distance?
5. Does only one eye squint when your child is in the sun?
6. Does your child tend to tilt his or her head to one side?

If you think that your child might have misaligned eyes, check with your doctor. It's never too early to have a child's vision tested for alignment. The key to diagnosing amblyopia in a young child is to identify a difference in vision between the eyes. An ophthalmologist can test your baby's vision by covering one eye and observing your child's responses to the movement of various objects. If one eye is amblyopic, the child might try to remove the patch, or he or she might object to having it over the better eye.

By age 3, vision usually can be measured accurately. Poor vision in one eye doesn't necessarily mean that a child has amblyopia. Poor vision may be due to nearsightedness, farsightedness, astigmatism or another disorder.

Treatment

Contrary to what many people believe, children don't outgrow strabismus and amblyopia, so prompt treatment is essential to prevent permanent visual impairment in the affected eye.

Optical approaches

If your child has strabismus associated with farsightedness — the eyes cross only when looking at close objects — eyeglasses may be enough to solve the problem. Sometimes, the lenses are bifocal or are specially designed to compensate for the defect in the eye.

Nonsurgical procedures

The nonsurgical treatment for amblyopia involves placing a patch over the normal eye to force use of the weak eye. This seems to help organize the nerve connections between that eye and the parts of the brain that process visual perception. Normally, this organization and coordination occur for both eyes in the first year of life.

Double Vision

Double vision (diplopia) generally results from a nerve or muscle problem. The problem may cause one eye to deviate from the other so that they don't focus in unison. The images the brain receives from the two eyes are positioned differently from each other, causing double vision.

If the eye and brain connections have already become well established, which usually happens by age 1 or 2, the brain interprets the signals just as it receives them and produces two images. The effect can be confusing and debilitating because objects appear twice in the field of vision.

Sometimes, double vision is a sign of a more serious underlying problem such as diabetes, myasthenia gravis, multiple sclerosis, Graves' disease or a brain injury. In these cases, the underlying disease affects the nerves between the brain and eye muscles or the nerves of the eye muscles themselves. Double vision is usually only one of several symptoms of these disorders.

If you develop double vision, have it checked out as soon as possible. In the meantime, you can alleviate the sensation temporarily by placing a patch over one eye.

Treatment of an underlying disorder may resolve the problem. Sometimes, double vision can be corrected with prescribed eyeglasses that contain prisms — special lenses that align the image seen by one eye with that seen by the other eye. Occasionally, the condition is treated surgically to improve alignment.

The same result sometimes may be achieved by treating the normal eye with medicated eyedrops called cycloplegics, which blur vision temporarily and dilate the pupil. Some children with strabismus may also be treated with eyedrops called miotics, which cause the pupil to constrict. These methods are most effective with young children.

Once vision in the weaker eye improves, treatment generally involves bringing the eyes into parallel position. Eyeglasses or surgery may be recommended. Some doctors prescribe eye exercises for strabismus and amblyopia, but most ophthalmologists believe they're of little value.

Surgery

Many children, particularly those with strabismus, require an operation to realign eye muscles. The surgeon makes a small incision in the tissue that covers the eye. One or more of the eye muscles are then repositioned to achieve proper alignment. Depending on the complexity of the problem, more than one operation may be necessary to bring the eye into normal position. When treatment is completed before age 5 or 6, vision often improves to near normal.

Conjunctivitis

Signs and symptoms

- A red eye
- A gritty feeling in an eye
- An itchy eye
- Discharge in an eye that forms a crust during the night
- Blurred vision and sensitivity to light

Conjunctivitis is an inflammation of the transparent membrane (conjunctiva) that lines the eyelids and covers the eyeball up to the edge of the cornea. Commonly known as pinkeye, conjunctivitis may result from a bacterial or viral infection, an allergic reaction or, in newborns, an incompletely opened tear duct. Newborns are also susceptible to certain bacteria acquired from the birth canal. This form of conjunctivitis (ophthalmia neonatorum) must be treated without delay to prevent loss of vision.

Viral and bacterial conjunctivitis are common among children and are often extremely infectious. Pinkeye can spread through a whole classroom of children in a few days. Although conjunctivitis can be irritating, it usually doesn't impair vision. Occasionally, severe conjunctivitis can cause corneal complications in adults.

All forms of conjunctivitis share certain signs and symptoms. The white of the eye becomes red or pink, and the eye feels gritty when you blink. The eye also produces a yellowish discharge that forms a crust during the night. This sticky crust can seal the eyes shut so that you have to pry the lids apart in the morning or soak off the crust.

Viral conjunctivitis usually produces a watery discharge, while the bacterial form often produces thicker matter. Allergic conjunctivitis usually causes intense itching, tearing and inflammation of the conjunctiva as well as some itching and watery discharge from the nose.

Treatment

You can soothe the discomfort of conjunctivitis by applying warm compresses to the affected eye or eyes. Soak a clean, lint-free cloth in warm water, squeeze the water out and apply the cloth to your eyes. You can wipe away discharge with a moistened, disposable tissue or clean cotton ball. Your doctor may prescribe antibiotic eyedrops if the infection is bacterial. Viral conjunctivitis clears up on its own.

Allergic conjunctivitis is often effectively treated with cool compresses. It may also be helped by eyedrops that contain both an antihistamine and an agent that constricts blood vessels.

Prevention

Because bacterial and viral conjunctivitis spread easily and quickly, good hygiene is the best way to prevent pinkeye from spreading. If someone in your family has it:

- Keep your hands away from your eyes.
- Wash your hands frequently.
- Change your towel and washcloth daily.
- Change your pillowcase each night. Wash sheets and pillowcases in hot water.
- Discard eye cosmetics, particularly mascara.
- Don't use other people's eye cosmetics.
- Don't share towels, washcloths, pillowcases, handkerchiefs, glasses or utensils with another person.
- Dispose of used tissues immediately.

Scleritis and episcleritis

Signs and symptoms

- Pain in one or both eyes
- Patchy redness on the eye
- Blurred vision
- Swelling of the eye

The sclera is a tough layer of tissue that forms the wall of the eyeball — the part commonly referred to as the white of the eye. The sclera, in turn, is covered by the episclera, a transparent tissue between the sclera and the outer membrane (conjunctiva). Occasionally, the episclera or the sclera becomes inflamed.

Inflammation of the episclera (episcleritis) is a mild, localized inflammation that generally occurs among young adults. Inflammation of the sclera (scleritis) is a less common but more serious disorder, often associated with inflammatory bowel disease or autoimmune diseases such as rheumatoid arthritis. Scleritis primarily affects people between the ages of 30 and 60.

Both scleritis and episcleritis are characterized by a red or violet patch on the eye or localized swelling on the eye. In both disorders, tiny blood vessels become inflamed. Scleritis may be accompanied by a dull pain. When scleritis

Question and Answer

What causes a red area on the eye?

The outer covering of the eyeball is filled with tiny blood vessels. Occasionally, one of them may break, appearing as a red spot or area of blood on the white of the eye. The blood from the broken vessel can travel through the space between the conjunctiva and sclera, causing what appears to be a bloody eye. This is called a subconjunctival hemorrhage. It can be alarming when you first see it, but it's nothing to worry about, unless your eye also hurts. If it does, see a doctor right away.

A blood vessel under the conjunctiva may break for no reason or when you cough, sneeze or vomit forcefully. An eye injury also can cause such a hemorrhage. Most subconjunctival hemorrhages disappear after 2 or 3 weeks. If hemorrhages recur, see your doctor, who may recommend a more thorough physical examination to detect a possible underlying problem.

occurs at the back of the eye, vision may be impaired.

Treatment

Episcleritis usually disappears on its own after a week or two but tends to recur from time to time. Your doctor may prescribe steroids in drop or ointment form to help reduce the inflammation of episcleritis or scleritis. Pupil-dilating drugs may be used to lessen the chance of damage to the iris and reduce discomfort. If you have scleritis, your doctor may have you undergo some tests to determine if the inflammation is associated with an underlying condition.

Uveitis and iritis

Signs and symptoms

- A red eye
- Blurred vision
- Sensitivity to light

Uveitis is an inflammation of the uvea, the layer of the eye immediately beneath the sclera. The uvea consists of the iris, the colored part of the eye, the ciliary body, which produces the fluid inside the eye and also helps control lens movement, and the choroid, which lies just within the sclera and lines the eyeball from the iris all the way around the eye. Thus, inflammation of the uvea may include the area at the back of the eye, the sides and the iris.

When the inflammation involves mainly the iris and ciliary body, it may be called anterior uveitis. When it involves mainly the choroid, it may be called either choroiditis or posterior uveitis. Iritis is inflammation of the iris.

Uveitis may result from an immune reaction provoked by a disease such as Crohn's disease, ulcerative colitis or sarcoidosis, or it may develop after a severe injury. It can also occur with herpes simplex or shingles (herpes zoster).

Treatment

Uveitis can be serious. Early diagnosis and treatment are important to prevent permanent damage. Uveitis and iritis can be treated with several medications. Your doctor may prescribe a cycloplegic drug that paralyzes the iris and keeps the pupil dilated. This relieves pain by preventing the inflamed iris from moving and lessens the chance of scars or adhesions between the lens and back of the iris. Steroid ointment or eyedrops may be prescribed to reduce inflammation. Aspirin or oral steroid medications also may be prescribed to reduce inflammation.

If inflammation from trauma-related uveitis persists for several weeks, complications can occur, including an immune reaction in the uninjured eye. The result may be inflammation of the uvea and, ultimately, a substantial loss of vision in both eyes. For this reason, an ophthalmologist may advise removal of the injured eye if the inflammation doesn't subside as expected.

Orbital cellulitis

Signs and symptoms

- Pain in one eye
- Decreased vision
- Displacement of the eye
- Swelling of the eyelid
- General malaise

Orbital cellulitis is a rare, acute infection of the eye socket. It primarily affects children, and its onset is rapid and severe. Bacteria enter the orbit, often from an infection in the sinuses, a foreign object in the eye or a boil on the eye or eyelid. The orbit's soft tissue contents become infected. In most cases, only one eye is affected.

The first signs of orbital cellulitis are usually swelling and redness of the eyelid, followed rapidly by pain and decreased vision. The eye may be noticeably displaced due to the swelling, so the eye seems to protrude from its socket. If your child has these signs or symptoms, go immediately to the nearest emergency department.

Diagnosis

Tests, including blood tests, may be conducted to determine the cause of the infection. A computerized tomography (CT) scan may be recommended to determine if the sinuses are involved or if a foreign object is present.

Treatment

Because orbital cellulitis is an acute and dangerous infection, hospitalization may be necessary. Antibiotics will likely be prescribed, based on the specific bacteria involved. Surgical drainage of an abscess may be necessary.

Corneal Transplantation

Transplantation of the cornea can restore good vision after severe corneal injury or scarring. Transplantation, however, isn't an option while there's any infection in your eye.

The cornea to be transplanted is obtained from a deceased person who, before dying, made arrangements to be a donor. Tissue typing can be done to help ensure a good match between the recipient and the donor cornea. Tissue typing is a way to identify proteins on the surface of white blood cells that serve as unique markers distinguishing one person from another.

Rejection is much less of a problem in corneal transplants than it is with organ transplants because the cornea has few blood vessels. However, if evidence of rejection develops following the procedure, corticosteroid drops usually control the problem.

The operation is performed by removing the central portion of the scarred cornea with a circular cutting instrument. Then a graft of the same size is fashioned from the donor cornea. The graft is placed over the removed portion of the recipient cornea and secured with very fine stitches (sutures).

Your surgeon will give you detailed instructions on caring for your eye after the operation and will watch closely for signs of rejection in the transplanted cornea. These include:

- Increased discharge or redness in the eye
- Pain in the eye
- Any marked change in vision
- Gray film over the field of vision
- Floaters in the field of vision

Corneal ulcers and infections

Signs and symptoms

- Impaired vision
- Eye pain
- A red eye
- A visible white patch on the cornea

A corneal ulcer is an open sore on the cornea. An ulcer can result from an infection by a virus, bacterium or fungus or, more commonly, from an abrasion that becomes infected. Viral infections are frequently caused by the herpes simplex virus. Eyelid problems, such as entropion and blepharitis, also can cause an ulcer. Retraction of the lids, as in Graves' disease or ectropion, may expose the cornea so that it's not bathed in tears. This also may result in ulceration.

The signs and symptoms of a bacterial ulcer are generally more severe than those of a viral one. A bacterial ulcer may be visible as a whitish patch on the cornea. An ulcer caused by the herpes simplex virus is usually invisible unless a staining solution is placed on the cornea. The ulcer that appears resembles the branches of a tree.

Treatment

Corneal ulcers are serious and should be treated as soon as possible. Once your doctor has determined what kind of ulcer you have, appropriate treatment can be prescribed. Bacterial ulcers usually are treated with antibiotic eyedrops. If the ulcer is severe, an antibiotic may be injected near the eye for faster absorption. Additional topical application of corticosteroid drops may lessen the inflammation.

If your infection is viral, antiviral drops or ointment may be prescribed. These will help control the ulcer. However, if it's due to the herpes virus, it may reappear.

Left untreated, an ulcer can permanently damage the cornea. A deep ulcer can even erode through the cornea and cause infection of the entire eyeball. If this happens you'll need surgery. A severely scarred cornea may require surgical replacement (corneal transplantation).

Glaucoma

Glaucoma is sometimes called a silent thief — it can steal your sight before you realize that anything is wrong. The most common form of the disease develops gradually, without warning signs. Many people aren't even aware they have an eye problem until their vision is already damaged extensively. In the United States, glaucoma is a leading cause of blindness and affects about 3 million people.

Glaucoma actually is a group of diseases. The common feature of these diseases is abnormally high pressure inside the eyeball. The space between the lens and cornea is filled with a fluid called the aqueous humor. This fluid circulates from behind the colored portion of the eye (iris) through the opening at the center of the eye (pupil) and into the space between the iris and cornea. Aqueous humor is produced constantly, so it must be drained constantly. Drainage is at the place where the iris and cornea meet, known as the drainage angle. From there the fluid is directed into a channel (Schlemm's canal) that leads to small veins outside the eye.

When the drainage angle doesn't function properly, fluid can't drain and pressure builds up within the eye. Pressure is also transmitted to the other fluid in the eye, the vitreous humor behind the lens. The vitreous humor in turn presses on the retina. This increased pressure affects the fibers of the optic nerve.

The optic nerve is a bundle of more than a million nerve fibers at the back of the eye. It's like a big electric cable made up of a million individual wires carrying images you see from the retina to the brain. When the optic nerve is damaged, blind spots develop in the visual field, usually starting with side (peripheral) vision. Over time, the

Are You at Risk?

Many people don't notice symptoms of chronic glaucoma until significant, permanent damage has occurred. For this reason, it's particularly important to be aware of the risk factors for the disease.

Age

Chronic glaucoma is rare before age 40. The risk of developing it nearly doubles every 10 years after age 50. Chronic glaucoma is most common in older women.

Race

Blacks are three to four times more likely than whites to get glaucoma and six times more likely to suffer permanent blindness as a result. The reasons for this difference aren't known, but blacks may be more susceptible to optic nerve damage or may not respond as well to current treatments. Asians, particularly people of Vietnamese descent, also are at increased risk.

Family history

Glaucoma runs in families. If one parent has glaucoma, you have about a 20 percent chance of developing the disease. If a sibling has it, your chance is 50 percent.

Medical conditions

If you have diabetes, your risk of developing glaucoma is about three times greater than that of people without diabetes. A history of high blood pressure or heart disease also can increase your risk. Other causes include eye inflammations, such as chronic uveitis and iritis, eye tumors and retinal detachment. Eye surgery also increases your risk.

Nearsightedness

An extensive study found that nearsighted (myopic) people had a two- or threefold greater risk of developing glaucoma compared with people who weren't nearsighted.

Physical injuries

Severe trauma, such as being hit in the eye, can result in increased eye pressure. Injury can also dislocate the lens, closing the drainage angle.

Prolonged corticosteroid use

Corticosteroids used for prolonged periods of time to treat another illness put you at increased risk of glaucoma.

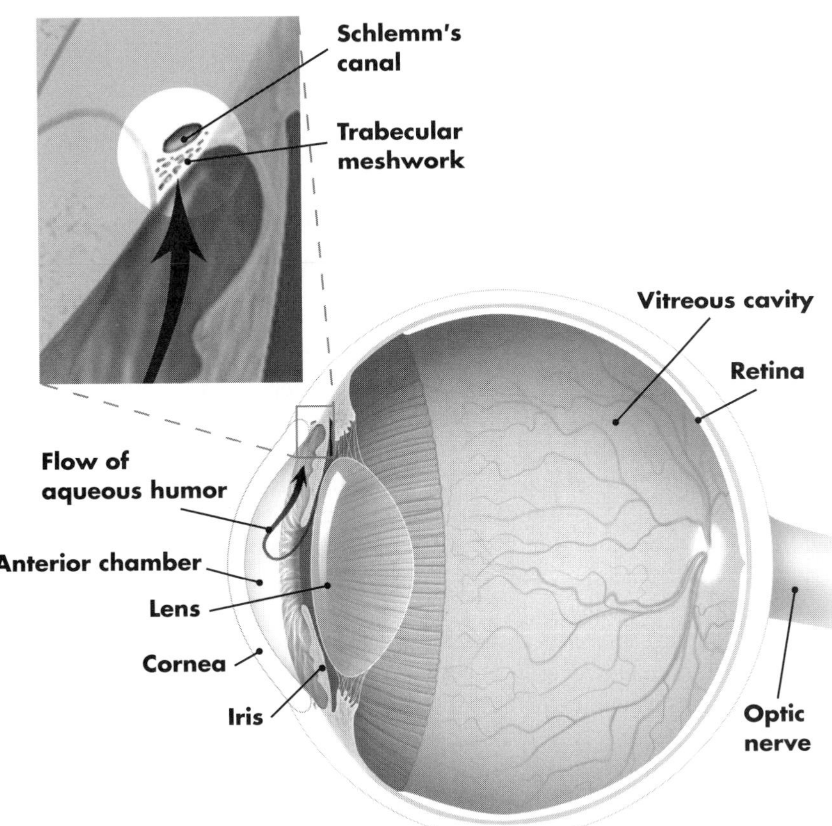

Vision loss caused by glaucoma results from the pressure of built-up fluid within the eye. Aqueous humor normally passes through a narrow space between your iris and lens (see inset), then drains out of your eye through Schlemm's canal. If this outward flow is blocked, pressure can damage your optic nerve and reduce vision.

result can be a marked loss of vision.

Fortunately, only a small percentage of people with glaucoma ever lose their sight. Recent advances have made it easier to diagnose and treat glaucoma. If detected and treated early, glaucoma need not cause severe vision loss. But it does mean you'll need to monitor the disease for the rest of your life.

Glaucoma can be divided into two forms, acute and chronic. The chronic form affects about 95 percent of people with glaucoma. In addition, there are several rare forms that don't fit into these two main categories.

Chronic glaucoma

Signs and symptoms

- Gradual loss of peripheral vision

Chronic (open-angle) glaucoma often goes undetected for years. With this condition, the drainage angle formed by the cornea and iris remains open, but the aqueous humor drains too slowly. This leads to gradual buildup of pressure within the eye. Damage to the optic nerve is so slow and painless that a large portion of your vision can be lost before you're even aware of it.

The cause of chronic glaucoma remains unknown. It may be that the aqueous humor drains or is absorbed less efficiently with age. However, not all older adults develop glaucoma.

Diagnosis

Chronic glaucoma has no early warning signs. The only way to detect glaucoma early is to have regular eye exams once you reach age 40. If you're at increased risk, your doctor may recommend even more frequent monitoring. Tests for glaucoma include:

Tonometry and ophthalmoscopy

Tonometry is an inexpensive and painless test that allows your doctor to determine the pressure within your eye. An ophthalmoscopic examination of the eye's interior can reveal damage to the optic nerve, a sign of glaucoma.

Visual field tests

These tests evaluate your peripheral as well as central vision. With a simple and quick test, a doctor can detect large defects in peripheral vision by asking you to count the number of fingers he or she is holding up while moving his or her hand around the periphery of your vision. Standard, more detailed visual field testing is done with computer-assisted devices.

Measuring the Pressure Within

Glaucoma is one of the leading causes of blindness in the United States. Early detection of the disease won't restore already lost vision, but prompt treatment can stop further deterioration and slow vision loss. A simple testing procedure, called tonometry, can alert your doctor to possible glaucoma.

Tonometry is a method of measuring the pressure within the eyeball. Normal eye pressure (intraocular pressure) is approximately 10 to 22 millimeters of mercury. If tonometry reveals higher pressure, further tests need to be done to determine if you have glaucoma.

Applanation tonometer

The applanation tonometer is a sophisticated device that's usually fitted to a slit lamp, a common instrument for eye examination. For this extremely accurate test, the doctor will numb your eyes with drops. You sit at the slit lamp and a small, plastic plunger pushes lightly against your eyeball. The force required to flatten (applanate) a small area of your cornea translates into a measure of your eye pressure. After the test, your eyes may feel scratchy for a short time.

Air-puff tonometer

An air-puff tonometer uses a puff of air to measure the force needed to indent your cornea. It's not as accurate as the applanation tonometer, but it has the advantage of not requiring the use of anesthetic drops because the instrument doesn't touch the eye.

Treatment

It's not always necessary to treat slightly increased eye pressure (intraocular pressure). If no evidence of optic nerve damage is found, your doctor may suggest careful monitoring of the condition by having an eye exam several times a year.

If you have elevated eye pressure, your optic nerve shows signs of damage and you've lost peripheral vision, treatment is generally necessary. If you have signs of optic nerve damage and visual field loss, even if your eye pressure is in the normal range, treatment is generally recommended to lower eye pressure further, which may help slow progression of glaucoma.

Glaucoma can be controlled with eyedrops, oral medications or surgical procedures.

Medication

Treatment for chronic glaucoma often starts with medicated eyedrops to help decrease pressure in the eye. For years, the most popular eyedrops to treat glaucoma were those containing adrenaline (epinephrine) or pilocarpine to increase the outflow of fluid. However, these medications sometimes cause troublesome side effects. As a result, other eyedrops have been developed and are now prescribed. The following list includes eyedrops and medications taken by mouth:

- *Beta blockers.* These eyedrop medications are remarkably effective and generally safe. Three drugs commonly used are timolol (Betimol, Timoptic), betaxolol (Betoptic) and levobunolol (AK-Beta, Betagan). Beta blockers can slow heart rhythm and worsen bronchial asthma symptoms. In some circumstances they can leave you feeling fatigued, drowsy, depressed or confused. They also can cause temporary impotence. If you have asthma, bronchitis or emphysema or if you have diabetes and use insulin, beta blockers usually should be avoided.
- *Other eyedrop medications.* These include alpha-adrenergic agents, such as apraclonidine (Iopidine) and brimonidine (Alphagan), carbonic anhydrase inhibitors, such as dorzolamide (Trusopt), prostaglandin analogues, such as latanoprost (Xalatan), and prostamides, such as bimatoprost (Lumigan). These medications work to lower eye pressure either by increasing the outflow of fluid from the eye or by reducing the

production of fluid. They all have various side effects.

- *Oral medications.* Another form of treatment involves medications taken by mouth. Certain drugs, such as acetazolamide (AK-Zol Diamox), can lower the pressure within your eye by decreasing the formation of normal eye fluid. This type of medicine can also cause general side effects. Long-term use of these drugs typically is avoided.

Your ophthalmologist understands the possible side effects of various medication options and will tell you what to look for. If you experience problems, your dosage may be adjusted or you may be switched to another treatment.

Surgery

If medication is unsuccessful in lowering intraocular pressure, your doctor may recommend an operation. Several options are available. In one procedure, a laser beam is used to open blocked drainage channels in the front chamber of the eye. For more severe cases, an operation known as a filtration procedure may be recommended. In this procedure, a drainage passage is surgically created between the interior of the eye and the conjunctiva to relieve pressure within the eye.

Acute glaucoma

Signs and symptoms

- Blurred vision, usually in one eye
- Halos appearing around lights
- Eye pain
- A red eye

Acute (closed-angle) glaucoma is less common than chronic glaucoma. This type of glaucoma occurs when the drainage angle formed by the cornea and iris closes or becomes blocked. The aqueous humor can't exit, resulting in an increase in eye pressure. The increase in pressure can occur suddenly or progress more gradually.

Most people with this type of glaucoma have a very narrow drainage angle, which may be an abnormality from birth. Acute glaucoma is more common among individuals who are farsighted. Normal aging also may cause angle blockage. As you age, the lens becomes larger, pushing your iris forward and narrowing the space between the iris and cornea.

A sudden increase in eye pressure can result from conditions that cause the pupils to become widely dilated. These may include:

- Darkness or dim light
- Stress or excitement
- Certain medications, such as antihistamines, tricyclic antidepressants and eyedrops used to dilate the pupil

Attacks of acute glaucoma can develop suddenly or follow warnings (preliminary attacks) weeks or months ahead. The attacks often occur in the evening when the light is dim and the pupils are dilated. Your vision may become blurred, you may see halos around lights, your eye becomes red and you may have pain. Although an acute attack often affects only one eye, the other eye is at risk as well.

In a severe attack, the symptoms are similar but more severe and persistent. The pain may be extreme, causing vomiting. The cornea may appear hazy, even gray. The eyeball may be painful and hard to the touch.

An attack of acute glaucoma is an emergency that should be treated immediately at your local emergency department. It can cause vision loss within hours of onset. Without treatment the eye can become blind in as little as 1 to 2 days.

PREVENTION TIP

It's very important to use glaucoma eyedrops exactly as prescribed to control eye pressure. Skipping even a few doses can cause glaucoma to worsen. You may need to apply the drops several times each day, although some are needed just once a day. If you're using more than one type of eyedrop, wait at least 5 to 10 minutes between applications.

To minimize absorption of the eyedrops into the bloodstream — and reduce the chance of side effects — close your eyes for 1 to 2 minutes after putting the drops in. Press lightly at the corner of your eye near your nose and wipe off any residual drops from your eyelid.

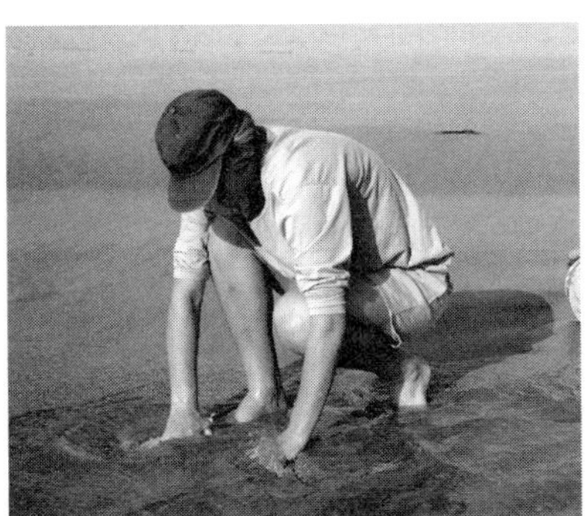
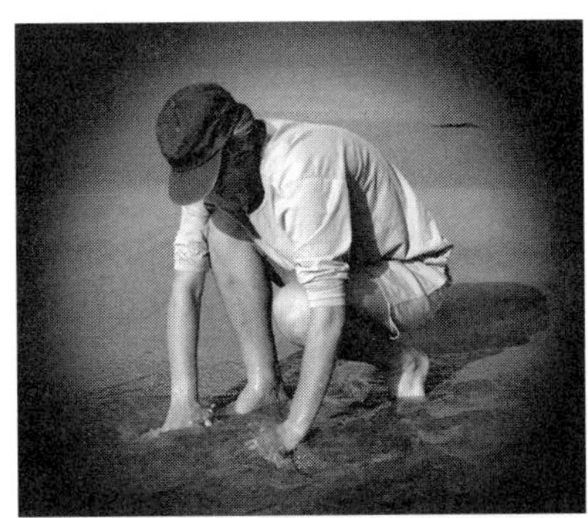
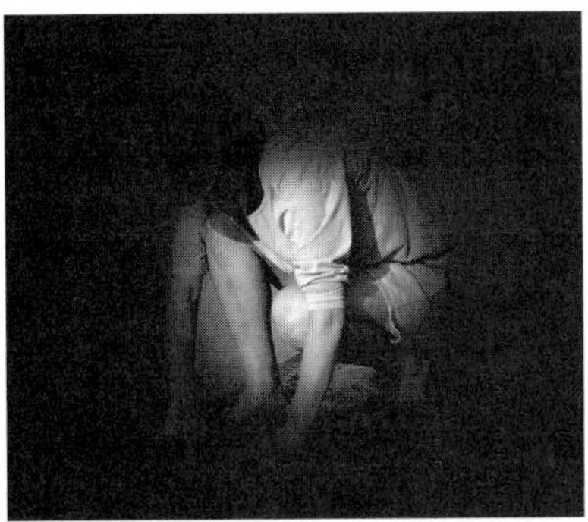

The gradual loss of peripheral vision associated with glaucoma is shown in this sequence from normal vision (left) to early-stage glaucoma (center) to advanced-stage glaucoma (right).

Are You at Risk?

Everyone is at risk of developing cataracts with increasing age. However, other factors also can increase your risk. Cataracts are more common in women than in men, and in blacks than in whites. Other factors that increase your risk of cataracts include:

- Diabetes
- A family history of cataracts
- Previous eye injury or inflammation
- Previous eye surgery
- Prolonged use of cortico-steroid medications
- Excessive consumption of alcohol
- Excessive exposure to sunlight
- Exposure to high levels of radiation, such as cancer therapy
- Smoking

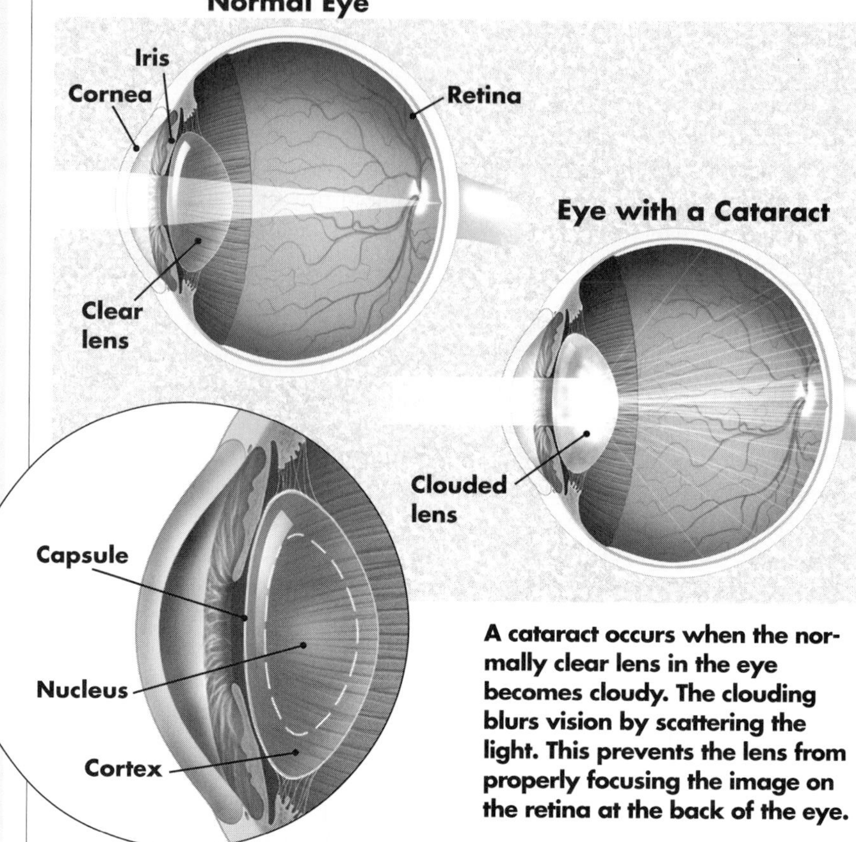

A cataract occurs when the normally clear lens in the eye becomes cloudy. The clouding blurs vision by scattering the light. This prevents the lens from properly focusing the image on the retina at the back of the eye.

A cataract can form in any one of the layers of the lens — the nucleus, cortex or capsule.

Treatment

Doctors may administer several medications to reduce eye pressure as quickly as possible.

Once your eye pressure is under control, you may need to have an operation called an iridotomy. In this procedure, an ophthalmologist uses a laser beam to create a small hole in the iris that allows aqueous humor to flow more freely within the aqueous cavity. With this technique, a surgeon can create a drainage hole without having to make a surgical incision, avoiding many of the risks generally associated with conventional surgery.

Many doctors will also perform an iridotomy on the other eye at a later date because of the high risk that it too will be affected by an acute attack within the next few years.

Cataracts

Signs and symptoms

- Clouded, blurred or dim vision
- Halos around lights
- Impaired vision at night or in bright light
- Sensitivity to bright light and glare
- A need for brighter light for reading and other activities
- Frequent changes in your eyeglass or contact lens prescription
- Fading or yellowing of colors
- Double vision or multiple vision in one eye

A cataract is a clouding of the normally clear lens of the eye. The lens, one of the two main focusing mechanisms of the eye, lies just behind the pupil. Clouding of the lens blocks the passage of light needed for sight. Although a cataract often starts in only one eye, usually both become involved. Cataracts are accompanied by changes in the chemical composition of the lens, but the cause of these alterations is unknown.

Cataracts are a major cause of vision loss worldwide. In the United States, more than 1.5 million cataract operations are performed each year. Many people find the idea of cataracts alarming — assuming that if they develop them, they'll become blind. In fact, cataracts are one of the least serious eye disorders because in most instances surgery can restore lost sight.

Everyone develops some clouding of the eye lenses with age. Most people older than age 60 have some degree of cataract formation. But age isn't the only factor in the development of cataracts. Certain diseases, such as diabetes, contribute to the formation of cataracts. People who take corticosteroid medications for a period of years, for diseases such as rheumatoid arthritis, may develop cataracts. People who are exposed to high amounts of ultraviolet radiation from the sun over a period of time also are at increased risk of developing cataracts.

Occasionally, a baby is born with cataracts or develops them shortly after birth. Certain eye disorders, such as iritis or an injury to the eyeball, can lead to the development of cataracts. Cataracts also tend to run in families.

There are three types of cataracts. The most common type, and the one associated with aging, is a nuclear cataract. It occurs in the middle of the lens. A cortical cataract begins as white, wedge-shaped streaks on the outer edge of the lens cortex. A subcapsular cataract starts as a small, opaque area just under the capsule or shell of the lens, usually at the back of the lens.

Most cataracts develop slowly and often don't disturb eyesight in early stages of the disease. Because almost everyone experiences changes in eyesight later in life, the gradual clouding of the lens resulting from cataracts is often ignored. But as the clouding progresses, eventually it can interfere significantly with your vision.

This change in vision is often described as a film-like covering over one or both eyes. You may seem to be looking through fog or a frosty window. Your vision may be worse in both dim and bright light, and you may have problems driving at night. Glare and halos around oncoming lights can make driving after dark especially uncomfortable and dangerous.

Some people experience an improvement in their near vision as the cataract progresses. They may find that they can read without their glasses, a condition known as second sight. In the early stages of development, a nuclear cataract increases the focusing power of the lens. People with a nuclear cataract may need more frequent changes in their prescription glasses. However, as the degree of clouding increases, the temporary improvement in reading ability decreases.

Diagnosis

If you notice changes in your vision, see your eye specialist for a complete examination. Cataracts often aren't visible until they're quite advanced. Tests to diagnose cataracts include a visual acuity test, a slit-lamp examination and a retinal exam. An ophthalmologist will likely dilate your pupil to examine the lens for signs of a cataract and determine how dense the clouding is.

Treatment

The only effective treatment for a cataract is surgery to remove the clouded lens and replace it with a lens implant.

Self-care

Medications, dietary supplements or optical devices can't cure cataracts. However, in the early stages of a cataract, when symptoms are mild, you can do a few things to deal with symptoms:

- Make sure your eyeglass or contact lens prescription is the most accurate possible.
- Improve the lighting in your home with more or brighter lamps.
- To reduce glare, wear sunglasses during the day when going outside. Some people also wear sunglasses at night to reduce glare from headlights.
- Limit or avoid night driving.
- Use magnifying glasses to read.

These measures may help temporarily, but as the cataract progresses, your vision deteriorates. When vision loss starts to interfere with everyday activities, you'll probably want to consider surgery.

Surgery

Cataract surgery usually is appropriate when failing vision seriously interferes with normal activities. The decision whether and when to have the operation varies with each individual, depending on age, occupation and lifestyle.

In some instances, surgery may be recommended early if there's a risk that the cataract may lead to other eye complications. Years ago, people with cataracts were often advised to postpone surgery until the cataract had "ripened," totally clouding the lens. Doctors no longer recommend waiting that long because allowing the cataract to become too advanced can cause complications.

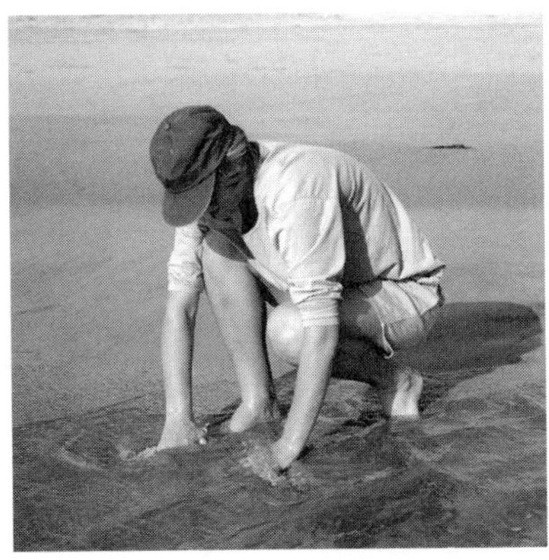

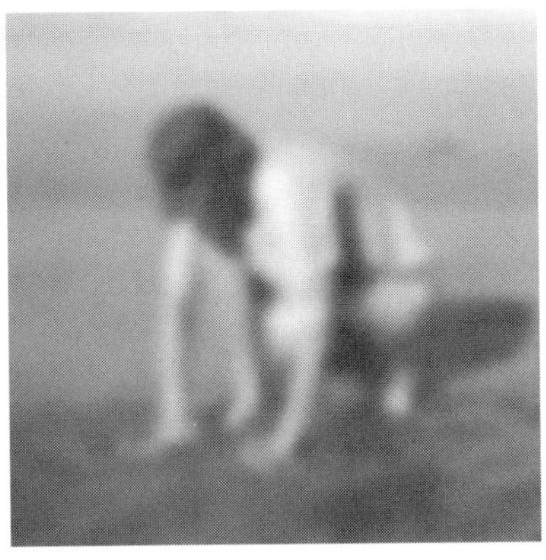

Normal vision (top) becomes blurred as a cataract forms (bottom).

Like all surgical techniques, cataract surgery is constantly being improved. Unlike years ago, when cataract surgery was a major operation, the surgery is often done now in an hour or less, without a hospital stay. The lens is removed from the eye and, in most cases, is replaced with an artificial lens (intraocular lens implant). More than 95 percent of people who have cataract surgery end up with improved vision.

The most common type of cataract surgery is phacoemulsification. In this procedure, the surgeon uses a microscope and ultrasound instruments to remove the cataract, leaving most of the lens capsule in place. The capsule helps support the lens implant. Phacoemulsification requires a very small incision, and the recovery period is short.

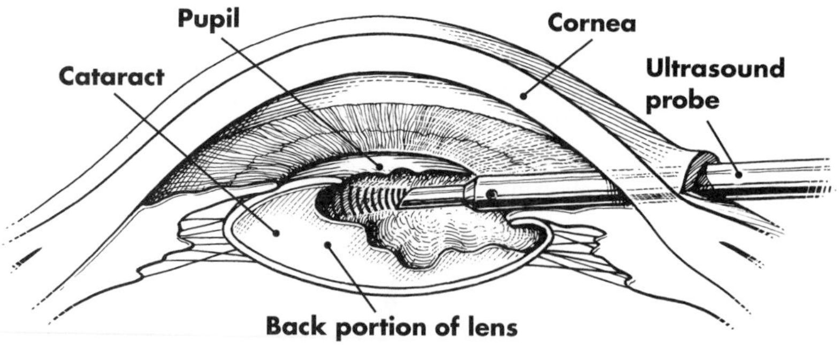

During phacoemulsification the rapidly vibrating tip of the ultrasound hand probe breaks up the cataract, which is then suctioned out.

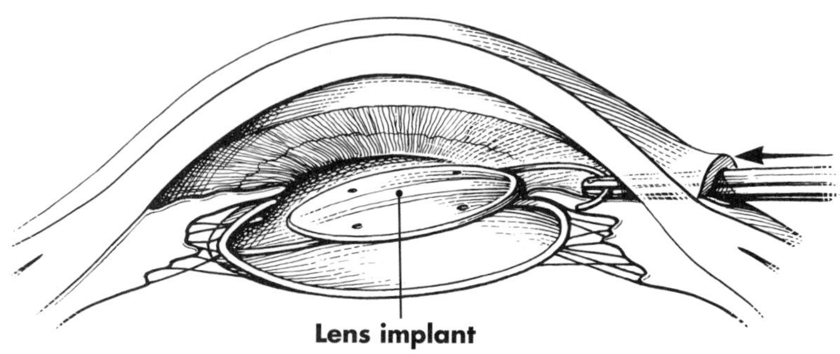

After removing the cataract, the surgeon inserts the lens implant into the empty capsule where the natural lens used to be.

An alternative procedure, called extracapsular cataract extraction, is similar to phacoemulsification but requires a larger incision. It may be needed if your cataract has progressed so far that phacoemulsification can't effectively break up the clouded lens.

After making an opening in the front part of the lens capsule, the surgeon removes the harder center of the lens in one piece and, with suction, removes the more peripheral cloudy lens material. The back portion of the lens capsule is left intact.

Rarely, a surgeon may use a procedure called intracapsular cataract extraction. This procedure involves removal of the entire lens, including the capsule. If a lens implant is performed, the lens will most likely be placed in front of the iris.

With phacoemulsification, surgical incisions are very small and no stitches (sutures) are required. Healing is fast, and vision starts to improve within a few days. If your surgery required a larger incision and sutures, full healing may take about 4 weeks.

Most people still need to wear glasses following cataract removal. In the small percentage of cases when cataract removal doesn't improve vision, it's often because of another disease, most often macular degeneration. Because cataracts can prevent your ophthalmologist from examining your retina and macula, he or she may not be able to diagnose vision-limiting problems in the back of the eye.

Other options

Alternatives to a lens implant include eyeglasses and contact lenses. Until the advent of lens implants, thick eyeglass lenses were the only way to correct vision after cataract surgery, if contact lenses weren't an option.

Although glasses are helpful, they do have significant drawbacks, including excessive magnification, reduced side vision and limited depth perception. Contact lenses usually provide better vision than do thick glasses. They're especially helpful if the lens of only one eye must be removed. However, some older adults don't care for contact lenses.

When Is Surgery the Right Choice?

Cataract surgery restores good vision to thousands of people every day — it's the most common surgery for Americans age 65 and older.

The decision when to have surgery is one that you and your ophthalmologist should make together. In general, consider surgery when your vision starts to hamper your lifestyle.

If you have cataracts and agree with one or more of the following statements, you may be a candidate for cataract surgery:

- Because of my vision, I don't feel confident when driving.
- Because of my vision, I can't do my best work.
- Because of my vision, I can't read comfortably.
- Because of my vision, I can't do things I enjoy.
- Because of my vision, I'm afraid I'll bump into something or trip and fall.
- Because of my vision, I'm not as independent as I'd like to be.

Age-related macular degeneration

Signs and symptoms

- A need for bright light when reading or doing close work
- Printed words become increasingly blurry
- Colors appear dull and washed out
- A gradual haziness of overall vision
- Increasingly blurred central vision

PREVENTION TIP

Most cataracts occur as a result of aging, so they can't be prevented altogether. Regular exams remain the key to early detection. However, you can take steps to help slow or prevent the development of cataracts:

- *Don't smoke.* Smokers are more likely to develop cataracts than are nonsmokers.
- *Protect your eyes from the sun.* Wear sunglasses that block out harmful ultraviolet light.
- *Eat a nutritionally balanced diet.* Research suggests that damage to the lens brought on by aging may be reduced by an increased dietary intake of antioxidants, substances that prevent oxidative damage to body tissue in the eye and elsewhere. Foods with antioxidants are those rich in vitamins A, C and E, found mainly in fruits and vegetables.
- *Limit alcohol.* Excessive alcohol use may increase your risk of developing cataracts.
- *Follow your doctor's treatment plan.* If you have diabetes, cardiovascular disease or other medical conditions, taking medication or other steps as recommended by your doctor may reduce your risk of cataracts.

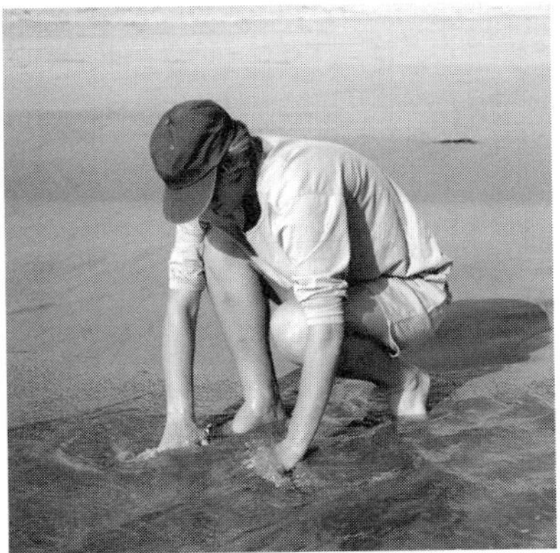

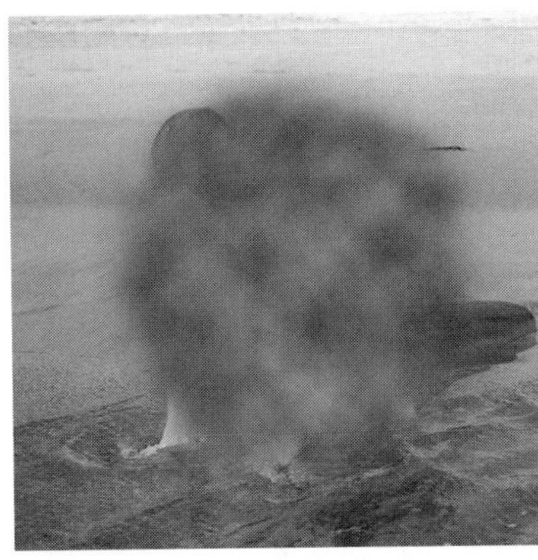

As macular degeneration develops, eyesight becomes impaired by general haziness and a blind spot at the center of the visual field.

- Visual distortions, such as straight lines appearing wavy or crooked

Age-related macular degeneration (AMD) is a chronic disease that occurs if tissue in the macula, the part of your retina that perceives central vision, deteriorates with aging. The result is blurred central vision or even a blind spot in the center of your visual field. Macular degeneration is the leading cause of severe vision loss in people age 50 and older.

The macula (Latin for "spot") is located in the center of the retina and is densely packed with light-sensitive cones and rods. In the early stages of macular degeneration, small deposits called drusen form in this area. As the disease progresses, abnormal blood vessels grow from the choroid, a layer rich in blood vessels under the retina. The retina's supporting tissue (retinal pigment epithelium) also disappears. Both processes damage the light-sensitive cells of the retina, causing loss of reading or central vision.

The first sign of macular degeneration may be a need for more light when you do close-up work. Fine newsprint and street signs may become more difficult to read. Eventually, you may notice that when you look at an object, what should be a smooth, straight line appears distorted or crooked. Gray or blank spots may mask the center of your visual field.

Macular degeneration affects your central vision but not your peripheral vision, so it doesn't cause total blindness. The damage caused by macular degeneration often can't be reversed. But early detection and treatment may help reduce the extent of vision loss.

Types

There are two types of macular degeneration: dry and wet.

Dry

Macular degeneration starts out as the dry form. This occurs when the supporting tissue of the retina begins to thin. The normally reddish-brown color of the macula takes on a mottled appearance, and drusen appear under the retina. Most people have the dry form. It may initially affect only one eye, but usually both eyes eventually become involved.

Wet

Wet macular degeneration develops when new blood vessels grow from the choroid underneath the macula. These abnormal vessels leak fluid or blood and cause your central vision to blur. All eyes with wet macular degeneration also show signs of the dry form (drusen and mottled pigmentation). Straight lines appear to be wavy or crooked, and blank spots appear in your field of vision. Vision loss is usually rapid and severe.

Another form of wet macular degeneration is called retinal pigment epithelial detachment. Fluid leaks from the choroid, although no abnormal blood vessels have started to grow there. The fluid collects under the retinal pigment epithelium, causing what looks like a blister under the macula. This type frequently develops abnormal blood vessels.

Diagnosis

Your eye specialist can test for macular degeneration during a routine examination. He or she may begin with a simple test of your central vision using an Amsler grid. If you have macular degeneration, some of the straight lines may seem faded, broken or distorted when you look at the grid. By noting

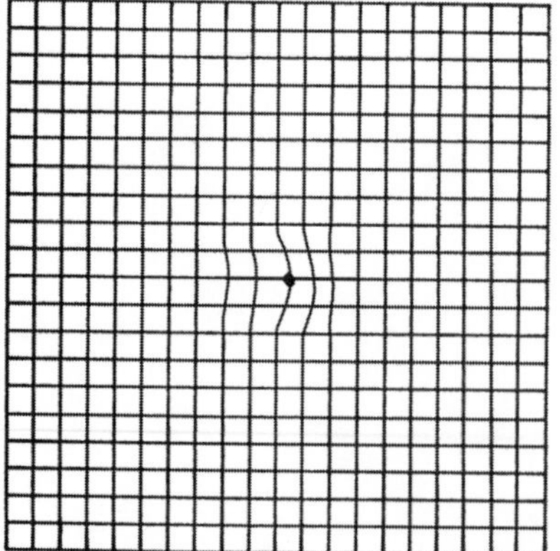
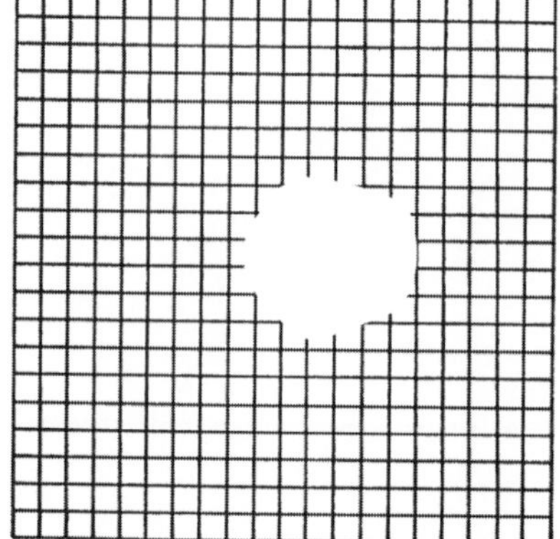

Someone in the early stages of macular degeneration may see distorted grid lines (left). Someone with a more advanced stage may see a blank spot at the center of the grid (right).

where the break or distortion occurs, your doctor can better determine the location and extent of the disease.

To evaluate the extent of damage to the macula, your doctor may also perform a test known as fluorescein angiography to look for abnormal blood vessels. In this test, a special dye is injected into a vein of your arm. The dye flows to the blood vessels in the eye. Photographs of the retina are taken and can identify problems with the macula.

Treatment

Currently, there's no treatment for dry macular degeneration. Because dry macular degeneration usually progresses slowly, many people with early-stage AMD are able to live relatively normal, productive lives.

For wet macular degeneration, some treatment options are available. The success of treatment generally depends on the location and extent of the abnormal blood vessels.

Successful treatment can halt further progress of the disease. In most cases, the damage already caused by macular degeneration can't be reversed.

Laser surgery

A form of laser surgery called photocoagulation can, in some cases, prevent further damage to the macula and halt progression of vision loss for some time. In this procedure, a special lens placed on the eye focuses laser light onto the retina to create small burns, which can seal off and destroy abnormal new blood vessels under your macula.

Whether this surgery is appropriate for you depends on the location and appearance of the blood vessels, the amount of blood that has leaked and the general health of your macula. Only about 20 percent of people with macular degeneration are candidates for laser treatment, and the results are often disappointing — it's successful only about 50 percent of the time, and new blood vessel growth may recur.

If you noticed a dark or gray spot in or near your central vision before laser treatment, the procedure will make vision in that spot completely and permanently blank. With time, you may not notice the blank spot any longer, especially when you use both eyes.

Photodynamic therapy

Photodynamic therapy (PDT) treats damaged areas at the center of the macula while still preserving some central vision. This procedure combines a cold laser and a light-sensitizing dye that's injected into your bloodstream. This dye concentrates in the abnormal blood vessels under the macula. When hit by cold laser light, the dye releases substances that seal the leaking vessels without damaging the macula. Overlying cones and rods are generally preserved. The treatment can be repeated if necessary.

Macular translocation surgery

Macular translocation surgery is an experimental treatment for wet macular degeneration. This surgery may be used if abnormal blood vessels are located directly under the center of the macula (fovea). The procedure shifts the fovea away from the damaged area and moves it over healthy tissue. The surgery is followed by laser treatment to destroy the abnormal blood vessels without damaging the fovea.

Are You at Risk?

Although researchers don't know the exact causes of macular degeneration, they've identified some contributing factors. These include:

- *Age and race.* The disease is most common in whites over age 50. It's less common among blacks, Asians and American Indians.
- *Family history.* If someone in your family has age-related macular degeneration, you're at greater risk.
- *Cigarette smoking.* Smokers are two to three times more likely than are nonsmokers to develop macular degeneration.
- *Exposure to sunlight.* Long-term exposure to ultraviolet light and blue light — the wavelength just above ultraviolet — increases your risk. This includes use of sunlamps as well as sunlight.
- *Cardiovascular disease.* This includes circulatory problems, stroke, heart attack and chest pain (angina). Cardiovascular disease that's not well controlled may contribute to the onset of macular degeneration.
- *Lighter eye color.* People with lighter colored eyes may be at greater risk than people with darker colored eyes.

COMPLEMENTARY MEDICINE

A growing body of evidence suggests that the foods you eat may help protect your eyesight. A large study — the Age-Related Eye Disease Study (AREDS) — showed the impact of dietary supplements on people at high risk of developing the advanced stages of macular degeneration. People in the study group were able to reduce the risk of progression of macular degeneration, as well as the risk of vision loss, by taking a combination of vitamin A (beta carotene), vitamin C, vitamin E, zinc and copper. This supplement didn't benefit people in the early stages of macular degeneration, nor did it affect the development of cataracts.

Vitamins C and E and carotenoids such as beta carotene are antioxidants. Antioxidants are vitamins, minerals and enzymes that help maintain healthy cells and tissues by combating free radicals, unstable oxygen molecules that damage normal cells in a process called oxidation. Oxidation is thought to play a role in the development of cataracts, macular degeneration and glaucoma, as well as many other diseases.

Scientists continue to look at the role that antioxidants may play in the prevention of eye disease. Another study found that people who regularly ate five servings or more a week of dark green leafy vegetables, which are rich in the carotenoids lutein and zeaxanthin, had a markedly lower risk of getting macular degeneration than did study participants who ate smaller amounts or none of these vegetables. However, there's little evidence that taking lutein in a pill or supplement form has a similar benefit.

Reducing your risk generally involves including foods that contain antioxidants in your diet for many years. Your best bet is simply to eat a variety of foods, especially fruits, vegetables and whole grains. Include deep green, dark yellow, red and orange fruits and vegetables. Good choices include collard greens, spinach, green and red peppers, carrots, kale, Swiss chard, cantaloupe, mango, squash, sweet potatoes, broccoli, Brussels sprouts, tomatoes, strawberries, oranges and other citrus fruits and watermelon.

If you eat a well-balanced diet, your body will get all of the nutrients it needs. It's fine to take a daily vitamin and mineral supplement, but supplements are no substitute for eating a variety of healthy foods. Excessive doses of vitamins can have dangerous side effects.

Retinal detachment

Signs and symptoms

- A sensation of flashing lights
- Many floaters — dark or light spots, specks or lines — in the field of vision
- Blurred vision
- A shadow over a portion of the field of vision

The retina is a thin, transparent membrane that lies smoothly against the inside back wall of your eye. It contains cells that are sensitive to light (cones and rods). It also contains the nerves that carry impulses from the cones and rods to the optic nerve. The optic nerve transports the signals to the brain. A thin layer of tiny blood vessels (choroid) lies under the retina. This layer supplies oxygen and nutrients to the retina, essential for it to function properly.

Retinal detachment results when the retina separates from this layer of blood vessels.

Most cases of retinal detachment are caused by a tear or hole in the retina. The defect may develop from changes in the eye's vitreous fluid caused by aging, or it may develop in weak patches of the retina. The tear allows fluid from the vitreous cavity to leak under the retina and lift it from the choroid.

Spots, Specks and Flashes

Just about everyone occasionally sees what appear to be specks, hairs and fine strings floating freely in the fluid of the eye. These vitreous floaters move in and out of your field of vision. They result from changes in the vitreous humor related to aging and from certain conditions such as nearsightedness (myopia) or inflammation.

As you age, you may notice more and different floaters because the vitreous humor in your eye may shrink and liquefy. The vitreous humor is a jelly-like substance that fills the inside of your eye. It's composed almost entirely of water and accounts for three-fourths of the weight of your eye. At the back of the eye, the vitreous cavity attaches to the retina, the light-sensitive tissue of the eye.

When the vitreous cavity shrinks, it gradually leads to the appearance of spots, specks, hairs or strings floating in the fluid. The floaters may be annoying, but they tend to become less conspicuous with time and only rarely affect vision.

If floaters develop or suddenly increase in number, this may signal a serious eye disorder. Consult your ophthalmologist immediately.

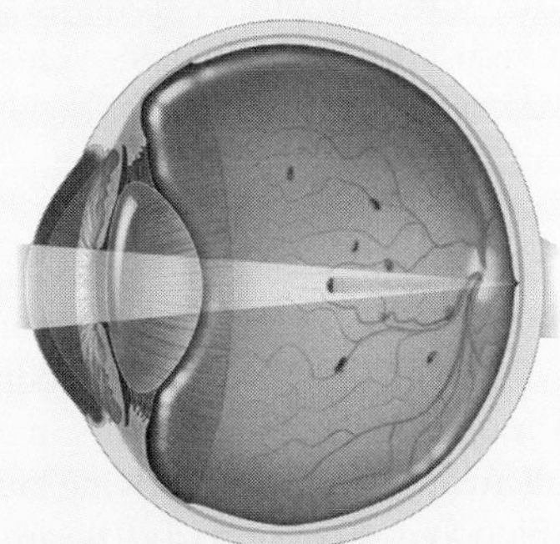

Floaters can interfere with vision by intercepting light entering the eye, casting a shadow on the retina.

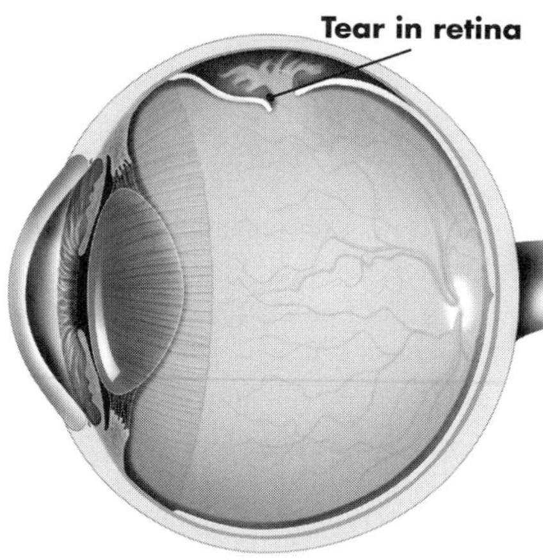

When vitreous humor leaks through holes in the retina, the retina may start to pull away from the underlying layer of blood vessels. As more liquid accumulates, the detachment may expand, and parts of the visual field may become blurred or lost.

This form of detachment is called rhegmatogenous detachment — caused by a retinal defect. Occasionally, a tumor or an inflammatory disorder affecting the back portion of the eye also can lead to a separation of the retina from the underlying choroid. Such a detachment is called secondary retinal detachment.

Each year, approximately 30,000 people in the United States suffer a rhegmatogenous retinal detachment. The condition almost always leads to blindness in the affected eye if it's not surgically repaired.

As the vitreous cavity shrinks and sags, it may tug on the retina, producing the sensation of flashing lights. If the tugging is strong enough to cause small holes or tears to develop in the retina, vitreous humor may seep under the retina. This causes hazy vision and the appearance of floaters — spots, specks or lines in the field of vision. As liquid collects, areas of the retina surrounding the holes or tears may pull away from the underlying layer of blood vessels (choroid). The areas where the retina is detached no longer function.

Not all tears and holes lead to retinal detachment. Sometimes, the retina remains attached to the choroid. But detachment that goes undetected and untreated can progress and eventually involve the entire retina, with complete loss of vision in that eye.

Diagnosis

An ophthalmologist can determine if you have a retinal hole, tear or detachment by carefully examining the retina with an ophthalmoscope. If blood in the vitreous humor prevents a clear view of the retina, he or she might use sound waves (ultrasound) to get an image of the retina.

Treatment

Surgery is the only effective therapy for retinal detachment. If a tear or hole is treated before detachment occurs or if a retinal detachment is treated before the portion of the retina responsible for central vision (macula) has detached, you'll probably retain much of your vision.

Surgery for a tear or hole

When a retinal tear or hole hasn't progressed to a detachment, your doctor may use one of two techniques:

- *Photocoagulation.* In this process a laser beam is directed to the area around the retinal defect. The treated area then forms a scar, which usually holds the retina to the underlying tissue.
- *Cryopexy.* This method uses intense cold to freeze the retina around the tear or hole. A freezing probe is applied to the outer surface of the eye directly over the retinal defect. It produces inflammation that leads to the formation of a scar, sealing the defect and holding the retina to the underlying tissue.

Surgery for retinal detachment

Three different surgical procedures are commonly used to repair a retinal detachment. Which of the procedures a surgeon chooses depends on the severity and complexity of the condition:

- *Pneumatic retinopexy.* This technique is used for an uncomplicated detachment in which the retinal defect is located in the upper part of the retina. After freezing the retinal defect (cryopexy), the surgeon injects a bubble of gas into the vitreous cavity. The bubble expands and seals the retinal defect and prevents any more vitreous humor from entering the space below the retina. Fluid that already has collected under the retina is absorbed, and the retina reattaches itself to the back wall of the eye.
- *Scleral buckling.* This is the most common surgery for repairing retinal detachment. First the surgeon treats the tears or holes with cryopexy. Then he or she indents (buckles) the sclera over the affected area by pressing in with a piece of silicone sutured to the outside of the wall of the eye (sclera). The silicone material is either solid or in the form of a soft sponge.

  The buckle closes the tear or hole and helps reduce the circumference of the eyeball, to prevent further pulling and separation. When there are several tears or holes or an extensive detachment, the surgeon may create a scleral buckle encircling the entire circumference of the eye. The buckle is stitched to the outer surface of the sclera, then covered with the conjunctiva. Once the incision heals, there's little evidence of the operation.

  This procedure works more than 80 percent of the time with one operation. The success rate exceeds 90 percent with additional operations, if necessary. But it doesn't guarantee normal vision. How well you see afterward depends on the severity of the problem before surgery. There's also a 10 percent chance of some loss of vision due to wrinkling or puckering of the macula.
- *Vitrectomy.* Sometimes, a doctor can't view a detached retina due to clouding of the vitreous by

hemorrhage or inflammation. In other instances, scar tissue in the vitreous makes it impossible to repair a retinal detachment with pneumatic retinopexy or scleral buckling alone. In such situations, a procedure called vitrectomy removes the clouded vitreous or scar tissue. The surgeon accomplishes this with a variety of delicate instruments inserted into the eyeball through small openings in the sclera. Following vitrectomy, a scleral buckling procedure may be performed.

In especially difficult cases, the surgeon may inject air, other gases or silicone oil into the vitreous cavity to help reposition the retina against the wall of the eye. Eventually, your eye absorbs the air or gas and replaces it with fluid that the eye normally produces. Silicone oil, however, isn't absorbed and has to be removed once the retina is reattached and completely healed.

Retinal vessel occlusion

Signs and symptoms

- Sudden blurring or loss of vision in part or all of one eye

The retina of the eye functions rather like the film in a camera, by capturing images that are focused by the cornea and lens and transmitting the information to the brain. The retina is nourished by arteries and veins. These retinal arteries and veins may become blocked (occluded) by a blood clot or fatty deposit.

If a retinal artery is blocked, the retina stops functioning, and partial or complete blindness can result in the affected eye. A retinal artery blockage is an emergency because without a blood supply, the inner layer of the retina will soon die. Blockage of a retinal vein is less threatening to sight than blockage of an artery. However, a blocked vein may rupture and spill blood and fluid into the retina. The blood blurs and clouds vision.

These conditions, known collectively as retinal vascular occlusion, are more common among older adults. Often, they're symptoms of another disorder, such as high blood pressure or diabetes.

Acute blurring of vision in one eye is the main symptom of retinal vessel occlusion. If the blockage is in an artery, the upper or lower field of vision may be abruptly affected. If a retinal vein becomes blocked, vision may blur and cloud more slowly over a period of hours or days.

Diagnosis

Regular eye examinations are most helpful for early detection of a possible problem. You may also undergo a general medical examination to identify any underlying disorder, such as high blood pressure, diabetes or narrowing of the major artery in your neck that supplies blood to your eyes and brain (carotid artery).

Treatment

Frequently, little can be done to treat retinal vascular occlusions. In some cases, the spilled blood may be reabsorbed by the eye and sight will improve. If the blood isn't reabsorbed, blurred vision likely will be permanent.

Laser therapy may be used to treat either glaucoma or swelling of the retina that can follow retinal vein occlusion. If the artery is involved, emergency treatment is the only chance of improving impaired vision. You may be given anticoagulant drugs to prevent further clotting. An operation to clean out the carotid artery might be suggested if the blockage originated in the carotid artery. Often, vision is only partially restored, if at all.

Optic neuritis

Signs and symptoms

- Acute loss of vision in one eye
- Pain when moving the eye

Optic neuritis is an inflammation of the optic nerve that may result from a viral illness or multiple sclerosis. When the condition affects the portion of the optic nerve visible through the ophthalmoscope, it's known as papillitis. An ophthalmoscope is an instrument that illuminates and allows viewing of the back of the eye. When the inflammation occurs in the portion of the optic nerve behind the eye, it's known as retrobulbar neuritis.

When the optic nerve swells, it blocks visual signals to the brain. The result is a gradual or sudden loss of vision. In the case of papillitis, loss of vision is usually the only symptom. With retrobulbar neuritis, loss of vision may be accompanied by pain when moving the eye.

Diagnosis

A series of tests will likely be conducted to determine the nature and extent of the problem. Because optic neuritis often is associated with multiple sclerosis in young adults, your doctor may recommend a thorough medical examination.

Treatment

In many cases, optic neuritis disappears on its own within 2 to 8 weeks, and sight returns. Corticosteroid medications may clear up the inflammation sooner, but such treatment is controversial. The condition can recur, especially when associated with multiple sclerosis, and each time may cause more damage.

Ischemic optic neuropathy

Ischemic optic neuropathy is a painless swelling of the optic nerve due to loss of blood supply to the nerve. It may be associated with inflammation of arteries in the scalp and head (temporal arteritis) or high blood pressure. Both eyes can be involved. The inflammation usually resolves. Treatment involves addressing the underlying condition and may include the use of corticosteroid medications for arteritis.

Coloboma

A coloboma is a rare congenital defect in the development of the eye. Parts of the iris, ciliary body, lens, retina, choroid and optic nerve may be absent.

Depending on the extent of the defect, there may be partial or even complete loss of vision in the affected eye. Sometimes, both eyes are affected. It's essential that a child with loss of vision from a coloboma wear protective glasses as soon as possible to protect the unaffected eye from injury.

Choroiditis

Signs and symptoms

- Blurred vision in one eye
- Pain or discomfort in the eye

The choroid is the layer between the retina and sclera of the eye. It's made up mainly of blood vessels, which nourish the retina. When this layer becomes inflamed (choroiditis), the retina may also become inflamed. This condition is then called chorioretinitis. When the inflammation subsides, the choroid and retina may be scarred. Vision may be impaired if the macula — the center part of the retina responsible for central vision — is involved.

Because the inflammation usually occurs in a spotty fashion, loss of vision is also spotty. Each scarred area will cause a corresponding blind spot, which can be discovered through testing. In many people, the scarring from choroiditis poses no handicap to vision because the blank spots (scotomata) are small and don't involve the macula.

The cause of this condition is often unknown. Occasionally, it may be associated with certain infections, such as histoplasmosis or toxoplasmosis.

Diagnosis

An ophthalmologist will examine the eye and may recommend fluorescein angiography. In this test, dye is injected into a vein of the arm and reaches the blood vessels of the eye. A series of photographs of the retina can reveal areas of inflammation. Your doctor may also recommend a general medical examination to rule out the possibility of a serious underlying disorder.

Treatment

Corticosteroid medications may be given in pill form or in an injection near the eye to reduce the inflammation. Treatment of any underlying disorder also may improve symptoms.

Retinitis pigmentosa

Signs and symptoms

- Difficulty seeing at night or in reduced light
- Poor central vision
- Loss of side (peripheral) vision

Retinitis pigmentosa is an inherited disorder in which the retina slowly degenerates in both eyes. The structures in the retina called rods are affected the most, causing defective night vision (night blindness). As the disease progresses, peripheral vision also may be lost, producing so-called tunnel vision.

The disease, which is uncommon, may lead to legal blindness. The main criterion for legal blindness is visual acuity of 20/200 or poorer in the better eye while wearing glasses.

Retinitis pigmentosa can be detected in childhood. Reduced night vision may become evident by age 10. If your family has a history of the disorder, have your child tested early.

Diagnosis

During an examination of your eye, an eye doctor may see dark pigmentation of the retina, hence the name pigmentosa. Tests to determine the presence and extent of the disease include a procedure that records the electric response of the retina to light (electroretinography) and another procedure to determine how well the eyes adjust to reduced illumination (dark adaptation).

Treatment

There's no known treatment to cure retinitis pigmentosa, although some research suggests that vitamin A supplements may slow progression of the disease. Use of low-vision aids can be helpful.

Some researchers suggest using sunglasses to protect the retina from the harmful effects of visible and ultraviolet light. Experimental devices that widen the field of vision may prove helpful in the future.

Retinoblastoma

Signs and symptoms

- A white reflection visible in the pupil
- Cross-eye
- A red, painful eye
- Poor vision
- Bleeding inside the eye
- A different-colored iris in each eye
- White spots on the iris

Tumors can develop anywhere in the body and may be either noncancerous (benign) or cancerous (malignant). Retinoblastoma is a malignant tumor found in children, usually those younger than 5 years. Tumors may occur in one or both eyes.

Retinoblastoma is hereditary in 30 percent to 40 percent of cases. The prognosis for retinoblastoma is good if it's treated early. If someone in your family has had retinoblastoma, be sure to have your children tested early and re-examined periodically.

Diagnosis

The key to diagnosis of retinoblastoma is a thorough examination by a specialist experienced in diagnosing and treating retinoblastoma. Examination is usually done with the child under general anesthesia in a hospital setting. The pupils are dilated widely so that the doctor can use indirect ophthalmoscopy to check for any growths. If a tumor is found, the ophthalmologist may order an ultrasound examination and recommend a computerized tomography (CT) scan of the head and eyes.

Treatment

Treatment of retinoblastoma depends on the number and size of tumors, their location and whether both eyes are involved. If a tumor is small and doesn't involve the macula or optic nerve, laser therapy or freezing (cryotherapy) may destroy it without damaging the eye. Larger tumors and those involving the optic nerve, the macula or both may be treated with chemotherapy, radiation or a combination of both. Multiple tumors also may be treated with chemotherapy or radiation. If a tumor is large and has already destroyed vision, or if it continues to grow despite treatment, the eye may be removed.

Melanoma of the eye

Signs and symptoms

Conjunctival melanoma

- A brown or black spot on the covering of the eye (conjunctiva)
- A spot on the eye that enlarges or changes color with time

Uveal melanoma

- A dark spot on the iris
- A change in iris color
- Decreased vision
- Visual field defects
- A flickering light sensation
- A red, painful eye

Melanoma is usually seen as a form of skin cancer, but it can also begin in the eye. Melanoma of the eye (ocular melanoma) is a cancer of the pigmented tissues of the eye. It can occur on the surface of the eye (conjunctival melanoma) or inside the eye (uveal melanoma), involving the iris, ciliary body, which produces the fluid inside the eye and helps control lens movement, or choroid, the layer of tissue between the retina and sclera.

Melanoma of the eye is a potentially deadly cancer. As with any type of cancer, early detection and treatment are essential. Melanoma of the eye almost always originates in the eye itself and rarely spreads there from elsewhere in the body.

Diagnosis

The key to diagnosis is a thorough examination by a specialist familiar with the features and variations of eye tumors. In addition to a thorough eye examination, diagnostic tests to determine the extent of the tumor may include an ultrasound examination, computerized tomography (CT) scan or magnetic resonance imaging (MRI).

Treatment

Treatment may depend on the size and location of the melanoma. Small, nongrowing tumors that cause no visual symptoms may be monitored closely with no immediate treatment.

Melanomas in the conjunctiva are often removed surgically, and the area around the tumor is treated with a freezing procedure (cryotherapy) to destroy any remaining cancer in the area. Small, limited tumors of the iris, ciliary body and choroid also may be treated with surgical removal.

When removing the tumor isn't possible, laser therapy (laser photocoagulation or transpupillary thermotherapy) may be used to destroy small, growing tumors.

The eye may have to be removed if the tumor is large, it has invaded other parts of the eye or other treatments are unsuccessful. Ocular melanoma, including cancerous cells that have spread to other organs, generally respond poorly to chemotherapy.

Other Diseases and Your Eyes

Some conditions and diseases that affect other parts of the body can also affect your sight. These include stroke, Graves' disease (a thyroid disorder), cranial arteritis (a circulatory problem), diabetes and high blood pressure.

Diabetic retinopathy

Signs and symptoms

- Blurred vision
- Fluctuating vision
- "Spiders," "cobwebs" or tiny specks floating in the eye
- Dark streaks or a red film that blocks vision
- A dark or empty spot in the center of your vision
- Poor night vision
- Difficulty adjusting from bright light to dim light
- Eye pain, in advanced cases

The most common and most serious eye complication of diabetes is diabetic retinopathy. *Retinopathy* is the medical term for damage to the many tiny blood vessels that nourish the retina. Increased blood sugar associated with diabetes can gradually damage the vessels.

The longer you have diabetes, the more likely it is that you'll develop diabetic retinopathy. The disease is most common in individuals with type 1 diabetes (formerly called juvenile or insulin-dependent diabetes) who have had diabetes for at least 20 years. Almost everyone who has diabetes shows signs of retinal damage after about 30 years of living with the disease.

Most people with diabetic retinopathy experience only mild vision problems. But the condition can progress and threaten vision. In fact, diabetic retinopathy is a leading cause of blindness among adults in the United States. Usually, both eyes are affected, although the disease may be more advanced in one eye than in the other.

Types

There are two types of diabetic retinopathy: nonproliferative and proliferative.

Nonproliferative

Nonproliferative diabetic retinopathy, also known as background

Question and Answer

How often should I have an eye exam if I have diabetes?

Eye exams are key to detecting problems from diabetic retinopathy. For this reason, regular eye examinations are crucial. The American Academy of Ophthalmology recommends the following:

- *People who received a diagnosis of diabetes before age 30.* This group should have a comprehensive eye exam when diabetes has been present for 5 years or when the individual is 10 years old, whichever is later.
- *People who received a diagnosis at age 30 or older.* This group should have a baseline exam at the time of diagnosis.
- *Women with diabetes who are pregnant or intending to become pregnant.* This group should have an exam before conception or early in the first trimester and thereafter every 3 months.

Following an initial exam, everyone with diabetes should have his or her eyes checked once a year. If you have other eye diseases, your eye specialist may recommend more frequent monitoring.

diabetic retinopathy, is the more common form. It's an early stage of the disease and symptoms are often mild.

In this condition, the walls of blood vessels in the retina weaken and tiny bulges (microaneurysms) protrude from the vessel walls. The vessels may leak fluid and blood into the retina. As the disease progresses, other signs of damage occur. These include patches of swollen nerve fibers, called cotton wool spots because they look like fluffy wisps of cotton.

Severe disease can cause the macula to swell or tiny capillaries to close, reducing blood flow to the macula and causing additional vision problems as central vision decreases.

Proliferative

Proliferative diabetic retinopathy is the more advanced form of the disease. Retinopathy becomes proliferative when abnormal new blood vessels grow (proliferate) on the retina or optic nerve. The blood vessels can also grow into the vitreous humor, the clear, jelly-like substance that fills the center of the eye.

This abnormal growth follows widespread closing of capillaries in the retina due to high blood sugar levels. The condition can cause vision loss affecting both central and peripheral vision. Other complications include retinal detachment and glaucoma.

Diagnosis

Diabetic retinopathy can develop with no initial visual problems. For this reason, annual eye examinations by an ophthalmologist are essential. Your ophthalmologist will examine the retina with an ophthalmoscope, which shines a bright light into the back of the eye and allows viewing of the retina. He or she will look for microaneurysms, hemorrhages, fatty deposits and newly formed blood vessels.

Fluorescein angiography, in which a dye is injected into a vein of your arm and a series of retinal photographs are taken, can detect leaky or newly formed blood vessels. This procedure is used in the evaluation of changes associated with nonproliferative and proliferative disease.

Treatment

Treatment of diabetic retinopathy begins with managing your diabetes. Tight control of blood sugar slows the onset and progression of retinopathy and lessens the need for surgery. Tight control means keeping blood sugar levels as close to normal as possible. Keeping your blood sugar in control may involve taking insulin or other diabetes medications, monitoring your blood sugar levels, following a healthy eating plan, getting regular exercise and maintaining a healthy weight.

Specific treatment for diabetic retinopathy depends on the severity of the condition and whether your vision is currently impaired or threatened. Mild nonproliferative retinopathy may not require immediate treatment. However, your ophthalmologist will closely monitor your retina for progression of retinopathy that may require treatment.

The two main treatments for diabetic retinopathy are photocoagulation and vitrectomy.

Photocoagulation

Photocoagulation is a laser treatment that's used to stop the leakage of blood and fluid in the retina to slow the progression of retinopathy. It may be recommended if you have macular edema (a swelling that involves the macula, an area in the center of the retina), severe nonproliferative retinopathy, proliferative retinopathy or glaucoma.

In photocoagulation, a laser beam creates small burns in the areas of the retina with abnormal blood vessels to seal any leaks. Even when laser surgery is successful in sealing the leaks, new areas of leakage may appear later. You may need additional laser treatments.

Immediately following laser surgery to treat macular edema, small spots may appear in your visual field. The spots generally fade and disappear with time. If you had blurred vision before surgery, you may not recover normal vision.

For proliferative diabetic retinopathy, a form of laser surgery called panretinal photocoagulation is used. With this technique, the entire retina, except the macula, is treated with randomly placed laser burns. The burns cause abnormal new blood vessels to shrink and disappear. Panretinal photocoagulation is usually done in two or more sessions. The treatment significantly reduces the risk of severe vision loss. However, if the treatment is extensive, you may notice some loss of peripheral vision afterward, as well as more difficulties with night vision and temporary blurring of central vision.

Vitrectomy

In proliferative diabetic retinopathy, new blood vessels may bleed (hemorrhage) into the vitreous. In severe cases, blood can completely fill the vitreous cavity and block all vision. Often a vitreous hemorrhage will clear up on its own. But if the hemorrhage is large and doesn't clear, photocoagulation treatment isn't possible. An operation called a vitrectomy is used to remove the blood-filled vitreous and restore clear vision. It is also used to remove scar tissue when it begins to pull the retina away from the wall of the eye (retinal detachment).

The surgeon performs the operation with a variety of delicate instruments inserted into the eyeball through small openings in the sclera. A light probe illuminates the inside of the eye. During vitrectomy, a surgeon may also perform panretinal photocoagulation with a laser probe to prevent renewed growth of abnormal blood vessels.

Recovery may take weeks. If you had extensive bleeding, some blood may remain in the eye, or fresh bleeding may occur for several weeks.

Vision improves in most people who have had a vitrectomy for vitreous hemorrhage or retinal detachment. However, visual recovery may be limited due to permanent retinal damage.

Third Nerve Palsy

Third nerve palsy is a common condition among people with diabetes. This disorder may involve a sudden onset of pain around the eye and double vision. The affected eye turns downward and outward. The pupil usually continues to react normally, enlarging in darkness and contracting in light. The upper eyelid often tends to droop (ptosis).

It's easy to think that these signs and symptoms might indicate a stroke — and in fact the disorder is the result of a temporary interruption of blood flow to the third cranial nerve. This nerve controls the action of some of the muscles that hold the eyeball in its normal position. The pain typically lasts a few days, and double vision and ptosis usually resolve in 2 to 3 months. If you have double vision, a droopy eyelid or pain around or in your eye, or if your eye fails to move properly in all directions, see an ophthalmologist promptly.

Graves' disease

Signs and symptoms

- Bulging or a feeling of pressure around the eyes
- Blurred or double vision
- Tearing
- Red or inflamed eyes
- Sensitivity to light
- Retraction of the eyelids
- Increased nervousness and heat intolerance
- Increased appetite, accompanied by weight loss

Graves' disease is a disorder of the thyroid gland in which too much of the hormone thyroxine is produced. An excess of thyroxine causes a wide range of signs and symptoms, including nervousness, heat intolerance, weight loss despite a healthy appetite, rapid and irregular pulse and a fine tremor of the hands. For more on Graves' disease, see page 1042.

Immune system abnormalities that stimulate the thyroid also can cause eye problems. Changes in the eyelids and in the muscles that control your eyes may cause double vision and a wide-eyed (bug-eyed) appearance. The eyes may also protrude because of an increase in muscle, fat and other tissues behind

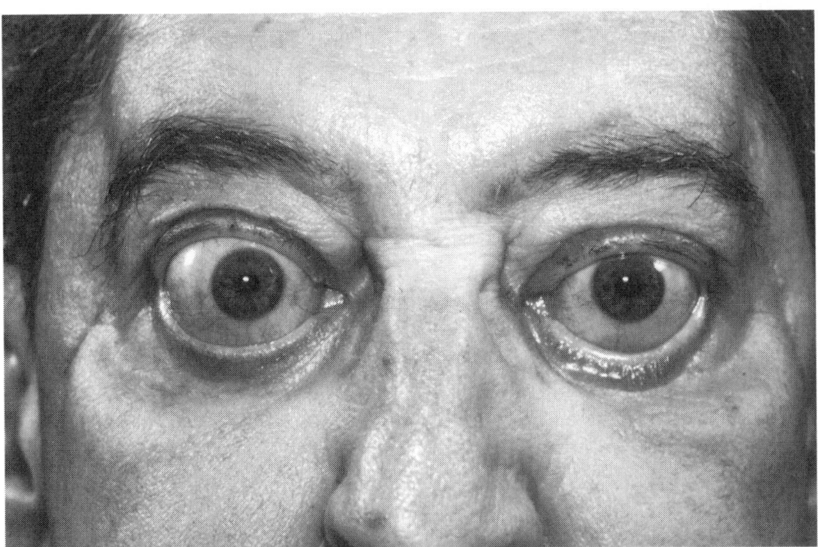

One of the most evident physical signs of Graves' disease is bulging eyes.

the eye. In some cases, enlarged tissues can compress and seriously threaten the optic nerve. Extreme retraction of the eyelids may expose the cornea enough to cause severe drying or a corneal ulcer.

Diagnosis

Eye changes may occur a year or more before or after the onset of the abnormal thyroid function. Protruding eyes and increased distance between the upper and lower eyelids are classic signs of Graves' disease. Sometimes, though, the eye changes are subtle and not readily apparent.

At times only one eye may seem to be affected, raising concerns about a tumor or sinus infection. Sometimes the most apparent symptom is irritation of the conjunctiva, which may be ascribed to conjunctivitis or an allergic reaction.

The degree of protrusion of the eye can be measured by an ophthalmologist with an exophthalmometer. This is more useful for determining whether the protrusion is worsening or improving than for establishing the diagnosis. A computerized tomography (CT) scan of the eye socket usually shows enlarged muscles within the socket and can eliminate the concern that a tumor or infection is causing the protrusion.

Treatment

Controlling overactivity of the thyroid gland is a key part of treatment to prevent the condition from worsening. If the treatment causes underactivity of the thyroid, you'll likely be given thyroxine tablets to replace the hormone.

Self-care

In many cases, the condition is a mild disorder that requires no treatment. Sleeping with your head elevated may decrease eyelid swelling. Topical ointments and artificial tears can help soothe eye irritation. Glasses with side guards help protect the eyes from irritating dust and wind.

Medication

Temporary treatment with corticosteroid medications can help relieve eye tissue swelling.

Surgery

In more severe cases, a surgeon may create extra space in a nearby sinus cavity to allow the eye to settle back into a more natural position within the orbit (socket). This procedure often corrects optic nerve changes, which can seriously threaten vision. The surgeon may also correct double vision by repositioning the enlarged muscles that control eye movement.

High blood pressure

Small blood vessels in the retina represent a sample of all of the blood vessels in the body, only they have the advantage of being readily visible. Narrowing of retinal arteries, small hemorrhages and protein deposits (exudates) that leak from affected blood vessels can be evidence of high blood pressure. It's very unusual for high blood pressure to impair vision, but reduced vision can occur during a hypertensive crisis, acute elevation of blood pressure that can be associated with neurologic and vascular symptoms. Retinal arteries may severely narrow and the retina may swell.

Stroke

The term *stroke* describes several disorders caused by a disturbance in the blood supply to the brain. The cause may be an insufficient supply of blood due to a blocked brain artery (ischemic stroke) or due to a rupture of an artery that causes bleeding into the brain (cerebral hemorrhage). In many cases, stroke has no warning signs. Only when you're experiencing one do you notice the signs and symptoms of headache, paralysis, sudden weakness and double vision or loss of vision.

If you experience a sudden loss of vision or double vision — or any other signs and symptoms such as sudden weakness on one side of the body, speech difficulty or lack of coordination — seek medical attention immediately. An ophthalmologist may check for deposits in retinal vessels (atherosclerosis) and measure the pressure and amount of blood flowing through the arteries of the eyes.

Treatment

Treatment may include medications or surgery. If atherosclerosis is detected, you may be given anticoagulant medication to keep blood from clotting. If the main arteries in your neck are narrowed by plaques that reduce blood supply to the brain and eyes, surgery may help restore blood flow.

Cranial arteritis

Cranial arteritis, also known as giant cell arteritis or temporal arteritis, is an inflammation of arteries in the head and scalp. The diagnosis is often made by removing a portion of a scalp artery (biopsy) and examining it microscopically for inflammation. The inflammation is thought to result from an abnormal immune reaction that thickens the lining of the affected arteries, reducing or blocking blood flow to various parts of the body, most commonly the eyes. Vision begins to diminish, and left untreated, the disorder can rapidly cause partial or total blindness in one or both eyes.

Cranial arteritis is most common in older women of Northern European ancestry. Blacks and Asians rarely develop the disease. Cranial arteritis can be treated and blindness prevented by treatment with oral corticosteroid medications. Symptoms usually improve soon after treatment begins. Treatment must be continued for a year or more and is monitored by blood tests and examinations. ■

CHAPTER 24 PART V

Ears, Nose and Throat

Your ears, nose and throat are responsible for a remarkable number of functions. Your ears and their associated nerve mechanisms enable you to hear and to keep your balance. Your nose makes it possible for you to inhale and filter air and to smell your surroundings. The structures of your throat enable you to eat, drink, speak and sing.

Your ears, nose and throat are interrelated in their functions and in the disorders that often affect them. An infection of your throat or nose, for example, can easily spread to your ears. An upper respiratory infection may affect your nose, throat and ears.

It's not surprising, then, that each of these is treated by the same specialist, an otorhinolaryngologist. The name derives from the Greek base words for ear (*otos*), nose (*rhinos*) and throat (*larynx*). More commonly, doctors who specialize in this area of medicine are referred to as ENT physicians.

Your Ears

The two main functions of your ears are hearing and balance. Each ear is composed of three parts: the outer ear, middle ear and inner ear.

Outer ear

Your outer ear is made up of the folds of skin and cartilage usually referred to as the ear (pinna), plus your outer ear canal. They carry sound waves to your eardrum and middle ear. The outer ear is the part of the ear you see. Within the outer ear canal are wax-producing glands and hairs that protect the middle ear.

Middle ear

The function of the middle ear is to deliver sound waves to your inner ear, where the vibrations are processed into a signal that your brain recognizes as sound. Your middle ear is a small cavity, with the eardrum (tympanic membrane) on one side and the entrance to your inner ear on the other.

Within your middle ear are three small bones (ossicles) known as the hammer (malleus), anvil (incus) and stirrup (stapes). The names reflect their shapes. These tiny bones act like a system of levers that conduct sound vibrations into your inner ear. The hammer is attached to the lining of your eardrum, the anvil is attached to the hammer, and the stirrup links the anvil to the opening of your inner ear, the oval window.

Your middle ear is connected to your throat by a narrow channel called the eustachian tube. The eustachian tube remains closed until you swallow or yawn, then it opens briefly to equalize the air pressure within your middle ear with the air pressure outside. You often feel a pop when this occurs.

Structures of Your Ear

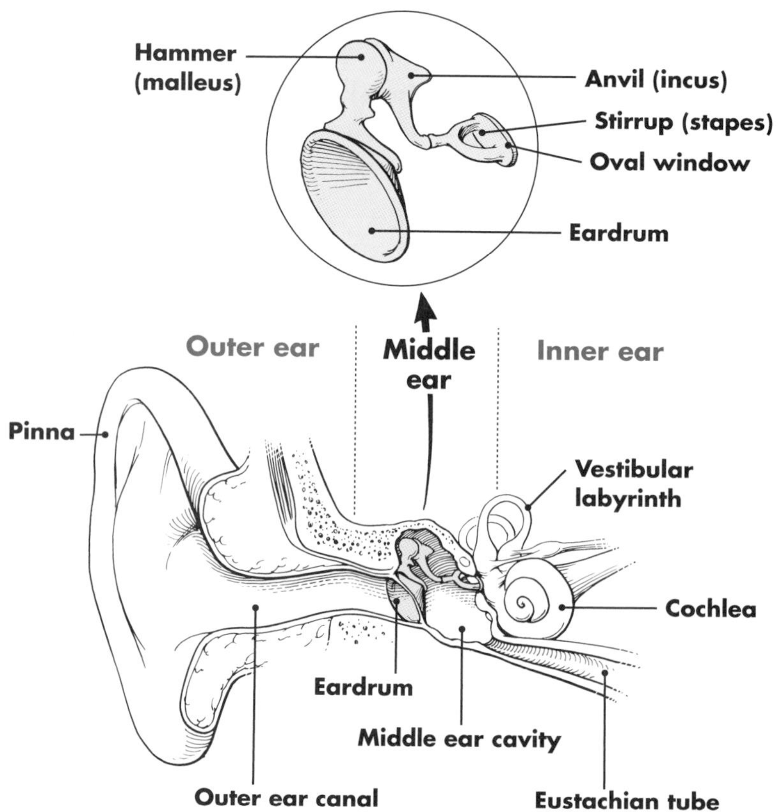

Inner ear

Your inner ear contains the most intricate parts of the hearing mechanism: two chambers called the vestibular labyrinth and cochlea. The vestibular labyrinth consists of elaborately formed canals — three semicircular tubes that connect to one another — that help control your sense of balance. The cochlea, which begins at the oval window, curves into a shape that resembles a snail shell. Tiny hairs attached to auditory nerve endings line the interior of the cochlea. Both the labyrinth and cochlea are filled with fluid.

Sound waves from the world outside cause your eardrum to vibrate. These vibrations continue passing through the bones of your middle ear and into your inner ear through the oval window. They're transmitted into the fluid of the cochlea, where the tiny hairs sense the vibration waves and convert them into electric impulses that are transmitted to your brain by your auditory nerve.

Your Nose

Your nose is a gateway to your respiratory system. Air that enters your nasal passages runs along the top of your palate, the structure that separates your nose from your mouth. As you inhale, air passes through to the intersection of your mouth and throat and continues its journey into your lower respiratory system.

Your nose is divided into two identical nostrils, which are separated by a partition (septum) composed of cartilage and bone and covered by mucous membrane. Thin bony structures covered by mucous membrane (turbinates) curve in from the outer part of your nose toward your septum and act as baffles in your nasal passages.

Your nasal passages also open into your sinuses, tiny air-filled cavities in your skull. Your adenoids are an aggregation of lymphatic tissue located behind your nasal passages.

Inside the front of your nose are protective hairs that help filter the air you breathe. The main cavity of your nose is lined with a mucous membrane that warms and moistens the air.

In addition to warming, moistening and filtering air, your nose is responsible for your sense of smell and, to a large degree, your sense of taste.

In fact, most of your ability to taste depends on your sense of smell. Smell begins in your olfactory structure, found in the upper part of your nose. This system contains very fine, sensitive fibers that transmit signals to your olfactory bulb, a structure located at the front of your brain, just above your nose.

Your Throat

Your throat (pharynx) is part of the system that delivers air to your lungs, food and drink to your esophagus and stomach, and sounds from your vocal cords to your mouth. Each time you inhale, air passes through your throat on its way to your windpipe (trachea) and lungs. When you swallow food, the muscles at the top of your throat help move the food from your mouth to your esophagus, which is connected to your stomach.

Several organs are located in your throat. Your voice box (larynx), which is above your trachea, contains your vocal cords, which are responsible for generating most of the sounds of speech. When you speak, your throat also helps you shape the sounds you make. Your tonsils are on both sides of the back of your mouth, and your adenoids are above them.

The epiglottis acts as a lid and diverter for your trachea, closing when you swallow and keeping water and food from "going down the wrong way" and entering your windpipe.

Structures of Your Nose

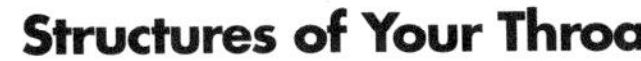

Structures of Your Throat

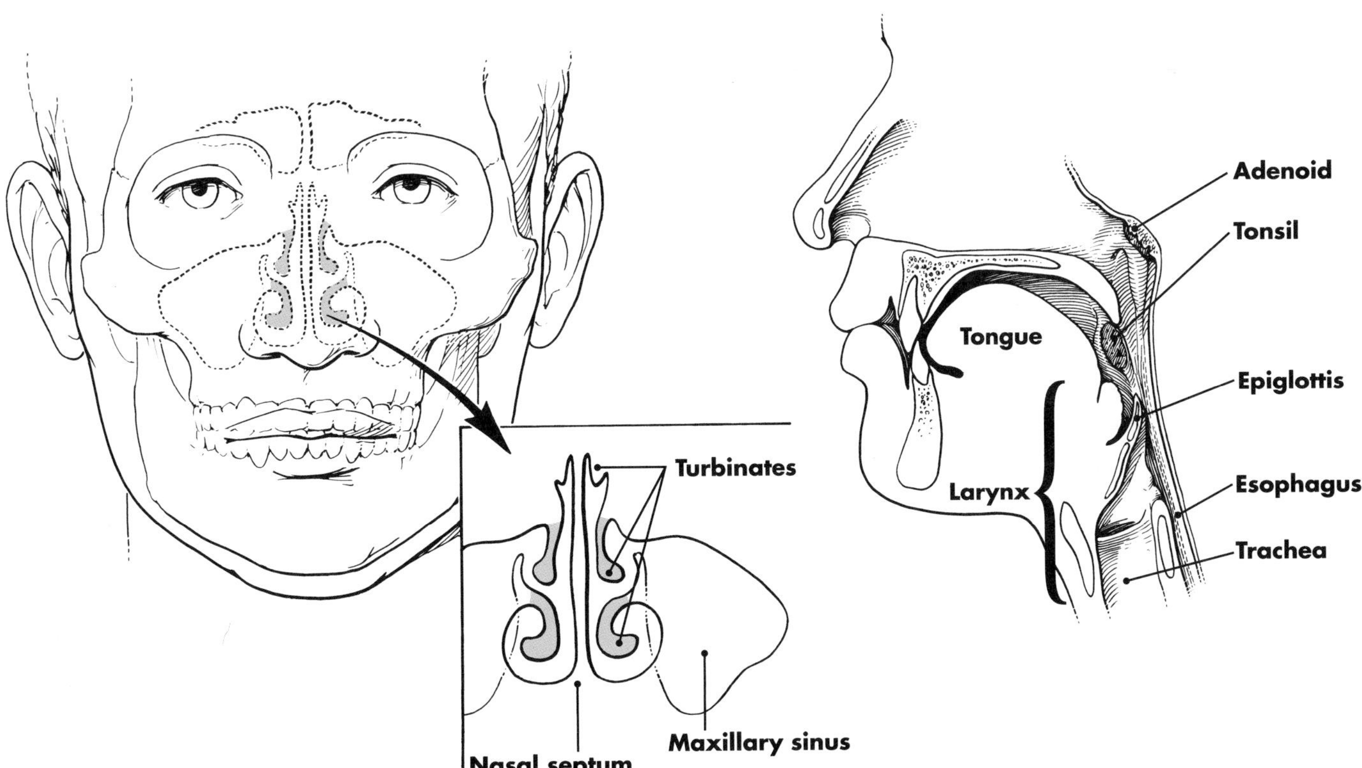

Disorders of the Ear

The ear is a structural marvel, but its complexity makes it susceptible to infections, congenital disorders and damage due to accident or noise exposure.

Outer ear infections

Signs and symptoms

- Pain in an ear
- Discharge of yellowish or yellowish-green, foul-smelling pus from an ear
- Hearing loss

An outer ear infection (external otitis) causes irritation and inflammation of your outer ear canal. It can occur at any age but most commonly affects young adults.

Under normal circumstances, earwax (cerumen) repels water from the surface of your outer ear canal. It also helps maintain a proper pH (acid-alkaline) balance in your ear to inhibit bacterial growth. If this balance is disrupted, infection may result.

A fungal, viral or bacterial infection can cause external otitis. Bacteria are the most common cause. This type of infection is sometimes referred to as swimmer's ear because it's often related to moisture problems in the ear canal.

Factors that may spur bacterial growth include:

- Excessive moisture in the ear canal. Repeated exposure to water may result in loss of earwax. Unprotected, the ear canal's skin retains moisture and becomes irritated. The normal pH balance also is disrupted, allowing bacteria to grow. Hearing aid use also may promote moisture buildup in the ear canal.
- Injury or irritation of the skin in the ear canal. Scratching the ear canal or removing wax with makeshift tools, such as paper clips or hairpins, can damage the skin — providing an entry for bacteria — and even your eardrum. Efforts to clean the canal with cotton-tipped swabs can backfire by forcing excess wax and debris deeper into the ear and causing injury.
- Chronic skin conditions or allergies. Skin conditions such as eczema and seborrhea may provide an entry point for bacteria. Allergies to hair dyes or sprays may irritate the skin and lead to infection.

Sometimes, a severe and aggressive infection may develop. This is more commonly seen in people with diabetes, especially older individuals. People with a weakened immune system also are at greater risk of developing this type of infection.

The infection usually begins as external otitis. But at some point, the bacteria spread from the ear canal skin into nearby tissues, including cartilage and bone. Nerve damage and even facial paralysis may occur.

Diagnosis

If you experience pain in an ear canal or notice yellowish or yellowish-green pus draining from an ear, see your doctor. Hearing loss can result if the pus or swelling blocks your ear canal.

Your doctor may use a hand-held instrument called an otoscope to examine your ear canal. If pus is present, a sample may be taken for laboratory analysis.

How serious are outer ear infections?

Most outer ear infections are bothersome, but if treated properly they're not usually dangerous to your general health. Severe external otitis that spreads to nearby tissues can damage underlying bones and cartilage. Left untreated, this condition can be life-threatening.

Treatment

If you suspect that you have external otitis, you can take steps to relieve the pain before you see your doctor. Placing a warm — not hot — heating pad over your ear may help. Acetaminophen (Tylenol, others), ibuprofen (Advil, Motrin, others) or aspirin may help relieve the pain. Aspirin isn't recommended for children because it can produce Reye's syndrome, a serious condition involving the brain, liver and blood.

After a diagnosis is made, your doctor will probably clean your ear canal with a suction device or a cotton-tipped probe. This will help relieve irritation and pain. Frequently, doctors prescribe eardrops containing a corticosteroid preparation to decrease inflammation and relieve symptoms, as well as an antibiotic to control infection. If you're in severe pain, your doctor may prescribe a painkiller. Try not to let any water get into your ear while it's healing, usually for 7 to 10 days.

If the infection doesn't show marked improvement after 3 or 4 days, your doctor may prescribe an oral antibiotic. He or she can select

PREVENTION TIP

An ounce of prevention can help you avoid an outer ear infection:

- Carefully dry your ears with a hair dryer or towel after bathing and swimming because moisture in an ear canal can make it susceptible to infection.
- Put several drops of a 50-50 mixture of water and vinegar or water and rubbing alcohol in the ear canal to aid drying after swimming.
- Avoid excessive ear canal cleaning. Simply wipe out whatever is at the opening of the ear canal.
- Cover your ear canals with cotton balls or something similar when applying hair spray or dye.

Question and Answer

Is it safe to pierce the upper area of the ear?

Generally, it's best to avoid piercing upper ear cartilage. An infection in the upper ear can lead to cartilage damage that can cause serious, permanent deformity of the ear.

Cartilage determines the shape of your outer ear. It's kept alive by absorbing nutrients from a special tissue that covers it. Inflammation and infection of that tissue lining can peel the nourishing layer off the cartilage, depriving it of nutrients. As a result, the cartilage can be destroyed. Making matters worse, antibiotics are often ineffective because the blood supply isn't adequate to deliver the medication to the cartilage. By contrast, the earlobe has its own blood supply and, if infected, generally responds well to antibiotics.

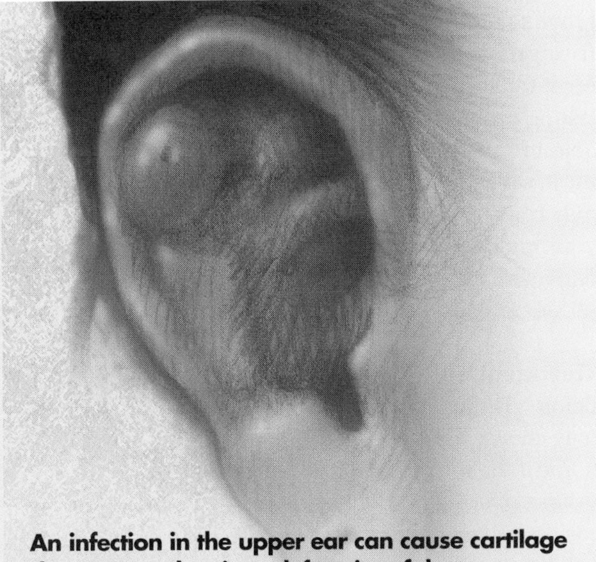

An infection in the upper ear can cause cartilage damage, and serious deformity of the ear may result.

a drug specifically for the organism causing your infection if a laboratory test has identified the organism. To treat an outer ear infection caused by a fungus, your doctor may prescribe acetic acid eardrops or an antifungal preparation.

Invasive external otitis is a serious infection of the outer ear and often requires intravenous antibiotics and hospitalization for several days. Sometimes, surgery is needed to remove dead or infected tissue and bone.

Following hospitalization, intravenous antibiotics may be continued, or oral antibiotics may be prescribed for several weeks. People who have diabetes or are immune suppressed require close monitoring.

Benign cysts and tumors

Signs and symptoms

- A lump in your ear canal or in front of or behind your ear
- Accumulation of earwax (cerumen)
- Discomfort in your ear
- Hearing loss

Sebaceous cysts are small sacs filled with cheesy material produced by your skin glands. They commonly develop behind your ear or in your scalp. The cysts are noncancerous (benign) and often aren't even noticeable. Benign tumors of the ear canal (exostoses), caused by an overgrowth of bone, also may occur. The tumors can grow large enough to block your ear canal, trap wax and interfere with hearing. Most exostoses grow very slowly and often present no problem.

Diagnosis

You may feel a semisoft lump on the bony protrusion behind your ear or in front of your ear. These cysts rarely cause discomfort, although they can become infected. If you detect such a cyst, visit your doctor.

In the case of a benign tumor, people are often unaware they have one, and the bony growth usually poses no problem. Occasionally, however, such a growth may partially obstruct an ear canal.

If your ear hurts or you experience hearing loss, consult your doctor. He or she typically will examine your ear canal with an otoscope, which allows full viewing of your outer canal.

Treatment

Benign cysts and tumors pose no general threat to health. If a benign tumor grows enough to block your outer ear canal, your doctor may recommend that it be surgically removed.

Foreign object in an ear

Signs and symptoms

- Pain in your ear
- Hearing loss
- The sensation of something present in your ear

The assortment of objects that doctors remove from ears is varied — marbles, tiny toys, jewelry, insects, seeds, bits of paper and plastic and even earplugs. Because of the complicated shape of your ear and ear canal, any small object that you place into your ear can become lodged there.

Diagnosis

Usually, you know when something is stuck in your ear. It hurts or feels full, and it may affect your ability to hear. The problem can be a little harder to diagnose when a small child is affected.

Don't attempt to remove the object unless it can be easily grasped with a tweezers. And don't attempt to dislodge an object by probing with a cotton-tipped swab, hairpin, paper clip or another tool. If the object can't easily be grasped, see a doctor.

How serious is a foreign object in an ear?

Most foreign objects don't cause a lasting problem. However, if an object is pushed into your eardrum, the eardrum (tympanic membrane) may rupture (tear) or perforate, and your middle and inner ear may be damaged, creating a potentially serious situation.

Treatment

Before visiting your doctor, you may choose to try these steps at home if the foreign object is clearly visible, pliable and can be grasped easily with a tweezers:

- If the object isn't an insect, use gravity to dislodge the object by tilting your head to the affected side. Don't strike your head, but shake it gently.
- If the foreign object is an insect, tilt your head so that the ear with the offending insect is upward. Try to float the insect out by pouring mineral oil, olive oil or baby oil into the ear canal. The oil should be warm but not hot. As you pour the oil in, ease the entry of the oil by gently pulling the earlobe backward and upward, which straightens the ear canal. The insect should suffocate and float out in the oil bath. Don't use oil to remove any object other than an insect. And don't use this method if you suspect a perforated eardrum, which is indicated by pain and bleeding or discharge from the ear.

If these methods fail or you continue to experience ear pain, reduced hearing or a sensation of something lodged in the ear, seek medical assistance.

Ruptured eardrum

Signs and symptoms

- Earache
- Partial hearing loss
- Bleeding or discharge from an ear

Risk of damaging your eardrum (tympanic membrane) is one reason not to place anything into your ear.

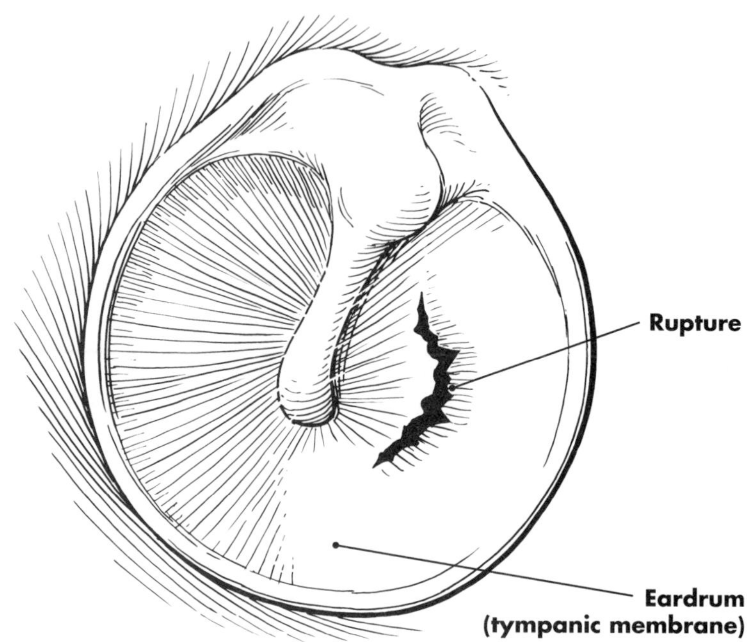

Pain in your ear, hearing loss and discharge from your ear may indicate a rupture (tear) of your eardrum (tympanic membrane).

You may puncture your eardrum when you clean or scratch your ear with a cotton-tipped swab or small, sharp object. Other causes of a punctured eardrum are a hard slap on your ear or an explosion, which can produce a sudden increase in air pressure in your ear.

A middle ear infection (otitis media) also can cause inflammation and, sometimes, perforation of part of an eardrum. This is the most common cause of a ruptured eardrum. Small holes may heal, but larger ones can stay open and permit infectious agents to enter your middle ear.

Diagnosis

If you experience increasing pain and hearing loss in your ear over a period of a day or so, followed by a discharge of blood or fluid — with subsequent relief of the pain — you may have a ruptured eardrum as a consequence of a middle ear infection. See a doctor promptly.

Your doctor will likely examine your ear with an otoscope, an instrument that allows full viewing of your ear canal. If your eardrum is punctured, your doctor should be able to see the ruptured area or the bones of your middle ear behind it.

How serious is a ruptured eardrum?

A ruptured eardrum can be painful, particularly at first. Most often the rupture heals by itself without complications and with little or no permanent hearing loss. Larger perforations may cause recurring inner ear infections and persistent hearing loss.

Treatment

If you suspect that you have ruptured an eardrum, see your doctor as soon as possible. You can relieve the pain by placing a warm — not hot — heating pad over your ear. Taking pain relievers such as acetaminophen (Tylenol, others), ibuprofen (Advil, Motrin, others) or aspirin may help. However, children shouldn't take aspirin because it can trigger Reye's syndrome, a serious condition involving the brain, liver and blood.

Your doctor may prescribe an antibiotic to prevent an infection from developing in your middle ear. Occasionally, a plastic or paper patch is placed over your eardrum to seal the opening. It's important to keep water out of your ear while the perforation heals.

Your eardrum may heal within 2 months. If it hasn't healed in that time, your doctor might recommend a surgical procedure to repair the tear.

Eustachian tube dysfunction

Signs and symptoms

- A plugged ear
- A sensation of fullness or pressure in the ear
- A popping noise in the ear
- Hearing loss

Many ear problems are the result of the eustachian tube not working properly. The eustachian tube has many roles. When you swallow or yawn, it opens briefly to equalize pressure in the ear with the air pressure outside. It also drains the middle ear of fluid.

Most of the time, though, the eustachian tube remains closed to prevent secretions from entering the middle ear. With eustachian tube dysfunction, the tube either doesn't open or close correctly or it's obstructed, preventing it from functioning properly.

Eustachian tube dysfunction can lead to problems with regulating pressure in the ear and problems with clearing the middle ear of secretions. It can cause such conditions as middle ear infection and cholesteatoma, a cyst-like, noncancerous tumor or collection of skin cells most commonly found in a bone behind your ear (mastoid process) or the middle ear.

This type of dysfunction has many possible causes. These include:

- Collapse of cartilage around the eustachian tube, which prevents the tube from opening
- Obstruction of the tube due to small growths (polyps)
- Swelling due to inflammation, infection or allergies
- Failure of the tube to open due to a cleft palate

Diagnosis

Your doctor may use any of several tests to determine whether you have eustachian tube dysfunction and, if so, its cause. For example, he or she may ask you to gently exhale while you hold your nostrils closed and keep your mouth shut. While you do so, your doctor will observe your ear through an otoscope to see if it reacts normally to the change in pressure.

A test called tympanometry evaluates the eardrum's reaction to positive, normal and negative air pressure. A special instrument is used to seal the ear canal and exert sound and pressure. The instrument measures how much sound is absorbed and determines if the eustachian tube is providing proper ventilation to allow the eardrum to vibrate properly.

Your doctor may also view the nasal opening of your eustachian tube using an endoscope, a thin, flexible tube with a fiber-optic light that's inserted through your nose.

Treatment

Treatment for eustachian tube dysfunction varies depending on the cause. It may involve decongestant medications or, in rare cases, surgery to treat the underlying cause.

Barotrauma

Signs and symptoms

- Moderate to severe pain in an ear
- A stuffy feeling in an ear
- Slight hearing loss
- Dizziness
- Noise such as a buzzing, ringing or roaring in your ears (tinnitus)

The air pressure in your middle ear usually is the same as that in your outer ear, thanks to the eustachian tube, a narrow channel that connects your middle ear to the top of your throat. When you swallow or yawn, it opens and allows air to flow into or out of your middle ear, equalizing the air pressure of your ear with the outside air pressure.

If a eustachian tube is blocked, differences in pressure occur between the two sides of the eardrum. This condition is known as barotrauma (barotitis media).

PREVENTION TIP

If you must fly when your nose and head feel congested, try these measures:

- Use a nasal decongestant spray and an oral decongestant an hour before takeoff and, if the flight is long, an hour before landing. This may prevent blockage of your eustachian tube.
- During your flight suck candy or chew gum to encourage swallowing. This helps open your eustachian tube to equalize pressure.
- Try using over-the-counter earplugs designed for air travel. They have a small filter to slow the rate of change in air pressure on the eardrum.
- For babies and young children, make sure they're swallowing during ascent and descent. Give the child a bottle or pacifier to encourage swallowing. Have a young child drink or suck on something or chew gum. You might also give the child acetaminophen (Tylenol, others) 30 minutes before takeoff to help control discomfort. Decongestants generally aren't recommended for young children.

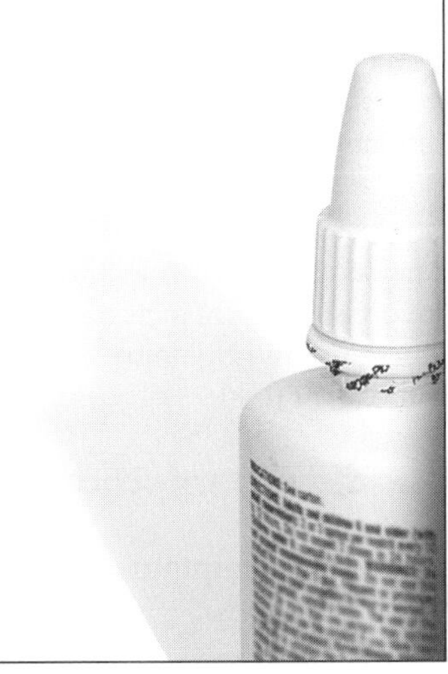

Diagnosis

If you fly in an airplane or scuba dive while you have a congested nose, you may experience the symptoms of barotrauma: ear pain, slight hearing loss and a stuffy feeling in your ears. The symptoms are caused by your eardrum bulging outward or retracting inward due to a change in air pressure.

A more severe problem can occur if the air pressure change is great or if a eustachian tube is entirely blocked. The small blood vessels (capillaries) of your middle ear may rupture and bleed, filling your ear with blood and producing hearing loss and a feeling similar to that of being underwater.

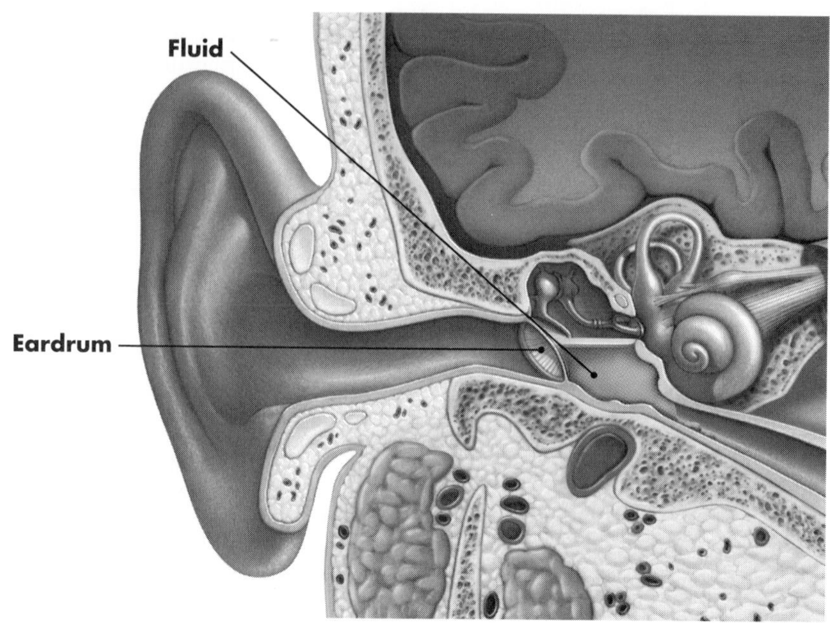

Fluid is trapped behind the eardrum (tympanic membrane).

How serious is barotrauma?

Symptoms of barotrauma usually disappear within a few minutes or hours after they begin. It usually isn't a serious condition and generally doesn't produce permanent hearing loss.

In some cases, severe pressure changes can cause bleeding into the middle ear and rupture the eardrum, which can lead to permanent hearing loss. If symptoms don't improve within a few hours after the incident, visit a doctor.

Treatment

If you experience barotrauma, gently blow air out of your nose while your mouth is closed and your nose is slightly pinched.

The symptoms usually clear up on their own. However, if they don't disappear within a few hours, you may be bleeding from the capillaries in your middle ear. See your doctor. Antibiotic treatment may be necessary to prevent infection. On rare occasions, treatment may also involve a surgical incision in your eardrum (myringotomy) and removal of fluid.

Middle ear infections

Signs and symptoms

- Severe earache
- Hearing loss
- A feeling of fullness in your ear
- Fever and chills

Middle ear infection (otitis media) results from inflammation or infection of the middle ear, which is located just behind the eardrum (tympanic membrane). Middle ear infections are one of the most common illnesses of infancy and early childhood, second only to the common cold.

Although middle ear infections can occur at any age, they're most common between 4 months and 5 years of age. Seventy percent of children have at least one ear infection by the age of 3. More than 90 percent have had at least one middle ear infection by age 7.

A middle ear infection often begins with a respiratory infection such as a cold. Colds cause swelling and inflammation in the sinuses and eustachian tubes. Children's eustachian tubes are shorter and narrower than those of adults. The small size increases the chances that inflammation will block the tube completely, trapping fluid in the middle ear. This trapped fluid may cause discomfort, and it creates an ideal environment for bacterial growth. The result can be a severe (acute) middle ear infection.

Sometimes, fluid stays trapped in the middle ear following treatment of an infection or because the eustachian tube is blocked. This can lead to chronic otitis media.

Occasionally, a more serious infection develops, called purulent otitis media. Pus fills the middle ear. The pressure of the pus may burst the eardrum, causing a discharge of blood and thick pus.

Is Your Child at Risk?

All children are susceptible to ear infections, but statistics show that certain groups of children are at higher risk:

- Boys
- Children whose siblings have a history of recurrent ear infections
- Children with a family history of asthma, allergies or eczema
- American Indian children and children of Alaskan or Canadian Eskimo heritage — possibly due to genetic factors that affect the shape of the eustachian tube

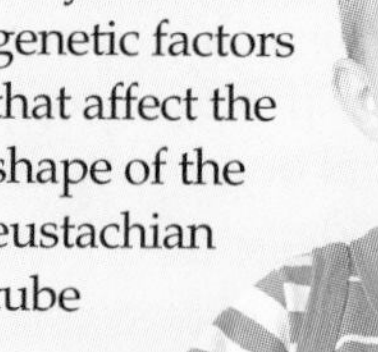

Diagnosis

Sharp, continuous pain in an ear, hearing loss and fever are common indications of a middle ear infection. Although very young children can't communicate this pain to parents, they often display signs that they're experiencing an ear infection. These include irritability, a sudden loss of appetite, the development of a fever a few days after the onset of a cold and a preference for sleeping in an upright position. Your child may also have discharge in the ear canal or may tug at his or her ear.

Your doctor can examine the eardrum with an otoscope to determine if there's fluid in the middle ear. The otoscope also allows a doctor to gently blow a small amount of air against the eardrum to see if it moves as freely as it should. If it doesn't, fluid may be in the middle ear. Your doctor will also examine the eardrum for bulging or change of color.

Testing a sample of the fluid can confirm that an infection is present and identify its specific cause, but this isn't practical with young children. The only way to obtain a sample is to use a small needle to penetrate the eardrum and draw off some of the fluid. Young children are unable to hold still long enough for the procedure to be done safely.

Without this type of fluid test, it may not be clear if you or your child has an ear infection or if the fluid in the middle ear has infectious organisms present. This is important because it influences treatment decisions. If the fluid is sterile, antibiotics won't help. If pus is draining into the ear canal, your doctor may take a sample to try to identify the organism that's causing the infection.

How serious are middle ear infections?

Most middle ear infections don't lead to permanent hearing loss. However, they can sometimes damage the eardrum, ear bones and inner ear structures, causing permanent hearing loss. Infections that aren't treated can spread to other parts of the ear, including the inner ear.

Treatment

Until you see a doctor, you can relieve some of the pain by placing a warm — not hot — heating pad over the ear. Pain medications such as acetaminophen (Tylenol, others), ibuprofen (Advil, Motrin, others) or aspirin also may help, but aspirin shouldn't be given to children because it can trigger Reye's syndrome. Your doctor may recommend one of the following:

Watchful waiting

In some situations, you and your doctor may decide to hold off on using antibiotics and check to see if the ear infection gets better or worse.

Watchful waiting is an option that's commonly used in other countries and is becoming more popular in the United States. If the fluid in the ear isn't infected or if the infection is viral rather than bacterial, antibiotics provide no benefit. Antibiotics won't help move fluid out of the ear, and they may cause side effects such as nausea, diarrhea or an allergic reaction. In addition, if antibiotics are used only when necessary, they're more likely to be effective when needed to fight future bacterial infections.

Even when there's an obvious ear infection, you may still want to consider watchful waiting as an option before giving antibiotics. Many middle ear infections clear up on their own without medical treatment.

If you and your doctor decide to hold off on antibiotics, watch for signs of increased pain or fever or hearing loss. Also be certain to schedule a follow-up visit to be sure the ear infection is improving.

Medication

If nasal allergies are contributing to development of a middle ear infection, your doctor may prescribe

PREVENTION TIP

Preventing middle ear infections in your child is difficult, but consider these approaches to help reduce your child's risk:

- Breast-feed rather than bottle-feed your baby. Breast milk passes along immunity that helps prevent middle ear infections.
- If you're bottle-feeding your baby, hold him or her in an upright position. Children of any age should never be allowed to feed from a bottle while lying down because this can lead to blocked eustachian tubes.
- Avoid exposure to tobacco smoke. If you or other members of your household smoke, your child is at greater risk of developing an ear infection. And if he or she does get an ear infection, recovery takes longer than it would in a smoke-free environment. Improperly vented wood or coal stoves also can contribute to this problem.
- If you use child care, select a facility with few children. Children who regularly attend large-group child care centers have more ear infections than do children who are cared for at home or in child care settings with few children. The more kids there are, the greater the chance that your child will catch a cold, which may lead to an ear infection.
- Immunize your child. A pneumococcal vaccine called Prevnar is available. It prevents the seven most common subtypes of *Streptococcus pneumoniae*, the bacterium often found in middle ear infections. This vaccine is given as a series of four shots at 2, 4, 6 and 12 to 15 months of age. Although the vaccine won't prevent all ear infections, you may want to talk to your doctor about having this vaccination for your child.

antihistamines or decongestants. Decongestants improve nasal breathing and increase airflow into and from the middle ear through the eustachian tube.

If the fluid is infected, your doctor may prescribe antibiotics to fight the infection. Unless the exact organism causing the infection has been determined, your doctor will probably prescribe an antibiotic that's effective against a range of bacteria most commonly associated with middle ear infections. If the infection doesn't respond to the first medication, your doctor may prescribe a different antibiotic.

Surgery

To rapidly relieve pain and pressure and restore hearing, a surgical incision in your eardrum (myringotomy) is sometimes used. In children, surgeons generally perform a myringotomy in the hospital under general anesthesia. The eardrum incision heals within 1 to 2 weeks.

Chronic ear infections

Signs and symptoms

- Earache
- Periodic drainage of pus from an ear
- Hearing loss

A chronic middle ear infection (chronic otitis media) can be more harmful than an acute infection because its slow, long-lasting effects can cause permanent ear damage. Unlike an acute infection, which develops suddenly, a chronic condition may not be noticed until it's well established.

Chronic otitis media may result from persistent swelling or inflammation of adenoid tissue behind your nasal passages. This can result in inflammation and blockage of the eustachian tubes.

Adenoid problems most often occur in children. In adults, blockage may stem from nasal allergies or from scarring of the eustachian tube from previous infections. It can also result from tumors in the back of the nose and throat.

In some cases, an initial acute infection never completely clears after treatment, and a low-level infection continues. It can spread to a bone behind your ear called the mastoid process.

Infection in the mastoid is more difficult to eradicate. A chronic infection can also cause perforation of your eardrum (tympanic membrane) or damage to the small bones in your middle ear.

Diagnosis

Seek medical attention if pus is seeping from the ear canal, if the ear continues to hurt or if there's a hearing loss.

An exam typically involves inspection of the ear with an otoscope to identify where the infection is. Your doctor may also arrange a computerized tomography (CT) scan of your head to determine if the infection has spread to the mastoid process.

How serious are chronic ear infections?

Chronic otitis media is uncomfortable and inconvenient, but it rarely causes permanent harm. However, uncorrected, active chronic otitis media can cause permanent hearing damage.

Treatment

The first line of treatment is generally medication. Another option is surgery.

Medication

Medication may be prescribed to treat a chronic ear infection or relieve nasal and sinus congestion if the condition is due to allergies.

If you or your child has had multiple or frequent ear infections — usually three or more ear infections in a 6-month period or four infections within 12 months — your doctor may suggest a low-dose antibiotic over a longer time (often

Ear Tubes in Children: The Pros and Cons

One way to treat recurrent middle ear infections (otitis media) is to surgically insert a small plastic tube through the eardrum (tympanic membrane), which helps drain fluid, ventilate the middle ear and equalize the pressure between the outer and middle ear. However, before embarking in this direction, discuss this procedure in detail with an ear, nose and throat specialist.

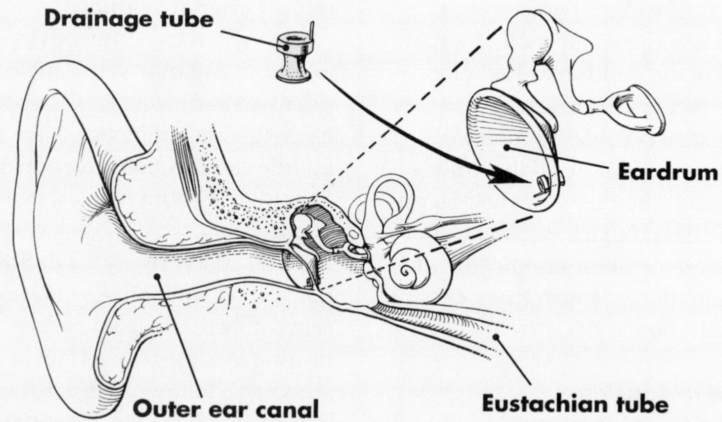

In persistent cases of ear infection, a doctor may insert a small tube into the eardrum (tympanic membrane) to help drain fluid, ventilate the middle ear and equalize the pressure between the outer and middle ear.

a few months) as a preventive measure. Preventive antibiotics won't help clear fluid from the middle ear, but they may prevent bacterial growth. Some studies have found that preventive use of antibiotics reduces the number of ear infections.

Unfortunately, the bacteria commonly responsible for ear infections are becoming increasingly resistant to antibiotics. Even while taking antibiotics, an ear infection can still occur. Because widespread and prolonged use of antibiotics contributes to the growth of drug-resistant bacteria, doctors don't agree on whether antibiotics should be used preventively.

Surgery

Recurrent ear infections that don't respond to antibiotics are sometimes treated by surgically inserting a small plastic tube through a hole made in the eardrum to drain and ventilate the middle ear. Surgery may also be done if fluid persists in the middle ear for more than 3 months, resulting in hearing loss. As with any surgery, consider the options before making a decision.

The operation is performed under general anesthesia, and the entire procedure usually takes less than 10 minutes. Working through the ear canal, the surgeon uses a microscope and very delicate instruments to make a small incision in the eardrum, remove any fluid, pus or blood with suction, and then insert a tiny metal or plastic tube into the hole. The procedure is usually performed on both ears. Hearing often improves immediately.

Generally, it's not necessary to come into the doctor's office to have the tube removed. It stays in the eardrum for about 10 months, although this can vary depending on the type of tube used. In a child, as the eardrum grows, the tube is eventually pushed out into the ear canal where it either falls out or is retrieved by the doctor. About 15 percent to 25 percent of children with ear tubes will need surgery to insert a second set of tubes. A small number of children may even need a third set.

When a tube is in the ear, the eardrum must not be exposed to water under pressure. This can be particularly difficult for children who like to swim. Your doctor may recommend special earplugs for water activities.

If the adenoids are thought to be contributing to the problem, your doctor may recommend surgically removing them (adenoidectomy). If the mastoid process becomes infected, your doctor may recommend a mastoidectomy, an operation in which the mastoid process is opened surgically to remove infected tissue and prevent recurrence or spread of the infection.

The pros

The benefits of tubes include:

- The operation provides ventilation and drainage of the middle ear to prevent fluid from accumulating. It also decreases the risk of permanent changes in the lining of the middle ear that can occur with prolonged infection.
- The procedure usually results in a decrease in the frequency and severity of episodes of middle ear infections.
- Hearing may improve immediately and aid speech development. Studies linking early hearing loss with long-term speech, language and cognitive skill problems have been the basis for a large number of ear tube procedures. However, a more recent study reported that tubes don't appear to have an effect on speech, language and development in children under age 3.

The cons

Reasons against the use of tubes include:

- Although small, a risk of infection and complications is associated with all surgery.
- Complications such as persistent drainage of fluid and perforation or scarring of the eardrum occur, although rarely.
- The tube itself can become infected.
- Future surgery to insert a new tube may be necessary.
- When swimming, special precautions are often recommended to protect the tubes.

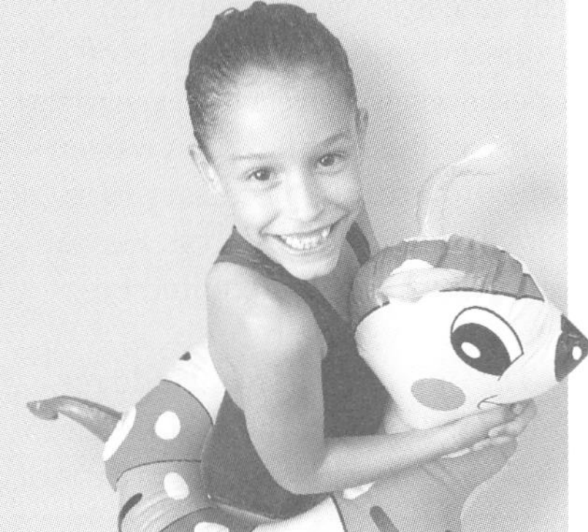

Mastoiditis

Signs and symptoms

- Redness, swelling and tenderness of the mastoid process
- Earache
- Fever
- Discharge of pus from your ear

If severe (acute) middle ear infection isn't treated, the infection may spread to the mastoid process, the bone located behind the outer ear that's connected to the middle ear. When mastoiditis occurs, the infection moves from your middle ear to the mucous membrane lining the mastoid process and the honeycomb-like bone within. If the infection is severe, it can destroy this bone and even spread farther.

Diagnosis

Your doctor may take a sample of any pus apparent in the ear canal and possibly arrange for a computerized tomography (CT) scan or magnetic resonance imaging (MRI) of the head to determine how far any infection has spread.

How serious is mastoiditis?
Before the availability of antibiotics, acute mastoiditis was a leading cause of death in children. Now it's treated successfully with antibiotics, and the health risk is vastly reduced.

Treatment
Antibiotics are used to treat mastoiditis. Curing this infection isn't easy because of the difficulty eradicating infected material from the many, small mastoid cells. It may take several weeks of high-dose antibiotic therapy to eliminate the infection. If antibiotic treatment doesn't solve the problem, your doctor may recommend a mastoidectomy, in which part or all of the mastoid bone is surgically removed.

Hereditary Deafness

Hereditary deafness is hearing loss due to a genetic defect that runs in families. In some cases, hereditary deafness occurs alone (nonsyndromic deafness). Other times, deafness is only one symptom of a syndrome (syndromic hearing loss). For example, Alport's syndrome is a kidney disorder accompanied by hearing loss. Deafness can also be associated with any number of inherited conditions, including an enlarged thyroid (Pendred's syndrome), malformation of the external ears, skin abnormalities, mental retardation and peripheral neuropathy.

Some causes of deafness are present at birth (congenital) but aren't hereditary. For example, if a mother has German measles (rubella) while pregnant, the newborn child runs a high risk of deafness. Other causes of early hearing loss include prematurity, lack of oxygen during or shortly after birth, blood incompatibilities and meningitis.

Cholesteatoma

Signs and symptoms
- Hearing loss
- Pus seeping from an ear
- Headache
- Earache
- Dizziness
- Weakness of facial muscles (uncommon)

Cholesteatoma is a cyst-like, noncancerous (benign) tumor most commonly found in the mastoid process — a bone behind your ear — and in the middle ear. It occurs as a complication of eustachian tube dysfunction in which the air pressure in your middle ear decreases and your eardrum (tympanic membrane) bends inward.

It can also occur when ear canal skin grows into the middle ear through a hole in your eardrum. In the middle ear, skin cells (epithelial tissue) that would normally be shed are caught, and then they form a cyst. The cyst can damage middle ear bones.

In some cases, cholesteatoma results from a congenital problem in which skin cells remain behind the eardrum during fetal development. When a cholesteatoma develops in the ear of a child, it may grow quickly. In adults, the problem usually develops more slowly.

Diagnosis
Your doctor may examine your ear with an otoscope, a small instrument that allows a full view of the ear canal. You may also receive a hearing test. A computerized tomography (CT) scan of the ear and mastoid may be done to determine the extent of the disease and to aid in planning possible surgery.

How serious is cholesteatoma?
A cholesteatoma isn't cancerous and won't spread to other sites. But it can cause permanent hearing loss and dizziness. If left untreated, it can affect your facial nerve and, rarely, cause meningitis, an infection and inflammation of your central nervous system.

Treatment
Cholesteatoma can only be treated surgically. A large or advanced cholesteatoma may require an extensive operation or series of operations to correct damage to the bones of the middle ear. A meticulous procedure is necessary to remove every bit of the cyst. Repeat operations may be required because the cyst can recur.

The operation may include rebuilding bones of the middle ear to restore hearing. Useable portions of natural bone or artificial (prosthetic) devices may be used to reconstruct the middle ear. In severe situations, a doctor may perform a radical mastoidectomy. This leaves a cavity that must be cleaned periodically. It doesn't restore hearing.

Otosclerosis

Signs and symptoms
- Gradual hearing loss in one or both ears
- Noise such as a buzzing, ringing or roaring in your ears (tinnitus)

In otosclerosis, the bony wall of the inner ear becomes disorganized due to abnormal growth of spongy bone in your inner ear. The stirrup, a tiny bone that vibrates to help pass sound waves into the inner ear, may become immobile, causing conductive hearing loss.

Conductive hearing loss is failure of the mechanism that passes vibrations through your middle ear via its three connected bones. Unlike nerve deafness (sensorineural deafness), conductive hearing loss often can be treated and reversed with surgery.

Otosclerosis is the most frequent middle ear cause of hearing loss in young adults. It affects about 10 percent of the American population to some degree. Otosclerosis runs in families and is more common in women than in men.

Symptoms usually become apparent between the ages of 15

and 35. The hearing loss tends to progress slowly, can affect one or both ears and may be mild or severe. In women with otosclerosis, the degree of hearing loss may increase during pregnancy.

Diagnosis

See your doctor if you notice that your hearing seems to be gradually worsening. He or she may examine your ears, conduct hearing tests and ask if any close relatives experienced early hearing loss.

How serious is otosclerosis?

Otosclerosis doesn't endanger your general health, and it may be corrected with treatment.

Treatment

Otosclerosis can often be treated successfully with stapedectomy, surgical removal of the stirrup (stapes). Medication may prevent further hearing loss and hearing aids may improve hearing.

Medication

Treatment with tablets of sodium fluoride, calcium and vitamin D may prevent progressive bony changes that cause further hearing loss by hardening the spongy bone. There's continuing debate about the value of this treatment.

Surgery

In stapedectomy, a surgeon cuts the skin of the ear canal and lifts the eardrum out of the way to replace the stirrup (stapes) with a tiny wire or prosthesis. The eardrum (tympanic membrane) is returned to its normal position, and the incision usually heals in a week or two.

In some instances, a doctor may use a laser to create a small hole in the bottom of the stirrup. This allows for placement of the wire or prosthesis.

You may experience temporary dizziness for some hours after the operation. Hearing usually improves quickly, and you may be able to resume normal activity within a few weeks. Occasionally, a blood clot blocks sound conduction. The clot usually disappears within a few weeks.

Stapedectomy helps most people with otosclerosis, but 1 percent to 2 percent of those who undergo the procedure lose all hearing in the ear. This is a matter to consider before proceeding with the operation. If you have otosclerosis in both ears, you might consider having surgery on one ear and then waiting a year to gauge the results before having the other ear done. If your inner ear is impaired, a stapedectomy may not improve hearing.

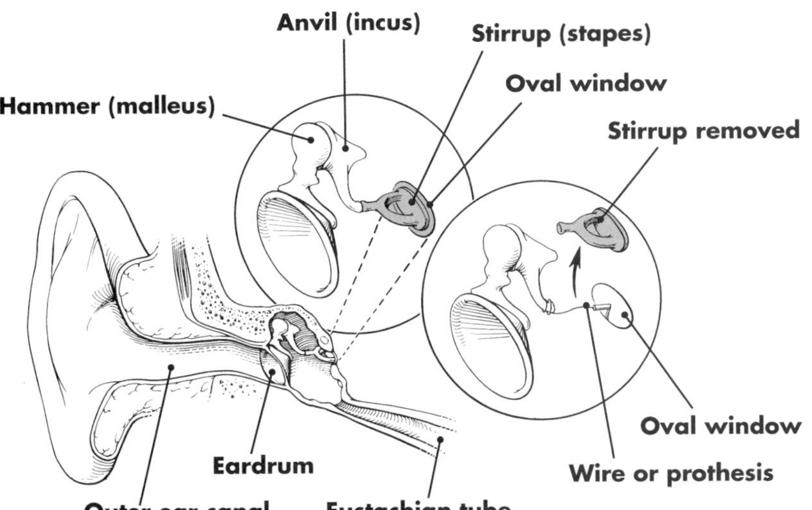

In a stapedectomy, the malfunctioning stirrup (stapes) of the middle ear is replaced with a tiny wire or prosthesis that transmits sound vibrations.

Noise-induced hearing loss

Signs and symptoms

- Progressive hearing loss
- Noise such as a buzzing, ringing or roaring in your ears (tinnitus)

Noise-induced hearing loss is common. It usually occurs as a result of cumulative exposure to loud sounds — 90 decibels or louder — over a period of years. The noise can be occupational, such as at a loud construction site, or recreational, as with snowmobiling or listening to loud music, including music from headphones. People at greatest risk have both a noisy job and a noisy hobby — for example, a mechanic who plays in a rock band.

Noise-induced hearing loss is a form of nerve deafness (sensorineural deafness), which is caused by damage to the cochlea or the sensory nerves. The intense vibration caused by loud sound waves damages the hair cells that line the cochlea of the inner ear. This damage prevents electrical impulses from reaching the auditory nerve, which normally transmits these impulses to the brain to be interpreted as sound.

Sensorineural deafness may also result from a blow to the head or a single exposure to loud impulse noise (acoustic trauma), such as gunfire or an explosion. Other causes include aging, illness, injury, infection, some medications and heredity.

It's crucial to use ear protection whenever possible during exposure to loud sounds. If you work in a noisy environment, your employer should regularly measure noise levels or provide protective devices. Noise-induced hearing loss is usually irreversible, and it often develops insidiously.

Diagnosis

If you notice that your hearing has worsened or you experience a ringing, buzzing or roaring sound in your ears (tinnitus), see an ear, nose

Identifying Dangerous Noise

Sounds are all around us. When sounds become uncomfortable or interfere with daily activities, they're commonly referred to as noise, the generic term for any unwanted sound. Exposure to loud noise levels over long periods of time can cause permanent and irreversible hearing loss. A single exposure to loud impulse noise, such as gunfire, also may result in irreversible damage to your hearing. Ringing, buzzing or roaring in your ears (tinnitus) after exposure to loud noise levels is an early indicator of hearing damage. It's crucial to protect your hearing when you're exposed to loud noise.

The loudness of sound (sound intensity) is measured in units called decibels (db). The pitch (frequency) of sound is measured in hertz (Hz). Loudness, pitch and length of exposure are all factors used to predict if noise is damaging to hearing.

Individuals who work in noisy environments fall under the guidelines of the Occupational Safety and Health Administration. OSHA requires that employers provide a hearing conservation program, including at least an annual hearing test, to workers exposed to noise that averages 85 db or more during an 8-hour workday. These workers should be offered the use of hearing protectors, such as earmuffs or earplugs. When workers are exposed to noise that averages more than 90 db during an 8-hour day, OSHA requires that they use hearing protectors.

The workplace isn't the only setting for noise exposure. Hazardous noise levels are also associated with commonplace household occurrences and recreational activities.

Noise source	Approximate decibels
Whisper	30
Normal conversation	60
Ringing telephone	80
Power lawn mower	90
Hair dryer	90
Bulldozer	105
Chain saw	110
Ambulance siren	120
Jet engine at takeoff	140
12-gauge shotgun blast	165

Source: National Institute for Occupational Safety and Health, Centers for Disease Control and Prevention, 2001.

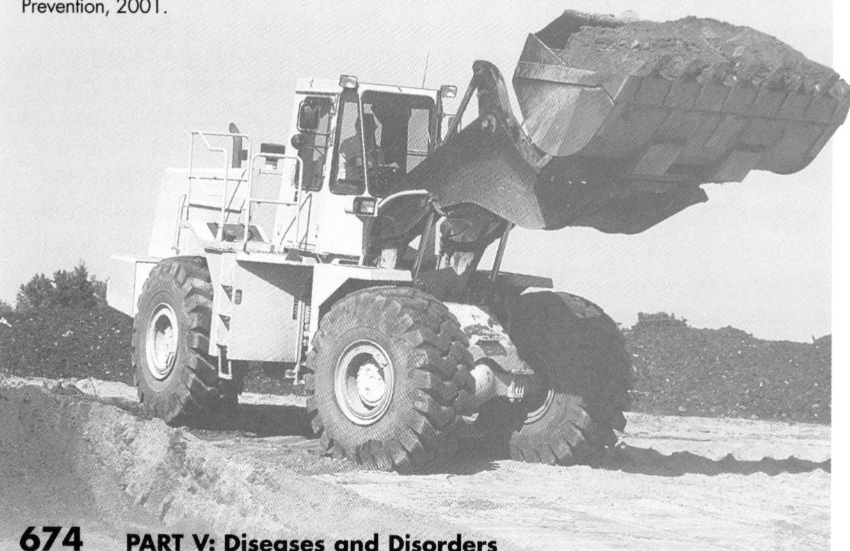

and throat (ENT) specialist and an audiologist. An ENT doctor will examine your ears, and the audiologist will perform a series of tests to determine the nature of your hearing loss. After these examinations, specialists can recommend a proper course of action.

Treatment

In many cases, the most effective treatment for severe sensorineural deafness caused by noise is a hearing aid (see page 676).

Age-related hearing loss

Signs and symptoms

- Gradual hearing loss
- Noise such as a ringing, buzzing or roaring in your ears (tinnitus)

Hearing impairment is common among people older than age 65. Almost a third of the people in this age group have noticeable hearing loss. Some lose very little hearing, and others become quite hard of hearing.

Hearing loss due to aging is called presbycusis, from the Latin words *presby*, meaning "old," and *cusis*, meaning "hearing." Typically, the hearing loss begins in middle age and progresses. It affects both ears, particularly for detecting high-frequency sounds. It affects men more often and more severely than women.

Presbycusis results from changes in the cochlea or the nerves attached to it. The cochlea, the snail-shaped cavity in the inner ear, has thousands of tiny hairs that convert sound vibrations into electric signals. The auditory nerve carries these signals to the brain, where they're interpreted as sound. When some of these hairs or the auditory nerve itself becomes damaged, signals aren't transmitted as efficiently, and hearing loss results. This damage is permanent and can't be reversed medically or surgically. Like noise-induced hearing loss, age-related hearing loss is a form of nerve deafness (sensorineural deafness).

Diagnosis

If you think that your hearing is diminishing, or a family member suggests that it might be, see your doctor. Often, people with hearing loss deny that a problem exists. Sometimes, people with presbycusis find that it's more difficult to hear the high-frequency voices of women and children than the lower voices of men. They may also find that it's more difficult to understand conversation in a group than conversation with a single individual. Severe hearing loss isn't a health threat, but it can interfere with work, cause isolation and be socially debilitating.

Treatment

Presbycusis can't be treated surgically or medically. A hearing aid is the only treatment (see page 676). You can also learn certain useful techniques.

These include reading lips, facing the speaker, decreasing background noise — for example, turning off the television or dishwasher and shutting the windows to avoid street noise — and making maximum use of nonauditory clues, such as gestures and facial expressions, to help understand what people are saying.

Tinnitus

Signs and symptoms

- Noise such as a buzzing, ringing or roaring in your ears

Tinnitus — an annoying sensation of noise in your ears when there's no source of such sound — is common. An estimated 40 million to 50 million adults in the United States have some degree of tinnitus.

Tinnitus can be a symptom of almost any ear disorder as well as other diseases, including cardiovascular disease, allergies and anemia. It may also result from high doses of aspirin, large amounts of caffeine or exposure to loud noise.

Scientists don't fully understand the mechanism that causes these

PREVENTION TIP

If you know you'll be exposed to loud noise, it's best to use specially designed ear protection. Hundreds of commercially produced hearing protectors are available, but the best protector is the one that's worn correctly 100 percent of the time when in the presence of loud noise. Earplugs must fit snugly to completely seal off the ear canal. Earmuff cushions must completely encircle the ear.

Commercially made devices that meet federal standards bring most loud sounds down to acceptable levels. You can obtain specially designed earmuffs or custom-molded earplugs made of foam, plastic or rubber. Some earmuffs close out the outside world. Others are fitted with earphones and a microphone that enable you to communicate with other workers. Active electronic hearing protectors, designed to use with firearms, use circuitry that shuts out loud noise almost instantaneously at the sound of gunfire.

Additional steps can be taken to protect your hearing. Identify the source of loud noise and try to reduce the volume. Or distance yourself from the noise. If that isn't possible, take breaks from the noise. Intermittent noise exposure is less damaging than continuous exposure because it gives the ears time to recover. However, even brief exposure to loud impulse noise, such as gunfire, may cause irreversible damage.

If someone in your home listens to loud music on a headset, use this simple test to determine if the sound is too loud for his or her health: If the individual is wearing the headset and you can identify the music being played, it's too loud. Suggest that he or she listen to the music at a lower volume or for shorter periods of time.

The arm's-length rule provides a good method for gauging potentially damaging noise exposures in everyday life. If you must raise the level of your voice to be heard by someone an arm's-length away, the noise is too loud.

Communication Tips

Here are a few suggestions for communicating effectively with someone who's hard of hearing:

- Make sure that you have the person's attention before talking. Simply saying the person's name directs his or her attention to you.
- Face the person to whom you're speaking.
- Speak at louder levels if listening conditions are difficult. Politely ask if you're being heard and understood.
- When listening conditions are difficult, talk naturally but a little more slowly and with a few more pauses.
- Stay within a few feet of the person with whom you're speaking.
- If possible, reduce background noise. For example, turn off the radio or television.
- If possible, talk on a one-to-one basis or in a small group.
- Alert your listener to changes in topics of conversation.
- Rephrase your comment if the listener is unsure about what was said.

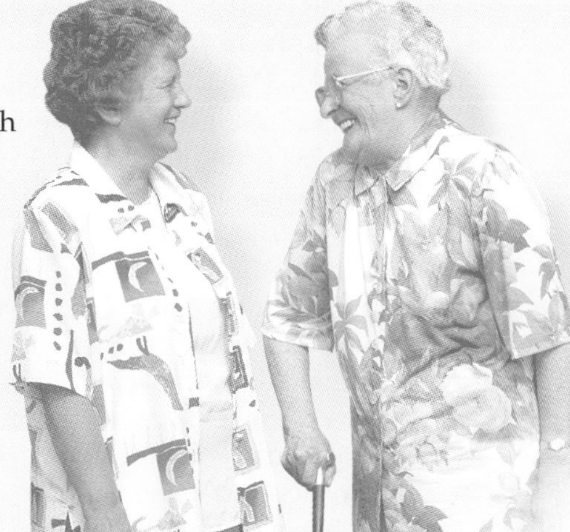

sounds. However, tinnitus is often associated with hearing loss, and it usually occurs in both ears instead of just one.

Diagnosis

If you hear ringing, buzzing, whistling or other sounds when there's no apparent source of such noises, you probably have tinnitus. These sounds may be continuous or intermittent, and they can vary in loudness. They may be in synchrony with your heartbeat.

When evaluating tinnitus your doctor looks for signs of an infectious disease, ear obstruction or hearing disorder. An audiologist may examine your ears, test your hearing and conduct a series of tests to determine the cause of noise in your ears.

In some cases, a computerized tomography (CT) scan or magnetic resonance imaging (MRI) is performed to check for structural abnormalities.

How serious is tinnitus?

Ear noise can be very annoying, but it's usually not a health threat.

However, if tinnitus occurs on one side only (unilateral), it could be a sign of a more serious condition, such as a form of cardiovascular disease or an auditory nerve tumor.

Treatment

In some cases, the cause of tinnitus is easily treated and the noise stops. In many cases, though, treating the underlying cause doesn't stop the noise.

If tinnitus is bothersome, one form of treatment is to cover up the unwanted noise with a competing sound, for example, sound from a radio or recorded environmental noise. Another option is a tinnitus masker, a device that's worn like a hearing aid and that produces a different, less annoying noise. In people who also have hearing loss, hearing aids may improve tinnitus.

Another method of treatment is learning how to cope with the condition through a relaxation process known as biofeedback. The idea is that the more relaxed you are, the better you're able to cope with chronic conditions such as tinnitus. Reducing exposure to loud noise and limiting intake of nicotine, aspirin, caffeine and alcohol also may help.

Hearing Aids

If you're thinking about trying a hearing aid for the first time or shopping for a new model, you may be happily surprised by new technology. Current models are small, simple to operate and technologically advanced.

Canal

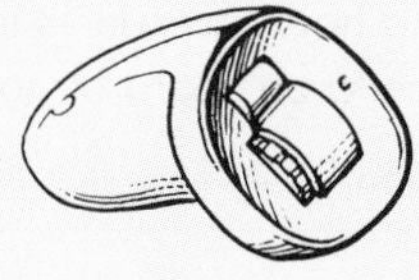

Low Profile

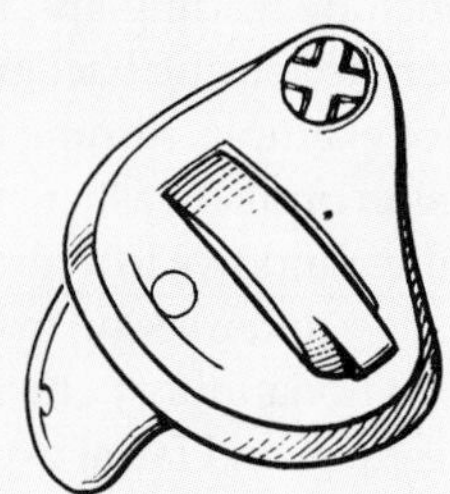

Styles

Hearing aids come in five basic styles, classified by where they're worn:

- Completely in the ear canal (canal)
- In the ear canal (low profile)
- All in the ear
- Behind the ear
- On the body

The canal styles appeal to individuals concerned with the appearance of a hearing aid. These styles are also easier to use with a telephone.

However, canal styles may not provide enough amplification if you have severe hearing loss. In addition, some people find the small controls on canal styles difficult to adjust — although some digital models work automatically after initial programming.

Generally, the smaller the hearing aid, the less powerful and more likely it is to produce feedback — a high-pitched squeal. These days, body-mounted hearing aids are rarely used. For those units, the earpiece is attached by a cord to a microphone and amplifier located in a small box that the user carries in his or her pocket.

If you have similar hearing loss in each ear, you may want to consider using two hearing aids. Your hearing will be more balanced, and it'll be easier to locate the source of sounds.

Conventional vs. digital

Conventional (analog) hearing aids work by amplifying all of the sound around you — sounds you want to hear as well as unwanted noise. Digital hearing aids offer more ability to fine-tune sound and reduce irritating background noise. They're programmed using a computer and can be adjusted to match your preferences. Fully digital devices are the most expensive.

Some analog hearing aids can be programmed digitally, resulting in a combination analog and digital device. Some come with a remote control unit that allows you to easily change to a program appropriate for the given conditions, such as conversation in a quiet setting or a loud restaurant.

Disposable hearing aids

Following the trend established by disposable contact lenses, dispos-

Meniere's disease

Signs and symptoms

- Severe attacks of dizziness (vertigo) accompanied by nausea and vomiting
- Hearing loss and distortion
- Noise such as a buzzing, ringing or roaring in your ears (tinnitus)
- Ear fullness, pressure

The symptoms of Meniere's disease were described more than a century ago by a Frenchman named Prosper Meniere. Symptoms include episodes of dizziness in which the room feels like it's spinning (vertigo), accompanied by fluctuating hearing loss, ringing in the ears and a sensation of pressure in an affected ear.

At first, meniere's disease usually affects one ear, but it eventually affects both ears in about 25 percent to 50 percent of people with the disease. Its cause is unknown, but the condition seems to be associated with an increase of fluid pressure in the inner ear.

The excess pressure is thought to cause tension upon the delicate membranes of the labyrinth — the fluid-filled chamber of the inner ear that controls balance and hearing — distorting and occasionally rupturing them. This trauma produces severe disruption in the senses of balance and hearing.

Diagnosis

Periodic attacks characterize Meniere's disease. Between attacks, which may last from several minutes to most of a day, there are far fewer symptoms.

Symptoms range from mild to serious but usually involve ear noise, hearing distortion, a feeling of fullness or pressure in the ear, and vertigo, which can be so severe as to cause nausea and vomiting. The attacks can become increasingly frequent and severe.

The first test you'll likely undergo to help establish the diagnosis is a hearing test. If it's inconclusive, you may need further tests. One such test, called electronystagmography, involves rinsing your ear with cool or warm water or air. Normally, this causes you to feel a whirling sensation that makes your eyes move rapidly from side to side. The responses to the stimulation of each ear are recorded and compared with each other and with normal responses to determine if

All in the Ear

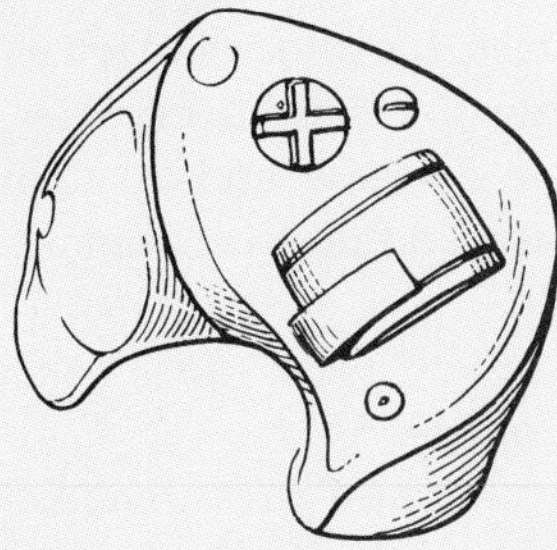

Behind the Ear

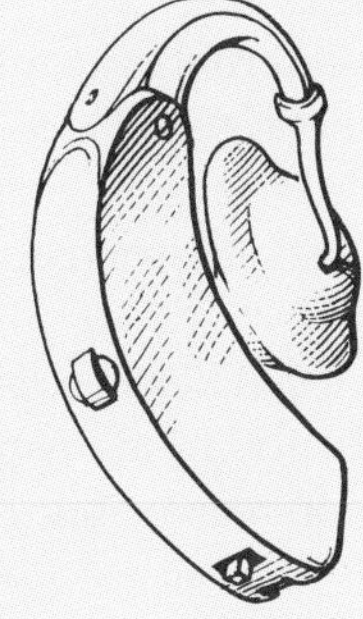

Body

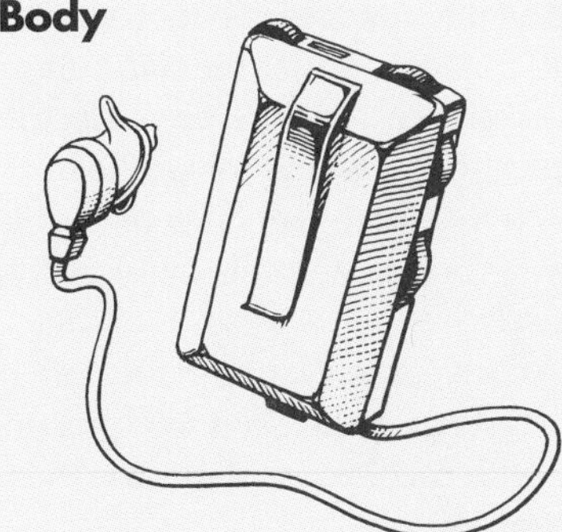

able hearing aids were introduced to provide a low-cost device with a relatively long battery life. By using disposable hearing aids, you avoid repair costs, and you don't have to commit to technology that may become obsolete.

A significant drawback is that these hearing aids aren't custom fitted, so they don't fit everyone comfortably.

Training

Getting used to a hearing aid takes time. The sound you hear is different because it's amplified. In addition, it takes practice to learn how to tune out background noise.

When you first get your hearing aid, try it in an ideal situation, such as listening to a radio or television in a quiet room. People often make the mistake of immediately using a hearing aid in a difficult listening condition, such as in a loud restaurant. This can be discouraging.

The best way to get accustomed to your hearing aid is to wear it daily, making it part of your routine. In addition, ask your audiologist about programs that teach listening skills, such as lip reading.

Shopping smart

A hearing aid can be an expensive purchase, so take steps to ensure that you choose a quality product. Begin by choosing a reputable audiologist. If you don't know one, ask your doctor for a referral.

Be cautious of "free" consultations from salespeople who sell only one brand. Also be alert to misleading claims. For years, some manufacturers claimed that their products eliminated background noise. No hearing aid can filter out the specific sound or voice you want to hear from other voices or sounds in a crowded room.

Make sure the hearing aid comes with a trial period and warranty. A typical trial period is 30 days. The warranty should extend for 1 to 2 years and cover both parts and labor.

If the hearing aid doesn't seem to improve your hearing or it's uncomfortable, ask your audiologist to adjust it. If you're not happy with it, return it for a refund.

Cochlear Implants

Some children and adults who have profound nerve deafness (sensorineural deafness) and who aren't helped by a hearing aid may benefit from a cochlear implant, an electronic device that's implanted under the skin behind the ear.

With nerve deafness the hair cells that line the cochlea of your inner ear have been damaged. Normally, these tiny hairs convert sound vibrations into electric impulses that are carried by the auditory nerve to the brain and then interpreted as sound.

A cochlear implant functions much like the hair cells did before they were damaged. It sends an electric signal via the remaining nerve fibers to the brain. This is altogether different from a hearing aid, which amplifies sound and directs it into the ear canal.

A cochlear implant consists of two sets of components: external and internal. The external component includes:

- A microphone to pick up sound
- A speech processor, which changes sound into a computer code
- A transmitter, which sends electric signals from the speech processor to an internal receiver

The external portion of some cochlear implants looks much like a conventional hearing aid. However, some devices require wearing the speech processor on your body.

The internal component consists of tiny devices that an ear surgeon (otologist) implants under the skin behind your ear. It includes:

- A receiver, which receives electric impulses from the external transmitter
- Electrodes, which collect the impulses from the internal receiver
- A transmitter, which sends the electric impulses to the brain

Your brain interprets the electric impulses as speech and environmental sounds.

A cochlear implant can't restore normal hearing, but it can help people understand speech and interpret environmental sounds. Today, many people with cochlear implants use the telephone and carry on reasonably good communication.

Before you decide to proceed with an implant, have a careful evaluation of your middle and inner ear, including X-ray imaging and a thorough hearing exam by an audiologist. After placement of the implant, you'll be trained in how to best use the device and interpret the sounds it produces.

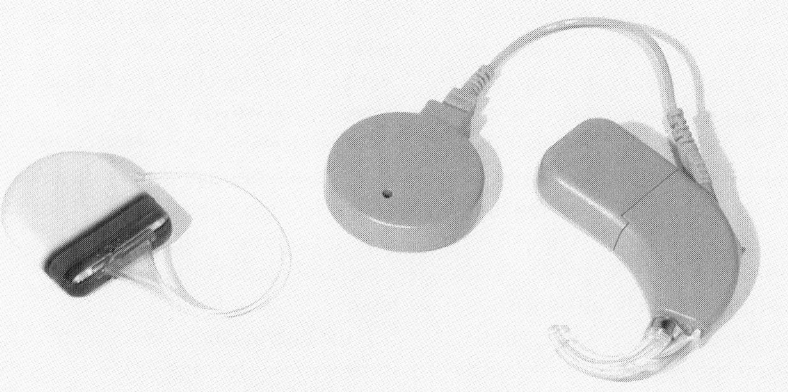

Newer cochlear implants use an externally worn speech processor that you can conceal behind your ear. The speech processor (right) sends signals to a surgically implanted electronic chip (left) that stimulates the hearing nerve.

the balancing system of the inner ear is operating normally.

How serious is Meniere's disease?

For most people, the attacks are infrequent, and the disorder is primarily an inconvenience. For a few, though, Meniere's disease can lead to complete deafness, and the vertigo and accompanying nausea can be frequent and debilitating.

Treatment

Treatment for Meniere's disease may include:

Medication

Your doctor may prescribe medication to combat the vertigo and its accompanying nausea and vomiting. Reducing body fluids with diuretic medications seems to help some people. Sometimes, a doctor prescribes a sedative to relieve the anxiety that can accompany a serious attack. It's difficult to tell if drug therapy is useful because Meniere's disease tends to go into remission and resolve spontaneously.

Other options

When other measures aren't helpful, a procedure may be performed in which gentamicin, an antibiotic that's toxic to your inner ear, is carefully injected through the eardrum and absorbed into the inner ear. This reduces the balancing function of that ear, and your other ear assumes responsibility for balance. The procedure, which can be performed with local anesthesia in your doctor's office, often reduces the frequency and severity of vertigo episodes.

Other treatments include cutting the nerve that controls balance. When hearing loss is severe or the condition is accompanied by severe vertigo, the entire inner ear can be destroyed. Again, your other ear takes over the balance function.

If you have Meniere's disease involving both ears, treatment is more difficult. You may have surgery on the more impaired ear to stop the most debilitating attacks.

Self-care
Some people find their attacks are reduced in frequency or severity when they reduce or avoid intake of caffeine, alcohol and nicotine.

Labyrinthitis

Signs and symptoms

- Extreme dizziness (vertigo)
- Nausea and vomiting
- Involuntary eye movement

Labyrinthitis is an inflammation of the labyrinth, the fluid-filled chamber of the inner ear that controls balance and hearing. The condition can result from a bacterial or viral infection.

Diagnosis

The diagnosis is usually made based on the presence of specific signs and symptoms: sensations of nausea and dizziness in which the room seems to be spinning, slow movement of your eyes to one side and then a quick move back to their original position, and the loss of hearing in an ear.

How serious is labyrinthitis?

Signs and symptoms of labyrinthitis can be frightening, but the condition itself generally isn't dangerous. However, if hearing loss accompanies the dizziness, then labyrinthitis may be permanent.

Treatment

If you have bacterial labyrinthitis, your doctor will typically prescribe antibiotics. For both bacterial and viral labyrinthitis, your doctor may recommend an antinausea drug and a sedative to combat the effects of vertigo. You may need to rest in bed for several days.

Symptoms of severe vertigo usually pass within a few days to a week. Feelings of imbalance may persist for several weeks or even months, particularly with quick movements of the head. Recurring episodes of labyrinthitis are rare.

Causes of Dizziness

Dizziness affects more than 50 percent of older adults and interferes with daily activities in 20 percent of those older than age 60. Between 15 percent and 30 percent of people — mostly women and older adults — will have an episode of dizziness some time in life that's so severe they'll seek medical attention.

But as common as this complaint is, it often presents a frustrating and complex puzzle to your doctor. Although dizziness may mean one thing to you, to your doctor it's an umbrella term that can signify one of several problems.

Spinning sensation

If you experience a spinning sensation (vertigo), the problem is likely related to the nerves and vestibular system — structures of your inner ear that sense position, movement and changes in your head position. Vertigo can also cause nausea and vomiting. It's almost always accompanied by involuntary, abnormal, rhythmic eye movement called nystagmus. The common causes of vertigo include:

- Meniere's disease
- Labyrinthitis
- Acoustic neuroma
- Benign paroxysmal positional vertigo
- Certain medications, including aspirin, streptomycin and gentamicin, and some medications taken for high blood pressure and heart disease
- Excess caffeine and alcohol

Feeling unsteady

Sometimes, an inner ear disorder can cause loss of balance or a feeling of unsteadiness when walking. A feeling of unsteadiness may also stem from certain medications, such as antiseizure drugs, sedatives and tranquilizers. Sensory deficits such as failing vision, nerve damage in the arms and legs, osteoarthritis and muscle weakness also can cause unsteadiness, as can disorders of the central nervous system.

Floating sensation

Many people refer to a sensation of floating as feeling woozy. This sensation is sometimes associated with hyperventilation or an anxiety disorder, such as a panic attack.

Feeling faint

Some people faint at the sight of blood or after hearing bad news or seeing a frightening sight. Feelings of faintness that occur for an unknown reason may be related to a cardiovascular problem. Possible causes include:

- A significant drop in systolic blood pressure on standing (orthostatic hypotension)
- Blocked arteries (ischemia)
- Disease of the heart muscle (cardiomyopathy)
- A rapid or slow heart rate (arrhythmia)

If you experience ongoing dizziness or your dizziness is accompanied by other symptoms, see your doctor. Only about 5 percent of cases stem from a serious condition, but it's important that the cause of your dizziness be identified and serious conditions be ruled out.

Acoustic neuroma

Signs and symptoms

- Mild dizziness
- Noise such as a buzzing, ringing or roaring in your ears (tinnitus)
- Hearing loss

An acoustic neuroma is a slow-growing, noncancerous (benign) tumor of the auditory nerve. It's usually located near the point where the nerve leaves the cranial cavity and enters the bone structures of your inner ear. Because this site is in an angle formed by two of your brain structures (the cerebellum and pons) and a part of your skull, an acoustic neuroma is sometimes called an angle tumor.

Diagnosis

If you experience mild dizziness, loss of balance, ringing or other noises in one ear and gradual hearing loss, you may have an acoustic neuroma. The dizziness usually is ongoing and doesn't occur in distinct episodes as it does in Meniere's disease.

Your doctor or audiologist may conduct an audiometry test to check the sharpness and range of your hearing. An audiometry test typically uses an electronic device to produce tones of varying intensity. When you hear a tone, you indicate this by raising your hand or pushing a button. The audiologist will also ask you to repeat a series of words to determine your ability to understand speech. Other diagnostic tests may include a balance test, a neurologic examination, a computerized tomography (CT) scan or magnetic resonance imaging (MRI) of your skull to see if a neuroma is present.

How serious is an acoustic neuroma?

Although benign in character and slow in growth, this tumor can be a serious threat because it's located next to a number of vital nerves and brain structures. As it grows, it can create pressure that can damage these structures.

Treatment

Depending on your age, general health and the size of the tumor, you and your doctor may decide to monitor the tumor's growth, remove it surgically or treat it with a form of stereotactic radiosurgery known as Gamma Knife radiosurgery. Stereotactic radiosurgery, commonly used to treat brain tumors, involves accurately delivering high-dose radiation using a computer's assistance. Your head is immobilized, and focused beams of radiation are aimed precisely at the tumor to avoid harming other parts of the brain. The Gamma Knife is an 18-ton machine that emits high-energy gamma radiation.

Surgical removal of an acoustic neuroma usually involves a surgical team that includes a neurosurgeon and a specially trained ear surgeon. The tumor is approached either through the mastoid and inner ear structures, from behind the mastoid region, from above the ear, or by using a combination of these approaches. An operating microscope and nerve monitors are used to help preserve the delicate nerves whenever possible. You usually remain in the hospital for 3 to 5 days after surgery and recover at home for a month or so.

Benign paroxysmal positional vertigo

Signs and symptoms

- Abrupt onset of dizziness when you move your head to certain positions
- Involuntary eye movements

Canalith Repositioning Procedure

To help relieve benign paroxysmal positional vertigo (BPPV), your doctor may instruct you in a series of maneuvers that move particles from the posterior semicircular canal into the utricle. The steps, each held for about 30 seconds, include the following (the movements shown are for the left ear):

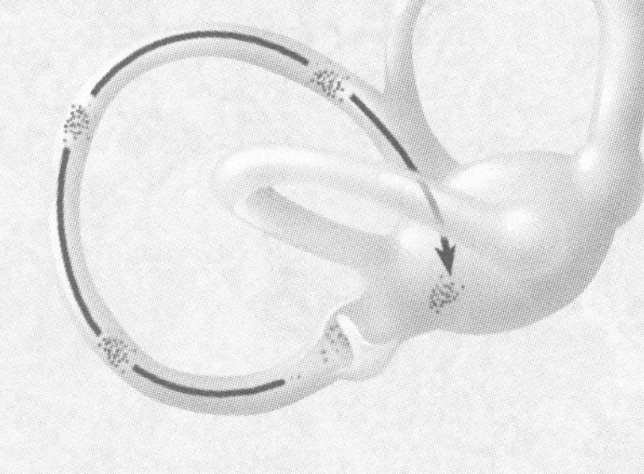

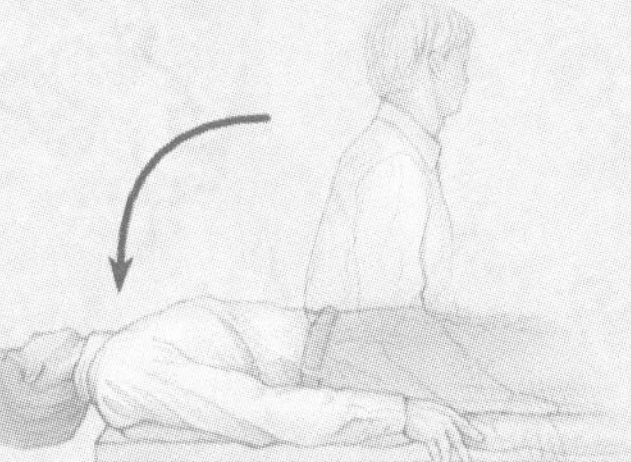

1. Move from a sitting to a reclining position. Your head is extended over the end of the table at a 45-degree angle.
2. Turn your head to the right.

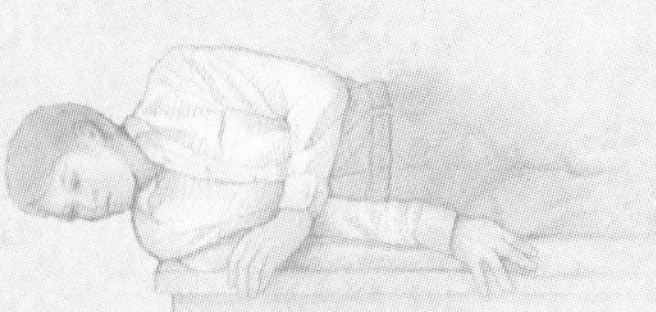

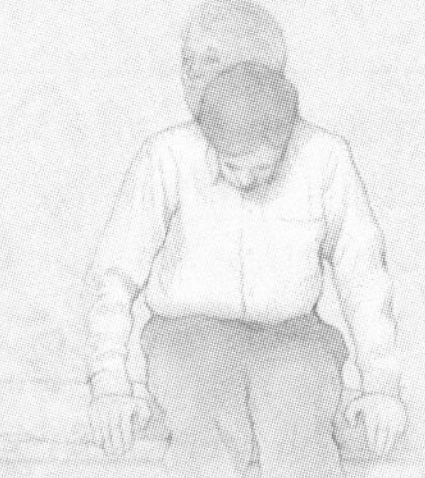

3. Roll over onto your side. Your head is slightly angled while you look down at the floor.
4. Return carefully to a sitting position and then tilt your chin down.

Benign paroxysmal positional vertigo (BPPV) disorder is characterized by a sudden, extreme sensation that the room is spinning (vertigo) when you move your head in a certain direction or lie in a certain position. It's the position of your head that causes the vertigo.

The problem lies in the vestibular labyrinth, the fluid-filled chamber of your inner ear that controls balance and hearing. Tiny granules or crystals, called otoliths and canaliths, within the semicircular canals of the labyrinth loosen and float in the fluid. In certain positions they can irritate the nerve endings associated with balance, giving a false signal of movement and causing a brief sensation of spinning.

What exactly causes these particles to loosen is unknown, but it's thought to be a natural result of aging. Sometimes, BPPV is preceded by a blow to the head.

Diagnosis

Your doctor may conduct a series of tests to determine what form of vertigo you have and whether your positional disorientation is a symptom of another disorder. Characteristics of BPPV include vertigo that occurs when you tip your head back or lie on a particular side when sleeping. The vertigo is generally accompanied by involuntary movement of your eyes from side to side. The symptoms usually decrease in less than a minute.

How serious is BPPV?

Positional vertigo is an inconvenience but rarely a serious problem, unless you're in an occupation in which even short episodes of vertigo may be disruptive.

Treatment

If BPPV is suspected, a simple office procedure may be able to end the spin cycle. The canalith repositioning procedure involves several simple maneuvers for positioning your head. The goal is to progressively move particles in the posterior semicircular canal back to a tiny bag-like structure called the utricle, where they don't cause trouble.

It may be necessary to repeat the procedure several times. After the procedure, you must keep your head upright for 48 hours, even as you sleep. This allows time for the particles to settle inside your utricle. You may need to wear a neck collar to prevent tilting your head.

Protruding ears

Signs and symptoms

- Ears that project an abnormally large distance from your head

Ears that protrude from the sides of your head are neither more efficient nor less efficient for hearing than are ears that lie flat against your head. Thus the problem is largely cosmetic.

The protrusion may vary from slight to extremely obvious. Sometimes, such ears may become the basis of an emotional problem, resulting in a sense of shame, ridicule or unattractiveness.

Treatment

A popularly held misconception about protruding ears is that you can train them to grow closer to your head by taping or strapping them to the sides of your head at night. It doesn't work. If you have mildly protruding ears, changing to a hairstyle that calls less attention to your ears is usually an effective approach to the problem.

Another option is cosmetic surgery. The surgeon makes an incision near the fold of skin behind your ear. He or she then removes a strip of skin and, in some cases, cartilage, pulls your ear flat against your head and closes the incision. Scars from the procedure are hidden behind your ear.

The procedure shouldn't be done in children under age 4 because their ears are still developing. Children who undergo this procedure usually do so just before beginning school so as to avoid teasing at school.

Wax blockage

Signs and symptoms

- A sensation that your ear is plugged
- Partial hearing loss

Your outer ear canal is lined with skin that contains hair follicles and glands that produce earwax (cerumen). These hairs and wax trap dust and other foreign particles to prevent them from entering your ear, thus protecting the delicate mechanisms of your ear.

Normally, the small amount of wax that forms makes its way over time to the opening of your ear, where it falls out or is removed as you wash.

Some people, however, produce or accumulate an excessive amount of wax. This extra wax can harden and block your ear canal. Hardened or impacted wax is one of the most common causes of hearing loss among people of all ages.

Diagnosis

If you experience progressive hearing loss over a period of a few weeks or months, your ears feel full, you have an earache or you hear constant or occasional noises such as ringing in your ears (tinnitus), your doctor will look for signs of earwax blockage.

Treatment

There's an old but wise saying: "Never put anything smaller than an elbow into your ear." Your ear canal and eardrum (tympanic membrane) are delicate, and you can damage them easily by poking around with common items such as cotton-tipped swabs, bobby pins or twisted pieces of paper. They usually don't remove problem wax and, more importantly, can easily damage your ear canal or eardrum.

If your ear is healthy and excessive earwax recurs, you can use an inexpensive home remedy to remove the wax. Over-the-counter preparations are available, but they're more expensive and often less effective.

Follow these steps:

1. Twice a day for several days, place a few drops of baby oil, mineral oil or glycerin in your ear with an eyedropper to loosen the wax. Once you soften the wax well, you can attempt to remove it.
2. Fill a 3-ounce rubber bulb syringe with water at body temperature. If the water is too cool or warm, the following procedure may cause severe, but brief, dizziness.
3. With your head tilted down, pull your outer ear up and back to straighten your ear canal. With the other hand, gently squirt water into the canal, exerting mild pressure but not causing pain.
4. Turn your head to allow the water to drain into a sink or bowl. You may need to flush your ear several times before the wax, usually in the form of a plug, falls out.
5. Dry your outer ear with a towel or a hand-held hair dryer.
6. Dry your ear canal by inserting one full eyedropper of rubbing alcohol into the canal. This will absorb the water and destroy bacteria and fungi. Tip your head to the side to drain the alcohol.

Your doctor may use a similar procedure to remove problem ear wax. Or he or she may use a special suction device or scoop the wax out with an instrument called a curet.

Disorders of the Nose and Sinuses

Your nose is the gateway to your respiratory system, with breathing beginning and ending at the nostrils. Normally, your nose filters, humidifies and warms the air as it moves from your nasal passages into your throat and lungs.

Occasionally, your nose is the site of conditions such as a nosebleed, a cold, hay fever (allergic rhinitis) or a sinus infection. Fortunately, most disorders of the nose and sinuses are temporary and easy to cure.

Nosebleeds

Signs and symptoms

Anterior nosebleed

- Sudden bleeding from one nostril

Posterior nosebleed

- Blood streaming down the throat

Most people experience a nosebleed at one time or another. Sometimes, the cause is a blow to the nose, but often a nosebleed is simply the result of a cold, a sinus infection, dry air or a scab being dislodged. Rarely, nosebleeds may be a sign of a serious underlying problem, such as high blood pressure, a bleeding disorder or leukemia.

Nosebleeds are typically thought of as a childhood problem, but they're actually more common in older adults — and they can be more serious the older you get.

Most nosebleeds begin on the septum, the wall of cartilage and bone that separates the two nasal chambers. This is called an anterior nosebleed. This form of nosebleed isn't serious and is usually easy to stop. The front of your septum, just inside your nostril, contains many fragile blood vessels. These vessels are easily damaged, either directly as from a blow or indirectly from crusting in your nose produced by breathing dry air. A head cold or an allergy also can cause crusting. Anticlotting medications, which include aspirin and anticoagulants, make you more susceptible to nosebleeds.

Posterior nosebleeds are more serious but less common. They occur when one of the large vessels in the inner (posterior) portion of your nose breaks. Blood streams down the nasal cavity into the throat rather than out the nostril, so blood loss is more difficult to monitor. Home treatment usually won't stop the bleeding, requiring a trip to the emergency department.

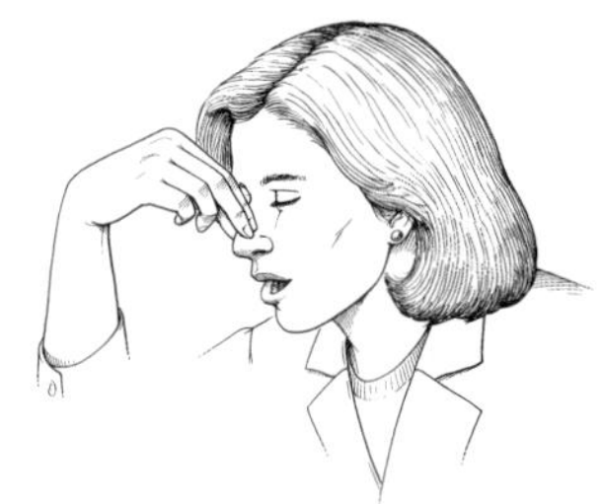

To stop a nosebleed, use your thumb and index finger to squeeze together the soft portion of your nose, located between the end of your nose and the hard, bony ridge.

Diagnosis

In most cases, you can stop an anterior nosebleed easily by leaning forward and pinching closed the collapsible portions of your nostrils for about 10 minutes. There's no need for further examination. But when bleeding is hard to stop or occurs frequently, see your doctor.

Your doctor may examine your nose with an endoscope, a flexible tube with a camera at the end, to see precisely where the problem lies. If the problem appears to be deep in your nose, your doctor may look for other, more serious, problems such as a tumor.

How serious are nosebleeds?

Most nosebleeds are just shirt-staining annoyances. But posterior and recurring anterior nosebleeds can be warning signs of a serious health problem, including thickening and hardening of artery walls (arteriosclerosis), high blood pressure, a bleeding disorder or leukemia. Frequent nosebleeds in children can be a sign of a noncancerous (benign) tumor (see page 684).

Treatment

Use these easy steps to stop an anterior nosebleed:

1. Sit up or stand. Don't lie down. An upright position decreases the blood pressure in the veins of your nose, which slows the flow of blood.

2. Pinch the front, soft part of your nose with your thumb and index finger and breathe through your mouth. Do this for about 10 or 15 minutes — the pressure on your bleeding septum should stop the flow of blood.

To prevent further bleeding, don't blow your nose for several days after the bleeding episode, and keep your head above the level of your heart. If further bleeding occurs, sniff in forcefully to clear your nose of blood clots, and spray both nostrils with a nasal decongestant (Afrin, Dristan, others). Pinch your nose and call your doctor.

If a nosebleed is difficult to stop or occurs frequently, your doctor may use a suction device to remove excess blood and place a medicated cotton ball in your nose. The medication anesthetizes and shrinks your nasal linings.

Cautery

If the bleeding continues, your doctor may recommend that you have the vessel that's causing the problem cauterized. This procedure creates a seal on the vessel by burning it with silver nitrate, electric current or a laser beam. For this procedure, your doctor applies a topical anesthetic to the inside of your nose.

If the bleeding persists after cautery, your doctor may gently pack your nostril with medicated gauze. The packing, which is left in place for several days, exerts pressure on the bleeding site to stop blood flow. When the packing is removed, your vessels may be cauterized again to discourage recurrence of the bleeding.

Surgery

In rare situations, doctors perform septoplasty, a surgical procedure that straightens the wall of cartilage between your nostrils. A bent (deviated) septum can cause anterior nosebleeds to recur.

For posterior nosebleeds and those caused by an underlying disease that are difficult to stop, one approach is to place a special pack in your nasal cavity. Its placement requires sedation. This procedure is

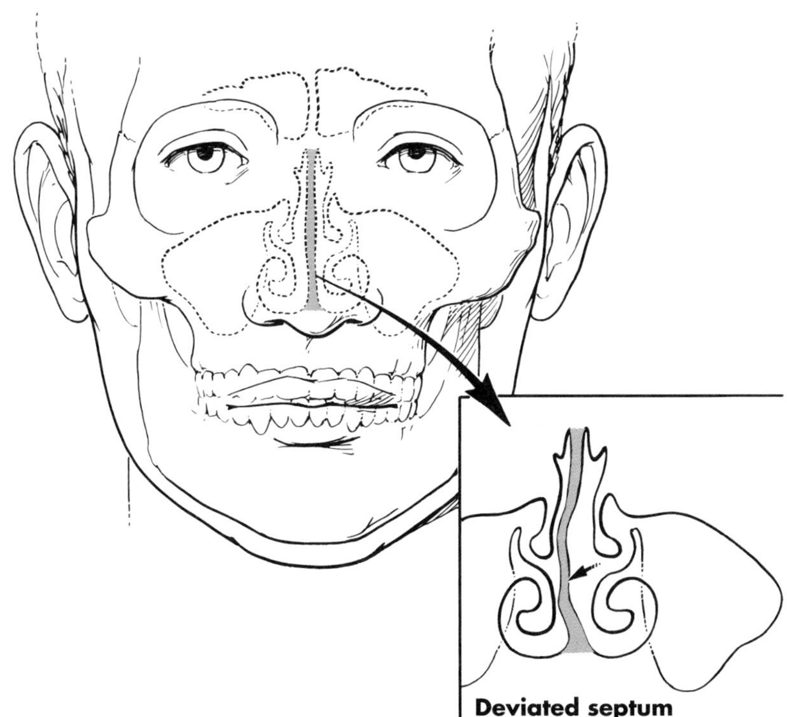

Your nasal septum separates your nasal chambers. A deviated septum may be a cause of nasal obstruction.

Nasal Decongestant Irritation

Your local drugstore sells many products designed to relieve nasal congestion, including decongestant nasal sprays and nose drops (Afrin, Dristan, others). These products provide quick relief by constricting blood vessels and thus shrinking the tissue in your nose. But use these products carefully and only for a limited period, if at all.

When used frequently over several days, decongestant nasal sprays and nose drops can have a rebound effect, causing your nasal tissues to become more swollen and even more congested between applications of the medication. As a result, you'll need greater and more frequent doses of the spray or drops. Use these products no more than three or four times a day over a period of no more than 3 to 4 days.

Prolonged use can irritate your mucous membranes, causing a stinging or burning in your nose and a chronic inflammation known as rhinitis medicamentosa.

The only way to treat the problem of nasal decongestant overuse is to stop using the sprays or drops. Your condition may become worse for a while, but over a period of weeks your breathing should approach normal as the ill effects of the nasal sprays or drops wear off. Your doctor may recommend a cortico-steroid nasal spray or, on occasion, a corticosteroid injection to reduce inflammation and make the transition easier.

done in a hospital and may involve a short stay for observation. The procedure may be uncomfortable, but it's usually effective in stopping the bleeding. In rare instances, when standard techniques don't work, a doctor may perform surgery to block the arteries that supply blood to the nosebleed site.

Prevention

If you have frequent nosebleeds, apply saline gel or petroleum jelly to your nasal septum once or twice each day. Increase the humidity of the air you breathe by using a humidifier or vaporizer. Don't pick your nose and avoid blowing your nose for several days after a nosebleed. Blowing your nose increases pressure on the damaged vessels and can lead to further bleeding.

Foreign Object in the Nose

If a foreign object becomes lodged in your nose, follow these steps:

1. Don't probe at the foreign object with a cotton-tipped swab or other tool, and don't try to inhale the object by forcefully breathing in. Breathe through the mouth until the object is removed.
2. Blow your nose gently to try to free the object, but don't blow hard or repeatedly.
3. If the object protrudes from the nose and can be easily grasped with tweezers, try to gently remove it.
4. If these methods fail, see your doctor immediately or go to an urgent care center or emergency department.

Nasal obstruction

Signs and symptoms

- An inability to breathe through your nose

Nasal obstruction occurs when the air passageways of your nose become blocked. Everyone experiences a certain amount of temporary blockage when suffering from a cold or an allergy.

Sometimes, nasal obstruction is caused by a deviated septum or excessive use of over-the-counter nasal sprays. Nasal tumors or polyps and enlarged adenoids are other causes. See page 531 for more information on nasal polyps.

Your septum is the cartilage and bony partition that separates your two nasal chambers. Few people have a septum that runs perfectly straight. Most variations are small, but in some people the septum veers significantly to one side or the other, creating the blockage. Such deviations are often the result of an injury such as a blow to your nose.

Diagnosis

In searching for the cause of the obstruction, your doctor may ask questions regarding possible injury, allergies and use of nasal sprays. He or she may use a lighted, flexible device that's inserted into your nose to assist in diagnosing the problem. A computerized tomography (CT) scan also can be helpful in some circumstances.

Treatment

For many people, a deviated septum poses little if any inconvenience. However, if the deviation causes a blockage that makes it difficult to breathe normally, a septoplasty may be necessary.

Septoplasty is a surgical procedure that realigns your septum. It usually can be done either under local or general anesthesia on an outpatient basis.

If the blockage is a result of overuse of nose drops or a nasal spray, you'll need to stop using the medication. If allergies are suspected, your doctor may refer you to an allergist for a series of tests to determine what you're allergic to. If the blockage is a result of polyps, enlarged adenoids or a tumor, surgery may be necessary to remove the blockage.

Juvenile angiofibroma

Signs and symptoms

- Frequent nosebleeds
- A nasal obstruction

An angiofibroma is a noncancerous (benign) tumor of the nose that occurs at puberty, particularly in boys. The tumor may shrink on its own after puberty, but it can grow rapidly, obstructing nasal passages and sinuses and causing frequent and often severe nosebleeds. Rarely, the tumor can put pressure on the brain.

Diagnosis

If your child has signs or symptoms suggestive of a juvenile angiofibroma, your doctor may examine the inside of his or her nose for evidence of a tumor. Magnetic resonance imaging (MRI) or a computerized tomography (CT) scan can help determine the size and location of the tumor. If the tumor doesn't shrink on its own, treatment is necessary.

Treatment

The most common treatment for an angiofibroma is surgery to remove the tumor. Occasionally, doctors use a procedure called embolization, either alone or just before surgery.

During embolization, a doctor injects pellets of a glue-like substance into the tumor's blood vessels. The pellets obstruct the blood vessels, cutting off blood supply to the tumor.

A Simple Remedy for a Stuffy Nose

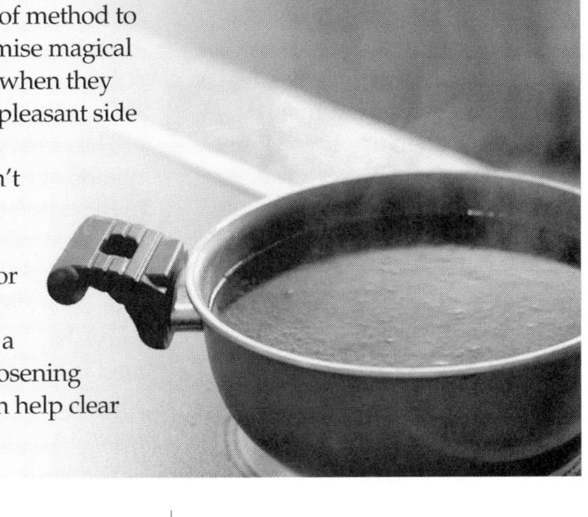

While in the throes of a cold, who doesn't yearn for a foolproof method to cure a congested nose? Dozens of ads tout products that promise magical cures, but such products rarely live up to their billings. Even when they do relieve the congestion in your nose, they may produce unpleasant side effects such as drowsiness or dry mouth.

One of the best temporary remedies for a stuffy nose doesn't cause complications or cost money. To loosen mucus in your nasal and sinus cavities and relieve congestion, inhale steam. Bring a kettle or pan of water to a boil and inhale the steam for several minutes, taking care not to get so close that you scald yourself. Some people place a towel over their head, making a tent while they inhale the steam. This method is useful for loosening the mucus in your chest too. Similarly, a steaming shower can help clear your head.

Rhinophyma

Signs and symptoms

- A nose that appears large, bulbous and ruddy

Rhinophyma, which results from a skin condition called rosacea (see page 1175), involves the upper layer of skin (epithelium) on the outer portion of the nose. The skin thickens, causing the nose to be large and bulbous. This is sometimes called a W.C. Fields nose after the famous comedy actor who had rhinophyma.

The cause isn't clearly understood. The condition was once thought to result from heavy drinking, but alcohol consumption isn't a factor. People who drink moderately or abstain from alcohol can develop rhinophyma.

Diagnosis

A diagnosis of rhinophyma is made based on the appearance of excessively thick skin on the outer portion of the nose, causing it to take on a large, bulbous shape.

Treatment

The only effective treatment for rhinophyma is surgery. In this procedure, the surgeon removes excess tissue from the outside of the nose using various surgical instruments or a laser. As it heals, the nose usually resumes its normal shape.

Loss of the sense of smell

Signs and symptoms

- Decreased ability to detect odors
- Decreased nasal breathing

Most people lose their sense of smell when suffering from a head cold, but sometimes the cause isn't so obvious. Loss of the sense of smell (anosmia) results when an obstruction in your nose prevents odors from reaching delicate nerve fibers in your nose that lead to the area of your brain dealing with smell (olfactory area).

Loss of the sense of smell may also occur if the olfactory area or its nerve fibers are damaged. A viral infection, allergies or a chronic nose infection can damage these nerves, as can a head injury, nasal surgery or a tumor. Another cause of loss of smell is nasal polyps, pearl-like lumps due to swelling of nasal membranes, which can block nasal passages.

Most people who have lost their sense of smell can still distinguish salty, sweet, sour and bitter tastes, which are sensed on the tongue. But they have trouble distinguishing more subtle flavors and sensations that require both taste and smell.

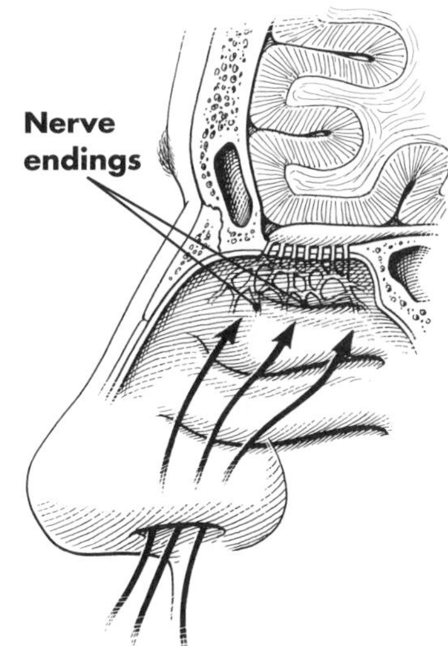

Your sense of smell and, to a large degree, your sense of taste begin with the olfactory nerve endings, found in the upper portion of your nose. These nerves contain sensitive fibers that transmit signals from the olfactory bulb to your brain.

Diagnosis

If you lose your sense of smell for no apparent reason, consult your doctor. Nasal polyps and chronic nasal allergies are the most common causes of anosmia. Your doctor may check for tumors of the nasal passages.

How serious is loss of the sense of smell?

Most often, anosmia is an inconvenience. Sometimes it can be a symptom of a more serious condition. You may need to have a computerized tomography (CT) scan or magnetic resonance imaging (MRI) to check for polyps, a tumor or signs of a head injury. If you lose your sense of smell after a concussion or other head injury, the blow may be the cause of your anosmia.

Loss of the sense of smell can pose certain dangers. If you have anosmia, be sure to have functioning smoke detectors in your home and workplace because you may not smell the smoke of a fire. In addition, carefully check for food expiration dates and refrigerate food appropriately to avoid ingesting spoiled food, which you may not detect through its smell.

Treatment

If your loss of the sense of smell is due to hay fever (allergic rhinitis) or nasal polyps, treating these conditions will often restore your sense of smell. When the cause isn't readily apparent, as is often the case when a virus is involved, your sense of smell may return when the tissues of your olfactory area regenerate on their own.

Vasomotor rhinitis

Signs and symptoms

- Stuffy or runny nose
- Frequent sneezing
- Coughing

The term rhinitis refers to inflammation of the mucous membranes of the nose. Rhinitis can occur for many reasons. The common cold causes nasal membrane inflammation. Allergies are another frequent cause. Nasal inflammation associated with allergies is called allergic rhinitis, commonly known as hay fever. To read about hay fever, see Chapter 21, "Allergies and Asthma."

Many people, however, experience nasal stuffiness — often accompanied by sneezing, a runny nose or phlegm in the throat — that isn't related to allergies or an infection, such as a cold. This form of rhinitis is commonly referred to as nonallergic, or vasomotor, rhinitis.

Vasomotor rhinitis stems from dilation of blood vessels in the nasal membranes. When the blood vessels expand (dilate), the membranes of the nose swell, taking up more space within an already limited area. This leads to nasal congestion — a stuffy nose.

Many factors may trigger vasomotor rhinitis. They include environmental irritants, such as smoke, dust, smog, dry air or certain odors, such as perfumes. Temperature changes or air conditioning can cause vasomotor rhinitis in some people. Other causes include hormonal changes, anxiety, exercise, spices, beer and wine.

Diagnosis

Rhinitis typically is diagnosed based on your signs and symptoms and when they occur. If you're bothered at a certain time of the year, such as the spring, fall or both, you may have allergic rhinitis. If your nasal congestion doesn't appear to be triggered by allergies, but other factors, your doctor may determine that you have vasomotor rhinitis.

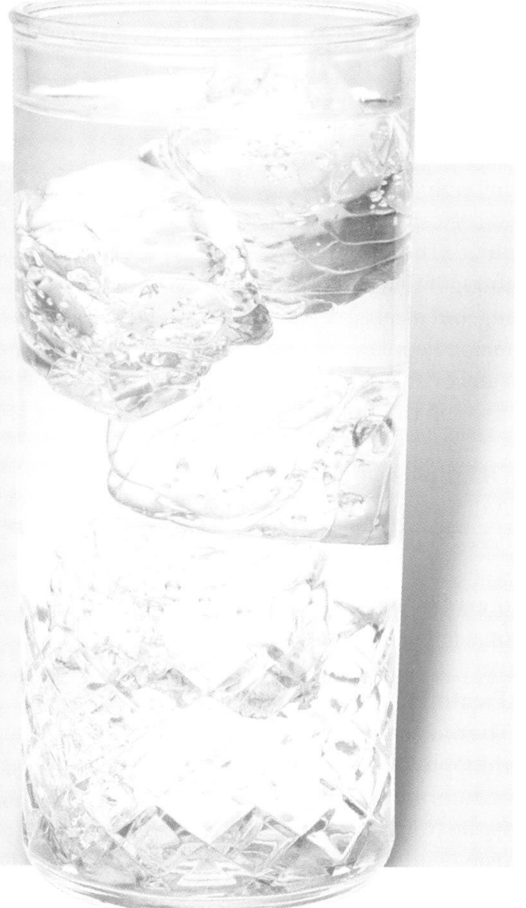

Postnasal Drip

Mucus produced in your nose and sinuses travels in a thin film to the back of your throat. There, it serves to protect your lungs by humidifying air and by trapping dust and other particles that you inhale. Generally, you're unaware of this process and swallow the mucus and impurities it captures. Swallowing this mucus isn't harmful.

Normally, your nose and sinuses produce a liter or more of mucus daily. However, when smoke or other irritants aggravate your nose, the amount may increase. The extra mucus, secreted to remove more irritants, is often the cause of the discomfort commonly referred to as postnasal drip.

You may become more conscious of mucus in your nose and throat when the air is dry because it may become thicker and more difficult to expel. Drinking plenty of water and humidifying the air you breathe will help keep the mucus thin. Corticosteroid nasal sprays available by prescription also may help relieve postnasal drip.

How serious is vasomotor rhinitis?

Although often annoying, vasomotor rhinitis isn't a worrisome condition. However, to manage your symptoms, you may have to take medication regularly or avoid certain situations, such as smoke-filled rooms or certain foods or beverages.

People with chronic vasomotor rhinitis can also develop nasal polyps and chronic sinusitis.

Treatment

Treatment of the disorder depends on its severity. For mild cases, no treatment may be appropriate. Simply avoiding those factors that seem to trigger the condition is often all that's needed.

Over-the-counter oral decongestants often help. Decongestant nasal sprays can provide temporary relief but they shouldn't be taken regularly because they actually can increase nasal congestion (see page 683).

Prescription corticosteroid nasal sprays are often effective in controlling moderate to severe vasomotor rhinitis. For some people, increased humidity at home and at work also is beneficial.

Sinusitis

Signs and symptoms

- Pain near the eyes or cheeks
- Tenderness of the sinus areas to pressure or touch
- Headache
- Swelling of the eyelids or tissues around the eyes
- Fever
- Obstructed nasal breathing
- Thick, yellowish-green nasal discharge
- Bad breath that's unrelated to dental problems
- Toothache (uncommon)

Your sinuses are cavities in the bones around your nose. There are four pairs of sinuses:

- Frontal sinuses, located in your forehead
- Ethmoid sinuses, located between your eyes
- Sphenoid sinuses, located deeper in your head, behind your nose
- Maxillary sinuses, located in your cheekbones

Each of these cavities has a tiny opening into your nose to allow for a free exchange of air and mucus. Your sinuses and nose are lined with a continuous mucous membrane. Consequently, anything that causes your nasal passages to swell and clog — such as a cold or an allergic reaction — can affect your sinuses in the same manner. The result is the pain and pressure that people commonly refer to as a sinus attack.

Sinusitis occurs when the lining of one or more of your sinuses becomes infected. The infection can be bacterial, viral or fungal.

About two-thirds of sinusitis cases are short-lived (acute). Bacteria take up residence in your sinus cavities and cause swelling of mucous membranes, production of thick, yellowish-green mucus, fever and facial pain. The swelling prevents mucus in your sinuses from draining properly into your nasal passages.

For some people, sinusitis becomes long-lasting (chronic). The symptoms never seem to go away, despite appropriate treatment. Some chronic sinusitis is thought to be related to a sensitivity to inhaled fungus. This type of sinusitis is frequently associated with polyps and asthma.

Causes

Acute and chronic sinusitis stem from a number of conditions, from simple to complex:

The Sinuses

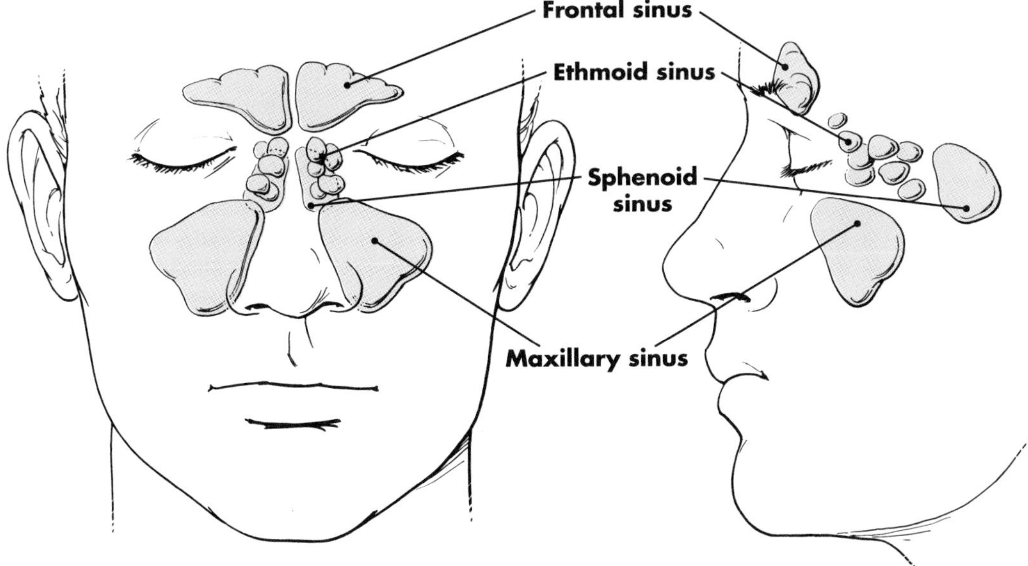

PREVENTION TIP

You may not be able to prevent all sinus problems, but you can take measures to reduce the number and severity of attacks and to help prevent an acute attack from becoming chronic.

- *Wash your hands.* When you've been near someone who has a cold, wash your hands with soap and water to reduce the chance that you'll catch a cold.
- *Keep your distance.* Minimize close contact with people who have colds.
- *Don't smoke.* Tobacco smoke can cause irritation and inflammation of the lining of the sinuses and nose. Inflammation can result in blocked nasal passages.
- *Avoid polluted air.* Contaminants in the air, whether indoors or outdoors, can irritate and inflame your lungs and nasal passageways.
- *Avoid known allergens.* These may include pollen, mold or cat dander. Attach an electrostatic filter to heating and air-conditioning equipment to help remove allergens from the air.
- *Use humidifiers.* This is especially important during the winter when heating systems can make indoor air dry. Be sure to keep humidifiers clean. Contaminated humidifiers can be a source of bacteria and fungi in the air.
- *Use decongestants before airplane travel.* Beware of antihistamine and decongestant drug combinations because antihistamines may cause drowsiness.
- *Talk to your doctor.* Ask your doctor about using a saline nasal spray to keep your nasal passages moist or a prescription medication to reduce inflammation.
- *Avoid alcohol.* It can cause nasal and sinus membranes to swell.

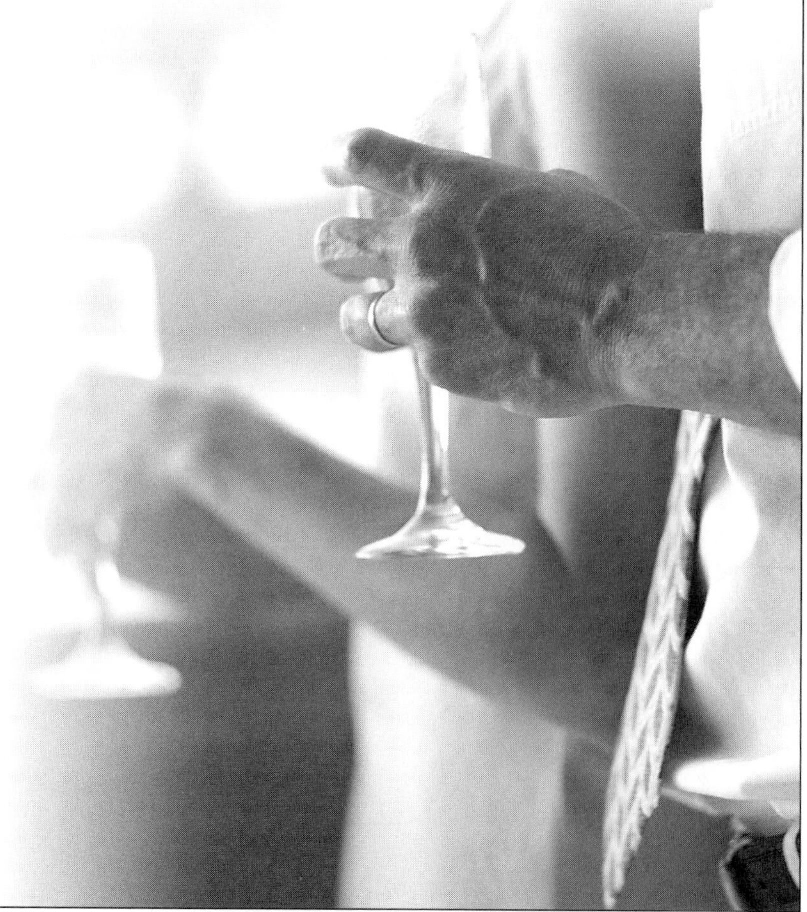

Colds

Most cases of sinusitis start with a cold virus. Sometimes, a cold produces so much mucus that your swollen and congested nasal passages become blocked. Bacteria, which normally reside in your sinuses in small numbers, can begin to multiply and cause bacterial sinusitis.

Allergies

If you're allergic to inhaled allergens such as pollen, pet dander or dust mites, your body mistakes these harmless particles as attackers. Your immune system fights back, causing well-known allergic symptoms, especially a stuffy nose and watery eyes. This immune response can lead to sinusitis. Because allergies are frequently persistent, they may cause chronic sinusitis.

Fungal infections

Some forms of chronic sinusitis stem from an immune system response to a fungus in nasal and sinus cavities. As long as the fungi remain, so will the irritation.

Structural abnormalities

Structural abnormalities of the nose include nasal polyps (see page 531) and a deviated septum, in which the cartilage separating the nasal cavities is bent toward one side. These problems can obstruct the flow of mucus from the sinuses, leading to chronic sinusitis.

Dental problems

Bacteria associated with dental infections or procedures can invade sinus cavities in the cheekbones. For example, a dental abscess can extend from the root of an upper tooth into a maxillary sinus cavity.

Diagnosis

Sinusitis may be difficult to diagnose because initially it closely resembles the common cold. If your symptoms disappear in 5 to 7 days, you probably had a cold. If symptoms persist and don't respond to over-the-counter decongestants, you may be dealing with a sinus infection. Your doctor may be able to determine if you have acute or chronic sinusitis by considering the duration and severity of your symptoms.

If you have repeated or chronic sinusitis, your doctor may perform a nasal endoscopy. A thin, flexible tube with a fiber-optic light (endoscope) is inserted through your nose, allowing your doctor to visually inspect the openings to your sinuses.

Your doctor may also order an X-ray or computerized tomography (CT) scan to see which sinuses are involved and if they appear obstructed or inflamed. If mucus or pus is present, a sample of it may be cultured in a laboratory and analyzed.

If allergies are suspected, allergy testing may yield important information about your allergic sensitivities (see page 525). These tests are safe and involve little if any discomfort.

How serious is sinusitis?

Most cases of sinusitis respond to antibiotics and are easily treated. Rarely, some people develop serious complications. The infection can spread to the bones around your eyes or into the membranes that protect your brain (meninges), causing meningitis, which can lead to brain damage. In a condition called cavernous sinus thrombosis, blood can clot in the veins around the sinuses, cutting off blood circulation to the brain, similar to a stroke.

Treatment

A few home remedies may improve the symptoms of sinusitis:

- Stay indoors in an even temperature.
- Refrain from bending over with your head down. This movement usually increases the pain.
- Try applying warm facial packs, inhaling steam from a kettle or basin of steaming water (be careful not to scald yourself) or taking a warm shower.
- Drink plenty of liquids to help dilute the mucous secretions. Don't drink alcohol, which can worsen nasal and sinus swelling.

Medication

Depending on the cause of your sinusitis and whether it's acute or chronic, your doctor may prescribe one or more of the following medications:

- *Allergy medications.* If allergies are causing your chronic sinusitis, your doctor may prescribe medications to reduce allergy symptoms and consequently reduce the number and severity of your sinus attacks.
- *Antibiotics.* If your infection is bacterial, your doctor may prescribe a course of oral antibiotic therapy lasting 10 to 14 days. Chronic sinusitis may require a long period of antibiotic treatment, often using broader-spectrum medications than those used for acute sinusitis. A broad-spectrum medication is one that is effective against a wide variety of bacteria.
- *Antifungal medications.* If your sinusitis is due to a fungal sensitivity or infection, your doctor may recommend use of an intranasal solution containing an antifungal agent. You squirt the solution into your nasal passages, allowing it to wash out (irrigate) your sinuses.
- *Corticosteroids.* For intense inflammation of the sinuses, your doctor may prescribe a corticosteroid medication. Nasal corticosteroid sprays are commonly used, but severe inflammatory sinusitis may require a corticosteroid injection or pills. After you've had a shot or pills, you might continue using a corticosteroid nasal spray to help prevent the swelling from recurring.
- *Decongestants.* Decongestants reduce stuffiness and help you breathe easier. However, over-the-counter nose drops or nasal sprays shouldn't be used for more than a few days. Otherwise, the medications can cause a rebound effect and lead to even more congestion and swelling. They can also raise your blood pressure and pulse rate.
- *Pain relievers.* Pain relievers include aspirin, ibuprofen (Advil, Motrin, others) and acetaminophen (Tylenol, others).

Surgery

Sometimes, sinusitis persists despite medical treatment. If this happens, a surgeon may perform endoscopic sinus surgery to restore nasal drainage. Endoscopes are fiber-optic instruments of various sizes, equipped with viewing devices. This type of surgery offers relief of symptoms, but results in no external incisions or scarring.

Most endoscopic sinus surgeries are done under general anesthesia. Your doctor inserts an endoscope and delicate cutting tools into your nostrils and blocked sinuses. Working with the aid of an image from the endoscope projected on a monitor, your doctor removes infected sinus membranes, polyps and small bone fragments that block your sinuses.

The surgeon may also enlarge sinus openings and use a small vacuum to drain trapped fluids. This typically requires no hospital stay, and you can sometimes return to work within a few days.

You may have a mild headache from the operation, and you may need to take antibiotics and pain medication afterward. During the first 2 weeks after surgery, it's normal to have some discomfort and bleeding from your nose. You'll also have to visit your doctor soon after surgery to have dried blood and other secretions removed from your nose.

Occasionally, sinus blockage redevelops, and surgery must be repeated. Complications, although rare, can be serious. They include eye damage, brain abscess and permanent facial numbness.

If a deviated septum is causing your sinusitis, your doctor may recommend a surgical procedure to realign your septum (septoplasty).

Disorders of the Throat

Like other parts of your respiratory system, your throat is susceptible to infection, both bacterial and viral. Your throat is also susceptible to abuse, including overuse while singing or speaking and damage from excessive alcohol consumption or smoking. Gastroesophageal reflux disease (GERD), a condition in which contents from your stomach reflux into your esophagus, also can affect your throat if the reflux is severe.

Sore throat

Signs and symptoms

- A scratchy or irritated sensation in your throat
- Difficulty swallowing due to pain
- Fever

Your pharynx is the segment between your adenoids and your voice box (larynx) — what you commonly think of as your throat. Thus, pharyngitis is another name for a sore throat. A tight, scratchy feeling in the throat is a familiar symptom of a cold or the flu.

Most sore throats are caused by either viral or bacterial infections. A sore throat and other accompanying signs and symptoms from a viral infection usually go away on their own in about a week, once your body's antibodies have destroyed the virus.

Bacterial infections are less common but more serious than most viral infections. Strep throat is the most common bacterial infection. It's caused by the streptococci bacteria and generally is spread by nose or throat secretions. Less commonly, infection may be transmitted through food, milk or water contaminated with these bacteria.

A sore throat can also stem from allergies and dry air. Constant irritation from smoking, breathing heavily polluted air or consuming too much alcohol can cause a chronic sore throat.

Diagnosis

If your sore throat is due to a viral infection, you may also experience coughing, sneezing, mild fever, hoarseness, runny nose and postnasal drip. If you have a bacterial throat infection, you may have a fever, and your tonsils and the lymph glands in your neck may be swollen and painful. The back of your throat may be bright red with white patches.

If your sore throat lasts more than a few days, consult your doctor. If you have symptoms of strep throat, your doctor or a nurse will likely take a culture to determine if you have a bacterial infection.

How serious is a sore throat?

A sore throat due to a viral infection isn't a serious threat. However, certain strains of streptococci bacteria, if left untreated, can lead to serious complications such as kidney inflammation (nephritis) or rheumatic fever.

Antibiotics are given to treat strep throat mainly to prevent these complications.

Treatment

If your sore throat is due to a viral infection, antibiotics won't cure it. Get plenty of rest and double your fluid intake. Fluids may keep your mucus thin and easy to clear.

You can help relieve the pain of a sore throat with acetaminophen (Tylenol, others), ibuprofen (Advil, Motrin, others) or aspirin, but don't give aspirin to children because it can trigger Reye's syndrome, a serious condition involving the blood, liver and brain.

Gargling with warm salt water — a half teaspoon of salt mixed in a glass of warm water — several times a day and using throat lozenges help relieve the pain to some degree.

You may want to switch to a soft or liquid diet to avoid irritating your throat. Avoid smoke and other air pollutants, including fumes from household cleaners or paint, which also can irritate a sore throat.

If you have a bacterial infection, your doctor will likely prescribe antibiotics to kill the bacteria.

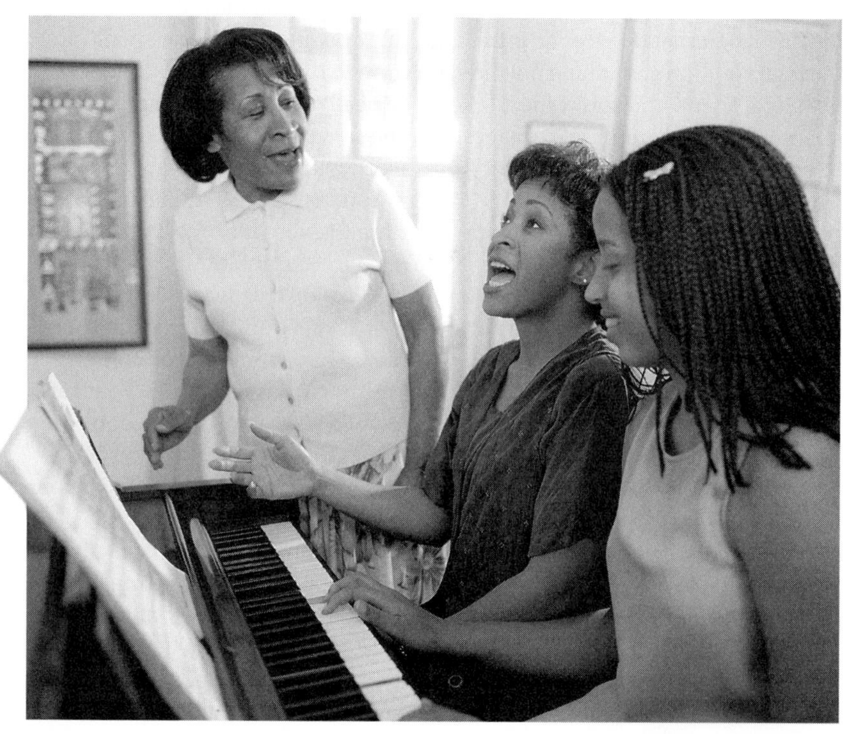

Removing the tonsils (tonsillectomy) may prevent recurrent strep infections.

Tonsillitis

Signs and symptoms

- A sore throat
- Headache
- Fever and chills
- Sore, enlarged glands in the jaw and neck

Your tonsils are composed primarily of lymph tissues. They're located at the back of your mouth, one on either side of your throat.

Among other functions, they filter out infectious microorganisms. When the tonsils become the site of a bacterial infection, they swell and become inflamed. This infection (tonsillitis) is common, especially in childhood.

Diagnosis

See your doctor if a sore throat, headache, fever and chills last more than 48 hours or if you have a history of tonsillitis. Your doctor may take a throat culture to determine if the cause of your symptoms is a bacterial infection.

Tonsillitis causes the tonsils to become visibly red and swollen. They may also have white specks on them. The lymph nodes under the jaw and in the neck may be enlarged and tender.

How serious is tonsillitis?

Left untreated, tonsillitis stemming from a bacterial infection can lead to an abscess in or around your tonsils.

In addition, certain strains of streptococci bacteria that cause tonsillitis may result in later complications, including kidney inflammation (nephritis) or rheumatic fever.

Treatment

If you have tonsillitis, get plenty of rest and drink soothing fluids. Gargling with warm salt water — a half teaspoon of salt mixed in a glass of warm water — several times a day often helps to decrease throat pain.

Acetaminophen (Tylenol, others), ibuprofen (Advil, Motrin, others) or aspirin may be helpful. However, don't give aspirin to children because it could trigger Reye's syndrome, a serious condition involving the blood, brain and liver.

Medication

If a bacterial infection is the cause of your tonsillitis, your doctor will likely prescribe an antibiotic. Signs and symptoms should disappear within a few days, but it's important that you take your full course of prescribed medications.

Epiglottitis

Signs and symptoms

- A sore throat
- Fever
- Difficulty swallowing due to severe pain
- Hoarseness

Adenoid and Tonsil Removal

Your adenoids and tonsils are composed primarily of lymph tissues. Your adenoids are located at the top of your throat just above the soft area at the back of the roof of your mouth (soft palate). Tonsils are located at the back of your mouth. Both act to filter infections from your body and are particularly useful in infants and children up to about 3 years old. In later childhood, the adenoids and tonsils shrink. By puberty, the adenoids have almost disappeared, and the tonsils shrink to the size of almonds.

Many young children and some adults develop bacterial tonsillitis. Occasionally, the adenoids also swell, giving the voice a nasal quality. If you or your child experiences frequent tonsillitis — four to six or more times a year — your doctor may recommend removing the tonsils and adenoids. This combined surgery is known as adenotonsillectomy.

In the past, most children with tonsillitis had their tonsils removed, and often their adenoids as well. Improved antibiotics have made the treatment of tonsillitis much easier and surgery less common. Surgery is still an option when the tonsils become so enlarged that they affect breathing and swallowing, or when an inflamed adenoid causes eustachian tube blockage, leading to a severe middle ear infection (otitis media) and nasal obstruction.

Following adenotonsillectomy, the tonsils don't grow back. Sometimes, small remnants of adenoid tissue can enlarge. This rarely causes another problem.

After surgery, the throat will be sore. This gradually gets better in 10 to 14 days. Adenotonsillectomy doesn't guarantee freedom from future infections, but the frequency of throat infections usually decreases.

Adenotonsillectomy may also be used to treat other conditions. In children, these conditions include:

- Mouth breathing and snoring (both of which are caused by chronic upper airway obstruction)
- Recurrent middle ear infection (otitis media)

Conditions that may prompt this type of surgery in an adult include:

- Snoring and sleep apnea
- An abnormal stony mass in a tonsil (tonsillar calculus)
- Recurrent inflammation of the tissues around the tonsils (peritonsillitis)

Emergency signs and symptoms
- Difficulty breathing
- Drooling
- A stiff or rigid neck and severe headache
- A fever of more than 102 F in adults or 103 F in children, or a fever that lasts more than 2 days
- A rash
- Persistent hoarseness or mouth ulcers lasting 2 weeks or more
- Recent exposure to strep throat

Epiglottitis is an inflammation of the lid-like structure that covers your vocal cords and windpipe (trachea). The condition is most common among children between ages 2 and 5, although adults can get it too. It's more common among males than females and among whites than other races.

Epiglottitis is usually the result of a bacterial infection. Certain conditions, such as Hodgkin's disease, leukemia and immunosuppressive disorders, predispose adults to epiglottitis.

Diagnosis
If your or your child's sore throat lasts more than a few days, see your doctor. He or she may check for a bacterial infection.

It's common for a person who has epiglottitis to spit into a cup to avoid the severe pain associated with swallowing. The person may also sit leaning forward, neck outstretched, to make breathing easier. If you or your child has difficulty breathing, call an ambulance or seek other emergency treatment.

How serious is epiglottitis?
Epiglottitis can begin swiftly and become serious within just hours. When your epiglottis swells, it can obstruct the entrance to your windpipe, making breathing difficult.

Treatment
Most cases of epiglottitis are treated with antibiotics to kill the bacterial organisms causing the infection. Severe difficulty breathing may require temporary insertion of a tube into the trachea (intubation or tracheotomy) to improve breathing.

Peritonsillar abscess

Signs and symptoms
- A sore throat and sore soft palate
- Severe pain on swallowing
- Fever
- Tendency to hold your head to one side, away from the pain
- Drooling
- Difficulty opening your mouth

Vocal Cord Problems

The two vocal cords in your larynx produce the sounds of speech by vibrating. The muscles of your voice box (larynx) control the length, position and tension of the vocal cords, which transmit vibrations to the column of air that passes through your larynx. Your vocal cords can also close, which helps prevent food and water from entering your lungs during swallowing. Like other organs, vocal cords are susceptible to various illnesses.

Vocal cord polyps
Polyps are small swellings that can develop in the mucous membranes covering your vocal cords. As they grow, they take on a rounded shape. Polyps may extend the full length of your vocal cords or be localized. Vocal polyps may stem from a chronic allergic reaction, or they may form as a result of breathing irritants such as cigarette smoke or industrial fumes.

Polyps can make your voice become breathy-sounding and harsh. Sometimes, a doctor is able to remove them during an examination of your throat with a laryngoscope. He or she may biopsy the polyp to be certain that it isn't cancerous (malignant).

Singer's nodules
People who use their voices a great deal, such as professional singers, teachers, auctioneers and members of the clergy, are prone to have nodules on their vocal cords. Such nodules result from excessive voice use.

When you have this condition, your voice may become breathy-sounding and hoarse. A nodule differs from a polyp in that it grows out of the epithelium that covers the mucous membrane, not out of the mucous membrane itself. Thus, it has a structural resemblance to a corn on a toe or a callus on your hand.

Resting your vocal cords by avoiding or minimizing speaking for several weeks may cause the nodules to shrink. Sometimes, surgical removal is necessary. Voice therapy may help eliminate speaking habits that sometimes are responsible for nodule formation.

Contact ulcers
Your vocal cords are subject to developing sores called contact ulcers. This condition results from trauma to your vocal cords. Causes include stomach content backing up into your esophagus and throat (gastroesophageal reflux disease, or GERD), a chronic cough or insertion of a tube through the mouth or nose into the throat (intubation).

Contact ulcers generally develop at the back of your vocal cords. Symptoms may include pain when swallowing or speaking, hoarseness and ear pain. Your doctor may take a sample (biopsy) of the ulcerated tissue to be certain no cancer is present. If GERD is the cause, treating the condition should promote healing of the ulcers.

Leukoplakia
Leukoplakia is the development of white patches on one or both vocal cords. The patches may be associated

Peritonsillar abscess (quinsy) is a complication of tonsillitis. It's most common in young adults. When a tonsil becomes infected, a collection of pus (abscess) forms between the tonsil and the soft tissues around it. The infection may even extend to the soft area at the back of the roof of your mouth (soft palate), making it possible for the abscess to cover a large area. The infection can also spread to your neck and even farther downward into your chest.

Diagnosis

A diagnosis often is based on displacement of an inflamed tonsil and swelling at the back of your palate.

How serious is a peritonsillar abscess?

In some cases, the swelling caused by a peritonsillar abscess can become so severe that the roof of your mouth is pushed against your tongue, blocking airflow and making breathing and swallowing very difficult.

Treatment

The infection is treated with antibiotics. If pus is present and the condition doesn't resolve quickly, your doctor may drain the abscess surgically. Because abscesses can recur, your doctor may also recommend a tonsillectomy at the time of the abscess or several weeks after the infection is cured.

Laryngitis

Signs and symptoms

- Hoarseness
- Tickling and rawness of your throat
- A constant need to clear your throat

Laryngitis is an infection or irritation of your voice box (larynx), which is attached to the top of your windpipe (trachea). When vocal cords become inflamed or irritated, they swell, causing distortion of the sounds produced by air passing over them. As a result, your voice sounds hoarse. In some cases, your voice can become so faint that it's undetectable.

Laryngitis may be short-lived (acute) or long-lasting (chronic). The symptoms and their treatment are often the same.

Acute laryngitis is usually caused by a virus, and the condition typically disappears without treatment. Acute laryngitis less commonly results from a bacterial infection. However, it often occurs in the

with cancer. Once the patches are discovered, your doctor can remove them and have them examined under a microscope to check for cancerous cells. Leukoplakia is often caused by smoking.

Laryngeal papillomatosis

Laryngeal papillomatosis is a disease caused by the human papillomavirus (HPV). These noncancerous (benign), warty tumors (papillomas) grow on the vocal cords, voice box (larynx) or the respiratory tract and cause problems with breathing and swallowing. Most laryngeal papillomas affect young children, usually before age 3.

The tumors may disappear at puberty. But they can be troublesome. The papillomas can grow quickly and in large quantities or clusters, making them difficult to remove without damaging the larynx. They may block the airway, causing severe difficulty breathing. In these cases, the tumors need to be treated quickly.

Laser treatment and powered-instrument shaving have become the primary treatments. Lasers vaporize tissue using intense beams of light. Shaving uses a small rotating blade to remove tissue. Removal of a papilloma is accomplished with the aid of a microscope in order to minimize injury to underlying tissues and prevent scarring of the vocal cords. Other options include chemotherapy or antiviral therapy. Because laryngeal papillomas frequently recur, repeat treatments are often necessary.

Another treatment under study is called photodynamic therapy. A dye that's sensitive to bright light is injected into the bloodstream. The dye concentrates in tumors and destroys them when activated by intense light of a certain wavelength.

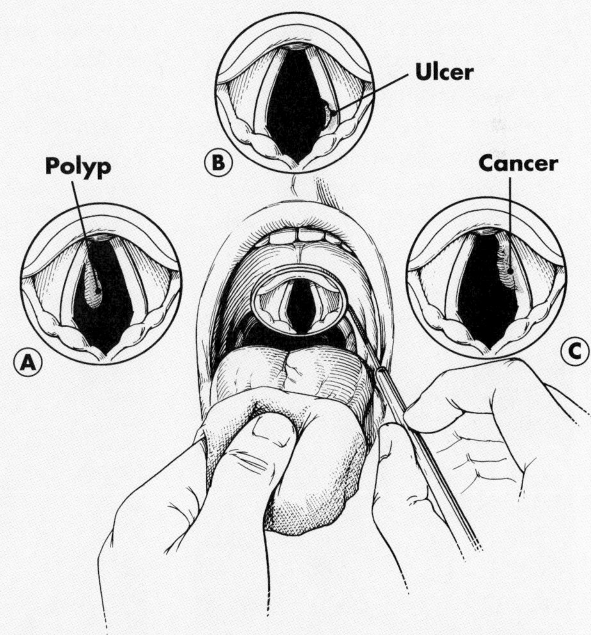

A small, angled mirror is used in performing indirect laryngoscopy, which provides a view of your vocal cords: (A) A vocal cord polyp. (B) A contact ulcer. (C) Vocal cord cancer.

Speech After Laryngectomy

If you've had your voice box (larynx) surgically removed, you must relearn how to speak.

After removal of the larynx (laryngectomy), you no longer breathe through your mouth and nose. Instead, you breathe through an opening at the front of the neck called a tracheostoma. This opening is created during a procedure called a tracheotomy.

This change in the way you breathe affects your ability to speak. It's still possible to speak, but your voice won't sound the same as it did before.

Artificial larynx

Using an artificial larynx is one method of vocal communication following a laryngectomy. These devices produce sound that can be transmitted into the throat or mouth. They're often used soon after surgery and in conjunction with speech therapy. Some people choose to use an artificial larynx as their only method of vocal communication after a laryngectomy.

The main kind of artificial larynx is a neck device. You hold the head of this battery-powered vibrating machine against your neck. The vibrations penetrate neck tissues and resonate in your throat and mouth, where you can convert them into speech by using your tongue, teeth, lips and palate.

Esophageal speech

Following a laryngectomy, some people learn to speak again by a technique called esophageal speech. You draw air into your esophagus, or pump air into your esophagus with your tongue, then immediately expel the air. The walls of your esophagus vibrate, making a low-pitched sound similar to a belch. You form this sound into words by using your tongue, teeth, lips and palate.

With training and much practice, some people become excellent esophageal speakers. Others are unable to produce the slightest sound because surgery or other procedures have changed the esophagus so that it can't vibrate.

Tracheoesophageal puncture and voice prosthesis

The most common method of vocal communication after laryngectomy is with a voice prosthesis. This device essentially provides a bridge between the trachea and the esophagus. Either at the time of the laryngectomy or later, your surgeon can make a small opening in the rear wall of your trachea and the front wall of your esophagus (tracheoesophageal puncture). After you heal, a speech pathologist places a small silicone tube (voice prosthesis) in the opening.

You produce voice by exhaling and placing your thumb or finger over your tracheal opening (tracheostoma). Air moves from your lungs, through the voice prosthesis and into your esophagus, which vibrates to produce voice. The prosthesis must be cleaned daily and replaced periodically.

A valve sometimes can be placed over the opening (stoma), allowing you to speak without using a thumb or finger. Not all people who have laryngectomies are candidates for this type of device.

Laryngeal transplantation

The first successful transplantation of a human larynx was done in 1998. Clinical trials are under way to determine if laryngeal transplantation is a feasible option to restore voice among otherwise healthy people who lost voice due to noncancerous (benign) conditions. More research is needed on people with cancer.

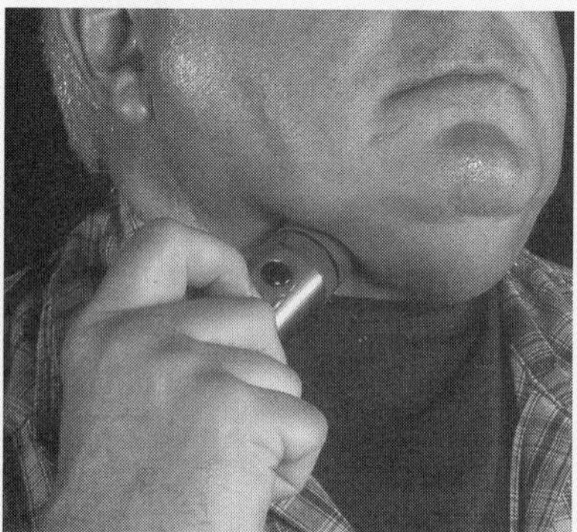

To talk, an artificial larynx is held against the neck. An artificial larynx is often used soon after laryngectomy surgery.

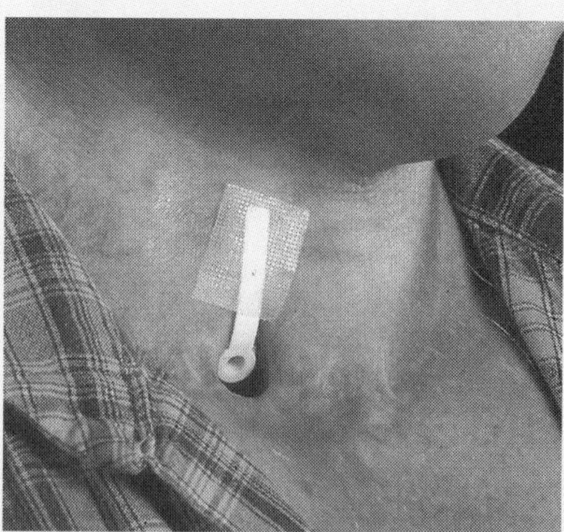

A voice prosthesis is positioned in an opening (stoma) in the neck. To speak, a person breathes in, covers the stoma with a finger, and then exhales and makes speech movements.

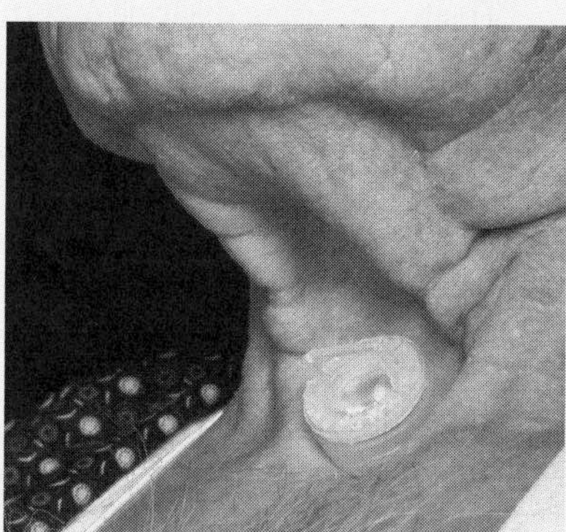

This type of voice prosthesis offers hands-free speaking following laryngectomy.

Structures of Your Larynx

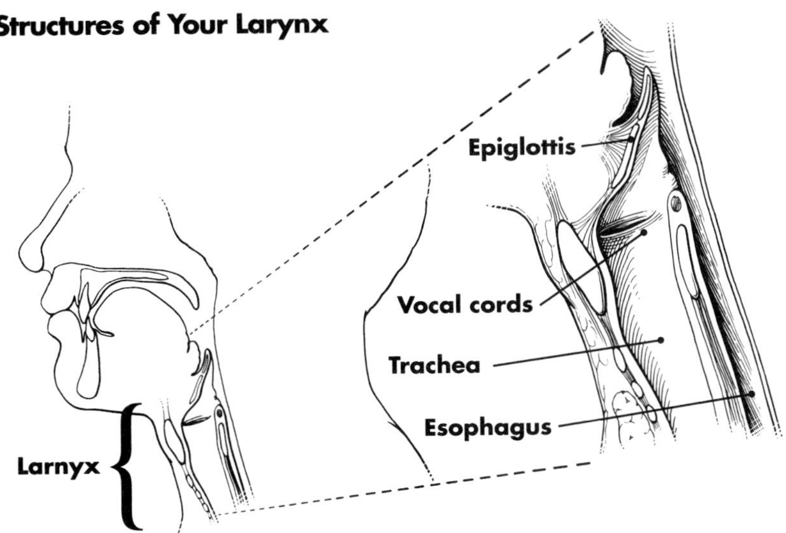

course of another illness such as an ordinary cold, flu or pneumonia.

Common causes of chronic laryngitis include constant irritation from excessive alcohol, heavy smoking or reflux of stomach acid into the esophagus and throat, a condition called gastroesophageal reflux disease (see page 850).

Irritations such as excessive talking or singing, allergies or the breathing in of irritating substances, such as tobacco smoke or chemicals, also can cause hoarseness and loss of your voice.

Diagnosis

The primary sign of laryngitis is hoarseness. Changes in voice can vary with the degree of infection or irritation, ranging from mild hoarseness to almost total loss of your voice. Your throat may tickle or feel raw, and you may have a frequent urge to clear your throat. If laryngitis persists for more than 5 to 7 days or you have additional symptoms, see your doctor.

How serious is laryngitis?

For most people, laryngitis is a temporary problem that either resolves itself or clears after treatment.

Treatment

Treatment depends on the type of laryngitis you experience. If you have bacterial laryngitis, your doctor may prescribe antibiotics. Signs and symptoms should disappear shortly after you take the drug.

For laryngitis caused by a virus or inhaled irritant, the best treatment is to rest your voice as much as possible, avoid clearing your throat and, if an inhaled irritant is to blame, avoid the irritant. It may also help to inhale steam from a bowl of hot water, teakettle or warm shower.

Drinking warm, noncaffeinated fluids helps keep your throat moist. A humidifier can help moisten the air, but if you use one, make sure you follow the manufacturer's instructions to clean the humidifier and prevent bacterial buildup.

To treat chronic laryngitis, you need to remove the underlying cause. If you smoke, stop. If alcohol consumption is responsible, you need to stop drinking.

Throat cancer

Signs and symptoms

- Hoarseness
- Difficulty swallowing due to pain
- Swelling in your neck

Most throat cancers occur as tumors on the vocal cords or in or around the voice box (larynx). Other forms of throat cancer can cause difficult and painful swallowing. They can also cause a large swelling in the neck.

If you smoke cigarettes, cigars or a pipe, or drink large quantities of alcohol, you're at greater risk of developing throat cancer. The combination of drinking and smoking poses an even greater risk.

Men are 10 times more likely than women to get throat cancer. The disease usually develops at around age 60.

Diagnosis

When hoarseness has no obvious cause and lasts more than 2 weeks, consult your doctor without delay. If swallowing is difficult or painful for several weeks or if you notice a swelling in your neck, see your doctor.

Your doctor may refer you to an ear, nose and throat specialist, who may conduct an examination called laryngoscopy. There are two kinds of laryngoscopies:

Indirect laryngoscopy

An indirect laryngoscopy involves looking at your throat using a mirror. This simple procedure can be done in your doctor's office. You're asked to open your mouth. Your tongue is pulled forward gently to help open your airway. A local anesthetic may be sprayed on the back of your throat and soft palate, particularly if you have a strong gag reflex. Your doctor then places the mirror toward the back of your throat. As you say ah and eee, your larynx will rise, and your doctor can view its interior, including the vocal cords, in the mirror. Most tumors or other abnormalities can be seen in the mirror.

Direct laryngoscopy

During direct laryngoscopy your doctor passes a small, flexible fiber-optic instrument through your nose to view your throat and voice box area. Surgical direct laryngoscopy is a more elaborate procedure that allows a more complete inspection of your larynx. It usually requires general anesthesia. During surgical direct laryngoscopy, a doctor inserts an instrument into your throat and often removes a tissue sample (biopsy) for laboratory analysis.

How serious is throat cancer?

Most cancers of the throat can be treated successfully if detected early. If symptoms are ignored, the cancer can spread to other parts of your throat and more widely.

Treatment

Throat cancer is treated in one of several ways. Radiation therapy may destroy the cancer, or the tumor may be removed surgically. A surgeon may be able to remove the tumor without removing your larynx. However, more advanced tumors may require complete removal of the larynx, a procedure known as a laryngectomy. Some advanced tumors may also be treated with radiation therapy, sometimes in combination with chemotherapy. You and your doctor will decide what is the most appropriate treatment.

If you require a laryngectomy, a prosthesis can help you speak, or you can work with a speech therapist to learn a new method of speaking. ■

CHAPTER 25 PART V

Teeth and Mouth

Few parts of your body play as many roles in everyday life as your oral cavity — your mouth and teeth. Many of the most important acts of self-expression, such as speaking, singing and simply smiling, utilize your teeth to shape the sounds you make and help form your appearance. Your mouth and teeth are also responsible for the first phase of the digestive process.

Your teeth may seem like only a minor health concern, but dental and oral disorders can disrupt many important aspects of your life.

Tooth Development

Most babies are born toothless, or so it appears. Actually, tooth development is well advanced by the third month of pregnancy, and by the fourth month enamel and dentin, the hard tissues of baby (primary) teeth, have begun to form.

The first teeth erupt in the mouth at about 6 months of age. The time when these first teeth emerge can vary greatly from child to child, but in most infants teeth have broken through the gums by age 1.

In general, the first teeth to emerge are the front teeth (incisors) in the lower jaw, followed by the front teeth in the upper jaw. Next come the first molars, followed by the canines (cuspids). The last to appear are the second molars. Most children have a full set of primary teeth by age 3 years.

Children have 20 primary teeth. Each primary tooth is normally replaced by a permanent tooth, incisor for incisor, canine for canine and premolar for molar. The permanent first molars erupt behind the primary molars.

For many children, the emergence of permanent teeth begins at about age 6. The lower front incisors tend to come in first, followed by the upper front incisors and first molars. Permanent premolars and canines emerge later.

The process of shedding primary teeth to be replaced by permanent teeth usually continues through the elementary school years. Around 14 years of age, 28 permanent teeth are usually in place. The last four molars, the wisdom teeth, usually emerge in early adulthood, to complete the permanent set of 32 teeth.

Your permanent teeth are divided equally between the top and bottom jaw. From the center of the mouth moving toward the back, they include 8 incisors (4 in each jaw), 4 canines (cuspids), 8 premolars and 12 molars.

Parts of a tooth

The basic structure of each tooth is essentially the same. At the center of the tooth lies the pulp chamber and pulp.

The pulp includes the nerves and blood vessels that feed and nourish the tooth. The nerves and blood vessels enter the tooth from the end of the roots.

The pulp is surrounded by hard dentin, the largest portion of the tooth. The dentin, composed of millions of tiny cells arranged in a tubular shape, is sensitive to temperature and touch.

The part of the tooth that's visible, the crown, extends from just beneath the gumline to the end of the tooth. It's covered with enamel, which is the hardest part of the tooth and protects the structures beneath. It has no sensation and can't heal after an injury.

The root, the part of the tooth below the gums (gingivae), is cov-

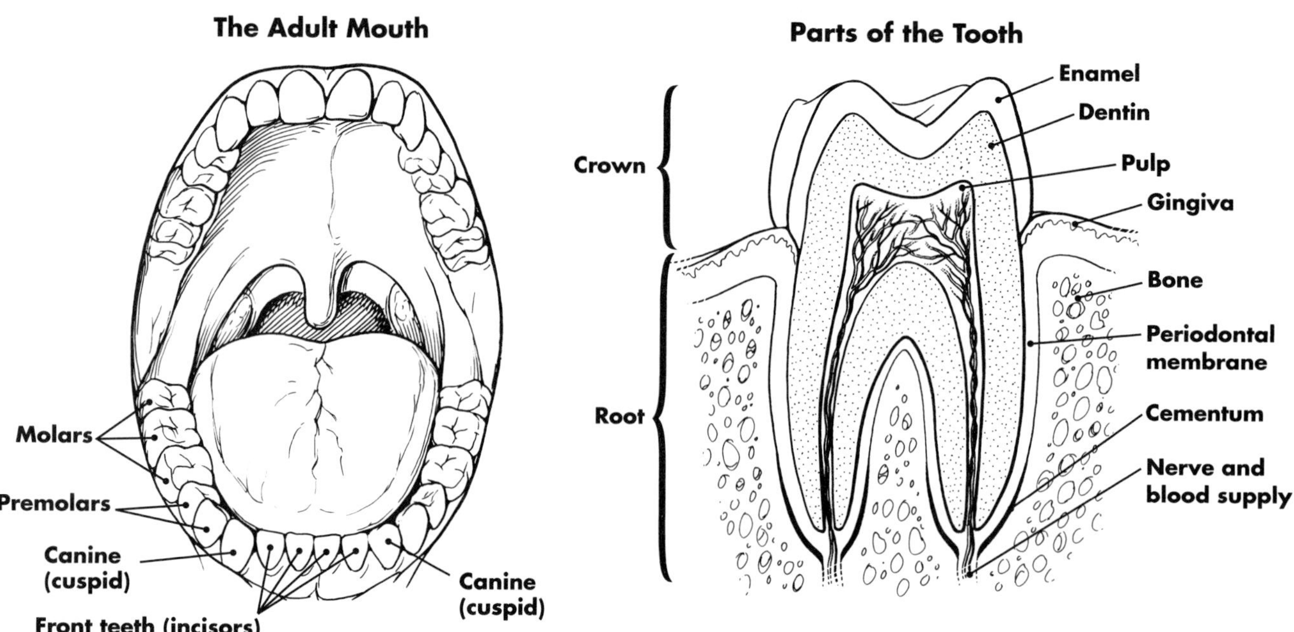

Soothing a Toothache

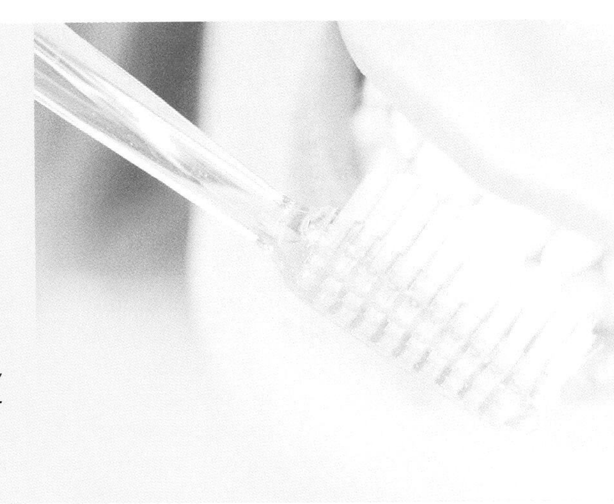

In most children and adults, tooth decay is the primary cause of toothaches. The first sign of decay may be a sensation of pain when you eat something sweet, cold or hot. Until you're able to see a dentist, try these self-care tips:

- Brush and floss to remove any food particles around and between the teeth. You may want to use warm water for brushing your teeth.
- Avoid foods and temperatures that trigger pain.
- Take an over-the-counter pain reliever such as acetaminophen (Tylenol, others), ibuprofen (Advil, Motrin, others) or aspirin. Or try an over-the-counter local anesthetic containing benzocaine (Anbesol, Orajel) or oil of cloves. These are available at most pharmacies.

ered with cementum, which is harder than bone but not as hard as enamel. This rigid connective tissue attaches to the periodontal ligament, which holds the tooth in its socket.

Tooth Decay

Tooth decay (caries) is a bacterial disease of teeth. It's one of the most common of all health disorders. Tooth decay affects children and young adults most frequently, although it remains a problem for many individuals throughout their life.

Decay is the primary cause of tooth loss. Almost half of all American children have some tooth decay by age 4, and many even earlier, despite great improvements in prevention through regular dental checkups, use of fluoride and improved oral hygiene (see Chapter 7, "Caring for Your Teeth").

Decades ago, few people still had their own teeth beyond middle age. Improved dental care and dentistry advances today make it possible for most people to keep their teeth much longer.

However, this has resulted in a new problem, called root caries. Root caries is the decay of a tooth's root. A lifelong program of appropriate dental care, preventive nutrition and good oral hygiene can help prevent root caries.

The decay process

Tooth decay is the result of three interacting factors: bacteria growth, dietary sugar and a vulnerable tooth surface.

Your mouth, like many other parts of your body, is host to bacteria. These bacteria convert some of the sugars and carbohydrates you eat into acid. The bacteria and acids they form become part of the sticky deposit — called dental plaque — that clings to the surface of teeth. In addition to bacteria, plaque is composed of saliva and food particles.

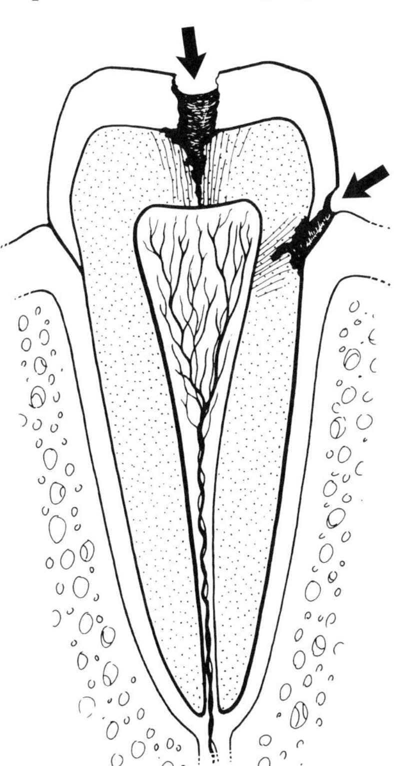

Dental cavities (see arrows) are a common cause of toothache and tooth loss.

You can feel the plaque when you pass your tongue over the surface of your teeth several hours after brushing. The texture is slightly rough and is particularly noticeable on the surfaces of back teeth. Plaque adheres most strongly in pits and grooves (fissures) of the molars and premolars, in the areas just above the gumline, between teeth and at the margins of fillings.

The decay-producing acid that forms in plaque attacks the minerals in the tooth's outer enamel surface. The erosion caused by the plaque leads to tiny openings (cavities) in the enamel, which you may not notice initially. The first sign of decay may be a sensation of pain when you eat something sweet, very cold or very hot.

Once the enamel is penetrated, the underlying softer dentin becomes vulnerable. The dentin contains tiny canals leading to the pulp at the core of the tooth.

If bacteria reach the sensitive pulp, the pulp becomes inflamed. Blood vessels within the pulp swell and, because there's no room within the rigid tooth to expand, you experience pain.

In addition, your body sends white blood cells to counteract bacterial invasion from the tooth into the surrounding tissues. This kind of bacterial infection may result in a tooth abscess.

Tooth decay takes time to develop, often 1 or 2 years in permanent teeth but less in primary teeth. The initial formation of acid occurs within the first 20 minutes after you eat. Fortunately, you're not totally vulnerable to the effects of acid and bacteria. The chemistry and the mechanics of your mouth provide a certain amount of protection: Your saliva and the actions of your tongue wash away some of the destructive material. Today's dentistry also can provide treatment and preventive measures to lessen the effects of dental cavities.

Cavities

Signs and symptoms

- Mild or sharp pain when eating or drinking something sweet, cold or hot
- Toothache

Most cavities are discovered during a dental examination. Detecting and treating tooth decay early can save pain, expense and, most importantly, your teeth. The sooner a cavity is detected, the less pain you'll experience because the outer parts of the tooth, the enamel and dentin, are far less sensitive to pain than is the pulp.

Diagnosis

Your dentist looks for signs of decay by using a dental explorer and a small mirror. Another way of detecting a cavity is with X-rays, which give the dentist information about the teeth and surrounding gums and bone.

Your dentist may find a cavity even if you haven't experienced symptoms. The early stages of tooth decay are often painless. Other times, you may experience mild pain in a tooth when eating something sweet, hot or cold. If you feel a sharp pain when eating such foods, you may have more serious tooth decay.

Treatment

Even if you have a seriously decayed tooth, it often can be saved through procedures such as dental fillings (restorations), crowns and root canals. Before such a procedure, a local anesthetic is typically injected into the nearby gum to deaden the nerve and prevent pain.

On occasion, some dentists offer nitrous oxide — sometimes called laughing gas — to decrease discomfort and anxiety. If you're taking any medications, mention this to your dentist before accepting any anesthetic because certain medications and anesthetics taken together can produce adverse reactions.

Fillings

The decay process usually can be halted by removing the decayed portion of the tooth and replacing it with a filling. Sometimes, when decay is extensive, a temporary filling is inserted to provide your dentist an opportunity to observe the tooth's response and sensitivity to treatment. After several weeks, if you've experienced no adverse signs or symptoms, your dentist removes this filling and replaces it with a permanent one.

The kind of filling used depends on the location and function of the tooth. Molars, which do most of the work of chewing, experience the most stress and require more durable materials than do front (anterior) teeth. If possible, a filling in a front tooth should blend in with the color of the tooth itself. This isn't as important with back teeth.

The most common restorative material is silver amalgam, which is used in back teeth. Such fillings are actually alloys of mercury, silver, copper and other metals. The addition of copper to the mixture makes the silver amalgam filling far more durable. Gold onlay, a more expensive restoration, is sometimes used in place of amalgam where more strength and support are necessary.

Fillings in front teeth need to be as invisible as possible. Silicate, a form of porcelain cement that resembles tooth enamel, was once the standard choice.

Now, composite resins are typically used in front teeth — and sometimes in back teeth if the decay is small and the area isn't used for heavy chewing. Composites, which can be tinted to match the color of your teeth, are made of plastic resin and a filler of finely ground glass-like particles.

Occasionally, gold foil is used as a restorative material for small cavities in front teeth. It's more expensive than white fillings but is more durable.

Crowns

If your tooth is so decayed that it can't support several small fillings or a large one without danger of breaking, your dentist may remove the decay and prepare the tooth to receive a crown over the tooth. The crown may be made of porcelain, metal or a combination of the two.

An impression of your tooth provides a model for the crown, which is made in a dental laboratory. The crown is then fitted, shaped and finally cemented in place on top of what's left of the original tooth.

Root canals

If you have a tooth that's severely infected or at risk of severe infection, your dentist or a dental specialist called an endodontist may

> **? Question and Answer**
>
> **Is a silver filling safe?**
>
> According to the American Dental Association, silver amalgam fillings are safe and haven't been linked to any medical disorder. In rare cases, a person may be allergic to the mercury used in amalgam fillings. Signs usually include a rash on the mouth and face, similar to other types of allergies. People who are allergic to amalgam often have a medical or family history of allergies to metals.

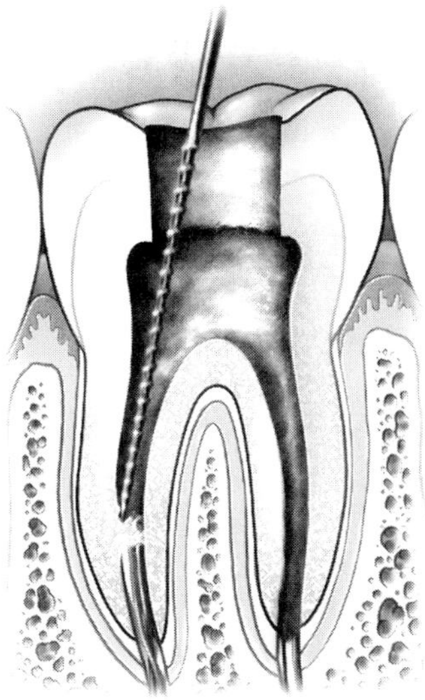
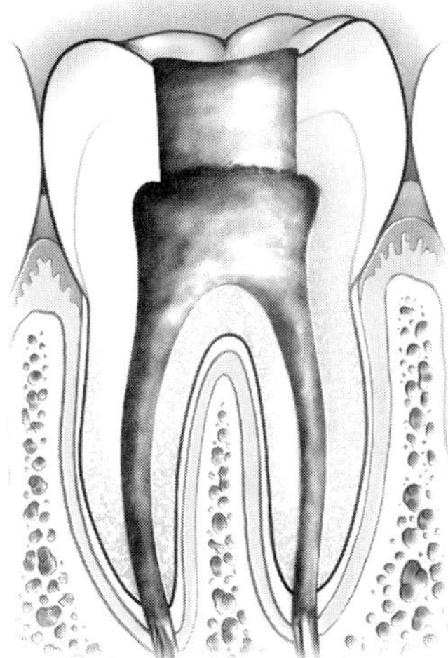
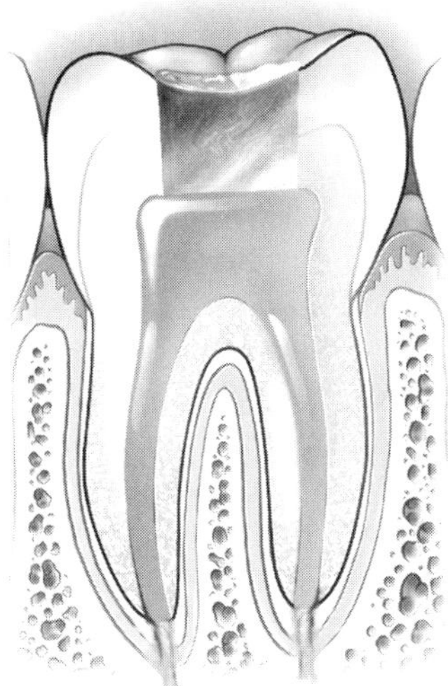

During a root canal, an opening is created into the pulp chamber (left), and the nerves and blood vessels are removed (center). The root canals are cleaned, enlarged, disinfected and filled (right).

perform a root canal. It involves removing the nerve and pulp, as well as any associated decayed material, from the root canal and pulp chamber.

In this multistage procedure, the pulp is removed and the opening that's created is disinfected and filled with an inert material (gutta-percha) and sealer. Once that's done, the remaining tooth structure is treated with a filling or crown.

Post and core procedures

Occasionally, when a tooth is fractured or severely damaged, it may need to be rebuilt into shape following a root canal. In this procedure, a post and core — a filling material — are cemented into the tooth before a crown is fitted.

Tooth abscesses

Signs and symptoms

- Persistent aching or throbbing pain in a tooth
- Sensitivity to sweet, hot or cold foods or liquids
- Pain when chewing
- Swollen lymph nodes in the neck
- A swollen area of the mouth, face or neck
- Fever and general malaise

If tooth decay isn't dealt with promptly and properly, it can lead to a tooth abscess. An abscess results when bacteria infect the pulp of a tooth, causing the pulp to become swollen and inflamed. Blood vessels in the pulp enlarge and may press on nerves in the area, producing pain.

The infection may spread to the root and into the surrounding bone and cause the tooth to loosen. Despite the body's efforts to fight it off, the infection can overwhelm the pulp, destroying the nerve and blood vessels. The pain may go away, but the infection may remain. The resulting breakdown material (pus) that forms as part of the infection can erode a channel through the jaw and form a swelling or boil on the gum.

Diagnosis

If you have persistent throbbing pain in a tooth, find chewing painful or are sensitive to sweet, hot or cold foods or liquids, you may have an abscessed tooth. You may have a slight fever and swollen lymph nodes in your neck and feel generally ill.

A swelling that forms on the gum near the sore tooth may at some point burst, releasing into your

Dental Specialists

Just as the medical field has various specialties, so does dentistry. General practitioner dentists may have special expertise in several areas, but for certain problems out of their area of expertise, you may elect to see or be referred to a specialist. These include the following:

- *Pediatric dentists.* Treat children from birth through adolescence
- *Orthodontists.* Diagnose and treat crowded and misaligned teeth and jaws
- *Endodontists.* Diagnose and treat diseases and injuries of the tooth pulp and surrounding tissues
- *Periodontists.* Diagnose and treat diseases of the tissues — gums and bone — that surround and support the teeth
- *Oral and maxillofacial surgeons.* Extract teeth and diagnose and treat injuries, diseases and defects of the jaw, face and mouth
- *Prosthodontists.* Create and fit artificial replacements for defective or missing teeth, including crowns, bridges (fixed partial dentures) and dentures

mouth a thick liquid with a foul taste and smell. Simultaneously, the pain may be relieved. If you experience any of these signs and symptoms, see your dentist.

Treatment

Before you see your dentist, you can help relieve the pain by taking acetaminophen (Tylenol, others), ibuprofen (Advil, Motrin, others) or aspirin. Rinsing your mouth with warm salt water — a half teaspoon of salt dissolved in an 8-ounce glass of warm water — every hour or so also may help soothe the pain.

Your dentist probably will prescribe an antibiotic to clear up the infection and keep it from spreading to other parts of your body. He or she can also prescribe pain relief medications to make you more comfortable.

At one time, the only treatment for an abscessed tooth was to remove (extract) it. Under certain conditions, extraction still is necessary. However, dentists today can often save an abscessed tooth by performing a root canal. Your dentist may anesthetize the area and then open a hole into the pulp chamber of the tooth. This releases the pressure. The pulp chamber can then be cleared out, disinfected and filled with an inert material.

Next, your dentist may place a temporary filling in your tooth. A permanent filling can be put in place after the infection has cleared. Your dentist most likely will want to see you again in a few months, at which time X-rays may be taken of the tooth to determine if gum and bone tissues are healing after the abscess.

If the tissues appear to be healthy, the treatment is finished. If the infection persists, additional treatment is necessary, and your dentist may refer you to a specialist who may perform a surgical procedure to remove the diseased tissue, sometimes including a small portion of the root tip.

If swelling persists after an abscessed tooth has been treated, your dentist may want to obtain special cultures or change your medication because of bacterial resistance or the presence of unusual bacteria.

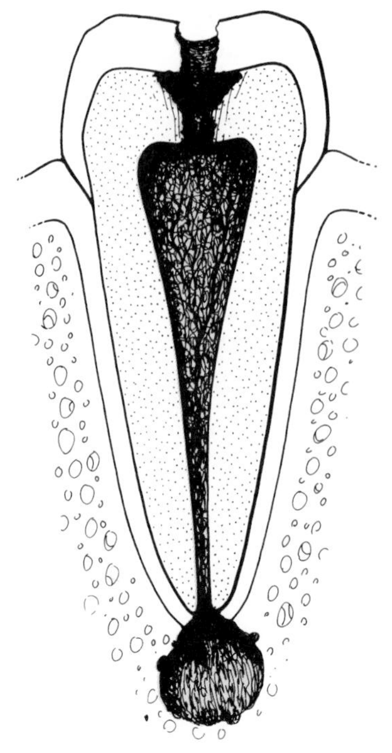

A tooth abscess occurs when bacteria enter through a decayed area and spread inward, infecting the pulp, root and even the bone surrounding the tooth.

Preventing tooth decay

A successful plan for preventing decay generally involves three steps: taking good care of your teeth, appropriately planning your diet and, in the case of children, applying fluoride and sealant to teeth.

Tooth care

Caring for your teeth includes brushing and flossing thoroughly on a daily basis and seeing your dentist regularly for checkups. In an ideal world, everyone would brush their teeth after all meals and snacks. A more realistic goal is to brush at least twice each day — in the morning and before going to bed — and floss at least once a day (see Chapter 7, "Caring for Your Teeth").

A key to developing lifelong good dental habits is to start early. Teach your children the ritual of brushing even before they have a full set of teeth. Similarly, your child's dentist or hygienist can demonstrate proper methods of flossing.

Diet

The concept that sugar contributes to tooth decay isn't new. But evidence points to all fermentable carbohydrates — not just sugar — as foods that cause tooth decay. Fermentable carbohydrates include all sugars and most cooked starches, including bread, crackers and potato chips.

Because carbohydrates are an important part of a healthy diet, don't cut down on them. And taking care of your teeth doesn't mean that you can't have ice cream, cake, pie or candy. The amount of sugar you eat is less important than how and when you eat it. Sweets eaten between meals do more harm than do those eaten with a meal.

Try to incorporate the following strategies into your eating habits and those of your children:

- *Avoid chewy, sticky, sugary foods, particularly as snacks.* Foods such as candy, candy-coated nuts, dry cereal, doughy bread, raisins and dry fruit cling to your teeth. When you do eat them, try to brush your teeth within 20 minutes afterward. Acid production by the bacteria that promote tooth decay is most active after this time. If you can't brush your teeth, rinse your mouth with water.
- *Choose snacks carefully.* Snacking on foods that promote tooth decay is worse than eating the same foods during meals. Nibbling on snacks throughout the day allows bacteria to produce a constant supply of acid on your teeth. Don't constantly sip sugar drinks, chew sugar gum or suck on hard candies, sugar-sweetened breath mints or cough drops.

If you do chew gum or suck on hard candies, select those that are sugarless. Sugarless products generally contain xylitol or aspartame, which can help reduce cavity-causing bacteria. Some also have a remineralizing agent that adds calcium and phosphates to teeth.

- *Don't give babies a bottle of milk or juice at bedtime.* Even babies are at risk of tooth decay, and milk and juice both contain sugar. If your baby needs a bottle to settle down, fill it with water. Don't allow your child to feed from a bottle while lying in bed because this can lead to blocked eustachian tubes and may increase your child's risk of ear infections.

Fluoride

People living in parts of the country where the public water supply naturally contains an optimal amount of fluoride have almost no dental cavities. Too high a fluoride content, however, can cause brown stains on the teeth.

Fluoride is especially helpful when it's ingested by children whose teeth are developing. The fluoride is incorporated into the enamel structure and offers continuing protection.

Many communities in the United States add small amounts of fluoride to their water supply because the water is deficient in fluoride. This approach is both cost-effective and safe.

There's no evidence that fluoride, whether added to water supplies or occurring naturally, is a health risk. If your municipal water supply isn't fluorinated or if you drink primarily bottled or filtered water, ask your dentist about supplemental fluoride rinses, pastes or tablets, which are available by prescription.

Children, teenagers and older adults are most susceptible to tooth decay. For these groups, topical application of fluoride, including fluoride toothpaste, is beneficial. Fluoride mouthwashes also can be useful. Many dentists also treat children's teeth with a fluoride solution as a part of regular checkups.

Fluoride is most effective in preventing cavities on the smooth, nonchewing surfaces of your teeth. Consequently, most cavities occur on the chewing surfaces. The reason: These surfaces of your back (posterior) teeth (premolars and molars) have pits and grooves (depressions and fissures) that are almost impossible to clean completely with a toothbrush.

Sealants

Besides good oral hygiene, the single best method to prevent decay on the chewing surfaces of back teeth is a dental sealant. The sealant covers the tooth surface with a thin, plastic-like coating that's usually clear or white.

Application of a sealant is painless and easy. First, your dentist cleans the chewing surface of your premolars and molars. Then these surfaces are etched with a mild acid to improve adhesion.

Next, the teeth are thoroughly washed and dried. Then your dentist paints the sealant onto each tooth in much the same way fingernail polish is applied. The sealant hardens into a shield that prevents accumulation of plaque in the pits and fissures.

A dental sealant can last up to 10 years, although various conditions may shorten its effectiveness. Regular visits to the dentist permit necessary touch ups to extend the life of the sealant.

If the sealant layer is lost, it can be replaced. If the sealant is damaged, the underlying tooth surface is at no greater risk of cavities than it would be if the sealant had never been applied.

Sealant protection is most appropriate for children. It should be applied when the first permanent molars erupt, at about age 6, and again when permanent second molars and premolars erupt, usually between ages 11 and 13. Older adults also may benefit from a dental sealant.

Developmental Disorders

In many people, teeth develop in a fairly orderly and normal manner. However, problems may occur due to improper prenatal development or environmental or genetic factors.

Fortunately, modern dentistry and oral surgery can often minimize the effects of the developmental disorders.

Impacted teeth

Signs and symptoms

- Pain in the gums
- Recurrent infection of a partially buried tooth
- Bad breath
- An unpleasant taste in your mouth

Teeth typically emerge through the gums at three times during life. The first time is when the baby (primary) teeth emerge. The second is when permanent teeth emerge during early school years. The third time is when the last teeth, the wisdom teeth (third molars) appear. This is generally during early adulthood.

Frequently, wisdom teeth have trouble emerging because the jaw is often too small. They may become rotated, displaced or tilted as they attempt to emerge. This can cause pain and occasionally infection when the tooth traps food debris in the soft gum tissue surrounding it. If the tooth comes in at an angle, it can push on and damage the adjacent tooth, causing pain and possibly shifting the bite.

Diagnosis

Impacted teeth don't always cause discomfort. But when they do, the experience is unpleasant. If you feel pain in your gums or have an unpleasant taste when you bite on or near where a wisdom or other unemerged tooth should be, you may have an impacted tooth.

The tooth may be partly visible, and the surrounding gums may be

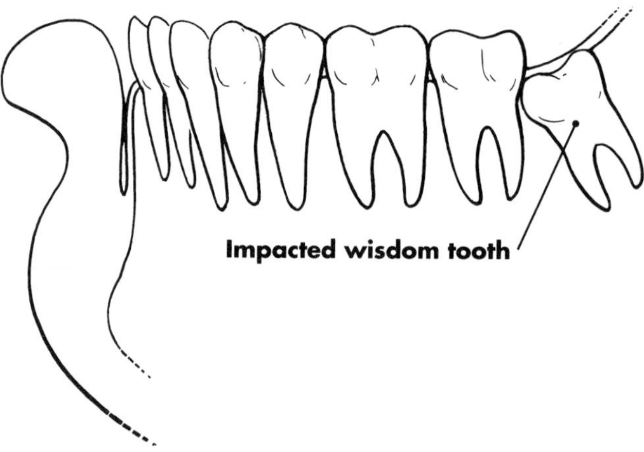

A tooth that doesn't emerge through the gum is called an impacted tooth. This most often occurs with the wisdom teeth at the back of the mouth.

infected. The impacted tooth may press on other teeth, causing pain.

Treatment

Over-the-counter pain relievers such as acetaminophen (Tylenol, others), ibuprofen (Advil, Motrin, others) or aspirin should help relive the pain from an impacted tooth. Rinsing your mouth with warm salt water — a mixture of a half teaspoon of salt and 8 ounces of warm water — also may help.

Your dentist can examine your mouth for signs of an impacted tooth. X-rays may be needed to determine the exact location and position of the tooth. If you have an infection around the tooth (pericoronitis) your dentist may prescribe an antibiotic.

The usual treatment for an impacted wisdom tooth is its removal. Wisdom teeth that emerge crooked can compromise your bite. Wisdom teeth are difficult to clean because they're far back in the mouth. This makes them prone to decay and gum disease.

Your dentist may remove the impacted tooth or teeth in the office under local anesthesia. If your case is more complicated, your dentist may refer you to an oral and maxillofacial surgeon. If an impacted tooth lies at a difficult angle or you have several of them, the procedure may be done in a hospital.

Misshapen or discolored teeth

Signs and symptoms

- Misshapen teeth
- Yellowish color on primary or secondary teeth

In rare cases, a child's teeth may not be normal in shape or color. Such abnormalities can result from many factors, including genetics, early illness or trauma or an environmental factor such as excessive fluoride in the drinking water or the mother's ingestion of tetracycline drugs during pregnancy and nursing. Enamel is completely formed on all but the wisdom teeth by about 8 years of age. Therefore, doctors don't prescribe a prolonged course of the antibiotic tetracycline for children under age 8 or pregnant women.

Other causes of misshapen or discolored teeth include infection, high fever or malnutrition during infancy or early childhood. In rare cases, misshapen teeth are related to serious disorders such as congenital syphilis or Down syndrome.

Most often, abnormalities affect both the primary and secondary teeth. The eight front teeth and the 6-year molars are the teeth most frequently affected because these develop first. The crowns of the teeth can be pitted or grooved and may be discolored.

Occasionally, the enamel covering the teeth will be imperfect. Although this can result from several factors, most often it's the result of a genetic trait that recurs in families. The enamel may be discolored, thin or even absent. Discoloration can also stem from drinking water with a fluoride content of more than 2 parts per million. In some areas, water naturally contains a high level of fluoride.

Treatment

Misshapen teeth often can be treated by adding a restorative material or by covering them with crowns. Teeth without a complete covering of enamel and some very discolored teeth also may be treated in this manner.

Sometimes this is done on primary teeth if the enamel is so malformed that serious cavities or wearing occurs. In these instances, the molar teeth often are fitted with stainless steel crowns.

Misaligned or crowded teeth

Signs and symptoms

- Lack of spacing between teeth
- Protruding (overt) upper front teeth (overbite)
- Upper and lower front (incisor) teeth that don't touch when biting (open bite)
- Upper teeth, either back or front, that bite inside the lower teeth (crossbite)
- A protruding lower jaw that causes the upper front teeth to bite behind the lower front teeth (underbite)

Few people have a perfect bite and symmetrical teeth. Your jaws may be slightly misaligned, perhaps where the upper and lower teeth clamp together to form the bite. Or your teeth may be crowded, sometimes in the front where they're most visible. The technical term for such problems is *malocclusion* (bad bite).

A minor amount of misalignment or crowding may require little or no attention. But a significant number of children and adults have problems that can benefit from treatment. The branch of dentistry that specializes in the diagnosis, prevention and treatment of dental and facial irregularities is called orthodontics. Orthodontists use appliances, such as braces, to properly align the teeth and jaws and produce an even bite.

In the ideal bite, the teeth of the upper jaw slightly overlap those of the lower jaw. The points of the molars fit into the grooves of the opposing molars. In the ideal jaw, there's room for all teeth to fit neatly, neither crowded nor spaced. There are no rotations of teeth or teeth that twist or lean forward or backward.

Straightening your teeth is important not just for the sake of appearance. When teeth don't fit together properly, they can cause chewing problems and eating and digestion difficulties. Crowded or crooked teeth make it more difficult to control plaque, which leaves you prone to cavities and periodontal disease.

Now more adults are seeking orthodontic correction of problems that weren't treated when they were younger (see page 706). Although the treatment time often is longer in adults because tooth movement is slower, the results are usually good. More corrective jaw surgery is performed on adults than on children.

Diagnosis

Dentists monitor the development of children's secondary teeth and recommend consultation with an orthodontist if problems seem imminent. Most alignment problems become apparent once the secondary teeth begin to erupt, often as early as age 6. In some instances, problems can be identified and appropriately treated even earlier.

Although teeth can be moved at any time, the American Association of Orthodontists recommends that children be screened by age 7. Some orthodontic problems are more easily corrected at a young age, before all the permanent teeth come in and before facial growth is complete.

Your orthodontist will examine your or your child's mouth thoroughly to help determine the best treatment. He or she may take a series of X-rays, some of which are used to determine the position of teeth — those that have erupted and those yet to erupt. Special X-rays of the head may help determine the size, position and relationship of the jaw and teeth.

Another diagnostic tool is a plaster model of the teeth. The dentist may ask you to bite down on a thin, wax-like material to make an impression. This impression is then used to position plaster models accurately to represent the actual bite of the upper and lower teeth.

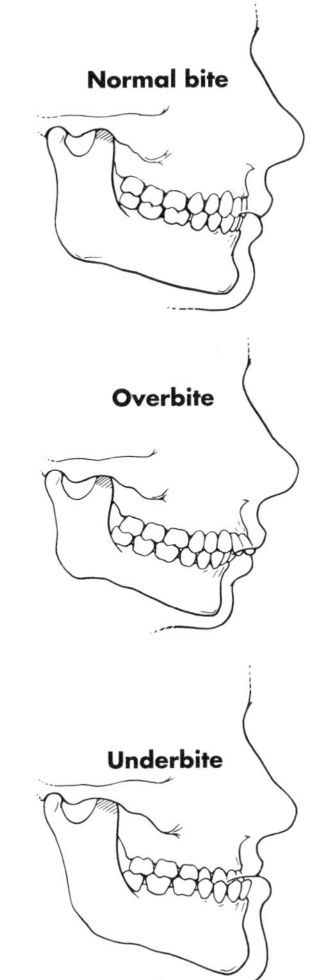

Photographs of the teeth and face and other measurements and recordings also may be needed to make an accurate diagnosis.

If the lower jaw is significantly smaller than the upper jaw, the upper teeth may protrude excessively over the lower (overbite). Similarly, if the lower jaw is larger than the upper, the upper front teeth may bite behind the lower ones (underbite).

When significant discrepancies exist between the upper and lower jaws, an operation called orthognathic surgery may be the best option. However, these problems often can be corrected with various appliances.

Treatment

Following a thorough examination, an orthodontist develops a treatment plan and designs corrective devices. Some devices are removable, and others are cemented or bonded to the teeth.

Braces

If severe overcrowding is the main problem, certain permanent teeth, usually premolars, can be extracted to create room, and the remaining teeth can then be realigned by fitting braces to them.

Fixed braces, which can be made of metal, ceramic or plastic, usually are either ring-like bands that encircle the molar teeth or brackets that are attached to the outside surfaces of the premolar and anterior teeth. Clear or tooth-colored braces are sometimes an option.

Wires, springs and other force-producing devices place pressure on the teeth and gradually shift them into new positions. The jaw responds to the pressure by dissolving bone in front of the moving tooth and laying down new bone behind it.

Occasionally, tension will be drawn from the opposite jaw. This usually is achieved with elastic bands placed on upper and lower teeth and connected to an opposite tooth.

Adult Orthodontics: It's Never Too Late

As many as 75 percent of adults have some misalignment in their teeth and could benefit from braces. Yet only about 15 percent to 20 percent of these adults seek orthodontic treatment. Many adults believe they're too old for braces, fear discomfort, think they'll be embarrassed or think they can't afford orthodontics.

Why get braces? Crowded or crooked teeth make it more difficult to control plaque, which leaves you prone to cavities and periodontal disease. If you need restorative work, such as crowns or bridges, having your teeth aligned can make these procedures easier.

Many adults get braces for cosmetic reasons. Aligned teeth look nicer than misaligned teeth. In addition, as you age your facial muscles normally become less taut, and your upper lip may sag. Skin may appear more taut after moving the teeth forward.

If you think you might benefit from braces, either because your teeth have shifted since you last wore braces or because you never had them, fear not. Braces aren't what they used to be. With advances in orthodontic materials, most adults' fears of wearing braces are unfounded. Here's why:

- Today's wires, made of nickel and titanium, don't need to be tightened as often as those used years ago did. Most adults report only mild discomfort for a day or two after each adjustment.
- Ceramic brackets that match your tooth enamel are less obvious than metal brackets. Even metal brackets are smaller and less noticeable than they used to be. Note, however, that ceramic brackets cost more and may result in longer treatment time.
- There's growing acceptance of adult orthodontics.
- The cost of treatment may be covered by insurance.

Other appliances

In growing children and teenagers, several other appliances can be used to direct forces that influence jaw growth and development. For example, headgear that directs pressure to the upper teeth and jaw may be used to influence the speed and direction of upper jaw growth. The appliance is attached to braces in the mouth, and pressure is applied with a strap that wraps around the head. The headgear is usually worn 10 to 12 hours each day, typically during the night.

A Herbst appliance is a device that can't be removed for the duration of the treatment. It's usually attached to the upper and lower molars. It holds the lower jaw forward to help correct severe overbite. A palatal expansion appliance is used when the upper teeth don't fit properly with the lower teeth. The appliance is fixed to the upper back teeth to widen the upper jaw.

Duration of treatment with braces and other appliances ranges from approximately 6 months to 3 years. The time varies depending on the growth of the face and mouth, the level of cooperation from the person wearing the braces and the severity of the problem.

Retainers

After braces are removed, treatment often isn't over. The teeth must be stabilized for months, years or sometimes indefinitely to prevent them from shifting. To accomplish this, the teeth are usually fitted with a retainer. Examples of retainers include:

- *Positioners.* These are rubber-like mouthpieces that you wear at night and bite into for a few hours during the day.
- *Removable retainers.* These are made of plastic material on the inside of the teeth and wires on the outside of the teeth.
- *Removable, clear plastic retainers.* These devices completely cover the sides and biting surfaces of the teeth.
- *Semirigid wires.* These devices most often are fitted to and bonded on the inside of the front teeth.

Corrective surgery

In extreme cases, when conventional orthodontic treatment isn't sufficient to correct a problem, your dentist may recommend corrective surgery. This is more common in adults than in children.

Protrusion of the upper or lower jaw can be corrected by removing a section of bone and setting the remainder in its correct position. Conversely, short jaws can be lengthened, or the height of the lower face can be shortened or lengthened to provide better facial aesthetics and function. Surgery can

PREVENTION TIP

Take special care to clean your teeth regularly during the course of orthodontic treatment. Food and plaque can accumulate around orthodontic appliances. If you don't remove these deposits, demineralization occurs and may leave permanent whitish marks (scars) or cavities on your teeth. Brush with a fluoride toothpaste and rinse with a fluoride mouthwash as recommended by your dentist. Although somewhat more difficult to do, flossing also is recommended.

be done to adjust misaligned bites that don't respond fully to orthodontic treatment alone. Surgery may also shorten the overall duration of orthodontic treatment.

Corrective surgery usually is performed under general anesthesia and requires hospitalization. It has a relatively short recuperation period. The jaws may be wired together for a few days to a few weeks during the initial healing to curtail movement of the jaws.

Gum Disease

You may have heard the adage, "To keep your teeth, take care of your gums." It's good advice. Gum (periodontal) disease is a major cause of tooth loss in adults. Most people experience periodontal disease in some form over the course of their life, but they don't necessarily lose teeth.

The tissue in which the disease occurs is called the periodontium. This includes the gums (gingivae), the periodontal ligament and the tooth sockets (alveolar bone). These structures support your teeth.

Gum disease results from a combination of factors involving bacterial plaque — the sticky substance found in everyone's mouth — and its long-term effects on the periodontium. It can take several forms, but the result is weakened tooth support. The two most common forms of gum disease are gingivitis, an inflammation of the gums, and periodontitis, which is a more advanced form with tissue destruction.

Gingivitis

Signs and symptoms

- Swollen, soft, red gums
- Gums that bleed easily, especially when brushing your teeth
- A change in gum color from pink to dusky red

The term *gingivitis* refers to inflammation of the gingivae, the part of your gums around the base of your teeth. The cause is plaque, a sticky, colorless film of bacteria that coats your teeth. If allowed to harden (become calcified), plaque turns into white-colored tartar (calculus) that darkens with time. Plaque and tartar buildup can irritate the gingivae. The buildup creates pockets of bacteria between your gums and teeth, which can cause your gums to inflame and bleed easily.

Risk factors

Many people first experience gingivitis during puberty and then at various degrees of severity throughout life. Mild forms of the disease are common among adults. The most common contributing factor is a long-term lack of attention to proper oral hygiene, but other factors can increase your risk (see page 709).

Diagnosis

Healthy gums are firm and pale pink. If you notice that your gums are swollen, very tender, bleed easily and are dusky red, you may have gingivitis.

Often, people first detect a change in their gums when they notice that the bristles of their toothbrush are pink after brushing, a sign that their gums are bleeding even with the gentle pressure of the bristles.

If you have signs and symptoms of gingivitis, consult your dentist. The key to determining the health of your gums is to measure the depth of the groove between your gums and your teeth — the gingival sulcus.

To do this, your dentist inserts a metal probe beneath your gum until it meets a slight resistance. A depth of 2 or 3 millimeters (mm) — about $\frac{1}{8}$ inch — indicates a healthy gum. A depth beyond 3 mm means a pocket has formed between your tooth and gum. The deeper the pocket, the more serious your gum disease. Dental X-rays also may help your dentist gauge the status

Complications of Gum Disease

Advanced gum disease (periodontitis) does more than just damage your gums. It also puts you at greater risk of:

- *Heart disease and stroke.* Research suggests a link between oral bacteria and clogged arteries and blood clots, which can lead to heart attack and stroke. Some evidence shows that people with gum disease are more likely to have a heart attack or stroke than are those with healthy mouths. The more severe the gum disease, the greater the risk.
- *Uncontrolled blood sugar.* Diabetes puts you at greater risk of developing gum disease, as well as other infections. In turn, oral infection makes blood sugar (glucose) levels harder to control.
- *Pneumonia.* If you have serious gum disease and lung problems, inhaling bacteria from your mouth into your lungs may result in pneumonia.
- *Osteoporosis.* Researchers suspect a link between the loss of bone mineral density from osteoporosis and an increased susceptibility to oral bacteria. If osteoporosis also causes the bones of your mouth to lose density, that may increase your risk of gum disease and tooth loss. Sometimes, gum disease or tooth loss may be an indication of osteoporosis.
- *Adverse pregnancy outcomes.* New research suggests that women who have gum disease during pregnancy are at increased risk of giving birth to low-weight, preterm babies.

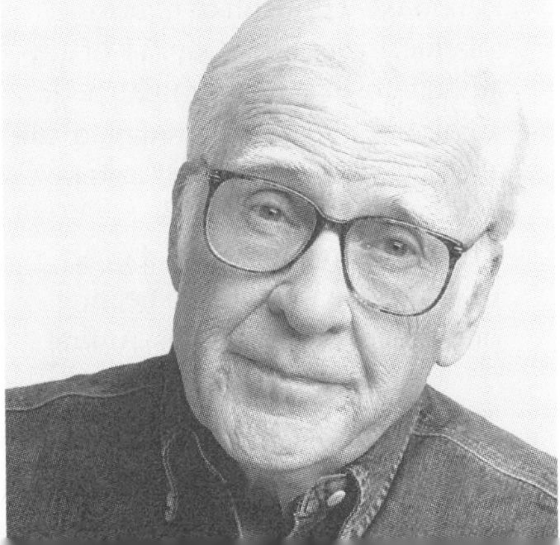

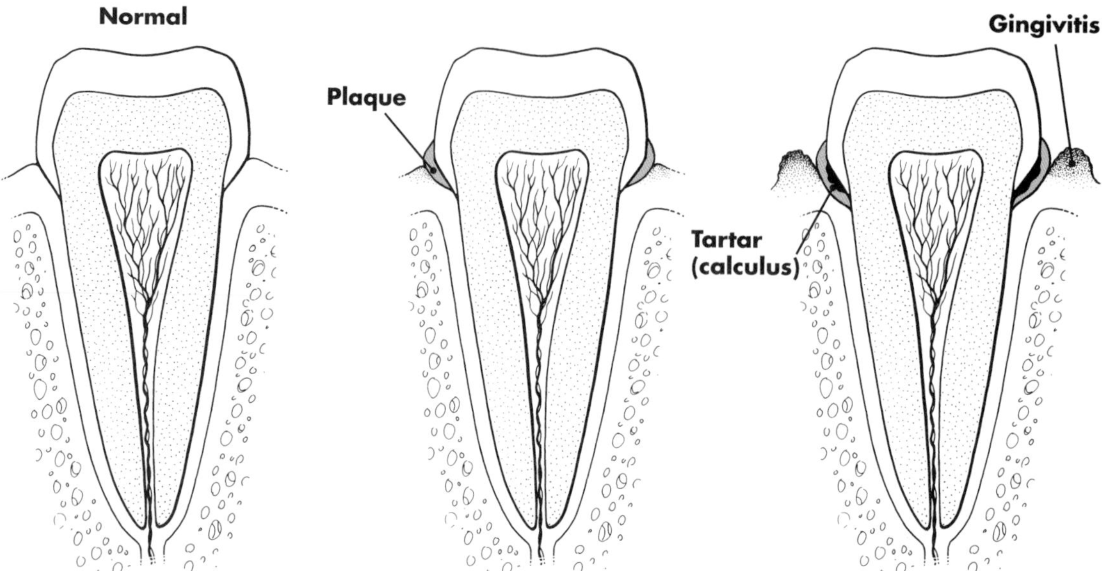

If plaque accumulates on a normal tooth and isn't removed promptly, it can harden into a mineral deposit called tartar (calculus). Gradually, the adjacent gums become inflamed and swollen, a disorder known as gingivitis.

of your gums by revealing bone loss associated with periodontitis.

How serious is gingivitis?

Gingivitis often is painless and goes unnoticed. If left unchecked, however, gingivitis can lead to periodontitis, a more serious disease that also affects other supporting structures of the teeth and leads to tooth loss.

Treatment

Your dentist may treat your gingivitis by using several techniques. The first step is to thoroughly clean your teeth, including removal of all plaque and tartar. This cleaning can be uncomfortable, particularly if your gums are sensitive or if your teeth are encrusted with plaque and tartar. The removal procedure is known as scaling.

Misaligned teeth, overhanging fillings or poorly contoured restorations such as crowns and bridges can make it difficult to remove plaque, increasing your risk of gingivitis. Teeth can be straightened to minimize plaque accumulation, fillings can be replaced, and restorations can be recontoured.

A long-term program of good oral hygiene is critical to treating and preventing gingivitis. At first your gums may bleed after brushing. This should last only a couple of days. Soon your gums should be pink and firm, a sign of their improved health. The program must be followed indefinitely for your gums to remain healthy.

Prevention

If you take good care of your teeth with thorough daily brushing, regular flossing and frequent professional cleaning, your chances of developing serious gingivitis are greatly decreased (see Chapter 7, "Caring for Your Teeth").

Periodontitis

Signs and symptoms

- Swollen or receding gums
- Bleeding gums
- An unpleasant taste in the mouth
- Bad breath
- Pain in a tooth when eating hot, cold or sweet foods
- Loose teeth
- A change in your bite
- Drainage of pus around one or more teeth

Periodontitis is an advanced stage of gum disease. Plaque-filled pockets form between your teeth and gums, and the gums become inflamed, enlarging the pockets and trapping increasing amounts of plaque. When plaque and tartar extend beneath your gumline, you may develop periodontitis. Gradually, your gums withdraw from around your teeth.

Pockets of infectious material (pus) can form in this dark, airless region and destroy tissue and your tooth sockets (alveolar bone). Left untreated, involved teeth eventually loosen and may fall out.

Periodontitis is usually painless. In some cases, however, an acute infection develops, causing an abscess in one or more of the pockets. This produces pain and erodes bone even more quickly than the chronic condition does. Generally speaking, the younger a person is when such bone loss begins, the less chance there is of saving the tooth.

Risk factors

Your greatest risk of periodontal disease comes from poor oral hygiene, but other factors increase your risk. People who smoke are more likely to develop periodontitis. They tend to have the problem more severely and respond poorly to treatment. People who grind their teeth also may have more periodontal problems.

Are You at Risk?

Everyone is susceptible to gum disease, but the most common contributing factor is long-term lack of attention to good oral hygiene. Other factors also can increase your risk:

- *Genetics.* Bacteria that lead to gingivitis are more harmful to some people's gums than to others. Those who are susceptible inherit a predisposition to gum disease.
- *Medications.* Some medications decrease the amount of saliva in your mouth, causing a dry mouth. Without the normal cleansing effect of saliva, plaque and tartar can more easily build up. Many antidepressants and cold remedies contain ingredients that decrease the production of saliva. Alcohol has a similar effect.
- *Smoking.* Smoking reduces your gums' ability to heal by inhibiting the replacement of tissues destroyed by bacteria.
- *Diabetes.* People with uncontrolled or poorly controlled diabetes are more susceptible to gum disease. Diabetes may cause a thickening of your small blood vessels, making them less able to carry nutrients to your gum tissue and remove wastes. This can leave your gums less healthy and more prone to infection.
- *Pregnancy.* Hormone changes during pregnancy make your gums more susceptible to the damaging effects of plaque.
- *Decreased immunity.* Some illnesses can impair your immune system and make you prone to infection, including gum disease.

Diagnosis

If you experience signs and symptoms of periodontitis, see your dentist. The sooner you do so, the better your chance of healing your gums and preventing loss of teeth.

To determine the health of your gums, your dentist may measure the depth of the groove between your gums and your teeth (gingival sulcus). The deeper the pocket, the more serious your gum disease. Dental X-rays also may help your dentist gauge the health of your gums by revealing bone loss.

In addition, your dentist may ask a series of questions to determine if a systemic disorder such as diabetes may be contributing to your condition.

Treatment

If you have pockets between your gums and your teeth that are 5 millimeters (mm) or less in depth, your dentist may recommend one of the following treatments:

Scaling and root planing

Scaling removes tartar and bacteria from your tooth surfaces and beneath your gums. Sometimes, scaling is done with an ultrasonic device. Root planing smoothes the root surfaces, reducing further accumulation of tartar. If followed by good daily oral hygiene, scaling and root planing may be all the treatment you'll need.

Antibiotics

Dentists can pinpoint the specific strains of bacteria that cause periodontal disease and prescribe antibiotics to deal with them.

Surgery

You may need surgery if you have advanced periodontitis — the depth of the pockets between your gums and teeth exceeds 5 mm. Options include:

- *Flap surgery.* If you have a deep pocket, your dentist can fold up a section of your gum surgically, exposing the roots for more effective scaling and planing. Antibiotics may help control infection.
- *Bone grafting.* If the bone surrounding your tooth root is destroyed, your dentist can obtain sterilized bone segments from a bone bank or synthetic bone grafts to fill the space and keep your tooth in place.
- *Guided tissue regeneration.* This technique allows bone previously destroyed by bacteria to regrow. Your dentist places a special piece of biocompatible fabric between existing bone and your tooth. This material prevents unwanted tissue from entering the healing area. It also stimulates bone to grow back. Sometimes, a bone graft is used in conjunction with the fabric.
- *Gingivectomy.* This procedure involves surgically removing gum (gingival) tissue to decrease the depth of the pockets. After the procedure, the gumline is covered with a protective putty-like packing that serves as a

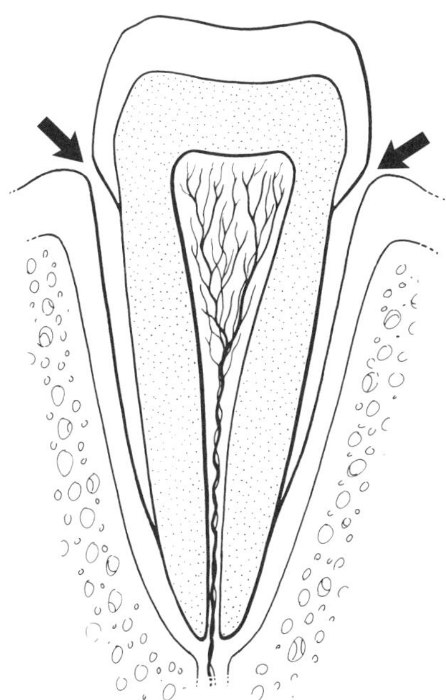

Left untreated, inflammation of the gums (gingivitis) can result in periodontitis, in which an inflamed gum gradually withdraws from the tooth, forming pockets (see arrows). As support for the tooth decreases, it loosens and may eventually fall out.

bandage. The dressing allows normal eating and drinking. Gingivoplasty, a surgical procedure to reshape gum tissue, also may be used. Although gingivectomy procedures were initially developed to treat periodontitis, today they're used more often for cosmetic surgery, such as when medications cause an overgrowth of the gums.

Orthodontics

If your teeth are misaligned and crowded, plaque accumulation is harder to remove. Orthodontic treatment can correct the positions of your teeth. Uneven biting and chewing surfaces can be recontoured to decrease pressure. If you grind your teeth during sleep (bruxism), you can be fitted with a device to protect your teeth from excessive pressure and damage.

Trench mouth

Signs and symptoms

- Profuse bleeding from and pain in the gums after slight pressure
- A grayish film on the gums

Trench mouth, also known as acute necrotizing ulcerative gingivitis or Vincent's gingivitis, is a painful form of gingivitis. It usually affects young adults and can range from mild to severe.

The condition received its name because during World War I it occurred in soldiers who were fighting in trenches under conditions of stress, poor hygiene and poor nutrition.

Trench mouth is characterized by profuse bleeding at the slightest pressure or irritation. The infection is caused by bacteria that normally inhabit your mouth. It's not passed from one person to another.

Onset of this disease is often sudden. The points of gum tissue between teeth (papillae) are usually damaged, leaving craters that collect plaque and food debris. The area is covered with a grayish layer of decomposing gum tissue. The inflammation and infection may involve other parts of the mouth.

Diagnosis

If you have gum pain and profuse bleeding after slight irritation or pressure on the gums, contact your dentist immediately.

Treatment

Good oral hygiene is crucial to cure the infection. This includes professional cleaning and proper brushing and flossing of your teeth, preferably after each meal and at bedtime.

Your dentist may begin by gently and thoroughly cleaning your teeth and gums. Irrigation of the mouth with salt or peroxide solution often helps to relieve symptoms. Your dentist may recommend a nonprescription pain reliever to lessen discomfort. You'll also be advised to get plenty of rest, eat a balanced diet and avoid irritation from smoking or eating spicy foods. Antibiotics may be prescribed if you have a high fever.

Preventing gum disease

As previously noted, gum disease is due in large part to poor dental hygiene. Inadequate care of your teeth allows plaque and tartar to form and anchor to your teeth.

Dental Care and Diabetes

If you have diabetes, you're at higher risk of gum disease and infections. Although plaque is the main cause of gum disease, diabetes may make things worse by decreasing your mouth's germ-fighting ability. Poor blood sugar control makes gum problems even more likely. The good news is that with proper care, your teeth can last a lifetime.

How often you need to see a dentist depends on many factors — your health, the types of medications you may take and the condition of your teeth and gums. Some people with diabetes should see a dentist every 3 months, but others may only need a yearly checkup. Talk to your dentist about what's appropriate for you.

See your dentist if you:

- Experience dry mouth, eating difficulty or tooth or mouth pain
- Haven't had a dental checkup for over a year
- Notice lesions, sores or lumps in your mouth

When you schedule your visit to a dentist, the American Diabetes Association recommends that you:

- Tell your dentist that you have diabetes, and talk to him or her about any problems you have with infections or controlling your blood sugar.
- Eat before you see your dentist. The best time for dental work is when your blood sugar is within a normal range and the action of your diabetes medication is low. For example, if you take insulin, a morning visit after a normal breakfast is best.
- Take your usual medications before your dental visit, unless your dentist or doctor tells you to change your dose before dental surgery. Your dentist may consult with your doctor about whether you need to adjust your diabetes medications or if you need an antibiotic before dental surgery to prevent infection.
- Wait to have dental surgery until your blood sugar is under control. If your dental needs are urgent and your blood sugar is poorly controlled, talk to your dentist and doctor about having dental procedures in a hospital or other setting where medical professionals can check on you during and after surgery.

Thorough brushing and flossing are your best defenses.

Brushing and flossing

Follow these tips to keep your gums healthy:

- *Pick the right toothbrush.* Select one with soft, rounded-end or polished bristles that's small enough to allow you to reach your back teeth as well as your front teeth. Replace your brush every 3 to 4 months, or sooner if the bristles become bent.
- *Use fluoride toothpaste.* Fluoride toothpaste helps remove plaque and protects against cavities.
- *Brush at least twice daily.* This should include just before bedtime and again each morning. During sleep, saliva flow lessens and allows bacteria to multiply.
- *Brush properly.* To clean the outer surfaces of your teeth and gums, use short, back-and-forth, then up-and-down strokes. Use vertical strokes to clean the inner surfaces. Be sure to clean the inside of your teeth, the teeth at the back of your mouth, your gums and your tongue. To clean the junction between your teeth and gums, hold your brush at a 45-degree angle to your teeth. This allows the bristles to clean the groove between your gums and your teeth.
- *Floss daily.* Hold the floss taut and bent around each tooth in a C shape and scrape up and down on the side of each tooth. Each stroke should go slightly below your gumline until you feel resistance. Flossing removes plaque between your teeth and helps massage your gums. If you have a bridge, be sure to floss the teeth around it as well as underneath the bridge.

Many toothpaste companies promote tartar-control products. The effectiveness of these products in preventing gum disease is unproved. Tartar-control toothpaste may reduce the formation of tartar on tooth surfaces and make your teeth more cosmetically appealing. However, these products don't help remove tartar below the gumline and between teeth, where gum disease develops.

Other devices

Some people develop plaque in unusual quantities or especially quickly. If you have this problem, your dentist may recommend special toothpicks, stimulators or electric toothbrushes.

Devices that irrigate with water under pressure can be used to flush out toxic products due to plaque between your teeth. These devices don't remove the plaque but can help prevent some of its effects.

Electric toothbrushes have been found to be superior to regular toothbrushes in removing plaque, but they can be expensive, and manual toothbrushes work well when used properly. Electric toothbrushes can be particularly useful to people with special needs. For example, they may benefit individuals whose manual dexterity is impaired by conditions such as arthritis or people who wear dental appliances, such as braces.

Mouth rinses

Over-the-counter mouth rinses that claim to decrease plaque haven't been proved more beneficial than brushing and flossing. The slick feel that some of these products impart to teeth isn't due to removing tartar and plaque but rather to the glycerine included in the rinse. If you use a rinse, do so in addition to brushing and flossing.

For people with chronic periodontal problems, the plaque-fighting rinse chlorhexidine (Peridex, PerioGard) is available by prescription. It's effective, but it isn't a cure for inflammation of the gums (gingivitis).

Side effects can include an unpleasant taste in your mouth, irritation of the soft tissues of your mouth and staining of your teeth. For these reasons, prolonged use of chlorhexidine products may be undesirable.

Dental cleanings

No matter how careful you are, you're bound to acquire some plaque and calculus. Visit your dentist every 6 to 12 months for dental cleanings. If you have periodontitis or you develop large amounts of tartar quickly, visit your dentist more often.

Prosthodontics

Among the many stories about the "Father of Our Country," one popular myth holds that George Washington had wooden teeth. Washington suffered from dental disease and tooth loss most of his life. At the time of his inauguration, only one tooth remained.

Dentures were an important part of Washington's life, but despite the folklore, they were never made from wood. Hippopotamus, walrus and elephant ivory and other materials such as cows' teeth were used to make his artificial teeth. They were fastened with metal springs that caused excruciating pain.

Before modern dentistry, losing your teeth was an inevitable part of aging. Rare was the person who by old age had any teeth left. In the 18th century, Washington's having dentures at all shows that he was one of the lucky few who were able to take advantage of the latest advances in dentistry. Today the story is different. Fewer people need to have their teeth removed and replaced with dentures.

Partial dentures

If a permanent tooth is lost, it should be replaced without delay. Your teeth are positioned such that every tooth has its own place and helps adjacent teeth retain their proper alignment. If you lose a tooth and don't replace it, teeth on either side gradually drift or tilt toward the open space. This can alter your bite, sometimes making it more difficult to chew.

Proper Care of Your Dentures

A denture or removable partial denture (dental prosthesis), can last from 6 months to 5 years or more, depending on the material, how well the denture fits, the condition of your jaw and how well you maintain the denture.

For a prosthesis to be comfortable and durable, you must care for it properly. Good maintenance isn't difficult, particularly if you:

1. Make sure your prosthesis fits properly. If it seems uncomfortable after the initial adjustment period, revisit your dentist or prosthodontist.
2. Remove your prosthesis each night at bedtime. Your gums need a period of rest to remain healthy.
3. Store your prosthesis in water and, when needed, add a denture-cleaning agent. Dentures not stored in water can warp, making them uncomfortable to wear.

   To avoid damage to the metal clasps of your dentures, don't soak removable dentures with metal bases in a cleansing solution for more than 15 minutes. Soaking them for more than 15 minutes may be fine if it's indicated on the label of the cleansing product.
4. Clean your prosthesis each day, according to your dentist's instructions. Food particles and plaque need to be removed regularly.
5. Each day, brush and floss any remaining natural teeth you have. It's imperative to keep remaining teeth and gums as healthy as possible, particularly if a partial denture is secured to these teeth.
6. Clean and massage your mouth and gums each day using a toothbrush, cloth or your finger. It's as important to keep the gums and soft tissues of your mouth clean and stimulated as it is to keep your teeth clean.

Your dentist will determine what sort of partial denture is best suited to meet your needs. If you have a healthy tooth on each side of the missing tooth or teeth, a fixed (nonremovable) partial denture or bridge may be an option. In this procedure, the healthy teeth on each side of the missing tooth or teeth are reshaped to receive a crown. The crowns and an artificial tooth (pontic) or teeth are then joined together, and the bridge is cemented to the two supporting teeth.

Another type of prosthetic device is known as a removable partial denture. This prosthesis has artificial teeth attached to a metal or plastic base. Clasps or other retainers are incorporated into the partial denture to secure it to the remaining natural teeth. Removable partial dentures are usually less costly than fixed partial dentures, and more teeth can be added to the denture if you lose adjacent teeth.

Partial dentures can trap food, particularly if they don't fit properly. Good oral hygiene is important because retained food particles lead to plaque, tartar, gum disease and decay of the natural teeth. If the partial denture is fixed, be sure to floss and brush it carefully. If it's removable, remove the prosthesis and brush it and the surrounding teeth carefully after every meal. Remove it at bedtime because it's important to allow the gum tissues to rest.

Dentures

If you must have all of your teeth removed as a consequence of serious gum disease or decay, your dentist or a specialist called a prosthodontist can make a set of artificial teeth (dentures).

Dentures can never replace the function and feeling of natural teeth, but they're certainly a better alternative to no teeth at all. You'll lose some of the sensations of eating because the roof of your mouth (hard palate) is covered by the upper denture. In addition, dentures may limit what foods you can eat. Foods such as corn on the cob, whole apples and hard candies may be difficult to eat because pressures exerted by biting or chewing these foods can cause dentures to loosen.

The chewing pressure you can exert with dentures is much less than you can exert with your natural teeth, which are anchored in your jaw. Well-fitted dentures usually don't require use of denture adhesives.

Fitting dentures

Two standard methods are used for fitting dentures. The teeth can be extracted and the gums and jaw allowed to heal before dentures are fitted. Or the dentures can be prepared in advance and inserted immediately after the extraction.

Not everyone is eligible for immediate dentures. Your dentist will be able to assess the conditions in your mouth and recommend the best approach for you. Immediate dentures save you the inconvenience of being without teeth for a period of time. However, they often must be refitted once the jaw heals, and occasionally new ones must be made if the jaw changes shape significantly after extraction.

A full set of dentures usually consists of complete upper and lower bases that fit over the gums.

Another option is an overdenture. When a few acceptable teeth remain in the jaw, the denture can be constructed to cover them. An overdenture may be somewhat more stable than a regular denture and, thus, reduce potential soreness in your mouth. It may be necessary to remove the nerves from the remaining teeth — a procedure called root canal — and then cover them with fillings before constructing the overdenture.

The remaining teeth under the denture must be carefully and regularly maintained to keep them healthy. Your dentist or prosthodontist can advise you on the possibility of using an overdenture.

Whatever kind of removable denture you have, it will need periodic adjustments to keep it comfortable and to help prevent bone loss and mouth sores.

Denture problems

Signs and symptoms

- A persistently loose denture
- Pain in the mouth while wearing dentures
- Inflamed gums
- Sores in the mouth at denture pressure points

President George Washington once returned an ill-fitting set of dentures to his dentist, writing: "I must once again resort to you for assistance. The teeth herewith enclosed have by degrees worked loose and, at length, two or three of them have given away altogether. I send them to you to be repaired .... they are both uneasy on the mouth and bulge my lips out."

Much like George Washington, many Americans suffer from ill-fitting dentures. Natural teeth are supported by a specialized type of bone in the upper and lower jaws. When teeth are lost, the supporting bone begins to shrink. This shrinkage may be accelerated by aging and also by wearing ill-fitting dentures. The result may be loose dentures, which can cause soreness during chewing. In addition, the dentures may become dislodged when you're talking or laughing.

Other problems include mouth sores and inflamed gums. If you're a new denture wearer, you may think that you should expect irritation or sores until you get used to your dentures. But you shouldn't. If you're having problems, your dentist should be able to adjust the denture to eliminate the source of irritation.

If you've worn dentures for a while and begin developing sores, the irritation may be due to a change in the denture or a change in the alignment of your mouth. Less commonly, denture sores can develop if food becomes trapped beneath the denture.

Problems are more common with a lower denture than an upper denture. The lower denture usually doesn't remain in place by itself, and successful use may depend on your ability to control a denture with the muscles of the tongue and cheeks.

Diagnosis

If your dentures are uncomfortable for more than the initial few minutes after you put them in, you experience pain when chewing or you notice that your gums are red and swollen or have sore, white patches, see your dentist.

How serious are denture problems?

Rarely, persistent or recurring mouth sores can signal a more serious health problem. Therefore, it's important to continue having yearly dental checkups, even if you have no natural teeth.

Treatment

Your dentist may be able to adjust your dentures to relieve the pressure on your gums. Or, if necessary, he or she can make a new set of dentures that conform to the current shape of your jawbone and gums.

If your jaw has shrunk and your dentist has trouble making dentures that fit well, several surgical techniques are now available that may provide a better foundation upon which a new denture can be constructed. These techniques include operations to build up the soft tissue of your gum or hard tissue of your jaw. Sometimes, a metallic support (dental implant) can be placed in the bone and can be used for tooth replacement.

If your gums are red and swollen because of a fungal infection, your dentist may prescribe an antifungal medication. Avoid using an over-the-counter ointment to numb denture-induced pain, unless directed to do so by your dentist. Using an ointment won't fix the cause of the sore, and it may mask a more serious problem.

Dental implants

Dental implants are an alternative to removable partial dentures, bridgework and missing teeth. They enable you to have permanent replacement teeth — a full mouth or just a few — that stay put when you eat, talk and laugh. Many people are rediscovering the joys of eating and interacting with others without the clicks and wobbles of dentures.

What are dental implants?

Dental implants, available in the United States since the 1980s, are metal — usually titanium — posts that are surgically secured in the jawbone beneath the gum tissue. These posts provide stable anchors, or "roots," for artificial replacement teeth, which look like natural teeth and are attached to the implants.

Dental implants are successful because of a natural process in which the bone grows around and attaches to the metal implant (osseointegration). This provides a solid foundation for artificial teeth. Dental implants feel and function very much like natural teeth.

Are dental implants right for you?

Anyone in good health who's missing teeth — be it one or all — can benefit from dental implants. Those who can't use conventional dentures or bridges because they're missing sections of their jaw might find implants the best option. Bone grafts can be used with implants to reconstruct the jaw and replace missing teeth.

However, implants might not be the best option if you smoke or have a disease such as diabetes. Tobacco use and some diseases can interfere with healing and your body's ability to resist or control

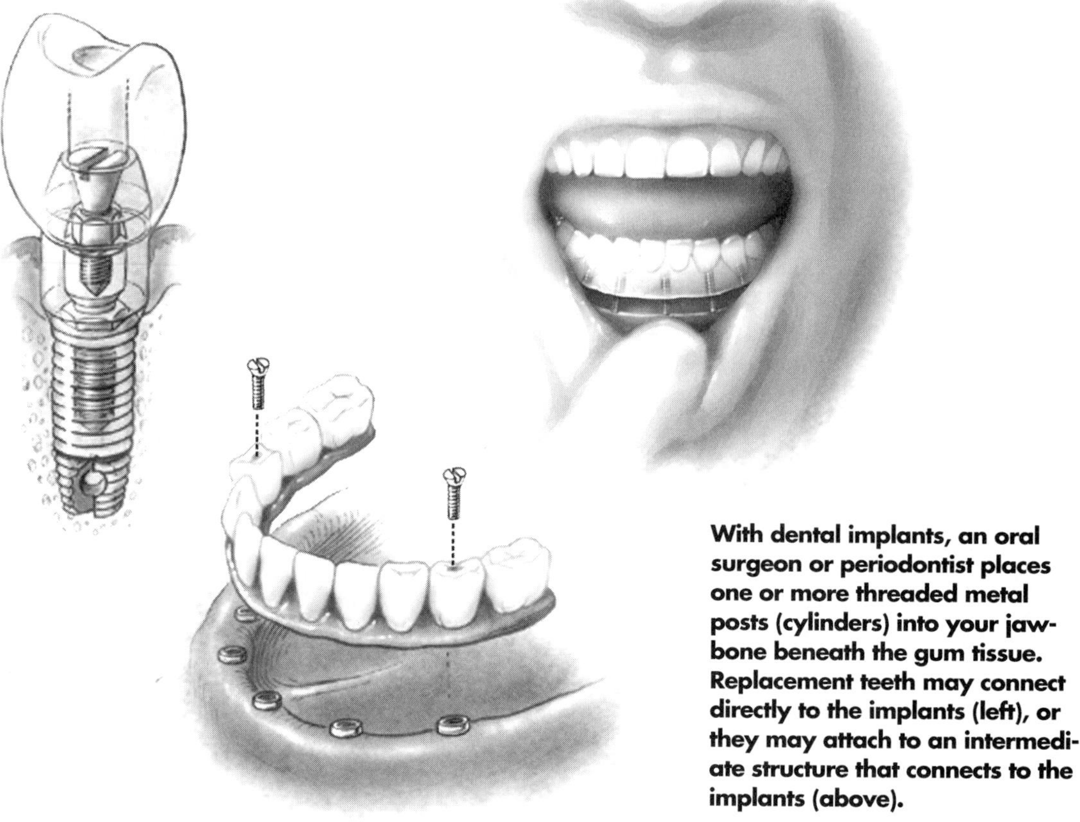

With dental implants, an oral surgeon or periodontist places one or more threaded metal posts (cylinders) into your jawbone beneath the gum tissue. Replacement teeth may connect directly to the implants (left), or they may attach to an intermediate structure that connects to the implants (above).

infection and cause a higher risk of implant failure. On average, about 1 in 20 dental implants fail. Other risks of implanted teeth include nerve damage from the surgery, infection or fracture of bone by implanted posts.

Dental implants are more expensive than conventional dentures. Weigh the pros and cons of implants before you decide which option is right for you.

Types

The two basic kinds of implants are endosteal and subperiosteal:

Endosteal

Endosteal means "within bone." This type of implant is similar in shape to the root of a natural tooth. It's placed directly into the jawbone, where it becomes solidly anchored through the process of osseointegration.

Subperiosteal

A subperiosteal implant fits over remaining bone and is used when the jaw structure is limited due to inadequate or weakened jawbone. This type of implant has an increased risk of nerve damage, lip numbness and infection. It's rarely used.

The procedure

Thorough oral examinations and consultations by a dentist and implant surgeon can determine if the procedure is appropriate for you. They use X-rays and models of your jaw in evaluating your situation.

Dental implant surgery is usually performed in an outpatient facility under local anesthesia. The procedure involves several steps over a number of months:

Placing the implants

Gum tissue is cut and lifted to expose the bone. Then precisely measured holes are drilled into the bone where each implant will be inserted. The implants are inserted in the holes, and stitches (sutures) are made to close the gum tissue over the bone and implants. The sutures will either dissolve or need to be removed by the doctor.

Swelling can be expected for up to 72 hours following the procedure, as well as some discoloration of the skin and gums for a few days. Use of an ice pack in the area during the first 24 hours after surgery may help reduce swelling. Your doctor may prescribe pain medication and antibiotics to control pain and prevent infection.

Minor bleeding is normal on the day of surgery, but report excessive bleeding to your doctor immediately. You'll likely be able to resume normal activity 1 or 2 days after surgery.

You'll be given special instructions that explain how you're to clean your mouth during the healing process following surgery. A soft diet is generally recommended to avoid undue pain and stress on the new implants. If you normally wear dentures, you can place a soft lining in them so that you can wear them with little discomfort. If spaces from missing teeth must be filled in during healing, your doctor may make temporary teeth for you.

Osseointegration occurs gradually as healing progresses. The implants are usually anchored firmly by bone within 3 to 6 months after placement.

Attaching metal posts

After healing is complete, the gums are reopened and small, metal posts (cylinders) are attached to the new implants. Each post has threads like a bolt that support the new artificial tooth. This stage of the implant procedure involves less pain and a healing time of only 1 to 2 days.

Making new teeth

When the gum tissue has recovered, impressions are made of your mouth, which are used to make models of the jaw and any remaining teeth. New artificial teeth (restorations, or prostheses) are based on these models.

Artificial teeth can be either removable, fixed (nonremovable) or a combination of both. A removable prosthesis is similar to a conventional denture, but it has the advantage of being fastened to the implant by clips or magnets. Fixed teeth are screwed into the implants and held firmly in place. They're designed to be removed only by a dentist.

Maintaining dental implants

Self-care is an important part of maintaining dental implants. The following guidelines are recommended by the American Association of Oral and Maxillofacial Surgeons:

- *Practice good oral hygiene.* Implants, artificial teeth and gum tissue must be kept clean. Home care aids such as special toothbrushes and floss holders can help.
- *Avoid damaging habits.* Smoking and excessive alcohol consumption as well as chewing hard items such as ice and hard candy may damage an implant.
- *Continue professional care.* Periodic checkup visits are necessary to ensure jawbone health and proper functioning of the implant.

Although the overall success rate of dental implants is 90 percent to 95 percent, a small percentage fail due to poor maintenance. The implants can also become infected or break.

Dental implantation is an extensive process that requires serious commitment from those who choose the procedure. For appropriate candidates, dental implants may make eating easier, improve speech and allow a more comfortable life.

Jaw Trauma and Disorders

When an accident happens, the most likely dental and oral injury is a dislocated or fractured jaw or loss of a tooth (tooth avulsion). Such injuries to the jaw are usually medical emergencies that should be treated without delay.

Broken or dislocated jaw

Signs and symptoms

- Misalignment of the teeth
- An inability to close your jaw
- Intense pain upon moving the jaw

Emergency signs and symptoms

- An obstructed airway
- Profuse bleeding

Most jaw trauma involves the lower jaw (mandible). If you sustain an injury to your mouth or face, seek immediate help from your doctor or the nearest emergency department. If breathing is difficult or considerable blood is present, call for emergency help.

Diagnosis

X-rays and an examination of the jaw are generally the first steps in determining if the bone is fractured. Computerized tomography (CT) scans may be obtained to see if other facial bones have been fractured. Blows that are strong enough to break other bones of your face may also damage your neck and back.

Your doctor may suspect a fracture if you're unable to close your mouth, your teeth are misaligned when your mouth is closed or you experience tenderness or numbness around your jaw. If you're unable to close your mouth, your jaw may be dislocated. Swelling and bruising are likely to accompany all jaw injuries.

Treatment

Treatment depends on whether you have a dislocation or a fracture:

Jaw dislocation

If your jaw is dislocated, your doctor may move it back into place by manually manipulating it. You may be given an anesthetic before this treatment.

Once the jaw is back in place, it may be stabilized with a bandage to keep your mouth from opening too wide and causing another dislocation. Avoid opening your mouth very wide for up to 6 weeks after the injury. When you feel a yawn coming on, place your fist under your chin to keep your mouth from opening wide.

If you've dislocated your jaw more than once, you may want to consult a surgeon who specializes in problems of the jaw and the bones of the face (an oral and maxillofacial surgeon) to discuss treatment options.

Jaw fracture

If your jaw is fractured, your doctor will immobilize the jaw with a bandage. In many cases, surgery is necessary to realign the bones and allow them to heal. Often after surgery, the jaw needs to be immobilized for 6 to 8 weeks. During this time, you'll be able to eat only soft or liquid foods, and talking may be difficult.

Loss of a tooth

When a permanent tooth is accidentally knocked out, appropriate emergency medical care is required, whether the tooth loss (tooth avulsion) happens to a child or an adult. Permanent teeth that are knocked out sometimes can be reimplanted if you act quickly. A broken tooth, however, can't be reattached. For more information, see page 369.

Temporomandibular joint disorders

Signs and symptoms

- Tenderness of your jaw muscles
- A dull aching pain in front of your ear
- A clicking sound or grating sensation when opening your mouth or chewing
- Locking of the joint, making it difficult to open or close your mouth
- Headache

The temporomandibular joints (TMJs) are the hinge-like joints that connect both sides of your lower jaw (mandible) to your skull. As with many other joints, the bony surfaces are covered with cartilage and are separated by a small disk that prevents the bones from rubbing against one another. Muscles that enable you to open and close your mouth also serve to stabilize these joints, which are located about a half inch in front of each ear canal.

When you open your mouth, the mandible moves downward and forward. For normal jaw function, both TMJs must work in synchrony. If the movement of both joints isn't coordinated, the disk that separates the lower jaw from the skull can slip out of position, resulting in jaw malfunction. Should your mouth be forced open rapidly or too far, the jaw can become dislocated.

As with other joints, the TMJ is susceptible to various disorders such as osteoarthritis, rheumatoid arthritis and other forms of inflammation. Other causes of TMJ pain include wear and tear on the joint, injury, stress, an improperly aligned bite and poorly fitting braces or other dental appliances. In rare instances, tumors may arise in this area.

Chronic tension and anxiety may cause you to habitually maintain a clenched jaw or grind your teeth — a condition called bruxism. Many people are unaware that they grind their teeth because it often happens while sleeping.

This overuse of your TMJ and supporting muscles may cause jaw pain and a headache when you awake in the morning. The pain associated with temporomandibular disorders can vary from minor to severe, and the condition can be temporary or chronic.

Diagnosis

Your doctor or dentist may listen for any sounds your jaw makes and observe its range of motion. Examining your bite can reveal abnormalities in the alignment of your teeth and in the movement of your jaw. Conditions such as a high filling, a tipped tooth, teeth displaced due to earlier loss of other teeth or certain inherited characteristics may produce misalignments and subsequent pain.

In addition, by examining wear patterns, your dentist can determine if you chronically grind your teeth. Feeling the joint while you move it also may help your dentist determine the cause of the condition. And an X-ray or magnetic resonance imaging (MRI) can help your doctor or dentist check for abnormalities.

Treatment

Aside from asking you to avoid overusing your jaw, your doctor or dentist may suggest one or more of the following treatments:

Anti-inflammatory medications
To reduce inflammation, your doctor or dentist may advise taking aspirin or another nonsteroidal anti-inflammatory drug (NSAID), such as ibuprofen (Motrin, Advil, others). For severe pain and inflammation, your doctor or dentist may inject a corticosteroid drug into the joint.

Corrective dental treatment
Your dentist may be able to improve your bite by balancing the

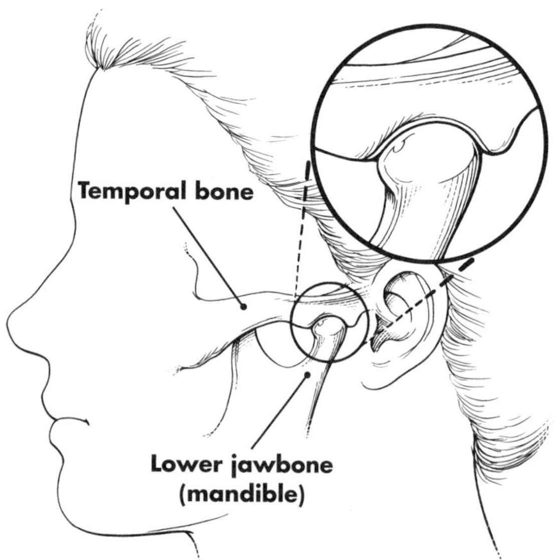

Your temporomandibular joints (TMJs) are hinged joints situated one on each side of your head where the lower jawbone (mandible) connects with the temporal bone of your skull. Inflammation, injury or dislocation of this joint can cause pain.

biting surfaces of your teeth or by replacing missing teeth, fillings or crowns.

Biteplate

If the temporomandibular joint is misaligned, your dentist may recommend a plastic biteplate (splint), worn over your teeth, to help align your upper and lower jaws.

Night guard

If you grind your teeth in your sleep, a night guard — a soft or firm device that you insert over your teeth — can help to protect your teeth during grinding.

Surgery

If other approaches don't work, surgery to repair or remove the disk between your mandible and temporal bone may be necessary, but this is rare.

Self-care

In addition to medical treatments, these self-care approaches can help prevent overuse and inflammation of your temporomandibular joint:

- Don't chew gum.
- Avoid sticky foods and foods that require a lot of chewing, such as caramels, tough meat and raw carrots and celery.
- When yawning, avoid opening your mouth too wide.
- If stress is causing you to habitually grind your teeth or clench your jaw, relaxation therapy or a night guard worn while you sleep may provide relief.

Teeth grinding

Signs and symptoms

- Severe or loud teeth grinding or clenching that occurs during sleep or during times of anxiety or stress
- Tips of teeth that are worn down, flattened or chipped
- Worn tooth enamel that exposes the inside of a tooth
- Increased tooth sensitivity
- Jaw clenching or muscle contractions
- Jaw pain or tightness in the jaw muscles
- Popping, clicking or locking of the jaw joint
- Earache due to jaw muscle contractions
- Dull morning headache
- Chronic facial pain
- Chewed tissue on the inside of the cheek

Bruxism is the term for grinding, gnashing or clenching of your teeth during sleep or situations that make you feel anxious or tense. The condition can be mild and occasional or frequent and violent.

Bruxism most often occurs in the early part of the night and can disturb sleep partners. Some people grind their teeth so loudly that they can't duplicate the sound while awake or relaxed. Others make no sound and deny having the condition, even when there's tooth or jaw damage.

Your bite (occlusion) affects the health of your teeth and jaw. Of an estimated 30 million to 40 million Americans affected by bruxism, 5 percent to 10 percent grind or clench their teeth with enough force to fracture dental fillings or crowns or cause other types of tooth damage. Severe bruxism may also cause tension-type headaches, facial pain and temporomandibular disorders, which occur in the temporomandibular joint (TMJ) located just in front of your ear.

Some people with bruxism clench their teeth only now and then. They might go days or weeks without doing so. People with bruxism may also habitually bite their fingernails, pencils or the inside of their cheeks.

Bruxism is a common sleep disorder. Research indicates that people who grind or gnash their teeth are more likely to snore, have pauses in breathing during sleep and develop sleep apnea. Bruxism is more prevalent in women than in men. In addition, women are more prone to tissue damage in the jaw joint resulting from teeth grinding and clenching.

Causes

Bruxism can stem from a variety of psychological and physical causes. These include:

- Abnormal alignment of upper and lower teeth (malocclusion)
- Anxiety, stress or tension
- Suppressed anger or frustration
- An aggressive, competitive or hyperactive personality type

Bruxism can sometimes occur as a complication of severe brain injury or as a symptom of rare neuromuscular diseases involving the face. It can also be caused by an uncommon side effect of some psychiatric medications, including antidepressants such as sertraline (Zoloft), paroxetine (Paxil) and fluoxetine (Prozac, Sarafem).

Stimulants such as tobacco and caffeine may cause your body to produce more adrenaline (epinephrine), which can worsen the condition. There's little evidence to support that bruxism is related to hereditary or genetic factors.

In children, bruxism may be related to growth and development. Some children grind or clench their teeth because their top and bottom teeth are misaligned. Others do so as a response to pain such as from an earache or teething.

Although most children outgrow bruxism, even short-term teeth grinding or clenching can damage permanent teeth. Of all children who grind their teeth between the ages of 3 and 10 years, more than half stop spontaneously by age 13.

Diagnosis

During regular dental exams, a dentist usually checks for evidence of bruxism. If your dentist notices signs, the condition may be observed over several visits to be sure of the problem before therapy is started.

Your dentist might ask about stresses in your life, your general dental health and any medications you take. He or she may also want to know whether you routinely drink beverages containing alcohol or caffeine, especially in the evening. Your dentist may want to ask your roommate or bed partner about your sleep habits, especially about any unusual grinding sounds heard during the night.

To evaluate the extent of the problem, your dentist or a specialist may perform a physical examination of your mouth and jaw. During this exam, he or she will check for tenderness in your jaw muscles and any obvious dental abnormalities, such as broken or missing teeth and poor teeth alignment.

In addition to checking your bite and examining your teeth, your dentist will check underlying bone and the inside of your cheeks for damage caused by bruxism. Mouth and jaw X-rays may be taken.

Treatment

The goal of treatment is to prevent permanent damage to your teeth and reduce pain caused by bruxism. Learning to rest your teeth, tongue and lips properly may help you to change your behavior and relieve bruxism. Resting your tongue upward with your teeth apart and lips closed can relieve discomfort by keeping your teeth from grinding or your jaw from clenching.

Other forms of treatment vary depending on the cause:

Stress

If your condition is stress related, strategies to help you relax may help reduce bruxism. You may also be prescribed a muscle relaxant medication to temporarily reduce the spasm in your clenched jaw.

Dental problems

If your bruxism is related to a dental problem, your dentist may treat it with orthodontic devices to correct misaligned teeth. In severe cases, he or she may need to use overlays or crowns to entirely reshape the chewing surfaces of your teeth. A mouth guard or protective dental appliance may be helpful if bruxism is severe enough to cause extensive tooth damage.

Brain injury or neuromuscular illness

Bruxism stemming from a brain injury or neuromuscular illness can be difficult to control. You may receive a mouth guard to help control bruxism.

Medication

If you develop bruxism as a side effect of medication, your doctor may change your medication or prescribe an additional medication to counteract your bruxism. Studies indicate that gabapentin (Neurontin) may successfully treat bruxism caused by antidepressant therapy.

Oral Infections and Diseases

Almost everyone experiences some sort of infection or disease of the mouth on occasion. Many times the problem is a passing irritation, such as an occasional canker sore. Other conditions are more debilitating or serious.

Canker sores

Signs and symptoms

- Small, painful, white ulcers in the mouth

Canker sores are common but annoying ulcers in the mouth. They occur singly or in clusters on the inside surface of the cheeks and lips, on the tongue, at the base of the gums and on the movable flesh at the back of the roof of the mouth (soft palate).

Despite a great deal of research, the cause of canker sores remains elusive. Current thinking suggests that either stress or tissue injury may cause common canker sores to erupt. Some researchers think certain foods — for example, citrus fruits, tomatoes and some nuts — may complicate the problem. A minor injury, such as biting the inside of your mouth, may trigger a canker sore.

Canker sores can be simple or complex. A simple type of canker sore may appear three or four times a year and last 4 to 7 days. The first occurrence is usually between the ages of 10 and 20, but it can occur in younger children.

As a person reaches adulthood, the sores occur less frequently and may stop developing altogether. Women seem to get them more often than men, and they seem to run in families.

Complex canker sores are less common but much more of a problem. People with this condition may have these sores 50 percent of the time. As old sores heal, new ones appear.

Treatment

There's no cure for either simple or complex canker sores, and effective treatments are limited. However, the following practices may provide temporary relief:

- Avoid abrasive, acidic or spicy foods, which may increase the pain.
- Apply ice to the canker sore.
- Brush your teeth carefully to avoid irritating the sore.
- Use an over-the-counter topical anesthetic.
- Rinse your mouth with over-the-counter preparations, such as diluted hydrogen peroxide.
- Use an over-the-counter pain reliever.

For severe attacks of canker sores, your dentist or doctor may prescribe an antibacterial paste called amlexanox (Aphthasol), an antibacterial mouthwash, a corticosteroid salve or an anesthetic solution containing viscous lidocaine (L-caine Viscous, Xylocaine Viscous). See your dentist if you have sharp tooth surfaces or dental appliances that may be causing the sores.

Gingivostomatitis

Signs and symptoms

- Mouth and gum sores
- Bad breath
- Fever and a feeling of malaise

Gingivostomatitis is a viral infection of the gingivae and oral mucus that occurs mostly in children. It often accompanies an upper respiratory infection such as a cold. Gingivostomatitis infections range from mild to severe and generally last about 2 weeks.

Diagnosis

Signs indicating gingivostomatitis include sores on the gums or on the insides of the cheeks, bad breath and a fever. A doctor or dentist may examine your child's mouth and check for any underlying infection, particularly of the chest or throat. A sample may be taken for culture.

Treatment

Treatment of an underlying infection or disorder may help clear the mouth infection. A medicated oral rinse may help relieve the pain and promote healing.

Good oral hygiene and a nutritious diet of soft foods and plenty of fluids are important. Using a mouthwash made of a half teaspoon of salt dissolved in 8 ounces of water, or an over-the-counter mouthwash, may be soothing.

Oral thrush

Signs and symptoms

- Creamy-white sore patches in the mouth or throat

Your mouth houses many different kinds of germs. One of them, the fungus *Candida albicans*, can reproduce uncontrollably, causing an infection known as oral thrush (candidiasis). The infection may extend downward into the esophagus.

This fungus is also responsible for vaginal yeast infections that many women experience. Oral thrush tends to occur most often when your natural resistance to disease has been weakened by illness or when your mouth's natural balance of microbes has been upset by medications such as antibiotics, immunosuppressants or corticosteroids.

Bad Breath

Everyone would like to have breath that's always "kissing sweet." Because fresh breath is important to most people, mints and mouthwashes constitute a multimillion-dollar industry.

Sad to say, these products don't always succeed in curing bad breath (halitosis), or their effects are only temporary. They actually may be less effective than simply rinsing your mouth with water and brushing and flossing your teeth.

What causes bad breath?

There are many causes of bad breath. First, your mouth itself may be the source. Bacterial decomposition of food particles and other debris in and around your teeth can produce a foul odor composed of volatile sulfur compounds. Pockets of infection, as in periodontitis, are obvious causes of odor. A dry mouth, such as occurs during sleep or as the result of some drugs or smoking, enables dead cells to accumulate on your tongue, gums and cheeks. These decompose and cause odor.

Another cause of bad breath is eating foods containing volatile oils with a strong, distinctive odor. Onions and garlic are the best-known examples, but other vegetables and spices also can cause bad breath. After such foods are digested, the volatile substances are absorbed into your bloodstream and carried to your lungs. Here they're exhaled in your breath. Alcohol behaves in the same fashion, thus allowing measurement of blood alcohol levels by breath tests.

Lung disease can cause bad breath, as can chronic infections in the lungs. If you have reduced action (impaired motility) in your stomach, you may have bad breath from fermentation of stomach contents. Belching may produce the odor. Gastroesophageal reflux disease also can cause bad breath.

Several general health problems can cause a distinctive breath odor. Kidney failure can cause a urine-like odor, and liver failure may cause an odor sometimes described as fishy. Acetone in the breath causes a fruity odor and may occur in people with diabetes who are developing excessive blood acids (ketoacidosis) or in ill children who have eaten poorly for several days.

Preventing bad breath

For most people, bad breath can be improved by:

- Brushing your teeth after every meal.
- Brushing your tongue to remove dead cells.
- Flossing once a day to remove food particles from between your teeth.
- Drinking plenty of water — not coffee, soda pop or alcohol — to keep your mouth moist.
- Avoiding strong foods that cause bad breath. Brushing your teeth or using a mouthwash only partially disguises odors of garlic or onion, which come from your lungs.
- Changing your toothbrush every 3 to 4 months.
- Rinsing your mouth after using inhaler medications.

In other situations, bad breath can be eliminated by treating the underlying condition, such as reflux, lung disease, liver failure or kidney failure.

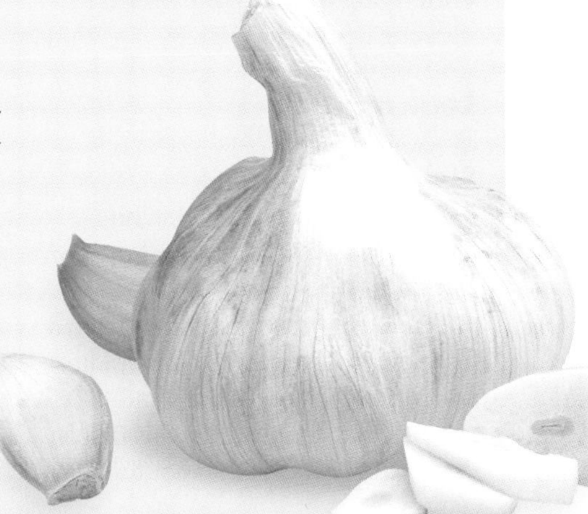

PREVENTION TIP

If you use an inhaled corticosteroid medication for asthma, you're at increased risk of oral thrush. After taking the medication, brush your teeth or thoroughly rinse your mouth with water and spit out the water. This will reduce your risk.

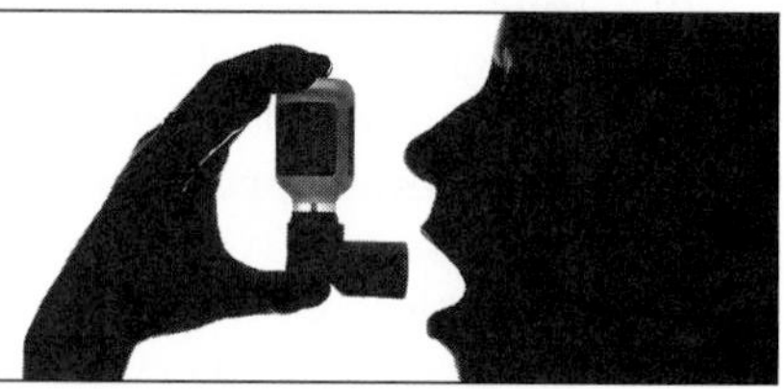

The infection is most common among babies, young children and older adults, although it can occur at any time of life. Thrush likes to develop in moist spots that may be chafed or sore, such as under poorly fitting dentures. You're also at increased risk if you smoke.

Diagnosis
If slightly raised, creamy-white painful patches develop in your mouth or on your tongue, you may have oral thrush. The patches may be brushed off when you clean your teeth or eat. Brushing may cause increased soreness and slight bleeding. The infection can spread to the roof of your mouth and your gums, tonsils and throat.

Your doctor or dentist will likely examine your mouth and throat to look for an underlying cause of the condition.

How serious is oral thrush?
Oral thrush can be painful, but ordinarily it's not a serious disorder. However, it can interfere with eating.

Treatment
Your doctor or dentist will likely prescribe a 7- to 10-day course of oral antifungal medication. Any underlying disorder, if present, must be treated as well.

Leukoplakia

Signs and symptoms
- A thickened, hardened, white patch on a cheek or your gums or tongue

The term *leukoplakia* comes from a Greek word meaning "white plate," an apt description of the white patches that characterize this disorder. Leukoplakia is the mouth's reaction to chronic irritation, such as from ill-fitting dentures or a rough tooth rubbing against a cheek or gum. Over the course of several weeks, you may notice a white or grayish patch developing on the inside of one cheek or on your tongue or gums (see the color illustration on page 440). At first it may not cause problems. After a while, it may become rough and sensitive to hot or spicy foods.

When a white patch develops in the mouth of a smoker, the condition is called smoker's keratosis. These patches are the body's natural protection against the heat of tobacco smoke. They also occur where a cud of chewing tobacco or snuff is held within the mouth for extended periods.

Leukoplakia is most common among older adults.

Diagnosis
Your doctor or dentist will likely examine the patch and try to determine the cause of the irritation. He or she may also take a specimen of the area for examination under a microscope (biopsy). About 5 percent of leukoplakias are either cancerous upon diagnosis or will develop into cancer within 10 years if not treated properly.

Treatment
Treating leukoplakia involves removing the source of irritation, if possible. If a rough tooth or denture is the cause, the offending tooth can probably be filed down or replaced. If the patch is linked to smoking or chewing tobacco, your best option for successful treatment is to quit the habit.

Once the source of irritation is removed, the patch usually clears up within weeks or months.

Oral lichen planus

Signs and symptoms
- Small, pale pimples that form a lacy network on the tongue or inside the cheeks
- Shiny, red, slightly raised patches on the tongue or cheeks
- A sore or burning mouth
- Dry mouth
- A metallic taste in your mouth

Oral lichen planus may be limited to a network of pale pimples or shiny, red, raised patches on the sides of the tongue or inside the cheeks, or it may advance into a painful erosive lesion. Your mouth may be sore and dry and have a metallic taste. Some people experience no symptoms other than the raised pimples or bumps.

The cause of oral lichen planus is uncertain. Emotional stress seems to trigger the response in some people. In others, it may be associated with any of a number of medications, such as antibiotics, diuretics, iodides, phenothiazines, chloroquine, quinacrine or quinidine.

Some cases have been linked to infections, such as hepatitis. Any adult can develop this rare disorder, but it affects middle-aged women more frequently than any other group.

There seems to be a relationship between the oral form and the skin form of lichen planus because almost half of those with the oral version also have it on the skin.

How serious is oral lichen planus?
Oral lichen planus usually isn't a serious condition. However, people with persistent oral lesions are at increased risk of squamous cell carcinoma — a form of skin cancer. In these cases, a doctor may advise

regular examinations to monitor any changes in the lesions. It's also important to stop any tobacco use, which raises your risk of squamous cell carcinoma.

Treatment

Treatment may not be necessary. If the cause is a certain medication, your doctor or dentist may advise you to stop using it and perhaps prescribe another medication instead.

Other treatments focus on relieving the itching. Your doctor or dentist may recommend:

- A corticosteroid ointment or cream
- Phototherapy with ultraviolet light, in some cases
- Oral corticosteroid medications, in severe cases
- Immune-modulating therapy, in severe cases

Tongue disorders

Signs and symptoms

- The tongue becomes smooth, dark red and sometimes sore
- The tongue becomes discolored, black or dark brown
- The tongue appears hairy or furry

A number of conditions can affect your tongue. Most are minor, but if the symptoms persist for more than 10 days, visit your doctor or dentist for an examination.

Inflammation of the tongue

Normally, the surface of your tongue is covered with small, hair-like projections of tissue called papillae. Inflammation of the tongue (glossitis) harms the papillae and may cause a range of other tongue changes to occur, including discoloration. Specifically, the tongue loses its usual pink and velvety character, and it may become sore.

Various factors can cause glossitis, including a bacterial or fungal infection, iron deficiency anemia and pernicious anemia, which is due to a vitamin B-12 deficiency.

Acute glossitis

Acute glossitis can occur as the result of a local infection, a burn or trauma. It may develop quickly with swelling and tenderness. It can interfere with chewing, swallowing and speaking.

If your tongue swells a great deal, it can obstruct your air passages. If this happens, immediately go to the nearest emergency department or call for emergency medical help. Immediate corticosteroid treatment usually relieves the swelling.

Geographic tongue

Geographic tongue is characterized by absence of papillae in patches, which makes the tongue appear smooth and bright red within those patches (see the color illustration on page 440). Soreness or burning may occur. The cause of this condition isn't completely understood.

Geographic tongue may vary from day to day or may be persistent. There's no specific treatment. Avoid hot or spicy foods, tobacco and alcohol.

? Question and Answer

Can oral piercing cause a serious infection?

The latest craze isn't always a healthy choice. Some people don't realize that oral piercing — piercing a tongue or lip — can land them in the doctor's office or the emergency room.

An oral piercing provides an opportunity for the millions of bacteria in your mouth to cause infection. Other complications include swelling, increased saliva flow, injuries to the gum tissue, uncontrollable bleeding and nerve damage.

Blood poisoning (septicemia) and blood clots also can occur. Tongue swelling is common and, if severe, can block the airway and obstruct breathing.

Black, hairy tongue

An overgrowth of bacteria normally present in the mouth can cause discoloration of the tongue (see the color illustration on page 440). These bacteria may accumulate on the papillae of the tongue. Some types of bacteria and yeast produce red blood cell pigments that may give the tongue a black appearance. In addition, the papillae can grow profusely, causing the tongue to look as though hair covers it.

The cause of this condition isn't clear, but it may be related to:

- Fungal growth following antibiotic treatment, which changes the normal bacterial content of the mouth
- Use of medications containing bismuth, such as Bismatrol and Pepto-Bismol
- Smoking or using chewing tobacco

Other possible causes for hairy tongue include excessive use of prescription mouthwashes that contain chlorhexidine, decreased saliva flow or poor oral hygiene.

The condition isn't serious, and it usually clears after discontinuing use of the offending medication or mouthwash. You can remove the discoloration and hair-like growths by gently brushing your tongue with your toothbrush twice a day.

Diluted hydrogen peroxide — 1 ounce hydrogen peroxide to 5 ounces water — may help bleach the color. You can gargle with it or apply it with a toothbrush. Avoid swallowing the solution. Rinse your mouth afterward. If this doesn't resolve the problem, consult your doctor or dentist.

Oral cancer

Signs and symptoms

- A mouth sore that doesn't heal or increases in size
- Persistent pain in your mouth
- Lumps or white, red or dark patches inside your mouth
- Thickening of your cheek
- Difficulty chewing or swallowing or moving your tongue

- Difficulty moving your jaw
- Swelling or pain in your jaw
- Soreness in your throat or a feeling that something is caught in your throat
- Numbness of your tongue or elsewhere in your mouth
- A lump in your neck
- A change in your voice

Each year, about 30,000 new cases of oral cancer — cancer of the lips, mouth, tongue, gums and salivary glands — and cancer of the upper throat (oropharyngeal cancer) occur in the United States. About 7,800 Americans die of these cancers annually.

About 80 percent of oral cancers arise on the tongue or on the floor of the mouth. They also may occur inside your cheeks, on your gums or on the roof of your mouth.

Periodic self-examination of your mouth is the best way to detect early signs of oral cancer. An early indication of oral cancer is one or more changes in the way the soft tissues of your mouth look or feel. When detected early and treated adequately, oral cancer is almost always curable. Unfortunately, more than half of all oral and upper throat cancers are advanced by the time a diagnosis is made.

Causes

Oral cancer appears to occur as a result of situations that damage the cells in your mouth so that they reproduce rapidly as cancer cells. A variety of factors that you can control increase your risk of oral cancer. They include:

Use of tobacco

Tobacco can damage cells in the lining of the oral cavity and upper throat. Smokers are six times more likely than nonsmokers to develop oral or upper throat cancers. About 90 percent of people who develop these cancers use some form of tobacco. People who use smokeless tobacco are at high risk of cancers of the cheek and inner surface of the lips. Oral cancer is twice as common in men as in women.

Excessive alcohol consumption

Alcohol can damage cells inside your mouth and upper throat. About 75 percent to 80 percent of people with oral and upper throat cancers are frequent drinkers of alcohol. The combination of alcohol and tobacco use increases risk.

Prolonged exposure to ultraviolet light

Too much ultraviolet light can damage the cells on your lips and increase your risk of lip cancer.

Leukoplakia

Most of the time leukoplakias, white patches on the inside of the cheek or tongue, aren't dangerous. But on occasion they may be early indicators of cancer. A large percentage of oral cancers occur in areas adjacent to leukoplakia. Leu-

Smokeless Doesn't Mean Harmless

If you think that spit tobacco won't hurt you, chew on this — one pinch held between your cheek and gum for 30 minutes puts the same amount of nicotine in your body as does smoking three cigarettes. Your body also absorbs several toxic chemicals including arsenic and formaldehyde.

Spit tobacco — also known as chew, snuff or dip — causes cancer. Each year, between 10 million and 16 million Americans put their health at risk by using spit tobacco. The risk of developing oral cancer among long-term spit tobacco users is up to 50 times higher than for nonusers.

Tobacco companies have coined the term *smokeless tobacco*, which implies to some that it's less harmful and less addictive than cigarettes. This might make an already dangerous product sound safer and more acceptable than other tobacco products.

Who uses it?

The majority of spit tobacco users are under age 18, despite the product being illegal for this age group in most states. High-school-aged boys are the biggest users. Contrary to popular belief, major-league baseball players aren't the only ones who use spit tobacco regularly. Other occupational groups have started using spit tobacco more frequently due to new "No smoking" regulations that prevent them from smoking on the job or at work sites.

What it does to you

Spit tobacco can get you hooked on nicotine. Research indicates that spit tobacco can be as addictive as morphine or cocaine.

Spit tobacco isn't made of only tobacco or natural products. Each time you use it, you absorb a number of toxic chemicals, many of which can cause cancer (carcinogens). These include:

- *Nitrosamines.* The most powerful cancer-causing chemicals known
- *Polonium.* Radioactive particles
- *Formaldehyde.* A chemical used in embalming fluid
- *Arsenic and cadmium.* Poisonous metals

As early as 1 week after you start using spit tobacco, you may develop small white patches called leukoplakia inside your mouth (see page 720). Within a few months of regular use, many spit tobacco users have these white patches, which can be an early sign of cancer. Red patches called erythroleukoplakia are even more likely to become cancerous.

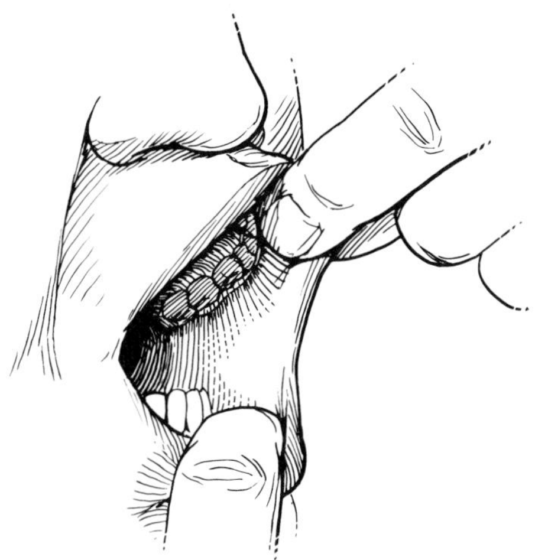
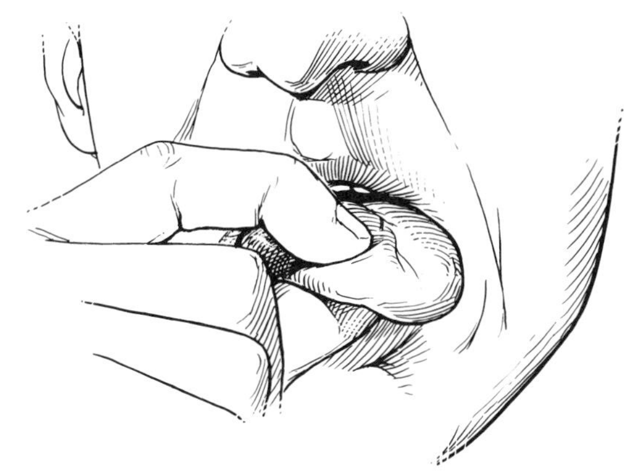

Routine self-examination of your mouth and tongue may enable you to see or feel an oral cancer when it's small and treatment is most effective.

koplakia may result from a variety of causes, including smoking or chewing tobacco products, ill-fitting dentures, a rough spot on an adjacent tooth or habitual cheek biting.

Diagnosis

To determine if a suspect area in your mouth is cancerous, your doctor will need to take a small tissue sample for examination under a microscope (biopsy).

Almost all oral cancers are of the squamous cell type. Squamous cells are firm and flat, and they form the lining of the oral cavity and upper throat as well as the surface of the skin. Squamous cell cancer begins with abnormal cells located only on the surface. As the cancer progresses, the malignant cells invade deeper layers of the oral cavity and upper throat and may spread to the lymph nodes as well as to other parts of the body.

For your doctor to determine whether or how far the cancer has

Other health risks

In addition to oral cancer, spit tobacco increases your risk of:

Tooth and gum disorders

To speed the delivery of nicotine into your blood, spit tobacco contains abrasives such as fiberglass and sand. These substances make tiny cuts in your gums causing you to lose gum tissue and even teeth. Gum recession isn't reversible and exposes the roots of your teeth, which makes them four times more prone to cavities.

Cardiovascular disease

Using spit tobacco increases your risk of high blood pressure, heart attack and stroke.

Other cancers

Using spit tobacco increases your risk of cancers of the esophagus, throat (pharynx), voice box (larynx), stomach, pancreas and prostate.

Quitting

Quitting is possible — either gradually or abruptly — and your doctor or dentist can help. Quitting spit tobacco use can be just as difficult as stopping smoking, and most people attempt it many times before quitting for good. You'll probably experience withdrawal symptoms: cravings, irritability and difficulty concentrating. These steps may help you kick your spit tobacco habit:

- *Pick a stop date.* Mark the date on your calendar and stick to it.
- *Use less.* Even before you quit, cut back on the number of times you dip each day, increase the time between each dip, and leave the dip in your mouth for less time.
- *Avoid peer pressure.* Surround yourself with people who support your decision.
- *Use spit tobacco substitutes.* Other products may help keep you from returning to spit tobacco use. Try sugarless gum or hard candy, sunflower seeds or beef jerky. Nontobacco chews and pouches (Oregon Mint), herbal chews (Golden Eagle) or dietary supplements (Winner's Edge) also may help curb your cravings.
- *Don't give in to cravings.* Each craving usually lasts only 3 to 5 minutes. During a craving, divert your attention with deep breathing, exercise or munching on substitutes.
- *Talk to your doctor or dentist.* Your doctor or dentist can help you plan a strategy.
- *Medication.* Studies have shown that bupropion (Zyban) may help people quit spit tobacco. Nicotine gum or a nicotine patch, inhaler or nasal spray also may be helpful. Consult your doctor about these products.

PREVENTION TIP

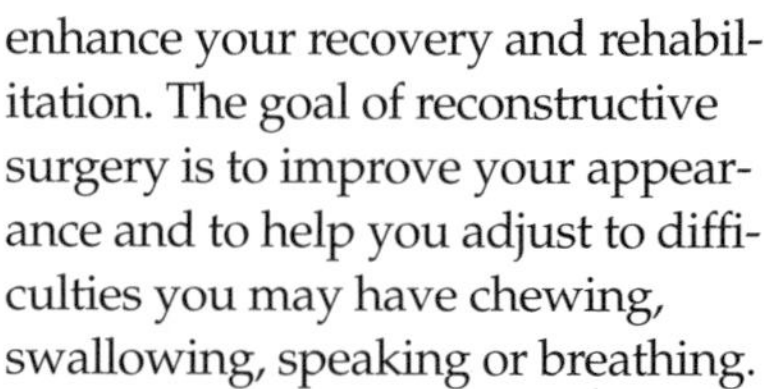

Tobacco and alcohol are by far the most important risk factors for oral cancer. You can greatly reduce your risk of oral cancer by not smoking and by limiting the amount of alcohol you drink or avoiding alcohol altogether. Here are other steps that you can take to help prevent oral cancer or to prevent its progression.

- If you wear dentures, make sure they fit well and clean them regularly. Oral irritation increases your risk of oral cancer.
- Don't chew the inside of your cheek or mouth.
- Limit sun exposure. When you're out in the sun, use lip balm with sunblock and a wide-brimmed hat to protect your face, including your lips.
- Check your mouth and tongue periodically. Standing in front of a mirror, use your forefinger and thumb to pull facial tissue aside to get a good view of the tissue on the inside of your lips, your cheeks and elsewhere inside your mouth. Look for bumps and changes in color. Use your thumbs and fingers to check for lumps and tender spots.
- If you notice changes, see your doctor or dentist as soon as possible. Oral cancer is curable, but treatment success depends on early detection.

spread, you may need dental X-rays, X-rays of your head and chest, a computerized tomography (CT) scan, magnetic resonance imaging (MRI) or an ultrasound scan. See Chapter 39, "Diagnostic Tests," for more on these tests.

Treatment

Surgery at an early stage provides the best chance for cure with the fewest side effects. If a tumor can't be completely removed, your doctor may recommend radiation. Sometimes, doctors recommend chemotherapy before surgery or in combination with radiation therapy.

Surgery

The type of surgery performed depends on the size and location of the tumor. Tumors that haven't invaded nearby tissues can be surgically removed with relatively few side effects. However, if the tumor has invaded nearby tissues, the surgery may be more extensive. Sometimes, surgeons need to remove bone from the jaw or tissue from the roof of the mouth.

To treat a cancer located on the tongue or upper part of your throat, a surgeon may need to remove tissues used for swallowing and, in some cases, the voice box (larynx). If the cancer has spread beyond the mouth, lymph nodes in the neck may also be removed.

Radiation

Radiation therapy uses X-rays to kill cancer cells. A doctor may advise treatment with radiation therapy if the tumor is small. Radiation may be used along with surgery to destroy small amounts of cancer cells that couldn't be removed during surgery.

Chemotherapy

Chemotherapy uses drugs to destroy cancer cells. You receive the medication either through your veins (intravenously) or orally. The type of drugs and the length of treatment depend on the size, type and location of the tumor. Chemotherapy may be used before surgery to shrink a tumor. In the case of a large and invasive tumor, it may be used in combination with radiation therapy instead of surgery.

Reconstructive surgery

Following removal of an extensive tumor, reconstructive surgery may enhance your recovery and rehabilitation. The goal of reconstructive surgery is to improve your appearance and to help you adjust to difficulties you may have chewing, swallowing, speaking or breathing.

Some people need grafts of skin or other tissue from other parts of their body to rebuild areas in the mouth, throat or jaw. You may also need to have a dental prosthesis implanted to replace a part of your jaw removed during surgery.

If you've had extensive neck surgery, you may need surgery to create a hole in your neck (tracheotomy) to help you breathe more easily. If muscles you need for swallowing have been removed, you'll need surgery to create access to your stomach (gastrostomy) in order to receive food directly through a feeding tube.

Salivary Gland Disorders

Saliva, produced by your salivary glands, serves several purposes. It helps clean your mouth and teeth, it aids in swallowing, and it contains enzymes that aid digestion and help control infection.

Three major sets of salivary glands as well as numerous smaller glands are located throughout your mouth. The parotid glands are located in each cheek. The submandibular glands are under your jaw, and the sublingual glands are in the floor of your mouth. Each gland has its own tube (duct) carrying saliva from the gland to your mouth.

Malfunctions of the salivary glands may cause either excessive secretion or decreased salivation. An excess of saliva is characteristic in childhood, when certain oral infections are present, and often in mentally disabled individuals. Too little saliva may result from aging, radiation treatment, certain diseases and use of certain drugs.

Dry mouth

Signs and symptoms

- A sensation of dryness in your mouth
- Saliva that seems thick and stringy
- Sores or cracked skin at the corners of your mouth
- Bad breath
- Difficulty speaking or swallowing
- A burning or tingling sensation on the tongue
- An altered sense of taste
- Increased plaque on your teeth
- Increased tooth decay or gum disease

Lack of saliva is a common problem that may seem little more than a nuisance. But don't ignore it. Persistent dry mouth can affect how your food tastes and even the health of your teeth. Although many things can cause dry mouth, it's often caused by a side effect of medication.

The saliva in your mouth serves many purposes. Most noticeably, saliva makes it easier to talk. It also enhances your ability to taste food, makes it easier to swallow and aids in digestion.

The minerals found in saliva help repair early tooth decay, and saliva helps prevent decay by:

- Washing away food and plaque from your teeth
- Limiting bacterial growth that can dissolve tooth enamel
- Neutralizing damaging acids in your mouth

Fluoride combines with saliva in your mouth to help enhance saliva's antidecay properties.

On any given day, a healthy adult produces about 3 pints of saliva. Saliva production generally goes unnoticed unless too little is produced. The result is dry mouth (xerostomia).

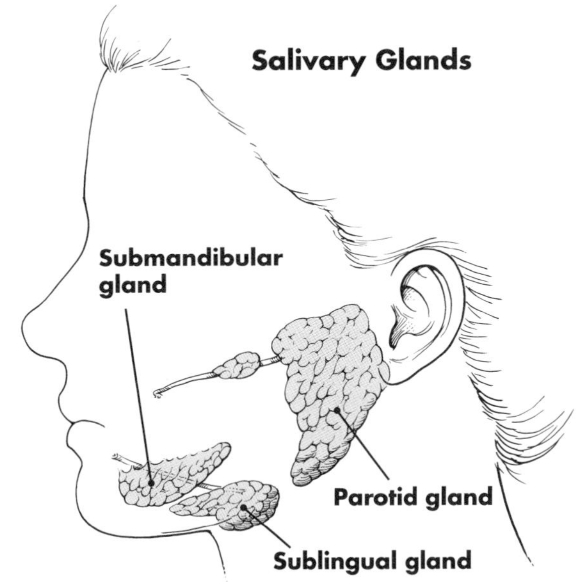

Causes

At one time, dry mouth was thought to be part of aging. It's now recognized that most cases of dry mouth are related to the medications taken by older adults rather than their age. Many common medications, including some over-the-counter drugs, produce dry mouth as a side effect.

Among the more likely drugs to cause problems are some depression and anxiety medications, antihistamines, high blood pressure medications, antidiarrheals, muscle relaxants, drugs for urinary incontinence and medications for Parkinson's disease.

Another cause of dry mouth is cancer therapy. Chemotherapy drugs can change the nature of saliva and the amount produced, and radiation treatments to the head and neck can damage salivary glands.

Nerve damage to the head and neck area from an injury or surgery also can result in dry mouth. Other conditions that can lead to dry mouth include salivary gland problems, endocrine disorders, Alzheimer's disease, stroke and Sjogren's syndrome, an autoimmune disorder.

In addition, smoking or chewing tobacco can affect saliva production, aggravating dry mouth. Snoring and breathing with your mouth open also can contribute to the problem.

Diagnosis

Your doctor or dentist likely will examine your mouth and go over your medical history. Sometimes, blood tests and imaging scans of the salivary glands are needed to identify the cause.

Treatment

If medication is believed to be the cause, your doctor may adjust your dosage or switch you to another medication that doesn't cause dry mouth. If a medical disorder is causing dry mouth, treating the underlying condition may help.

When the cause of the problem can't be detected or changed, saliva flow may be improved by sucking on sugar-free hard candy or chewing sugar-free gum. Avoid lemon-flavored hard candy because it makes saliva acidic, increasing the risk of tooth decay. Your doctor may also consider prescribing the drug pilocarpine (Salagen) to stimulate saliva production.

In addition, you might try:

- Sipping water regularly throughout the day
- Over-the-counter saliva substitutes, which are typically liquids or gels that are sprayed or rubbed in the mouth to add moisture

- Breathing through your nose, not your mouth
- Adding moisture to the air at night with a bedroom humidifier

Salivary gland infections

Signs and symptoms

- Swelling in the floor of the mouth, under the jaw or in front of the ears
- Decreased saliva flow
- Peculiar tastes in the mouth
- Pain in the mouth

Infection of the salivary glands isn't uncommon. Viral infections, such as mumps, commonly affect the salivary glands. Bacterial infections may occur following obstruction of a salivary gland or may be associated with poor oral hygiene.

The enlarged gland may be quite painful and may limit your ability to open your mouth widely. Your doctor or dentist may also notice pus at the opening of the duct.

Treatment generally involves antibiotics to clear the infection. Warm saltwater rinses — a half teaspoon of salt mixed in 8 ounces of warm water — can often aid in removing the pus.

Salivary gland stones

Signs and symptoms

- Swelling under the chin or in front of the ear, particularly at mealtimes
- Lack of saliva, particularly when eating
- Pain in the mouth

Sialolithiasis is the medical term for a stone or stones in a salivary gland or its duct. Caused by chemicals from the saliva that harden (calcify) into a solid material, these stones can block the submandibular, sublingual or the parotid glands.

When the stone partially blocks a duct, you may experience pain, particularly during mealtimes when large quantities of saliva are needed. The engorged gland may become swollen and lead to gland infection.

Diagnosis

Your doctor may check for swelling under your chin or in front of your ear, indicating a blocked salivary duct. Other indications are lack of saliva and pain in the bottom of your mouth. An X-ray of your mouth can often help identify a blocked duct.

Treatment

A stone in a salivary duct can be removed by one of two methods: manipulation or excision. Your doctor may be able to push the stone out of the salivary duct. If not, the stone can be removed by a surgical procedure. Occasionally, a gland that has had repeated infections and recurrent salivary duct stones may need to be removed surgically.

Salivary duct tumors

Signs and symptoms

- Swelling under the jaw or in front of your ear

Rarely, cells in one of the salivary glands — usually one of the parotid glands in the cheeks or submandibular glands under the jaw — multiply to form a tumor. In most cases, the growth is noncancerous (benign) and self-contained. These tumors develop over a period of years and cause the gland to gradually swell.

People who've had radiation exposure to the jaw or neck are at increased risk of cancerous tumors in the salivary glands. Tobacco use also may increase your risk.

Diagnosis

A special X-ray called a sialogram (ptylogram) is most often used to detect a salivary gland tumor. This test detects dye that's injected into the gland, revealing the flow of saliva into the mouth. Removal of some tumor tissue for examination (biopsy) is the only way to establish a cancer diagnosis.

Treatment

Treatment usually involves surgical removal of the involved gland. If the tumor is malignant, radiation therapy or additional surgery may be recommended, as well, to help prevent spread of the cancer. ■

CHAPTER 26 PART V

Heart and Blood Vessels

About the size of your fist, your heart is a hollow, muscular organ located under your rib cage beneath and to the left of your breastbone. Hard-working and powerful, the heart pumps blood to all parts of the body — each cell, muscle, bone and organ.

Every minute of your life, your heart beats approximately once a second and considerably more often when you're engaging in physical activity. It weighs about a pound yet pumps 5 or more quarts of blood a minute. Each day, your heart pumps the equivalent of about 2,000 gallons of blood through your circulatory system.

The blood your heart pumps provides individual cells with the oxygen and nutrients they need. The circulatory system through which your blood passes consists of two main types of vessels. Arteries and their branches carry freshly oxygenated blood away from the heart to tissues throughout the body. Veins and their branches carry blood containing waste products, such as carbon dioxide, back to the heart and then to the lungs. The lungs remove the carbon dioxide and provide a fresh supply of oxygen.

If the pumping of your heart, and the resultant circulation of blood, stops for more than a few minutes, life ends. In fact, all too often the first sign of heart and blood vessel (cardiovascular) disease is sudden death. This is a major reason so much emphasis is given to prevention of cardiovascular disease.

Your Heart

Your heart lies inside a thin sac of fibrous tissue called the pericardium. It has three layers of tissue: the epicardium, myocardium and endocardium.

The epicardium is a thin, shiny membrane covering the surface of the heart. Under the epicardium is a thick layer of muscle called the myocardium. The inside of the heart is covered with a smooth, shiny membrane called the endocardium. It covers the inside of the chambers of the heart, the heart valves and muscles in the heart chambers that attach to the valves.

The heart is made up of four chambers. The top two chambers are called the right and left atria (plural for atrium). The two lower chambers, the ventricles, are larger, thick-walled chambers that do the work of pumping blood to the lungs and the rest of the body.

The septum is a muscular wall that divides the right atrium from the left atrium and the right ventricle from the left ventricle. The septum prevents blood from passing from one side of the heart to the other. The right atrium and right ventricle are referred to as the right heart. The left atrium and left ventricle together are called the left heart.

Four flexible structures called valves keep blood flowing in the proper direction through the heart, to the lungs and then to the body.

Double pump

You might think of your heart as a double pump operating in a parallel fashion. One pump, the right heart, receives blood from all parts of the body through two large veins called the superior vena cava and inferior vena cava. Blood headed for the right heart has just delivered oxygen and nutrients to the body. Because it has less oxygen, this blood is called deoxygenated blood. The right heart pumps this blood to

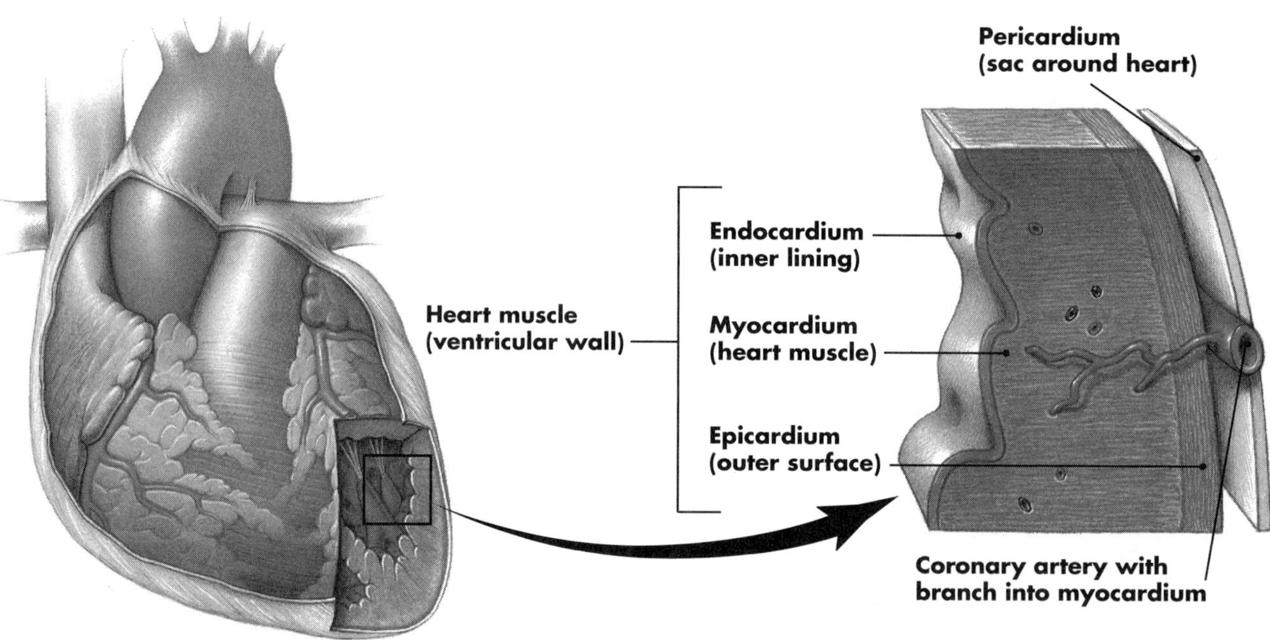

the lungs, where it picks up additional oxygen from air sacs (alveoli). Blood then leaves the lungs and returns to the heart, arriving into the left atrium. From there it's pumped to the body by way of the aorta, the largest blood vessel in the body. The aorta divides into several branches to supply blood to various parts of the body.

These parts of the heart work together to create the double-pump action of the heart. It receives blood from veins, pumps it to the lungs, receives it back from the lungs and pumps it into the body by way of arteries. This cycle is repeated thousands of times each day.

Cardiac cycle

On the right side of the heart, the tricuspid valve allows blood to flow from the right atrium into the right ventricle and prevents blood from flowing in the opposite direction.

From the right ventricle, the blood is pumped through the pulmonary valve to the lungs, where it picks up oxygen from and disposes of carbon dioxide and other waste products into the air sacs.

From the left atrium, the blood flows through the mitral valve into the left ventricle. From the left ventricle, the blood is pumped through the aortic valve and then to the rest of your body, including your brain, other organs and extremities.

In this cycle, the atria serve as the priming pumps and the ventricles as the main pumps responsible for circulating blood. While many people can live without effective atrial function, death ensues within minutes if the ventricles cease to function.

Systole and diastole

Contraction of the ventricles, which forces blood out to the lungs and other parts of the body, is called systole. Relaxation of the ventricles to allow blood to enter the heart is referred to as diastole. The right and left chambers contract and relax simultaneously.

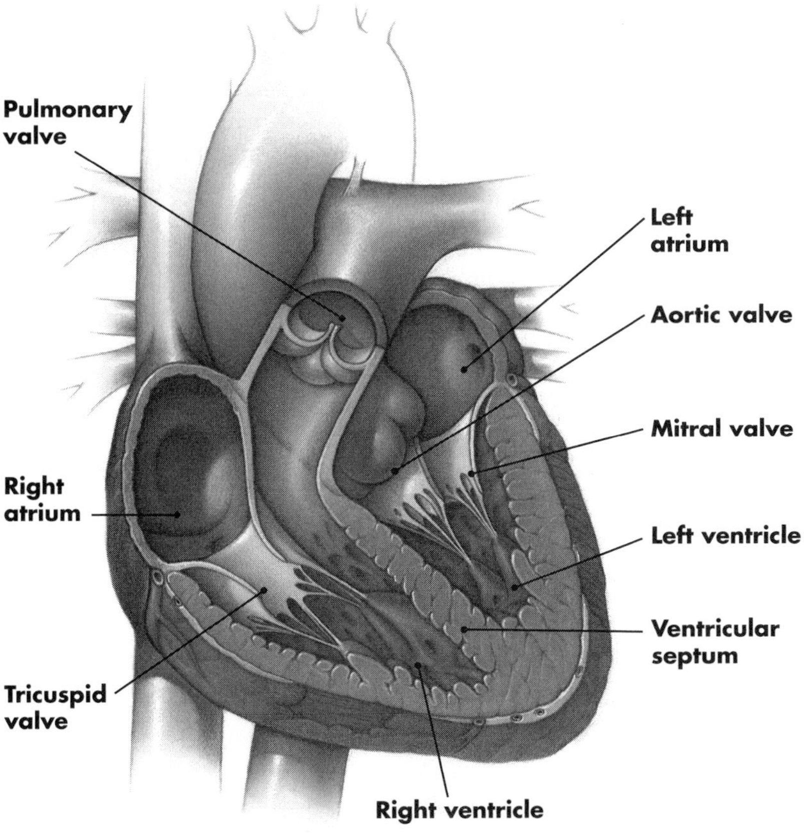

Pulmonary valve
Left atrium
Aortic valve
Mitral valve
Right atrium
Left ventricle
Ventricular septum
Tricuspid valve
Right ventricle

The rate at which the heart contracts and relaxes varies, depending on your body's activities at the moment. When you're at rest, your heart pumps more slowly. When you run or climb stairs, the pace of your heart increases to provide your muscles and other tissues with additional oxygen.

Natural pacemaker

Unlike other muscles in your body, which rely on brain or spinal cord nerve connections to receive the electrical stimulation they need to function, your heart has its own electrical stimulator — a natural pacemaker that transmits electric impulses signaling the heart to beat.

These electric impulses course through a network of specialized fibers within the heart, stimulating the atria to contract and move blood into the ventricles, and the ventricles to contract and force blood out to the lungs and the rest of the body.

With each heartbeat, blood circulates to all parts of the body. The typical heart rate is about 72 beats a minute, and with each beat 2 to 3 ounces of blood are pumped into the arterial system. At this rate, the heart beats about 104,000 times daily.

Your Blood Vessels

Your vascular system consists of the blood vessels in your body. Its name comes from the Latin word *vasculum* for "a small vessel."

The farther blood vessels extend from the heart, the smaller they become. The aorta, the principal blood vessel in your body, delivers blood from your heart to the larger arteries. These arteries, in turn, branch into smaller arteries, which become tiny arterioles. These eventually become so small that they allow only a single blood cell to

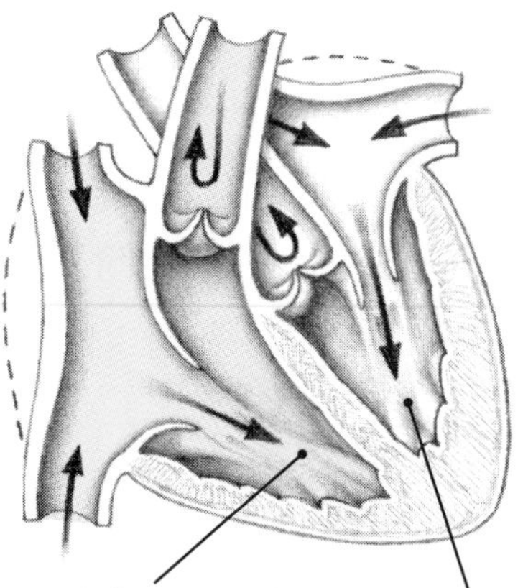

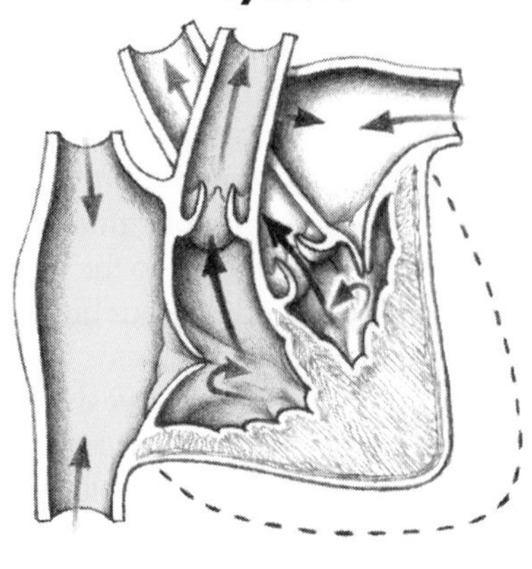

The heart pumps in two stages. The ventricles relax during diastole so that blood can enter the heart. They contract during systole to pump blood out.

pass through at a time. These smallest vessels are called capillaries. Capillaries deliver oxygen and nutrients to your tissues and pick up waste, such as carbon dioxide, from your cells.

Blood begins its return trip to your heart through tiny veins called venules. Blood flows from venules to larger and larger veins until it reaches the right atrium. Your veins, which are under less pressure, aren't as muscular and elastic as your arteries.

Like all muscles in your body, your heart needs oxygen and nutrients from blood to survive. Thus, it has its own pair of arteries, called coronary arteries. These special heart vessels branch off the aorta just as it leaves the heart. The right coronary artery supplies blood to the bottom and back of the heart. The left coronary artery supplies the top, front and left sides, as well as an area of the back of the heart (see the color illustration on page 408).

Blood pressure

To keep blood moving, there must be pressure in your blood vessels at

Interpreting Your Heartbeat

For most of us, the feel of a stethoscope on our chest is familiar. Less familiar is the bass drum heart thumping your doctor hears through the other end of the hearing device. Heart sounds can provide your doctor with considerable information about your heart and your health.

When listening to your heart, your doctor may ask you to breathe in and out naturally or perhaps in a deliberately rhythmic fashion. He or she may move the stethoscope in small steps from one location to another over your chest.

A normal heartbeat has a consistent pattern represented by the syllables *lubb* and *dubb*. These sounds correspond to closure of the heart valves. *Lubb* is followed by a short pause, and *dubb* is followed by a longer pause.

Differences in the intensity of these heart sounds may provide clues to disease involving your heart or lungs. Obesity, emphysema or fluid around the heart can muffle the heart's pumping sounds.

Other sounds also may be detected. Murmurs are the result of turbulence in the blood during the heartbeat. Depending on the location and character of the murmur and its relationship to the lubb-dubb sounds, your doctor can often identify a structural change in the heart that's responsible for the turbulence.

The presence of abnormal sounds during the relaxation (diastole) phase of your heart rhythm suggests an alteration in the function of the heart muscle. Sounds heard during the contraction (systole) phase, often called clicks, combined with a murmur identify specific types of valve abnormalities.

A heart murmur may be a sign of anemia, a leaky valve or other problems. Some murmurs are benign and aren't associated with a heart condition. In children, murmurs that aren't the result of a structural abnormality can sometimes be heard. Called innocent murmurs, they're typically faint, heard only intermittently and detected in only a small area of the chest. Innocent murmurs are harmless and may disappear by adulthood.

When your doctor listens to your heartbeat, he or she is gathering clues to the health of your heart.

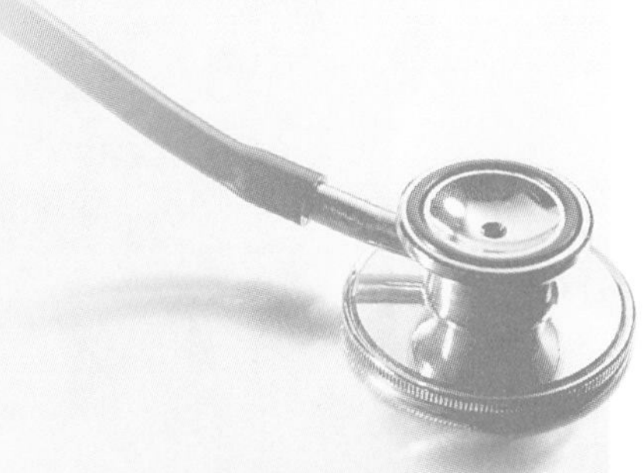

all times. During the contraction (systole) phase — when the left ventricle pumps blood into the arteries — the pressure rises (systolic pressure). This is the moment of highest pressure. During the relaxation (diastole) phase — between heartbeats while the left ventricle is refilling — the pressure falls (diastolic pressure). This is the moment of lowest pressure.

A blood pressure cuff (sphygmomanometer) is the instrument used to measure blood pressure in units of millimeters of mercury (mm Hg). Your blood pressure is written like a fraction — the systolic number is on the top, and the diastolic number is on the bottom. When stated verbally, the word *over* is generally used to separate the two numbers. For example, a blood pressure reading of 120/80 mm Hg would be stated as "120 over 80."

> **?** **Question and Answer**
>
> **How is cardiovascular disease different from heart disease?**
>
> The phrase *cardiovascular disease* is often used interchangeably with *heart disease*. However, *cardiovascular* is a more inclusive term than *heart* because it takes into account not only the heart but also all of the arteries, capillaries and veins that are directly or indirectly connected to the heart. In this sense, the term *cardiovascular disease* includes not only diseases of the heart but also of the blood vessels, such as a stroke.

Risk Factors

Heart and blood vessel (cardiovascular) disease has been the No. 1 killer in the United States every year since 1900, except for 1918 when an influenza epidemic briefly claimed its spot. Cardiovascular disease claims more lives each year than the next six leading causes of death combined, including cancer and accidents.

About one in five American men and women have some form of cardiovascular disease, whether it's high blood pressure, coronary artery disease, stroke or congestive heart failure.

Because of its serious nature and wide prevalence, a tremendous amount of research is being directed at improving doctors' understanding of cardiovascular disease, which should continue to result in better treatments and, perhaps more important, prevention.

Researchers continue to investigate the cause-and-effect relationships between our behavior, genes and aging processes and the ways our hearts function and malfunction. Many ongoing, long-term medical studies, such as the Multiple Risk Factor Intervention Trial and the Framingham Heart Study, have brought about a new level of understanding as to why cardiovascular disease is so common.

The findings are persuasive. A remarkably high percentage of people with cardiovascular disease have a history of certain risk factors. Risk factors are lifestyle habits or family characteristics that increase your likelihood of developing a certain disease.

Risk factors for cardiovascular disease include some things in life over which you have no control — sex, age and heredity — and aspects of your life that you can control — tobacco use, body weight, physical activity, blood cholesterol levels, high blood pressure and elevated blood sugar (glucose).

As you read through the following pages, remember that ways of controlling cardiovascular disease are constantly evolving. As investigators search for the best forms of prevention and treatment, conflicting findings sometimes result.

Some studies suggest that causal relationships exist between certain dietary habits and cardiovascular disease, and others conclude there's no clear-cut evidence of this. Still, studies are consistently finding that your lifestyle habits are likely to have an important effect on the health of your heart and blood vessels.

Also keep in mind that risk refers to odds or chances, not to inevitability. Risk factors can affect your chances of having cardiovascular disease, but they don't automatically guarantee that you'll develop it.

Smoking

About four decades ago, the U.S. Surgeon General announced that smoking tobacco is a health hazard. Subsequently, cigarette manufacturers were required to put a printed warning of the hazards of smoking on every package of cigarettes sold in the United States. In the years since, that warning has been made more emphatic — and an immense amount of clinical, statistical and other research has reinforced the original point.

Smoking is harmful — not only because of the association between smoking and lung cancer but also because smoking is high on the list of risk factors for cardiovascular disease.

If you smoke cigarettes, your risk of a heart attack or stroke is at least double that of nonsmokers. The risk increases with the number of cigarettes you smoke each day. Cigarette smokers who have a heart attack are more likely to die and die suddenly — within an hour — than are nonsmokers. Cigars, pipes and chewing tobacco seem to increase your risk as well, but to a lesser degree.

When smoking is combined with other risk factors, such as high blood pressure, high blood cholesterol or a family history of heart problems, the risk of cardiovascular disease appears to be greatly increased.

Complications

Smoking a cigarette causes your adrenal glands to secrete a hormone that temporarily increases your blood pressure and makes your heart work harder. In addition, smoking decreases the amount of oxygen available to your heart. As a result, every cigarette places a small but unnecessary load on your heart and blood vessels.

Smokers also have more fatty deposits (plaques) in their arteries (atherosclerosis) than nonsmokers do. This is probably because smoke increases the clumping of certain blood cells (platelets), which stimulates the deposit of cholesterol in arteries. Because the process of atherosclerosis is accelerated by both high blood pressure and smoking, probably as a result of the harmful effects of nicotine and carbon monoxide on blood vessels, a smoker who has high blood pressure is at much greater risk of atherosclerosis.

Tobacco smoke contains carbon monoxide gas. When inhaled, carbon monoxide binds to hemoglobin, the oxygen-carrying pigment in blood, and takes the place of oxygen. The result is that blood traveling to all parts of your body carries less oxygen to your cells. Often, as much as 8 percent of a smoker's hemoglobin may be occupied by carbon monoxide, making it unable to carry out its normal function of transporting oxygen.

Research suggests that carbon monoxide may have a direct, degenerative effect on the heart muscle itself, on the blood vessels and perhaps even on the clotting of your blood. Low-tar, low-nicotine cigarettes also can produce carbon monoxide and thus can't be considered safe.

Benefits of quitting smoking

The cumulative harmful effects of smoking on your body's organs argue convincingly for quitting. Furthermore, quitting smoking may actually reverse some of the damage smoking caused initially.

After 1 year of not using tobacco, your risk of coronary artery disease, including heart attack and chest pain (angina), is reduced by half. After 15 years of abstinence, your risk is similar to that of someone who has never smoked. And the earlier you quit, the more years you can expect to add to your life.

It's not easy to quit tobacco. It generally takes most people three to four attempts at stopping before they're successful. However, each try increases your chances of success. For specific advice on how to break the tobacco habit, see page 81.

Obesity

If your weight exceeds a "desirable" weight for your height and sex by 20 percent or more, you're generally considered to be seriously overweight (obese).

Defining *overweight* and *obese*

Doctors define desirable weight by means of body mass index (BMI). Your BMI is a sex-based estimate of body fat that's calculated from your weight and height. It's a better measure of your health risks than your weight alone or than weight tables based only on your height. See the BMI chart on page 39.

A BMI between 25 to 29 is considered overweight. Obesity is defined as a BMI of 30 or more. If you're very muscular, you may be an exception because BMI doesn't account for heavily muscled people with relatively little body fat.

By BMI definitions, close to 107 million Americans age 20 and older are overweight, and more than 43 million are obese. In addition, 13 percent to 14 percent of children are estimated to be overweight. These numbers are considered to be of epidemic proportions.

Complications

As you put on weight, you gain mostly fatty tissue. Just like other parts of your body, this tissue requires oxygen and nutrients from your blood. As demands for oxygen and nutrients increase, the amount of blood circulating through your body also must increase. Being overweight or obese increases your risk of high blood pressure.

Excess fat is also associated with elevated blood levels of low-density lipoprotein (LDL) cholesterol (the "bad" cholesterol) and triglycerides and a reduced level of high-density lipoprotein (HDL) cholesterol (the "good" cholesterol). Over time, these changes in blood fats can contribute to the buildup of fatty deposits (plaques) in your arteries, a condition called atherosclerosis. Atherosclerosis puts you at risk of coronary artery disease and stroke.

Obesity has many other harmful effects. It's a major cause of type 2 diabetes (formerly called adult-onset or noninsulin-dependent diabetes) and gallstones, and it can worsen sleep apnea and degenerative joint disease. Several types of cancer are associated with being overweight as well. In women, these include cancer of the breast, uterus, colon and gallbladder. Overweight men have a higher risk of colon and prostate cancer.

Benefits of losing weight

Even small amounts of weight loss are beneficial. The amount of weight you need to lose to improve your health may be much less than what you feel you need to lose. Losing just 10 percent of your current weight if you're obese can have a positive effect on your health. Slow and steady weight loss of 1 or 2 pounds a week is considered the safest way to lose weight and keep it off. For more information on healthy weight loss, see Chapter 3, "Controlling Your Weight."

Physical inactivity

Physical inactivity is a major risk factor for cardiovascular disease. It also contributes to other risk factors, including obesity, diabetes, high blood pressure and a low level of high-density lipoprotein (HDL) cholesterol (the "good" cholesterol).

Complications

Being inactive approximately doubles your risk of coronary artery disease and is comparable to the risk observed with high blood cholesterol, high blood pressure or cigarette smoking. In addition, sedentary people have a 30 percent to 50 percent greater risk of developing high blood pressure.

Are You an Apple or a Pear?

If you're overweight, observing where your fat is concentrated can help you assess your risk of obesity-related diseases. If your weight is concentrated around your abdomen, giving you an apple shape, your risk may be higher than if your weight is concentrated around your hips and thighs, resembling a pear shape.

To find out if you're an apple or a pear, measure your waist circumference just above your hipbones and your hip circumference at the widest part of your buttocks. Then divide your waist measurement by your hip measurement. A waist-to-hip ratio greater than 0.95 for men or 0.80 for women indicates an apple shape.

Benefits of physical activity

Regular, moderate-to-vigorous exercise plays a significant role in preventing cardiovascular disease. Even modest levels of physical activity are beneficial if done regularly and over the long term.

Daily physical activity can decrease your risk of cardiovascular disease. It increases the amount of "good" cholesterol in your blood, decreases the levels of "bad" cholesterol and triglycerides, reduces high blood pressure, improves the efficiency of your heart muscle and helps you control your weight. Regular exercise can also reduce the risk of a second heart attack and death.

In addition to benefiting your heart and blood vessels, physical activity benefits other parts of your body. It builds healthy bones, muscles and joints and reduces the risk of colon cancer. Physical activity also brings psychological benefits. It reduces feelings of depression and anxiety, improves mood and promotes a feeling of well-being.

Aerobic and anaerobic exercise

Not all types of exercise have the same effect on your body. Aerobic exercise, which includes activities like moderate paced walking, jogging, bicycling and swimming, improves cardiovascular fitness by causing your body to continuously use extra oxygen and calories while exercising.

Your heart rate and depth of breathing increase, and your body becomes warm. If the exercise is sufficiently long and vigorous, you'll perspire.

Anaerobic exercise, such as weight training, strengthens and tones your muscles through short periods of intense exercise. Anaerobic activities generally aren't as beneficial to your heart because they often don't challenge your heart and lungs to deliver oxygen in a sustained fashion to your body's tissues.

To benefit from regular physical activity, you don't need to develop a formal fitness plan or sign up for an organized activity — unless, of course, that's the only way you'll commit to regular conditioning. What's important is regular exercise, which should include three parts: warm-up, aerobic conditioning and cool-down.

Choose an exercise routine that's frequent enough, intense enough, of sufficient duration and of the appropriate type to gradually improve your health. Many people do a lot of walking at work or frequently move about during the day. However, for exercise to be of benefit, it needs to be uninterrupted and of adequate duration.

In general, try to burn about 1,000 to 2,000 calories a week with exercise. Walking 10 to 20 miles a week accomplishes that goal for the average person. Unless you're trying to lose weight, there's no evidence that you'll reduce your cardiovascular risks further by burning off more than 2,000 calories a week. For more information on how to develop a fitness program, see Chapter 4, "Keeping Active."

Undesirable blood fats

Cholesterol is a type of fat found in the bloodstream and in all of your body's cells. It's an important part of a healthy body because it's used to form cell membranes, some hormones and other needed tissues. But an undesirable blood cholesterol level is a major risk factor for coronary artery disease, which can lead to a heart attack.

Cholesterol comes from two sources. It's produced in your body, primarily by the liver, and it's found in foods that come from animals, such as meats, poultry, fish, seafood and dairy products. Fish is generally lower in cholesterol than other meats. Foods from plants, such as fruits, vegetables, grains, nuts and seeds, don't contain cholesterol.

Triglycerides are another form of fat that circulate in your blood and are a source of energy. A high level of triglycerides is linked to coronary artery disease and possibly inflammation of the pancreas (pancreatitis).

Types

There are several types of blood fats (lipids):

Low-density lipoprotein

Low-density lipoprotein (LDL) cholesterol is the major cholesterol carrier in the blood. LDL transports

Before You Start

For most people, the health advantages of regular physical activity far outweigh possible risks. However, if you have a chronic health condition or several risk factors for cardiovascular disease, some special precautions might apply. Check with your doctor before you begin an exercise program if you:

- Have heart, lung or kidney disease, diabetes or arthritis
- Are age 40 or older
- Are obese
- Have parents or siblings who've experienced coronary artery disease before age 55
- Are unsure of your health status

Your doctor may advise you to have an exercise stress test to help determine if physical activity is likely to cause an insufficient supply of blood and oxygen to reach your heart or to provoke heart rhythm abnormalities (see page 764). Discuss with your doctor any exercise limitations that he or she would suggest because of a health condition that you have.

If you've previously been sedentary, start with 5- to 10-minute sessions of physical activity and gradually build up to your desired level of activity. Your doctor can help you determine a desirable (target) heart rate to strive for while exercising. Achieving this target heart rate brings you the maximum benefit from the activity. As your fitness improves, your target heart rate may change.

cholesterol to sites throughout your body, where it's either deposited or used to repair cell membranes. But like hard water that causes lime to build up inside plumbing, LDL cholesterol promotes accumulation of cholesterol in the arteries feeding your heart and brain.

Combined with other substances, LDL cholesterol can form thick, hard deposits (plaques) that clog the arteries and cause them to narrow (atherosclerosis), increasing your risk of heart attack and stroke. This is why LDL cholesterol is often called the "bad" cholesterol.

High-density lipoprotein

Think of high-density lipoprotein (HDL) as a scavenger or cleanup form of cholesterol. It helps decrease the amount of LDL cholesterol in your blood. For this reason, HDL cholesterol is commonly thought of as the "good" cholesterol.

Higher values of HDL cholesterol mean a lower risk of atherosclerosis. Your HDL cholesterol level tends to increase with exercise and weight loss, but considerable amounts of exercise may be needed before significant results are seen.

Triglycerides

Triglycerides are another type of blood fat. An excess amount of triglycerides in your blood is called hypertriglyceridemia. This condition is thought to favor development of atherosclerosis, but this relationship isn't nearly as clear as that for LDL cholesterol and total cholesterol values.

Causes

Some people appear to have a genetic predisposition to an abnormal cholesterol or triglyceride level. One rare hereditary disorder, called familial hypercholesterolemia, causes such high levels of cholesterol that the affected person may experience a heart attack in childhood. Those who inherit a lesser form of this disorder have very high cholesterol levels and often have heart attacks by midife or earlier. The trend to a high triglyceride level may also be in one's genetic makeup.

Diseases such as hypothyroidism, diabetes and kidney failure may influence blood fat levels. Some medications may have an adverse effect. For many people, though, abnormal blood fat levels are a result of an unhealthy diet and too little exercise.

Measuring blood fats

Early detection of high blood cholesterol or triglycerides allows you to take steps to improve your health and prevent cardiovascular disease. The only way to find out your cholesterol and triglyceride levels is by having them measured with a blood test. To get the best results, it's important to fast prior to having a cholesterol test.

A typical lipids test measures total cholesterol, HDL cholesterol and triglycerides. Tests that measure only total cholesterol can be misleading because some people have a low level of HDL cholesterol and a high level of triglycerides but a normal or even high level of LDL cholesterol. In these cases, a total cholesterol measurement might appear normal, and you and your doctor would be unaware of cardiovascular disease risks posed by the abnormal levels that weren't measured. Even with a desirable total cholesterol level, if you have a low HDL level, you may be at increased risk of heart disease.

Desirable ranges for cholesterol levels depend on your age, sex, family history and overall health status. There's no magic number that separates risky levels from safe levels. Rather, researchers and doctors have identified lipid levels above which your risk of developing heart and blood vessel complications is high enough to warrant lifestyle changes.

Benefits of managing blood fats

If you have a family history of high cholesterol and triglyceride levels, heart attack or stroke at an early age, you're at greater risk of developing atherosclerosis. You can't do anything to change your heredity, but you can take precautions by having your blood cholesterol measured regularly as recommended by your doctor, following a healthy diet, controlling your weight and avoiding tobacco.

In 2001, the National Cholesterol Education Program (NCEP), a branch of the National Institutes of Health, issued a new set of guidelines for cholesterol management. These guidelines are stricter than earlier recommendations, calling for a more aggressive approach to lowering cholesterol and better identification of individuals at risk of a heart attack.

The guidelines also contain a risk assessment tool that can help doctors predict a person's chance of having a heart attack within 10 years. This tool takes into account such factors as age, weight, sex, blood pressure, total cholesterol and smoking habits.

The primary goal of cholesterol management is to reduce an abnormally high level of LDL cholesterol. After assessing your cholesterol levels, major cardiovascular risk factors and your 10-year risk, your doctor can help you establish an LDL goal.

In general, the higher your risk of cardiovascular disease, the lower the goal for your LDL cholesterol level. If you have only one or no risk factors, NCEP guidelines recommend an LDL goal of less than 160 milligrams per deciliter (mg/dL).

If you have two or more risk factors, such as smoking combined with high blood pressure, the recommended LDL goal is less than 130 mg/dL. If you have coronary artery disease, the recommended LDL goal is less than 100 mg/dL.

Lifestyle changes are usually the first line of treatment. If they don't suffice or if your LDL cholesterol is very high, medication is recommended.

What Do the Numbers Mean?

Results from a blood fat test are listed as a set of numbers in milligrams per deciliter (mg/dL) indicating total, low-density lipoprotein (LDL) cholesterol (the "bad" cholesterol) and high-density (HDL) cholesterol (the "good" cholesterol) and triglyceride levels. The National Cholesterol Education Program, a branch of the National Institutes of Health, has developed a set of guidelines to help determine which numbers are acceptable and which ones carry increased risk. As you compare your numbers with these values, remember that numbers alone don't tell the whole story. Ask your doctor to interpret your test results.

Cholesterol and Triglyceride Classifications

Total cholesterol

*Mg/dL**	*What your level means*
<200	Desirable
200-239	Borderline high
≥240	High

LDL ("bad") cholesterol

Mg/dL	*What your level means*
<100	Optimal
100-129	Near optimal
130-159	Borderline high
160-189	High
≥190	Very high

HDL ("good") cholesterol

Mg/dL	*What your level means*
<40	Low
≥60	High

HDL cholesterol protects against cardiovascular disease, so for HDL, higher numbers are better.

Triglycerides

Mg/dL	*What your level means*
<150	Normal
150-199	Borderline high
200-499	High
≥500	Very high

*Milligrams per deciliter

Source: National Cholesterol Education Program, Adult Treatment Panel III, 2001

Know Your Fats

Foods contain several different kinds of fats.

Saturated fats
Most saturated fats come from foods of animal origin — meats, milk and milk products. Plant sources of fat include the tropical oils: coconut oil, palm kernel oil, palm oil and cocoa butter. Unlike other plant oils, tropical oils are composed predominantly of saturated fatty acids. They're common ingredients in commercial cakes, cookies and other snack foods. Saturated fats contribute to low-density lipoprotein (LDL) cholesterol (the "bad" cholesterol).

Monounsaturated fats
Olive, peanut and canola oils are sources of monounsaturated fats. Unlike saturated fats, monounsaturated fats, in recommended amounts, help lower total blood cholesterol and resist oxidation, the process that enables cells in your arteries to absorb fats and cholesterol.

Polyunsaturated fats
Like monounsaturated fats, polyunsaturated fats are found in many vegetable oils and help to lower your total and LDL blood cholesterol levels. Unlike monounsaturated fats, however, polyunsaturated fats are vulnerable to oxidation.

Trans fats
Trans fats (trans fatty acids) are produced when polyunsaturated fats undergo the chemical process of hydrogenation. One example is margarine. When it's hydrogenated, some of its polyunsaturated fatty acids are converted to saturated fats or trans fats. This process makes the fat more solid. The greater the degree of hydrogenation, the more saturated the fat becomes.

Research indicates that trans fats may raise your total cholesterol and "bad" cholesterol level, and lower your high-density lipoprotein (HDL) cholesterol (the "good" cholesterol) level. Some of the main sources of trans fats include margarine and vegetable shortening, as well as products made from them, such as cookies, desserts, crackers and other prepared foods.

Reduce fat and cholesterol intake
Keep all types of fat — saturated, polyunsaturated, monounsaturated and trans fats — within a range of 25 percent to 30 percent of your daily calories. Use monounsaturated and polyunsaturated fats, which can help lower your LDL cholesterol level, to replace saturated fats.

In addition, limit your daily cholesterol intake to less than 200 milligrams. You can accomplish this goal by limiting or avoiding concentrated sources of cholesterol, such as fatty or heavily processed meats, egg yolks and whole milk products.

Try fat substitutes
Foods containing a certain type of micronutrient found in fruits and vegetables (plant sterols) may be useful in lowering cholesterol, when consumed as part of a diet low in saturated fat and cholesterol. These plant extracts imitate the role cholesterol plays in the molecular structure of foods but reduce the absorption of blood cholesterol in your body.

In 2000, the Food and Drug Administration approved the use of plant sterols in foods for the prevention of coronary artery disease. Several margarines that contain plant sterols or derivatives of plant sterols (plant stanols) are currently available.

Eat foods with soluble fiber
Soluble fiber can help lower your total blood cholesterol level. Foods high in soluble fiber include oat bran, oatmeal, beans, peas, rice bran, barley, citrus fruits, strawberries and apple pulp.

Consider soy products
Soy compounds called isoflavones mimic human hormones that regulate cholesterol levels. Eating soy proteins can lower total cholesterol, LDL cholesterol and triglycerides. It may also raise the level of potentially protective HDL cholesterol.

Eat more foods with antioxidants
Antioxidants may help prevent damage to the lining of your arteries by slowing oxidation, a chemical process that enables cells in your arteries to easily absorb fatty acids and LDL cholesterol. Antioxidants are found in many fruits and vegetables. A healthy diet should provide an adequate amount.

Drink alcohol in moderation, if at all
Moderate consumption of alcohol may raise your level of HDL cholesterol. On the other hand, alcohol increases your blood triglyceride level, so avoid it if you have a high level of triglycerides. If you do drink alcohol, limit yourself to one drink daily if you're a woman or no more than two a day if you're a man.

Exercise regularly
Regular physical activity, such as brisk walking, jogging, bicycling or cross-country skiing, helps increase

your level of HDL cholesterol. An exercise program can also help you lose weight, which in turn decreases your risk of cardiovascular disease.

Don't smoke
Cigarette smoking damages the walls of your blood vessels, making it easier for cholesterol to accumulate. It may also lower your level of HDL cholesterol.

Atherosclerosis

When fatty deposits (plaques) and other substances accumulate in your arteries and cause them to narrow, blood flow becomes restricted. This condition is called atherosclerosis. It's a leading cause of blockage of the blood vessels to your heart (coronary arteries), which can result in a heart attack or chest pain (angina).

When the inner wall of an artery is injured, blood cells called platelets often clump at microscopic sites of injury. At these sites, fatty deposits also collect. Initially, the deposits are only streaks of fat-containing cells, but as they progress, they invade some deeper layers of the arterial walls, causing scarring and calcium deposits. Larger accumulations of plaques are the principal characteristic of atherosclerosis.

Complications
The greatest danger from these deposits is the narrowing of the channel through which the blood flows. When this occurs, body tissues supplied by an affected artery don't receive their full quota of blood, particularly during exercise, when demand is greatest. Pieces of the fatty deposits may dislodge, travel with the blood flow and obstruct an artery at some distant point — a condition called arterial embolism.

Atherosclerosis is one form of arteriosclerosis, but the two terms are often used interchangeably. The term *arteriosclerosis* refers to hardening of the arteries. As calcium is

Cholesterol Medications

If lifestyle changes aren't sufficient to lower your total cholesterol, especially your low-density lipoprotein (LDL) cholesterol (the "bad" cholesterol), to a desirable level, your doctor may recommend a prescription medication.

In making such a recommendation, a doctor often weighs many variables — your lifestyle, age, current health and the medication's side effects. After treatment begins, your doctor will likely monitor your blood fat levels with periodic blood tests to judge the treatment's effectiveness and to determine if additional measures are needed, such as increasing your medication dosage or changing the type of medication.

Medications used to lower cholesterol and triglycerides include:

Statins
Statins interfere with the body's synthesis of cholesterol by blocking a substance your liver needs to make cholesterol. This depletes cholesterol in your liver cells, which causes them to remove cholesterol from your blood. These medications are particularly effective in reducing total cholesterol and LDL cholesterol. Statins may even promote the reabsorption of existing cholesterol deposits, which would help to unplug clogged arteries.

Statins include fluvastatin (Lescol), lovastatin (Mevacor), simvastatin (Zocor), pravastatin (Pravachol) and atorvastatin (Lipitor). These medications are generally safe, effective and well tolerated. However, they aren't recommended if you have significant liver disease.

Bile acid sequestrants
The medications cholestyramine (Questran), colestipol (Colestid) and colesevelam (Welchol) lower cholesterol by binding to bile acids in the intestinal tract, thereby causing the liver to increase its manufacture of bile acids. Because the liver uses cholesterol to make bile acids, increased production of bile acids means an increased need for cholesterol by the liver. This, in turn, means that less cholesterol remains in your blood.

Like all medications intended for control of blood fats, these must be used daily, for months and years, to have a favorable effect on atherosclerosis. These medications tend to cause constipation and bloating.

Nicotinic acid
Nicotinic acid (niacin) is one of the vitamin B complex. When taken in amounts far higher than needed for its vitamin function, it becomes a medication. It has a favorable effect on triglycerides, high-density lipoprotein (HDL) cholesterol and LDL cholesterol. It's inexpensive but has the drawbacks of causing flushing, changes in liver function test results and a tendency toward diabetes and gout. Taking aspirin 20 to 30 minutes before taking nicotinic acid may lessen flushing.

Fibric acids
Fibric acids include gemfibrozil (Lopid) and fenofibrate (Tricor). These medications are more convenient to take than nicotinic acid and, like nicotinic acid, have a favorable effect on HDL cholesterol, triglycerides and LDL cholesterol. Side effects may include some adverse intestinal effects. These medications generally shouldn't be taken with statins, as the combination of the two increases the risk of muscle inflammation.

Cardiovascular Disease: Men vs. Women

Women sometimes think that concerns about cardiovascular disease don't really affect them. True, men tend to develop heart disease earlier than women do. However, over time, women and men are equally likely to die of a heart attack.

Until puberty, males and females have roughly the same level of "good" — high-density lipoprotein (HDL) — cholesterol. However, during puberty, the level of HDL cholesterol in males decreases, making them more susceptible to cardiovascular disease.

In females, the hormone estrogen tends to increase the level of "good" cholesterol and lower the level of "bad" — low-density lipoprotein (LDL) — cholesterol, thus providing a potentially protective effect against cardiovascular disease. Following menopause, when estrogen levels are decreased, women become increasingly likely to have heart attacks and related problems.

Before the age of 60, men are the most likely candidates for heart attack. After age 60, the difference in risk between men and women narrows. However, these patterns could change. Due to an increase in the number of women who smoke, women are beginning to experience heart attacks at earlier ages.

deposited in an artery, its walls may become more rigid or hardened. Sometimes, arteries in the forearms can be felt and may resemble small, hard pipes.

To some extent, your body can protect itself from narrowing of an artery by gradually developing additional arterial connections that detour blood around the narrowed point. This is called collateral circulation.

If you have a significant amount of atherosclerosis in one part of your body, you're more likely to have some degree of the disease in another part. For instance, a person who has poor arterial circulation in his or her legs is more vulnerable to angina or a heart attack because of similar narrowing of the coronary arteries.

For more information on the treatment of atherosclerosis, see page 753. Treatment may involve procedures to open narrowed segments of your arteries or surgery to bypass the plaques, as well as steps to control further accumulations of plaques through dietary measures and, possibly, use of medication.

High blood pressure

Your blood pressure is the force that's exerted on your artery walls as blood passes through. You might compare it to the pressure inside a garden hose. Your heart, arteries and kidneys all work together to control the amount of pressure put on your artery walls. When this complex system malfunctions, too much pressure can develop within your arteries. If this condition continues on a persistent basis, it's called high blood pressure (hypertension). Often, high blood pressure causes no symptoms.

Complications

High blood pressure is an important risk factor for cardiovascular disease. Left uncontrolled over a period of years, high blood pressure can damage arteries throughout your body so that their walls become thickened and stiff (arteriosclerosis) and obstructed (atherosclerosis), thus decreasing blood flow to vital organs.

Your body responds to this threat by increasing blood pressure to maintain an adequate flow of blood. The increase in blood pressure in turn results in further blood vessel damage, setting a vicious cycle in motion. This cycle exacts a toll on your heart, too, because your heart is forced to work harder. The heart muscle may thicken — called cardiac hypertrophy — to accommodate its added load. Aside from affecting your heart, long-term complications of high blood pressure can affect your kidneys, eyes and brain.

For information on diagnosis and treatment of high blood pressure,

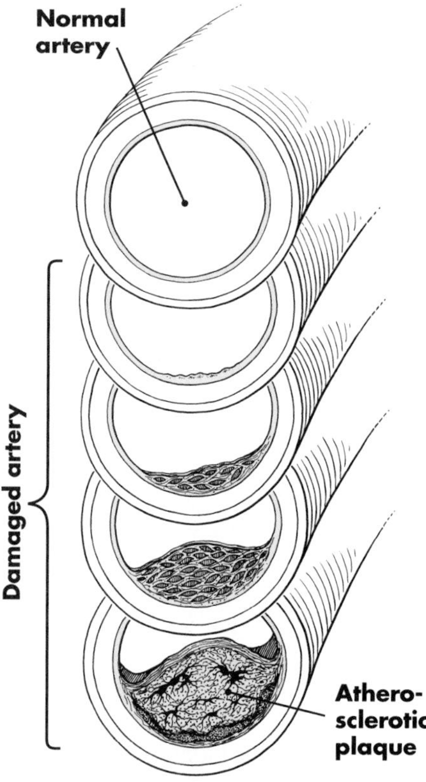

Atherosclerotic fatty deposits (plaques) gradually develop in the lining of the arteries. As plaques form, blood circulation decreases. This increases the risk of heart attack, stroke and other serious vascular problems.

see page 740. Many of its complications can be avoided with proper management, which may include medications and lifestyle changes.

Diabetes

Diabetes is characterized by a lack of insulin or your body's resistance to this hormone, resulting in the body's inability to process sugars found in your diet. The use of insulin and other medications has made the disease manageable, but diabetes remains an important risk factor for cardiovascular disease.

Complications

Increased blood sugar (glucose) levels are often accompanied by increased blood fat levels and blood vessel problems. Men with diabetes have about twice the normal risk of coronary artery disease, and women with diabetes have five times the risk. An individual with diabetes who smokes is at particularly high risk of cardiovascular disease.

If you have diabetes, careful management of your blood sugar levels can reduce your risk of heart and blood vessel problems. For more information on diabetes, see Chapter 32, "Endocrine System."

Family history

Your genes help determine your risk of developing cardiovascular disease, but heredity factors are complex. In simple terms, if one of your parents or another close relative had a heart attack at a young age — for a man, younger than age 55, and for a woman, younger than age 65 — then your risk of coronary artery disease is significantly greater than that of someone with no family history of cardiac problems. This doesn't mean that you're destined to suffer the same fate. It argues strongly, though, for taking every preventive advantage offered to minimize the risk factors that you can control.

If you don't have a family history of cardiovascular disease, you can still develop the condition. Therefore, individuals without a strong genetic link also need to pay attention to cardiovascular risk factors.

Emerging risk factors

As researchers gain a better understanding of cardiovascular disease and its causes and treatment, other potential risk factors are emerging. If you have a strong family history of cardiovascular disease, your doctor may recommend monitoring one or more of the following blood substances:

Homocysteine

Homocysteine is a natural byproduct of your body's use of protein. Research indicates a relationship between high homocysteine levels in your blood and increased risk of coronary artery disease. Folic acid and vitamins B-6 and B-12 can help lower homocysteine levels, although it hasn't yet been proved that such treatment decreases risk of coronary artery disease.

Lipoprotein lipase

Lipoprotein lipase is an enzyme that regulates the metabolism of lipids and lipoproteins. The way it operates isn't well understood. Some evidence links elevated levels of lipoprotein lipase in the blood to premature heart attack.

C-reactive protein

The level of C-reactive protein (CRP) in your blood increases when inflammation is present. Some studies show that the process of inflammation — your body's reaction to injury — plays a role in the buildup of fatty deposits (plaques) in your arteries (atherosclerosis). If this is true, then an elevated CRP level may be an indicator of atherosclerosis and a potential predictor for first heart attacks.

Fibrinogen

Fibrinogen is a protein made by the liver that's important in blood clotting. In some studies, an elevated

? Question and Answer

Should I take a daily aspirin to reduce my risk of heart problems?

It's well-known that aspirin inhibits platelets, blood cells that contribute to clotting. By doing this, aspirin reduces the tendency of blood to clot. Thus, it may help reduce or prevent narrowing of your blood vessels due to atherosclerosis. Your doctor may recommend that you take an aspirin daily:

- If you have a cardiovascular condition such as atherosclerosis, angina, high blood pressure or atrial fibrillation, each of which puts you at increased risk of a heart attack or stroke
- To avoid a second heart attack
- If you've had a coronary artery bypass operation, to reduce the likelihood that the bypass grafts will become blocked by a blood clot and accumulation of plaques

Taken in low doses, aspirin is inexpensive, generally safe and easy to take. But if you don't have cardiovascular disease, it's not clear that aspirin offers any benefits for your heart and blood vessels. Aspirin can cause stomach irritation and bleeding, although that's uncommon when it's taken in low doses. This risk can be decreased by taking coated aspirin, which dissolves in your small intestine rather than your stomach. Discuss daily aspirin use with your doctor.

level of fibrinogen in the blood has been associated with a greater risk of cardiovascular disease. Other cardiovascular risk factors, including smoking, advancing age, obesity, physical inactivity and high cholesterol levels, seem to increase the fibrinogen level. This indicates that controlling other risk factors may also help to control the level of fibrinogen.

Although these factors seem to provide new information about cardiovascular disease, more research is needed to establish their relationship with the workings of the heart and blood vessels. In addition, the methods used to measure these substances in the blood require further investigation and fine-tuning.

High Blood Pressure

Throughout this book, medical disorders are generally accompanied by a list of their signs and symptoms. With high blood pressure, that approach doesn't work. Most people with high blood pressure have no symptoms. Even a doctor can't readily tell that you have high blood pressure until he or she actually measures the pressure of the blood flow in your arteries. Some people think that headaches, dizziness and nosebleeds are signs and symptoms of high blood pressure, but this isn't necessarily true.

High blood pressure and *hypertension* are interchangeable terms that refer to a condition in which your blood is traveling through your arteries at a pressure that's too high for good health. The incidence of high blood pressure increases with age. High blood pressure is more common in blacks than in whites or Hispanics. More men than women have high blood pressure in young adulthood and early middle age. Thereafter the situation reverses.

Although high blood pressure generally doesn't produce any symptoms, this doesn't mean that it's not dangerous. High blood pressure is often called the silent killer because about one in four adult Americans have it, but a third of them aren't aware of their condition. The risk lies in the long-term damage the ailment can produce. High blood pressure is a leading cause of stroke, heart attack, heart failure, kidney failure, dementia and premature death.

The past 30 years have brought important advances in detecting and treating high blood pressure. Greater attention to this illness is one of the main reasons that deaths from stroke have gone down about 60 percent and deaths from heart and blood vessel (cardiovascular) disease are down more than 50 percent. Still, only half of all Americans with high blood pressure are receiving treatment, and only about a fourth have their blood pressure under control.

There's no cure for high blood pressure, but the condition is both preventable and treatable. Lifestyle adjustments and medication, if necessary, can help you control your blood pressure and keep it at a safe level.

? Question and Answer

What causes an adrenaline rush?

One of the most significant hormones to affect blood pressure is adrenaline (epinephrine). Adrenaline is released into your body during periods of high stress or tension, such as when you're frightened or in a hurry. When this happens, your arteries narrow, and your heart contractions become stronger and faster, increasing pressure in your arteries. The feeling created by the release of this hormone is often referred to as an adrenaline rush.

Blood pressure basics

Blood pressure is determined by the amount of blood your heart pumps out and the resistance to this blood flow within your arteries. Organs and substances that help to regulate blood pressure include:

Your heart

The pumping action of your heart needs to create a certain amount of force in order to eject blood into your main artery (aorta). The harder your heart muscle has to work to eject the blood, the greater the force exerted on your arteries.

Your arteries

To accommodate the surge of blood with each heartbeat, your arteries are lined with smooth muscles that allow them to expand and then contract as blood courses through. The more elastic your arteries are, the less resistant they are to the flow of blood and the less force that's exerted on their walls. When arteries lose their elasticity or they become narrowed, resistance to blood flow increases, and additional force is needed to push blood through the vessels.

Your kidneys

Your kidneys regulate the amount of sodium your body retains and hence the volume of water circulating in your body. Sodium retains water. Therefore, the more sodium that's in your body, the more water that's contained in your blood. This extra fluid in blood can increase blood pressure.

Others

Other organs and substances that influence blood pressure include your central nervous system and many hormones and enzymes. Within the walls of your heart and various blood vessels, tiny structures called baroreceptors continuously monitor your blood flow and send signals to your brain regarding the status of your blood pressure. The brain responds by

Blood Pressure Classifications

	Systolic pressure (mm Hg*)		Diastolic pressure (mm Hg)
Optimal†	lower than 120	and	lower than 80
Normal	lower than 130	and	lower than 85
High-normal	130-139	or	85-89
High			
Stage 1‡	140-159	or	90-99
Stage 2‡	160-179	or	100-109
Stage 3‡	180 or higher	or	110 or higher

*Millimeters of mercury
†Optimal pressure with respect to cardiovascular risk.
‡Based on the average of two or more readings taken at each of two or more visits after an initial screening.

signaling the release of hormones and enzymes that affect the functioning of your heart, blood vessels and kidneys.

Measuring your blood pressure

Your blood pressure is measured with a sphygmomanometer. The device includes an inflatable cuff that's wrapped around your upper arm, an air pump and a standardized pressure gauge or electronic meter.

Blood pressure is expressed as two numbers in units of millimeters of mercury (mm Hg). For example, a blood pressure below 120/80 mm Hg (120 over 80) is ideal (optimal). The number on top is the systolic pressure — the amount of pressure in your arteries when your heart contracts and forces blood into the aorta. The number on the bottom is the diastolic pressure, the pressure that remains in your arteries between beats when your heart muscle is relaxing and filling with blood. During this time, your blood pressure decreases.

Your blood pressure normally fluctuates throughout the day. It increases during periods of activity and decreases when your body is at rest. Before you receive a diagnosis of high blood pressure, usually your doctor determines your average blood pressure by taking two or more readings at each of two or more visits after an initial screening.

Normal vs. high blood pressure
A newborn's blood pressure is usually about 90/60 mm Hg. During childhood, it slowly increases. For an adult, the normal range of blood pressure extends from 120/80 mm Hg up to 139/89 mm Hg. However, a systolic blood pressure between 130 and 139 mm Hg and a diastolic pressure between 85 and 89 mm Hg are considered high-normal. High-normal blood pressure can increase your risk of cardiovascular disease.

Your blood pressure is considered high if your systolic pressure is consistently 140 mm Hg or higher or your diastolic pressure is consistently 90 mm Hg or higher, or both. In the past, diastolic pressure was assumed to be a better indicator of potential heath risks than systolic pressure. But recent long-term studies have shown that a high systolic reading is an equally important — if not more serious — risk factor, especially in older adults.

High blood pressure is separated into three stages, based on increasing severity, with stage 3 being the most serious. The terms *mild* and *moderate* are no longer used to describe levels of high blood pressure so that people won't mistakenly dismiss mild or moderate high blood pressure as not a serious health threat.

High blood pressure usually develops gradually. In most instances, people start out with normal blood pressure that slowly progress to high-normal blood pressure and, eventually, to stage 1 high blood pressure.

If untreated, this excessive pressure can damage many of your organs and tissues. The higher your blood pressure stage, the greater the risk that damage will occur. However, even stage 1 high blood pressure can be harmful if it continues over months to years.

Causes

In about 95 percent of people with high blood pressure, no cause can be found. The condition of these people is categorized as essential hypertension.

In the few cases where the cause can be clearly established, the term *secondary hypertension* is used because the increased pressure is the result of some other condition or factor. These might include:

- Over-the-counter cold remedies, nasal decongestants, appetite suppressants, nonsteroidal anti-inflammatory drugs (NSAIDs) and prescription medications such as oral contraceptives, steroids, tricyclic antidepressants and sibutramine (Meridia) taken for obesity.
- Kidney disorders such as kidney failure, kidney artery narrowing (stenosis) and inflammation of the glomeruli (glomerulonephritis)
- Adrenal gland overactivity
- Thyroid problems
- Blood vessel abnormalities
- Preeclampsia, a complication of pregnancy
- Illicit drug use

Sometimes, if the primary problem is taken care of, the secondary hypertension goes away.

Complications

The symptoms of high blood pressure are silent, but the dangers are very real. Left untreated over a period of years, high blood pressure can damage various body organs. Heart attack, heart failure, kidney failure, stroke, dementia and loss of vision are some of the complications that can result.

Coronary artery disease

The major cause of death in people with high blood pressure is coronary artery disease. High blood pressure accelerates the buildup of fatty deposits (plaques) in your arteries and leads to narrowing of these blood vessels (atherosclerosis). If the arteries that supply blood to the heart muscle become obstructed, the heart muscle is deprived of oxygen, and a heart attack may occur.

When blood pressure is elevated, the heart is forced to work harder to maintain blood flow to the tissues. Over time, the heart muscle may thicken (hypertrophy) in order to keep pushing blood out of the heart against increased resistance.

The left ventricle is the chamber of the heart that pumps blood to other parts of the body, except for the lungs. Thus, this muscle thickening is called left ventricular hypertrophy. Left ventricular hypertrophy is associated with a higher risk of sudden death and heart attack.

Over time, high blood pressure can also cause the heart muscle (myocardium) to wear out, and congestive heart failure may result. With this condition, your heart can't push forward all of the fluid returning to it from your veins. Fluid accumulates in your lungs, legs and other tissues.

Controlling your blood pressure can greatly reduce your risk of these cardiovascular diseases. If blood pressure is controlled for at least 5 years, your risk of heart attack decreases by about 20 percent, and your risk of heart failure by more than 50 percent.

Stroke

A stroke is when a blood vessel in the brain ruptures (cerebral hemorrhage) or a fragment of an atherosclerotic plaque breaks free and blocks blood flow to part of the brain (cerebral embolism) or a clot forms in an artery in the brain (cerebral thrombosis).

Strokes are much more common in people with high blood pressure. In fact, high blood pressure is the most important risk factor for stroke. When blood pressure is decreased by appropriate treatment, the risk of stroke is decreased as well — about 40 percent over 2 to 5 years.

Dementia

Research indicates that high blood pressure can lead to significant memory impairment (dementia). Studies reveal that the onset of dementia varies from a few years to several decades following diagnosis of high blood pressure. There's increasing evidence that drug treatment to lower elevated blood pressure may lower this risk. Further research is still necessary to confirm an association between high blood pressure and dementia.

Isolated Systolic Hypertension

If the top number in your blood pressure reading (systolic blood pressure) is consistently high (140 mm Hg or above) but your bottom number (diastolic blood pressure) is in the normal range (lower than 85 mm Hg), you may have isolated systolic hypertension (ISH). This condition affects about two-thirds of the people over age 60 with high blood pressure.

Doctors once thought that ISH was a harmless result of aging and were reluctant to treat it because of a lack of evidence of benefits and the risk of possible side effects, along with the cost of treatment. However, several studies have shown that treating this form of high blood pressure can prevent thousands of strokes and other severe cardiovascular problems each year.

If you've received a diagnosis of ISH, get accurate, regular readings of your blood pressure. Ask your doctor about medications to control the problem and follow the prescription carefully. Address the lifestyle factors that can add to your risk of ISH: smoking, obesity, a high-sodium diet, lack of regular exercise and the use of alcohol.

Kidney disease

About one-fifth of the blood dispersed to your body with each pump of your heart goes to your kidneys. The kidneys filter waste products from the blood and help to maintain a proper balance of salts, acids and water in your blood.

High blood pressure can injure your kidneys and impair their ability to perform normal functions, one of which is to help control blood pressure. So damage to these organs can worsen high blood pressure. This leads to a destructive cycle that, ultimately, results in increasing blood pressure and less ability of the kidneys to remove impurities from the blood.

Lifestyle changes

Although the precise cause of high blood pressure many times remains

Risk Factors

Certain genetic traits and lifestyle habits can increase your chances of developing high blood pressure. Generally, the more of these risk factors that you have, the greater your odds of having high blood pressure during your lifetime. By managing risk factors that are controllable, you can reduce your risk.

Uncontrollable risk factors

Risk factors you can't change include:

Race

High blood pressure occurs more frequently in blacks than in whites and Hispanics. In blacks, high blood pressure generally develops at an earlier age, is more severe and tends to progress more rapidly.

Age

Your risk of high blood pressure increases with age, particularly among Americans age 65 and older.

Family history

If high blood pressure is common in your family, your chances of developing it are increased.

Sex

Among young and middle-aged adults, men are more likely to have high blood pressure than women are. After about age 50, when most women are beyond menopause, high blood pressure becomes more common in women than in men.

Controllable risk factors

Risk factors that you can change include:

Obesity

Excess body mass requires more blood to supply tissues with oxygen and nutrients. More blood flowing through your blood vessels creates extra force on artery walls.

Inactivity

Lack of physical activity increases your risk of being overweight, which increases your risk of high blood pressure. People who are inactive also tend to have higher heart rates, and their hearts work harder to pump blood.

Tobacco use

Nicotine makes your heart work harder by temporarily constricting your blood vessels and increasing your heart rate and blood pressure. In addition, carbon monoxide in cigarette smoke replaces oxygen in your blood, causing your heart to work harder to supply adequate oxygen to your body's organs and tissues.

Sensitivity to sodium

People who are sodium sensitive retain sodium more easily, leading to fluid retention and increased blood pressure. Salt is a major source of sodium.

Low potassium intake

Potassium helps balance the amount of sodium in your body. If your diet doesn't include enough potassium or your body isn't able to retain a proper amount, too much sodium can accumulate, increasing your risk of high blood pressure.

Excessive alcohol consumption

Excessive alcohol use contributes to about 8 percent of all cases of high blood pressure. How or why it increases blood pressure isn't clear.

Stress

Stress doesn't cause persistent high blood pressure, but a high level of stress can lead to temporary, dramatic increases in blood pressure. If these temporary episodes occur often enough, they can eventually damage your blood vessels, heart and kidneys in the same manner as persistent high blood pressure.

Chronic illness

Certain illnesses can contribute to increased blood pressure or make high blood pressure more difficult to control. These include atherosclerosis, diabetes, sleep apnea and heart failure.

unknown, the condition can often be effectively treated. With proper medical attention and advice, most or all of the potentially dire consequences of high blood pressure can be avoided

Depending on your blood pressure, your doctor may begin your treatment by recommending lifestyle changes alone or lifestyle changes with medication.

Even with drug treatment, making changes in your daily habits are important to managing your disease. Lifestyle adjustments may include losing weight, adjusting your diet, restricting use of alcohol and caffeine, quitting smoking and increasing your level of physical activity.

Physical activity

Physical activity is important in controlling your blood pressure because it makes your heart stronger. Your heart is able to pump more blood with less effort. The less your heart has to work to pump blood, the less force that's exerted on your arteries.

Aerobic activity that increases your heart rate and need for oxygen has the greatest beneficial effect on blood pressure. As your body becomes accustomed to this level of activity, your heart becomes stronger, and your blood pressure drops. Regular aerobic activity can reduce your blood pressure by 5 to 10 mm Hg. It can also help with weight loss.

For more information on becoming more physically active, see Chapter 4, "Keeping Active."

Diet

Eating a nutritionally balanced diet also benefits your blood pressure. And eating well doesn't mean focusing on calories and giving up all of your favorite foods. Rather, it means enjoying a variety of foods that help to ensure the right mix of nutrients your body needs to be healthy. Emphasizing plenty of grains, fruits, vegetables and low-fat dairy foods can help you control your blood pressure and possibly avoid the need for medication.

The DASH diet

A 1997 study called Dietary Approaches to Stop Hypertension (DASH) compared three diets among 459 people. The group included people with high blood pressure and those with high-normal blood pressure at risk of developing high blood pressure.

Of the three diets in the study, one matched the typical American diet — low in fruits, vegetables and dairy products, and a fat content that accounted for 37 percent of total calories. Another diet stressed fruits and vegetables but didn't control intake of dairy products or fat. The third diet, called the combination diet, stressed fruits and vegetables plus ample grains and low-fat dairy products. Fat was kept to less than 30 percent of calories.

By the end of the study, both the fruit-and-vegetable diet and the combination diet lowered blood

Stocking Your Kitchen

You'll be able to find everything you need for the DASH diet at a well-stocked supermarket. Having the right ingredients at your fingertips makes it easier to whip up healthy dishes. Here are some examples of foods to stock up on:

Dairy products
- Low-fat or fat-free milk
- Low-fat or reduced-fat cottage cheese or ricotta
- Reduced-fat cheeses
- Reduced-fat or fat-free sour cream
- Tub or squeeze margarine

Grains
- Bread, bagels and pita bread
- Low-fat flour tortillas
- Plain cereal
- Brown or white rice
- Pasta

Fruit
- Standard fresh varieties
- Seasonal fresh fruits
- Canned fruit in juice or water
- Frozen fruit without added sugar
- Dried fruit

Vegetables
- Standard fresh varieties
- Seasonal fresh vegetables
- Frozen vegetables without added butter or sauces
- Canned tomato products low in sodium
- Canned vegetables or vegetable soups low in sodium

Legumes
- Lentils
- Black beans
- Red (kidney) beans
- Navy beans
- Chickpeas (garbanzos)

Meat
- White meat, skinless chicken and turkey
- Unbreaded fish
- Pork tenderloin
- Extra-lean ground beef
- Round or sirloin beef cuts

Baking items
- Imitation butter, flakes or buds
- Nonstick cooking spray
- Canned evaporated milk, fat-free or reduced-fat
- Cocoa powder, unsweetened
- Angel food cake mix

Condiments, seasonings and spreads
- Low-fat or fat-free salad dressings
- Herbs
- Spices
- Flavored vinegars
- Salsa or picante sauce

The DASH Diet

Food	Benefits	Serving examples
Grains 7-8 daily servings*	Grains include breads, cereals, rice and pasta. In addition to being low in fat, grains are rich in complex carbohydrates and nutrients. Whole grains provide even more fiber and nutrients than refined varieties do. Avoid adding high-fat toppings to your breads and pasta, such as butter and sauces made with cream and cheese. Instead, choose fruit spreads or honey for your breads and use fresh vegetable or tomato-based toppings for your pasta.	• ½ cup (3 oz.) cooked cereal, rice or pasta • ½ cup (1 oz.) ready-to-eat cereal • 1 slice whole-grain sandwich bread • ½ bagel or English muffin
Fruits and vegetables 8-10 daily servings	Fruits and vegetables are virtually fat-free and low in calories, so load up on these. They also provide fiber and a variety of nutrients, including potassium and magnesium, as well as phytochemicals, substances that can reduce your risk of cardiovascular disease and some cancers. Replacing high-fat, high-calorie foods with fruits and vegetables is an easy way to improve your diet without cutting back on your portions. Just don't smother them with dips or sauces that contain a lot of fat.	• ¼ cup (1½ oz.) raisins • ¾ cup (6 fl. oz.) 100% fruit juice • 1 medium apple, banana or other fruit • 12 grapes • 1 cup (2 oz.) raw leafy green vegetables • ½ cup (3 oz.) cooked vegetables • 1 medium potato
Dairy products 2-3 daily servings	Dairy products are key sources of calcium, vitamin D and protein, but they can be high in fat. Choose low-fat or fat-free varieties. This way you'll get the health benefits minus the fat.	• 1 cup (8 fl. oz.) low-fat or fat-free milk or 1 cup (8 oz.) yogurt • 1½ oz. reduced-fat or fat-free cheese
Meat, poultry and fish 2 or fewer daily servings	Meat, poultry and fish are rich in protein, B vitamins, iron and zinc. Choose lean cuts, such as tenderloin, round or sirloin. Remove all visible fat from meats and skin from poultry. Fish is one of the leanest animal proteins you can choose. The fat it does contain is mainly omega-3 fatty acids, which may help lower your blood pressure, thin your blood and reduce your risk of blood clots.	• 2-3 oz. cooked skinless poultry, seafood or lean meat
Legumes, nuts and seeds 4-5 servings a week	Legumes include beans, dried peas and lentils, which are low in fat, contain no cholesterol and are an excellent source of protein. They also provide a variety of nutrients, including magnesium, potassium, phytochemicals and fiber. Although nuts and seeds contain fat, most of it is monounsaturated, the type that may help protect against coronary artery disease.	• ½ cup (3½ oz.) cooked legumes • ¼ cup (1 oz.) seeds • ⅓ cup (1 oz.) nuts

*Serving amounts are based on a diet of 2,000 calories a day. Most Americans need between 1,600 and 2,400 calories daily, depending on age and activity. To include fewer or more servings, talk to a registered dietitian.

Source: Adapted from National Institutes of Health, 1997

Shaking Out the Sodium

Here are some ways to reduce sodium in your diet:

- *Eat more fresh and fewer processed foods.* Fresh foods usually have less sodium than processed foods.
- *Look for lower-sodium products.* Some processed foods that are typically high in sodium, such as soups, broths, canned vegetables and condiments, are also prepared in lower-sodium versions.
- *Read labels.* Read the nutrition facts labels on food products that you're considering purchasing or consuming. Each label tells you how much sodium is in a serving of that particular product.
- *Don't add salt to food.* If you think your food needs more flavor, try another seasoning, such as lemon, pepper, cilantro or other herbs and spices.
- *Limit your use of condiments.* Salad dressings, sauces, dips, ketchup, mustard and relish all contain sodium. So do pickles and olives.
- *Rinse canned foods.* Rinsing canned vegetables and meats helps to remove about one-third of the sodium.

Before you try a salt substitute, check with your doctor. Some salt substitutes or "lite" salts contain a mixture of sodium chloride (salt) and other compounds. To achieve that familiar salty taste, you may end up using more of the salt substitute than you do regular salt and not reducing your sodium intake.

In addition, potassium chloride is a common ingredient in salt substitutes. Too much potassium can be harmful if you have kidney problems or if you're taking certain high blood pressure or heart failure medications. Check with your doctor before using a salt substitute.

pressure. But the combination produced the most dramatic results. People with high blood pressure on the combination diet experienced an average decrease of 11.4 mm Hg in systolic pressure and 5.5 mm Hg in diastolic pressure, which is about the same effect as achieved with some medications.

Although researchers aren't certain why the combination diet fared better, they believe it may be because the diet promotes weight loss and because it's rich in potassium, calcium and magnesium, minerals linked with lower blood pressure.

A follow-up study called the DASH-Sodium study found that reductions in sodium consumption reduced blood pressure even further.

Reducing sodium

Sodium plays a critical role in maintaining the right balance of fluids in the body. It also helps to transmit nerve impulses that influence contraction and relaxation of muscles.

If too much sodium accumulates in your blood, blood volume increases because sodium attracts and holds water. Your heart has to work harder to move the increased volume of blood through blood vessels, increasing pressure on your arteries. Some people are simply more sensitive to high levels of sodium in their blood. You're more likely to be sodium sensitive if you're black, age 65 or older or have diabetes.

There's been some controversy over whether salt restriction can help to reduce blood pressure. Some studies have found little to support this theory. Other studies, including the DASH-Sodium study published in 2001, indicate that reducing sodium does reduce blood pressure.

The National High Blood Pressure Education Program, sponsored by the National Institutes of Health, recommends that all Americans limit sodium to no more than 2,400 milligrams a day. Its position is that the bulk of evidence suggests that limiting sodium is reasonable and safe. Many health professionals and organizations also support a reduced-sodium diet.

If you have high blood pressure and you're sodium sensitive, consuming less sodium can help lower your blood pressure. Limiting sodium in combination with other lifestyle changes may be enough to keep you off medication. Even if you take blood pressure medication, limiting sodium can help the medication be more effective.

Weight control

If you have high blood pressure — or if you're at increased risk of it — it's not critical that you become "thin." But you should try to achieve and maintain a weight that improves control of your blood pressure and lessens your risk of other health problems. In general, blood pressure increases with weight gain and decreases with weight loss.

If your body mass index (BMI) is 25 or more, try to lose some weight (see BMI chart on page 39). Losing as few as 10 pounds may reduce your blood pressure significantly. For some people, weight loss alone is enough to avoid blood pressure medication.

To learn more about achieving a healthy weight, see Chapter 3, "Controlling Your Weight."

Tobacco, alcohol and caffeine

High blood pressure combined with tobacco use increases the risk of fatty deposits in your arteries (atherosclerosis), a major risk factor for a heart attack.

Reducing use of alcohol may reduce your blood pressure. If you drink alcohol, limit your consumption to a moderate level. For most men, that generally means no more than two drinks a day. Moderate consumption for women is no more than one drink a day. For small-framed men and men older than age 65, a moderate level of alcohol is no more than one drink a day.

Caffeine may increase your blood pressure. If you have high blood pressure, limit daily caffeine to no more than two cups of coffee, four cups of tea or four cans of caffeinated soda. Also avoid caffeine right before activities that naturally increase your blood pressure, such as exercise or hard physical labor.

Stress

The effects of stress are usually only temporary. But if you experience stress regularly, it can produce increases in blood pressure that may gradually damage your arteries, heart, brain, kidneys and eyes. Changes in your daily routine and use of relaxation techniques may help you avoid or better cope with stress (see Chapter 5, "Managing Stress").

Medications

If you need medication to control your blood pressure, your doctor can determine which medication or combination of medications may be best suited for you.

Your doctor will take into consideration how a particular medication works and the fact that some medications work better than others in people of different ages or races. In addition, he or she will consider drug side effects, possible interactions with other medications and cost.

Diuretics

The first choice of medication, especially if you have stage 1 high blood pressure, may be a diuretic. Diuretics act on the kidneys to help your body eliminate sodium and water. This results in a smaller volume of blood pushing through your arteries and thus less pressure on your artery walls.

Diuretics have two distinct advantages: They've been proved effective over many years, and they're the least expensive of all the blood pressure medications. The three types of diuretics are thiazides, loop and potassium sparing.

Thiazides are the most common and include hydrochlorothiazide (Hydrodiuril, Microzide) and chlorothiazide (Diuril). Loop diuretics are more powerful and may be recommend if a thiazide isn't effective. They include bumetanide (Bumex), furosemide (Lasix) and torsemide (Demadex).

Potassium-sparing diuretics keep your body from losing too much potassium, but they aren't as powerful as the other two. They're often used in combination with thiazides and loop diuretics. Potassium-sparing diuretics include amiloride (Midamor), spironolactone (Aldactone) and eplerenone (Inspra).

A common effect of diuretics is increased urination. Other side effects may include dizziness and dehydration. High doses of thiazides can lead to slight increases in blood sugar (glucose) and total blood cholesterol.

If you have kidney disease, check with your doctor before taking potassium-sparing diuretics because they can raise your level of potassium, which could possibly lead to heart rhythm irregularities and other problems from excessive potassium.

Beta blockers

Beta blockers have been used for many years and are often a medication of choice for high blood pressure. They work by blocking many of the effects of adrenaline (epinephrine) in your body. The result is that your heart beats more slowly and less forcefully. In addition, they may provide a protective effect against repeat heart attacks.

A number of different types of beta blockers are used. Some common ones are atenolol (Tenormin), carvedilol (Coreg), metoprolol (Lopressor, Toprol), and propranolol (Inderal).

A common side effect of beta blockers is lethargy and fatigue. Certain beta blockers may slightly decrease your high-density lipoprotein (HDL) cholesterol (the "good" cholesterol).

Angiotensin-converting enzyme (ACE) inhibitors

Angiotensin-converting enzyme (ACE) inhibitors work by preventing the kidney's production of angiotensin II (A-II), a substance that constricts your blood vessels and potentially increases your blood pressure. By limiting the production of A-II, ACE inhibitors allow your blood vessels to dilate, and thus your blood pressure is decreased.

ACE inhibitors include captopril (Capoten), enalapril (Vasotec), lisinopril (Prinivil, Zestril) and quinapril (Accupril).

ACE inhibitors are often prescribed for people who also have impaired heart function because this type of drug can also reduce the risk of heart attack, stroke, heart failure and death due to cardiovascular disease. ACE inhibitors can also reduce the risk of diabetes and diabetes complications.

ACE inhibitors generally cause few side effects, but a number of people develop a dry, nagging cough. Other possible side effects of the medication include a rash, an altered sense of taste, reduced appetite and an elevated blood potassium level.

Swelling (edema) of deep skin tissues (angioedema) is a rare side effect and may be life-threatening if it affects the face or throat. ACE inhibitors aren't recommended if you're pregnant or plan to become pregnant because they can cause serious birth defects.

Angiotensin II receptor blockers

Angiotensin II (A-II) receptor blockers help relax and dilate blood vessels by blocking the action of A-II rather than its formation. They are effective in reducing kidney damage, stroke, left ventricular hypertrophy and other cardiovascular

Hypotension

Hypotension is low blood pressure. If blood pressure falls to dangerously low levels and blood can't be effectively circulated to vital tissues, shock occurs, a condition that can be life-threatening. Shock may result from significant loss of fluid or blood and, rarely, from serious infections. A major goal of emergency treatment for hypotension is to increase your blood pressure to more normal levels.

Chronic low blood pressure — when your blood pressure is below average but not symptomatically or dangerously so — isn't uncommon. It can be a normal finding or may result from medications given for high blood pressure. Conditions such as pregnancy, diabetes or arteriosclerosis also can produce low blood pressure.

One potentially dangerous type of low blood pressure is called postural hypotension. Dizziness or faintness that occurs on standing up quickly from a seated position is the key symptom. Typically, this type of low blood pressure isn't serious, but it may increase the risk of falls and injury. Taking precautions can help you to avoid danger: Stand up slowly from a seated position and wait a few seconds before walking. If episodes seem to occur after you've been in the sun for prolonged periods or after fasting, avoid such circumstances.

complications and the incidence of diabetes. Sometimes, A-II receptor blockers and ACE inhibitors are used in combination. An added benefit of A-II receptor blockers is that they don't produce a dry cough as often as ACE inhibitors do.

A-II receptor blockers include candesartan (Atacand), irbesartan (Avapro), losartan (Cozaar) and valsartan (Diovan).

Side effects are uncommon, but in a few cases the medication may cause dizziness, nasal congestion, back and leg pain, diarrhea, indigestion or insomnia. Like ACE inhibitors, these medications shouldn't be taken if you have severe kidney disease, are pregnant or are contemplating becoming pregnant.

Calcium channel blockers

These medications function by blocking the entry of calcium into your cells. This decreases the tendency of your small arteries to constrict. Some of these medications slow your heart rate as well.

There are two types of calcium channel blockers: short acting and long acting. Short-acting calcium channel blockers aren't recommended for treating high blood pressure because they generally don't control blood pressure as well as other drugs, and they've been linked to other health conditions.

Long-acting calcium channel blockers may not be as effective as other medications, and studies are underway to clarify their safety and effectiveness. Long-acting calcium channel blockers include amlodipine (Norvasc), felodipine (Plendil), nifedipine (Adalat, Procardia), diltiazem (Cardizem, Dilacor) and verapamil (Calan, Isoptin).

Possible side effects include constipation, headache, rapid heartbeat, rash and swelling in your lower extremities and gums. Don't drink grapefruit juice if you're taking calcium channel blockers. A substance in the juice interferes with your liver's ability to eliminate these medications from your body, which might allow them to build up to a toxic level.

Alpha blockers

Alpha blockers prevent muscle contractions in smaller arteries and reduce the effects of naturally occurring body chemicals that narrow blood vessels. The use of these medications is being re-evaluated because researchers found that the alpha blocker doxazosin (Cardura) provided less benefit than traditional diuretics, and a higher percentage of people taking doxazosin developed congestive heart failure.

It's recommended that alpha blockers be taken in combination with another blood pressure medication. Other alpha blockers are prazosin (Minipress) and terazosin (Hytrin). Side effects of alpha blockers include dizziness, headache, pounding heartbeat, nausea and weakness.

Central-acting agents

Central-acting agents prevent your brain from signaling your nervous system to increase your heart rate and constrict your blood vessels.

They aren't used as often as they once were because they can produce severe side effects. However, your doctor may recommend a central-acting agent if you're prone to panic attacks or you're going through alcohol or drug withdrawal. The medications can help reduce symptoms of these conditions.

Central-acting agents include clonidine (Catapres), guanfacine (Tenex) and methyldopa (Aldomet). Side effects may include extreme fatigue, impotence, dry mouth, headaches, weight gain, impaired thinking and depression.

Direct vasodilators

Direct vasodilators work directly on the muscles in the walls of your arteries, preventing the muscles from contracting and your arteries from narrowing. They're used mainly to treat severe high blood pressure that doesn't respond well to other medications. They include hydralazine and minoxidil (Loniten).

Common side effects of these medications include a fast heartbeat and retention of water. Because these effects are undesirable if you have high blood pressure, doctors often prescribe direct vasodilators with another medication such as a beta blocker and a diuretic, which can reduce symptoms.

Home monitoring

If you have high blood pressure, monitoring your blood pressure at home may be a necessary part of your treatment. A variety of devices to measure blood pressure (sphygmomanometers) are available. You can purchase a sphygmomanometer at a medical supply store or, usually, at a pharmacy.

When you're taking your blood pressure, it's important that you use proper technique. To get an accurate reading with an upper arm device, make sure that the cuff fits properly.

Before you purchase a sphygmomanometer, have your doctor or other health care professional measure your arm to determine the correct cuff size for you. Then after you buy one, bring it to your next appointment and ask your doctor or one of his or her staff to show you how to use it and make sure that it's working properly. Some health care facilities offer classes in home blood pressure monitoring.

If you use a home blood pressure monitor, verify its accuracy yearly. To do this, bring it to your doctor's office. If the reading is off more than 3 mm Hg, replace the unit.

Benefits

There are various benefits to monitoring your blood pressure yourself. For starters, it can help:

- *Track your treatment.* Because high blood pressure has no symptoms, the only way to make sure lifestyle changes or medications are working is to check your blood pressure regularly.
- *Promote better control.* When you take the initiative to measure your own blood pressure, this responsible act tends to rub off on other areas. It can give you added incentive to eat more healthfully, increase your activity level and take your medication properly.
- *Identify white-coat hypertension.* Simply going to a doctor's office can create stress in some people and increase their blood pressure (white-coat hypertension). Home monitoring can help determine if you have true high blood pressure or white-coat hypertension.
- *Save money.* Monitoring your blood pressure at home may save you the cost of going to your doctor's office to have your blood pressure taken. This is especially true when you first start to take medication or your doctor adjusts your medication. In these cases, frequent measurements help ensure better control.

Types of monitors

Not all blood pressure monitors are the same. Some are easier to use. Others are more reliable, and some are inaccurate and a waste of money.

Spring-gauge monitors

Spring-gauge monitors (aneroid manometers) are fitted over your upper arm and feature a round dial activated by a spring-pressure gauge. Each scale for the needle is set to match millimeters of mercury (mm Hg). They're the type most often used by your doctor or nurse.

Spring-gauge models are generally inexpensive and easy to transport. Some gauges are extra large, for easier reading, and some models have a built-in stethoscope for easier use.

Standard spring-gauge monitors aren't recommended if you have trouble hearing or if you have poor dexterity in your hands, because they require that you listen to a stethoscope and operate a bulb pump simultaneously.

Electronic monitors

Electronic (digital) monitors are the most popular and the easiest to use. They're also the most expensive, although the price is declining.

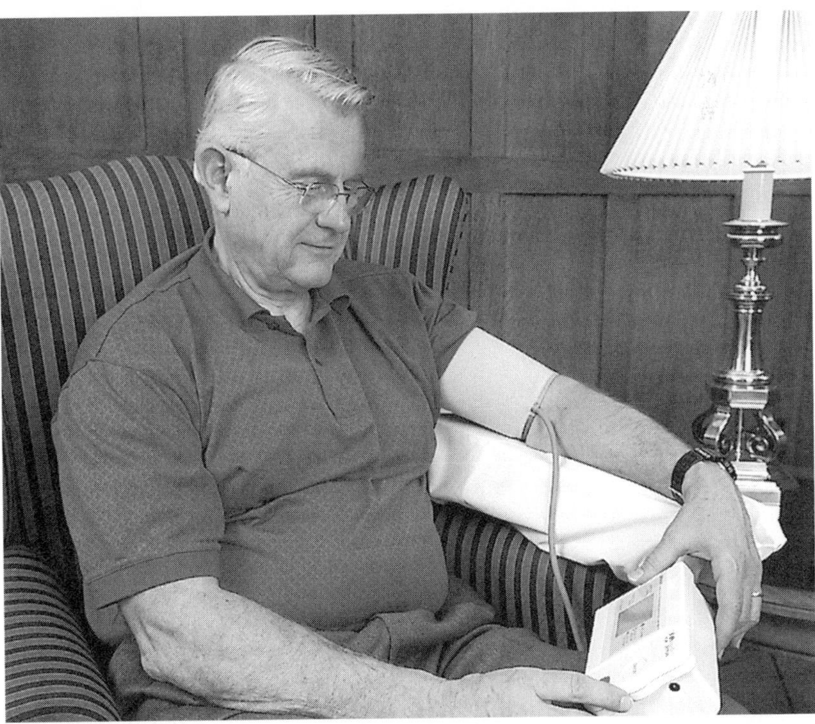

An electronic blood pressure monitor enables you to take your own blood pressure without the use of a stethoscope. Your blood pressure reading appears on a digital screen.

Taking Your Own Blood Pressure

Learning to take your blood pressure correctly isn't hard, but it takes training and a little practice. Here are some tips to improve the accuracy of your measurements:

- Don't measure your blood pressure right after you get up in the morning. Wait until after you've been active for an hour or more. If you exercise after you awaken, check your blood pressure before you exercise.
- Wait to measure your blood pressure for at least a half-hour after you've eaten, smoked or used caffeine or alcohol. All of these factors can increase your blood pressure.
- Empty your bladder first. A full bladder increases your blood pressure slightly.
- Sit quietly for about 5 minutes before taking a reading. Repeat once after several minutes.
- Remember that your blood pressure varies throughout the day. Readings are often a little higher in the morning. Your mood also can affect your blood pressure. If you've had a difficult day, don't be alarmed if your blood pressure reflects it.
- Measure your blood pressure at work as well as at home, to ensure that it remains in your target range. Keep in mind, though, that measurements taken at places other than at home tend to be slightly higher.

Electronic blood pressure monitors generally require that you do just two things: Put the cuff on your arm and push a button. The cuff automatically inflates with air and slowly deflates. Unlike spring-gauge models, electronic monitors detect artery motion, not sound. Your blood pressure measurements are displayed as numbers on a screen.

If you have an irregular heart rhythm, check with your doctor before purchasing an electronic monitor. It may give you inaccurate readings.

Finger or wrist monitors
Some models are available that measure blood pressure in your wrist or finger instead of your upper arm. This makes them more compact and easier to use but not as precise. Avoid the finger monitors because they're inaccurate. Wrist monitors are fairly accurate as long as you make sure your wrist is supported at the level of your heart when you take your measurement. It's more difficult to validate the accuracy of wrist monitors.

Coronary Artery Disease

Coronary artery disease causes more deaths, disability and economic loss than any other form of heart and blood vessel (cardiovascular) disease.

The condition often develops gradually and silently, typically over many years. In fact, it can go virtually unnoticed until it suddenly produces a heart attack. Approximately 1 million Americans have a heart attack each year,

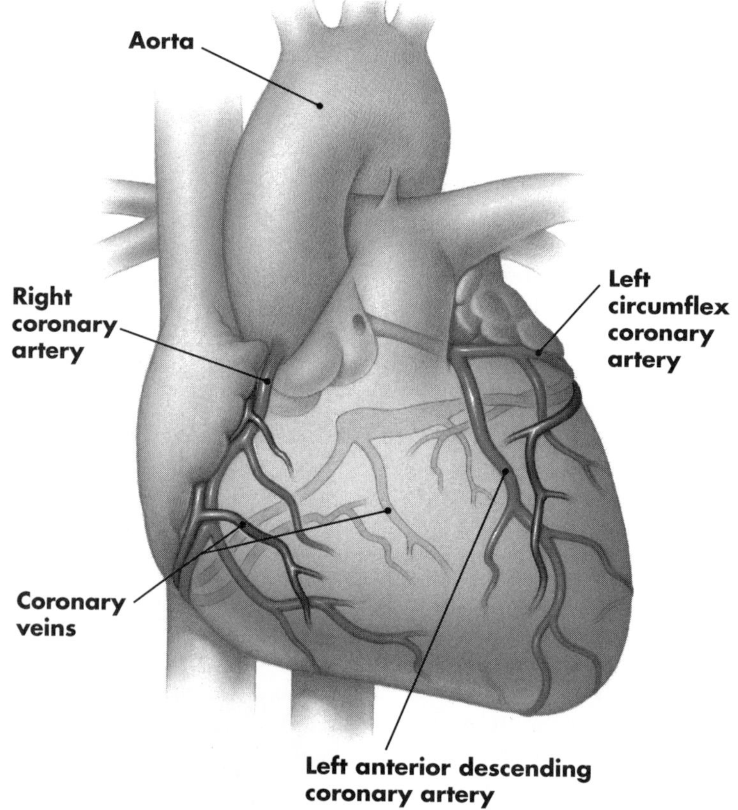

The coronary arteries emerge from the aorta and extend along the surface of your heart. Branches extend into your heart's wall to supply cells with oxygen and nourishment. The blood returns to your heart through your coronary veins.

Heart Glossary

angina. Chest pain or pressure that results from myocardial ischemia.

cardiovascular disease. Any disease that affects the heart or blood vessels.

coronary artery disease. Disease in the coronary arteries, which supply blood to the heart.

heart attack (myocardial infarction). Myocardial ischemia that lasts long enough to cause death in the area of the heart muscle supplied by a blocked coronary artery.

myocardial ischemia. Insufficient blood and oxygen reaching the heart muscle due to blockage of the coronary arteries.

silent ischemia. Myocardial ischemia that causes no symptoms.

of which about 40 percent of these are fatal.

The coronary arteries are part of your heart's own circulatory system. They provide the muscles of your heart with a steady supply of blood carrying oxygen and nutrients. The coronary arteries encircle the heart like a crown and send branches downward to the tip of the heart. When disease develops or damage occurs in these arteries, the condition is known as coronary artery disease.

The diagnosis and treatment of coronary artery disease have seen a great deal of innovation in recent years. Newer and better tests to identify coronary artery disease — particularly in its early stages — are continuously being developed.

Treatments also are improving. Specialized procedures can open narrowed coronary arteries. Bypass operations to direct blood around narrowed or blocked arteries also continue to be refined. In addition, the introduction of new medications to improve the flow of blood to the heart muscle have proved helpful in minimizing symptoms and have contributed to longer life in those who have coronary artery disease.

Despite these advances, you still play a critical role. Greater awareness of the disease and better control of its risk factors are likely behind the decreased death rate from coronary artery disease.

Common cause

Coronary artery disease usually results from accumulation of fatty deposits (plaques) in the lining of arteries. Plaques contain substances such as cholesterol, scar tissue and calcium. They narrow the arteries and create a condition called atherosclerosis. As plaques increase within the arteries, the flow of blood is progressively blocked. This often occurs in an irregular fashion, with considerably more blockage at some points than at others.

Plaques also increase the chances that a blood clot will develop. When a clot blocks the flow of blood through a coronary artery, your heart muscle doesn't receive its proper supply of blood, oxygen and nutrients. This is called myocardial ischemia. If death of heart muscle tissue occurs, this is a heart attack (myocardial infarction).

Symptoms such as chest pain (angina) and fatigue are more likely to occur during exercise than at rest, at least initially. When you stop and rest, the discomfort usually resolves in a few minutes. However, blockages can be so severe that even resting your muscles doesn't allow adequate blood flow, and you may experience symptoms such as claudication or angina with minimal exertion. On the other hand, many people experience no symptoms until serious complications arise.

Factors that contribute to the development of atherosclerosis include high blood cholesterol levels, high blood pressure, diabetes and tobacco use.

Diagnosis and detection

One of the challenges faced by doctors is detecting coronary artery disease before serious signs and symptoms or complications occur. Your doctor can't detect blocked coronary arteries simply by listening to your heart with a stethoscope. To diagnose coronary artery disease, more specialized tests are generally needed.

Electrocardiogram

The electrical activity of your heart is characterized by a pattern of changing impulses. These can be recorded through electrodes attached to the surface of your body. The electrical activity of the heart — represented by characteristic waves — can be evaluated instantaneously on a monitor or studied later on graph paper printouts.

The electrocardiogram (ECG) procedure is safe and painless. While you're relaxing on a bed or examining table, 12 to 15 electrodes are attached to the skin of your legs, arms, neck and trunk. The recording process then takes only a few minutes.

Analysis of an ECG involves looking for indications of heart rhythm abnormalities, a past heart attack or a heart attack in progress. If you have narrowed arteries but haven't had a heart attack, an exercise ECG (cardiac stress test) may be helpful. Your doctor may want to record an ECG of your heart

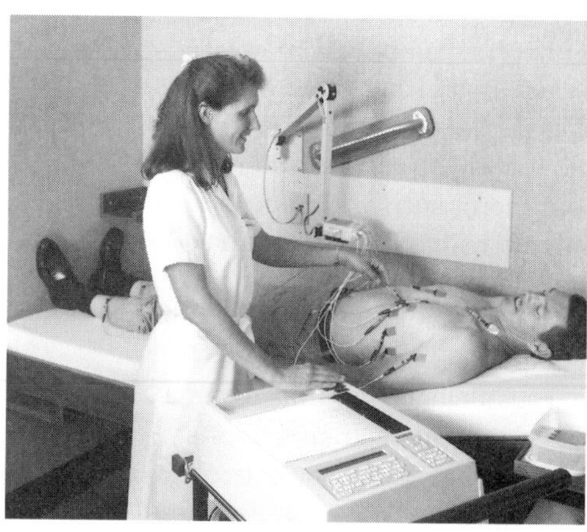

An electrocardiogram (ECG) records electrical activity of your heart. Electrodes convey impulses to a device that produces a graphic representation of your heart's activity. This can be studied for patterns and abnormalities.

when you're between 30 and 40 years old and in good health to provide a basis for comparison later if any heart problems develop.

ECG recordings taken continuously over a 24-hour period or longer may help detect conditions such as rhythm disturbances or inadequate blood flow to the heart muscle (myocardial ischemia). This technique, called Holter monitoring (ambulatory electrocardiography monitoring), involves use of a portable monitor that's slightly larger in size than a deck of cards.

Electrodes attached to your chest are connected to the monitor, which is hooked to your belt or carried on a shoulder strap. You wear the monitor for 24 hours as you go about your normal activities. Information on your heart's activity is stored in the monitor and retrieved later by medical personnel.

Blood tests

A sample of your blood may be taken for analysis. Your doctor may want an analysis of your cholesterol levels.

Too much low-density lipoprotein (LDL) cholesterol or too little high-density lipoprotein (HDL) cholesterol puts you at greater risk of atherosclerosis, an accumulation of fatty deposits in your blood vessels.

Other tests may include measurement of your blood sugar (glucose) for indications of diabetes, and of thyroid hormone — abnormal levels of these substances can increase your risk of cardiovascular disease. Elevated levels of certain enzymes in the bloodstream that are released from injured or dying heart muscle tissues, such as creatine kinase and troponin, also may indicate heart damage during a heart attack.

Cardiac stress test

A cardiac stress test helps measure how well your heart muscle is functioning and whether it's receiving an adequate blood supply. A stress test may be used to evaluate symptoms such as chest pain or shortness of breath during exertion. In some individuals with several risk factors for coronary artery disease, the test may be used as a screening tool.

A stress test accurately identifies the presence of significant coronary artery disease, and it also helps identify people who don't have significant coronary artery disease.

If you've had a heart attack, your doctor may order a stress test to determine the extent of your coronary artery disease. Stress tests are also recommended before you begin a program of vigorous exercise, particularly if you have any cardiovascular risk factors. Before you enter a cardiac rehabilitation program, you'll likely undergo a stress test.

The two main types of stress tests are exercise and nonexercise (pharmacologic). A pharmacologic test may be combined with imaging tests done before and after it to visualize your heart under a workload.

Exercise stress test

With an exercise stress test, electrodes are placed on various parts of your chest, and a blood pressure cuff is placed on your arm. You then walk on a treadmill while an

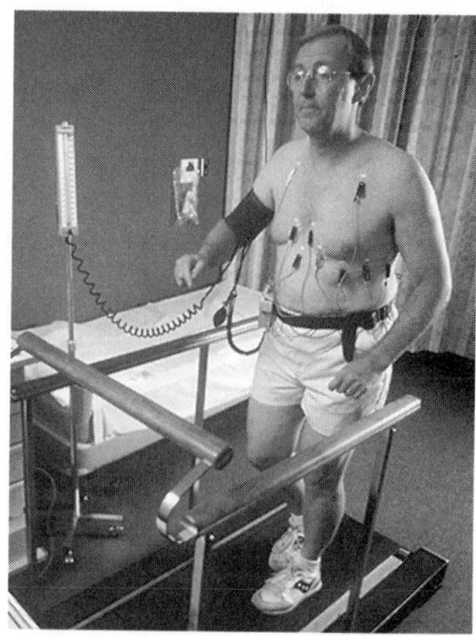

A treadmill test measures the activity of your heart while you exercise.

ECG records your heart's response to an increasing workload. As the speed and grade of the treadmill is gradually increased and the workout becomes more demanding, your heart rate increases.

Problems rarely occur during the test because doctors recommend these tests only for people in whom they believe the testing will be safe. In addition, the health care professional overseeing the test will be monitoring your heart rate, blood pressure and electrocardiographic tracings.

If a problem should occur, a medical facility is probably the safest place to have it happen, because the condition can be diagnosed and treated appropriately and quickly. For individuals who can't walk on a treadmill, other forms of exercise, such as pedaling a stationary bicycle or doing arm exercises, are sometimes used instead.

Nonexercise stress test

A nonexercise (pharmacologic) stress test is used with individuals who can't exercise due to conditions such as arthritis in the hip or knee. A medication is injected into your bloodstream that stresses your heart, mimicking the effects of exercise. The effects of the medication are observed with imaging tests.

If the test indicates that your heart's activity was unaffected by the stress, the chances are excellent that your heart will function properly when you work out on your own. If the test shows signs of problems, the test results can be useful in establishing exercise limits and developing a specialized fitness program. If the test produces any abnormal patterns on the electrocardiographic tracings or other special images ordered, your doctor may advise additional evaluations.

Chest X-ray

A chest X-ray produces a picture that includes your heart and blood vessels. It can be useful in identifying the presence of an enlarged heart, which may develop after a heart attack or during heart failure. It can also show calcium deposits in some of the large arteries. A chest X-ray may also detect changes in your lungs that are related to abnormal functioning of your heart.

Coronary angiography

Coronary angiography has long been considered the definitive test for coronary artery disease. This test reveals specific sites of narrowing in the coronary arteries. A hollow, flexible tube (catheter) is inserted into an artery in your groin or wrist and is threaded back through your main artery (aorta) into your heart. The tip of the catheter is then guided into a coronary artery. A dye (contrast agent) is injected through the catheter. As the dye flows through coronary arteries, your doctor can see narrowed segments and blockages with the help of X-ray movies (angiogram).

Angiography can be performed on many other blood vessels in the body. When it's done on the coronary arteries, the test is called coronary angiography. A variation of this procedure also is used to treat narrowed coronary arteries (see page 754).

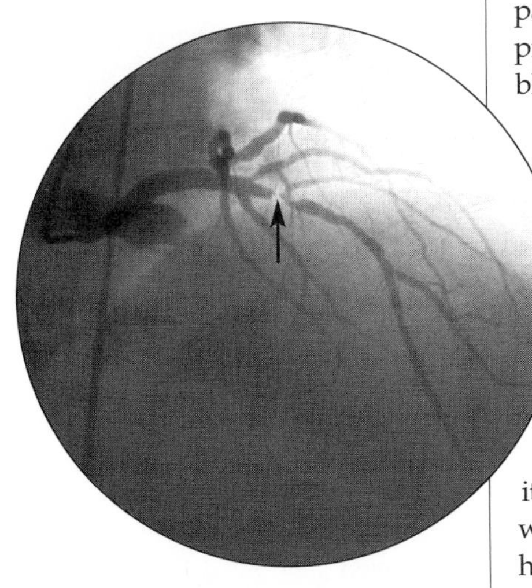

A coronary angiogram outlines the major arteries of the heart. It can show a blockage in an artery (see arrow) due to accumulation of atherosclerotic fatty deposits (plaques).

Nuclear scan

A nuclear scan is a noninvasive test that helps identify blood flow problems to your heart. The procedure involves injecting a trace amount of radioactive material, such as thallium, into your bloodstream, often during a treadmill test. A special scanning device then records a series of pictures registering the locations of the radioactive material in the heart muscle. Dark areas on the scans indicate portions of your heart to which blood flow is impaired. However, this test doesn't provide an image of the actual blocked artery.

Echocardiography

Echocardiography, another noninvasive test, uses ultrasound sound waves that reflect (echo) off the surfaces of your heart's structure (see the illustration on page 777). A computer then constructs an image of your heart or analyzes its blood flow. By assessing how well that area moves with each heartbeat, it can help identify whether an area of your heart muscle has been damaged.

When combined with a stress test, echocardiography can help identify areas of diminished blood flow to the heart. For example, when a portion of the heart muscle receives insufficient blood flow during exercise, it develops an abnormal weakened contraction pattern that can be recognized by comparing the images of the contractions at rest before exercise and immediately following exercise.

Electron beam computerized tomography

Electron beam computerized tomography (EBCT) can detect calcium deposits within coronary arteries. Calcium deposits (calcifications) are indicators of atherosclerosis, the leading cause of coronary artery disease. If a substantial amount of calcium is discovered, coronary artery disease is likely. Calcium deposits appear as light spots on the scans and can be measured. However, the presence of coronary calcium doesn't necessarily mean you'll have a heart attack, nor does the absence of calcium deposits exclude coronary artery disease.

The role of EBCT in diagnosing coronary artery disease is still being defined.

Treatment

Treatment of coronary artery disease involves treating the underlying cause — in most cases, atherosclerosis.

Changing your daily habits may be the single most effective way to treat atherosclerosis and prevent coronary artery disease from progressing.

The most beneficial changes that you can make include:

- *Diet.* Eating a diet low in fat — especially saturated fat — and cholesterol helps reduce high blood cholesterol, a primary cause of atherosclerosis. In fact, maintaining healthy cholesterol levels following a heart attack helps lower your risk of having another one. Eating less fat can also help you lose weight. If you're overweight, losing weight can help you further lower blood cholesterol. For more on blood cholesterol, see page 733.

- *Exercise.* A program of regular walking can stimulate the formation of collateral vessels around a narrowed artery, thus bypassing the blockage and increasing circulation. Although collateral vessels won't return circulation to normal, they may reduce symptoms enough to eliminate or delay the need for more aggressive treatment.
- *Quitting smoking.* Smoking increases the tendency for blood to clot and obstruct the flow of blood. It also reduces your high-density lipoprotein (HDL) cholesterol — the "good" kind — and deprives your heart muscle of the oxygen it needs to function properly. Quitting smoking dramatically lowers your risk of complications from atherosclerosis.

Medication

Cholesterol-lowering medications can help treat atherosclerosis. If lifestyle changes alone aren't enough to improve atherosclerosis, your doctor may advise you to take one or more medications (see page 737).

Revascularization procedures

In some cases, medications don't provide adequate relief, and the blocked artery must be widened (dilated) to allow adequate blood flow. This is done with a procedure called coronary angioplasty, which most often uses a balloon-tipped tube (catheter) to inflate the narrowed section of the artery.

Surgery

Severe blockages or those in places that are too difficult to reach using a catheter may require surgery. In these cases, a doctor may recommend an operation to bypass the arteries, thereby providing an alternate route for blood flow (see page 759).

Angina

Signs and symptoms

- Pain — a tight, band-like, crushing, suffocating sensation — that's usually centered beneath the breastbone (sternum) and may spread to the throat, jaw or arm
- A sensation of heaviness or tightness in the chest that is less than pain

Coronary Angioplasty

Narrowed or blocked coronary arteries can produce a heart attack, angina or other heart-related problems. In some cases, diet, medication or both may be the best treatment. In other instances, a procedure to open obstructed arteries, called coronary angioplasty, may be the preferred treatment.

The full name for coronary angioplasty is percutaneous transluminal coronary angioplasty (PTCA). It's also referred to as percutaneous coronary intervention (PCI) or balloon angioplasty.

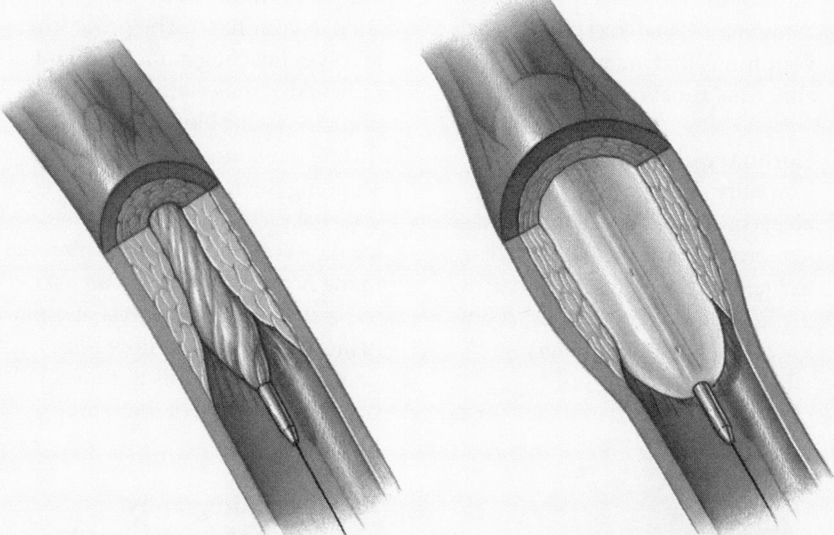

During coronary angioplasty, a balloon-tipped tube is inserted through a catheter and directed to the narrowed portion of the artery (left). The balloon is inflated, compressing deposits and widening the artery (right).

Procedure

After injection of a local anesthetic into the groin or arm, a doctor inserts a flexible tube (guide catheter) into a leg or arm artery.

Aided by images on a monitor, your doctor guides the catheter to the blocked artery in your heart. A contrast dye may be injected through the catheter to enhance the image's clarity and confirm the exact location of the blockage.

A second, narrower catheter with a balloon at its tip is then threaded through the guide catheter. When the tip reaches the obstruction in the coronary artery, the balloon is inflated for about half a minute to widen (dilate) the narrowed portion of the artery. While it's inflated, you may feel chest pain. When it deflates, the pain will fade. Several inflations and deflations usually are necessary. Then the balloon catheter is removed, and more images are taken to see how blood flow has improved.

Angioplasty was revolutionized by a device called a stent — a small, metallic mesh tube that's positioned in an artery following dilation of the blocked area.

- Chest pain brought on by exercise or emotional stress

Angina pectoris, the medical term for angina, gets its name from the nature of the pain. The Latin *angere*, for "choke," describes the characteristic suffocating sensation, and the term *pectoralis*, for "chest," indicates where it's located.

Angina is a symptom, not a disease. It can result from spasm of the coronary arteries. More likely, it's the result of atherosclerosis, in which arteries are narrowed by fatty deposits (plaques). Thus, angina is often one of the warning signs of coronary artery disease. When the attacks come frequently and without physical activity, they may be warning signs of an impending heart attack and require urgent treatment.

The discomfort usually lasts from 2 to 15 minutes. The pain may be severe and may be accompanied by a constricting feeling behind the breastbone and extending into the throat, jaw or arm. People sometimes describe it as mild heaviness, tightness or burning discomfort. Angina pain may be referred, which means that your brain confuses the pain impulses, causing you to feel the discomfort in your throat, jaw or arm rather than in your chest.

Angina is usually brought on by exertion such as heavy lifting, sexual activity or strenuous exercise. It's generally relieved by rest. Extreme cold or emotions such as intense fear, anger, grief and frustration can bring on the pain, as can ingestion of a heavy meal.

Angina is the direct result of insufficient blood reaching your heart muscle (myocardial ischemia). When you exert yourself, your heart requires more oxygen to do the extra work. When the coronary arteries that serve your heart are narrow and unable to provide the increase in blood flow demanded by the exercise, nerves in your heart transmit pain messages to your brain.

Angina related to blocked coronary arteries can be subdivided according to whether it occurs in a predictable pattern over a long time (stable angina) or is new or increasing (unstable angina). Unstable angina — particularly when it occurs at rest — may be a warning of an impending heart attack. You should seek medical attention

Approximately 90 percent of people who undergo PTCA are candidates for stent placement.

The stent acts as a scaffold to hold the vessel open. It's intended to be permanent and reduce the likelihood that the artery will narrow again. This condition, called restenosis, is a common problem following angioplasty. Stents often are coated with medication to help keep them open.

Some people with stents require medications for 4 to 8 weeks after the procedure to reduce the risk of blood clotting in the stent. Many people take a daily aspirin indefinitely as a form of prevention.

The entire procedure usually takes 30 minutes to 2 hours and often requires a 1-day hospital stay. This procedure may also be used to treat blocked arteries elsewhere in the body, including the legs.

Results

Hoped-for results are improved blood flow, an increase in blood pressure in the affected artery, compression or splitting apart of the blockage itself and enlargement of a portion of the artery wall. In a very small percentage of cases, the procedure is unsuccessful, and bypass surgery is necessary. Usually, a surgical team is available to proceed immediately. When the angioplasty is successful, the costs are considerably less and the hospital stay is shorter.

For 24 hours after the angioplasty, your heart rate and rhythm and other vital signs will be closely monitored. Many people go back to work a week after the procedure.

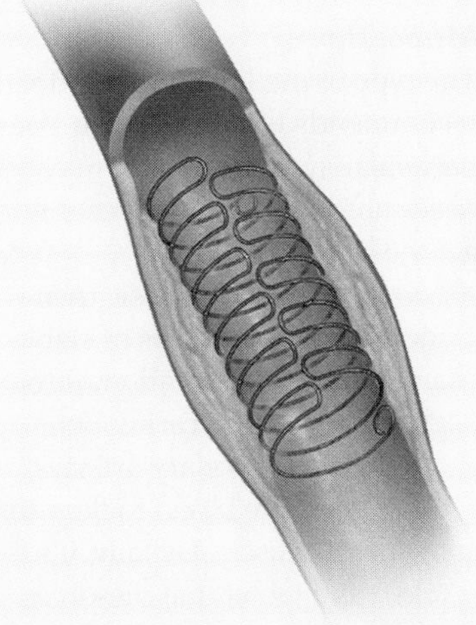

After angioplasty, a fine, metallic mesh tube (stent) is often placed in the artery to prevent renarrowing (restenosis).

Who's a candidate?

The decision to recommend angioplasty over bypass surgery is generally based on the location, number and severity of blockages, as well as on the overall function of the heart. The procedure doesn't cure the underlying disease, and it may have to be repeated to reopen the same or other coronary arteries that become blocked. Use of medication is important to help prevent disease progression.

Variations

Other techniques may be used to treat narrowed arteries. However, their use has become less common.

Use of a rotating blade that resembles a drill is one such procedure. It may be used if a coronary blockage is very hard due to calcification. The drill pulverizes the plaque into fragments that are removed through the catheter. Smaller microparticles wash downstream in the circulation.

immediately. A third type of angina, called variant angina, is caused by a spasm of the muscles in the wall of the coronary arteries.

Diagnosis

A diagnosis of angina is usually suspected based on a person's history of chest discomfort and the setting in which it occurs. There's no specific laboratory test for the diagnosis of angina. Your doctor may want to obtain an electrocardiogram to see if a heart attack has occurred or is occurring. He or she may also order certain blood tests to rule out heart damage, thyroid abnormalities or anemia. These disorders may force your heart to beat faster, use more oxygen and, therefore, precipitate angina. A stress test can measure how your heart and blood vessels respond to exertion, which may indicate if your pain is related to your heart (see page 752).

How serious is angina?

The decrease in blood flow to your heart caused by angina is partial and temporary, so muscle damage doesn't occur. This is in contrast to complete blockage of a heart artery that can cause permanent damage to a part of the heart muscle. In some cases, angina may serve as a warning of a future or impending heart attack. If you have angina, see your doctor.

Treatment

If you experience angina, try to stop the activity that precipitated the attack. This should lessen the load on your heart and reduce its need for increased oxygen. Your pain and other symptoms will probably improve within a few minutes. If the discomfort doesn't stop within several minutes or if the frequency or severity of the attacks increases, seek prompt medical attention.

One of the first steps in treating angina is to modify factors that may trigger or worsen the condition. If you smoke, stop. If you're overweight, lose the extra pounds. Eliminating obesity or smoking may decrease or even eliminate your symptoms. Exercise and a low-fat, low-cholesterol diet may help keep your arteries from further narrowing.

Exercise

Having angina doesn't need to make you sedentary. In fact, exercise is a key part of managing your condition. The exercise must be compatible with the limitations imposed by your pain and is often suggested after your angina is under control with medications. Your symptoms and your doctor will help you determine how much exercise is appropriate.

If you have unstable angina — pain that's becoming more frequent, more easily provoked or more intense or prolonged — don't begin an exercise program before consulting your doctor.

Medication

The type of medication your doctor recommends will depend on your particular symptoms. You may need more than one medication to get the best effect.

- *Nitroglycerin.* The classic treatment for acute attacks of stable angina is the medication nitroglycerin. Nitroglycerin opens (dilates) the coronary arteries, allowing more blood to flow to the heart muscle. Usually, it's taken as a tablet that dissolves under your tongue. A form of nitroglycerin that's sprayed under the tongue also is available. Often within a few minutes, the discomfort of angina eases.

  If your doctor prescribes nitroglycerin, keep your medication supply fresh because the tablet form loses potency in a matter of months. In addition, keep the tablets out of direct sunlight, which causes loss of potency.

  One side effect of nitroglycerin is that it can cause headaches and dizziness. Usually, the headaches are brief and mild. In case of dizziness, sit down before taking the medication.

  Long-acting nitrites, medications that are similar to nitroglycerin, also may be helpful in decreasing the frequency of angina attacks.
- *Aspirin.* Your doctor may recommend that you take a low-dose aspirin daily. Aspirin decreases the tendency of blood to clot, thus reducing the risk of a blood clot forming in a coronary artery and causing a heart attack.
- *Beta blockers.* Beta adrenergic blockers decrease your heart rate and blood pressure. Both effects are useful in reducing the workload of your heart and thus the symptoms of angina.
- *Calcium channel blockers.* These medications interrupt the normal flow of calcium through channels in your cells. This produces a widening (dilation) of the coronary arteries and other arteries in your vascular system, increasing blood flow to the heart muscle. Work required of the heart is also decreased, and its demands for oxygen are lessened. Calcium channel blockers also decrease blood pressure and some decrease your heart rate.
- *Cholesterol medications.* Individuals with angina usually have atherosclerosis, a condition where arteries are narrowed by the buildup of plaques containing cholesterol, scar tissue and calcium. Because of this, people with angina are often advised to reduce their low-density lipoprotein (LDL or "bad") cholesterol level to less than 100 milligrams per deciliter.

  Some people may be able to achieve this with a low-fat, low-cholesterol diet, but often people need the help of cholesterol-lowering medication (see page 737).

Surgery and other procedures

If angina continues despite the use of medications or occurs more often or with greater intensity (unstable angina), your doctor may consider coronary angiography to look at the anatomy of your coronary vessels.

This test can help your doctor evaluate whether you're a candidate for coronary angioplasty (see page 754) or coronary artery bypass surgery (see page 759).

Heart attack

Emergency signs and symptoms

- Intense, prolonged chest pain (heavy pressure)
- Pain that extends beyond the chest to the left shoulder and arm, the back and even the teeth and jaw
- Prolonged pain in the upper abdomen
- Shortness of breath
- Loss of consciousness
- Nausea and vomiting
- Perspiration
- Frequent angina attacks that aren't due to physical exertion

A heart attack causes injury to your heart muscle from loss of blood supply. It usually occurs when a blood clot blocks blood flow through a coronary artery. Lack of blood flow to your heart muscle can cause damage or death to part of the heart. It can also be fatal.

The medical term for heart attack is *myocardial infarction*. *Myo* means "muscle," *kardia* means "heart," and *infarct* refers to an area of dead tissue that's caused by lack of oxygen.

Most often the clot that causes a heart attack forms in a coronary artery narrowed by an accumulation of cholesterol and other fatty deposits in atherosclerotic plaques.

A plaque consists of a firm shell that may contain calcium with areas of fatty material. The center consists of soft cholesterol. The shell may crack or fissure, exposing the inner portion. When this happens, a blood clot tends to develop at that site. If the clot blocks blood flow in a coronary artery for longer than 20 minutes to 2 hours, it causes a heart attack.

Rarely, a heart attack can occur when a blood clot from inside a diseased heart breaks loose and lodges in a coronary artery. Another uncommon cause of a heart attack is a spasm of a coronary artery that shuts down blood flow to the heart. Drugs such as cocaine can cause such a life-threatening spasm.

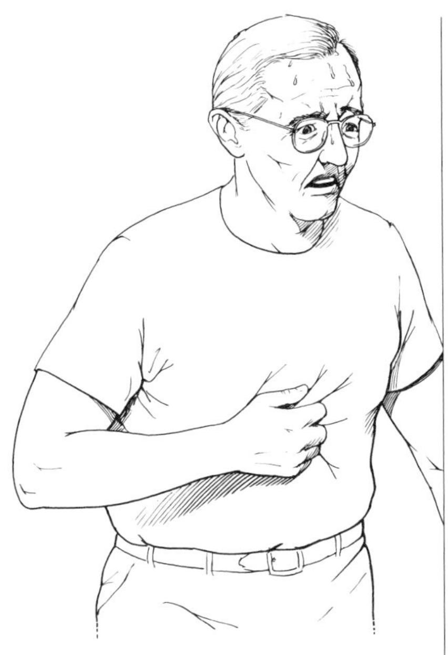

The pain of a heart attack varies from person to person, but typically you'll experience a profound squeezing sensation in the chest, accompanied by profuse perspiration. Pain may radiate to the left shoulder and arm, to the back and even to the jaw and teeth.

A heart attack isn't a static, one-time event. It's a dynamic process that typically evolves over 4 to 6 hours. With each passing minute, more heart tissue is deprived of oxygen and deteriorates or dies, forming scar tissue and causing pain and pressure. If blood flow can be restored quickly, damage to the heart can be prevented or limited.

Thus, a heart attack is a medical emergency: If you think that you or someone you're with is having a heart attack, call for emergency medical assistance or take the sick person to the nearest hospital emergency department. Don't delay in seeking medical help. In this situation, time equals heart muscle. Delay is a mistake that takes thousands of lives every year. Some people think the pain will disappear of its own accord. At other times, a heart attack can be confused with indigestion.

A powerful squeezing sensation in your chest may be the chief symptom. Some people describe it as the feeling of an enormous hand enclosing and squeezing their heart. Many recall an accompanying sense of doom. The pain may be similar to that of angina, but it's sustained and responds very little to nitroglycerin, if at all. The pain may be a discomfort or an inexplicable tightening or crushing sensation as though an elephant has stepped on your chest.

A heart attack may be preceded by a series of angina attacks, or it may occur suddenly with no advance warning. Unlike angina, however, the pain doesn't cease when the exercise or stress that caused it is discontinued.

The pain may be constant, or it may come and go. Any prolonged or severe pain in your chest or upper abdomen is cause for concern. Get to a hospital emergency department right away.

Occasionally, the pain doesn't fit any particular pattern. This is especially true in older adults and people with diabetes. In these individuals, it's not unusual for a heart attack to occur with no symptoms. These silent heart attacks may be detected only when a routine electrocardiogram reveals a change in the pattern of transmission of electric impulses through the heart.

In some people, a primary symptom of a heart attack is sudden onset of shortness of breath, which may or may not be associated with chest pain. In approximately 10 percent of people who experience heart attach, the only symptom is a sudden fainting spell.

Diagnosis

In the emergency vehicle or when you reach the hospital, your blood pressure will be taken and you'll likely have an electrocardiogram (ECG) taken. At the hospital, other tests may be ordered, including blood tests for enzymes that are released by damaged heart tissue, scans to look for heart damage and

What to Do in Case of a Heart Attack

If you think you or someone you're with is having a heart attack, promptly take the following steps:

1. *Seek urgent medical attention.* Call for emergency medical help or take the sick person to the nearest emergency department. Each year thousands of people die because they didn't seek medical help in time. Don't worry about confusing a heart attack with indigestion or something else. If in doubt, don't wait before calling for help.
2. *Have the sick person chew an aspirin.* Aspirin prevents blood from clotting and may help restore blood flow through clogged arteries, significantly improving the odds of surviving. Chewing the aspirin instead of swallowing it whole speeds absorption into the system.
3. *Use cardiopulmonary resuscitation (CPR).* If you're with someone who stops breathing, begin CPR immediately. After a person stops breathing, he or she can live only a few minutes without CPR.

angiography to check for narrowed coronary arteries.

How serious is a heart attack?
A heart attack may lead to sudden death, either because so much of the heart tissue dies that the heart no longer can function or because a fatal heart rhythm disorder develops. Most people who die of a heart attack have severe blockages of more than one coronary artery. But approximately 60 percent of those who have a heart attack survive.

If the area of damaged tissue is small and the electrical system that controls your heart isn't damaged, your chances of surviving a heart attack are good. The sooner you get to a hospital, the more that can be done to limit the amount of heart muscle damage.

In general, damage to only a small portion of the ventricle muscle may lead to a decrease in the amount of blood that your heart can eject during each contraction. The reduction in heart function is mild, so you can usually expect a return to a reasonably normal lifestyle.

If a moderate amount of heart muscle is damaged, congestive heart failure may develop. If a significant amount of the heart muscle is damaged — close to half the muscle, or more — shock or death may occur.

Complications

Any heart attack can lead to further complications, including:

Abnormal heart rhythms
The system that controls your heartbeat is electrical. In some people, damage to heart tissue from a heart attack can result in electrical short circuits, causing abnormal heart rhythms (cardiac arrhythmias) such as ventricular fibrillation. In this condition, rapid, uncoordinated contractions of the ventricles result in loss of significant blood flow to vital organs.

In other people, the arrhythmia may be a heartbeat that's too slow. This may require temporary or permanent placement of a pacemaker.

Congestive heart failure
Sometimes, the amount of damaged heart tissue is so extensive that the remaining heart muscle can't do an adequate job of pumping the blood out of the heart. Blood flow to tissues and organs throughout your body is decreased, producing shortness of breath, fatigue and swelling in your ankles and feet.

If the heart muscle recovers, congestive heart failure may occur only during the time surrounding the heart attack. If a significant part of the heart muscle is permanently damaged or destroyed, the heart failure may persist.

Treatment

As early as the initial minutes of a heart attack, ventricular fibrillation can occur. This unstable heart rhythm produces an ineffective heartbeat, and the heart muscle quivers uselessly.

Without immediate treatment, ventricular fibrillation leads to sudden death. Use of automatic external defibrillators (AEDs) that can shock the heart back into a normal rhythm can provide emergency treatment before reaching the hospital.

These lifesaving, portable devices are increasingly available in ambulances, police cars, commercial airplanes and some public facilities. They come with plainly worded instructions and require little training to use.

At the hospital, diagnostic tests are initiated. Oxygen may also be given. In some cases, medication may be administered to restore blood flow to the heart. In other cases, an urgent angiogram may be performed, and blood flow is returned using angioplasty techniques.

Medication
Initial treatment of a heart attack may involve medications such as:

Bypass Surgery

Heart attacks, angina and other heart-related problems can occur as the result of narrowed or blocked coronary arteries that supply blood to the heart muscle. In certain situations, coronary artery bypass surgery may provide an alternate route for blood flow to your heart muscle. Bypass surgery is most often performed when your symptoms don't respond to other medical treatment or when you have multiple blockages of the coronary arteries.

Procedure

To create a bypass, a surgeon transplants (grafts) a blood vessel from another part of your body to a coronary artery. He or she may use one of three blood vessels: the internal mammary artery from the chest, the saphenous vein from the inner side of the leg or the radial artery from the forearm. These are blood vessels that your body doesn't need. Some doctors may use a combination of these grafts.

In most cases, the internal mammary artery is used as the bypass. This artery lies inside the front wall of the chest. There's one on each side of the breastbone. The lower end of this artery is freed from the inside surface of the chest wall and sewn to the coronary artery beyond the blockage. The other end is left attached and blood is rerouted into the coronary arteries. The major advantage of this type of graft is its tendency to resist later formation of fatty deposits (plaques).

To create a bypass graft with the saphenous vein or the radial artery, a segment of the vein or artery is removed. One end of the vein or artery is attached to the aorta above the blocked coronary artery. The other end of the vein or artery is connected to the coronary artery beyond the blocked area. Thus, the diseased part of the artery is bypassed.

For a portion of the operation, the functions of your heart and lungs are assumed by a heart-lung machine.

Results

The goal of bypass surgery is adequate blood flow to the heart muscle, which generally is re-established. Improved blood flow often relieves angina or other coronary artery problems.

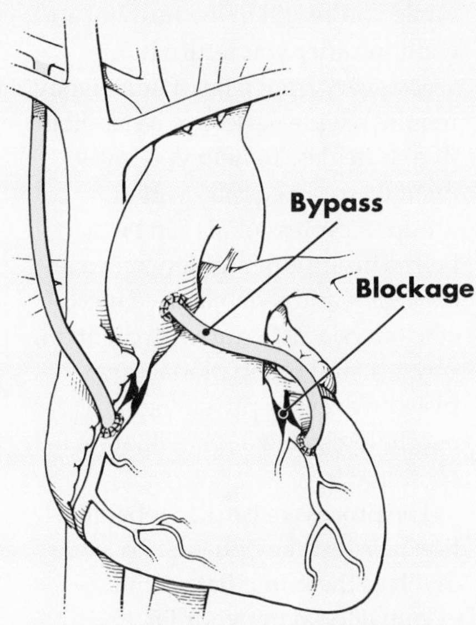

Bypasses around blockage sites can be surgically constructed out of blood vessels taken from the leg (saphenous veins) or forearm (radial arteries) or from arteries arising near the collarbone (internal mammary arteries).

Bypass operations are done frequently by experienced surgical teams. However, as with any operation, there are risks. In general, if you're under age 65, you have a normal left ventricle — the heart's major pumping chamber — and you're in relatively good health, your chance of surviving the operation and recovery is 99 percent.

Recovery and rehabilitation

A 5- to 7-day stay in the hospital is usual following bypass surgery. Immediately after the operation, you may spend 24 to 36 hours in a special coronary (cardiac) care unit (CCU) or intensive care unit (ICU). There the rate and rhythm of your heart and other vital signs are closely monitored.

Your doctor or surgeon will advise you about the degree of exertion your activities can involve for the next several weeks of recovery and the gradual resumption of normal activities.

Who's a candidate?

If you have mild angina on exertion or have recovered from a heart attack with no continuing symptoms, you may be best treated with medication or by other means.

Bypass surgery is generally considered appropriate for the following people:

- Individuals with a blocked left main coronary artery
- Individuals with disease in multiple arteries and poor function of the left ventricle
- Individuals with incapacitating angina

For such people, a bypass procedure is of clear value and life is prolonged in most cases.

- *Thrombolytics.* These are the most common medications used to treat a heart attack. They're also called clot-busters because they help dissolve a blood clot that's blocking an artery and blood flow to your heart. The earlier you receive a thrombolytic medication following a heart attack, the greater the chance you'll survive and the less the damage to your heart.
- *Angiotensin-converting enzyme (ACE) inhibitors.* These medications widen (dilate) arteries and decrease resistance to the flow of blood being pumped from the heart. The result is lower blood pressure for the heart to pump against.
- *Anticoagulants.* Medications such as aspirin or heparin make your blood less likely to form additional dangerous clots.

- *Painkillers.* If your condition is stable but your pain is great, you may be given an analgesic medication to relieve the pain.
- *Nitrates.* Nitrates work by decreasing the oxygen requirement of your heart muscle. The best known of them, nitroglycerin, is placed under your tongue at the onset of angina pain. It can also be given through a vein during or after a heart attack to decrease the heart's oxygen demand and improve blood flow through the coronary arteries.
- *Statins.* Statins reduce the low-density lipoprotein (LDL) cholesterol (the "bad" cholesterol) level in people for whom diet and activity alone aren't sufficient. Over time they can help prevent further narrowing of your arteries and reduce the risk of a second heart attack.
- *Beta adrenergic blockers.* These medications block the stimulating effect of the hormone adrenaline (epinephrine) on your heart. The result is that your heart beats more slowly and less forcefully and thus requires less oxygen to continue its work.

Invasive procedures

In addition to receiving medication, you may undergo one of the following procedures:

- *Angioplasty.* During this procedure, a doctor gently inserts a long, thin tube (catheter) through an artery in your groin or shoulder and threads it to the blocked artery in your heart. Another tube with a balloon at its tip is inserted inside the catheter and threaded through to the blockage. Once in position, the balloon tip is briefly inflated, sometimes repeatedly, to open up a blocked coronary artery, restoring blood flow to the heart (see page 754). A metal mesh device (stent) may be inserted into the artery to help keep it open.
- *Bypass surgery.* In rare cases, emergency bypass surgery may be performed at the time of a heart attack. Bypass surgery involves attaching veins or arteries at a site beyond a blocked artery, directing blood flow around (bypassing) the narrowed section (see page 759).

Recovery and rehabilitation

Emergency treatment of a heart attack is designed to restore blood flow and save heart muscle. Subsequent treatment is designed to promote healing of your heart and prevent another attack.

Remember that following a heart attack, you aren't necessarily disabled. In fact, regular exercise — within the guidelines set by your doctor — can contribute to the return of good health. Cardiac rehabilitation programs can help with recovery. Many programs begin while you're still in the hospital and continue after you return home.

Recovery from a heart attack may require a wide variety of rehabilitative strategies. To help you implement them, an equally varied group of professionals can be of help. This group might include cardiologists and rehabilitative medicine (physiatrist), nurses, a dietitian, physical and occupational therapists, an exercise physiologist, a psychologist and a rehabilitation coordinator.

The process of cardiac rehabilitation has three key phases. Phase 1 involves the immediate activities essential to saving your life and over which you have little control. Phase 2 is the ongoing medical attention, including medication and perhaps surgery. You and your doctor make most of the decisions concerning this part of the process.

In phase 3, which may include lifestyle readjustments, you're the one in charge. This stage usually begins with mentally and emotionally adjusting to your situation and carries through to changes in exercise and diet. It may also include quitting smoking or avoiding alcohol.

You don't need to go it alone, however. The rehabilitation team can assist you, particularly as you begin to learn and implement new habits.

Stress

The psychological aspects of cardiovascular disease are still somewhat of a mystery, but there's a clear consensus that many people exert unnecessary stress on themselves as they go about their life. After a heart attack, try your best to minimize such stress.

Recovering from a heart attack doesn't necessarily mean you should change your job, avoid all of life's challenges or make other radical changes. Decreasing the stress in your day-to-day activities may involve simply rethinking work habits, avoiding frustrating commutes or high-pressure deadlines and working to minimize stressful events in your life.

Many individuals temporarily experience insecurity and even depression following a heart attack or coronary artery bypass surgery. A cardiac rehabilitation team is experienced in these issues and can help you deal with these emotions.

Exercise

As you recover, your heart gradually grows stronger. Exercise can enhance this process. In the beginning, you may be given an exercise stress test (see page 752) to assess your heart's responses to physical activity. Members of your rehab team will advise you on how much and what types of exercise to do.

You won't resume full-speed activities on day one, but enrolling in a cardiac conditioning course may help you get started. If you were sedentary before your heart attack, a carefully planned exercise program is especially important. Ask for help in planning and establishing new exercise patterns appropriate to your lifestyle and condition.

Diet and weight control

If it was true before your heart attack, it's even more true now:

Sex Following a Heart Attack

Having a heart attack doesn't mean that you'll never be able to have sex again. Usually, all that's required is a sensible lapse, perhaps of a few weeks after your heart attack.

The demands placed on your heart when you have sexual relations are roughly the same as taking a brisk walk or climbing a flight or two of stairs. Your heart rate, breathing rate and blood pressure increase. Therefore, sexual activities need to be approached as any other physical activities: sensibly, with caution but without fear.

Take it easy
In order to minimize the stress on your heart, it may help to resume sexual activity with your partner under circumstances you're already accustomed to: You'll probably feel more relaxed making love in a familiar setting. If you find certain positions less strenuous than others, choose the less taxing route.

Communicate
Talk to your partner, both before and after sexual activity, to reassure yourself and your partner. Shared fears and concerns may be alleviated if lines of communication are open. Talk to your doctor if you have any questions. It's quite normal for your needs to change temporarily. You may experience either increased or reduced desire for sexual activity.

Be aware
If you experience chest pain, extreme shortness of breath or an irregular heart rhythm during sexual activity, stop. Men should avoid the use of sildenafil (Viagra), a medication taken for erectile dysfunction, until their doctor has approved its use. Using Viagra while also taking nitrates, such as nitroglycerin or isosorbide (Imdur, Isordil), may increase the chance of serious cardiovascular events and a severe drop in blood pressure.

Keeping your weight at a healthy level and avoiding saturated fats and cholesterol-rich foods are very important. Losing excess pounds reduces the stress on your heart. A change in eating habits to avoid fats also helps limit further disease in your arteries.

Discuss your eating habits with a registered dietitian. A dietitian can help you draw up a plan to decrease your consumption of fat and help you eat more nutritiously (see Chapter 2, "Eating Right," and Chapter 3, "Controlling Your Weight").

Smoking
Every cigarette you smoke affects your blood pressure and heart rate, and smoking can accelerate the process of atherosclerosis. Use the experience you have just had as an impetus to quit smoking.

Heart Failure

Heart failure is a serious problem, but it doesn't mean that the heart isn't working at all. Heart failure has various degrees of severity, depending on what the problem is and how long it has existed.

Congestive heart failure

Signs and symptoms

- Weakness and fatigue
- Breathlessness
- Swelling in the ankles

In congestive heart failure, your heart is still working but isn't circulating enough blood to meet your body's needs.

Congestive heart failure mainly affects older adults. It's usually the end result of long-standing cardiovascular disease. It can also be a complication of a heart attack or uncontrolled high blood pressure.

If failure occurs in the left pumping chambers of your heart, blood collects in your lungs, which causes them to become congested with fluid. This congestion is responsible for the sensation of breathlessness that's common in congestive heart failure.

If the right side of your heart fails, blood backs up into your legs and into your liver, which become congested. This produces swelling (edema) that's usually most obvious in the lower legs and ankles. Often, both the left and right sides of the heart fail simultaneously. Lack of adequate blood flow to the kidneys also leads to excess fluid and water in your body, an additional factor that increases the edema.

Inadequate blood flow to the muscles reduces endurance. Therefore, people with congestive heart failure often experience fatigue when they exert themselves physically.

The heart's loss of pumping efficiency in congestive heart failure may be the result of:

- Narrowed coronary arteries (coronary artery disease)
- Weakened heart muscle tissue from a heart attack
- Diseases directly affecting the heart muscle, such as cardiomyopathy
- Mechanical problems in the valves of the heart
- Prolonged high blood pressure
- Stiffening and constriction of the sac that surrounds the heart (pericardium), which may occur after inflammation of the pericardium (pericarditis)

Diagnosis

At first, congestive heart failure causes weakness, fatigue and breathlessness. Routine physical activities may become more and more difficult to perform. Initially, breathlessness may occur only after exercise. But as the disease progresses, shortness of breath may occur while resting or after going to bed. Breathing may be more difficult when you lie down so that you need to elevate your head on several pillows in order to sleep.

If your doctor suspects heart failure, he or she will likely listen to your heart and lungs with a stethoscope to detect sounds associated with heart failure. Your doctor will probably also look for swollen or distended neck veins, an enlarged liver and swelling of the feet, all of which may be signs of heart failure. Blood and urine tests can reveal whether your kidneys are functioning properly.

Your doctor may recommend an electrocardiogram (ECG) to evaluate your heart's rhythm and to look for evidence of a previous heart attack. A chest X-ray may be ordered to look for enlargement of the heart and excess fluid in the lungs. Echocardiography may be performed to check for valve problems and evaluate function of the heart muscle (see page 776).

How serious is congestive heart failure?

Untreated congestive heart failure can be fatal. However, lifestyle adjustments and proper medication treatment can improve heart function, relieve symptoms and prolong life. Although medications can't cure the condition, their long-term use may permit a nearly normal lifestyle.

Treatment

In some cases, congestive heart failure can be corrected by treating the underlying cause. For example, controlling a fast heart rhythm may lead to recovery from heart failure and restoration of the heart's strength. But many times the problem can't be eliminated. Then the goal of treatment is to prevent further damage to your heart and help it pump as efficiently as possible. Proper self-care is important in anyone with congestive heart failure. Other treatment options are medication, assistive devices and surgery.

Self-care

Your doctor may recommend that you make it a habit to get plenty of rest to help you conserve energy. However, this doesn't mean that you should retire to your bed. On the contrary, maintaining your mobility and an exercise regimen can be a key component of the treatment program. Motion improves circulation.

Your doctor may also give you specific nutritional guidelines to follow. In general, you restrict the amount of sodium you consume to help reduce accumulation of fluid. A dietitian may advise you to eat salt-free or reduced-sodium foods. You may also need to avoid alcoholic beverages and, if you're overweight, to lose weight.

Medication

Medications used to treat congestive heart failure include:

- *Angiotensin-converting enzyme (ACE) inhibitors.* In people with heart failure, ACE inhibitors can reduce the need for subsequent hospitalization for heart failure and prolong life. ACE inhibitors lower blood pressure to decrease your heart's workload. They also blunt some of the effects of excess adrenaline (epinephrine).

  Examples of these medications include enalapril (Vasotec), lisinopril (Prinivil, Zestril) and captopril (Capoten). A common side effect of these medications is a persistent cough. In addition, while you're on these medications, your kidney function and the level of potassium in your blood may need monitoring on a regular basis. Although the medications generally work to protect your kidneys, in some situations they can worsen kidney failure in people with kidney disease and cause an elevated level of potassium.
- *Angiotensin II (A-II) receptor blockers.* These medications may be an alternative for people who can't tolerate ACE inhibitors. They have many of the same effects as ACE inhibitors but are less likely to cause a cough. However, they haven't been studied as extensively in people with heart failure. Examples of these medications include losartan (Cozaar), valsartan (Diovan) and candesartan (Atacand).
- *Diuretics.* Often called water pills, these medications increase the rate at which your body eliminates urine and sodium. This can decrease the congestion in your lungs and fluid accumulation in your legs. Diuretics have few side effects, although you may urinate more frequently, especially after consuming fluids. In addition to sodium loss, potassium and magnesium also are eliminated. Your doctor may need to monitor your blood levels of these minerals and perhaps prescribe a potassium or magnesium supplement.

  Although a weak diuretic, spironolactone (Aldactone) has been shown to improve survival for people with significant heart failure, but it can raise the potassium level in your blood, so your doctor will want to monitor your blood potassium level. Occasionally, the medication can cause breast swelling and soreness in men (gynecomastia).
- *Digitalis.* This medication increases the strength of the heart's pumping action and seems to work best in people who have severe heart failure. It's also useful if your heart failure is the result of certain disturbances of heart rhythm because it can slow a rapid heart rate associated with some disturbances.
- *Beta blockers.* These medications were initially regarded as inappropriate therapy for people with congestive heart failure. How-

Kawasaki Syndrome

Kawasaki syndrome is named for the Japanese doctor, Tomisaku Kawasaki, who first described this childhood illness. This condition is capable of producing coronary artery disease in children, and rarely it can cause heart attacks and death. The number of children affected by the illness has increased, and it's now one of the leading causes of acquired heart disease in children — a position once occupied by rheumatic fever.

Four of every five people who acquire Kawasaki disease are less than 4 years old. People of Asian descent, even if they've lived in the United States for generations, are more susceptible than are people of other ethnicities.

Signs and symptoms include:

- A high, spiking fever for more than 5 days
- Swollen, watery eyes
- Reddened, cracked and swollen surfaces on the lips, tongue, mouth and throat
- Swollen, reddened hands and feet, followed by peeling of the skin in these areas
- A measles-like rash
- Swollen lymph glands of the neck

No one is certain what causes the syndrome. No infectious agent has been identified with it, although it tends to occur in outbreaks, especially in winter and spring. Some experts suspect that an unusual virus or other germ may be the cause or that toxic agents may be involved. Most of the hallmarks of Kawasaki syndrome are related to inflammation, and the damage that sometimes occurs in the coronary arteries or heart muscle may be an immune response.

In about one out of five children with Kawasaki syndrome who aren't treated, heart-related problems develop. The most common is expansion of sections of coronary arteries (aneurysms). In some children, an aneurysm can become obstructed by a blood clot and cause a heart attack. However, this is rare, especially when the condition has been treated.

Although the illness can be harrowing, and despite its effect on the coronary arteries, Kawasaki syndrome is usually a self-limited illness. The death rate in treated children is well below 1 percent. Even among those in whom coronary problems develop, most have substantial improvement with time.

The goal of treatment is to reduce inflammation and prevent damage to the heart and coronary arteries. This may be accomplished with anti-inflammatory medications and injections of purified human antibodies (immunoglobin).

ever, large studies suggest that these medications are safe and beneficial. By preventing the adverse actions of adrenaline on the cardiovascular system, beta blockers may prevent progressive heart enlargement and a decline in pump function. Sometimes, cardiac function actually improves.

Like ACE inhibitors, these medications may reduce symptoms and prolong life. Beta blockers shouldn't be prescribed in certain situations, such as if blood pressure or heart rate is too low. Use of the medications requires a consultation with your doctor.

- *Nesiritide.* Nesiritide (Natrecor) is a synthetic version of a naturally occurring hormone in the body called B-type natriuretic peptide. BNP is secreted in high levels by the heart when it's overloaded with pressure and its volume is expanded. BNP causes the body to excrete excess fluid, helping to combat the effects of congestive heart failure. Nesitiride may benefit people who have very severe congestive heart failure.

Whatever medication you're prescribed, it's extremely important to take the recommended doses regularly.

Assistive devices

Special mechanical devices have been developed to help people with congestive heart failure.

- *Biventricular pacing system.* In 2001, the Food and Drug Administration (FDA) approved a type of pacemaker designed to treat moderate to severe congestive heart failure. The device, called a biventricular pacing system, simultaneously stimulates both the left and right ventricles of the heart by sending specially timed electric impulses to the heart's lower chambers.

  By coordinating the heart's electric signals, the heart beats more efficiently. Such a device may be recommended for individuals who haven't been helped by medications and whose ventricles aren't synchronized correctly.

  In May 2002, the FDA approved a device that accomplished two goals: jump-starting the heart when it needs it and resynchronizing the left and right ventricles. The device combines an implantable cardioverter defibrillator and cardiac resynchronization therapy. It's intended for people with advanced heart failure whose symptoms don't improve with medication.
- *Heart pumps.* These devices, called ventricular assist devices (VADs), are attached to a weakened heart to help it pump. Heart pumps are used to keep heart

transplant candidates alive while waiting for a donor heart. Studies are ongoing to examine their role as an alternative to transplantation.

Surgery
Occasionally, surgery is required. For example, if you have a defective heart valve or an area of damaged cardiac muscle, surgical repair may be appropriate. For individuals who can't be helped by medications or other treatments, heart transplantation may be an option (see page 782).

Pulmonary edema

Emergency signs and symptoms
- Severe shortness of breath
- Restlessness, anxiety and a feeling of suffocating
- Pink, frothy sputum
- Perspiration
- Pallor

Pulmonary edema occurs when increased pressure in the veins and capillaries of your lungs forces fluid out of the capillaries and into the lungs' air sacs (alveoli). The result is that your lungs are filled with fluid, making it difficult for them to supply your body with oxygen and eliminate carbon dioxide. This is an emergency situation and requires urgent care.

Pulmonary edema is usually caused by heart problems such as an extensive heart attack or disease of the heart valves. Rarely, it may result from noncardiac causes such as high-altitude exposure or a high blood pressure crisis.

Diagnosis
Severe shortness of breath is the primary symptom of pulmonary edema. You may feel as if you're starving for air or drowning. This feeling of suffocation is often accompanied by anxiety and restlessness.

Other signs and symptoms include sweating, pallor and a cough that commonly brings up pink, frothy sputum. In some people, the fluid also causes wheezing (cardiac asthma).

Chest X-rays can detect engorgement in your lungs' blood vessels. X-rays don't pass through fluid as easily as they pass through air, so fluid that has leaked into lung tissue is visible on an X-ray image.

How serious is pulmonary edema?
Pulmonary edema is a life-threatening condition. Immediate hospitalization and treatment are required.

Treatment
Treatment typically consists of receiving supplemental oxygen. If you're having extreme difficulty breathing, it may be necessary to insert a breathing tube into your trachea and provide temporary mechanical ventilation.

Medication
A diuretic medication is usually given intravenously to remove fluid from your lungs. Morphine sulfate also may relieve pulmonary congestion. If pulmonary edema is due to a decrease in the pumping function of your heart, medications that strengthen the heart muscle may be given intravenously. If high blood pressure is present, your doctor may prescribe an intravenous vasodilator medication, which causes the walls of your blood vessels to relax, thus lowering your blood pressure.

Heart Rate and Rhythm Disorders

The pumping of your heart must be continuous. If the process becomes disordered or interrupted, your heart may fail to deliver the blood that your tissues require for life.

Your heart consists of four chambers — two upper chambers (atria) and two lower chambers (ventricles). Within the upper-right chamber (right atrium) is a group of cells called the sinus node. The sinus

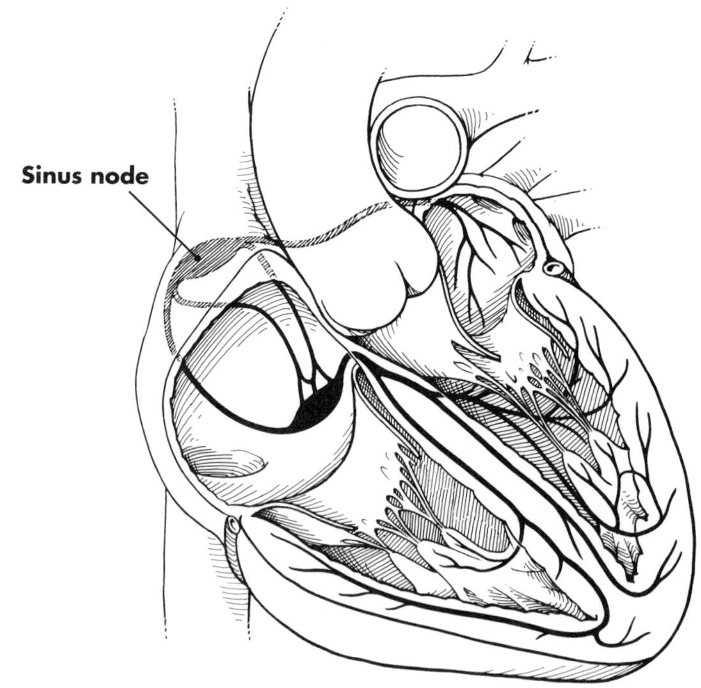

The sinus node, located in the right atrium, acts as your heart's pacemaker, controlling its contractions by issuing nerve impulses along electrical pathways throughout the heart.

node acts as your heart's natural pacemaker, producing electric impulses that cause the heart muscle to contract and pump blood. This contraction is heard as a heart beat.

The rate at which your heart muscle pumps (beats) varies depending on your activity at any given moment.

When you're at rest, your heart pumps more slowly and at a regular rate, about 60 to 80 beats a minute. When you run, climb stairs or otherwise exert yourself, the sinus node issues electric stimuli that increase the pace of your heart in order to provide your muscles and other tissues with additional blood and oxygen. Depending on your age and level of fitness, your heart rate may increase to 200 beats a minute if you exert yourself strenuously.

If something goes wrong with the functioning of the sinus node, disturbing the normal pacing of your heart, one of a number of disorders of the heart rhythm may occur. Too rapid a heartbeat is called tachycardia. Too slow a heart rate is bradycardia.

Arrhythmias

Signs and symptoms

- Often, none
- Fluttering in your chest
- A racing heartbeat
- A slow heartbeat
- Chest pain
- Shortness of breath
- Lightheadedness
- Dizziness
- Fainting or near fainting

Cardiac arrhythmia, also called dysrhythmia, is an abnormal heart rhythm. The heart may beat irregularly, too fast or too slowly.

The electric impulse sent out by the heart's sinus node to start each heartbeat travels first through the upper chambers (atria) then through a connecting electrical pathway between the upper and lower chambers of the heart called the atrioventricular (AV) node.

As the signal passes through the atria, they contract, pumping blood from the atria into the ventricles. A split second later, as the signal passes through the AV node to the ventricles, the ventricles contract, pumping blood to the lungs and the rest of the body.

Each contraction represents one heartbeat. At rest, the heart typically beats 60 to 100 times a minute, which is detectable by taking your pulse. Any disruption in the electrical conducting system can cause an abnormal heart rhythm.

Nearly everyone has felt their heart skip a beat, race or flutter inside their chest. Occasional heart palpitations are common and harmless, even though they're considered arrhythmias. However, more than 4 million Americans, mainly older adults, experience recurrent or symptom-producing heart arrhythmias that may require treatment. Recurrent heart arrhythmias may cause frequent heart palpitations, chest pain and lightheadedness. Some produce no symptoms but are detected during a physical or heart checkup.

Causes

Arrythmias may occur for no reason, or they may be produced by something that stimulates your heart, such as stress, tobacco, alcohol, caffeine, appetite suppressants or cold and cough medicines that contain caffeine or other stimulants. If you have an otherwise normal heart, occasional heart palpitations are rarely cause for alarm, and most don't require medical treatment. If they're bothersome, you might have success in eliminating the problem by limiting or avoiding what prompted the palpitations.

Some people are born with an electrical short circuit in their heart, which may not occur until years later. Other than the circuitry problem, their heart is normal.

Many things can damage your heart's electrical pacing and conducting system and lead to an electrical problem. Coronary artery disease, high blood pressure and a leaky heart valve can weaken your heart muscle, impairing its ability to pump properly. With age, natural weakening of the heart also can lead to an arrhythmia.

An arrhythmia can develop after a heart attack because scar tissue that forms during an attack can disrupt the flow of electricity through the heart. In addition, certain heart medications can produce an arrhythmia as a side effect.

Other health problems not specifically related to your heart also can lead to an arrhythmia. These may include an overactive thyroid gland or an imbalance in your blood chemistry. The use of certain illegal drugs, such as cocaine, also can disrupt your heart's electrical system and produce potentially fatal arrhythmias.

Types

Arrhythmias are categorized by their speed and rhythm. Bradycardia refers to a slow heart rate. Tachycardia refers to a fast heart rate. Fibrillation refers to rapid, uncoordinated beats.

Arrhythmias are also categorized by where the electrical problem originates in the heart. Arrhythmias that start in your heart's upper chambers (atria) are called atrial or supraventricular arrhythmias. Those that stem from your heart's lower chambers (ventricles) are called ventricular arrhythmias and tend to be more serious. Types of arrhythmias include:

- *Supraventricular tachycardia.* This type of arrhythmia is characterized by bursts of rapid heartbeats that originate in your heart's upper chambers. The bursts usually begin and end suddenly. Episodes can last seconds to days.

  A condition called Wolff-Parkinson-White syndrome is a common form of supraventricular tachycardia that tends to run in families. Wolff-Parkinson-White syndrome is associated with an extra electrical pathway

Supraventricular Tachycardia

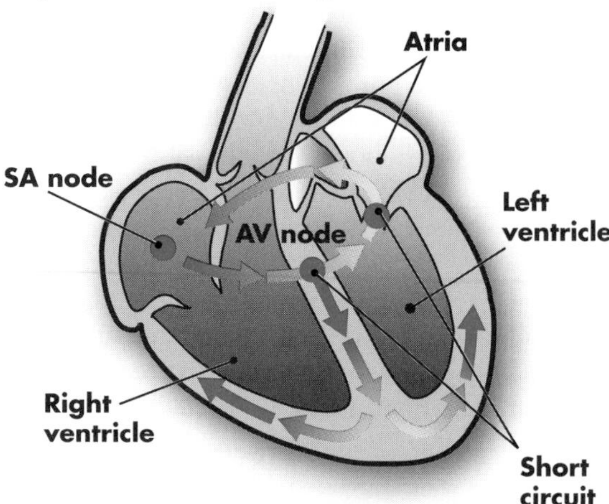

In some supraventricular tachycardias, a short circuit stops some of the electrical signals before they reach the ventricles.

Atrial Fibrillation

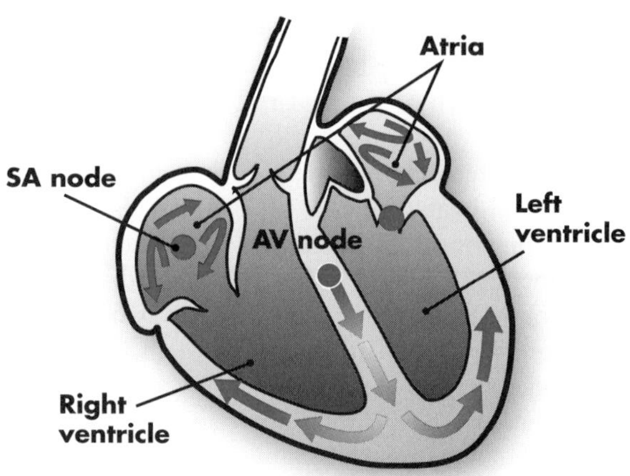

In atrial fibrillation, the upper chambers of the heart (atria) quiver due to chaotic, uncoordinated electrical activity.

that develops between the heart's upper and lower chambers. This pathway allows too many electric impulses to reach the ventricles, speeding up the heart rate.

- *Atrial flutter.* As the name implies, in this condition the heart's upper chambers flutter, creating a regular, rapid beat — as many as 300 beats a minute. Some of these beats transmit to the lower chambers, often resulting in a regular pulse of 100 to 150 beats a minute.
- *Atrial fibrillation.* This is a common arrhythmia, affecting mainly older adults. In atrial fibrillation, the heart's upper chambers beat fast — 300 to 600 beats a minute — and chaotically. The ventricles also speed up, resulting in an irregular and rapid heart rhythm.
- *Ventricular tachycardia.* In this type of arrhythmia, faulty electric signals that arise from your heart's lower chambers cause your ventricles to beat too fast. Ventricular tachycardia is almost always associated with heart disease or recent heart attack and can change into the most serious of arrythmias — ventricular fibrillation. Rarely, the condition occurs in an otherwise normal heart, in which the prognosis is much better.
- *Ventricular fibrillation.* This arrhythmia is a medical emergency. Chaotic electric signals through your heart's lower chambers cause your heart to suddenly quiver and cease pumping. Because blood doesn't get pumped to the brain, most people lose consciousness within seconds and require some type of immediate emergency medical assistance, such as cardiopulmonary resuscitation (CPR). Unless the heart is shocked back into a normal rhythm by a device called a defibrillator, ventricular fibrillation results in sudden death.
- *Long QT syndrome.* This disease is caused by a defect in the ventricles. It's associated with a high risk of arrythmia — usually a variant of ventricular fibrillation. QT refers to a pattern seen on an electrocardiogram (ECG). The different peaks and valleys of waves that appear on an ECG are designated by letters — P, Q, R, S and T. The Q-to-T interval represents the electrical firing and resting of the ventricles during each heartbeat. Doctors measure this interval and can tell if a QT interval takes a normal amount of time or takes too long and results in rapid heartbeats.
- *Sick sinus syndrome.* If your heart's sinus node isn't firing right, your heart rate slows down or slows down and then speeds up. Sick sinus syndrome, which is common in older adults, is considered a type of bradycardia. This arrhythmia sometimes is accompanied by atrial fibrillation.
- *Heart block.* This arrhythmia occurs when the electrical pathways that run between your heart's upper and lower chambers and through your heart's lower chambers become blocked, slowing the transmission of electric impulses through the heart. The result is a slow heart rate (bradycardia).

Minor heart palpitations — that feeling that your heart has skipped a beat — are known as premature atrial contractions (PACs) or premature ventricular contractions (PVCs). In reality, the heart doesn't skip a beat. Instead, an extra beat occurs sooner than normal. PACs and PVCs seldom are due to a serious problem, and they seldom lead to one. They're often produced by something that stimulates your heart, such as stress, tobacco, alcohol, caffeine, appetite suppressants

Ventricular Fibrillation

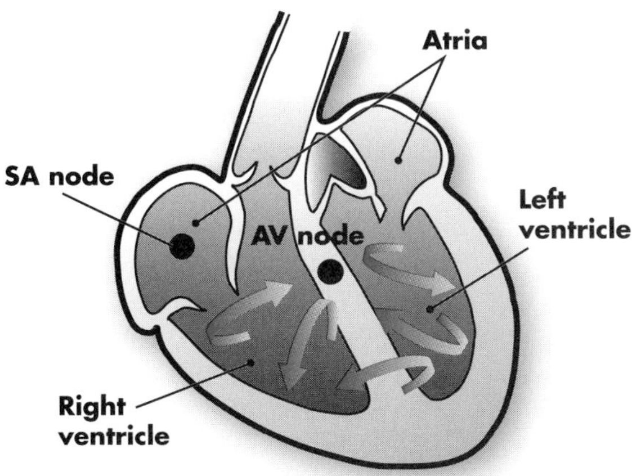

Ventricular fibrillation is associated with chaotic activity of the ventricles, which requires immediate treatment.

Heart Block

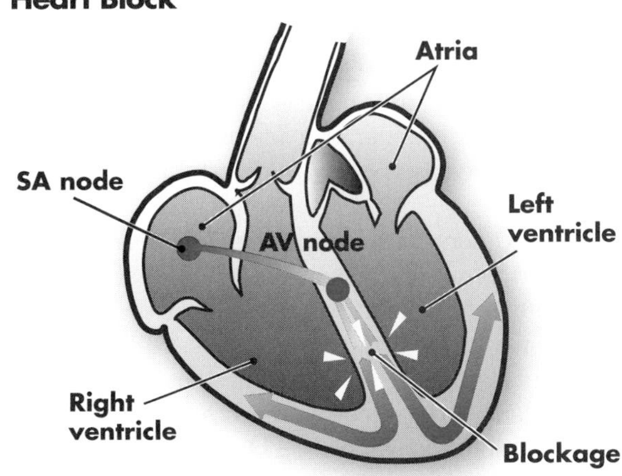

Slow heart rates can result from defects in the heart's conduction system that prevent electric impulses from reaching the ventricles. This is called heart block.

or cold and cough medicines that contain caffeine or other stimulants. An overactive thyroid can sometimes cause premature heartbeats. Rarely, PACs and PVCs can indicate more serious structural heart disease.

Diagnosis

Doctors may use a variety of methods to diagnose arrhythmias. An electrocardiogram (ECG) is often the initial step in diagnosis (see page 751). Other tests may include:

Holter monitor

A Holter monitor is a portable version of a continuous ECG. It's especially useful in diagnosing heart rhythm disturbances that occur at unpredictable times. The monitor is worn under your clothing. It records important information about the electrical activity of your heart as you go about your normal activities for a day or two.

Event monitor

For arrhythmias that occur sporadically, your doctor may ask you to wear a portable device called an event monitor. Two types exist. One type, called a loop recorder, is like a Holter monitor but is worn for a longer period of time. When you experience symptoms of an arrhythmia, you push a button on the device to record your heart's rhythm.

The other type of event monitor is a credit-card-shaped device that you place on the skin over your heart whenever you experience symptoms. The card records your heart rhythm. Both devices help your doctor determine if abnormal heart rhythms may be the cause of your symptoms.

Cardiac stress test

Your heart naturally speeds up during exercise or excitement, which can trigger an arrhythmia. Stress tests, which come in many variations, are used to help identify arrhythmias triggered by exertion. In one type of stress test, you may be asked to walk on a treadmill while hooked up to an ECG. In another, you may be connected to an ECG and then given a medication that stimulates your heart to beat faster in a manner similar to exercise (see page 752.)

Electrophysiologic testing

In a procedure called electrophysiologic (EP) testing, electrodes attached to a long, thin tube (catheter) are threaded through a vein in your arm or leg to your heart. Once in place, these electrodes can map the spread of electric impulses within your heart. These electrodes can also give off electric impulses of their own to pace your heart and see how it reacts.

This type of testing is useful in determining what type of arrhythmia you may have and where the problem occurs in the heart. During the procedure, many arrhythmias can be treated by means of catheter radiofrequency ablation — a procedure used to destroy (catheterize) heart muscle cells responsible for an arrhythmia (see page 771.)

Tilt table

A tilt-table exam is a way to test for other causes of fainting, which could mimic an arrhythmia. Your heart rate and blood pressure are monitored as you lie flat on a table. The table is then tilted. The changing angle puts stress on the part of your nervous system that regulates your heart rate and blood pressure. Doctors can see how your heart responds to the change in angle — similar to the change when you go from lying down to standing up.

How serious are arrythmias?

Many arrhythmias rarely cause complications. However, some can be serious, especially if untreated. A heart that's not beating normally

Sick Sinus Syndrome

The function of the sinus node is to regulate your heartbeat. Sometimes the sinus node fails to perform adequately in its role as your heart's pacemaker. When this occurs, the condition is called sick sinus syndrome.

In this condition, the sinus node initiates heartbeats too slowly, pauses too long between beats or stops producing beats. If it stops producing beats, a different part of the heart must take over the pacemaker function, which it usually does at a rate that's substantially slower than normal.

To further complicate the situation, sinus nodes that are sick may also have a tendency to beat too fast at times, and occasionally they beat in an irregular fashion, such as in atrial fibrillation. Thus, the symptoms of sick sinus syndrome can be those associated with slow heartbeats, such as fatigue, lightheadedness and blackouts, alternating with symptoms of fast heartbeats, such as palpitations. Either the slow or fast rhythms can cause shortness of breath, lightheadedness, blackouts and fatigue.

Therapy for sick sinus syndrome can be complex because the condition often involves slow and fast components. Medications may be given to slow the rapid heartbeat. In addition, a pacemaker may be required to prevent the slow heartbeats. Giving medication without the pacemaker may slow the heartbeats even more and lead to worse symptoms.

may not be able to pump blood efficiently. If blood flow to the brain is inadequate, you can faint. A heart that beats very fast for a prolonged period may become weakened, leading to congestive heart failure.

Certain arrhythmias, such as atrial fibrillation, may allow small blood clots to form in a chamber of your heart.

If one or more clots break loose and are carried by way of your bloodstream to your brain, they could cause a stroke. Your risk of stroke depends on your age, the type of arrhythmia you have and whether you have any other cardiovascular risk factors for stroke, such as high blood pressure.

Ventricular arrhythmias may be fatal in people with structural heart disease, such as a weakened heart muscle from a previous heart attack.

Artificial Cardiac Pacemakers

If your heart is unable to maintain a fast enough heartbeat or if it occasionally pauses, the solution may be an artificial cardiac pacemaker. This may be either a short-term treatment or a permanent solution.

Symptoms that may suggest a problem requiring a pacemaker include blackout spells, near faints, shortness of breath (especially during physical activity) and undue fatigue. A slow heartbeat or pauses can occur with various types of heart disease and even in an otherwise apparently normal heart.

An artificial pacemaker is an electric device that causes the heart to beat with a series of electric discharges. It replaces the function of your heart's own control system, the sinus node and conduction system. An implanted pacemaker mimics the electric impulses of a healthy heart and restores a sufficiently fast heartbeat. At times, your heartbeat may be fast enough on its own. When this occurs, the pacemaker automatically goes on standby.

Equipment

The pacemaker itself is small, weighing about $1\frac{1}{2}$ ounces, and is powered by a lithium battery that lasts up to 10 years.

Other models that are generally used only for short periods aren't implanted but instead are carried outside the body (external pacemakers).

Procedure

The pacemaker usually is implanted beneath the skin just below your collarbone. The device is connected to one or two insulated, flexible wire leads. These are usually passed into the right side of the heart by way of a large vein beneath the collarbone. There, an electric contact (electrode) discharges impulses to the inner surface of the right side of the heart to stimulate its contractions when the heart rate slows.

Applications

An artificial cardiac pacemaker isn't a solution to all heart problems, but it can be used to treat a number of heart disorders. Its primary application is to control or prevent slow arrhythmias of the ventricles. Many pacemakers are designed to increase the heart rate automatically during activity or stress, just as in the normal heart.

Two-wire pacemakers — with one wire located in the top chamber (atrium) of the heart and one wire in the bottom chamber (ventricle) — are called dual chamber devices. They ensure that the heart beats in a normal sequence. When medications aren't effective, some specialized devices can treat specific types of fast arrhythmias. Some pacemakers have three wires. They're generally used to treat heart failure.

Living with a pacemaker

Modern pacemakers may be affected by outside electric interference in some circumstances. If you have a pacemaker, talk to your doc-

In people with healthy hearts, life-threatening arrhythmias are exceedingly rare. In general, arrhythmias are more serious if you have other heart-related conditions.

Treatment

Once an arrhythmia has been diagnosed, your doctor will try to determine what type it is and where the rhythm problem originates in your heart.

Some arrhythmias don't require treatment. However, if an arrhythmia is causing symptoms or putting you at risk of more serious arrhythmias, treatment is usually required.

There are several treatments for arrhythmia. These include medications, implantable devices, external defibrillators, catheter techniques and surgery.

Medication

Several kinds of prescription medications are used to treat arrhythmias. Your doctor may prescribe one or more of the following medications, called anti-arrhythmic medications. They're usually taken daily for life.

- *Digitalis.* This medication slows the transmission of the heart's electric impulses, slowing a fast heart rate. It's also used to increase the pumping efficiency of the heart.
- *Calcium channel blockers.* These heart medications decrease the frequency and force of your heart's contractions, reducing the likelihood of some types of arrhythmia. Like digitalis, they also slow the heart's electrical conduction system. Two commonly prescribed calcium channel blockers are diltiazem (Cardizem, Dilacor) and verapamil (Calan, Isoptin).
- *Beta blockers.* Beta blockers slow the speed at which electric impulses travel from your sinus node to the rest of your heart muscle, reducing the likelihood of some types of arrhythmia. They also block the stimulating effect of the hormone adrenaline (epinephrine) on your heart.

  Some commonly prescribed beta blockers include carvedilol (Coreg), metoprolol (Lopressor, Toprol), nadolol (Corgard) and propranolol (Inderal).
- *Adenosine.* This drug slows conduction in the atrioventricular node and is used to terminate paroxysmal atrial tachycardia. It's administered intravenously.
- *Anticoagulants.* In people with atrial fibrillation, an anticoagulant, such as warfarin

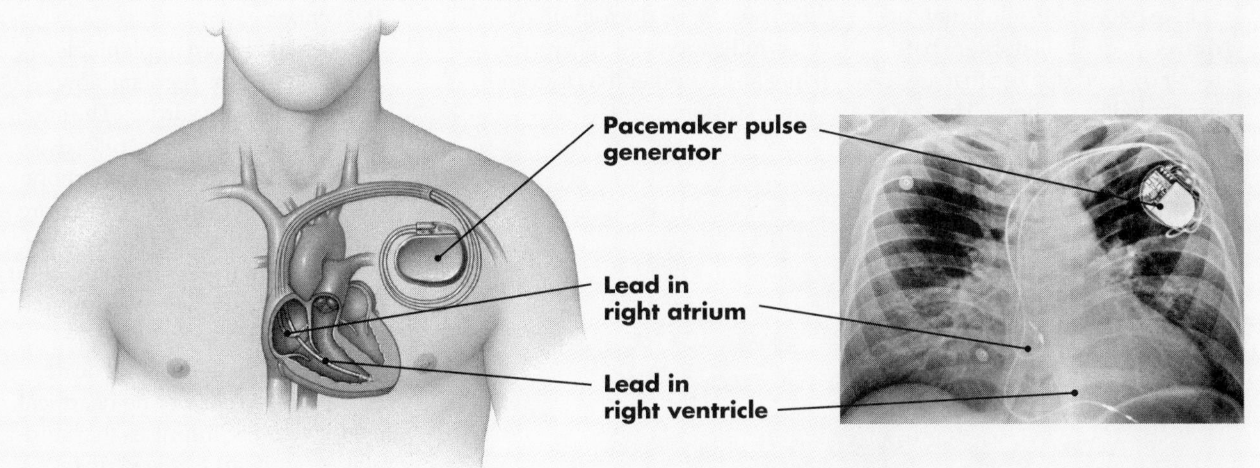

If your heart's internal pacing system fails to control your heartbeat, an artificial pacemaker may be surgically implanted. The battery-powered device is inserted beneath the skin of your chest. Flexible wire leads are threaded into the right side of the heart to deliver electric impulses.

tor before doing arc welding or mechanical work on a running car engine, because electromagnetic fields may interfere with your pacemaker's function. Although cell phones rarely cause problems, if you use one, it's best to hold it to the ear farthest from your pacemaker and to not carry it in a pocket over your pacemaker. In addition, avoid electromagnetic fields such as those found near high-voltage transmission lines or substations. Don't linger in doorways armed with electromagnetic anti-theft or surveillance devices.

Pacemakers can also pose problems during a magnetic resonance imaging (MRI) scan or an operation in which electrocautery is used to control bleeding. If you need one of these procedures, be sure to tell your doctor you have a pacemaker. Avoid hard contact to the pacemaker, such as might occur while playing football or firing a rifle from the shoulder near the pacemaker. Modern pacemakers aren't affected by microwave ovens.

Internal Cardioverter Defibrillator

Ventricular fibrillation is a life-threatening rhythm disturbance. Unfortunately, people who experience ventricular fibrillation are at risk of recurrence. In addition, individuals with ventricular tachycardia may have serious symptoms, such as loss of consciousness. And the tachycardia may proceed to the more dangerous ventricular fibrillation.

Because no medication is 100 percent effective for preventing or treating any recurrence, special measures are often warranted. Internal cardioverter defibrillators are increasingly being used to fulfill this need.

Like pacemakers, internal cardioverter defibrillators are battery-powered devices that are implanted in the body. They're implanted beneath the skin of the upper chest. The devices can also function like a regular pacemaker, should the need arise.

Wire electrodes that are inserted through veins attach the pulse generator to the heart. Internal cardioverter defibrillators continuously sense the heart's rhythm and respond in a fashion that's designed to convert the heart to a normal rhythm.

Some of these devices can detect when ventricular tachycardia occurs and then attempt to correct the rhythm with a small electric pacing current. If several of these attempts are unsuccessful, or if ventricular fibrillation develops, then the internal cardioverter defibrillator shocks the heart directly.

The shock may feel different for each person in each event. It may feel like a kick or a thump in the chest. Your doctor will discuss indications for this procedure and its potential risks and complications.

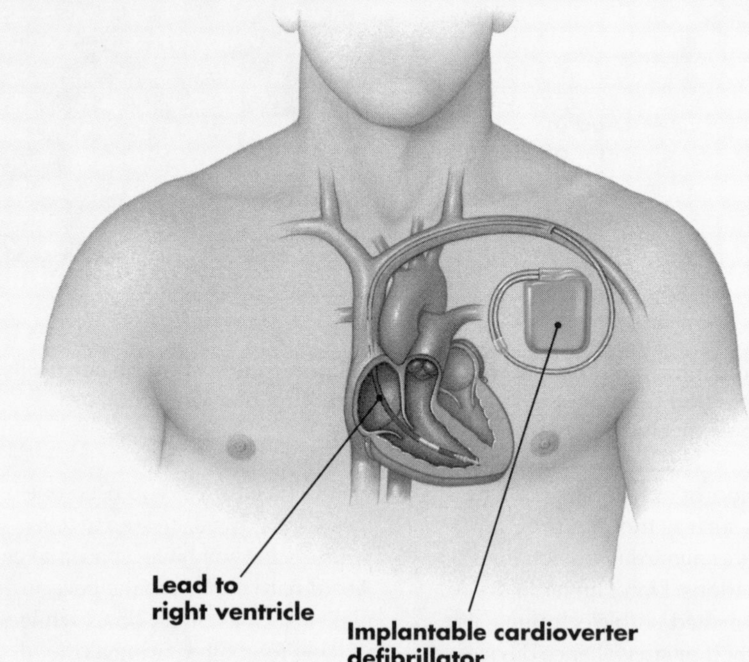

Implantable cardioverter defibrillators can both pace and deliver shocks that can treat ventricular fibrillation or ventricular tachycardia.

(Coumadin) or aspirin, may be taken to reduce the risk of blood clots and stroke.

- *Others.* The medications that can slow rapid heart rhythms and normalize irregular ones, such as in atrial fibrillation, include quinidine (Quinidex), disopyramide (Norpace), propafenone (Rythmol), sotalol (Betapace), amiodarone (Cordarone, Pacerone) and dofetilide (Tikosyn). The choice of medication usually depends on the type of arrythmia.

Anti-arrhythmic medications can cause side effects. Sometimes, they can actually make arrhythmias worse, so their use has to be carefully monitored. To test your medication's effectiveness and safety, your doctor may give you the medication while you're connected to a monitor or, occasionally, during electrophysiologic testing.

Pacemaker

A pacemaker is an implantable device that helps regulate slow heartbeats (bradycardia). The small battery-driven device is placed under the skin near the collarbone during a minor surgical procedure (see page 768). An insulated wire extends from the device to the right side of the heart, where it's permanently anchored.

If a pacemaker detects a heart rate that's too slow or no heartbeat, it emits electric impulses that stimulate your heart to speed up or begin beating again. Most pacemakers have a sensing device that turns them off when the heart rate is above a certain level. It turns back on when the heart rate drops too low.

Implantable defibrillator

An internal cardioverter defibrillator (ICD) is a device used to treat ventricular tachycardia or ventricular fibrillation. An ICD is a small, battery-driven device that's implanted under the skin, usually near the left collarbone. One, two or three thin wires run from the ICD through veins to the chambers of the heart.

The device delivers an electrical shock to the heart when it senses an accelerated or chaotic rhythm. The shock restores a normal rhythm. ICDs can also act like pacemakers, regulating slow heartbeats if necessary. In addition, they also can deliver fast pacing pulses to treat some tachycardias.

Automatic external defibrillator
An automatic external defibrillator (AED) does the same job as an ICD except that it's an external device. AEDs are mainly used by emergency response teams and in hospitals to shock a heart in ventricular fibrillation back into a normal rhythm. The device, which is about the size of a laptop computer, sends a jolt of electricity through the chest wall to the heart by way of small pads that are applied to the chest.

AEDs are also being placed in many public places, such as stadiums, casinos, airports, airplanes, shopping malls, offices and health clubs so that in an emergency situation people don't have to wait for a medical professional to receive life-saving assistance. The devices provide audible instructions and can automatically determine if an abnormal rhythm is present that requires a shock.

Individuals who are treated with AEDs may later need an internal cardioverter defibrillator implanted to prevent life-threatening heart rhythms from recurring.

Catheter radiofrequency ablation
Catheter radiofrequency ablation is the preferred treatment for many types of arrhythmias, including most supraventricular tachycardias.

In catheter ablation, a doctor guides a long, thin tube (catheter) through a vein in your arm or leg to your heart. The catheter is then positioned in the area of your heart responsible for the arrhythmia. Electrodes at the tip of the catheter emit a radiofrequency energy pulse similar to microwave heat. This pulse destroys the heart muscle cells responsible for the arrhythmia.

Catheter radiofrequency ablation can be effective for many arrhythmias and has a low risk of complications. It causes little or no discomfort and can usually be done under mild sedation with a local anesthesia. Most people resume normal activities a few days after the procedure.

Surgery
When an arrhythmia can't be controlled by other treatments, doctors may surgically remove or destroy heart tissue that's causing the arrhythmia. For example, rhythms such as ventricular tachycardia have their source in a specific heart muscle site, which can be surgically removed.

In some people with atrial fibrillation, maze surgery is effective. In this procedure, a surgeon makes multiple incisions in the right and left upper chambers of the heart (atria). The tiny holes create a path (maze) for electric impulses to follow through the upper chambers of the heart, helping to eliminate atrial fibrillation. The corridors that remain are too narrow for fibrillation, forcing electrical signals to follow an orderly pattern.

Heart surgery may also be used to treat underlying heart disease, such as coronary artery blockage, that's contributing to an arrhythmia.

Conduction system disease

Signs and symptoms

- Often, none
- Breathlessness and a feeling of exhaustion

Emergency signs and symptoms

- Extreme breathlessness and weakness
- Loss of consciousness, convulsions

Your heart rate is controlled by electric impulses issued by the sinus node in the right atrium. These pacemaker cells produce electric impulses that travel throughout both atria, causing the muscular walls of the atria to contract. The electric impulses travel from the atria through a small bed of specialized tissue called the atrioventricular node to a band of specialized fibers (the bundle of His) that conducts the impulses to the muscle fibers of the ventricles. These muscles then contract.

In conduction system disease (heart block), the electric impulse passes through the atrioventricular node and the bundle of His slowly, intermittently or not at all. This condition can result from various causes:

- Scarring in the path of the specialized conduction fibers
- Coronary artery disease, including a heart attack
- Congenital heart disease
- Effects of certain medications, including digitalis and the beta adrenergic and calcium channel blockers
- Infections such as Lyme disease and mononucleosis

Diagnosis

Many people with heart block have no obvious symptoms. In severe cases, you may experience a sudden loss of consciousness due to dramatic slowing of your heart rate.

Heart block is classified by degrees. First-degree heart block causes no symptoms (asymptomatic) and is evident only on an electrocardiogram as a delay in the transmission of the impulse from the atria to the ventricles. It requires no treatment.

In second-degree heart block, some of the impulses fail to reach the ventricles. The result is an irregular pulse. In many cases, second degree heart block is a result of excessive medications, and the heartbeat often returns to normal with the withdrawal of the medication. Sometimes, use of a pacemaker is necessary.

In third-degree heart block, no impulses reach the ventricles, and

Fainting Spells

A fainting spell can be frightening. Often, however, there's no reason to panic.

A fainting spell (syncope) is a symptom, not a disorder. When you faint, it means that your brain isn't getting sufficient oxygen to function properly. The signs of impending syncope may include nausea, perspiration or a graying-out of your vision. The key sign, however, is a loss of consciousness.

What are the causes?

Fainting is generally classified into three broad categories:

- *Vasodepressive.* Fainting due to a temporary internal nervous system (autonomic) imbalance.
- *Cardiac.* Fainting that results from an electrical or mechanical problem in the heart.
- *Neurologic.* Fainting related to a seizure or, less commonly, a stroke.

In healthy individuals, most fainting spells are harmless and often due to a temporary autonomic imbalance, such as standing too quickly. Syncope can also be triggered by the sight of blood and nausea. In people with heart and blood vessel (cardiovascular) disease, the cause may be more serious and should be evaluated by a doctor.

What are the risks?

Once you're lying flat, blood flow is quickly restored, and you usually regain consciousness. Recovering consciousness quickly after a fainting spell means that little or no damage is sustained by your brain due to the shortage of oxygen. In fact, the most serious risk of syncope is usually from the fall itself. Fractures or head injuries may result.

What should you do?

If you experience a fainting spell that doesn't have an apparent cause — such as extreme heat or a suddenly moving from a lying position to a standing position — consult your doctor. He or she may perform some tests to try to determine a cause and treat the condition appropriately.

the ventricles are forced to beat with their own intrinsic rhythm. The beating of the heart at this intrinsic rate is often so slow that the flow of blood to the brain and other parts of the body is insufficient. Loss of consciousness may result.

Treatment

First degree heart block and many forms of second degree heart block aren't serious conditions. Observation, or withdrawing or reducing the medication responsible, may be all the treatment that's necessary. When the heart is no longer able to pace itself, an artificial cardiac pacemaker is required (see page 768).

Sudden cardiac death

Signs and symptoms

- Immediate loss of consciousness for no apparent cause
- No pulse

Approximately 70 percent to 80 percent of people who experience sudden cardiac death have significant coronary artery disease, even if they don't experience any symptoms. Reducing risk factors for coronary artery disease reduces your risk of sudden cardiac death.

The ventricles are the lower two chambers of the heart and are largely responsible for pumping the blood to all parts of the body. When the control system of the heart malfunctions and causes the ventricles to quiver rapidly and ineffectively (fibrillate), the blood flow stops and sudden cardiac death can result. Coronary artery disease is often the cause. In some cases, the cause can't be determined.

When ventricular fibrillation occurs in a hospital and prompt treatment is available, this rhythm disturbance sometimes can be corrected. However, in most cases of sudden cardiac death, the event occurs beyond the immediate reach of appropriate care, and the person dies before treatment can be given.

Treatment

If the heart ceases to function, cardiopulmonary resuscitation (CPR) is required to maintain some oxygenation of the blood and some flow of blood to the brain.

CPR temporarily restores circulation, but an electrical shock delivered to the heart is required to restore a spontaneous heartbeat. A defibrillator is used to shock the heart, which stops the ventricular fibrillation and allows a normal heart rhythm to return. After resuscitation, anti-arrhythmic medications may be used to prevent recurrent episodes.

Most individuals who survive receive an implantable cardioverter defibrillator (see page 770), which monitors the heart rhythm. If it detects ventricular tachycardia or ventricular fibrillation, the device delivers a shock to terminate the arrhythmia.

Prevention

As doctors learn more about the causes of sudden cardiac death, it's apparent that some people at high risk can be identified.

These include individuals who've experienced a pervious heart attack, those with a weakened heart muscle and some individuals with specific hereditary disorders. These individuals can be treated with a defibrillator before a life-threatening arrhythmia occurs.

Because many cases of ventricular fibrillation stem from coronary artery disease, one of the most important preventive steps is to take care of your heart health. Quit smoking, lose weight if you're overweight, stay physically active and limit dietary fat and cholesterol.

Heart Valve Disorders

The human heart consists of four chambers and four valves. Two of the valves — the mitral and tricuspid valves — regulate the flow of blood from the upper chambers (atria) to the lower chambers (ventricles). The other two valves — aortic and pulmonary valves — regulate the flow of blood out of the ventricles for circulation to other parts of the body.

The mitral valve links the atrium to the ventricle on the heart's left side. The aortic valve, which is also on the left, opens to allow blood to flow from the left ventricle into the body's main artery (aorta).

On the right side, the tricuspid valve regulates flow from the atrium to the ventricle, and the pulmonary valve allows blood to exit from the heart's right ventricle into the lungs by way of the pulmonary artery (see the color illustration on page 409).

The valves allow blood to flow in only one direction. Each valve consists of two or three strong, thin flaps (leaflets) of tissue. When closed, a valve prevents blood from flowing to the next chamber or from returning to the previous one.

When the valve opening becomes narrowed and flow through it is limited, the condition is called stenosis. Each of the heart's valves may be subject to stenosis or obstruction. In addition, a valve may lose its shape and begin to bulge (prolapse) or fail to close completely (leak), causing a backflow of blood (regurgitation).

Valve problems may occur as a result of infection, a congenital abnormality, heart attack, a disease of the heart muscle or deterioration due to aging.

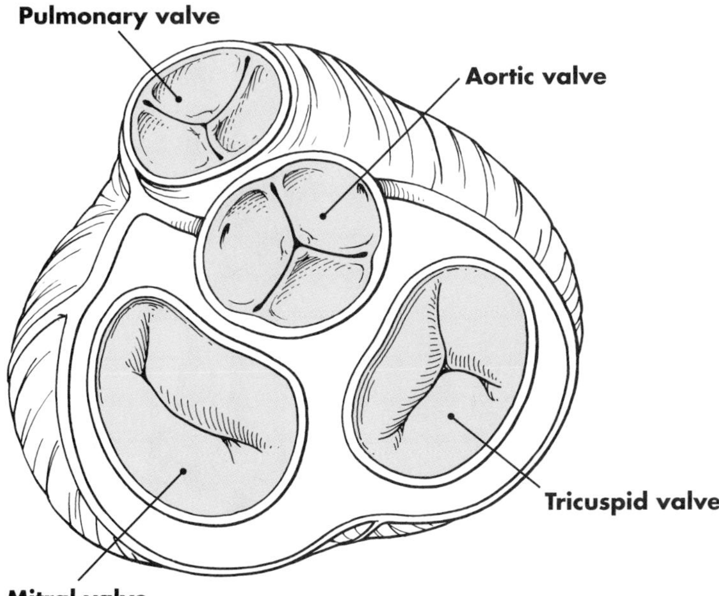

Each heart valve consists of two or three flaps (leaflets) of tissue. When closed, a valve prevents blood from flowing to the next chamber or from returning to the previous one. When open, blood flows freely.

Mitral valve problems

Signs and symptoms

- Often, none
- Breathlessness, especially after exercise
- Fatigue
- Frequent bouts of bronchitis
- Chest discomfort or palpitations

On the left side of your heart, the mitral valve links the upper chamber (atrium) to the lower chamber (ventricle). When the opening of the mitral valve becomes narrowed and the passage of blood through it is restricted, the condition is termed mitral valve stenosis. When the mitral valve fails to close properly and blood leaks back into the atrium from the ventricle, the disorder is called mitral valve regurgitation or incompetence.

Mitral valve stenosis

When the mitral valve narrows and blood flow is restricted, too much blood accumulates in the left atrium. Pressure builds up in the left atrium and the chamber may enlarge. Blood may back up into the lungs, leading to lung congestion (pulmonary edema). Mitral valve stenosis commonly leads to a heart rhythm irregularity called atrial fibrillation.

Mitral valve stenosis is almost always due to rheumatic fever, a complication of streptococcal throat infection (strep throat). But some babies are born with an already narrowed mitral valve and develop mitral stenosis early in life. These babies usually require heart surgery to correct the valve. Others are born with a malformed mitral valve that puts them at risk of developing mitral valve stenosis when they're older.

Mitral valve prolapse

Located on the left side of your heart, the mitral valve, which consists of two strong, thin flaps (leaflets) of tissue, links the upper chamber (atrium) to the lower chamber (ventricle). When functioning normally, the mitral valve controls the movement of blood between the chambers. In some people, however, one or both valve leaflets bulge (prolapse) into the left atrium like a parachute during the heart's contraction. The prolapse of the valve may result in clicking sounds that your doctor can detect when listening to your heart with a stethoscope.

The condition may also result in failure of the valves to close properly, and blood may leak back (regurgitate) into the atrium during pumping by the ventricle. This flow of blood back into the atrium produces a sound called a murmur.

This generally harmless condition may be found in as many as 1 in 10 Americans, more often in women than in men. It's also more common in women who have scoliosis or certain other skeletal abnormalities. It appears to occur more often in some families than others.

Mitral valve regurgitation

In this condition, regurgitation of blood into the atrium causes blood flow to the rest of the body to decrease. The left ventricle, the main pumping chamber, then pumps harder in an attempt to compensate for the decreased blood flow. Consequently, the left ventricle may become enlarged and eventually may fail.

Mitral valve regurgitation has several possible causes. It can be the result of damage sustained during a bout of rheumatic fever. It can be present from birth. Or it can result from a ballooning out (prolapsing) of the mitral valve or from damage to the cords that anchor the flaps (leaflets) of the mitral valve to the heart wall. Other causes include an infection of the heart's inner lining (endocarditis), age-related wear and tear and a prior heart attack.

Diagnosis

Breathlessness, especially on mild exertion or at night, is a common symptom of mitral valve problems. In advanced cases, backing up of blood may lead to accumulation of fluid (edema) in the ankles, causing them to swell.

Many of the signs and symptoms of mitral valve regurgitation are similar to those of mitral valve stenosis. To confirm the diagnosis, your doctor will likely listen to your heart to try to detect the sound of a characteristic heart murmur. A chest X-ray also can help your doctor determine if the left ventricle is enlarged. Lung congestion also is visible on an X-ray.

Often, mitral valve prolapse is discovered during a routine stethoscope examination of your heart. Your doctor may confirm the diagnosis with a test called an echocardiogram.

An electrocardiogram can help detect heart rhythm irregularities. A test called an echocardiogram can define the configuration of the valve along with abnormalities of blood flow through it (see page 776). Tests such as a transesophageal echocardiogram or cardiac catheterization can provide even more detailed information about the state of your heart valves.

How serious are mitral valve problems?

If your valve disease is mild, you may remain well or have only minimal symptoms for decades.

Severe valve disease can weaken your heart to the point where it's

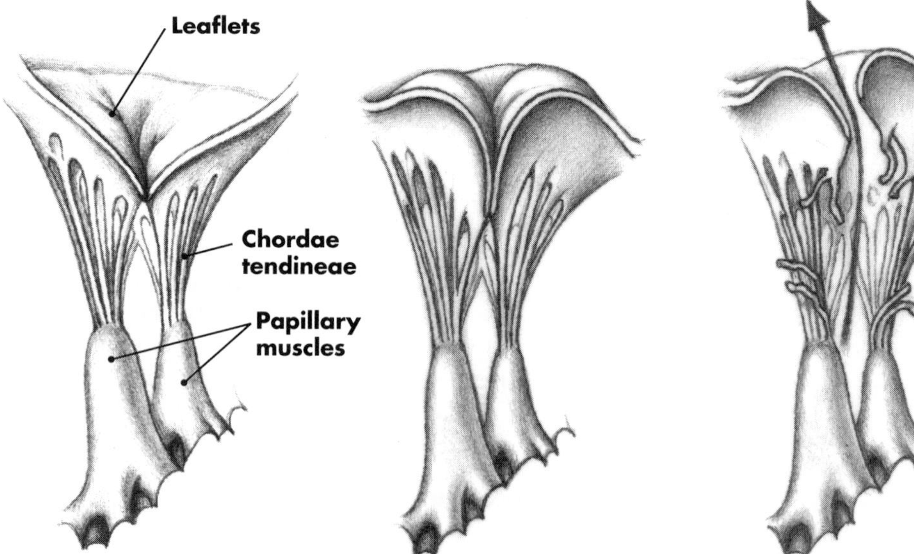

A normal mitral valve (left) closes tightly to prevent leakage of blood. A prolapsed mitral valve (center) causes the thin flaps (leaflets) of tissue that control the flow of blood to bulge (prolapse) upward during closure. This may occur because the leaflets are too large or the valve's tendons are too long. Mitral valve regurgitation (right) may result if some of the valve's tendons break, causing leaflets to flail and allowing blood to leak back into the atrium.

Balloon Valvuloplasty

A narrowed heart valve (stenosis) can limit blood flow and lead to complications such as heart failure. The problem may be treated by open heart surgery or a procedure called balloon valvuloplasty.

The decision to proceed with valvuloplasty is based on the risk of the procedure versus the risk of surgery. Less calcified and less severely deformed valves carry a very low risk for balloon valvuloplasty. Balloon valvuloplasty is more commonly used for mitral valve stenosis than aortic valve stenosis. In the case of aortic valve stenosis, balloon valvuloplasty is generally used only if aortic valve surgery is thought to be too risky for you or if you have some other serious medical problem that requires treatment before aortic valve replacement.

Procedure

During balloon valvuloplasty of the mitral valve, a catheter is inserted through a vein, most often in the groin area. The catheter is guided through your blood vessels to the right side of the heart and to the mitral valve. A balloon at the tip of the catheter is gently inflated to widen the valve opening, thus improving blood flow. Sometimes, two balloons are inflated.

The procedure for aortic valvuloplasty is similar except that a catheter is inserted into an artery and advanced backward across the aortic valve. When the tip is in the opening of the diseased valve, the balloon is inflated.

Recovery

As with any heart procedure, there are risks. But the result may be immediate relief of symptoms such as breathlessness. The hospital stay and recovery time for balloon valvuloplasty are substantially less than for open heart surgery.

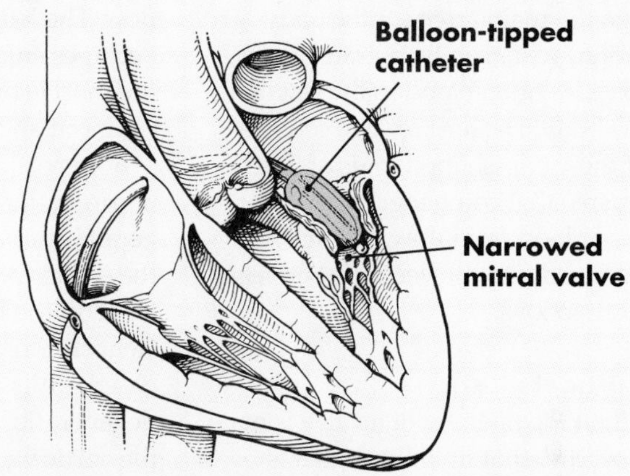

Mitral valve stenosis may be effectively treated by threading a catheter with an inflatable balloon through a vein and across the atrial septum. The balloon is positioned through the tight mitral opening and then inflated, forcing the valve leaflets apart to produce a wider opening.

unable to pump enough blood to meet your body's needs, a condition called congestive heart failure. There's also risk of atrial fibrillation, in which the heart beats in a rapid and uncoordinated fashion. This can lead to the dangerous formation of a blood clot (thrombus) that can travel to other parts of the body (embolism) and cause serious damage. Mitral valve problems also put you at risk of infection of your heart's inner lining (endocarditis).

Treatment

Treatment depends on the severity and progression of your condition. In general, the focus is on maximizing your heart's function, minimizing your signs and symptoms and avoiding future complications.

Most people with mitral valve prolapse have normal life expectancies and aren't required to make adjustments in their lifestyle. For most, the condition is best regarded as nothing more than a harmless variation from normal.

Medication

Excess accumulation of fluid in your lungs or lower extremities (edema) may be treated with a diuretic medication. Often called water pills, these medications increase the rate and volume of your urine formation, helping to decrease excess fluid in your body. Other medications, such as angiotensin-converting enzyme (ACE) inhibitors, may be used to help your heart to pump blood more efficiently.

If you experience atrial fibrillation, a medication such as digoxin, a calcium channel blocker or a beta blocker may be prescribed to slow the rapid heart rate. An anticoagulant medication may be prescribed to prevent blood clots or emboli.

Surgery

In mitral valve stenosis, when other treatments are unsuccessful, your doctor may recommend balloon valvuloplasty. In this procedure, the constricted valve opening is enlarged using a catheter with a balloon on its tip. If the valve is too hardened (calcified), the balloon procedure may not be safe or feasible, and the valve will need to be replaced surgically (see page 778).

A complication of mitral valve prolapse, particularly in middle-age or older adults, is rupture of one or more of the supporting tendons, causing a valve leaflet to flail and allow a greater backflow of blood into the atrium. This generally requires surgery.

With mitral valve regurgitation, the valve may be repaired surgically. Other times, the valve may have to be replaced with an artificial valve.

Aortic valve problems

Signs and symptoms

- Often, none
- Weakness on exertion
- Breathlessness
- Chest pain (angina)
- Fainting spells

The aortic valve controls the flow of blood out of the heart's main pumping chamber (left ventricle) into the main artery of the body (aorta) which, in turn, transports oxygen-laden blood to the rest of the body. The aortic valve consists of three cup-shaped folds of tissue (cusps) that come together to prevent blood from flowing back from the aorta into the ventricle between contractions.

Aortic stenosis

When the opening of a valve is narrowed so that flow through it is limited, the condition is termed stenosis. Such a narrowing in the aortic valve requires the left ventricle to pump harder to maintain normal blood output. This often results in thickening of the muscle of the left ventricle, a condition called left ventricular hypertrophy. Over time, the left ventricle muscle becomes less efficient, enlarged and flabby.

Aortic regurgitation

A different sort of problem occurs when the aortic valve fails to shut tightly between contractions. Called aortic regurgitation, this condition allows blood to leak back into the ventricle. Consequently, flow of blood to the rest of the body decreases, and the heart must pump harder in an attempt to compensate for the decreased blood flow. The left ventricle often becomes enlarged over time, and the muscle of the ventricle may wear out and become flabby.

Both aortic stenosis and aortic regurgitation can result from a congenital abnormality or damage to the aortic valve from rheumatic fever. In the United States, aortic stenosis most commonly occurs in older adults and results from degeneration and calcification of the aortic valve.

Diagnosis

Your doctor may suspect either of these disorders while listening to your heart with a stethoscope. He or she may order one or several tests, including a chest X-ray, electrocardiogram, echocardiogram and cardiac catheterization. These tests can help your doctor determine how damaged your aortic valve may be and how well your heart is pumping.

How serious are aortic valve problems?

The most serious risk with aortic valve problems is posed by overwork of the left ventricle. This can result in angina, congestive heart failure or fainting spells. Aortic valve disorders can also lead to heart rhythm abnormalities.

Aortic valve problems put you at greater risk of infection of your heart's inner lining (endocarditis). As a precaution, preventive use of antibiotics before dental and certain surgical procedures is usually recommended.

Aortic valve problems may develop and progress without symptoms until they reach a hazardous phase. Prompt treatment, such as aortic valve surgery, may then be necessary.

Treatment

In most cases, neither aortic stenosis nor aortic regurgitation means that you need to adopt a passive lifestyle. While you many need to avoid strenuous activity, reasonable physical activity is usually encour-

Echocardiogram

Before the development of echocardiography, a doctor generally had to rely on a medical history, a physical examination, an electrocardiogram and an X-ray to evaluate how well an individual's heart was functioning. Now it's possible to "look" directly at a person's heart without ever penetrating the skin.

Echocardiography is a special application of ultrasonography, or ultrasound. The concept behind ultrasound is the same as that used in depth finders on boats.

A wand-like device called a transducer sends sound waves into your body and receives echoes from the surfaces of internal structures, such as your heart muscle and heart valves. A machine called an echocardiograph analyzes the waves to determine how far away the structures are from the transducer. Using this information, a computer calculates the time it takes the sound waves to travel to and from your heart and then reconstructs an image of the heart. The image (echocardiogram) of your heart is displayed on a monitor and can be recorded on videotape or printed on paper.

Echocardiography allows the heart to be seen in action and can be used to diagnose various heart disorders. On the screen, your doctor can observe the heart's main pumping chamber, its movement (contractility), the shape and thickness of the chamber walls, the valves, the heart's external covering (pericardium), and the large veins and arteries that lead into and out of the heart. The velocity and direction of blood flow through the heart valves and chambers also can be recorded by a technique called a Doppler ultrasound to determine narrowing and leakage of the valves.

Procedure

When you undergo echocardiography, you lie on your back and perhaps turn slightly to your left. A special jelly is applied to your

aged. Follow an exercise program within guidelines recommended by your doctor.

Medication
Because aortic valve disease can reduce the heart's pumping efficiency and lead to heart failure, you may need medications to augment contraction of the ventricles, to control fluid retention or to reduce the workload on your heart. Aortic valve disease can also lead to heart rhythm problems, requiring antiarrythmic medications to control your heart rhythm.

If your condition is complicated by atrial fibrillation, heart failure or blood clots, you may need anticoagulant medications to reduce the risk of blood clot formation.

Surgery
If your aortic valve malfunction is severe, the only long-term solution may be surgical repair or replacement of the valve (see page 778).

Tricuspid and pulmonary valve problems

Signs and symptoms

- Often, none
- Fatigue
- Breathlessness
- Lightheadedness
- Fainting
- Fluid retention
- Swelling in the arms, legs and liver
- Discomfort in the upper-right abdomen
- Nausea and vomiting

The valves on the right side of the heart (tricuspid and pulmonary) are much less frequently affected by disease than those on the left side, and when they are, the problem is often better tolerated.

Blood returning from the body flows into the right atrium, through the tricuspid valve to the right ventricle below. Then it exits from the right ventricle through the pulmonary valve to the pulmonary artery, which carries the blood to the lungs for oxygenation.

The tricuspid and pulmonary valves, like the aortic and mitral valves, can have problems in which the valve opening narrows, restricting the flow of blood (tricuspid stenosis and pulmonary stenosis). In some cases, the valve fails to close properly, allowing blood to flow back through the valve when it's supposed to be closed (regurgitation).

Tricuspid and pulmonary valve problems are usually caused by rheumatic fever or congenital abnormalities.

Diagnosis

Often, these conditions are discovered by doctors during routine examinations. Your doctor may recommend tests — such as a chest X-ray, electrocardiogram and echocardiogram — to determine the status of blood flow and your heart's pumping ability.

How serious are tricuspid and pulmonary valve problems?

Tricuspid and pulmonary valve disorders are usually associated with other mitral or aortic valve problems, which will determine how serious the condition may be. In some cases, right-sided heart failure may develop. In pulmonary stenosis, which is almost always a congenital problem, failure of the right ventricle can lead to death before 30 years of age. Therefore, most people with pulmonary stenosis require treatment to correct the problem.

These valve problems may also put you at greater risk of endocarditis, an infection of the heart's

chest to increase the conductivity of the ultrasound waves. The transducer is maneuvered to different locations and in different positions on your chest to view your heart from various angles.

Although the test is noninvasive and usually painless, you may feel some pressure as the transducer occasionally must be held firmly against your chest. A thorough examination may take from 15 minutes to more than an hour, depending on the complexity of the problem.

Advantages

The procedure requires no X-ray exposure. The equipment is portable, so the test can be done in your hospital room, in your doctor's office or even in the operating room.

Variation

If your doctor needs a clearer picture, he or she may request a variation of the test called transesophageal echocardiography. In this test, a transducer is threaded down your throat into your esophagus. The proximity of the esophagus to the heart and major blood vessel in your chest (aorta) can overcome some limitations — such as body shape and weight — that accompany traditional echocardiography, and provide an even better view of the heart.

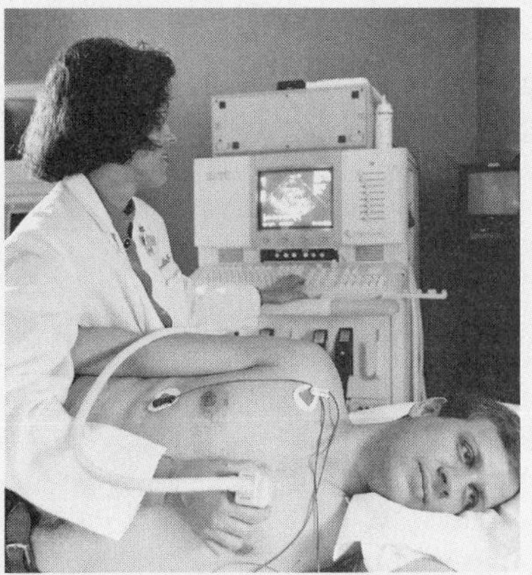

During an echocardiogram, a technician or doctor holds a wand-like device (transducer) over your chest wall. The transducer produces images of your heart that can be seen on a monitor.

lining. As a precaution, preventive use of antibiotics before dental and certain surgical procedures is appropriate.

Treatment
Treatment may not be required. However, if the valve is badly deteriorated, valve repair or replacement may be necessary. In certain situations, the valve may be opened by stretching it with a balloon catheter inserted through a vein in the leg and advanced to the heart.

Rheumatic fever

Signs and symptoms
Major
Two of the following must be present:
- Inflammation of the heart, sometimes manifested by weakness and shortness of breath
- Arthritis that tends to migrate from one joint to another
- Uncontrolled movement of limbs and face
- Raised, red patches on the skin
- Lumps under the skin

Minor
Presence of one major and two minor criteria and evidence of a throat infection:
- Joint aches without inflammation
- Fever
- Previous rheumatic fever or evidence of rheumatic heart disease
- Abnormal heartbeat on electrocardiogram (ECG)
- A blood test indicating presence of inflammation

Rheumatic fever is a serious inflammatory condition that appears to be the result of an immune reaction of the body to specific strains of streptococcal bacteria. A week or two after a streptococcal throat infection (strep throat), symptoms of rheumatic fever may appear.

Prompt and appropriate antibiotic treatment of strep throat will largely prevent the occurrence of rheumatic fever. In fact, prevention of rheumatic fever is the main reason antibiotics are prescribed for strep throat.

One of the problems in preventing rheumatic fever, however, is that sore throats that result from harmless viral infections are often difficult to distinguish from those caused by streptococci. To be sure that strep throat infections are treated properly, throat cultures are obtained to identify the organisms. If the culture is positive, the doctor will likely prescribe an antibiotic.

Rheumatic fever is relatively rare. It isn't as common in the United States today as it was 40 years ago, before the widespread use of penicillin. But several outbreaks were reported in U.S. cities during the late 1980s. Rheumatic fever is still common in developing countries.

Most strep throat infections don't lead to rheumatic fever. When

Heart Valve Surgery

In some cases, open heart surgery may be the best option for individuals with heart valve problems. The term *open heart surgery* implies opening the chest and using a heart-lung machine to support the patient's breathing and blood flow while the abnormality of the heart is being repaired. Open heart procedures include coronary artery bypass surgery, correction of congenital abnormalities of the heart, heart valve surgery and removal of some heart tumors.

Valve repair
If you need valve surgery, your doctor will, if possible, repair the natural valve rather than insert an artificial (prosthetic) valve because the results with natural valve repair are usually better and longer-lasting. And with this type of surgery, you may not need to take anticoagulant medications, as is necessary with artificial valves. A surgeon may repair the valve by reconnecting the valve leaflets to the tendons that anchor the valve to the heart muscle or by cutting out excess tissue so that the leaflets can close snugly. Sometimes, repair includes cinching the surrounding ring of heart tissue tighter to ensure that the leaflets close adequately.

Valve replacement
Replacement of the mitral valve with an artificial valve is necessary if either repair or balloon valvuloplasty is unlikely to provide a satisfactory result. Valve replacement is also the preferred treatment for aortic valve disease that needs treatment beyond medication. To replace a damaged heart valve, the surgeon removes it and sutures an artificial valve in its place.

Your doctor will discuss with you what type of prosthetic valve would be best for you. Each type has some advantages and disadvantages. Mechanical prosthetic valves are constructed from metal and synthetic materials. These are extremely durable, but if you have one implanted, you'll need to take an anticoagulant such as warfarin (Coumadin) for the rest of your life because blood has a tendency to clot on the valve.

Bioprostheses are made from animal or human tissue. An animal tissue bioprosthesis is usually made from a pig's heart valve, or it is fashioned from the pericardium or outer lining of the heart of a cow. A human tissue bioprosthesis (homograft) consists of a heart valve obtained from someone who has died. The advantage of bioprostheses is that they rarely require anticoagulation medication. However, they're not as durable as mechanical valves.

Procedure
When you undergo heart valve surgery, you'll be given a general anes-

rheumatic fever does occur, it usually occurs in children.

Diagnosis

No laboratory test can confirm that your child has rheumatic fever. A diagnosis is generally based on his or her symptoms, classified by the several major and minor criteria listed above.

The most common major criteria are pain and swelling that migrate from joint to joint and inflammation of the heart. In some cases, your child's doctor may take a blood sample to test for the presence of antibodies to streptococcal bacteria. He or she may also recommend an ECG to check for any abnormal heart rhythms.

How serious is rheumatic fever?

Rheumatic fever can result in inflammation in one or several organs. Most often, several joints are affected with arthritic swelling, redness and the sensation of heat.

Between 40 percent and 60 percent of people having a first attack of rheumatic fever have heart inflammation, which may resolve with no permanent damage. In some cases, however, permanent scarring of one or more heart valves may occur, which can cause obstruction to blood flow (stenosis) or backflow of blood (regurgitation).

Over a period of months or years, valve function may be seriously compromised, and surgery ultimately may be necessary to repair or replace the damaged heart valve or valves. In rare instances, the heart muscle becomes overwhelmed by the inflammation (myocarditis) and death from heart failure occurs.

If acute rheumatic fever affects the brain, uncoordinated or uncontrolled movements of the limbs or facial muscles (chorea) may occur. Rheumatic fever can also produce disk-like raised and red areas on the skin (erythema marginatum). Lumps or nodules may form beneath normal-appearing skin.

Treatment

Antibiotics are given to eliminate any remaining streptococcal organisms. Administration of low-dose penicillin, orally or by monthly injection, effectively prevents recurrences of rheumatic fever.

Nonsteroidal anti-inflammatory drugs (NSAIDs) can help reduce inflammation of the heart or joints. For severe heart inflammation, a corticosteroid medication, such as prednisone, can help reduce the inflammation.

Endocarditis

Signs and symptoms

- Fever
- A heart murmur

thetic. Through an incision the length of your breastbone (sternum), your heart is exposed and connected to a heart-lung machine that takes over the functions of breathing and maintains blood circulation during the procedure. The damaged heart valve is repaired or replaced.

Recovery

After the operation, you'll likely spend one or more days in an intensive care unit (ICU). During recuperation, therapists, dietitians, patient educators and your doctor will assist your recovery and return to a productive life.

All prosthetic valves are prone to infection, which is difficult to treat with antibiotics once it develops. If you have a prosthetic valve, it's extremely important to take appropriate precautions, which generally involve taking antibiotics before any dental or surgical procedure.

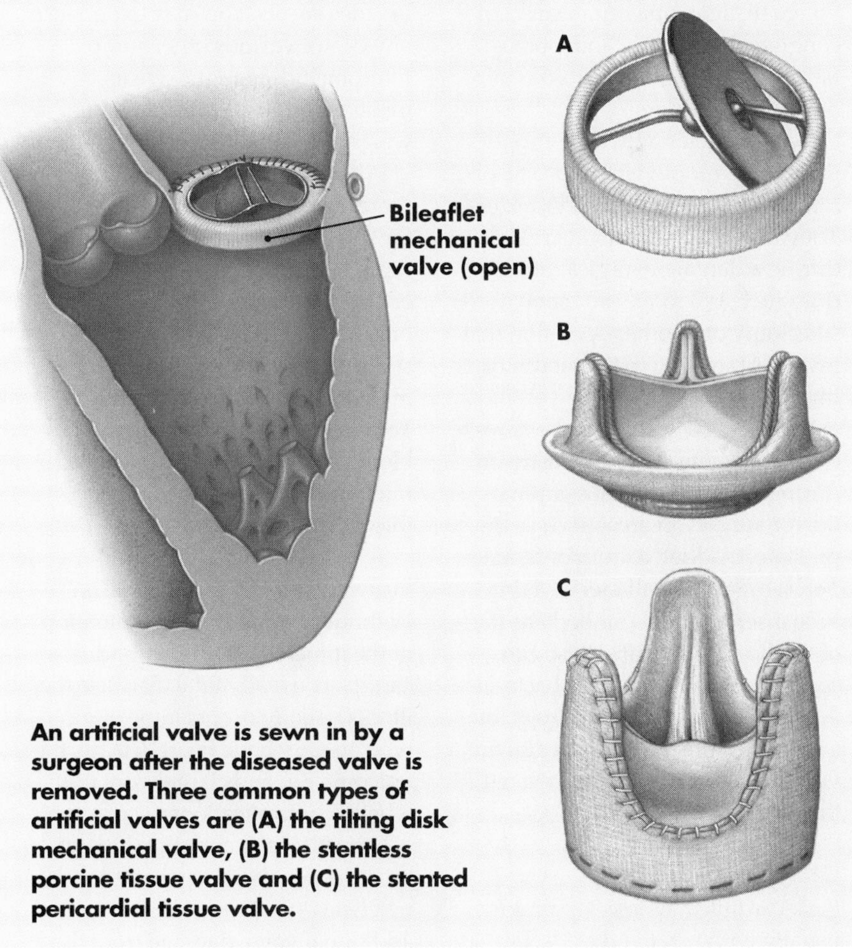

An artificial valve is sewn in by a surgeon after the diseased valve is removed. Three common types of artificial valves are (A) the tilting disk mechanical valve, (B) the stentless porcine tissue valve and (C) the stented pericardial tissue valve.

- Unusual fatigue or loss of appetite
- Night sweats, chills

Endocarditis is an infection of your heart's inner lining (endocardium). Typically, the infection involves one of your heart valves. It occurs when germs enter your bloodstream and travel to your heart, where they adhere to abnormal tissue inside the heart and attack that tissue. Bacteria or fungi can cause the infection. Most cases are caused by bacteria and referred to as bacterial endocarditis.

If you have a normal, healthy heart, you're unlikely to contract endocarditis. Usually, your immune system destroys bacteria that enter into your bloodstream. In addition, bacteria may pass through a normal heart and never cause an infection.

However, you're at risk of this disease if you have a diseased or damaged heart valve because you may have a roughened and abnormal surface within your heart where the infecting organisms can congregate, multiply and, potentially, spread to other parts of your body.

Certain bacteria that commonly inhabit the mouth and upper respiratory tract may cause endocarditis. They may enter the bloodstream during a dental or surgical procedure such as a tooth extraction, tonsillectomy or another operation that involves bleeding in the mouth or throat.

Intestinal bacteria, called enterococci, may enter your bloodstream during an instrumental examination or surgery in areas such as the prostate, bladder, rectum or female pelvic organs. A catheter — a thin tube inserted into your body as part of medical treatment — also can serve as an entry point for bacteria.

Individuals who inject drugs into a vein with unsterilized needles are vulnerable to endocarditis, even if they have normal valves.

Diagnosis

Endocarditis may develop rapidly, usually with fever and chills, but this isn't always the case, especially in older adults. You may experience any one of various other symptoms, including night sweats, malaise, fatigue, loss of appetite, weight loss and joint inflammation.

When the infection develops more slowly, your doctor will look for such signs as an abnormally rapid heart rate (tachycardia), an enlarged spleen, pallor or a yellow-brown color to the skin, tiny red spots on the skin and mucous membranes and heart murmurs. Your doctor may order a series of blood cultures to determine which microorganism is causing the infection.

> **PREVENTION TIP**
>
> Rheumatic fever is avoidable. Pay close attention whenever your child develops a sore throat. Consult your child's doctor if a sore throat persists for more than 24 hours and is accompanied by a fever. If your child's doctor suspects a streptococcal throat infection (strep throat), he or she will probably order a throat culture for your child. If the culture results are positive, your doctor will likely prescribe an antibiotic medication to kill the streptococcal bacteria and prevent complications such as rheumatic fever.
>
> Even if your child's throat begins to feel better after just a couple of days, make sure he or she takes all of the medication as prescribed.

How serious is endocarditis?

Without treatment and elimination of the infecting organism, endocarditis is usually fatal. Because the illness usually occurs in people who already have heart disease, the outcome depends largely on whether complications occur.

Even if you're cured of the bacterial infection, you may have continued heart symptoms due to additional valve damage from the infection. Complications such as cardiac or renal failure may develop as well.

A more common danger with endocarditis is that clumps of bacteria and cellular debris (vegetations) may form in your heart at the site of the infection. These clumps may break loose and block blood vessels elsewhere in your body, causing a variety of problems including stroke or other organ damage.

Treatment

Even with the availability of powerful modern antibiotics, treatment of endocarditis can be difficult and the results uncertain. Furthermore, many types of bacteria have become resistant to antibiotics. Thus, prevention is still the best approach.

Medication

Antibiotic therapy depends on the type of microorganism causing the disease. Blood cultures are used to determine which antibiotic is most appropriate. Often, a combination is used, with penicillin commonly being one of them. The medication is often given through a vein continually over a period of several weeks to eradicate the infection.

Surgery

If the infection causes major damage to the heart valves, valve replacement may be necessary.

Diseases of the Heart Muscle and Lining

The heart wall has three layers:

- The epicardium, a thin, smooth covering on the outside of the heart
- The myocardium, the heart muscle itself
- The endocardium, the smooth inner lining of the heart that's in contact with the blood

Endocarditis: Protection and Prevention

Antibiotics offer protection from endocarditis by destroying or controlling bacteria. Use of such medications may be advisable before and after certain medical and dental procedures during which bacteria could enter your bloodstream, travel to your heart and cause an infection.

Who's at risk?
The following conditions put you at greater risk of endocarditis:
- Heart valves scarred by rheumatic fever
- Congenital heart or heart valve defects
- Other heart valve problems, such as mitral valve prolapse
- An artificial heart valve
- Thickening of the heart muscle (hypertrophic cardiomyopathy)
- A history of previous endocarditis

Which procedures carry the greatest risk?
Procedures that may put certain individuals at risk of endocarditis include:
- Any procedure on your mouth or throat that may cause bleeding
- Professional teeth cleaning
- A bladder operation
- Prostate removal
- Gynecologic procedures
- Gastrointestinal procedures, including gallbladder removal, hemorrhoid removal, polyp removal or colon surgery

Antibiotics may be recommended before other types of procedures, even nonmedical ones such as body piercing and tattooing. Your doctor may also prescribe antibiotics if you develop a lung or skin infection.

What should you do?
If you're at risk of endocarditis, it's vital to let medical and dental professionals know of that risk. Many people carry a card prepared by the American Heart Association for this purpose. To secure a copy, contact your local chapter or visit the association's Web site (see page 1380).

You can also help prevent endocarditis by taking good care of yourself and avoiding infections in general. In particular, take care of your teeth and gums because your mouth can be a reservoir for germs. Routinely floss and brush your teeth and gums and get regular dental checkups.

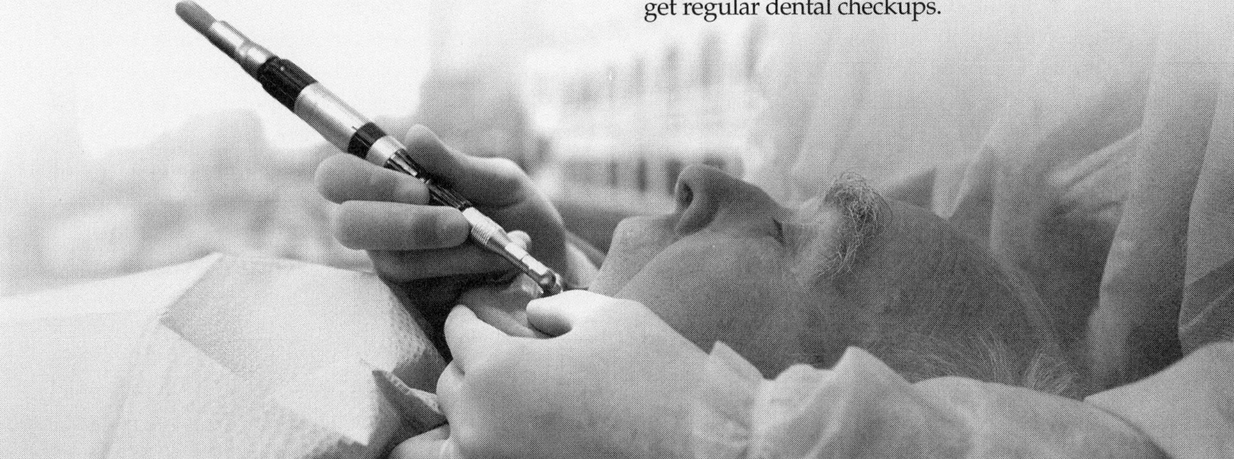

Surrounding the heart on the outside is the pericardium, a fibrous sac.

Like the rest of your body, the heart muscle and its associated linings are subject to disease. Although relatively rare, diseases that can damage the heart muscle and the heart's linings do occur. These diseases may develop as isolated problems or they may be consequences of disorders that affect other organs.

Cardiomyopathy

Signs and symptoms
- Episodes of rapid heartbeat (palpitations)
- Breathlessness
- Weakness
- Chest pain and pressure (angina)
- Fainting
- Fluid retention

When the muscle of the heart is damaged or defective, the disorder is termed *cardiomyopathy*. The term comes from Greek roots for "heart" *(kardia)*, "muscle" *(myo)* and "disease" *(pathos)*.

Types
Cardiomyopathy may appear in one of several forms:

Dilated cardiomyopathy
In dilated cardiomyopathy, also referred to as congestive cardiomyopathy, the heart muscle is weakened and is unable to pump

efficiently. This may produce symptoms of congestive heart failure, including breathlessness and retention of water, which results in swelling (edema) that's most prominent in the feet and ankles.

Dilated cardiomyopathy also causes enlarged heart chambers and may lead to the formation of clots within the chambers. The clots may travel to other parts of the body and cause an embolism.

Dilated cardiomyopathy occurs at any age and seems to run in families. Alcoholics may develop dilated cardiomyopathy after consuming large quantities of alcohol over many years. If the problem hasn't advanced to the point of heart failure, avoiding alcohol may halt progression of the disease. Dilated cardiomyopathy may also develop after a viral illness.

Hypertrophic cardiomyopathy
Hypertrophic cardiomyopathy occurs when the heart muscle thickens. This thickening reduces the size of the pumping chambers and may cause obstruction of the blood flow out of the heart. It also prevents the heart from relaxing between beats. This doesn't allow the heart to fill properly, further decreasing the volume of blood pumped out of the body.

Because hypertrophic cardiomyopathy may be inherited, it's advisable to have all close relatives of a person with the condition tested for the disorder, even if they have no symptoms.

Heart Transplantation

In some situations, the heart becomes so damaged or weak that conventional medical treatment can do little to improve its functioning. In such cases, a heart transplant may be considered.

During the past 30 years, heart transplantation has become a relatively common procedure in many medical centers. Approximately 2,300 heart transplants are done each year in the United States. Results have improved so that current 1-year survival rates at experienced medical centers are from 85 percent to 95 percent. Survival without a transplant in this group is dismal. Most people who undergo a transplant enjoy a full and active life, and many return to full-time employment.

Who qualifies?

Almost anyone from a newborn infant with a serious congenital heart defect to an older adult with end-stage heart disease can be considered for heart transplantation. Potential heart transplant candidates should be motivated for transplantation and have good function of all other vital organs, including the liver, kidneys and lungs. Candidates need to be free of other noncardiac diseases, such as blood disorders, severe diabetes or cancers that reduce life expectancy.

People most likely to benefit are usually those younger than age 65 with irreversible heart disease in which the life expectancy without transplantation would be less than 2 or 3 years.

Available organs

Unfortunately, nearly one-third of the people waiting for a heart transplant die before a donor heart becomes available because of the shortage of hearts for transplant. Educational efforts to inform the public of the need for more donor hearts is a high priority. Although no one should want another person to die so that a heart will be available for transplantation, when deaths occur, families often find comfort in helping others through organ donation.

Procedure

Before a heart transplant operation, a donor heart must be available. Most often, this heart comes from a healthy person who died of an accident that didn't damage the heart. A nationally maintained waiting list uses a computer to match a patient in the region of the donor with a compatible blood type and acceptable size range for the donor heart. Once doctors remove the heart from the donor, ideally it should be transplanted into the recipient within 4 hours.

The donated heart is transported in a special cold solution to the recipient hospital. The recipient's chest cavity is opened, and the diseased heart is removed. During this portion of the procedure, the supply of oxygenated blood to the recipient is maintained by a heart-lung machine, as is done in many other types of heart surgery. The donated heart is then placed into the recipient's chest cavity and delicately connected to the major blood vessels.

Rejection

All transplanted organs are susceptible to rejection. The body's immune system recognizes the transplanted tissue as foreign and produces antibodies to attack it, just as the immune system might attack a virus or bacterium.

To minimize the risk of rejection of a transplanted heart, medications that suppress the body's normal immune response are needed. Some of these immunosuppressant medications are used for only a short time after the operation. Others must be taken for the rest of a person's life.

Immunosuppressant medications also decrease your body's ability to recognize and resist infections. Dosages must be monitored carefully to minimize side effects. Periodic biopsies of your heart tissue can aid your doctor in assessing rejection. The biopsy specimen is

Restrictive cardiomyopathy
Restrictive cardiomyopathy is characterized by stiffening of the heart muscle and decreased ability of the heart to expand and fill with blood between contractions. Development of blood clots within the heart chambers, water retention and a tender liver are other common signs.

The condition is rare in industrialized nations, but in other parts of the world, such as Central Africa, it's common.

Diagnosis
In diagnosing cardiomyopathy, your doctor will consider your symptoms and may perform X-ray and electrocardiographic examinations.

Your doctor will likely recommend an ultrasound procedure (echocardiography) to observe the motions of your heart at work (see page 776). An echocardiogram often can determine what form of cardiomyopathy is present. In some cases, a procedure called heart catheterization may be needed. During this procedure, your doctor may also obtain a tissue sample (biopsy) from the heart for microscopic examination.

How serious is cardiomyopathy?
In most cases, cardiomyopathy poses no symptoms until the disease is quite advanced. Rarely, the condition causes sudden death.

Certain forms of cardiomyopathy may put you at greater risk of an

obtained by way of a catheter that's placed in a vein and advanced to the heart.

Recovery
Most people who have had a successful heart transplant can live a relatively normal life. Many live for more than a decade and some for more than 20 years following their heart transplant.

Long-term complications
Now that transplant recipients are living longer, doctors have found that some problems appear years after transplantation. The transplanted heart's coronary arteries may develop widespread narrowing (atherosclerosis). Because the nerves have been cut in the transplanted heart, recipients don't usually feel chest pain (angina) when their coronary arteries don't supply enough oxygen to the heart muscle. Therefore, doctors may perform annual coronary angiography and intracoronary ultrasound to look for possible narrowing of the coronary arteries.

Doctors also continue to examine recipients for any evidence of tumor formation, especially of the skin and lymph glands, because immunosuppressant medications can increase the chances of these types of cancers (malignancies).

Recent developments
The greatest challenge in heart transplantation is solving the serious donor shortage. It doesn't appear that there will ever be enough human donors to satisfy the need, therefore alternative strategies are being explored:

Ventricular assist devices
One such effort involves the use of a left ventricular assist device to perform the work of the main pumping chamber of the heart (left ventricle). Weakness of the left ventricle is the cause of heart failure symptoms in most people. Assist devices are currently being used in many major centers to keep heart transplant candidates alive while they wait for a donor heart. Several ventricular assist devices and full artificial hearts have been studied as an alternative to transplantation among individuals who aren't candidates for transplantation. The devices are proving effective and ultimately may offer hope for long-term treatment of people with heart failure.

Xenotransplantation
Another approach is developing animals, particularly pigs, whose organs have been genetically engineered to be used for human transplantation (xenotransplantation). This work is still in its early phases. If this research is successful, this type of transplantation could prove to be a long-term solution to the donor shortage.

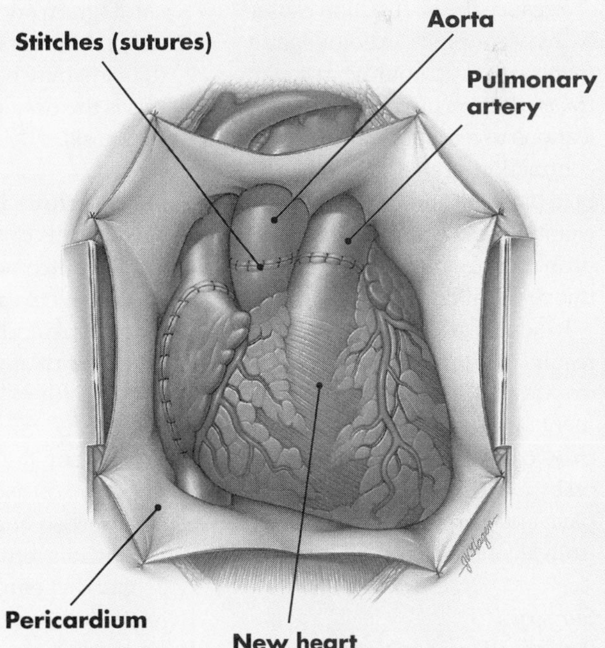

During a heart transplant operation, the ventricles and part of the atria, together with the heart valves and coronary arteries, are transplanted.

infection of your heart's inner lining (endocarditis). As a precaution, preventive use of antibiotics before dental and certain surgical procedures may be appropriate.

Treatment

Treatment is individualized to the type of cardiomyopathy. Often, treatments can ease the symptoms and improve life expectancy. In some instances, surgery may be necessary.

Medication

The choice of medications depends on the type of cardiomyopathy present. Possible drugs include those commonly used to treat heart failure, including angiotensin-converting enzyme (ACE) inhibitors, to improve your heart's pumping efficiency, diuretics to reduce fluid retention, beta blockers to counteract the effects of adrenaline (epinephrine), and anticoagulants to prevent blood clots. These medications have side effects that should be discussed with your doctor before beginning a treatment regimen.

Because the obstruction caused by hypertrophic cardiomyopathy increases when your heart contracts, doctors often prescribe medications to reduce the heart's contraction strength. These include beta blockers and certain calcium channel blockers. When rhythm problems are present, anti-arrhythmic medications may be needed.

In some cases, cardiomyopathy results from another ailment and may improve after effective treatment of the primary problem. In cases of cardiomyopathy brought on by excessive alcohol use, complete and permanent abstinence from alcohol is essential.

Surgery

If medications don't adequately relieve the symptoms of hypertrophic cardiomyopathy, doctors may suggest removal of the portion of overgrown heart muscle that's blocking blood flow. This procedure is called a myotomy-myectomy. Like all surgical procedures, it carries certain risks and needs to be carefully considered.

When the heart function is irreversibly impaired, heart transplantation may be an option.

Myocarditis

Signs and symptoms

- Fever
- Vague chest pain
- Joint pain
- A rapid heartbeat
- Breathlessness
- Fluid retention

The muscular layer of heart tissue is the myocardium. Acute myocarditis is an inflammation of that muscle and usually occurs as a complication of an infectious disease, such as the coxsackievirus or rheumatic fever, or exposure to radiation or certain chemicals or medications. Accompanying pericarditis also may develop.

Diagnosis

In diagnosing myocarditis, your doctor may recommend an electrocardiogram and an X-ray. Examination of heart muscle tissue (biopsy) may be performed because this is the only way to confirm the diagnosis.

How serious is myocarditis?

Myocarditis can be very serious, but the outcome depends on the cause. Severe cases can lead to cardiac failure and death, but most often the inflammation clears and good health follows.

Treatment

Therapy consists of avoiding vigorous exercise until the heart's functioning has returned to normal. A proper diet emphasizing salt restriction and treatment of the underlying cause, if it can be identified, are important.

If your doctor observes abnormalities in your heart rhythm, he or she may recommend hospitalization, electrocardiographic monitoring of your heart and appropriate anti-arrhythmia medications until your heartbeat returns to normal. In severe situations, your doctor may recommend heart transplantation.

Pericarditis

Signs and symptoms

- Sharp, piercing pain over the center or left side of the chest, which may extend to the left shoulder and worsen when you take a deep breath or lie down
- Breathlessness
- A general feeling of being sick
- Low-grade fever
- Swelling of the abdomen

The pericardium is a sac that encloses the heart. It's has a smooth inside surface. Outside is the tough (fibrous) parietal pericardium.

Pericarditis is an inflammation of the pericardium that may be caused by bacterial or viral infection. It occurs primarily in men between the ages of 20 and 50, often after a respiratory infection. As a result of the inflammation, pain is felt when the pericardium and the outer layer of the heart rub against each other. There may be an accumulation of excess fluid between the pericardium and the heart (pericardial effusion).

If a great deal of fluid accumulates in the pericardium and presses on the heart, preventing it from filling properly, the condition is called cardiac tamponade. Injury to the pericardium during surgery or in an accident can cause an accumulation of blood leading to cardiac tamponade. Tuberculosis, tumors or acute viral infections may result in fluid accumulation and cardiac tamponade. The result can be a restriction of blood flow to the lungs and the rest of the body. Acute cardiac tamponade is a medical emergency.

One of the aftereffects of some cases of pericarditis is a permanent thickening, scarring and contracture of the pericardium. Occasionally, a previous inflammation may be responsible for decreasing the ability of the heart muscle to expand between contractions and fill with blood (constrictive pericarditis).

Diagnosis

Your doctor may have you undergo an X-ray, electrocardiogram and echocardiogram in order to differentiate pericarditis from a heart attack. Blood tests also may be obtained. Although recurrences are common, most episodes of pericarditis last 2 to 6 weeks and resolve without further problems. The diagnosis of constrictive pericarditis may require additional tests, such as a computerized tomography (CT) scan of the chest and heart angiography.

For both diagnosis and treatment of cardiac tamponade, a procedure called pericardiocentesis may be of benefit. This involves draining excess fluid from the pericardial cavity using a small tube (catheter).

Treatment

Treatment of pericarditis may include an anti-inflammatory analgesic to relieve the pain and quell inflammation. If water retention and swelling are present, diuretic medications may be recommended. If an underlying cause such as tuberculosis or another bacterial infection is identified, antibiotic medications may be prescribed.

In some cases of constrictive pericarditis, surgery may be necessary to cut out portions of the pericardium that have grown stiff and are limiting the working of the heart. This procedure is called pericardiectomy. Your heart will continue to function normally even if the entire pericardial sac is removed.

Circulatory Problems

Your circulatory (vascular) system, the circuit through which your blood travels, consists of all the blood vessels in your body. It has two loops. The shorter loop handles lung (pulmonary) circulation. It begins at the right side of your heart, delivers blood to your lungs and then returns the oxygenated blood to your heart.

The longer loop is for whole-body (systemic) circulation. It begins at the left side of the heart, which receives blood that was oxygenated in the lungs. From the left side, this blood is pumped to the tissues of your body through a series of arteries that become smaller and smaller: arteries branch into smaller arterioles, and the arterioles branch into tiny capillaries that deliver blood to the tissues. After the blood in the capillaries collects carbon dioxide and other waste products from the tissues, it begins its trip back to your heart by way of small venules and, eventually, veins.

The total amount of blood within your body is relatively constant — about 7 percent of your body weight. The distribution of blood within blood vessels varies considerably with exercise and exposure to heat and cold. During exercise, for example, blood flow to active muscles is increased. After you eat, your stomach and intestines require more blood to assist in the digestive process.

Changes in the surrounding temperature also affect the flow of blood. Warmer temperatures produce increased flow to the outer layers of your skin, which helps you to get rid of heat. Alternatively, your body responds to cold by redistributing blood flow into the inner vessels, to conserve heat.

This complex yet flexible system is subject to a wide range of malfunctions. Some are the result of heart disorders, others occur because of disorders that directly affect the blood vessels, such as diabetes. The problems range from a weakened artery wall that balloons out (aneurysm) to clot development and inflammation in veins (thrombophlebitis).

? Question and Answer

What's the difference between arteriosclerosis and atherosclerosis?

The distinction between the two terms isn't always clear. *Arteriosclerosis* refers to the abnormal thickening and hardening of the walls of your arteries.

Atherosclerosis is one form of arteriosclerosis, but it's often used to describe many forms of arteriosclerosis. *Atherosclerosis* refers to the accumulation of fatty deposits (plaques) in your arteries. Atherosclerosis that occurs in your coronary arteries is called coronary artery disease.

Arteriosclerosis

Signs and symptoms

- Pain in the feet, legs, buttocks or hips that develops during activity and resolves after the activity is stopped
- Numbness or pain in the feet or toes when at rest
- Ulcers or gangrene on the feet or toes

Arteriosclerosis is a disease of the arteries, the blood vessels that carry oxygen and nutrients from your heart to the rest of your body. In arteriosclerosis, the walls of your arteries lose their elasticity and become thick and stiff. As a result, blood flow may be reduced, and your organs and tissues don't receive the necessary amount of nourishment.

The effects of arteriosclerosis generally appear first in your legs or feet. The major arteries that deliver blood to your legs and feet become narrowed, and blood flow decreases. Smaller blood vessels assume some of the load, but the physical activity of walking even a block or two can create an unmet need for increased blood flow and produce pain in your legs or feet. The discomfort often disappears within a few minutes after you discontinue the exercise. This sequence of walk-pain-rest is called intermittent claudication.

With the form of claudication called arteriosclerosis obliterans, some of the blood vessels actually become blocked (occluded). Sometimes, the blockage develops gradually, and your foot may become vulnerable to minor injury and infection. If the blockage occurs suddenly, as when a fragment of a fatty deposit (plaque) or clot lodges at a fork of your leg artery (a condition called arterial embolism), you may experience sudden and severe pain and your leg may become pale and cold below the level of the blockage.

The limited blood supply will often cause inflammation and damage to the nerves (neuritis), which is manifested by burning, pain and numbness in the leg or foot. In severe cases, gangrene may occur. Gangrene is a condition in which tissue dies. The affected tissue usually appears as an area of black, shrunken skin near the tips of your toes or your heel. In some instances, it can affect the whole foot or an entire lower leg.

Circulation problems are common in people with diabetes. In addition, people with diabetes may have nerve damage (diabetic neuropathy). The decreased sensitivity to touch that often accompanies diabetic neuropathy makes the person more likely to injure the affected foot.

Diagnosis

A key aspect to diagnosis of arteriosclerosis is observing the nature and timing of your discomfort. Does the pain occur only with exercise? Is it relieved by rest? Does it recur when activity is resumed? If so, your doctor may suspect arteriosclerosis. He or she may take your blood pressure in an ankle and compare it with the blood pressure in your arm. If pressure in your ankle is much less than in your arm, it may indicate that the arteries in your legs are narrowed.

Other tests, including an ultrasound scan, may be ordered. Angiography can help your doctor determine where the blockage is and if surgical repair should be considered. For this procedure, an X-ray is taken during and after a dye is injected into the artery that supplies the affected area.

How serious is arteriosclerosis?

For many people, arteriosclerosis in one or both legs can be serious because it may be an indication of problems elsewhere in the body. For example, it may suggest coronary artery disease or an increased risk of stroke. Appropriate care can prevent severe disability or loss of a limb. Among people with diabetes, circulatory problems are more common. Poor arterial circulation can blunt sensation to heat or cold, making you more susceptible to damage from both burns and freezing. If gangrene develops, surgical amputation may be necessary.

Treatment

In many cases, you can take control of your own treatment by making certain modifications in your lifestyle. Other times, medication may be appropriate. In severe cases, surgery may be necessary.

Self-care

With few exceptions, physical activity is a useful element in treatment of limited arterial blood supply to the legs. Your doctor can help you devise an appropriate regimen of daily walking or other exercise. Improvement in circulation occurs as collateral vessels that bypass the blocked segment develop. Walk, climb stairs or ride a stationary bicycle — but only to the point where you start feeling pain. This is not a pain that you should "exercise through" to cure.

Over time, the pain that occurs with physical activity will decrease, and you'll gradually be able to exercise for extended periods of time.

Smokers are at particular risk of arteriosclerosis. Smoking reduces the amount of oxygen in your blood and may contribute to the harmful depositing of blood platelets on the inner layer of arteries (atherosclerosis). If you have limited arterial circulation, stopping smoking can improve your blood flow.

Other steps you can take to control cardiovascular risk factors include maintaining a healthy weight, lowering the amount of fat in your diet and reducing stress in your life.

Foot care is essential for people with arteriosclerosis of the legs or feet. Wear shoes that fit properly. Even minor cuts or scrapes require

Are You at Risk?

Your risk of arteriosclerosis of the legs and feet increases if you:

- Smoke
- Are a man
- Are a woman past menopause
- Are at least 60 years old
- Have high blood pressure
- Have high blood cholesterol
- Are overweight
- Are sedentary
- Have diabetes

Not smoking is the best way to prevent or reduce this condition. Regular exercise can improve blood flow in the smaller arteries of your legs and condition your muscles so that they require less oxygen.

Gangrene

When the supply of blood to any tissue is severely impaired, the supply of oxygen and nutrients is also restricted. If blood flow isn't restored, the tissue may die. This condition is called gangrene.

Blood flow to the legs can cease abruptly or slowly. In either situation, the foot becomes pale and cold. The pain is variable.

Forms of gangrene

The two main types of gangrene are dry and wet. With dry gangrene, the tissue has died but has not become infected. With wet gangrene, the tissue has died and become infected with bacteria.

Dry gangrene

Tissue affected with dry gangrene is cold to the touch and gradually becomes black. At first, it's painful, but as the affected tissue dies, the pain decreases. Over time, the tissues dry and drop off, but the gangrene doesn't usually spread. However, there's some risk of wet gangrene developing.

Dry gangrene is more prone to occur in people who've had diabetes for a long time, hardening of the arteries (arteriosclerosis) or a recent case of severe frostbite.

Wet gangrene

Wet gangrene, which is also called moist gangrene, involves a bacterial infection. At first, the involved tissues may be red and hot as a result of inflammation. With time, the tissues become cold and blue and pus may ooze from the area. Eventually, the tissues begin to slough off.

Wet gangrene tends to spread rapidly as the bacteria contribute to tissue breakdown. If the bacteria produce a gas that has a strong, disagreeable odor as it destroys the tissue, the condition is called gas gangrene. If not promptly treated, a person with gas gangrene may die in a matter of days.

Prevention

If you have diabetes or advanced arteriosclerosis, proper care of your extremities, especially your feet, is essential. Even minor injuries must be treated with special attention. Careful control of blood sugar (glucose) level is important if you have diabetes. If you smoke, choose to stop. Every cigarette causes additional damage to blood vessels.

If you sustain a wound or injury, be sure it's properly treated. If virulent bacteria are present, wet gangrene may result from even a minor limb injury in which the blood supply is decreased.

Treatment

If you think you may have gangrene, consult your doctor right away. Treatment should be initiated immediately. Surgery to open or bypass blocked arteries may be possible. Tissues affected by dry gangrene may shrivel up and not be a problem, but surgical removal of the dead tissue often is needed.

Antibiotic medications are usually prescribed to prevent or treat wet gangrene. Tissue affected by wet gangrene may need to be removed surgically.

immediate attention because decreased circulation means that the tissues heal more slowly. If left untreated, even a minor injury to the skin of your lower leg or foot can lead to infection, gangrene and possibly amputation.

Medication

Your doctor may prescribe aspirin or another analgesic if the pain continues even at rest. If your condition doesn't respond to lifestyle changes, your doctor may prescribe pentoxifylline (Trental) to improve circulation.

A potentially bothersome side effect of this medication is nausea. The medication cilostazol (Pletal) may help by working to widen leg arteries and keep blood from clotting.

If you have diabetes or high blood pressure, carefully following your prescribed medication regimen can help improve blood flow.

Surgery and other procedures

Surgery may be appropriate if one of the larger arteries in your leg becomes blocked. In some cases, your doctor may recommend a procedure that uses a balloon device to expand the narrowed artery (balloon angioplasty). Occasionally, lasers and other devices are used to open blocked arteries.

Surgery to clean out the damaged artery or to bypass it with an artificial vessel may be required. Surgery is usually reserved for individuals with pain, impaired ability to walk or breakdown of skin, or for those at high risk of losing a limb.

Arterial embolism

Signs and symptoms

- Pain
- Pale, cool skin
- Numbness

An embolus is a clot that has moved from its point of origin to a new location and is blocking the flow of blood. An embolus isn't the same as a thrombus. A thrombus is a clot that forms in the vessel and remains stationary.

Emboli may be multiple and small, or they may be single and massive. Emboli can be life-threatening, such as when they lodge in the brain and cause a stroke, or they can lead to tissue death in an arm or leg if not treated within a few hours. Arterial emboli may originate in the left atrium of the heart among people experiencing an abnormal heart rhythm (atrial fibrillation) or in the left ventricle following a heart attack.

When embolization occurs, the flow of blood to the affected areas may stop abruptly or can slow gradually over weeks and months. If a clot or debris from a fatty deposit (plaque) in the aorta is carried with the flow of blood through an artery in the thigh, it may plug the artery at the level of the knee, where the larger artery splits into several small ones. This obstruction causes sudden pain and pallor in the lower leg and foot.

Diagnosis

Your doctor will measure the blood pressure in the affected limb and also may try to locate the embolus with an ultrasound examination or arteriography, a test in which dye is injected into the affected blood vessels and X-rays are taken.

How serious is an arterial embolism?

If the clot or debris isn't removed by surgery within a matter of hours, the tissue below that level may die and amputation may be necessary.

When embolism occurs, it's important to protect the limb from any injury by wrapping it loosely with a soft blanket and gauze. It's tempting to apply heat, but this may worsen already damaged tissue. However, protecting the limb from loss of heat by using a blanket, gauze or other wrap is safe and important.

Treatment

Once a diagnosis of an arterial embolism is reached, clot-dissolving medication may be given to try to break up the embolus, perhaps delivering it directly to the affected artery through the use of a catheter. This is called thrombolysis. Long-term use of aspirin or another anticoagulant medication may be appropriate in order to prevent the development of more clots.

If the health of a limb is in danger, immediate surgical removal of the clot may be attempted. This is usually done with a balloon-tipped catheter inserted into the artery. As it's being withdrawn, the inflated balloon pulls the clot out. Occasionally, replacement or bypass of the blocked vessel is necessary.

Aortic aneurysm

Signs and symptoms

- Often, none
- A pulsating mass in the abdomen

Emergency signs and symptoms

- Shock and loss of consciousness

An aneurysm is an abnormal widening of a blood vessel. A weakened wall of a vessel is stretched as the blood flows through it, often creating an egg-shaped ballooning.

An aneurysm can occur in any blood vessel, including major vessels in the brain and minor vessels anywhere in the body. However, an aneurysm is most likely to occur in an artery, particularly the aorta, the main blood vessel that carries blood from the heart. A common site for an aortic aneurysm is immediately below the kidneys but above the junction of the abdominal aorta and arteries to the legs.

Abdominal aneurysms are thought to be largely the result of damage to artery walls due to atherosclerosis. Complicating factors such as high blood pressure may contribute to the development of an aneurysm.

In addition to the expansion of the arterial wall, an aneurysm characteristically has an accumulation of cholesterol, calcium and even small blood clots. The weakened muscle fibers of the artery wall become fragmented and are replaced by scar tissue. Despite all these changes, the size of the artery's central channel may remain fairly normal.

Abdominal aortic aneurysms most often occur after age 55, and men are more commonly affected than women. In addition, an injury or an infection can weaken blood

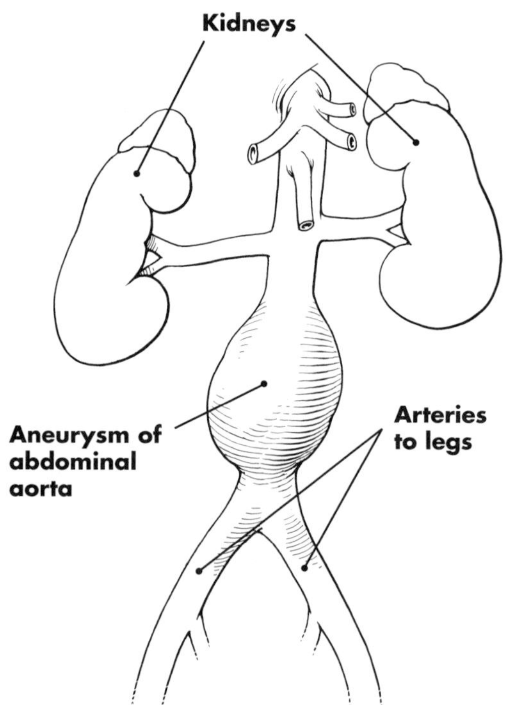

An aneurysm, an abnormal widening of an artery, can occur in any location, but commonly occurs in the abdominal aorta just below the kidneys. The weakened wall of the aorta balloons out over time, usually growing at a rate of 1/8 to 1/4 inch a year.

vessels, as can some congenital conditions. Abdominal aneurysms tend to run in families.

Diagnosis

Often, aortic aneurysms have no symptoms. In advanced cases, pain may be present in the abdomen and lower back. Aneurysms tend to grow at a rate of about 1/8 to 1/4 inch a year and often don't cause symptoms until blood begins to leak from the ballooning wall of the artery. If the aneurysm ruptures, massive bleeding may lead to shock, loss of consciousness and death.

Your doctor may detect the pulsating vessel on routine examination of your abdomen. In some cases, an X-ray taken for another reason will reveal an aneurysm. Its presence is usually confirmed with an ultrasound examination or a computerized tomography (CT) scan.

How serious is an aortic aneurysm?

An abdominal aortic aneurysm can be life-threatening. All too often, it's discovered during an autopsy. Like high blood pressure and some forms of coronary artery disease, an abdominal aortic aneurysm can be a silent killer. If discovered in time, surgical procedures are available to treat this disorder.

In some people, the layers of tissue that compose the wall of the aorta separate (dissect). Immediate treatment is required for this disorder. Often surgical removal of the affected artery is necessary.

Treatment

Medications aren't of value in treating an abdominal aortic aneurysm.

Watchful waiting

If the aneurysm is small and no symptoms are apparent at the time it's discovered, your doctor may recommend a watch-and-wait approach. No changes are required in your physical activities, but periodic ultrasound examinations or computerized tomography (CT) scans are done to determine if the aneurysm is expanding. In general, people with small abdominal aneurysms (less than 2 inches in diameter) can be safely monitored and don't require surgery until the estimated risk of rupture outweighs the risk of surgery.

Surgery

In an emergency, or as a preventive measure, your doctor may recommend an operation to replace the diseased portion of aorta. A traditional operation on an aortic aneurysm involves opening the abdomen or chest and stopping blood flow in the aorta so that the damaged section can be replaced with a synthetic tube. Although this surgery is generally successful, it requires an incision in the abdomen or chest, and recovery may take several weeks.

A new, minimally invasive procedure called endovascular surgery uses a synthetic graft attached to the end of a catheter. The catheter usually is inserted into your bloodstream through an artery in your leg. It's threaded upstream to your aorta and used to position the graft at the site of the aneurysm. Once in place, the graft is expanded and fastened with small hooks or pins. The graft reduces pressure on the walls of the aorta. This type of surgery reduces recovery time to a few days.

The risk of the aneurysm rupturing, a potentially life-threatening event, increases as the aneurysm enlarges. Surgery is relatively safe when performed before rupture, but less than half of the individuals operated on after an aneurysm ruptures survive.

PREVENTION TIP

Sitting during a long airplane flight or automobile ride commonly causes swollen ankles. The inactivity also increases your risk of thrombosis in the veins of your legs. To help prevent a blood clot from forming:

- Take a walk around the airplane cabin once an hour or so. If you're driving, stop every hour and walk around to stretch your legs.
- While seated, flex your ankles.
- Wear support hose (compression stockings). They help compress your leg veins to promote blood flow. Wear them if you're prone to swollen legs and ankles.
- If you're not allergic to aspirin, consider taking one just before a long trip. It may help prevent clot formation. Before using aspirin on a regular basis, consult your doctor.

Thrombophlebitis

Signs and symptoms

- Tenderness and pain
- Redness and swelling

Thrombophlebitis is the medical term for a blood clot and inflammation in a vein. The name comes from Greek words for "clot" (*thrombos*), "vein" (*phleb*) and "inflammation" (*itis*). Often, the name is shortened to *phlebitis*. If the inflammatory component of the condition is minor, it may be termed venous thrombosis.

Phlebitis usually occurs in an extremity and is most common in leg veins. It may affect either the deep or the superficial veins. Potential causes include prolonged bed rest after an operation, paralysis, a cancerous tumor or the use of the hormone estrogen. Sometimes, prolonged sitting during a long car or airplane ride causes venous thrombosis.

Diagnosis

When the clot and inflammation occur in a vein near the surface of the skin (superficial phlebitis), your doctor can make the preliminary diagnosis on the basis of discomfort in the area and a hard, usually

Lymphedema

Lymphedema is an abnormal accumulation of lymph fluid in the extremities. It causes painless swelling, which usually starts in the toes and feet and progresses toward the trunk. This form of swelling (edema) may initially improve with bed rest and elevation of the leg, but as it progresses, the improvement may be minimal.

In some situations, the cause is obvious. For example, it occurs after some types of traumatic injury, operations and radiation therapy. It might also result from an infection, particularly in tropical climates. A more serious cause of lymphedema is a cancer that obstructs the flow of lymph fluid back into the abdominal cavity. Thus, if you develop lymphedema for unexplained reasons in an extremity, your doctor may perform tests to rule out cancer.

tender, cord-like clot that can be felt and seen. Superficial phlebitis is most often seen in varicose veins.

When thrombophlebitis occurs in a deep vein in the leg or, more rarely, in the arm, the condition is called deep vein thrombosis. To confirm this diagnosis, your doctor may perform one or more special tests including an ultrasound examination or venography, in which dye is injected into the affected blood veins and X-rays are taken.

How serious is thrombophlebitis?

Superficial thrombophlebitis rarely leads to serious complications. With deep vein thrombosis, the principal danger is the clot breaking loose, moving upstream and lodging in a blood vessel in your lungs — a condition called pulmonary embolism. A less dangerous but bothersome complication called post-phlebitic syndrome — an obstruction in the vein with persistent leg swelling — may occur after one or more episodes of deep vein thrombosis.

Treatment

Treatment of superficial thrombophlebitis usually is limited to the application of heat to the affected area, elevation of the limb and use of an anti-inflammatory drug. Deep vein thrombosis is generally treated with anticoagulant medications and elevation of the leg if it's swollen. Hospitalization may be required.

Medication

An anticoagulant medication such as heparin is typically prescribed to treat deep vein thrombosis. It's likely to be administered intravenously, although a type of heparin called low molecular weight heparin may permit injection treatment without hospitalization. Following heparin treatment, an oral anticoagulant, warfarin (Coumadin), may be given for several months or longer. The purpose of the anticoagulant therapy is to prevent further clot formation while your own body works to dissolve the existing clot. Sometimes, medications to dissolve the blood clot may be needed.

Filters

On rare occasions, filters can be inserted into the main vein in the abdomen (inferior vena cava) to prevent movement of a blood clot from the legs to the lungs. Filters are often used in people who are actively bleeding and can't take anticoagulant medications but have an acute deep vein thrombus. Once a filter is set in place, it usually remains in the vena cava indefinitely. Newer filters are being developed that can be removed when no longer needed.

Varicose veins

Signs and symptoms

- Enlarged, often bulging veins visible under the skin of the legs
- Brownish-gray skin discoloration on the ankle
- Skin ulcers near the ankles

Varicose veins are twisted and enlarged veins close to the surface of the skin. The name comes from the Latin root *varix*, meaning "twisted." Any vein may become varicose, but the areas most likely to be affected are the legs and feet.

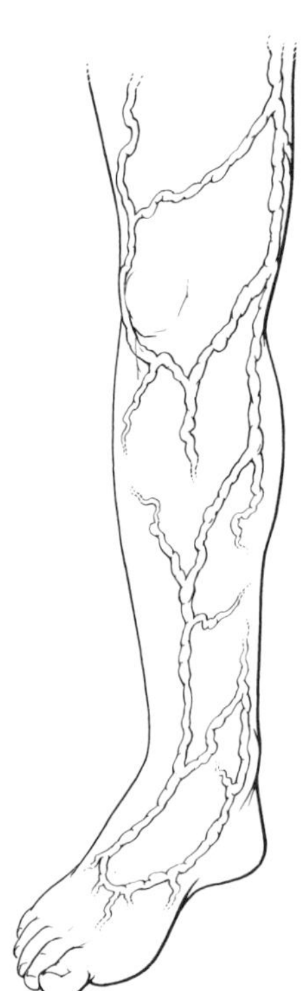

Varicose veins are enlarged veins that are easily seen beneath the surface of the skin of the legs and feet. These twisted veins may be caused by incompetent valves, which allow blood to flow backward.

About 40 million Americans have varicose veins. Women are about twice as likely as men to have this disorder.

Varicose veins occur as a result of a malfunction of the valves in the veins. Normally, the valves help prevent blood from flowing backward, but they can become stretched as a result of pregnancy, thrombophlebitis, congenital weakness, obesity or standing for long periods of time. When the valves are weakened and are no longer able to close normally, blood pools in the veins. As a result, the veins enlarge and become varicose.

Spider veins are a mild version of varicose veins. They're smaller, closer to the surface and may look like a spider web. They're not medically serious, but they may be of cosmetic concern.

Diagnosis

Superficial varicose veins are dilated, twisted and appear dark blue. You may or may not have mild aching of your legs.

Occasionally, veins deep within the legs are involved, causing significant swelling and, sometimes, skin ulcers. This is known as vein (venous) insufficiency.

Your doctor will examine your legs while you're upright and look for swelling, another indication of malfunction of the veins' valves.

Ulcers caused by varicose veins or malfunction of the valves within a vein ordinarily are located near the ankles and are the result of long-term waterlogging of ankle tissues due to diminished outflow of venous blood. Brownish pigmentation usually precedes the development of an ulcer.

How serious are varicose veins?

Varicose veins aren't life-threatening, but they tend to increase over time. If you're concerned about how your veins look and feel, talk to your doctor. In severe cases, the skin near a varicose vein may become itchy or ulcerated or the pigmentation may change. If skin ulcers develop, contact your doctor. Ulcers require medical attention.

Treatment

Self-help measures may limit the progression and discomfort of varicose veins. In some cases, surgery may be required to correct severe varicose veins and ulcers.

Self-care

Avoid standing or sitting for long periods. If your lifestyle is essentially sedentary, be sure to flex your legs and ankles frequently — get up and walk around. At the end of the day, you may find that elevating your legs at least 12 inches above the level of your heart helps relieve any swelling.

Mild aching and swelling of the lower legs due to vein insufficiency is most often treated with knee-high support (compression) stockings. These stockings provide outside pressure over the lower legs and prevent severe swelling, which can lead to thickened skin and ulcerations.

Regular exercise also is valuable. Activities such as walking, biking or swimming will help decrease pressure in the veins and may ease discomfort.

Surgery

If self-help measures don't suffice, your doctor may recommend one of the following treatments. Most of them are done on an outpatient basis.

- *Sclerotherapy.* Small- and medium-sized varicose veins are injected with a solution that scars the veins. The scarring process closes the dilated veins and the blood reroutes to healthier veins.
- *Ambulatory phlebectomy.* Smaller varicose veins are removed through a series of tiny skin punctures. Local anesthesia is generally sufficient, and scarring is minimal.
- *Vein stripping.* Long segments of vein are removed through small incisions. Usually, you're able to resume normal activities in 2 weeks or less.
- *Endoscopic vein surgery.* A flexible tube (endoscope) with a tiny video camera in it is inserted in your leg to help the surgeon visualize and close the veins. Only small incisions are needed. You might benefit from this operation if you have severe varicose veins with skin ulcers.
- *Laser surgery.* Smaller varicose veins and spider veins are closed off with a laser. Doctors are increasingly using lasers and other heat devices for treatment of varicose veins.

PREVENTION TIP

If you have varicose veins or a malfunction in the valves of your deep veins, a component of your treatment may involve wearing the right clothing. An appropriate type of support hose (compression stockings) may provide immediate and lasting relief. Use of compression stockings may also be appropriate during pregnancy. They steadily squeeze your legs, providing support and helping veins and leg muscles move blood more efficiently.

Compression stockings are sold at medical supply stores. Put them on first thing in the morning, even before you get out of bed. They're worn throughout the day. Make sure, however, that the stockings you wear are not too tight around your upper thigh or the calf of your leg.

Vascular skin ulcers

Signs and symptoms

- Swelling in legs or feet
- A wound or sore that doesn't heal on a leg or foot
- An aching or burning sensation at the sore site

- Paleness of a leg or foot or discoloration of a foot
- Numbness or tingling in a leg, foot or toes

Vascular skin ulcers usually start out as a small sore on the foot or an itchy patch of skin near the ankle from which fluid eventually seeps. These ulcers result from impaired circulation in the arteries or veins in your feet and legs, which may be caused by conditions such as atherosclerosis, diabetes, excess weight or pregnancy.

The two main types of vascular skin ulcers are venous ulcers and ischemic ulcers:

- *Venous ulcers.* Venous ulcers are the most common type of vascular skin ulcers. They're associated with circulatory problems in veins, and they typically develop on the inside area of your leg's lower calf or near your ankle. One-way valves that keep blood from flowing backward in the veins may become stretched or damaged, allowing blood to pool. Swelling (edema) may result and weaken surrounding tissues. Skin may take on a bluish or brownish color and become leathery before it gives way to an open wound. The sore may drain clear or blood-tinged fluid.

  Your risk of a venous ulcer is greater if you're older than age 60, others in your family have had them, you have varicose veins or you've been pregnant.
- *Ischemic ulcers.* Ischemic skin ulcers can occur when the flow of oxygenated blood is reduced in arteries serving the legs and feet. The main cause of ischemic ulcers is atherosclerosis. As arteries become progressively more narrow, blood flow to the legs and feet may be significantly reduced. This can lead to temporary cramping or pain in your muscles after walking (intermittent claudication).

Diagnosis
Tests may be needed to determine the cause of the ulcer and its severity. These may include the use of blood pressure cuffs on your legs and ultrasound imaging. If surgery is being considered, your doctor may use X-ray imaging with a contrast dye to view your veins (venogram) or your arteries (arteriogram).

How serious are vascular skin ulcers?
Once recognized, most vascular ulcers can be treated, and they eventually heal. Left untreated, a skin ulcer has the potential to become very deep — affecting fat tissue, muscle and even bone.

Treatment
Regular cleaning and dressing changes are an important part of treatment. For venous ulcers, elastic compressive wraps also may be used to improve blood flow while the ulcer heals.

Other options
If an ulcer isn't responding to such standard treatment, is recurrent or particularly deep, more intensive measures may be needed. These include:

- *Mechanical pumps.* A sleeve attached to a small pump fits over your leg. The sleeve compresses intermittently, forcing blood and fluid out of swollen tissues to promote venous blood flow.
- *Hyperbaric oxygen.* This treatment involves periodically spending about 90 minutes in a chamber where you breathe pure oxygen at high pressure to promote wound healing.
- *Human growth factors.* A topical paste that contains growth factors found in human blood platelets is applied to a wound. The growth factors help stimulate new tissue formation.
- *Skin grafting.* Skin grafting involves removing healthy skin from another area of your body and grafting it to the area affected by the ulcer. Or your doctor may use artificial skin (human skin equivalent), a cellular skin substitute that includes cells derived from human tissues. It provides wound protection and fosters growth of new skin.

Surgery
Only about 10 percent to 20 percent of people with venous ulcers are candidates for surgery. Most people with ischemic ulcers can be helped by some type of treatment to improve blood flow. This may include vein stripping to treat varicose veins or balloon angioplasty, in which a balloon-tipped catheter is used to open a narrowed artery. A stent — a small metallic mesh tube that's positioned in an artery following dilation of the blocked area — also may be placed in the artery to keep it open.

Other options may include surgery to remove fatty deposits (plaques) and blood clots in blocked arteries, or bypass surgery, which uses a vein or a synthetic graft to bypass a blockage.

Raynaud's disease

Signs and symptoms
- White fingers or toes on exposure to cold, with an accompanying stinging pain
- Blue or red skin

Named after Maurice Raynaud, the French doctor who described it more than a century ago, this disease results from changes in circulation in your hands or feet. It's normal for the blood vessels in your extremities to constrict when exposed to cold temperatures. However, for unknown reasons, in people with Raynaud's disease, this response to cold is exaggerated.

In Raynaud's, arteries to the fingers and toes go into what's called vasospasm. This constricts the vessels, temporarily but dramatically limiting blood supply. Over time, these same small arteries may thicken slightly, further limiting blood flow. The result is that affected skin turns pale and dusky-colored due to the lack of blood flow to the area. Once the spasms subside and blood returns to the area, the tissue may turn red or blue (a condition called acrocyanosis) before returning to a normal color.

Women are more likely to develop the problem than are men. Typically, the first episode occurs before age 40.

You can have Raynaud's without any underlying disease associated with it, in which case it's called Raynaud's disease or primary Raynaud's. Or you can have it as part of another disease, in which case doctors may refer to it as Raynaud's phenomenon or secondary Raynaud's. Raynaud's phenomenon may be a consequence of:

- Connective tissue diseases, such as scleroderma or lupus
- Use of certain medications, including beta blockers, which are used to treat high blood pressure, ergotamine preparations, which are used to treat migraines, and over-the-counter cold remedies, narcotics, and others that cause constriction of your blood vessels
- Exposure to certain agents in cancer chemotherapy
- Exposure to certain chemicals, especially vinyl chloride, used in the rubber industry
- Long-term use of vibrating tools such as pneumatic drills, jackhammers or chain saws.

Another related disorder, acrocyanosis, involves persistent coldness of the fingers, toes or other affected tissues. Like Raynaud's disease, it's not a consequence of another disorder, but the affected areas are almost always cold. Excessive perspiration often accompanies the feeling of coldness.

Diagnosis

Your doctor may be able to diagnose Raynaud's disease by examining affected parts, such as your fingers and toes for characteristic changes. Over time, Raynaud's disease can lead to decreased blood flow to the affected area, causing your extremities to become smooth and shiny and your nails to grow slowly. Blood tests may also be performed to check for certain antibodies found in people with autoimmune disorders, such as scleroderma or lupus, and for inflammation. A cold stimulation test may be performed to observe how your fingers and toes react to low temperatures.

How serious is Raynaud's disease?

For most people, Raynaud's disease is more of a nuisance than a disability. But people with secondary Raynaud's phenomenon may experience complications including skin ulcers and even tissue death (gangrene).

Treatment

Prevention is key to reducing the number and severity of attacks of Raynaud's disease. In some cases, medication may be prescribed. Rarely is surgery performed.

Prevention

To avoid attacks of Raynaud's disease, adequate protection from the cold is essential. Dress warmly when exposed to the cold, protecting your entire body.

Other preventive steps you can take include the following:

- Don't smoke. Nicotine in tobacco decreases blood flow in your skin.
- Use insulated glasses for cold drinks.
- Keep a pair of mittens or gloves next to the freezer to use when handling cold containers.
- Warm up your car for a few minutes before driving in cold weather.
- Stress may trigger attacks, so do your best to avoid stressful situations.
- Exercise. Doing so can increase your sense of well-being and energy level and improve your blood flow.
- Avoid over-the-counter cold remedies, which can worsen symptoms. If you use birth control pills, switch to another method of contraception because these medications affect your circulation and may make you more prone to attacks.

In cases of acrocyanosis, these steps are often all that's needed to prevent symptoms.

Medication

If self-help measures aren't sufficient, your doctor may prescribe a medication, such as a calcium channel blocker or vasodilator, to relax smooth muscle, dilate small blood vessels and prevent the blood vessel spasm that characterizes Raynaud's disease. Women who are pregnant or trying to become pregnant should avoid medications used to treat Raynaud's disease as they may affect the fetus.

Surgery

In extreme cases, a surgical procedure to cut the sympathetic nerves that control the blood vessels (sympathectomy) may be performed, but the operation isn't always successful.

A similar procedure called sympathetic blockade can be performed by injecting certain chemicals into the appropriate nerves.

Buerger's disease

Signs and symptoms

- Pain or tenderness in the hands or feet
- Pain in the legs, ankles or feet
- Ulcers in the hands or feet
- Pale, red or bluish skin of affected areas
- Cold hands or feet

Buerger's disease is named after American doctor Leo Buerger, who first described it in 1908.

It's a rare disorder in which the blood vessels of the hands and feet become diseased. The skin of the hands and feet becomes tender and, over time, pain and ulcers develop and amputation is often needed. This occurs because of blockages that form in the smaller vessels supplying blood to the extremities.

The disease characteristically strikes men between ages 20 and 40. For unexplained reasons, there appears to be a direct link between tobacco use and Buerger's disease.

Diagnosis

Your doctor may be able to diagnose Buerger's disease by looking at the affected hands or feet. Usually, two or more limbs are affected. Tests may be needed to check for blockage of blood vessels in an arm or leg.

How serious is Buerger's disease?

If you smoke but choose to quit, symptoms of the disease may disappear. In some cases, particularly if tobacco isn't avoided, gangrene may develop and amputation of the affected limb may be necessary.

Treatment

Eliminating the use of tobacco usually results in a cure. Avoid cold temperatures and other conditions that may impair circulation.

Warmth and gentle exercise may increase circulation. Medications to relax the muscles in the walls of blood vessels (vasodilators) may be prescribed. A surgical procedure to cut the sympathetic nerves that control the blood vessels (sympathectomy) may be performed, though the operation isn't always successful. ■

CHAPTER 27 PART V

Lungs and Respiratory System

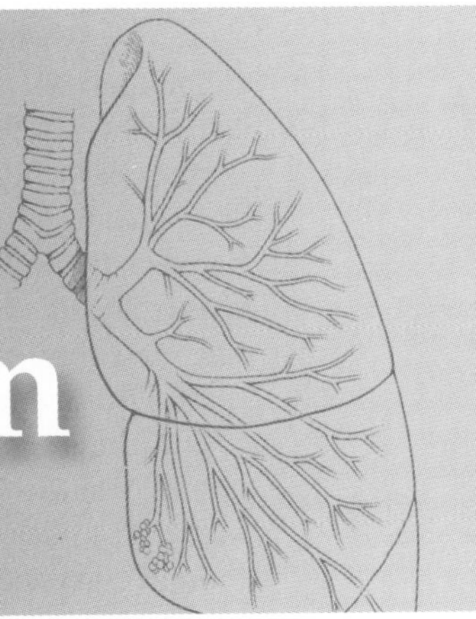

Your lungs are part of your respiratory system. This system includes a network of organs and nerves that enable you to breathe. Your lungs are enclosed by the chest wall, which is made up of ribs, cartilage and the muscle between them. The diaphragm consists of sheets of muscle that separate your chest cavity (thoracic cavity) from your abdominal cavity.

The lungs are soft and spongy. If you're healthy, they're usually a mottled pinkish-gray color, although even healthy lungs can become blackened from carbon particles in polluted air. Your right lung is divided into three sections (lobes), and your left into two lobes. Your heart is between your lungs.

The pleura is a membrane with lubricating fluid between its two layers. The pleura covers the surface of each lung and the inside of the chest wall. The slippery pleural surfaces allow your lungs to move easily within the chest cavity as you breathe.

Your windpipe (trachea) branches into two main airways, called bronchial tubes. Each bronchial tube then branches into smaller passageways that divide several times more, finally forming much smaller tubes called bronchioles. The branching gives the airways of your respiratory system the appearance of an upside-down tree.

The smallest bronchioles end in tiny closed elastic air sacs (alveoli). Your lungs contain approximately 300 million alveoli. If they all could be stretched out on a flat surface, they would cover an area approximately the size of a tennis court.

Tiny blood vessels carry blood to the alveoli. The vessels, called pulmonary capillaries, release carbon dioxide from your blood into the air sacs to be exhaled and absorb inhaled oxygen from the air sacs into your blood.

How Your Lungs Work

The primary function of your lungs is to supply oxygen to and remove carbon dioxide from your blood. To reach your lungs, air enters through your mouth and nose, travels through the back of your throat (pharynx), through your voice box (larynx) and down your windpipe (trachea) and into air passages called bronchi.

When you inhale, the muscles between your ribs contract, causing your ribs to move upward and outward. At the same time, your diaphragm contracts, pushing down toward your abdomen. These two actions increase the size of your chest cavity, causing your lungs to expand so that air is sucked into them. Individual alveoli also fill with air. During normal breathing, a healthy adult draws about a pint of air into the lungs with each breath. However, during deep breathing, you can draw as much as 3 to 6 quarts of air into your lungs.

When you exhale, your diaphragm and rib muscles relax and return to their original positions. This decreases the size of your chest cavity, compressing your lungs slightly and forcing stale air — now carrying carbon dioxide — out of your body. The whole process of breathing in and out occurs automatically without your having to think about it.

Your lungs are connected to your heart by the pulmonary arteries and veins. The term *pulmonary* comes from the Latin word *pulmo,* for "lung." After traveling through your body, blood returns to the right side of your heart, where the bottom-right chamber (right ventricle) pumps it through the pulmonary artery to your lungs. Blood then passes through the arteries of the lungs into smaller and smaller vessels, similar to the branching of the bronchi. Finally, it flows into the smallest blood vessels (capillaries), which are situated in the walls of the alveoli.

After gases are exchanged in the alveoli, blood — now carrying oxygen — passes into the smallest veins. These veins merge to form larger vessels until the pulmonary veins reach the heart. The pulmonary veins carry oxygen-rich blood from the lungs back to the lower-left side of your heart (left ventricle). The left ventricle then pumps the blood back to the cells and organs of your body.

The Chest Cavity

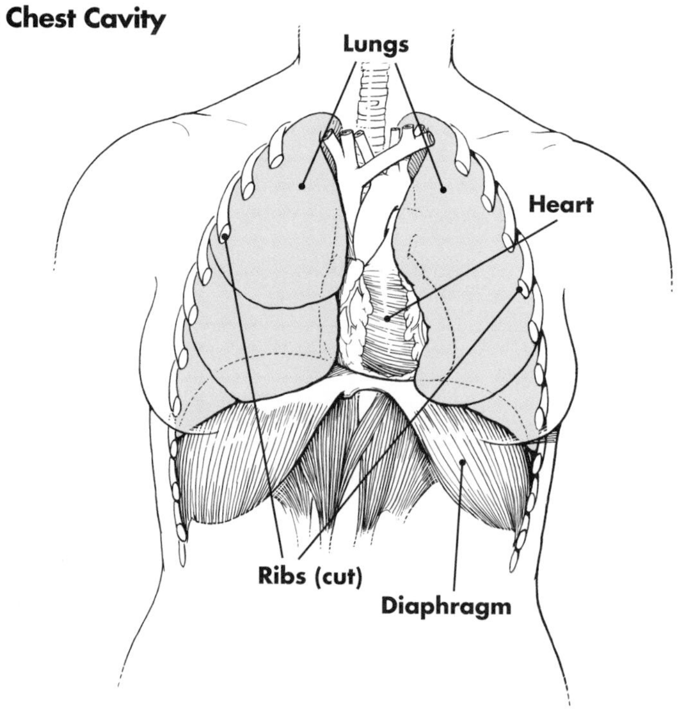

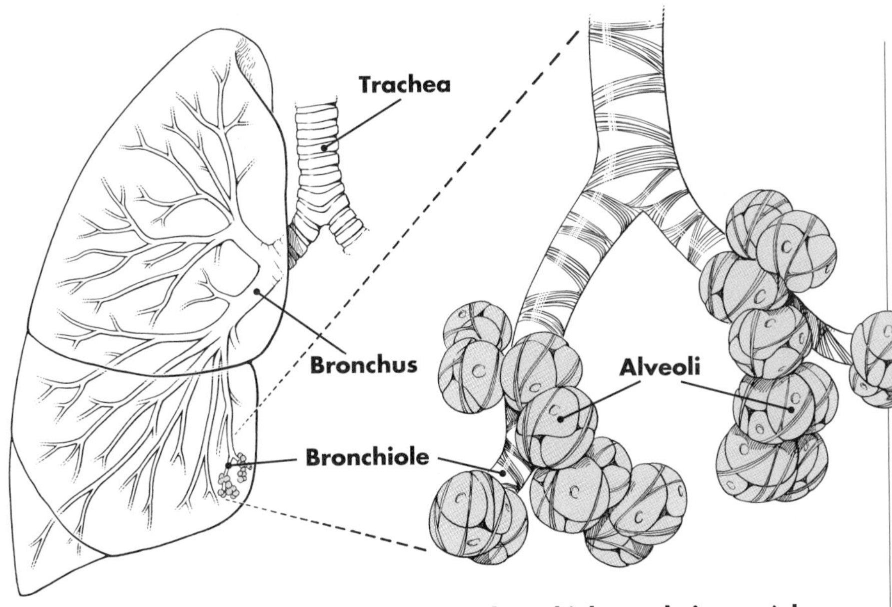

Enlargement of a lung segment shows bronchioles and air sacs (alveoli). Within these air sacs, your blood releases carbon dioxide as it absorbs oxygen.

Natural defenses

Your respiratory system has several defense mechanisms that prevent foreign material from entering your lungs. The hairs and mucus in your nose trap larger particles. Special cells in your trachea and bronchial tubes secrete mucus that helps keep the airways moist and lubricated. The mucus also traps bacteria, dust and other foreign material.

Cilia are microscopic hair-like projections that line your airways. The cilia continuously beat so that mucus moves upward, away from your lungs and toward your throat, to help keep air passageways clean. Some substances, such as cigarette smoke, interfere with their function. Inhaling cigarette smoke causes cilia to stop beating and increases mucus production.

Respiratory Infections

If bacteria, viruses or fungi enter the lungs and become established there, they can cause several diseases, ranging from common and usually benign illnesses such as a chest cold to more serious illnesses such as bronchiolitis, pneumonia and tuberculosis.

Bronchiolitis

Signs and symptoms

- Wheezing
- Exhaling heavily
- Rapid breathing and rapid heartbeat
- A sputum-producing cough
- Fever
- Bluish skin

A respiratory infection such as that caused by the flu (influenza) virus or a bacterium may cause the small airways in the lungs (bronchioles) to become inflamed and to secrete an excessive amount of mucus. This is bronchiolitis. Bronchiolitis is fairly common, especially during the winter, in children younger than age 2, but under certain circumstances it can also occur in young adults. It's usually caused by a viral infection, often contracted from someone in the child's household. In infants or families with a history of allergies or in infants with recurring bronchiolitis, an allergic reaction may be an underlying factor.

Diagnosis

Usually, bronchiolitis is preceded by mild nasal congestion for a day or two. Gradually, breathing becomes more difficult and may become rapid with more vigorous exhalation. Wheezing, a rapid heartbeat and a cough also may develop. Fever might be present. In some cases, the infant's lips and fingernail beds become blue — a condition called cyanosis — due to a decrease in blood oxygen.

How serious is bronchiolitis?

Bronchiolitis usually isn't serious in older children and adults, but it can be serious in infants because their air passages are much narrower than those of adults. The air passages of an infant may become partly or completely blocked, making it difficult for him or her to breathe.

Treatment

Hospitalization may be necessary, especially for an infant younger than 2 months who has cyanosis, has had repeated attacks of bronchiolitis or is breathing rapidly and shallowly. Treatment consists of providing warm, moist air, perhaps with extra oxygen. Use of medications depends on the nature and severity of the illness.

Most infants recover within 2 days to a week, although in rare cases the condition can be fatal. About half of all children who contract bronchiolitis have later episodes of wheezing and may become more susceptible to respiratory infections.

Acute bronchitis

Signs and symptoms

- Soreness and a feeling of constriction in the chest
- Difficulty breathing
- Wheezing
- Coughing
- Production of sputum
- Chills
- Malaise and a slight fever

When mucous membranes that line the main air passageways of the lungs (trachea and large bronchi) become inflamed, the con-

A Cough

Coughing is both normal and common. Often more annoying than serious, a cough is a normal protective reflex, designed to defend your respiratory system against irritants.

However, a forceful or nagging cough can be painful and bothersome. Some of these coughs need your doctor's attention. Others respond to simple self-care techniques and nonprescription medicine.

What causes a cough?

The mucus that lines your nose and airways increases in response to irritants so that it can trap them. The irritants stimulate the cough receptors in your nose, throat or chest, and the receptors send messages to your brain that lead to coughing to help clear out the irritants by expelling the mucus.

Cold and flu viruses are the most common causes of cough. Generally, the cough goes away when the infection clears. Other coughs may be triggered by:

- *Postnasal drip.* Overproduction of mucus that slowly trickles from the back of your nose down into your throat may be due to allergies, inflamed mucous membranes within sinuses (sinusitis) or other causes.
- *Environmental irritants.* These may include cigarette smoke, smog, dust, home aerosol sprays and other scents and cold or dry air.
- *Asthma.* Because asthma inflames and constricts air passages, it could cause you to cough, especially if attacks occur during the night, after exercise or when you're exposed to irritants. Although wheezing is a common symptom of asthma, many people with this condition cough but don't wheeze.
- *Gastroesophageal reflux disease.* GERD is the result of acid from your stomach working its way up the esophagus — and in rare cases into your lungs — when you lie down. Although heartburn is the most common symptom of GERD, some people develop a cough instead.
- *Some medications.* These include angiotensin-converting enzyme (ACE) inhibitors and some beta blockers prescribed for high blood pressure or heart disease.
- *A foreign body in a bronchial tube.* Rarely, a foreign body, such as a piece of food, can lodge in a bronchial tube, producing a cough.
- *Coughing itself.* Some people cough out of habit. There's no medical explanation for their coughing, and sometimes they're not even aware they're doing it. For some, it may be a way of releasing nervous tension or expressing anger. Whatever the reason, one cough can irritate your throat and lead to another, setting up a vicious cycle.

Treatment

Treatment depends on the type of cough you're experiencing.

Dry, hacking coughs

Dry, hacking coughs generally go away within 1 to 2 weeks. Drinking fluids, especially water, keeps your throat lubricated. If a persistent cough irritates your throat, suck on hard candy or throat lozenges or drink hot tea sweetened with honey to soothe your throat. Because long-term use of these products isn't good for your teeth and the extra calories from the sugar can cause weight gain, consider using sugar-free candy and throat lozenges.

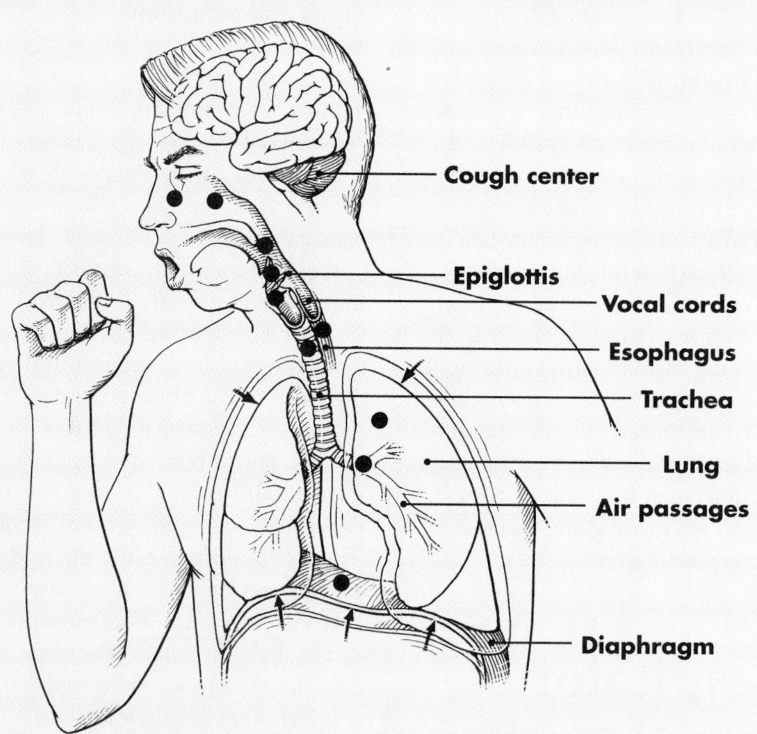

A cough begins when irritants reach one of the cough receptors in your nose, throat or chest (see large dots). The receptor sends a message to the cough center in your brain, signaling your body to cough. After you inhale, your epiglottis and vocal cords close tightly, trapping air within your lungs. Your abdominal and chest muscles contract forcefully, pushing against your diaphragm (see arrows). Finally, your vocal cords and epiglottis open suddenly, allowing trapped air to rush outward.

If a cough caused by GERD disrupts your sleep, try antacids and raise the head of your bed 6 to 8 inches by putting blocks under the legs. If symptoms persist, see your doctor, who may prescribe medication to prevent reflux.

To temporarily reduce the frequency of your cough, take an over-the-counter cough suppressant. Although codeine is one of the most effective cough suppressants, it's a narcotic, so in most states cough formulas containing codeine are available only by prescription. Dextromethorphan is nearly as effective as codeine, with less risk of side effects. It's listed on the label of over-the-counter cough suppressants that contain it.

Productive coughs

Productive coughs are those that raise mucus to help remove irritants from your lungs and air passages. It's best not to suppress a productive cough. Drinking fluids, especially water, helps thin and loosen mucus to make your cough more productive. However, if your cough continually disrupts your sleep, then you can take just enough suppressant to decrease the frequency and severity of your cough but not enough to get rid of it altogether.

Antihistamines may help dry up secretions associated with allergies, sinusitis and postnasal drip, but they can make you sleepy. Don't take antihistamines in combination with alcohol or tranquilizers or when you need to stay alert.

Chronic coughs

If your cough lasts longer than 2 or 3 weeks, becomes progressively worse or is accompanied by wheezing, fever, night sweats, weight loss or bloody mucus, you may have a chronic cough. See your doctor. Managing a chronic cough requires careful evaluation and identification of the cause, when possible.

dition is called acute bronchitis or tracheobronchitis. Virtually everyone experiences bronchitis at some time, just as everyone catches the common cold. So it's reasonable to expect that you may have acute bronchitis occasionally.

In most cases, this common ailment is caused by a viral infection similar to those that cause the common cold. The infection spreads to the bronchi, producing a deep cough that, in turn, tends to bring up yellowish-gray sputum from your lungs.

Diagnosis

If you have a fever, experience chest discomfort that leaves you breathless or cough up blood or yellow or green sputum, see your doctor. He or she may listen to your chest using a stethoscope and may request a chest X-ray, sputum culture or other tests to rule out other causes. If you have chronic lung or heart problems, such as asthma, emphysema, chronic bronchitis or congestive heart failure, and think you have bronchitis, it's especially important that you see your doctor.

How serious is acute bronchitis?

In virtually all cases, this temporary but severe form of bronchitis improves in a matter of days with no lasting effects. However, a pattern of recurring bronchitis may be associated with a more serious health concern.

Treatment

Because bronchitis is most often the result of a viral infection, your doctor may not be able to do much to hasten your recovery. Getting plenty of rest, drinking adequate fluids, taking acetaminophen (Tylenol, others) for fever and taking a nonprescription cough medicine are the cornerstones of treatment for most acute bronchitis.

In addition, avoid other irritants to the airways, such as tobacco smoke. You don't have to confine yourself to bed while you have acute bronchitis, but it's wise to remain in a warm environment in which the air is somewhat humid, perhaps from the use of a vaporizer.

Your doctor may prescribe a bronchodilator drug to help open narrowed passages in your lungs. Yellow or green sputum may indicate a bacterial infection, for which your doctor may prescribe an antibiotic.

Prevention

If you have repeated attacks of bronchitis, you may be able to trace their occurrence to conditions in which you live. For example, cold, damp environments combined with excessive air pollution can make you more susceptible to acute bronchitis.

Respiratory syncytial virus

Signs and symptoms

- Wheezing
- A congested or runny nose
- Coughing
- Low-grade fever
- Rapid or labored breathing
- Bluish skin

Respiratory syncytial virus (RSV) is a common respiratory infection in children under age 4. Adults also may become infected. RSV may affect the upper or lower respiratory tract.

Caused by a virus that enters the body through the eyes, nose or mouth, RSV spreads easily. If you inhale infectious respiratory secretions, such as those spewed by coughs or sneezes, or touch objects contaminated with oral or nasal secretions and then touch your mouth, nose or eyes, you're likely to acquire the virus.

The peak season for catching the virus typically begins in the fall and ends in the spring.

Diagnosis

Your child's doctor may suspect respiratory syncytial virus based on a physical exam, during which he or she may listen to your child's lungs with a stethoscope to check for wheezing or other abnormal sounds. The doctor may also order blood tests to check the white cell count or to look for the presence of viruses, bacteria or other organisms, as well as chest X-rays to rule out pneumonia or other diseases. He or she may collect respiratory secretions for analysis by inserting a swab into the nose.

How serious is respiratory syncytial virus?

In adults and older, otherwise healthy children, the infection typically mimics the common cold. Symptoms usually improve in 7 to 10 days.

In some infants, children with underlying conditions such as congenital heart defects or lung disease, or children who were born prematurely, the infection may be more severe, even life-threatening, and the child may require hospitalization.

Of infants and young children infected for the first time, about 25 percent to 40 percent also develop symptoms of pneumonia and bronchiolitis. Middle ear infection (otitis media) is another complication.

Treatment

Because respiratory syncytial virus causes a viral infection, antibiotics are of no use unless a bacterial condition also is present, such as an inner ear infection or bacterial pneumonia.

In cases of severe infection, infants and children may need hospitalization so that they can be treated with humidified oxygen to get sufficient oxygen to the blood, intravenous fluids to prevent dehydration and, sometimes, a ventilator to support breathing.

Medication

Over-the-counter medications such as acetaminophen (Tylenol, others) may reduce symptoms. In severe cases, a doctor might prescribe a bronchodilator or ribavirin (Virazole), an antiviral medicine inhaled through a mist, nebulizer or face mask. The effectiveness of bronchodilators and ribavirin is uncertain.

Self-care

To help ease breathing, use a cool mist humidifier or vaporizer to humidify air. Be sure to keep the humidifier clean to prevent the growth of bacteria and molds. Sitting upright makes breathing easier. Offer the sick person plenty of fluids to drink, including warm ones such as soup. Over-the-counter saline nasal drops may ease congestion.

Prevention

There's no vaccine against this disease, but intravenous respiratory syncytial virus immune globulin (RespiGam) and palivizumab (Synagis) may decrease the risk of hospitalization and limit the severity of the illness. They may be given monthly to high-risk individuals for about 5 months during the peak season for the infection.

Pneumonia

Signs and symptoms

- Coughing that may produce colored or bloody sputum
- High fever and chills with shaking
- Difficulty breathing
- Chest pain that increases with deep breathing and coughing
- Headache
- Loss of appetite
- Nausea and vomiting
- Bluish skin
- Fatigue
- Mental confusion

Pneumonia is a common, potentially serious inflammation of the lungs that causes difficulty breathing. In the United States, it affects about 1 out of 100 people each year.

There are many types of pneumonia. They range in severity from mild to life-threatening. Pneumonia can affect one or both lungs. Inflammation of both lungs is sometimes called double pneumonia.

Causes

Pneumonia has more than 50 causes. Infectious pneumonia can be caused by viruses, bacteria such as pneumococci, staphylococci and streptococci, or other organisms. Viruses, including those that cause the flu (influenza), are responsible for half of all cases of pneumonia.

Chemical irritants, parasites and certain types of fungus also can cause pneumonia. Mycoplasma pneumonia organisms cause symptoms similar to both viral and bacterial pneumonia, although the symptoms appear more gradually and often are milder.

Pneumonia is sometimes classified according to where or how you're exposed to the disease. These classifications include:

Community-acquired pneumonia

Community-acquired pneumonia gets its name from the way it's acquired — from the community at large rather than in the hospital. Common causes of community-acquired pneumonia are pneumococci bacteria, mycoplasmas and the influenza virus.

Hospital-acquired pneumonia

Your risk of developing pneumonia increases if you're hospitalized, especially if you are on a mechanical ventilator, in an intensive care unit (ICU) or have a compromised immune system. In a hospital, many types of potentially infectious organisms are present, and they may be more severe than those you encounter in everyday life. Hospital-acquired pneumonia can be extremely serious, especially for older adults and young children.

Aspiration pneumonia

Aspiration pneumonia is the result of inhaling (aspirating) foreign matter into the lungs. This commonly occurs when stomach contents enter your lungs after you vomit.

Opportunistic pneumonia

Pneumonia caused by opportunistic organisms strikes people with a compromised immune system. Opportunistic organisms don't ordinarily cause illness in healthy people but can be extremely dangerous to those with human immunodeficiency virus (HIV) or AIDs, sickle cell disease and other conditions that impair the immune system. Medications that suppress your immune system, such as corticosteroids, or treatments for certain cancers also can put you at increased risk of opportunistic pneumonia.

Diagnosis

Because pneumonia often mimics a cold or the flu, many people don't realize they have it. Symptoms can vary depending on the organism causing the pneumonia.

Your doctor listens to your lungs with a stethoscope to check for abnormal bubbling or crackling sounds (rales) and for rumblings (rhonchi). These sounds may indicate inflammation caused by infection. Your doctor may order a chest X-ray to determine the location and extent of the infection.

If your immune system is compromised or the X-ray isn't definitive, you may have a more sophisticated imaging test known as a computerized tomography (CT) scan of your chest.

A sample of your sputum may be tested to help identify the infecting agent. Usually, you can produce a sample that's sufficient for the test by coughing. In some cases, it may be necessary to use other means to obtain a sputum sample, including inserting a bronchoscope into your airway. Your doctor may also request blood tests to check your white cell count or to look for the presence of viruses, bacteria or other organisms.

How serious is pneumonia?

In the United States, more than 40,000 people die of pneumonia every year. It's likely that everyone inhales certain organisms that can cause pneumonia. The seriousness of this disorder depends largely on your overall health and the type of pneumonia you contract. Healthy people generally have sufficient defense mechanisms to neutralize most infectious agents. In young people, pneumonia might be a mild, undiagnosed illness that's regarded as simply a cold.

If alcoholism, aging, injury, use of immunosuppressant drugs or other medical conditions have impaired your natural defense mechanisms, you may be more susceptible to pneumonia. In older adults and people weakened by disease — especially people with heart failure or lung disease, such as asthma or emphysema — pneumonia can be fatal.

Pneumonia becomes deadly when inflammation from the disease fills so many of the air sacs within your lungs (alveoli) that it interferes with your ability to breathe. In some cases, the inflammation enters your bloodstream — a condition called invasive bacteremia. It can then spread widely and quickly to other organs, where it may create pus-filled abscesses.

Sometimes, fluid accumulates between the layers of the pleural membrane, which covers the surface of the lung and lines the inside of the chest wall. This condition is known as pleural effusion. When your lungs are infected, fluid can accumulate and become infected.

> **?** **Question and Answer**
>
> **What's walking pneumonia?**
>
> *Walking pneumonia* isn't a specific medical term. It's typically used to describe pneumonia that isn't severe enough to cause confinement to bed. Many people don't feel sick enough to seek medical care.
>
> If you've been told that you have walking pneumonia, it may be due to a tiny organism called mycoplasma. This community-acquired pneumonia spreads easily among people who spend a lot of time together, such as school-aged children. It usually affects people under age 40. Although this pneumonia isn't a true bacterial infection, it typically responds well to antibiotics.
>
> Mycoplasma causes symptoms similar to those of both bacterial and viral pneumonia, although the symptoms appear more slowly and often are milder.

Treatment

When you have pneumonia, proper medical care, bed rest and careful monitoring are essential. The treatment your doctor recommends depends on the cause and severity of your pneumonia. In viral pneumonia, for example, antibiotics aren't effective unless you have a secondary bacterial infection.

Medication

When the cause of your pneumonia is bacterial or mycoplasmal, your doctor will likely prescribe an antibiotic. Whatever the cause, your doctor may recommend over-the-counter medications to reduce fever, treat your aches and pains and relieve your coughing.

If you have what's called a productive cough — that is, one that raises mucus when you cough to help remove irritants from your lungs and air passages — don't completely suppress it. If you use a cough suppressant, use the lowest dose that enables you to rest.

Other therapies

Hospitalization may be necessary in severe cases, for instance, if your breathing is labored. You may receive intravenous (IV) antibiotics and supplemental oxygen. If you develop pleural effusion, the fluid may need to be drained with a needle or chest tube.

Prevention
Because pneumonia can be a complication of influenza, getting a yearly flu shot can reduce your risk of pneumonia. An injection of a pneumococcal polysaccharide vaccine (PPV) also reduces your risk of getting a common type of bacterial pneumonia called pneumococcal pneumonia. A pneumococcal vaccine is recommended for:

- Healthy adults age 65 and older
- People with diabetes or cancer
- Adults who have chronic heart, lung, kidney or liver disease
- People with alcoholism
- People who've had their spleen removed
- People with an impaired immune system
- People who live in a nursing home or long-term-care facility
- People who have received an organ transplant

If you're in one of these groups, ask your doctor about getting vaccinated. You may need a second dose after 5 years.

A vaccine known as pneumococcal conjugate vaccine (PCV) can help protect young children against pneumonia. It's recommended that the vaccine be given to all children in four doses between ages 2 and 15 months. The vaccine is also recommended for children between ages 2 and 5 years who haven't had pneumococcal vaccine and are at high risk of the disease, such as those with an immune system deficiency, asthma, chronic heart or lung disease or sickle cell disease.

Other measures that may help reduce the risk of pneumonia include regular and thorough hand washing, not smoking, eating a healthy diet and exercising regularly.

Syndromes that Can Mimic Pneumonia

Some rare lung disorders that aren't caused by infectious agents may mimic pneumonia. These include:

Pulmonary alveolar proteinosis
Pulmonary alveolar proteinosis occurs when fluid builds up within the air sacs of the lungs (alveoli). It occurs primarily in men between the ages of 20 and 50 who aren't known to have lung disease. The cause is unknown.

In pulmonary alveolar proteinosis, fluid-filled alveoli inhibit the lung's ability to transfer oxygen to the blood, causing shortness of breath with exertion and sometimes at rest. Most nonsmokers with this disorder also develop an unproductive cough, and smokers develop a cough that produces sputum. A chest X-ray may reveal shadowy areas on both lungs.

People with few symptoms or none require no treatment. For others, a procedure called whole-lung lavage, performed while you're under general anesthesia, may be used to rinse material within the alveoli from the lung.

People with this disease usually recover, although occasionally the disorder may recur.

Goodpasture's syndrome
The precise cause of Goodpasture's syndrome is unknown, although it's more likely to occur in young, male smokers. It causes bleeding (hemorrhage) of the lungs and a type of kidney inflammation called glomerulonephritis (see page 937).

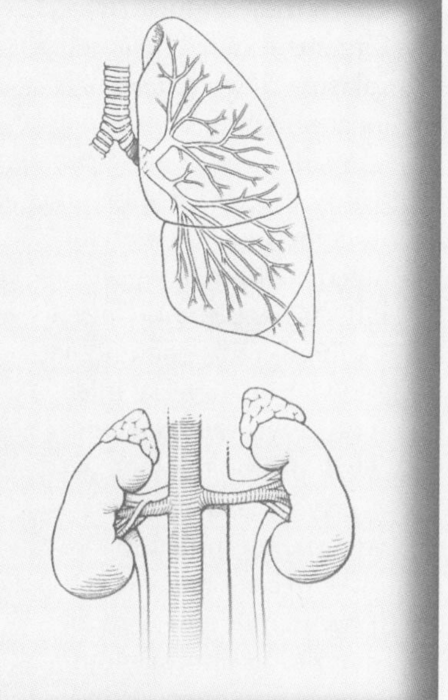

Although lung hemorrhage can be life-threatening, the effect on the lung can range from mild to severe. The diagnosis is made by a biopsy of either the lung or kidney. The course of the disease varies considerably.

Your doctor may prescribe corticosteroids or cyclophosphamide (Cytoxan) to control the disorder. In addition, your doctor might recommend removing antibodies from your blood that may play a role in causing this disease.

Tuberculosis

Signs and symptoms

- Persistent coughing that may produce discolored or bloody sputum
- Slight fever
- Fatigue
- Loss of appetite and weight
- Night sweats
- Pain with breathing or coughing
- Pain in the spine or large joints

Tuberculosis (TB) has been present since antiquity. Although its incidence declined greatly during most of the last century, there has been a significant increase since the 1980s. This has been especially evident among homeless people living in inner cities and people infected with the human immunodeficiency virus (HIV). The disease has also been occurring more frequently in certain areas of the country, where it has been linked to the arrival of refugees from Asia, Africa and Central America.

TB is a long-lasting (chronic) bacterial infection. You can get it if you inhale droplets sprayed into the air by a person with the disease who sneezes or coughs. Your risk of contracting TB varies directly with the frequency and intensity of your contacts with people who are infected. TB results from the bacterium *Mycobacterium tuberculosis.* These bacteria can attack any part of your body, but most commonly invade your lungs.

Diagnosis

If you're exposed to the TB bacterium, the organism may gain entry to your lungs. You can become infected but have no symptoms initially, or you may develop only a mild cough and slight fever.

The TB organism can spread through your lymph nodes and blood to almost any part of your body. Areas commonly affected include the lungs and the membranes that cover the lungs (pleural membranes), the spine or large joints and your kidneys. If your kidneys are involved, you may experience symptoms similar to those of a bladder infection.

The tuberculin skin test can determine whether you've ever been infected with the TB organism. This test involves injecting a small amount of tuberculin purified protein derivative into your skin. If you've been infected by the TB organism, this injection causes a reaction in your skin within 48 to 72 hours. Your doctor or a nurse will interpret the results of this test 2 to 3 days after the injection. If you have a very active infection or if your immune system is suppressed, the tuberculin test reaction may be falsely negative.

A preliminary diagnosis of TB is often based on a chest X-ray, where changes may appear within 2 to 3 months after the initial infection. In addition, your doctor may have you collect sputum for staining and examination under the microscope. He or she may also use a molecular technique called polymerase chain reaction to see if you've been infected with the TB organism.

The diagnosis is confirmed by growing (culturing) the organism in the laboratory. Your sputum is usually the easiest sample to obtain for culture. Other common sources are urine and stomach secretions. Stomach secretions are collected by passing a small tube through the nose, down the back of the throat, through the esophagus and into the stomach. Your doctor may get preliminary results from a staining test within 24 hours, but culture results may not be available for up to 6 to 8 weeks because the TB bacterium grows slowly.

Culture results can also provide important information as to how well or poorly the bacterium may respond to treatment. Some strains of the TB organism require different or more intensive treatments than other strains.

How serious is tuberculosis?

In the United States, more than 95 percent of individuals with a TB infection recover completely. You'll show no subsequent evidence of disease except for changes seen on a chest X-ray and a positive tuberculin skin test. Once you have TB, your skin test remains positive even after the disease is cured.

Sometimes, tuberculosis develops within weeks after initial exposure. However, the TB organism may lie dormant for years before the disease becomes apparent. The disease may be reactivated under conditions that weaken your immune system, including advancing age, malnutrition, alcoholism, the use of immunosuppressant medications or the presence of certain illnesses, such as HIV or AIDS, or certain cancers.

Treatment

Drugs offer the most effective therapy for TB. In recent years, though, an increasing number of TB organisms have become resistant to drugs commonly used in treatment. It's important to determine the sensitivity to antituberculosis drugs in every newly diagnosed case so that each case is treated with the most effective medications.

If you have active TB, treatment commonly starts with four drugs — isoniazid (Laniazid, Nydrazid), rifampin (Rifadin), pyrazinamide — which can be combined in one tablet (Rifater) — and ethambutol (Myambutol).

To determine the bacteria's sensitivity or resistance to each drug, cultures of sputum or other body secretions or tissues are evaluated in the laboratory. When the culture results are available in 6 to 8 weeks, your doctor may replace ineffective drugs with other medications. Or your treatment may continue with fewer than four drugs. Wearing a hospital mask in public until you're no longer contagious, generally after 2 to 3 weeks of treatment, helps keep you from spreading the disease.

Once a drug regimen is started, improvement in your symptoms often occurs within 2 to 3 weeks, followed by improvement on chest X-rays. Successful drug therapy, however, may require taking drugs for 6 to 12 months to completely destroy the TB bacteria.

All medications used for TB have some potential toxicity. Both rifampin and isoniazid may cause a noninfectious form of hepatitis and jaundice. These effects are generally reversible after you stop taking the medication. Rifampin may cause urine, sweat and tears to take on an orange or brownish color.

Prevention

If you have a positive tuberculin skin test, especially if you've recently been in close contact with a person with TB, your doctor may consider giving you isoniazid to decrease your risk of developing active TB. The drug must be taken for 9 months. In addition, your doctor may consider giving the medication or a similar one to others in your household.

Legionnaires' disease

Signs and symptoms

- Malaise
- Slight headache
- Fever and shaking chills
- Shortness of breath

- Coughing that produces mucus or blood
- Chest, muscle and abdominal pain
- Nausea and vomiting
- Diarrhea

Legionnaires' disease was first identified when a sudden, virulent outbreak of pneumonia occurred primarily among delegates attending an American Legion convention at a hotel in Philadelphia in July 1976 — hence its name. More than 200 people became ill with severe pneumonia of unknown cause, and 34 died.

The cause eventually was identified as a previously unknown bacterium that was later named *Legionella pneumophila.* The bacterium was identified in retrospect as the one responsible for several earlier, smaller outbreaks of pneumonia. Children have developed the disease, but most cases have occurred in middle-aged or older adults, particularly those who smoke or have chronic lung disease.

Although Legionnaires' disease is uncommon, legionella bacteria have been identified in stagnant, warm water — such as air conditioning cooling towers, whirlpool spas and showers — all over the world. They can thrive in air-circulation systems of large buildings and travel through air ducts. Breathing the mist from the water spreads the bacteria to humans.

Diagnosis

Legionnaires' disease usually begins with headache and malaise, followed by a rapidly rising temperature. Within 24 to 48 hours, the fever reaches 104 F in about half of those affected, causing chills.

A mild, dry cough usually begins early and gets worse over several days. Then the cough generally produces mucus. About 20 percent of those affected have blood in their sputum. About 25 percent have gastrointestinal symptoms.

The disease tends to get progressively worse during the first 4 to 6 days. Another 4 or 5 days may pass before recovery begins, although some people get a milder version. In most cases, the lungs continue to be congested for some days after the fever disappears.

Pneumonia may show up on a chest X-ray, but other tests not usually used for pneumonia, such as a sputum culture and a urinary antigen test, are needed to pinpoint Legionnaires' disease. Blood samples generally are taken twice, 3 to 6 weeks apart, to compare legionella antibody levels.

How serious is Legionnaires' disease?

Typically, Legionnaires' disease is extremely virulent, causing pneumonia severe enough to require hospitalization. Although most people recover fully, about 15 percent of those who get the disease die of respiratory failure.

Treatment

Hospitalization may be required, and you may need intravenous (IV) fluids because the high fever can cause dehydration. Supplemental oxygen may be necessary to help you breathe.

Medication

Various antibiotics appear to be effective against Legionnaires' disease. Erythromycins seem to be the safest and most effective.

Bronchiectasis

Signs and symptoms

- Persistent mild or severe coughing that may produce thick, foul-smelling sputum, usually gray-green, that may contain blood
- Loss of appetite and weight
- Anemia and general weakness
- Recurring attacks of pneumonia

Inhalation Anthrax

Anthrax is a disease caused by the bacterium *Bacillus anthracis,* which is housed in a hardy spore. The disease usually affects livestock, but it can affect humans as well. A naturally occurring disease that has been around since biblical times, anthrax has become a biological weapon of great concern.

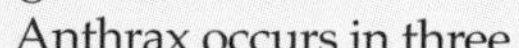

Anthrax occurs in three forms: skin (cutaneous), intestinal and inhalation (pulmonary), which infects your lungs. Inhalation anthrax is the deadliest form. It's caused by inhaling sufficient quantities of anthrax spores to cause infection. Once the infection spreads, inhalation anthrax is fatal in the majority of cases.

After lodging in the respiratory tract, the spores can take from a day to 2 months to become active, at which time signs and symptoms develop. Initially, the infection may feel like a cold or the flu, with a sore throat, muscle aches and mild chest discomfort. These first symptoms may last for a few hours to a few days before they may seem to briefly subside. However, within a few days of the onset of symptoms, the disease leads to a high fever and breathing problems. The disease destroys lung tissue and may spread to the brain, causing meningitis.

Fortunately, all three forms can be prevented or treated with antibiotics. With inhalation anthrax, antibiotics can reduce the risk of death, especially if started within the first few days of symptoms.

For more information on anthrax see page 517.

Bronchiectasis is long-lasting, abnormal expansion (dilation) of the walls of bronchial tubes. This dilation can also result from chronic bronchitis, but the dilation is more pronounced in bronchiectasis.

Some people are born with the condition, but most people with bronchiectasis develop it as a complication of cystic fibrosis or from diseases such as whooping cough, pneumonia and tuberculosis. Rare causes of bronchiectasis include defects of the microscopic hair-like projections (cilia) lining the breathing (bronchial) tubes and low levels of blood antibodies (gamma globulin). Bronchiectasis occurs primarily

Postural Drainage and Chest Percussion

Respiratory conditions such as bronchiectasis, cystic fibrosis and lung abscess may cause a large volume of secretions to accumulate in your lungs. Postural drainage and chest percussion help empty your lungs of the unwanted secretions. These therapies are especially important for individuals with cystic fibrosis. Your doctor may recommend a sequence that combines both methods for maximum effect.

Postural drainage

Postural drainage uses gravity to help clear your lungs of secretions. You position yourself to allow the secretions move to your windpipe (trachea) so that you can cough them out. Because the branches of your lungs point in various directions, it may be necessary for you to assume various positions to drain different areas of the lungs.

Some doctors recommend a time-consuming series of positional changes for individuals with cystic fibrosis. Others have found that compliance with these instructions tends to decrease as the child who has cystic fibrosis gets older. Therefore, the recommended positions may be limited to those that drain areas of the lungs where secretions are most likely to lodge, usually the lower portions of the lungs.

Cystic fibrosis

If you have cystic fibrosis, your doctor or a trained therapist can provide you with specific instructions on postural drainage. Remember to cough during each position change to aid in raising the sputum.

Bronchiectasis

Bronchiectasis is uncommon in the upper lobes of the lungs because they drain well when you're in an upright position. Therefore, postural drainage for bronchiectasis may be simpler than it is for some other conditions. You can drain lower portions of your lungs quite well by kneeling or lying facedown on a bed or couch and putting your hands on the floor. Stay in this position for about 10 minutes, coughing periodically.

Collect the expectorated sputum and note its color and approximate amount. You may stop postural drainage when you produce no more sputum, and resume it later when you notice that you're producing sputum again. This is a valuable technique because antibiotics work better and remain effective longer if you keep your airways as free of secretions as possible.

Chest percussion

To use chest percussion to loosen secretions in your lungs, lie on your back on a firm surface. Cup your hands and rapidly strike your chest wall with one hand and then with the other. You may want to protect your skin with a bath towel. Be careful not to strike the heart area, breasts, lower ribs, shoulders or kidneys.

This technique may be more effective applied to the back. Parents and others concerned with a child's care should learn this technique. Adults also may need someone to help them use this technique on their back.

Some people loosen secretions with the aid of an electric chest clapper, known as a mechanical percussor. Some use an inflatable vest with a machine attached that vibrates at high frequency to help the user cough up secretions.

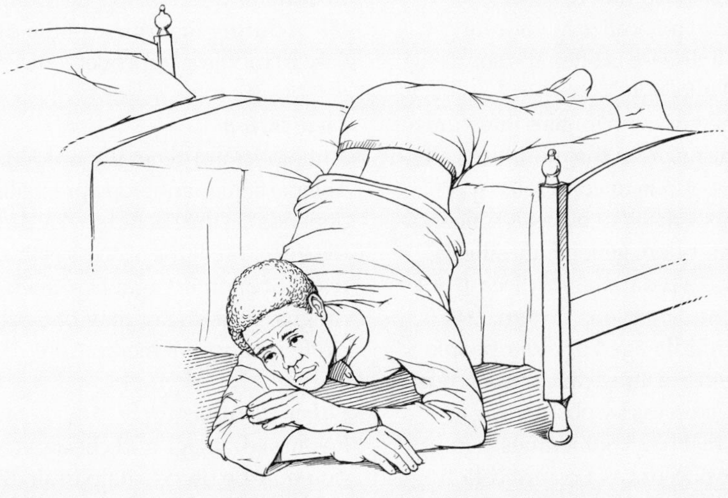

The postural drainage technique uses gravity to help clear your lungs of unwanted secretions. The position shown here is designed to clear the lower lungs.

in children and young adults under 21. It has become much less common since the introduction of antibiotic treatment of pneumonia.

Diagnosis

A doctor may have you undergo X-rays or a high-resolution computerized tomography (CT) scan to confirm the diagnosis.

How serious is bronchiectasis?

The damage to the walls of the bronchial tubes is irreversible and areas of the bronchial walls may be destroyed. Severe cases can lead to scarring and loss of lung blood vessels, which can affect the heart.

Treatment

Your doctor may suggest chest physiotherapy to help treat the condition. This includes positioning the body to help lung drainage (postural drainage) and vibrating the chest wall (chest percussion), as discussed on page 805. Breathing exercises also can help improve the functioning of your lungs. Avoid dust, smoke and other respiratory irritants. Get plenty of exercise because deep breathing helps raise secretions. Eat a nutritious diet. Drinking fluids helps to dilute the sputum in your lungs.

Unless your doctor advises against it, get a pneumococcal vaccine and a yearly flu shot. You may need a second pneumonia vaccine after 5 years.

Medication

Because bacterial infections are associated with production of pus in bronchiectasis, your doctor will likely prescribe an antibiotic. Unless a specific antibiotic is indicated by tests of your sputum, ampicillin, tetracycline or a similar drug is usually given. Your doctor may also prescribe a bronchodilator to relieve spasms in your bronchial tubes.

Antibiotics usually are prescribed for intermittent use to prevent lung infection. A common regimen requires taking the antibiotic for 7 to 10 consecutive days each month. It's generally not advisable to use an antibiotic continuously. At times, it may be advisable to take two or three kinds of antibiotics on a rotating basis. Alternating medications can help prevent the development of an antibiotic-resistant bacterial strain.

Surgery

If you have inadequate response to other treatments or if you're coughing up blood, surgical removal of the affected portions of the lungs may be necessary. However, this is an option only if the disease is localized in one or two areas of the lungs and there's adequate lung function to allow removal of part of your lungs.

Lung abscess

Signs and symptoms

- A high and irregular fever
- Sweats and chills
- Shortness of breath
- Coughing that produces sputum containing pus and sometimes blood
- Malaise
- Loss of appetite and weight
- Chest pain

A lung abscess is a cavity that develops in your lungs and fills with pus. Usually, inhaling infectious material from your mouth or throat (aspiration) causes the infection to localize in your lungs. Dental disease is often the source of the infection.

A person who inhales infectious organisms from the mouth usually does so while unconscious, typically as a result of excessive alcohol consumption, general anesthesia, excessive sedation or a disease of the central nervous system.

In middle-aged or older people who smoke, lung cancer may cause a lung abscess by obstructing a bronchial tube. Sometimes, a lung abscess occurs as a complication of pneumonia. More rare causes of lung abscess are infections caused by tuberculosis or by fungal or parasitic organisms.

In most cases, a single abscess develops in one lung, although occasionally multiple abscesses appear.

Diagnosis

Signs and symptoms of a lung abscess develop slowly over several days or weeks. Initially, they're similar to those of pneumonia. A cough develops after the abscess ruptures into a bronchial tube. Depending on the type of organism causing the infection, the sputum may be foul smelling.

In addition to giving you a physical examination, your doctor may request a chest X-ray and a computerized tomography (CT) scan of the lung and may take a sample of your sputum to check for bacteria or other organisms if he or she suspects a lung abscess. Such information can lead to more effective treatment with specific antibiotics or other therapy.

How serious is a lung abscess?

A lung abscess is generally a temporary (acute) disease, although if not treated adequately it can become long-term (chronic). With treatment, most people with an acute abscess recover completely without surgery.

Treatment

A combination of medication and drainage techniques is the usual treatment. Chest X-rays are often taken during the course of the disease to monitor improvement.

Medication

Antibiotics are generally needed. The particular antibiotic prescribed depends on the bacterium causing the infection. If the abscess is the result of another organism, such a fungus, your doctor may prescribe a different type of medication.

Other therapies

Postural drainage and chest percussion may be used to help drain the lung abscess. If your lung abscess doesn't respond to antibiotics or drainage and percussion, bronchoscopy may be recommended (see page 819). If the abscess has been present for several weeks, if it has a thick wall or if it has spread into the space between the membranous layers surrounding your lungs (pleural space), surgery may be necessary.

Empyema

Signs and symptoms

- A dry or productive cough
- Fever and night sweats
- Weight loss
- Shortness of breath
- Chest pain on deep breathing

Normally, only a tiny amount of clear, lubricating fluid is present between the membranous layers surrounding your lungs (pleural space). In empyema, pus collects in the pleural space as the result of an infection. It's typically a complication of bacterial pneumonia, a lung abscess, an open wound in the chest or chest surgery.

Diagnosis

You may experience chest pain due to inflammation in the plural space (pleurisy) early in the course of the disease. But as fluid accumulates in the pleural space, the pain may gradually disappear. A collection of infected fluid — up to 1 pint or more — can compress your lungs.

To confirm a diagnosis of empyema, your doctor may perform thoracentesis. In this procedure, a needle is inserted between your ribs to remove fluid from your pleural cavity.

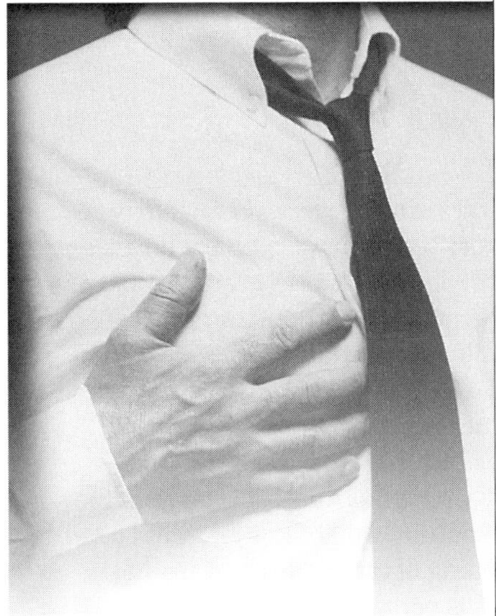

Treatment

Treatment consists of antibiotic therapy and drainage of the infected fluid from the chest.

If the fluid in the pleural space flows through a needle, repeated thoracentesis may remove it. However, to achieve adequate fluid removal, tube thoracostomy is often necessary. For this procedure, you're given local anesthesia, and a doctor makes a small incision in your chest wall and inserts a chest tube for drainage.

If thoracostomy is unsuccessful, you may need a thoracotomy. While you're under general anesthesia, an opening is made in the chest wall to remove all of the infected fluid. If thickening of the pleura restricts expansion of your lung, surgical removal of the thickening may be advisable to enable your lungs to expand.

Pleurisy and pleural effusion

Signs and symptoms

- Shortness of breath
- Chest pain
- A dry cough
- Fever and chills

Pleurisy is inflammation that involves the pleura, the membrane that lines your chest cavity and surrounds each of your lungs. Pleural effusions are accumulations of fluid in the pleural space, the space between the membranous layers surrounding each lung and lining the chest wall.

Pleurisy and pleural effusions occur as complications of an underlying disease such as tuberculosis, pneumonia, pulmonary embolism, pancreatitis, cancer or congestive heart failure, as well as from trauma to the chest.

In pleurisy, the two inflamed layers of the pleural membrane rub against each other when you inhale and exhale. This produces sharp, stabbing pains in your chest that are made worse by coughing, sneezing, moving and deep breathing. The pain of pleurisy is relieved when you breathe shallowly or, sometimes, when you apply pressure over the painful area to restrict motion.

If a pleural effusion develops, the pain usually improves as fluid separates the pleural surfaces. However, if enough fluid accumulates, it compresses the lung, causing shortness of breath. Sometimes you develop a dry cough, fever and chills, particularly if the fluid in the pleural space is infected.

Diagnosis

Your doctor may suspect pleurisy or plural effusion based on your symptoms, findings on examination of your chest with a stethoscope and the results of a chest X-ray.

Sometimes, a doctor numbs the skin over the chest with a local anesthetic and inserts a needle through the chest wall and between the ribs to remove fluid for laboratory analysis. Your doctor may also obtain a tiny sample of lung tissue for microscopic study, to rule out lung cancer or another lung condition, such as tuberculosis or sarcoidosis.

How serious are pleurisy and pleural effusion?

The outcome of these conditions primarily depends on the seriousness of the underlying disease. If the underlying disease can be treated effectively, pleurisy and pleural effusion generally resolve.

Treatment

First, it's important to treat the underlying condition or illness causing the pleurisy or pleural effusion. In some cases, a pleural effusion needs to be drained through a chest tube for several days.

Pain relievers (analgesics) and anti-inflammatory medications are generally prescribed. Sometimes, codeine is prescribed to suppress coughing.

Fungal Diseases of the Lungs

If yeast and the spores of certain fungi are inhaled, they can infect the lungs, causing disease. Most of these ailments cause fever, cough and malaise.

Histoplasmosis

Signs and symptoms

- Fever
- Coughing
- Malaise
- Enlargement of the liver, lymph nodes or spleen
- Oral or gastrointestinal ulcers
- Difficulty breathing

Histoplasmosis results from inhaling dust — particularly from chicken houses, bat-infested caves and pigeon droppings — that contains the spores of the fungus *Histoplasma capsulatum.* Men are more likely to contract this disease than are women. In the United States, histoplasmosis is most commonly seen in the Mississippi and Ohio River valleys.

Histoplasmosis can range from mild, which may be indistinguishable from diseases such as the common cold, to severe. If the fungus spreads from the lungs through the blood, it may cause enlargement of the liver, lymph nodes or spleen and, less frequently, oral or gastrointestinal ulcers.

Histoplasmosis can become long-lasting (chronic), producing an illness similar to chronic tuberculosis. At its most severe, histoplasmosis spreads (disseminates) throughout the body. People with a weakened immune system are at highest risk of disseminated histoplasmosis.

Diagnosis

To confirm the diagnosis of histoplasmosis, your doctor likely will obtain specimens of sputum, lymph nodes, bone marrow, liver, blood, urine or oral ulcerations to check for the fungus. In people who have had histoplasmosis, it's common to see evidence of it on a chest X-ray.

How serious is histoplasmosis?

Mild histoplasmosis usually is benign and requires no treatment. Severe forms of the disease can be fatal.

Treatment

If you have no symptoms, treatment may be unnecessary. If you experience symptoms, your doctor may prescribe an oral antifungal agent such as itraconazole (Sporanox) or a related drug. For severe infections, it may be necessary to administer amphotericin B (Amphocin), which must be given intravenously. If your lungs are affected, treatment eliminates the fungus, but the lesions it produces on your lungs remain. Normally, they calcify and don't cause any long-term problems.

Cryptococcosis

Signs and symptoms

- Low-grade fever
- Chest pain
- Coughing that may produce sputum
- Malaise
- Lesions in the lungs
- Increasingly severe headaches
- Nausea
- Vertigo
- Loss of appetite
- Vision disorders
- Mental deterioration

Cryptococcosis is caused by the yeast *Cryptococcus neoformans,* which lives in soil and on pigeon droppings. Disease results when a person inhales the organism. The yeast may remain in the lungs, or it may spread, particularly to the central nervous system. Some pulmonary cases produce only mild symptoms. More serious cases resemble bronchitis, and lesions develop in the lungs.

Diagnosis

Your doctor may request a chest X-ray and samples of sputum, pus or spinal fluid to check for presence of the yeast.

How serious is cryptococcosis?

People who have a weakened immune system — such as those with leukemia, Hodgkin's disease or AIDS — or individuals taking immunosuppressant drugs such as corticosteroids are most susceptible to the disease. Some mild cases resolve without treatment, but for people with a weakened immune system, cryptococcosis can lead to death, especially if it spreads beyond the lungs.

Treatment

Treatment includes medication and possibly surgery. Milder cases may respond to oral antifungal medications. For individuals with a sup-

Aspergillosis

Aspergillus is a genus of fungi that's found virtually everywhere. It may be present in nasal discharges and respiratory secretions of people who are exposed to it regularly from the soil or farm dust, but it rarely causes problems.

In people with asthma, however, aspergillus can produce an allergic response. In other susceptible individuals, such as those with a weakened immune system, it can cause an unusual form of pneumonia. Both of these conditions, called aspergillosis, can be treated effectively with corticosteroids or antifungal medication, such as itraconazole (Sporanox).

In people whose lungs are damaged, aspergillus may collect within the lungs and cause coughing and bloody sputum, weight loss and mild fever. Often, surgery is needed to control bleeding. If aspergillosis occurs in an individual with leukemia, the prognosis is poor.

pressed immune system, treatment may require the intravenous IV antifungal drug amphotericin B (Amphocin) or the oral medication flucytosine (Ancobon). In some cases, surgery to remove nodules that form in the lungs is recommended.

Coccidioidomycosis

Signs and symptoms

- Fever and chills
- Malaise
- Backache
- Headache
- Chest pain
- A red, spotty rash
- Swelling of the knees and ankles
- Coughing
- Nasal congestion

Coccidioidomycosis is caused by inhaling spores of the fungus *Coccidioides immitis,* which lives in the soil in certain arid parts of the southwestern United States, Mexico and Central and South America. In the United States, the fungus is prevalent in California's San Joaquin Valley, hence its more popular names, San Joaquin fever and valley fever.

Nine of every 10 people who move to the desert areas of the southwestern part of the United States test positive for this fungus within 4 to 5 years. Most often, coccidioidomycosis causes no symptoms.

But approximately 10 percent of infected people develop chest pain, which usually begins 10 to 30 days after exposure to the fungus. Fever, chills and other flu-like symptoms often accompany the pain. Nasal congestion and a mild cough may be followed by bronchitis. One to 2 days after the fever begins, a red, spotty rash, similar to that of the measles, may appear, and your knees and ankles may swell.

Coccidioidomycosis can affect anyone, but pregnant women and people with a weakened immune system are especially vulnerable. The disease tends to be more serious in dark-skinned people.

Diagnosis

Your doctor may order a chest X-ray and tests of blood, sputum and spinal fluid to determine the presence of the fungus.

How serious is coccidioidomycosis?

Usually, the disease clears without complications, although in some cases lesions formed in the lungs can be difficult to cure. In rare cases, the disease may recur after weeks or months. Occasionally, the infection spreads throughout the body, causing lesions in the bones and other organs as well.

Treatment

If you have no symptoms, treatment usually is unnecessary. For flu-like symptoms, your doctor may recommend over-the-counter medications to relieve the signs and symptoms and bed rest until the fever disappears.

If you have a more severe illness, your doctor may give you the intravenous IV medication amphotericin B (Amphocin), which is often effective. Ketoconazole (Nizoral) or a similar medication taken orally may be used in localized pulmonary disease. Surgical drainage of lung abscesses or pleural fluids is sometimes necessary.

Chronic Lung Conditions

Three common chronic lung disorders restrict the flow of air out of the bronchial passages: chronic bronchitis, emphysema and asthma.

Chronic bronchitis causes a persistent inflammation of the lining of the bronchial tubes, which are the two main branches of the windpipe (trachea). Emphysema is characterized by enlargement of the air sacs (alveoli) and the destruction of the walls between them. Some degree of bronchitis is usually associated with emphysema. Doctors often refer to emphysema and chronic bronchitis as chronic obstructive lung disease (COLD) or chronic obstructive pulmonary disease (COPD) because these conditions both commonly obstruct the outflow of air.

COPD affects 17 million Americans and is the fourth leading

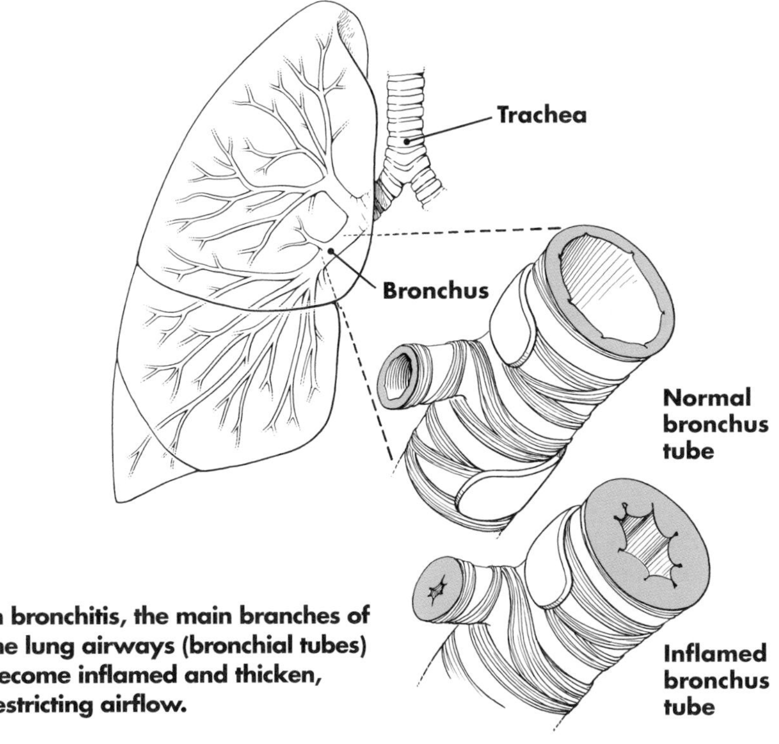

In bronchitis, the main branches of the lung airways (bronchial tubes) become inflamed and thicken, restricting airflow.

cause of death in the United States. Smoking is the most common cause of COPD.

The third disorder, asthma, involves inflammation of the airways and excess mucus production that contribute to airway obstruction. With asthma, the bronchial passages narrow too much and too easily in response to a wide variety of provoking stimuli. Obstruction of the outflow of air tends to be variable and episodic, often occurring in attacks of wheezing and shortness of breath.

What It Feels Like to Have COPD

To get an idea of what if feels like to have chronic obstructive pulmonary disease (COPD), try this exercise with a thin straw, but only if your lungs are healthy: First, inhale normally without the straw, then exhale fully through the straw. Likely you'll feel the need to inhale again before you're done exhaling. If you continue the exercise, you won't be able to empty your lungs, your breathing will become shallow, and you'll become short of breath.

Chronic obstructive pulmonary disease

Signs and symptoms

- Chronic coughing that usually produces mucus
- Shortness of breath
- Possibly, chest enlargement

Chronic obstructive pulmonary disease (COPD) is the overall term for a group of long-standing (chronic) conditions that result in obstruction of the lungs' airways. The term generally refers to two disorders — chronic bronchitis and emphysema. You can develop either condition independently, but most people with COPD have both. Sometimes, several other lung disorders — cystic fibrosis, bronchiolitis, bronchiectasis and, especially, asthma — are classified as COPD because they have similar and overlapping features.

COPD develops gradually and produces few symptoms in its early stages. In addition, because people typically become less active as they get older, it becomes easier to blame COPD symptoms on age or being out of shape.

Chronic bronchitis

Chronic bronchitis is a chronic inflammation and thickening of the lining of the bronchial tubes. This disorder can narrow air passages enough to interfere with breathing and induce spells of coughing. The inflammation also causes the glands of the bronchial tubes to produce excessive amounts of mucus, increasing lung congestion that further hampers breathing. It's a chronic and recurring disease, but it may become persistent and be fatal.

Chronic bronchitis is defined as having a cough and sputum on most days for at least 3 months in at least 2 consecutive years. As the disease worsens, relapses of the cough become more frequent and more severe. Shortness of breath develops late in the course of the disease, especially if smoking has caused significant lung damage.

Emphysema

Lungs normally contain about 300 million elastic air sacs (alveoli), where oxygen is added to the blood and carbon dioxide is removed. The inflammation from emphysema damages the walls of the alveoli, causing them to lose elasticity, become overstretched and rupture. Several adjacent alveoli may rupture, forming one large space instead of many small ones. Larger spaces can combine into an even bigger cavity, called a bulla.

Damage to alveoli means fewer and less elastic sacs are helping force air out of the lungs. It also means that less outward tension is placed on the small passageways (bronchioles) connected to the alveoli, so the tubes can collapse and obstruct airflow. Air that you aren't able to exhale before you need to inhale again gets trapped in your lungs, and you become short of breath. The effort it takes to force air out of your lungs when exhaling can be exhausting. In addition, damage to alveoli walls can disrupt the oxygen and carbon dioxide transfer.

Emphysema usually produces no symptoms until the disease is far advanced. At that point, shortness of breath may occur, along with less capacity for exertion.

The shortness of breath from emphysema typically isn't due to poor transfer of oxygen and carbon dioxide within the lungs. Rather, it's a result of decreased efficiency

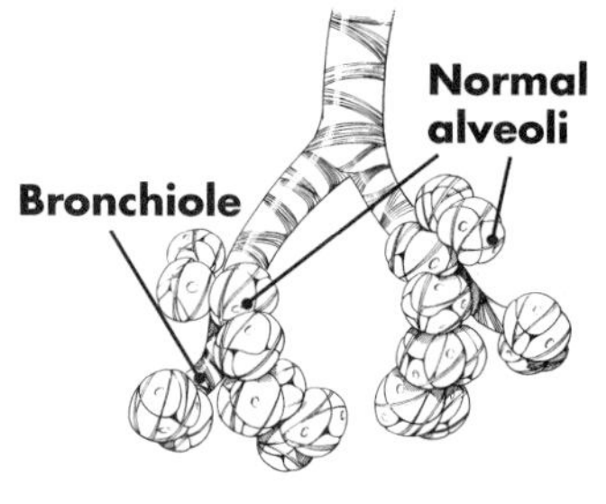

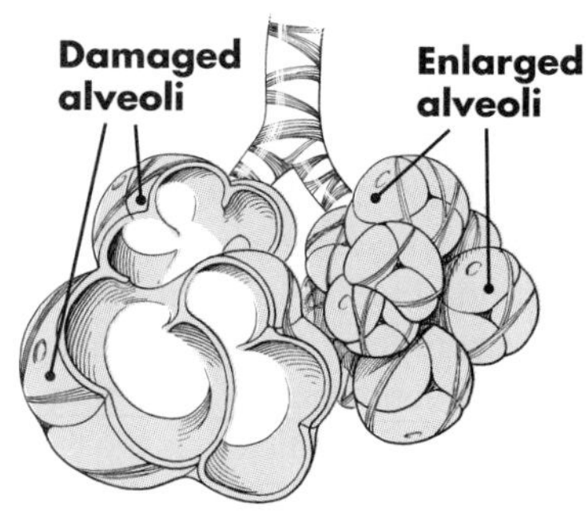

In emphysema, the air sacs of the lungs (alveoli) lose elasticity, enlarge and may rupture. This decreases the exchange of oxygen and carbon dioxide in your blood.

of breathing and a resultant increase in the effort to breathe. This explains why supplemental oxygen is neither necessary nor particularly useful for treating shortness of breath in this disease, unless you also have a significantly reduced blood oxygen level.

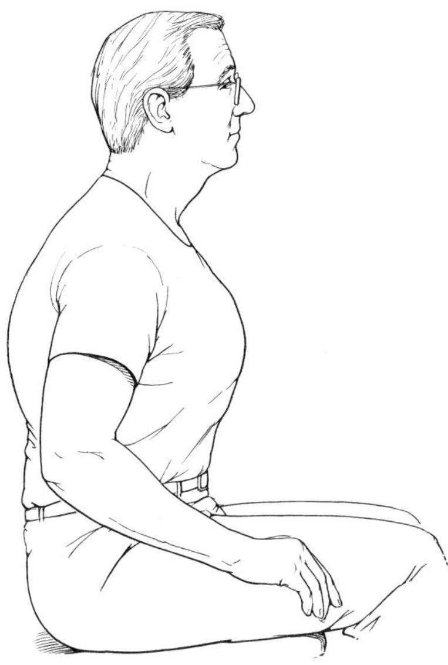

An enlarged chest is one characteristic sign of emphysema.

Cause

If you smoke, you have a one in four to one in six chance of getting COPD. Inhaled tobacco smoke paralyzes the microscopic hairs (cilia) that line the bronchial tubes. As a result, irritants and germs caught in mucus remain in the bronchial tubes because the cilia can't sweep them out. This results in the inflammation of bronchial membranes, eventually resulting in chronic obstruction.

Research indicates that exposure to secondhand smoke may contribute to COPD when combined with other risk factors — for example, past smoking or continuous exposure to air pollution.

Although smoking is the most common cause of COPD, occupational exposure to chemical fumes or dusts from grain, cotton, wood, coal or other sources also can put you at risk. In addition, air pollution and toxic gases in the environment, such as smog, can contribute to the development of COPD in smokers.

COPD was once more prevalent in men than in women. Unfortunately, more women are smoking, so almost as many women as men now have COPD. And the incidence among women is increasing.

Diagnosis

To determine if you have COPD, your doctor will likely ask about your symptoms and perform a physical examination. He or she will want to know if you are or have been a smoker and whether you're regularly exposed to pollutants, such as dust or chemicals, or have been in the past.

A number of tests can help your doctor evaluate your condition and determine the best course of treat-

Smoking and Genetics

Smoking is clearly the primary risk factor for emphysema. There's also a rare inherited condition known as alpha-1-antitrypsin deficiency that can cause the disorder.

Alpha-1-antitrypsin is a protein in the blood that circulates to the lungs, where it limits damage to the air sacs (alveoli) during episodes of infection or inflammation. If you're deficient in this protein, this protection is lacking, so you're more likely to develop emphysema at a young age — usually in your 30s and 40s — if you smoke. If you don't smoke and you have this genetic deficiency, you may not develop emphysema until much later in life, if at all.

About 1 in 2,500 people have alpha-1-antitrypsin deficiency, which can be detected with a blood test. The test isn't performed routinely, but if you have family members who weren't smokers but developed COPD or who smoked and developed the disease at a young age, you might want to discuss this testing with your doctor.

How Smoking Damages Your Lungs

Tobacco smoke contains thousands of substances, including chemicals, gases and tiny droplets of tar, many of which can cause cancer. Irritants in tobacco smoke cause your air passages to constrict and your bronchial tubes to produce excess mucus. These irritants may also impair the function of the immune system cells in your lungs and upset the normal balance of pulmonary enzymes, making you more susceptible to respiratory disease. Finally, inhaled tobacco smoke stops the movement of the tiny hair-like projections (cilia) in your windpipe (trachea) and bronchial tubes that help expel foreign material from your lungs.

Tobacco smoke also contains carbon monoxide, a toxic gas that combines with hemoglobin to form carboxyhemoglobin, which blocks the transport of needed oxygen to your tissues. Many smokers have carboxyhemoglobin levels of 8 percent to 10 percent in their blood, whereas a nonsmoker commonly has only up to 1.5 percent.

Because some cigar and pipe smokers don't inhale smoke directly, many believe they have a lower risk of developing lung disease than cigarette smokers do. This is only partly true. Smoking-related diseases are also more common in cigar and pipe smokers than in nonsmokers.

ment. They include a chest X-ray and a chest computerized tomography (CT) scan. A pulmonary function test determines how well your lungs are functioning by measuring how much air you can breathe in and how fast you can blow it out. Arterial blood gas analysis is a test that measures how well your lungs bring oxygen into your blood and remove carbon dioxide from it. Pulse oximetry uses a small device that attaches to your fingertip to measure the amount of oxygen in your blood. Your doctor might also obtain a sample of your sputum for laboratory analysis.

How serious is COPD?

COPD is extremely serious. A severe case is likely to shorten your life span. If the disease is detected early and you stop smoking if you're a smoker, your outlook improves greatly. If you stop smoking before you experience symptoms, you may prevent further progression of the disease.

As COPD progressively decreases lung function, some people don't get enough oxygen in their blood, a condition called hypoxemia. Common signs and symptoms of hypoxemia include decreased ability to exercise, fatigue, memory loss, depression, confusion and poor nighttime sleep with frequent awakenings.

People with COPD are particularly prone to pneumonia, acute bronchitis and other serious respiratory diseases.

Treatment

COPD can't be cured. However, proper treatment, beginning with quitting smoking if you're a smoker, may prevent further damage and occasionally leads to improvement in lung function. It's important for you to take an active role in your treatment and preserve the lung function you still have.

Smoking cessation

By the time signs and symptoms of COPD appear — typically, cough, shortness of breath and difficulty exercising — your lungs are already damaged. If you don't stop smoking, your disease will get worse. Stopping smoking can help prevent progression of COPD, although it can't fully repair damage already done.

Other therapies

The therapy your doctor recommends will depend on the severity of your disease. The goals of therapy include:

- Preventing or treating respiratory infections
- Relieving any reversible airway obstruction
- Controlling your cough
- Increasing your physical fitness
- Controlling complications, such as high blood pressure in the lungs (pulmonary hypertension) and cardiovascular problems related to low blood oxygen

Some people are able to improve their tolerance for exercise by improving the strength and endurance of the muscles that control breathing (see page 813). A balanced diet gives your body the nutrients it needs to maintain energy and normal cell functioning. Achieving and maintaining a healthy weight may help you feel better. Carrying extra weight demands more oxygen and being underweight may reduce your strength. If the effort to eat taxes you, try eating smaller meals more frequently.

See your doctor promptly if your symptoms increase or if you develop a respiratory infection.

Protecting Your Lungs From Everyday Hazards

If you have COPD, you need to protect yourself from hazards in the air and exposure to infectious agents. Here are some suggestions:

Eliminate smoke from your environment

- Don't let anyone smoke in your home.
- When in public, look for no smoking establishments or sit in no smoking areas.
- Avoid wood smoke and cooking smoke.

Prevent respiratory infections

- As much as possible, avoid exposure to anyone who has a cold or the flu (influenza). Avoid crowds when colds and flu are common.
- Wash your hands frequently, especially before you eat or take medicine, because viruses are often passed from hand to mouth.
- Unless your doctor advises against it, get a yearly flu shot and a pneumococcal pneumonia vaccination. You may need a second pneumonia vaccination 5 years following your first one.

Limit pollutants in your home

- Change your furnace and air conditioner filters according to manufacturers' instructions.
- Keep windows closed when it's dusty or smoky outside.
- Keep the humidity level in your home at 40 percent to 50 percent. If you use a humidifier, clean it frequently to prevent molds and bacteria from growing and potentially aggravating your lung condition.
- Limit your use of cleaning chemicals and avoid aerosol sprays and irritants such as paint fumes.
- Wear a dust mask when cleaning.

Signs and symptoms include a change in the amount, color or consistency of your sputum, increased coughing, wheezing or shortness of breath, a fever, swelling of the ankles or hands or the need to sleep in an upright position.

Medication

Changes in the color, volume or thickness of your sputum may indicate a respiratory infection. Your doctor may prescribe a 7- to 10-day course of an antibiotic. If lung tests indicate that you have spasms of your bronchial tubes (bronchospasms), your doctor may also prescribe a bronchodilator to relax and open airways.

Your doctor may prescribe oral or inhaled corticosteroids to reduce inflammation and swelling in your airways and reduce mucus production. Expectorants in liquid or tablet form can help liquefy and remove mucus from your airways.

If your body's ability to move oxygen from your lungs into your blood is significantly impaired, causing low blood oxygen, home oxygen therapy may be beneficial. Supplemental oxygen can improve low blood oxygen levels, as well as

Question and Answer

What are pulmonary function tests?

Pulmonary function tests detect lung disease and indicate its severity. The tests typically involve use of a device called a spirometer that you blow into to determine how much air you can take into your lungs and how fast you can blow it out.

You may be asked to blow into a spirometer before and after you use inhaled medications to test your response to them. Such tests may include inhalants such as albuterol (Proventil, Ventolin), which can open bronchial tubes, or methacholine (Provocholine), which can constrict your bronchial tubes briefly and indicate if your airways have an asthma-type reaction.

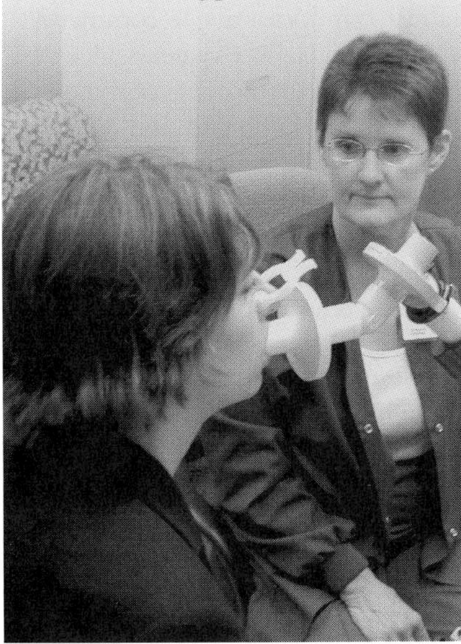

Diaphragmatic Breathing

If you have chronic obstructive pulmonary disease (COPD) or another chronic lung disorder, a regular program of aerobic exercise, such as walking or bicycling, is the most effective way to improve your lung function — after you quit smoking, that is. In addition to exercise, practicing diaphragmatic breathing also may be helpful. The following exercise can help you learn to breathe more efficiently. You might want to practice this breathing exercise at least once a day.

1. Lie on your back with your head and knees supported by pillows. Begin the exercise by breathing in and out slowly and smoothly in a rhythmic pattern. Relax.
2. Place the fingertips of one or both hands on your abdomen, just below the base of your rib cage. As you inhale slowly, you should feel your diaphragm lifting your hand.
3. Practice pushing your abdomen against your hand as your chest becomes filled with air. Make sure your chest remains motionless as you inhale through your mouth for a slow count of 3. Then purse your lips, which helps to increase the amount of air that can be exhaled, and exhale through your mouth while counting slowly to 6.
4. After you can take 10 to 15 consecutive breaths in one session without tiring, practice the exercise while lying on your side, and then on your other side. Progress to doing the exercise while sitting in a chair, while standing up, while walking and, finally, while climbing stairs.

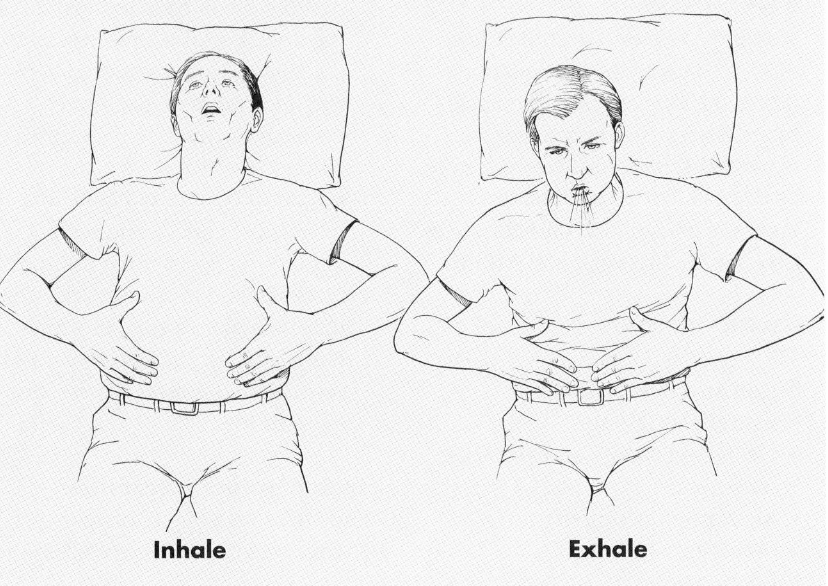

improve your ability to function both physically and mentally. You may need continuous supplemental oxygen, or you may need it only at certain times, such as when exercising. Portable oxygen units keep you from being confined to your home.

Surgery
Although uncommon, expensive and not covered by insurance, surgery may be an option for severe emphysema. One possibility is replacing a damaged lung with a healthy lung from a donor (lung transplant). Unfortunately, few donor organs are available.

Another treatment involves removing some of the damaged lung tissue to allow healthier lung tissue to expand and function better. Lung volume reduction surgery is being studied to determine its role in COPD treatment.

Asthma

Signs and symptoms

- Shortness of breath
- Coughing
- Tightness in the chest
- Wheezing

Emergency signs and symptoms

- Extreme difficulty breathing
- Bluish lips and nails
- Severe shortness of breath
- Increased pulse rate
- Sweating
- Severe coughing

Asthma is a form of chronic lung disease characterized by inflammation of the lung airways (bronchial tubes) that causes them to narrow. Signs and symptoms of asthma may be persistent or occur periodically. For more information on asthma, see Chapter 21, "Allergies and Asthma."

Cystic fibrosis

Signs and symptoms

- Chronic coughing
- Decreased energy and exercise intolerance
- Recurring pneumonia
- Shortness of breath
- Poor appetite

Supplemental Oxygen

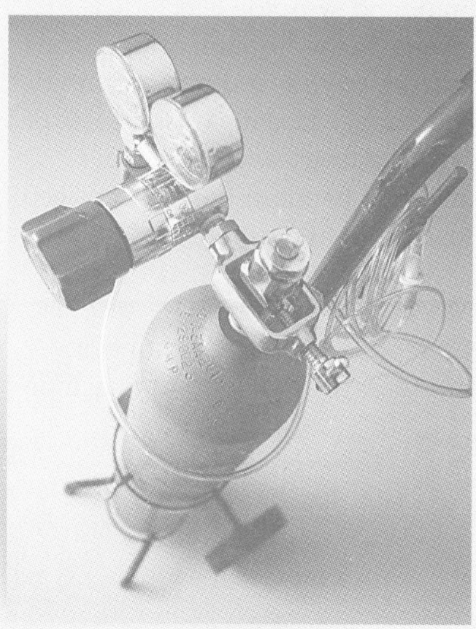

If you have a chronic lung disease and appropriate testing reveals a significant lack of oxygen in your blood, your doctor may prescribe supplemental oxygen.

Supplemental oxygen may decrease shortness of breath and improve your sense of well-being, but it's prescribed primarily to support the heart because inadequate blood oxygen can seriously disturb heart function.

You might need oxygen only at certain times, such as when you exercise or sleep, or you may need to use it all of the time. Three sources of supplemental oxygen are available. Your doctor will help you determine which type is best for you.

- Compressed oxygen comes in a tank with a flow meter and a regulator attached so that you can adjust the flow. The oxygen is stored under pressure, so you must handle the tank carefully. This may be your best choice if you don't need supplemental oxygen all of the time.
- An oxygen concentrator, which operates on electricity, takes oxygen from the air and concentrates it for your use. This may be your best bet if you need oxygen all of the time. Portable units are available for use in recreational vehicles and campers. Backup is necessary in case of an electrical outage.
- Liquid oxygen is available in a tank. Most tanks come with a light, portable unit that you can fill easily and take with you. The most portable option, this may work best for you if you want to stay active but need oxygen during activity.

Taking proper precautions

Fire burns faster in an oxygen-rich environment, so take special care when using oxygen in your home. Keep objects that produce sparks, flames or intense heat well away from the area where you keep oxygen equipment. Keep flammable materials away from the area too. Never expose the oxygen tank and its attachments to temperatures above 125 F.

Be sure that the oxygen cylinders are well secured to prevent them from tipping over. When not in use, seal the tank's connections properly with protective caps.

When installing the regulator, follow instructions precisely. Before the regulator is attached, open the valve slightly and then close it immediately. This clears out dust or combustible material.

If you require oxygen 24 hours a day, your doctor may recommend use of a portable oxygen device that allows you to travel beyond the reach of the large tank and its hose. The rules and regulations cited above apply equally to portable tanks.

Portable containers carry only a limited amount of oxygen. Longer trips require preparation to ensure a continuous oxygen supply. Plan where you'll need to stop to refill your tanks and check to make sure you can get a refill when you need it. Your oxygen supplier can help you determine your oxygen needs for travel.

- Chronic diarrhea and malnutrition
- Salt (sodium) depletion and heat exhaustion in hot weather

Cystic fibrosis affects both the respiratory and digestive systems and is one of the more common causes of chronic lung disease in children. It's the most common potentially fatal hereditary disease among white children in the United States, affecting approximately 1 in every 2,000 infants. It occurs in boys and girls equally.

Cystic fibrosis is inherited recessively, which means that a child can have the disease only if both parents are carriers of the gene. The parents may have no symptoms themselves, or they may have the disease too.

The disease affects the body's mucus and sweat glands. The first indication of cystic fibrosis in a newborn may be blockage of the intestine due to abnormally thick meconium, the material present in an infant's intestine that makes up its first stool.

As the infant grows older, chronic respiratory disease may develop, including bronchitis, bronchiectasis, pneumonia, a collapsed lung or fibrosis of the lung. These problems occur because the mucus in the child's lungs is unusually thick and sticky. Instead of serving as a lubricant, it clogs the respiratory system and allows bacteria and other microorganisms to grow in it, impairing the body's natural defenses.

The child's pancreas may not produce the enzymes needed to completely digest fats and proteins, resulting in chronic diarrhea and malnutrition. The child's sweat glands also are affected, causing the sweat to contain excessive salt.

Diagnosis

If your child has chronic respiratory or digestive problems, your physician may perform lung function or stool tests. He or she may also order a sweat test to measure the amount of salt in your child's perspiration. A blood test is available to detect the genetic defect that causes the disease.

How serious is cystic fibrosis?

Cystic fibrosis is very serious and may be fatal. About half of the individuals with this disease live beyond age 30. As techniques for treating cystic fibrosis improve, many people are living much longer. Mild forms of the disease may not produce symptoms until adulthood.

Treatment

Treatment is a long-term process, and frequent checkups with a doctor are important.

Exercises

Because the most common cause of death with cystic fibrosis is respiratory failure, aggressive respiratory management is essential.

Special exercises are used to loosen and promote drainage of mucus from the lungs (see page 805). These exercises should be done at least once a day. A health professional can provide instruction on how to do them correctly. A mechanical chest compression vest also may help with this process.

Supplements

If digestive or bowel symptoms are present, pancreatic enzyme supplements may be necessary, but usually no special diet is required.

Medication

Cystic fibrosis decreases immune defenses against respiratory disease, so it's important to receive available vaccines against respiratory diseases, including flu (influenza) and pneumococcal pneumonia.

Antibiotics may be prescribed for flares of bronchitis and other respiratory infections. Resistant bacteria are common, sometimes resulting in the need for more powerful antibiotics that are often administered intravenously for long periods. Occasionally, supplemental oxygen is used.

Treatment with medications that can dissolve the mucus is being tested.

Prevention

If a couple has a child with cystic fibrosis, each subsequent child of that couple has a 25 percent chance of having the disease, a 50 percent chance of being a carrier and a 25 percent chance of having normal genes. Specialists in cystic fibrosis and genetics can advise you on the latest developments in screening and help you determine if genetic testing may be of benefit to you.

Sarcoidosis

Signs and symptoms

- Malaise
- Fever
- Shortness of breath, especially with exertion
- Weight loss
- A dry cough
- Raised skin eruptions

Sarcoidosis is a chronic disease characterized by abnormal collections of inflammatory cells (granulomas) that can form in any part of the body, including the skin, eyes, peripheral nerves, liver, lymph nodes and heart. In 90 percent of cases, sarcoidosis affects the lungs.

In the United States, sarcoidosis is more common in blacks and people of Scandinavian descent. Women are affected more often than men. It occurs primarily in individuals between the ages of 20 and 40, although it can develop in children and older adults.

The cause of sarcoidosis is unknown, but researchers suspect it's an immune system reaction to something an affected individual has inhaled or come into contact with.

In this disease, helper T cells, a type of white blood cell that protects your body from disease, seem to overrespond, causing a buildup of inflammatory cells. This accumulation of cells distorts the walls of the small air sacs (alveoli), bronchial tubes and blood vessels, reducing the transfer of oxygen from your lungs to your blood.

Diagnosis
A routine chest X-ray may reveal inflamed patches in the lungs or lymph node enlargement. To confirm the diagnosis, your doctor may perform a lung biopsy using a fiber-optic bronchoscope to obtain tissue for examination (see page 819).

If the skin, lymph nodes or sclera of the eye are involved, tissue may be taken from these organs instead because the retrieval process is less invasive.

Sarcoidosis may cause an abnormally high level of calcium in your blood. Your doctor may request other tests, including blood tests, to rule out other diseases that can mimic sarcoidosis.

How serious is sarcoidosis?
Sarcoidosis often is a temporary condition, but it may be long-lasting (chronic). Most people recover completely or have only minor lingering effects, even without treatment. Some, though, have chronic disease that stays active or comes and goes intermittently for many years. Rarely, sarcoidosis leads to death, usually after many years.

Treatment
Often, no treatment is necessary. If you have pronounced symptoms or if the disease doesn't resolve spontaneously after 4 to 6 months, your doctor may prescribe corticosteroids.

As the condition improves — as demonstrated by chest X-rays or other tests — your doctor may taper you off the medications. This may take several months or even years. If the disease recurs, you may need another, longer course of corticosteroids.

A number of other immunosuppressant medications have been used for treating more severe forms of the disease, and several new medications are being developed.

Interstitial lung disease

Signs and symptoms
- Shortness of breath, particularly with exertion
- Nonproductive coughing with chest discomfort
- Fatigue and malaise
- Loss of appetite and weight

Interstitial lung disease refers to a large group of diseases that are long-lasting (chronic) but aren't cancerous or infectious. These diseases are characterized by infiltration of inflammatory cells into the air sacs of your lungs (alveoli). The result is formation of scar tissue in the connective tissues that support the alveoli, impairing the transfer of oxygen to the blood. If the disease progresses, the scarring can proliferate to the point of destroying the lungs.

Interstitial lung disorders most often occur in people older than age 50. Their causes aren't known. The course of the disease depends on the type. Some are progressive and ultimately fatal. Others resolve spontaneously or stabilize. Some have a fluctuating course.

Sarcoidosis is the most common form of interstitial lung disease (see page 815). Another form is idiopathic pulmonary fibrosis.

Idiopathic pulmonary fibrosis
This chronic disorder causes progressive shortness of breath. Average duration of life after the onset of symptoms is 3 to 5 years, but many people live much longer. Males and females get the disorder in equal numbers. It commonly develops in the middle years of life, but it can occur at any age.

With idiopathic pulmonary fibrosis, the air sacs become inflamed and eventually damaged and scarred. The sacs behave like stiff balloons — they thicken and won't inflate well. It takes more effort to breathe as scar tissue interferes with oxygen transfer.

A variant of this disorder is desquamative interstitial pneumonia, which has the same symptoms, but the lung tissue, when seen under a microscope, looks different. Lymphoid interstitial pneumonia, another variant, generally affects the lower lobes of the lung. It tends to develop in people with Sjogren's syndrome and sometimes in children and adults with human immunodeficiency virus (HIV) infection.

Certain typical sounds heard through a stethoscope, characteristic patterns seen on a chest X-ray and results of lung function tests can be of help in the diagnosis. However, lung biopsy by a bronchoscope or open surgery also may be required. If the affected person has a history of occupational exposure to asbestos, there is increased risk of lung cancer.

Treatment may include corticosteroids, but they help only a small percentage of individuals. Other medications that may be prescribed include immunosuppressants or the drug colchicine, typically used to treat gout. Some people require lung transplantation for this disorder.

Lung collapse

Signs and symptoms
- Usually, none
- Shortness of breath
- Fever
- Decreased blood pressure and a rapid heartbeat
- Shock
- Pain on the side of the affected lung
- A severe, hacking cough

Atelectasis is the medical term for collapse of portions of a lung or, rarely, an entire lung. The collapse can occur slowly when it's due to a growing tumor, or it may happen suddenly.

The collapse may result from an infection, from an obstruction of bronchial passages in the lungs — commonly by a plug of thick mucus — by accidental inhalation of a foreign object, by outside pressure from a tumor, aneurysm, or enlarged lymph node or from

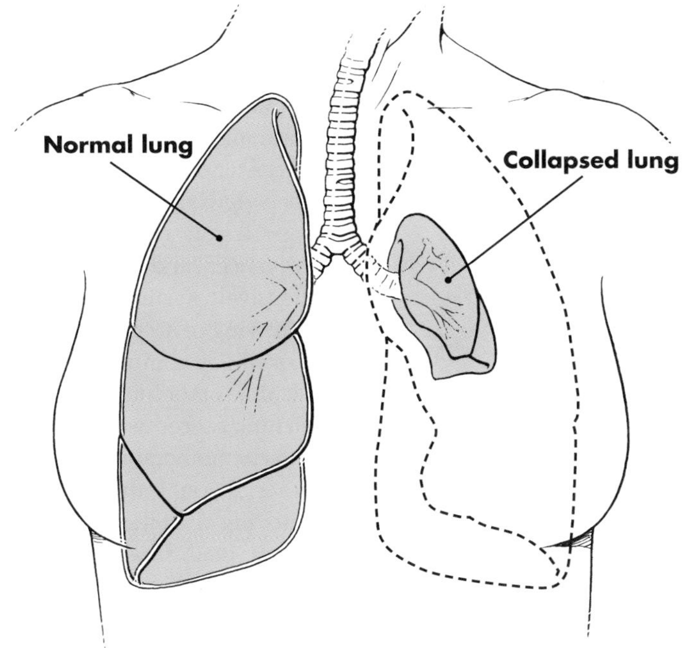

A portion of a lung or, rarely, an entire lung may collapse for a variety of reasons, including an obstruction of lung airways, an infection or a complication of surgery.

pneumothorax. Sometimes, atelectasis occurs as a complication after abdominal or lung surgery, when breathing is shallow and portions of the lung don't expand.

Diagnosis

A chest X-ray will show an airless portion of the lung.

Treatment

If the collapse is due to an obstruction, the first goal is to remove the cause of the obstruction when possible. If coughing, suctioning or other therapeutic measures don't work, a doctor may perform bronchoscopy (see page 819). If your doctor suspects that you have an infection, he or she may prescribe antibiotics.

Prevention

Lung collapse is much less likely to occur following surgery if during recovery you get up and walk around as soon as possible and take frequent deep breaths. You may be given a device to help you draw more air into your lungs rapidly and forcefully.

Pneumothorax

Signs and symptoms

- Difficulty breathing
- Chest pain

Pneumothorax is the presence of air in the pleural space between the lung and chest wall. When the condition occurs spontaneously, it's commonly due to the rupture of a blister containing air (bleb) on the surface of the lung. Spontaneous pneumothorax is most frequent in people younger than age 40.

Air can also enter the pleural space by other means. It can enter the space in the center of the chest between the lungs (mediastinum), especially during an asthma attack, and then rupture into the pleural space, causing pneumothorax. In addition, pneumothorax can result from tests and treatments, such as a lung biopsy or removal of fluid from the pleural space. The procedures may penetrate the pleura lining the lung, causing an air leak.

Diagnosis

If the pneumothorax is small — meaning there's only a small amount of air in the pleural space — you may have no signs or symptoms. When signs or symptoms are present, your doctor may request a chest X-ray or a computerized tomography (CT) scan to confirm the diagnosis and to determine the amount of air present.

Treatment

If your lung is less than 20 percent to 25 percent collapsed due to pneumothorax, your doctor may monitor your condition with a series of chest X-rays until the air is completely absorbed and the lung is re-expanded.

If collapse of the lung exceeds 25 percent or if you're short of breath at rest, your doctor may recommend removing the air by inserting a tube through the chest wall to provide constant suction for several hours or longer. Recurrent pneumothorax may require more aggressive surgical treatment to repair the air leak in the lung.

Lung cancer

Lung cancer is the leading cause of cancer deaths in the United States in both men and women. According to the American Cancer Society, about 89,200 men and 65,700 women die of lung cancer each year, and the incidence is increasing rapidly. The number of women dying of lung cancer is increasing because of increased smoking in this group over the past 30 years. Lung cancer occurs mainly in people between the ages of 45 and 70.

Signs and symptoms

Lung cancer usually doesn't cause any symptoms until the disease is advanced. When symptoms do occur, they may include:

- Coughing that produces sputum that may contain pus and sometimes blood
- Shortness of breath
- Loss of appetite and weight

Normal Lung

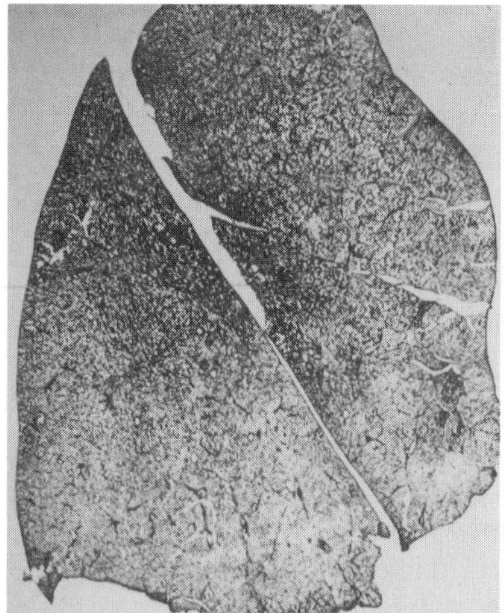

Cancerous Lung

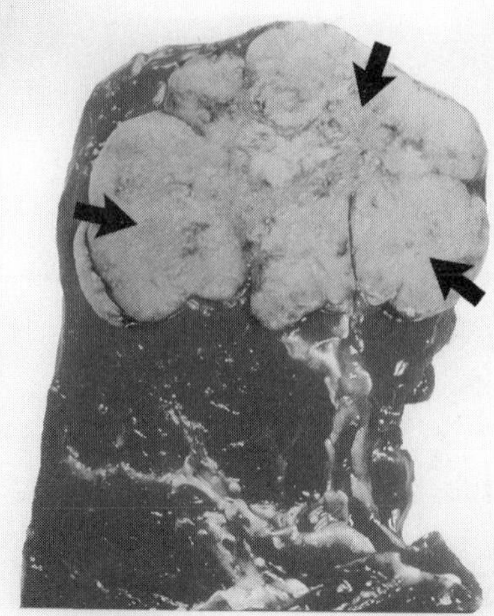

- Chest pain
- Hoarseness
- Fever

Lung cancer is among the most preventable of all cancers. Cigarette smoking causes at least 85 percent to 90 percent of lung cancers. Other risk factors for lung cancer include secondhand smoke, exposure to asbestos and other occupational carcinogens and high concentrations of radon.

Cancer that develops in the lungs (primary lung cancer) is uncommon in nonsmokers. Secondary lung cancer — cancer that spreads (metastasizes) to the lungs from other organs, such as the breast, colon, prostate, testicle, kidney, thyroid or bone — can occur in smokers and nonsmokers.

Types of tumors

Noncancerous (benign) tumors can develop in the lungs. A benign tumor is a mass of abnormal tissue that doesn't spread and can be removed surgically if it's causing symptoms or if the diagnosis is uncertain.

A cancerous (malignant) tumor is an abnormal growth of cells that can invade and destroy nearby tissue and organs and can spread to other parts of the body. The two main types of lung cancer are small cell and non-small cell.

Small cell lung cancer

Small cell lung cancer, also called oat cell carcinoma, develops in the central areas of the lung. Named for the small, round or oval shape of the cancer cells that resemble oats when viewed under the microscope, it's one of the more aggressive cancers and is found almost exclusively in smokers. It can cause narrowing of air passageways (bronchi) by compressing them.

Unlike other lung cancers, small cell lung cancer usually is treated with chemotherapy instead of surgery, because the chance of removing all of the cancer surgically is small. Small cell lung cancer accounts for 20 percent of lung cancers.

Non-small cell lung cancer

Non-small cell lung cancer is the most common type of lung cancer. The three major categories of this type are adenocarcinoma, squamous cell cancer and large cell carcinoma.

- *Adenocarcinoma.* Adenocarcinoma is the most common type of lung cancer in women and people who have never smoked. It usually develops in the mucus-producing cells of the lung. It may spread to the lymph nodes in that area of the lung or through the bloodstream to other organs.

Smoking and Lung Cancer

Approximately 85 percent to 90 percent of the cases of lung cancer can be traced to smoking. People who smoke more than one pack of cigarettes a day have a 20 times greater risk of developing lung cancer than do people who never smoked. A person who smokes two packs of cigarettes or more daily for 20 years has a 60- to 70-fold increase in risk of developing lung cancer compared with a nonsmoker.

Because some cigar and pipe smokers don't inhale smoke directly, many believe that they have a lower risk of developing lung cancer than cigarette smokers do. This is only partly true. Smoking-related diseases are also more common in cigar and pipe smokers than in nonsmokers.

Currently, lung cancer is more common in men than in women. Unfortunately, more women are smoking, so their incidence of lung cancer is increasing rapidly. Lung cancer now surpasses breast cancer as the most common cause of cancer deaths in American women.

The tar in cigarette smoke contains numerous substances that cause cancer (carcinogens) as well as substances that accelerate the production of cancer cells (cocarcinogens). Small cell lung cancer and squamous cell cancer are most strongly associated with cigarette smoking.

Cancer risk decreases when you quit smoking. Ten years after quitting, individuals who smoked more than 20 cigarettes a day can expect their early death rate to decrease by two-thirds. Unfortunately, many people don't quit until they've already developed symptoms of respiratory disease or have lung cancer.

Because adenocarcinoma tends to arise in the periphery of the lung, it's most often detected by chest X-ray or computerized tomography (CT) scan. A subtype of adenocarcinoma, bronchioalveolar carcinoma, accounts for less than 5 percent of cases.

- *Squamous cell cancer.* Squamous cell cancer accounts for 25 percent to 30 percent of cancers that originate in the lung. It's the most common type of lung cancer in men. The majority of squamous cell cancers arise from cells lining the largest air passages of the lungs (central bronchi). Diagnosis can be made through an examination of your sputum or by bronchoscopy.
- *Large cell carcinoma.* Large cell carcinoma appears in the periphery of the lung and spreads through the bloodstream. It accounts for 15 percent to 20 percent of lung cancers.

Diagnosis

Some lung cancers are discovered on a routine chest X-ray or one taken for other disorders. However, chest X-rays aren't an effective screening tool for identifying early-stage lung cancer, and such screening isn't recommended, even in high-risk individuals. A computerized tomography (CT) scan may reveal very small lesions and show whether the cancer has spread to other areas. Magnetic resonance imaging (MRI) and positron emission tomography (PET) also are proving effective in detecting the spread of cancer.

Examination of the sputum for cancer cells may sometimes detect lung cancer before symptoms appear, but this, too, has been disappointing as a screening tool.

In many cases, a cough develops as a growing cancer begins to block an air passageway. Streaks of blood may also appear in sputum. Coughing up large amounts of blood is rare, but when it happens, it indicates that the cancer has invaded a blood vessel.

Persistent chest pain suggests that the tumor has invaded the chest wall. Infection in a lung because of blockage of an airway (obstructive pneumonia) may cause a fever, chest pain and weight loss. If large bronchi are blocked by a tumor, that portion of the lung may partially or fully collapse. Various other symptoms may develop as the cancer spreads to other organs.

Physical signs and symptoms consistent with lung cancer or an abnormal mass on a chest X-ray may be an indication of lung cancer. Your doctor may request a computerized tomography (CT) scan to look for small lesions on the lungs and determine if the cancer has spread to other sites. In a procedure called bronchoscopy, your doctor can view air passages in the lungs and obtain a specimen of tissue for microscopic examination (biopsy) to determine if cancer is present and, if so, what type.

Other methods of obtaining a tissue sample include mediastinoscopy, thoracentesis and video thoracoscopy.

Mediastinoscopy

While you're under anesthesia, an instrument is passed through a small incision at the base of your neck, allowing doctors to take a biopsy of lymph nodes in your chest. This enables a surgeon to define the extent of the tumor and

Bronchoscopy

Bronchoscopy is a procedure in which a specially designed tube is passed down your airway to allow your doctor to see the inside of your air passages. Bronchoscopy enables your doctor to look for tumors, foreign objects, areas of internal bleeding and abnormalities of your lungs and air passageways. A bronchoscope also has an open channel through which a doctor can remove secretions and obtain biopsy specimens.

There are two types of bronchoscopes: the fiber-optic bronchoscope, which is flexible and 3 to 7 millimeters in diameter, and the rigid bronchoscope, which is larger and more difficult to use. The flexible fiber-optic bronchoscope is used more often. It contains glass fibers that transmit light and return a magnified picture of the passageways of your lungs. Your doctor watches the progress of the bronchoscope through an eye piece or on a small television-like monitor.

You shouldn't eat for at least 6 to 12 hours before you undergo bronchoscopy. Just before the procedure, you may be given a local anesthesia, or general anesthesia may be used. The anesthetic agent, which depresses your cough and swallowing reflexes, is usually administered through your nostrils or mouth. Your doctor may also give you a sedative to help you relax.

During the procedure, you'll either be sitting or lying down. The bronchoscope is inserted through your mouth or nose. Lidocaine jelly serves as an oral anesthetic and a lubricant to protect your air passages.

Flexible bronchoscopy usually is painless and seldom causes complications. After the procedure, you shouldn't eat or drink anything for about an hour, until your swallowing and coughing reflexes return to normal.

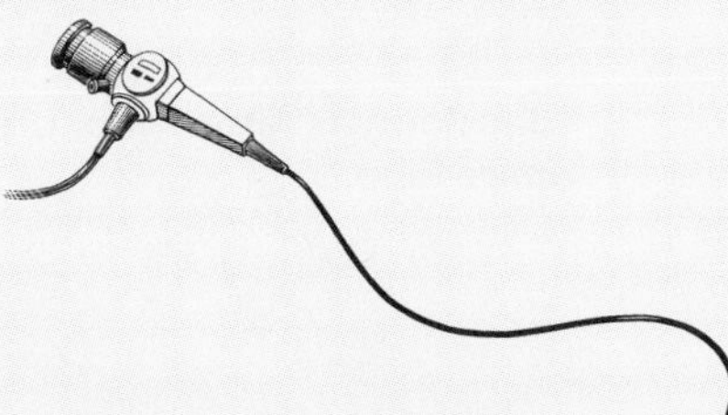

During a procedure called bronchoscopy, your doctor can see the inside of your airways by passing a flexible tube (bronchoscope) into them.

determine whether it's reasonable to attempt surgery.

Thoracentesis

If fluid is present in your chest cavity, your doctor can remove a sample by inserting a thin needle into your chest between the ribs. This fluid can then be examined in the laboratory for presence of cancer cells.

Video thoracoscopy

In this procedure, your doctor inserts a tube (endoscope) through a small incision to collapse one of your lungs. This creates a space through which a pen-sized instrument with a video device may enter your chest wall. Your doctor then can remove fluid and perform biopsies of nodules or masses while watching the procedure on a video screen.

Prognosis

Lung cancer is a very serious disease that often has a poor prognosis. Overall, only about 14 percent of people with the disease survive for 5 years. However, the outcome depends on a number of factors, including the extent of the disease when discovered, your general health and age, the type of cancer, how rapidly it grows and the therapy used.

Only about 10 percent to 15 percent of lung cancers are detected before the cancer has spread. Seventy-five percent of the people with lung cancer indentified at this stage live 5 or more years after diagnosis and treatment.

Once signs or symptoms of lung cancer appear, the disease may be advanced and not treatable by surgery. In fact, only 20 percent to 25 percent of all lung cancers can be removed surgically at the time of initial diagnosis.

Of those for whom surgery is an option, approximately one-third of people with squamous cell cancer and one-fourth of those with adenocarcinoma or large cell carcinoma survive 5 years.

Lung Cancer Surgery

Surgical removal (resection) of a cancerous tumor commonly is used for people who have lung cancer that hasn't spread to other parts of the body. Depending on the extent of the cancer, people with squamous cell cancer, large cell carcinoma or adenocarcinoma are candidates for surgical treatment. Surgery is seldom performed for small cell lung cancer because it spreads too rapidly and too extensively to be removed completely with surgery.

The procedure

The surgeon removes the tumor and the tissue that's immediately surrounding it. The most common surgery is lobectomy, in which the involved lobe is removed. Other types of lung surgery include a wedge resection, in which a small portion of a lobe is removed, a segment resection, which involves removal of a larger portion of a lobe, and pneumonectomy, removal of the entire lung. Usually, the surgeon also removes those lymph nodes that drain the involved lung.

The hospital stay following the surgery usually lasts 5 to 7 days, although it'll take longer for you to recover completely. Many people are able to resume their normal activities in 4 to 6 weeks. However, the rate and degree of recovery depend on the general condition of your lungs, the amount of lung tissue removed and your overall health.

The outlook

Of individuals whose cancer is detected early, approximately 80 percent survive 1 year, and 75 percent are alive at 5 years after the operation. After surgery, it's important to have regular medical checkups to detect possible recurrence of the cancer, either within the lung or in other parts of your body. If the cancer recurs, chemotherapy or radiation therapy may decrease the size of the tumor, prolong life and relieve pain and other symptoms.

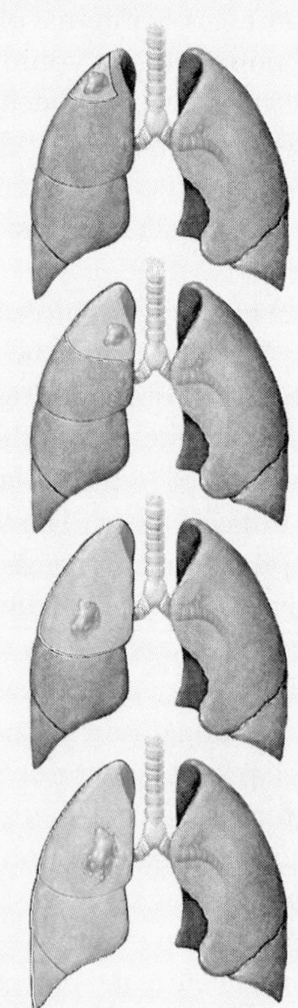

Wedge resection is removal of a small portion of a lobe.

Segment resection is removal of a larger portion of a lobe.

Lobectomy is removal of an entire lobe.

Pneumonectomy is removal of an entire lung.

Small cell lung cancer is extremely serious because of its tendency to spread before signs or symptoms are apparent. The 5-year survival rate following diagnosis is approximately 5 percent.

Treatment

Basically, the treatment options for lung cancer are surgical removal of the tumor and surrounding tissue, chemotherapy, radiation therapy or some combination of these. Laser surgery may be used to improve breathing when tumors obstruct central air passageways and removal of the cancer isn't possible.

Surgery

Surgery generally involves removal of the entire portion or lobe of the lung in which the cancer is located. However, because lung cancer commonly occurs in people who have smoked heavily for many years, the other lung may be severely damaged by emphysema and not healthy enough to meet the person's oxygen needs. Breathing tests before the operation may help determine the function of the noncancerous lung.

Chemotherapy

Chemotherapy involves a regimen of anticancer drugs taken by mouth or intravenously. The drugs are designed to reach tissues throughout the entire body in an effort to destroy any cancer that may have spread beyond the lung.

Some newer chemotherapy agents cause fewer complications than did anticancer drugs of the past. Medications to combat the nausea that usually accompanies chemotherapy also have markedly improved compared with treatments available even a decade ago. Chemotherapy usually is the preferred treatment for people with small cell lung cancer.

Radiation

With this treatment method, a beam of high-energy radiation is aimed at the tumor to destroy cancer cells. Radiation therapy may also be used to relieve lung cancer signs and symptoms, including pain, bleeding and difficulty swallowing.

Advances in targeting the radiation to the cancerous tissue have reduced complications associated with its use. However, radiation may cause inflammation of the lung, scarring and decreased lung function.

Occupation-Related Lung Disease

Over time, hazardous materials in the workplace that are inhaled on a regular or significant basis can cause lung disease. Perhaps the best known of these diseases are asbestosis, coal miner's disease and silicosis. In addition, various industrial and agricultural dusts and some fungi cause lung diseases, which are usually named after the occupation in which they're most likely to occur or the type of dust inhaled.

Asbestosis

Signs and symptoms

- Shortness of breath
- Decreased exercise tolerance
- Coughing
- Chest pain

Asbestos was used extensively as insulation in building construction for many years until 1975, when it was replaced by other materials, such as fiberglass and slag wool. There are four types of asbestos fibers that can cause respiratory disease if large amounts of fine asbestos fibers accumulate in your lungs.

More than 9 million workers are estimated to be at risk of asbestosis. People exposed to asbestos include workers in mining, milling, manufacturing of asbestos and its products and those who installed asbestos products. People who installed asbestos products include pipe fitters, boilermakers, shipbuilders and construction workers.

Asbestos was once sprayed on steel girders of buildings to prevent

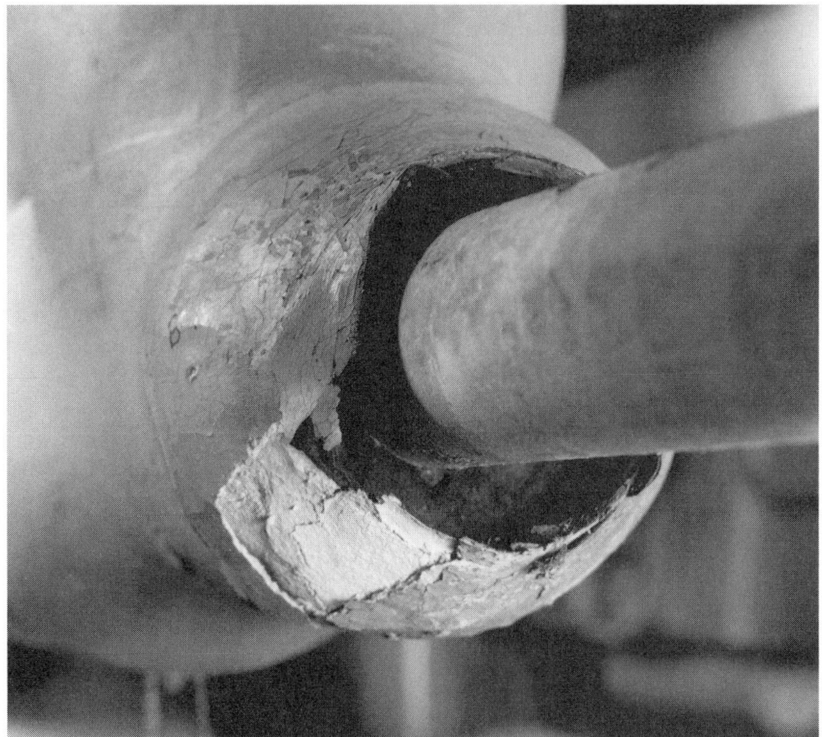

Asbestos used in this pipe covering can be hazardous to your health. Removal requires care and expertise.

Mesothelioma

In addition to impairing lung function, asbestosis can increase your risk of a rare cancer of the lining of the lung called mesothelioma.

Mesothelioma may develop 20 to 40 years after exposure to asbestos fibers and can occur even if you were exposed only for 1 or 2 years or less. Some people with mesothelioma have no history of exposure to asbestos.

Signs and symptoms include significant chest pain, shortness of breath and weight loss. In about half of those with mesothelioma, the disease spreads, producing tumors in other parts of the body. In other cases, the tumors are limited to the chest. Accumulation of fluid between the two layers of the pleural membrane (pleural effusion) often contributes to shortness of breath and chest pain.

The chance of recovery depends on the size and location of the cancer, whether and how far it has spread and how it responds to treatment. Mesothelioma is usually treated with surgery to remove the cancer, radiation therapy, chemotherapy or some combination of these therapies.

them from buckling in a fire. It also was used in fire-smothering blankets and safety clothing, as filler for plastic materials, in brake and clutch linings and in cement and some floor tiles.

The problem with asbestos is that its particles flake off. When disturbed during routine maintenance work, the tiny fibers easily release from the surface. These loose fibers may stay airborne for some time. The vast majority of the people who work in or go into buildings containing friable asbestos have a very small risk of contracting respiratory illness from the fibers, but the safe level of asbestos exposure is uncertain.

You don't need to handle the material yourself to be exposed to the fibers. Electricians, painters and others who worked next to the person handling asbestos are at risk, as are people who handle and wash the clothes of someone who works with or near it.

Various federal, state and local government regulations now require asbestos control or removal, particularly in schools. Many insurance companies won't cover buildings that contain asbestos.

Asbestosis generally results when asbestos fibers accumulate around small air passageways in the lungs (bronchioles). Your lungs react to the fibers by forming small masses of scar tissue (fibrosis). Symptoms appear when the scar tissue causes your lungs to lose their elasticity. The first symptom of asbestosis may be the gradual onset of shortness of breath on exertion.

On a chest X-ray, the scar tissue may appear as small, scattered, opaque areas. These areas are generally first evident in the lower parts of the lung, but gradually spread upward as the disease progresses. Eventually, your entire lung may be affected, giving it a honeycomb appearance on an X-ray.

The severity of the disease is directly related to the amount and duration of exposure. Usually, you must have at least 10 years of moderate to severe exposure before symptoms of asbestosis appear.

Another result of prolonged exposure to asbestos may be the development of pleural plaques around your lungs. These areas of thickening of the membrane that surrounds your lungs (pleura) usually occur along the lower part of the chest wall or near the diaphragm. The presence of pleural plaques is strong evidence that you've been exposed to asbestos, but it doesn't mean that your lungs are impaired, unless you have other signs and symptoms.

Diagnosis

Provide your doctor with a detailed history of your work activities and any other sources of possible exposure to toxic dusts. Tell your doctor about the availability and use of dust masks and other respiratory protection devices in your workplace.

An abnormal chest X-ray may suggest that you have been exposed to asbestos, but it doesn't necessarily mean you have asbestosis. Physical findings and symptoms of debilitating pulmonary fibrosis, including the abnormal development of scar tissue, are also necessary in making a diagnosis.

Treatment

Treatment is usually for easing symptoms. Oxygen therapy or draining fluid from around the lungs may improve your breathing. Occasionally, lung transplantation may be used to treat asbestosis.

Black lung and silicosis

Signs and symptoms

- Shortness of breath
- Coughing that produces sputum

Black lung (coal workers' pneumoconiosis) and silicosis result from inhaling industrial particles that become permanently lodged in the lungs. Black lung is caused by inhaling coal dust for prolonged periods, usually for at least 10 years. The disease is much more common in miners of anthracite coal — which, in the United States, is mined primarily in the East — than in miners of bituminous coal, which is mined primarily in the West.

Silicosis is caused by the inhalation of free silica (crystalline quartz). Free silica exposure occurs in occupations such as mining, stonecutting, quarrying (especially of granite), sandblasting, rock blasting, road building and industries that manufacture abrasives. It usually takes 15 to 20 years of exposure before symptoms develop.

Unprotected workers in occupations with intense exposure to silica — such as sandblasting in confined spaces, tunneling through rock with a high quartz content or manufacturing of abrasive soaps — may develop silicosis in less than a year.

Diagnosis

In most cases, both black lung and silicosis cause no respiratory symptoms, unless you smoke cigarettes. The diseases are generally diagnosed when small, irregular, opaque areas are seen on a chest X-ray, and they can be attributed to a history of exposure to coal dust or silica. With long-term exposure, the irregular areas become larger and combine into rounded nodules.

Both black lung and silicosis may develop into significant scarring of lung tissue, called progressive massive fibrosis. Only a small percentage of individuals with black lung develop massive fibrosis, but individuals with silicosis are likely to develop it. The mechanism that causes it is unknown.

Fibrosis is diagnosed when an opaque area with a diameter larger than ½ inch is seen over smaller opaque areas on a chest X-ray. The opaque areas may combine and cover an entire lobe of the lung. At this stage, the disease causes shortness of breath and a cough that produces mucus. Symptoms often are more severe than the chest X-ray appearance might suggest.

How serious are black lung and silicosis?

In their early stages, black lung and silicosis don't cause respiratory impairment, which usually occurs with development of massive fibrosis. Despite avoidance of further exposure, massive fibrosis can cause death. Survival time may be less than 2 years. In addition, people with silicosis have a three times greater-than-average risk of tuberculosis.

Treatment

There's no specific treatment for either of these diseases, although lung transplantation may be an option in some cases.

If you have either condition, avoid additional exposure to the causative dust. If you smoke, stop. In addition, limit exposure to respiratory irritants such as irritating fumes or cold, dry or extremely humid air. If you have silicosis and your tuberculin skin test is positive, you'll need treatment for tuberculosis, even if you have no symptoms.

Occupational asthma

Signs and symptoms

- Shortness of breath
- Coughing
- Tightness in the chest
- Wheezing

Emergency signs and symptoms

- Extreme difficulty breathing
- Bluish lips and nails
- Severe shortness of breath
- Increased pulse rate
- Sweating
- Severe coughing

In 2 percent to 5 percent of people with asthma, the cause is related to their occupation or environment.

Some agents known to cause asthma are paints, wood dust, grain dust, pollens, synthetic dyes, gum arabic and rosin (soldering flux). Inhalation of one of these agents doesn't mean you'll develop asthma, but in some individuals they can trigger the disease.

Industrial Bronchitis

Bronchitis that occurs in coal miners and workers exposed to cotton, flax or hemp dust is called industrial bronchitis. Fumes from ammonia, strong acids, certain organic solvents, chlorine, hydrogen sulfide, sulfur dioxide and bromine also may cause bronchitis.

Common signs and symptoms include shortness of breath and a chronic cough that produces sputum.

It's not clear whether exposure to the dusts causes bronchitis in these workers or whether the exposure aggravates bronchitis from other causes, such as smoking. The disease generally clears up with rest, drinking plenty of liquids and eliminating exposure to the irritant that caused it. Sometimes, use of a humidifier or vaporizer is helpful.

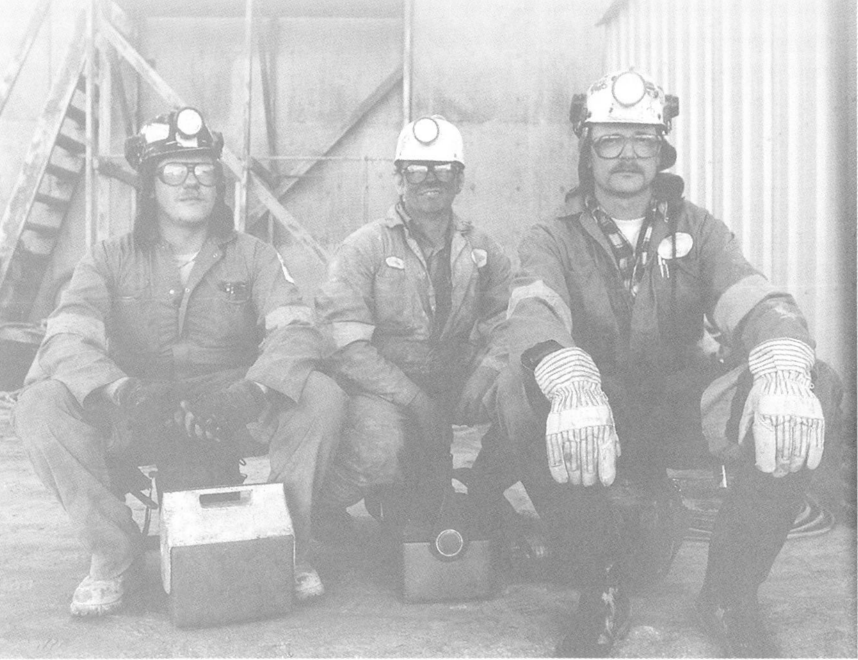

Diagnosis

The signs and symptoms of occupational asthma are the same as those of nonoccupational asthma. A diagnosis is based primarily on your medical history and the results of pulmonary function tests. Testing may include a bronchial provocation test, in which you're exposed to the suspected allergen or irritating substance in a laboratory so that your airway reaction to it can be measured.

Treatment

Treatment generally consists of bronchodilators and anti-inflammatory medications, such as corticosteroids, to help keep your airways open. Avoiding the substance that causes your asthma is also important. You may have symptoms of asthma for years after you stop coming into contact with the offending agent. For more information on asthma, see Chapter 21, "Allergies and Asthma."

Allergic alveolitis

Signs and symptoms

- Persistent coughing that produces large amounts of sputum
- Wheezing
- Shortness of breath
- Decreased pulmonary function

Causes

This disease is caused by exposure to organic dusts. It goes by many names, usually relating to the occupation in which it's acquired:

- Farmer's lung, caused by exposure to dust from moldy hay
- Byssinosis, caused by dust from cotton or, to a lesser extent, flax, jute or hemp yarn or rope
- Humidifier lung, caused by dust or moisture from humidifiers, heating systems and air conditioners contaminated by a fungus
- Bagassosis, caused by fungi in moldy sugar cane fiber (bagasse)
- Suberosis, caused by inhaling cork dust
- Sequoiosis, caused by redwood sawdust
- Maple bark stripper's disease, caused by dust from rotting maple tree logs and bark
- Mushroom worker's lung, caused by dust from moldy compost
- Detergent worker's lung, caused by dust from enzyme additives

PREVENTION TIP

Prevention is the best course of action. If you work in an occupation that puts you at risk of developing a work-related lung disease, always wear a dust mask and take other steps to prevent exposure to dust.

Diagnosis

All of these dusts cause the same symptoms in individuals who are sensitive to them. Pulmonary function tests can help the doctor in making the diagnosis.

How serious is allergic alveolitis?

People who smoke are more susceptible to all of these conditions and have more serious complications than do nonsmokers with the same disease.

Treatment

Avoiding the irritating dust usually relieves the symptoms. Drink plenty of liquids. Use a humidifier to reduce dust indoors. Clean the humidifier regularly to keep it free of mold and bacteria. If necessary, your doctor may prescribe medications, such as a bronchodilator or possibly a corticosteroid medication.

Byssinosis

Signs and symptoms

- Tightness in the chest

Byssinosis is an asthma-like disease that's sometimes found in workers who produce cotton or, to a lesser extent, flax, jute or hemp yarn or rope. Also known as brown lung and Monday fever — a misnomer because it doesn't cause a fever — byssinosis results from inhaling dust from the raw plant bales. Those who work with cotton and other fibers during the cleaning processes — blowing, mixing and carding (straightening) — that precede spinning are at greatest risk.

Diagnosis

The disease may develop right after first exposure or after years of working in the industry. You may feel tightness in your chest toward the end of the day on Monday, the first day after the weekend, assuming you had the weekend off.

At first, the symptoms don't appear during the rest of the week, but in 10 percent to 25 percent of those affected, the chest tightness eventually persists for several days, then throughout the week and into the weekend and vacation periods.

How serious is byssinosis?

Byssinosis generally isn't serious. But if the disease persists or gets worse, it can lead to chronic illness such as emphysema or chronic bronchitis. To avoid damage to your lungs, stop working in that industry. When you stop being exposed to the fibers, the illness resolves.

Treatment

Bronchodilators and antihistamines help control the symptoms.

Farmer's lung

Signs and symptoms

- Fever
- Chills
- Coughing that produces sputum
- Worsening shortness of breath on exertion
- Fatigue
- Nausea and vomiting
- Loss of appetite and weight

Farmer's lung is a type of lung disease caused by repeated inhalation of dust from moldy hay that

Fumes, Gases, Smoke and Air Pollution

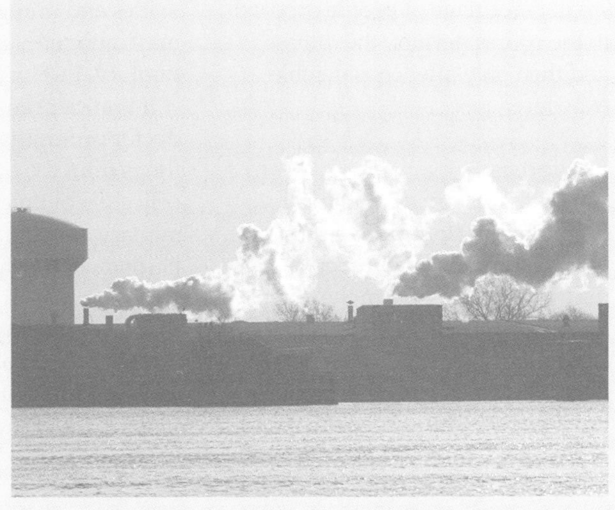

Exposure to high concentrations of toxic fumes and gases, indoor and outdoor air pollutants, and smoke can cause various respiratory symptoms.

Industrial fumes and gases

Long-term, low-level exposure or accidental exposure to high levels of industrial toxic chemicals can cause various temporary (acute) and, sometimes, long-lasting (chronic) respiratory problems. Usually, the lower respiratory tract is affected, causing symptoms such as shortness of breath and coughing and possibly leading to chronic bronchitis. A sampling of toxic chemicals includes ammonia, cyanides, formaldehyde, hydrogen sulfide, diazomethane, halides, nitrogen dioxide, isocyanates, ozone, phosgene, phthalic anhydride and sulfur dioxide.

The industrial process of heating certain metals, such as cadmium, chromium, nickel and beryllium, to high temperatures and quickly cooling them releases fumes that can cause various respiratory diseases if inhaled. Signs and symptoms usually appear several hours after exposure and clear up within 24 hours, only to return with repeat exposure.

If you work in an industrial trade that uses high heat, such as welding, brazing, smelting, pottery making and furnace work, you may be at risk. Using nonhazardous compounds, ensuring adequate ventilation and using safe machinery and work practices can help prevent exposure to toxic fumes.

Workers exposed to these fumes and gases and who also smoke have a greatly increased risk of developing lung cancer.

Outdoor air pollutants

Air pollution, such as that caused by automobiles, power plants and factories, can increase levels of ozone and sulfur dioxide in the air. Exposure to this pollution can cause wheezing in people who have asthma and may cause shortness of breath in older adults, young children and people with chronic cardiopulmonary disease. On days when the ozone level is high, usually after a long stretch of hot, humid weather, it may be best for individuals at risk to stay indoors.

Indoor air pollutants

Energy efficiency concerns have led to the construction of houses that are more tightly sealed than older houses were, and many codes now require outside air intake into heating and air-conditioning systems. Therefore, fumes that once were of little concern may build up in the house instead of escaping to the outside. One example is cigarette smoke, which, besides having major health effects on the smoker, also affects nonsmokers who are exposed to it. Secondhand (passive) cigarette smoke has been shown to increase respiratory infections and decrease lung function in children whose parents smoke.

For people with asthma, poorly ventilated areas, wood smoke from wood-burning furnaces and fumes from kerosene floor heaters can aggravate symptoms.

Another potentially hazardous agent is formaldehyde. It's present in urethane foam insulation and in some types of flooring used in construction of new houses, mobile homes and furniture. New products made with formaldehyde may have a pungent odor due to formaldehyde fumes, which may irritate the eyes, nose, throat and airways. The formaldehyde gradually evaporates within a few months, after which it should cause no problem. But before it evaporates, it may worsen symptoms for people with respiratory disease.

Smoke

Whenever anything containing carbon burns, it produces carbon monoxide that, when inhaled, interferes with transportation of oxygen by the blood. All smoke contains some of this odorless gas. Be careful, therefore, when you have any fire indoors, such as from a wood-burning stove or fireplace. The effects of inhaling carbon monoxide are so subtle as to be unnoticeable, and you can become unconscious without realizing anything is wrong. Smoke that contains a heavy concentration of floating particles also irritates the lungs.

Many plastics, polyurethanes and other synthetic materials used in home furnishings give off toxic gases when they burn. They're particularly harmful to the lungs and may cause severe, temporary illness. Firefighters and others who have long-term exposure to smoke may have an increased risk of chronic illness, although this is difficult to measure.

contains spores of a fungus. Only a small percentage of people exposed to the spores develop the disease, and then only after considerable exposure.

Diagnosis

A medical history and physical examination, along with a chest X-ray and pulmonary function tests may be used to confirm the diagnosis. The results of blood tests for antibodies associated with the disease can strongly suggest farmer's lung, but the results aren't diagnostic.

How serious is farmer's lung?

In temporary (acute) cases, avoiding exposure to moldy hay usually reduces the severity of symptoms within hours, although it may take weeks for a complete recovery. The disease can also be long-lasting (chronic), particularly if you're continually exposed to low levels of the fungus over long periods.

Treatment

Avoiding exposure to the dust from moldy hay is the only sure way to prevent progression to chronic lung disease. If you can't avoid contact with moldy hay, your doctor may recommend a special type of protective dust mask. If you have a severe case of the disease, your doctor may prescribe a corticosteroid medication.

Silo filler's lung

Signs and symptoms

- An irritated, runny nose
- Coughing
- Shortness of breath

Silo filler's lung is an acute illness that results from inhalation of nitrous oxide fumes given off by moist silage. When inhaled, the gas irritates the bronchi and lungs.

How serious is silo filler's lung?

The severity of the illness depends on the length of exposure. A farmer can die after spending an extended period of time in a silo filled with the yellowish gas and acrid odor of oxides and nitrogen. Less exposure may cause only irritation of the respiratory tract.

If you've been exposed, see your doctor promptly. Irritation to the lungs from the fumes can lead to a collection of fluid in the lungs (pulmonary edema), which can result in permanent lung damage or be fatal. Exposure may also cause inflammation of the tiny airways near the alveoli (bronchiolitis), which can cause permanent damage to your lungs if you don't seek prompt treatment.

Treatment

A doctor may prescribe a corticosteroid medication to prevent permanent damage to the lungs.

Your Lungs and Cardiovascular System

The workings of your heart and lungs are interrelated. Blood travels from your heart through your lungs to be oxygenated.

If a blood clot forms in your veins and travels through your bloodstream, the clot may eventually become lodged in an artery in your lungs (pulmonary embolism). Chronic lung disease also can lead to heart failure of the right ventrical (cor pulmonale).

Pulmonary embolism

Signs and symptoms

- Sudden shortness of breath
- Anxiety
- Coughing that produces bloody or blood-streaked sputum
- Excessive perspiration
- Rapid heartbeat

Emergency signs and symptoms

- Sudden loss of consciousness

The term *embolism* refers to blockage in an artery caused by an embolus. Usually, an embolus is a clot of blood, but sometimes it may be a globule of fat, an air bubble, tissue from a tumor or a clump of bacteria. This clot is carried into a blood vessel in the lungs, where it becomes lodged and interrupts blood flow.

Most emboli originate from blood clots (thrombi) in the veins of the lower extremities or pelvis. The veins carry them up through the right side of the heart to a lung. Emboli may also arise from the walls of the heart. If a clot arises in the left side of the heart, then the embolus will go to the brain or some other part of the body, rather than to the lung. Tissue death (infarction) occurs when the clot blocks blood supply to tissues.

An embolism can occur in any small artery, but the lungs are particularly vulnerable because all of the blood in your body passes through them every time it circulates.

Signs and symptoms resulting from the blockage depend on the size of the embolus and the health of your cardiopulmonary system.

Diagnosis

A pulmonary embolism can be difficult to diagnose, especially in people with underlying lung or heart disease. Your doctor may order a chest X-ray, a specialized computerized tomography (CT) scan of the chest, a lung scan or pulmonary angiogram to detect the clot.

A lung scan called a ventilation-perfusion scan uses small amounts of radioactive tracers (radioisotopes) to study air flow and blood flow in your lungs. The radioisotopes are attached to substances known as radiopharmaceuticals so that a special device (gamma camera) can show images of the movement of air in your lungs and the movement of blood in the lungs' blood vessels.

This scan can be useful in diagnosing pulmonary embolism. However, the findings of about half of all such lung scans are indeterminate.

Pulmonary angiography is the most accurate test for detecting emboli in the lung. During a pulmonary angiogram, a dye is injected into a vein of an arm or leg. As it circulates into the arteries of the lung, the arteries are highlighted so that they show up better on an X-ray and clots, if present, can be seen. Your doctor may recommend other tests as well.

How serious is a pulmonary embolism?

A pulmonary embolism causes death within an hour in about 10 percent of those who develop one. If you survive and have appropriate diagnosis and treatment, the outlook is good. You should return to normal health within a few weeks unless you have another serious disease.

Each year, the condition affects as many as 500,000 people in the United States and causes as many as 50,000 deaths. Once you've had a pulmonary embolism, you're at increased risk of another, which has up to a 50 percent chance of being fatal.

Surgery, prolonged bed rest or inactivity, stroke, heart attack, obesity and a hip or leg fracture increase your risk of pulmonary embolism. In addition, any increase in the tendency of your blood to clot makes you more susceptible.

Treatment

Treatment most often involves medication.

Medication

Your doctor may prescribe anticoagulant therapy to prevent further blood clots from forming or to keep an existing clot from enlarging. Intravenous (IV) heparin may be prescribed initially, often in conjunction with oral warfarin (Coumadin).

If you experience a massive pulmonary embolism or recurring emboli, have pre-existing cardiopulmonary disease or if other treatments aren't effective, clot-dissolving (thrombolytic) therapy may be an option.

Rather than simply preventing clot formation, medications such as streptokinase (Streptase), urokinase (Abbokinase) and the tissue plasminogen activator alteplase (Activase) dissolve clots.

All of these medications have side effects and require close monitoring by a doctor.

Surgery

Surgery is rarely necessary, but a vein filter may help people with recurring emboli that have become fibrous and obstruct the lung vessels.

To prevent clots from being carried into the pulmonary artery, a doctor may surgically place a filter in the main vein (inferior vena cava) in the abdomen leading from your legs and pelvis to the right side of your heart.

Prevention

After any type of surgery, you'll be encouraged to get up and move around as soon as possible or to perform active and passive leg exercises to help prevent formation of a blood clot.

When sitting for long periods, such as on an airplane or in a car, make sure to walk periodically or at least wiggle your toes and move your feet. If you're immobilized, elevate your legs and perhaps wear support stockings. All of these can help prevent pooling and clotting of blood in your leg veins, a frequent cause of emboli.

Lung and Heart Transplantation

Lung transplants were first performed in the early 1960s, but later discontinued because of poor results. The introduction in the late 1970s of a new immunosuppressant drug called cyclosporine (Neoral, Sandimmune) revived the possibility of performing lung transplants successfully. But animal studies found that the supply of blood to the new lungs was insufficient and that the transplanted lungs didn't heal adequately.

In the 1980s, researchers found a solution. They discovered that transplanting the lungs with the heart helps ensure that the new lungs receive enough blood. In 1981, the first successful heart-lung transplantation was performed.

This procedure has many problems and limitations. Finding donor lungs and hearts is very difficult because the lungs of brain-dead accident victims often are damaged. To be usable, lungs also must match the recipient's body size, blood type and tissue type.

However, progress is being made. Using new immunosuppressant drugs and new procedures, many double-lung and single-lung transplantations have been performed successfully without transplanting the heart as well. This opens up the possibility that a donated heart and both lungs can help save the lives of up to three people instead of only one. If a lung transplant recipient's heart is healthy, the donor heart often can be used for someone else.

Lung transplantation may be considered for people with idiopathic pulmonary fibrosis, a chronic scarring of the lungs for which there's no known cause. The quality of life and life span of a person with pulmonary fibrosis can be increased with a lung transplant. Sometimes, a lung transplant may be considered for individuals with emphysema. The decision to undertake the risks of lung transplantation in people with emphysema is based on possible improvement in quality of life.

A lung transplant is a risky and complicated procedure. Most recipients of successful lung transplants recover to carry on relatively normal lives in the short term. The long-term outcome isn't yet known.

If you're at risk of a recurrent pulmonary embolism, heparin, warfarin or an antiplatelet drug such as aspirin may be prescribed.

Cor pulmonale

Signs and symptoms

- Swelling of the lower extremities
- Shortness of breath during exertion
- Bulging of the veins in the neck
- An enlarged and tender liver
- Weakness and fatigue

Cor pulmonale is enlargement and eventual failure of the lower right chamber of the heart (right ventricle) due to pulmonary disease. Because the heart and lungs are closely associated in function, diseases of the lungs often affect the heart as well.

Blood goes from the right side of the heart into the lungs, where carbon dioxide is removed and oxygen added to it. Normally, it doesn't take a great deal of pressure to move blood into the lungs, so the muscular walls of the right ventricle aren't as strong as those on the left side, which pumps blood under high pressure to the rest of the body. However, when emphysema, fibrosis or other severe chronic lung disease impairs your lungs, it requires more pressure to pump blood into them. Although the heart may compensate for a while, eventually it fails.

Diagnosis

Tests used to help diagnose cor pulmonale may include a pulmonary function test, chest X-ray, electrocardiogram and echocardiogram.

How serious is cor pulmonale?

Once symptoms of cor pulmonale appear, survival on average is 2 to 5 years. If the underlying cause is uncomplicated emphysema, survival may be considerably longer.

Treatment

An important step is to treat the underlying disease causing cor pulmonale, when possible. In addition, your doctor may advise the use of oxygen and restriction of salt and fluids. He or she might prescribe diuretic medications to control fluid accumulation in tissues. ■

CHAPTER 28 PART V

Breast Conditions

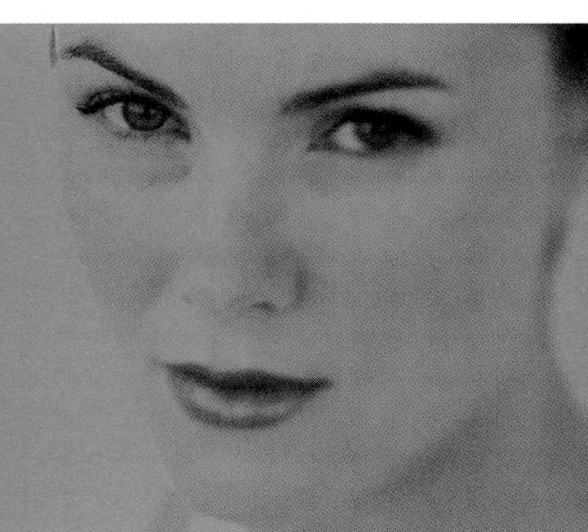

The structure of the human female breast is remarkable and complex. For the most part, a woman's breasts consist of fat and connective tissue. This tissue houses a network of blood vessels and milk-producing glands called lobules.

During lactation, these glands secrete milk into a system of ducts — milk passages that connect the lobules to the nipples. The breasts are attached to the muscles of the chest wall (pectoral muscles) by connective tissue.

Nipples may be flat, but they contain tissue that becomes erect (protrudes) with certain types of stimulation, such as when they're cold, during sexual arousal or when something brushes against them. Some women's nipples are always erect, and other women's are turned inward (inverted). Having any of the three types of nipples is perfectly normal.

Encircling the nipple is the areola, a ring of tissue colored the same as the nipple. Oil glands in the areola lubricate the nipple during breast-feeding. In some women, these glands are visible as small bumps. Many women have hairs growing at the edges of the areola. Taking birth control pills may increase hair growth in that area.

Some women are self-conscious about their breasts. They think that their breasts are either too small or too large, or they're concerned because one is larger than the other.

Actually, breast size makes no difference either in a woman's sexual responsiveness or in her ability to nurse a baby. Women who have small breasts are as responsive as women with large breasts, and they can nurse an infant just as successfully. Furthermore, it's normal for a pair of breasts to differ somewhat from each other in size and shape. Usually, the right breast is smaller than the left.

Normal Breast Changes

To understand the diseases and conditions that can affect breasts, it's helpful for you to know how a normal breast functions. Hormones play a major role both in breast development and in the changes breasts undergo at different stages of life.

From puberty until after menopause, a woman's breasts change as her hormones fluctuate. At puberty, when a girl's body first produces estrogen in quantity, her breasts rapidly develop both a framework of connective tissue (stroma) and a system of glands, ducts, blood vessels, lymph channels and nerves. At the same time, breasts develop fat cells, which make up the bulk of breast tissue.

The lymph system is made up of lymph, lymphatic vessels and lymph nodes. Lymph is a clear fluid that contains tissue waste products and immune system cells. Lymphatic vessels are similar to very small veins but carry lymph instead of blood. Most of the lymphatic vessels of the breast drain into underarm (axillary) lymph nodes, which are collections of immune system cells.

After puberty, a woman's breasts change each month. During the first half of the menstrual cycle, her ovaries release estrogen, which causes new cells to grow in glands, ducts and other breast tissue. Blood flow to the breasts also increases.

During the second half of the cycle, after ovulation, glands in the breasts are stimulated by progesterone as well as estrogen, and they begin to secrete substances that are the precursors of breast milk. Unless the woman becomes pregnant, these hormone levels decrease, her body absorbs both the secretions

The Breast

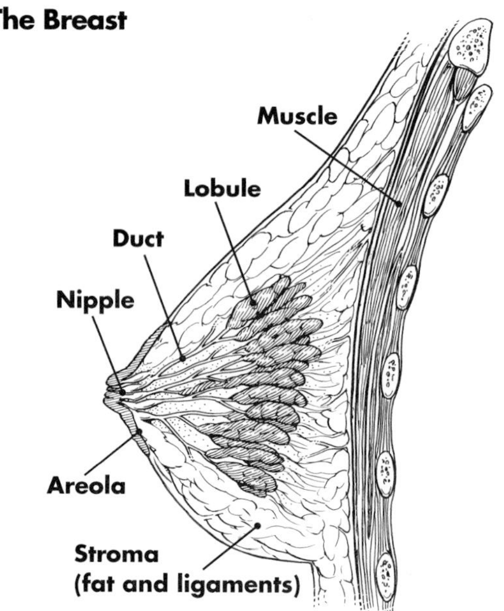

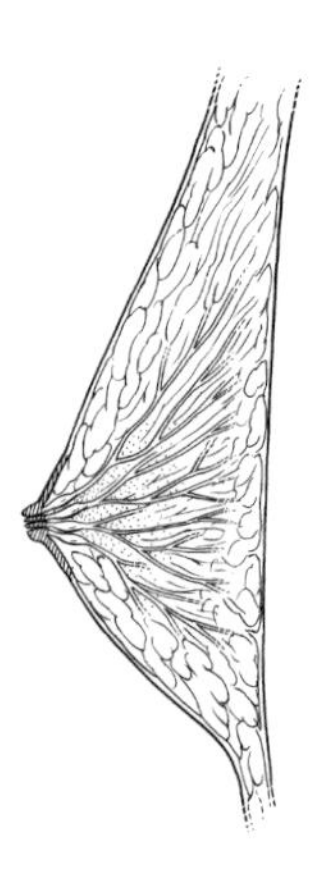

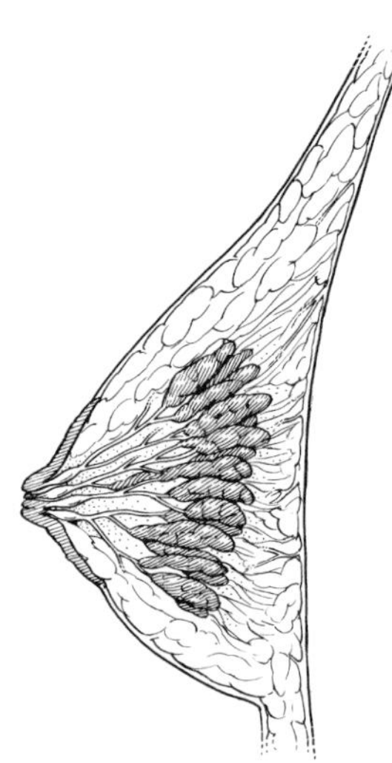

During puberty, the female breast rapidly develops fat and ligaments (stroma). The adult breast (right) has more fatty tissue and changes in response to monthly variations in hormone levels.

Breast Reduction

The size of a woman's breasts can be much more than a cosmetic issue. Very large breasts can cause a host of problems, including:

- Chronic upper back, neck and shoulder pain
- Poor posture
- Persistent skin rash under the breasts
- Grooves worn in shoulders from bra straps
- Difficulty exercising

Such problems may be one reason why breast reduction surgery (reduction mammoplasty) has increased by 88 percent since 1997.

An analysis of 29 studies involving more than 4,000 women who had breast reduction surgery indicated that the procedure significantly improved their physical symptoms and, for most of the women, their quality of life. Benefits included decreased headache, back, neck, shoulder and breast pain, and reduced hand pain and numbness caused by pressure on the shoulders from bra straps.

The most commonly used technique for breast reduction surgery involves making an incision around the dark part of the breast (areola) and down to the crease under the breast so that the surgeon can remove tissue. Typically, the surgeon removes 1 to 3 pounds of breast tissue from each breast. The surgery leaves permanent scars, which can be covered by a bra or swimsuit.

As with any surgery, breast reduction surgery has a small risk of infection and adverse reaction to anesthesia. You may end up with breasts of slightly different sizes or unevenly positioned nipples. You may experience a permanent loss of sensation in the nipples and breasts.

Some breast reduction techniques can preserve enough of the milk duct system to allow future breast-feeding.

Recovery usually takes about 6 weeks. Breast reduction surgery may be medically indicated and covered by medical insurance, but it usually requires prior authorization from the insurance company.

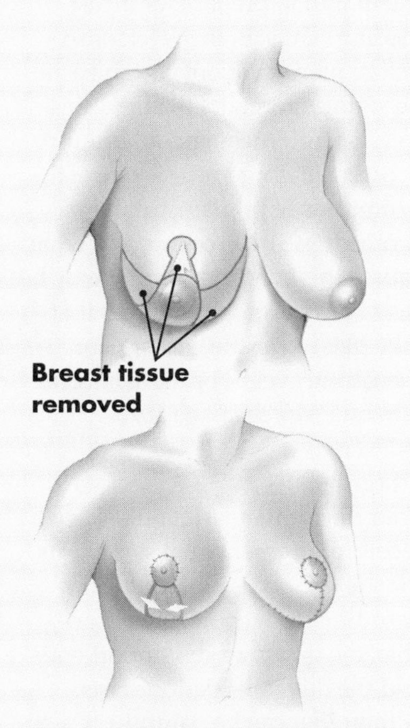

The most commonly used breast reduction technique involves making an incision around the dark part of the breast (areola) and down to the crease under the breast. Typically, the surgeon removes 1 to 3 pounds of tissue from each breast.

and the new cells, and the blood supply to the breasts diminishes.

Some women's breasts become painfully engorged just before their menstrual period. Others have cysts in their breasts that enlarge at that time. Birth control pills also can cause breast tenderness and swelling, although most women who take birth control pills don't experience these side effects.

During pregnancy, the breasts gradually enlarge. Together they may gain as much as a pound. The breasts' duct systems, stimulated by hormones produced by the placenta and the pituitary gland, grows and branches.

The body creates more cells in the stroma and adds fat cells. The nipple and areola are apt to grow larger and become darker, changes that are often permanent.

Once the baby is born, additional hormones affect the breasts. Prolactin, produced by the pituitary gland, regulates milk production. Even before the baby is weaned and breast stimulation ends, prolactin production tapers off.

After the baby is weaned, the flow of breast milk ceases, and the breasts return to nearly their prepregnancy state.

At menopause, the breast changes that occurred during the menstrual cycle cease. Some problems, such as cystic breast lumps, diminish or disappear. However, the risk of breast cancer increases with age.

It's important to do a breast self-examination (see page 836) once a month at every age. Breast self-exam becomes even more important after menopause.

Breast Disorders

Breast conditions range from the uncomfortable but harmless swelling and tenderness many women experience before menstruation to breast cancer.

Premenstrual tenderness and swelling

Signs and symptoms

- Swelling in the breast
- Lumpiness in the breast
- Breast discomfort

During each menstrual cycle, you may experience temporary changes in your breasts. Just as the uterine lining thickens each month in preparation for a possible pregnancy, breasts develop new cells in their glands and ducts over the course of the month to prepare for breast-feeding. Thus, in the week or so before menstruation, your breasts become engorged. For some, this causes tenderness and discomfort.

Breast engorgement is one of the symptoms of premenstrual syndrome (PMS). No one knows what causes this syndrome, but it may be related to hormonal changes that take place near the end of your menstrual cycle. For more information on PMS, see page 1075.

Diagnosis

Your doctor may ask you to keep a record of premenstrual symptoms for a few months, noting the day your breasts become uncomfortable, the day your discomfort ends and the day your period starts. Although it can be painful, premenstrual breast engorgement isn't considered serious.

Treatment

Medications and self-care techniques may ease the discomfort of premenstrual symptoms.

Medication

Your doctor may prescribe a diuretic drug to reduce fluid retention. It can be taken for the 10 days before the onset of your period or starting 1 or 2 days before your symptoms usually appear.

If you have severe breast pain, taking a nonsteroidal anti-inflammatory drug (NSAID), such as ibuprofen (Advil, Motrin, others), before your period begins may provide some relief.

Self-care

You may feel more comfortable if you cut down on salt before the end of your cycle because salt causes tissues to retain more fluid and increases engorgement. Caffeine may contribute to breast tenderness, so you might want to cut your intake or switch to decaffeinated products. A comfortable bra worn 24 hours a day may help too. An underwire bra can irritate tender breasts. If you wear that type, try switching to one without an underwire during this time of the month.

COMPLEMENTARY MEDICINE

For breast tenderness and pain, some women find vitamin E supplements helpful. However, small-scale studies haven't found that the supplements reduce breast pain. Oral supplements of evening primrose oil have been shown to benefit some women who take them for cyclical pain. Ask your doctor about the appropriate dosage.

Breast infections

Signs and symptoms

- Tenderness and redness of the skin on the breast
- Painful swelling or a lump in your breast
- Swelling of nearby lymph glands in your underarm area
- Flu-like symptoms
- Fever (uncommon)

Breast infection (mastitis) is common in women who are nursing a baby or who have recently stopped breast-feeding. Bacteria that enter one or both breasts are the cause.

If the infection is severe, it can form an abscess. Surrounding tissues protect themselves by secreting a substance that creates a wall around the infection. Pus collects inside.

Diagnosis

In a woman who is breast-feeding, the signs and symptoms listed above strongly suggest mastitis. Breast infections may also develop in women who aren't breast-feeding. Your doctor will likely want to see you in a few weeks after the initial diagnosis and treatment to make sure that the infection has cleared up.

Persistent or frequent recurrences of a breast infection require evaluation to rule out cancer. Evaluation may include a mammogram, an ultrasound and a biopsy procedure.

How serious are breast infections?

Breast infections usually respond quickly to treatment. If they don't, an abscess may form, which must be drained.

Treatment

Medication will usually clear up an infection. However, sometimes surgery is necessary.

Medication

Your doctor will likely prescribe an antibiotic and perhaps an analgesic for pain and fever. If you're breast-feeding, continue to do so. These

? Question and Answer

What is a yeast infection of the breast?

Yeast (candida) is a fungal organism that may infect your nipples and breasts during breast-feeding. You may experience pain in your nipple or breast, even when your baby is correctly positioned and sucking properly. The pain can be in one nipple or breast or in both.

Signs and symptoms include red, itchy, flaky skin on the nipple or the dark area surrounding it (areola). Cracked nipples that don't heal may be due to a yeast infection. Other symptoms may include a burning, throbbing pain in your breast during or after feeding. Your baby may have no signs or symptoms or may have thrush or a diaper rash caused by a yeast infection.

Yeast outbreaks can occur after antibiotic treatment. See your doctor for diagnosis and treatment.

PREVENTION TIP

If you're breast-feeding, preventing entry of bacteria into your breasts can help prevent an infection. Keep your nipples clean and dry between feedings. Avoid clothing that chafes or irritates your nipples.

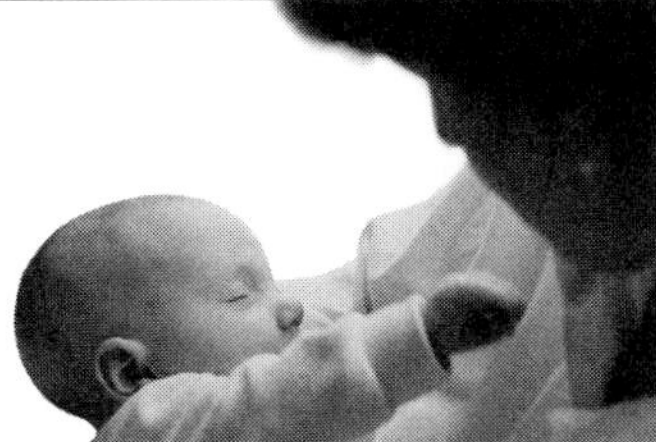

drugs shouldn't have any harmful effects on your milk supply or on your baby.

Self-care
Get adequate rest and increase your intake of fluids. Applying heat to the affected area also may help reduce pain.

Surgery
Usually, an antibiotic is sufficient treatment, but if an abscess forms, it needs to be drained. Your doctor may aspirate the abscess with a needle or drain it by making a small incision in it.

Nipple disorders

Signs and symptoms

- Discharge from your nipple
- A nipple that's newly inverted
- Lumps in the area surrounding your nipple (areola)
- Scaling of your nipple

It's wise to pay attention to changes in your nipples. Although most often the cause is noncancerous (benign), some changes are cancer related.

Yellow, green, brown or gray fluid that leaks from multiple ducts in both your nipples is likely due to either fibrocystic changes of the breasts (see page 835) or dilated ducts (mammary duct ectasia). Whitish fluid from multiple ducts is probably breast milk, especially if it comes from both nipples.

A discharge that's dark red or black contains blood. It may indicate a tiny, benign tumor growing in a milk duct, although breast cancer also is a remote possibility. A discharge that's clear (watery) also can indicate an underlying cancer.

Inverted nipples are normal if you've had them since puberty. A nipple that inverts later in life can be a sign of cancer.

Small lumps in your areola generally are cysts caused by blocked oil glands. If an infection develops, a cyst may turn into a boil. Scaling of a nipple is usually due to benign changes.

If scaling persists, you may need a biopsy to rule out an underlying cancer. Paget's disease of the breast is a type of breast cancer that usually appears first as a red, scaly or itchy nipple. It may be misdiagnosed as eczema, a type of skin disease.

Diagnosis

If you notice any unusual changes in your nipples or breasts, see your doctor for a breast examination. In case of nipple discharge, he or she may gather a sample of the discharge for laboratory analysis. For a newly inverted nipple or a bloody discharge, tests for cancer are often necessary, which may include a mammogram.

How serious are nipple disorders?

Nipple discharge and inverted nipples are rarely serious. However, they can be an indication of cancer, so it's important to have an evaluation by your doctor to determine the cause.

Treatment

If the changes aren't cancer related, you may not need treatment. If an infected cyst evolves into a boil, your doctor will probably prescribe an antibiotic. Whether surgery is necessary depends on the underlying problem.

Galactorrhea

Signs and symptoms

- Whitish discharge from your nipples, usually from both breasts
- Missed menstrual periods (amenorrhea)

Normally, you produce breast milk only after giving birth — for as long as you continue breast-feeding — and perhaps for a few days beforehand. If your nipples leak milk at other times, you have an uncommon condition called galactorrhea. The name comes from the Greek words *gala*, for "milk," and *rhoia*, for "flow."

Galactorrhea is at times something of a mystery. Researchers report that in about 50 percent of the cases, a cause can't be found for it. Approximately 25 percent of women with the condition have a type of pituitary tumor called a prolactinoma. The tumor is usually noncancerous (benign) but secretes prolactin, the hormone that regulates production of breast milk.

In the remaining 25 percent of cases, galactorrhea has various causes. For instance, it can be a sign of an underactive thyroid (hypothyroidism) or a side effect of a medication.

Drugs that can cause galactorrhea include methyldopa (used for high blood pressure), phenotiazines (a class of tranquilizers), several types of antidepressant medications and dextroamphetamine (Dexedrine), a psychostimulant used to treat conditions such as attention-deficit/hyperactivity disorder and narcolepsy.

Diagnosis

If you're experiencing signs and symptoms, see your doctor for a breast examination. He or she will likely take a sample of the fluid your breast is producing to make sure it isn't associated with breast cancer.

To help determine the cause of the problem, your doctor may also test you for conditions such as hypothyroidism. Other tests may

Breast-feeding

Women choose to breast-feed because of the health benefit to their babies and for the mother-baby bonding opportunity it offers. Breast milk is biologically complex. It provides your baby with unique protection against infections and stimulates the development of the baby's immune system.

The sticky, yellowish fluid secreted by your breasts for the first several days after you give birth (colostrum) contains hormones and antibodies that benefit your baby. After 3 to 5 days, your pituitary gland directs your breasts to produce mature milk, which contains essential nutrients. The removal of milk from your breasts sustains your milk production.

The let-down reflex controls the flow of breast milk. When a baby suckles, the nipples respond by sending sensory impulses to the brain. The pituitary gland releases hormones, principally oxytocin, into the bloodstream. When the hormones reach the breasts, they cause the cells surrounding the cavities where milk is produced (alveoli) to contract, expressing milk into the ducts.

Initially, this process may take several minutes. Once you establish breast-feeding, the let-down reflex triggers easily, often merely in response to your baby's cry.

Expect some temporary nipple tenderness initially. You shouldn't experience pain, which is generally a sign that something is wrong. Make sure your baby's mouth is centered on the nipple area. You can help avoid nipple injury by positioning your baby properly while nursing.

Breast-feeding should be enjoyable for both you and your baby. Using a breast pump intermittently can enable you to have a more flexible lifestyle.

You may experience a plugged milk duct when you breast-feed, or you may develop a breast lump that's hot and painful. For relief, try heat, rest, massage and prolonged, frequent nursing. If the lump does not get better with these measures, you may have mastitis.

Mastitis is a breast infection usually caused by bacteria. Signs and symptoms include fever, flu-like symptoms and breast pain and redness. For relief, increase fluids, get more rest and apply heat to the affected area. In addition, notify your doctor, who may prescribe an antibiotic.

Weaning your child from breast milk should be a gradual process. Abrupt weaning can be difficult for you and your baby and can result in engorged breasts. Starting your baby on solid food at about 6 months can begin the weaning process.

Prolactin, the hormone that helps prepare your breasts for breast-feeding, also offers some protection from pregnancy. But don't rely on it for birth control. You may ovulate while breast-feeding even if you don't menstruate.

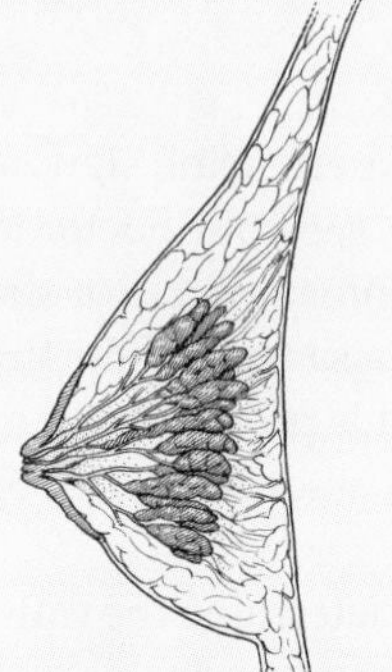

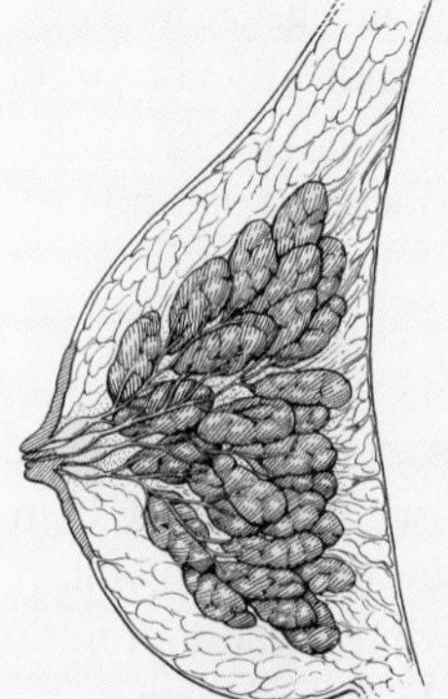

When breast-feeding, the system of ducts and glands within the breast expands as milk is produced, a process called lactation.

include blood tests to check your prolactin level and magnetic resonance imaging (MRI) of your hypothalamus and pituitary gland.

How serious is galactorrhea?
Galactorrhea isn't threatening to your health unless it's caused by a pituitary tumor. Such tumors grow slowly, and some eventually stabilize. They often can be treated successfully with medication. If that fails, your doctor may recommend surgery or radiation.

Treatment
The type of treatment used for galactorrhea depends on the cause of the disease.

Medication
For hypothyroidism, your doctor is likely to prescribe the medication thyroxine (Levothroid, Synthroid, others). If you have a pituitary tumor that's causing the problem, or tests find no explanation for your galactorrhea, your doctor may prescribe the medication bromocriptine (Apo-Bromocriptine, Parlodel). This medication can shrink a tumor and reduce prolactin levels. In addition, bromocriptine often suppresses galactorrhea even when its cause remains unknown.

Surgery
For a large pituitary tumor, surgery may be necessary. Because such tumors tend to recur, you may need long-term treatment with bromocriptine or a course of radiation.

Intraductal papilloma

Signs and symptoms
- Watery or bloody discharge from your nipple
- A very small lump beneath your nipple

An intraductal papilloma is a tiny, noncancerous (benign) tumor that grows within a milk duct of your breast at the point near the nipple. These uncommon tumors are often too small to feel. An intraductal papilloma can be detected on examination of the breast in fewer than half of the cases.

Diagnosis

Your doctor will likely go through diagnostic procedures to make sure you don't have breast cancer. He or she may apply gentle pressure in the area around your nipple to try to determine which duct may contain a papilloma. Although intraductal papillomas are benign, they should be removed to be sure the lump is a papilloma and not cancer.

Treatment

Surgery is necessary in most cases of intraductal papilloma. If your doctor can feel a lump or see it on a mammogram or ultrasound image, a surgeon can remove it. When no lump is present, but the discharge is persistent from a single duct, your doctor may recommend a procedure called a duct exploration, in which milk ducts are removed. If the discharge occurred only once, careful follow-up, including regular mammograms, is advisable.

Breast lumps

Signs and symptoms

- A change in breast tissue that makes it feel different from surrounding tissue
- One or more lumps in a breast, which may or may not be painful
- Sometimes, a retracted nipple, dimpling of the skin, or a greenish or straw-colored discharge from your nipple

Most breast lumps aren't cancerous. But some are, so it's important to have breast lumps evaluated.

Cysts

A breast lump that occurs late in your menstrual cycle often is a harmless cyst. After menstruation, this type of lump often disappears. A breast cyst is a fluid-filled sac that tends to enlarge near the end of your menstrual cycle, when your body is retaining more fluid. Some cysts are tiny, but others can be as large as an egg. If squeezed, a cyst may change shape slightly, and most can be moved under the skin.

Obstruction or dilation of ducts in the underlying breast tissue may be the cause of the cysts. You're most likely to develop cysts when in your 40s, years before menopause. Because cysts generally disappear after menopause, changes in ovarian hormones probably cause the fluctuations in size.

Normal Breast

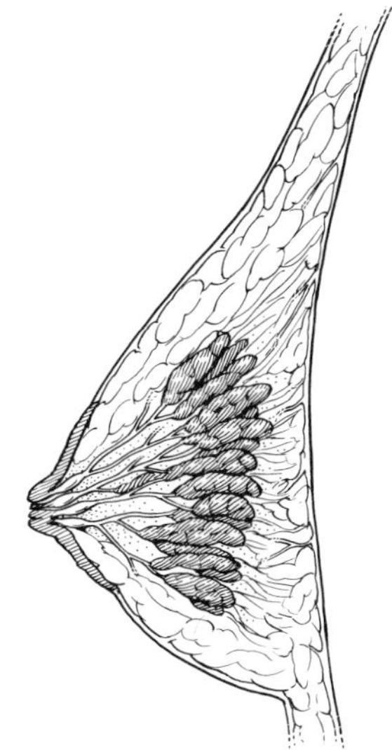

Fibrocystic Breast

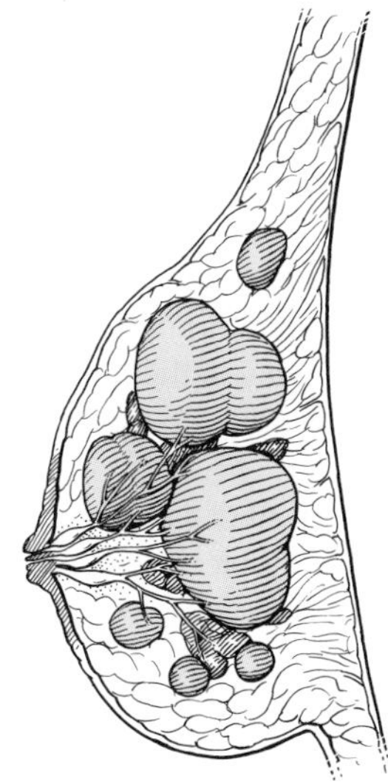

Fibrocystic breasts

Fibrocystic breasts are more common in women in their 20s and 30s. This condition is also called fibrocystic changes, chronic cystic mastitis or benign breast disease.

In this condition, growth or proliferation of fibrous connective tissue and ducts, in combination with cyst development, causes glandular breast tissue to thicken. The thickened tissue usually is more prominent in the upper, outer region of your breast. This condition is also associated with variations in hormonal levels during your menstrual cycle and can be painful.

Fibroadenomas

Breast lumps that are neither cysts nor cancer are most likely to be fibroadenomas (adenofibromas). These noncancerous (benign) tumors most often develop in women in the first half of their childbearing years. A fibroadenoma has a firm, smooth, rubbery feeling and a well-defined shape. It can be moved about under the skin. It develops when connective tissue grows within the glands or lobules of the breast.

Others

Other types of breast lumps include those caused by infection or by bleeding from an injury (hematoma). A lump caused by a tumor of the fatty tissues is called a lipoma. Or a lump can be caused by an intraductal papilloma, especially if it's blocking a duct, causing a cyst. None of these conditions are cancerous (malignant).

Diagnosis

Your doctor's main focus will be on making sure the lumps in your breast aren't cancerous. If you have a single lump that feels like a cyst, your doctor may try to draw (aspirate) fluid from it by using a thin needle. If fluid can be aspirated, the lump may disappear, an indication that it was a cyst.

The fluid found in cysts is straw-colored or yellow and may not need to be analyzed. If the fluid appears bloody or abnormal, or if the lump doesn't disappear after the fluid is aspirated, then your

Breast Self-Examination

Regular breast self-examination (BSE) can be lifesaving because it can alert you to cancerous (malignant) breast lumps. Most breast lumps — about 75 percent — are noncancerous (benign), but if you find one, see your doctor to rule out cancer if possible. If your lump is cancerous, treatment for breast cancer is most successful when it's found in the early stages.

All women should examine their breasts once a month. If you haven't reached menopause, the best time is a few days after your period ends because your breasts are less likely to be tender or swollen then. If you're no longer menstruating, then pick a day of the month and do the examination regularly on that date each month.

A BSE takes a little bit of time, but it isn't difficult. Here's how to do it:

1. Stand nude in front of a mirror. With your arms at your sides, look at your breasts for puckering or dimpling or for changes in their size or shape. Unless your nipples are normally inverted, make sure they haven't turned inward. Rest your hands on your hips, then place them behind your head. Check for the same signs in each position.

2. Next, step into the shower and wet and soap your breasts. Place your left hand behind your head and examine your left breast with your right hand. Think of your breast as the face of a clock and place your right hand at 12 o'clock, at the top of the breast, approximately $\frac{1}{2}$ inch below your collarbone. Hold your hand flat, fingertips pressed together, and, using the pads of your three middle fingers (not the fingertips), make a tiny circling motion, feeling for lumps. Apply light pressure, moderate pressure and deep pressure at each position. Move your hand to 1 o'clock, to 2 o'clock, and so on. When you return to the 12 o'clock position, slide your fingertips closer to your nipple (about $\frac{1}{2}$ inch) and repeat the same motions, going around the clock in a circle within the first circle, then make an even smaller circle. Continue using the same pattern until you have checked every part of your breast, including the nipple.

3. To check for nipple discharge, make a V shape with your thumb and first finger and place to the left and right of your nipple. Push down on the areola and gently pull up once. Then change the position of the V shape so that the thumb and finger lie on the areola above and below the nipple. Push down and gently pull up.

4. Finish by examining the area adjacent to your breast, under your armpit, because it also contains breast tissue and lymph nodes that drain the lymph channels in the breast tissue.

5. Repeat the whole procedure using your left hand on your right breast.

6. After you're done with your shower, lie on your back and examine your breasts again. To examine your right breast, put a pillow under your right shoulder and place your right hand under your head and apply pressure in a circular motion as described above. To examine your left breast, place the pillow under your left shoulder and your left hand under your head and again thoroughly feel the entire breast for lumps.

7. If your breasts are normally lumpy because of fibrocystic changes, make a note of how many lumps you have, where they're situated and approximately what size they are. Each month, check for changes. Once you know what's normal for your breasts, if you find a new lump or lumps that persist for two or three menstrual cycles or increase in size, see your doctor.

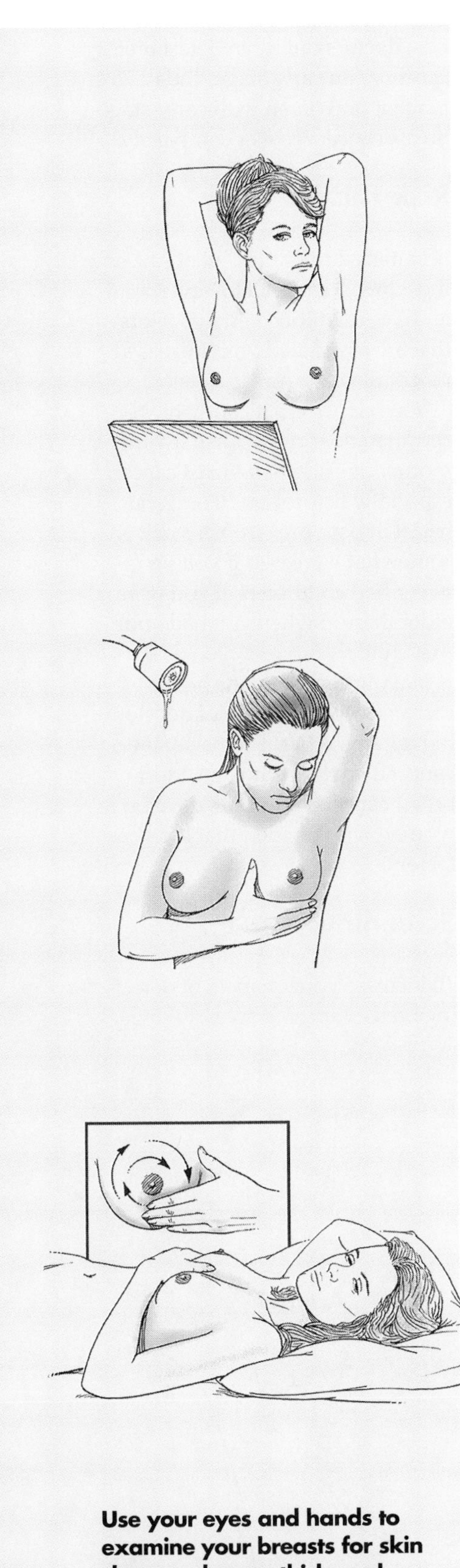

Use your eyes and hands to examine your breasts for skin changes, lumps, thickened areas or swelling. Feel for lumps in your breasts while you're standing and again while lying down.

doctor may send the fluid to a laboratory to be analyzed for evidence of cancer. Your doctor also may recommend further evaluation with ultrasound and mammography.

Ultrasound may also be used in an initial evaluation of a lump. When performed by an experienced operator, an ultrasound exam can reliably detect a cyst. If confirmed by ultrasound, a cyst doesn't need to be aspirated as long as you have no symptoms. However, if your cyst is painful, then aspiration may relieve your discomfort.

If aspiration fails to find fluid in a lump, your doctor may recommend a mammogram. If a mammogram indicates a lump, or if an ultrasound procedure shows a solid area rather than a fluid-filled cyst, then the next step may be a biopsy to remove some or all of the lump and examine it under a microscope.

Several types of needle biopsies, including fine-needle aspiration (FNA), core biopsy and stereotactic biopsy, can be used to help evaluate a breast lump. FNA tends to be the least accurate because it's usually not done with imaging guidance and therefore carries risk of not sampling the lump accurately. In addition, the technique only samples cells and doesn't help indicate the structure of the tissue.

A core biopsy, performed by a radiologist using ultrasound guidance, is considered very accurate. The procedure is done under local anesthesia. A stereotactic biopsy, also performed by a radiologist and under local anesthesia, involves use of special mammogram imaging for guidance.

A surgical biopsy (excisional biopsy, or lumpectomy), which involves removing the whole lump, is another way to determine the cause of a lump. A surgical biopsy is done in a hospital or an outpatient surgical facility, using either local or general anesthesia.

How serious are breast lumps?

The majority of lumps aren't cancerous. Benign lumps usually aren't harmful beyond causing occasional discomfort. All lumps, though, need to be taken seriously until cancer has been excluded.

Some breast lumps, such as complex fibroadenomas, are associated with an increased risk of breast cancer. According to recent studies, most fibrocystic changes don't increase breast cancer risk. However, women with lumpy breasts may have more trouble detecting a cancerous tumor, if one were to develop. Check for changes or thickening when you do your monthly breast self-examination. If you find anything suspicious, notify your doctor.

Treatment

Depending on the type of lumps you have, they may be treated with medication or surgery. Self-care measures also may prove useful.

Medication

Some women take mild pain relievers, such as aspirin or ibuprofen (Advil, Motrin, others), for pain associated with cysts or fibrocystic breast changes. The medications danazol (Danocrine) and bromocriptine (Apo-Bromocriptine, Parlodel) often relieve breast pain, but both can have unpleasant side effects and are expensive.

Some women take vitamin E for their symptoms, but there's no solid evidence that it works. Evening primrose oil has been shown to relieve pain for some women with cyclical breast pain.

Self-care

Good breast support with a well-fitted bra, worn even at night, can be effective at relieving some breast discomfort. If you smoke, then having breast lumps is just one more health reason to quit. If you drink caffeinated beverages, you may want to cut down or switch to decaffeinated products. Although the evidence is inconclusive, some women report that their lumps subsided after they stopped smoking or gave up caffeine.

Surgery
Your doctor may aspirate your cysts to relieve the pain. Otherwise, they don't need to be removed or treated unless they're filled with blood or they recur or enlarge following aspiration.

Any solid-appearing lump, even if it has a benign appearance on an ultrasound image or a mammogram, is typically biopsied to exclude cancer. A lump that has been confirmed by biopsy to be a fibroadenoma may be left in place unless it's uncomfortable. You and your doctor will want to check it at regular intervals to see whether it continues to grow.

A fibroadenoma that continues to grow is usually removed surgically because of a small risk of cancer.

Breast Cancer

Signs and symptoms

- A lump or thickening in your breast, which may not be painful
- Clear or bloody discharge from a nipple
- An inverted nipple — if it isn't normally inverted
- A change in the contours of your breasts
- Any dimpling or puckering of the skin of your breast
- Skin redness on your breast

An estimated 175,000 new cases of female breast cancer are diagnosed yearly in the United States. Adult women in the United States who live to be 85 have a one in eight chance of developing breast cancer during their lifetime.

Among American women, breast cancer is the most frequently diagnosed life-threatening cancer, and the second leading cause of cancer death, after lung cancer. Age is a factor — approximately 78 percent of breast cancers are found in women older than age 50.

Breast cancer can kill by spreading (metastasizing) through your lymph system and bloodstream to other parts of your body. If the cancer is detected and treated early — while it's confined to your breast duct, while the tumor is small and before malignant cells have spread to neighboring lymph nodes — there's a 90 percent to 95 percent chance of successful treatment.

With the greater use of mammography and other screening methods, doctors often can detect breast cancer at an early stage. Today, 75 percent of women with early-stage breast cancer recover completely.

Risk factors

Scientists don't know what causes most breast cancer. However, studies have identified certain factors that are associated with increased risk of developing the disease.

You have a significantly higher risk than do most women if your mother or sister had breast cancer, especially before age 50 or if she had it in both breasts. Your risk is somewhat increased if you've never had children or if you were older than 35 when you had your first child.

Having cancer in one breast increases your chances of developing it in the other. The risk of breast cancer also rises with age. Most breast cancers, however, develop in women with no identifiable risk factors.

Screening

To increase your chances of detecting breast cancer at an early stage,

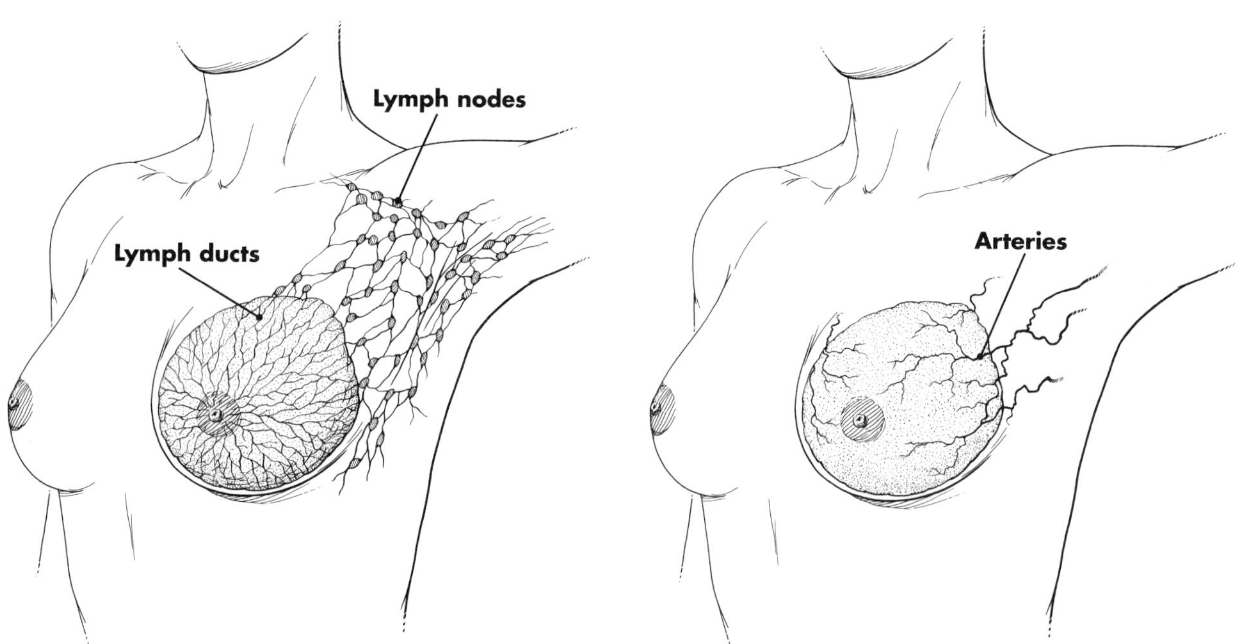

Breast cancer cells may spread (metastasize) through your lymph system and through your blood vessels.

when chances of successful treatment are highest, it's important to be screened. Early detection of breast cancer, while the tumor is small and before it spreads, is key to survival. Screening includes:

Clinical breast exam
If you're between 20 and 40 years old, have your doctor examine your breasts at least once every 3 years. If you're older than 40 years, have a clinical breast examination once a year. During a clinical exam, your doctor examines your breasts for lumps or hard spots.

Breast self-exam
By performing breast self-examinations (see page 836), you increase your chances of finding breast changes that may develop between medical checkups. You should do a self-exam once a month throughout your life.

Mammography
A mammogram, a breast X-ray that uses low doses of radiation, can detect tumors even before you or your doctor can feel them.

Mammography saves lives by identifying breast cancer at a stage when it's most curable. However, the test isn't infallible. Occasionally, it fails to show a tumor, and at other times it indicates a problem when none exists.

It's best to combine screening by mammography with regular clinical breast examinations done by your doctor and with breast self-examinations.

Screening mammography, designed for women without new concerns or lumps, consists of two standard views. A concern or lump that needs to be evaluated more closely often requires additional

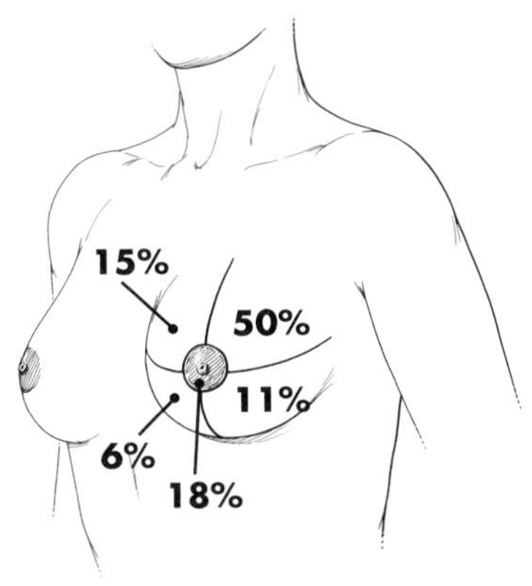

Cancer develops more frequently in some areas of the breast than in others.

Inherited Breast Cancer: Are You at Risk?

An estimated 10 percent to 15 percent of breast cancer is inherited. Some inherited breast cancer is linked to breast cancer genes 1 and 2 (BRCA1 and BRCA2). A blood test may be helpful in assessing your risk if you have a strong family history of breast cancer — that is, if you have two or more close relatives with the disease, especially if their cancer developed before the age of 50.

Having an alteration on one of the two genes doesn't mean you'll get cancer, but your risk is greater. Research is looking at different therapies to prevent breast cancer caused by gene abnormalities. In the meantime, if you have an alteration, then you can be more vigilant about monitoring for signs of breast cancer. Be sure to conduct monthly breast self-exams and discuss with your doctor how often you should have clinical breast exams and mammograms.

Some women at high risk choose to have their breasts removed (radical mastectomy). This preventive procedure is called prophylactic surgery. It reduces the risk of breast cancer but doesn't eliminate it entirely because some breast tissue remains (see page 843).

Lifestyle and Breast Cancer

Can the decisions you make about exercise, alcohol use and managing your weight affect your risk of developing breast cancer? Growing evidence suggests they may.

Exercise
One study of 25,624 women found that the risk of breast cancer was lowest in lean women — those with a body mass index less than 22.8 — who exercised at least 4 hours a week.

For more information on how to determine your body mass index, see page 38.

Alcohol
An analysis of several studies found that women who consumed two to five drinks a day were at increased risk of breast cancer compared with nondrinkers.

Weight
A study involving a large group of women found that weight gain after age 18 was associated with 16 percent of breast cancers in women who were beyond menopause. No association was found between weight gain after age 18 and breast cancer in women who hadn't yet reached menopause.

More study is needed to confirm these relationships. However, experts say that making healthy dietary and exercise decisions certainly can't hurt because they result in many other known health benefits.

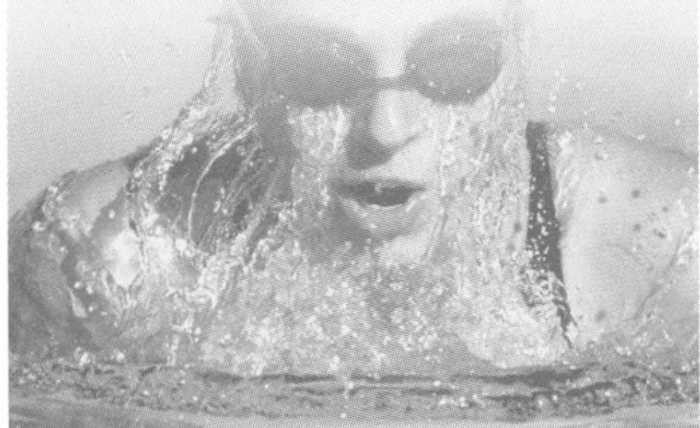

views, called magnification views, to better define the lump.

During mammography, it's necessary to compress the breast between two plates on the X-ray device. This compression can cause some discomfort, but it smoothes the breast tissue, making it easier for the radiologist to detect abnormalities.

In addition, a compressed breast receives less radiation, and compression reduces movement, which can create a blurry image. If the breast is inadequately compressed, then overlapping normal breast tissue can create the appearance of an abnormality where none exists.

There's disagreement within the medical profession about the age at which women should begin having regular mammograms. Young women rarely develop breast cancer, and their breasts usually are so dense that they don't X-ray well. Most medical experts agree that women younger than 35 who aren't in a high-risk category need not have mammograms and that women older than 50 should have them annually.

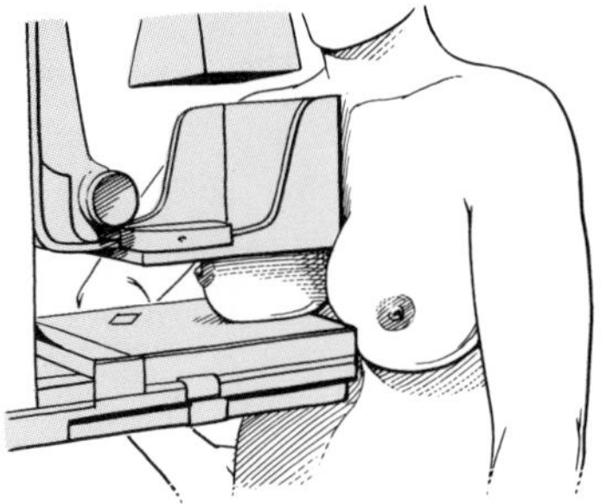

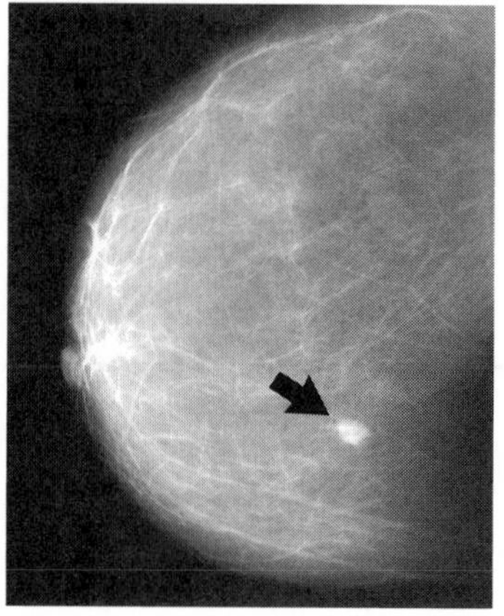

Mammograms are produced by a special X-ray device (top) that can detect tumors before you or your doctor can feel them. This mammogram (right) shows breast cancer (see arrow).

Controversy has centered on whether screening is necessary for women in their 40s and on whether a woman should have a baseline mammogram at age 35 to establish a norm for her breasts. Recent studies indicate that regular mammograms do save lives among women in their 40s, but the value of the earlier baseline X-ray remains questionable.

Advances in Detection

Mammography combined with clinical breast examinations remains the most commonly used method of screening and early detection.

Standard mammography, however, can miss about 15 percent of cancers, especially in women with dense breast tissue. And three out of four areas that look like a cause for concern on a mammogram will end up being noncancerous (benign).

Promising advances in screening include the following:

Computer-aided detection

After a radiologist reviews the mammogram, a sophisticated computer technology — mammography enhanced by computer-aided detection (CAD) — scans the film for suspicious areas and highlights them for a closer look. Research indicates that CAD identifies more suspicious areas than does standard mammography, but many of the suspicious areas often prove to be normal.

Digital mammography

A mammogram image on a computer screen — as opposed to a film image — allows for the contrast and darkness of the image to be adjusted. This enhances the radiologist's ability to identify subtle differences in tissues.

Another advantage is that the image can be stored and transmitted electronically. One benefit of this technology is that women who live in remote areas can have their mammograms more easily and quickly transmitted to and read by an expert who's situated elsewhere. Digital mammography may improve detection of breast cancer, but studies have yet to prove it's more effective than conventional mammography.

Magnetic resonance imaging

Magnetic resonance imaging (MRI) can reveal tumors that are too small to be detected through physical examination and are difficult to see on conventional mammograms. In addition, it can also help distinguish between noncancerous and cancerous (malignant) tumors.

Using a magnet linked to a computer, MRI takes pictures of the inside of the breast. Unlike mammography, it doesn't pick up microcalcifications, tiny calcium deposits that serve as one early sign of breast cancer.

Although MRI isn't used for routine screening, studies are evaluating whether it may be a valuable screening tool for women who are at high risk of developing breast cancer.

Ductal lavage

Ductal lavage is the latest early detection technique for women at high risk of developing breast cancer. It involves injecting saline through the nipple into a breast duct, withdrawing the solution and then examining it for abnormal cells.

Chemoprevention

Advances in breast cancer research have led to the use of natural or synthetic drugs to reduce the risk of cancer. For example, the drug tamoxifen (Nolvadex) can reduce the risk of breast cancer in high-risk women. Tamoxifen belongs to a class of drugs known as selective estrogen receptor modulators (SERMs), which block the effects of estrogen on the breast. Unfortunately, tamoxifen has an estrogen-like effect on the uterus, increasing the risk of uterine cancer.

As a result, researchers are seeking other SERMs with the benefits of tamoxifen but without the potentially harmful side effects. Raloxifene (Evista) is one such drug under study.

Presently, the best advice:

- If you're younger than age 40, you probably don't need a mammogram unless you develop a breast problem or you're at high risk.

  Women with a family history of breast cancer should begin having regular mammograms 5 to 10 years before the age when the youngest relative to develop breast cancer received her diagnosis.
- If you're between the ages of 40 and 49, talk with your doctor about how often you should have a mammogram based on your risk factors and preferences.
- If you're age 50 or older, have a mammogram yearly.

Diagnosis

Diagnosis of breast cancer often begins with a breast examination. Your doctor may also squeeze your areola area gently to see if any discharge comes from the ducts leading to the nipple, and feel your armpits for signs that your lymph nodes might be involved. Breast cancer commonly spreads through the lymph channels.

A mammogram is generally the next step. A suspicious lesion may correspond to a lump that your doctor can feel (palpable lump). A mammogram may also reveal a suspicious area that doesn't correspond to a palpable lump. Mammograms can't detect all breast cancers.

Your doctor may also request an ultrasound scan to determine whether a lesion appears cystic (filled with fluid). If the lesion doesn't appear to be a simple benign cyst, he or she may use a thin needle to try to draw (aspirate) fluid from it. This fluid is analyzed for cancerous (malignant) cells.

If the lump disappears after the fluid is withdrawn, then chances are that it was simply a cyst. However, even if the aspirated fluid shows no evidence of cancer, you'll want to follow up with another exam, usually in 6 months, to make sure the lump hasn't continued to grow.

If a lump can't be aspirated, it could be evaluated with a needle biopsy. Even if the biopsy result is benign, a 6-month follow-up is important to determine whether that lump has grown. If it has, surgical removal of the lump is usually done because of the risk that the lump wasn't adequately sampled in the needle biopsy.

A lump can also be biopsied surgically. A surgical biopsy usually involves removing the entire lump to determine whether it's malignant. Your doctor probably will advise such a biopsy if fluid can't be drawn from the lump, if the lump doesn't collapse after the fluid has been drawn out, if the lump recurs or if the fluid contains blood or malignant cells.

Stereotactic breast biopsy is a nonsurgical procedure in which your doctor views mammograms

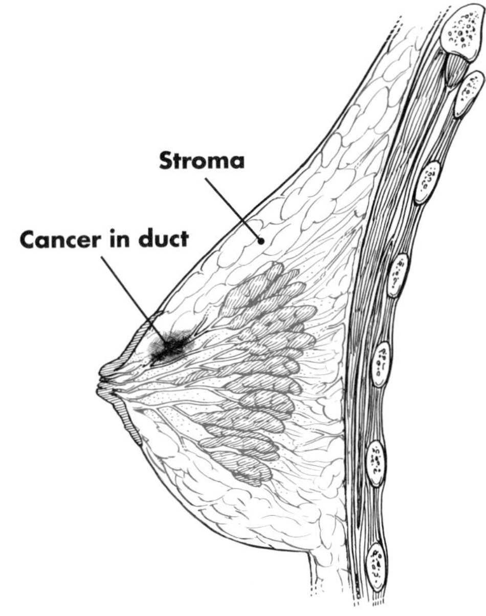

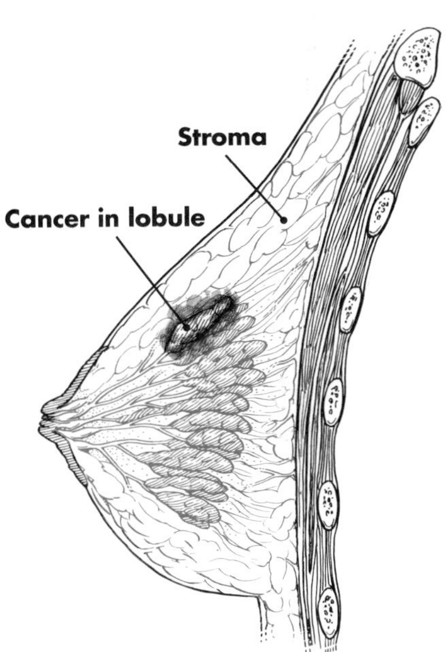

Breast cancer often begins in one of two locations. More commonly, it originates as an abnormal growth in a milk duct (top) that breaks through the duct wall and invades fatty tissue and connective tissue (stroma). About 70 percent of breast cancers are this type. Breast cancer may also develop in a milk-producing lobule (bottom) and spread to nearby stroma.

taken from different angles to determine the precise location of a suspicious area. A computer aligns a needle with the area, allowing a radiologist to remove a small amount of tissue. The tissue is sent to the lab for microscopic examination to rule out cancer. Stereotactic biopsy takes about 30 to 45 minutes and is performed under local anesthesia. It leaves only a tiny scar, costs about one-third that of a surgical biopsy, and studies indicate it may be as accurate.

Your diagnostic work-up may also include hormone receptor tests to determine if estrogen or progesterone causes the tumor to grow and a HER-2-neu test to predict the response of the tumor to certain drugs.

Breast Cancer Staging

Stage refers to how far a cancer has spread. Determined by exams and diagnostic tests such as blood tests, bone scans, computerized tomography (CT) scans and X-rays, staging is one of the most important factors in determining optimum treatment, and the most significant factor in predicting prognosis or outcome.

Breast cancer can be grouped into five stages:

- **Stage 0** (noninvasive, or *in situ*)**.** This is very early breast cancer that hasn't spread within the breast. This includes lobular carcinoma *in situ* (LCIS), in which the cancer is confined to the lobule, and ductal carcinoma *in situ* (DCIS), in which abnormal cells remain within the duct.

- **Stage I.** The diameter of the tumor is less than 2 centimeters (cm) — 2.5 cm equal 1 inch — and the cancer hasn't spread beyond the breast.

- **Stage II.** This stage is divided into two substages. In stage IIA, the tumor is smaller than 2 cm, but the cancer has spread to the lymph nodes under the arm, or the tumor is between 2 and 5 cm, but the cancer hasn't spread to the lymph nodes under the arm.

  In stage IIB, the tumor is between 2 and 5 cm, and the cancer has spread to the lymph nodes under the arm, or the tumor is larger than 5 cm, but the cancer hasn't spread to the lymph nodes under the arm.

- **Stage III.** This stage also is divided into substages. In stage IIIA, the tumor is smaller than 5 cm (2 inches), and the cancer has spread to lymph nodes under the arm in a way that the lymph nodes are matted together, or the tumor is tumor is larger than 5 cm, and the cancer has spread just to lymph nodes under the arm.

  Stage IIIB signifies a tumor of any size in which the cancer has spread to tissues near the breast — skin, chest wall, muscles or ribs — or has spread to lymph nodes inside the chest wall along the breastbone.

- **Stage IV.** The cancer, regardless of its size, has spread (metastasized) to distant sites, such as bones, the lungs or lymph nodes not near the breast.

Questions to Ask Your Doctor

To be an active partner with your doctor in determining the best form of treatment for your cancer, you need to know as much as you can about what you're facing.

Cancer experts recommend asking your doctor a number of questions, including the following:

1. What type of cancer do I have?
2. How large is my cancer, and where is it located?
3. How many tumors do I have, and how large are they?
4. What stage and grade of cancer do I have?
5. Has the cancer spread to my lymph nodes? If so, where?
6. How does my age and menopausal status affect my treatment?
7. Should my tumor be tested for genetic mutations?
8. Should I get a second opinion?

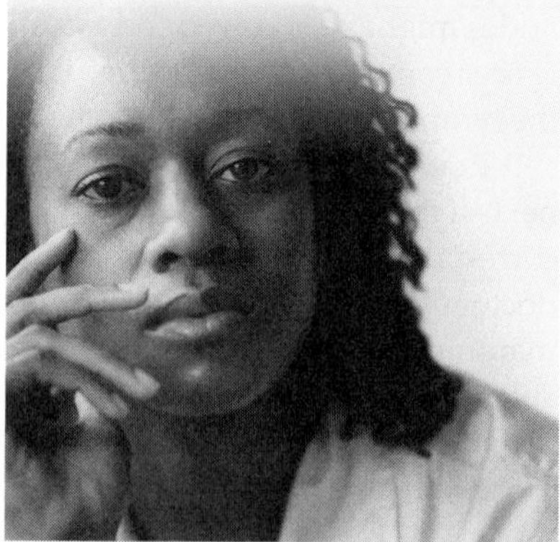

Treatment

Treatment for breast cancer depends on several factors, but it usually involves some combination of surgery, radiation therapy, hormone therapy or chemotherapy.

Surgery

Routine mammography and heightened awareness among women and their doctors about breast cancer have contributed to an increase in the number of people who receive an earlier diagnosis of the disease.

When discovered at its earliest stage, breast cancer is highly curable with surgery. And with the development of a technique called sentinel node biopsy, surgeons may be able to more accurately determine how much tissue needs to be removed.

Surgical procedures for breast cancer include:

Lumpectomy

A lumpectomy involves removing the tumor and some of the surrounding tissue. Some lymph nodes under the arm also may be removed. For a small tumor that's detected early, a lumpectomy to remove the tumor may be all the surgery that's necessary. If the tumor is larger or the cancer has spread, additional surgery may be required.

Radical mastectomy

Rarely performed today, radical mastectomy involves removing the entire breast, including a portion of skin containing the nipple and areola, as well as the underlying chest wall (pectoral) muscles. This procedure used to also involve the removal of numerous lymph nodes underneath your armpit (axilla) in an attempt to halt the spread of cancer, but sentinel node biopsy has all but eliminated this procedure.

Commonly performed until 20 years ago, radical mastectomy is disfiguring and it may result in significant arm swelling (lymphedema) as well as diminished arm mobility.

Today, surgeons usually resort to this procedure only for large, locally advanced tumors invading large segments of your chest wall muscles. Often, they'll first try to shrink the tumors with preoperative (neoadjuvant) chemotherapy. Reducing the size of a breast tumor with chemotherapy before surgery may offer a woman an option other than radical mastectomy, that is, one that saves her breast.

Modified radical mastectomy

As doctors gain more knowledge about the biologic behavior of breast cancer, it has become apparent that less radical operations than radical mastectomy are as effective in treating the primary tumor and are much less debilitating and disfiguring.

A modified radical mastectomy is similar to radical mastectomy, but it spares the chest wall muscles. Maintaining your chest wall (pectoralis) muscles facilitates breast reconstruction, if you choose to have it. Sentinel node biopsy may help determine the degree of lymph node removal necessary in a modified radical mastectomy.

Simple mastectomy

A simple mastectomy is similar to modified radical mastectomy, but

Sentinel Node Biopsy

In cases of invasive breast cancer, which has a tendency to spread to lymph nodes and the bloodstream, doctors used to routinely remove the underarm (axillary) lymph nodes. This requires more extensive surgery and sometimes leads to complications, including fluid buildup in the arm (lymphedema), infection and numbness.

Today, many doctors rely on a procedure called sentinel node biopsy to determine if the cancer has spread to the lymphatic system. The sentinel lymph node is the first lymph node to which a tumor drains, and therefore the first place to which the cancer is likely to spread. By finding the sentinel node before surgery, doctors can remove the node for study during surgery.

Early research indicates that if the sentinel node is free of cancer, then the cancer isn't likely to have spread. If the sentinel node is free of cancer, further removal of lymph nodes is typically unnecessary. The presence or absence of cancer in the lymph glands of your armpit is also important for determining treatment after the operation.

One way to find the sentinel node is to inject blue dye near the tumor. The dye travels to and accumulates in the sentinel node (see the color illustration on page 424). Another method is to inject a bit of radioactive solution near the tumor and use an instrument called a gamma detector to see where the radioactivity accumulates. Sometimes, both methods are used together. Once the sentinel node is found, it's removed during a lumpectomy or mastectomy and sent to a laboratory for examination.

Studies indicate that sentinel node biopsy delivers accurate information about the spread of the cancer. This makes the standard practice of removing several if not all of the axillary nodes in the underarm area generally unnecessary if the sentinel node shows no sign of cancer. If the sentinel node is malignant, further node dissection is necessary to determine the stage of lymph node involvement. Further node dissection is also necessary if the sentinel lymph node can't be identified by either of the two techniques above.

Although further research on this procedure continues, many doctors now perform sentinel node biopsy on some of their breast cancer patients.

Breast Conservation Therapy

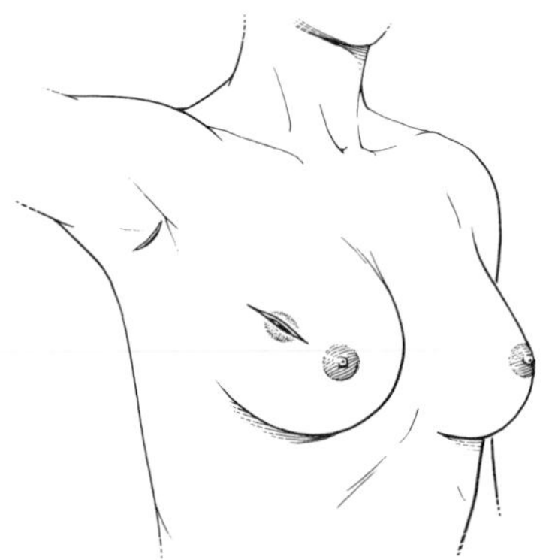

Breast conservation therapy preserves your breast following a lumpectomy and underarm (axillary) node sampling by radiating remaining breast tissue.

Modified Radical Mastectomy

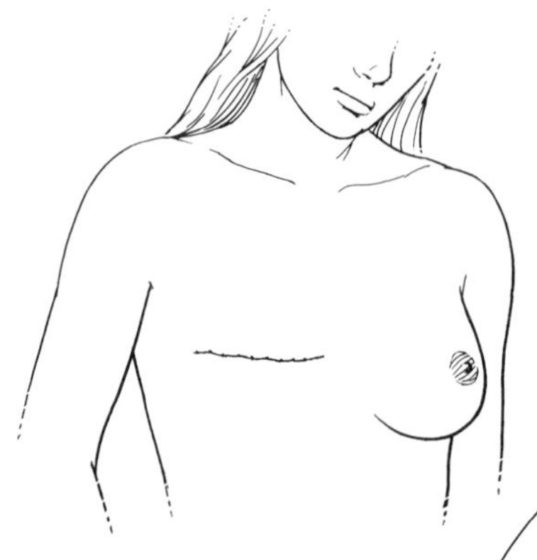

In a modified radical mastectomy, your entire breast is removed, along with one or more lymph nodes from your adjacent armpit. Chest muscles remain intact.

Breast Reconstruction

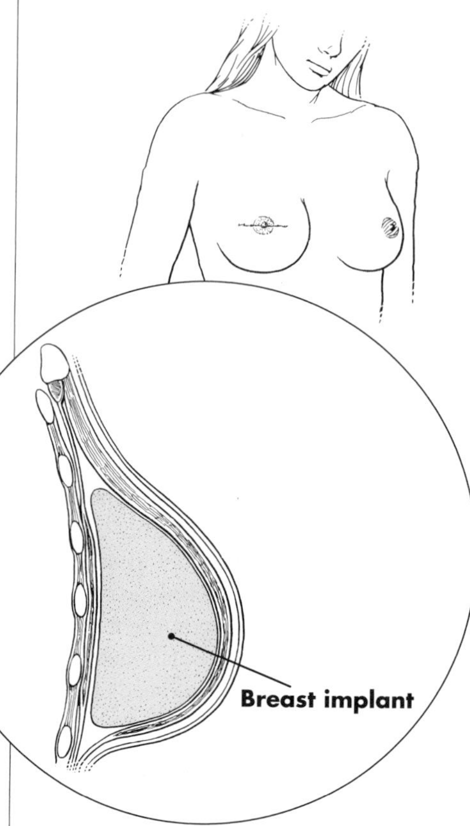

In breast reconstruction, a breast implant may be inserted beneath your chest wall muscles. The surgeon may also reconstruct the nipple and areola.

without the removal of underarm (axillary) lymph nodes. The operation is most appropriate when the cancer is in multiple sites within the breast but is confined to the ducts (carcinoma *in situ*). In this case, the risk of the cancer spreading to the lymph nodes is negligible.

Mammography isn't necessary after simple mastectomy because not enough breast tissue remains to screen. Breast self-exams and clinical breast exams are important.

Breast conservation therapy
More recent investigations have shown that the success rates for breast conservation surgery are similar to those of modified radical mastectomy. Breast conservation therapy involves removing the tumor and a small rim of normal breast tissue — a lumpectomy with a wide local excision — followed by a 6-week course of radiation to the remaining breast tissue and the lumpectomy site. With this procedure, your surgeon samples one or more underarm (axillary) lymph nodes through a separate small armpit incision, possibly using the sentinel node biopsy technique.

Subcutaneous mastectomy
In this procedure, a surgeon removes only breast tissue, sparing the skin, nipple, areola, chest wall muscles and lymph nodes. This is one of several surgical procedures plastic surgeons may perform as a preventive measure for people at high risk of breast cancer. It's less commonly used today because it leaves more breast tissue than does simple mastectomy.

Surgeons often couple this operation with placement of a breast implant to re-establish breast contour. Because of the residual breast tissue, you still need to have yearly screening mammograms.

Breast reconstruction
Many women who undergo mastectomy have breast reconstruction. Although controversy exists about the safety of prosthetic silicone implants, most studies haven't found a relationship between them and systemic disease. The Food and Drug Administration has approved the use of saline-filled silicone implants for post-mastectomy reconstruction. Tens of thousands of women have had excellent results from such procedures.

If you're reluctant to have a prosthetic implant but want reconstruction, your surgeon may reconstruct your breast from skin, fat and muscle taken from your abdominal wall or chest. This is a much more complex operation that isn't an option for everyone.

You can have breast reconstruction at the time of your mastectomy or as a separate procedure at a later time, depending on your preference and that of your surgeon. In any case, it's not a good idea to use your own nipple for reconstruction after a mastectomy for cancer because the cancer may recur in the nipple.

Plastic surgeons can reconstruct and pigment a new nipple and areola. Reconstruction doesn't interfere with chemotherapy or hormone therapy, nor does it hide cancer recurrences or increase the likelihood that your cancer will recur.

Palliative surgery
If you have widespread cancer that has gone beyond the confines of your breast and underarm area, such as to your bones, brain or liver,

a procedure called palliative surgery is done to provide tissue for laboratory analysis and some degree of tumor control.

The intent of this surgery isn't to cure the cancer but to control the growth and reduce complications. When tumors are large and ulcerating, a simple mastectomy may provide relief from pain, infection and bleeding.

Radiation therapy

If you have breast conservation surgery, you'll also need breast radiation. If you've had a mastectomy, radiation to your chest wall or underarm area may be necessary to kill any cancer cells that may have escaped surgical removal. If the breast cancer has spread to your bone, your doctor may use radiation to relieve pain.

Radiation therapy uses a high-energy X-ray focused on the area of the cancer to kill cancer cells. It's also used to shrink tumors that can't be removed surgically or, sometimes, before surgical removal.

Hormone therapy

After your surgery, you and your doctor can talk about whether you would benefit from additional therapy to prevent the growth of any cancer cells that might have spread but are undetectable. Radiation is one option.

Some cancers also respond to treatment with medications that counteract the effects of your hormones, primarily the hormone estrogen. The medication most often prescribed for breast cancer is tamoxifen (Nolvadex).

If a breast cancer is hormone receptor positive (as determined by a hormone receptor test), estrogen or, sometimes, progesterone may encourage the growth of the cancer cells. For this reason, women who are using estrogen-containing hormone replacement therapy at the time of their cancer diagnosis are usually advised to discontinue it. Drugs such as tamoxifen have an antiestrogen effect by binding to hormone receptors, thus keeping estrogen from binding to them and feeding the cancer.

Therapy to interfere with the action of hormones can stop a tumor from growing or actually cause it to shrink. If one hormone medication stops working, another may help. In this way, doctors can frequently stall the disease for years. When hormone-related therapy is no longer effective, your doctor may try another approach, usually chemotherapy.

Chemotherapy

The anticancer drugs given in chemotherapy are toxic but are beneficial for many people with breast cancer. After your initial surgery, your doctor will assess the risk of

Selecting a Surgical Procedure

It's important that you and your doctor thoroughly discuss the options available for removing your cancer and reconstructing your breast. To help you make the best decisions, check out available reading materials and, if you're still uncertain, request another opinion.

Once you've had breast cancer surgery, several self-help groups can assist you. They include Reach to Recovery, a program sponsored by the American Cancer Society. In locations where this program is in place, volunteers visit you in the hospital to provide moral support and practical advice on topics such as exercises and breast prostheses.

Monoclonal Antibodies

Biological therapy is an area of research that shows promise for treatment of cancer. Cancer may develop when your immune system functions inadequately or breaks down. Biological therapies, also known as immunotherapies, are targeted at repairing or stimulating your immune response to fight the cancer.

One type of biological therapy, called monoclonal antibodies (MOABs), includes the medication trastuzumab (Herceptin). This drug has been approved by the Food and Drug Administration for the treatment of metastatic breast cancer. It's effective on tumors that overexpress, which means that they produce excess amounts of a protein called HER-2-neu found on the surface of cancer cells. Approximately 25 percent of breast cancer tumors overproduce HER-2-neu. Herceptin, which is made in a laboratory, is given intravenously and may be used alone or with other chemotherapy agents.

MOABs may enhance the immune system of a person with cancer, interfere with the growth of cancer cells and work with anticancer drugs to deliver toxin directly to the tumor in an effort to destroy it. For more information on cancer treatment advances, see Chapter 19, "Cancer."

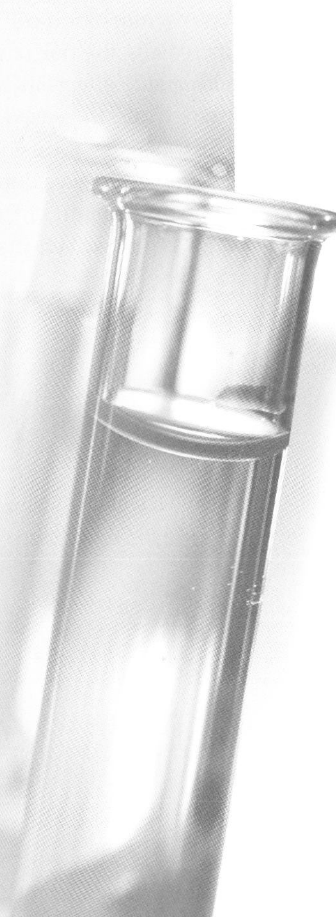

Breast Cancer in Men

Although male breast cancer is rare, it happens. Having a father or brother with the disease puts you at higher risk, whether you're male or female. To learn more about breast disorders in men, see Chapter 32, "Endocrine System."

recurrence of your breast cancer and whether you may benefit from chemotherapy. The goal of chemotherapy is to kill any breast cancer cells that might have spread to other parts of your body.

If your breast cancer recurs, then chemotherapy may stop tumor growth or cause shrinkage. This can slow the progression of your disease and relieve symptoms.

Chemotherapy frequently has unpleasant side effects. It can lower your white blood cell count, thus increasing the risk of infection. Other side effects include hair loss, nausea and increased fatigue. Doctors use various drugs in different combinations, depending on your prior treatment, overall health and risk of side effects. ■

CHAPTER 29 PART V

Digestive System

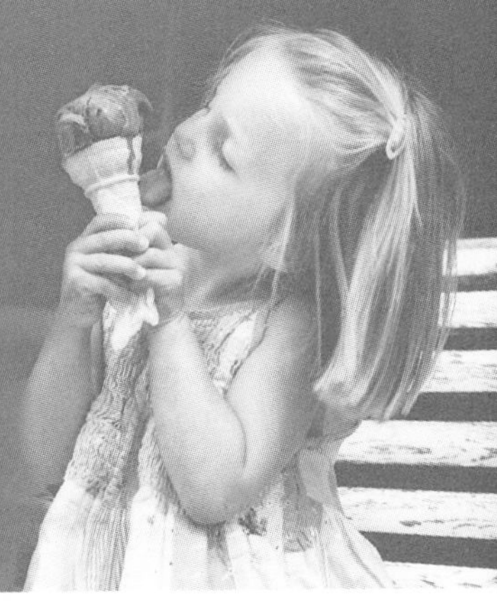

Heartburn, cramps, nausea, diarrhea, constipation — these are just a few of the ways the organs that make up your digestive system let you know when they aren't well. Most people experience these signs and symptoms on occasion. Often, they last just a day or two and then disappear. For many people, though, digestive signs and symptoms linger and become a daily annoyance.

It's estimated that one in every three Americans — perhaps even more — regularly battle some kind of digestive problem. You can see the evidence in your local drug, grocery or discount store. Shelves are lined with an increasing array of medicines for digestive conditions: antacids, acid blockers, laxatives, fiber supplements and antidiarrheals.

A general overview of how digestion works might help you understand why digestive problems are so common.

Your digestive system is much more than your stomach and intestines. It's a complex system of organs that conveys and converts the food you eat into the energy you need. Because of this, digestion is one of the critical functions your body performs.

Your Digestive System at Work

Digestion begins even before you take your first bite. The aroma of the food you're about to eat — or even the mere thought of eating — is enough to start saliva flowing in your mouth.

Once you take a bite, your salivary glands kick into high gear pumping out juices that begin to chemically break down the food. Not all of the work is chemical, though. Your teeth crunch and grind the food, while your tongue mixes it with saliva.

Your saliva contains the enzyme ptyalin that begins to change starches (carbohydrates) into sugars. Chewing reduces the food to a mushy consistency. When you swallow, the food is propelled into the back part of your throat, past the opening of the voice box (larynx), and into the upper part of your esophagus.

Food is prevented from entering your larynx and air passages by a flap of soft tissue (epiglottis) that closes as food passes into the esophagus. If the epiglottis fails to close completely, a brief coughing fit may result, commonly referred to as food having "gone down the wrong way." This coughing has a protective function in that it brings food and saliva back into your mouth, preventing this material from going down your windpipe (trachea) and into your lungs.

Esophagus

The esophagus is a tube approximately 10 inches long that leads directly into the stomach. The food is moved into your esophagus by muscles in the back of your throat (pharynx). When it enters the main part of the esophagus, muscles there undergo a series of wave-like contractions, called peristalsis, to move the food into your stomach. Peristalsis is also the mechanism by which the food moves throughout the remainder of its trip through your digestive tract until the waste products reach the muscles of the anus.

A muscle that encircles the bottom portion of the esophagus (lower esophageal sphincter) is critical in the passage of food into your stomach. When this valve-like sphincter relaxes, it opens and permits food to enter your stomach. It then closes, preventing food from re-entering your esophagus (regurgitating). When this sphincter fails to work properly and acidic stomach contents regurgitate into the esophagus, the sensitive lining of your esophagus is damaged. If this occurs, you may experience the symptoms of heartburn. Frequent heartburn is a symptom of a common condition called gastroesophageal reflux disease (GERD).

Stomach

The walls of your stomach consist primarily of various layers of powerful muscles. These muscles cause the stomach to churn, breaking food into smaller and smaller pieces. At the same time, gastric juices manufactured by glands that line your stomach mix with the food particles. These juices contain pepsin, a digestive enzyme that breaks down proteins in the mixture, and hydrochloric acid, which provides pepsin with the proper chemical environment.

There's a delicate balance in your stomach between the acid produced by its glands and the resistance of your stomach lining to that acid. If this balance is upset, the result may be damage to the stomach lining, causing a peptic ulcer or a diffuse inflammation known as gastritis.

Food leaves your stomach in two phases. The upper portion of your stomach contracts first, pushing liquid material into your small intestine. The more solid contents leave later, primarily by the action of the muscles in the lower part of your stomach. This partially processed food (chyme) then travels through the adjoining pyloric canal into the first portion of your small intestine, called the duodenum. Very little food is actually absorbed by your stomach — only small amounts of alcohol, simple sugars and some medications.

Small intestine

The small intestine (small bowel) is a tube whose length in adults varies from 12 to 22 feet, depending on the tone of its muscular wall and the way it's measured.

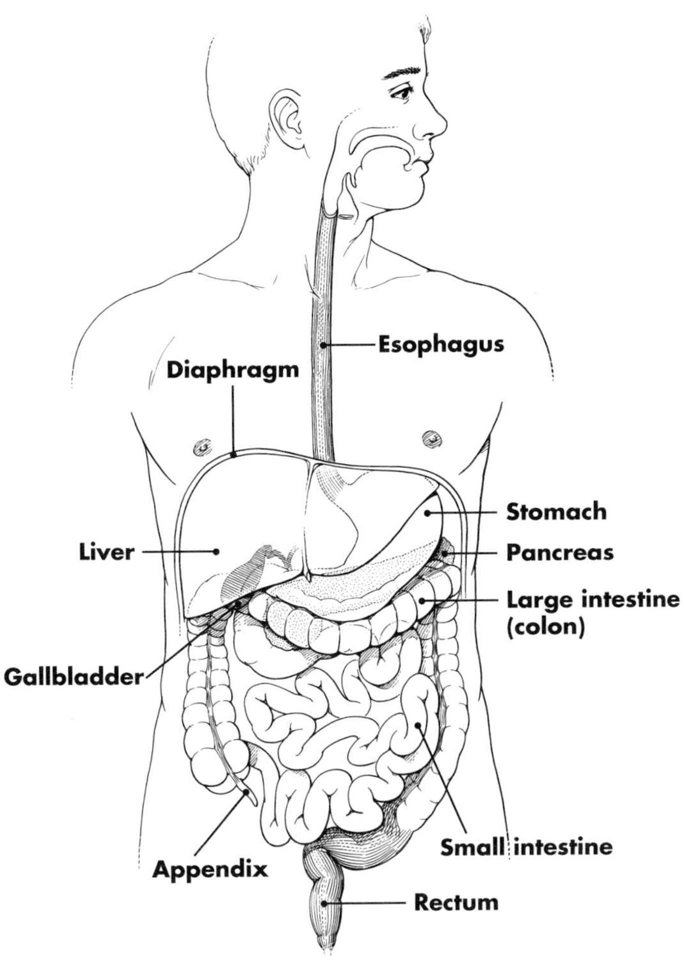

The small intestine is divided into three parts. The duodenum is the first and shortest part, and it's here that the absorption process truly begins. The jejunum, the middle and largest portion of the small intestine, is where the majority of absorption takes place. The final section of the small intestine, the ileum, also has important absorptive functions (vitamin B-12, for example). It's also responsible for the passage of food into the large intestine.

The duodenum contributes to the mixing of food material and also neutralizes acid coming from your stomach. Bile tubes (ducts) from the liver and gallbladder and the pancreatic duct from the pancreas empty their digestive juices into the duodenum to prepare the chyme for maximum absorption.

As the semisolid food continues its movement through your small intestine, it undergoes further digestion by various enzymes. In this process, the food is broken into smaller components that can be absorbed through the lining of the small intestine and enter your bloodstream. Starches are converted to simple sugars, and proteins are broken down into amino acids. Fats are broken down by enzymes from the pancreas. Because of their detergent-like properties, bile acids from the liver make the fat molecules soluble in water so that they can then be absorbed into your bloodstream. In addition, minerals, vitamins, water and electrolytes, such as sodium and calcium, are absorbed through the wall of the small intestine and into your bloodstream.

By the time the food is ready to pass into your large intestine, most of its nutrients have already been absorbed.

Large intestine

Once food residue reaches the large intestine (large bowel, or colon), the role of your digestive system changes. Now its job is to process the waste, consisting mainly of undigested and nonabsorbed food, fiber and water.

Liquid (primarily water) from the small intestine is carried into the colon where most of it is absorbed into the bloodstream. Your colon is extremely efficient at this. Of the approximately 1 quart of fluid that enters it every day, nearly 80 percent is absorbed before reaching the anus.

The rest of the waste material moves through the three major segments of your colon — right (ascending), transverse and left (descending) colon — then into the S-shaped sigmoid colon located in the lower-left abdomen. Finally the waste material moves into the last 4 to 6 inches of the colon (rectum). It's here that the material collects until defecation.

Liver

Your liver produces bile, a fluid containing cholesterol and bile acids. Bile flows from the liver and through the cystic duct into your gallbladder, where it's concentrated and stored. Bile is eventually emptied into the duodenum following meals, where it performs its major function of assisting in the absorption of fats through the lining of the small intestine into the bloodstream. Bile acids are then reabsorbed by the small intestine — mostly in the ileum — and recycled into the liver to be used again.

The liver has other functions as well. One of these is the storage of glycogen, a complex carbohydrate that's converted to sugar for release into your bloodstream when your blood sugar level falls. Glycogen is deposited in the liver when the level of sugar in the blood increases. Many proteins are synthesized in the liver.

The liver also helps determine the amount of nutrients that are sent to the rest of your body. It serves as a clearinghouse to eliminate some foods and substances that have served their purpose and are no longer useful. In addition, your liver breaks down some medications to enable them to be eliminated in the stool. Alcohol is metabolized in the liver to supply energy or to be deposited as fat.

Gallbladder

The gallbladder is a pear-shaped organ that sits beneath the liver. It's a storage site for much of the bile produced in the liver. Bile enters the gallbladder through the cystic duct and is stored there until needed for the digestion of fats.

Although the gallbladder serves a useful function, it's not vital to maintaining normal body functions because bile can be delivered directly from the liver ducts into the duodenum.

Pancreas

Shaped somewhat like a banana only wider, the pancreas stretches from your duodenum, to which its head is attached, to the spleen. This organ produces two kinds of secretions — those that are released into the duodenum and those that pass directly into your bloodstream. The first type is called pancreatic juice. It aids in the digestion of fats, proteins and some carbohydrates. The other type includes the hormones insulin and glucagon, which regulate the metabolism of blood sugar (glucose).

Esophageal Disorders

Your esophagus is the muscular tube that leads directly into your stomach, transporting food from your throat to your stomach. Many conditions can affect the esophagus and interfere with swallowing or the transport of food from your mouth to your stomach.

Gastroesophageal reflux disease

Signs and symptoms

- A burning sensation in the chest, often beginning in the upper abdomen and radiating into the neck
- Regurgitation of sour or bitter-tasting material into the throat and mouth, especially when lying down
- Chest pain
- Persistent coughing
- Bleeding
- Difficulty swallowing

Nearly everyone experiences heartburn, that burning sensation in the chest — and sometimes the throat — from stomach acid that washes back into the esophagus. An occasional episode of heartburn is generally nothing to worry about. Many people, though, battle heartburn regularly, even daily. Frequent heartburn can be a serious problem, and it deserves medical attention. Most often, frequent heartburn is a symptom of gastroesophageal reflux disease (GERD).

When you eat, food travels down your esophagus to a muscular valve that separates your lower esophagus and stomach. Called the lower esophageal sphincter, this valve opens to allow food to pass into your stomach and then closes again.

Sometimes, though, the sphincter muscle relaxes (opens) at the wrong time, allowing acidic stomach contents to re-enter the esophagus, producing the symptoms commonly referred to as heartburn. When the acid regurgitates into your upper esophagus, it leaves a sour taste

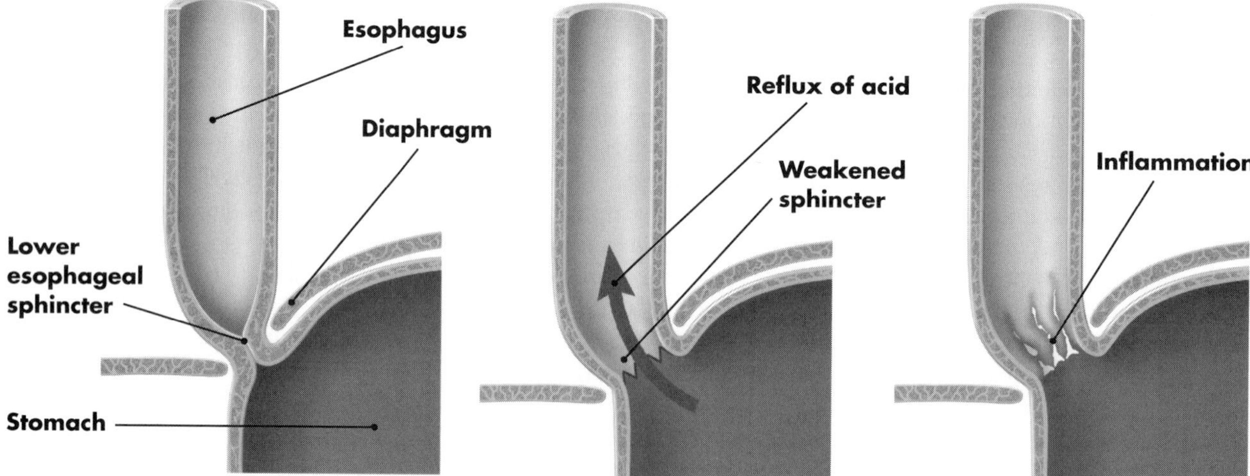

Normally, the lower esophageal sphincter remains closed, preventing acidic stomach contents from washing into the esophagus. If the sphincter weakens or relaxes, stomach contents can enter the esophagus, causing heartburn and tissue inflammation.

Hiatal Hernia

Your chest is separated from your abdomen by a dome-shaped sheet of muscle called the diaphragm. To reach your stomach, your esophagus has to pass through an opening (hiatus) in the diaphragm.

When tissues around the hiatus weaken, part of the stomach may protrude through the opening into the chest cavity. This is termed hiatal hernia. Hiatal hernia is thought to result from a weakening of the anchoring tissues at the junction to the diaphragm, possibly due to increased pressure within the abdomen, such as with obesity.

Hiatal hernias are common. About 25 percent of all people older than age 50 have a hiatal hernia. Because the majority of these hernias produce no signs or symptoms, they usually go undetected. In fact, they're often found incidentally on a chest X-ray where part of the stomach can be seen in the chest cavity. Hiatal hernias are frequently found in people with heartburn who undergo barium X-ray studies. It's unlikely that a small hiatal hernia will cause serious problems, and by itself it isn't a dangerous ailment.

Large hernias, in which a substantial portion of the stomach is above the diaphragm, can cause slow bleeding and iron deficiency anemia. One potential but extremely rare danger of a very large hernia is strangulation of the stomach, in which the herniated stomach becomes so tightly constricted that its blood supply is severely reduced. Symptoms typically include persistent chest pain and difficulty swallowing. This is a medical emergency and may require prompt surgery.

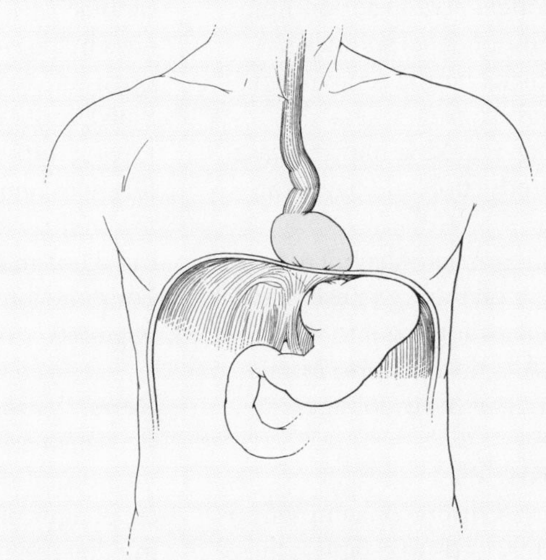

In hiatal hernia, a portion of the stomach protrudes through the diaphragm into the chest cavity.

in your mouth and may cause you to cough.

The constant backwash of acid can irritate the lining of the esophagus causing it to inflame, a condition called esophagitis.

Over time, the inflammation can narrow or erode the esophagus, producing bleeding, difficulty swallowing or chest pain. Gastroesophageal reflux disease is the name for chronic acid reflux that causes esophagitis.

Anyone can have GERD, even children and infants. However, the condition is more common in people older than age 40. The condition is also common in pregnant women because of hormonal changes and increased pressure within the abdomen.

Factors that can significantly increase GERD include:

- *Being overweight.* Many, but not all, people with GERD are overweight. Excess weight puts extra pressure on your stomach and diaphragm, the large muscle that separates your chest and abdomen, forcing open the lower esophageal sphincter. Eating very large or high-fat meals may produce similar effects.
- *Family history.* Mayo Clinic researchers believe that a genetic link predisposes some people to the disease. If your parents or siblings have or had GERD, your chances of having the condition increase.
- *Hiatal hernia.* Hiatal hernia is a condition in which part of your stomach protrudes into your

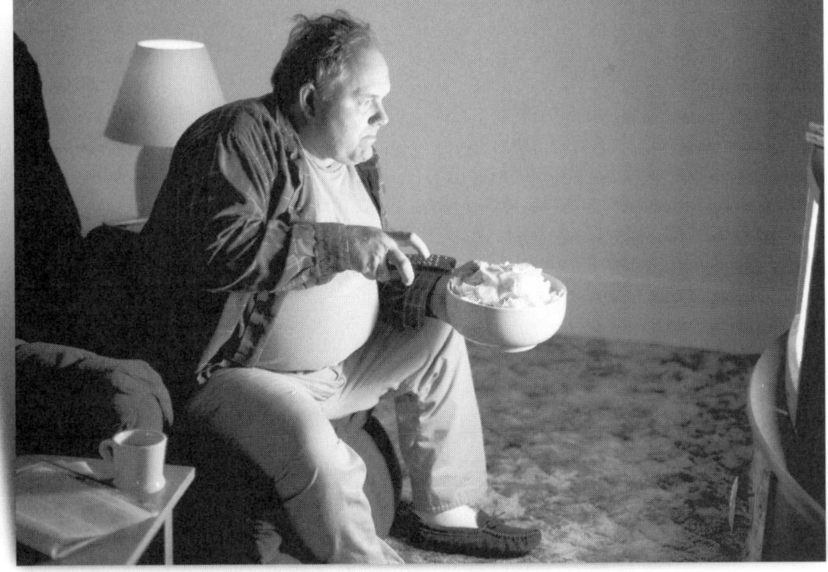

lower chest, and your diaphragm is no longer able to support the lower esophageal sphincter. A large hiatal hernia can worsen acid reflux.
- *Smoking.* Smoking may increase acid production and aggravate reflux.
- *Excessive alcohol.* Alcohol reduces pressure on the lower esophageal sphincter, allowing it to relax and open. Alcohol may also irritate the lining of the esophagus.

Diagnosis

Often, a description of symptoms is all a doctor needs to establish the diagnosis of GERD. However, if symptoms are particularly severe or don't respond to treatment, tests such as a barium X-ray of the esophagus and stomach or an endoscopic examination of your upper gastrointestinal tract may be necessary. An ambulatory acid (pH) probe also may be done to measure the acid levels in your upper and lower esophagus. See Chapter 39, "Diagnostic Tests," for more information on these tests.

How serious is gastro-esophageal reflux disease?

Occasional heartburn can be uncomfortable, but it generally isn't a serious problem. GERD, however, is a serious condition that requires treatment. Left untreated it can lead to one or more of the following complications:

Esophageal narrowing

Esophageal narrowing (stricture) occurs in about 10 percent of people with GERD. Damage to cells in the lower esophagus from acid exposure leads to formation of scar tissue. The scar tissue narrows the food pathway and can interfere with swallowing, causing food to get caught in the narrowing.

Treatment for stricture typically consists of a procedure that stretches tissues and widens the esophagus followed by acid-suppressing medication to help prevent renarrowing.

Ulcer

Stomach acid can severely erode tissues in the esophagus, causing an open sore to form. The ulcer may bleed, cause pain and make swallowing difficult. Medication and lifestyle changes to control stomach acid reflux can cure an ulcer by giving damaged tissues time to heal. For more information on ulcers, see page 860.

Barrett's esophagus

Persistent acid reflux can damage the normal skin-like lining of the esophagus, replacing it with a lining that resembles that of the stomach or small intestine. This abnormal development of tissue is called metaplasia.

Metaplasia is brought on by repeated and long-term exposure to stomach acid and is associated with an increased risk of esophageal cancer. About 5 percent of people with GERD have Barrett's esophagus. Once you have it, your chances of having esophageal cancer are significantly higher than that of the general population.

Treatment for Barrett's esophagus generally includes lifestyle changes and medication to control acid reflux. Your doctor may also want to periodically examine the lining of your esophagus to increase the chance of detecting and treating abnormal (precancerous) cells at an early stage.

If tests indicate that you have a precancerous condition known as high-grade dysplasia, your doctor may recommend treatment to prevent the development of cancer. Treatment may involve burning away the abnormal tissue or surgery to remove a portion of the esophagus.

Other

Other complications of GERD include laryngitis, bronchitis and aspiration pneumonia.

Treatment

Regardless of the severity of the disease, the first step in managing GERD is to change certain lifestyle habits. For mild symptoms, a change in habits may be all that's needed to manage the disease. For more severe symptoms, lifestyle changes can make your condition easier to control with medication.

Self-care

You can take several steps to help relieve GERD symptoms:
- *Don't smoke.* Smoking increases acid reflux and dries your saliva. Saliva helps protect your esophagus from stomach acid.

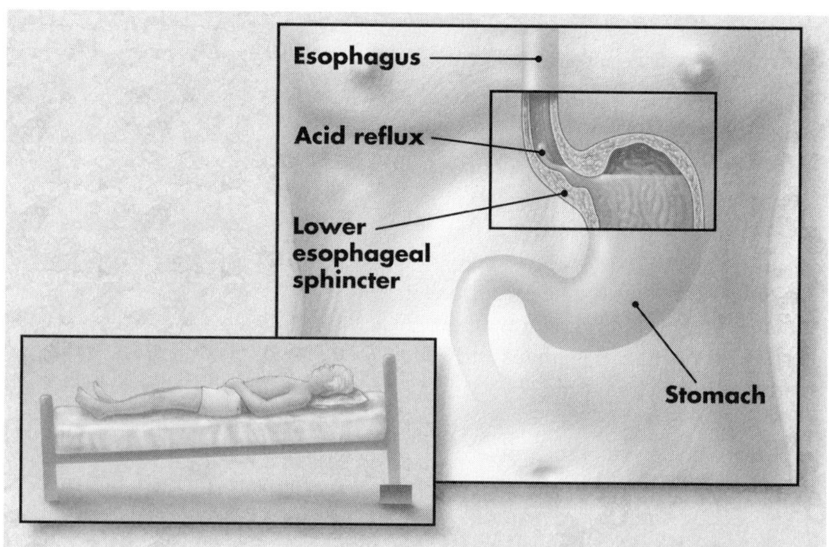

Raising the head of your bed helps keep acid in your stomach while you sleep. Place a 4-inch block under the feet at the head of the bed.

- *Eat smaller meals.* This reduces pressure on the lower esophageal sphincter, helping to prevent the valve from opening and acid from washing back into your esophagus.
- *Sit up after you eat.* After eating wait at least 3 hours before going to bed or taking a nap. By then most of the food in your stomach will have emptied into the small intestine, so it can't flow back into your esophagus.
- *Don't exercise immediately after a meal.* After a meal wait 2 to 3 hours before engaging in strenuous activity.
- *Limit fatty foods.* Studies show a potentially strong link between consumption of fat and GERD. Fatty foods relax the lower esophageal sphincter, allowing stomach acid into the esophagus. Fat also slows stomach emptying, increasing the length of time acid can regurgitate.
- *Avoid problem foods and beverages.* These may include caffeinated drinks, chocolate, onions, spicy foods and mint. They tend to increase production of stomach acid and relax the lower esophageal sphincter. Also limit citrus fruits and tomatoes and tomato-based foods. They're acidic and can irritate an inflamed esophagus, making GERD symptoms worse.
- *Limit or avoid alcohol.* Alcohol relaxes the lower esophageal sphincter and may irritate the esophagus, worsening symptoms.
- *Lose excess weight.* Heartburn and acid regurgitation are more likely to occur when there's added pressure on your stomach from excess weight.
- *Elevate the head of your bed.* Raise the head of your bed 6 to 9 inches. This provides a gradual incline from your feet to your head and helps prevent acid from flowing back into your esophagus as you sleep. Place a foam wedge under the mattress to raise it. Or put blocks of wood under the legs at the head of your bed.
- *Avoid tight-fitting clothes.* They put pressure on your stomach.
- *Take time to relax.* When you're under stress, digestion slows, worsening GERD symptoms. Although not scientifically proved, relaxation techniques, such as deep breathing, meditation and yoga, may improve GERD by reducing stress.

Medication

For people with more severe symptoms, medication is generally the main line of treatment. Drugs used to treat GERD include:

- *Antacids.* Available over-the-counter, antacids (Maalox, Rolaids, others) neutralize gastric acid and provide quick, temporary relief. Antacids can relieve your symptoms, but they don't eliminate all reflux. These products are generally safe, but if taken regularly they can cause side effects such as diarrhea and constipation. Some of them can also interfere with other medications taken for kidney or heart disease.
- *Acid blockers.* Also known as histamine (H-2) blockers, these medications are available both over-the-counter and by prescription. Instead of neutralizing acid, they reduce acid secretion. Acid blockers include cimetidine (Tagamet), ranitidine (Zantac), famotidine (Pepcid) and nizatidine (Axid). The advantage of acid blockers is that they help prevent acid secretion, rather than just neutralizing acid. Acid blockers are generally safe, but some may interact with other medications. Check with your doctor or pharmacist for possible drug interactions.
- *Proton pump inhibitors.* These medications are most often prescribed for severe symptoms. They're the most effective in preventing acid secretion and in treatment of GERD. Examples of proton pump inhibitors include lansoprazole (Prevacid), omeprazole (Prilosec), rabeprazole (Aciphex), pantoprazole (Protonix) and esomeprazole (Nexium). They inhibit acid production and allow time for damaged esophageal tissue to heal. In clinical trials, proton pump inhibitors have been found safe to use for at least 10 years. Using the lowest effective dosage can help prevent side effects of the medication, such as abdominal pain, diarrhea and headache.

Surgery

Only about 5 percent of adults with GERD continue to have severe symptoms or have complications despite medication and lifestyle changes. Few require surgery anymore.

The most common type of surgery for GERD is a procedure called Nissen fundoplication. It involves tightening the lower esophageal sphincter to prevent reflux by wrapping the very top portion of the stomach around the outside of the lower esophagus. Often, this surgery can be performed laparoscopically — a less invasive form of surgery in which a few small incisions are made in the abdomen instead of one large one.

Two other procedures used to treat GERD may become alternatives to medications and more invasive surgery. One of the procedures involves the use of a device that works like a miniature sewing machine to place stitches (sutures) near the weakened sphincter. The suturing material is then tied together, creating barriers to

Hiccups

Holding your breath, swallowing water from the wrong side of the glass, breathing in and out of a paper bag, eating a spoonful of sugar or having someone startle you. These all are common — and not necessarily successful — methods of getting rid of the hiccups, a generally minor complaint that afflicts almost everyone from time to time.

For the most part, hiccups are harmless and resolve in a short time. On rare occasions, hiccups may persist for days or even weeks. When this occurs, they can interfere with eating and sleeping. Following major surgery, a prolonged case of the hiccups can impede the healing of an abdominal wound. In a few instances, persistent hiccups can be a sign of a serious disorder.

Although almost everyone has had hiccups, few people know exactly what they are. Very simply, hiccups are repeated, involuntary contractions of your diaphragm, the muscle that separates the chest from the abdomen. The phrenic nerves control the smooth, coordinated, normal contraction of the two flaps of the diaphragm for breathing. The phrenic nerves extend from the neck to the chest. Hiccups may result from irritation anywhere along the path of a phrenic nerve. Reflex contraction of the diaphragm similarly can be the result of irritation to nerves.

Hiccups are more likely to occur when your stomach is distended, typically after eating a big meal or drinking an overabundance of alcohol. As for a cure, try this: Massage the back portion of the roof of your mouth with a cotton-tipped swab, moving the swab gently back and forth for a minute or so. There's no guarantee this method will work, but it often does.

prevent stomach contents from washing into the esophagus.

The other procedure uses controlled radiofrequency energy to heat and coagulate tissues within the portion of the esophagus that contains the malfunctioning valve. The procedure causes scarring that can help tighten the valve.

These procedures take an hour or less to perform, don't require incisions and allow you to go home the same day. Neither are recommended if you have a hiatal hernia or Barrett's esophagus.

Other causes of esophagitis

In addition to GERD, other disorders can cause inflammation of the esophagus.

Scleroderma of the esophagus

Scleroderma is a disease characterized by an overgrowth of scar-like tissue, causing stiffening and hardening of tissues. This condition can weaken the lower esophageal sphincter, allowing acid to reflux into the esophagus and causing symptoms and complications similar to those of GERD.

Your doctor may prescribe an acid-blocking medication to reduce acid reflux. He or she may also instruct you in self-care measures to prevent reflux (see page 852). If constriction of the esophagus prevents or retards the passage of food, a procedure to widen (dilate) the esophagus may be necessary.

Herpes simplex esophagitis

Infection from the herpes simplex virus can cause inflammation and ulcers in the esophagus. People who develop this condition are often debilitated from another disease or have a weakened immune system. The antiviral drug acyclovir (Zovirax) may be helpful in treating herpes simplex esophagitis.

Candida esophagitis

The fungus candida growing in the esophagus can cause inflammation and painful swallowing. This is called candida esophagitis. Such an infection often occurs in people whose immune systems are weakened, for example, as a result of medications used to fight cancer. Several antifungal medications can treat candida esophagitis.

Radiation esophagitis

Inflammation of the esophagus can result from radiation treatment for cancer, most commonly lung or esophageal cancer. Symptoms include heartburn and pain when swallowing. The likelihood of this disorder increases in direct relation to the amount of radiation received. With the help of medication, the inflammation usually resolves once the radiation treatment is stopped.

Pill esophagitis

Acute pain in the front of the chest made worse by swallowing can result from pills or capsules that stick in the esophagus and dissolve or break open before entering the stomach. Common culprits include tetracycline antibiotics, potassium, vitamin C and iron medications and some arthritis drugs. The condition is preventable by taking medications with plenty of water and not lying down right after taking a medication. Pill esophagitis usually gets better on its own within a few days.

Swallowing difficulties

Signs and symptoms

- Liquids and solid foods stick in the throat or chest
- Regurgitation of food
- A gurgling sound in the throat
- Chest discomfort on swallowing

Emergency signs and symptoms

- An inability to swallow liquids or solids
- Drooling saliva

The causes of persistent swallowing problems vary. Damage or malfunction of the muscles in the wall of the throat or esophagus can cause swallowing difficulties. Ulcers or scar tissue in the esophagus as the result of stomach acid reflux can be another cause.

Pouches (diverticula) may form in the esophageal lining and interfere with the movement of food down the esophagus. Sometimes, swallowing difficulties are associated with diseases such as myasthenia gravis and cancer. In addition, the muscles that line your esophagus and propel food to your stomach can weaken with age, making it more difficult for you to swallow.

Swallowing difficulty may be transient and unimportant, but it's always possible that the problem is an indication of a serious medical condition. Therefore, see your doctor if you continue to have painful or difficult swallowing.

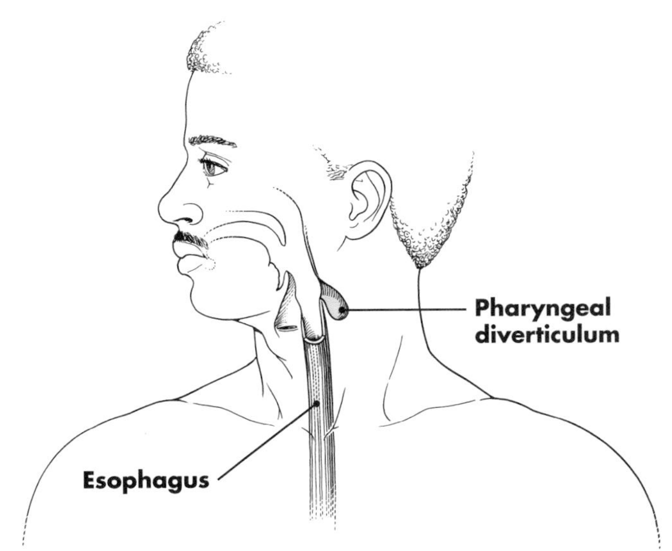

When the muscular wall of your throat (pharynx) weakens, a small pouch, called a pharyngeal diverticulum, may form and trap food or liquids.

Achalasia

Achalasia is a rare disorder of the esophagus caused by lack of coordinated movement of the muscles of the esophagus and the sphincter muscle at the lower end of the esophagus. The disorder makes it very difficult for food and liquids to pass into the stomach.

People with achalasia often regurgitate food. Sometimes, particularly in the early stages, drinking a large amount of liquid helps to push the food into the stomach. Eventually, however, this fails to help. Some chest discomfort or pain also may occur, although heartburn is unusual. The underlying cause of the condition isn't fully known.

If you have signs or symptoms of achalasia, your doctor may order a series of tests, possibly including a barium X-ray or an esophageal muscle test, to determine if the esophageal muscles are functioning properly. A procedure called upper endoscopy also may be done to rule out cancer. See Chapter 39, "Diagnostic Tests" for more information on these tests.

If achalasia is left untreated for several decades, esophageal cancer may develop. Malnutrition, weight loss and aspiration of food into the lungs, leading to pneumonia, are other problems associated with achalasia. Medication can be helpful in some instances, but it often has little effect. Sometimes, a muscle relaxant derived from botulinum toxin (Botox) can be injected by endoscopy into the lower end of the esophagus, allowing food to pass more easily.

A form of treatment for achalasia involves mechanical stretching of the esophageal muscles. A slender tube with a balloon attached is passed down the esophagus to the narrowed area. The balloon is filled with water or air under pressure to expand the balloon and stretch open (dilate) the passageway. Balloon dilation weakens the lower esophageal sphincter so that food can pass down the esophagus by gravity. Following this treatment, coordinated contractions in the esophagus don't return to normal, but most people can swallow better.

A surgical procedure called esophagomyotomy is another option. In this procedure, a surgeon opens the chest and partially cuts the muscles at the lower end of the esophagus to allow easier passage of food. Risks of this operation are low, and long-term results generally are good. Some newer techniques involve less invasive (laparoscopic) surgery, allowing speedier recovery and earlier return to normal activities.

Diffuse spasm

Diffuse spasm is the term for multiple high-pressure, poorly coordinated contractions of the esophagus that usually occur after swallowing. This is another rare disorder of unknown cause that affects the smooth (involuntary) muscles in the walls of the lower esophagus.

Signs and symptoms can be mild and may even disappear without treatment. You may mistake the symptoms for simple heartburn. Sometimes, acid reflux can trigger spasm. With this condition, signs and symptoms often occur intermittently over a period of years and then become more severe. A procedure called balloon dilation can widen (dilate) the esophagus and may produce relief initially. Occasionally surgery is necessary.

Pharyngeal diverticula

When muscles in the wall of the throat (pharynx) weaken, especially with aging, pouches called diverticula can form, sometimes becoming large enough to trap food. This is especially true when the upper esophageal sphincter doesn't function properly.

With pharyngeal diverticula, also known as Zenker's diverticulum, your throat may become irritated, you may notice a gurgling sound, and you may regurgitate food particles shortly after eating. As the pouches grow larger, food that's retained for days may give you bad breath. There's also a risk that fluid and regurgitated food will be inhaled into the lungs (aspirated), increasing the risk of a lung infection, such as pneumonia.

For large diverticula that produce troublesome symptoms, surgical removal of the diverticula, often combined with surgery to the upper esophageal sphincter, is the most common treatment. Diverticula can also occur in the esophagus, but they rarely cause problems.

Pharyngeal paralysis

The principal characteristics of pharyngeal paralysis are weakness and lack of coordination of the muscles of the throat (pharynx), which cause swallowing difficulty. People with this problem have trouble getting food from their mouth into their throat and esophagus. In addition to swallowing difficulty and throat discomfort, this disorder may result in inhalation of food or fluids (aspiration) into the windpipe (trachea) or regurgitation of food or fluids into the nose.

The symptoms are thought to be the result of faulty transmission of nerve impulses to the muscles in the pharynx and are often due to one of several neurologic disorders.

Tests to establish a diagnosis of pharyngeal paralysis may include a barium X-ray or an esophageal motility study. A procedure called upper gastrointestinal endoscopy may be performed to eliminate other possible causes. See Chapter 39, "Diagnostic Tests," for more information on these tests.

If the paralysis is due to a neurologic disease, it may respond to treatment for the disease. People recovering from a stroke often experience improvement over time. Surgery is rarely effective.

Gastrostomy

When the swallowing mechanism of your throat (pharynx) or upper esophagus is disabled, you may be unable to eat properly, preventing you from getting adequate nutrition. Another method is needed to deliver food to your stomach.

This can be done by placement of a tube into the stomach, a procedure called gastrostomy. The tube bypasses the pharynx and esophagus, allowing nutrients to go directly into the stomach, where they pass into the small intestine for digestion and absorption. Sometimes, an extension of this tube is placed directly into the small intestine.

With this type of feeding mechanism, often referred to as a feeding tube, you can receive adequate calories to maintain nutrition.

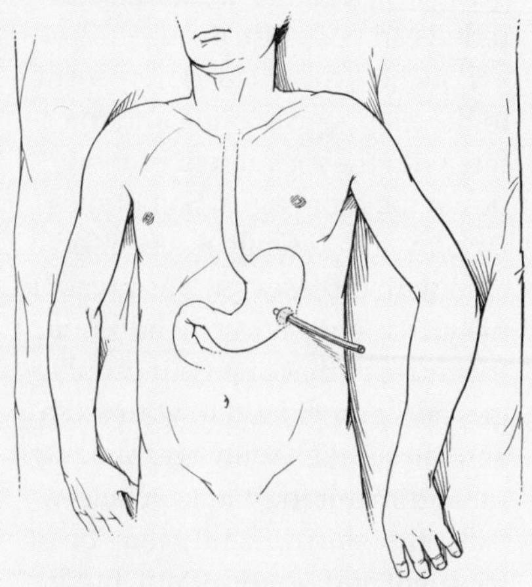

A gastrostomy (feeding) tube allows an individual to receive food directly into the stomach.

Your doctor or dietitian will instruct you in proper feeding techniques, including the amount of calories to be infused to ensure adequate nutrition.

If the ability to swallow returns, the feeding tube can be removed.

Many people with pharyngeal paralysis require a temporary feeding tube (nasogastric tube), which runs through the nose to the stomach. Sometimes, a feeding tube is placed directly through the abdominal wall into the stomach, a procedure called gastrostomy. This bypasses the affected area in the pharynx or esophagus and allows use of the remaining gastrointestinal tract for proper digestion.

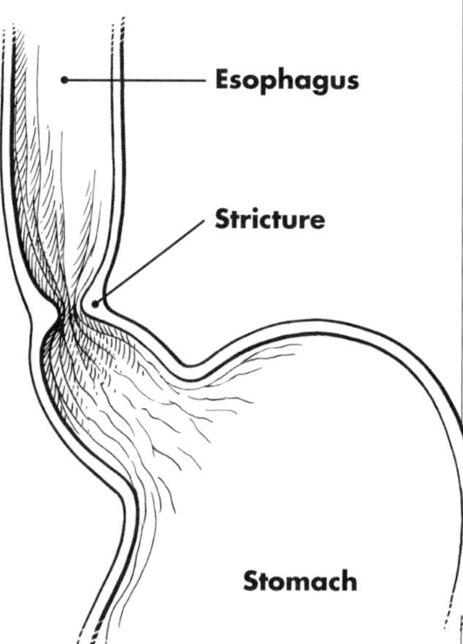

Narrowing of the passageway of the esophagus is called an esophageal stricture. This can cause difficulty in swallowing.

Globus

Some people experience the sensation of a lump in their throat without having any problem swallowing their food. This disorder is called globus. At times, it may be the result of stress.

If your doctor suspects globus, as part of your examination he or she may ask you to identify any possible source of stress in your life. Often times, relief of stress eliminates the problem.

Esophageal stricture

Signs and symptoms

- Difficulty swallowing

Esophageal stricture is a narrowing of the passageway of the esophagus, so food and even liquids can't pass through without difficulty. The main cause of a stricture in adults is scar tissue caused by reflux of stomach acids (see page 850). Scar tissue can also result from other causes, including radiation, previous esophageal surgery or ingestion of caustic chemicals.

An esophageal web, a network of thin membranes across the esophagus, also can narrow the upper end of the esophagus. For unknown reasons, this condition is more likely to appear in middle-aged women and may be associated with iron deficiency.

Difficulty in swallowing is usually noted with solids only. Another condition that can cause esophageal constriction is a mucosal ring. This may occur near the lower esophageal sphincter. This disorder also causes difficulty in swallowing solids.

Diagnosis

To determine the cause of your swallowing difficulty and to identify the stricture, your doctor may perform a variety of tests, including an upper endoscopic examination and a barium X-ray. For more information on these tests, see Chapter 39, "Diagnostic Tests."

Treatment

One form of treatment for an esophageal stricture is a procedure in which the narrowed passageway is opened with a dilator. The dilator stretches the scar tissue, web or ring.

Before this procedure, you need to fast for at least 6 to 8 hours. A topical anesthetic is generally applied to the lining of your throat. You may also receive a sedative. A thin, flexible instrument called a fiber-optic endoscope is inserted into your esophagus to perform the procedure.

In one method, a guide wire is inserted through the endoscope and then the endoscope is withdrawn. Progressively larger dilators are threaded along the length of the wire and through the stricture, to force open the passageway. At times, balloons are attached to the guide wire and are moved to the point of the narrowing. There they are inflated, helping to open the passageway.

Dilation is generally quite safe, but for a few hours after the procedure you may feel a little tightness or discomfort in your chest or some pain when you swallow. The benefit of dilation is that it permits blocked food and fluids to move freely through the esophagus and into the stomach. Repeat dilations may be necessary from time to time. Surgery is rarely necessary to treat a stricture.

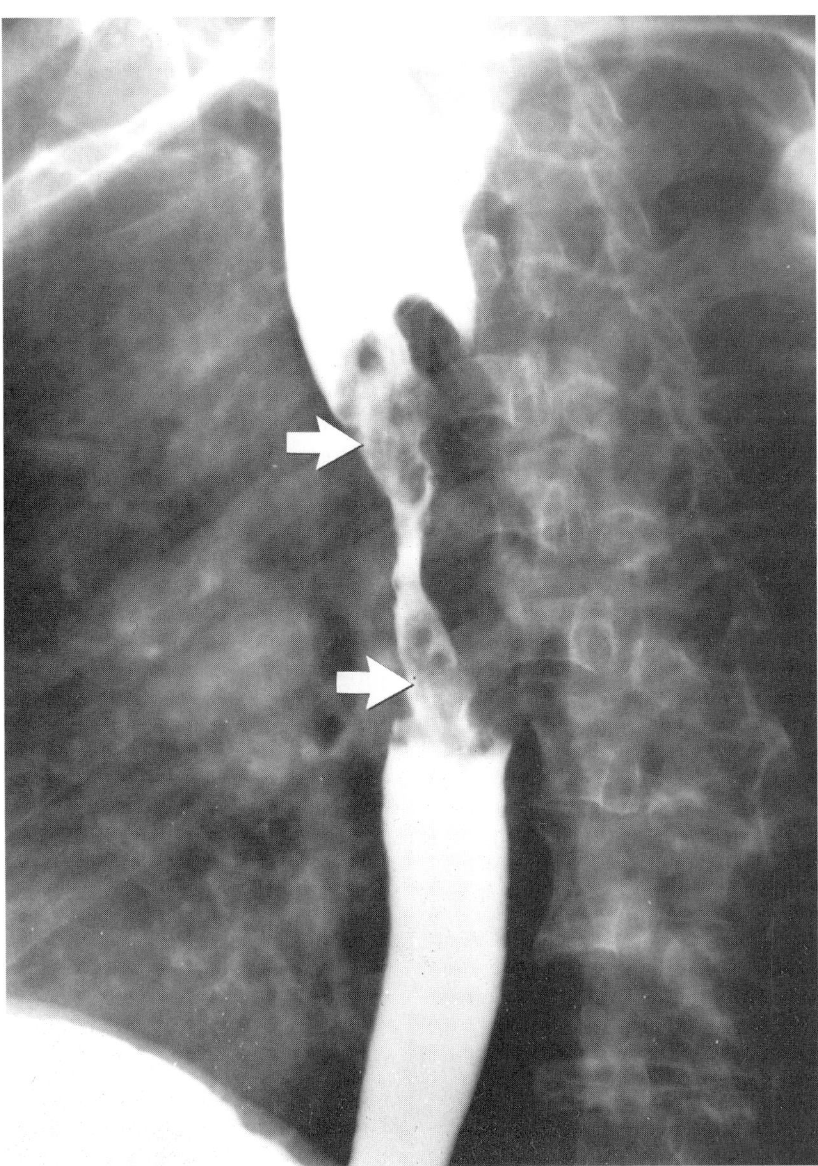

A barium X-ray reveals narrowing of the esophagus (see arrows) caused by a cancerous tumor.

Foreign bodies

Signs and symptoms

- Difficulty swallowing
- A complete inability to swallow liquids or solids
- Drooling saliva

Emergency signs and symptoms

- Inability to breathe or to utter a sound
- Pale and clammy skin

Sometimes, food, such as a large piece of meat or bone, or another object can become lodged in your throat or esophagus. Older adults with dentures and people who have difficulty chewing their food properly are prone to obstruction of the throat or esophagus. Children are prone to swallowing pins, coins, pieces of their toys or other small objects that can become stuck.

Blockage of the throat may cut off the airway, prompting a medical emergency. The Heimlich maneuver (see page 344) should be performed to dislodge the offending piece of food or object. A more common situation occurs when food is stuck farther down the esophagus, where it blocks the passage into your stomach. If the obstruction is partial, you may still be able to drink liquids. If the obstruction is total, you may spit up saliva.

Many foreign objects actually may pass into the stomach and through the gastrointestinal tract without complications. However, if the object is sharp-edged, it may scratch or perforate the esophagus, stomach or intestine on its way through.

If an obstruction causes an inability to swallow or interferes with your ability to breath, call for emergency help or have someone take you to the nearest emergency department immediately. If you're able to breath satisfactorily but have difficulty swallowing water or food, go to the emergency department right away.

Diagnosis

Your doctor may use a variety of tests, including endoscopy, in which a fiber-optic tube is inserted down your throat, to identify the location and severity of the obstruction. Before the instrument is inserted, you may receive a sedative, and your throat (pharynx) may be anesthetized.

Treatment

Often, a doctor can retrieve a foreign object lodged in the throat or esophagus with an endoscope. Or he or she might push the object into the stomach if it's something that will likely pass all the way through the digestive tract. Once the object has been removed from the esophagus and the swelling subsides, your doctor may want to inspect your esophagus to determine if some type of abnormality contributed to the obstruction.

Esophageal tumors

Signs and symptoms

- Progressive difficulty in swallowing
- Weight loss
- Regurgitation
- Blood in vomit or stool

Most esophageal tumors form in the middle or lower portion of the esophagus, and nearly 90 percent of them are cancerous (malignant). The principal symptom of an esophageal tumor, whether noncancerous (benign) or malignant, is progressive difficulty in swallowing. The difficulty often begins with solid foods but eventually includes liquids. As the condition worsens, weight loss, regurgitation of food and foul-smelling breath often occur.

Because swallowing becomes progressively worse over a relatively long period of time, many people delay seeing a doctor. Consequently, in many cases by the time the person receives a diagnosis of esophageal tumor, the tumor is large enough to fill about half the diameter of the esophagus.

Malignant tumors are twice as likely to occur in men as in women. Individuals at the highest risk are those between the ages of 50 and 60 who are heavy smokers and drink excessive amounts of alcohol.

Diagnosis

Diagnostic tests used to identify an esophageal tumor may include a barium X-ray and an upper endoscopic examination. If a tumor is found, a sample of tissue (biopsy) may be removed and analyzed in a laboratory. Your doctor may also order a computerized tomography (CT) scan or an endoscopic ultrasound exam to determine the extent of the tumor. See Chapter 39, "Diagnostic Tests," for more information on these tests.

How serious are esophageal tumors?

Most tumors in the esophagus are malignant. And because the disease is often far along in its development before the cancer is identified, the cure rate is poor. Early detection is key to successful treatment.

Treatment

The most common surgical treatment for esophageal cancer is to remove the cancerous section of the esophagus and reconnect the remaining healthy sections.

If a large portion of your esophagus is removed, your surgeon may form a new passageway from your throat to your stomach using a segment of your intestine. This type of surgery often reduces signs and symptoms and it can prolong survival, but it doesn't always lead to a cure.

Chemotherapy and radiation are sometimes used, alone or in combination, to ease signs and symptoms, shrink the tumor or kill cancerous cells that have spread beyond the esophagus. A relatively new treatment, called photodynamic therapy, uses medications that make cancer cells sensitive to laser light, in an attempt to destroy the cancer (see page 469).

To improve swallowing, sometimes a hollow, plastic tube (stent) is inserted into the esophagus. The tube helps increase the opening through the obstructing cancer, making eating easier.

Esophageal varices

Signs and symptoms

- Vomiting of blood
- Faintness, sweating and pallor

With esophageal varices, veins that line the esophagus become abnormally enlarged (varicose). Pressure within the expanded varicose veins (varices) of the esophagus can cause them to rupture. Heavy bleeding can result in shock. Esophageal varices occur infrequently and usually result as a complication of liver disease.

How serious are esophageal varices?

Although uncommon, esophageal varices are serious. The bleeding can be life-threatening.

Treatment

Treatment depends in large part on the location of the bleeding and how severe it is. Often, drugs are used initially to control the bleeding. Your doctor may place a special tube into the stomach that may temporarily stop the bleeding. This tube (Sengstaken-Blakemore tube) has balloons attached at the levels of the esophagus and the stomach. When in place, one or both balloons may be inflated to compress the varices.

Other options include placing small rubber bands over the enlarged veins to stop the bleeding, or injecting into the vein a solution that initially obliterates and then inflames and scars the varicose vein, a process called variceal sclerotherapy. These methods often stop the bleeding but may need to be repeated.

Yet another procedure, called transjugular intrahepatic portosystemic shunt (TIPS), involves placing a metal mesh tube (stent) between your liver (hepatic) vein and your portal vein to shunt blood away from the portal vein and reduce pressure on the connecting esophageal veins. Blockage of portal vein outflow due to liver disease is often the cause of increased pressure in your esophageal veins.

If these methods fail, surgery may be necessary to shunt blood away from the ruptured veins.

Esophageal trauma

Signs and symptoms

- Chest pain
- Rapid, shallow breathing
- Sweating
- Vomiting blood

A tear or puncture can sometimes occur in the esophagus. The injury may result from swallowing a foreign object or from a diagnostic procedure in which an instrument is inserted into the esophagus. It may also be a complication of another disorder or, rarely, a result of an episode of forceful vomiting.

Esophageal trauma may produce some blood in vomit. In more severe cases, such as a large perforation, breathing can become shallow and rapid, accompanied by severe chest pain.

Treatment

The first step typically involves diagnostic tests to determine the location and source of the bleeding. If the trauma is severe, such as a large perforation, surgery is often necessary to repair the esophagus. For less serious injuries, such as a superficial tear, the condition may be treated with intravenous (IV) fluids and antibiotics until the injury heals.

Stomach Disorders

A hollow, J-shaped sac, the stomach rests in the left-central section of your upper abdomen, just below your rib cage. It receives food from the esophagus, reducing it to a semiliquid mixture. Most of the stomach's contents trickle into the small intestine for further digestion and absorption.

The stomach is a remarkable organ, but it doesn't always function smoothly. Problems primarily affecting the lining of the stomach can lead to illness. The lining of the stomach generally is resistant to injury, but at times its resistance can break down.

Indigestion

Signs and symptoms

- Discomfort or a feeling of fullness in the upper abdomen
- Nausea
- A sensation of bloating, often relieved by belching

Indigestion (dyspepsia) is a nonspecific term used to describe many symptoms associated with abdominal distress, particularly after eating. Most commonly, though, people associate indigestion with stomach pain or discomfort. Indigestion itself isn't a disease. Rather, it's a symptom that most people experience at some point.

Some people experience indigestion only after eating certain foods or drinking excessive amounts of alcohol. Others have indigestion daily. Sometimes it's caused by an ulcer or inflammation of the stomach lining (gastritis). Often, no specific cause is found. Indigestion is commonly associated with a condition called nonulcer dyspepsia. In this condition, symptoms often mimic an ulcer, but no ulcer can be found. Nonulcer dyspepsia may result for many reasons:

Reaction to drugs and supplements

Nonsteroidal anti-inflammatory drugs (NSAIDs) such as aspirin, ibuprofen (Advil, Motrin, others) and naproxen (Aleve, Naprosyn, others) can cause ulcers and gastritis. These medications may irritate your digestive system without producing visible stomach or intestinal damage. The same may be true for other medications and supplements, including antibiotics, steroids, minerals and herbs.

Overproduction of stomach acid

Acid-secreting cells in the stomach may produce higher-than-normal amounts of digestive juices that irritate gastric tissues.

Stomach disorder

For unknown reasons, your stomach may not function or empty normally. This sometimes happens after certain viral infections.

Acid sensitivity

Tissues in the stomach and duodenum may be overly sensitive to normal acid levels and become easily irritated.

Food sensitivity
Your stomach or intestines may be overly sensitive to certain foods, food ingredients or beverages. Often, but not always, these include certain spices, citrus fruits and vegetables that contain moderate to high levels of acid. Some people also find that coffee seems to increase their symptoms.

Overreaction to normal stimuli
Nerve signals between your stomach and brain may be altered, causing an exaggerated response to normal changes that take place during digestion.

Stress
Indigestion may be your body's way of responding to stress.

Psychological factors
Depression, anxiety or some other factor affecting your emotional health may play a role.

Diagnosis

Because *indigestion* can be a vague term, it's important that you be specific about your symptoms when describing them to your doctor. Where is the discomfort located? Does it occur before, during, shortly after or several hours after a meal? Because indigestion can be caused by problems anywhere in the digestive system, answers to these questions can help your doctor pinpoint the affected area.

Once your doctor has determined the pattern of your symptoms, diagnostic tests that he or she may recommend will depend on the nature and severity of your specific symptoms and your age. Tests may include an upper endoscopic examination, a barium X-ray or an ultrasound or computerized tomography (CT) scan of your pancreas, liver and gallbladder. See Chapter 39, "Diagnostic Tests," for more information on these tests.

How serious is indigestion?

In itself, indigestion is more of a discomfort than a serious problem. However, because it can be a symptom of a major underlying disease, treat your indigestion seriously, particularly if it's of recent onset. It's important to see a doctor so that more serious problems can be ruled out.

Treatment

If a specific cause such as a peptic ulcer or gastritis is responsible for your indigestion, treating that condition will likely relieve the symptoms. When a cause can't be found, lifestyle adjustments and medication are often the most common treatments for indigestion.

Self-care
Your doctor may advise you to eliminate or limit certain foods or beverages that may be causing your indigestion. He or she might also discourage the use of cigarettes, alcohol or NSAIDs, which can contribute to indigestion.

In addition, your doctor may suggest techniques to help reduce stress, if stress appears to be a possible cause of your symptoms. Efforts should be directed at changing those factors that may relieve your symptoms.

Medication
Your doctor may elect to have you try a few weeks of treatment with an antacid (Maalox, Rolaids, others) or an acid blocker, such as cimetidine (Tagamet), ranitidine (Zantac), nizatidine (Axid) or famotidine (Pepcid), and see if symptoms improve.

Your doctor may also recommend a medication such as sucralfate (Carafate), which works by protecting the lining of the stomach. A medication called metoclopramide (Reglan) is sometimes prescribed to enhance emptying of the stomach. These medications have various degrees of success.

Peptic ulcers

Signs and symptoms

- A burning, aching, gnawing or hunger discomfort in the upper abdomen or lower chest that's relieved by milk, food or antacids
- Black, tarry, foul-smelling stools
- A bloated feeling after meals
- Nausea and vomiting

Emergency signs and symptoms
- Cold, clammy skin and fainting, suggesting excessive blood loss
- Vomiting of bright red blood

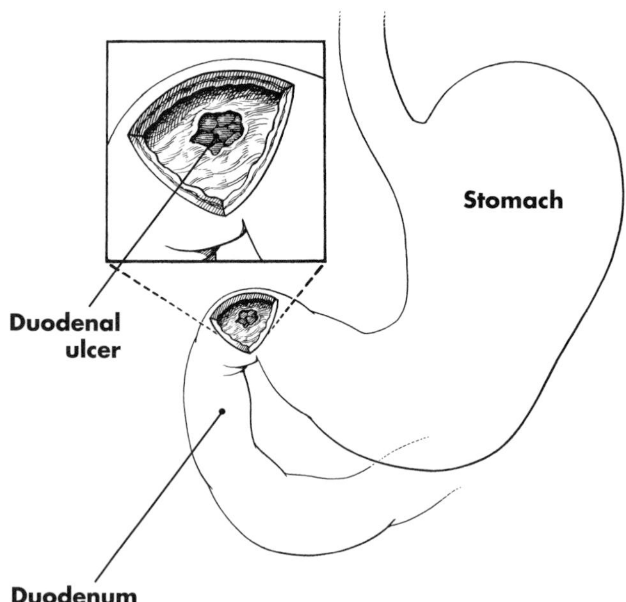

A peptic ulcer that occurs in the upper portion of the small intestine (duodenum) is called a duodenal ulcer.

Peptic ulcers are open sores in the inner lining of the esophagus, stomach or duodenum. Peptic ulcers are not uncommon in our society. Statistics suggest that 1 of every 10 people will have a peptic ulcer at some point.

Causes

Exactly how peptic ulcers develop isn't fully known. The lining of the esophagus, stomach and duodenum is normally resistant to injury and kept intact by a balance of stomach acid. When the balance breaks down, the result may be a peptic ulcer.

In the United States, the bacterium *Helicobacter pylori* is a common cause of peptic ulcers, especially in areas characterized by crowded conditions and a low socioeconomic standard of living.

Regular use of nonsteroidal anti-inflammatory drugs (NSAIDs), such as naproxen (Aleve, Naprosyn, others) or ibuprofen (Advil, Motrin, others), also can irritate or inflame the lining of your stomach and small intestine and lead to an ulcer. About 20 percent of people who take NSAIDs on a regular basis develop an ulcer.

Smoking and excessive alcohol also increase your risk of developing an ulcer. Nicotine increases both the volume and concentration of stomach acid. Alcohol can irritate and erode the mucous lining of your stomach and small intestine.

Types

The most common peptic ulcer is a duodenal ulcer. It appears in the first part of the small intestine (duodenum). A gastric ulcer (stomach ulcer) is usually found on the lower portion of the stomach, and an esophageal ulcer is usually located in the lower section of the esophagus.

Duodenal ulcer

There's no one symptom that will tell you that you have a duodenal ulcer. A possible indication, however, is a burning, aching, gnawing or hungry sensation in the upper middle section of your upper abdomen or a pain under the lower part of your breastbone that comes and goes. If the ulcer is located on the back wall of your duodenum, you may feel pain in your midback. At times you may feel bloated and nauseated after meals. If scarring results from a long-standing ulcer, it can obstruct the outlet of the stomach (pylorus). Your stomach may feel distended after meals, and you may vomit or regurgitate stomach acids.

Some people don't experience any pain with an ulcer. Bleeding may be the only sign. The stools may be black, tarry and foul smelling or maroon colored. Vomiting of red blood or blood that looks like coffee grounds is a bleeding emergency.

Duodenal ulcers are more likely to develop in heavy smokers and are less likely to heal as quickly as in nonsmokers. The relationship between smoking and ulcer formation isn't fully understood, but it's thought that nicotine may inhibit alkaline secretions of the pancreas that help neutralize stomach acid. In rare instances, a tumor called a gastrinoma, located in the pancreas or duodenum (Zollinger-Ellison syndrome), can cause a duodenal ulcer.

Gastric ulcer

Excessive gastric acid may contribute to the formation of a gastric ulcer. However, in most cases it's believed that a gastric ulcer develops because the mucus and protective lining of the stomach are defective and unable to resist the usual amount of stomach acid. Because excess acid secretion isn't the primary cause of a gastric ulcer, smaller doses of either liquid antacids or acid-reducing medications than are required for duodenal ulcers may be effective. Certain medications, including pain relievers such as aspirin, ibuprofen (Advil, Motrin, others) and naproxen (Aleve, Naprosyn, others)

? Question and Answer

What if my ulcer won't heal?

Approximately 90 percent of all peptic ulcers heal within 1 to 3 months of beginning treatment. Those that don't are called refractory ulcers.

Ulcers fail to heal for many reasons. Not taking medications properly is one reason. In ulcers caused by the bacterium *Helicobacter pylori*, a failure to heal may be due to bacterial resistance to antibiotics. Other factors that can interfere with the healing of an ulcer include regular use of tobacco, alcohol or nonsteroidal anti-inflammatory drugs (NSAIDs). Sometimes, people are unaware that a medication they're taking even contains an NSAID.

In rare cases, refractory ulcers may be a result of an extreme overproduction of stomach acid as in Zollinger-Ellison syndrome, an infection other than *H. pylori*, or other digestive diseases, including Crohn's disease or cancer.

Treatment of refractory ulcers generally involves eliminating all of the factors that may interfere with healing, along with taking larger doses of medication. Sometimes, additional medications may be needed. Surgery to help heal an ulcer is rarely necessary and only needed when the ulcer doesn't respond to aggressive medical treatment.

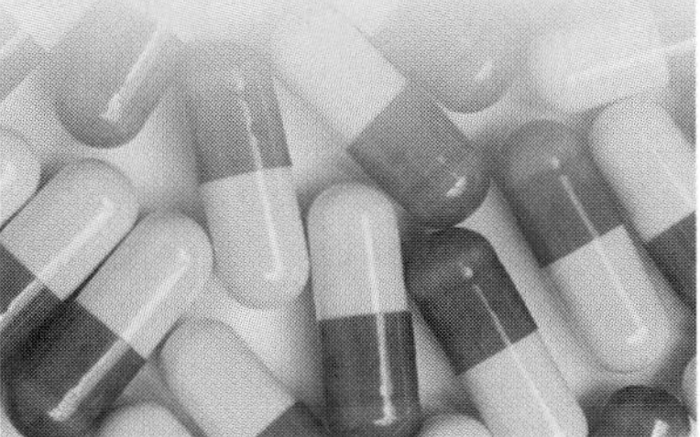

can cause gastric ulcers. These drugs inhibit production of the enzyme cyclooxygenase, which produces hormone-like substances (prostaglandins) that help protect your stomach lining from chemical and physical injury.

It's not easy to distinguish between a duodenal ulcer and gastric ulcer on the basis of symptoms. The pain from a gastric ulcer may be less likely to be relieved by eating. In some cases, eating actually increases the pain of a gastric ulcer.

Diagnosis

If your doctor suspects that you have an ulcer, he or she may conduct several diagnostic tests. The two most common tests are an upper endoscopic examination and a barium X-ray. See Chapter 39, "Diagnostic Tests," for more information on these tests. If the ulcer is in your stomach, your doctor may take a sample of tissue (biopsy) through an endoscope for laboratory analysis to check for cancer. Duodenal ulcers are rarely cancerous (malignant).

In addition to a biopsy, other tests also can determine if the cause of your ulcer is *H. pylori* infection. These include a blood test, breath test and stool antigen test.

How serious are peptic ulcers?

With early detection and proper treatment, most people recover from an ulcer within a few weeks. However, early treatment doesn't guarantee a cure because some people treated for ulcers have a recurrence.

Several potentially serious complications are associated with peptic ulcers. Sometimes, an ulcer will bleed (hemorrhage), necessitating hospitalization. One danger of severe bleeding is shock. If the bleeding is only slight but continues over a period of time, iron deficiency anemia may develop.

Perforation, another serious complication, occurs when the ulcer erodes through the wall of the stomach or duodenum into the abdominal cavity. This produces sudden onset of intense, persistent abdominal pain. A long-standing ulcer may cause an obstruction at the outlet of the stomach.

What About Diet and Stress?

Before the bacterium *Helicobacter pylori* was discovered and the association was made with NSAIDs, ulcers were thought to be a result of certain lifestyle factors, such as diet and stress.

There's no clear evidence that people who are under a lot of stress or eat hurried, irregular meals or spicy foods are more likely to have ulcers. And now that these factors have been eliminated as causes, they no longer figure in treatment. For example, following a bland diet with plenty of milk is no longer advised. In fact, drinking large quantities of milk is discouraged because foods rich in protein and calcium tend to stimulate acid production.

It's still a good idea, though, to avoid spicy foods and reduce stress while an ulcer is healing. Even though stress and food don't cause an ulcer, they can exacerbate ulcer pain. Stress also slows digestion, allowing food and digestive acids to remain in your stomach and intestines for a longer period.

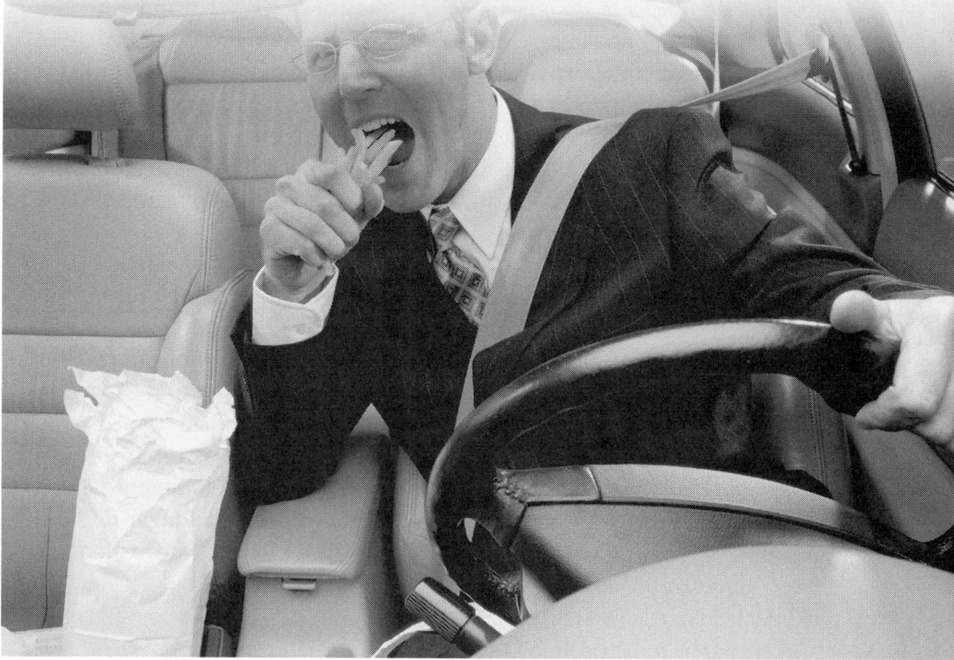

Treatment

Because many ulcers stem from *H. pylori* bacteria, treatment usually is aimed at achieving two objectives. One objective is to kill the bacteria. The second is to reduce the level of acid in your digestive system to relieve pain and encourage healing. Accomplishing these objectives requires a combination of medications such as antibiotics, acid blockers, proton pump inhibitors and antacids.

Several combinations of antibiotics are effective against *H. pylori*. Those most commonly prescribed include amoxicillin (Amoxil, Trimox), clarithromycin (Biaxin), metronidazole (Flagyl) and tetracycline (Achromycin V, Sumycin). Antibiotics are taken for 1 to 2 weeks, depending on the type and number of antibiotics you're taking. Other medications prescribed in conjunction with antibiotics generally are taken for a longer period.

Acid blockers — histamine (H-2) blockers — reduce the amount of acid secreted by your stomach to relieve ulcer pain and encourage healing. These medications include cimetidine (Tagamet), ranitidine (Zantac), nizatidine (Axid) and famotidine (Pepcid). Your doctor may also consider a more powerful acid-suppressing agent, such as omeprazole (Prilosec), lansoprazole (Prevacid), rabeprazole (Aciphex) or esomeprazole (Nexium), which belong to a class of medications called proton pump inhibitors. Pantoprazole (Protonix) can be taken orally or administered intravenously in the hospital. Proton pump inhibitors also appear to inhibit *H. pylori*.

Once your ulcer has healed, your doctor may advise you to take a smaller dose of an acid suppressor on a daily basis, particularly if you've had recurrent ulcers in the past. Other useful medications include cytoprotective agents that aid in protecting the lining of your stomach and duodenum, such as sucralfate (Carafate) and misoprostol (Cytotec). Antacids sometimes are used to supplement these medications. Instead of reducing acid secretion, antacids neutralize existing stomach acid and can provide rapid pain relief.

Surgery may be an option in cases where the ulcer doesn't respond to treatment or serious complications arise, such as hemorrhage, obstruction or perforation. With the advent of newer medications and a better understanding of what causes most ulcers, surgical treatment of peptic ulcer is now uncommon.

Prevention

The delicate balance of acid in your stomach and gastrointestinal tract can be disrupted by aspirin and other pain relievers. If you need to take pain relievers on a regular basis, ask your doctor about acetaminophen (Tylenol, others). It doesn't cause ulcers and stomach upset as do other pain relievers. Anti-inflammatory prescription medications called COX-2 inhibitors (Bextra, Celebrex, Vioxx) may be less damaging to your digestive system.

Smoking and drinking excessive amounts of alcohol contribute to the development of ulcers and retard or prevent healing in people who have ulcers.

If you have a history of ulcers, mention this whenever a doctor prescribes a medication for you. If an ulcer-provoking drug is absolutely necessary to treat another condition, your doctor can prescribe a second medication to reduce the risk of a recurrent ulcer.

Zollinger-Ellison syndrome

Signs and symptoms

- Ulcer-like symptoms in the upper abdomen
- Severe, persistent ulcer-like symptoms that aren't relieved by antacids
- Diarrhea

Zollinger-Ellison syndrome is a rare condition in which tumors, called gastrinomas, form in the body, most commonly in the pancreas or duodenum. The tumors secrete a substance called gastrin, which stimulates excessive acid secretion by the stomach.

As a result, most people with Zollinger-Ellison syndrome have a peptic ulcer at some point during their disease. Ulcers associated with Zollinger-Ellison syndrome are typically more persistent and less responsive to treatment than usual peptic ulcers are. The syndrome may occur at any age, but signs and symptoms are more likely to appear between the ages of 30 and 60.

Diagnosis

If you have symptoms that suggest Zollinger-Ellison syndrome, your doctor may perform blood tests to see if the gastrin level in your blood is increased. Generally, a person with Zollinger-Ellison syndrome has an abnormally high serum gastrin level, which causes production of excessive amounts of stomach acid. Your doctor may also order an upper endoscopic examination or a barium X-ray of your stomach to search for evidence of ulcers.

Gastrinomas are often small and difficult to locate, but recent advances in diagnostic techniques have improved identification and localization of these tumors. Techniques include ultrasound that can be used in the operating room and nuclear medicine scans, which use a tiny dose of radioactive material that binds to the tumor and shows as a hot spot on the scan.

How serious is Zollinger-Ellison syndrome?

Zollinger-Ellison syndrome can be a serious disease. The tumors may spread slowly, most commonly to the lymph nodes and liver. In addition, ulcers associated with the syndrome are usually severe and not easily treated with conventional medication or surgery. As with most serious diseases, the earlier you receive a diagnosis, the better the chances of a favorable outcome.

Treatment

Ulcers associated with Zollinger-Ellison syndrome typically are resistant to standard doses of ulcer medication. Especially if you're young and in good health, your doctor may elect to perform an operation to identify and remove the one or more tumors responsible for the excess production of acid. Sometimes, these tumors are so small or multiple in nature that they can't be identified and removed.

If your surgeon is unable to remove the gastrinomas, you'll need to take an acid-reducing medication. The most effective drug is a proton pump inhibitor, such as omeprazole (Prilosec), lansoprazole (Prevacid), rabeprazole (Aciphex), pantoprazole (Protonix) or esomeprazole (Nexium), which has the advantage of virtually eliminating acid production for a period of time. With this type ulcer, you may need to take larger and more frequent doses than you would for an ordinary peptic ulcer. Usually, these medications are taken indefinitely to prevent recurrence of signs and symptoms.

You'll also need follow-up examinations to watch carefully for growth or spread of the tumors.

Gastritis

Signs and symptoms

- Upper abdominal discomfort
- Nausea and, occasionally, vomiting
- Bleeding

Gastritis means "inflammation of the lining of the stomach." It can result from a number of causes, each of which may produce somewhat different signs and symptoms. Gastritis can occur as a result of acid-induced damage to the lining of the stomach when no ulcer is present. Excessive smoking or alcohol consumption is known to produce gastritis or to aggravate existing signs and symptoms.

Gastritis can also be a side effect of a number of prescription drugs. One form, erosive gastritis, is often associated with the ingestion of aspirin or similar pain medications, such as ibuprofen (Advil, Motrin, others) or naproxen (Aleve, Naprosyn, others). Severe stress due to burns, trauma, surgery or shock may produce stress gastritis.

Interestingly, gastritis is sometimes seen in people whose stomachs don't produce acid. In such cases, the lining of the stomach is atrophied. This condition, called atrophic gastritis, may be associated with vitamin B-12 deficiency and occurs in many older adults.

Diagnosis

Your doctor may be able to make a diagnosis based on a description of your symptoms. Your doctor may inquire about your eating habits and use of medications. He or she may also want to know if you're a heavy drinker or smoke regularly.

In addition, your doctor may request a barium X-ray of your stomach. However, the results of this study are often normal. A diagnosis of gastritis can best be confirmed with an upper endoscopy examination, which reveals typical lesions. A biopsy of stomach tissues also can be helpful.

How serious is gastritis?

In most cases, symptoms of gastritis are relatively mild and short-lived, pose no real danger and have no lasting effect, especially if you receive an early diagnosis and the condition is treated. Occasionally, gastritis may cause bleeding.

Treatment

Antacids in liquid or tablet form are a suitable and common treatment for mild gastritis. If antacids fail to provide relief, your doctor may prescribe a medication such as cimetidine (Tagamet), ranitidine (Zantac), nizatidine (Axid) or famotidine (Pepcid), which decreases the amount of acid produced by your stomach. Medication to protect the lining of the stomach, such as sucralfate (Carafate) or misoprostol (Cytotec), also may be used.

If the gastritis is associated with vitamin B-12 deficiency, you may need to take vitamin B-12 injections on a monthly basis for the rest of your life.

If your condition is associated with use of alcohol, cigarettes or pain medications, it's critical that you avoid the offending agent.

Gastrointestinal tract bleeding

Signs and symptoms

- Red blood in the stool
- Black, tarry stool
- Vomiting of blood

Gastrointestinal tract bleeding may result from a variety of conditions, including a peptic ulcer, gastritis, esophageal varices, esophageal trauma, ulcerative colitis, cancerous (malignant) tumors, diverticulitis and hemorrhoids.

Red or maroon stool can indicate several problems, such as colon polyps, cancer, Crohn's disease or ulcerative colitis. One of the more common explanations for heavy bleeding in stool in people older than age 60 is bleeding from pouches (diverticula) or blood vessels in the colon.

Red blood in the stool may also indicate blood loss from the stomach or duodenum, particularly if the bleeding is heavy and rapid. Slow bleeding that occurs in the stomach or duodenum and passes through the gastrointestinal tract causes black and sticky stools that resemble tar. Licorice or ingestion of iron or bismuth subsalicylate (such as Pepto-Bismol) also may turn your stool black.

If you notice blood in your stool or in the toilet bowl, consult your doctor promptly. The source of the blood may be as simple as hemorrhoids, but you want to be sure to rule out other more serious conditions such as colon cancer.

Vomited blood, on the other hand, suggests that the bleeding is from the esophagus, stomach or upper small intestine (duodenum). Blood that enters the intestines below the duodenum usually doesn't reflux back into the stomach but passes in stool.

Vomiting of bright red blood indicates that the bleeding began shortly before you vomited. Blood that has been in your stomach for a longer time is generally dark red or brown in color or has the texture and color of old coffee grounds.

Diagnosis

For bleeding that occurs in the upper portion of the gastrointestinal tract, your doctor may perform a procedure called upper gastrointestinal endoscopy, in which a small fiber-optic tube is inserted down your esophagus and into your stomach to look for the source of the bleeding. For bleeding in the lower gastrointestinal tract, your doctor may perform a colonoscopy, which is similar to upper endoscopy only the tube is inserted through the rectum and threaded up through the colon.

Often, blood in the stool can be detected only by diagnostic tests because the amount is too small to see. This is termed hidden (occult) blood.

Treatment

Treatment depends on the cause and severity of the bleeding. For variceal bleeding in the esophagus, various techniques may be used to stop the bleeding. If the bleeding is from a diverticulum, injecting medication directly into the artery that supplies blood to the diverticulum may stop the bleeding.

For bleeding related to an ulcer, gastritis, polyps or hemorrhoids, treating the condition will often stop the bleeding. At times, the use of an electric current or laser light delivered through an endoscope may stop bleeding in the stomach, duodenum or colon. In some cases, such as if the bleeding resists these treatments, surgery may be required.

Stomach cancer

Signs and symptoms

- Discomfort in the upper or middle regions of the abdomen
- Black, tarry stools
- Vomiting of blood
- Vomiting after meals
- Weight loss
- Anemia
- A bloated feeling after meals

Most tumors that develop in the stomach are noncancerous (benign) growths (polyps) that have little if any potential to turn cancerous. Much less common are adenomas, which infrequently become cancerous as they grow in size. Stomach cancer affects twice as many men as women, usually between the ages of 50 and 70. It's rare to find this type of cancer in people younger than age 40.

The cause of cancerous stomach tumors isn't certain. Since the discovery of *Helicobacter pylori* bacteria as a common cause of peptic ulcers, researchers have wondered if there might be a connection between the bacteria and stomach cancer as well. One long-term study of this theory, done in Japan, concluded that chronic *H. pylori* infection does indeed increase the risk of stomach cancer.

Genetic factors also may have some influence. Stomach tumors are two to four times more common in members of the immediate family of people with the disease. In addition, stomach cancer is much more common in some countries, such as Japan. It's interesting to note, though, that the children of Japanese parents who migrate to the United States have a much lower incidence of stomach cancer, suggesting that environmental influences, such as diet, also may be potential causes.

Diagnosis

No one symptom suggests that you may have stomach cancer. Some people with cancerous stomach tumors have symptoms similar to individuals with peptic ulcers.

If persistent indigestion develops for the first time in your life, along with unexplained weight loss and nausea, your doctor may want to perform an upper endoscopic examination or barium X-ray to determine if your symptoms are due to cancer or to some other abnormality. During an endoscopic examination, your doctor may remove a small piece of tissue from your stomach for laboratory analysis (biopsy). If cancer is found, he or she may also want to obtain a computerized tomography (CT) scan or endoscopic ultrasound examination to determine if the cancer has spread (metastasized). See Chapter 39, "Diagnostic Tests," for more information on these tests.

How serious is stomach cancer?

Stomach cancer can be difficult to treat. If the cancer is confined to the stomach, chances of successful treatment are good. If the disease has spread, the chance of cure is significantly decreased.

Treatment

Surgical removal offers the best chance for treating stomach cancer. The likelihood of success depends almost exclusively on whether the cancer has spread to other organs or areas of the body. If the cancer is detected early and surgery can remove all of the affected areas, full recovery is possible. Even when surgery may not offer a cure, treatment with chemotherapy and radiation therapy can prolong survival. Chemotherapy and radiation may also prevent recurrence of the cancer following surgery.

Even when a cure isn't possible, surgery still may help alleviate pain, bleeding or obstruction.

Menetrier's disease

Signs and symptoms

- Stomach pain
- Nausea and vomiting
- Weight loss
- Intestinal bleeding
- Swelling of the hands, feet or legs

Menetrier's disease is of unknown origin. It usually develops after age 50.

In this condition, the lining of the stomach overdevelops (hypertrophies) and creates large folds, which may have tiny breaks (erosions). Some erosions can develop into ulcers and lead to bleeding from the stomach. Protein may be lost from the folds, causing low blood proteins and swelling in the extremities (edema).

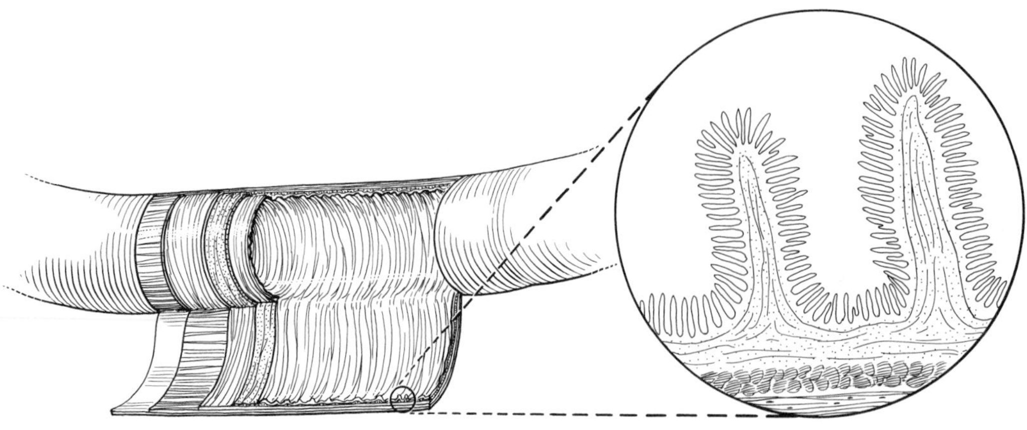

The wall of the small intestine is lined with many small projections called villi (see inset). Villi increase the surface area through which nutrients can be absorbed.

X-rays can reveal the enlarged stomach folds. To rule out any possibility of cancer, your doctor may perform other tests such as an upper gastrointestinal endoscopic examination or an endoscopic ultrasound exam. Under certain conditions, a doctor may opt to make a small surgical opening in the abdomen (laparotomy) to confirm the diagnosis.

There's no single treatment for all people with this disease. Your doctor may urge you to eat a high-protein diet to compensate for any protein loss. If you develop associated problems such as ulcers or protein deficiency, they also need to be treated. The use of acid-suppressing medications may be helpful, particularly if erosions or ulcers are present. A variety of other medications can sometimes be helpful. In severe cases, surgery may be necessary to remove at least a portion of the stomach.

Eosinophilic gastroenteritis

Signs and symptoms

- Abdominal pain
- Nausea and vomiting
- Intermittent diarrhea, possibly bloody
- Weight loss and a failure to thrive and grow

This is a rare disease in which the lining of the stomach and the intestinal tract become infiltrated with a type of white blood cell (eosinophils). A diagnosis can be made by a biopsy of tissue in the stomach and intestinal tract.

Treatment

Corticosteroid medications are usually effective in treating the disease.

Intestinal Disorders

The small intestine consists of three parts: the duodenum, the jejunum and the ileum. This organ continues the processes of digestion and absorption that began in your stomach. Bile from the liver and juices from the pancreas enter the small intestine to aid in the process of digestion.

Most of the nutrients from the food you eat are absorbed into your bloodstream by the small intestine. The wall of the small intestine is lined with numerous small projections called villi. These projections significantly increase the surface area through which food can be absorbed.

The small intestine is connected to the large intestine at the ileocecal valve. Through this valve, the semiliquid material from the small intestine passes into the first part of the large intestine (cecum). The shape of the large intestine resembles an upside-down U in that it runs up, across and down in the abdomen.

The ascending colon starts on the right side of the abdomen at the cecum and moves up near the liver. The portion of the colon that crosses the abdomen from right to left is the transverse colon. The descending colon is the section on the left that extends to the sigmoid colon. Shaped like the letter S, the sigmoid colon curves into the pelvis, where it joins the rectum. The rectum is a relatively straight 4- to 6-inch tube that leads to the anus.

In the large intestine, food waste is solidified and prepared for excretion. What passes from the small intestine into the large intestine is generally a mixture of unabsorbed fiber, water and electrolytes, such as sodium. As this mixture proceeds through the large intestine, much of the water and salt are absorbed through the lining of the large intestine. Once the water is removed, the residue becomes a semisolid mass that's passed out the anus as stool (feces). By the time waste products reach the anus, about 80 percent of the liquid that originally entered the colon has been absorbed.

Gastrointestinal infections

Signs and symptoms

- Watery, sometimes bloody, diarrhea
- Cramping abdominal pain
- Fever
- Nausea and vomiting
- Muscle aches and headache

Emergency signs and symptoms

- Profuse diarrhea to the point of dehydration

Gastrointestinal tract infections are extremely common throughout the world. In developing countries, diarrhea caused by infection is among the leading causes of death in children. Improvements in sanitation and hygiene have had a significant impact on preventing many of these infections, particularly those transmitted by contaminated food and water. Even so, the Centers for Disease Control and Prevention estimates that foodborne diseases cause approximately 76 million illnesses and 5,000 deaths in the United States each year.

Viruses account for well over half the infections of the gastrointestinal tract. Other gastrointestinal infections are the result of bacteria and parasites.

Viral infections

Acute viral gastroenteritis — the stomach flu — is the second most common disease in the United States, with upper respiratory tract infections being the most common. Signs and symptoms usually include diarrhea, nausea, vomiting, a low-grade fever, abdominal cramps and muscle pains.

Viral gastroenteritis is often the cause of considerable discomfort and of time lost from school or work. In some people — especially in infants, older individuals and individuals whose immune systems are suppressed by disease or certain medications — signs and symptoms can be severe.

Many of viruses responsible for acute viral gastroenteritis are passed by fecal-oral transmission. Hand washing is a key to preventing transmission of the virus to others. Generally, the infection resolves over time. Antibiotics are not effective. Antidiarrheal medications are generally avoided because they may prevent elimination of the virus and actually prolong the infection.

Many types of viruses can cause acute viral gastroenteritis. However, the most common are those caused by the rotavirus and the Norwalk virus.

The Large Intestine

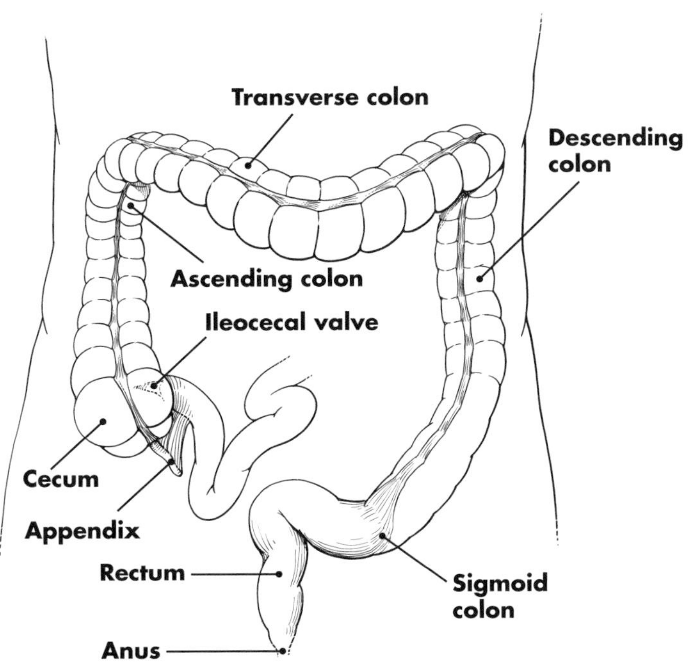

Rotavirus

Rotavirus is the most common cause of infectious diarrhea in developed countries such as the United States. It's frequently identified as the cause of diarrhea in children younger than 2 years. It's also the most common source of diarrhea in children attending child care centers. Rotavirus occasionally causes epidemics of infection among older adults in nursing homes. The peak frequency of rotavirus infections in the United States is during the winter. The virus is transmitted from one person to another.

The incubation period is 1 to 3 days. Typical signs and symptoms include watery, nonbloody diarrhea, vomiting and a low-grade fever lasting 5 to 8 days. There's no specific treatment for rotavirus gastroenteritis. Current research centers on the development of a vaccine.

Norwalk virus

The Norwalk virus is an important cause of outbreaks of gastroenteritis in families and communities, particularly in older children and adults. This ailment is also called winter vomiting disease. In addition to diarrhea, nausea and vomiting, many people with this disorder experience muscle aches.

This virus usually is acquired by ingesting contaminated food or water. The incubation period from the time of ingestion of the contaminated food or water to the onset of signs and symptoms ranges from 4 to 72 hours.

Other causes

Cytomegalovirus is a common cause of diarrhea in people with a weak (immunosuppressed) immune system. A medication called ganciclovir (Cytovene) may be effective in treating cytomegalovirus-induced diarrhea.

Gastrointestinal infections with herpes simplex virus are frequent in individuals who engage in anal intercourse, especially the receptive

PREVENTION TIP

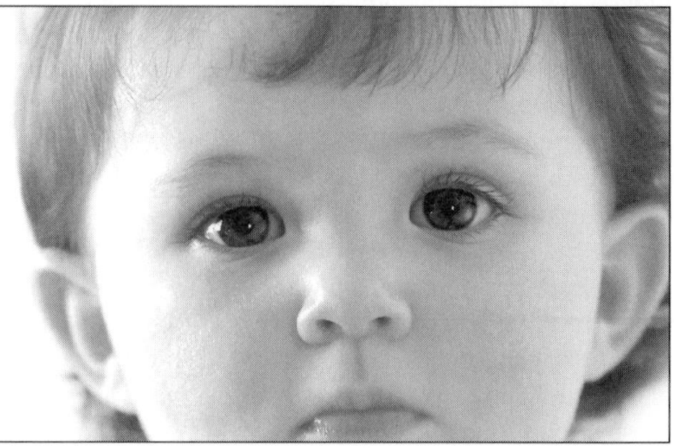

Dehydration is the main complication of diarrhea-causing diseases such as gastrointestinal infections. In infants and children, dehydration can be fatal in a matter of days. If you have diarrhea, be sure to drink plenty of fluids, and if your child has it, keep him or her hydrated. Water usually doesn't supply all of the needed minerals lost in diarrhea, so a sports drink or electrolyte solution may be a better alternative.

In case of severe diarrhea or persistent vomiting, fluids may need to be administered intravenously in a hospital.

participant, and in immunosuppressed individuals. Generally, people infected with the herpes simplex virus experience anal pain, constipation and sometimes mild, bloody diarrhea. These people may also develop neurologic symptoms, including pain in and numbness or tingling of the buttocks, upper thighs or anal area.

Treatment generally consists of soaking in a warm bath and taking pain relievers and stool softeners. The antiviral drug acyclovir (Zovirax) can decrease the severity of the initial attack and the chance of later relapses.

Bacterial infections

Gastrointestinal infections resulting from bacteria often are easier to identify than are viral causes. Bacterial infections are commonly referred to as food poisoning because they generally result from contaminated food. The illness generally improves on its own without need for specific treatment. In some cases, antibiotics are useful.

Campylobacter

Campylobacter infections occur in all age groups, but most occur in children younger than 1 year and in young adults. Campylobacter may be the most common bacterial cause of infectious diarrhea in young adults. Infections with this organism generally occur in the summer and fall.

The most common source of campylobacter appears to be contaminated food, particularly poultry and unpasteurized milk. The incubation period from exposure to onset of signs and symptoms is 2 to 4 days. The illness may have an abrupt onset, with the appearance of abdominal pain, nausea, a low-grade fever, headache and muscle pains. You may experience many loose bowel movements each day. In severe cases, the stools may be bloody.

This illness rarely lasts longer than 1 week. Occasionally, you may experience a relapse or a prolongation of your illness. Antidiarrheal agents aren't recommended because they may delay clearing of the organism from your system and prolong the illness. Antibiotic treatment often isn't necessary, but an antibiotic such as erythromycin or tetracycline can be given if signs and symptoms are severe.

Salmonella

Salmonella has been implicated as responsible for about one-third of cases of diarrhea from contaminated food. Salmonella generally originates from contamination of the food itself, as opposed to the hands of infected food handlers. About two-thirds of people infected by this type of bacteria are under the age of 20. Salmonella infections generally occur in the summer and fall.

Some evidence suggests that salmonella may occur in animals treated with antibiotics, possibly increasing the risk of salmonella infection in individuals who consume meats from these animals. The potential risk to consumers is an area of intense investigation.

Salmonella bacteria are commonly are found in meats, poultry, eggs, unpasteurized cheese and milk, chocolate made from contaminated cocoa beans and contaminated marijuana. Some pets, such as turtles, iguanas, lizards and snakes, also can be a source of infection. The disease can be passed by the fecal-oral route. For example, if you change your infected baby's diaper, fail to wash your hands properly and then sit down to dinner, you could become infected.

When salmonella-infected food isn't cooked adequately or thawed properly, you may acquire the infection directly from the food. Signs and symptoms of salmonella infection include abdominal cramps, diarrhea, nausea, vomiting and fever.

In most cases, the infection clears on its own and only supportive treatment, such as drinking plenty of fluids, is needed. In some people, salmonella can cause a severe and prolonged illness, and antibiotic treatment may be necessary. In these cases, the stool is often tested to make sure that an effective antibiotic is chosen for the particular type of salmonella the person has.

Shigella

Shigella is an important cause of bacterial gastroenteritis in the developing world and in travelers to these areas. It also occasionally occurs in outbreaks in the United

States. The ailment is most common in children ages 1 through 5.

Shigella is transmitted primarily from person to person by the fecal-oral route. Outbreaks can occur in child care centers. Occasionally, outbreaks can be caused by contamination of food by infected food handlers. The usual signs and symptoms are watery diarrhea associated with cramping abdominal pain, fever and, sometimes, blood and mucus in the stool.

Generally, the disease improves on its own. Antibiotics may be effective in shortening the duration of the diarrhea and in eliminating shigella from the gastrointestinal tract. The usual drug of choice is ampicillin (Omnipen, Principen), and it can be given orally after appropriate stool cultures have been obtained. Other possible medications include trimethoprim and sulfamethoxazole (Bactrim, Septra), ciprofloxacin (Cipro) and chloramphenicol (Chloromycetin).

Escherichia coli

The organism called *Escherichia coli* has various subgroups. The source of this infection usually is contaminated food and water. A particular strain of this bacterium named *E. coli* 0157:H7 is sometimes found in undercooked beef, particularly ground beef, and in infected produce. In about 2 percent to 7 percent of cases, particularly in the very young and the very old, *E. coli* 0157:H7 can lead to a serious complication called hemolytic uremic syndrome. A potentially fatal condition, this syndrome destroys red blood cells and causes kidney failure.

If the diarrhea is mild, generally no treatment is necessary other than rehydration. For more severe or prolonged signs and symptoms, an antibiotic such as trimethoprim and sulfamethoxazole (Bactrim, Septra) or ciprofloxacin (Cipro) is often prescribed. Anti-diarrheal medications generally are not used because they delay elimination of the organism.

Cooking meats properly, especially ground meat, can help prevent an *E. coli* 0157:H7 infection. It's also important to wash hands and cooking utensils after working with raw meat and to avoid having the meat come into contact with other foods. For more on *E. Coli* 0157:H7, see page 493.

Clostridium perfringens

Another common cause of food poisoning is the bacterium *Clostridium perfringens* and its toxin. The infection is usually acquired by ingesting contaminated food — particularly inadequately cooked and refrigerated meat that has been insufficiently reheated before consumption.

Signs and symptoms include severe abdominal cramps and diarrhea, which begin about 8 to 24 hours after consuming foods containing large amounts of the bacteria. Diagnosis is obtained by identifying the bacteria in an infected person's stool. The illness usually resolves on its own and usually lasts no more than a day. During the illness it's important to drink plenty of fluids to prevent dehydration, a potential complication of diarrhea.

Outbreaks most often occur in places such as school cafeterias, nursing homes and hospitals where large quantities of food are prepared ahead of time and stored for future meals. A potentially fatal type of this bacterial infection is known as pig-bel disease (enteritis necroticans), but it's very rare in the United States.

Staphylococcus

Staphylococcal food poisoning often results from eating foods such as egg, dairy and poultry products, sandwich fillings and egg, chicken, tuna, potato and macaroni salads, which are commonly found to harbor the bacteria. The bacteria

Food Poisoning

Food poisoning is caused by the ingestion of contaminated food. Its signs and symptoms usually include diarrhea and nausea. Vomiting and abdominal pain also may occur.

The most common cause of food poisoning is the toxin produced by the bacterium *Staphylococcus aureus.* When this organism contaminates certain foods — especially cream pastries, mayonnaise-containing foods or potato, chicken, egg or tuna salad — it multiplies rapidly. This explains why staphylococcal food poisoning often occurs in outbreaks. Contamination most often occurs from the hands of a food handler.

What to do?

Usually, the discomforts of food poisoning pass in a few hours. After the vomiting or diarrhea ends, consume clear liquids for the first 12 hours. Then limit food intake to bland foods for the next 24 hours. For very young children, older adults and individuals who have other ailments, consult a doctor.

Prevention

The best strategy is to avoid contaminated food. Keep all meats and leftovers refrigerated. Don't allow food to come into contact with uncooked meat juices. Wash fruits and vegetables thoroughly.

are usually transmitted through the food handler and thrive when the food hasn't been kept hot or cold enough.

Onset of signs and symptoms, including nausea, vomiting, diarrhea, loss of appetite and fever, is usually swift following the ingestion of contaminated food. Presence of the bacteria in a stool sample confirms the diagnosis. The illness may last from 24 to 48 hours, but typically resolves on its own. Antidiarrheal medication generally isn't necessary and may prolong the infection by preventing elimination of the bacteria. To avoid dehydration, consume plenty of fluids.

Careful washing of your hands and food utensils before and after food preparation can help prevent infection. In addition, don't let food sit out. Instead, refrigerate it promptly.

Parasitic infestations

Parasitic infestations are the least common of the three major causes of diarrheal diseases:

Giardia lamblia

This parasitic organism causes giardiasis, which is probably the most common parasitic cause of diarrhea in the United States. Outbreaks of giardiasis can occur in communities where the water supply is contaminated by raw sewage. Giardiasis may also be contracted by bathing in pools, lakes and water parks or by drinking water from lakes or mountain streams.

As many as two-thirds of people with giardiasis have no signs or symptoms. However, they may pass the infestation to others. Those who do develop signs and symptoms typically have watery diarrhea, abdominal cramps and, sometimes, weight loss. Generally, these signs and symptoms occur 1 to 3 weeks after exposure. The stools may be foul smelling, greasy looking and floating. Bloating and distention also may occur. A low-grade fever may be present. These signs and symptoms usually last for 5 to 7 days, although some people have problems for months.

Diagnostic tests may identify the parasite. Giardiasis is usually treated with metronidazole (Flagyl) or, occasionally, quinacrine. Follow-up stool examinations are important because the medications may not eliminate the parasite entirely.

Entamoeba histolytica

Entamoeba histolytica is a common cause of diarrheal disease throughout the world, although it's relatively uncommon in the United States. Infection generally occurs from person to person through the fecal-oral route. Your doctor may treat the infection with metronidazole. Other drugs are sometimes used.

Cryptosporidium

Cryptosporidium is a common cause of diarrhea in people with AIDS. It can also cause illness in otherwise healthy people. Epidemics have occurred as a result of contaminated public water supplies. Signs include prolonged watery diarrhea with up to 25 bowel movements a day. In otherwise healthy individuals, the infection resolves without treatment in 1 to 2 weeks.

In people with AIDS, the infection usually is chronic. There's no effective treatment, although several promising drugs currently are undergoing study.

Treatment

The initial danger of gastrointestinal infections is dehydration following the loss of fluids and electrolytes in stool. Therefore, the primary goal of treatment is replacement of fluids and essential electrolytes.

For most infections, the use of antidiarrheal agents isn't recommended because they may delay the elimination of the causative organism and prolong the disease. Most parasitic infections require specific treatments to eradicate the organism.

Antibiotic-associated diarrhea

Signs and symptoms

- Diarrhea occurring during or shortly after antibiotic therapy
- Abdominal cramps
- Fever

Antibiotics, especially clindamycin (Cleocin), ampicillin (Omnipen, Polycillin), cephalosporins and the aminoglycosides, can cause diarrhea. Usually, the diarrhea is a result of the antibiotic having altered the environment of the bowel, which permits certain bacteria to flourish. This can cause inflammation of the colon.

Antibiotic-associated diarrhea is fairly common, affecting up to 25 percent of clindamycin users and up to 10 percent of those who take ampicillin. The most serious form of antibiotic-related diarrhea is pseudomembranous colitis, caused by a toxin secreted from an organism called *Clostridium difficile.*

Typically, diarrhea begins 4 to 10 days after the antibiotic treatment is started and the signs and symptoms usually abate after the drug is discontinued. However, in as many as 25 percent of people, signs and symptoms don't develop until the antibiotic has been discontinued.

Diagnosis

If your doctor suspects that your diarrhea is related to the use of antibiotics, he or she may perform tests on a sample of stool.

How serious is antibiotic-associated diarrhea?

Many people improve after discontinuing the antibiotic. Others become extremely ill and have persistent diarrhea and dehydration. On occasion, pseudomembranous colitis can develop into a life-threatening situation.

Treatment

Your doctor will likely stop treatment with the antibiotic that may be causing your diarrhea. The medications metronidazole (Flagyl) or vancomycin (Vancocin) can be used for treatment, if necessary. Another option is the medication cholestyramine (Questran), which binds to and eliminates the offending toxin of the *C. difficile* organism.

Malabsorption disorders

Signs and symptoms

- Weight loss
- Diarrhea
- Abdominal cramps, gas and bloating
- Weakness
- Foul-smelling and yellowish stools that may be fatty or oily

During digestion the nutrients contained in the food you eat must be broken down (digested) into molecules that can be absorbed into your bloodstream. For various reasons, these nutrients may not be completely digested and their absorption is impaired. When this occurs, vital nutrients needed by your body are instead eliminated in stool. The result of this malabsorption can be malnutrition.

Malabsorption can stem from many different problems. In the case of pancreatic disease, enzymes necessary to digest certain foods may be absent. This is often called maldigestion. Maldigestion can also occur with chronic liver disease.

A principal sign of malabsorption is fatty (steatorrheal) stools. This results from fat not being properly digested and absorbed during digestion and being eliminated in stool. Stool may be yellow or pale and somewhat larger than normal. The excessive fat content may cause stool to be more malodorous than normal. In addition to fat, protein also may be lost in stool, resulting in wasting of the body's tissues. Malabsorption can also lead to deficiencies in vitamins A, B-12, D, E, K and folate.

Celiac disease

Celiac disease, also known as celiac sprue, is a common cause of malabsorption. This disease is caused by sensitivity to gluten, a protein found in wheat, and similar-acting proteins found in rye, oats and barley. The intolerance to gluten causes the lining of the intestine to lose its tiny folds (villi) through which nutrients are absorbed.

Signs and symptoms include foul-smelling diarrheal stools, bloating, weight loss and anemia. In mild cases, signs and symptoms may be limited to anemia or early-onset osteoporosis and not include any digestive signs or symptoms. Sometimes, celiac disease may mimic irritable bowel syndrome.

Celiac disease often occurs in children. The most dramatic signs are weight loss and failure to grow. Bony changes similar to those in rickets may be seen in some children. In adults, demineralization of bone (osteomalacia) may occur with bone pain and tenderness.

In addition to examining your stool for excessive amounts of fat, your doctor may order a barium X-ray of your small bowel if he or she suspects the disease. Biopsy of the lining of the small intestine can provide a supporting diagnosis. It's generally done by inserting a small device (endoscope) through your mouth and into the small intestine. The tissue specimen is examined under the microscope for the characteristic changes of sprue. Specific blood tests also may be helpful but aren't diagnostic by themselves.

Celiac disease is treated by eliminating foods from your diet that contain gluten. Your doctor or a dietitian will instruct you in how to follow a gluten-free diet. Either may be able to give you the names of gluten-free diet cookbooks and of support groups in your area. If a gluten-free diet is carefully followed, the villi of the small intestine will resume their normal shape and regain their absorption ability over a period of several months. Your stools should return to normal, and you should stop losing weight. To correct certain nutrient deficiencies, initially you may be given vitamin and mineral supplements.

Tropical sprue

Tropical sprue is a disease that affects visitors to tropical regions of the world, particularly in the Caribbean and Southeast Asia. People with tropical sprue may experience diarrhea, weight loss, anemia and an inability to gain weight.

Signs and symptoms can appear many months or even years after you return from the area. The cause of this disease is uncertain, but it may be an infectious microorganism.

Diagnostic tests are basically the same as those for celiac sprue. Treatment for tropical sprue generally consists of vitamin supplementation and an antibiotic such as tetracycline. Usually, no special diet is required. Depending on the severity of the disease, you may be on antibiotics for as long as 6 months.

Bacterial overgrowth

Normally, overgrowth of bacteria in the small intestine isn't a problem because the constant muscular movement of the intestine (peristalsis) removes the bacteria.

However, under certain conditions, intestinal bacteria may grow to a point where they cause malabsorption.

This condition can occur in people with diabetes. Other conditions that may predispose a person to this sort of bacterial overgrowth include the development of pouches (diverticula) in the small intestine, narrowed areas (strictures) of the small intestine and radiation damage to the intestine (radiation enteropathy).

Bacterial overgrowth may also be seen after bowel surgery in which segments of the small bowel are bypassed. The diagnosis is made by samples taken from the small bowel or sometimes by indirect tests that involve collections of blood, breath or urine. The treatment is antibiotics, often given intermittently, such as 1 week out of each month.

Scleroderma

When scleroderma affects the intestine, it causes shrinking (atrophy) of its muscular walls, which can impair absorption of nutrients and affect peristalsis. Because the disease is progressive and can spread to other organs, medically it's known as progressive systemic sclerosis (PSS). The cause of this long-term (chronic) disease is unknown. PSS may cause pouches (diverticula) to form in the intestine, and it may restrain peristalsis in the small bowel, leading to an overgrowth of bacteria. This overgrowth may, in turn, lead to severe diarrhea. Antibiotics given in cyclical fashion, often 1 week each month, may be helpful.

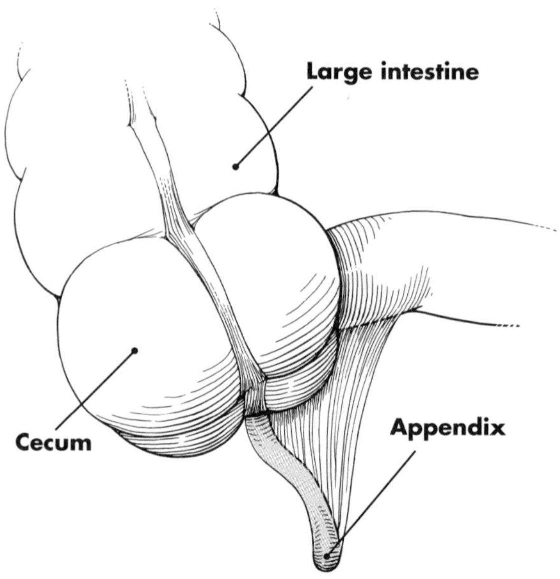

The worm-shaped appendix is attached to the cecum. The appendix can become inflamed and, without prompt treatment, burst.

AIDS

Acquired immunodeficiency syndrome (AIDS) also can cause malabsorption. The primary signs, diarrhea and weight loss, are thought to be the result of infections in the small intestine and colon.

Whipple's disease

Whipple's disease is an extremely rare malabsorption disorder that primarily affects men older than age 45. The disease is likely caused by a recently identified infectious organism, the *Tropheryma whippelii* bacterium. Signs and symptoms such as diarrhea, abdominal pain, progressive weight loss and a darkening of the skin may occur. The infection also may cause a low-grade fever.

A diagnosis is made by a biopsy of the small bowel, in which a sample of tissue is taken for laboratory examination. Long-term — 12- to 18-month — use of antibiotics typically is effective in correcting malabsorption due to Whipple's disease.

Amyloidosis

Amyloidosis is a disease produced by a protein — amyloid — present in excessive amounts in various tissues and locations. Depending on where the deposits of this protein occur in the body, the consequences can range from insignificant to severe. For example, amyloid in the small intestine will make the lining rubbery, firm and waxy and result in serious malabsorption.

Diagnosis of this condition is made by a small bowel biopsy. There's no method of preventing the formation of amyloid deposits. Treatment is geared toward relieving signs and symptoms or treating an underlying disorder that sometimes is responsible for the condition. Such disorders include tuberculosis, Hodgkin's disease and rheumatoid arthritis.

Lactose intolerance

Lactose, the principal sugar in cows' milk, requires the enzyme lactase for its digestion. Lactose intolerance occurs when the lining of your small intestine produces reduced amounts of this enzyme.

Lactose intolerance causes abdominal cramps, bloating, diarrhea and excessive gas when more than a certain amount of milk or milk products is ingested. Small amounts of milk usually don't produce signs and symptoms.

Approximately 70 percent of the world's population is thought to

Diabetic Intestinal Disorders

Long-standing diabetes can cause decreased function of the autonomic nerves that control the muscular activity of the stomach. A condition called diabetic gastroparesis diminishes the mixing and propelling activity by the stomach. Gradually, the stomach begins to resemble a limp bag and enlarges. Signs include vomiting rather large amounts of fluid and partially digested food that was eaten as long as a day or two before. Medications such as metoclopramide (Reglan) or erythromycin sometimes are effective in treating this disorder.

Similar deterioration of nerves in the intestines can impair the propulsive action of the intestines. Diarrhea tends to occur at night, and because of impaired sensation and function of the anal sphincter, there may be fecal incontinence especially during sleep. Some degree of malabsorption also may be seen.

have a low level of lactase in the lining of the small intestine. More than 30 million Americans may have some degree of lactose intolerance.

Low lactase levels may occur in association with other malabsorptive diseases, such as celiac or tropical sprue, viral or bacterial infections of the small intestine and cystic fibrosis.

If you have lactose intolerance, you don't need to eliminate all dairy products from your diet unless your signs and symptoms are severe. Rather, decrease your consumption of milk products. Drink milk only during meals and try to get your calcium from cheese and yogurt, dairy products lower in lactose than milk. Another alternative is to buy a commercial lactase preparation, such as Lactaid or Dairy Ease, which can be mixed into your milk. These preparations convert lactose into simple sugars that are easily absorbed.

Short-bowel syndrome

A number of situations can reduce the surface area of your small intestine. Surgical removal of a significant portion of the intestine is one of the most common. Damage from radiation therapy or a disease that affects the intestine also can reduce the length of your bowel.

Because of reduced surface area, absorption of nutrients may be impaired. In some people, this can lead to malabsorption problems, called short-bowel syndrome.

Because different nutrients are absorbed in different areas of the small intestine, the type of malabsorption depends on how much and what part of the intestine was removed.

For example, removal of the last portion of the small intestine — the main location for bile acid and vitamin B-12 absorption — may lead to excess bile acids spilling over into the colon and vitamin B-12 deficiency. If bile acids enter the colon, they may irritate or inflame the lining of the colon, causing watery diarrhea.

Appendicitis

Signs and symptoms

- Abdominal pain, usually starting around the navel and settling in the lower right side of the abdomen
- Loss of appetite
- Nausea and, sometimes, vomiting
- An unusual urge to pass stool or gas
- Mild fever

The appendix, a hollow worm-shaped structure that's attached to the first section of the large intestine (cecum), is about 3½ inches long. It's not certain exactly what its function is, but it may play a role in bowel immunity. It's not always clear why the appendix can become inflamed, swollen and fill with pus, but many times appendicitis is associated with an obstruction.

Individuals most likely to have acute appendicitis are between the ages of 10 and 30, although it can occur at almost any age. Appendicitis can be especially difficult to diagnose in infants and people who are very old.

Diagnosis

Your doctor may ask you questions about your symptoms, including your appetite, location of the pain and an unusual urge to pass gas or move your bowels. On examination of your abdomen, tenderness is an important sign. Depending on your symptoms, a blood test and an ultrasound or computerized tomography (CT) scan of the abdomen may be done.

How serious is appendicitis?

Most cases of appendicitis aren't life-threatening, but the condition warrants prompt treatment. Peritonitis, a serious infection of the abdominal cavity, may develop if the appendix bursts.

Treatment

The standard procedure is to remove the infected appendix surgically. This can sometimes be done with a less invasive form of surgery called laparoscopy.

Meckel's diverticulum

A diverticulum is a pouch that develops in tubular organs such as the bowel. Meckel's diverticulum is a specific type of diverticulum present at birth. The pouch generally forms in the lower part of the small intestine (ileum) and is typically about 2 inches long.

Although this fairly common disorder frequently causes no signs and symptoms, the pouch can become inflamed and bleed. In some cases, especially among young children, bleeding may occur as the result of an ulcer that has formed at the same site.

If inflammation of a Meckel's diverticulum becomes severe, it can perforate the intestinal wall. A Meckel's diverticulum may also twist or herniate, causing a bowel obstruction. Treatment of any of these complications generally includes surgical removal of the diverticulum.

Intussusception

Signs and symptoms

- Sudden, severe abdominal pain
- Weakness and lethargy
- Vomiting, often with bile
- Bloody stools that may resemble currant jelly
- Shallow breathing
- Faintness, sweating and pallor

Intussusception is a rare disorder in which a portion of the intestine, usually the small intestine, telescopes into another segment of the intestine. It's the most common cause of intestinal obstruction in children between the ages of 3 months and 6 years. The cause is unknown, but in some cases there may be a correlation between intussusception and certain viral infections.

Typically, intussusception strikes abruptly in a previously well child. The child suddenly has a severe, colicky abdominal pain that occurs at frequent intervals. At first, the child may play normally between the pains but soon becomes weaker and lethargic.

Intussusception in adults is uncommon and, unlike in children, usually associated with an intestinal disease.

Diagnosis

If your child has these signs and symptoms, don't delay in calling your doctor. The signs and symptoms and physical findings may be sufficient to establish a diagnosis, but often further tests, such as an abdominal X-ray and a barium X-ray, may be needed. See Chapter 39, "Diagnostic Tests" for more on these tests.

How serious is intussusception?

If untreated, the condition may be very serious. Most children recover if treatment is begun within 24 hours after the initial signs and symptoms.

Treatment

A barium enema used for diagnosis may be sufficient to push the telescoped intestine back into its proper place. The recurrence rate, however, can be as high as 10 percent. In many cases, surgery is necessary. Generally, there's no recurrence following surgery.

Protein-losing enteropathy

Signs and symptoms

- Blood in the stool
- Generalized swelling of tissues

Some gastrointestinal disorders cause protein in the blood (plasma protein) to leak into the gastrointestinal tract and be excreted in the stool. Plasma protein may pass into the gastrointestinal tract through an inflamed or ulcerated intestinal lining, as with the diseases regional enteritis and ulcerative colitis. The result is low blood protein, which in turn can cause generalized swelling (edema) of tissues.

Intestinal lymphangiectasia is a type of protein-losing intestinal disease in which swelling of the lymph channels of the small intestine leads to loss of protein and fat from these lymph channels into the intestines. Children and young adults are most commonly affected by this disorder. The principal treatment is a low-fat diet.

Inflammatory bowel disease

Inflammatory bowel disease is a term generally used to describe two similar disorders that involve the gastrointestinal tract and for which no cause has been found. These disorders are Crohn's disease and ulcerative colitis.

Signs and symptoms of Crohn's disease

- Long-term (chronic) diarrhea
- Abdominal cramps and pain
- Blood in the stool
- Fever
- Fatigue
- Weight loss
- Joint pain
- Skin lesions

Crohn's disease, sometimes referred to as ileitis, regional enteritis or granulomatous colitis, is a chronic inflammation of the intestine. It often involves the lower part of the small intestine (ileum). However, it can also affect the colon or any other part of the digestive tract. The inflammation often affects the entire thickness of the bowel wall.

Crohn's disease develops in about 7 out of 100,000 people every year. Anyone may be affected, but people with this disease typically first receive a diagnosis between the ages of 15 and 35. Heredity or environmental influences may play a role in the development of Crohn's disease. About 1 out of 5 people with Crohn's disease have a relative with Crohn's or ulcerative colitis. Jewish people of European descent also are more likely to develop inflammatory bowel disease.

Diagnosis

Signs and symptoms of Crohn's disease may include persistent diarrhea, abdominal pain, fever and general fatigue. Occasionally, there may be blood in the stool. Significant weight loss is common.

A barium X-ray of the small intestine may reveal abnormal-looking areas. Segments of intestine may appear irregular and less flexible than normal. Sometimes, a doctor performs a procedure called colonoscopy to examine the lining of the colon and the last several inches of the ileum. A computerized tomography (CT) scan may show fibrotic masses or an abscess.

How serious is Crohn's disease?

The course of Crohn's disease varies greatly from one person to another. Some people with Crohn's disease remain without signs and symptoms (asymptomatic) after the initial one or two episodes. Others have recurrent episodes of abdominal pain, diarrhea and fever. Crohn's disease is usually long-term (chronic), but you may have long periods of remission.

The diarrhea can be debilitating to the point of significant malnutrition. Episodes of abdominal pain after eating, due to gradually increasing bowel obstruction, may cause you to avoid eating because of discomfort.

The complications of Crohn's disease are many and varied. Progressive obstruction, particularly of the small bowel, is the most common reason for surgical treatment of Crohn's disease. Obstructive symptoms generally develop gradually over a long period.

Fistulas and fissures in and around anal and rectal areas are common. A fistula is an abnormal passage between two segments of the intestine or from the intestine to the skin. Fistulas can also develop from the intestine to the vagina or bladder. An anal fissure is a crack or cleft in the anus or skin around the anus.

When internal fistulas develop, food bypasses areas of the bowel necessary for absorption. With external fistulas, there can be continuous drainage of bowel contents to the skin, sometimes causing infection. Intestinal bleeding also may occur with Crohn's disease.

If you have Crohn's disease, you may have signs and symptoms not related to the digestive tract. These may include arthritis, particularly of large joints, or inflammation involving an eye or your skin. Occasionally, you may experience inflammation of the bile ducts (primary sclerosing cholangitis). In addition, the development of kidney stones and gallstones is common with Crohn's disease.

Treatment

There's no cure for Crohn's disease. The goal of treatment is to reduce the inflammation that triggers its signs and symptoms. At times, this can lead not only to symptom relief but also to long-term remission. Treatment usually involves medication or surgery. If your Crohn's disease is asymptomatic or in remission, treatment may be unnecessary.

Medication

The medication you may receive depends on the type and severity of your signs and symptoms. If they primarily involve several loose stools each day, your doctor may prescribe antidiarrheal medication or a bulking agent that contains vegetable fibers. If your disease is more active, your doctor may consider anti-inflammatory medications, such as sulfasalazine (Azulfidine). Sulfasalazine has been prescribed for nearly 60 years to treat both Crohn's disease and ulcerative colitis. It's often effective but can have several side effects, such as loss of appetite, nausea, vomiting, skin rashes and headache.

If sulfasalazine isn't effective or you don't tolerate it well, newer medications that work similarly, such as mesalamine (Asacol, Rowaza) or olsalazine (Dipentum), may be used. Both produce fewer side effects. Mesalamine is also available as a suppository and as an enema, both of which are useful when the disease is limited to the lower part of the colon or rectum.

Corticosteroids, another type of anti-inflammatory medication, are prescribed mainly for moderate to severe disease that doesn't respond to other treatment. Corticosteroids are often effective, but they can cause numerous side effects, including a puffy face, acne, excessive facial hair, night sweats, insomnia, irritability and hyperactivity. More serious side effects include high blood pressure, diabetes, osteoporosis, cataracts and reduced resistance to infections.

Some of the more commonly used corticosteroids are prednisone (Deltasone, Sterapred) methylprednisolone (Medrol) and hydrocortisone (Cortef, Hydrocortone). Newer and slower-acting drugs, such as budesonide (Entocort), are proving safer and more effective for mild to moderate Crohn's disease of the small intestine. Corticosteroids are most commonly taken orally, although they can be administered rectally as a suppository, enema or foam.

Investigators are studying new corticosteroid preparations and other medications that have fewer side effects and more potent anti-inflammatory activity.

Some doctors recommend a course of immunosuppressive therapy. Immunosuppressant drugs target your immune system, which may be causing or contributing to the inflammation. Drugs such as azathioprine (Imuran) or 6-mercaptopurine (6-MP) are the most widely used immunosuppressants. However, it can take up to 3 months before these medications are effective. Infliximab (Remicade), a more recently developed immunosuppressant, is designed to neutralize a natural protein, called

Nutrition and Crohn's Disease

The ability to absorb adequate nutrients is often limited in people with Crohn's disease, particularly if the disease affects significant portions of the small bowel or if portions of the small bowel have been surgically removed.

Your doctor may advise specific replacement of certain vitamins or minerals if there's evidence of a deficiency. It's not uncommon for people with Crohn's disease to have a deficiency of vitamin B-12, which is absorbed in the lowest segment of the small bowel (ileum). Vitamin B-12 can be easily replaced with monthly injections.

Bile acids also are absorbed in this portion of the small bowel. If bile acids aren't absorbed from the small bowel, they may cause diarrhea by irritating the colon lining and interfering with the absorption of water. A bile acid binder, such as cholestyramine (Questran), may decrease the amount of free bile acid in stool.

Avoiding foods and beverages that aggravate signs and symptoms is helpful, especially during a flare-up of the disease. Other dietary suggestions include limiting dairy products, trying low-fat foods, eating small meals and drinking plenty of liquids that aren't caffeinated, alcoholic or carbonated.

Some doctors advocate the use of elemental diets consisting of liquid preparations containing simple sugars, amino acids and minerals, particularly for people with active Crohn's disease who are malnourished. Some people need to receive all of their nutrition intravenously for weeks, or even months, during severe bouts of Crohn's disease.

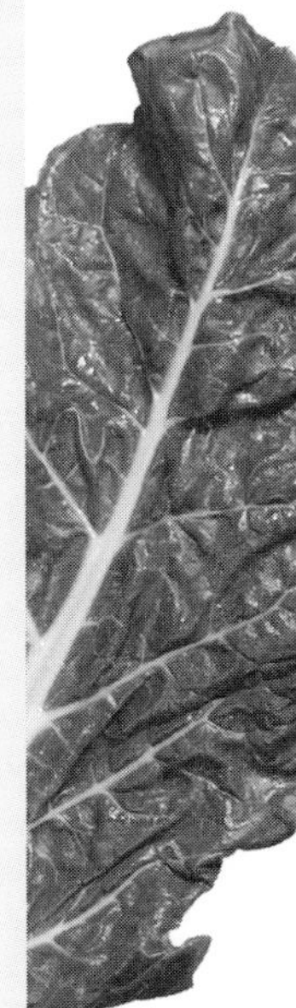

tumor necrosis factor, that causes inflammation. Methotrexate (Rheumatrex) and cyclosporine (Neoral, Sandimmune) are sometimes recommended for people who don't respond well to other medications, but long-term use of these drugs can have significant side effects.

Antibiotics such as metronidazole (Flagyl) also may be effective, particularly for fistulas or abscesses in the anal region. Generally, this medication needs to be taken indefinitely not only to heal the fistula or abscess but also to prevent recurrence. At times, metronidazole is used for Crohn's disease of the colon. Metronidazole may cause numbness or tingling in the fingers and toes if used for many months at a time. If this occurs, discuss it with your doctor. An alternative to metronidazole is ciprofloxacin (Cipro), which causes fewer side effects and is gaining in popularity.

Surgery

Approximately 70 percent of people with Crohn's disease require at least one operation at some point. These operations usually are performed for complications of the disease, such as continued bleeding, obstruction, abscesses or bowel perforation.

Surgery typically involves removing the diseased segment of bowel and rejoining the two ends of healthy intestine.

Sometimes, the obstructed segment may be bypassed rather than removed. Your surgeon may also close fistulas or remove scar tissue that's formed and is blocking or

Colostomy, Ileostomy and Ileoanal Anastomosis

Colostomy, ileostomy and ileoanal anastomosis are surgical treatments for diseases such as Crohn's disease, ulcerative colitis and colon cancer. All three procedures alter the normal route for the elimination of waste.

Colostomy

During a colostomy, the surgeon makes an incision to examine the colon and possibly remove diseased areas. Sometimes, the anus and rectum are removed and the anal area permanently closed. A separate incision is made in the abdomen, and a section of colon is pulled through this opening (stoma). A small bag is securely fastened over the opening. The feces then flow into the bag, which is emptied periodically.

Colostomies are identified by the portion of the colon that's brought out through the stoma. For example, a sigmoid colostomy involves the sigmoid colon. The consistency of the stool also depends on where the intestine has been interrupted. If the initial portion of the colon empties into the pouch, the stool will be loose. If the lower end of the colon is brought through the stoma, the stool will be more formed because more liquid has been absorbed in the colon.

Although many colostomies are permanent, sometimes a temporary colostomy is done to allow a portion of the bowel to heal after injury or disease. After the area is healed, the stoma is closed and the bowel is reconnected so that the normal waste elimination can continue.

Ileostomy

This procedure usually follows the entire removal of the colon and rectum. During a conventional ileostomy, a portion of the small intestine is brought out through the stoma created in the abdominal wall. As with a colostomy, an ileostomy requires that a bag be worn over the stoma to collect the waste, which in this case has a liquid consistency because the colon has been removed, where much of the liquid normally is absorbed. Sometimes, a colostomy may be a temporary procedure to allow the bowel time to heal.

A variation of the standard ileostomy is called a continent ileostomy (Kock pouch), which uses a portion of the small intestine to construct an internal pouch and valve for waste. This pouch can store your waste internally for several hours at a time, eliminating the need for an outside bag. You can then drain the pouch at your convenience using a thin tube (catheter) inserted into the stoma.

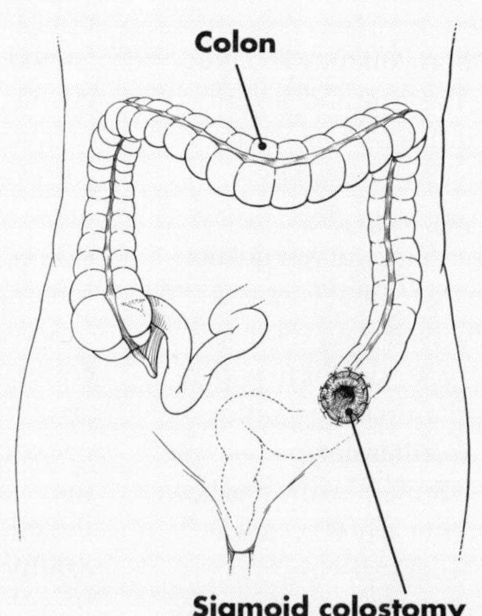

In performing a sigmoid colostomy, the surgeon alters the normal route for waste excretion. The remaining intestine is brought through an opening (stoma) in the abdominal wall. Stool is eliminated into a small bag worn securely over the opening.

narrowing the intestinal passageway. But surgery often times isn't a cure. Crohn's disease may come back elsewhere in your intestinal tract.

In some cases, an ileostomy may be done. In this operation, the entire colon, rectum and anus may be removed. The last section of the small intestine is brought out through an opening (stoma) in the abdominal wall for the passage of stool. A plastic pouch into which the stool is evacuated is attached to the skin around the stoma.

Signs and symptoms of ulcerative colitis

- Bloody diarrhea that may contain mucus
- Abdominal pain
- Painful, urgent bowel movements
- Fever
- Weight loss
- Joint pain
- Skin lesions

Unlike Crohn's disease, which can involve any portion of the intestinal tract, ulcerative colitis is confined to the colon. Similar to Crohn's disease, the cause of ulcerative colitis is largely unknown.

Ulcerative colitis is a long-term (chronic) condition in which an inflammatory reaction characterized by tiny ulcers and small abscesses occurs in the inner lining of the colon. The reactions almost always involve the rectum and may extend into the entire colon. The amount of colon affected varies from person to person. If the inflammation is limited to the rectum, the term *ulcerative proctitis* may be used.

The ileostomy and Kock pouch procedures are being done less frequently, having been replaced in large part by ileoanal anastomosis.

Recovery

With either colostomy or ileostomy, there's a period of adjustment. A stomal therapist can be helpful in this period.

- During the 6 to 8 weeks immediately after the operation, avoid lifting, pushing or pulling more than 5 to 10 pounds. In general, simple exercises such as walking and swimming are good activities to firm your muscles and keep your digestive tract working properly.

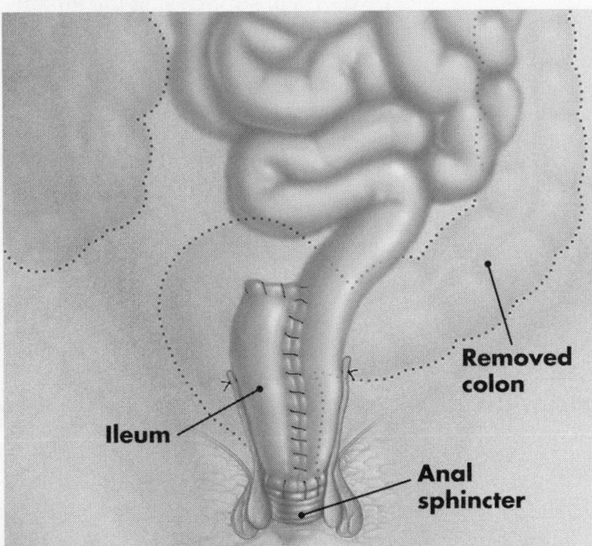

In ileoanal anastomosis, a surgeon removes the colon and innermost lining of the rectum, creates a J-shaped pouch out of the last section of the small intestine (ileum), then reattaches the pouch near the anal sphincter. Leaving the anal sphincter and rectal muscles intact preserves near-normal passage of stool.

- Most doctors advise abstaining from sexual activity for a while after this operation. Sexual dysfunction may occur immediately after the operation. If pain in the vagina or an inability to achieve erection occurs, it may be temporary. If the problem persists, discuss it with your doctor.

Ileoanal anastomosis

An ileoanal anastomosis is the most common surgical procedure for ulcerative colitis. It involves the removal of the colon and rectum through an incision in the abdomen. The surgeon removes the inner lining from the anus but carefully preserves the sphincter muscles. A small J-shaped pouch is made from the end of the ileum to collect fecal material to decrease the number of bowel movements you have. A temporary ileostomy is necessary to divert feces away from the ileal pouch until this new area of intestine has time to heal — about 2 to 3 months.

Recovery

After some initial pain, you'll likely start feeling better soon. Many people debilitated by their disease are surprised to notice weight gain and increased strength so quickly following their operation. By the time they return to the hospital to have the ileostomy closed, they often feel better than they have in years.

Once the ileostomy is closed, expect to have frequent bowel movements for several months. Usually, the first bowel movement occurs about 3 days after the stoma is closed. The pouch made at the end of the ileum slowly increases in size. As this pouch becomes larger, it can store more stool and the number of bowel movements a day decreases.

If incontinence is a problem, your doctor may prescribe a medication to slow down your bowel and thicken the consistency of the stool.

Although ulcerative colitis can strike at any time of life, it's most common between the ages of 15 and 35. It can occur in people of all races and ethnicities, but the risk seems to be higher among whites. Ulcerative colitis also tends to run in families.

Diagnosis

Ulcerative colitis is often identified during a procedure called colonoscopy, in which a thin, flexible tube with an attached camera is inserted into the colon. If tissues are inflamed, bowel walls will bleed even when gently touched by the probe. A tissue specimen may be taken from the area for analysis (biopsy). A similar procedure called a flexible sigmoidoscopy may be performed in place of a colonoscopy. It examines just the lowest part of the colon. Blood tests or X-rays also may be done.

How serious is ulcerative colitis?

At times, ulcerative colitis may be without signs and symptoms. At other times, inflammation of the colon may occur, causing bloody diarrhea. Such flare-ups may alternate with periods of remission.

In approximately 15 percent of people with ulcerative colitis, the disease involves the entire colon and may cause severe bloody diarrhea, fever and abdominal pain. Signs and symptoms that progressively worsen may even constitute a medical emergency because of risk of dilation of the colon (toxic megacolon) and perforation of the markedly inflamed colon.

Ulcerative colitis may cause various signs and symptoms in other areas of the body. These may include pain or inflammation of large joints, most often the knees, ankles and wrists. Skin abnormalities that can occur with ulcerative colitis include chronic skin ulcers (pyoderma gangrenosum) and tender, red bumps that turn into dark areas that look like bruises (erythema nodosum). Acute eye inflammation also may develop. Although uncommon, the disease can also affect the flow of bile from the liver, a condition called primary sclerosing cholangitis.

Among people who've had the disease for at least 8 to 10 years and in whom more than half of their colon is affected, there's also increased risk of colon cancer.

In people who have lesser degrees of involvement, risk of colon cancer is less and not apparent until 15 to 20 years after the onset of colitis. Risk of colon cancer increases with time. However, cancer can develop even if signs and symptoms are minimal.

Your doctor may suggest periodic colon examination with biopsies of colon tissue to look for changes suggesting a transformation to cancerous (malignant) cells. If such changes are found, an option is removal of the colon to prevent cancer.

Treatment

The goal of treatment is to control the inflammatory process, relieve signs and symptoms and prevent complications.

Medication

The principal drugs used in the treatment of ulcerative colitis are the anti-inflammatory agents. Sulfasalazine (Azulfadine) is generally used for minor flare-ups of the disease and in maintaining remissions. Mesalamine (Asacol, Rowasa), olsalazine (Dipentum) and balsalazide (Colazal) are derivatives of sulfasalazine and contain the active ingredient 5-ASA. These drugs may be used if you can't tolerate sulfasalazine or if it's ineffective. Mesalamine is also available as a suppository or enema.

Corticosteroids are generally reserved for those with more severe signs and symptoms because the medications can cause several side effects, including a puffy face, acne, excessive facial hair, night sweats, insomnia, irritability and hyperactivity. More serious side effects, especially if the medications are used long term, include high blood pressure, diabetes, osteoporosis, cataracts and an increased susceptibility to infections. If the inflammatory process is confined to the rectum, a corticosteroid enema may be useful in suppressing the inflam-

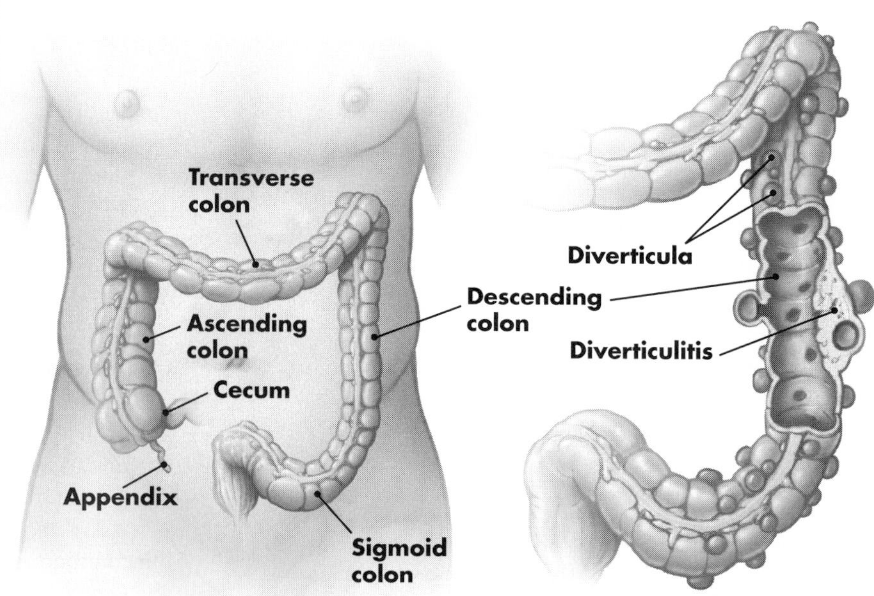

The most common location for development of small pouches (diverticula) is the large intestine (colon). When a pouch becomes inflamed or infected, the condition is called diverticulitis.

mation and alleviating signs and symptoms.

Immunosuppressive therapy may be helpful for severe disease. Cyclosporine (Neoral, Sandimmune), a potent immunosuppressant agent, has shown promise in the treatment of selected cases of severe ulcerative colitis. Cyclosporine, however, can produce significant side effects, including high blood pressure and liver and kidney damage, and use of it requires careful supervision by your doctor.

Surgery

Approximately 25 percent to 40 percent of people with ulcerative colitis require surgery at some time. Surgery is often necessary when the disease doesn't respond to medication or produces severe complications.

The present trend is to perform surgery earlier in the disease, when it appears the inflammation is unresponsive to medication, instead of waiting until the individual becomes debilitated. Cancer risk may be an indication for surgery as well. After about 10 years, risk of colon cancer increases, especially if the colitis affects most of or all of the colon.

The operation most commonly done is total removal of the colon and rectum with ileoanal anastomosis. Unlike other surgical techniques, ileoanal anastomosis isn't as disfiguring because it permits the passage of stool through the anus and is usually well tolerated.

Nutrition

No food has been shown to make ulcerative colitis better or worse, although it's best to avoid foods that aggravate signs and symptoms of the disease.

Diverticulosis and diverticulitis

Signs and symptoms

- Pain
- Abdominal tenderness
- Fever
- Bleeding
- Constipation or diarrhea

Diverticulosis is the name for the development of small pouches (diverticula) in the colon wall. Most people with diverticulosis experience no signs or symptoms, and typically the condition goes undiscovered or is identified when diagnostic tests are performed for other reasons. Occasionally, a pouch will bleed, alerting a doctor to the condition.

When inflammation occurs in or around one or more pouches, the condition is called diverticulitis. Diverticulitis is more likely to occur in the lower (sigmoid) portion of your colon and may result from undigested food and bacteria lodging in a pouch. The inflammation can compromise the blood supply to the pouch, making it susceptible to an invasion by bacteria. The result can range from a small abscess to a massive infection or perforation. The process resembles that of appendicitis except that it occurs in the lower-left side of the colon.

Symptoms of diverticulitis include cramping pains, which are usually most severe on the left side. Fever and nausea also may be present. Sometimes, an inflamed diverticulum can rupture, spilling intestinal material into the abdominal cavity. This can cause peritonitis, a medical emergency.

Causes

The cause of diverticulosis is unknown, but diverticular problems are much more common in industrialized nations such as the United States, leading some doctors to speculate that low fiber intake in the Western diet may be a major factor.

Risk of diverticular disease increases with age, perhaps because the outer muscular wall of the colon thickens over time, narrowing the internal passageway and increasing pressure in the colon. Pressure on the colon wall can also be increased by straining to pass hard stools, which may result from a low-fiber diet. Increased pressure can cause weak spots in the colon wall to bulge out, forming pouches.

Treatment

For diverticulosis without signs and symptoms, treatment is generally unnecessary. A high-fiber diet with plenty of fluid may reduce the risk of complications and the development of more diverticula. In some instances, an antispasmodic medication may be prescribed.

Treatment for diverticulitis often involves bed rest, stool softeners, a liquid diet and oral antibiotics if the inflammation is mild and the diverticulum hasn't ruptured. In case of a rupture or widespread infection, intravenous (IV) antibiotic therapy in a hospital may be required. Surgery also may be necessary to remove the diseased segment of colon. For severe signs and symptoms, a temporary colostomy (see page 876) may be necessary while the colon heals. Later, after healing has occurred, a second operation to reconnect the colon is performed.

Irritable bowel syndrome

Signs and symptoms

- Abdominal pain or discomfort
- Bloating or gas
- Diarrhea
- Constipation
- Mucus in the stool

Approximately 20 percent of Americans periodically have signs and symptoms of irritable bowel syndrome. Because the signs and symptoms are often common digestive complaints and can occur intermittently, many people never seek medical attention. However, this condition is one of the leading causes of lost work and school time. Irritable bowel syndrome often begins in adolescence or in young adulthood. It occurs more frequently in women than in men.

Abdominal pain and a change in bowel habits are the main signs and symptoms. The pain can occur anywhere in your abdomen, and it can be severe. Indigestion, heartburn and nausea also may sometimes occur. Typically, the signs and symptoms occur after a meal and are temporarily relieved by a bowel movement. People with irritable bowel syndrome frequently complain of feeling bloated and passing an excessive amount of gas, which also relieves the discomfort.

Constipation also is a frequent complaint. The bowel movement may be pellet-like or in small balls or ribbons. Diarrhea also may occur and is a predominant sign among many people.

Causes

Irritable bowel syndrome is often called spastic colon because it's thought to result from abnormal muscular activity of the intestinal wall.

The causes of this abnormal activity are unknown. At times, the condition may be aggravated by a specific food, but in many people chronic stress and depression worsen signs and symptoms.

Diagnosis

A diagnosis of irritable bowel syndrome depends largely on a complete medical history and physical examination to exclude more serious signs and symptoms. Your doctor may also recommend conducting several tests, including stool studies to check for infection or malabsorption problems. He or she may perform a flexible sigmoidoscopy or colonoscopy. These tests help rule out more serious conditions, such as ulcerative colitis, Crohn's disease and colorectal cancer. See Chapter 39, "Diagnostic Tests," for more information on these tests.

You may also have tests to determine whether you're lactose intolerant. Lactase is an enzyme needed to digest the sugar found in dairy products. If you lack this enzyme, you may have signs and symptoms similar to those caused by irritable bowel syndrome, including abdominal pain, gas and diarrhea. Lactose intolerance may coexist with irritable bowel syndrome.

Because there are usually no physical signs of disease in irritable bowel syndrome, diagnosis is often a process of elimination. To help in this process, researchers have developed diagnostic criteria, known as Rome criteria, for irritable bowel syndrome and other functional gastrointestinal disorders — conditions in which the bowel appears normal but doesn't function normally.

According to these criteria, you must have certain signs and symptoms before receiving a diagnosis of irritable bowel syndrome. The most important are abdominal pain and diarrhea or constipation lasting at least 3 months. You also need to have at least two of the following signs and symptoms a quarter or more of the time:

- A change in the frequency or consistency of your stool. For example, you may change from having one normal, formed stool every day to several loose stools. Or you may have only one hard stool every 3 to 4 days.
- Straining, urgency or a feeling that you can't empty your bowels completely.
- Mucus in your stool.
- Bloating or abdominal swelling.

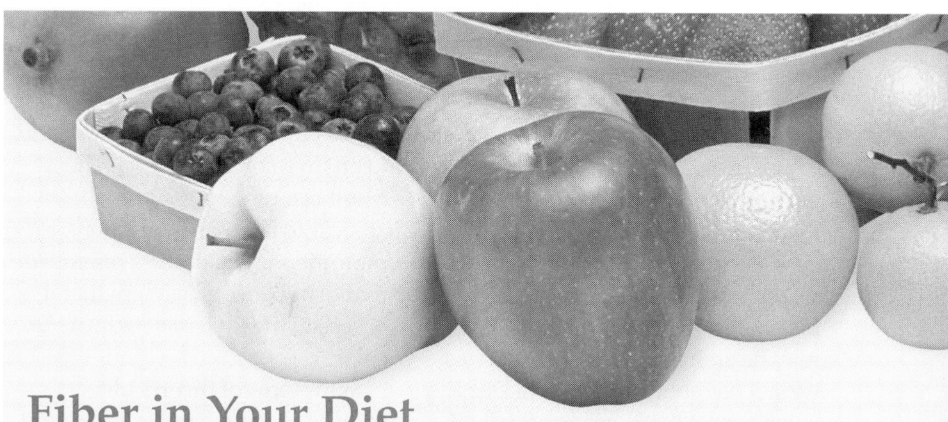

Fiber in Your Diet

In recent years, Americans have become increasingly aware of the need for more fiber in their diets. A high-fiber diet helps to prevent constipation, and it may lower your risk of specific disorders, such as hemorrhoids, diverticular disease and irritable bowel syndrome. Other benefits of fiber include a possible lowering of cholesterol and, in people with diabetes, a slowing of sugar absorption, which may decrease the need for insulin.

The role of fiber in the prevention of colon cancer remains unclear. Some studies suggest a high-fiber diet reduces the risk of colon cancer, but other studies don't show evidence of benefit.

Fiber and digestion

High-fiber foods — often referred to as bulk or roughage — include whole-grain products, fruits, vegetables and legumes, such as beans and lentils. These may be better sources of fiber than fiber supplements.

Unlike most components of food, fiber isn't affected by digestive enzymes. It passes virtually unchanged through the stomach and small intestine and into the colon. In the colon, some forms of fiber are fermented by bacteria. Others resist fermentation and are eliminated in stool unchanged, which increases the weight and size of the stool, in addition to softening it. A bulky stool is easier to pass, decreasing the chance of constipation. If you have loose, watery stools, fiber may help to solidify the stool because it absorbs water and adds bulk to stool.

Treatment

Irritable bowel syndrome is a chronic condition that may occur on and off throughout your life, but you can take steps to minimize the signs and symptoms:

See your doctor

The signs and symptoms of irritable bowel syndrome may mimic those of a serious disease. It's important that you undergo a complete examination, particularly if the symptoms have appeared only recently, to be sure your problem isn't caused by something more serious. Knowing that your symptoms aren't due to a serious disease may ease your mind — and possibly decrease stress that may be contributing to your condition.

Select foods carefully

If a specific food appears to trigger symptoms, eliminate it from your diet. Sometimes, a high-fiber diet including consumption of fresh fruits, vegetables and fiber supplements is helpful. In some people, however, the same diet can increase bloating and gas.

But don't eliminate a food just because it appears to cause signs or symptoms on a single occasion. A varied diet is important. Be sure that the food produces signs or

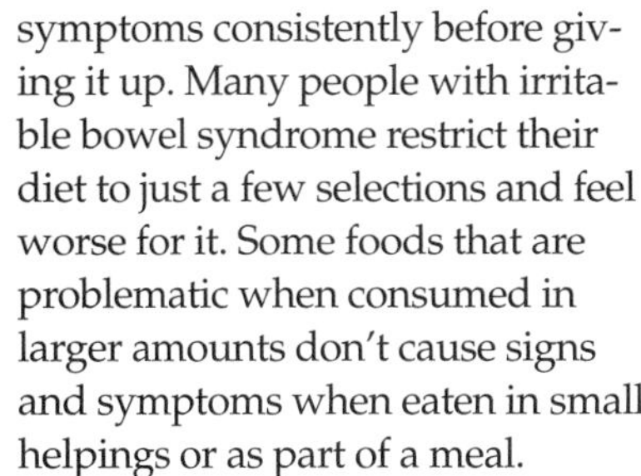

symptoms consistently before giving it up. Many people with irritable bowel syndrome restrict their diet to just a few selections and feel worse for it. Some foods that are problematic when consumed in larger amounts don't cause signs and symptoms when eaten in small helpings or as part of a meal.

Drink plenty of liquids

Liquids help relieve constipation and replace body fluids absorbed by fiber. Water is best. Beverages containing caffeine and alcohol cause you to urinate more and lose fluid. They can also worsen diarrhea by stimulating or irritating your intestines. Carbonated beverages can produce gas.

Eat at regular times

Don't skip meals, and try to eat about the same time each day to help regulate bowel function. If you have diarrhea, you may find that eating small, frequent meals makes you feel better. But if you're constipated, eating larger amounts of high-fiber foods and consuming plenty of fluid may help move food through your intestines.

Exercise daily

Exercise helps relieve depression and stress, stimulates normal contractions of your intestines and can help you feel better about yourself. Aim for 30 minutes of exercise most days. If you've been inactive, start slowly and gradually increase the amount of time you exercise.

Use supplements, if necessary

Fiber supplements can be convenient and are sometimes even necessary, especially for people who have trouble eating foods rich in fiber because they cause abdominal pain, cramping and gas. Although these symptoms tend to disappear after a few weeks, fiber supplements may be an alternative if you can't tolerate high-fiber foods.

Bulk formers, which generally contain either a tasteless powder called methylcellulose or the

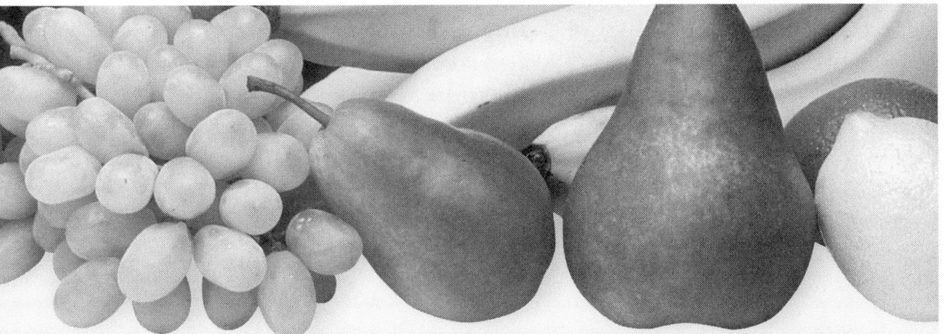

Fiber does have some disadvantages too. It frequently causes excess gas. In people with inflammatory bowel disease, fiber can make diarrhea, pain and gas worse. In addition, some sources of fiber — oat bran and wheat fiber, for example — can remove minerals such as calcium, iron and zinc from your body. If you eat a balanced diet and consume a reasonable amount of milk with your oat bran or high-fiber cereals, this usually isn't a problem.

Fueling up on fiber

Americans typically consume 10 to 15 grams of fiber daily. Dietary guidelines recommend twice that amount. To help ensure adequate dietary fiber, follow these suggestions:

- *Get your fiber from food.* Sometimes, people assume that if they take a fiber supplement, they need not pay attention to their diet. A supplement may be helpful, but natural fiber found in food may be better.
- *Eat a varied diet.* Include high-fiber foods such as grains, vegetables, fresh fruits and legumes. High-fiber snack foods include nuts, seeds, popcorn, fresh and dried fruits and whole-grain crackers.
- *Limit your consumption of processed foods.* These often contain little fiber. The refining process often removes the outer coat (bran) from grain. This is why whole-grain products are higher in fiber content than those made of refined flour. In a similar fashion, removing the skin from fruits and vegetables decreases their fiber content.
- *Increase your fiber intake gradually.* This will help your digestive system adjust to the increased levels of this bulking agent. A gradual increase will also help prevent problems with bloating and gas.

Laxative Abuse

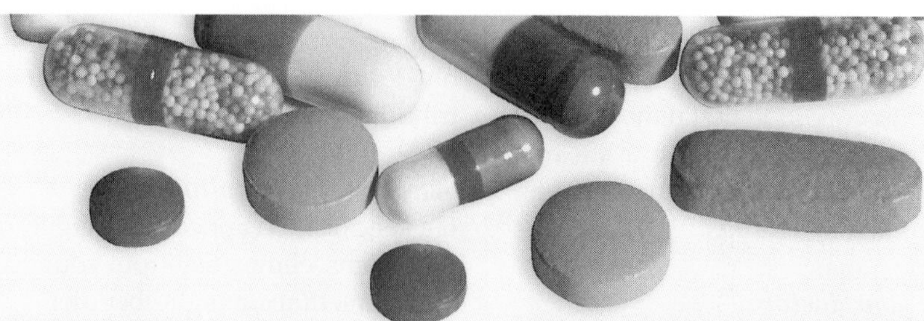

It's rare for anyone to need a laxative on a daily basis, yet many people use them regularly. Some people take laxatives to fight constipation. Others take them regularly as a preventive measure even though they aren't really constipated. Still others take laxatives in an attempt to lose weight.

Kinds of laxatives

One of the oldest laxatives is castor oil. It undergoes chemical transformation within the small intestine to become an acid that stimulates intestinal activity and prevents the intestinal wall from absorbing water. Prolonged use of castor oil can damage the cells that line your intestinal tract.

Some laxatives act by inhibiting water absorption. Other laxatives work by increasing water content within your colon and are less irritating to your bowel. These include milk of magnesia and stool softeners.

Bulk-forming agents or so-called natural laxatives (psyllium and methylcellulose) don't stimulate your digestive system. Instead, they expand when they come into contact with water in the colon. These agents generally are safe for long-term use and can help prevent the formation of hard stools.

What are the risks of overuse?

When taken in excess, laxatives may flush out necessary vitamins and other nutrients before they can be fully absorbed. Laxatives also contribute to an excessive excretion of water, sodium and potassium. In addition, habitual use of laxatives tends to weaken intestinal muscles and make them less able to function properly. As a result, once you stop taking a laxative regularly, your constipation not only will return but may be worse.

Excessive use of laxatives can induce lazy bowel syndrome. This is a condition in which the bowels fail to function properly because they've begun to rely on the laxative to do the work of elimination. Laxatives can also interfere with the effectiveness of other medications your doctor might prescribe.

natural vegetable fiber psyllium, are available without a prescription. They may help relieve both constipation and diarrhea. However, they can be constipating themselves if you don't take the supplements with plenty of water (8 ounces) and continue drinking fluids throughout the day.

Ask your doctor about medication

Loperamide (Imodium) slows the rate at which food moves through your intestines and increases intestinal water and ion (sodium) absorption to help solidify stool. Discuss the use of these medications with your doctor. Overuse can cause or increase constipation.

For moderate to severe signs and symptoms, your doctor may recommend an antispasmodic (anticholinergic) medication to relax intestinal muscles and relieve muscle spasms. However, the data supporting their use for irritable bowel syndrome are limited and these medications aren't approved by the Food and Drug Administration for treatment of irritable bowel syndrome.

Antidepressants can help relieve depression associated with irritable bowel syndrome. Side effects of these medications may also help relieve abdominal pain and diarrhea or constipation.

Chronic constipation

Signs and symptoms

- Passage of hard stools less than three times a week
- Occasionally, abdominal bloating and discomfort

Many people believe that constipation is the inability to have a daily bowel movement. In fact, it's not necessary to have a bowel movement every day. For some, regularity means having a bowel movement three times a week. For others, it may be three times a day. Chronic constipation refers to bowel movements that occur infrequently — generally less than three times a week — and in which the stool is hard and difficult to pass.

Alterations in the speed at which waste passes through the colon or in the amount of water removed from the waste can affect normal bowel function and cause chronic constipation. The condition can also occur from use of medications, including some used to treat Parkinson's disease, depression, hypertension and some heart disorders. In addition, constipation often becomes more common with age.

Diagnosis

If your constipation is a recent development or your stool habits differ from what you consider normal, see your doctor. He or she will first want to rule out other causes, such as an obstruction to the passage of stool. Diagnostic tests may include a colonoscopy or sigmoidoscopy examination and a barium X-ray. See Chapter 39, "Diagnostic Tests," for more information on these tests.

Treatment

Treatment of constipation generally involves changes in eating and lifestyle habits:

- Drink at least six to eight glasses of water or other liquids every day.
- Gradually increase fiber in your diet by eating more fresh fruits and vegetables. If you're intolerant of high-fiber foods, talk to your doctor about using a bulk former that contains methylcellulose or the vegetable fiber psyllium.
- Incorporate regular physical exercise into your daily regimen. Exercise helps to stimulate bowel contractions.
- Set aside a specific time every day for a bowel movement. Even if you don't feel like you have to have a bowel movement, try.
- Don't resist the urge to have a bowel movement.
- Avoid enemas. Thorough "cleansing" of the colon, by either repeated enemas or laxatives, can remove minerals from your body, which may be harmful. Many people with constipation rely heavily on laxatives to relieve their problem. However, laxatives can lead to even more constipation. They can also damage your bowel and disrupt your body's normal balance of minerals.
- If your constipation doesn't improve, see your doctor.

Fecal impaction

Signs and symptoms

- An intense urge to have a bowel movement
- An inability to have a bowel movement
- Rectal pain and abdominal cramping
- Nausea and vomiting

A fecal impaction is a mass of stool that can't be eliminated by a normal bowel movement. It can occur following an extended period of constipation and most often poses a problem for older adults, especially those who are bedridden, and young children.

Symptoms may include an intense desire to have a bowel movement and pain in the anal region, rectum and center of the abdomen. Nausea, vomiting and loss of appetite also may occur.

Causes

Inadequate consumption of dietary fiber and liquids can lead to a fecal impaction. Other possible causes include:

- Medications such as codeine-containing pain relievers, antidepressants and aluminum-containing antacids
- Excessive laxative use
- Immobility, especially bed rest
- Chronic health problems such as hemorrhoids, kidney disease, cancer, cardiovascular disease and neurologic disorders
- Failing to heed the call when your body tells you it's time for a trip to the bathroom, a habit that is most common among young children

Treatment

A fecal impaction can generally be removed manually by a doctor or other medical professional. To prevent recurrence:

- Drink two or more glasses of water with each meal and one between meals.
- Eat a high-fiber diet.
- Heed the first urge to go to the bathroom.
- Don't use laxatives on a regular basis.
- If possible, avoid prolonged bed rest and medications that increase your risk of fecal impaction.

Megacolon

Signs and symptoms

- Severe constipation
- Malnutrition

From either congenital or acquired causes, the colon can become so enlarged that it becomes unable to move stool, a condition referred to as megacolon or giant colon. Nerve damage or deficiencies in the colon or rectum frequently are the cause of megacolon.

Hirschsprung's disease is a congenital disorder in which babies are born without normal nerve cells in a segment of their rectum. These infants are unable to have a bowel movement because the segment of the colon nearest the anus is unable to relax to permit the passage of feces. Signs and symptoms may include massive abdominal distention, absence of bowel movements and impaired nutrition. Hirschsprung's disease occurs more often in males than in females and often runs in families.

A type of acquired megacolon is psychogenic megacolon, which usually develops at the time of toilet training, causing severe and chronic constipation. In Central and South America, an infection called Chagas' disease causes megacolon. The infection destroys the ganglion nerve cells of the colon to create a condition similar to Hirschsprung's disease that occurs in adults rather than in children.

Other conditions that can cause megacolon are severe neurologic disorders such as a spinal cord injury or Parkinson's disease and some medications, including narcotics.

Diagnosis

Diagnosis of this condition generally involves an examination of the rectum, and possibly a test called anorectal manometry. For this test a balloon is dilated in the rectum to check for the rectoanal inhibitory reflex, which is absent in someone with Hirschsprung's disease.

Treatment

The most effective treatment for Hirschsprung's disease is surgery to remove the affected portion of the colon. This usually restores normal bowel movements. For acquired causes, the key is education on proper bowel habits, such as drinking plenty of fluids, increasing the fiber content of your diet and not resisting the urge to have a bowel movement.

Your doctor may suggest treatments to help retrain your bowel. Decreasing the use of narcotic-containing medication also may be recommended.

Peritonitis

Signs and symptoms

- Increasing abdominal pain
- A distended and tender abdomen
- Nausea and vomiting
- An inability to pass feces or gas
- Fever
- Low blood pressure
- Thirst

Peritonitis is an inflammation, either confined or widespread, of the peritoneum, the membrane that covers the abdominal organs and lines the abdominal cavity.

Peritonitis most often is due to bacterial infection of the peritoneal cavity. Typically, the bacteria enter from a perforation in the gastrointestinal tract, such as that owing to a ruptured appendix or trauma to the abdomen, as with a penetrating wound. Peritonitis can also result from a severe reaction related to the release of pancreatic enzymes, digestive enzymes or bile. People with systemic lupus erythematosus sometimes have bouts of peritonitis.

The most frequent causes of peritonitis are perforations related to appendicitis, diverticulitis or a peptic ulcer. Obstruction of the bowel with subsequent gangrene and bowel perforation also can cause peritonitis.

How serious is peritonitis?

Peritonitis is a medical emergency that must be treated immediately. Blood tests and X-rays may be done to help establish the diagnosis.

Treatment

Surgery is usually necessary, either to remove the cause of the problem, such as a ruptured appendix, or to repair an injury, such as a perforation in the stomach or intestine. Antibiotics are given to fight the infection. Because the intestines don't function during peritonitis, a tube may be inserted through your nose into the stomach to drain secretions and air that accumulate.

Intestinal obstruction

Signs and symptoms

- Abdominal distention
- Spasmodic pain or cramping, usually in the midabdomen
- Vomiting
- An inability to pass feces or intestinal gas

An intestinal obstruction is a partial or complete blockage in either the small intestine or colon. It prevents contents from completing their journey through the intestines.

If you have a blockage in your small intestine, you may feel cramp-like pain in the middle of your abdomen and have bouts of vomiting. Failure to pass feces can occur no matter how high up the obstruction is located. If your intestine is totally blocked, you may not be able to pass gas. A partial intestinal obstruction may stimulate your intestines to contract and secrete more fluid than can be absorbed, which may result in diarrhea.

A dramatic feature of intestinal obstruction is abdominal distention. The abdomen will protrude more and more as the condition worsens. The swelling is produced by intestinal gas and fluid trapped within the obstructed segment of the intestine.

Several things can cause an obstruction. The most common cause in the small intestine is scar tissue (adhesion) from a prior operation. Hernias and a knotted or twisted intestine (volvulus) also are common causes of small bowel obstruction. In the colon, a tumor may create a blockage. These are called mechanical obstructions because they physically block movement of contents through the bowel.

Sometimes, abdominal swelling (distention) and an inability to have a bowel movement result not from a physical blockage but from failure of the intestines to move waste along the digestive tract. This is called adynamic (paralytic) ileus and sometimes occurs after an abdominal injury or operation. Other causes include pancreatitis, peritonitis, injury to the abdominal blood supply and metabolic disturbances, such as low blood potassium levels. Narcotics such as morphine also may result in adynamic ileus.

Diagnosis

If your doctor believes that your signs and symptoms suggest an intestinal obstruction, he or she may order various tests, possibly including abdominal X-rays, sigmoidoscopy, colonoscopy or a barium X-ray. See Chapter 39, "Diagnostic Tests," for more information on these tests.

How serious is an intestinal obstruction?

If the obstruction blocks the blood supply to the intestine, the tissue may begin to die. This increases the possibility of gangrene or perforation of the intestine. Both are life-threatening.

Treatment

Your doctor may begin treatment by placing a small tube through your nose and into your stomach or small intestine. Suction is applied to remove intestinal secretions and air through the tube (nasogastric suction). This often relieves distention of the abdomen. Lost fluids are replaced with intravenous (IV) feedings.

Sometimes, the cause of an obstruction resolves spontaneously after the swelling has been relieved. If the obstruction doesn't resolve, surgery may be necessary to correct the blockage, such as removal of scar tissue or untwisting an intestinal knot. An underlying cause may then be identified.

Primary intestinal pseudo-obstruction

Signs and symptoms

- Sudden attacks of abdominal pain
- Abdominal swelling
- Nausea and vomiting
- Weight loss

Primary (idiopathic) intestinal pseudo-obstruction isn't a true intestinal obstruction. Rather, it's a motility disturbance that causes intestinal malfunction similar to an actual obstruction. The intestines become distended, and you may experience sudden, severe (acute) attacks of abdominal pain, nausea and vomiting. Malabsorption may accompany this disorder, with subsequent weight loss.

Because the cause of the condition is unknown, doctors sometimes call this condition idiopathic intestinal pseudo-obstruction — the term *idiopathic* refers to a disease with no recognizable cause, and *pseudo* means "false." When an underlying disease such as scleroderma or diabetes is the cause, the term *secondary intestinal pseudo-obstruction* is used.

Treatment of intestinal pseudo-obstruction is difficult. Special diets are ineffective. If the disorder is severe, liquid nutrients can sometimes be administered into a vein (intravenously), thus bypassing the intestines. Intravenous (IV) feedings can be done on a temporary basis in the hospital or on a permanent basis at home (home parenteral nutrition).

Vascular problems of the bowel

A vast network of blood vessels nourishes the organs located in your abdomen. Sometimes, a blood vessel (vascular) or abdominal disorder can reduce the blood supply to the intestines. When this happens, the affected area becomes deficient in nutrients and oxygen, and the result can be tissue death. Three vascular problems of the bowel are mesenteric ischemia, ischemic colitis and angiodysplasia of the colon.

Mesenteric ischemia

This disorder is characterized by a partial or complete lack of blood flow to the intestines. This vascular obstruction may occur gradually from accumulation of cholesterol-containing deposits (plaques) in the linings of arteries supplying oxygen to the intestines. The main symptom is severe, midabdominal pain. The pain is usually aggravated by eating and relieved by fasting.

Another type of vascular obstruction is a blood clot (embolus) that passes from the heart into the arteries supplying blood to the intestines. The result is sudden, complete blockage of blood flow to a portion of the intestines. The condition often causes severe and sudden abdominal pain and is a medical emergency.

Examination of blood vessels in the abdomen (angiography) can determine the site of vascular obstruction. This is generally followed by an operation to remove the segment of intestine that has lost its blood supply. If there hasn't been permanent damage, the clot can be removed or the affected artery reconstructed or bypassed.

Ischemic colitis

In ischemic colitis, blood supply to the colon is decreased, often stemming from congestive heart failure or low blood pressure (hypotension). The condition most often affects older adults. Signs and symptoms include cramping lower abdominal pain and rectal bleeding.

Surgery may be required in severe cases, but most often the problem resolves spontaneously as heart failure or low blood pressure is corrected. A narrowing of the colon (stricture) can occur later at the site of the prior ischemia.

Angiodysplasia of the colon

This condition is characterized by dilation, distortion or thinning of blood vessels in the inner wall of the colon. It's most common in older adults. Rectal bleeding is a common symptom, which is often managed with cautery or laser treatment. Severe bleeding (hemorrhage) is infrequent. It often can be halted by blocking the affected vessel during a diagnostic procedure called arteriography. For massive bleeding or bleeding from multiple sites, surgical removal of the affected portion of the colon may be necessary.

Carcinoid syndrome

Signs and symptoms

- Flushing of the skin
- Diarrhea

Carcinoid tumors are slow growing, potentially cancer-causing growths that usually occur in the appendix or ileum, the lowest section of the small intestine. These tumors may spread (metastasize) to the liver, lungs and other organs. Occasionally, they can cause flushing of the skin, asthma and diarrhea, called carcinoid syndrome. Excessive levels of a normal body chemical or metabolite in urine is an important biochemical indicator of carcinoid tumors.

The objective of treatment is to decrease the mass of one or more tumors by either chemotherapy or surgery. Treatment generally relieves the signs and symptoms of carcinoid syndrome. Some people recover fully after surgery, depending on how soon the cancer is detected and where it's located. In the case of advanced cancer, medication such as octreotide (Sandostatin) may be used to control the episodes of flushing and diarrhea and to try to retard tumor growth.

Tumors of the small intestine

Signs and symptoms

- Abdominal cramps and pain
- Nausea and vomiting
- Weight loss
- Bloody stools

It's uncommon for tumors to occur in the small intestine — they represent only 3 percent to 6 percent of all abnormal growths in the gastrointestinal tract. Most tumors of the small bowel are noncancerous (benign), and they're usually discovered between the ages of 40 and 60. The most frequent signs and symptoms are pain, bloody stools and nausea and vomiting.

There are several types of benign tumors, including lipomas, leiomyomas, angiomas and adenomas. These tumors don't spread. Often, they're found when an X-ray is taken related to another condition.

A small percentage of tumors of the small intestine are cancerous (malignant). The most common malignant types are adenocarcinoma, leiomyosarcoma, carcinoid tumor and lymphoma.

Signs and symptoms of a malignant tumor may include weight loss, abdominal pain, bloody stools and nausea and vomiting. Your doctor may feel an abdominal mass during a physical examination. Bleeding, perforation and obstruction are commonly associated with a leiomyosarcoma. A carcinoid tumor may cause no signs and symptoms before it spreads.

Diagnosis

A barium X-ray and computerized tomography (CT) scan are procedures used to detect small intestinal tumors. Sometimes, the diagnostic image can't distinguish a benign from a malignant tumor, and surgical exploration of the abdomen may be necessary to establish the diagnosis. Occasionally, the tumors are identified by accident during testing for another condition.

How serious are tumors of the small intestine?

Benign tumors aren't life-threatening, but they can cause dangerous signs and symptoms, such as bleeding and obstruction. Malignant tumors are dangerous, can be life-threatening and require prompt treatment.

Treatment

Surgery is usually recommended for all benign tumors that cause signs and symptoms and for malignant tumors that haven't become too widespread. When a tumor has spread (metastasized) to such an extent that surgery isn't effective, some medications, as well as chemotherapy and radiation — either individually or in combination — may be used.

Colon polyps

Signs and symptoms

- Most often, none
- A recent change in bowel movements
- Blood in stool, often in microscopic amounts
- Mucus discharged from the anus

Benign (noncancerous) tumors of the large intestine are common. It's estimated that 4 of every 10 Americans older than age 60 have mushroom-like growths (polyps) in their colon.

Polyps arise from the lining of the colon. They usually cause no signs and symptoms and are discovered incidentally, often during a screening test for colorectal cancer or during a test to diagnose another disorder. However, polyps should be removed because they can sometimes become cancerous if left untreated.

Types

Several varieties of polyps are found in the colon:

Hyperplastic polyps

The most common type of polyp is a hyperplastic polyp, which is generally less than $1/4$ inch in diameter. These tiny polyps typically are not a health risk, but if they grow to larger than $1/2$ inch in diameter, they should be removed for examination to make certain they aren't cancerous or precancerous.

Adenomatous polyps

Adenomatous polyps (adenomas) also are quite common. They're

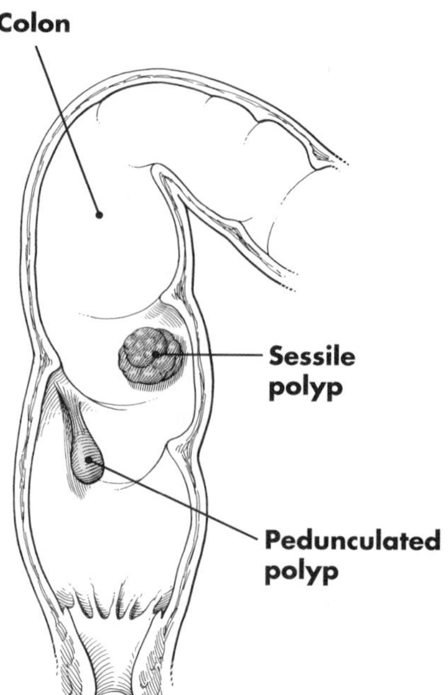

Polyps are small growths that may appear in the colon and rectum. In most cases, they're noncancerous (benign). They may assume various shapes. Polyps that grow on fleshy stalks are called pedunculated. Those that have a broad base are sessile polyps.

classified into three varieties based on their microscopic features: tubular, tubulovillous and villous. The most common are tubular adenomas, which generally are less than $1/2$ inch in diameter. Villous adenomas are less common. More than half of them are at least 1 inch in diameter. Tubulovillous adenomas contain characteristics of the other two.

Nearly 50 percent of Americans develop an adenoma at some time in their life, an occurrence that becomes more common with age. Adenomatous polyps have the potential to become cancerous (malignant). The potential usually increases as the size of the polyp increases and when more villous characteristics become present.

These polyps should be removed to prevent transformation into cancer. Most often removal is done by colonoscopy, in which a thin, flexible fiber-optic tube is inserted into the rectum and threaded into the colon. Even if a polyp shows microscopic cancer in a few cells, removal of the polyp by colonoscopy often can successfully treat the cancer. If there's concern the cancer may have spread from the polyp, your doctor may recommend an operation to remove the section of the colon that had included the polyp, along with surrounding tissue and lymph nodes.

Inflammatory polyps

Inflammatory polyps are thought to result from injury to or inflammation of the lining of the colon, such as in ulcerative colitis. These are uncommon and typically not a significant health risk.

Juvenile polyps

Juvenile polyps are uncommon and tend to occur during childhood. These polyps can easily be removed during a colonoscopy procedure. Juvenile polyps and similar ones associated with Peutz-Jeghers syndrome are an inherited condition.

Hereditary polyps

Most polyps that develop in the colon aren't hereditary. But hereditary polyps can occur in some families. One disorder that causes colon polyps is believed to be strongly hereditary. Called familial adenomatous polyposis (FAP), this rare disorder is characterized by the appearance of numerous — at least 100 and often 1,000 or more — polyps throughout the entire colon. These polyps may not cause signs and symptoms (asymptomatic), or they may cause rectal bleeding. Polyps may also develop in the small intestine. Typically, the condition appears during adolescence.

Gardner's syndrome is FAP along with other nonmalignant tumors in other regions of the body.

Cancer of the colon inevitably occurs with FAP. The condition accounts for about 1 percent of all cases of colorectal cancer. Removal of the entire colon is often advised as soon as a diagnosis is made. It's also important for blood relatives to be examined starting at a relatively young age — approximately 10 to 12 years — so that they can receive appropriate evaluation and treatment.

Diagnosis

Colon polyps are most frequently found during a colon screening examination or during an evaluation of the colon to identify the cause of rectal bleeding, a change in bowel habits or abdominal pain. Depending on the type of polyps detected, your doctor may recommend periodic checkups or removal of the polyps.

How serious are colon polyps?

An adenomatous polyp has the potential to become cancerous. Most, if not all, colorectal cancers seem to develop from adenomas. In addition, sometimes colon polyps may cause problems such as bleeding and obstruction.

Treatment

Many polyps are removed when detected because this eliminates the chance that they'll ever become malignant. For most, their removal is a relatively simple procedure. If the tumor can't be removed during colonoscopy, minimally invasive surgery may be necessary. If you've previously had adenomatous polyps, you're at risk of growing additional polyps, so your doctor will likely recommend periodic examinations of the colon to identify and remove any new polyps.

For people with hereditary polyps, the likelihood of colorectal cancer approaches nearly 100 percent by age 40. Therefore, doctors will usually recommend that the entire colon be removed to prevent cancer. This may require a surgical procedure that provides you with an alternative method of expelling stool (see page 876).

Colorectal cancer

Signs and symptoms

- Sometimes, none
- Rectal bleeding
- A change in bowel habits
- Abdominal pain or cramping
- Unexplained anemia
- Unexplained weight loss

Colorectal cancer (cancer of the colon and rectum) is one of the most common forms of cancer in adult men and women. Each year, more than 130,000 Americans receive a diagnosis of this disease, and close to 60,000 die of it.

A complex mix of factors, including lifestyle, environment and genetics, may be responsible. Researchers theorize that most people have dormant genes that can produce cancerous cells. These genes stay dormant until they're activated by an outside agent, such

Genetic Testing

If you have a family history of colorectal cancer, you may be a candidate for genetic testing. A blood test may help determine if you're at increased risk of a hereditary form of colorectal cancer. Knowing that you are may lead to more frequent screening tests and perhaps early detection of cancer, while chances for successful treatment are good.

But genetic testing also has drawbacks. The presence of a defective gene doesn't always mean that you'll develop cancer. And not having the gene doesn't guarantee you'll be cancer-free. It's also important to consider the psychological impact. How will you cope with the knowledge that you're likely to develop cancer, if that's what the test results determine? Therefore, genetic counseling is very important before genetic testing is undertaken. For more on genetic testing, see Chapter 18, "Genetics and Disease."

as an infection, tobacco or pollutants in food, air or water.

Most gastrointestinal cancers occur in the colon and rectum, where food residue moves more slowly and toxins linger. Colorectal cancer risk appears to be more common in people who eat a high proportion of animal fat and small amounts of fresh fruits and vegetables. Risk of colorectal cancer is also higher in individuals who smoke, consume large amounts of alcohol and are physically inactive.

A small percentage of colorectal cancer — between 5 percent and 10 percent — is considered hereditary. One type of inherited cancer is called hereditary nonpolyposis colorectal cancer (HNPCC). People with this disorder have a 50 percent chance of passing on the gene to their children. They also have an 80 percent chance of developing colon cancer, and at a younger age than normal. Another inherited condition called familial adenomatous polyposis (FAP) produces hundreds, even thousands, of tiny precancerous growths (polyps) in the colon and rectum. Cancer almost always develops in one or more of these polyps, typically between the ages of 30 and 50.

Are you at risk?

The following factors generally determine colorectal cancer risk:

Age

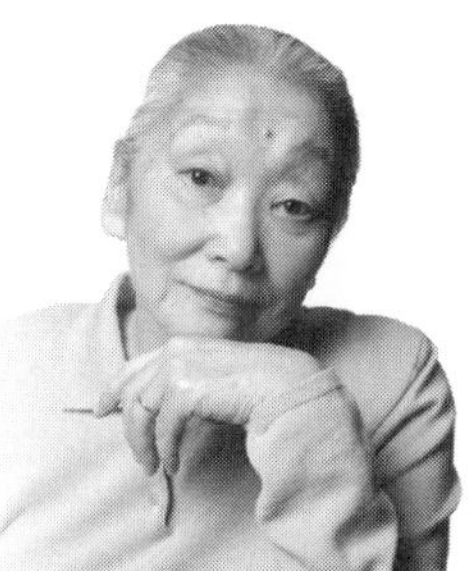

About 90 percent of people with colorectal cancer are age 50 or older. Many health organizations recommend that average-risk adults begin a colorectal

Screening for Colorectal Cancer

A number of tests can identify early colorectal cancer or potential cancer-causing polyps (adenomas) before they produce signs and symptoms. The American Cancer Society recommends that all adults have one or a combination of the following screening tests beginning at age 50. Screening may be done earlier for individuals at higher-than-average risk.

Digital rectal exam

In this simple office exam, your doctor inserts a gloved finger into your rectum to feel for polyps or masses. Although simple and safe, this test is limited to examination of your rectum. Thus, it's usually done in conjunction with other screening tests.

Fecal occult blood test

A fecal occult (hidden) blood test checks for microscopic amounts of blood in stool. It can be performed in a doctor's office or at home. The problem is that some cancers and most polyps don't bleed and aren't detected with this test. In addition, positive test results don't necessarily mean that you have cancer or polyps. The bleeding may be from other sources, such as hemorrhoids or gastritis. For these reasons, many doctors recommend alternative or additional screening methods. A fecal occult blood test is often combined with sigmoidoscopy.

Sigmoidoscopy

A sigmoidoscopy allows your doctor to see and inspect the lower portion of your colon (sigmoid and rectum). The test requires one or two enemas for preparation. It doesn't require sedation, and it takes about 5 to 10 minutes to perform. A flexible, lighted tube with a fiber-optic camera (sigmoidoscope) is inserted into your rectum and threaded through your rectum and sigmoid colon (see illustration on page 1280). About one-third to one-half of all colorectal cancers or polyps can be seen during such an examination. If a polyp or suspicious area is identified, a biopsy is performed, in which samples of tissue are taken with the instrument for microscopic examination.

Colonoscopy

A colonoscopy is considered the gold standard of colorectal cancer screening. In general, it's the preferred test for individuals at higher-than-average risk of colorectal cancer. A flexible, lighted tube with a tiny camera attached is used to examine your entire colon and rectum. The tube is inserted into your rectum and threaded through the rectum and entire length of your colon. If polyps or suspicious areas are detected, your doctor can painlessly remove them and take tissue samples for laboratory analysis (biopsy). Preparation for the test generally involves a clear liquid diet, a special laxative preparation and, sometimes, enemas to cleanse the colon for better viewing. Most people also receive mild sedation just before the examination.

Barium enema

A barium enema allows your doctor to view your large intestine on an X-ray. Barium, a chalk-like contrast medium, is inserted into your colon. The barium coats the lining of the colon, creating a clear silhouette of your colon, and then an X-ray is taken. The test takes about 20 minutes. A barium enema is often combined with sigmoidoscopy.

What test is best?

The best screening methods for you depends on your age, your overall health and if you have other risk fac-

screening program at age 50. Earlier or more frequent screening may be needed if you have other risk factors of colorectal cancer that put you at higher risk.

Family or personal history
If you or a close family member has a history of colorectal cancer or you or a close family member has received a diagnosis of FAP, you're at greater than average risk of developing colorectal cancer. Screening should begin earlier than age 50 and be done more frequently.

Racial group
Black men and women are at increased risk of colorectal cancer.

A history of inflammatory bowel disease
A long-term history of ulcerative colitis or Crohn's disease of the colon increases your risk of colorectal cancer. Screening for this cancer should start earlier and be more frequent.

Smoking
Research shows higher rates of colon cancer among people who use tobacco. The longer you smoke and the more tobacco you use, the greater the risk.

Diet
People who eat a high-fat diet, especially one that contains a lot of red meat, such as beef, pork and lamb, are at higher risk.

A diet high in fiber has long been considered a way to lower your risk of colorectal cancer. The role of fiber, however, is controversial. Some studies suggest that fiber doesn't protect against colorectal cancer.

tors that put you at higher-than-average risk of colorectal cancer. Discuss these with your doctor, and together the two of you can determine the best course of action. Proper screening and early detection can go a long way in preventing and treating this disease.

Future screening
Several innovations on the horizon could improve the effectiveness and lower the cost of colorectal cancer screening. Stool tests that identify specific substances shed from cancers or polyps, rather than detect blood, may increase the accuracy of early detection.

Improved techniques may also allow more complete and comfortable visualization of the colon and rectum. These include special noninvasive radiologic procedures called virtual colonoscopy.

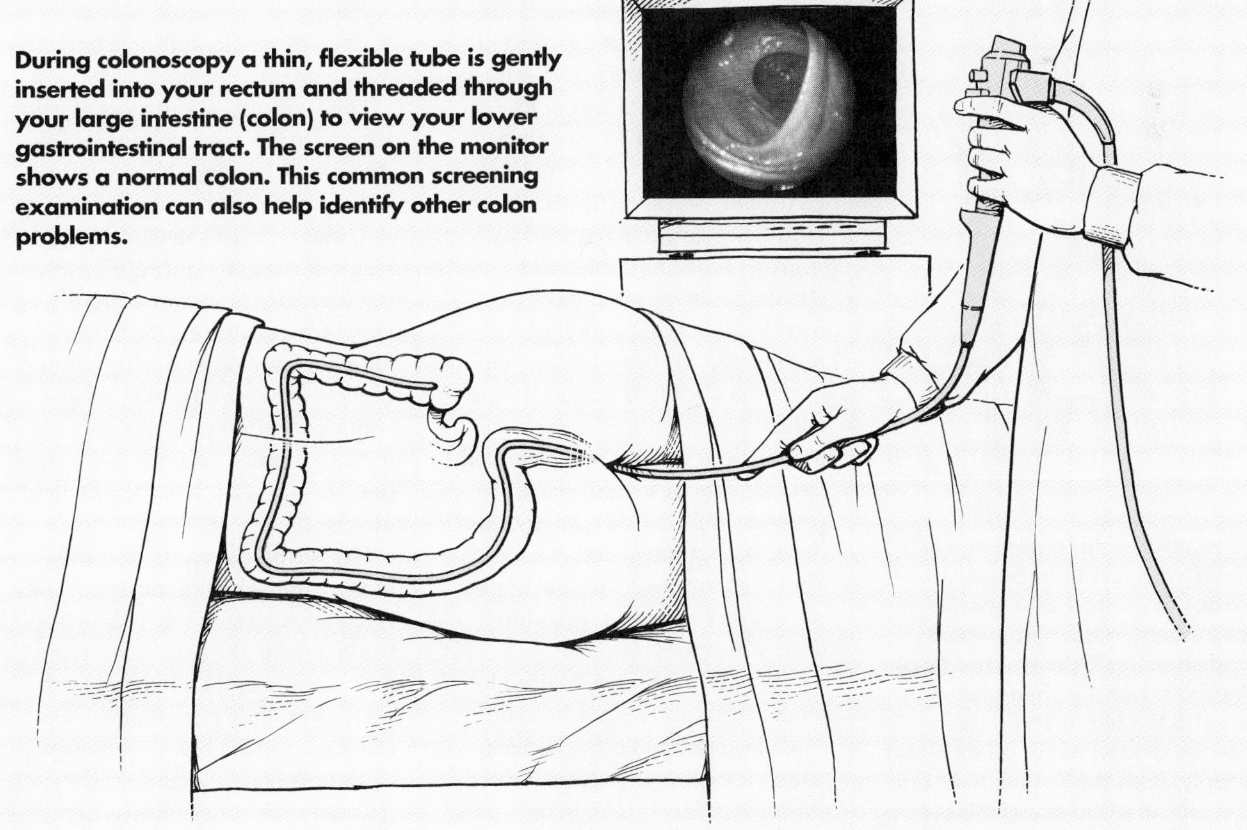

During colonoscopy a thin, flexible tube is gently inserted into your rectum and threaded through your large intestine (colon) to view your lower gastrointestinal tract. The screen on the monitor shows a normal colon. This common screening examination can also help identify other colon problems.

Exercise
People who are inactive tend to be at increased risk of colorectal cancer.

Diagnosis
Colorectal cancer increasingly is being detected by periodic screening examinations. Rectal bleeding, a change in bowel habits, unexplained weight loss and abdominal pain also can be warnings of the disease. If you experience these signs and symptoms, your doctor may advise diagnostic tests such as colonoscopy, sigmoidoscopy or a barium enema.

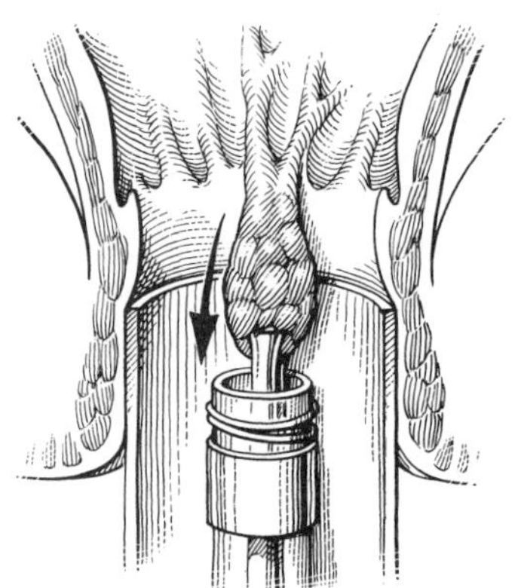

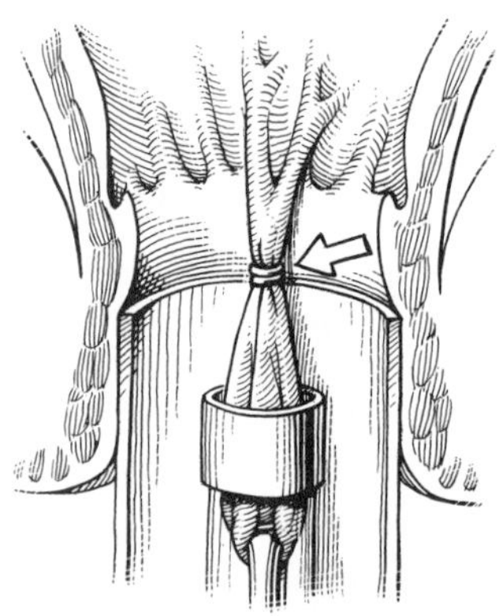

To remove an internal hemorrhoid with a rubber band, a doctor first attaches a special instrument to the hemorrhoid and stretches it downward (top). A rubber band is then placed around the hemorrhoid (see bottom arrow) to cut off its blood supply. Both the hemorrhoid and the rubber band are eliminated later with stool.

If cancer is identified, other tests, including blood tests and a computerized tomography (CT) scan, may be done to determine if it has spread to adjacent tissues or other organs. See Chapter 39, "Diagnostic Tests," for more information on these tests.

How serious is colorectal cancer?
Colorectal cancer is the third most common cancer in men and women in the United States and accounts for about 10 percent of cancer deaths. When detected and treated at an early stage, chances for cure are high. Mortality rates for colorectal cancer have declined in the past 20 years, probably due to increased screening and polyp removal. Unfortunately, many people still don't seek medical attention even when such warning signs as rectal bleeding and a change in bowel habits occur.

Treatment
Surgery is the most common treatment for colorectal cancer. In about half of all cases, surgery can cure this form of cancer. If the cancer is advanced and widespread, surgery may not be advised except to relieve obstruction or bleeding.

Among people at high risk of recurrence of colorectal cancer, or in whom the cancer has spread to nearby tissue or lymph nodes, chemotherapy is often recommended following surgery. Radiation and chemotherapy are sometimes advised for rectal cancer, either before or after surgery. Medications such as 5-fluorouracil (5-FU, Adrucil), levamisole, or leucovorin (Wellcovorin) can decrease the chance of tumor recurrence. They also improve survival in people whose cancer has spread to nearby lymph nodes.

Chemotherapy may be used to relieve signs and symptoms and extend survival among people in whom the cancer has spread too extensively for surgery to be effective.

In case of an obstruction or bleeding, laser therapy may help relieve signs and symptoms. Sometimes an obstruction can be relieved by placing a small, expandable tube (stent) in the narrowed section.

Anorectal Disorders

The anus is the muscular canal that's the outlet for the rectum. It's a relatively simple structure, in contrast to the other parts of the digestive system. However, it too can be a site for significant problems, collectively referred to as anorectal disorders.

Hemorrhoids

Signs and symptoms

- Bright red blood on the toilet paper, in the water of the toilet bowl or on the stool after a bowel movement
- Protrusion of soft tissue at the anus
- Pain, especially during a bowel movement

Hemorrhoids are clusters of veins located in the anus, just under the membrane that lines the lowest part of the rectum and anus.

These veins can swell, often as a result of straining during a bowel movement. And because these veins are thin and easily ruptured, bleeding may occur during a bowel movement. Hemorrhoids are also common during pregnancy due to increased pressure in the veins from the size and weight of the pregnant uterus.

Hemorrhoids can occur internally near the beginning of the anal canal or externally, where they protrude outside the anus. Both types are common and both may bleed.

Hemorrhoids can become especially painful if a blood clot forms in a swollen vein, a condition referred to as a thrombosed hemorrhoid. These clots generally occur in

Rectal Bleeding

Rectal bleeding can be a sign of cancer, but more often it indicates a bowel problem that isn't life-threatening and responds well to treatment. Other causes of bleeding in the lower gastrointestinal tract include:

- Proctitis or colitis, an inflammation of the inner lining of the rectum or colon
- Colon or rectal polyps, small noncancerous (benign) growths in the lining of the lower intestine
- Hemorrhoids, enlarged veins in the lining of the anus
- Anal fissure, a tear in the lining of your anus
- Anal fistula, an abnormal channel between the anal canal and the skin around the opening to the anus
- Rectal prolapse, a condition in which a portion of the rectum protrudes through the anus
- Diverticular disease, small pouches (diverticula) that form in the large intestine
- Angiodysplasia, weakened blood vessels in the colon lining

Rectal bleeding requires prompt evaluation by your doctor to establish its cause and, more importantly, to exclude cancer.

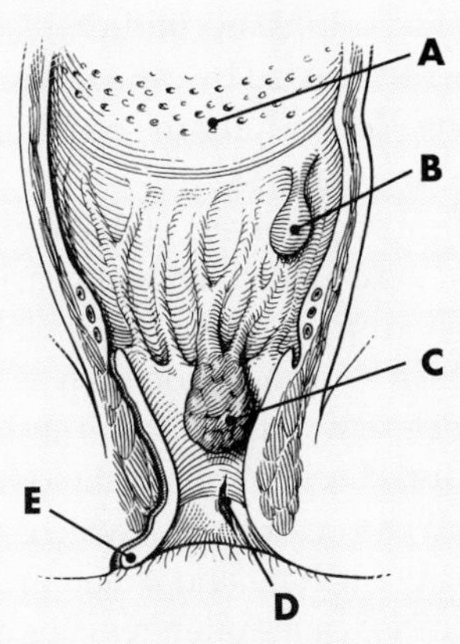

This cross-sectional view of the anus and rectum shows some common causes of rectal bleeding: (A) proctitis, (B) polyp, (C) hemorrhoids, (D) anal fissure and (E) anal fistula.

external hemorrhoids and cause a painful lump at the anal opening.

Itching and anal pain generally aren't symptoms of hemorrhoids but can occur with a complication such as thrombosis or irritation or inflammation of the skin surrounding the anus.

Diagnosis

Visual examination of the anus by a doctor usually reveals external hemorrhoids. The interior of the anus can be examined with a rubber-gloved finger, but because hemorrhoids are very soft, a definite diagnosis may not be made. Sometimes, a doctor will use a thin scope to view inside the anus and rectum.

All episodes of rectal bleeding should be investigated. Don't assume that rectal bleeding is from hemorrhoids until other potential sources of bleeding, such as a colon polyp or colorectal cancer, have been excluded.

Treatment

Most people with hemorrhoids are bothered so little by the problem that they ignore it. For others, however, the symptoms are too annoying to easily dismiss.

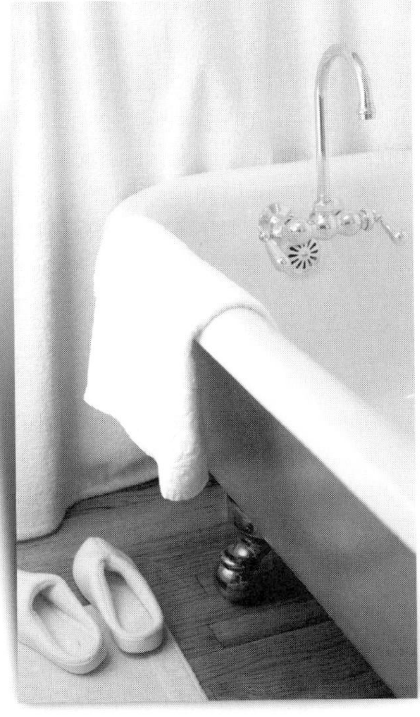

For mild discomfort, a doctor may suggest over-the-counter creams, ointments or pads containing the astringent witch hazel, or a topical anesthetic agent, to relieve symptoms. Other steps that might help include daily warm baths and consumption of additional liquids and fiber to help soften stool and reduce constipation and straining. If possible, avoid prolonged periods of standing or sitting.

If you have moderate to severe bleeding or discomfort caused by an internal hemorrhoid, your doctor may perform a corrective procedure that involves tying off the hemorrhoid with a rubber band. In a few days, the hemorrhoid painlessly falls off. This method is effective in about 75 percent of cases. If a blood clot has formed within an external hemorrhoid, your doctor may remove the clot to provide prompt relief.

Other techniques for treating hemorrhoids include injecting them with a shrinking agent, freezing them (cryosurgery) or destroying them with infrared photocoagulation, a technique that cuts off circulation to the affected veins.

Large hemorrhoids can be removed surgically in a procedure called hemorrhoidectomy. The more hemorrhoidal tissue that's removed, the less chance of recurrence but the greater the discomfort from the surgery.

Anal itch

Anal itching (pruritus ani) is a common, distracting and potentially embarrassing problem. Almost everyone is afflicted at one time or another. A persistent anal itch is a more common problem for children and older adults. In children, it's frequently caused by pinworms. Among older adults, the cause usually is dry, aging skin.

For most of the rest of the population, the cause isn't always easily identified. Your doctor will look for signs of a skin condition such as psoriasis or a yeast infection and may also check for hemorrhoids or an anal fissure or fistula, which may cause itching and irritation. The precise cause often remains a mystery, but usually isn't due to any serious disorder.

Additional factors also can cause anal itching:

- Some people scrub their anus with a harsh soap and rough washcloth. This can cause irritation and itching. On the other hand, inadequate cleansing following a bowel movement also can cause irritation and itching.
- Some people use over-the-counter products to relieve anal itching. They may actually increase itching by irritating and sensitizing the skin.
- Some doctors believe that stress may be a factor.
- Sometimes, the muscles and sphincter that normally keep the anus closed can become lax, allowing stool to seep out and irritate the surrounding skin.

Treatment

If anal itching is a problem for you, try the following measures. If they don't help, see your doctor for an evaluation.

Stop scratching

As hard as this may be, summon your willpower and try it. Continued scratching leads to persistent inflammation and damage to the delicate tissue. The more you scratch, the more you itch.

Keep the area clean

Cleanse the area gently in the morning, in the evening and after a bowel movement. Use moistened, unscented, white toilet paper or cotton balls. Pat the area dry rather than rubbing it, then dry it thoroughly with a hair dryer set to its lowest heat setting.

After a bath or bowel movement, dab the anus with cotton moistened with a perianal cleansing lotion (Balneol).

Pad the area

To prevent skin irritation caused by leakage of stool, place a cotton pad between your buttocks, up against the anus. Replace the pad as necessary.

Drink extra fluid

Try to drink six 8-ounce glasses of water each day. This will help make your stool soft and bulky. A hard stool can irritate your anus further.

Take a stool-bulking supplement

Once or twice a day, take a stool-bulking supplement (Citrucel, Metamucil, others) mixed with water to prevent your stool from being uncomfortably hard.

Avoid certain foods and beverages

Try eliminating alcohol, coffee, tea, soda, nuts, popcorn, chocolate, tomatoes, citrus juices and milk from your diet for about a month. Then reintroduce these items one at a time into your diet. If resumption of the itching corresponds to consumption of an item, avoid the item.

Use hydrocortisone

Try a cold pack and a 0.5 percent hydrocortisone cream or ointment (available without a prescription) to relieve the discomfort.

Anal Pain

Have you ever been awakened from a sound sleep by a sharp, severe pain in your anus and rectum? This condition is called proctalgia fugax, which means fleeting rectal pain. Its cause isn't well understood, but the pain is believed to be the result of an intense spasm of muscles in the lower pelvis and rectum. The pain resembles the discomfort you experience from a cramp in your calf.

Typically, the pain begins at night during sleep. Within a few minutes to half an hour, the pain subsides. It may recur at irregular intervals, with the frequency varying from twice a week to a few times a year. Sometimes the spells disappear entirely.

Although proctalgia can be frightening, rest assured that the pain probably isn't serious. However, it's a good idea to see your doctor. He or she can perform some diagnostic tests to rule out a more serious cause.

Here are some tips to try the next time you have this sort of pain:

- Sit in a bathtub full of warm water.
- Try to have a bowel movement. This sometimes eliminates the pain.
- Drink warm water or eat crackers. This may stimulate normal contractions in the intestines that will relieve the spasm.

Anal fissures and fistulas

Signs and symptoms

- Pain during and after bowel movements
- Bright red blood in the stool or on the toilet paper

Anal fissure

An anal fissure is a relatively minor cut or crack in the lining of the anal canal in an area adjacent to the tailbone, scrotum or vagina. It starts at the anal opening and extends up into the canal.

Adding more fiber to your diet and using stool softeners or bulking agents can often help heal a temporary (acute) anal fissure. If the cut is deep, the pain may be more

Sexually Transmitted Rectal Infections

Several infectious diseases are transmitted through anal intercourse. Inflammation of the rectum (proctitis) may result from gonorrhea and the herpes simplex virus. Anal warts also can be acquired through anal intercourse.

Sexually transmitted rectal infections can be serious because of the risk of complications, such as bleeding, later development of a narrowing (stricture) in the rectum or, rarely, cancer.

Many bacterial infections pose no threat to other systems of the body. However, if you experience signs and symptoms of any sexually transmitted infection, see your doctor for proper treatment. Your doctor may want to screen for the human immunodeficiency virus (HIV) and other diseases if a sexually transmitted infection of the rectum is present.

intense, both during and after passage of stool because the affected tissue may cause the anal sphincter muscle to spasm. Again, the addition of more fiber, a stool softener or a bulking agent will often help relieve the pain. A warm bath can relax the sphincter muscle and reduce painful muscle spasm. For severe pain, your doctor may recommend a nitropaste or nitroglycerin ointment. An operation to repair the cut is generally performed if other measures fail. This is usually a minor surgical procedure.

Anal fistula

An anal fistula is an abnormal tube-like passageway from the anal canal to a hole in the skin around the opening to the anus. A fistula usually results from an anorectal abscess that has drained, although it may result from inflammation of the lower colon or a previous surgery involving the lower colon. Sometimes, an anal fistula or anorectal abscess is due to Crohn's disease.

Pus and debris can collect in the fistula tract, causing pain and swelling. This often drains spontaneously, and signs and symptoms resolve until the opening again becomes clogged.

Treatment of fistulas usually consists of making an incision through the skin, fat and muscle overlying the fistula tract. This is usually done with a local anesthesia. The wound is left open and usually heals in 4 to 6 weeks. An abscess may be drained by lancing the skin overlying the collection of pus.

Anorectal abscess

Signs and symptoms

- Discomfort in or around the anal opening
- Swelling and redness near the anus
- Discharge of pus
- Fever

Anorectal abscesses affect the area immediately around the anus. Most are the result of infected tissue around the anus and rectum.

An abscess that's easily accessible near the anus can be pierced and drained, either in your doctor's office or at a hospital outpatient service. Deep abscesses are less accessible, their diagnosis is more difficult, and potential complications are more serious. Deep rectal abscesses warrant careful attention because they may stem from a fistula due to Crohn's disease or from diverticulitis. In addition to draining the abscess, your doctor may give you antibiotic and pain medication if needed. If a fistula is present, it may need to be treated at a later time.

Proctitis

Signs and symptoms

- Blood, mucus or pus in the stool
- Constipation
- Diarrhea
- Severe rectal pain
- Fever

Proctitis is an inflammation of the rectum that may result from a bacterial or viral infection or be a feature of ulcerative colitis or Crohn's disease.

In some instances, proctitis can stem from a sexually transmitted disease (STD) acquired by anal intercourse. An individual with proctitis from an STD can spread the disease to other sexual partners. Radiation treatment, such as for prostate cancer, also can cause proctitis, as can reduced blood flow to the rectum (ischemia).

A repeated urge to defecate or an inability to move your bowels may occur. If the inflammation is higher in your bowel (proctocolitis), signs and symptoms may be more severe.

Diagnosis

Sometimes, signs and symptoms associated with proctitis are a clue to the possible cause of the infection. Mucus, blood or pus in your stool may suggest an inflammation caused by gonorrhea.

If herpes simplex virus has caused the infection, you may experience extreme anal pain and ulcers or blister-like elevations around the anus. In both cases, skin around your anus may burn and itch.

Your doctor may examine the skin around your anus, analyze the stool for infection and conduct an examination of the rectum using a flexible, fiber-optic tube (endoscope) inserted into the rectum.

How serious is proctitis?

Depending on the cause, the inflammation may or may not be easily treated. Bacterial infections usually respond to antibiotics, but viral infections don't.

Treatment
Treatment for a bacterial infection generally includes an antibiotic. Other forms of proctitis may be treated with enemas that contain anti-inflammatory medications.

There's no medication available to cure proctitis caused by the herpes virus, although your doctor may prescribe agents that can control the spread of the infection and ease the signs and symptoms. For proctitis caused by other STDs, such as gonorrhea, appropriate treatment of the disease helps cure the proctitis.

Proctitis associated with Crohn's disease or ulcerative colitis can be treated with 5-aminosalicylic acid (5-ASA) or corticosteroid suppositories. These agents can also be used in radiation-induced proctitis, although it can be difficult to treat. If bleeding persists, laser treatment may be used to seal the affected blood vessels.

Fecal incontinence

Fecal incontinence refers to the inability to retain stool between bowel movements. The problem is usually due to an underlying condition such as an abscess or inflammation in the rectum, anus or perianal area.

It can also result from a previous operation in the area or, in women, from trauma to the anal sphincter during childbirth. In some cases, fecal incontinence is related to a spinal cord injury or nervous system disorder.

In older adults, fecal incontinence may result from the aging of the sphincter and pelvic floor muscles and ligaments. Fecal impaction, which is more common in older adults, is another possible cause of fecal incontinence.

To determine a cause, your doctor may ask a number of questions, including if the incontinence occurs with sneezing or coughing or if it occurs only at night. He or she may examine your anal sphincter to see if the sphincter muscles are intact and order tests to determine various pressures in the rectal and anal regions.

Treatment
In some adults, a bowel retraining program can improve fecal continence, particularly if the anal sphincter is intact.

Your doctor may advise you to take time each day to have a bowel movement. This often results in continence during the remainder of the day. He or she may also advise you to eat more fresh fruits and vegetables. This sometimes helps produce a more normal stool and decreases the number of times you have to pass stool.

If the sphincter muscle has been damaged by trauma, childbirth or prior surgery, an operation may be necessary to repair the damage.

Hernias

A hernia occurs when one part of your body — usually the small intestine — protrudes through a gap or weak spot into another part of your body. Several types of hernias can affect the abdomen: inguinal, femoral, umbilical, hiatal and incisional. A hiatal hernia (see page 851) is a protrusion of part of the stomach through the esophageal opening (hiatus) of the diaphragm.

People tend to associate hernias with heavy lifting, but in fact, hernias often have no apparent cause, and even a baby can be born with one.

Inguinal hernia

In men, a hernia commonly develops in the groin — the region where the spermatic cord and blood vessels to the testicles pass out of the abdominal cavity and into the scro-

Hernia Surgery

Surgery is the preferred treatment for most abdominal hernias, with the exception of an umbilical hernia in an infant, which usually corrects itself in 1 or 2 years.

The procedure
Hernia surgery consists of replacing any protruding intestine into the abdomen and surgically repairing the weakened or torn tissues to prevent the intestine from breaking through again.

Surgery may be postponed if you have a cold and cough because the spasmodic pressure in the abdomen may weaken the incision before it can heal properly.

Before the operation you'll be given some type of anesthetic — local, spinal or general, depending on the type and severity of the hernia. A small incision is then made in the area of the hernia, and the herniated tissue is returned to the abdominal cavity. This type of surgery is called a herniorrhaphy. If the herniated intestine is strangulated and gangrenous, that section of the intestine will be removed (resected), and the healthy ends will be sutured together. The operation is concluded by repairing the tissues of the abdominal wall. Your surgeon may elect to strengthen a weakened abdominal wall by placing a synthetic mesh patch over the tissue to keep it from protruding again. This procedure is called a hernioplasty.

Sometimes, hernia repair is performed laparoscopically. Instead of making a large incision in your abdomen, the surgeon makes several small incisions of ½ to 1 inch in length. Flexible, tube-like instruments (laparoscopes), one of which has an attached miniature camera, are inserted through the incisions, allowing the surgeon to

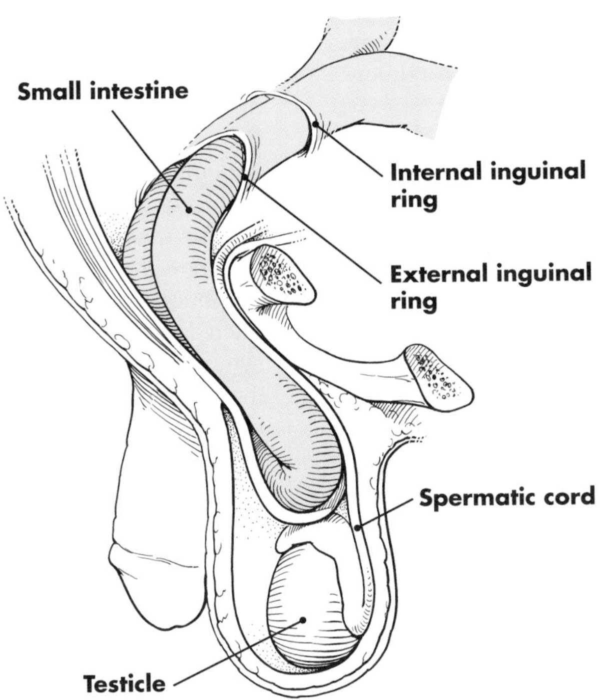

In an inguinal hernia, the small intestine protrudes into the scrotum. It commonly occurs in men at the point where the spermatic cord that suspends the testicles passes out of the abdomen into the scrotum.

tum. The area where these structures pass through the abdominal muscles is called the inguinal canal.

When a loop of bowel passes out of the abdomen along with the spermatic cord, this is called an indirect inguinal hernia. A bulge directly through the abdominal wall in this area is called a direct inguinal hernia. Both indirect and direct inguinal hernias probably account for four of every five hernias in men. Less often, an inguinal hernia can develop in a woman at the point where the connective tissue supporting the uterus exits from the abdomen to join with the tissue near the vaginal opening.

Signs and symptoms of an inguinal hernia include discomfort while bending or lifting and a tender lump in the groin area. In men, the protruding intestine sometimes enters the scrotum, causing pain and swelling of the scrotum.

Diagnosis

Usually, a doctor can diagnose an inguinal hernia by examination. Many hernias cause a noticeable bulge adjacent to the pubic bone. Many minor hernias are detected during routine physical examinations.

How serious is an inguinal hernia?

A hernia that can't be replaced into the abdomen by application of gentle pressure may be trapped (incarcerated). Without treatment, the hernia can strangulate and cut off the blood supply to the intestine. This can cause gangrene in a section of the bowel, a life-threatening condition requiring immediate surgical attention. If the bulge is accompanied by nausea and vomiting, the hernia may have become obstructed or strangulated.

Treatment

The best treatment for an inguinal hernia that's causing signs and symptoms is an operation in which the intestine is pushed back into the abdomen and the weakened

see inside your abdomen, guide the protruding intestine back into place and repair weakened tissue and muscle. Because only small incisions are made, the procedure often results in a quicker recovery than with conventional surgery.

Recovery

Hernia surgery is usually done on an outpatient basis. After the operation you'll be urged to move about as soon as you're able, usually within the first day. Some soreness is typical, but many people go back to work within a few days. Recovery may last anywhere from 1 to 6 weeks, depending on the type of surgery you had and your occupation.

Your doctor may offer recommendations on any restrictions of activity, but in general it's best to avoid contact sports and heavy lifting or straining for at least 3 weeks to allow the incision to heal properly.

If you notice any redness or discomfort around the site of the incision, report it to your doctor. It may be a sign of infection.

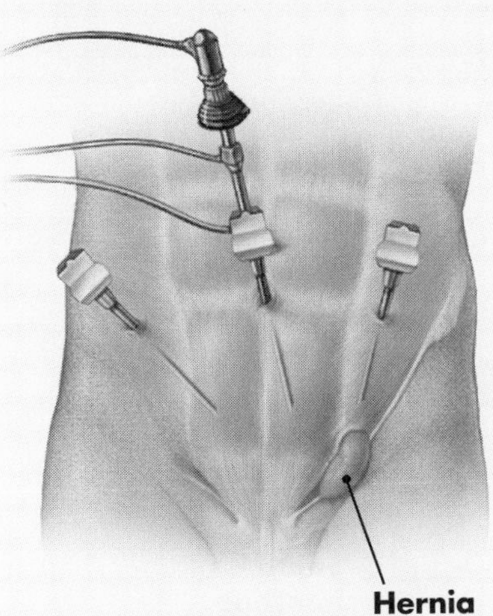

Laparoscopic surgery involves inserting instruments through several small incisions. Traditional surgery uses one larger incision.

muscles in the abdominal wall are sewn together. This is called a herniorrhaphy.

In some cases, your doctor may elect to do a hernioplasty, which involves using a prosthetic mesh patch to reinforce the weakened area. This type of surgery may be performed using a minimally invasive technique called laparoscopy, in which a few small incisions are made in the abdomen instead of one large incision. This type of surgery reduces symptoms, such as pain, following surgery and it speeds recovery.

Wearing a truss doesn't provide a good long-term solution for a hernia. However, your doctor may suggest that you wear one before surgery to prevent the condition from getting worse.

Femoral hernia

A femoral hernia forms along the canal that carries the principal blood vessels (femoral artery and vein) into the thigh. This hernia usually produces a bulge that's slightly lower than where an inguinal hernia tends to appear.

Femoral hernias are more common in women than in men, and these types of hernias are more likely to become strangulated.

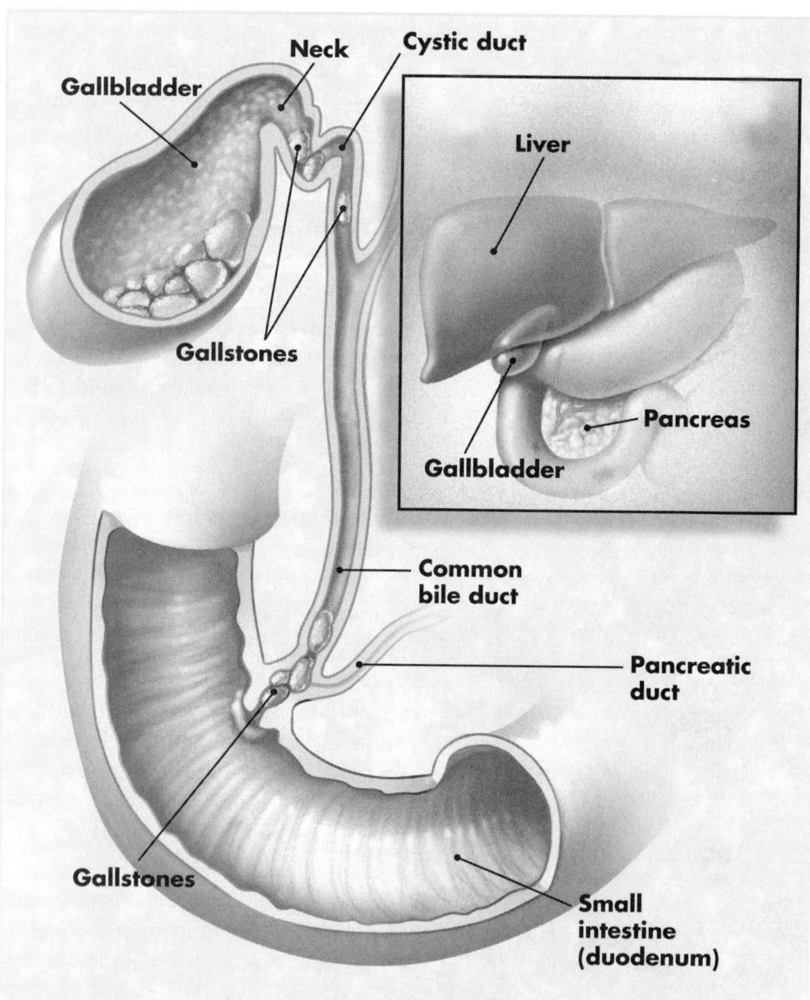

The gallbladder is located behind the liver on the right side of the upper abdomen. A gallbladder attack occurs when stones that form in the gallbladder lodge in the neck of the gallbladder or the cystic duct leading to the main (common) bile duct. Gallstones that obstruct the common bile duct or pancreatic duct can cause inflammation of the bile ducts (cholingitis) or pancreatitis.

Umbilical hernia

With this type of hernia, a bulge appears at the navel (umbilicus) because of a weakness in the abdominal wall surrounding the umbilicus. Some newborn children have an umbilical hernia. Part of their bowel has remained outside of the abdominal cavity. These hernias often don't cause any signs and symptoms and may resolve on their own. In adults, umbilical hernias sometimes become sore or painful and should be repaired.

Incisional hernia

A surgical incision in the abdominal wall can lead to an incisional hernia. Incisional hernias usually pose only a minor risk of complications, although at times portions of your intestine may protrude (prolapse) through the hernia and cause discomfort.

Gallbladder and Bile Duct Disorders

The gallbladder is a pear-shaped sac 3 to 4 inches long and roughly 1 inch in diameter that's attached to the underside of the liver on your right side. The gallbladder stores bile that's produced in your liver and discharges it into the upper part of your small intestine (duodenum) after a meal. Bile facilitates the digestion of fats. Several conditions can affect the gallbladder and bile ducts.

Gallstones

Signs and symptoms

- Intense and sudden pain in the upper abdomen
- Abdominal pain that lasts 30 minutes to several hours
- Pain that moves around to the right shoulder blade area

Detecting Duct Obstructions

Bile and pancreatic ducts are small and located deep in the abdomen, so standard diagnostic tests often aren't beneficial in examining them. To identify a possible obstruction in a duct, a doctor may use one of the following procedures:

Endoscopic ultrasound

Endoscopic ultrasound (EUS) involves the use of a small ultrasound probe that's attached to a thin, flexible instrument called an endoscope. While you're sedated the endoscope is inserted through your mouth and threaded down your throat to your stomach and upper small intestine (duodenum).

The ultrasound probe is used to view internal organs and structures that are adjacent to the stomach and intestines, including the gallbladder, pancreas and liver. EUS can help diagnose disorders affecting these organs, including obstructions in the pancreatic and bile ducts. This procedure provides clear pictures without having to inject contrast materials into the ducts, reducing the risk of complications. If a growth is detected, tissue samples can be taken (biopsies) for laboratory analysis.

Endoscopic retrograde cholangiopancreatography

Endoscopic retrograde cholangiopancreatography is another procedure used to identify the cause of a bile duct obstruction, such as a gallstone, damaged bile duct tissue or tumor.

While you're sedated, an endoscope is threaded into your mouth, down your throat, through your stomach and into the first part of your small intestine (duodenum). Air is injected to inflate the duodenum to help identify the tiny opening through which the bile and pancreatic ducts drain. Once this opening is found, a hollow tube (catheter) is passed through the endoscope and into the bile and pancreatic ducts. A dye or contrast solution is injected through this catheter into the ducts. X-rays are then taken of the ducts.

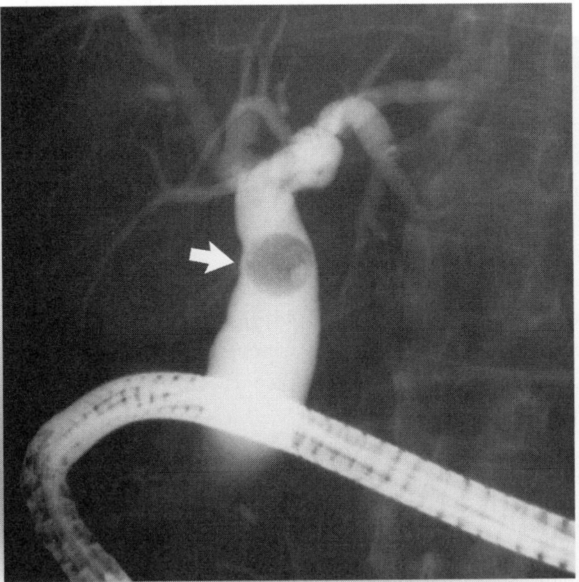

This X-ray image taken during an endoscopic retrograde cholangiopancreatography procedure shows a dilated common bile duct containing a gallstone (see arrow).

Other types of catheters may be placed through the endoscope to take tissue samples or treat specific abnormalities identified on the X-rays.

Percutaneous transhepatic cholangiography

Percutaneous transhepatic cholangiography is an X-ray procedure that uses a contrast material to provide pictures of the bile duct. Before the test you lie down on an X-ray table that can be rotated into vertical and horizontal positions. A tube is inserted into a vein in your arm for administration of a sedative and antibiotic. The skin over your liver is cleansed with an antiseptic, and a local anesthetic is injected below the skin.

Once the area where the anesthetic was injected becomes numb, a long, thin needle is inserted into your liver. Most people don't feel the needle pass into the liver. When X-ray images indicate that the needle has reached the bile duct, a contrast medium is injected through the needle. A series of X-rays is taken as you're rotated into different positions to provide varying views of your liver. You may need to stay in the hospital overnight for monitoring in case bleeding or infection develops.

- Nausea and, sometimes, vomiting

Gallstones are crystalline structures that can be as small as a grain of sand or larger than a golf ball. They can be smooth and round or irregular with many edges. Some people have only one gallstone, and others have hundreds. Gallstones are common, affecting about 10 percent of all adults in the United States.

A gallstone that obstructs the cystic duct leading from the gallbladder to the main (common) bile duct may cause pain and, sometimes, gallbladder inflammation. The common bile duct is a conduit into the duodenum from both the liver and gallbladder. Although gallstones develop in many people, they usually don't cause signs and symptoms. The chance of signs and symptoms or complications developing from gallstones is probably less than 20 percent over a period of years. In a small percentage of cases, they can cause a gallbladder attack.

The pain of a gallbladder attack often begins quite suddenly and may persist for several hours. Typically, it's severe and constant and may be accompanied by nausea and vomiting. As the pain subsides, you may have a mild aching sensation or soreness in the upper abdomen, which may last for up to a day.

Gallbladder attacks can be infrequent, occurring no more than a few times a year. People often blame gallstones for their belching, bloating, intolerance to fatty foods and frequent abdominal pain, but generally these signs and symptoms aren't due to gallstones.

Yellowing of your skin and eyes (jaundice), especially if it's accompanied by pain, suggests that a stone may have migrated into the common bile duct. The presence of a high fever or shaking chills usually indicates a complication such as inflammation of the gallbladder (cholecystitis), acute pancreatitis or infection in the bile duct (cholangitis) due to an obstruction.

Sometimes, signs and symptoms of gallbladder disease occur after eating, but they can occur any time, even while you're sleeping.

Autopsies show that gallstones develop in 20 percent to 30 percent of women by the age of 70, more than twice the number found in men. The likelihood of gallstones increases with age and obesity. Extreme, rapid weight loss also is associated with gallstone formation.

Types

Not all gallstones are made of the same material. Most contain a mixture of substances. Among Americans, 80 percent of the stones are composed primarily of cholesterol. The remaining 20 percent contain mostly calcium salts of bile pigment.

Normally, bile acids and phospholipids, such as lecithin, keep cholesterol from becoming too concentrated and forming gallstones. However, if the amount of cholesterol in bile increases beyond the ability of bile acids and lecithin to maintain this balance, the cholesterol can crystallize and form into stones.

Diagnosis

If a severe, persistent pain develops in your upper abdomen, your doctor may want to check for gallstones. Your doctor may palpate your abdomen to see if your gallbladder is tender or has become swollen (distended) because of obstruction of the duct. Tests used to diagnose gallstones generally include a blood test and an ultrasound examination of the gallbladder, which can detect stones inside. Other tests that may be used are a computerized tomography (CT) scan and radionuclide scan. See Chapter 39, "Diagnostic Tests," for more information on these tests.

Treatment

If you have gallstones but aren't bothered by signs or symptoms, your doctor may not recommend any specific treatment but rather advise you to watch and wait. If you have gallbladder pain or have had one or more episodes of inflammation of the pancreas, your doctor may recommend treatment.

Surgery

Surgical removal of the gallbladder (cholecystectomy) is the preferred treatment for most people with gallbladder disease. Often, this surgery can be performed using a procedure called laparoscopy, which is less invasive than traditional surgery because it involves a few small abdominal incisions instead of one large one. In some cases, a procedure called endoscopic retrograde cholangiopancreatography may be used. This procedure involves threading a flexible tube with an attached camera (endoscope) through the digestive tract to the opening of the common bile duct. If a stone is discovered in the duct, it can be removed immediately with tools attached to the endoscope.

Stone dissolution

Stone dissolution is a form of gallstone treatment developed in the 1970s. It can dissolve cholesterol stones, but because of its limitations, it's now used infrequently. A bile acid (ursodeoxycholic acid) is taken by mouth in tablet form. The medication decreases the cholesterol concentration within the gallbladder, allowing bile acids to return solid cholesterol stones to a solution mixture. The drug works best if the cholesterol stones are small and don't show detectable calcium on a CT scan.

Dosage of the medication is based on body weight and can be costly. It generally takes many months or even years for bile acids to dissolve the stones. Therefore, this approach isn't practical if you're having frequent bouts of gallbladder pain. In addition, if drug therapy is discontinued, you have at least a 50 percent chance of developing more gallstones because the underlying problem of excess secretion of cholesterol is still present.

Bile duct obstruction

Signs and symptoms

- Pain in the upper abdomen
- Yellowing of the skin and eyes
- Itching
- High fever with chills
- Light gray or tan stools
- Tea- or coffee-colored urine

Emergency signs and symptoms

- Cold, clammy, pale skin and a weak or rapid pulse
- Mental confusion

An obstruction in the main passageway for transport of bile into the duodenum (common bile duct) can occur for several reasons:

Gallstones

The most common cause of a bile duct obstruction is a gallstone that has lodged in the duct. One or more stones may obstruct the narrow duct and cause episodic pain in the upper abdomen. Spiking fevers with shaking chills and yellowing of your skin and eyes (jaundice) may signal a severe (acute) bile duct obstruction.

An obstruction in the common bile duct at the location where it's joined by the pancreatic duct can cause inflammation of the pancreas (pancreatitis). Pancreatic enzymes aren't able to flow out of the pancreas and become trapped inside, damaging the organ. Obstruction of the common bile duct can lead to a medical emergency requiring immediate relief of the obstruction.

Narrowing of a duct

Narrowing (stricture) of the common bile duct is a potential complication of gallbladder or bile duct surgery. The stricture may develop immediately after surgery or several years later. Strictures may also develop following a gallstone obstruction. An operation can often correct the problem.

Hemobilia

Blood in the bile duct (hemobilia) can clot and obstruct the duct. Hemobilia is a rare condition that may occur as a result of trauma to the liver or bile duct during surgery. People with hemobilia often have abdominal pain, jaundice and blood in stool. Often, the clot dissolves spontaneously, but it might need to be removed with a surgical or nonsurgical procedure.

Primary sclerosing cholangitis

The term *sclerosis* refers to hardening and thickening of tissue. A chronic disorder called primary sclerosing cholangitis causes tissues in the bile duct wall to harden and thicken. This can partially block the duct and lead to formation of bile duct stones. Either the obstruction or resulting stones can cause the same signs and symptoms as gallstones in the bile duct, including jaundice, itching, pain in the right side of the abdomen and episodes of fever and chills.

Primary sclerosing cholangitis can also lead to cirrhosis, liver failure, bile duct cancer or bleeding from veins in the esophagus. Frequently, sclerosing cholangitis is associated with an underlying disease such as ulcerative colitis.

Bile duct cancer

A cancerous (malignant) tumor in the bile duct can cause obstruction. Signs and symptoms of bile duct cancer may include jaundice, weight loss, light-colored stools and abdominal pain.

Other disorders

Sometimes, the common bile duct can become partially or completely obstructed by external pressure. This can occur as a complication of pancreatitis, pancreatic cancer, lymphoma or cancer that has spread (metastasized) from another part of the body. The principal sign is jaundice. Treatment is directed at the underlying disorder.

Diagnosis

Because the early signs and symptoms of a bile duct obstruction are similar, regardless of the cause, your doctor may use many of the same diagnostic tests used to identify gallstones. Two other diagnostic procedures, called percutaneous transhepatic cholangiography and endoscopic retrograde cholangiopancreatography, involve injection of a contrast material into the common bile duct (see page 897).

How serious is a bile duct obstruction?

Bile duct blockage is a serious and even life-threatening problem that requires prompt treatment. Blood cultures during episodes of fever may reveal the presence of bacteria that have entered into the bloodstream from the obstructed and infected bile duct. Blood infection (sepsis) can lead to shock.

Treatment

The principle goal of treatment is to relieve the blockage.

Surgery

If the cause of the obstruction is one or more gallstones within the bile duct and you have gallstones in your gallbladder, your doctor may recommend surgical removal of the gallbladder and the stones lodged in the duct. Sometimes, a doctor prefers to remove stones in the bile ducts before surgery, using other techniques.

If the obstruction is due to narrowing (stricture) of the bile duct, a surgeon skilled in biliary tract repair may reconstruct the bile duct. If previous attempts at bile duct repair have been unsuccessful, the duct may be widened and a tiny tube (stent) inserted into the narrowed area to help keep the duct open and permit passage of bile.

Because late-stage primary sclerosing cholangitis typically causes multiple narrowings that can't be treated with stents or by other means, presently there's no specific treatment. If the disorder results in severe liver failure, liver transplantation may be an option.

Endoscopic retrograde cholangiopancreatography

Endoscopic retrograde cholangiopancreatography (ERCP) is a procedure in which a flexible tube (endoscope) is threaded into your digestive tract to where the common bile duct enters into the upper portion of the small intestine (duodenum). A cutting device attached to the tube can be inserted through the entrance of the bile duct, enlarging the entrance to permit passage of the obstructing stone. A tiny mesh tube may be placed in the duct to keep it open.

Medication

Itching is often a predominant symptom with chronic obstruction of the bile ducts. It can be successfully managed with medication. Your doctor may also prescribe vitamins A, D, E and K, which are poorly absorbed in people with bile duct obstruction. If fever and chills are present, you may be given an antibiotic.

Choledochal cysts

Cysts can sometimes form in the bile duct. Those due to a birth defect that causes expansion of the duct are called choledochal cysts. A choledochal cyst can lead to obstruction or infection of the bile duct, which causes a narrowing (stricture) of the duct. Because the process is gradual, many people experience occasional symptoms of abdominal pain and irritation for years before an obstruction develops.

Once such a cyst is identified, it's generally removed surgically. People who have had a choledochal cyst have an increased risk of developing bile duct cancer.

Pancreatic Disorders

The pancreas lies horizontally behind the lower part of the stomach. Its head rests against the wall of the first portion of the small intestine (duodenum), and its tail extends toward the spleen. The pancreas is a gland, meaning that it has the ability to manufacture a secretion used in another part of the body. The pancreas has two parts and produces several secretions.

The pancreas produces and secretes digestive enzymes and alkaline material (sodium bicarbonate) into the pancreatic duct, which then flow into the duodenum. The alkaline secretion makes it possible for digestive enzymes to break down nutrients into smaller units, enabling them to be absorbed into the bloodstream by the small bowel.

The pancreas also produces and secretes the hormones insulin and glucagon into the bloodstream. These hormones are important to help regulate your metabolism, including your level of blood sugar (glucose).

Infections, injury and tumors can damage the pancreas and affect its functions. If, for example, secretion of the hormone insulin is diminished, diabetes may result.

Acute pancreatitis

Signs and symptoms

- Intense, continuous abdominal pain, possibly radiating to the back and chest
- Pain that may begin after a large meal or bout of heavy drinking
- Fever
- Nausea or vomiting
- Abdominal swelling and tenderness

Acute pancreatitis is a severe but temporary inflammation of the pancreas. Factors associated with acute pancreatitis include alcohol use, gallstones, increased blood triglyceride or calcium levels, viral and bacterial infections and certain drugs. The mechanisms by which these conditions trigger pancreatic inflammation aren't well-known. However, several theories exist.

A principal theory is that acute pancreatitis results when enzymes of the pancreas damage the gland itself, a process called autodigestion. Powerful digestive enzymes normally are secreted by the pancreas in inactive forms, and they become active only after they enter the small intestine. During acute pancreatitis these enzymes may become activated inside the gland. As a result the enzymes begin to digest the tissue of the pancreas. In addition, certain enzymes may set off a chain reaction by activating other enzymes, increasing the number of enzymes involved in the destructive process.

Autodigestion causes swelling (edema), inflammation and bleeding due to damage to pancreatic blood vessels. If unchecked, this series of events can produce a serious problem.

Diagnosis

Acute pancreatitis is characterized by intense, constant pain in the upper abdomen that may radiate to the back or chest. The pain is often worse when lying flat and relieved when sitting up and bending forward. Other signs and symptoms include a swollen (distended) and tender abdomen.

During a physical examination, your doctor may elicit pain by pressing the abdominal area. A sample of your blood may be taken to check for specific abnormalities, such as excessive levels of certain pancreatic enzymes, a high white blood cell count, high blood sugar

The Pancreas

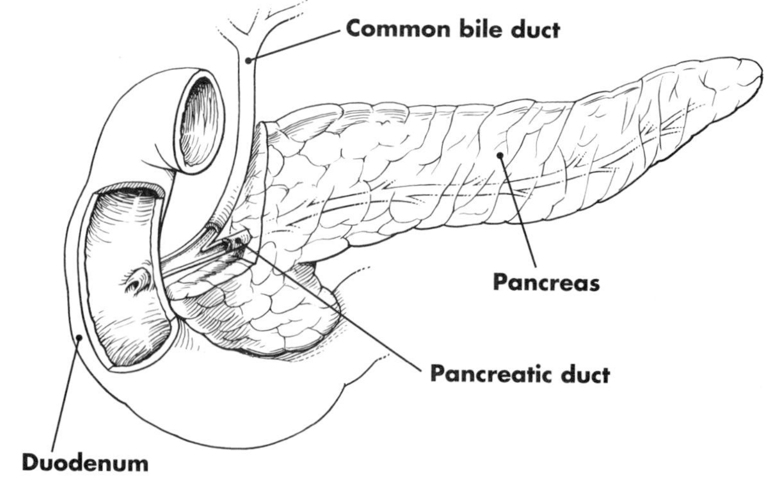

(hyperglycemia) and low calcium levels (hypocalcemia). Other tests may include an abdominal X-ray, an endoscopic ultrasound examination or a computerized tomography (CT) scan. See Chapter 39, "Diagnostic Tests," for more information on these tests.

How serious is acute pancreatitis?

In most cases, signs and symptoms of mild acute pancreatitis subside within a week. Severe pancreatitis, however, can be life-threatening. Major complications include extensive destruction of the gland, development of an abscess or a cyst in the pancreas (pseudocyst) and leakage of pancreatic fluid into the abdomen.

Treatment

Treatment of mild acute pancreatitis centers on decreasing the flow of pancreatic enzymes. An important part of treatment is to prevent or reduce the release of pancreatic enzymes and thus protect the pancreas from further damage. Because eating may increase secretions, you may be given nourishment intravenously until signs and symptoms improve. You shouldn't drink any alcohol.

Medication

To ease the pain, a pain reliever is usually prescribed. Antibiotics may be given if an infection is present or suspected.

Surgery

If the underlying cause of the pancreatitis is gallbladder disease or an obstructed pancreatic duct, surgery may be necessary to remove a gallstone or relieve the obstruction. But this usually is done after the pancreatitis has been brought under control. If a stone is present at the entrance into the small intestine from the common bile and pancreatic ducts, your doctor may consider a procedure called endoscopic retrograde cholangiopancreatography, in which a thin, flexible fiber-optic tube (endoscope) is inserted through your mouth and digestive tract until it reaches the small intestine. The opening of the ducts is enlarged and the obstructing stone removed, using instruments passed through the endoscope (see page 897).

Chronic pancreatitis

Signs and symptoms

- Persistent or recurrent abdominal pain, possibly intense and radiating to the back and chest
- Excessively foul, bulky stools
- Weight loss
- Onset of diabetes

Chronic pancreatitis differs from acute pancreatitis in that it develops over a period of years. A person with chronic pancreatitis may have both recurrent attacks of acute pain and chronic persistent pain. The acute attacks may be accompanied by nausea, vomiting and abdominal swelling (distention). Many people with chronic pancreatitis have a history of alcohol abuse. In some cases, the cause is unknown.

If you have chronic pancreatitis, your pancreas gradually becomes less able to secrete the enzymes needed for proper digestion and absorption of dietary fats. This is called pancreatic exocrine insufficiency. Among adults, alcoholism is the most common cause of this insufficiency. In children, cystic fibrosis is the most common cause.

Unlike the persistent pain of acute pancreatitis, the pain of chronic pancreatitis can vary — it may be constant, occasional, intermittent or absent altogether. Pancreatic insufficiency may also cause weight loss and pale-colored, foul, bulky, fat-containing stools (steatorrhea). Severe scarring of the pancreas from chronic pancreatitis can lead to diabetes.

Another sign of chronic pancreatitis is small, hard deposits that form in the pancreatic duct or tissue. This condition, called pancreatic calcification, can be seen on an X-ray or abdominal computerized tomography (CT) scan. Alcohol-induced pancreatitis is a common cause of this kind of calcification. Even moderate but consistent social drinking over the years may produce significant pancreatic calcification. Smoking may increase the rate of calcifications.

Diagnosis

To confirm a diagnosis of chronic pancreatitis, your doctor will likely take a stool and blood sample. People with chronic pancreatitis often have a high fat content in their stool because fat isn't being absorbed by the intestine.

Abnormal levels of pancreatic enzymes in your bloodstream are another indication that your pancreas may be diseased or damaged.

Other tests may include a CT scan of the abdomen, endoscopic ultrasound examination (see page 1276) or endoscopic retrograde cholangiopancreatography (see page 897). These tests can identify evidence of pancreatic duct damage or obstruction of the pancreatic or common bile duct.

Your doctor may also order a pancreatic stimulation test. It involves administering a solution through a tube that passes through the nose into the stomach and then into the duodenum, to stimulate the pancreas to secrete digestive juices. A stimulating hormone may be given. Secretions into the duodenum are then withdrawn and analyzed over a period of 2 hours. Abnormal secretions suggest that the function of the pancreas may be impaired.

Treatment

The therapy for chronic pancreatitis usually centers on its two main problems: pain and malabsorption. If diabetes is identified, it also needs to be treated.

Medication

If you have intermittent pain, you may be given a non-narcotic pain reliever (analgesic) to help control

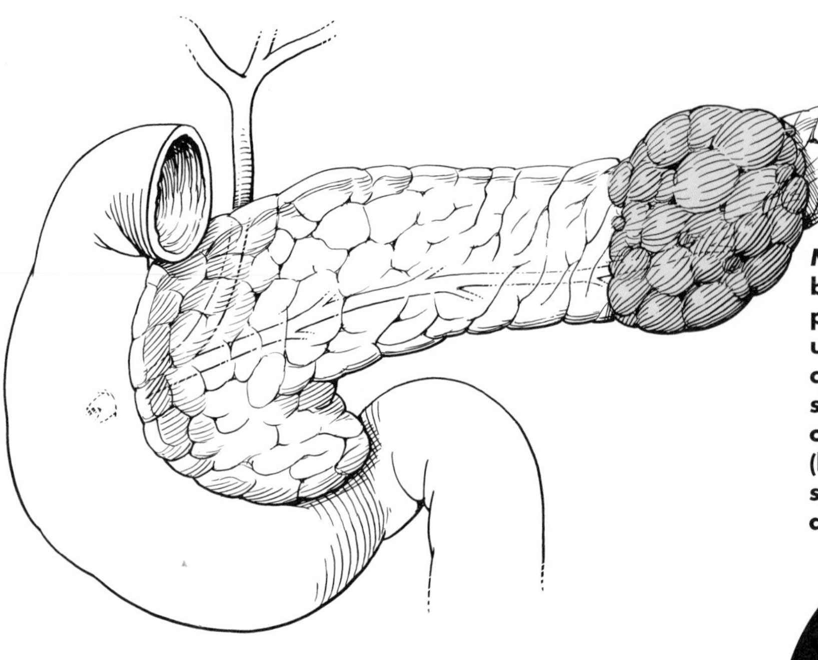

Most pancreatic cancer begins in the lining of the pancreatic ducts and grows undetected for years. The computerized tomography scan below shows a cancerous tumor in the pancreas (black arrow) that has spread to the liver (white arrow).

the pain. Malabsorption is generally treated with a pancreatic enzyme preparation that you take to replace enzymes that aren't being secreted into the duodenum by your pancreas. The tablets are taken with meals and snacks. Enzyme therapy may also help relieve the pain.

Diet
You'll be directed to abstain from drinking alcohol and, most likely, to avoid foods high in fat content.

Surgery and other procedures
For severe pain that can't be controlled, treatment options include endoscopy or surgery to relieve obstructed ducts or remove damaged tissue or procedures to block pain signals or deaden the nerves that are transmitting the pain.

Pancreatic cancer

Signs and symptoms

- Sometimes, none
- Abdominal pain, possibly radiating to the back
- Loss of appetite and weight
- Yellowing of the skin and eyes
- Itching
- Nausea and vomiting
- Intestinal bleeding

Although pancreatic cancer accounts for only a small percentage of all cancers in the United States, it's the fourth leading cause of cancer deaths. The reason it's so deadly is that it's usually diagnosed too late — this cancer typically produces no signs and symptoms until it's advanced and incurable. When signs and symptoms do develop, the most common are abdominal pain, weight loss and yellowing of the skin and eyes (jaundice). Weight loss usually is significant, averaging about 25 pounds. Jaundice occurs if the cancer blocks the common bile duct.

Much about why or how this cancer develops is unclear. Several factors may increase your risk:

- *Smoking.* Cigarette smokers are two to three times more likely to get pancreatic cancer than are nonsmokers.
- *Family history.* Cancer of the pancreas seems to run in families.
- *Age.* Most people are between ages 60 and 80 when they receive a diagnosis of this disease.
- *Sex.* Men are about 30 percent more likely to get pancreatic cancer than are women.
- *Race.* Blacks are more likely to get the disease than are people of other racial groups.
- *Chronic pancreatitis.* Some studies suggest that people with long-term inflammation of the pancreas (chronic pancreatitis) may have an increased risk of developing pancreatic cancer.

Diagnosis

Because the pancreas is located deep in the abdomen and behind other organs, it's almost impossible for a doctor to feel a lump on examination. Possible evidence of pancreatic cancer on physical examination includes abdominal tenderness, jaundice or liver enlargement.

Tests used to help diagnose pancreatic cancer include an endoscopic ultrasound (EUS) examination and abdominal computerized tomography (CT) scan. Tissue samples of the pancreas may be obtained by biopsy during an EUS exam or by biopsy using a CT scan for guidance. See Chapter 39, "Diagnostic Tests," for more information on these tests.

Occasionally, a procedure called endoscopic retrograde cholangiopancreatography may be helpful (see page 897). At times, exploratory surgery is required to establish the diagnosis.

How serious is pancreatic cancer?

The survival rate with pancreatic cancer is generally poor. By the time the cancer is identified, it often has spread (metastasized) beyond the pancreas. The median survival of advanced pancreatic cancer is about 3 to 6 months from the time of the diagnosis.

Treatment

If the cancer is found early and confined to the pancreas, surgically removing all or part of the pancreas may be successful. The most common operation is called the Whipple procedure. It includes removal of part of the pancreas, part of the stomach and the first portion of the small intestine, along with the gallbladder. It's a complex and difficult operation with a long recovery period.

Radiation and chemotherapy may help extend survival but can't cure the cancer. Painkillers are commonly prescribed to control the pain. Another option is a nerve block (celiac ganglionic block), which destroys the nerves leading to the pancreas. Pancreatic enzyme therapy may help reduce malabsorption and weight loss.

Congenital pancreatic abnormalities

Occasionally, problems with the pancreas occur at birth.

Annular pancreas

An annular pancreas is a rare, ring-shaped formation of pancreatic tissue that surrounds the first portion of the small intestine (duodenum) and may cause an intestinal obstruction. The condition can cause symptoms in children and, rarely, adults.

You may feel exceptionally full after meals and later have pain in the pit of your stomach that may cause nausea and vomiting. Because the symptoms may be mild and tolerable, many people go for years before they receive a diagnosis of this condition.

In addition to intestinal obstruction, individuals with annular pancreas may have complications such as pancreatitis or a peptic ulcer. Once you receive a diagnosis of this condition, the potential for complications requires that the problem be corrected surgically.

Pancreas divisum

Pancreas divisum is a congenital defect in which two parts of the pancreas fail to grow together. As a result, the pancreas must drain its secretions through a smaller secondary duct. Most people with this condition have no signs and symptoms, but some develop inflammation of the pancreas (pancreatitis).

Liver Disorders

The liver is the largest single internal organ, and the most complex. Weighing as much as 4 pounds, the liver performs many complicated tasks essential to proper functioning of the entire body. These functions may be grouped into three categories: regulation, metabolism and detoxification.

- *Regulation.* The liver regulates the composition of your blood, in particular the amounts of sugar (glucose), protein and fat that enter the bloodstream. The liver also removes a substance called bilirubin from the blood. Bilirubin comes from the breakdown of red blood cells. Once bilirubin enters the liver, it's chemically changed so that it becomes soluble in water, added to bile and eliminated in the stool.
- *Metabolism.* The liver processes most of the nutrients absorbed from the intestines. In addition to converting many nutrients into forms that can be used by the body, the liver serves as a storage center for other nutrients, such as vitamin A and iron. It also manufactures cholesterol, blood clotting substances, specific proteins and bile, a fluid that facilitates the digestion of fat.
- *Detoxification.* The liver detoxifies blood. It removes some drugs and potentially harmful metabolites or chemicals from the bloodstream and converts them so that they can be excreted in bile, and subsequently in stool.

Because of its complexity and exposure to many potentially harmful substances, the liver is especially vulnerable to injury. However, nature protects the organ in two key ways. First, the liver is capable of regeneration — it can heal itself by repairing or replacing injured tissue. Second, it has many units that are responsible for the same task. Thus, if tissue in one section of the organ is injured, other cells can perform the functions of the injured section indefinitely or until the damage has been repaired.

Hepatitis

Signs and symptoms

- Fatigue
- Loss of appetite
- Nausea and, occasionally, vomiting
- Yellowing of the skin and eyes
- Low-grade fever
- Mild abdominal discomfort

The most common disease to affect the liver is hepatitis, inflammation of the liver. It can take several forms:

Alcohol- or drug-induced hepatitis

Alcohol- or drug-induced hepatitis is the most common form of this disease, occurring in people who drink excessive alcohol or take certain medications.

Acute vs. Chronic Hepatitis

Hepatitis signs and symptoms may last for a short period of time and then disappear (acute hepatitis), or they may persist indefinitely (chronic hepatitis).

Acute hepatitis

Acute hepatitis generally causes little or no permanent liver damage. It may develop suddenly or gradually, but it usually subsides in 6 months or less. As your body's defenses overcome the virus, liver inflammation and associated signs and symptoms gradually subside and disappear. Hepatitis A and E are acute forms. Hepatitis B also is acute, but in a few cases the inflammation can become chronic. Infants born with hepatitis B usually have chronic disease.

Chronic hepatitis

In chronic hepatitis, the liver remains inflamed even though you may have no signs and symptoms. Some people have hepatitis for more than 20 years without realizing it. In others, the inflammation may gradually cause formation of scar tissue in the liver (cirrhosis) and lead to liver failure. People with chronic hepatitis are at increased risk of liver cancer.

Nonalcoholic steatohepatitis is a common cause of chronic hepatitis. Hepatitis C may begin as an acute infection but often becomes chronic.

Chronic hepatitis can take different routes. It may progress very slowly with limited damage, or it may progress rapidly, causing extensive liver damage.

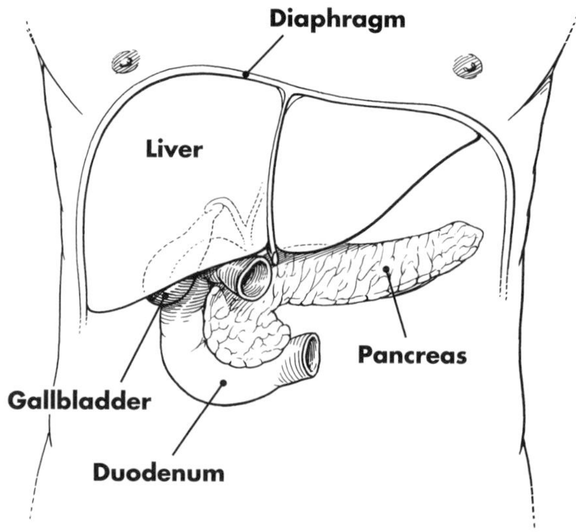

The inflammation stems from toxic chemicals that your body produces as it breaks down alcohol and drugs. Over time, these chemicals can damage liver cells and interfere with your liver's ability to do its job.

Approximately 10 percent to 35 percent of heavy drinkers get alcoholic hepatitis. Someone with a severe case of alcoholic hepatitis may run a high fever and develop an enlarged, painful liver. Recovery often is slow, even after complete abstinence from alcohol.

Medications that most commonly lead to drug-induced hepatitis are nonprescription pain relievers, especially if the medications are taken frequently or they're combined with alcohol. Nonprescription pain relievers include acetaminophen (Tylenol, others) and nonsteroidal anti-inflammatory drugs (NSAIDs), such as aspirin (Bayer, Bufferin, others), ibuprofen (Advil, Motrin, others), naproxen (Aleve, Naprosyn, others) and ketoprofen (Orudis).

Prescription medications also can lead to liver disease, including hepatitis. In most people, the following medications don't cause any problems. But in some people with liver disease or other health problems, they can cause or increase liver injury:

- Isoniazid, used for treatment of tuberculosis
- Valproic acid, an antiseizure medication
- Methotrexate, a cancer medication that's also used to treat psoriasis and rheumatoid arthritis
- The statin family of cholesterol medications, including atorvastatin (Lipitor), lovastatin (Mevacor), pravastatin (Pravachol) and simvastatin (Zocor)
- Certain high blood pressure medications, including calcium channel blockers and angiotensin-converting enzyme (ACE) inhibitors
- Certain antibiotics
- Some diabetes medications

If you have any signs and symptoms or laboratory findings that suggest hepatitis, your doctor will likely want to know if you've been taking any medication — including nonprescription drugs — during recent months.

Hepatitis A

Hepatitis A is caused by a virus most commonly encountered during international travel. This highly infectious disease is transmitted mainly by contaminated food or water. The virus may be present in your stools, blood and bile for 2 to 3 weeks before any signs and symptoms develop. The virus disappears once yellowing of the skin and eyes (jaundice) develops or within 2 to 3 weeks afterward.

Are You at Risk?

A simple screening test can pinpoint hepatitis C antibodies in blood, often identifying the disease before signs and symptoms develop and serious liver damage occurs. Have a screening test if you:

- Are using or have used, even once, illicit intravenous (IV) or intranasal drugs
- Received a blood transfusion before 1992
- Received a transplanted organ before 1992
- Received blood-clotting factor before 1987
- Have been accidentally exposed to the blood of others
- Are undergoing or have undergone hemodialysis
- Have hemophilia
- Have had sexual relations or have shared razors, toothbrushes or nail clippers with someone who has hepatitis C

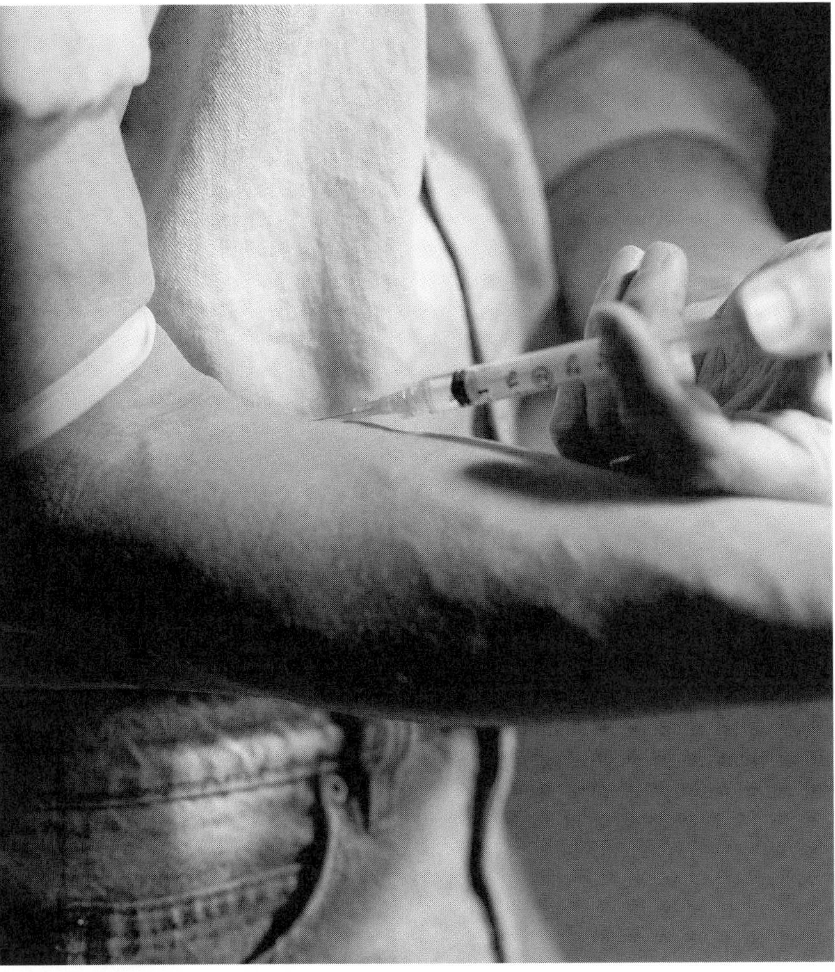

The vast majority of people with hepatitis A recover completely. The liver is often entirely healed within 1 to 2 months. In a few cases, especially in older adults, hepatitis A may cause severe signs and symptoms requiring medical therapy and perhaps hospitalization. In rare cases, it can be fatal.

Hepatitis B

Hepatitis B is a more serious form of viral liver infection. About 1 million people in the United States have hepatitis B infection. Worldwide, about 350 million people have this form of hepatitis, most of them men.

Its signs and symptoms are much the same as those of hepatitis A, but this disease can be more severe and last longer. As a result, there's a greater possibility of liver damage. Up to 10 percent of people with hepatitis B eventually develop chronic hepatitis.

Hepatitis B is highly contagious. It's found in blood, semen, vaginal fluid and saliva and can survive for 7 days or more outside the body. It's most often transmitted through sexual contact, contaminated syringes and needles and blood products. People at greatest risk of the disease are users of illicit drugs, those who practice unprotected sexual intercourse and hospital workers who are exposed to blood and blood products.

Some people (carriers) infected with the virus never experience signs and symptoms but are still capable of passing the virus to others. Approximately 90 percent of people with uncomplicated hepatitis B recover within 4 to 5 months.

Hepatitis C

Hepatitis C is the most common cause of viral hepatitis in the United States, affecting more than 3 million people. It may produce signs and symptoms similar to those of hepatitis A and B, except that often they're less severe and don't include jaundice. In fact, the majority of people with hepatitis C are without signs and symptoms or have only mild fatigue. Often, an abnormal result on a routine liver test alerts a doctor to the possibility of hepatitis C.

Hepatitis C is spread through blood and blood products and contaminated needles. Users of illicit intravenous (IV) or intranasal drugs who share paraphernalia account for approximately 60 percent of new infections. People who received blood transfusions before 1992, when blood banks began screening for the virus, also are at increased risk of hepatitis C. The virus can now be identified with a simple blood test.

Commonly, hepatitis C may lead to chronic liver diseases such as cirrhosis — an irreversible

PREVENTION TIP

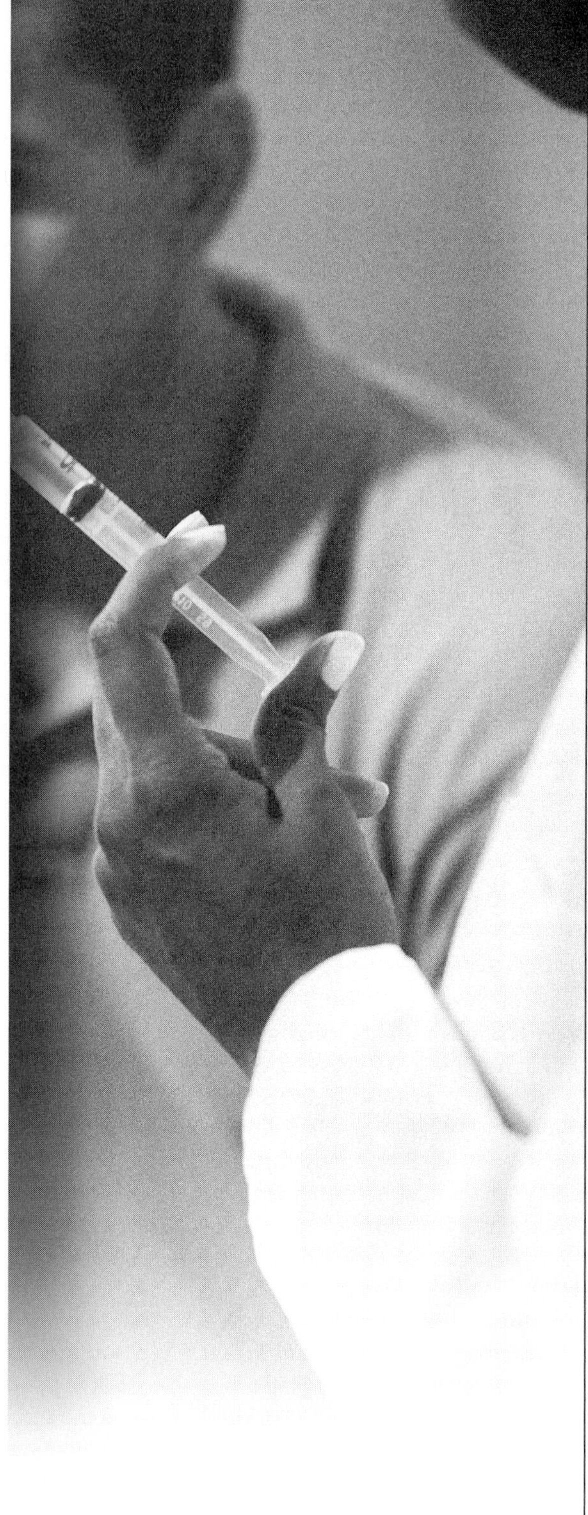

You can take a number of precautions to avoid viral forms of hepatitis:

Immunization

Effective vaccines for preventing hepatitis A and B are available. Depending on the type of vaccine used, a series of two or three injections offers about 20 years of protection from hepatitis A. A series of three or four injections protects you for at least 10 years against hepatitis B.

Americans considered to be at high risk of hepatitis B virus infection include:

- Individuals who inject illicit drugs with needles
- Individuals with multiple sex partners
- Sexually active homosexual and bisexual men
- Sexual partners of individuals with hepatitis B
- People with hemophilia
- People who undergo hemodialysis for kidney failure
- Dental and medical health professionals
- Male prison inmates

Most infants now receive hepatitis B vaccination as part of their routine childhood immunization series. Preadolescents, adolescents, college students and young adults also should receive the vaccine if they haven't been previously immunized.

The Occupational Safety and Health Administration (OSHA) requires some employers to offer hepatitis B vaccine at no cost to employees such as health care workers, public safety personnel and others who might be exposed to blood in the course of their work.

Food preparation

Follow these safe food-handling tips:

- Always wash fruits and vegetables.
- Cook foods thoroughly.
- When in developing countries, use only bottled water or boil tap water for at least 10 minutes, even for brushing your teeth. Avoid ice cubes.

Workplace precautions

In health care settings, follow all infection control procedures, including washing your hands and wearing gloves. In child care settings, wash your hands thoroughly after changing or handling diapers.

Other precautions

Practice good health habits:

- Follow safe sex practices. If you have sexual relations with multiple partners, use a latex condom with each sexual contact.
- Don't share drug syringes.
- If you undergo acupuncture, body piercing or tattooing, make sure the needles are sterilized.
- Don't share toothbrushes, razors or other items that may come into contact with blood.

and potentially fatal scarring of the liver — liver cancer and liver failure. It ranks close to alcoholism as the main cause of liver disease and is the leading reason for liver transplants in the United States.

Hepatitis D

To get this blood-borne virus, you must already have had hepatitis B. The hepatitis D virus survives and replicates by attaching itself to the hepatitis B virus. Hepatitis D isn't common in the United States, except among users of illicit drugs.

Hepatitis E

A food-borne virus similar to that of hepatitis A, the hepatitis E virus is prevalent in Asia and South America. Most cases of hepatitis E reported in the United States are in travelers to parts of the world where the virus is common.

Autoimmune hepatitis

Autoimmune hepatitis is believed to result from an agent that triggers the immune system to attack liver cells. Suspected triggers include the measles virus, the Epstein-Barr virus (the cause of mononucleosis) and viral hepatitis. The disease is more common among women than among men and typically occurs between ages 15 and 40.

Nonalcoholic steatohepatitis

With nonalcoholic steatohepatitis (NASH), your liver contains excessive fatty deposits, similar to alcohol-induced hepatitis. But the condition isn't associated with alcohol abuse.

NASH most often occurs in people who are obese or who have diabetes, high cholesterol levels or thyroid problems. It can also occur in people who take steroids or are malnourished. NASH is a common cause of abnormal liver test results and is a common cause of chronic hepatitis.

Diagnosis

To determine the type of hepatitis you may have, your doctor will likely ask you a number of questions about medications you're taking, whether you've traveled outside the United States, whether you had any blood transfusions before 1992 and your sex life.

A physical examination may reveal an enlarged, shrunken or hardened liver. Blood tests and imaging tests can help identify liver disease, including hepatitis.

To confirm the diagnosis, your doctor may remove and examine a sample of liver tissue (biopsy). A biopsy specimen also helps your doctor to identify the specific type of hepatitis you have and determine the severity of the inflammation and the extent of any permanent liver damage.

How serious is hepatitis?

Nearly all people who are healthy before contracting hepatitis A recover from the illness, and it doesn't become chronic. Approximately 90 percent of individuals with hepatitis B also recover. Hepatitis C and nonalcoholic steatohepatitis often give rise to chronic hepatitis.

In alcohol- or drug-induced hepatitis, if the individual stops drinking early enough or avoids the medications causing the condition, the liver can heal itself. But, recovery is often long and requires complete abstinence from alcohol.

If you're older or you have medical problems such as diabetes, congestive heart failure or severe anemia, recovery may take longer, and the risk of complications is greater.

Treatment

Treatment depends on the type of hepatitis you have. If you have hepatitis A, you probably won't need medications. However, you may be asked to abstain from any alcohol, at least during your recovery, because alcohol and some drugs can cause more injury to the already damaged liver.

Hospitalization may be required if you're pregnant, an older adult,

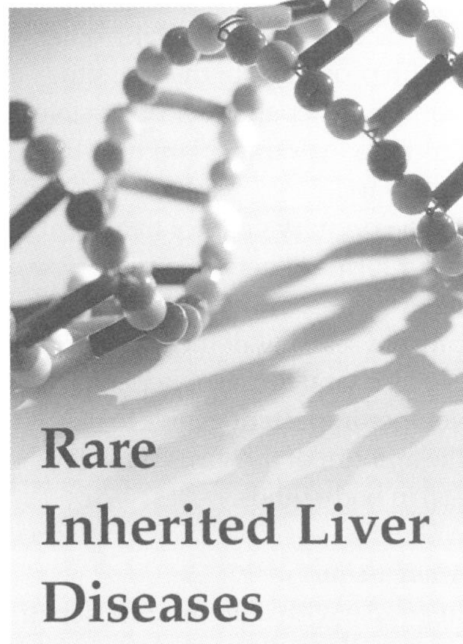

Rare Inherited Liver Diseases

Two uncommon inherited liver disorders that can affect digestion are Wilson's disease and alpha-1-antitrypsin deficiency.

Wilson's disease

Wilson's disease is an inherited disorder in which copper accumulates in various organs of the body, especially the brain, eyes, kidney and liver. It may be characterized by tremors, a copper ring near the cornea of the eye and signs and symptoms of chronic hepatitis. If untreated, cirrhosis and neurologic problems may result.

Treatment involves removing the deposits of copper with use of medication. This treatment usually is continued for life. If you have Wilson's disease, your blood relatives should be screened for evidence of the disease.

Alpha-1-antitrypsin deficiency

Alpha-1-antitrypsin deficiency results from a genetic defect that causes your body to produce abnormal forms of alpha-1-antitrypsin, an enzyme inhibitor. The deficiency may lead to liver and lung disease. A liver transplant is the only treatment that can halt the liver damage.

dehydrated or experiencing other health problems. In the rare situation when hepatitis A leads to liver failure, a liver transplant may be necessary.

The primary goals of treatment of other forms of hepatitis are to relieve signs and symptoms and prevent scarring of the liver (cirrhosis). For viral forms of hepatitis, another important goal is to reduce the amount of the virus (viral levels) in body fluids.

Medication

In people with autoimmune hepatitis, corticosteroids relieve signs and symptoms (cause remission) about 80 percent of the time. Steroids reduce liver inflammation by suppressing the immune system. The two most commonly prescribed are prednisone and prednisolone. Because of the side effects associated with corticosteroids, your doctor may gradually reduce the dosage to the lowest possible amount needed. Corticosteroids aren't prescribed for viral forms of hepatitis because suppressing your immune system may allow the virus to multiply more rapidly.

Chronic hepatitis B and C may be treated with interferon, a natural protein that inhibits viral replication. Sometimes, interferon is combined with ribavirin, an oral antiviral agent. Although interferon can lower viral levels, it's seldom possible to completely eliminate a hepatitis virus. In nearly all cases, the virus recurs and requires additional treatment.

Side effects such as fatigue, depression and lowered blood cell counts make treatment with interferon difficult, especially for people with a history of major depression, hyperthyroidism, low blood cell counts or autoimmune disease, or people who abuse alcohol or drugs.

Lamivudine, a drug originally approved to treat AIDS, can effectively reduce liver inflammation and hepatitis B viral levels. But over time the virus may become resistant to the medication.

A Liver Biopsy

In the course of evaluating liver disease, your doctor may perform a liver biopsy. This is a diagnostic procedure that's used in various liver disorders, including cirrhosis, hepatitis and tumors.

You'll be positioned flat on your back and given a local anesthetic. A thin needle is inserted between or below your ribs into your liver to remove small samples of tissue for laboratory analysis. This is often done with the help of ultrasound guidance. Infrequently, there's some discomfort following the procedure.

Laboratory tests on the liver tissue may reveal the presence or absence of certain disorders. Liver biopsy can be helpful in evaluating the progress of disease.

Liver transplantation

When liver damage is extensive and medications are no longer helpful, your doctor may discuss the possibility of a liver transplant (see page 912). Hepatitis C now leads to 30 percent of all liver transplants. If you have hepatitis C or B, the hepatitis virus might recur in the transplanted liver. Immunoglobulin injections and medication may reduce this risk.

Hemochromatosis

Signs and symptoms

- Fatigue
- Joint pain
- Impotence or loss of sex drive
- Increased skin pigmentation (bronzing)
- Increased thirst and urination

Hemochromatosis is due to a genetic abnormality that causes your intestines to absorb too much iron, leading to iron overload. The extra iron enters the bloodstream and builds up in certain organs, primarily the liver.

In rare cases, iron overload results from repeated blood transfusions or overconsumption of dietary iron. But by far the most common cause of the disease is a flawed gene discovered in 1996, called the HFE gene. Exactly how the gene causes iron overload isn't known. Researchers speculate that it holds the blueprint for a faulty protein that leads your intestines to absorb excessive amounts of iron.

It's estimated that approximately 1 in 10 Americans, most commonly those of Northern European descent, carry a flawed HFE gene. People with just one copy of the abnormal gene generally don't experience problems. Hemochromatosis tends to develop among people with two abnormal copies, usually inheriting an abnormal gene from each parent.

Diagnosis

A blood test called a transferrin saturation test is often the first step in diagnosing hemochromatosis. If the test shows that you have too much iron in your blood, your doctor may order additional blood tests to further assess iron amounts and the status of your liver. A genetic test can be done to see if you carry two abnormal copies of the HFE gene. To determine the extent of your disease, your doctor may recommend a liver biopsy.

Some doctors recommend that all adults have a transferrin saturation test at least once during their lifetime, preferably in early adulthood, to check for iron overload.

How serious is hemochromatosis?

Left untreated, hemochromatosis can lead to organ damage including cirrhosis and diabetes. The good news is that hemochromatosis is easily treated. If discovered early, permanent damage can usually be prevented.

Treatment

The most common treatment is to remove the excess iron from your blood by withdrawing about a pint of blood, a process called phlebotomy, once a week. Blood is withdrawn in the same manner as when donating blood. Sometimes, this treatment may be necessary for 1 to 2 years until the iron level decreases to normal. After reaching a normal iron level, most people need to have blood withdrawn four to eight times a year to keep iron from building up.

If the disease has damaged your liver or other organs, you may also need treatment to prevent further organ damage. This may include medication or surgery.

It's not necessary to remove all iron from your diet, but avoid consuming more than the recommended daily amount, 18 milligrams. Products highest in iron are iron supplements and some multivitamins. In addition, you may want to limit excessive consumption of vitamin C. Vitamin C facilitates iron absorption. In addition, avoid alcohol because it can aggravate liver disease.

Cirrhosis

Signs and symptoms

- Sometimes, none
- Loss of appetite
- Weight loss
- Fatigue and weakness
- Yellowing of the skin and eyes
- Abdominal swelling

Cirrhosis is characterized by progressive and irreversible damage to the liver, often due to alcohol abuse, infection, toxins or other diseases. The damage causes scarring within the organ, keeping it from functioning normally.

Causes

Cirrhosis can result for various reasons:

Alcohol abuse

In the United States, alcoholic cirrhosis is the most common type. It usually occurs after many years of excessive drinking and develops in as many as 15 percent of alcoholics.

Typically, people who develop cirrhosis from alcohol abuse have consumed a pint or more of liquor or several quarts of wine daily for at least 10 years. Women may be more susceptible to liver injury than men are. However, as little as 3 ounces of 100-proof whiskey (45 grams of alcohol) daily for several years may cause cirrhosis in some people, suggesting that other factors probably play a role as well.

Chronic viral hepatitis

Chronic inflammation resulting from hepatitis B or C may cause cirrhosis. Viruses that cause hepatitis inflame liver cells, injuring or destroying them. Attempts at healing result in scarring and cirrhosis.

Inherited diseases

Inherited diseases that can cause cirrhosis include hemochromatosis, Wilson's disease and alpha-1-antitrypsin deficiency.

Bile duct inflammation or blockage

Biliary cirrhosis is characterized by chronic inflammation and scarring of the liver bile ducts. The bile ducts and surrounding liver tissue are progressively destroyed and scarring (cirrhosis) develops.

Diagnosis

Visible signs of cirrhosis — yellowing of the skin and eyes (jaundice), abdominal swelling (distention) and weight loss — aren't always present. But even without such recognizable evidence, your doctor may detect liver damage during a routine medical examination.

By examining your abdomen, your doctor may be able to determine if your liver is enlarged and firm, a sign that you may have liver disease. As cirrhosis progresses, however, your liver may shrink. When that happens, blood flow may be impaired, resulting in an enlarged spleen. Abnormal blood test results may be the first sign of liver injury.

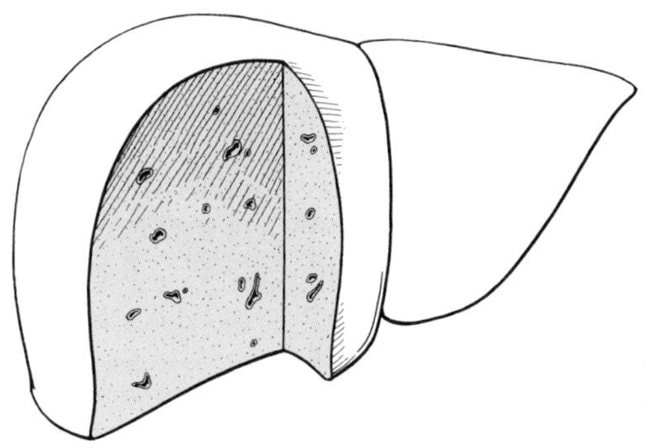

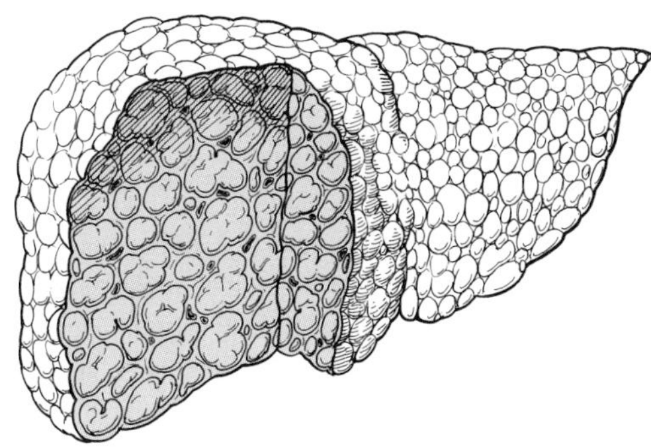

These cross-sectional illustrations show a normal liver (top) with no sign of scarring, and a cirrhotic liver (bottom) with extensive scarring.

To determine the extent of your disease, your doctor may want to evaluate your liver with ultrasound, computerized tomography (CT) or magnetic resonance imaging (MRI). A definitive diagnosis of cirrhosis requires a sample of liver tissue (biopsy) for microscopic examination. This can reveal the extent and possibly the cause of the liver damage.

How serious is cirrhosis?

There's no cure for cirrhosis as it causes irreversible liver damage. The good news is that it often progresses slowly. In the United States, cirrhosis results in about 25,000 deaths annually. People with cirrhosis have an increased risk of a certain type of liver cancer (hepatocellular cancer).

Cirrhosis may lead to several serious complications:

Portal hypertension

Internal bleeding and ascites obstruct blood flow to the liver. Increased pressure in the portal system causes enlargement of the spleen and the development of dilated veins (varices) in the esophagus and stomach.

Bleeding may result from rupture of esophageal or gastric varices, a complication that occurs in about two-thirds of people with cirrhosis. This can be a life-threatening emergency that requires immediate attention.

Ascites is an accumulation of excess fluid within the abdominal cavity due to portal hypertension and low serum albumin (a protein), resulting from impaired liver function. Treatment often includes a salt-restricted diet and the use of diuretics to eliminate excess water and salt. Repeated removal of fluid (paracentesis) and intravenous (IV) infusion of albumin may be of benefit in some cases.

Spontaneous bacterial peritonitis

This condition occurs when ascites fluid becomes infected. Abdominal pain along with a low-grade fever may result. The condition is treated with antibiotics.

Hepatic encephalopathy

When the liver is damaged, it can no longer filter toxic elements from blood, resulting in a higher concentration of ammonia and other metabolites. Hepatic encephalopathy affects brain function, causing mental confusion, drowsiness and trembling, and may lead to coma.

Treatment

The main focus of medical care often is treating and preventing complications. Self-care measures and medication can help decrease further damage to the liver. If liver failure occurs, liver transplantation may be an option.

Self-care

Although the damage caused by cirrhosis is irreversible, you can do things to reduce further liver damage:

- *Stop using alcohol.* Some of the chemicals contained in alcohol are toxic to your liver.
- *Limit medications.* Your damaged liver is unable to detoxify and eliminate medications normally from your system. Discuss all medications that you take, including nonprescription ones, with your doctor. Don't combine pain relievers with alcohol, as this can be especially damaging to your liver.
- *Take measures to prevent yourself from getting sick.* When your liver is damaged, you're unable to fight off infections as well as healthy people. Avoid sick people and get vaccinated for hepatitis A and B, flu (influenza) and pneumococcal pneumonia.
- *Eat plenty of fresh fruits, vegetables and whole grains.* These foods are high in nutrients, including vitamins A, C and E. Cirrhosis tends to deplete these important vitamins. Your doctor may prescribe supplemental vitamins K, A and D, which may be depleted in your body as well.
- *Restrict salt.* Reducing salt can help reduce fluid buildup.
- *Monitor dietary protein.* If your cirrhosis is advanced, excessive protein may lead to the complication hepatic encephalopathy.

Medication

In an attempt to prevent esophageal and gastric varices from rupturing and bleeding, your doctor may recommend a medication to lower the pressure within the varices. Other options include a procedure to help prevent blood from flowing into them or a procedure to destroy them.

Diuretics help reduce accumulation of excess abdominal fluid. To reduce fluid retention, your doctor may ask you to avoid salt.

Sometimes, abdominal fluid may become infected, causing pain and fever. If this occurs, your doctor may insert a long, thin tube (catheter) into your abdomen to remove a fluid sample so that the infecting organism can be identified (cultured) and the proper antibiotic prescribed.

Cholestyramine (Questran) and rifampin (Rifadin, Rimactane) are often prescribed to reduce itching caused by metabolites in the blood.

The medication lactulose (Cholac, Duphalac) can help lower blood ammonia levels. Your doctor may also recommend an antibiotic to reduce the level of bacteria in your intestines that produce ammonia.

Liver transplantation

A liver transplant is generally considered when the disease has advanced to the point when the liver can no longer function. The success rate of liver transplantation continues to improve, and more than 90 percent of people who receive transplants are still alive 1 year later. The problem is, when cirrhosis is related to viral hepatitis, there's a chance the disease will recur in the new liver. For more information on transplantation, see page 912.

Liver cancer

Signs and symptoms

- Sometimes, none
- Loss of appetite and weight
- Abdominal pain
- General fatigue and weakness
- Enlarged liver
- Abdominal swelling
- Yellowing of the skin and eyes

Most liver cancers start elsewhere in the body and spread (metastasize) to the liver. These cancers are called secondary liver cancer. The liver is especially vulnerable to invasion by cancerous cells and, with the exception of lymph nodes, is the most common site of abdominal metastasis.

Cancer that originates in liver or bile duct cells is called primary liver cancer (hepatocellular carcinoma or cholangiocarcinoma). In the United States, primary liver cancers account for only 1 percent to 2 percent of all cancerous (malignant) tumors found during autopsy. Primary liver cancer is about twice as common in men as it is in women.

Factors that increase risk of primary liver cancer include chronic liver disease, such as cirrhosis, hepatitis B or C infection, hemochromatosis, long-term use of anabolic steroids and exposure to certain toxins, such as aflatoxin and vinyl chloride.

Diagnosis

A thorough physical examination and blood tests are generally the first steps in diagnosing liver cancer. Additional tests may include images of the liver by a computerized tomography (CT) scan or ultrasound examination. Either can detect masses within the liver. See Chapter 39, "Diagnostic Tests," for more information on these tests.

A liver biopsy, in which a sample of liver tissue is removed for laboratory analysis, can provide even more information. If a liver biopsy doesn't provide a definitive diagnosis, an abdominal operation may be necessary.

How serious is liver cancer?

Both primary and secondary liver cancer often are fatal, especially secondary liver cancer, which is a sign that the primary cancer has already spread (metastasized). Early detection poses the best chances for successful treatment.

Treatment

Surgery is the most effective treatment for primary liver cancer. If the cancer is small enough, your doctor may be able to remove the tumor and successfully treat the cancer. For a limited group of people who meet specific health criteria, a liver transplant may be an option.

Other treatments for liver cancer often aren't curative, but they may relieve signs and symptoms and extend survival. These include:

- *Embolization.* This procedure involves blocking the blood supply to the tumor by surgically tying the artery that feeds the cancer, or injecting materials that obstruct the artery.
- *Chemoembolization.* This procedure involves blocking the blood supply to the tumor and instilling

Liver Cysts and Noncancerous Tumors

Liver cysts are common and usually are detected in the course of examining the liver by computerized tomography (CT) or ultrasonography for another condition. Liver cysts don't become cancerous (malignant) and rarely cause signs and symptoms. Treatment is unnecessary except in the rare instances when they cause significant abdominal discomfort.

Some liver tumors are noncancerous (benign). The most common is hemangioma. Often, hemangiomas are discovered incidentally during study of the liver for another reason. Hepatic adenoma, another benign tumor, can occur in women who have taken oral contraceptives for a long time. When the birth control pill is discontinued, the tumors may become smaller. Hepatic adenomas may cause pain or rupture and require surgical removal.

Benign liver tumors often don't cause signs and symptoms or require treatment.

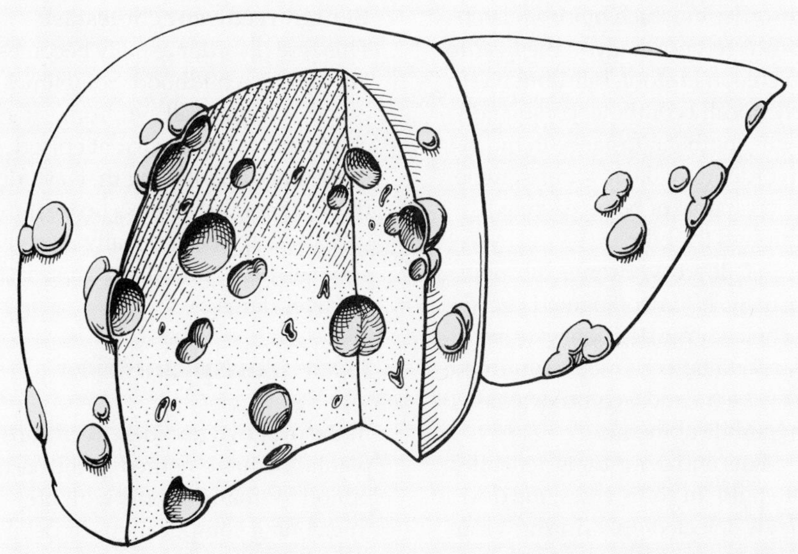

Cysts commonly occur in the liver. Most often they're harmless.

a chemotherapeutic drug in the sealed off artery.
- *Ethanol ablation.* This procedure involves injecting concentrated alcohol into the tumor to destroy cancer cells.
- *Cryosurgery.* This procedure involves destroying the tumor by freezing it.
- *Radiofrequency ablation.* This procedure involves targeting the tumor with energy from high-frequency radio waves.

Traditional chemotherapy and radiation may temporarily shrink malignant liver tumors, but these therapies generally don't improve survival.

Liver abscesses

Signs and symptoms

- Persistent fever
- Chills
- Nausea and vomiting
- Weakness
- Weight loss
- A tender liver
- Yellowing of the skin and eyes

Abscesses — fluid- or pus-filled cavities — sometimes form within the liver as a result of infection by a bacterium or parasite. Those of bacterial origin generally have a more rapid course with fever and chills. An abscess from a parasite tends to develop more slowly.

Diagnosis

Liver abscesses can generally be identified with a computerized tomography (CT) scan or ultrasound examination of your liver. From the image produced, a doctor often can determine the size, location and number of abscesses. Blood tests also may be helpful, particularly if your doctor suspects the abscess may be caused by a parasite.

Fluid from the abscess can often be obtained for examination by insertion of a needle into the abscess, using ultrasound or a CT scan for guidance. However, if your doctor suspects that the abscess is caused by a parasite such as amoeba, other testing is preferred to avoid spreading the infection.

How serious are liver abscesses?

A liver abscess, particularly one caused by bacteria, is potentially fatal and requires immediate treatment.

Treatment

If the abscess is the result of a bacterial infection, your doctor may advise drainage of the abscess with a tube (catheter) and intravenous (IV) antibiotics to kill the infection. Antibiotics may be required for several weeks.

Sometimes, surgical drainage of the abscess or even removal of the portion of the liver containing the abscess is required.

If the cause is a parasite, your doctor may advise treatment with medications aimed at eliminating the parasite.

Genetic liver disorders

Some inherited liver abnormalities cause increased concentrations of bilirubin in the blood (hyperbilirubinemia) and produce yellowing of the eyes and skin (jaundice).

Gilbert syndrome

Gilbert syndrome is an inherited disorder in which bilirubin isn't processed normally in the liver for excretion in stool. Bilirubin has to chemically combine (conjugate) with another substance in the liver in order to make it water-soluble and capable of being excreted through the bile.

In Gilbert syndrome, bilirubin is usually left unconjugated because of an enzyme deficiency or liver function defect. Gilbert syndrome may be the most common cause of hyperbilirubinemia.

Signs and symptoms generally are mild. In some cases, the disorder is detected only during a routine blood test. Gilbert syndrome doesn't lead to liver damage, and no treatment is necessary.

Crigler-Najjar syndrome

This rare disorder causes two types of hyperbilirubinemia: type 1 and type 2. Type 1, the most severe form, is also due to an absence of an enzyme needed to conjugate the bilirubin. Type 2 involves only a partial enzyme deficiency and is less severe.

Crigler-Najjar syndrome is caused by a different genetic mutation than Gilbert syndrome and is generally much more severe.

There's no treatment that will cure type 1 Crigler-Najjar syndrome. An infant born with the condition usually dies within the first year. Type 2 hyperbilirubinemia, however, can be treated successfully with medication.

Dubin-Johnson syndrome

Some genetic disorders cause elevated concentrations of predominately conjugated (chemically combined, water-soluble) bilirubin. One such inherited disorder is Dubin-Johnson syndrome, also known as chronic idiopathic jaundice. People with this disorder often will have either no signs and symptoms or vague gastrointestinal symptoms. In some cases, the liver is enlarged and pigmented. This disorder generally requires no treatment.

Benign recurrent cholestasis

This rare disorder usually becomes apparent in childhood. Sometimes called Summerskill syndrome, it's characterized by recurrent episodes of jaundice and itching that last for days or months. There's no treatment, but episodes usually resolve spontaneously and don't cause lasting liver damage.

Liver transplantation

In the past two decades, liver transplantation has emerged as the best option for many people with life-threatening complications or debilitating signs and symptoms of severe liver disease. The survival rate for people who receive a liver transplant is steadily improving. Based on today's national averages, almost 90 percent of people who receive a liver transplant are alive 1 year later, and about 75 percent are alive 5 years after the procedure.

Advances in the preservation of donor organs have improved survival rates, as have refinements in surgical techniques, antirejection medications and postoperative care. This success has led to a wider application of this procedure. For example, in the past, liver transplantation wasn't an option for people with cancer. Now, transplantation is sometimes considered for individuals with a certain type of liver cancer (hepatocellular carcinoma) and for individuals with some neuroendocrine cancers — tumors that originate in the complex body system where nervous and endocrine systems interact — that have spread to the liver.

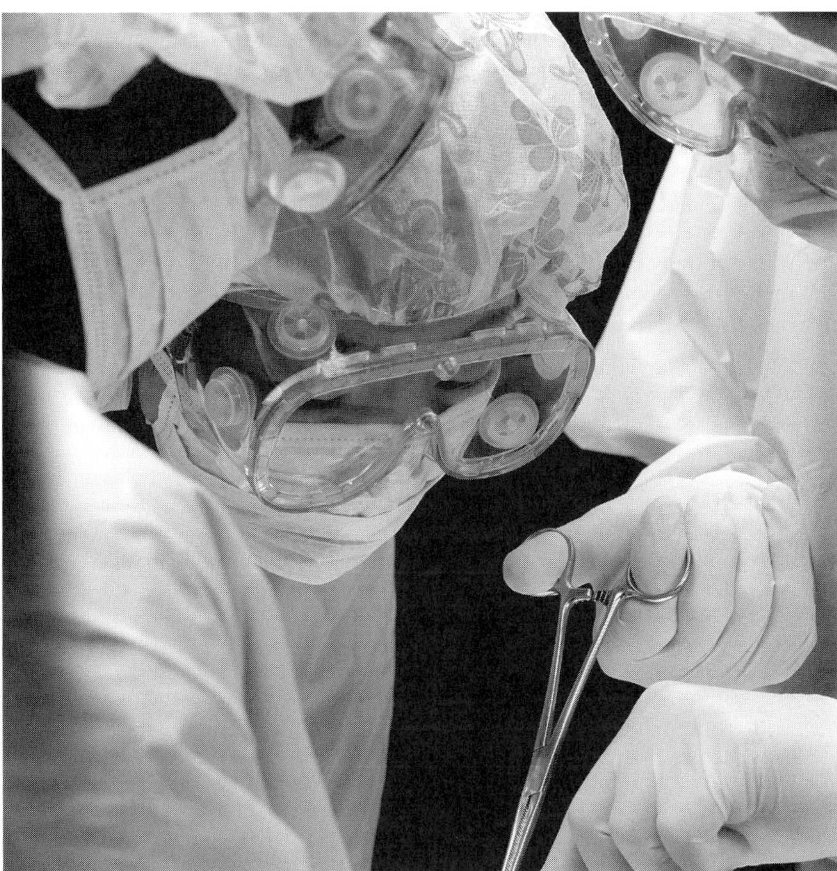

New methods of transplantation

The main factor that limits use of liver transplantation is a shortage of donor organs. The waiting time has increased from about a month to more than a year. In the meantime, many people become increasingly ill, and some die while waiting for a donor liver.

Thus, alternatives to traditional liver transplantation are being pursued. In one procedure, about 60 percent of a healthy liver is removed from a living donor, generally a relative. In the person with liver disease, the failing liver is removed and replaced with portions of healthy liver. Because liver tissue normally regenerates, within a few weeks to a few months the liver usually returns to normal size in both the donor and the recipient.

Living donor liver transplantation achieved initial success in children in the early 1990s. Today, approximately 50 percent of pediatric transplantations are done using living donors. Studies of adult-to-adult living donor liver transplantations have been positive, and this method is now becoming acceptable therapy. Adults require more liver mass than children do, but even so, the graft regenerates rapidly in the recipient, as does the remaining portion left in the donor.

The risks to recipients of living donor liver transplantation are similar to those of traditional transplantation, such as bleeding, poor function of the transplanted liver, infection and rejection of the new organ. Risk to the donor is generally minimal. Immediately after removal of a portion of their liver, donors may experience temporary jaundice, and it may take longer for blood to clot. Bile leakage also is a risk. But the liver usually returns to full size in 2 to 4 weeks. As with all major surgeries, there is a very small risk of fatality for both the recipient and donor.

Medication

Important advances in medications used to prevent transplant rejection also have improved outcomes. Cyclosporine (Neoral, Sandimmune) decreases the body's natural tendency to reject a donated organ by suppressing the effectiveness of the immune system. Specifically, cyclosporine prevents certain white blood cells (lymphocytes) from attacking the transplanted liver.

More recently, tacrolimus (Prograf) has been added to the expanding list of immunosuppressant medications. This drug enables doctors to more rapidly reduce doses of corticosteroids, which are also used to prevent rejection.

Newer antibiotic and antiviral drugs are playing important roles in preventing and treating infection of the transplanted liver. Ganciclovir (Cytovene), for example, can be used to prevent or treat cytomegalovirus infection.

Who's a candidate?

Adults under age 65 and children are the best candidates. Individuals selected for transplantation generally have liver disease that's progressive and incurable by other medical or surgical treatments and don't have other life-threatening illnesses.

The procedure

Liver transplantation is a complex procedure and may involve two operations if there is a living donor. The procedure can take 3 to 5 hours and is performed mainly in large medical centers where experienced personnel and extensive facilities can yield the best results.

Recovery

Rehabilitation may take up to 4 months. Lifelong therapy with immunosuppressant drugs to prevent organ rejection is necessary. Use of these drugs also requires lifelong monitoring for complications. ■

CHAPTER 30 PART V

Kidneys and Urinary Tract

The kidneys are part of the urinary tract, a complex system whose primary function is to remove excess fluid and waste material from blood. In addition, the kidneys function as endocrine glands — releasing hormones important to the production of red blood cells, regulation of blood pressure and formation of bone.

In addition to the kidneys, the urinary system includes two ureters, a bladder and a urethra. The kidneys, a pair of bean-shaped organs, are located against the back of the abdominal wall, one on each side of the spine at the level of the lowest ribs. Each kidney is generally about the size of your fist.

The ureters are muscular tubes that propel urine from each kidney to the bladder. The bladder is a muscular bag that stores urine. The urethra is the narrow tube through which urine leaves the bladder during urination.

The kidneys vary their activities from day to day in response to changes in the kinds and amounts of food and fluids you consume. For example, suppose that one day you drink large amounts of water and juice and on the next you drink almost none. Your kidneys adapt accordingly, allowing your tissues to be neither flooded nor depleted. They do this by carefully controlling the amount of fluid and salts excreted in your urine. Although other organs, such as the skin, lungs and intestines, also remove fluid, the kidneys are by far the most important organ for fluid excretion.

Blood enters each kidney from its renal artery, a major branch of the aorta, the body's main artery. Although the kidneys account for less than 1 percent of the body's weight, 20 percent of the blood pumped from the heart passes through them.

Within the kidney, blood passes through filtering systems called nephrons. These are the main functioning units of the kidney. Each kidney contains more than 1 million nephrons, each consisting of a tuft of small blood vessels (glomerulus) and attached small tubes (renal tubules).

As blood passes through the glomeruli, blood cells, proteins, large particles and some water remain in the bloodstream. Everything else, including a large percentage of the water, filters out and passes into the tubules.

Waste products, such as urea, creatinine and uric acid, along with excess salts and water, remain within the tubules. Cells that make up the walls of the tubules absorb and return other substances to the bloodstream in precisely the right amounts needed by the body. Thus, the composition of urine is determined by both the need to get rid of unwanted substances and the need to retain other substances.

Urine that emerges from the lower end of each tubule enters the renal pelvis, then the ureter and then the bladder, where it's stored. When the nerves of the bladder signal a feeling of fullness, urine is voided through the urethra, usually voluntarily. On average, about $1\frac{1}{2}$ quarts of urine are excreted every day. This is only a small fraction of the fluid initially filtered through the glomeruli into the tubules.

Blood that leaves the kidneys contains salts, protein, sugar, calcium and other substances vital to maintaining normal body function. This blood travels through the renal vein and back to the heart to recirculate throughout the body.

The Kidneys and Urinary Tract

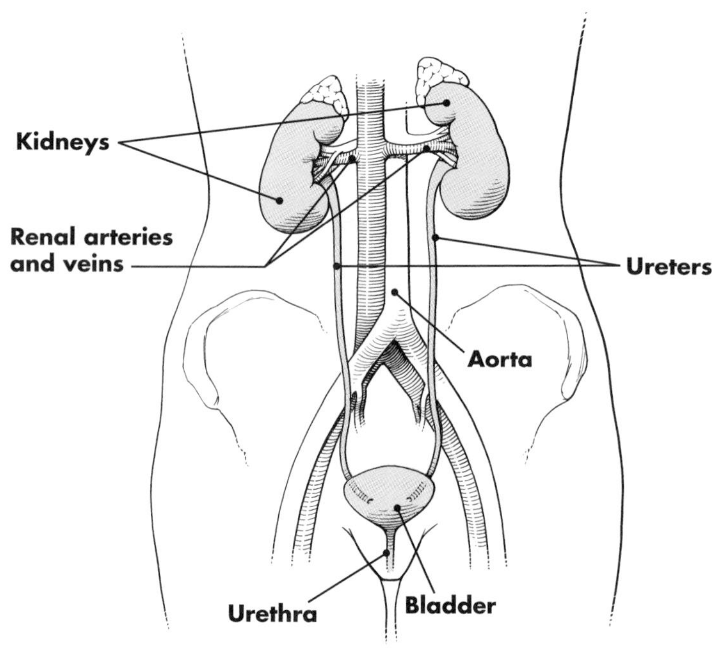

Cross Section of a Kidney

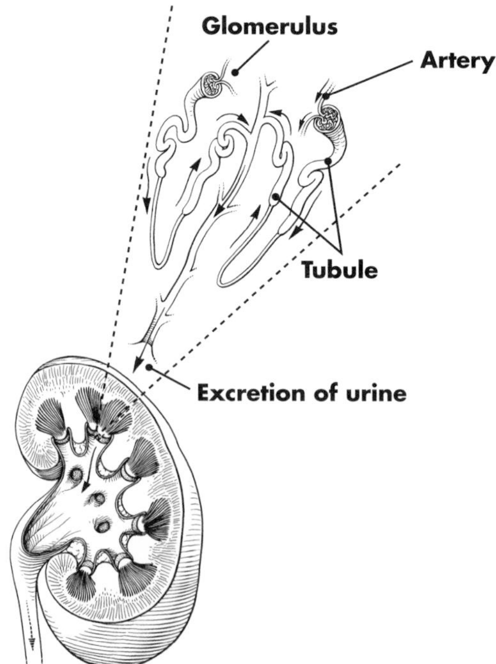

Most of the time this complex process is performed flawlessly. Sometimes, however, problems impair the kidneys' ability to filter. For example, if the tubules are defective, valuable substances that should be returned to the bloodstream may be excreted in urine. Or glomeruli may leak enough protein into the urine to cause a condition called nephrotic syndrome.

Diabetes, trauma, high blood pressure, toxins, kidney stones, tumors, some drugs and even infections in other parts of the body can cause kidney damage. Unfortunately, many kidney diseases cause no notable symptoms until substantial and even irreparable damage has occurred.

Congenital Kidney Disorders

Some infants are born with an abnormal kidney that doesn't function properly, or even with only one kidney. Fortunately, human beings can lead normal lives with just one functioning kidney. Many of the following anatomic abnormalities cause no symptoms and may go undetected, at least initially. They're typically diagnosed when tests are done for other purposes.

Medullary sponge kidney

Signs and symptoms

- Pain in the side
- Burning pain during urination
- Blood in the urine
- Kidney infection or stones

Medullary sponge kidney results from an abnormal widening of the ducts (papillary ducts) that drain into the urine-collecting portion of the kidney (renal pelvis). Often this condition produces no signs or symptoms in the people who have it. If it does, the signs or symptoms typically occur in adolescence or early adulthood. In many cases, the condition can be diagnosed with a kidney X-ray.

Treatment

Treatment involves relieving symptoms, if some are present. If you have the condition but are experiencing no symptoms, your doctor will likely recommend that you drink adequate quantities of water. This reduces the chance of kidney infection and the chance of kidney stone formation.

Vesicoureteral reflux

Signs and symptoms

- Recurrent urinary tract infections
- A scarred or small kidney on a kidney X-ray
- Excess protein in the urine
- High blood pressure

Vesicoureteral reflux, the abnormal flow of urine from the bladder back into the ureters, is the single most common urinary tract problem in children. It often results from anatomic abnormalities of the valve that normally prevents the backflow of urine from the bladder.

Diagnosis

A doctor may suspect vesicoureteral reflux if a child has recurrent urinary tract infections. Reflux can sometimes be detected with the help of a kidney X-ray or intravenous pyelography (see page 918). However, the definitive test for this problem is voiding cystourethrography (see page 918). It shows if fluid stays in the bladder or flows back up (refluxes) to the kidney. A related test called radionuclide cystography also may be used.

If your child has reflux, additional tests may be performed to determine if the kidneys have been scarred or sustained any other damage.

How serious is vesicoureteral reflux?

The reflux can be mild, moderate or severe. If your child has mild reflux, there's a good chance that the problem will disappear as he or she grows. Moderate or severe reflux is less likely to disappear with time.

Kidney damage is a real danger with this condition, particularly in infants and children younger than age 5. Reflux can be harmful to the kidneys because it creates abnormal pressure and, most important, it may introduce bacteria from the bladder into the kidneys. The kidneys can become infected and, ultimately, damaged.

Reflux is one of the most common causes of severe high blood pressure and end-stage kidney (renal) failure in children and young adults. It's responsible for about 6 percent of all end-stage kidney failure in children and young adults.

Treatment

Treatment for the condition depends on its severity.

Medication

Initially — particularly if the reflux is mild to moderate — low doses of antibiotics may be prescribed to keep the urine free of bacteria, thus preventing the refluxed urine from infecting the kidneys. Urine samples may be taken at regular intervals to ensure no bacteria are present.

Surgery

An operation to correct vesicoureteral reflux may be considered if:

- A child has severe reflux.
- A child has moderate reflux that over time shows no sign of resolving.
- Urinary infections occur despite continuous antibiotic treatment.
- Other urinary abnormalities make the resolution of reflux unlikely.

The operation involves reimplanting the ureter into the bladder. In 95 percent of cases, this cures the reflux. However, urinary tract infections continue to occur in a small number of cases despite an apparently successful operation. Children who undergo this operation often receive antibiotics for several months after the operation.

Other anatomic abnormalities

Additional kidney abnormalities that may be present at birth include:

Solitary kidney

Solitary kidney is a condition in which one kidney is missing at birth. The lone kidney performs the work of two. Usually this disorder doesn't pose any problems.

Horseshoe kidney

Horseshoe kidney is a condition in which the lower ends of the two kidneys are connected, forming a horseshoe appearance. Horseshoe kidney often goes undetected until diagnostic tests are performed for another condition or because of signs and symptoms.

Blood in urine, kidney stones, urinary obstruction and increased susceptibility to infection are complications of horseshoe kidney. These signs and symptoms can be treated if they occur. The condition itself rarely leads to kidney (renal) failure.

Kidney duplication

Kidney duplication is a condition in which the urine-collecting portion of the kidney (renal pelvis) is divided into separate compartments, each with its own ureter. This may occur in one or both kidneys.

People with this condition may not have any signs or symptoms, but the disorder carries with it an increased risk of infection and urinary obstruction.

Floating kidney

Floating kidney is an unusual condition in which one of your kidneys moves up or down in your side area between your ribs and hip, depending on body position. A floating kidney usually isn't a matter of concern and doesn't require further testing or treatment.

Kidney and Bladder X-Rays

X-rays can help your doctor detect abnormalities in your urinary tract. The following two types of X-rays are commonly used to detect a kidney or bladder condition:

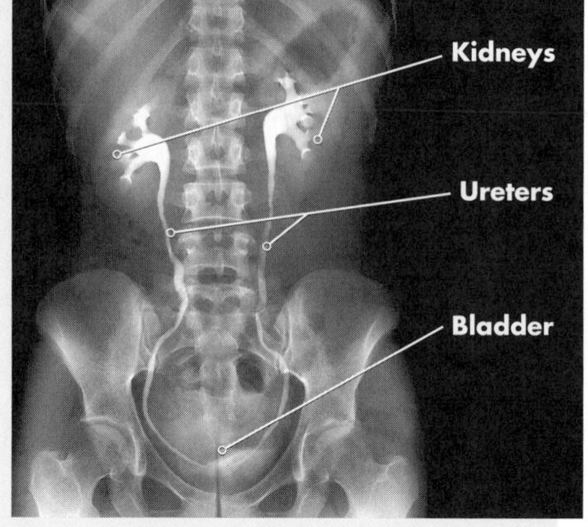

Intravenous pyelography

Intravenous pyelography (IVP, or excretory urography) is an X-ray examination that provides a detailed picture of the kidneys and lower urinary tract.

Individuals who undergo IVP are instructed not to eat or drink for 6 hours before the test. They may also be given a laxative to empty the colon, making it easier to see the kidneys on the X-ray.

The examination begins with the injection of a contrast agent into a vein in your arm. This substance makes the kidneys and urinary tract visible on X-rays. The bloodstream rapidly delivers the contrast agent to the kidneys, where it's filtered through the glomeruli and into the renal tubules. It then flows throughout the kidneys, down the ureters and finally into the bladder. Throughout this approximately hour-long procedure, a series of X-rays is taken of the various structures.

If your doctor suspects an abnormality of your urinary tract, IVP is often one of the first radiologic tests done. It's also useful for determining the presence of congenital abnormalities, tumors, scarring of the kidneys and stones in the urinary tract. An ultrasound or computerized tomography (CT) scan is often used to further define any abnormal IVP findings.

The success of IVP depends on the ability of each kidney to concentrate the contrast agent and move it throughout the urinary system. Thus, it's difficult to obtain a good IVP study when the kidneys don't filter properly.

Most of the time, people who undergo IVP experience no side effects, although some people report nausea, vomiting or pain in the arm where the injection was made. Allergic reactions to substances injected into the body occasionally occur, so before the procedure be sure to tell your doctor about any allergies you have.

Voiding cystourethrography

Voiding cystourethrography is a procedure in which X-rays are taken while the bladder is filled with X-ray contrast fluid and subsequently emptied during urination. In order to introduce the contrast fluid into the bladder, a small, flexible tube (catheter) is inserted through the urethra into the bladder. This test reveals whether any of the fluid flows back (refluxes) into the ureters or kidneys.

Voiding cystourethrography is most often performed to check the structure and function of the bladder and urethra. It can detect faulty bladder emptying or an anatomic abnormality. In males with noncancerous enlargement of the prostate gland (benign prostatic hyperplasia), it can identify narrowing in the urethra at the location where the tube is surrounded by the prostate gland. The procedure usually doesn't cause any side effects.

Congenital ureteropelvic junction obstruction

Congenital ureteropelvic junction obstruction is a disorder that involves an obstruction in the area where the ureter leaves the kidney. Typically, this occurs on one side.

Abdominal pain or infection may lead to the diagnosis. The obstruction is sometimes detected after the passage of bloody urine, often after a blow to the kidney area. Sometimes, this disorder is detected in a fetus during a prenatal ultrasound.

Pressure from obstructed drainage can lead to scarring of the kidney and cause loss of function on the affected side. Surgery may be required to eliminate the obstruction and prevent further kidney damage. Newer technologies that remove the obstruction internally may soon replace surgery.

Multicystic dysplasia

Multicystic dysplasia is a disorder caused by abnormal growth of tissue in the kidney. It's characterized by multiple fluid-filled sacs (cysts).

Sometimes, this disorder is detected in a fetus during a prenatal ultrasound. On an X-ray, the affected kidney often resembles a bunch of grapes. It commonly functions poorly, if at all.

Multicystic dysplasia may spontaneously regress with time. The other kidney typically functions satisfactorily, so this condition doesn't interfere with normal growth and development.

Inherited Kidney Disorders

Some kidney disorders run in families. If a doctor diagnoses an inherited kidney disease in a family member, he or she may also perform tests on other family members — even if they have no symptoms — to see if they also have the disease.

Polycystic kidney disease

Signs and symptoms

- Pain in the side
- Blood in the urine
- Excessive urination at night
- Kidney stones
- Anemia (in children)
- High blood pressure

In polycystic kidney disease, the kidneys contain clusters of round, hollow, fluid-filled sacs (cysts) that interfere with kidney function and enlarge the kidneys. The disease can occur in children and adults but is much more common in adults.

It usually doesn't cause problems until the second or third decade of life or later. It's estimated that 1 in 400 to 1 in 1,000 Americans have this disease.

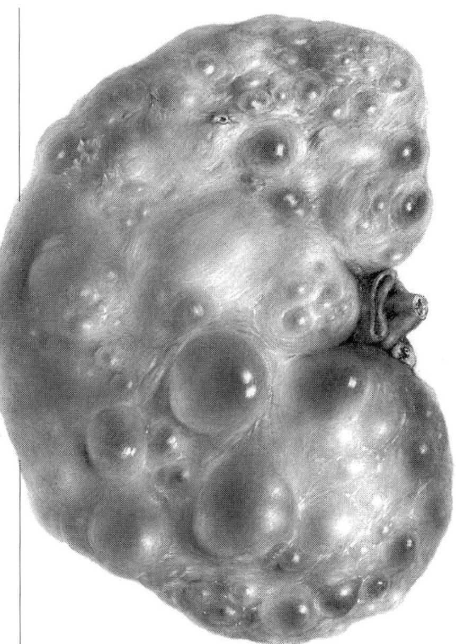

Development of many fluid-filled sacs (cysts) in kidney tissues causes polycystic kidneys, which may progress to kidney failure.

Types

The two types of polycystic kidney disease are caused by different genetic flaws.

Autosomal dominant

Autosomal dominant polycystic kidney disease accounts for approximately 95 percent of all adult polycystic kidney disease. Symptoms often develop between the ages of 30 and 50. It's termed autosomal dominant because a single dominant faulty gene inherited from either parent can cause the disease.

Autosomal recessive

Autosomal recessive polycystic kidney disease is less common. Abnormal recessive genes must be inherited from both parents in order to produce this disease. Symptoms often appear shortly after birth but can be delayed until later in childhood or adolescence.

Diagnosis

An ultrasound examination, computerized tomography (CT) or magnetic resonance imaging (MRI) is used to diagnose the disease (see Chapter 39, "Diagnostic Tests"). Your doctor may also recommend genetic testing to determine if you carry the gene associated with polycystic kidney disease.

How serious is polycystic kidney disease?

With the adult form of the disease, high blood pressure and progressive loss of kidney function often develop during adulthood. Most people with the severe form of this disease reach end-stage kidney (renal) disease by the time they're in their 40s or 50s, but some experience it earlier. Others may have only a mild to moderate loss of renal function throughout life. Once end-stage kidney disease is reached, either kidney dialysis or kidney transplantation is necessary to sustain life.

Many adults with this disease also have liver problems, including cysts that can become infected and cause fever and other symptoms. The childhood form of the disease is very serious and may result in death in infancy or childhood.

Treatment

No treatment is available to prevent the cysts from forming and enlarging, but measures can alleviate the symptoms and complications of polycystic kidney disease. If you have high blood pressure, your doctor will help you manage it in order to help preserve remaining kidney function. If you get a urinary tract infection, seek prompt treatment to prevent additional kidney damage.

Sometimes, a doctor punctures and drains the cysts because of pain, bleeding, infection or obstruction or because massive enlargement of the kidneys is affecting other abdominal organs. Occasionally, this procedure is done in an attempt to improve or stabilize kidney function.

When end-stage kidney disease ensues, kidney dialysis or transplantation is generally your best option for successful treatment.

The childhood form of the disease requires careful and consistent medical attention to monitor any complications. High blood pressure is common and usually requires medication.

Most children with polycystic kidney disease reach end-stage kidney disease during childhood. Thus, dialysis or transplantation is used much earlier than in the adult form. Associated liver disease is often severe, as well.

Cystinuria

Signs and symptoms

- Blood in the urine
- Pain
- Kidney stones

Cystinuria causes the kidneys' tubules to not reabsorb certain amino acids (protein elements) adequately. Excessive amounts of the amino acids lysine, arginine, ornithine and cystine are excreted in the urine. This inheritable disorder occurs in 1 of every 10,000 people and is characterized by stones in the kidneys, ureters and bladder.

Diagnosis

A chemical analysis of the urine can reveal the presence of excessive amounts of amino acids. If you pass a kidney stone, your doctor may have it tested to determine its composition. If the stone contains cystine, it's likely that you have cystinuria.

How serious is cystinuria?

Cystinuria is a long-lasting (chronic) disease. People with it are likely to form cystine stones, which may damage the kidneys by causing ureteral obstruction or infection. Some people produce many such stones and need surgical operations to remove them. Occasionally, cystinuria can cause kidney failure and lead to other organ damage.

Treatment

If you have cystinuria, drink plenty of water — up to a gallon every 24

Blood in Urine

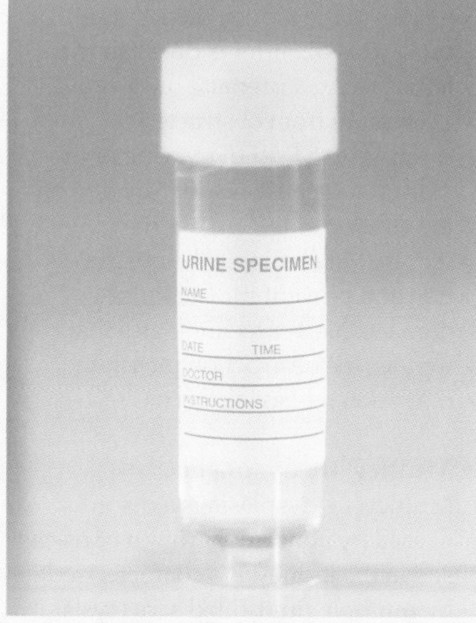

Blood in urine (hematuria) may be visible to the eye or apparent only when the urine is examined under a microscope. Hematuria is often detected when a urinalysis is performed for some other reason, such as a screening test at the time of a routine physical examination.

Hematuria may result from a wide variety of kidney or urinary tract problems, such as infection, stones, cysts or tumors. However, many people with hematuria have no evidence of any of these problems, despite careful evaluation. They have what's called benign hematuria, which isn't associated with kidney damage.

Benign hematuria has two forms: recurrent (sporadic) and familial (inherited). Benign recurrent hematuria typically is detected in childhood but may not become apparent until later in life.

Aside from the presence of blood in the urine, all other findings related to the urine, blood and kidneys are normal. Treatment is unnecessary, and in many cases the blood disappears with time.

Benign recurrent hematuria is fairly common among athletes, particularly long-distance runners. The exact cause of blood in the urine isn't clear, but the incidence of exercise-induced hematuria is directly related to the duration and intensity of physical activity. The hematuria usually goes away within 24 hours after exercise stops.

The familial form is acquired from a parent — a single gene inherited from either parent is capable of causing the disorder. If one parent has the condition, his or her child has a 50 percent chance of inheriting it. In such situations, several members of a family are usually affected.

In many cases, a kidney biopsy is necessary to confirm the diagnosis of benign familial hematuria and distinguish it from other conditions. Benign familial hematuria commonly is recognized in childhood. Typically, it persists throughout life but causes no kidney damage or other problems.

No treatment is necessary. In some children with isolated hematuria, a high concentration of calcium is found in the urine (hypercalciuria) and is believed to be the cause of the hematuria. These children may have an increased risk of kidney stones.

hours — with a third of it being drunk at night. This isn't always easy to do, but it'll help dilute the concentration of cystine in your urine.

Because cystine is more soluble in an alkaline solution, your doctor may also advise you to ingest a sodium bicarbonate or sodium citrate solution to keep the urine alkaline. If you don't respond to treatment with water and alkaline salts, your doctor may prescribe other medications that decrease cystine excretion. However, because of possible adverse effects, these are used only if other methods fail.

Renal tubular defects

In some cases of inherited kidney disease, the small tubes (tubules) contained in the kidneys' microscopic filtering units (nephrons) are the main parts affected. Renal tubules play a key role in your kidneys' absorption of nutrients and removal of waste.

Renal tubular acidosis

Renal tubular acidosis refers to several inherited disorders that cause the kidneys to not remove enough acid from the bloodstream or to eliminate a base such as bicarbonate in excessive amounts. This disrupts the normal acid-base balance (pH) of the body.

Under these circumstances, the kidneys often lose an abnormal amount of potassium, calcium and sodium in the urine. The blood becomes acidic, and chloride levels increase in the blood.

In children, such tubular defects are often manifested by impaired growth. In adults, kidney stones may result. Treatment generally consists of giving enough sodium bicarbonate or potassium citrate to keep the blood within its normal range of alkalinity.

Vitamin D-resistant hypophosphatemic rickets

Vitamin D-resistant hypophosphatemic rickets is an inherited disorder in which the kidneys are unable to retain phosphate normally. The result is impaired growth, rickets and shortened adult stature.

Bartter's and Gitelman syndromes

Bartter's and Gitelman syndromes are rare conditions. They're known as urinary wasting disorders.

Bartter's syndrome is generally diagnosed in childhood. It's characterized by an excessive amount of potassium in the urine. The condition is thought to result from a defect in the kidneys' ability to reabsorb potassium. Signs and symptoms include muscle cramping and weakness, constipation, increased urination and growth failure.

Gitelman syndrome is similar in many respects to Bartter's syndrome. However, it also causes loss of magnesium in urine. In addition, it's usually diagnosed in adulthood and is often milder than Bartter's syndrome.

Alport's syndrome

Alport's syndrome is an inherited disease due to a defect in the gene for collagen, a substance that helps to form the basement membranes of cells in many body organs, including the kidneys and the hearing apparatus of the inner ear. The syndrome causes kidney damage and possibly loss of hearing. It affects men more severely than women.

In males, the usual course of the syndrome is progressive loss of kidney function. Eventually, dialysis or kidney transplantation is necessary, usually between adolescence and age 40. Females may have minimal symptoms, if any, but can pass on the genetic defect to their children.

Congenital nephrotic syndrome

Congenital nephrotic syndrome is evident shortly after birth and is most commonly found in children of Finnish origin. Its manifestations are low birth weight, large amounts of protein in the urine (proteinuria) and massive fluid retention.

Infection, malnutrition or kidney failure can result in death during the first year of life. Early treatment, including kidney transplantation, has been successful therapy for some children.

Sickle cell disease

People with sickle cell disease have a blood abnormality and can experience a delay in growth, and in infants, failure to thrive. It occurs most frequently in blacks. Associated kidney problems include susceptibility to urinary tract infection, blood in urine and loss of the kidneys' ability to concentrate urine, which causes dehydration.

Progressive loss of kidney function can occur in older adults. The condition is generally treated with kidney dialysis or transplantation.

People who inherit only one gene for the disease carry the sickle cell trait but don't develop the disease, although they may notice blood in their urine. See page 1142 for more on sickle cell disease.

Blood Vessel Problems

The aorta is the largest blood vessel in the body, originating directly from the heart. Its branches carry blood to different parts of the body. Each kidney receives blood from one or more branches of the renal arteries. Twenty percent of the volume of blood pumped from the heart at any given time passes through the kidneys.

After the kidneys perform their filtering function, the blood returns by way of the renal veins to the vena cava inferior, the major vessel that carries blood from all parts of the body back to the heart.

Disorders of either the renal arteries or the renal veins not only can affect the way the kidneys function, but also can be a major cause of high blood pressure.

Acute arterial occlusion

Signs and symptoms

- Abrupt onset of side or abdominal pain
- Blood in the urine

Acute arterial occlusion of the kidney occurs when a renal artery is obstructed by a blood clot (thrombus). It usually occurs in people with known cardiovascular disease, primarily mitral or aortic valve disease or atrial fibrillation.

Diagnosis

A diagnostic test called arteriography can help pinpoint the location of the obstruction in the renal artery. In this test, a small, flexible tube (catheter) is inserted through the groin into the aorta and manipulated into the renal artery. Then a contrast agent is injected and X-rays are taken.

Occasionally, a diagnosis is made using a renal scan. This is a procedure that uses tiny amounts of radioactive materials called tracers (radiopharmaceuticals). These tracers emit radiation that is detected by a special camera. The camera produces detailed images of the kidneys and measures blood flow to the kidneys.

How serious is acute arterial occlusion?

The danger of acute arterial occlusion is that the affected kidney may cease to function. The other kidney can take over the process of eliminating wastes, but if arterial occlusion occurs in a person with only one kidney, or if it affects both kidneys, kidney failure may occur.

Treatment

Sometimes the blood clot dissolves spontaneously. If the artery has been blocked for only a few hours, your doctor may give you clot-dissolving medications or anticoagulant medications that prevent your blood from clotting.

In some cases, the blockage may be removed using a catheter that can be threaded through the arterial system into the affected artery. Occasionally, surgery is necessary to repair the artery.

Renal artery stenosis

Signs and symptoms

- High blood pressure
- A history of hard-to-control blood pressure

Renal artery stenosis is a narrowing or blockage of the renal artery before it enters the kidney. The narrowing or blockage impedes blood flow to the kidney and can cause chronic kidney failure or high blood pressure. Renal artery stenosis is responsible for 1 percent to 2 percent of all cases of high blood pressure.

In older adults, renal artery stenosis most often develops as a result of a buildup of fatty deposits (atherosclerotic plaques) in the renal artery. Renal artery blockage also can occur as a result of bead-like thickening of the artery wall (fibromuscular dysplasia), a condition most commonly seen in women 20 to 40 years of age.

Diagnosis

Your doctor may suspect renal artery stenosis if he or she hears a sound called a bruit when listening with a stethoscope over your kidneys. Tests may include a special kidney X-ray called intravenous pyelography (see page 918).

A kidney ultrasound examination, which measures blood flow, may be helpful in identifying narrowing of the arteries. Or an X-ray test called arteriography may be used to determine the exact location and extent of the blockage. In this test, a small, flexible tube (catheter) is inserted through the groin into the aorta and manipulated into the renal artery. Then a contrast agent is injected and X-rays are taken.

Treatment

Sometimes, surgery may be needed to remove or bypass the obstruction or narrowing of the renal artery. This surgery is done to prevent progressive renal failure and to improve control of high blood pressure. Another treatment consists of passing a special catheter into the renal artery and then inflating the

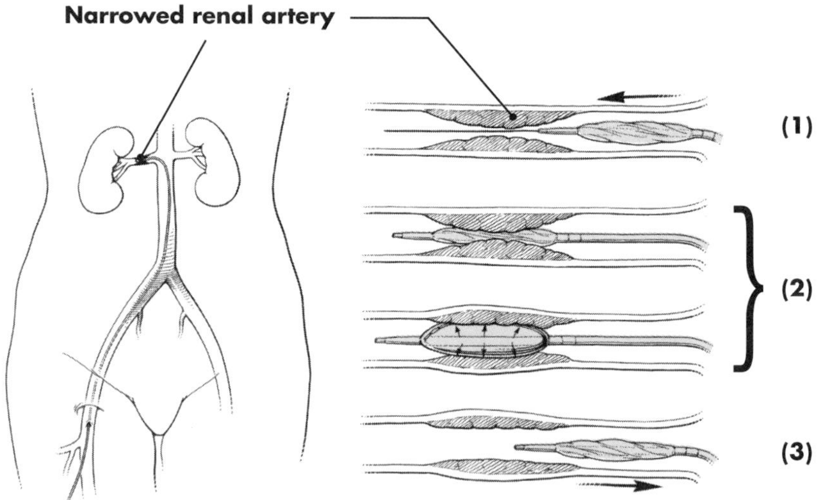

Percutaneous transluminal angioplasty (balloon angioplasty) may be used to open a narrowed renal artery. During the procedure, a catheter is threaded up an artery in the thigh and into the narrowed renal artery (1). The artery is dilated by inflating a balloon situated at the tip of the catheter (2), and then the catheter is removed (3).

balloon at the tip of the catheter to open the artery (percutaneous transluminal angioplasty, also called balloon angioplasty). This has been particularly successful in women with fibromuscular dysplasia. Some people need medication to control high blood pressure.

Renal vein thrombosis

Signs and symptoms

- Severe pain in the lower back and side
- Large quantities of protein in the urine

In this condition, a blood clot (thrombus) develops in the vein leaving the kidney. The blood clot may develop shortly after significant trauma to the abdomen or back.

Renal vein thrombosis may also be the result of a tumor blocking blood flow in the renal vein, or it may be associated with congenital nephrotic syndrome. In some cases, particularly in infants, severe dehydration may be responsible for the condition.

Diagnosis

Your doctor may use arteriography, a test in which a contrast agent is injected through the groin into the major vein that returns blood from the lower part of your body to your heart (vena cava inferior), and then into the renal vein. This agent may outline the blood clot in the renal vein, allowing it to show up on an X-ray.

Sometimes, a doctor can make a diagnosis with the use of an ultrasound technique called Doppler imaging, which can detect evidence of a blood clot in the vein.

Treatment

Most often, the treatment for renal vein thrombosis consists of anticoagulant medications that prevent blood from clotting. Generally, over time the renal vein reopens unless the obstruction is due to tumor growth into the vein from extension of a kidney cancer.

Kidney Failure

Kidney (renal) failure occurs when the kidneys are unable to adequately perform their task of filtering waste out of the blood. This may happen suddenly (acute renal failure), such as with a blood vessel obstruction, or as a result of the slow and silent destruction of nephrons, the kidneys' filtering units (chronic renal failure).

Because the kidneys have so many nephrons — approximately 1 million — symptoms of chronic kidney failure may go unrecognized until substantial damage has occurred. Kidney function must drop from normal by at least 80 percent before serious complications result.

Diabetes and high blood pressure, when untreated or uncontrolled, cause almost two-thirds of adult cases of kidney failure. Other causes of kidney failure include infection, injury, exposure to toxins and drugs, and various kidney diseases.

In addition, systemic lupus erythematosus, sickle cell anemia, cancer and obstruction of urine flow can cause kidney failure.

Acute kidney failure

Signs and symptoms

- Fluid retention
- Bleeding in the stomach or intestines
- Seizures
- Coma

Acute kidney (renal) failure is a condition in which the kidneys rapidly lose their ability to remove enough waste products from your blood. It often follows a severe drop in blood pressure, which can occur for a variety of reasons.

Although acute kidney failure is a potentially serious condition that may require hospitalization and intensive care, the kidneys generally are able to resume normal function over a period of several weeks to a few months following the onset. If untreated, it can be lethal.

Causes

Many theories are used to explain how kidney shutdown occurs. Some believe that cell debris obstructs the tubules, interfering with their ability to filter waste products. Others theorize that a combination of several of the following factors diminish blood flow through the glomeruli:

Blood vessel obstruction or constriction

Reduced blood flow to the kidneys (renal ischemia) is the most common direct cause of acute kidney failure. The condition results from an obstruction or constriction of a blood vessel.

Complicated surgery or severe trauma

Many cases of acute kidney failure are related to surgery or trauma with severe bleeding, dehydration or shock. In such cases, acute kidney failure often results from a severe drop in blood pressure that prevents blood from reaching the kidneys. In addition, when muscles are crushed in severe injuries, they release myoglobin, which lodges in the kidneys' tubules and blocks the flow of urine.

Drugs

Many drugs can precipitate acute kidney failure. Exposure to contrast dyes, such as those used in diagnostic tests for cardiovascular disease and stroke (arteriography), can lead to acute kidney failure, particularly in people with diabetic kidney disease.

Occasionally, a person with a life-threatening infection who receives an antibiotic such as streptomycin or gentamicin may go into acute kidney failure. The risk of kidney failure resulting from an antibiotic is much greater for older adults, people who use a diuretic or other drug toxic to the kidneys, and people with underlying kidney disease, potassium depletion or liver disease.

In addition, nonsteroidal anti-inflammatory drugs (NSAIDs),

even if used for a relatively short time, occasionally can cause acute kidney failure.

Heatstroke and excessive exercise
Heatstroke, a condition that occurs when your body can't cope with heat stress, combined with extreme exercise can lead to acute kidney failure. Severe dehydration often plays a key role in kidney failure that develops in this manner.

Toxins
Exposure to toxic substances, including excessive amounts of alcohol, heavy metals such as lead, or various solvents such as carbon tetrachloride, can induce acute kidney failure.

Multiple organ failure
In some people, acute kidney failure is a result of multiple organ failure in which the heart, lungs, liver, brain and kidneys totally or partially fail. This organ failure most often results from major trauma or an overwhelming infection that spreads throughout the body's circulatory system and prevents adequate blood flow to all organs (sepsis).

Obstruction of urine flow
Obstruction of the flow of urine out of a kidney may result from a stricture, tumor or, rarely, noncancerous enlargement of the prostate (benign prostatic hyperplasia).

Release of plaques
Fatty deposits (atherosclerotic plaques) can accumulate in arteries and harden in a process called atherosclerosis. Material in a plaque can break away from the vessel wall and lodge in a renal artery, reducing blood flow to the kidney.

Hemolytic uremic syndrome
Hemolytic uremic syndrome is a complex condition caused by certain strains of *Escherichia coli (E. coli)* bacteria. It's the leading cause of acute kidney failure in infants and young children. This condition occurs less often in adolescents and rarely strikes adults.

Kidney disease
Acute kidney failure may result from diseases characterized by inflammation of the spaces between the glomeruli and the tubules (interstitial nephritis) and inflammation of the glomeruli (glomerulonephritis).

Diagnosis

If your doctor suspects kidney failure, he or she will likely request blood and urine tests to check for abnormal levels of waste products normally removed from your blood. Excess protein in the urine (proteinuria) is a common sign of damaged nephrons in the kidneys.

You may also have an X-ray to check for fluid in your lungs (pulmonary edema), as well as tests to rule out other potential causes of your signs and symptoms, such as a urinary tract infection.

An abdominal ultrasound examination may be necessary to evaluate kidney failure or to rule out an obstruction. In some cases, computerized tomography (CT) or magnetic resonance imaging (MRI) also may be used (see Chapter 39, "Diagnostic Tests").

How serious is acute kidney failure?

Acute kidney failure can be life-threatening and requires intensive treatment. Unlike chronic kidney failure, however, the acute form of the disease is often reversible and many people recover in 1 to 2 months. Some take as long as a year to regain normal kidney function. In some people, acute kidney failure may progress to chronic kidney failure.

Mortality rates are highest for people whose acute renal failure followed an operation or a traumatic accident, or among people with severe chronic medical problems. In addition, individuals with acute kidney failure who have recently had a stroke typically don't recover as well. Other factors that can adversely affect the outcome of acute kidney failure are old age, infection and gastrointestinal bleeding.

Treatment

The first goal of treatment for acute kidney failure is to address the illness or injury that originally damaged the kidneys. When that's under control, the focus is directed toward preventing excess fluids and waste products from accumulating in your blood while your kidneys heal.

One way to accomplish this is by limiting the amount of fluids you consume and by following a low-potassium, high-carbohydrate diet. Too much potassium can be dangerous to your heart, and a high-carbohydrate diet can provide necessary calories while limiting fat and protein.

At one time, doctors recommended a low-protein diet because protein produces a waste called urea. Now most doctors believe that high-quality proteins, which don't produce as much waste as other proteins, are important to proper nourishment. Examples of high-quality proteins include meat, poultry, fish and eggs.

If your nutritional status is poor, you may be given essential amino acids and glucose intravenously. Your salt intake may be restricted because salt tends to make you want to drink more.

Your overall health will be monitored for evidence of complications such as infection, cardiac or neurologic problems, high blood pressure or gastrointestinal bleeding. Laboratory tests can indicate the development of uremic poisoning or other chemical imbalances. Your doctor may prescribe medications, such as calcium, glucose or sodium polystyrene sulfonate (Kionex, Kayexalate), to prevent excessive levels of potassium from accumulating in your blood. You might need dialysis to help remove toxins and excess fluids from your body while your kidneys are healing.

Chronic kidney failure

Signs and symptoms

- An abnormal urinalysis
- High blood pressure
- Loss of weight
- Nausea and vomiting
- A general sense of discomfort and unease (malaise)
- Headache
- Decreased urine output
- Fatigue
- Difficulty concentrating, confusion
- Muscle twitches and cramps
- Gastrointestinal bleeding
- A yellowish-brown cast to the skin
- Itching

Chronic kidney (renal) failure is due to a slow, progressive loss of kidney function resulting in the buildup of wastes and fluid in the blood, which a properly functioning kidney would excrete into the urine. It's usually a result of chronic conditions such as diabetes and high blood pressure.

Unlike acute kidney failure, chronic kidney failure generally develops over a number of years as the kidneys' filtering units (nephrons) are progressively destroyed. A person with chronic kidney failure is said to have *uremia,* a term used to describe the toxic condition the body falls into when the blood is contaminated by excessive waste products.

Often this disease causes no signs or symptoms in its early stages. In many cases, no symptoms are apparent until kidney function has decreased to less than 25 percent of what's considered normal.

Causes

The following conditions can lead to chronic kidney failure:

Diabetes

Type 1 diabetes — formerly called juvenile or insulin-dependent diabetes — is a leading cause of chronic kidney failure. In the United States, it accounts for about 35 percent of new cases each year.

Approximately 5 percent to 10 percent of people who have had type 2 diabetes — formerly called adult-onset or noninsulin-dependent diabetes — for at least 20 years develop kidney disease. Because of the large number of people with type 2 diabetes, this disease accounts for a large number of cases of chronic kidney failure.

High blood pressure

Uncontrolled high blood pressure is another leading cause of chronic kidney failure. Added force exerted on the tiny blood vessels (glomeruli) within your kidneys' nephrons can cause damage and scarring. When this happens, the nephrons lose their ability to filter waste from your blood.

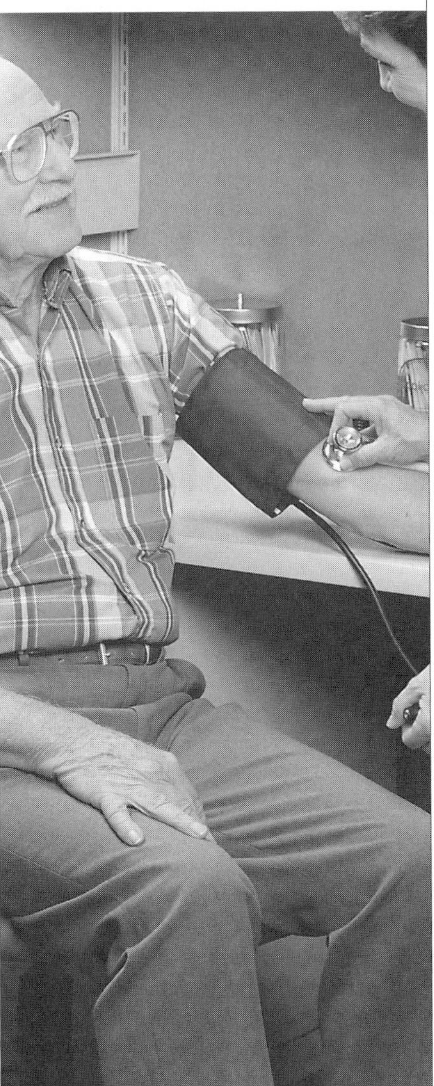

Analgesic nephropathy

Long-term use of aspirin or other nonsteroidal anti-inflammatory drugs (NSAIDs) can cause injury to the kidneys, leading to kidney failure. Taking large amounts of acetaminophen (Tylenol, others) also may harm the kidneys, especially in children.

Kidney disease

Several kidney diseases can lead to chronic kidney failure. These include an inherited condition in which the kidneys contain numerous clusters of cysts (polycystic kidney disease), a kidney infection (pyelonephritis) and an inflammation of the glomeruli (glomerulonephritis).

Renal artery stenosis

Blockage of the renal artery before it enters your kidney can lead to kidney failure. In older adults, such a blockage often results when hardened fatty deposits (atherosclerotic plaques) accumulate in the arteries.

Renal artery stenosis can also affect young women who have fibromuscular dysplasia. This is a condition that causes the walls of the arteries to become thicker and the arteries narrower. Atherosclerosis and fibromuscular dysplasia are almost always associated with high blood pressure.

Toxins

Long-term exposure to fuels and solvents, such as carbon tetrachloride, and lead (lead poisoning) can cause chronic renal failure.

Diagnosis

If you have diabetes, your doctor may schedule an annual test to measure small amounts of protein in your urine (microalbuminuria). This can screen for early signs of kidney damage related to diabetes (diabetic nephropathy). If you have another chronic condition that increases risk of kidney failure, such as high blood pressure, your doctor may want to monitor your kidney function on a regular basis.

Blood tests and urine analyses are the most common tests used to measure kidney function. Blood tests can detect elevated amounts of waste products such as creatinine in blood. Excess protein found in a urine sample is generally a sign of damaged nephrons.

Urine studies may also be done over a 24-hour period to measure protein leakage into the urine over the course of a day and to compare the urine creatinine level over 24 hours with the creatinine level in the blood. This creatinine comparison allows your doctor to measure how much blood the kidneys are filtering per minute.

If blood and urine tests indicate inadequate functioning of the kidneys, your doctor may request an ultrasound examination of your kidneys. Ultrasound images can indicate the shape and structure of the kidneys and reveal obstructions contributing to the problem.

Your doctor may also have you undergo other imaging tests, such as computerized tomography (CT) or magnetic resonance imaging (MRI). In some cases, your doctor may recommend that a small sample of kidney tissue be taken for study in a laboratory (biopsied).

How serious is chronic kidney failure?
Chronic kidney failure affects almost all of the body systems. Fluid retention from the disease can cause congestive heart failure and swelling of body tissues (edema).

Healthy kidneys produce a hormone called erythropoietin that stimulates your bone marrow to produce new red blood cells. Red blood cells carry oxygen to all of the tissues and organs in your body. When the kidneys are damaged, they may not be able to make enough erythropoietin, causing a decreased production of red blood cells. This results in anemia.

Other problems that may occur include stomach ulcers, miscarriage, changes in skin color and weakening of the bones, which makes them susceptible to fracture. Even the central nervous system can be affected so that individuals

Kidney Dialysis

Dialysis is an artificial means of removing waste products and extra fluid from blood. For many people with irreversible kidney failure, kidney dialysis provides the opportunity to live long after their kidneys have ceased to function. In the United States, more than 230,000 people are on dialysis.

The different forms of dialysis are as follows:

Hemodialysis
Hemodialysis is the most common form. It uses a machine (kidney dialyzer) to remove extra fluid, chemicals and waste from your blood.

Before you can undergo hemodialysis, a surgeon must create an access point in your blood vessels for blood to leave and re-enter your body during dialysis. Usually, the access is in the forearm. The procedure increases blood flow by enlarging a blood vessel or creating an artificial one.

When you're connected to the dialysis machine, your blood is pumped from the access point into the machine, where it flows across membranes that let waste compounds filter through. A solution in the machine helps remove excess fluid and regulates substances left in the blood. The blood then flows back into you. Less than 1 cup of blood is outside your body at a time.

As a rule, most people on dialysis require 6 to 12 hours of dialysis a week. These are usually divided into three sessions.

Peritoneal dialysis
When you undergo peritoneal dialysis, instead of using a dialyzer, you use the vast network of capillaries located in your abdomen (peritoneal cavity) to filter your blood.

First, an access is created to this network of capillaries, either in your arm or abdomen. Then a slender, flexible tube (catheter) is inserted into your abdominal cavity. Dialysis solution is introduced into the abdominal cavity through this catheter. Small blood vessels in the inside lining of your abdomen filter waste products and water from your blood into the dialysis solution. After 4 to 6 hours, the solution is drained out of your abdomen, taking with it excess waste and fluid.

Each of these cycles is called an exchange. You need several exchanges each day. Exchanges can be done as you go through your daily routine, or at night if you have a home peritoneal dialysis machine. The machine fills and empties fluid automatically while you sleep.

Continuous ambulatory peritoneal dialysis
You can perform continuous ambulatory peritoneal dialysis (CAPD) at home by using a permanently implanted catheter in your abdomen to exchange the dialysis solution four times a day, 7 days a week. In this way, the solution is in your abdomen continuously. In between exchange sessions, you're not attached to anything, so you can move about freely while the dialysis solution is in the peritoneal cavity.

Continuous cyclical peritoneal dialysis
Continuous cyclical peritoneal dialysis (CCPD), also called nocturnal cyclical periotoneal dialysis (NCPD), uses a machine that automatically infuses dialysis solution into your peritoneal cavity — through an implanted catheter — and drains several times over the course of the night while you sleep. This allows your days to be free, but you need to be attached to the machine at night.

with chronic kidney failure find it difficult to concentrate or to remember and have problems with the nerves and muscles in their arms and legs.

Chronic kidney failure eventually can progress to end-stage kidney disease. When this occurs, the kidneys aren't capable of sustaining life and either dialysis or kidney transplantation is the only option to preserve life.

Complications in children

In children, one of the most serious consequences of chronic kidney failure is failure to grow properly. In addition to regulating fluids and ridding the body of waste, the kidneys regulate the interaction of calcium and vitamin D, both of which are essential for bone growth.

Complications during pregnancy

Women with chronic kidney failure who become pregnant face a number of potential complications because the kidneys must work especially hard to deal with the demands of pregnancy. This can lead to worsening high blood pressure and an increase in waste products circulating in the blood.

Chronic high blood pressure can decrease the amount of blood the baby receives through the placenta, which can seriously affect fetal development. And waste products in the mother's bloodstream also may harm the baby's health.

Pregnant women with chronic kidney failure are also at high risk of preeclampsia, a serious complication of late pregnancy. Preeclampsia causes a dangerous rise in blood pressure. If not treated, it can lead to hemorrhages in the brain, liver or kidneys and may be fatal to both mother and baby.

Treatment

Although chronic kidney failure isn't curable, you and your doctor can take steps to control the symptoms, minimize the complications and slow its progression.

Address underlying causes

The first priority in treating chronic kidney failure is, whenever possible,

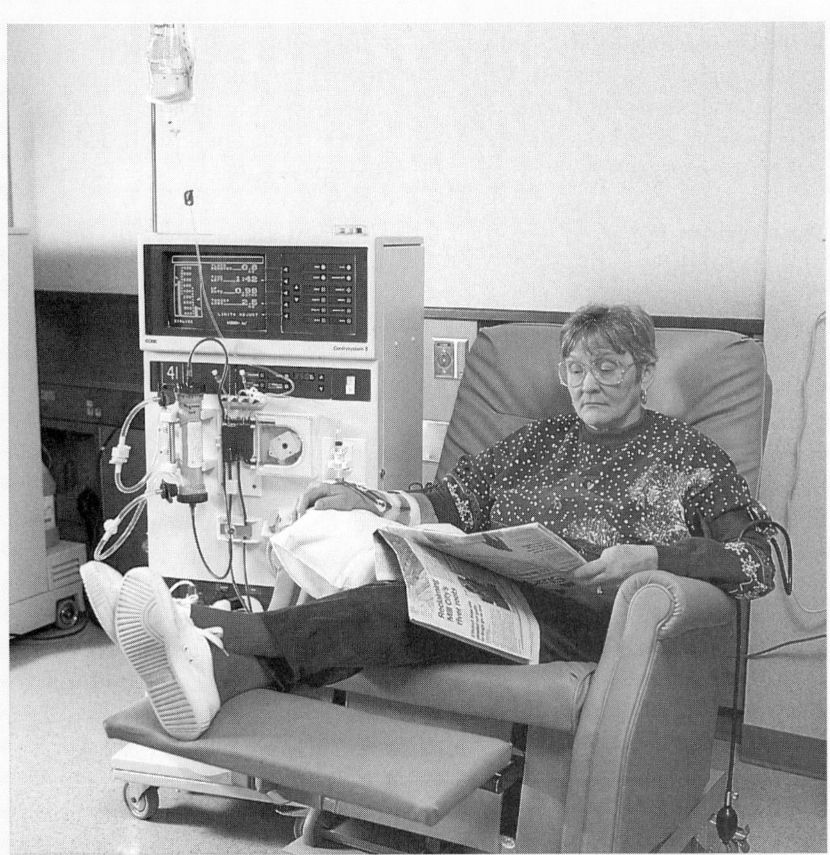

A dialysis machine (kidney dialyzer) artificially cleanses waste products from the blood of people whose kidneys are no longer able to do so.

Your doctor can help you decide which type of dialysis is best for you. Mostly it depends on your particular needs and what's available in your community.

Dialysis can be used as a temporary measure during acute kidney (renal) failure, preventing the buildup of waste in blood while the kidneys heal. In acute situations, dialysis may be performed in a hospital dialysis unit or in an intensive care unit. Dialysis may also be a temporary measure for young and otherwise healthy individuals awaiting a kidney transplant.

Dialysis may be a permanent form of treatment for individuals with chronic kidney failure in whom transplantation isn't an option because of age or other medical problems. When does a person with chronic kidney failure need dialysis? Every one is different. As a rule, most doctors try to manage chronic kidney failure for as long as possible with conservative measures, such as dietary modifications and medication.

Inevitably, though, there comes a time when the potential benefits of dialysis outweigh the risks. Complications associated with various forms of dialysis include malfunction of the dialysis machine, infection of the access point and nutritional deficiencies.

to control the condition causing the problem. If you have diabetes or high blood pressure, carefully follow your doctor's advice about diet, exercise and medications. If you have congestive heart failure, urinary tract infections, kidney stones, urinary tract problems or glomerulonephritis, these also need to be appropriately treated.

Nutrition

A proper diet is extremely important so that you receive sufficient calories to avoid malnutrition. Limiting the amount of protein you eat may help slow the progression of chronic kidney failure by reducing the amount of waste handled by the kidneys. A low-protein diet is especially helpful in chronic renal failure due to diabetes.

Restricting salt intake can help control high blood pressure. To avoid fluid buildup, you may also need to restrict the amount of liquids you drink. As the disease progresses, you may need to restrict your intake of phosphate and potassium to prevent excessive levels of these substances in your blood.

Medication

Blood pressure medications known as angiotensin-converting enzyme (ACE) inhibitors can help slow the rate of kidney decline. Anemia may require supplements of the hormone erythropoietin to induce production of more red blood cells. In addition, a form of vitamin D (calcitriol) may be administered to prevent bone disease, which can accompany kidney failure.

Phosphate-binding medication also may be prescribed to lower the amount of phosphate in the blood. Phosphate can reduce calcium in your bones, making them weak and vulnerable to fracture.

End-stage kidney disease

Signs and symptoms

- Kidney function permanently deteriorates to a level unable to sustain life
- Uremia and many resulting complications, which may include high blood pressure, congestive heart failure, anemia, bone disease, gastrointestinal problems, urinary tract infection and dementia

When kidney function deteriorates to only 5 percent to 10 percent of normal capacity, the condition is called end-stage kidney (renal) disease. This means that the kidneys are incapable of sustaining life and that their function must be replaced by kidney dialysis or a kidney transplant. More than 230,000 people in the United States are on kidney dialysis and more than 100,000 people are living now because they had kidney transplant surgery.

Diabetes is the most common cause of end-stage kidney disease in the United States. Other causes include high blood pressure, various kidney diseases and a urinary tract problem called vesicoureteral reflux (see page 917).

How serious is end-stage kidney disease?

End-stage kidney disease is fatal unless dialysis is initiated or kidney transplantation is performed. But both of these treatments also have risks that can be life-threatening.

Treatment

Once a person has progressed to end-stage kidney disease, conservative measures used to manage chronic kidney failure — treating the underlying cause, dietary restrictions and medications — no longer suffice. If kidney transplantation isn't in the best interest of the individual because of poor general health, dialysis is the only option.

Stones, Cysts and Tumors

Kidney stones can develop in overly concentrated urine. Bladder stones, which occur mostly in men, are usually the result of urinary tract blockage. Kidney cysts — hollow, fluid-filled, benign lesions — are common and typically produce no symptoms. More than half of Americans over age 50 have at least one kidney cyst. Malignant tumors also can develop in or invade the kidneys, ureters or bladder, but they're much less common.

Kidney stones

Signs and symptoms

- Pain that usually begins in the side and moves downward to the groin, vulva or testicles as the stone moves down the ureter
- A persistent urge to urinate
- Blood in the urine

Few who have passed a kidney stone ever forget the experience. Most people who have gone through it agree that it was one of the most painful episodes in their life. Occasionally, though, a kidney stone passes with minimal or no symptoms.

Kidney stones are relatively common. Evidence indicates that these stones have plagued humans for thousands of years — scientists have detected the presence of kidney stones in mummies more than 7,000 years old. Today, more than 1 million cases are reported each year in the United States. On average, your chance of passing at least one kidney stone in your lifetime is about 10 percent.

Certain types of stones tend to run in families. In addition, some kidney stones are associated with other medical conditions, such as overactive parathyroid glands, renal tubule defects, cystic kidney disease, chronic urinary tract infections and rare metabolic disorders.

Gout, inflammatory bowel disease, blockage of the urinary tract and too much vitamin D also can increase your risk of developing kidney stones, as can certain AIDS medications, diuretics and calcium-based antacids. However, the exact cause of kidney stone formation often remains unknown.

Kidney Transplantation

In the past 15 years, more than 100,000 kidney transplants have been performed in the United States. Kidney transplantation provides the best alternative for most individuals with end-stage kidney (renal) failure. With the increased use of living donor organs for this procedure, many people today can receive a transplant before they need kidney dialysis.

Who's eligible?

Most people with end-stage renal disease are candidates for kidney transplantation. But those with a recent history of cancer or another severe medical condition may not be considered suitable for a transplant. Today, kidney transplantation — especially with a kidney from a living donor — is a relatively safe procedure that can be performed even among people with significant medical problems, such as cardiovascular disease or diabetes.

Living vs. cadaver donor

The surgical technique used to perform a kidney transplant has been well established for years. With the development of new immunosuppressant medications designed to prevent organ rejection, only a relatively small number of kidney transplant patients have significant problems with rejection.

During an evaluation, the person receiving the transplant is generally presented with two options — receiving a kidney transplant from a living donor or joining the cadaver waiting list and waiting until a cadaver kidney becomes available. The best option, when available, is a living donor because a living donor presents the possibility for an immediate transplant, reducing or, in many cases, completely eliminating the need for dialysis.

Compatibility and matching between the donor's and the recipient's tissue types has become less important in recent years. This is due to significant improvements in antirejection medications. Currently, it's common to perform kidney transplants between husband and wife, where one spouse is the donor and the other is the recipient. Because no genetic relationship exists between the two, the tissue types are usually completely different (mismatched). This hasn't been associated with worse outcomes. Success rates are comparable to those of people who receive a kidney transplant from a sibling.

Finding a donor

The primary qualification to be a kidney donor is to be healthy, with no relevant medical problems that may put you at risk of complications during or after the surgery. Generally, the blood type of the donor and of the recipient has to be compatible to prevent hyperacute rejection at the time of the transplant. However, some medical centers, including Mayo Clinic, are performing kidney transplants between friends and relatives of incompatible blood types. This requires special techniques, which include removal of blood antibodies by a process called plasmapheresis. This is a good option for individuals whose only potential donor happens to have an incompatible blood type.

When a living donor isn't available, the person in need of a transplant gets placed on a transplant waiting list and is called when an organ becomes available. The waiting time for a person on a cadaver kidney waiting list is on average 3 to 5 years. Once a kidney is located, it's usually transplanted within 48 hours of removal from the donor.

Following transplantation

Individuals undergoing kidney transplantation usually stay in the hospital for 4 to 6 days following the surgery. Kidney rejection used to be a significant hurdle during the days following the surgery, but with new immunosuppressant drugs this has become less of a problem. Kidney transplant success rates at 1 year are in the neighborhood of 95 percent for living donor transplants and 90 percent for cadaver transplants.

The medications administered following the transplant can have some side effects. Your doctor will look for and address the side effects if they appear. A combination of immunosuppressant medications must be taken for life. In addition, anti-lymphocytic preparations are sometimes used during the first few days following the transplant. During the first few weeks or months following transplantation, most people receive antibiotics and antiviral and antifungal drugs. These medications help prevent some of the most common infections that tend to occur in transplant recipients.

Recent advances

The development of the laparoscopic donor nephrectomy technique has resulted in a significant increase in the number of kidney transplantations performed in recent years. This technique allows for removal of the living donor kidney through a very small incision and a quick recovery time for the person donating the kidney.

Some people develop what's known as high antibody titers following multiple blood transfusions, a previous transplant or childbirth. This makes a kidney transplant almost impossible because these circulating antibodies would destroy the new kidney within minutes following the transplant. Today, these individuals can receive a transplant with a method called positive cross-match transplant. It involves cleaning the antibodies from the recipient's blood (plasmapheresis) before the transplant. Positive cross-match transplants make it possible for some people who otherwise would have to remain indefinitely on dialysis to receive a kidney transplant.

A kidney stone is the result of a crystal formation that occurs when urine becomes too concentrated. Calcium salts, uric acid, cystine and other substances in the urine can crystallize to form a hard, mineral deposit, often the size of a pebble.

The pain usually occurs when the stone dislodges and leaves the kidney to work its way down the ureter. This can cause an intense, colicky pain that fluctuates in intensity over a period of 5 to 15 minutes. The pain starts in your back or your side just below your lower ribs. As the stone moves toward your bladder, the pain may radiate down to your groin. If the stone stops moving, the pain may stop too. Many stones in the kidney produce no symptoms and are discovered during an X-ray for an unrelated problem.

Types

Several different types of stones may develop in the kidneys:

Calcium stones

Calcium stones, which account for 75 percent to 85 percent of all kidney stones, are more common in men than in women. Once you've had one calcium stone, unless you're treated for the condition, you're likely to have another.

A number of factors can cause high calcium concentrations in urine, including:

- Excess intake of vitamin D, which may cause your body to absorb too much calcium
- Drugs such as thyroid hormones
- Certain diuretics
- Certain cancers
- Other kidney conditions
- Overactive parathyroid glands, which regulate calcium in the body

In the past, people who formed calcium stones were told to avoid high-calcium foods, such as dairy products, but more recent studies have shown that high-calcium foods actually help to prevent this type of kidney stone. Calcium pills, on the other hand, may increase your risk of calcium stones.

Calcium stones usually form when calcium combines with chemicals such as oxalate, phosphate or carbonate. The most common type is that which combines calcium and oxalate, a substance found in many vegetables, fruits and grains. In addition, some people with inflammatory bowel disease have an increased tendency to form oxalate stones.

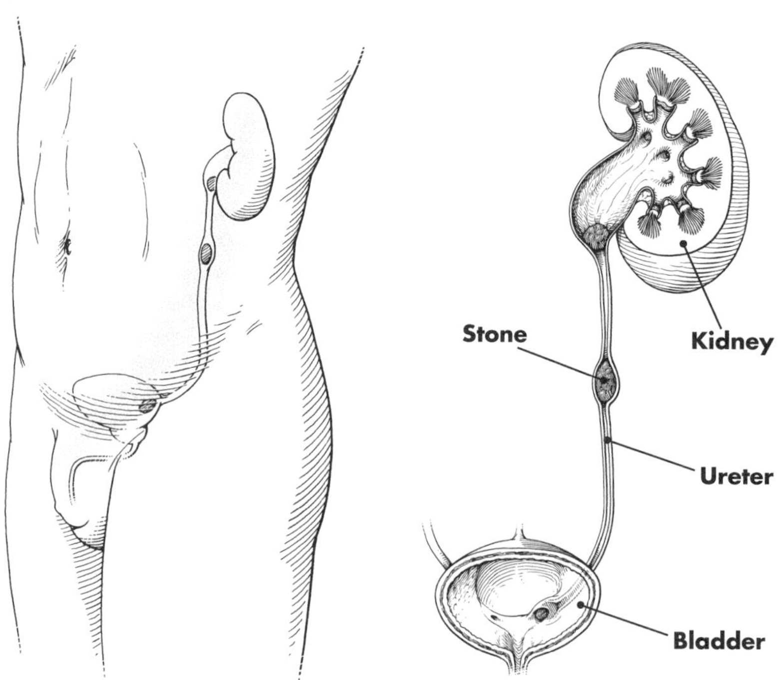

The blue-tinted zone on the torso is where the pain of kidney stones most often occurs. Stones originate in the kidneys and can travel down into the ureters and bladder.

Uric acid stones

Uric acid stones are formed of uric acid, a byproduct of protein metabolism. A diet rich in meat can cause an increased amount of uric acid in your urine. You may also have high levels of uric acid in your blood and urine if you have gout or are receiving chemotherapy.

Struvite stones

Found mainly in women, struvite stones are the result of a bacterial urinary tract infection that produces specific enzymes. The enzymes increase the amount of ammonia in the urine, which contributes to the formation of crystals in struvite stones. These stones can grow large. They can obstruct the urinary tract and cause kidney damage.

Cystine stones

People who have the hereditary disorder cystinuria excrete excessive amounts of certain amino acids and form cystine stones in the kidneys. Men and women are equally likely to have cystine stones. They account for only 1 percent of kidney stones.

Diagnosis

Tests that may be used to diagnose a kidney stone include an ultrasound exam, a computerized tomography (CT) scan or a special kidney X-ray called intravenous pyelography (see page 918). Your doctor will send your stone to the laboratory for analysis to determine its composition. This information may suggest the cause of the problem and help your doctor plan your treatment.

If you have recurrent or multiple stones, your doctor may request a chemical analysis of your blood and a 24-hour collection of urine to measure the clearance of waste products from the kidneys.

How serious are kidney stones?
Although passing a stone is painful, most kidney stones pass through the ureter and into the bladder without causing permanent damage. If complications develop, such as ureteral obstruction or urinary tract infection, kidney damage may result.

Treatment
Treatment depends on the type, size and location of the stone and on whether your condition has any complicating factors.

Nutrition
Some dietary excesses or deficiencies — such as too much vitamin D, sodium or meat — may contribute to stone formation. Your doctor may suggest appropriate dietary modifications.

People with kidney stones, regardless of the type, need to drink at least six to eight glasses of water daily, including one at bedtime. Adequate fluid intake dilutes urine, thus making it less likely that crystals will form.

Medication
Whether you'll need to take a medication that can inhibit the growth of stones depends on the severity of your disease and the type of stones you've developed.

- *Calcium stones.* With certain types of calcium stones, a thiazide diuretic is often successful in preventing or decreasing formation of new stones. A phosphate-containing preparation also may inhibit stone formation. Calcium stone formation that results from a defect in the ability of the kidney tubules to filter acids may be prevented by taking sodium

Kidney Stone Lithotripsy

Thousands of kidney stone operations are avoided each year because of a technique called kidney stone lithotripsy. This procedure, developed in Germany, was approved for use in the United States in 1984.

The procedure produces shock waves that pulverize the stones, allowing the fragments to be passed in the urine. Several variations on lithotripsy treatment exist.

Extracorporeal shock wave lithotripsy
Extracorporeal shock wave lithotripsy is generally used for stones within the kidney or the upper end of the ureter. In some cases, you may be lowered into a large tub of water so that your body is submerged up to your shoulders. In others cases, you may lie on a surgical bed. High-energy shock waves are emitted from a machine (lithotripter) positioned below your back.

X-rays or ultrasound help determine the position of your stones and monitor their status during treatment. You may feel a tapping on your back as the procedure begins. You're given some type of anesthetic, either local or general, to help you lie still and reduce any discomfort that may occur. Typically, a stone begins to crumble after 200 to 400 shock waves. As many as 2,000 shock waves may be given during the treatment.

After the anesthetic wears off, you're encouraged to walk around and drink lots of water to help wash out the small stone fragments. You may experience some discomfort as the fragments pass, and you may notice blood in your urine for a few days.

Kidney stone lithotripsy with a bath

Percutaneous ultrasonic lithotripsy
A stone that can't be fragmented using the extracorporeal method often can be treated in other ways. In percutaneous ultrasonic lithotripsy, a small incision is made in the skin through which a small, flexible tube is passed into the kidney. A small ultrasound-producing unit is inserted into the tube to apply sound waves to the stone. The doctor can remove the resulting fragments through the same tube.

Other variations
In endoscopic lithotripsy, a small instrument that includes an ultrasound-producing unit is passed up through the bladder and into the ureter. Other techniques to break stones in the ureter include laser lithotripsy and electrohydraulic lithotripsy, which uses sparks to create shock waves in a fluid environment. These work particularly well on ureteral stones that aren't accessible by other lithotripsy methods.

bicarbonate or potassium bicarbonate medications.

- *Uric acid stones.* If you have uric acid stones, your doctor may prescribe allopurinol (Aloprim, Zyloprim) and a medicine to keep the urine alkaline.
- *Struvite stones.* When a struvite stone is found, the first task is to suppress the infection that caused it. Several types of antibiotics may be of benefit.
- *Cystine stones.* Cystine stones are the most difficult to treat. Your doctor may prescribe medication only when all other approaches have failed.

Surgery

A kidney stone that causes an obstruction, infection or intractable pain is often removed surgically. Typically, a stone is removed by passing a small instrument up the ureter through a cystoscope in the bladder or by using shock waves to fragment the stone.

For calcium stones caused by abnormally active parathyroid glands, removal of parathyroid tissue is often necessary to avoid further stone formation and kidney damage.

Bladder stones

Signs and symptoms

- A urinary tract infection
- Interruption of urine flow
- Pain in the penis
- An inability to urinate except in certain positions
- Blood in the urine

Most bladder stones are the result of an underlying urologic problem, most commonly a bladder outlet obstruction due to an enlarged prostate gland.

Sometimes, bladder stones are caused by long-term use of catheters that are left in place, causing an associated infection. The vast majority of bladder stones occur in men.

Diagnosis

If you have a bladder stone, a urinalysis will usually reveal blood in the urine and an infection. Generally, a stone can be seen on an X-ray.

How serious are bladder stones?

Bladder stones may pass without intervention if they're small. If they don't pass, they should be removed. Your doctor will also want to identify and treat the underlying cause of the bladder stones in order to prevent recurrence.

Treatment

Small bladder stones can be removed with a thin, flexible fiber-optic tube (cystoscope) that is inserted into the bladder through the urethra. A larger stone may require a fragmentation procedure, such as electrohydraulic lithotripsy, to fragment the stone without injuring surrounding tissues. In electrohydraulic lithotripsy, an instrument that emits shock waves is placed in the bladder through the urethra. The shock waves break up the stone and the fragments pass out with urine.

Kidney cysts

Signs and symptoms

- Pain in the side
- Blood in the urine

Kidney cysts are noncancerous (benign) lesions of the kidney. They're usually round and contain water-like fluid. They can vary from small to large cysts that contain quarts of fluid. Unlike cancer, a cyst generally enlarges slowly and stops growing when it attains a certain size.

Cysts in the kidney are common. Some research has reported a higher incidence of cysts in women than in men. The fact that infants and children rarely have cysts suggests that the cysts aren't inherited.

Diagnosis

You doctor can usually distinguish between benign cysts and cancer of the kidney by using ultrasound, computerized tomography (CT) or magnetic resonance imaging (MRI).

How serious are kidney cysts?

Most kidney cysts don't cause symptoms. Only when a cyst is extremely large will it impair renal function. Bleeding may occur within the cyst. An infection or, rarely, cancer can develop in a cyst. Cysts rupture very infrequently.

Treatment

Usually, no treatment is required. In rare instances, fluid must be removed from a cyst by way of an operation or aspiration to relieve pressure or pain and to prevent damage to the kidney.

Kidney or ureter cancer

Signs and symptoms

- Blood in the urine
- Pain in the side
- An abdominal mass felt during examination
- Loss of weight
- Fatigue
- Intermittent fever

The kidneys and ureters can sometimes develop cancer. Unfortunately, kidney cancer often gives no warning signs in its early stages. As the tumor grows, your doctor may feel a mass in the kidney during a physical examination of the abdomen, and blood may be detected in your urine.

Kidney cancer is diagnosed in more than 31,000 Americans each year, and nearly 12,000 die of the disease annually. Yet if kidney cancer is detected and treated early, the chances for a full recovery are good. Cancer that originates in the ureters is relatively rare, accounting for less than 5 percent of renal tumors.

Types

The most common types of cancer of the kidneys or ureters include:

Renal cell carcinoma

Renal cell carcinoma is the most common kidney cancer. It's also called renal adenocarcinoma or hypernephroma. It begins in the cells that line the small tubes (renal tubules) attached to the small blood vessels (glomeruli) of the kidney. Renal cell carcinoma occurs twice as often in men as in women. The age at diagnosis is usually between 50 and 70 years. Smokers are at a slightly greater risk of renal cell carcinoma than are nonsmokers.

In some instances, the disease appears to be hereditary. A large percentage of people with von Hippel-Lindau disease, a rare, inherited condition affecting the capillaries in a particular area of the brain, also develop renal cell carcinoma.

Other factors that may increase your risk of this type of cancer include high blood pressure, especially in men, obesity, radiation exposure, certain environmental toxins — such as asbestos — and long-term kidney dialysis.

Transitional cell cancer

Transitional cell cancer can occur in the lining of the kidneys or ureters and accounts for 10 percent of all urinary tract cancers. People who have bladder cancer also are at increased risk of developing transitional cell cancer of the ureters and kidneys. The painless passage of blood in the urine may be the only sign of this disorder.

Wilms' tumor

Children with cancer of the kidney usually have Wilms' tumor. It accounts for 95 percent of the renal cancers in children under age 14 and occurs in approximately 8 of every 1 million children. The majority of the children with Wilms' tumor are less than 7 years old at the time they receive a diagnosis. The tumor usually causes no symptoms and is found when a doctor feels a mass in the child's abdomen.

Diagnosis

Tests that might be used to diagnose kidney or ureter cancer include a special kidney X-ray procedure call intravenous pyelography (see page 918), computerized tomography (CT), magnetic resonance imaging (MRI) or ultrasound (see Chapter 39, "Diagnostic Tests"). Occasionally, additional tests are required. Procedures such as a chest X-ray, a bone scan or liver tests may be used to determine if the cancer has spread to other organs or tissues. A special examination of urine (cytology) may reveal cancer cells shed in the urine.

How serious is cancer of the kidney or ureter?

The outcome in individuals with renal cell carcinoma depends on the extent to which the tumor has spread. If the tumor is in its earliest stage, 85 percent to 95 percent of affected people survive for at least 5 years. If the lymph nodes around the kidney have been infiltrated, the 5-year survival rate drops to 5 percent to 15 percent. When the cancer has spread to other organs, fewer than 5 percent survive for 5 years.

If a transitional cell cancer hasn't spread, 5-year survival rates are very high. If the cancer has spread, the chance of surviving the next 5 years is significantly diminished.

Children with Wilms' tumor generally have a good chance of survival if the disease hasn't spread. Overall, more than 90 percent survive for at least 5 years.

Treatment

Small tumors within the kidney may be treated by removing only the affected part of the kidney and the surrounding tissues (partial nephrectomy). Larger, localized tumors or tumors near the kidney's blood vessels require removal of the entire kidney. Some surgeons also advocate removing the adjacent lymph nodes.

If the disease has spread, there's no universally agreed-upon treatment. Chemotherapy and immunotherapy for kidney cancer are still under study but have been effective in some cases. Experimental therapy is reasonable for some people with advanced kidney cancer.

In transitional cell cancers, the kidney and ureter are removed along with the portion of the bladder that connects to the ureter, which decreases the risk of transitional cell cancer reoccurring. Chemotherapy or radiation or both also may be used.

A combination of treatments is used for Wilms' tumor. The mass is generally removed, followed by chemotherapy. Sometimes, radiation therapy may be used.

Bladder cancer

Signs and symptoms

- Blood in the urine
- Pelvic pain
- Difficulty urinating

Nearly 55,000 new cases of bladder cancer are diagnosed annually in the United States. This disease is responsible for more than 12,000 deaths each year. Bladder cancer rarely occurs in people younger than age 40. It's four times more common in men than in women and twice as common in whites as it is in blacks.

Bladder cancer appears to be related at least partially to environmental factors. The disease is more prevalent among smokers, as several carcinogens that are inhaled are concentrated in the urine. Exposure to certain chemicals once used in the dye, chemical, leather and rubber industries was associated with an increased risk of bladder cancer. Such substances have been banned by the Environmental Protection Agency and largely removed from the environment.

Diagnosis

Blood in the urine, without pain or discomfort, is the most frequent early symptom. A common error is to presume that blood is due to a bladder infection (cystitis).

Your doctor may have a sample of urine examined for malignant cells (cytology). Other procedures may include a kidney X-ray procedure called intravenous pyelography (see page 918) and a cystoscopic examination in which your doctor inserts a thin, flexible fiberoptic tube through the urethra and into the bladder so that he or she can see inside. During a cystoscopic examination, a sample of the bladder lining can be removed and examined for cancerous cells (biopsy).

If cancer is found, your doctor may order a computerized tomography (CT) scan or magnetic resonance imaging (MRI) of the abdomen or pelvis to help determine the extent of the cancer and whether it has spread. Other tests may include a chest X-ray and blood studies.

How serious is bladder cancer?

If the tumor is superficial — that is, it's small and hasn't invaded deeply tissues within the bladder wall — the chances of recovery are excellent. About 74 percent of bladder cancers are detected at this early stage. The chance of surviving the next 5 years is about 93 percent.

About half the people whose cancer has already invaded muscle or fat live at least 5 years following treatment. The 5-year survival rate for people whose bladder cancer has spread to other organs is only about 6 percent.

Treatment

Treatment varies with the extent of the disease.

Superficial cancer

For a superficial bladder cancer, treatment usually consists of removing the tumor itself. A major operation often isn't necessary for superficial bladder cancer because the surgeon is able to remove the tumor through a specialized cystoscope (resectoscope), which is inserted into the bladder while the person is anesthetized.

Following removal of a superficial tumor, cystoscopic evaluation is repeated every 3 to 6 months for many years to check for recurrence of the cancer.

Approximately 60 percent of the people with bladder cancer eventually will have new tumors appear. If only superficial disease recurs, the tumor can again be removed cystoscopically. This time, the bladder may be infused with cancer-fighting drugs to decrease the chance of future tumors.

Localized cancer

If the disease has progressed to invade bladder muscle and fat but hasn't spread beyond the bladder, surgery to remove the bladder is the most common form of treatment. In men, the prostate gland also is removed.

Removal of the bladder requires creation of an opening through which urine can pass. In one of the more successful techniques, the ureters are connected to an artificial bladder made from a piece of intestine. The new bladder is attached inside the body near the navel. An opening (ostomy) is created through the abdominal wall so that urine can drain into a plastic pouch worn against the body under the clothes. This is the ileal conduit procedure.

Increasingly, bladders are being fashioned from sections of the large or small intestines, which are then connected to the urethra. A bladder made in this way is called a neobladder. There's no ostomy. People with cancers that aren't near the

Cystoscopy

Cystoscopy is an important technique for direct examination of the urethra, the inside of the bladder and, in men, the prostate gland. In adults, the procedure is done under local anesthesia, meaning that just before the procedure, the area around your urethral opening is anesthetized, and you remain awake during the examination. Children are usually given a general anesthetic. The cystoscope, a flexible, narrow tube made of metal or rubber, is inserted through the urethra into your bladder. This tube carries a lens and a fiber-optic light so that your doctor can examine the structures through which the scope passes.

It may be necessary to remove a sample of bladder tissue for examination for cancer or other diseases (biopsy), or even to remove a small stone. All of this can be done through the cystoscope. Cystoscopy is useful for evaluating a range of bladder problems, including recurring infection, painful urination and cancer. In men, the procedure sometimes is used to evaluate the degree of obstruction resulting from an enlarged prostate gland.

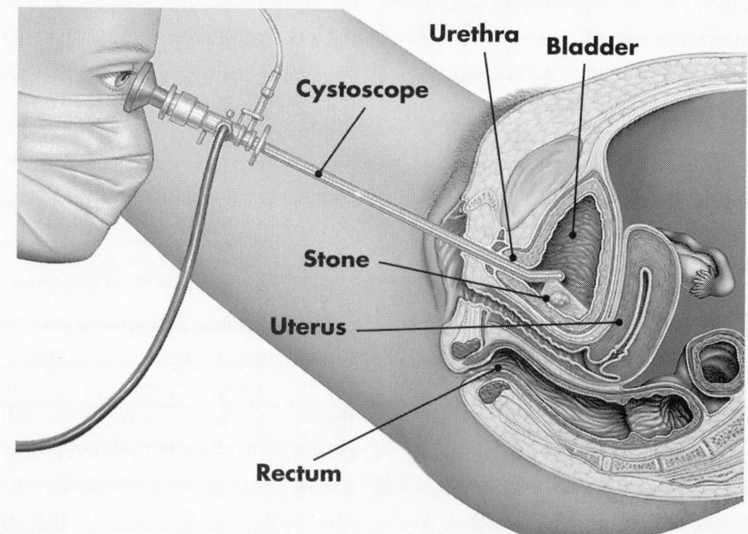

Cystoscopic examination can reveal a stone in the bladder. It can also help identify other diseases, such as cancer. This simple procedure is usually done under local anesthesia.

bladder neck or urethra may be candidates for this procedure.

Chemotherapy may be given following the surgery as a precautionary measure to increase chances of a full recovery.

Invasive cancer
In 30 percent to 70 percent of the people with bladder cancer that has spread to other organs, chemotherapy is helpful in halting or slowing the spread of cancer and alleviating pain. However, the benefit usually isn't permanent and the cancer continues to progress. In some cases, surgery is performed to remove the bladder and adjacent tissues and possibly other organs.

Injury and Inflammation

The kidneys and other parts of the urinary tract are subject to many types of injuries and inflammations. Because of the kidneys' protected location within the body, direct traumatic injury to them is uncommon, but they are quite susceptible to injury by toxic substances. Inflammation of the urinary tract, including the kidneys, can be associated with drugs, an infection or disorders of other organs.

Injury of the kidney

Signs and symptoms

- A history or evidence of physical injury
- Blood in the urine
- Severe pain in the side
- Nausea and vomiting
- Swelling of the abdomen
- Fever
- Internal bleeding
- Shock

Traumatic injury to the kidney occurs mainly from athletic activities or industrial or traffic accidents. Such injuries are relatively rare because the kidneys are protected by the rib cage and large back muscles.

Diagnosis
If you have signs or symptoms of kidney injury, your doctor will likely have your blood and urine examined in a laboratory. He or she may also have you undergo a kidney X-ray, computerized tomography (CT), magnetic resonance imaging (MRI) or an X-ray of the arteries leading to your kidneys. This last test is useful in determining whether blood flow to your kidneys is blocked or reduced.

How serious is kidney trauma?
When a kidney is injured, most often it's merely bruised, and the bleeding stops spontaneously.

The Kidneys and Toxic Injury

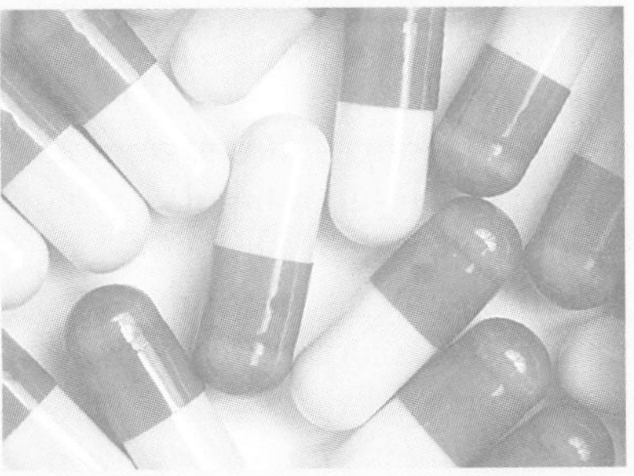

The kidneys are particularly vulnerable to toxic injury because of the vast quantity of blood circulating through them at any given time. If you've been exposed to a toxin, the effect may be greater on your kidneys than on any other organs. The four most common types of toxic injury to the kidney are:

Analgesic nephropathy
Analgesic nephropathy results from long-term, excessive use of nonsteroidal anti-inflammatory drugs (NSAIDs) — such as phenylbutazone (Butatab), indomethacin (Indocin) and ibuprofen (Advil, Motrin, others) — and long-term, excessive use of phenacetin-containing medications, which are no longer produced in the United States. Some doctors believe that excessive amounts of acetaminophen (Tylenol, others) also may damage the kidneys, but this hasn't been definitely proved.

Analgesic nephropathy occurs more often in women than in men. The incidence of analgesic nephropathy has decreased significantly since phenacetin was removed from most over-the-counter drugs. Signs and symptoms of analgesic nephropathy include pus in the urine, anemia and high blood pressure.

Lead nephropathy
In children, lead nephropathy usually results from ingestion of lead-based paint. Adults generally are poisoned from inhaling vapors produced when metal covered with lead-based paint is welded. Alcohol illegally distilled in an apparatus made from car radiators is another source of lead poisoning.

In children, signs and symptoms of lead poisoning may include irritability, weight loss, sluggishness and abdominal pain. Signs and symptoms of lead poisoning in adults may include gouty arthritis, high blood pressure, abdominal pain and anemia.

Acute uric acid nephropathy
Acute uric acid nephropathy results from overproduction of uric acid. It most often occurs in individuals with bone marrow and lymph node malignancies who've been treated with certain cancer medications. Signs and symptoms include diminished urine output and the presence of blood and uric acid crystals in the urine.

Solvent and fuels nephropathy
Carbon tetrachloride and other solvents and fuels have the potential for causing kidney damage. This is the reason for the warning on many commercial cleaners and sprays stating that they be used only in well-ventilated environments.

Sometimes, however, complications such as severe hemorrhage, infection and shock develop. After an injury to its blood vessels, a kidney's ability to function may be lost within just a few hours. In most cases, kidney injuries require hospitalization.

Treatment

In some cases, treatment for kidney trauma includes bed rest, pain relievers and intravenous (IV) administration of fluids to control blood pressure and stimulate urine production. Within 6 to 12 weeks after the injury, a CT scan may be done to make sure that the kidney is properly healed.

If the kidney is more severely injured, it may need to be repaired or removed. Drainage of the space surrounding the kidney and repair of lacerations or a torn ureter also may be necessary. Up to 20 percent of people with traumatic injuries to the kidneys require emergency surgery to control massive bleeding.

Injury of the bladder or urethra

Signs and symptoms

- A history of trauma
- An inability to urinate
- Blood in the urine
- Pain in the lower abdomen
- Shock

Direct traumatic injury to the bladder is uncommon because of the organ's location deep within the pelvis. The bladder may be ruptured by bone fragments following pelvic fracture, an injury that might be sustained, for example, in an auto accident. The bladder also may be injured during an operation such as hernia repair.

Rupture of the urethra, the narrow tube that carries urine from the bladder, is rare but requires immediate realignment or placement of a special tube. In men, most injuries to the urethra occur when a catheter is passed into an obstructed urethra for bladder drainage. In women, urethral damage is rare.

Diagnosis

If your signs and symptoms suggest a bladder or urethral injury, your doctor likely will perform a thorough examination of your abdomen and rectum. He or she may also order an X-ray to help determine if your bladder or urethra is torn.

Your doctor may also do a cystoscopic examination, which involves passing a thin, flexible fiber-optic tube up the urethra and into the bladder. Cystoscopy permits your doctor to visually inspect this part of the lower urinary tract.

How serious is injury of the bladder or urethra?

The most serious situation is a ruptured bladder that leaks urine into the abdominal cavity. This is a life-threatening situation because of the risk of infection, and it requires emergency surgery to repair the bladder wall and to remove the urine from the abdominal cavity.

A long-term complication of urethral injury is formation of a stricture. This is a severe narrowing of the urethra produced by stiffening of scar tissue. The scar tissue develops during an injury and remains after it has healed. In men, a stricture may also cause partial or total impotence.

Treatment

The first step is to treat shock or bleeding that may accompany the injury. These are treated by blood transfusions and fluid replacement given through a vein (intravenously). Antibiotics may be given to prevent infection.

If the bladder is ruptured, you'll need surgery. If your urethra is injured, your doctor may need to pass a thin, flexible tube (catheter) through the urethra into the bladder to provide an exit route for urine while you heal. The catheter can usually be removed after several days or weeks. Urethral injuries sometimes require immediate repair, but often treatment of the injury is delayed.

Acute interstitial nephritis

Signs and symptoms

- Blood in the urine
- Excess protein in the urine
- High blood pressure
- Fever
- A rash
- Weight gain
- Fluid retention

Acute interstitial nephritis is an inflammation of the kidney that affects the tubules and small blood vessels (glomeruli) of the nephrons and the spaces between these structures (see the illustration on page 916). Most often, the inflammation is confined to the spaces.

Acute interstitial nephritis is generally associated with an allergic reaction to a drug or to a kidney condition called analgesic nephropathy (see page 925). Some commonly prescribed drugs that may cause acute interstitial nephritis include penicillin, ampicillin (Omnipen, Polycillin) and nonsteroidal anti-inflammatory drugs such as indomethacin (Indocin), ibuprofen (Advil, Motrin, others) and naproxen (Aleve, Naprosyn, others).

Diagnosis

In this condition, damage to the kidneys allows red blood cells and proteins to leak into the urine. Thus, a urine analysis is the first step toward making the diagnosis. Your doctor likely will also order blood tests to help him or her assess your kidney function. He or she may also perform a kidney biopsy to confirm the diagnosis and to evaluate the nature and extent of the damage.

How serious is acute interstitial nephritis?

Kidney damage that results from acute interstitial nephritis is often reversible. If the condition stems from use of a drug, discontinuing use of that drug usually allows the kidney to heal. Sometimes, short-term dialysis is needed (see page 926). Complete recovery is the rule, although progression to chronic kidney failure may occur in rare cases.

Treatment

The first step in your treatment is to avoid drugs known to cause acute interstitial nephritis. You can reduce fluid retention and swelling by restricting your intake of salt, water and other beverages. Your doctor may prescribe medication for high blood pressure. You may need dialysis for a short time if you experience acute kidney failure. In some cases, corticosteroid drugs such as prednisone are beneficial.

Acute glomerulonephritis

Signs and symptoms

- Cola- or tea-colored urine
- Foamy urine
- High blood pressure
- Fluid retention
- Protein and red blood cells in urine
- Mild anemia
- Headache
- Blurred vision
- Generalized aches and pains

Glomerulonephritis is a medical term for inflammation of the small blood vessels (glomeruli) of the kidneys' filtering structures (nephrons). The inflammation damages the membrane of the glomeruli, allowing some of the proteins and red blood cells that flow through them to be lost in the urine. It can also interfere with the glomeruli's filtering of waste products, increasing waste products in the blood.

Acute vs. chronic

The two main categories of glomerulonephritis are acute and chronic. Acute glomerulonephritis is a sudden attack of inflammation of the glomeruli. Chronic glomerulonephritis is characterized by persistent inflammation of the glomeruli and is associated with gradual kidney failure.

Associated diseases

Several diseases can lead to inflammation of the glomeruli. Some of them are diseases in which your body's immune system attacks itself (autoimmune diseases). These include systemic lupus erythematosus, various types of inflammations of blood vessels (vasculitis) and a condition called Berger's disease (IgA nephropathy), which leads to protein deposits in the glomeruli.

Some infections in other parts of the body also can be followed by glomerulonephritis. The most common one that may lead to acute glomerulonephritis is caused by the streptococcal bacteria. Although the bacteria don't attack the kidneys, the body's immune response to the bacteria sometimes creates an excess of antibodies. These antibodies eventually may be deposited in the kidneys, where they damage the glomeruli. Other infections that may affect the kidneys include infection of a heart valve (endocarditis), typhoid fever, syphilis and malaria.

In addition, glomerulonephritis may be triggered by viruses such as those that cause AIDS, mononucleosis, mumps, measles or hepatitis, by echovirus or by coxsackievirus.

Poststreptococcal glomerulonephritis

Acute glomerulonephritis may follow a streptococcal infection such as strep throat or, rarely, strep skin infection (impetigo). It usually happens in children ages 6 to 10. Typically, the infection develops a few weeks after the person is over the acute infection.

In cases of strep throat, it may take from 2 to 6 weeks after the cessation of throat symptoms for acute glomerulonephritis to develop. For strep skin infection, the average latency period is about 2 weeks. Only a few types (strains) of streptococci have the potential to cause glomerulonephritis. In addition, not everyone who gets acute glomerulonephritis has symptoms.

In families who have experienced an outbreak of strep infection by a strain that can cause glomerulonephritis, for every one who had symptoms, three or four didn't.

Schonlein-Henoch purpura

Schonlein-Henoch purpura is a cause of acute glomerulonephritis in children. Signs and symptoms include a characteristic rash that's prominent on the legs and buttocks, pain in joints (especially in the ankles and knees) with or without swelling or tenderness, and abdominal pain. Some children also have blood in their stools.

The condition can cause fluid retention, high blood pressure and blood and protein in the urine. The cause of Schonlein-Henoch purpura is unknown, but the condition may be associated with a drug sensitivity or respiratory infection.

Most people with Schonlein-Henoch purpura recover without kidney damage, although, if urinary abnormalities persist, kidney function may continue to deteriorate. Most children recover completely without specific treatment, but many adults are left with permanent kidney damage. In some cases, corticosteroid medications are prescribed.

Hemolytic uremic syndrome

Hemolytic uremic syndrome is seen mainly in infants and young children. It occurs much less often in older children and rarely in adults. In its typical form, an illness accompanied by diarrhea — often caused by a certain type of *Escherichia coli (E. coli)* bacteria — is quickly followed by a decrease in the red blood cell count and rapid loss of kidney function. Other systems may be affected as well.

Often, fever, low platelet count and mental status changes are associated with the condition. Dialysis and blood transfusions are often required during the acute phase of the illness.

Most children with this syndrome recover completely, but some are left with chronic kidney damage or damage to some other organs. In some cases, death may occur.

Diagnosis

If your doctor suspects that you or your child has acute glomerulonephritis, he or she may take a throat or skin culture to determine if streptococcal organisms are present. Your doctor might order blood studies that measure the levels of waste products such as creatinine and urea nitrogen in the blood. With this information, your doctor can assess the filtering capacity of your kidneys.

He or she may also order a urine analysis to determine blood cell and protein content. If these tests point to glomerulonephritis, your doctor may need to do a kidney biopsy.

How serious is acute glomerulonephritis?

In some cases of acute glomerulonephritis, particularly those that follow strep infection, fluid retention and high blood pressure may resolve within a week. Abnormal urinary analysis findings may persist for several months.

Most children make a complete recovery and show no evidence of chronic renal disease later in life, although a very small percentage of them develop the chronic form of glomerulonephritis that may end in renal failure.

Adults don't do as well as children following acute glomerulonephritis. The reasons for this are unclear. Adults who've had a particularly severe initial acute form that leads to high blood pressure or large amounts of protein in the urine are more prone to chronic kidney failure. Those who've had one attack of the disease generally recover once the kidneys heal.

Although recurrent attacks are unusual, one-third to one-half of those who do experience repeated attacks progress to renal failure.

Treatment

The treatment and outcome of acute glomerulonephritis depend on the underlying cause of the disease. Your doctor may advise bed rest. Your salt and water intake may be restricted to prevent or minimize fluid retention and swelling.

You may need medication for high blood pressure and a special diet to restrict protein intake. In some cases, protein can increase your creatinine or urea nitrogen levels to undesirable levels.

If you have an active strep infection or your glomerulonephritis is caused by bacteria other than streptococci, your doctor will likely prescribe an appropriate antibiotic. Some types of acute glomerulonephritis are treated with steroid medications or other immunosuppressive drugs.

Chronic glomerulonephritis

Signs and symptoms

- Protein in the urine
- Blood in the urine
- High blood pressure
- Gradual kidney failure

Chronic glomerulonephritis refers to persistent inflammation of the small blood vessels (glomeruli) in the kidneys that frequently leads to progressive loss of renal function. The kidneys' ability to retain protein and red blood cells is impaired.

Causes

Several diseases may lead to chronic glomerulonephritis:

Membranous glomerulonephritis

In this condition, irregular deposits of immune-related protein develop along the walls of the glomeruli. More than 80 percent of people with this disease have sufficient loss of protein in the urine to cause swelling and weight gain from fluid and sodium retention.

Spontaneous remission of membranous glomerulonephritis is common in children but occurs in only 20 percent to 25 percent of adults with the disease. Renal failure is most likely to occur within a few years after diagnosis. About 30 percent to 40 percent of people with membranous glomerulonephritis require either dialysis or kidney transplantation within 10 years after their diagnosis.

Berger's disease

Berger's disease (IgA nephropathy) is characterized by recurrent episodes of blood in the urine. It results from deposits of the immunoglobulin A (IgA) protein in the glomeruli.

Young men are most often affected, but the condition can occur in all people at any age. Berger's disease usually progresses slowly, if at all. In the majority of cases, renal function is well preserved for years. About a quarter of people with this disease develop end-stage kidney (renal) failure within 25 years after diagnosis.

Individuals with high blood pressure, large amounts of protein in their urine and excess urea in their blood tend to have a worse outcome than do those with more moderate signs and symptoms.

Focal segmental glomerulosclerosis

Focal segmental glomerulosclerosis is characterized by scattered scarring of some of the glomeruli. It may result from another disease or occur for no known reason. Both children and adults are affected. Males are slightly more likely to have this disorder than are females.

Children with focal segmental glomerulosclerosis occasionally have spontaneous remission of the disease. In adults, however, that isn't likely. Most adults and children with this disease have a progressive decline in renal function. Those with an aggressive form of the disease may progress to end-stage kidney (renal) failure within 2 to 3 years after the diagnosis.

Corticosteroids and immunosuppressant medications may decrease levels of protein in the blood (proteinuria) and improve kidney function in some people, but the results aren't consistent. Treatment often focuses on controlling blood pressure and cholesterol, which may contribute to scarring.

Mesangial proliferative glomerulonephritis
Mesangial proliferative glomerulonephritis is a rare, chronic disease in which portions of the glomeruli are enlarged. Older children and young adults are most commonly affected by this disease, and it occurs slightly more often in males.

Mesangial proliferative glomerulonephritis might progress to end-stage kidney (renal) failure, but if leakage of protein into the urine can be controlled, there's a good chance of avoiding long-term kidney damage. If you don't respond to medication and your symptoms persist, often the condition will progress to end-stage kidney disease.

Diabetic nephropathy
Diabetic nephropathy may be the most common cause of end-stage kidney disease in the United States. The longer you have diabetes, the higher your risk of kidney damage. Elevated blood sugar (glucose) levels that characterize diabetes can lead to scarring and increased blood flow into the kidneys. This creates additional strain on the glomeruli and raises blood pressure.

Controlling high blood pressure with a class of medications called angiotensin-converting enzyme (ACE) inhibitors may delay the development of end-stage kidney disease. Once there's a significant amount of protein in the urine, end-stage kidney disease usually follows within 5 to 10 years.

Other diseases
Several diseases that affect other organ systems also can damage the glomeruli. These include systemic lupus erythematosus, amyloidosis, high blood pressure, cancer, hepatitis C and AIDS.

Diagnosis
Chronic glomerulonephritis is often diagnosed after a doctor discovers high blood pressure or urine abnormalities during a routine physical examination or an examination for an unrelated illness.

If your doctor thinks that you may have the disease, he or she may have you undergo blood and urine tests and diagnostic studies to visualize the kidney, such as a kidney X-ray, an ultrasound examination or a computerized tomography (CT) scan (see Chapter 39, "Diagnostic Tests"). Your doctor may also remove a small sample of tissue (biopsy) to determine the cause of the inflammation.

How serious is chronic glomerulonephritis?
The outlook for you depends on the cause of your disease and the severity of your complications, particularly high blood pressure and protein loss in the urine.

Most forms of chronic glomerulonephritis develop slowly and gradually lead to the loss of kidney function (chronic kidney failure). Chronic kidney failure often can be delayed through management of symptoms.

Treatment
If you have high blood pressure, you'll likely be given medication to treat it. Your doctor may also recommend reducing protein and salt, a dietary adjustment that will help meet the needs of your impaired kidneys.

If you have diabetic nephropathy, good control of your blood sugar (glucose) level and your blood pressure is essential. If the cause of your glomerulonephritis is hepatitis C, your doctor may recommend treatment with interferon therapy.

In some people, glomerulonephritis is treated with corticosteroids and immune-suppressing drugs designed to reduce inflammation. But the disease doesn't always respond to this type of treatment.

If you're approaching end-stage kidney disease, you and your doctor will want to give careful consideration to dialysis or kidney transplantation. Either of these options may enable you to lead a productive, active life.

Nephrotic syndrome

Signs and symptoms
- Large amounts of protein in the urine
- Swelling of the eyelids, feet and abdomen
- Fluid retention
- Poor appetite
- High cholesterol
- Low blood protein

Nephrotic syndrome isn't a disease but rather a group of signs and symptoms that often accompany many diseases that affect the filtering function of the kidneys' glomeruli. The syndrome is characterized by high levels of protein in urine and low levels of protein in blood, high cholesterol and swelling of the eyelids, feet and abdomen.

The most common causes of nephrotic syndrome are diabetes, nonsteroidal anti-inflammatory drugs (NSAIDs), multiple myeloma, glomerulonephritis and systemic lupus erythematosus.

In children, the average age at onset is 3 to 4 years. The majority of these children have a form of nephrotic syndrome called minimal change disease (also known as lipid nephrosis, nil disease and foot process disease).

Minimal change disease is characterized by the signs and symptoms of nephrotic syndrome but little or no changes in the structure of the glomeruli when examined by a standard microscope. About 15 percent to 20 percent of the adults who have nephrotic syndrome have this form of the syndrome.

Diagnosis
Diagnostic tests for nephrotic syndrome include blood and urine studies. If these show large amounts of protein in the urine, your doctor may recommend removal of a sample of kidney tissue (biopsy) for evidence of a specific cause and for formulating the best treatment plan. Children less often require a renal biopsy.

How serious is nephrotic syndrome?
The seriousness of this syndrome depends on its cause and complications. As a rule, if you have minimal change disease, you can expect both remissions and relapses of excessive protein in urine. The vast majority of children and adults with minimal change disease don't progress to kidney failure.

When the syndrome is caused by infection or drugs, it often resolves after the infection is cured or the drug is discontinued. Some of the other causes don't have such a favorable outcome. The more persistent the nephrotic syndrome, the worse the long-term outcome.

Treatment
Treatment of nephrotic syndrome is aimed at alleviating symptoms and preventing complications. Predictors of a good outcome depend on how well your treatment:

- Reduces or eliminates high protein levels in your urine
- Controls your high blood pressure
- Controls or improves your decreased renal function

Several medications may be useful in reaching these goals. Corticosteroids such as prednisone are often prescribed to decrease the protein content of urine. In minimal change disease, corticosteroid therapy enhances the body's tendency toward natural remission.

Treatment usually consists of daily oral doses of prednisone for 2 months. When you're ready to discontinue the medication, your doctor may reduce the dosage gradually to prevent relapse.

Prednisone is a potent drug with significant side effects, the most common being increased appetite, weight gain and facial puffiness. Some children may require so much of the drug that their growth is temporarily retarded.

Immunosuppressive drugs such as cyclophosphamide (Cytoxan, Neosar) may be given if there's no improvement with prednisone. However, this medication can cause bone marrow problems, bladder irritation or, occasionally, reproductive problems.

Angiotensin-converting enzyme (ACE) inhibitors also may be prescribed. Other treatment measures include a salt-restricted diet and diuretic drugs to control fluid retention and high blood pressure.

Urinary Tract Infections

Urinary tract infections (UTIs) are common — especially among women — and lead to about 8 million medical office visits annually in the United States. In fact, one in five women will develop a UTI during their lifetime, and many will have more than one. Young girls — as well as men — also are at risk of developing UTIs.

The majority of urinary tract infections affect the lower urinary tract (bladder and urethra). Most bacteria enter the urinary tract by way of the urethra.

Under normal circumstances, these bacteria are flushed out during urination or controlled by the antibacterial properties of urine. However, certain factors increase the chance that these bacteria will take hold and multiply into a full-blown infection.

Urinary Tract Infections and Sexual Intercourse

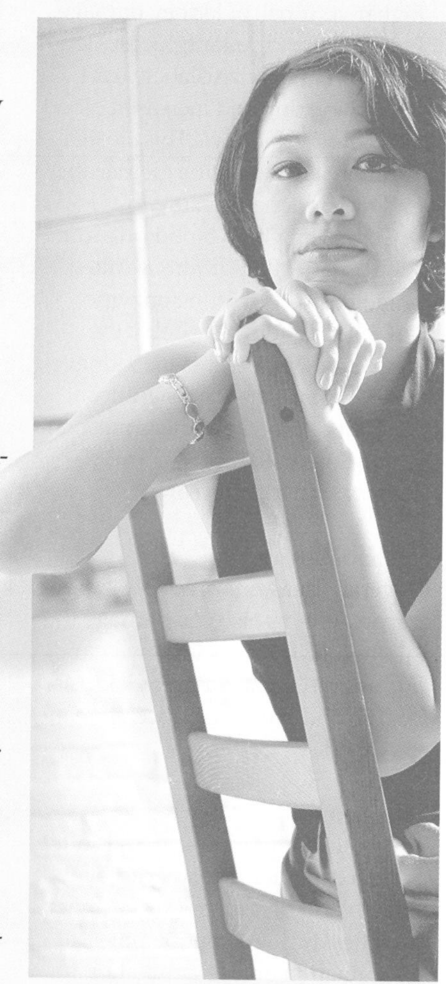

Some women experience frequent, painful urination following sexual intercourse. The symptoms generally last for a day or two and then disappear, only to recur the next time they have sex.

This problem is sometimes called honeymoon cystitis (bladder infection), although it's actually a form of chronic urethral infection (urethritis). It's generally the urethra, not the bladder, that's inflamed. Sometimes laboratory tests don't reveal any microorganisms that could be responsible, and some women, even after treatment with an antibiotic, continue to have symptoms whenever they have intercourse. In such cases, a doctor may suggest preventive measures, such as taking a low dose of an antibiotic, such as trimethoprim sulfamethoxazole (Bactrim, Septra), after sexual activity.

To make these infections less likely, after intercourse, empty your bladder immediately to flush bacteria out of your urethra. Use a water-soluble lubricant during intercourse to make penetration easier and urethral inflammation less likely.

Sexual intercourse, pregnancy, urinary obstruction and the virulent nature of some bacteria all contribute to the likelihood of an infection.

The general term urinary tract infection is often used to describe infections that begin in the bladder (cystitis), kidney (pyelonephritis) or urethra (urethritis).

Bladder infection

Signs and symptoms

- Frequent and urgent urination
- Burning during urination
- Pressure in the lower abdomen
- Blood in the urine
- Malodorous urine

Bladder infection (cystitis) refers to inflammation of the bladder, usually from an infection. Cystitis commonly occurs in women after sexual intercourse.

During sexual activity, bacteria that are frequently present in the lower urethral and vaginal areas are pushed up into the bladder. Once inside the bladder, the bacteria begin to multiply. Usually, the body can remove such bacteria by urination, but when it can't, cystitis may occur.

Although sexually active women between 20 and 50 years of age are the most likely to acquire cystitis, even young girls are susceptible to lower urinary tract infections because the anus, a constant source of bacteria, is so close to the female urethral opening. More than 90 percent of cystitis episodes are due to *Escherichia coli (E. coli)*, a species of bacteria commonly found in the colon and rectum.

Bladder infections are uncommon in men because of the male anatomy — the urethra is much longer in men than in women, making it more difficult for bacteria to reach the bladder. When men do develop cystitis, it's often related to a problem with emptying of the bladder, such as with an enlarged prostate.

? Question and Answer

Can drinking cranberry juice prevent urinary tract infections?

For many years, people have linked cranberries with urinary tract health, believing that eating cranberries — or drinking their juice — made urine more acidic and provided protection from infection. Research now indicates that there may be some benefit.

The *Escherichia coli (E. coli)* bacterium is a common cause of urinary tract infection (UTI). At best, this type of infection is a nuisance. At its worst, it can cause kidney damage. So it makes sense to promptly treat a UTI. However, with the concerns about overuse of antibiotics, attention has turned to preventing infection in the first place.

In 1994, researchers at Harvard University demonstrated that cranberry juice did decrease growth of *E. coli* in the urinary tract, but they weren't sure why.

Then a 1998 study from Tulane University found that cranberry juice changed the shape of *E. coli* by inhibiting the growth of hair-like filaments that otherwise allow the bacteria to attach to the lining of the bladder. This anti-adhesion mechanism permitted bacteria to be naturally flushed away through urination.

That same year, researchers at Rutgers University identified the substances, called concentrated tannins (proanthocyanidins), that prevent *E. coli* bacteria from attaching to the lining of the urinary tract. They concluded that a daily 10-ounce glass of cranberry juice cocktail provided the needed protection.

Diagnosis

A urine sample is generally used to diagnose cystitis. To collect a urine sample for laboratory analysis, you wash the vaginal area or the tip of the penis with a disinfectant, pass a small amount of urine into the toilet to flush out the urethra and then collect the next portion of voided urine midstream in a sterile cup for examination. This is called a midstream collection.

A urine culture can reveal an abnormal bacterial count and determine the type of bacteria present so that appropriate treatment can be initiated.

How serious is a bladder infection?

Although a bladder infection is uncomfortable and annoying, it isn't a serious disease.

Treatment

Some minor cases of bladder infection resolve without treatment. Most people are treated with a 3- to 5-day course of oral antibiotics. The symptoms usually improve within 24 to 48 hours after the first dose. More severe cases may require treatment for 7 to 10 days before there's improvement.

Individuals who have more than three infections within 6 months may benefit from low-dose antibiotic therapy as a way to decrease the number of infections. Some women who are prone to bladder infection may further reduce their risk by taking a low dose of an antibiotic following sexual intercourse.

Urethral infection

Signs and symptoms

- Frequent urination
- Burning pain during urination
- Pus in the urine
- In men, penile discharge

The urethra is the tube that drains urine from the bladder during urination. Urethral infection (urethritis) can be caused by the same organisms that infect the bladder, including *Escherichia coli (E. coli)* bacteria.

In addition, some sexually transmitted diseases cause urethral infection. In women, because of the urethra's proximity to the vagina, infections caused by the herpes simplex virus or chlamydia bacteria are possible.

In men, gonococci and chlamydia bacteria cause most urethral infections. Reiter's syndrome is a combination of urethritis, arthritis and conjunctivitis (an eye inflammation) that's usually acquired through sexual contact.

Diagnosis

In women, it's difficult to differentiate a urethral infection from a bladder infection (cystitis) because the signs and symptoms of these conditions are similar. A urine sample can help in the diagnosis.

Approximately 30 percent of women with painful and frequent urination don't have a significant number of bacteria in their urine. This indicates that the inflammation may be in the urethra or that it may not be the result of an infection.

Your doctor will question you about your signs and symptoms. Bloody urine, a sudden onset of illness of short duration and a history of previous similar infections suggest that a bacterial infection is causing the inflammation. If the illness began gradually more than 7 days before the examination and no blood is in your urine, the symptoms may be from chlamydia infection, particularly if you've recently changed sex partners.

How serious is a urethral infection?

In most cases of urethritis, the infection goes away after treatment. When urethritis caused by gonorrheal or chlamydial infection is left untreated, it can lead to much more serious problems, such as pelvic inflammatory disease, stricture of the urethra, prostatitis, epididymitis, sterility, arthritis, meningitis and inflammation of the heart.

Chlamydia and gonorrhea are sexually transmitted diseases. If you have them, notify your sexual partner or partners. During treatment, abstinence or the use of condoms can help prevent spread of the infection.

Treatment

Treatment for urethritis depends on the cause of the infection. For chlamydia infection, an antibiotic such as tetracycline may be taken for a week or so. For gonorrhea, penicillin is usually prescribed. Some strains of gonorrhea are resistant to penicillin. If laboratory tests indicate that this is the case, a different medication is prescribed. Antibiotics may also be prescribed for other bacterial infections. In some situations, your doctor may advise that your sexual partner also be treated.

Acute kidney infection

Signs and symptoms

- Pain in the side
- High fever
- Shaking chills
- Vomiting
- Burning pain during urination
- Increased frequency of urination

Sometimes bacteria travel up the ureters to the upper urinary tract, which includes the kidneys, causing an acute kidney infection (acute pyelonephritis).

Diagnosis

A culture of a urine sample should reveal if you have a bacterial infection. There's no simple test to differentiate a kidney infection from a lower urinary tract infection, but the presence of fever and side pain suggests that the infection extends into the kidney.

How serious is an acute kidney infection?

When properly treated, acute kidney infection rarely progresses to chronic kidney (renal) disease, but it can lead to blood infection (sepsis) and be life-threatening in an older adult in poor health or an individual with a weakened immune system. It can also recur if the bacteria aren't totally eradicated.

Treatment

Antibiotics are the first line of treatment. When recurrences are frequent or the kidney infection becomes chronic, your doctor may suspect an underlying problem, such as urine flowing backward from the bladder into the ureter (vesicoureteral reflux). He or she may use a computerized tomography (CT) scan, an ultrasound examination or other diagnostic tests to search for a hidden cause.

Other Urinary Disorders

Although urinary tract infections are the most common urinary disorders, other conditions also can cause urinary problems.

Urinary incontinence

Signs and symptoms

- Involuntary urination
- Small amounts of urine escaping under pressure, such as during a cough or sneeze

Urinary incontinence refers to the inability to keep urine in your bladder until you decide to void, resulting in an accident.

Urinary incontinence can have several causes. The muscular and neurologic systems that control the retention and release of urine are complex. These systems can be affected by illness, medications, urinary tract infections, prostate gland problems or complications of an operation. Neurologic disorders such as Alzheimer's disease, Parkinson's disease and stroke are some of the conditions that can cause incontinence.

In children, bed-wetting is common. After puberty, however, urinary incontinence is rare until the later decades of life. It's estimated that 1 out of 10 people age 65 and older experience incontinence. In general, urinary incontinence is more frequent in women than in men.

Types

In most cases, incontinence occurs either because your bladder muscle contracts involuntarily, causing urine to leak, or because your pelvic muscles and tissues are too weak to withstand the pressures in the bladder. The two main types of urinary incontinence are stress incontinence and urge incontinence.

Stress incontinence

With stress incontinence, leakage occurs in response to some kind of physical activity, such as sneezing, coughing or lifting something heavy, that increases pressure on your abdominal area.

Women past menopause and those who have given birth are especially susceptible to stress incontinence. It's often associated with a loss of strength in pelvis support tissues. This weakening can result in a downward displacement (prolapse) of the uterus and vaginal tissues or a shift of the bladder. Being overweight and some chronic medical conditions also can cause stress incontinence.

Urge incontinence

With urge incontinence, leakage occurs when your bladder contracts on its own and overpowers your urinary sphincter, which is the circular band of muscle fibers in your urethra that holds back urine flow. Prevalence of this condition increases with age. This type of incontinence may also stem from a low-grade urinary infection or an abnormality of the bladder muscle.

Diagnosis

Your doctor may examine your urethral opening, rectum and abdominal area and request a urine specimen for analysis. Depending on what your doctor suspects as the cause of your incontinence, other tests may include an ultrasound examination, a special X-ray called an intravenous pyelogram (see page 918), a cystoscopic examination (see page 934) or a procedure to measure pressure inside your bladder at rest and when filling (urodynamic studies).

To perform urodynamic studies, a doctor or nurse inserts a catheter into your urethra and bladder. The catheter is used to fill your bladder with water. As your bladder is filled, pressure within your bladder is recorded. Normally, pressure increases slowly. However, in some people with incontinence, the bladder goes into spasms as it fills. This test also helps your doctor measure the strength of your bladder muscle.

Urinary Tract Infections in Men

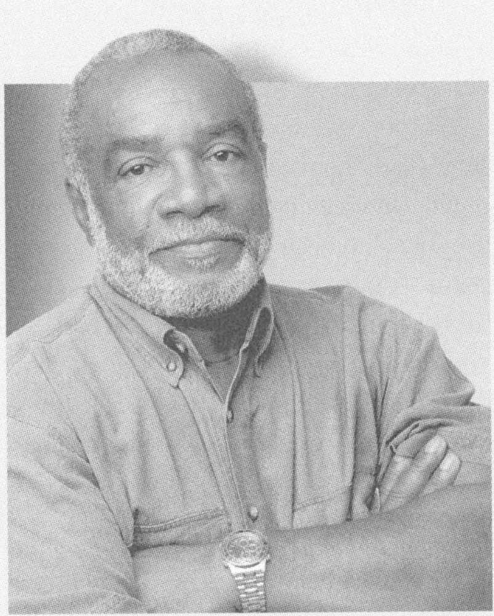

Although urinary tract infections (UTIs) are more common in women, they also affect men.

The classic symptoms are a painful sensation when you urinate and difficulty urinating. Even when you feel the urge, you may not be able to pass urine freely, or you release only a small amount. The urge quickly returns. Most UTIs aren't dangerous if you get proper care. If you have pain in your abdomen or back, chills, fever or vomiting, your kidneys may be infected. A kidney infection is a more serious medical condition requiring prompt treatment.

The most common cause of UTIs is the *Escherichia coli (E. coli)* bacterium. It resides in your intestinal tract and may migrate through your lymph system to your bladder. Inflammation of the bladder (cystitis) is frequently due to infection with *E. coli*. Other factors also can promote urinary tract infections in men:

Prostate problems

Your prostate gland is walnut sized and situated below your bladder, surrounding your urethra. A urinary tract infection can occur if your prostate gland enlarges and constricts your urethra, preventing your bladder from emptying completely. Leftover (residual) urine creates a breeding ground for bacteria. Enlargement of the prostate gland is a normal part of aging, but infection isn't.

Invasive medical procedures

A catheter inserted into the urethra can introduce bacteria, especially if the catheter stays in place for several days.

Narrowed urethra

Frequent inflammation of your urethra (urethritis) can lead to scarring of your urethra (urethral stricture). In years past, strictures were usually associated with recurrent bouts of a sexually transmitted disease, such as gonorrhea. Today, they're more commonly associated with trauma from catheters or instruments used to evaluate or treat urologic problems.

Dehydration

An inadequate intake of fluids can lead to stagnant (concentrated) urine and possibly a UTI.

How serious is urinary incontinence?

Although bothersome, urinary incontinence generally isn't medically serious. But by trying to determine the cause of the leakage, your doctor may find underlying disorders that may require treatment.

Treatment

Treatments for urinary incontinence are available. In many cases, bladder control can be regained by treating the underlying cause or by modifying daily habits. Your doctor may advise specific exercises to strengthen the pelvic area or bladder-training techniques to regain control of urination. Sometimes, simple adjustments in your daily routine, such as remembering to go to the bathroom regularly or limiting fluids before bedtime, can make the difference.

If urinary incontinence persists, medications, special aids or surgery may help manage the problem.

Medication

For symptoms of urge incontinence, medications called anticholinergics (Detrol, Ditropan) may help relax your bladder and prevent involuntary contractions.

Special aids

Absorbent undergarments are available that neutralize the odor of urine and keep the skin fairly dry.

Women may be fitted with a pessary, a device that encircles the cervix, to wear in the vagina during the day. A pessary helps support the pelvic organs to prevent leakage. A urethral insert is another device that you can put directly into the urethra. You remove the small plug-like device to urinate and then replace it until you're ready to void again. Urine seals are small foam pads you place over the urethral opening to keep urine from leaking out. You throw away the discardable seals when you're ready to urinate.

Men may use devices designed to catch urine, such as a type of condom that fits over the penis and drains urine through a tube into a plastic bag. Another device is a foam rubber clamp that can be worn around the penis. For more difficult cases, a catheter is placed through the penis to the bladder, which allows urine to drain into an external plastic bag.

Surgery

Some underlying causes of incontinence, such as a prostate gland problem, can be corrected with surgery. In some types of incontinence, a urologist may recommend a sur-

Training Your Bladder

If you urinate involuntarily at times, it may be a result of weakened muscles. Exercise can improve pelvic muscle condition and tone, allowing you greater control over your bladder.

Although these exercises are best taught by a doctor, nurse or therapist, here are some tips on how to do them.

Women

Bladder training exercises for women are sometimes called Kegel exercises, after the physician who developed them in the 1950s.

- Starting with an empty bladder, contract the muscles that you use when you try to stop urine flow. When you contract them, you should feel a pulling. An effective Kegel exercise will cause the vagina to tighten.
- Pull in the muscles and hold for a count of three. Then relax for a count of three. Work up to 10 to 15 repetitions each session.
- For best results, do the exercises at least three times a day in different positions — standing, lying and sitting.

It may take 3 to 6 weeks to notice an improvement in bladder control. As the tone in your pelvic floor muscles increases, you should have better bladder control. As a bonus, many women find that they also become more sexually responsive.

Men

Weakened pelvic muscles in men sometimes occur following prostate surgery.

To improve your bladder control, you need to exercise two groups of muscles: those that you tighten when you want to stop a bowel movement or hold back gas in the rectum and those at the base of the penis that you use to expel final drops of urine or ejaculate semen.

- Tighten the muscles you use to stop a bowel movement.
- While tightening these muscles, tighten muscles at the base of the penis. You may feel your penis pull in slightly toward your body.
- Hold both sets of muscles as tight as possible for a count of 10.
- Relax muscles and rest for 1 minute.
- Repeat the exercise six times.
- Perform this exercise once a day before going to bed, preferably in a sitting position. Don't overexercise, as your muscles may become tired and you may experience more leakage.
- Holding these muscles tight while rising from a sitting position or while lifting can help prevent urinary leakage.
- Once you achieve urinary control, continue to perform this exercise to keep these muscles in good condition.

gically implanted artificial urethral sphincter, which allows you to control its open (voiding) and closed (continent) settings.

Surgery also may help tighten weakened pelvic floor tissues. But about 60 percent to 75 percent of women find that muscle exercises alone improve leakage so significantly that they don't need surgery.

Chronic urethral infection

Signs and symptoms

- Discomfort during urination that persists or recurs
- Frequent urination

Sometimes the urethra may remain irritated and inflamed for weeks or months, with or without evidence of a bacterial infection. This is known as chronic urethral infection (chronic urethritis). You may feel the need to urinate frequently, and urinating is uncomfortable. As your chronically inflamed urethra undergoes periods of healing, it may gradually narrow.

Inflammation that extends into the bottom of your bladder is called trigonitis.

Diagnosis

In order to determine whether you have chronic urethritis and trigonitis, your doctor will probably insert a thin, flexible fiber-optic tube (cystoscope) into your urethra and bladder. A urinalysis can indicate the presence of bacteria. Your doctor may also ask you if you use any douches, washes or laundry detergents that may contain irritating chemicals.

How serious is chronic urethral infection?

Untreated, chronic urethral infection may eventually lead to narrowing of the urethra and kidney infection. Most of the time, a cause can be identified and the condition properly treated.

Treatment

If an infection is present, your doctor may prescribe antibiotics or sulfa drugs. If no infection is evidence, your doctor may prescribe phenazopyridine (Baridium, Pyridium) to relieve your discomfort. Your doctor may also advise you to discontinue using any possible irritants to see if your condition improves.

Interstitial cystitis

Signs and symptoms

- Pelvic pain
- Frequent urination
- Burning pain during urination

Interstitial cystitis is an inflammation of the bladder wall, but with no apparent cause. This uncommon condition usually affects women in their childbearing years. The symptoms are similar to those of a bladder infection (cystitis), including a frequent urge to urinate and burning or cramping while voiding. Intercourse may be painful as well. The condition isn't the result of an infection, however, nor is it a more serious problem such as cancer.

Diagnosis

A diagnosis of interstitial cystitis is generally arrived at by ruling out all other possible causes for the symptoms, such as infection, cancer or bladder overactivity. Your doctor may examine your bladder lining and determine your bladder's capacity with a thin, flexible fiber-optic instrument called a cystoscope. In some cases, he or she may do a biopsy, that is, take a sample of tissue for microscopic analysis.

How serious is interstitial cystitis?

Interstitial cystitis isn't life-threatening, but the difficulty in identifying the disorder and the lack of a specific treatment can make it a disabling condition.

Treatment

Treatment is aimed primarily at relieving pain and urination symptoms. Many people notice improvement after a bladder distention, which may help by increasing the bladder's capacity and interfering with pain-conducting nerve pathways. Following a schedule for voiding may help by reducing the frequency of urination.

Medication directed to control chronic pain, such as an antidepressant, may be prescribed. Pentosan (Elmiron) is an oral anti-inflammatory medication that's helpful for some people. Dietary modifications also are often helpful in relieving symptoms.

In case of severe symptoms, your doctor may administer a medication called dimethyl sulfoxide (Rimso-50) directly into your bladder to reduce inflammation. Initial symptoms rarely worsen and may improve with time.

Overactive bladder

Signs and symptoms

- A sudden and sometimes uncontrollable urge to urinate (urgency)
- A frequent need to urinate during the night (nocturia)

An overactive (unstable) bladder is one that at times contracts uncontrollably. It's one of the causes of urge incontinence. You may need to urinate so suddenly and urgently that you can't make it to the bathroom. This problem is fairly common. Sometimes, an infection is to blame, but often the cause remains unclear, although aging is frequently suggested as a primary cause.

Diagnosis

The first step in diagnosing overactive bladder is to rule out other causes of urinary leakage, such as infection. To do this, your doctor will likely want a urine specimen for laboratory analysis. You may also have a special kind of X-ray (voiding cystogram) taken while you're urinating.

Other tests may include viewing the bladder with a lighted instrument (cystoscope) inserted into the bladder by way of the urethra and measuring the pressure and function of the bladder (urodynamic studies).

How serious is an overactive bladder?
An overactive bladder can be distressing, but it isn't dangerous.

Treatment
If an infection is responsible for your symptoms, your doctor will likely prescribe an antibiotic. Medications called anticholinergics (Detrol, Ditropan) can help relax the muscles that make your bladder contract. Other medications can reduce the activity of the nerves that lead to the contraction.

Sometimes, bladder-training techniques can help improve symptoms (see page 944). Reducing your intake of irritants such as caffeine, citrus juices and acidic foods also may help.

Urethral stricture

Signs and symptoms
- A slow, weak urine stream
- Dribbling

A urethral stricture is a narrowing of the tube that transports urine from the bladder to the outside. In men, this tube also transports semen. In extreme instances, the urethra can become totally obstructed. The condition is most common in men. Causes of urethral stricture include an infection or disease that produces scar tissue in the urethra and, in men, injury to the penis. Urethral stricture may develop years after an acute episode of gonorrhea.

Diagnosis
A number of conditions other than urethral stricture can produce similar symptoms. Your doctor will likely perform various tests to rule out other causes, including examination of the urethra with a thin, flexible instrument called a cystoscope.

How serious is urethral stricture?
The stricture may narrow to the point that it blocks urine flow, causing acute urinary retention. This requires quick relief. Treatment usually works very well, but recurrence of the stricture is common.

Treatment
Often, the first approach is to stretch the urethra by dilating it with progressively wider instruments that are inserted into the urethra. This treatment often must be repeated a number of times. If the passageway doesn't remain open after repeated dilations, surgery may be necessary.

One surgical procedure can be performed by passing an instrument with a sharp knife attached at the end through a cystoscope. The surgeon uses the knife to cut away the fibrous tissue that's blocking the urethra.

The other option is open surgery to remove the affected section of the urethra. The healthy ends are then reattached or a graft is used to replace the damaged urethra. ■

PREVENTION TIP

Although no direct link has been shown between what you eat and drink and urinary problems, some foods and beverages may be more irritating to your bladder than others. The National Association for Continence offers the following list of items that may contribute to bladder problems:
- Alcoholic beverages
- Beverages and medications with caffeine
- Carbonated drinks
- Dairy products
- Citrus juice and fruits
- Tomatoes and tomato-based products
- Spicy foods
- Sugar
- Honey
- Chocolate
- Corn syrup
- Artificial sweetener

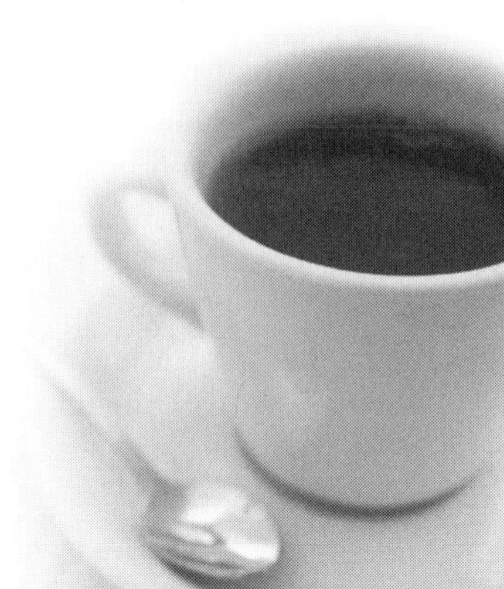

CHAPTER **31** PART V

Bones, Joints and Muscles

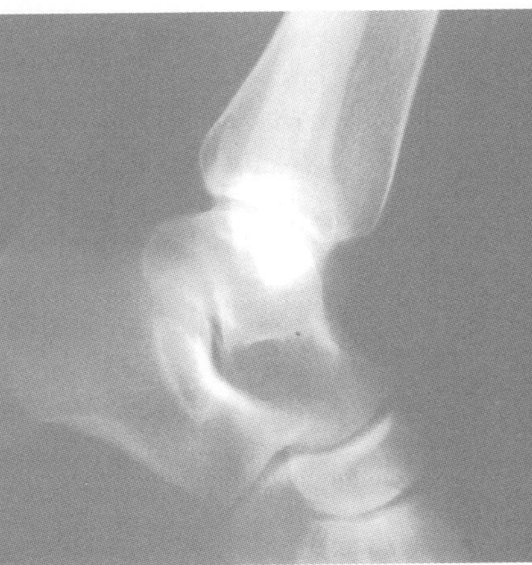

How Your Bones, Joints and Muscles Work

The musculoskeletal system is a marvel of mechanics. Made up of muscles, bones, ligaments and tendons, it allows you to move in myriad ways — walking, running, bending, stretching, sitting and much more.

Most bones in this remarkable system are interconnected by joints, essentially hinges that allow the bones to move. Some joints move differently. The hip and shoulder are ball-and-socket joints, and the backbone (vertebral column) has limited movement.

Besides providing mobility, your musculoskeletal system also protects your internal organs. Your ribs surround your lungs and heart, your skull protects your brain, and your spine protects your spinal cord.

Until this amazing system breaks down — whether due to accident, disease or general wear and tear over time — it's easy to take the workings of your bones, muscles and joints for granted. Breakdowns can occur at any time and for various reasons.

Your bones are living tissue and are always changing. They provide support for your body and function as your body's depository for important minerals.

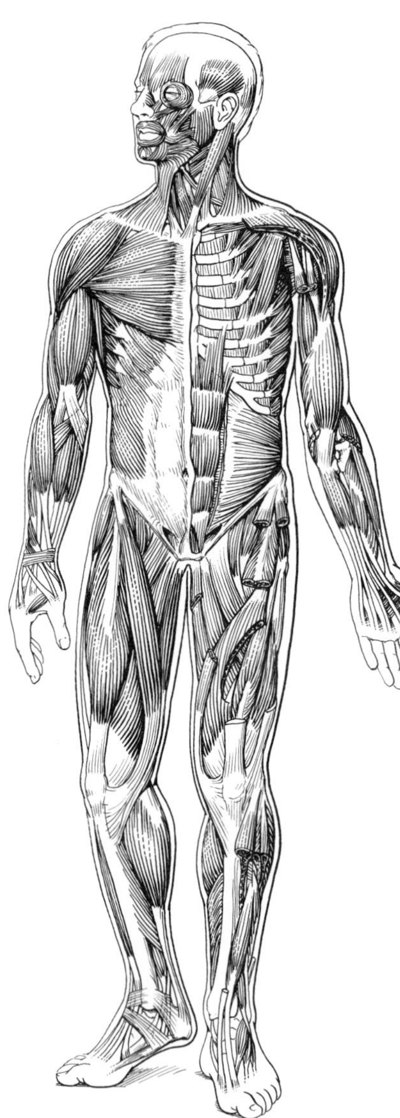

Many of your skeletal muscles are paired, enabling your body to move. Tendons connect skeletal muscles to your bones.

Components of your musculoskeletal system work together to keep the human body functioning. Here's a look at the various roles they play.

Bones

Your body houses 206 bones. They're composed of osseous tissue, which is made of various substances, including proteins, minerals and bone cells. The proteins form a framework into which minerals — especially calcium and phosphate — become incorporated.

Bone is made up of two types of tissue. The spongy inner layer is called cancellous bone. The hard outer layer is known as cortical bone.

Despite its stable appearance, bone is always changing in a process called remodeling. It's constantly being torn down by cells called osteoclasts, reabsorbed and then rebuilt by cells called osteoblasts.

Your bones provide support for your body and function as your body's storehouse for important minerals. Inside certain bones is the marrow, a soft core that manufactures blood cells.

Joints

The ends of bones that meet in a joint are cushioned with a layer of cartilage, which absorbs some of the shock or weight involved in movement.

Your joints also contain a liquid called synovial fluid, a membrane, a protective casing called the capsule and bands of fibrous tissue called ligaments. Ligaments join bones together and help make the joint stable.

Musculoskeletal Specialists

Several types of medical specialists deal with problems of the musculoskeletal system. These include rheumatologists, orthopedists, physiatrists and physical and occupational therapists.

Rheumatologists
A rheumatologist is a doctor who has special training in diagnosing and treating diseases of the muscles and joints, especially inflammatory or autoimmune illnesses, such as rheumatoid arthritis or lupus erythematosus.

Orthopedists
An orthopedist is a surgeon who has special training in managing disorders of the body's moving parts, including the skeleton, joints, muscles, ligaments and cartilage. An orthopedist may recommend nonsurgical or surgical treatment.

Physiatrists
A physiatrist is a specialist in physical medicine and rehabilitation — a doctor who is specially trained to help restore and maximize the function of injured or damaged joints, muscles and limbs. Physiatrists also teach methods to condition the musculoskeletal system and protect joints from further injury. Physiatrists provide nonsurgical management of musculoskeletal injuries and often work closely with physical and occupational therapists.

Physical therapists
A physical therapist is a licensed professional who designs programs — including therapeutic exercise and pain management strategies — to help in rehabilitation and recovery after an injury or illness. Physical therapists aren't medical doctors, and they can't prescribe medications.

Occupational therapists
An occupational therapist is a licensed professional who focuses on the function of the upper limbs. Often, occupational therapists work in collaboration with physical therapists. Occupational therapists offer training in how to perform daily tasks following an injury or illness that has impaired upper body movement.

Muscles

Some 650 muscles primarily help move your body. Your muscles are made of fibers that can contract, which enables them to shorten and lengthen, producing movement. Tendons connect your muscles to your bones.

Most muscles are paired with another muscle that works in opposition to it, such as the biceps and triceps muscles in your arm. When you bend your arm at the elbow, your biceps contract, and when you extend your arm, the opposing triceps contract.

Not all muscles move your skeleton. In addition to the skeletal (striated) muscles, you have smooth (nonstriated) muscles. You can find smooth muscles in internal organs, such as the stomach, uterus and bladder, and in the walls of blood vessels. They're usually arranged in sheets. Doctors call them involuntary muscles because they're under autonomic rather than conscious control. The heart (myocardium) is a special type of involuntary muscle. Smooth muscles and the heart muscle aren't part of the musculoskeletal system.

Common Injuries

Although the body's musculoskeletal system is extremely durable, muscle and bone injuries are common. A fall or an accident can stress and break a bone, overstretch muscles and extend a joint beyond its usual range of motion. Whether from falling out of the backyard apple tree as a child or tripping while playing tennis as an adult, most people experience a variety of musculoskeletal injuries during their lifetime.

Bone fracture

Signs and symptoms

- A swelling or bruising over a bone
- Deformity of a limb
- Localized pain that intensifies when the affected area is moved or pressed
- Loss of function in the area of the injury
- A bone that perforates the skin

When a bone can't withstand the physical force exerted on it, it breaks (fractures). Fractures are common. Most people sustain one or more during their lifetime.

Fractures can be classified into several categories. A simple fracture is one in which the bone breaks into two pieces. A comminuted fracture is one in which the bone fragments into several pieces. When the bone protrudes through the skin, it's called an open (compound) fracture (see page 362).

Fractures are also categorized according to the way the bone breaks. If the bone snaps completely into two or more parts, it's called a complete fracture. If the bone cracks but doesn't separate, it's an incomplete fracture. If one fragment of bone is embedded into another fragment of bone, it's called an impacted fracture.

Another type of fracture occurs in people with bones weakened by disease. When diseased, bones may fracture spontaneously or with only minor stress exerted on them. Such breaks are termed pathologic fractures because the principal cause is an underlying disease, such as osteoporosis or a cancer that has spread to the bone.

Severity of fractures often increases with age. Children's skeletons are flexible, so their bones are more likely to bend than to break. As a result, when a child fractures a bone, it's often an incomplete fracture. Conversely, falls or other accidents that generally don't affect younger bones can cause complete fractures in older adults, whose bones are more likely to be brittle.

A stress fracture, another type of break, is really a hairline crack that often is invisible on an X-ray for up to 6 weeks after the onset of pain.

When a bone breaks, damaged blood vessels between the ends of the broken bone will clot, which prevents further bleeding. Cells called osteoclasts reabsorb the damaged bone. A soft callus made of fibrous protein (collagen) develops as the bone begins to regenerate with the help of cells called osteoblasts. These cells build a mesh of spongy bone on the collagen, creating an internal splint that links the fractured bone ends. Eventually, this mesh is replaced by denser bone, resulting in a healed fracture.

Diagnosis

A bone protruding from the flesh makes the diagnosis obvious. In some instances, though, identifying a fracture isn't easy. Soft tissue injuries and fractures often produce similar signs and symptoms.

An X-ray taken from two or more angles helps confirm the diagnosis (see image on page 1273). In the case of suspected skull fracture or the fracture of a vertebra, a doctor may order a computerized tomography (CT) scan or magnetic resonance imaging (MRI). An MRI or

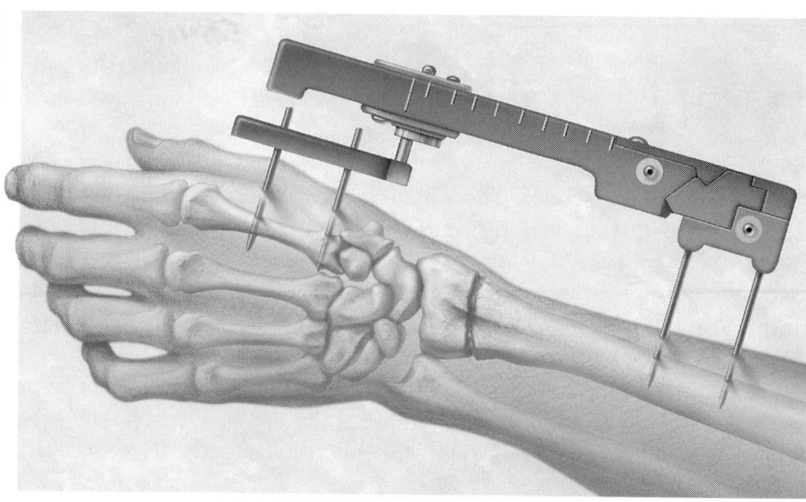

Some fractures heal best with pins inserted through the skin and into the fractured bone. The pins are attached to an external frame that holds the fracture in place while it heals.

bone scan is sometimes used to detect a stress fracture.

How serious is a bone fracture?

The seriousness of a bone fracture depends on the location of the break and the damage to the bone and adjacent tissues. Some fractures require only temporary protection, such as using crutches to bear weight or a splint to immobilize the broken bone. For more serious fractures, dangerous complications can occur if you don't receive medical treatment.

With any fracture, your doctor should examine the adjacent area carefully to establish if there's additional damage to nerves or blood vessels. Injuries to the skull or spine might put you at risk of brain injury or spinal cord damage.

The time it takes a broken bone to heal varies with the age and health of the person with the fracture and the nature and location of the fracture. In children, a minor break may heal within a few weeks. In older adults, a serious fracture often requires months to heal. Sometimes a fracture that's healing particularly slowly may require a procedure in which tissue taken from another bone is grafted onto the fracture to fill in bone and stimulate healing. The source of bone for a graft is often the pelvis (iliac bone). With prompt and proper treatment and a good rehabilitation program, you can usually expect a complete recovery.

Treatment

All suspected fractures should be treated with proper first aid and evaluated by a doctor. To heal properly, a bone that has been displaced must be put back (set) in its proper position. Setting (realignment) of the bone is called reduction. When this can be done without surgery, it's called a closed reduction. You're given an anesthetic to numb the area so that your doctor can reposition the bone using X-rays as a guide.

Surgery

When surgery is necessary to set or repair a fracture, the procedure is called an open reduction. You're given an anesthetic, and the doctor makes an incision to gain access to the broken bone so that it can be restored to its proper position.

A fracture that's unstable or one that's immediately adjacent to or extending into a joint may require a device such as a rod, pin, plate or screw to hold it in place. During a surgical procedure, an orthopedic surgeon fastens the device to the bone to position and stabilize the broken parts. Advantages of this approach include early mobility of the joint and some use of the injured limb within weeks rather than months.

In rare instances, it's better to insert an artificial joint, especially in an older adult with osteoporosis or another disorder that has led to deterioration of the bone or joint.

Casts and splints

If you have a broken arm or leg, your doctor may put a cast on it to immobilize it. Preventing motion between the two ends of the bone reduces pain and facilitates healing.

First, a layer of soft material is applied to cover your arm or leg, protecting the skin from irritation. Next, the arm or leg is covered with a layer of bandages saturated with plaster, fiberglass or plastic. As the cast dries, it becomes rigid. Be careful to avoid changing the cast's shape while it dries. Because flattening the cast can put pressure on your skin beneath the plaster, don't rest the cast on a flat surface. Use pillows instead.

Casts made of fiberglass or plastic — which are more commonly used today than plaster of Paris — dry more quickly and are lighter and stronger than those made of plaster.

For some fractures, a doctor may apply a splint. This device immobilizes and supports an injured, displaced or deformed limb or joint. Often, splints are used instead of a cast to prevent motion of a dislocated joint or of the ends of a fractured joint.

In some cases, no device is needed. The mass of chest muscles that surround a broken rib, for example, hold it in place. With a broken finger, your doctor may simply tape it to an adjacent finger.

Ultrasound

If a fracture isn't healing properly, your doctor may use low-intensity ultrasound, applied to the skin over a fracture through a wand-like transducer for about 20 minutes a day. The sound wave pulses jiggle the bone, a motion that is believed to promote healing.

Electromagnetic stimulation

Although controversial, electromagnetic stimulation may be another way to aid healing. An electromagnetic current is directed to the area over the fracture site for several hours a day. At the same time, a cast is usually worn for several months to stabilize the fracture. People with a fracture that fails to heal may opt for electromagnetic stimulation in the hopes of avoiding surgery.

Traction

Some femur fractures in children are treated with a mechanical system of weights that temporarily hold broken parts of the bones in the proper position. The force created by this system, called traction, is especially useful for fractures in which surrounding muscles tend to pull ends of the broken bone over one another.

Rehabilitation

After the bone has been set in its proper position and immobilized, the next step in treatment is rehabilitation. This process begins as soon as possible, even with the broken bone still in a cast.

A rehabilitation program generally follows the principle of relative rest, meaning the injured tissue rests while the rest of your body engages in exercise or activity. Movement of adjacent tissues increases blood flow, enhances healing and prevents the formation of potentially dangerous blood clots, which can form in the vessels of immobilized limbs. Movement also helps maintain muscle tone. And it can limit wasting (atrophy) of muscles and withering of bones from prolonged immobilization. Rehabilitation also helps prevent stiffness that can occur in unused joints.

Medication

In most cases, a doctor will prescribe medication to relieve pain and, on occasion, antibiotics to reduce the risk of infection.

Hip fracture

Signs and symptoms

- Severe pain in your hip or groin
- Inability to bear weight on your injured leg
- Bruising and swelling in and around your hip area
- Shorter leg on the side of your injured hip
- Turning inward or outward of your leg on the side of your injured hip

You can break your hip at any age, but 90 percent of hospitalizations for hip fractures are for people older than age 65. As you age, your bones slowly lose minerals and become less dense. Gradual loss of density weakens bones and makes them more likely to fracture.

More than 320,000 Americans are hospitalized each year because of a hip fracture. Doctors expect that number to grow as the U.S. population ages. If you're a woman, you're two to three times more likely than a man to fracture a hip. That's because women lose bone density at a greater rate than men do. The drop in estrogen levels in women during and after menopause accelerates bone loss and increases the risk of hip fractures.

The direct cause of a hip fracture often is an accident or a fall, even a relatively minor fall. The underlying cause, especially as you get older, is likely to be osteoporosis.

In osteoporosis, your bones don't contain adequate calcium and other minerals and your bone structure weakens. Loss of bone strength tends to be greatest in your spine, lower forearms and upper thighbones (femurs), the site of hip fractures.

Diagnosis

Often, your doctor can determine that you have a hip fracture based on a history of injury, your symptoms, and by observing the abnormal position of your hip and leg. An X-ray can confirm that you have a fracture and show exactly what part of your hip is fractured.

Ninety percent of hip fractures occur in one of two locations along your femur, the long bone that extends from your pelvis to your knee:

- *The femoral neck.* The femoral neck is located in the upper portion of your femur, the ball part of the ball-and-socket joint.
- *The intertrochanteric region.* This region is the portion of your upper femur that juts outward.

How serious is a hip fracture?
A hip fracture is a serious injury, particularly if you're older. Although the fracture itself is treatable, complications can be life-threatening, especially in older adults.

Doctors rarely treat unstable (displaced) hip fractures without surgery because bed rest or traction are associated with serious complications. The risk of traction is that it keeps you immobile for a long period, during which you can develop blood clots in one or both legs. You can also develop a blood clot in a leg after hip surgery, especially if you don't get up and move around. This blood clot can break off and travel to and become lodged in a lung artery, blocking blood flow to lung tissue. This condition, called pulmonary embolism, can be fatal unless treated promptly.

Fortunately, surgery to repair a hip fracture is usually very effective, although recovery often requires time and patience. Most people, even those older than age 80, make a good recovery from a hip fracture. Generally, the better your health and mobility, the better your chances for a full recovery.

Hip Fractures
Most hip fractures occur in one of two locations — the femoral neck or the intertrochanteric region.

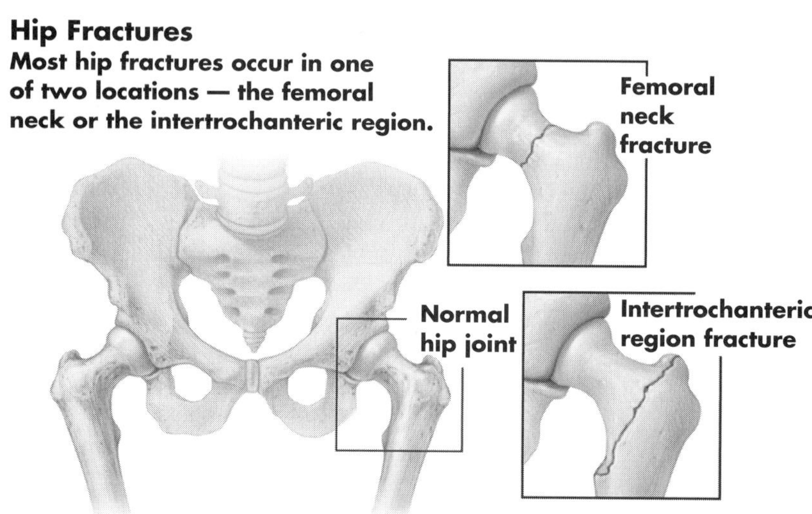

Hip Fracture Repair Techniques
For a fracture in the femoral neck, partial hip replacement or internal fixation may be used. A hip compression screw may be used for a fracture in the intertrochanteric region.

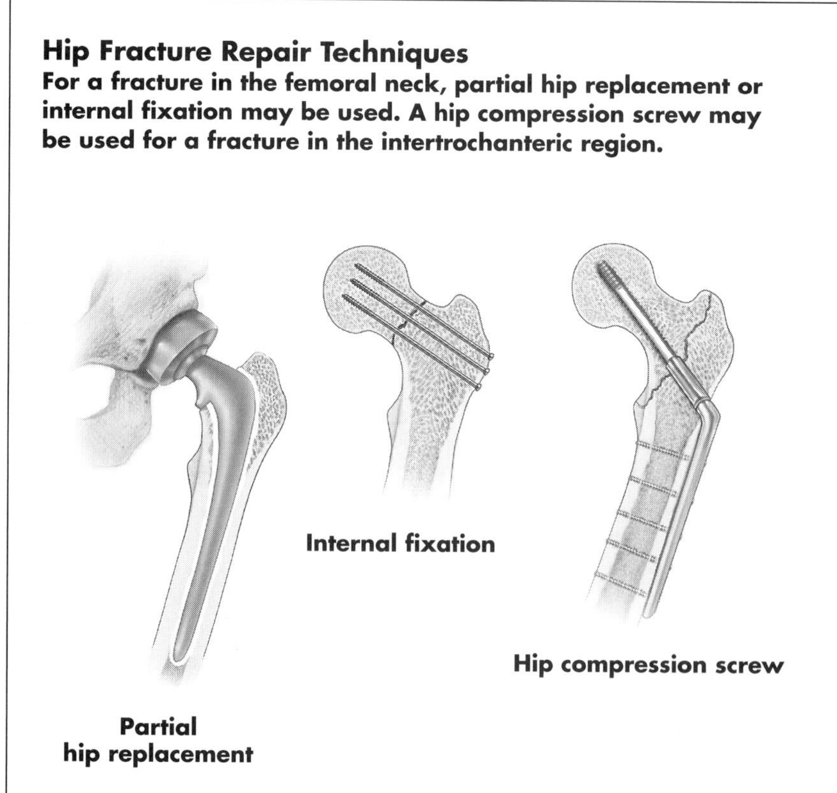

Treatment

Surgery is almost always the best way to repair a broken hip. Doctors typically use nonsurgical alternatives only if the fracture is stable or you have other medical problems that make surgery too risky. The type of surgery you have generally depends on the nature and severity of the hip fracture and your age.

Femoral neck fractures

Surgeons generally repair this type of fracture by one of three methods:

- *Internal fixation.* If, following the break, bones can be properly aligned, your doctor may insert metal screws or a plate and screws into the bone to hold it together while the fracture heals. This is called internal fixation.
- *Partial hip replacement.* If the ends of the broken bone are severely damaged and the blood supply to the femoral head is compromised, your doctor may remove the head of the femur and replace it with a metal prosthesis. This is known as hemi-arthroplasty.
- *Total hip replacement.* This procedure involves replacing your upper femur and the socket in your pelvic bone with artificial prostheses. Total hip replacement

Hip Protectors

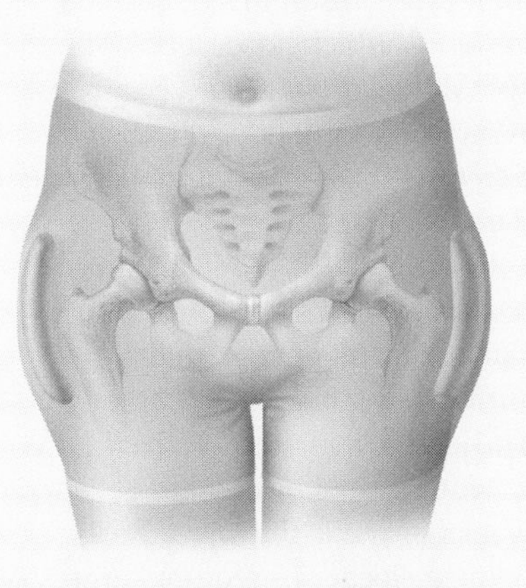

An effective step that won't prevent you from falling but may protect you if you do is to wear a hip protector. These padded, externally worn protectors are similar to what hockey players wear to avoid injury. One study involving active older adults found that wearing hip protectors reduced the risk of a hip fracture from a fall by more than 60 percent.

The protectors are small enough that they can be worn under a skirt or pants, and they don't limit activity such as walking or sitting.

is a common operation to treat severe arthritis of the hip joint, but it's rarely used to treat a hip fracture.

In general, the more complex the fracture and the older you are, the more likely you are to receive a hip prosthesis. Internal fixation is used more in younger people and for fractures that are less complex and well aligned.

Intertrochanteric region fractures
To repair this type of fracture, a doctor usually inserts a metal plate and screw device (compression hip screw) to fix the fracture. The screw is attached to a plate that runs down alongside the femur and is attached with other screws to help keep the bone stable. As the bone heals, the screw allows the bone pieces to compress, so the edges grow together.

Recovery
Recovering from a hip fracture involves a lengthy period of rehabilitation. The goal of rehabilitation is to help you regain full mobility. You'll learn how to gradually place more weight on your hip until it can bear your full weight. You'll also learn how to sit, stand and walk so that you don't re-injure your hip or damage your prosthesis, if you have one.

Following a hip fracture, you'll likely need the help of a walking aid, such as a cane, walker or crutches, for several months. You may also need help getting around your home and doing daily tasks. About half of people older than age 65 who break a hip enter an extended-care facility for at least part of their recuperation because they need assistance that's unavailable at home.

Prevention
These steps can help you guard against hip fracture by reducing your risk of falls:

- *Fall-proof your home.* Keep your home well lit and free of situations that might cause you to trip and fall. Avoid area rugs and exposed electrical cords. Place furniture where you're unlikely to bump into it. Consider installing grab bars in your bathroom, stair treads on steps and handrails along stairways.
- *Wear sensible shoes.* If you're older, wear thinner, hard-soled, flat shoes. Resilient-soled athletic shoes may impair your balance and contribute to falls. Avoid wearing high heels or sandals with light straps. Avoid wearing shoes that are either too slippery or too sticky.
- *Avoid dangerous activities.* Be careful doing tasks that require you to climb a ladder or stepladder. Ask for help. Avoid lifting heavy objects, climbing and engaging in unusually vigorous activities.
- *See your eye doctor.* Poor eyesight is a common cause of falls. If you're having trouble seeing, have your eyes checked. Wearing proper glasses and being able to see well around your home makes it more likely that you'll see objects that you might trip over.
- *Be mindful of medication side effects.* Feeling weak or dizzy is a side effect of many medications. This can increase your risk of falling. Talk to your doctor about possible side effects caused by your medications.

Joint dislocation

Signs and symptoms

- A joint that slips out of place after being subjected to a blow, fall or other trauma
- Swelling, intense pain and, frequently, immobility of the affected joint

A joint dislocates when the ends of bones are forced from their normal positions. As a result, the joint no longer functions properly. In addition, the displaced bones may damage the structure in or around

Nursemaid's Elbow

Nursemaid's elbow is a common and often misdiagnosed dislocation of the elbow. It typically occurs in children younger than age 5, usually when an adult or another child pulls or jerks a child's arm. The immature elbow dislocates easily because it can't withstand the stress.

The child typically experiences pain and limited mobility in the elbow. An X-ray may be taken to rule out any other problems. When the bones are returned to their proper position, the pain resolves.

the joint, including muscles, ligaments, nerves and blood vessels.

In some cases, the cause of a dislocation is an underlying disease or disorder, such as rheumatoid arthritis or a defective ligament. Some people who sustain repeated dislocations have such a congenital weakness, which may allow some joints to dislocate spontaneously.

Diagnosis

After you sustain a dislocation, it becomes difficult, if not impossible, to move your joint. Trying to move it is likely to intensify the pain. Usually, you can see a change in the alignment of the joint and there's swelling.

If your doctor suspects a dislocation, an X-ray usually helps him or her confirm the diagnosis and determine if you also have an accompanying fracture.

How serious is a joint dislocation?

It depends on which joint is affected. A serious neck or back injury may result in a dislocated vertebra, which poses a risk of spinal cord damage and paralysis. A serious shoulder or hip dislocation can possibly result in nerve damage.

In many cases, a doctor can correct a simple dislocation nonsurgically without damage to the surrounding nerves and tissues. The joint is then immobilized for a short time — typically about 2 weeks — while the injury heals. Some dislocations require surgery to repair or reconstruct damaged ligaments.

Treatment

Any suspected dislocation should be examined by a doctor. If you suspect someone has a dislocated vertebra because of a serious neck or back injury, don't move the injured person. Wait for emergency medical personnel to arrive.

A dislocation usually needs treatment as quickly as possible. The displaced bones in the joint must be returned to their proper position by a procedure called reduction. If the injury remains untreated for more than half an hour, increased swelling and pain often makes it more difficult to reduce the dislocation.

Immobilize the affected area and transport the injured person to a doctor or hospital emergency room. It's important that only a person with proper training provides treatment because improper attempts at repositioning the joint can cause additional damage to the joint and adjacent structures.

Immobilization

After a joint has been returned to its normal position, it may be necessary to immobilize it. Most often a splint is used.

Rehabilitation

Rehabilitation begins after the joint is back in its proper position and immobilized, even if the joint is in a cast. Movement stimulates blood flow in adjacent tissues and enhances the healing process.

Absence or Loss of a Limb

Some people are born without one or more of their limbs, generally because of a developmental defect. Other individuals lose a limb because of an injury or disease. Doctors perform surgical amputations for a variety of reasons. Some people with advanced diabetes develop poor circulation in their extremities that can result in ulcers and gangrene and necessitate amputation of a foot or leg.

The best treatment for certain bone cancers may require amputation of an arm or leg. Removing a limb through amputation is a major operation. In addition to drawing on the body's healing capacity, an amputation also requires significant psychological adjustment — learning to live with altered physical capacities and an altered body image.

Risks

Amputation that results from an accident has additional risks, including blood loss and shock. As with any invasive procedure, there's also the risk of infection, which is greater if a limb is severed in an accident than if it's removed surgically.

In most cases, though, an amputation isn't life-threatening. The biggest challenge often is dealing with the consequences of the amputation, which range from coping with the pain of the surgery to making major adjustments to your lifestyle.

Surgical removal of a body part can also be emotionally demanding. There may be pain in the residual limb or the sensation that the limb or part of the limb is still present (phantom limb sensation). In addition, amputation can affect an individual's self-image, self-confidence and sense of self-worth.

Reattaching a severed body part

Surgeons have made remarkable advances in recent years in reattaching severed fingers, hands and even limbs. With the help of a microscope, surgical repairs and reattachments of tiny structures, such as blood vessels and nerves, are possible. The results depend on many factors, but tend to be more successful for hand or finger reattachments than for arms, and more successful for arms than for legs.

If the severed body part has had proper care and a trained surgeon is readily available, chances of a successful reattachment are good. The function of the reattached finger, hand or limb varies from person to

Movement also helps maintain muscle tone and limits the wasting of muscles and weakening of bone from prolonged immobilization. It also helps prevent the joint stiffness that extended disuse may cause.

Be sure to follow your doctor's advice about limiting physical activity of the affected joint. Returning to full activity too soon increases your risk of re-injuring the joint.

Medication

To manage the pain, your doctor may recommend that you take a pain reliever.

Severed tendon

Signs and symptoms

- A deep cut in a hand, foot, forearm or calf
- An inability to move a finger, toe or whatever joint is near the cut

A deep cut in a hand, foot, forearm or calf can damage tendons, the fibrous tissues that connect muscle to bone. Severing a tendon may result in an inability to move the affected joint.

A severed tendon requires two kinds of attention. First, the wound must be closed to aid healing and prevent infection. Second, the tendon must be repaired surgically. Sometimes, both can be done in one procedure, when the wound is treated. However, in some cases, the cut should heal before an operation to repair a tendon is performed. Generally, reattachment is done within a week of the injury.

Diagnosis

The key sign suggesting a severed tendon is an inability to move a finger, toe or other joint in the area of an injury. Your doctor may want an X-ray of the affected area in case you also have a fracture.

How serious is a severed tendon?

In most cases, timely repair of a severed tendon allows the affected area to return to nearly normal. However, you may experience stiffness and a decrease in the range of movement of a related joint.

Treatment

A severed tendon usually requires surgery and rehabilitation.

Surgery

When a tendon is severed, one part may retract and be difficult for a surgeon to retrieve. As a result, a long surgical incision may be required. In some instances, doctors use tissue from another tendon to repair the damaged one.

Rehabilitation

Following an operation, the area you've injured probably will be immobilized. Your doctor may recommend an exercise program when it's time for you to resume physical activity.

Doctors often recommend passive exercise during the recovery period to help prevent long-term stiffness. These exercises involve movements that place minimal stress on the injured tendon.

person. In some instances, the reattached part regains most or all of its usefulness. In others, sensitivity, flexibility and strength remain impaired.

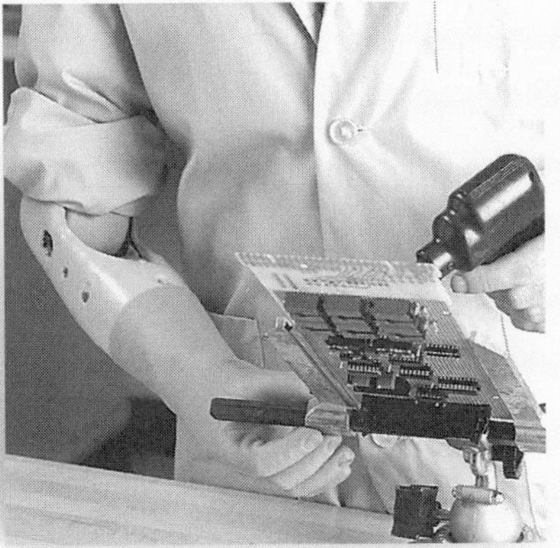

Use of a prosthesis

If a severed limb can't be reattached or if your limb is amputated due to disease, a replacement part (prosthesis) is generally the next best option. A prosthesis can never replicate the movement, flexibility, strength and sensitivity of your original body part. Yet once you adjust to it, a prosthesis can help you live more fully.

As the surgical wounds heal, exercises are important for keeping your remaining muscles in condition and your joints mobile. Then the process of fitting you for a prosthesis begins, starting with a temporary one. A training process helps you master the different movements involved in using the prosthesis.

Gradually, you'll be able to wear the prosthesis all day. After you've adjusted to the temporary prosthesis, a specially designed prosthesis can be fabricated. A permanent prosthesis is tailored to meet your specific needs. It can strike a balance between physical demands for mobility and strength and concern with appearance.

In general, leg prostheses work better than arm prostheses. A person with a prosthetic leg is more likely to use his or her prosthesis than is someone with a prosthetic arm.

Rehabilitation

Following an amputation, a doctor or physical therapist can outline a program of rehabilitation. Frequently, it's a team approach that involves physical and occupational therapists under the guidance of a physiatrist, a physician who specializes in physical medicine and rehabilitation.

The goal of rehabilitation is to help you achieve as normal a life as possible. The program may include exercises to help you maintain or increase the strength of your remaining muscles. If you need a prosthesis or other equipment, the program may include additional exercises. Other components generally include counseling, detailed instruction on proper use of a prosthesis and learning new ways to perform daily tasks.

Sports Injuries

Most injuries that occur during athletic activity result from unusual demands placed on bones, muscles or other tissues. A novice runner who completes 5 miles the first day will likely have undreamed-of aches and pains the next morning. The over-40 former athlete who comes out of retirement for the company softball game is an excellent candidate for sprains and strains.

You can't expect to go through life without injury. However, a few sensible rules will help you avoid inconvenient, painful, expensive and, at times, disabling injuries.

Warm up first

Give your muscles a chance to warm up before you exercise. Before you start running, for instance, walk or march in place for 5 minutes and then stretch your muscles for another 5 minutes. Don't stretch cold muscles before warming them up. The increased blood flow reduces tension in your muscles, improves their range of motion and flexibility and may even increase your level of performance. This reduces your risk of muscle strains and other injuries.

Cool down afterward

It's just as important to cool down your muscles after a workout as it is to warm them up before you exercise. The muscles you use contract during a workout, and repetitive activities can cause them to shorten. Stretching after the workout is critical for maintaining flexibility.

Muscles that aren't kept flexible through stretching are more likely to sustain strains.

Pace yourself

Sudden and unfamiliar exertion increases the risk of injuries. If you want to improve your performance, do so at a sensible pace. Don't increase your distance or the duration of your exercise by more than 10 percent a week. Develop a program that allows your body to adjust gradually to the challenges you're giving it.

Select an appropriate activity

If you have a painful back or perpetually sore knees, the pounding of running isn't for you. You might try swimming or riding a stationary bicycle instead. Whatever activity you choose, make sure your technique is as good as possible. Take lessons and have an expert watch you perform. Imperfect technique and overuse often lead to injury.

Make it a habit

Working out only once a week, no matter how vigorous the activity, fails to provide you with maximal aerobic and conditioning benefits and puts you at risk of injury. Try to establish a schedule of at least 30 minutes of activity most days of the week. And keep this advice in mind: Don't play your sport to get in shape. Get in shape to play your sport.

Give injuries their due

If you do sprain an ankle or twist a knee, get medical advice. Then follow it. A key to recovery is what doctors commonly refer to as the tincture of time. Allow the injury to heal before you use that body part too vigorously. Make sure the injury is properly rehabilitated and ready to withstand the stresses of your sport or activity.

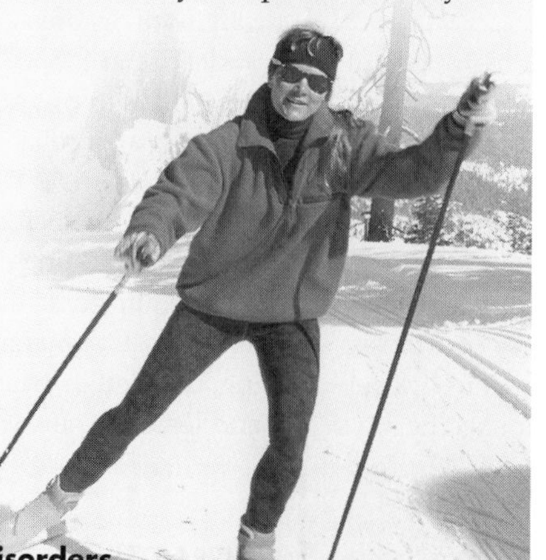

Muscle strain

Signs and symptoms

- Localized pain when a muscle injury occurs, followed by tenderness and possibly swelling
- Stiffness or tenderness a day after you overwork the muscles in an area of your body
- An inability to use the muscle

Excessive demand on a muscle may strain it. This is also known as a pulled muscle. Overstretching or overworking a certain area of your body may cause minor muscle strains. The muscle doesn't lose strength, but it's sore.

A more serious muscle strain occurs when some of the fibers of a muscle actually tear, causing your muscle to contract and bleed internally. Occasionally, the muscle may rupture, either partially or, in rare instances, entirely.

One of the most common muscle strains occurs in the group of muscles at the back of the thigh (the hamstrings), especially in people who run or water-ski.

The hamstrings enable you to flex your knee and extend your thigh, motions used in running. Pain or muscle weakness at the back of your thigh may indicate an injury to your hamstrings.

A second common muscle injury is a groin pull. When you sustain a groin pull, the tendons and muscles in your groin — including the lower abdominal, leg and pelvic muscles — may be stretched or torn. This may result from repetitive overuse or a single injury and cause pain or muscle spasms in the groin area.

Diagnosis

Discomfort in the involved area, which may include tenderness, muscle spasms and swelling, is the key to diagnosis. An X-ray can rule out bone injury as a cause of the problem.

How serious is a muscle strain?

Muscle strains often respond well to rest and simple self-care measures. However, if you suspect that a muscle has ruptured or that a bone is fractured, or if the pain persists for more than a few days, see a doctor.

Treatment

Apply ice or cold packs to the injured area for about 20 minutes at a time several times a day for the first 48 hours after injury. You may be able to prevent or reduce swelling by elevating the injured limb and using a compression wrap such as an elastic bandage. Don't bind it tightly. Try not to use the injured muscle until the pain subsides.

Medication

For minor muscle pulls, acetaminophen (Tylenol, others) or an over-the-counter nonsteroidal anti-inflammatory drug (NSAID), such as ibuprofen (Advil, Motrin, others) or aspirin, may help reduce the pain. Use aspirin only if there's no sign of bleeding. For moderate or more severe muscle strains, your doctor may prescribe an anti-inflammatory drug, a muscle relaxant or a prescription pain reliever, depending on the injury.

Surgery

If the injury is severe enough to rupture the muscle, surgical repair is usually needed.

Prevention

You can avoid many muscle strains with appropriate conditioning that includes warming up before exercising and stretching afterward. If you experience recurrent muscle pulls, then you may benefit from a program of muscle development to strengthen weak muscles.

Heat vs. Cold

After you sprain a ligament or strain a muscle, it's best to use cold treatment for 1 to 3 days after the injury to reduce swelling and inflammation. Swelling damages cells by decreasing the oxygen supply to surrounding tissues. Cold applications slow metabolism of cells within the area and allow the tissue to survive a temporary lack of oxygen. This promotes the renewal or repair of cells and speeds healing. Cold also constricts blood vessels to minimize bleeding and relieves pain by acting as a local anesthetic. Most bleeding associated with acute inflammation resolves within 1 to 3 days.

To relieve muscle spasms, minor sprains and strains, apply cold treatment intermittently for 24 to 72 hours. After this time period, some people find that heat lessens pain from the injury and improves stiffness. If you try heat, apply it only after swelling and bleeding have stopped. The heat may complicate your early recovery by causing more swelling and bleeding. For chronic symptoms, use either heat or ice, whichever feels better.

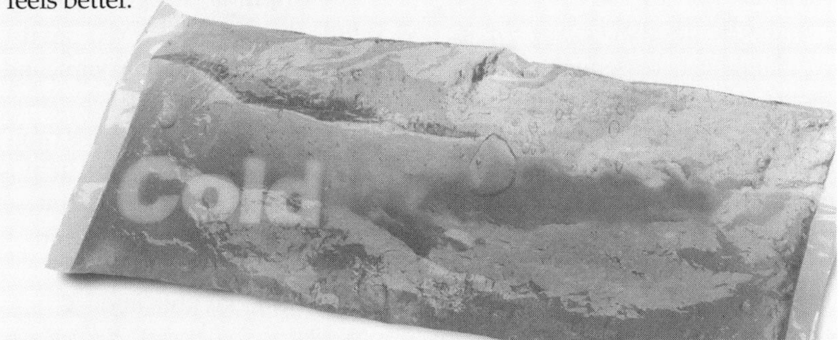

Sprain

Signs and symptoms

- Rapid swelling, sometimes accompanied by discoloration of the skin
- Impaired joint function or a feeling of instability
- Pain and tenderness in the affected area
- An audible popping sound
- Difficulty using the joint

A wide range of injuries are referred to as sprains, but a true sprain involves damage to the ligaments, the tough bands of connective tissue that attach bone to bone in a joint. Sprains most commonly occur in the ankles and knees.

A sprain occurs when a traumatic event, such as a fall, stumble or collision, causes your joint to move beyond its normal range of movement and a ligament stretches or tears.

Diagnosis

You can sprain any joint. With a sprain, the joint may be able to function or may feel unstable. Movement and pressure over the ligament are painful.

If the joint can't function, the injury may also involve a fracture or dislocation. If you suspect a

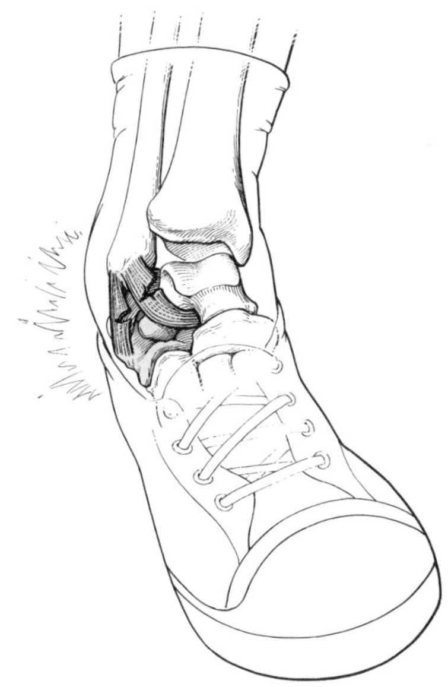

An ankle sprain occurs when ligaments that support your ankle stretch or tear. The anterior talofibular ligament (see highlighting) is the one most likely to be injured.

PRICE

If you sustain a minor soft-tissue injury, remember these words — *protection, rest, ice, compression, elevation* — and their acronym, *PRICE.* PRICE is a self-help treatment that can help speed your recovery. Follow these steps:

Protection
Immobilize the affected area to promote healing and protect it from further injury. Use elastic wraps, slings, splints, crutches or canes as necessary.

Rest
Avoid activities that cause pain or swelling. Rest is essential to promote tissue healing in the injured body part, but try to keep uninjured body parts moving and active to prevent significant deconditioning.

Ice
To decrease pain, swelling or muscle spasm, immediately apply ice to the injured area. Ice packs, slush baths and ice massage to smaller areas of injury are all useful. Reapply ice periodically as long as the swelling lasts.

Compression
Swelling can result in loss of motion in an injured joint. To control swelling, compress the injured area with wraps or elastic bandages until the swelling has stopped.

Elevation
Raise the swollen arm or leg above the level of your heart, to reduce swelling. This is especially important at night.

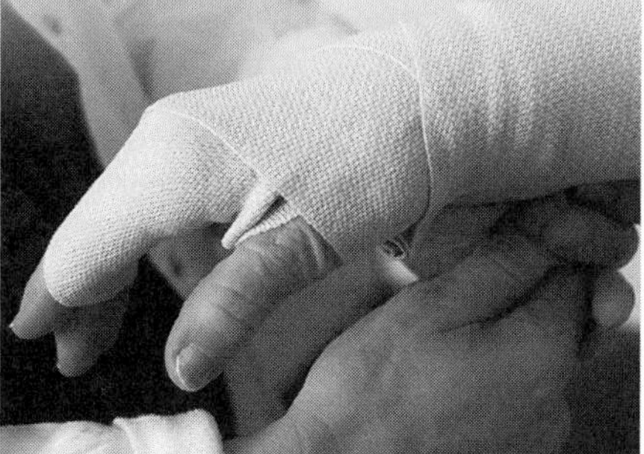

fracture or serious ligament damage in the joint — or if the pain and your difficulty in moving the joint don't go away within 2 or 3 days — seek medical care. Your doctor may order an X-ray to check for a fracture.

How serious is a sprain?
In general, the greater the pain, the more serious the injury. Sprains range in severity from minor to severe.

- *Mild sprain.* A mild sprain occurs when fibers within ligaments overstretch or tear slightly. You may feel minor to considerable pain and tenderness when you touch or move the joint. There's little or no swelling. You can usually put weight on the joint, and X-rays are normal.

  Repeated minor sprains can lead to a weakened joint. In most cases, a mildly sprained joint will be able to bear weight within approximately 24 hours and be fully healed within about 2 weeks.
- *Moderate sprain.* When ligament fibers tear without rupturing completely, you have a moderate sprain. Pain and tenderness are moderate, but you may hesitate to use the injured part because of a feeling of instability. You may experience some swelling and black-and-blue discoloration.
- *Severe sprain.* If one or more ligaments tear completely, you have a severe sprain. The area is painful, swollen and black-and-blue. You can't move your joint normally or stress it. If you try to use it, the joint may feel or be unstable.

Treatment
For a simple sprain, apply ice during the first 24 hours after the injury to reduce swelling. Support the joint with a supportive wrap such as an elastic bandage and rest it in an elevated position.

Slowly resume normal activity, testing the injured joint gradually after a day or more has passed.

Medication
You may want to take acetaminophen (Tylenol, others) for pain or a nonsteroidal anti-inflammatory drug (NSAID), such as ibuprofen (Advil, Motrin, others), to relieve pain accompanied by swelling. Be aware, however, that use of aspirin and many other NSAIDs may increase bleeding because they affect platelet function.

Surgery
If your sprain is serious enough that the joint is unstable, you may need an operation to repair ligaments that are torn or detached from the bone. Your doctor may also elect to immobilize the area of the sprained joint in a cast or splint. Be sure to follow your doctor's advice on rehabilitation. This may involve a supervised physical therapy program and an exercise program to strengthen the muscles surrounding the sprained joint.

Prevention
Taping, bracing or wrapping knees, ankles, wrists or elbows hasn't been shown to effectively prevent a sprain, but these tools may be used in rehabilitating injuries. Exercises, especially stability training, are critical for strengthening muscles weakened by recurrent injury and for stabilizing a joint to help prevent recurrent injury.

Shin splints

Signs and symptoms
- Pain over the front part of the leg above the ankle and below the knee
- Occasionally, swelling

Pain on the front, inside portion of the tibia, the large bone of your lower leg, may be the result of shin splints. Shin splints occur when fibers of the membrane that ties muscles to the front and side of your tibia become irritated and inflamed, producing pain and occasional swelling. Often, shin splints occur when you stress and overload the inner portion of the tibia,

Neck Pain

Your neck supports a weight equivalent to that of a bowling ball year after year. No wonder it occasionally becomes stiff and sore.

When your neck muscles stiffen and movement becomes painful, your muscles automatically tense to prevent further movement. But tense neck muscles can cause painful spasms, strain your ligaments and cause radiating pain.

Sometimes, tight neck muscles can irritate or impinge on scalp (occipital) nerves that are in close proximity to the muscles. This can cause pain to radiate up the back of the neck, behind an ear and to the side of the scalp, a condition called occipital neuralgia. To combat a flare-up of neck pain, try the following approaches.

Medication

Acetaminophen (Tylenol, others) or a nonsteroidal anti-inflammatory drug (NSAID), such as aspirin, ibuprofen (Advil, Motrin, others) or naproxen (Aleve, Anaprox, others), may provide temporary relief.

Rest

Lie down during the day to ease neck strain. But avoid prolonged inactivity. It can increase stiffness.

Cold and heat

A cold pack often dulls the pain for the first day or two. Apply a cold pack to the back of your neck several times a day for 20 minutes or less each time. After that, use either heat or cold to relieve discomfort. Don't use cold or hot packs if you have severe heart or circulation problems.

Exercises

Certain exercises can help you maintain proper posture and reduce neck pain and stiffness. Exercises can also improve your overall fitness, which may help prevent recurrence of neck pain. Try the following:

- *Shoulder squeeze.* Squeeze your shoulder blades together and hold for about 3 seconds. Repeat as often as is comfortable.
- *Shoulder shrug.* Gently raise your shoulders tightly to your neck, hold for 5 to 10 seconds, then slowly relax to a normal position.
- *Seated rowing.* Sit on the floor or on a stool or weight bench and pull your arms back and forth in a rowing motion.
- *Fly.* Grasp light dumbbells (1 to 2 pounds), bend forward at your hips keeping your back straight and let your arms hang straight down. Gently raise and lower the weights as if you were flying. If you can't keep your back straight, lie on your stomach on a table or weight bench.

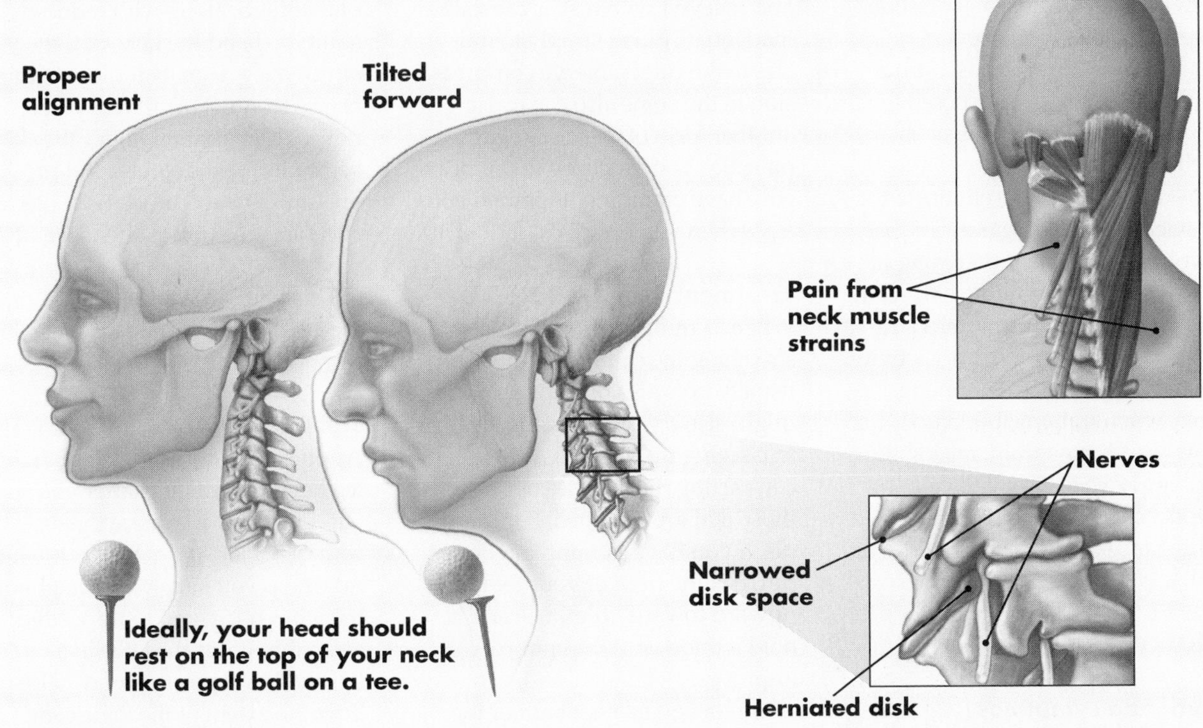

A variety of factors can cause neck pain, including improper alignment, muscle strains, narrowed disk spaces, herniated disks and pinched nerves.

but the stress isn't enough to cause a stress fracture. Doctors call this condition medial tibia stress syndrome.

Shin splints usually result from repeated pounding on hard surfaces during activities such as running, marching for long periods or playing basketball, soccer or tennis.

Diagnosis

In addition to examining your leg, your doctor may order an X-ray to check for a hairline crack of the tibia or a magnetic resonance imaging (MRI) scan or bone scan to rule out a stress fracture.

Treatment

Similar to other minor musculoskeletal injuries, shin splints are treated with rest and ice. Acetaminophen (Tylenol, others) or an over-the-counter anti-inflammatory medication may help reduce pain.

Other therapies

In some cases, putting a soft insert in your shoe can reduce some of the shock during vigorous physical activity. Your doctor may prescribe a specially fabricated device (orthotic) if your foot has a structural factor that's predisposed to injury, such as an excessively high arch or a flatfoot.

You may be able to eliminate the problem by avoiding exercise that involves a persistent pounding of the legs, such as running or basketball, for 2 weeks to 2 months and substituting a lower impact activity, such as bicycling or swimming. Also, when training, build up slowly and cross-train, mixing the low-impact exercise with your impact exercise. Avoid adding time or distance to your routine too quickly.

Muscle cramp

Signs and symptoms

- A sudden and sharp muscle pain, often in the legs
- A lump of muscle tissue visible beneath the skin

A cramp — sometimes called a charley horse — is actually a spasm in which a muscle contracts, producing sudden and intense pain. A common variety of muscle cramp occurs in your calf muscles during sleep. Overuse of a muscle, dehydration, injury, muscle strain or simply holding a position for prolonged periods may result in a muscle cramp. Athletes who become fatigued and dehydrated while participating in warm-weather sports frequently develop muscle cramps.

How serious is a muscle cramp?

Almost everyone experiences a muscle cramp at some time. For most people, cramps are only an occasional inconvenience. For some individuals, though, muscle cramps, especially at night, are recurrent and severe. If you experience frequent and severe cramps that interfere with sleep, consult a doctor.

Intermittent claudication, a distinct form of cramp-like discomfort in the legs associated with exercise and relieved with rest, is caused by inadequate blood supply to muscles in the calves. Nerve compression in the spine also can cause another form of exercise-related pain. See your doctor if you repeatedly have cramping or pain in your legs when you exercise.

Treatment

When a cramp occurs, gently stretching the contracted muscle usually provides prompt relief. You might also try compressing and massaging the affected muscle or contracting the muscles opposite those that are cramped. For example, if you have a cramp in your calf, flex the front of your foot upward toward your knee and hold it there until the cramp improves.

Immersion in a hot bath or the use of a heating pad may provide relief. Cold packs also may reduce muscle spasm or relax a tense muscle.

If recurrent cramps disturb your sleep, your doctor may prescribe a medication to relax your muscles and help you sleep.

Prevention

To reduce risk of muscle cramps, drink plenty of water to avoid dehydration, warm up before your workouts, cool down afterward and don't overfatigue your muscles. If you get cramps at night, stretch your legs before going to bed.

Thigh bruise

Signs and symptoms

- Sudden pain and tenderness in the muscles at the front of the thigh from a blow to the thigh
- Discomfort aggravated by movement

Physical contact can cause you to bruise the muscles on the front of your thigh that allow you to extend your leg at the knee (quadriceps).

Diagnosis

Pain and swelling of the front part of the thigh, along with reduced ability to bend the knee of the affected leg, usually indicate a thigh bruise (contusion). Often, you'll notice discoloration under the skin, beginning with redness and progressing to the characteristic black-and-blue of a bruise after several days.

This injury may take a week or months to heal. X-rays can rule out a bone fracture.

Treatment

Applying ice to the bruise with the leg bent immediately after you sustain the injury may ease the discomfort. Short-term use of crutches may help you keep your weight off the injured leg, and a supportive wrap that holds the knee in a tightly flexed position may help limit the extent of the injury and speed recovery. Supportive wraps or tape can provide some protection when you resume normal activities.

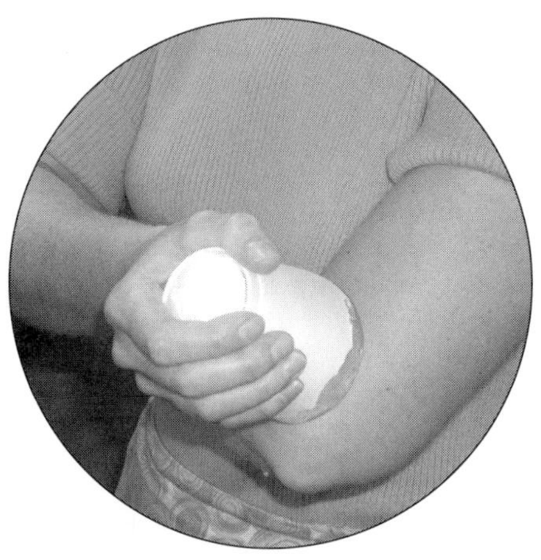

To help relieve pain, freeze water in a Styrofoam cup, peel away the top of the cup and rub the ice over the affected area.

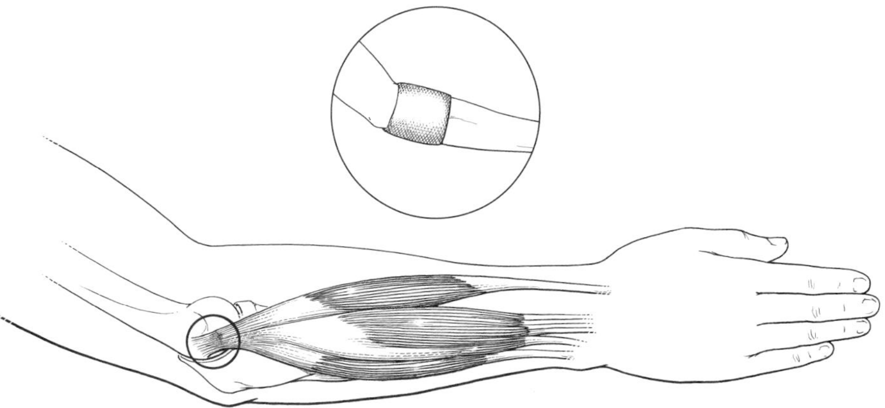

Tennis elbow produces pain on the outside of your forearm near your elbow when you exercise the joint. Tiny tears in tendon tissue cause the discomfort (see small circle). In some cases, you can get relief from a forearm support band (see inset) worn just below your elbow.

Tennis elbow

Signs and symptoms

- Recurrent pain on the outside of the upper forearm below the crease of the elbow
- Sometimes, pain extending down the forearm toward the wrist

Tennis elbow is a misnomer because you don't have to play tennis to experience it. Both tennis elbow and a related ailment called Little League elbow are pains that likely result from repeated, tiny tears in the tendons that attach the muscles of your lower arm at the elbow.

The tears can result from a wide variety of activities that involve a repeated rotary motion of the forearm and repeated wrist movement. Hitting a backhand in tennis, painting a house or twisting a screwdriver all can precipitate tennis elbow. Little League elbow usually affects the inside of the elbow in youngsters and is often brought on by the strain of throwing a baseball.

In adults, tendinitis over the inside of the elbow is called golfer's elbow because a golf swing, especially with improper technique, may strain these tendons.

Diagnosis

To rule out other possible causes of your symptoms, your doctor may order an X-ray of the painful area.

How serious is tennis elbow?

In most cases, the discomfort of tennis elbow improves in 6 to 12 weeks. Youngsters with Little League elbow shouldn't use the arm in ways that cause pain because doing so can injure the growth plate.

Treatment

Apply ice to the injured elbow. One way to do this is to freeze water in a Styrofoam cup, peel away the top of the cup, exposing the ice, and then rub the ice over the affected area.

Massaging the area, stretching the forearm muscles and taking a break from the activity that provoked the condition also are appropriate. Depending on the severity of your injury, your doctor may refer you to a physical therapist.

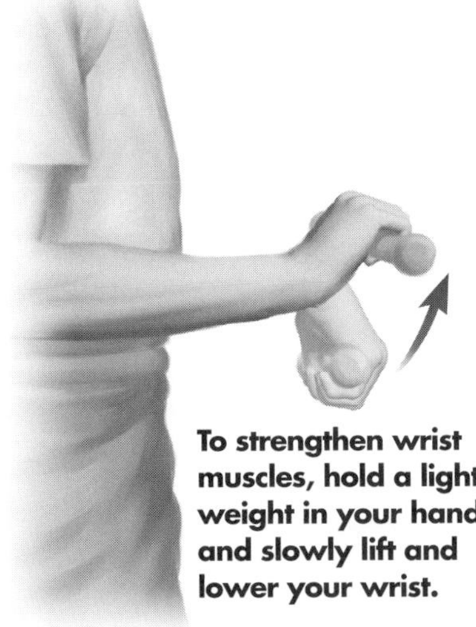

To strengthen wrist muscles, hold a light weight in your hand and slowly lift and lower your wrist.

Exercise

Exercise can strengthen the wrist muscles to speed healing and may prevent a recurrence. Once the pain has subsided, you can do strengthening exercises with a light hand weight. Holding the weight in your hand, with your elbow bent and your palm down, lift and slowly lower your wrist.

Medication

Acetaminophen (Tylenol, others) or an over-the-counter nonsteroidal anti-inflammatory drug (NSAID) can reduce the pain of tennis elbow. In certain cases, your doctor may inject a corticosteroid drug into the painful area to help reduce the swelling.

Prevention

To avoid recurring episodes of tennis elbow, pay special attention to your technique when engaging in the particular activity that provoked the injury. A stable wrist position in sports and other activities is critical.

Baseball finger

Signs and symptoms

- Swelling and pain in the last joint of a finger
- An inability to straighten a finger

Rehabilitation from an Athletic Injury

The goal of a sports rehabilitation program is to return the injured athlete to normal physical activity, good health and full function. Various factors, including your age, level of physical activity, body structure and conditioning program at the time of injury, influence the approach of rehabilitation and determine how quickly you'll recover from the injury.

The rehabilitative process generally has four stages. Skipping any of them may put you at risk of re-injury or prolong your recovery.

Stage 1

Stage 1 involves controlling the inflammation and pain of the acute injury, usually through PRICE — protection, rest, ice, compression and elevation.

Stage 2

Stage 2 involves restoring the full range of motion to the injured joint. A physical therapist may recommend exercises that you can do alone or with an assistant moving the extremity at the injured joint. Muscle strengthening exercises follow — usually beginning with isometrics, in which you tighten and release the muscles without moving the extremity. This may be followed by light resistance training.

When you've regained substantial strength and normal range of joint motion, additional exercises, including ones that promote agility and stability, may be added. You'll also begin a general cardiovascular endurance program, perhaps involving long-distance biking, swimming or running, to prevent deconditioning.

Stage 3

In stage 3 you return to movement patterns related to your specific sport. For example, a baseball pitcher recovering from an operation on the arm would resume throwing a baseball.

Stage 4

When you regain your pre-injury level of conditioning and can resume normal activity, your doctor or physical therapist may prescribe a program to enable you to maintain and improve flexibility, strength and endurance.

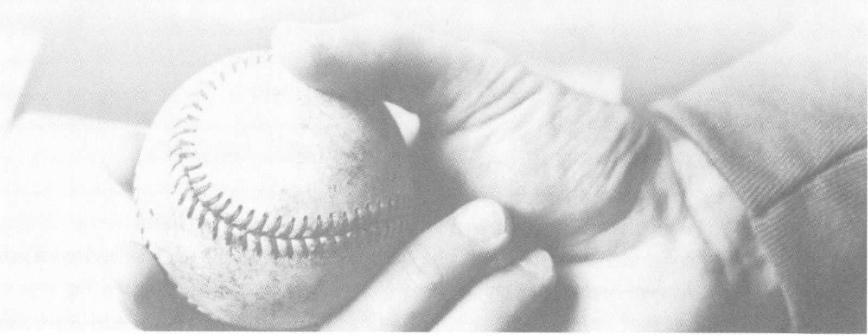

Baseball finger, also known as mallet finger, occurs when the tendon that connects the muscles to the end of your finger is forcibly separated from the bone. This often results when a thrown or batted baseball strikes the tip of a finger.

Diagnosis

Typically, this injury is the result of trauma to the finger, so your doctor will likely order an X-ray of the injured joint to rule out a fracture.

How serious is baseball finger?

With proper treatment, you should be able to use the injured finger normally within approximately 8 weeks. However, your finger may be permanently deformed.

Treatment

Treatment generally involves immobilizing the finger and taking medication to control the pain. Surgery usually is necessary only when a bone is fractured.

To immobilize the affected finger, your doctor will probably splint the last joint in an extended position for about 6 weeks to allow the tendon to repair itself. After the splint is removed, gradually try to return the finger to its normal position. Your doctor may recommend gentle range-of-motion exercises.

Runner's or jumper's knee

Signs and symptoms

- Pain at the front of the knee
- Pain with pressure to the tendon just below the kneecap (patella)
- Swelling

Many athletes develop pain at the front of the knee known as patellar tendinitis — commonly called runner's knee or jumper's knee.

Inflammation of tendons (tendinitis) in the knee causes the pain, which may occur in one or both knees. Knee inflammation is usually the result of overuse or misuse rather than a single traumatic event. The pain usually isn't constant, but occurs when you jump, run, squat or climb stairs.

Diagnosis
A doctor often makes a diagnosis on the basis of a physical examination and the degree of discomfort.

How serious is runner's or jumper's knee?
Given proper rest and treatment, pain from patellar tendinitis usually disappears within a matter of weeks. However, if you don't address the cause of the problem, it may recur.

Treatment
Apply ice to the sore knee and avoid the activity that caused the discomfort. Avoid jumping, repetitive stair climbing and running until symptoms subside. Acetaminophen (Tylenol, others) and anti-inflammatory drugs can reduce the pain.

Prevention
The most common causes of anterior knee pain are overuse and improper training. You may prevent recurrences by reviewing your training program with someone knowledgeable about sports medicine. It may be necessary to change your exercise program.

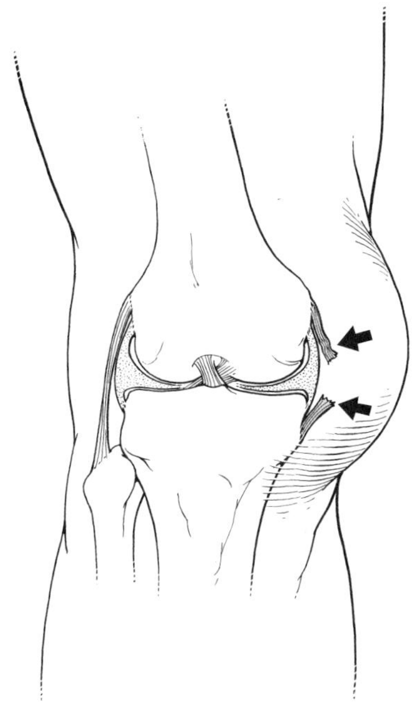

A torn ligament (see arrows) is a common form of knee injury. The knee swells, and the joint becomes unstable.

Some people switch from running to swimming or bicycling, activities that put less stress on their knees. Orthotic devices may help correct flatfeet or other alignment problems in your legs. If alignment problems seem to be causing your symptoms, your doctor may refer you to a physiatrist, podiatrist or physical therapist.

Support for your kneecap in the form of a light brace also may help. A strap across your patellar tendon may help reduce the pressure. Another important strategy is to stretch and strengthen the quadriceps, the muscles at the front of your thigh.

Knee injury

Signs and symptoms

- Pain and swelling in your knee
- Instability of the knee
- A popping sound, a snapping sensation or locking of the joint

Three key factors make the knee joint susceptible to injury. First, its

Knee Braces

If your knee is swollen or unstable, your doctor may recommend that you wear a knee brace, especially when you're participating in activities that may stress the joint.

One type of brace available in medical supply stores is a rubbery neoprene or elastic sleeve that slips over your knee. Be aware, though, that the brace may seem to offer more support than it actually does. The warmth and compression the brace provides can make your knee feel better, but it doesn't necessarily protect you from injury. Some braces — especially those designed for medial and lateral support — may even increase your risk of injury. It's best to avoid them even if they ease discomfort.

Your doctor might also recommend another type of brace if you have osteoarthritis of the knee. It shifts the load on your knee, protecting the joint and helping to ease discomfort.

If you tear your anterior cruciate ligament (ACL) — the most common knee ligament injury — and you don't choose surgical reconstruction, your doctor may prescribe a functional brace to help stabilize your knee during certain activities. A knee brace can't take the place of a fully functioning ACL, but it can keep your knee properly aligned during activities such as skiing, playing tennis or hiking. These braces usually are custom fitted or custom tailored, so they can be costly. Depending on your situation, your insurance provider may or may not cover the cost. Check with your insurance provider.

Factors a doctor considers in deciding if you need a brace include your age, lifestyle and injury. With the aid of a brace, most people can continue to participate in many of their favorite activities that don't involve jumping, turning sharply and pivoting. People who wear knee braces report fewer episodes of instability or giving way. But your knee may continue to be unstable during certain types of activities, even with a brace. Repeated episodes of instability can damage the knee further.

The best way to protect your knees against further injury is to strengthen the muscles in the thighs — hamstring and quadriceps — because these strong muscles support your knees.

location leaves it exposed to trauma. Second, you use it constantly. Third, the structure of your knee is complex. More than a hinge, a knee's range of motion is unique among body joints. It must slide, glide and swivel, as well as bend.

Knee injuries result from a variety of causes. Acute knee injuries often occur during sports. Wear and tear over time can produce chronic knee problems, such as osteoarthritis in a knee joint. Knee injuries also can result from an accident or simply a mistaken step that causes the joint to extend beyond its normal range of motion.

Diagnosis

If you sustain a knee injury, your doctor will likely examine your knee in a variety of positions to assess the joint's internal structure and the damage it has sustained.

Traditional X-rays are one method of evaluating a knee injury. Magnetic resonance imaging (MRI) provides much more detailed images of the structures of the knee, including its soft tissues.

Another diagnostic tool is arthroscopy, a procedure in which a doctor examines the interior of your knee joint by inserting a small tube containing a fiber-optic camera through a small incision in the knee.

How serious is a knee injury?

The severity of a knee injury depends on the type of damage the joint has sustained.

Most knee injuries fall into one of three classifications: meniscal tears, a torn ligament or loose bodies. Each of these types of injuries can produce pain and swelling of the knee joint.

Meniscal tears

The meniscus is the crescent-shaped cartilage in your knee situated between the ends of the bones of your thigh and lower leg. Certain types of impact and twisting injuries can produce tears in the meniscus, causing pain in the joint.

Other Causes of Knee Pain

Your knee is a complex, vulnerable joint, and many factors can cause knee pain. The most common sources of knee pain are injuries, the constant stress of excess weight on your knees and general wear and tear. Osteoarthritis commonly affects the knees as the cartilage in the knee joint gradually deteriorates.

Another source of knee pain is chondromalacia, softening and the loss of smooth cartilage that covers the backside of the kneecap. This condition can be aggravated by a tracking malalignment, a condition in which the kneecap slides over leg bones when bending or straightening the knee. Chondromalacia causes pain when you move your knee, especially when you kneel or go down stairs.

When the fluid membrane that lubricates your knee joint (synovium) becomes inflamed, a bulging cyst may form behind your knee. This is a popliteal cyst, also called a Baker's cyst (see page 1001).

Arthroscopy

Before the development of the arthroscope in 1972, injuries of the knee and other joints often required traditional surgery through a long incision. This type of surgery often involved an extended hospital stay and a long, painful period of recuperation. Although some joint conditions still require incisions to open and reconstruct the joint, doctors can now correct many injuries by using an arthroscope.

Arthroscope comes from the terms *arthro* for "joint" and *scope*, meaning "to view." The device consists of a slender tube, an optical system of magnifying lenses and a fiber-optic light source.

Before the procedure, you're given a local or general anesthetic. The surgeon then makes a small incision into the affected joint to

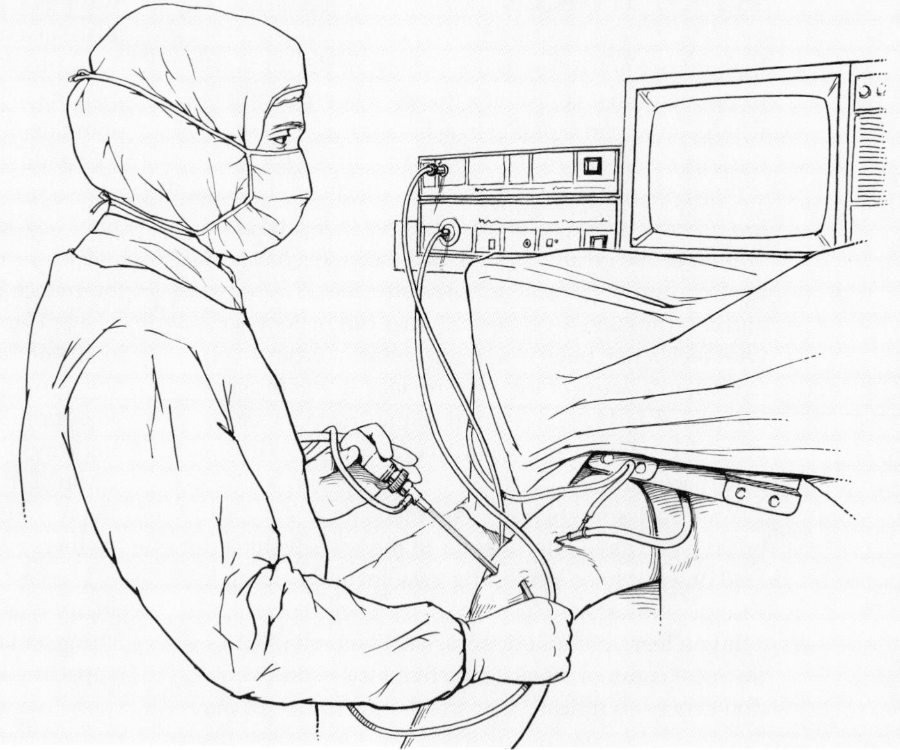

Knee Swelling

Occasionally, a knee may swell for no clear reason. The swelling is sometimes associated with pain when you move your knee, and your knee may be tender and appear red or inflamed. Knee swelling may also occur without pain, tenderness or inflammation. Regardless, the swelling should prompt you to see your doctor to determine the cause.

If your knee is inflamed, you have a fever and it hurts to move your knee, see your doctor right away. These signs and symptoms may indicate infection in the joint. Occasionally, knee swelling, tenderness and pain may be initial manifestations of gout. If you have pain most of the time or with certain movements, you may have injured the cartilage or ligaments that support your knee.

Sometimes, isolated knee swelling may be an initial symptom of a physical illness, such as inflammatory bowel disease, or a systemic disease, such as rheumatoid arthritis.

insert the arthroscope. Other small incisions are made, as needed, to insert surgical instruments. Often, the incisions are so small that stitches aren't required.

Sterile fluid may be injected into the joint space to enlarge it and enhance visibility before inserting the arthroscope. Once the arthroscope is in place, the surgeon can view the inside of your joint on a monitor. Small instruments can be inserted into the joint to remove floating bits of cartilage or bone, repair the meniscus or reconstruct ligaments.

Recovery from an arthroscopic procedure generally requires much less time than recovery from traditional surgery. Many people go home the same day. Be careful not to subject the joint to vigorous physical activity for several weeks after surgery. Many people can, however, resume most normal activities within a few days.

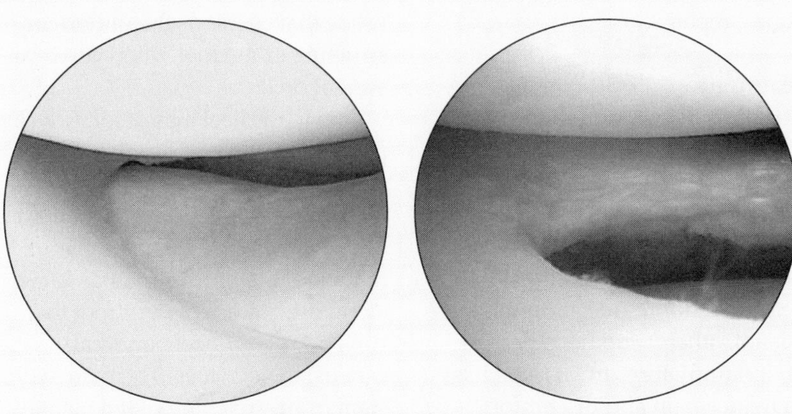

Using an arthroscope, a surgeon can see inside your knee or another joint to examine the joint or repair it without major surgery. Above are arthroscopic views of a normal meniscus (left) and a partial tear of the meniscus (right).

Sometimes, you hear a popping sound at the moment of injury.

Often, a meniscal tear causes you to collapse due to acute, severe knee pain. In some cases, you'll be able to get up and even resume activity, but more likely the tear will cause swelling and persistent pain. The pain may subside over a period of weeks, but symptoms may recur if you participate in activities that involve rotating or pivoting the knee joint.

Torn ligament

Ligaments are dense bands of tissue that surround a joint and provide stability. Occasionally, a ligament in a knee may stretch and tear, causing immediate pain, tenderness over the site of injury and swelling of the knee.

Loose bodies

Some knee injuries involve pieces of cartilage or bone that are torn from their proper positions and float about in the joint space. The effect is similar to a pencil being caught in a door hinge. Even a small piece of loose cartilage can become pinched in the knee joint, locking the joint or causing pain.

Treatment

The treatment for a knee injury depends on the injury. For relatively minor knee injuries, the proper treatment approach is PRICE: protection, rest, ice, compression and elevation (see page 958). Stop using your knee after you injure it. Use ice and compression to limit swelling, and keep your leg elevated to help reduce pain and swelling.

If your knee joint has sustained major damage, you may need reconstructive surgery. A dislocated or fractured bone may need to be reset. A ruptured ligament may need to be reattached. Often, the damage can be repaired surgically with an endoscopic procedure called arthroscopy, which requires small incisions in the knee rather than a large incision. Arthroscopy causes less tissue disruption than traditional surgery, and it can mean more rapid rehabilitation.

Rehabilitation
Following surgery, your doctor may apply a splint or brace to the knee for a brief period. Once you're allowed to move your knee, you'll likely receive a program of exercises to restore range of motion to your joint and to strengthen it. You may be referred to a physical medicine and rehabilitation specialist or to a physical therapist who will oversee your rehabilitation.

Problems of the Feet

Your feet are highly specialized structures. Each foot has 26 bones held together with ligaments, muscles and tendons. As you walk, your muscles work the bones like levers, making movement possible.

As long as your feet take you where you want to go without pain, you probably don't think much about them. You may even mistreat them unwittingly by squeezing them into too-tight shoes, often with high heels and pointy toes. However, if you're lucky and you wear properly fitted, comfortable footwear, your feet will cause you little worry.

When your feet are sore, walking can be painful. If you develop foot problems, you may want to seek guidance from your doctor, an orthopedist or a podiatrist. A podiatrist, although not a medical doctor, is a licensed professional whose area of expertise is the diagnosis, prevention and treatment of foot disorders.

Achilles tendinitis

Signs and symptoms

- A dull ache or pain in the Achilles tendon, especially when running or jumping
- Mild swelling or tenderness over the tendon
- Severe pain and inability to move the foot

Achilles tendinitis is an inflammation of a tendon known as the heel cord or Achilles tendon. This tendon links your leg muscles to the back of your heel bone. Pain and inflammation result from tiny tears in the tendon that can occur during strenuous exercise. More severe injury results when the tendon is torn more extensively or fully torn (ruptured).

Diagnosis

Your doctor will examine your foot and may take an X-ray of the area to rule out other causes of the pain.

How serious is Achilles tendinitis?

Unless the Achilles tendon ruptures, conservative treatments such as rest, ice and perhaps a change in your exercise program should allow the tendon to repair itself over a period of weeks. If left untreated and if the tendon continues to sustain small tears through exercise and repeated movement, it can rupture. A ruptured tendon is a serious injury that affects your ability to walk and usually requires surgical repair.

Treatment

Resting your foot is often the best treatment for Achilles tendinitis. Applying ice to the tendon can provide relief. A temporary orthotic device that elevates the heel within the shoe may relieve strain on the stretched tendon. Acetaminophen (Tylenol, others) and nonsteroidal anti-inflammatory drugs (NSAIDs) can reduce pain and discomfort.

Once the pain is gone, gently stretch the heel cord and the hamstring muscles at the back of your thigh. Strengthening the calf muscles is key to healing and preventing recurrence. Until the tendon is fully healed, it may be best to take part in nonimpact or low-impact exercises.

Surgery
A complete rupture of an Achilles tendon usually requires surgery. The procedure generally involves making an incision in the back of the leg and stitching the torn tendon together. Recovery involves spending about 6 to 12 weeks with your leg in a walking boot, cast, brace or splint.

If the tendon is only partially torn, treatment may involve wearing a cast or walking boot and allowing the ends of the torn tendon to reattach without surgery. Studies indicate that this method can be effective and doesn't have the same risk of complications, such as infection, that can occur with surgery. However, the incidence of re-rupture is higher with the nonsurgical approach, and recovery can take longer.

Heel pain

Signs and symptoms

- Pain in the bottom of the heel of the foot when you bear weight on the foot
- Pain that's worse with the first few steps after awakening or when climbing stairs or standing on tiptoe

The heel pad consists of fibrous tissue that cushions the underlying structure of the foot when you bear weight on it.

Pain in the heel may result from a pinched nerve or a chronic condition, such as arthritis. But the common cause of heel pain is a condition called plantar fasciitis, an inflammation of the fibrous plantar fascia along the bottom of your foot that runs from your heel bone (calcaneus) to your toes. The pain may stem from stretching of the plantar fascia, causing inflammation or tears in the tissue.

Heel pain usually develops gradually, but it can come on suddenly and be severe. It tends to be worse when you get out of bed in the morning. Although both feet can be affected, it usually occurs in only one foot.

Exercises that Help Strengthen the Heel

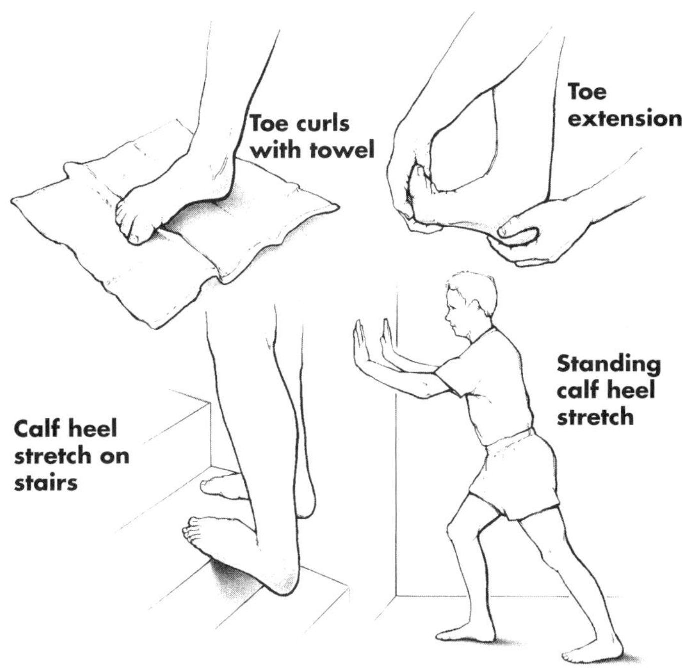

These exercises stretch or strengthen your plantar fascia, Achilles tendon and calf muscles. Hold each for 20 to 30 seconds and do one or two repetitions two to three times a day.

Heel pain may result from small tears or inflammation of your heel pad where the tissue attaches to your heel bone (see highlighting). Bone spurs may form but rarely cause pain.

The pain generally subsides once your foot limbers up, but it can recur if you stand or sit too long. Climbing stairs or standing on tiptoe may be painful. Tension on your heel bone from this condition can cause a bone spur to form. However, the spur usually is painless.

Anyone can develop plantar fasciitis, but it tends to become more common with age as the arch of your foot begins to sag.

Carrying excess weight, wearing improperly fitting shoes, having a foot abnormality and engaging in activities that place added pressure on your feet, such as running, increase your risk of plantar fasciitis.

Diagnosis

Your doctor will ask if the pain is constant or occurs only when you put weight on your heel. An X-ray may rule out a stress fracture. However, a stress fracture often isn't apparent on an X-ray for up to 6 weeks after an injury. If your doctor suspects an acute stress fracture, a magnetic resonance imaging (MRI) scan or bone scan may be obtained.

Sometimes, an X-ray shows a spur of bone projecting forward from the heel bone. In the past, bone spurs often were blamed for heel pain and removed surgically, but doctors have found that they're typically not the cause of pain. Surgery to remove such a spur is rare today.

How serious is heel pain?

In most cases, the pain will gradually improve or disappear. It can recur, though, especially if you walk barefoot or wear poorly fitted shoes or shoes that lack cushioning at the heel when performing weight-bearing exercise.

Some people find that the only way to avoid a recurring problem is to modify their activity, switching from running or playing tennis to swimming or bicycling, for instance. For most people, though, a complete recovery is often possible with appropriate treatment.

Treatment

Self-care measures may help to relieve the pain and inflammation, but recovery may take 6 months or longer. If self-care measures are ineffective, your doctor may refer you to a physical therapist.

Medication

To relieve pain, try acetaminophen (Tylenol, others) or an over-the-counter nonsteroidal anti-inflammatory drug (NSAID). If that doesn't help, your doctor may inject your heel with an anti-inflammatory steroid drug such as cortisone. However, these drugs usually are used only when other measures are ineffective. Multiple injections aren't recommended because they can weaken your plantar fascia, as well as shrink the fat pad covering your heel bone.

Self-care

You can take several self-care steps to treat plantar fasciitis:

Shopping for Shoes

Improperly fitted shoes are the source of many foot problems. Choosing shoes carefully can help you avoid many problems with your feet. When buying shoes, look for the following:

- *Wide toe box.* Buy shoes with a wide toe box that provides adequate toe room. Pointy, narrow-toed shoes can cramp your feet and lead to ingrown toenails, calluses, corns and bunions.
- *Low heels.* Select shoes with heels of no more than 2 inches. High heels place extra stress on your knees and back. They force you to lean back to compensate for the forward tilt of your heel. High heels can contribute to tightness of the Achilles tendon and toe pain.
- *Laces.* Lace-up shoes generally offer more room and adjustable support.
- *Breathable materials.* Soft leather or suede allows perspiration to evaporate from your feet, whereas vinyl and plastic inhibit evaporation of perspiration.

Shop for shoes in the afternoon to get a fit that accommodates your feet as they swell throughout the day. However, you don't want a shoe to be so roomy that your foot slips around inside. Measure the size of both of your feet. As you age or gain weight, your shoe size may increase.

Don't buy shoes that need breaking in. If they're not comfortable in the store, they're not likely to be comfortable later on. Ask to have the shoes stretched at any pressure point.

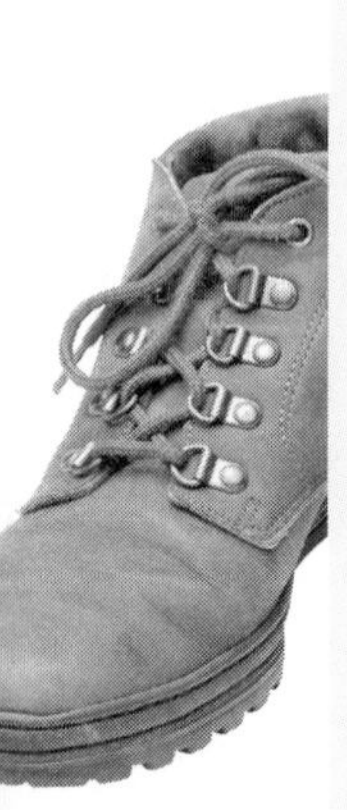

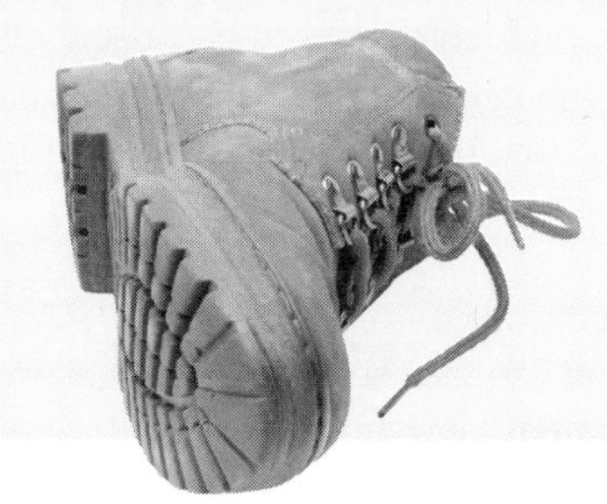

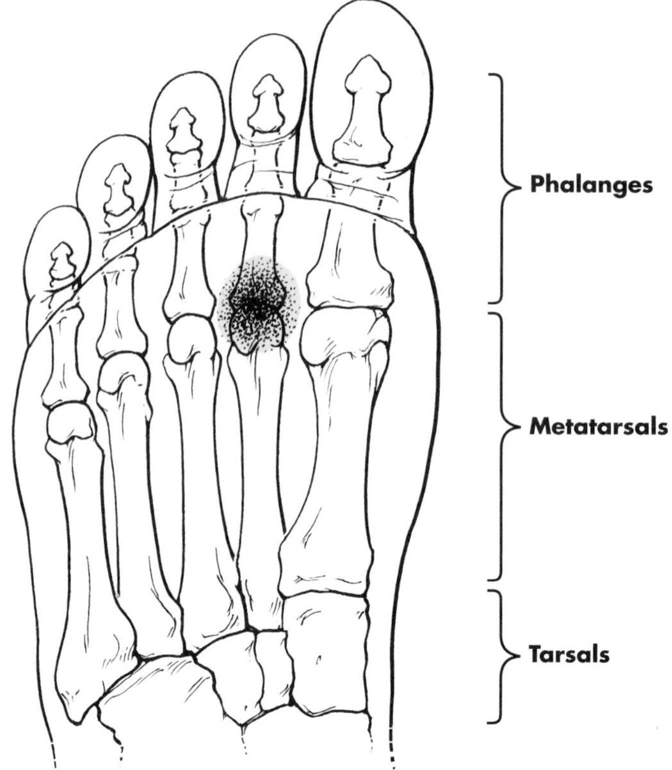

The pain of metatarsalgia can occur at any of the joints that separate the phalangeal and metatarsal bones in your foot. The highlighted area shows the joint most commonly affected.

- Apply ice to your sore heel for up to 20 minutes after an activity that causes pain.
- Massage and gently stretch the arch and calf muscles. Stretching increases flexibility in the plantar fascia, Achilles tendon and calf muscles. Stretching your foot as soon as you wake up also helps reverse the tightening of the plantar fascia that sets in overnight.
- Do daily exercises to strengthen your arch and the muscles in your foot (see page 967).
- Wear soft-soled shoes when running. Your health care provider may prescribe an arch support to wear in your shoes or a night splint to stretch the arch and calf overnight.
- For everyday wear, buy shoes with a low to moderate heel (no higher than 2 inches), good arch support and shock absorbency.
- Deep heat from ultrasound or a corticosteroid solution applied through the skin via electrical particles (iontophoresis) may be used by your physical therapist to help improve the pain.

Surgery

When pain is severe and all else fails, surgery is sometimes performed to detach the plantar fascia from the heel bone. Side effects include a weakening of the arch in the foot.

Metatarsalgia

Signs and symptoms

- Pain in the ball of the foot
- The sensation of walking on pebbles

The term *metatarsalgia* means pain in the ball (metatarsal area) of your foot.

You have five metatarsal bones in each foot. Each metatarsal bone has a narrow shaft and a rounded tip. The bones link your ankle and heel bones (tarsals) with the bones in your toes (phalanges). Hinge joints between the metatarsals and phalanges let your toes move up and down and, to a lesser extent, sideways.

Although metatarsalgia may affect males and females from adolescence to older adulthood, the condition is most common among middle-aged women. This condition has multiple causes. Having narrow, high-arched feet can put excessive stress on the balls of your feet, as can certain types of flatfeet. If your legs are unequal in length, the metatarsal-phalangeal joints of the shorter leg receive additional stress. Other contributing factors include rheumatoid arthritis, stress fractures, fluid accumulation, muscle fatigue, excess weight from pregnancy or obesity and prolonged standing or walking.

Diagnosis

Your doctor or podiatrist will likely examine your feet and legs and ask about your pain. He or she may want to know if the pain tends to occur in certain circumstances or with certain activities.

Treatment

Simple self-care measures usually reduce the pain. Avoid wearing tight, thin-soled or high-heeled shoes. Your doctor might suggest that you wear a foot pad or arch support, a type of orthotic device, that relieves pressure under the painful area.

An over-the-counter pain medication can often help relieve the pain. Your doctor may inject a corticosteroid medication into the tender area. Surgery is seldom necessary.

Burning feet

Signs and symptoms

- Nearly constant burning and stinging in the feet

This condition tends to be most common among people older than age 65. The discomfort ranges from mild irritation to severe pain. Possible culprits include irritating fabrics, poorly fitted shoes or a fungal infection, such as athlete's foot.

To avoid an ingrown toenail (A), don't clip your toenails too short. Clip them straight across. When a toe takes on a claw-like, clenched appearance, the condition is called hammertoe (B). Hammertoe most often affects the second toe, which frequently develops a corn due to pressure from shoes. To help avoid hammertoe, ingrown toenails and other foot problems, wear shoes that fit properly.

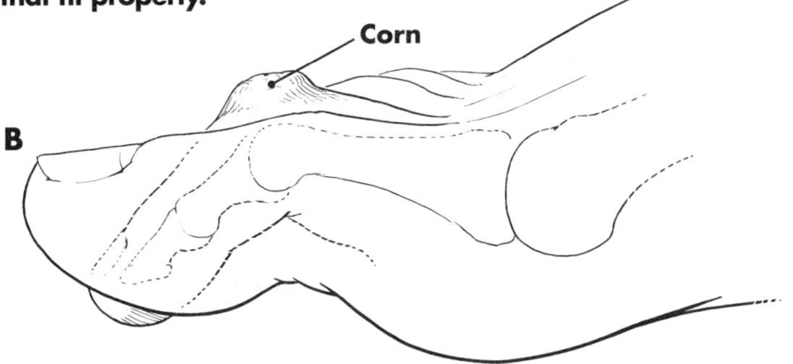

Diagnosis

The cause of burning feet is often difficult to pinpoint. If a nerve or blood disorder is responsible, you may also have a prickling feeling in your feet, weakness or change of sensation in your legs, nausea, diarrhea, loss of urine or bowel control or impotence.

Damaged peripheral nerves (neuropathy) can cause persistent burning or tingling. Peripheral neuropathy has many possible causes, including inherited disorders, diabetes, pernicious anemia, malnutrition, side effects of medications, exposure to toxins, chronic kidney failure and liver disease.

How serious are burning feet?

Although generally not serious, this condition can signal a serious underlying problem.

Treatment

Self-help measures may help improve your symptoms. Wear socks made from synthetic fibers such as acrylic or polypropylene. Select well-fitting shoes made of natural materials that breathe. Reduce or eliminate activities that aggravate your condition, such as standing in one place for a long period. Cool your feet in cool tap water for 15 minutes twice a day. Or soak your feet in cool water and then in hot water, a method called contrast foot soaks.

If nerve damage is the cause, your symptoms may take months to subside because nerves heal slowly. Prescription and over-the-counter pain relievers may provide pain relief.

Morton's neuroma

Signs and symptoms

- Burning pain in the ball of the foot that may radiate into the toes
- Numbness in the toes

Morton's neuroma is a noncancerous (benign) tumor of a nerve. Also called plantar neuroma, it's actually a thickening of the tissue that surrounds the digital nerve leading to the toes. This condition may occur in response to irritation, pressure or injury. Morton's neuroma is more common in women than in men.

Diagnosis

Typically, there's no outward sign of this condition, such as a lump. A doctor may feel a palpable mass or notice a clicking between the bones upon examination of the affected foot.

How serious is Morton's neuroma?

The condition causes discomfort but otherwise isn't serious.

Treatment

Usually, treatment involves self-care. Wear sandals or well-fitting shoes with adequate room in the toe box. Avoid high heels. Custom shoe inserts or pads may help reduce pressure on the nerve.

A doctor may recommend injections with steroid medications to reduce swelling and inflammation of the nerve. In rare cases, surgery to remove the benign growth may be indicated.

Ingrown toenail

Signs and symptoms

- Pain
- Swelling and redness around a toenail

An ingrown toenail is a condition in which the toenail grows into the flesh of a toe, often the big toe. This can result from unusually curved toenails, poorly fitted shoes or toenails that are cut improperly. The tissue around the nail may become infected.

Treatment

If the tissue around the nail is infected, your doctor may prescribe an antibiotic and trim the portion of the nail that has grown into the toe. This minor procedure can be done in a doctor's office. Your doctor may recommend soaking your foot in warm water and resting the foot.

Prevention

To avoid chronic recurrence of ingrown toenails, don't clip your nails too short. Cut them straight across rather than curving them to match the shape of your toes.

It's also important to wear socks and shoes that fit properly without putting excessive pressure on your feet and toes.

Question and Answer

How can I get rid of an ugly corn or callus?

Apply over-the-counter pads to protect areas where corns and calluses develop. Be careful using over-the-counter liquid corn removers or medicated corn pads. These contain salicylic acid, which can irritate skin and cause infection, especially in people with diabetes or poor circulation.

You can gradually thin some of the thickened skin of a corn or callus by rubbing it with a pumice stone or washcloth during or after a shower or bath. Soaking your foot in water and using an alkaline soap may soften your skin enough for you to rub off the upper layers. Never cut or shave corns or calluses. You could introduce an infection.

If you have diabetes or poor circulation, call your doctor before self-treating corns or calluses. Even a relatively minor injury to your foot could lead to an open sore (foot ulcer) that's difficult to heal.

Corns and calluses

Signs and symptoms

- A thickened layer of skin
- With corns, pain

Corns and calluses are the result of pressure or friction, causing the skin to protect itself by thickening and hardening. Corns typically are smaller — less than a quarter-inch in diameter — than calluses and have a hard center. They usually develop on the tops and sides of your toes and can be painful. Calluses, which may be rough but are rarely painful, usually develop on your soles and palms.

Shoes that fit poorly are often the cause of corns or calluses on your feet. Calluses on your hands usually result from the pressure or friction of hand tools. For instance, over time daily use of a shovel will line your hands with calluses.

How serious are corns and calluses?

Although corns and calluses can be unsightly, they need treatment only if they cause discomfort. If you have diabetes, you're at increased risk of complications from a corn or callus. See your doctor if a corn or callus becomes painful or ulcerated.

Treatment

In most cases, you can prevent corns and calluses by wearing properly fitted shoes or protecting your hands by wearing gloves when using tools. Often, you can treat corns or calluses on your own. If a large corn persists or is painful, your doctor may pare it down.

The problem can be more serious if you have an underlying foot deformity. Your doctor may be able to correct the situation with surgery or with custom-made padded shoe inserts (orthotics), which prevent recurring corns.

Hammertoe and mallet toe

Signs and symptoms

- A claw-like or mallet-like clenched appearance of a toe
- Pain and difficulty moving the toe

Unlike a bunion, which affects only the big toe, hammertoe can affect any toe. Most commonly, it occurs in the second toe. Generally, both toe joints are affected, causing the toe to bend upward in the middle, giving it a claw-like appearance. Wearing shoes that are too short can cause hammertoe. The condition tends to run in some families. The deformity may occur in people with muscle and nerve damage from diabetes. A mallet toe is characterized by a deformity at the end of the toe that gives it a mallet-like appearance.

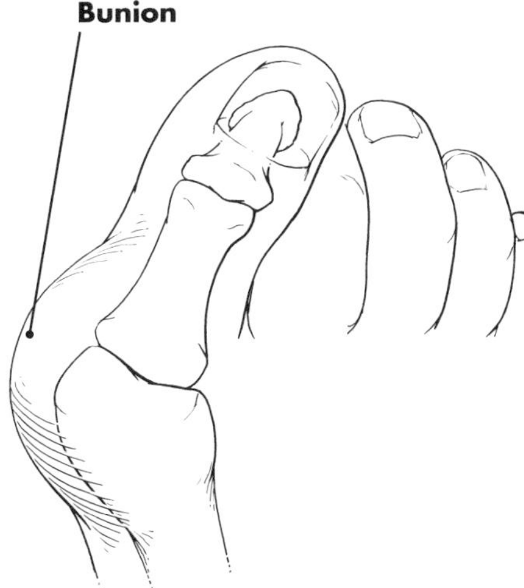

When the base of your big toe extends beyond the normal profile of your foot, the bump that results is called a bunion. To prevent a bunion, avoid shoes with narrow toes or high heels.

How serious are hammertoe and mallet toe?

Both conditions can cause pain with walking and other movements.

Treatment

Your doctor or a podiatrist may prescribe an orthotic device to reposition the toe and relieve the pressure and pain. It's also important to wear shoes that fit properly and that have a wide toe box. In severe cases, the condition may require surgery.

Bunions

Signs and symptoms

- A bony protrusion at the base of your big toe
- Pain and limitation of motion

A bunion develops when the big toe bends toward the next toe or overlaps it, causing deformity of the foot. The base of the big toe juts out beyond the normal profile of the foot, producing a bump known as a bunion. A bunion is often subjected to constant rubbing that, in turn, results in thickening of the skin.

Women are seven times more likely to develop this common problem than are men. Some people are genetically predisposed to getting bunions, but the problem can also develop as a result of wearing tight, high-heeled shoes with pointed toes.

Diagnosis

Your doctor may be able to diagnose a bunion simply by looking at your foot. However, he or she may request X-rays to evaluate the problem and treatment options.

How serious is a bunion?

Typically, a bunion causes only minor discomfort, but sometimes the pain can be severe. Accompanying bursitis or osteoarthritis can develop in the toe joint, causing pain and stiffness. Because a bunion distorts the shape of your foot, finding suitable shoes can be difficult.

Treatment

The best way to relieve a painful bunion — or to prevent the condition — is to wear shoes that fit properly, with a wide toe box that provides ample room for your toes. To provide more room in a leather shoe for a bunion deformity, take your shoes to a shoe repair shop and have them stretched.

Treating corns and calluses in the area of the bunion may reduce discomfort. If you develop bursitis, wearing an old shoe with a hole cut in the area over the bunion may provide relief. Felt pads also may be helpful.

Surgery generally isn't necessary unless the deformity is severe or causes severe pain. During surgery, a surgeon realigns the bones by removing excess bone.

Flatfeet

Signs and symptoms

- No visible arches in your feet when you place your weight on them

The intricate alignment of bones, muscles, ligaments and tendons in your feet form side-to-side (metatarsal) and lengthwise (longitudinal) arches. As you walk, these springy, elastic arches help distribute your body weight evenly across each of your feet. Your arches play an integral role in how you walk. They act as rigid levels for proper mobility but are resilient and flexible to adapt to various surfaces.

Everyone has flatfeet at birth. Your arches usually develop fully by age 12 or 13 years. But some people's arches never form properly. Many people with flatfeet have no problems because alignment elsewhere in their lower extremities compensates for their flatfeet.

Some people with flatfeet, however, experience inflammation and pain in the ligaments in the bottoms of their feet, Achilles tendinitis, stress fractures, shin splints, bunions and calluses. For them, flatfeet can lead to muscular imbalances and joint problems in their ankles, knees, hips and lower back.

Most flatfooted people develop arch problems as a result of continual stress on the feet. Excessive weight, postural abnormalities, weakened supportive tissue or overuse may weaken the ligaments and muscles supporting the arch that runs lengthwise in your foot, causing it to fall. Prolonged stress on the balls of your feet or walking, standing or exercising on hard surfaces may weaken or flatten the metatarsal arch at the front of your foot. This places additional pressure on nerves and blood vessels in the area, causing pain and irritation.

Diagnosis

A doctor or podiatrist can diagnose flatfeet by examining your feet.

Treatment

If you experience chronic pain as a result of flatfeet, wearing a custom-designed arch support might provide relief. You slip this orthotic device into your shoe, and it helps support and re-form the arch of your foot.

Corrective orthotic devices help align your foot in a better weight-bearing position. They also absorb shock and help control excessive inward or outward rotation (pronation or supination) of your longitudinal arch when you walk. To get custom-made orthotic devices, you need to see your doctor or podiatrist. Flexible models are available for people who can't tolerate the more rigid corrective orthotic devices.

Foot ulcer

Signs and symptoms

- An open sore on the skin surrounded by inflamed tissue
- Pus from the ulcer, if the tissue is infected

A foot ulcer can result from a foot wound or from skin irritation caused by wearing improperly fitting shoes. They're most common in individuals with diminished circulation or nerve deterioration due to diabetes.

See your doctor if you develop a foot ulcer. Several treatments are available to treat the condition and only rarely is surgery necessary. For more information on foot ulcers, see page 1025.

Back Pain

The spine is one of the strongest parts of the body. It's made up of more than 26 bones, 24 of which are called vertebrae. You have 7 cervical vertebrae in your neck, 12 thoracic vertebrae in the middle of your back behind your chest and 5 lumbar vertebrae in your lower back. The other 2 bones are the sacrum, made up of 5 fused vertebrae between your pelvic bones, and your tailbone (coccyx), which is made up of 3 to 5 fused bones at the end of your spinal column.

Your vertebrae stack on top of one another to form your backbone, the flexible column that runs from the base of your skull to your tailbone. Between your vertebrae are spongy cushions called disks. They have a strong, fibrous outer covering that protects a gel on the inside. The joints of your vertebrae are reinforced by strong ligaments and surrounded by many sturdy muscles.

The intricate structure of your back bends and twists and bears the weight of your body and the loads you carry. Your backbone also protects your spinal cord.

The complex structure of your spine contributes to its potential for problems. Seemingly minor changes in the alignment or balance of any part — whether a disk, vertebra, joint or muscle — can make movements painful. When the nerves or spinal cord that travels through your backbone (spinal canal) are affected, there's a risk of pain or numbness in parts of your body. A serious back injury can cause permanent damage to your spinal cord and paralysis (see page 606).

Fortunately, it's difficult to damage the spine. Usually, when your back hurts, there's an irritation of one of the spine's components. For example, your disks may have a poor blood supply. As a result, adults are susceptible to disk cracking and dehydration (degeneration) over time. All adults' disks degenerate to some degree as they age.

Risk factors that may make some people more prone to back problems and slow recovery are lack of physical activity, poor posture, being overweight and being under physical or mental stress. Work-related risk factors include heavy physical labor, frequent bending or twisting or static work postures, such as standing still, sitting in one place or bending over for long periods of time.

Back strain and spasm

Signs and symptoms

- Back pain and stiffness
- Difficulty moving

Back problems are among the most common human ailments. Young or old, male or female, short or tall, most people experience back discomfort in their lifetime. Most often, back pain is caused by straining a muscle in your back — a pulled muscle — or stretching a ligament. Lifting a barbell improperly can lead to back pain. So can a sneeze. Sometimes there's no apparent cause.

Back pain can occur at any part of your spine, but it's most commonly in the lower back. About 1 percent of low back pain has a potentially serious underlying cause, such as fracture of the spine due to trauma, a herniated disk, infection or tumor of the spine. The other 99 percent is related to everyday wear and tear.

Sometimes, you may feel pain at the moment you strain the muscle or sprain the ligament. At other times, soreness may develop gradually. You may awaken with the discomfort. Regardless of how the pain develops, it's often difficult for your doctor to determine the exact cause.

Diagnosis

Your doctor will likely review your medical history, ask if you have a history of back problems and perform a physical examination. If there's reason to suspect a spinal problem, he or she may recommend diagnostic tests to rule out problems such as a herniated disk or spondylosis.

How serious are back strain and spasm?

There's no ignoring the discomfort that accompanies a sore back. Performing daily tasks can be agonizing, and severe pain may immobilize you.

In most cases, the problem subsides given time and rest. Unfortunately, recurring episodes of back discomfort are the rule rather than the exception.

See a doctor if you experience any of the following:

- Severe pain
- Fever, chills, night sweats or unexplained weight loss — these

Structures of Your Spine

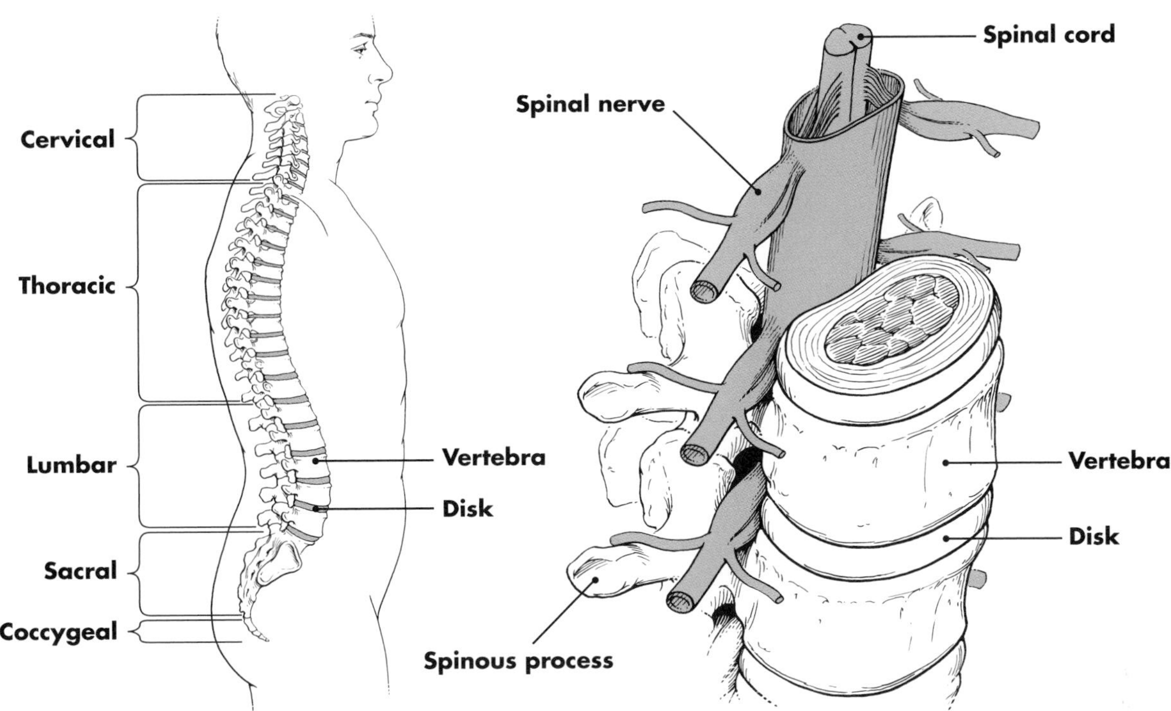

signs and symptoms may indicate a spinal infection or tumor

- Pain that radiates down one of your legs and associated weakness in the leg or a bowel or bladder change
- Pain that severely limits your day-to-day activities
- Signs or symptoms that don't improve within 1 to 2 weeks

Diagnosing the cause of back pain often isn't easy, but it's important to rule out certain underlying causes. Once that's done, knowing precisely what's causing the pain probably won't change the approach to treatment.

Treatment

Ninety percent of back pain resolves in 4 to 6 weeks with or without treatment. In the other 10 percent of cases, there's a more protracted recovery of 6 to 12 weeks or longer, especially if the pain involves sprained ligaments or severe muscle strain. People with back and leg pain may have an even longer recovery time. But with time and proper care, symptoms usually resolve.

Self-care

Self-care that you can perform at home is the most common approach to resolving back pain. Sources of heat and cold — hot baths, hot and cold compresses — can soothe sore and inflamed muscles. Use cold treatments first, several times a day, for no longer than 20 minutes each time to avoid injury to the skin. Use ice wrapped in a plastic bag and then in a cloth or towel to protect your skin. Check your skin every 5 minutes or so during treatment. It will redden with the use of ice. If it begins to lose its redness, stop icing the area because the loss of color may indicate frostbite.

After severe pain subsides — usually in 1 or 2 days — apply heat with a heating pad or heat lamp. Avoid falling asleep while using a heating pad because the pad may get hotter the longer it's on. You don't want to burn yourself. Limit heat applications to 20 minutes.

Avoid using heat or ice on areas of skin with decreased sensation or poor circulation or if you have severe heart disease.

Exercise

Exercise is one of the keys to recovery. Do whatever you can do, such as walking, riding an exercise bike or swimming. Start with a small amount of exercise and increase by small increments.

Rest

In the past, doctors recommended staying on your back in bed for 2 to 6 weeks. Now the recommendation is for, at most, 1 to 2 days, and only in severe cases. Prolonged bed rest is generally not good for your back because it decreases strength and endurance.

Medication

Over-the-counter pain relievers such as acetaminophen (Tylenol, others) or nonsteroidal anti-inflammatory drugs (NSAIDs), such as ibuprofen (Advil, Motrin, others) or aspirin, can help ease your pain. Depending on the cause and your pain level, your doctor may prescribe stronger painkillers or muscle relaxants. Narcotic medications rarely are prescribed for back pain, and if they are, they should be taken only for a limited time. For localized back pain, a doctor may inject a corticosteroid drug into the painful area to reduce inflammation.

Physical therapy
Physical therapy programs have been shown to be effective in people with chronic low back pain. Physical therapy may also be used after resolution of acute back pain to restore back fitness, coordination of muscular contraction and flexibility. Exercises to stretch and strengthen the muscles of your back reduce the risk of future problems.

For people with severe symptoms, physical therapists may use heat treatment and gentle massage. For some disorders, braces, corsets or mechanical traction can help. Manipulation of the back, such as that done by a chiropractor, physical therapist or some osteopathic physicians, may help in some instances, as well.

Surgery
In general, surgery isn't recommended for low back pain because the pain is likely to resolve given time and because surgery may not relieve symptoms. In fact, surgery is recommended in less than 1 percent of all cases of back pain. It's more often used to treat a herniated disk that causes leg pain due to a pinched nerve. Surgery is also used to decompress the spine if a bony narrowing of the spine pinches one or more nerves.

Prevention

The best way to deal with back pain is to prevent it. If you've already had episodes of back pain, you may be able to prevent a recurrence. If your pain does recur, you may be able to lessen its duration and severity.

Exercise daily
Regular exercise is your most potent weapon against back problems. Activity can increase your aerobic capacity, improve your overall fitness, strengthen back and abdominal muscles and help you shed excess pounds, which can stress your back. Stretching and strengthening your muscles also can help reduce wear and tear on your back.

Stretching after warm up and again after you exercise reduces your risk of injury by increasing flexibility in your muscles. Strengthening your arms, legs, abdomen and lower body can help prevent or relieve back pain and decrease your risk of falls and other injuries.

If you have the bone-thinning disease osteoporosis, back-strengthening exercises may help prevent small fractures in the bones of the spine (vertebral compression fractures).

Ask your doctor or a physical therapist for advice before beginning an exercise program, especially if you've hurt your back before or if you have other health problems, such as osteoporosis.

If you're out of condition from lack of activity, your back muscles may be weak and susceptible to injury. Start slowly and pace yourself. As you become stronger, work up to 30 minutes of exercise daily.

Swimming and other water exercises place minimal strain on your lower back. Using a stationary bike, treadmill, elliptical trainer or cross-country ski machine will jar your back less than running on hard surfaces. Bicycling is a good option too. However, be sure to adjust the height of the seat and handlebars so that you maintain good posture while pedaling. You might consider riding a recumbent bike, which gives more support to your back.

If you play golf, your swing puts added strain on your back. The best way to avoid injuries from a poor swing is to take lessons to make sure you're using proper form, which can help you avoid putting undue stress on your back or other parts of your body.

You may need to avoid or modify some activities. Avoid movements that overstretch your muscles. For example, don't try to touch your toes with your legs straight. Contact sports and activities that involve a lot of twisting and quick stops and starts pose the greatest risks to your back.

Practice good posture
Poor posture can lead to back pain, inhibit your breathing and fatigue your muscles. Good posture supports and protects all parts of your body. By keeping your muscles, ligaments, tendons and bones in their

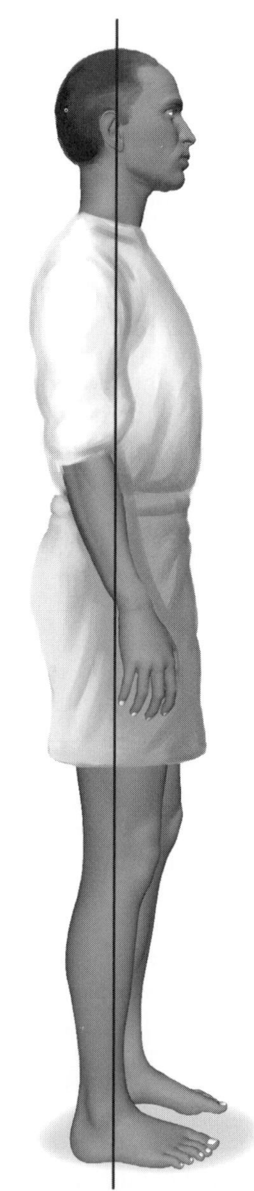

For proper posture, stand straight and imagine that a string extends from your earlobe to your instep.

Back-Strengthening Exercises

The following exercises can help stretch and strengthen the muscles in your back and prevent spinal fractures.

Hamstring Stretch

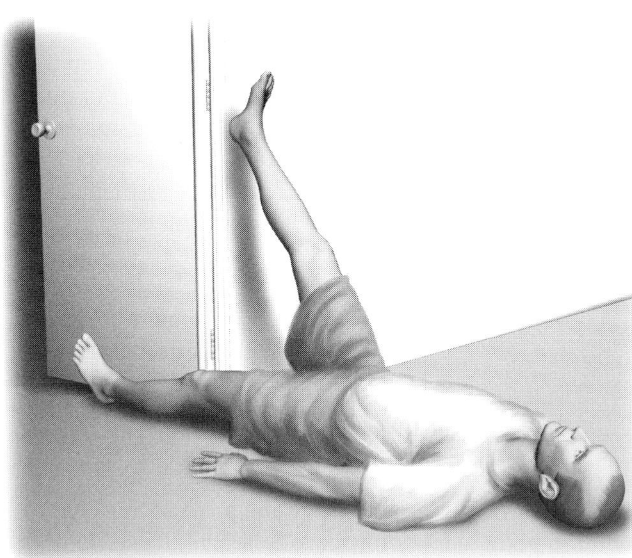

Lie on the floor in front of a doorway and extend your left leg across the threshold. Slide into the door-frame with the leg to be stretched up against the wall and straighten the leg. Hold for 30 seconds. Repeat, reversing leg positions. Don't lock your knee.

Knee-to-Chest Stretch

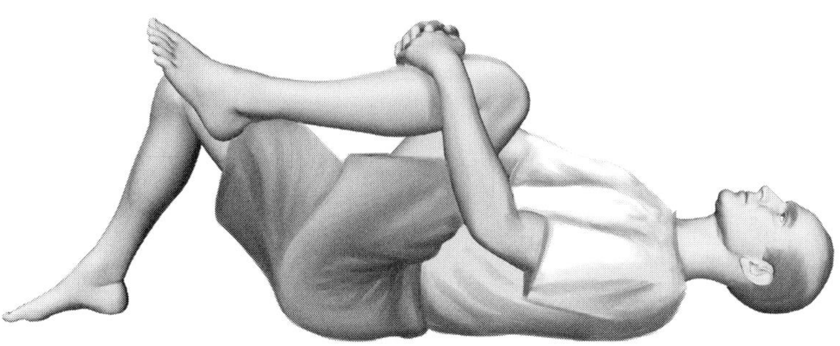

Lie with your knees bent and feet flat on the floor. Pull your left knee toward your chest with both hands. Hold for 30 seconds. Switch legs. Repeat four times with each leg.

Bridging

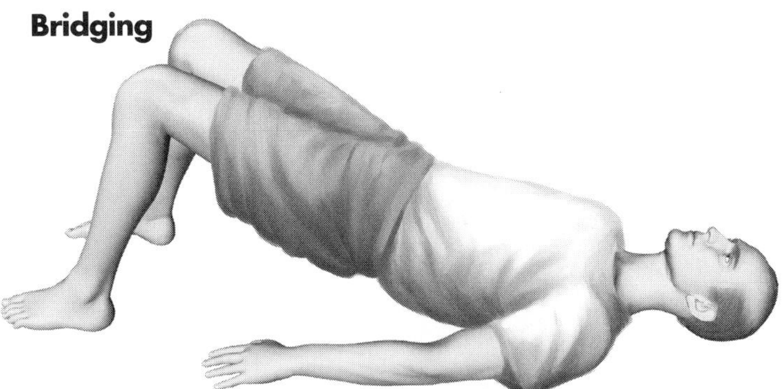

Lie on a mat with your feet flat, about shoulder-width apart. Raise your buttocks off the mat, keeping a level line from your knees to your hips. Keep your shoulders, head and neck relaxed on the mat. Hold the position until you become fatigued and can no longer comfortably keep your knees and hips in a straight line.

Mountain Pose

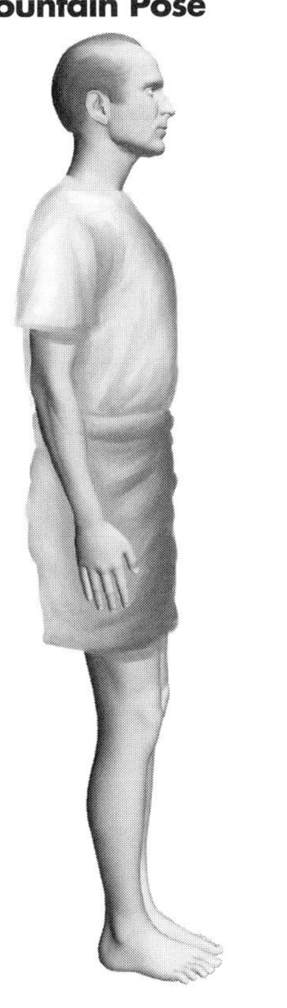

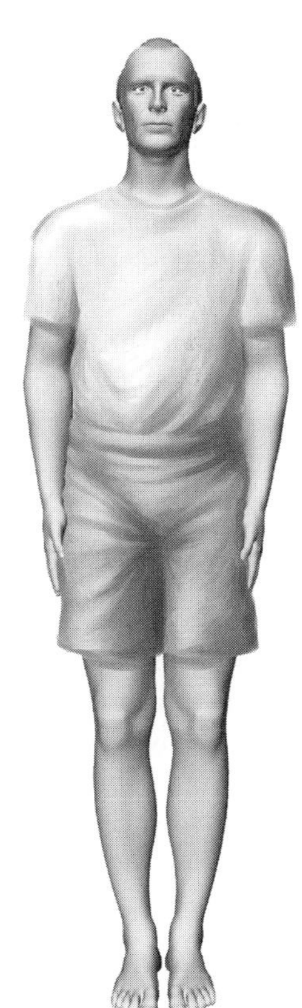

Stand with your feet together, toes forward and heels slightly apart. Keep your arms at your sides, your shoulders relaxed and your chin parallel to the floor. Contract your thigh muscles, buttocks and abdominals and lift your chest. Drop your shoulders away from your earlobes, lower your chin slightly and lift the crown of your head. Hold for several breaths.

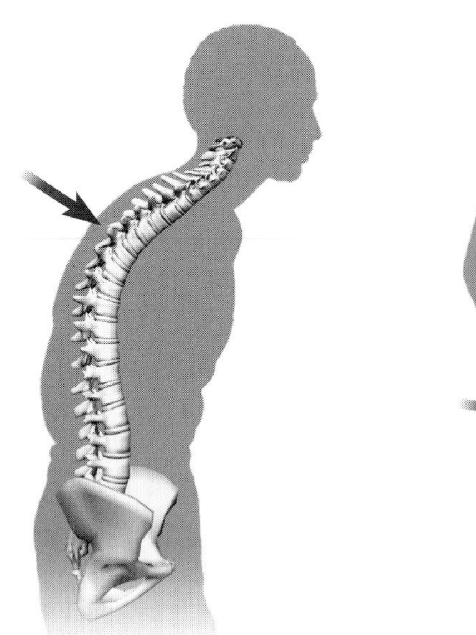

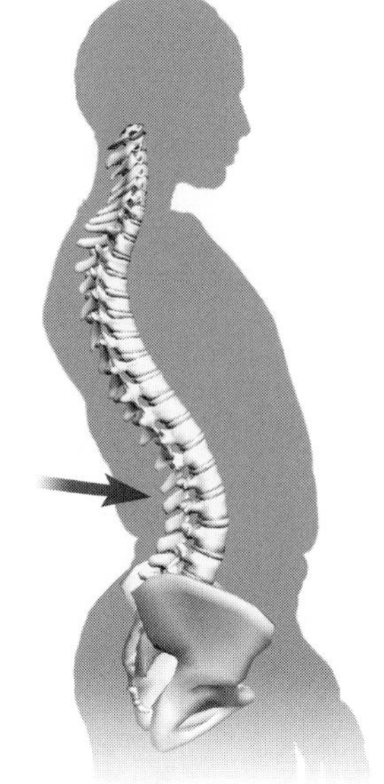

Two common forms of improper posture are slouching your shoulders (kyphosis), left, in which shoulders roll forward, and swayback (lordosis), right, in which your abdomen sticks out too far in front and your buttocks too far in back.

natural positions, you reduce stress on your back.

You normally have three spinal curves: an inward (forward) curve at the neck, an outward curve at the upper back and an inward curve at the lower back. Slouching or rolling your shoulders forward (kyphosis) shortens your chest muscles and reduces their flexibility. Swayback (lordosis) causes your abdomen to stick out in front and your buttocks to stick out in back, creating an exaggerated curve between your pelvis and ribs and stressing your lower back.

Many posture problems are the result of having to sit for long periods. Sitting is harder on the back than standing is. Wearing poorly fitting shoes or high heels also can cause posture problems. So can carrying excess weight.

Practice good posture by becoming aware of how you sit and stand and correcting your position when necessary. When standing, keep your shoulders back and your head high. Pull in your abdomen and buttocks, and tuck in your chin. When sitting, make sure your thighs are parallel to the ground and that your head isn't slumped forward.

If you're not sure whether you're using good posture, imagine a string that extends from your earlobe to your instep. When you're standing straight, the string should extend up the side of your leg, just behind your kneecap, across the middle of your thigh and past the tip of your shoulder.

Strengthening and stretching exercises that target specific muscles also can contribute to improved posture. Some examples are shown on the previous page. If you practice them regularly — once a day is good — they'll help support and align your back. Because your posture is ingrained, it won't improve overnight. Keep doing your exercises and concentrate on maintaining good posture at all times.

Lift correctly

When lifting, bend your knees, not your back. Whether the object you want to pick up weighs a fraction of an ounce or 50 pounds, squat with your back straight and let your legs do the lifting. Hold the load close to your body and increase the tension on your muscles gradually. Don't jerk or lunge to lift the load.

Sleep on your side

Don't sleep on your stomach unless you cushion your abdomen with a pillow. The best position for sleeping is on your side with your legs bent and drawn up slightly toward your chest and with a pillow between your knees. If you sleep on your back, put a pillow under your knees to keep a slight bend in your

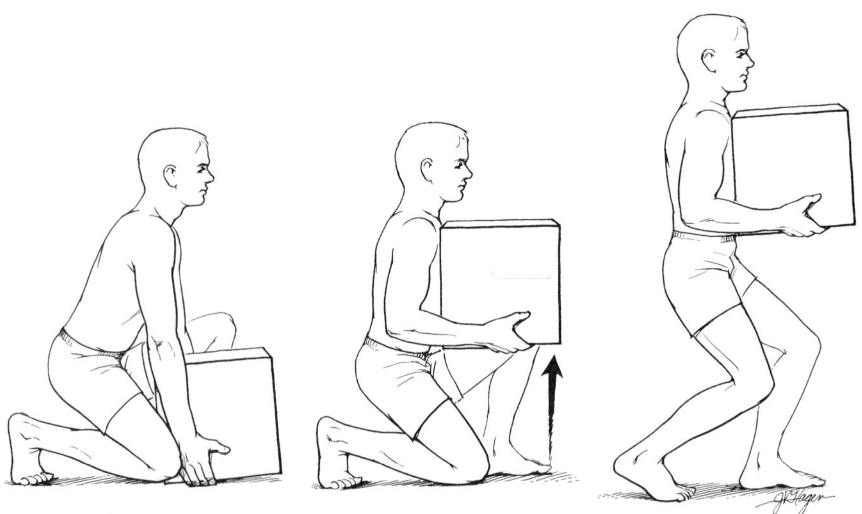

When lifting any object, let your legs do the work. Bend your knees rather than your back. Hold the object close to your body and lift gently. Avoid jerking or lunging upward.

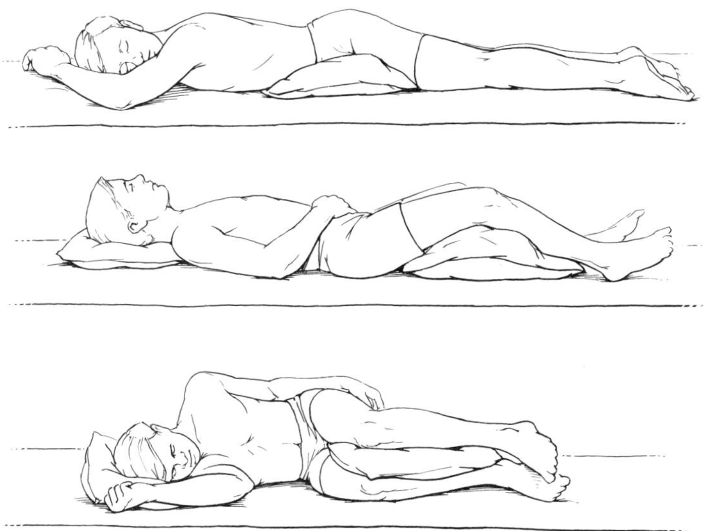

If you have back problems, to avoid aggravating your backache when you sleep or lie down, don't sleep on your stomach unless you cushion your abdomen with a pillow (top). If you sleep on your back, use pillows to support your knees and neck (middle). The best option is to sleep on your side with your legs drawn up slightly toward your chest (bottom) and with a pillow between your knees.

legs. Make sure your mattress provides your back with proper support. If your mattress is too soft or sags, place a board of $^1/_2$-inch plywood under the mattress.

Avoid stiffness
If you sit at a desk, stand in one position or drive a vehicle for hours every day, you're at risk of stiffness and muscle fatigue. Make a point of breaking your routine at frequent intervals.

When standing, periodically shift your weight from one foot to the other. When sitting, get up — if only for a few seconds — and walk or stretch. Take frequent breaks when driving. A small pillow placed at the base of your back can help support your spine while you drive.

Maintain a healthy weight
A major cause of backache is being overweight. Extra pounds at the midriff stress your back. If you're overweight, try to achieve and maintain a healthy weight and establish an exercise program.

Back Braces

Custom-fitted back braces (corsets) are available by prescription. Some are sold over-the-counter at most full-service pharmacies and medical supply stores. Worn properly, they relieve muscle strain by restricting motion in your lower back when you sit or stand. They can provide warmth, comfort and support to your back.

Unfortunately, many back braces have stiff stays and uncomfortable shoulder straps. They can also be unattractive and expensive. More important, because the support comes from the brace rather than from your own muscles, a back brace may actually weaken your back muscles, especially if you wear it for long periods. Most doctors recommend using a back brace only for short periods during back-straining activities or after some types of back surgeries.

Herniated disk

Signs and symptoms

- Mild to severe pain in your neck or back
- Numbness or weakness of an arm or hand and serious neck, shoulder and upper extremity pain, which might indicate a herniated disk in the neck
- Numbness or weakness in the buttocks, legs or feet, which might indicate a herniated disk in the middle or lower part of the back
- Shooting pain during coughing, sneezing or straining
- Usually, one arm or one leg affected significantly more than the other
- Sudden change in bowel or bladder function, such as incontinence

Disks, situated between the bones (vertebrae) of your spine, contain a soft, jelly-like substance. When a disk bulges or ruptures, the resulting condition is called a herniated disk. Other names for this disorder include a prolapsed or slipped disk, although there's no actual slippage.

Age or excess strain may cause a disk to herniate. This places pressure on nearby nerves, causing pain, numbness or weakness. A herniated disk is most likely to occur in the lower back, although any disk can be affected. The condition rarely occurs in children.

Diagnosis

Your doctor will take your medical history and perform a physical exam. Then he or she may order a series of X-rays, a computerized tomography (CT) scan or magnetic resonance imaging (MRI). The material protruding from the disk isn't visible on routine X-rays but sometimes can be seen on an MRI or CT scan (see image on page 1278). These tests help determine the extent of the injury and rule out other conditions that cause similar symptoms, such as a spinal tumor or circulatory problem.

A type of X-ray called myelography may be used (see page 610). It involves injection of a dye into your spinal column to help define a suspected abnormality. Myelography is helpful in planning surgery. Electromyography, a study of nerve conduction pathways, can confirm nerve compression caused by a herniated disk or spinal stenosis (see page 979).

To check for a bone tumor or a compression fracture, your doctor may recommend a bone scan. For this test, a radioactive substance called a tracer is injected into a vein, which is followed by a scan with a special camera.

How serious is a herniated disk?

In many people, a herniated disk will repair itself given time — usually 2 to 6 weeks — and proper rest. In some instances, an operation is necessary.

Treatment

The most common treatment for a herniated disk is decreased activity and, rarely, bed rest. Your doctor may recommend 1 or 2 weeks of decreased activity, after which you may slowly resume activity. Pain medication and physical therapy measures such as the use of heat or ice, massage, gentle exercises and, sometimes, traction may be helpful.

Surgery

Sometimes nerve compression from a herniated disk doesn't resolve with decreased activity or you have significant or progressive weakness in a muscle supplied by the involved nerve or a change in your bowel or bladder function. In such cases, a doctor may recommend a laminotomy or laminectomy and a diskectomy. A laminotomy is a surgical procedure that removes a portion of a bone over the spinal canal (lamina). A laminectomy removes all of the lamina. Removing all or part of the lamina gives the surgeon access to the affected disk. A diskectomy involves removing a portion of the disk to relieve pressure on the nerve.

In the lower back, a diskectomy usually involves making an incision, removing a small amount of bone and removing part of the disk. The whole disk isn't removed. A similar procedure may be done in the neck or upper back.

If the surgeon needs to reach the front of the spine, the incision will be made in the abdomen or the front of the neck. This approach eliminates the need to remove bone and enables the doctor to remove a larger amount of disk.

Other therapies

To avoid surgery and decrease recovery time, your doctor may try an epidural injection to relieve the pain.

If the disk is torn but not herniated, your doctor may use a procedure called intradiskal electrothermal therapy (IDET). A needle is inserted into the damaged area. A wire is passed through the needle and into the torn disk. The wire is heated, bonding collagen in the disk to stimulate healing. Collagen is a fibrous protein that occurs naturally in the body, primarily in skin. The heat also deadens nerves in the disk that may be causing pain.

Another procedure, called percutaneous diskectomy, allows the disk to be removed from between the vertebrae with a mechanical device inserted through a large needle. The surgeon inserts the needle through the skin into the disk.

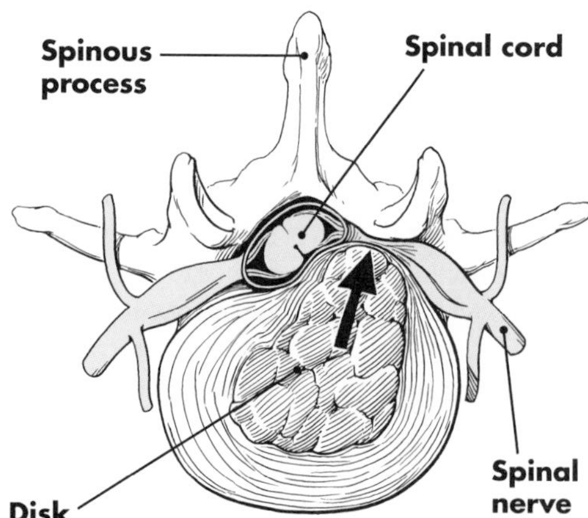

If a disk in your back ruptures, a portion of its jelly-like interior may protrude, putting pressure on a spinal nerve (see arrow) or on the spinal cord.

Spondylosis

Signs and symptoms

- Back pain and tenderness
- Difficulty moving your back

Sciatica

Inflammation of a nerve or compression of a nerve root in your lower back can cause sciatica. The condition is named after the sciatic nerve that extends down each leg from your hip to your heel. Only 1 percent or 2 percent of people with back pain have sciatica.

The disorder is characterized by pain radiating from your lower back down through your buttock to your lower leg. The nerve compression can also cause tingling, numbness or muscle weakness. Coughing, sneezing and other activities that exert pressure on your spine can aggravate sciatica.

Usually, the pain resolves on its own. However, severe nerve compression can cause progressive weakness of affected muscles and require surgical intervention.

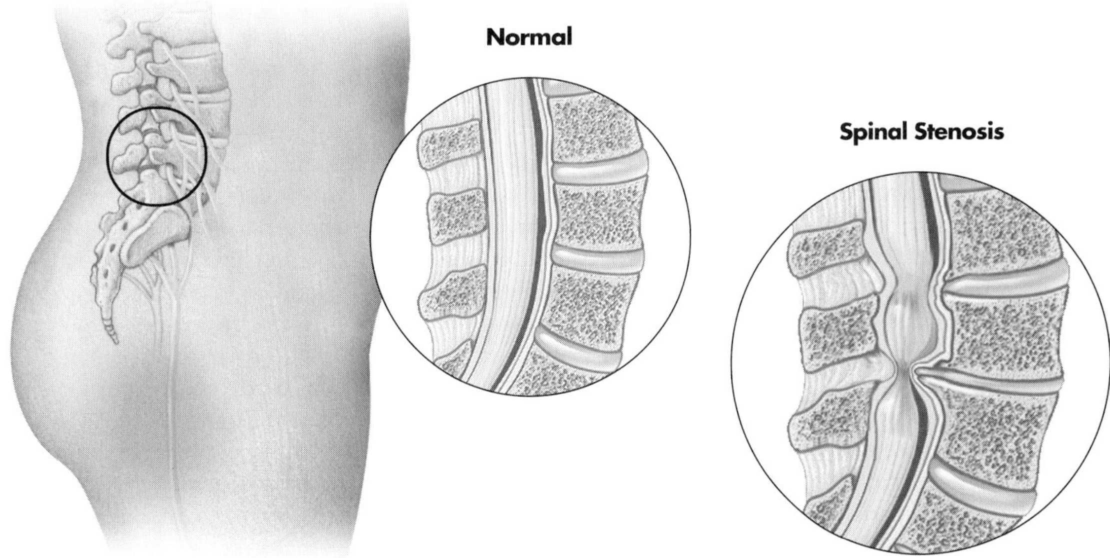

In spinal stenosis, an area of the spinal canal is narrowed, often from a herniated disk. The narrowing may place pressure on the spinal cord and compress nerve roots.

- Pain in the back of your thighs when standing
- In mild cases, none

Spondylosis is a disorder in which, over time, the spine becomes stiff and loses its flexibility. Spondylosis may result from excessive wear and tear, an injury or simply aging.

Whatever the cause, the disks between the vertebrae become worn, and the spaces between them narrow. The facet joints of the spine are usually affected as well, and bone spurs may develop. The result is pain and stiffness.

Spondylosis is sometimes referred to as degenerative joint disease or osteoarthritis of the spine. It's not the same condition as ankylosing spondylitis (see page 1005).

Diagnosis

An X-ray of your spine can often reveal the condition of your vertebrae. If you've had a herniated disk, you may be more susceptible to spondylosis.

How serious is spondylosis?

For many people, the condition isn't serious, but learning to deal with the discomfort can take time.

In rare cases, spondylosis in the lower back can lead to difficulty with bladder and bowel control and with walking.

Treatment

Depending on the severity of the condition and your symptoms, your doctor may recommend a combination of physical therapy, self-care measures such as heat, cold and gentle massage, and pain relievers.

Spinal stenosis

Signs and symptoms

- Pain in the lower back, buttock, thigh and calf associated with walking and standing
- Improvement in pain with sitting, bending forward or leaning on something for support
- Difficulty walking, especially downhill
- Progressive numbness or weakness in your leg
- Trouble with bladder and bowel control

Spinal stenosis is a narrowing of an area in your spinal canal that can cause compression of your spinal cord and nerve roots. You may first notice an ache in a buttock, thigh and calf when you walk or stand.

If you bend forward at your waist or sit for a few moments, the pain goes away. These symptoms suggest spinal stenosis. Symptoms are often subtle and similar to those associated with other causes of back and leg pain.

Spinal stenosis typically affects adults beyond age 50. It can develop because of a congenital defect, but it usually results from osteoarthritis.

Wear and tear, a previous injury, or aging can slowly deteriorate the protective tissue (cartilage) covering joint surfaces in your spine. Disks between vertebrae in your spine may become worn, and spaces between vertebrae may narrow. Bony outgrowths (spurs) also may develop. These changes can cause vertebrae and soft tissue to move inward into the spinal canal, compressing nerves.

Pressure may develop on roots of your sciatic nerve. This may cause pain to radiate from your lower back down your buttock to your calf. Numbness or weakness in your legs may eventually develop. Occasionally, nerves to the bladder and bowel become compressed, which leads to incontinence.

Bending forward at your waist or sitting relieves the pain because these positions increase the diameter of your spinal canal, reducing pressure on spinal nerves. In severe cases of narrowing, the pain may persist regardless of activity or position.

Diagnosis

Before a diagnosis is made, your doctor will likely perform tests to rule out other conditions that can cause leg pain or numbness, such as a spinal tumor or a circulatory problem. A herniated ("slipped") disk also can cause similar symptoms.

Additional tests to diagnose narrowing of your spinal canal may include a computerized tomography (CT) scan or myelography (see page 610).

Pain from spinal stenosis tends to be more noticeable when you walk downhill and persists when you stand. It's relieved with sitting. Pain caused by poor circulation, on the other hand, is usually worse when you walk uphill and subsides when you stand.

How serious is spinal stenosis?

Symptoms differ depending on what part of your spine is involved and how large an area it affects. If the pressure on your nerve roots can be effectively relieved with treatment, symptoms may not progress any further and may even improve.

In some cases, spinal stenosis can lead to disabling pain or other symptoms that require surgery.

Treatment

For mild to moderate spinal stenosis, medication and physical therapy may be all the treatment you'll need. Bed rest was once the mainstay of treatment for acute back pain. Now it's recommended for only a few days if the pain is severe. Prolonged bed rest can reduce muscle strength and lead to further disability.

Medication

Nonsteroidal anti-inflammatory drugs and muscle relaxants can relieve pain and reduce inflammation. Over-the-counter pain medications also may help. Corticosteroid medications may be injected for temporary relief, but they don't cure spinal stenosis.

Physical therapy

For acute pain, applications of heat or cold or a gentle massage performed by a physical therapist may help. Once the pain subsides, your therapist can design an exercise program to improve your flexibility, strengthen your back and abdominal muscles and improve your posture.

A brace worn around your lower back also can improve your posture. Limit use of back supports to activities that put extra stress on back muscles. Extended use of back supports can lead to muscle weakness in your back and abdomen.

Surgery

Your doctor may recommend a surgical procedure if you have disabling pain, progressive weakness in your legs or reduced control of your bladder or bowel. During this operation, called a laminectomy, a surgeon removes bone and soft tissues that protrude into your spinal canal or that put pressure on your spinal nerves.

If you have spondylolisthesis, a condition in which vertebrae slip forward and create pressure on spinal nerves or the spinal cord, some vertebrae in your lower back may be fused.

Laminectomy often improves or eliminates pain in the buttocks and legs, but it may not relieve low back pain that's associated with an underlying condition such as osteoarthritis.

Within a few months of surgery, you'll be able to resume most of your daily activities with the exception of heavy physical labor. Your recovery and rehabilitation may take longer if spinal fusion was required.

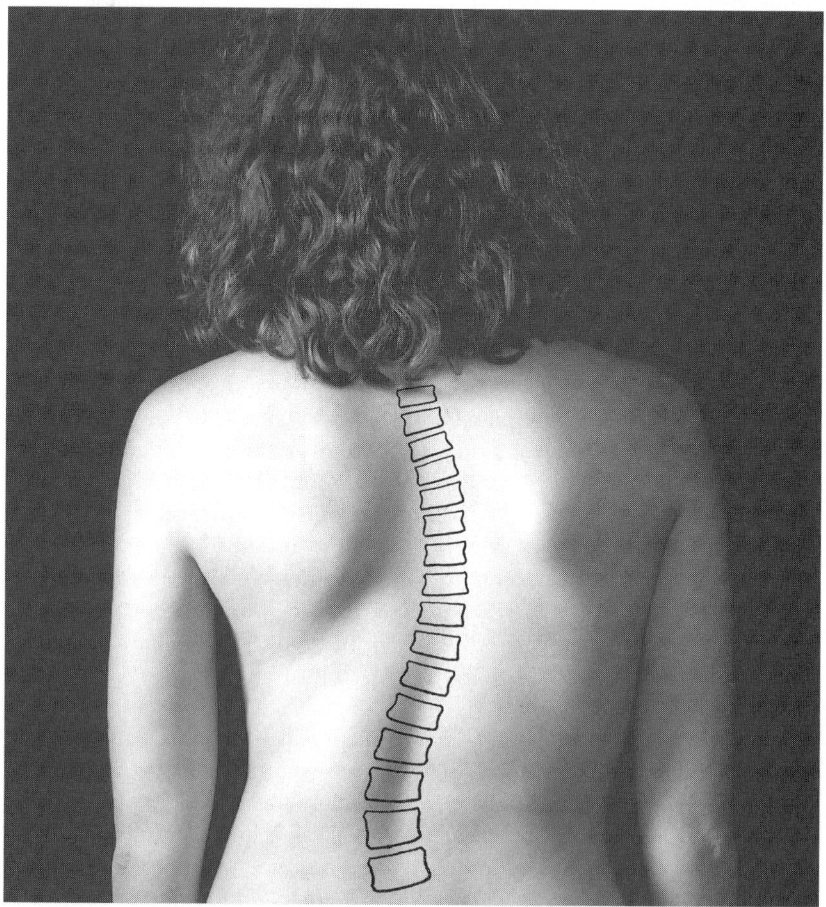

A sideways curvature of the spine is called scoliosis.

Bone Density Testing

Bone density can be measured in several painless and noninvasive ways. Various types of bone density tests include:

- *Central dual energy X-ray absorptiometry.* Called DEXA or DXA, this test uses low-level X-rays to assess your spine, hip or total body. This is the preferred method, but it may be available only in a hospital or clinic.
- *Peripheral dual energy X-ray absorptiometry.* Called pDEXA or pDXA, this test uses low-level X-rays to measure bone mass in your wrist, finger or heel. Your doctor's office may be more likely to offer this than a central DEXA, making it more accessible.
- *Quantitative ultrasound.* A QUS test transmits sound waves through your heel, shinbone and kneecap. This equipment is portable and inexpensive, which makes it potentially accessible to more people. Its accuracy compared with DEXA is being studied.
- *Quantitative computerized tomography.* A QCT test is most commonly used to measure your spine.

How often you need repeat testing depends on the results. If you're taking medication for osteoporosis or osteopenia, you may have measurements every 2 to 3 years to determine the effectiveness of your treatment.

Scoliosis

Signs and symptoms

- A sideways curvature of the spine
- An asymmetric rib cage with one shoulder blade protruding

Scoliosis is a painless, abnormal curvature of the spine. Usually, a curve to one side develops, followed by a compensating bend in the opposite direction, forming an S-like configuration — as seen from the back.

A small percentage of cases result from a congenital spinal defect. The cause of most cases is unknown, although heredity may play a role. The deformity may begin during infancy or in the preschool or early grade school years, but often the condition is detected in adolescence. Because the onset is gradual and the condition doesn't cause pain, significant curvature can develop without the child or parent noticing it. Many schools have screening programs to detect scoliosis.

Diagnosis

A visual examination of the spine is usually sufficient to identify scoliosis, although your doctor may want an X-ray of your spine to help determine the extent of the curvature.

How serious is scoliosis?

Mild cases generally cause few problems and don't require treatment, but they need close monitoring because the condition can worsen.

In more severe scoliosis, involved vertebrae may rotate, resulting in widely separated ribs on one side of the body and narrowed spaces on the other. Lung problems may develop as a result of the disease.

Treatment

Small curves don't require treatment. More pronounced curves may require treatment with a brace, especially in growing adolescents. The brace helps correct the deformity and straighten the spine. More severe curvature may require surgery. In general, exercises have no effect on scoliosis.

Bone Diseases

Your bones are living, changing tissues. The marrow within the bones produces blood cells, and the bones act as a storehouse for the minerals calcium and phosphate. Some of the diseases that affect bone, such as osteoporosis, are common, and others are rare.

Osteoporosis

Signs and symptoms

- Initially, none
- Back pain
- Loss of height with stooped posture
- A bone fracture, including a vertebral compression fracture

The National Osteoporosis Foundation estimates that approximately 44 million people in the United States age 50 and older have osteoporosis or are at increased risk of the disease. Sixty-eight percent of them are women. The number of cases in both women and men is on the rise.

Osteoporosis is a condition in which your bones become less dense and more porous. The amount of calcium stored in your bones decreases, causing your skeleton to weaken and your risk of fractures to increase. Most cases of osteoporosis are due to an acceleration of normal bodily changes. Approximately 1 of every 4 women older than age 45 and 9 of 10 women older than age 75 have osteoporosis. The condition is more prevalent after the onset of menopause. Compared with women, men start with a larger reserve of bone minerals and they tend to lose less bone mass.

Risk factors for osteoporosis include aging, a family history of osteoporosis, inadequate calcium in the diet, a sedentary lifestyle, smoking, excessive alcohol use and eating disorders, such as anorexia and bulimia.

Osteoporosis may accompany endocrine disorders such as acromegaly and Cushing's syndrome, or it may result from use of some prescription medications, such as corticosteroids and antiseizure medications. In these cases, treating the underlying disease or

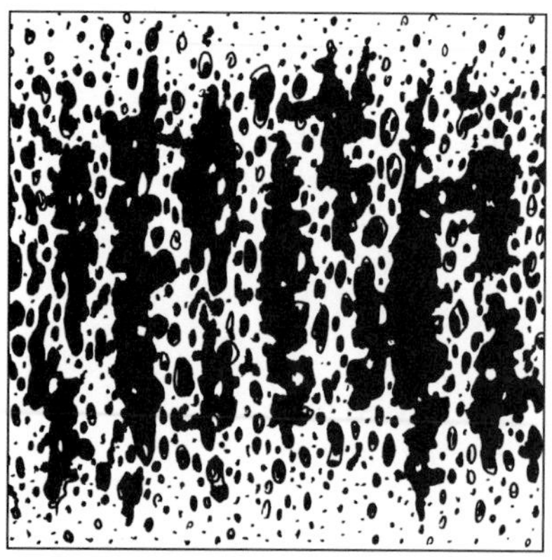

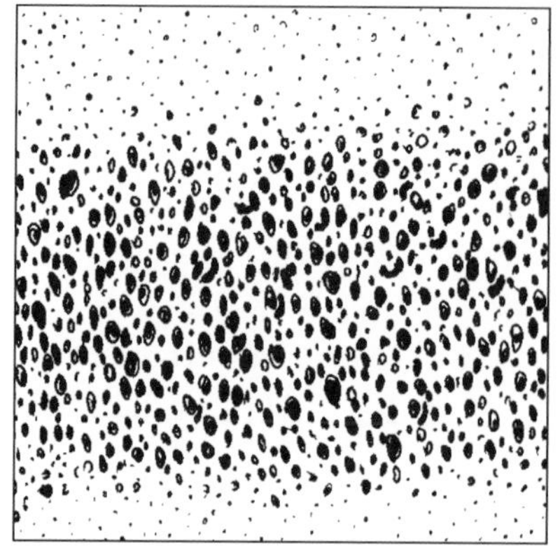

Osteoporotic bone (left) is weaker, more porous and more prone to fracture than is normal bone (right).

stopping use of a particular medication may improve the condition.

Diagnosis

You may not know that you have osteoporosis until you fracture a bone. Your doctor may recommend a painless, noninvasive bone density test — most commonly at the spine, hip or wrist.

The test results are compared with two standards — average bone density for someone your age, sex and size and optimal peak bone density of a healthy young adult of the same sex.

Results are reported in T-scores, which reflect the difference between your bone density and that of a healthy, young adult. The lower your bone density, the higher your risk of fractures.

If your T-score is greater than -1, you have normal bone mass. A reading between -1 and -2.4 means that you have osteopenia, a somewhat low bone density that puts you at greater risk of developing osteoporosis. A T-score at or below –2.5 indicates osteoporosis.

There's lack of agreement among medical organizations and doctors as to who should have a bone mineral density test. Generally, the test is recommended for:

- All women by the age of 65
- All adults with conditions known to lower bone mass
- All individuals who are going to take — or are taking — glucocorticoid medications
- All young adults who have low levels of the hormones estrogen or testosterone
- Any adult over age 40 who has had a fracture and is willing to undergo osteoporosis treatment.

How serious is osteoporosis?

Fractures are the most common consequence of osteoporosis.

Vertebroplasty

Vertebroplasty is a procedure used to relieve pain that can accompany compression fractures of the vertebrae. It entails injecting bone cement into the involved vertebrae. The cement hardens within hours, stabilizing the fractures and relieving pain.

Spinal compression fractures are most often the result of acute stress on bones weakened by osteoporosis. Less frequently, the fractures are the result of cancerous (malignant) tumors that involve the spine.

Vertebroplasty often provides pain relief when standard care for compression fractures — which includes rest, pain medications and a brace — doesn't. It may be most effective in fractures that are less than 6 months old.

A similar procedure is kyphoplasty, in which a balloon-like device is inserted into a compressed vertebra to expand the vertebra before the cement is injected. More than 80 percent of people who undergo vertebroplasty experience significant pain relief within 48 hours.

Who's a candidate?

Many people with compression fractures get significant pain relief after several weeks of standard care. But for some, pain persists, limiting mobility and interfering with daily activities. For them, vertebroplasty may be a good alternative.

If you're a candidate for the procedure, you'll likely need to have spinal X-rays as well as more specialized radiographic imaging such as magnetic resonance imaging (MRI) or a bone scan to help determine which vertebrae are involved and the age of the fractures.

People who may not be good candidates for vertebroplasty are those who have medical conditions that prevent them from lying on their stomachs for up to 2 hours and those who have bleeding disorders or who can't be taken off anticoagulant medication.

What does the procedure involve?

You'll be asked to lie on your stomach, and you'll receive a sedative. An injection of a local anesthetic will numb the skin over the affected vertebra. Some individuals may receive general anesthesia.

A radiologist — a doctor who specializes in the use of X-rays and other radiographic procedures — inserts a specially designed needle into the involved vertebra, using X-ray to provide guidance. When the needle is in the correct position in the vertebra, the radiologist injects the bone cement.

Following the procedure, you'll be asked to lie flat on your back for about 3 hours while the cement

Osteoporotic bones can break with little or no unusual stress. Osteoporosis also affects your lifestyle. For many people, living with osteoporosis means changing dietary and exercise habits to minimize future bone loss. It also means taking a common-sense approach to daily activities to avoid putting your bones at avoidable risk.

Vertebral compression fractures due to osteoporosis rarely require surgical treatment. Commonly, severe pain begins abruptly, centers on your back, possibly radiates around the trunk, is aggravated by movement and relieved by heat, and gradually subsides within 1 to 2 months. Over a period of years, however, a sequence of spinal compression fractures can lead to dowager's hump (widow's hump) and an increasingly stooped posture.

If your bones are severely weakened, osteoporosis can be disabling. The disorder is associated with approximately 40,000 deaths annually, largely from complications of hip fractures.

Treatment

A number of treatments may be used to treat or prevent reduced bone density. Lifestyle factors also play a significant role.

Medication

Your doctor may prescribe one of the following medications, depending on your age, health, sex and the cause of your disease.

- *SERM.* Raloxifene (Evista) is a selective estrogen receptor modulator (SERM) used to prevent and treat osteoporosis. Unlike estrogens, raloxifene doesn't appear to stimulate uterine or breast tissues, but studies are ongoing.
- *Bisphosphonates.* The medications alendronate (Fosamax) and risedronate (Actonel) belong to a class of drugs known as bisphosphonates. They help reduce bone

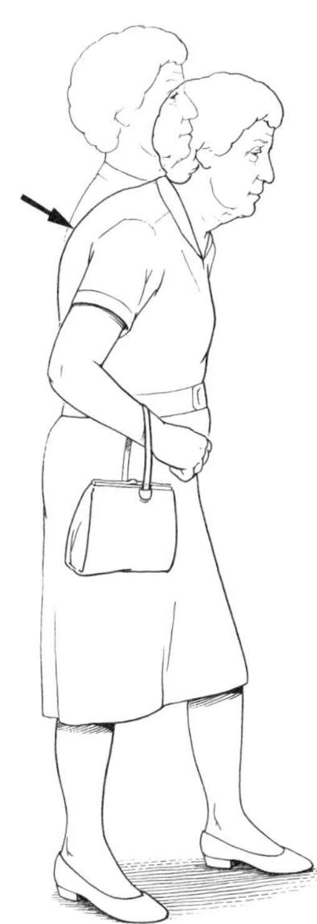

One of the possible long-term effects of osteoporosis is a series of vertebral compression fractures that can produce a stooped posture and the appearance of an upper-back hump.

hardens. You may return home either later that day or the next morning.

What are the risks?

The primary risk associated with vertebroplasty is that bone cement may leak into surrounding tissues and vessels and put pressure on the spinal cord or nerve roots, causing pain and weakness. Another risk is that if bone cement enters blood vessels, it could travel to the lung and lodge in a lung artery (pulmonary embolism), causing chest pain and breathing difficulties. Both of these risks are rare, however.

A person with soft bones may fracture a rib by lying stomach-down during the procedure. Other possible risks include infection, bleeding and further injury to the vertebra from needle placement.

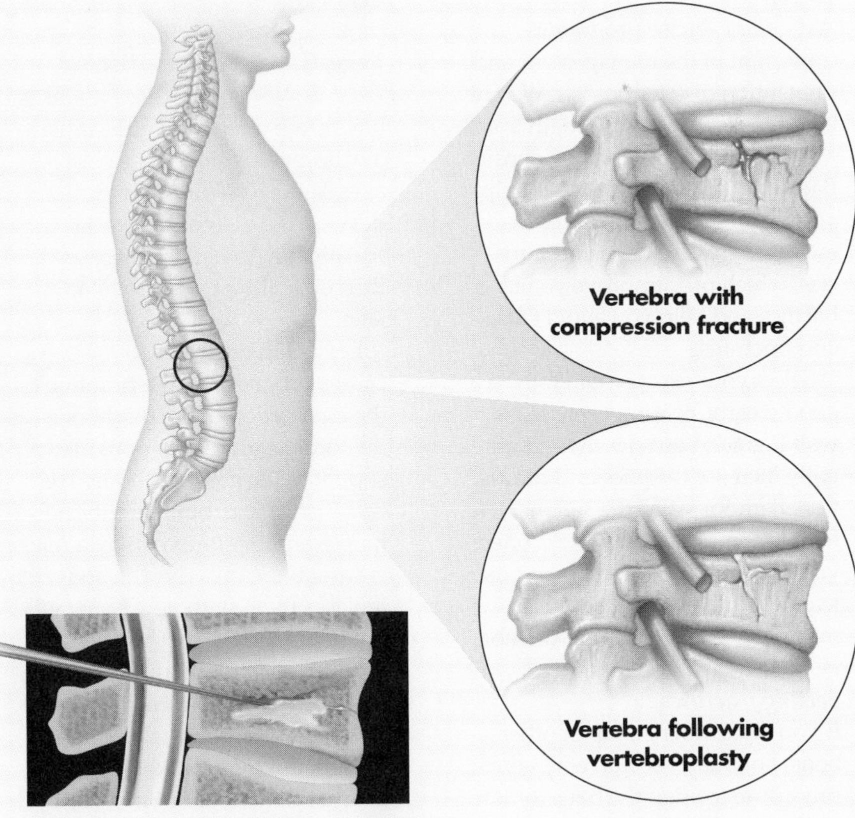

Vertebra injected with bone cement

loss and increase bone density. These drugs are used to treat osteoporosis in men and in people taking corticosteroids.

- *Hormone replacement therapy.* If you're a postmenopausal woman, your doctor may recommend hormone replacement therapy, which usually involves taking a combination of the hormones estrogen and progestin. Estrogen may reduce bone loss and increase bone density. Progestin has other benefits and risks which should be discussed with your doctor. If you've had a hysterectomy, you only need estrogen.
- *Other hormones.* Calcitonin, a naturally occurring hormone involved in calcium regulation and bone metabolism, is sometimes prescribed for women 5 years past menopause to slow bone loss and increase bone density in the spine. Calcitonin is administered by injection or in the form of a nasal spray (Miacalcin).

Exercise

A regular exercise program is important in the management and prevention of osteoporosis. Weight-bearing exercise and strength training can help maintain bone density. Back-strengthening exercises help you maintain good posture. Exercise also strengthens your muscles, which may improve your balance and help you avoid falls and fractures.

Select your exercise carefully. A good weight-bearing exercise is walking. Start out slowly, and gradually increase the pace and duration. Paradoxically, the serious female competitive runner is often vulnerable to osteoporosis because leanness and excessive exercise may decrease estrogen production.

Setting fractures

If you break a wrist, hip or other bone, you may need an emergency procedure to align the bone for it to heal correctly. Fractures of vertebrae may require a procedure known as vertebroplasty to stabilize the bone. Physical therapy is often a key part of the recovery from any fracture.

Prevention

Indications are that the more calcium a woman has stored in her skeleton before menopause, the less risk she's at of developing significant osteoporosis. So starting at a young age, women should eat a calcium-rich diet with adequate vitamin D to aid absorption of calcium.

Foods high in calcium include dairy products, leafy green vegetables, beans, nuts and whole-grain cereals. Many doctors advise taking a calcium supplement to ensure that you get adequate calcium in your diet. A calcium intake of at least 1,000 milligrams (mg) a day from your diet or a supplement may help you maintain maximal calcium status. If you're older, especially if you have osteoporosis, the recommended amount is 1,200 mg to 1,500 mg a day.

Regular weight-bearing and strength-training exercises are important for prevention of osteoporosis. Weight-bearing exercises include running, walking, tennis, dancing, cross-country skiing,

Skeletal Disorders of Childhood

Numerous skeletal problems are peculiar to children. Fortunately, most of them are rare. These disorders include:

Legg-Calvé-Perthes disease

Legg-Calvé-Perthes disease affects boys more often than girls. It usually becomes evident between ages 3 and 10. Children who develop the disease before age 6 usually have a better outcome than do children who develop it later.

Legg-Calvé-Perthes disease causes progressive deterioration of the top portion of the thighbone (femoral head) due to poor blood supply to the growing bone. The cause isn't clear, but heredity, hormones and injury may play a role.

After bone cells die, the body replaces them with new bone cells. But while these new bone cells are forming, the bone is unstable and may break and become deformed.

A child may complain of pain in the hip and may walk with a limp. Because a number of other childhood conditions may cause hip pain and a limp, it's important to identify the cause.

The focus of treatment is to protect the bone and joint from further stress and injury during the natural healing process, which may last $1\frac{1}{2}$ to 3 years. Treatment depends on the severity of the disease, but may include bed rest, range of motion exercises, crutches and nonsteroidal anti-inflammatory drugs (NSAIDs). Traction on the bone to immobilize it and help it heal, bracing and surgery may be necessary.

Most children with this disorder resume normal function. However, they may continue to limp for several years. Children with severe cases are more likely to develop osteoarthritis of the hip joint.

Slipped capital femoral epiphysis

During the growth spurt just before puberty, the growth plate of the ball of the hip may slip. The thighbone rotates outward and slides upward relative to the ball of the hip. This unusual condition is called a slipped capital femoral epiphysis.

Common symptoms are pain in the knee, thigh or hip and a limp that involves lurching to the side and turning the foot outward.

weightlifting and almost any activity that combines movement with stress on your limbs.

Additional precautions also may be beneficial. Don't smoke, limit caffeine consumption to no more than three cups of coffee a day and avoid consuming large amounts of protein and excessive amounts of alcohol.

Osteomalacia and rickets

Signs and symptoms

- Pain in the bones of your arms, legs, spine and pelvis
- Progressive weakness
- Bowlegs, projection of the chest (pigeon breast) and, in children, protrusion of the stomach

Osteomalacia means softening of the bones. The softening stems from an inability of the skeleton to incorporate adequate minerals into the bones. The bones become flexible so that body weight and other forces gradually mold them, often resulting in deformities. In children, osteomalacia is known as rickets.

One of the most common causes of osteomalacia is malabsorption of fat, a condition called steatorrhea. Instead of being absorbed in the small intestine, fat passes out of the body in your stool. As a result, vitamin D, a fat-soluble vitamin, is poorly absorbed. This, in turn, hinders the intestinal absorption of the minerals calcium and phosphorus, which rely on vitamin D for their absorption. Digestive disorders such as nontropical sprue and short-bowel syndrome can cause malabsorption of fat.

Another cause of osteomalacia is a dietary deficiency of vitamin D. In the United States, people get vitamin D by drinking milk, which is supplemented with it. In addition, your body naturally produces vitamin D when your skin is exposed to sunlight. Inadequate vitamin D is most common in countries where the vitamin isn't added to foods or where people get little sun exposure.

A rare cause of osteomalacia is an increased amount of acid in the body fluids due to abnormal kidney function. This problem, called renal tubular acidosis, occurs in people with congenital or acquired kidney disorders. The increased acid gradually dissolves the skeleton, just as vinegar softens an eggshell.

There's also a rare hereditary form of rickets that leads to shortened adult stature, often called vitamin D-resistant rickets.

Diagnosis

Blood tests to measure levels of calcium and phosphorus and X-rays of the affected bones are often the first steps in a diagnosis of osteomalacia or rickets. Infrequently, a tiny piece of bone is removed (biopsied) for examination in a laboratory.

Once osteomalacia is diagnosed, typically the next step is to determine the cause, such as an intestinal problem (malabsorption) or a kidney defect.

How serious are osteomalacia and rickets?

In many cases, correcting the mineral deficiency eliminates the signs and symptoms. In children and

Symptoms usually evolve gradually over weeks or months, but they can also appear suddenly in association with an injury.

The condition is most common in boys between ages 11 and 14, particularly those who are overweight. In one-fourth of cases, it affects both hips.

A slipped capital femoral epiphysis requires surgery to correct the problem or prevent further displacement. If the slip progresses until it's severe, it can deform the hip and interfere with normal walking.

Osgood-Schlatter disease

Osgood-Schlatter disease affects children between 11 and 15 years of age, especially boys, and is characterized by pain and swelling at the bony protuberance on the shinbone (tibia), just below the kneecap. This is where the tendon from the kneecap attaches to the tibia. This disease is associated with overuse and is much more common than other conditions discussed in this section.

Icing, stretching and rest from impact activities such as running and jumping are usually the best treatment for Osgood-Schlatter disease. A strap across the kneecap tendon can help take the force away from the bony protuberance. Anti-inflammatory medications, such as ibuprofen (Advil, Motrin, others), also may be helpful. The condition usually resolves as the skeleton matures.

Congenital dislocation of the hip

Congenital dislocation of the hip, also called developmental dysplasia of the hip, is caused by a hip socket that's too shallow at birth, making the joint especially susceptible to dislocation. The problem can lead to an altered shape of the bones of the joint, which may require surgery later in life.

Even if a baby appears to be entirely healthy, a doctor should be on the alert for this condition during the first year of a child's life. Early diagnosis allows for simple treatment with splinting, which is usually successful. Congenital dislocation of the hip tends to recur in families, so alert your doctor if you or your spouse had the condition.

Clubfoot

Clubfoot, technically known as talipes equinovarus, is a deformity of the foot present at birth. It may be hereditary. It can be treated with casts or splints in the first few weeks of life, often with good results (see page 182).

adults, appropriate treatment can correct most of the mineral depletion in the bones, and the skeletal deformities may improve over time.

Treatment

Usually, treatment is directed at correcting the underlying problem. Sometimes, calcium, phosphorus and vitamin D supplements are necessary. In vitamin D-resistant rickets, skeletal deformities may require surgical correction.

Paget's disease

Signs and symptoms

- Sometimes, none
- Pain, ranging from mild discomfort to more severe if it's near a joint
- Warmth in the skin over the affected area
- Neurologic problems, such as hearing loss, blindness, headache and weakness
- Bowing of a leg

Paget's disease is a metabolic bone disease named after a mid-19th-century English surgeon. Paget's disease of the bone isn't related to Paget's disease of the breast, which is a type of breast cancer.

Many people think the human skeleton stops changing once it reaches full growth. That's not true. Bone is living tissue engaged in a continuous process of renewal. Paget's disease disrupts the normal process of bone loss and formation, resulting in the breakdown of excess bone tissue and increased new bone formation. This leads to an abnormal structure in the affected bone because new bone is laid down in a disordered pattern and may be softer and weaker than normal bone.

The cause of Paget's disease isn't clear. Some experts believe that it may be due to a viral infection of certain bone cells called osteoclasts. In addition, some people may be genetically predisposed to the disease.

Endocrine Disorders and the Bones

Your endocrine system is made up of hormone-secreting glands that affect virtually all body functions and parts, including bones. The following endocrine disorders affect your bones. For more information on these conditions, see Chapter 32, "Endocrine System."

Acromegaly

This condition is the result of the pituitary gland secreting too much growth hormone in adults. People with acromegaly have characteristically large hands and feet, as well as a large jawbone and skull.

Gigantism

Gigantism is a rare condition caused by too much growth hormone before a child reaches full growth. The condition causes accelerated growth resulting in excessive height.

Hypopituitarism

Hypopituitarism occurs when the pituitary gland produces too few or no hormones. When a child with the disorder receives too little growth hormone, dwarfism results.

Hyperparathyroidism

In this condition, your body produces too much parathyroid hormone. Your bones then release too much calcium, causing a weakening of the skeleton.

People older than age 40 are the most likely to develop Paget's disease, although in rare instances it occurs in younger adults. Occasionally, it runs in families. The disease frequently affects the skull, arms, legs and spine. It may affect only one or two areas within the skeleton, or it may be widespread.

Diagnosis

Often, the first indication of this condition is an elevated alkaline phosphatase level found through routine blood testing. Alkaline phosphatase is an enzyme involved in bone breakdown. If you haven't had a blood test and your doctor suspects Paget's disease, he or she will probably order one. Your doctor may also order X-rays and bone scans. A sample of affected bone tissue (biopsy) may be obtained for laboratory analysis.

How serious is Paget's disease?

Most people with the disease have no symptoms. Among people with symptoms, usually only one area of the body is affected, most commonly the spine, skull, pelvis, thighs or lower legs. However, multiple sites can be involved. The affected bones can become deformed and subject to fracture. In most cases, the disease progresses very slowly.

In rare cases, serious, long-term complications occur. These range from deafness to congestive heart failure or spinal cord injury. Rarely, a bone cancer known as osteosarcoma may develop in bones affected by Paget's disease.

Treatment

If you don't have symptoms, you probably won't need treatment. If you have symptoms, your doctor may recommend medication.

In its early stages, Paget's disease may require treatment to reduce pain and inflammation. Pain relievers such as acetaminophen (Tylenol, others) and nonsteroidal anti-inflammatory drugs (NSAIDs), such as ibuprofen (Advil, Motrin, others) or aspirin, often suffice.

If the disease progresses, your doctor may prescribe a biphosphonate drug such as pamidronate (Aredia), alendronate (Fosamax), risedronate (Actonel), tiludronate (Skelid) or etidronate (Didronel) to help reduce bone loss and increase bone density. They're usually taken for several months. Calcitonin (Miacalcin), a naturally occurring hormone involved in calcium regulation and bone metabolism, is another effective medication. Rarely, surgery is necessary to repair deformities.

Fibrous dysplasia

Signs and symptoms

- Bone pain, especially in the lower leg
- Difficulty walking
- Rarely, fractures and multiple bone deformities
- Often, none

Fibrous dysplasia resembles Paget's disease in that it's characterized by abnormal growth of bone tissue. In the case of fibrous dysplasia, however, the bone tissue is fibrous rather than bony. The condition typically first appears in childhood and affects one or more bones. The abnormal growth usually stops at puberty.

The cause of fibrous dysplasia is unknown. Severe cases in which bones deform or fracture can seriously affect quality of life. One form of the disease, called Albright's syndrome, is associated with premature sexual maturation in girls.

Diagnosis

The presence of fibrous dysplasia generally is confirmed with X-rays of your bones or by removing samples of bone for laboratory analysis (biopsy).

Treatment

Although fibrous dysplasia isn't curable, surgery to remove fibrous growths from affected bones may help.

Osteogenesis imperfecta

Signs and symptoms

- Fragile bones resulting in fractures
- Bluish coloration in the white part of the eye (sclera)
- Limb deformities, particularly bowing
- Flatfeet
- Short stature

Osteogenesis imperfecta is a rare, inherited disease in which bones are abnormally brittle and fragile. Fractures may be present at birth or occur later when the child begins to walk. Hearing impairment also is common.

Diagnosis

X-ray studies of the bones often can confirm the diagnosis.

How serious is osteogenesis imperfecta?

This disease takes several forms. The most severe often are fatal. In less severe forms, the number of fractures decreases markedly once a child reaches adolescence.

Treatment

The treatment for less severe forms of this disease involves reducing the risk of fractures. It's important to set all fractures promptly and to correct skeletal deformities. Parents of an affected child might consider genetic counseling before another pregnancy.

Osteomyelitis

Signs and symptoms

- Intense pain and increased heat over the affected bone
- Tenderness and swelling
- Fever
- Fatigue

Osteomyelitis is a bone infection caused by bacteria or, rarely, fungi. The infectious organism may be acquired through a wound, fracture or other injury and carried to the bone by the blood. It can lead to destruction of bone and surrounding tissue.

Osteomyelitis is rare in the United States and is more common in children than in adults. It's usually treated successfully with antibiotics, but it can recur.

Diagnosis

If your doctor suspects osteomyelitis, blood tests or imaging tests may help with the diagnosis. Your doctor may also perform a biopsy, in which a sample of bone, pus or other tissue is removed for analysis and culture.

Treatment

An extended course of antibiotics is the usual treatment, along with bed rest. In some instances, it may be necessary to surgically remove the infected tissue.

Bone tumors

Signs and symptoms

- A hard lump on the surface of a bone
- Pain
- Fracture of the involved bone

Tumors that begin in bones are rare. The majority of bone tumors are noncancerous (benign), but some are cancerous (malignant). Both types may grow and impinge on healthy bone tissue, but benign tumors don't spread and rarely are life-threatening.

If the tumor is cancerous, most often the cancer has spread to the bone from elsewhere in the body (metastasized). Exceptions are a type of blood cancer called multiple myeloma that begins in bone marrow and osteosarcoma, the most common primary bone cancer. Osteosarcoma develops in new tissue in growing bones, most commonly in the knees, upper legs and upper arms. It occurs mostly in children, adolescents and young adults ages 10 to 25.

The exact cause of bone cancer is unknown. Children and young adults who've had radiation or chemotherapy treatments for other conditions are at increased risk of developing osteosarcoma. Adults with Paget's disease of the bone also may be at increased risk.

Diagnosis

Many times, X-rays are helpful in diagnosing a bone tumor, but they may not provide a conclusive diagnosis. Your doctor may perform a biopsy, in which a small sample of the tissue is removed for laboratory examination.

How serious is a bone tumor?

A benign growth rarely presents a serious health risk. If the tumor is a cancer that originated in bone (primary tumor) and hasn't spread, it may be curable with a combination of treatments. Bone cancer that has spread to another site or cancer that has metastasized to bone from another site is rarely curable.

Treatment

Benign tumors may require no treatment, but some are removed surgically if they cause pain or other symptoms. A cancerous tumor may require a combination of treatments, including surgery, radiation and chemotherapy. Amputation of the affected limb sometimes is necessary, but preoperative and postoperative chemotherapy has made it possible in many cases for the surgeon to preserve the limb by removing only the diseased portion of the bone and reconstructing the extremity. A program of rehabilitation follows.

For cancer that has spread, generally the focus is on relieving pain and maintaining quality of life.

Muscle, Tendon and Soft Tissue Disorders

Your muscle fibers are elongated and contractible. When you move a limb, one muscle contracts to produce the movement. To return the limb to its original position, the opposite muscle must contract.

Equally important to movement are tendons, which connect muscles to bones. In most parts of your body, tendons either intertwine with the muscles or take the form of short connectors between the ends of the muscles and bones. Tendons in your hands and feet are long and cord-like. Throughout your body fibrous tendons convey the movement of the muscles to the bones. Contract a muscle and it causes the attached tendons and bones to move.

Your muscles, tendons and soft tissues can be affected by a number of common disorders, from the discomfort of tendinitis to the crippling effects of muscular dystrophy.

Tenosynovitis

Signs and symptoms

- Tenderness and pain
- Movements accompanied by a crackling sound or feeling
- Pain when you move the affected area
- A joint that's hot and inflamed

Long, cable-like tendons run through your hand and into each finger. Each tendon is enclosed within a sheath lined with a membrane called the synovium. The synovium secretes fluid to lubricate the joints and the tendon sheaths and to nourish cartilage.

The function of the tendon sheath is to keep the tendon from adhering to tissues along its path. In tenosynovitis, the synovium becomes inflamed or infected.

Tenosynovitis may be related to underlying arthritis, but most often the cause is unknown or is related to overuse or overload of the tendon and its corresponding muscle. The condition may be aggravated by repetitive activity, but it occurs no more frequently in people who perform repetitive tasks, such as factory workers and computer keyboard operators, than in those who don't.

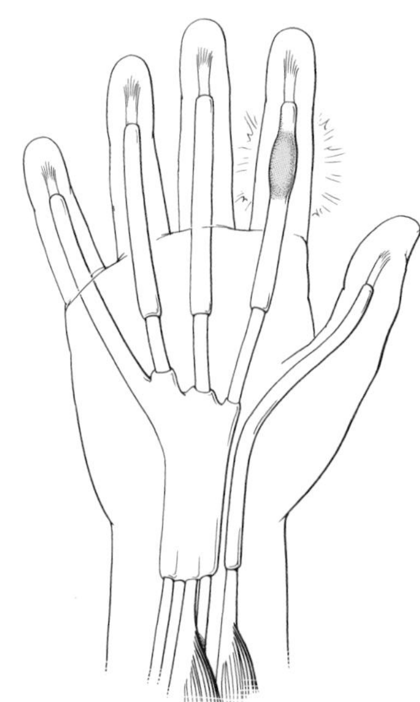

Each of the cable-like tendons in your hand is surrounded by a protective sheath called the synovium. When the synovial membrane is inflamed or infected (see highlighting), tenosynovitis results. Treatment varies but may include rest, medication or even surgery.

Tenosynovitis can occur in the wrist, hand, ankle and, more commonly, the bicipital tendon in the shoulder. It's most common in women at or beyond middle age.

Diagnosis

Your doctor will examine the affected area to determine if the synovium is infected. He or she may order an X-ray to rule out other bone problems, such as a bone growth or deformity, that may be causing your symptoms.

How serious is tenosynovitis?

If an infection is causing tenosynovitis, it's important to receive treatment immediately because the infection can permanently damage tissues and affect function.

Treatment

Medication and, in some cases, surgery may relieve your discomfort and restore function to the affected area. When tenosynovitis is aggravated by overuse, treatment may include resting and modifying your activities. Proper technique in sport and work activities is important to preventing overload of the tissue.

Medication
For noninfectious tenosynovitis, a pain reliever, such as acetaminophen (Tylenol, others) or a nonsteroidal anti-inflammatory drug (NSAID), such as ibuprofen (Advil, Motrin, others) or aspirin, may reduce the pain. If an infection is causing the discomfort, your doctor will likely prescribe an antibiotic.

Injection of a steroid drug, such as cortisone, may relieve symptoms. An injection is most often used when more conservative measures aren't helpful.

Splint
A protective splint that limits movement can provide needed rest and support for a hand or wrist affected by tenosynovitis.

Surgery
In some cases of infectious tenosynovitis, surgery is performed to drain pus at the infection site and limit spread of the infection.

Carpal tunnel syndrome

Signs and symptoms

- A numbness or tingling sensation in your fingers and hand, especially your thumb and index and middle fingers
- Wrist pain that may extend into your forearm, the palm of your hand or your fingers
- Numbness or pain that worsens at night and may be severe enough to awaken you
- Hand weakness

The eight wrist (carpal) bones and the tendons that overlay them form a tunnel-like structure in your wrist. Bounded by bones and ligaments, the carpal tunnel protects the nerves and tendons that extend into your hand.

Swelling or inflammation of tissues within the tunnel can compress the median nerve. The median nerve provides sensation to your thumb, index and middle fingers and part of your ring finger. Pressure on the nerve produces a specific pattern of numbness and pain that characterizes carpal tunnel syndrome. Many times it affects both wrists.

Although carpal tunnel syndrome often develops without a specific cause, a number of factors can predispose you to developing it. They include arthritis, obesity, smoking, pregnancy and certain occupations that require forceful repetitive hand motions.

Carpal tunnel syndrome may affect carpenters, meat cutters, pianists, mechanics and, occasionally, hobbyists such as golfers, canoeists and bicyclists. The common factor is performing repetitive, forceful motions with the wrist flexed.

Carpal tunnel syndrome may accompany some endocrine disorders, such as diabetes, acromegaly and, rarely, hypothyroidism, as well as rheumatoid arthritis. In general, women approaching middle age are most likely to develop carpal tunnel syndrome.

Diagnosis

A key symptom that helps in making a diagnosis is that the numbness in your fingers doesn't include the little finger. Your doctor may perform certain tests to determine if electric impulses traveling along the median nerve slow in the carpal tunnel, indicating that the nerve is being compressed.

Tingling or shooting pain into your hand or forearm when tapping on the palm side of your wrist also may be an indication of carpal tunnel syndrome. In addition, you may have loss of bulk in the muscles of your thumb.

How serious is carpal tunnel syndrome?

Proper treatment can relieve the pain and numbness and usually prevent permanent damage to your hand and wrist. Untreated, the syndrome can lead to permanent nerve and muscle damage.

Trigger Finger

A condition sometimes confused with tenosynovitis is a more common condition called trigger finger. The characteristic symptom is a clicking sensation in the finger as you bend or straighten it. In addition, when you try to point your finger, rather than responding smoothly, it seems to hesitate, then suddenly straightens with a snap. Left untreated, the condition can lead to an inability to straighten the finger.

The usual cause of trigger finger is a thickening and narrowing of the sheath that protects the tendon and helps guide it as it moves. What causes the sheath to thicken is unknown, but the condition is more common in older adults and people with diabetes.

Corticosteroid injections usually are effective in treating trigger finger. A protective splint that limits movement of the affected finger may be used in mild cases. Sometimes, surgery is necessary. An incision is made in the tendon sheath of the affected finger. This often relieves the constriction and restores full movement.

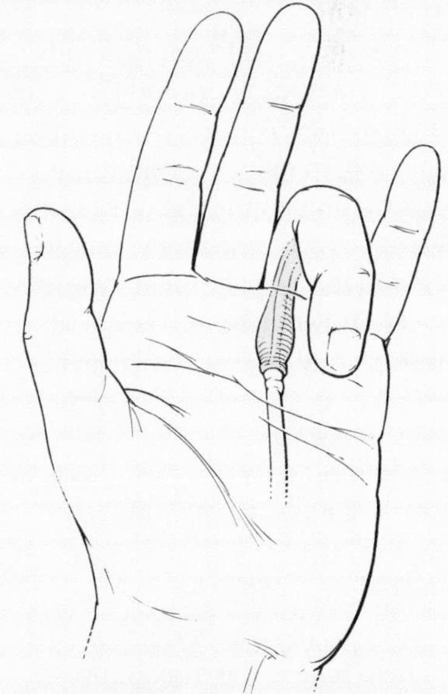

A condition sometimes confused with tenosynovitis is called trigger finger. The sheath that protects the tendon thickens, making it difficult to straighten the affected finger.

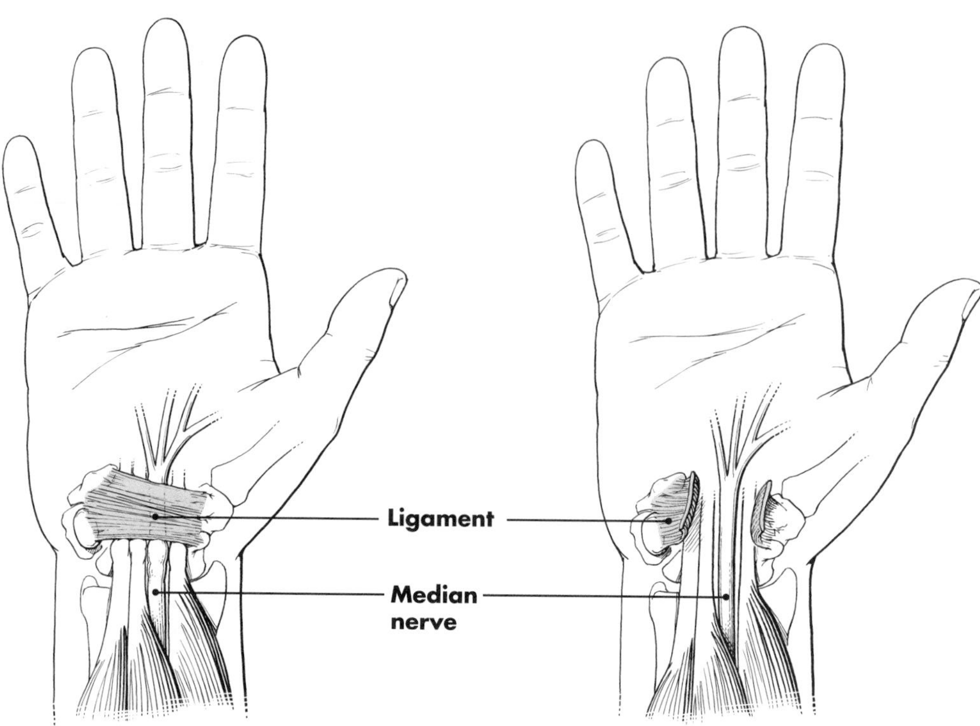

A narrow tunnel through your wrist — the carpal tunnel — protects the median nerve, which provides sensation to your thumb, index and middle fingers and a portion of your ring finger. Swelling or inflammation of tendon sheaths within the carpal tunnel or swelling of tissues around the carpal tunnel can compress the median nerve, producing pain and numbness. If conservative treatment isn't effective, the carpal tunnel may be surgically cut (right) to relieve the compression.

Treatment

Conservative treatment generally involves avoiding or modifying certain activities. A splint often helps, especially in relieving nighttime pain, by preventing the wrist from flexing, which pinches the median nerve in the carpal tunnel. Applying ice and stretching your wrist muscles may relieve symptoms.

Medication

Acetaminophen (Tylenol, others) or nonsteroidal anti-inflammatory drugs (NSAIDs), such as ibuprofen (Motrin, Advil, others), naproxen (Anaprox, Aleve, others) or aspirin, can help relieve the discomfort.

If more conservative strategies fail, your doctor may inject the affected area with a steroid drug, such as cortisone. If the problem continues to recur, your doctor may recommend an operation.

Surgery

When the symptoms of carpal tunnel syndrome persist despite other treatments, an operation to open the tunnel and create more room for the median nerve may be the best option. Frequently, this surgery can be done through a small instrument called an endoscope. Full use of the wrist and hand usually returns within a few weeks to months.

In some cases, though, some numbness may persist, and it's not uncommon to continue to experience discomfort with certain activities.

Prevention

When engaging in activities that require repetitive, forceful motion with your wrists flexed, take some precautions. Stop every 15 to 20 minutes and gently stretch and bend your hands and fingers. If possible, change activities and do something else for several minutes every hour. Avoid gripping too hard when driving, writing or using small hand tools. Using oversized, soft grip adapters on pens, pencils and tools may help.

Ganglion cyst

Signs and symptoms

- A generally painless lump on your wrist, usually near a joint
- Possible pain, especially when your wrist is extended or flexed

A ganglion cyst is a swelling that appears beneath your skin, usually on the back of your wrist. In some instances, it may occur on the top of your foot, on the front of your wrist or on your fingers. Ganglion cysts are formed by an accumulation of a jelly-like substance from a joint or tendon sheath. Usually rubbery to the touch, ganglion cysts vary in size.

Diagnosis

Your doctor will feel the lump and may order an X-ray or other tests to rule out other problems. An ultrasound examination may help to confirm the diagnosis.

How serious is a ganglion cyst?

A ganglion cyst is essentially harmless. However, if you find a lump on your wrist or foot, consult your doctor so that he or she can check for more serious causes.

Treatment

If a ganglion cyst is painful, your doctor may take steps to relieve the discomfort. In most cases, the lump doesn't interfere with your lifestyle and requires no treatment. Sometimes, a doctor may inject a ganglion cyst with a corticosteroid drug or drain it with a needle. Often, though, it recurs after the drainage.

Surgery

If a ganglion cyst is painful and doesn't respond to drainage, it can be removed surgically.

Dupuytren's contracture

Signs and symptoms

- A small lump, cord or area of tightness in the palm of your hand
- Dimpling of the skin over the affected area
- An inability to straighten one or several fingers

Named after the early 19th-century French surgeon Guillaume Dupuytren, this disorder is characterized by a hardening of tissue beneath the skin of the palm of the hand (palmar fascia). The condition can lead to an involuntary, fixed contraction of one or more fingers.

Dupuytren's contracture usually isn't painful, but it may progressively deform your hand. A similar hardening and shrinkage of tissue

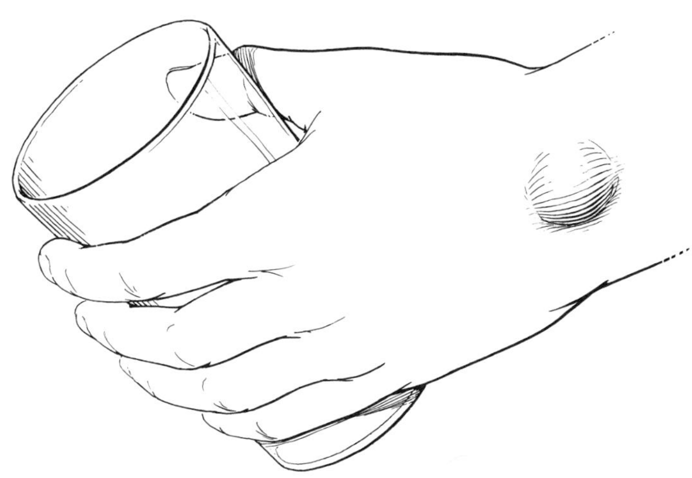

A ganglion cyst is a harmless swelling beneath the skin, usually on the back of the wrist.

Ulnar Nerve Dysfunction

If you've ever hit your "funny bone" on your elbow and felt a tingling sensation down your arm into your hand, you've bumped your ulnar nerve. The ulnar nerve travels down the arm and aids in sensation and movement of the wrist and hand. At the elbow, the nerve passes close to the skin surface. Because of this vulnerable location, this nerve is easily damaged by repeated leaning on or trauma to the elbow. It also is stretched every time you bend your elbow. Over time, this repeated stretching can cause problems with the ulnar nerve. Sometimes, abnormal bone growth in the elbow or swollen tendons or ligaments can compress the ulnar nerve, damaging its protective covering (myelin sheath) or the nerve itself.

Ulnar nerve dysfunction is the result of ulnar nerve damage, whether from direct pressure or stretching. The most characteristic problem is numbness and tingling in the ring and little fingers, aggravated by leaning on your elbow, or holding your elbow bent for a long period of time, such as when talking on the telephone or sleeping. You may also have difficulty moving your ring and little fingers, and you may experience tenderness along the inside of the elbow. Persistent ulnar nerve dysfunction (ulnar neuropathy) can lead to muscle degeneration (atrophy) in the affected hand and some difficulty fully straightening the ring and little fingers.

Treatment depends on the cause. Often, no treatment is required except to avoid pressure on the elbow. Recovery is spontaneous. In case of trauma, a splint or elbow pad may be used to prevent further injury and to allow the nerve to heal. In some cases, surgery may be necessary to relieve the pressure on the ulnar nerve. To eliminate the effect of stretching, the surgeon may shift the path of the nerve from behind to in front of the elbow.

Ulnar nerve dysfunction can result in complete loss of sensation in the hand or fingers and complete loss of hand or wrist movement. However, if the cause of the dysfunction can be identified and successfully treated, full recovery is possible. Early diagnosis and treatment increase the chances of successful treatment.

may affect the soles of your feet. Dupuytren's contracture most commonly involves the ring and little fingers, but it can affect any finger, the thumb or the feet.

The cause of Dupuytren's contracture isn't known, but there appears to be a strong genetic component. Many people with the condition are middle-aged men of Scottish, Irish or Scandinavian descent.

There also appears to be some predisposition associated with alcoholism and epilepsy, although the reason for the linkage is unknown. The condition isn't related to a traumatic event.

Diagnosis

A physical examination usually is adequate to diagnose Dupuytren's contracture. Dimpling of the skin over the affected area is characteristic of the disorder. A cord of immobile tissue may lie beneath the skin.

Your doctor may ask you to place your hand palm down on a tabletop or other flat surface. If you're unable to hold your fingers and hand flat, you may need treatment. Even if you can perform this task, you should repeat it periodically to monitor the progression of the condition. If the result indicates that your condition has worsened, surgery may be advisable.

How serious is Dupuytren's contracture?

Although this common disorder is rarely painful, the decreasing flexibility of your fingers can be gradually debilitating. Many times, surgery can restore most, if not all, normal movement, although the problem may recur.

Treatment

In many cases, treatment isn't required. When treatment is necessary, surgery is usually recommended.

Medication

A corticosteroid injection may shrink the nodules. Some doctors are experimenting with the injection of enzymes or other medications to treat Dupuytren's contracture.

Surgery

Surgical treatment involves removing the thickened tissue. Extreme cases may require skin grafting or other surgical intervention.

Your hand will be bandaged with your fingers straight for a few days or weeks, after which you may begin physical therapy that includes finger and hand exercises. Usually, the hand is splinted at night for several months after surgery, as well.

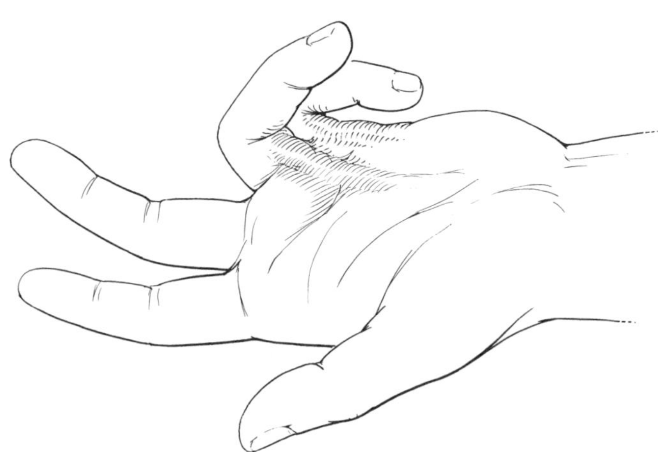

Thickening and hardening of tissue beneath the skin on the palm of the hand (palmar fascia) can lead to an involuntary, fixed contraction of one or more fingers, called Dupuytren's contracture.

Tendinitis

Signs and symptoms

- Pain, tenderness and stiffness near a joint
- Pain aggravated by movement
- A fever
- Redness, swelling or warmth over the affected area

Tendinitis is inflammation or irritation of a tendon. The condition — which causes pain and tenderness just outside a joint — is most common around the shoulders, elbows and knees, but it can also affect the hips, back of the ankles and wrists.

Tendons are thick, fibrous cords that attach muscles to bone. Usually, a tendon is surrounded by a sheath of tissue (synovium) similar to the lining of the joints. The most common cause of tendinitis is injury or overuse from work or recreational activities. Rarely, an infection within the tendon sheath causes the inflammation. Tendinitis also may be associated with diseases such as rheumatoid arthritis.

Diagnosis

If pain interferes with your normal activities or doesn't improve after 2 weeks, see your doctor. An X-ray of the area of soreness and other tests may reveal the cause of the problem.

How serious is tendinitis?

Tendinitis may become a chronic problem and can cause permanent damage to or rupture of a tendon. If the overuse that causes the soreness continues, then what was a vague discomfort at age 30 can lead to a loss of flexibility and decreased strength due to tissue scarring later in life. The natural tendency to favor the painful area can lead to stiffness in the joint.

Sometimes the discomfort of tendinitis disappears within a few weeks, especially if you rest the affected joint. In individuals who continue to overuse the affected area and in older adults, the condition tends to heal more slowly or progress to a chronic problem. The ligaments and tendons around your shoulder may gradually stiffen, which leads to a loss of movement. Severe loss of range of motion in a shoulder is called frozen shoulder (see page 1009).

Treatment

The goals of treatment are to relieve pain and reduce inflammation.

Medication

An over-the-counter nonsteroidal anti-inflammatory drug (NSAID), such as aspirin or ibuprofen (Advil, Motrin, others), may help reduce your discomfort. If symptoms persist, your doctor may inject the area with a steroid drug, such as cortisone, to reduce the inflammation.

Self-care

Don't use the affected area for several days, but move other parts of your body. Elevating and applying ice to the area may help reduce discomfort and swelling.

Although rest is a key part of treating tendinitis, prolonged inactivity can cause stiffness in your joint. After you've rested the injured area completely for a few days, do gentle range-of-motion exercises four times a day to help you maintain flexibility in the joint. Movement is especially important for the shoulder, which tends to lose mobility quickly when it isn't used.

Surgery

Surgeons can repair tendon tears to reduce pain, restore function and, in some cases, prevent complete tendon rupture. Surgery may also be necessary to clean inflamed tissue out of the tendon sheath or relieve pressure on the tendon by removing a portion of bone.

Prevention

To reduce your chance of developing acute or recurrent tendinitis, warm up before you exercise or engage in physical labor and cool down afterward. Avoid activities that place excessive stress on your tendons. Strengthening exercises may also help.

Consider taking lessons or getting professional instruction when starting a new sport or using exercise equipment. Improper technique in either a sport or a work activity is one of the most common causes of tendinitis. An ergonomic arrangement that fits your workspace to your body may prevent your stressing or overloading any one tendon.

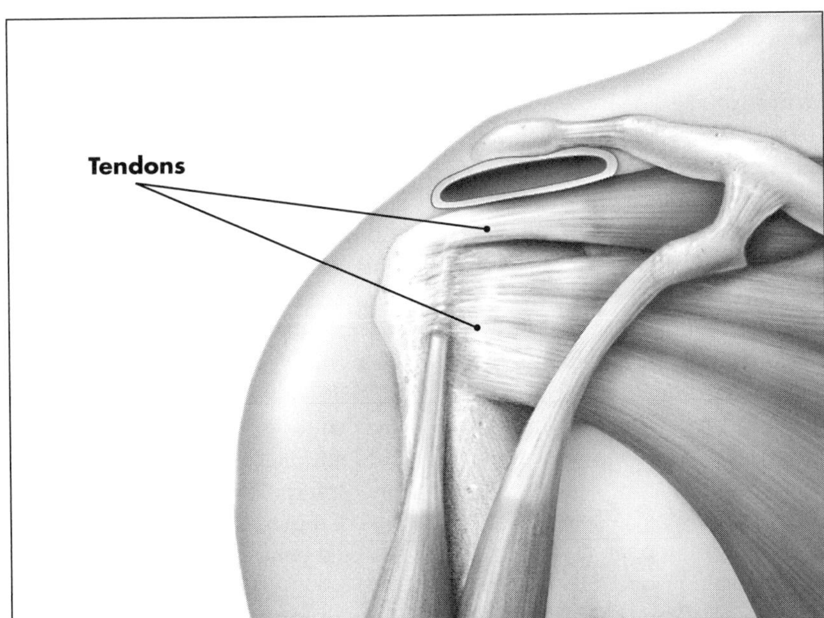

The shoulder joint is a complex structure. Strong tendons attach muscle to bone. Inflammation or irritation of a tendon causes tendinitis.

Fibromyalgia

Signs and symptoms

- Multiple tender points in soft tissue that become intensely painful when pressed
- Fatigue, associated with disordered sleep

Fibromyalgia is characterized by widespread aches and pains in your muscles, ligaments and tendons. The pain may vary from a deep muscle ache to a burning, throbbing, shooting or stabbing sensation. Aside from tenderness with pressure at various locations, there are no related physical abnormalities.

Tender points that occur with the disorder are generally located around your shoulders and elbows, the outsides of your hips, the insides of your knees, near the buttocks, the back muscles alongside your vertebrae and the back of your head. Pain and soreness may result from muscle fatigue or prolonged tension, and the pain may be aggravated by motion. Symptoms may persist for years or may go away only to recur.

Researchers don't believe there's one single cause of fibromyalgia. Rather, it may result from a number of contributing factors, including chemical changes in the brain that affect the regulation of certain brain chemicals, particularly substance P. Environmental toxins haven't been found to cause fibromyalgia, but about 50 percent of people who have the condition also complain of sensitivity to odors, noise, bright lights, various foods and the weather.

Conditions sometimes associated with fibromyalgia include irritable bowel syndrome, chronic headache and facial pain.

Diagnosis

A diagnosis of fibromyalgia is based on characteristic symptoms and the absence of evidence of any other disease that could account for the symptoms. According to criteria set by the American College of

Rheumatology, you must have at least 11 of 18 specific areas of your body — called tender points — that are intensely painful when pressed. In addition, the widespread pain must persist for at least 3 months.

Not all doctors agree with the diagnostic criteria. Some believe the criteria are too rigid and that you can have the condition even if you have fewer than 11 tender points. Others question the validity of tender points as a diagnostic tool.

No laboratory tests can confirm or exclude a diagnosis of fibromyalgia, but your doctor may order laboratory tests to look for other causes of the symptoms.

How serious is fibromyalgia?

The disorder is chronic but not progressive, crippling or life-threatening. It shouldn't lead to disability, and it generally doesn't lead to other, more serious disorders. However, it can cause depression and interfere with sleep. Pain associated with fibromyalgia can also affect your self-esteem and your overall quality of life.

Treatment

Treatment generally involves a combination of therapies:

Self-care

Regular physical activity is important to ease sore muscles and maintain range of motion. If you don't already exercise regularly, start slowly and build up. Swimming, walking, stretching, participating in water aerobics and stationary bicycling are all good choices.

Establishing a regular sleep routine and getting adequate sleep each night also are important. You may need occasional rest breaks throughout the day. If you're overweight, achieving a healthy weight may reduce the pain.

Many people find stress management techniques and complementary forms of medicine, such as meditation or biofeedback, to be helpful. For more information, see Chapter 5, "Managing Stress," and Chapter 43, "Complementary and Alternative Medicine."

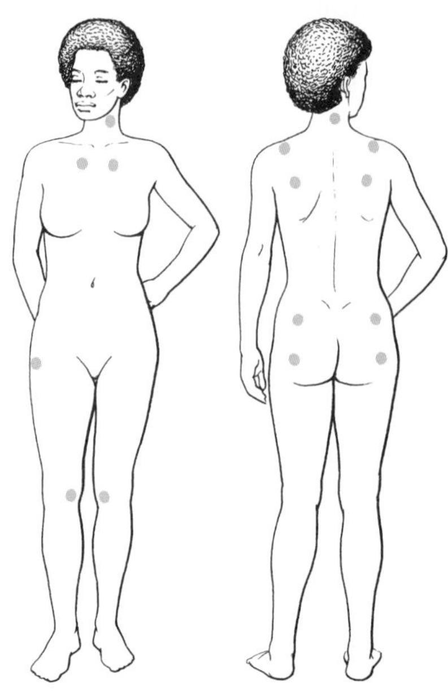

Before making a diagnosis of fibromyalgia, your doctor may check your body for tender (trigger) points — locations that are intensely painful when pressed (highlighted above).

Physical therapy

Physical therapy that includes posture and movement training, application of ice and heat and use of ultrasound may help relieve discomfort.

Medication

To boost your serotonin levels and help improve your sleep, your doctor may prescribe a low dose of an antidepressant, either a tricyclic antidepressant such as amitriptyline (Elavil) or nortriptyline (Aventyl, Pamelor), or a selective serotonin reuptake inhibitor (SSRI), such as fluoxetine (Prozac), venlafaxine (Effexor) or sertraline (Zoloft). The SSRIs may be better tolerated.

Your doctor may also recommend acetaminophen (Tylenol, others) or a nonsteroidal anti-inflammatory drug (NSAID), such as ibuprofen (Advil, Motrin, others) or aspirin, for treating certain symptoms of fibromyalgia, but these medications may not provide much overall benefit.

Complex regional pain syndrome

Signs and symptoms

- Pain and tenderness in a hand or foot that develops weeks or months after an injury, heart attack or stroke
- Tender, thin or shiny skin in the affected area, accompanied by increased sweating and hair growth

Formerly called reflex sympathetic dystrophy syndrome, complex regional pain syndrome usually affects a hand or foot. It causes burning pain and often swelling due to water retention and tenderness in your joints. The skin will likely be tender. Sometimes, the pain is so severe that any skin contact, even the touch of a gentle breeze, can hurt.

The syndrome usually advances over a period of months to a second phase in which the skin becomes cool and shiny. Some people also have limited mobility in the affected area.

An injury, heart attack or stroke precipitates complex regional pain in approximately two-thirds of the cases. In other cases, no specific precipitating event can be identified and the cause is unknown. The syndrome can occur at any age and is more common in women.

Diagnosis

Tests that measure perspiration, temperature or circulation can help confirm the diagnosis by showing abnormal patterns in response to cold or other stimuli. A bone scan may show increased circulation to the joints in the affected area. In later stages, X-rays may reveal a loss of minerals (osteopenia) in affected bones.

Treatment

The focus in treatment is to provide pain relief and to get the affected joints moving. Maintaining range of motion is essential. A physical therapy program that includes heat and cold and exercise may help relieve pain and tenderness.

Your doctor may recommend a pain reliever or a prescription medication to help control the pain. Medications sometimes used include an antidepressant, antiseizure medication or a corticosteroid drug. Sometimes, injections of an anesthetic are used to block nerves that transmit pain messages to affected areas. Surgery is rarely helpful and may actually worsen symptoms.

Chest wall pain

Signs and symptoms

- Pain in the front of the chest where your ribs join your breastbone (sternum)
- Pain that intensifies when you push on your sternum
- Sometimes, swelling at the site of the pain

Chest wall pain (costochondritis) is an inflammation of the cartilage of the rib cage that causes pain and soreness. It's most likely to affect the cartilage that joins your rib cage to your sternum. A blow or other trauma to the rib cage, physical exertion or upper body strain may cause the inflammation, but often the cause is unknown. Movement of the ribs and pressure exerted directly on the affected area often intensify the pain.

The pain associated with this condition is often mistaken for a heart attack because it can be intense and come on suddenly. The difference between chest wall pain and a heart attack is that with chest wall pain, it hurts when you push on your sternum or on your ribs near your sternum. Chest wall pain isn't a medical emergency, but the sudden onset of severe chest pain should be evaluated by a doctor to rule out a heart attack.

Diagnosis

Tenderness at the junction of the ribs and breastbone suggests chest wall pain, but without actual swelling that you or your doctor can feel, it's difficult to be sure. Your doctor may have you undergo chest X-rays, electrocardiograms, blood tests and other tests to exclude other unrelated disorders that could produce similar pain.

Treatment

Given time and rest, the symptoms may disappear. In the meantime, applying ice or heat may help ease your discomfort. Exercise may aggravate the symptoms, so avoid activities that worsen the pain. Your doctor may refer you to a physical therapist for guidance on use of ice and heat and proper exercises.

Acetaminophen (Tylenol, others) and nonsteroidal anti-inflammatory drugs (NSAIDs), such as ibuprofen (Advil, Motrin, others), may reduce your discomfort. Sometimes, a doctor will inject a steroid drug, such as cortisone, into the affected area.

Abdominal wall pain

Signs and symptoms

- Sharp pain in the abdomen
- Increased pain when you push directly over a tender spot
- Increased pain and tenderness when abdominal muscles are tensed and improvement when the muscles are relaxed

Abdominal wall pain is a chronic pain that originates in the abdominal wall. Often the source of the pain is a strained muscle or an irritated nerve ending. The pain may also result from structural conditions, such as lesions associated with endometriosis, an abdominal wall hernia or a muscle tear.

The abdomen typically is tender to the touch in a specific location. Pushing on that spot (trigger point) produces moderate to severe pain. Movements that tense the abdominal muscles — such as when moving from a lying to a sitting position or when doing leg lifts or sit-ups — increase pain and tenderness. Symptoms generally improve when the muscles are relaxed.

Diagnosis

A diagnosis is often based on your medical history and an examination of your abdomen. Increased pain in an area of the abdomen when you lift your head and shoulders off the examining table, or pain when a doctor pushes on the trigger point while your muscles are tensed, generally are positive indications of the condition.

Treatment

Given time and rest, the symptoms may disappear. In the meantime, applying ice or heat may help ease your discomfort. Acetaminophen (Tylenol, others) and nonsteroidal anti-inflammatory drugs (NSAIDs), such as ibuprofen (Advil, Motrin, others), may reduce pain. Sometimes, a doctor will inject a steroid drug, such as cortisone, into the affected area. Reassurance that there's nothing seriously wrong is often treatment in and of itself.

Muscle tumors

Signs and symptoms

- A lump in a muscle, perceptible on the surface of the skin
- Pain in the affected area
- Rapid growth of a lump in a muscle

Most lumps located under the skin are lipomas, which consist of fat and are situated between the skin and the muscle layer. Often they're easy to identify because they move readily with slight finger pressure. They're rubbery to the touch and usually not tender. It's not unusual to have several lipomas.

Muscle tumors are rare. Most muscle tumors are noncancerous (benign), but some can be cancerous (malignant). A malignant muscle tumor (rhabdomyosarcoma) can be life-threatening and requires prompt treatment.

Diagnosis

Your doctor will examine the lump and may order an X-ray, magnetic resonance imaging (MRI) scan or a

PREVENTION TIP

Although much still remains to be learned about muscular dystrophies, it's clear that they're usually inherited disorders. Because females carry the affected genes for Duchenne's and Becker's muscular dystrophies — the two most common forms of the disease — women with a family history of muscular dystrophy should seek genetic counseling before deciding on pregnancy. The odds are half of all the male children of a carrier will have the devastating disorder.

computerized tomography (CT) scan of the area. A biopsy of the lump, in which a sample of tissue is removed for laboratory analysis, also may be necessary.

How serious are muscle tumors?

A benign tumor isn't serious. A malignant tumor requires prompt treatment.

Treatment

A benign tumor may be left alone or surgically removed. A cancerous tumor requires removal, which may be followed by radiation or chemotherapy.

Muscular dystrophy

Signs and symptoms

- Muscle weakness
- Lack of coordination of motor movements
- A clumsy gait
- An inability to lift the arms overhead
- Progressive muscle weakening, causing loss of mobility and an inability to do everyday tasks

Muscular dystrophy is a rare, progressive disease involving mostly the voluntary muscles. The most common and severe form of the disease is Duchenne's muscular dystrophy (pseudohypertrophic muscular dystrophy). In this disease, muscles appear to be deficient in the protein dystrophin, which is essential to muscle function. Without this protein, the muscles grow progressively weaker, but may appear larger than normal because fat and connective tissue replace lost muscle fibers.

An inherited disorder that strikes only males, Duchenne's muscular dystrophy may be passed from mother to son through one of the mother's genes. It usually begins at an early age, often before age 5.

Becker's muscular dystrophy, a milder form of the disease, usually strikes older boys and young men. Also passed from mother to son, it progresses more slowly, usually over several decades.

There are many other less common types of muscular dystrophy characterized by different patterns of muscle weakness. Some are passed along in the same inheritance pattern that marks Duchenne's and Becker's muscular dystrophies. Other types may be handed from one generation to the next, affecting males and females alike. Still others require a defective gene from both parents.

Diagnosis

In a toddler, loss of mobility — such as difficulty walking, climbing stairs or rising to a standing position — or difficulty in lifting his or her arms head high may be signs of muscular dystrophy. Your child's doctor may review your family's health history, perform an examination and order blood tests.

Electromyography, in which a needle electrode is inserted through the skin into the muscle to measure electrical activity, can confirm a muscle disease. Your doctor may also order a biopsy of the muscle, in which a small sample of tissue is removed for analysis. Some forms of muscular dystrophy can be diagnosed by analyzing a blood sample for an abnormal gene.

How serious is muscular dystrophy?

Duchenne's muscular dystrophy is a crippling disease. In most cases, the arms, legs and spine become progressively deformed. By their teenage years, most girls and boys with Duchenne's muscular dystrophy need a wheelchair. Increased susceptibility to respiratory infections often causes early death.

Other forms of muscular dystrophy are less severe, and they generally don't have such a devastating affect on physical functioning and survival.

Treatment

There's no cure for muscular dystrophy. Treatment may include a combination of medication and physical therapy. If respiratory muscles become weakened, a ventilator may become necessary.

Medications

Anti-inflammatory corticosteroid medications may be used in an attempt to slow the progression of Duchenne's muscular dystrophy. Because respiratory infections can become a problem in later stages of muscle diseases, vaccinations against pneumonia and flu (influenza) are important.

Physical therapy

Physical therapy can help maximize muscle function. Exercises can prevent contractures of muscles and joints and may reduce or delay curvature of the spine. Occupational therapy can help people with the disease maintain independence.

Arthritis and Other Joint Disorders

In every joint, a layer of cartilage cushions the ends of your bones. Cartilage has a smooth surface, allowing for uninhibited movement of bones within a joint. Surrounding the joint space is a membrane called the synovial membrane. It produces synovial fluid that lubricates the joint. Encasing the synovial membrane is a fibrous, protective layer called the joint capsule. Bands of fibrous tissue called ligaments bind the parts of a joint together and help keep the joint stable.

A problem in a joint may be the result of mechanical failure, or it may stem from inflammation produced by infection, disease or some unknown cause.

Osteoarthritis

Signs and symptoms

- Pain in a joint during or after use or following periods of inactivity
- Stiffness in one or more joints, especially in the morning after sleep
- Sometimes, development of lumps on finger joints or around the knees

Osteoarthritis, also known as degenerative joint disease, is one of the most common disorders known to humankind. It affects tens of millions of Americans, and the figure is climbing. More than 50 percent of people older than age 65 have osteoarthritis in varying degrees of severity. Seventy-five percent of them are women. Many of those it affects have a family history of osteoarthritis.

Osteoarthritis may initially strike only one joint, such as a knee or hip, or it may involve multiple joints, such as the joints of the fingers. Wear and tear on cartilage in a joint, affecting the joint's mobility, is a principal feature of the disease.

With age, slippery, lubricated cartilage that normally cushions the ends of the bones in a joint gradually changes. Cartilage may lose its elasticity, making the joint more vulnerable to damage from injury or overuse. The smooth surface also roughens and loses its cushioning effect. The breakdown of cartilage causes the lining in a joint (synovium) to become inflamed. The inflamed tissue releases enzymes that further damage cartilage. As the ends of the bones become exposed from cartilage loss, they thicken and form bony growths (spurs or osteophytes), and bone rubs against bone. Each of the steps in this process produces pain.

Normal joint deterioration, however, doesn't necessarily result in osteoarthritis, and osteoarthritis isn't an inevitable part of aging.

In addition to age, injury to a joint is another factor in the development of osteoarthritis. People with joint injuries due to sports, work-related activity or accidents may be at increased risk of developing osteoarthritis. A major factor that leads to arthritis of the knees is obesity. Genetics also plays a role in development of osteoarthritis, particularly in the hands. Some people are born with defective cartilage or with slight defects in the way their joints fit together. As they age, these defects can cause early cartilage breakdown in the joint.

Osteoarthritis commonly occurs in your neck or back. The usual progression involves the breakdown of disks in the spine and the development of bone spurs on the sides of a damaged vertebra. Osteoarthritis also commonly affects the knee and hip, and it can strike hands and feet. It affects wrists, elbows and ankles less often. In young people, osteoarthritis is relatively rare.

Diagnosis

Pain in one or more joints is a prominent symptom of osteoarthritis. Your doctor will likely ask you about your symptoms and examine your joints. An X-ray may be taken to confirm the diagnosis.

Many people who have osteoarthritis don't realize it until their

Anatomy of a Joint

The joints in your body are made of tissues designed for a lifetime of service. Bones in your joints are capped with shock-absorbing cartilage. Cartilage is a tough, smooth, slippery material that prevents bone-against-bone contact.

The joint is surrounded and lubricated by the synovial membrane, which forms and releases lubricating fluid. The joint capsule is tough, fibrous tissue that attaches to bone on either side of a joint. It helps stabilize the joint. Ligaments — short cords of strong fiber that attach bone to bone — contribute to joint alignment and stability. Muscles end in tendons that attach to bone above or below the joint capsule.

Near many joints are small fluid-filled sacs called bursae. Bursae are located between muscles or between muscles, tendons and bone. They help reduce friction around joints.

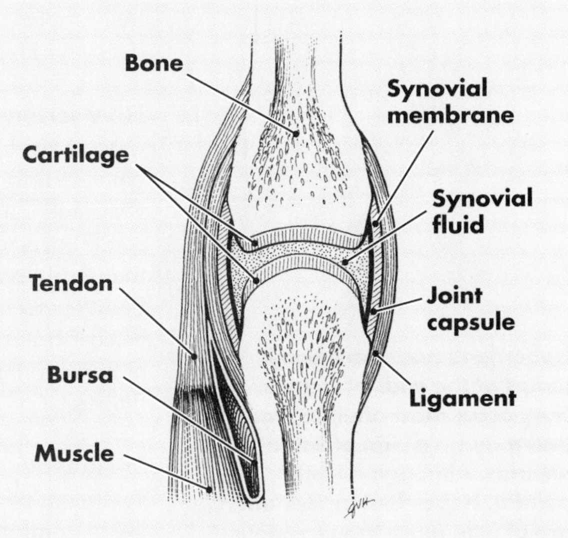

Corticosteroid Medications

Corticosteroid medications (glucocorticoids) are modified forms of two hormones — cortisone and hydrocortisone — naturally produced by your adrenal glands. This class of steroid medications is useful in treating a variety of problems.

Uses

Corticosteroids have a strong anti-inflammatory effect that can reduce swelling, pain, redness and warmth of inflamed joints.

In addition to their obvious value in treating deficiency disorders of the adrenal glands, corticosteroids can be invaluable remedies for a wide range of other ailments, including skin diseases, autoimmune diseases, allergies, certain tumors and several types of arthritis and other musculoskeletal disorders. Corticosteroids are also used to prevent rejection of a transplanted organ.

Corticosteroids are available in tablet form, topical form, as eyedrops and as injections. The drug can be injected directly into a muscle, joint or bursa, a fluid-filled sac between bone.

Corticosteroid medications aren't the same as anabolic steroid preparations (male sex hormones) that some athletes use inappropriately to increase muscle bulk.

Doses

The risk of side effects from corticosteroid drugs increases over time, especially with higher doses. Up to 7.5 milligrams (mg) a day of the corticosteroid prednisone is considered a low dosage, comparable to what's normally present in your body.

Some people with rheumatic diseases take corticosteroid medications for years with minimal side effects. Even so, long-term use of these drugs requires careful monitoring.

A daily dose from 7.5 mg to 20 mg is considered an intermediate-level dose and presents a moderate risk of side effects. The risk is small in the first month or so, but increases over time.

If you take 20 mg to 60 mg a day, your risk of side effects increases dramatically. Such a high dosage ideally should be used only for short periods, then reduced as quickly as possible.

A dosage above 100 mg a day is extremely high and should be used only in extreme circumstances.

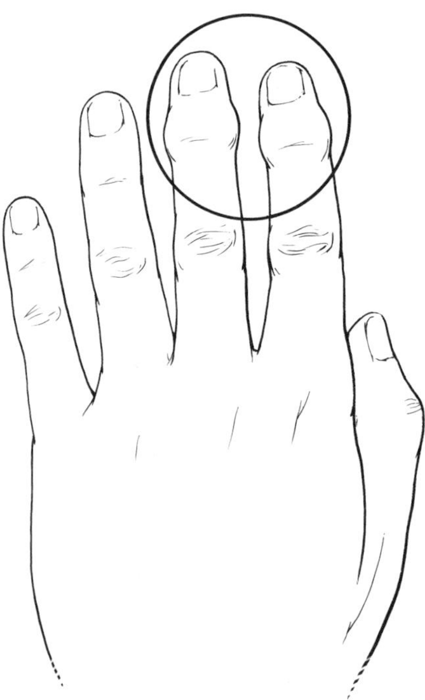

Heberden's nodes are bony lumps at the ends of fingers. They occur most often in women and may be a sign of osteoarthritis. Although initially painful, Heberden's nodes often are of little more than cosmetic concern.

doctor spots it on a routine X-ray. Bone spurs (osteophytes), an indication of osteoarthritis, may show up in an X-ray of an affected joint.

Another clue may be Heberden's or Bouchard's nodes. Not really nodes, these are bony lumps that appear over a period of years in the end and middle joints of your fingers. Your doctor may ask if your parents also had them because there appears to be a genetic tendency for Heberden's nodes.

How serious is osteoarthritis?

Osteoarthritis doesn't go away. The pain tends to increase over the years and may limit activity. The condition is responsible for more than 7 million doctor visits a year. Eighty percent of people with osteoarthritis report some form of limitation in movement or activities.

Treatment

Treatment generally focuses on easing discomfort and, if possible, improving joint mobility through exercise, medication or surgery, among other therapies.

Exercise

Appropriate exercise is important for keeping joints flexible and building muscle strength. Range-of-motion and muscle-strengthening exercises can help you prevent progression and reduce stiffness. A doctor or physical therapist can advise you on a proper exercise program.

Another benefit of exercise is that it can help you lose weight and maintain a weight that's healthy. Excessive weight puts unnecessary pressure on many joints, such as the spine, knee and hip, and it can exacerbate osteoarthritis. In fact, every pound of weight adds as much as 4 pounds of load on each knee.

In addition, exercise can strengthen the muscles of your trunk to help you maintain good posture. Good posture is important, especially if you have osteoarthritis of the spine.

Side effects

With sustained, long-term use, the risk of side effects is high. The adrenal glands tend to shrink (atrophy). Other effects include weight gain, a loss of bone mineral (osteoporosis), muscle weakness, water retention, acne, slow healing of cuts and wounds, increased risk of infection, redistribution of body fat and a rounding of the facial features (moonface), thinning of the skin, diabetes and cataracts. Additional side effects include high blood pressure, elevated blood sugar and stomach irritation, especially when the drug is taken with other anti-inflammatory medications.

Few, if any, people experience all of these side effects, and with short-term use and a low dosage, you have a good chance of having none. The risks with topically applied corticosteroid medications are regarded as so small that you can obtain some preparations without a prescription. However, long-term use of corticosteroid creams can cause your skin to thin.

If you take enough prednisone daily for 3 to 6 months or longer, your adrenal glands atrophy. If this happens and you go off the drug abruptly, your adrenal glands can't produce the amount of hydrocortisone your body needs to face the stress of severe infection, injury or surgery. Lack of adrenal hormone may be fatal. When people whose bodies no longer produce enough hydrocortisone have a surgical procedure or sustain injury, doctors may prescribe prednisone or another corticosteroid drug to provide for the temporary increase in hormonal needs.

When it's time to stop taking prednisone, your doctor will work with you to slowly taper the dose so that you don't become sick. If you have taken prednisone daily or have taken it for a few months and stopped, be sure to mention it to your doctors for a year after your last dose, especially if you need surgery or invasive diagnostic tests or if you become seriously ill.

Cortisone injections

Cortisone injections have remarkable effects for the treatment of acute conditions such as bursitis and tendinitis. They're also beneficial for relieving pain and swelling in individual joints affected by osteoarthritis or rheumatoid arthritis. Often, a single injection will relieve a severe (acute) condition permanently, but subsequent injections can be given if necessary. However, as few as six injections within a 12-month period can damage bone and joint structures, so your doctor may be unwilling to administer more than three or four injections within a calendar year.

Medication

Nonsteroidal anti-inflammatory drugs (NSAIDs), such as aspirin and ibuprofen (Advil, Motrin, others), have been the treatment of choice. For pain without inflammation, acetaminophen (Tylenol, others) may provide relief.

Other NSAIDs used to treat osteoarthritis are the selective COX-2 inhibitors. They include the medications rofecoxib (Vioxx), celecoxib (Celebrex) and valdecoxib (Betra). An advantage of these prescription drugs is that they may cause less gastrointestinal pain and bleeding than traditional NSAIDs.

Hyaluronate is a substance found naturally in joint fluid. Preparations of this substance include hyaluronate (Hyalgan) and hyaluronate derivative (Synvisc). A series of injections of one of these medications may provide pain relief for osteoarthritis of the knee. Your doctor may also recommend an injection of a corticosteroid medication into a joint that's inflamed and not responding to other treatments.

Other therapies

Some people find pain relief from use of ice, heating pads, hot water bottles and hot baths.

Joint protection devices may help prevent strain and stress on painful joints. For instance, if you have osteoarthritis in your neck, your doctor may prescribe a cervical collar to wear during episodes of severe (acute) pain.

Surgery

If you have long-term deterioration, your doctor may recommend replacing the joint with an artificial joint. Replacement surgery is most often performed on hip and knee joints (see page 1002). If the joints in your hands have deteriorated significantly, an operation may help relieve pain and increase finger mobility.

Other surgical techniques are designed to remove loose fragments of bone or cartilage that may cause pain or mechanical symptoms such as "locking." The procedure is usually done with an arthroscope, a small tube inserted into the joint through which the surgeon works.

A 2002 study evaluated some types of arthroscopic procedures in people with osteoarthritis of the knees. The study showed no significant difference in pain relief or improved knee function 2 years after surgery among those who underwent arthroscopic surgery and those who underwent a sham (placebo) procedure. Additional studies are needed to better evaluate the results of this study.

Arthritis of the thumb

Signs and symptoms

- Pain at the base of your thumb, commonly aggravated by simple activities such as writing, opening a jar or turning a key in a lock
- Swelling and deformity
- Difficulty holding small objects due to pain

Often the first indication of osteoarthritis is pain in a thumb, which may be accompanied by

COMPLEMENTARY MEDICINE

People with osteoarthritis spend millions of dollars each year on nontraditional therapies, including herbal preparations, acupuncture and nutritional supplements. Many turn to alternative treatments either because the medications they take offer little relief or because they can't tolerate the side effects of the medications. Some people use nontraditional treatments to complement a traditional treatment regimen.

There's evidence that some non-traditional treatments may be helpful:

Glucosamine and chondroitin sulfate

Two of the most popular nontraditional treatments for osteoarthritis are glucosamine and chondroitin sulfate supplements. People may take them because the supplements supposedly maintain existing cartilage and stimulate growth of new cartilage, easing symptoms and slowing progression of the disease.

Your body naturally produces glucosamine, which helps give cartilage its strength and rigidity. The supplements sold in stores are a synthetic version of this substance.

Although promising, studies so far have tended to be small and of short duration. Furthermore, scientists don't know if the results from a study on a knee joint, for instance, can be applied to other joints. In addition, doctors know little about tolerance for and long-term toxicity of these supplements.

Talk to your doctor about the supplements. If you have an allergy to shellfish, you shouldn't take glucosamine. It may also raise blood sugar levels in people with diabetes. If you take an anticoagulant medication, such as warfarin (Coumadin), chondroitin sulfate may interfere with the effects of the medication.

Relaxation techniques

Meditation, when practiced regularly, helps some people enter a deep, restful state that reduces the body's stress responses. Meditating can relax breathing, slow brain waves and decrease muscle tension and heart rate. In this way, it may help you manage arthritis pain.

You might also experiment with other relaxation techniques, such as guided imagery and hypnosis (see Chapter 43,"Complementary and Alternative Medicine"). Another option is biofeedback, in which you learn how to control certain body functions, such as your heart rate, breathing patterns and body temperature. Managing these functions may help you cope with pain.

Acupuncture

Acupuncture is an ancient Chinese healing art that involves the insertion of thin needles into your skin at specific points in your body, called meridians. Acupuncture is based on the belief that good health is related to the free flow of qi (CHEE), the body's life force. Inserting needles into specific meridians is intended to stimulate the flow of qi. Western scientists believe the procedure may stimulate the release of endorphins, the body's natural painkillers.

Acupuncture has been shown to be effective for some conditions. The National Institutes of Health found that acupuncture may be a reasonable pain management option for osteoarthritis. More recently, however, the American College of Rheumatology reported that acupuncture works no better than a placebo. Future research may help define which individuals might benefit from acupuncture.

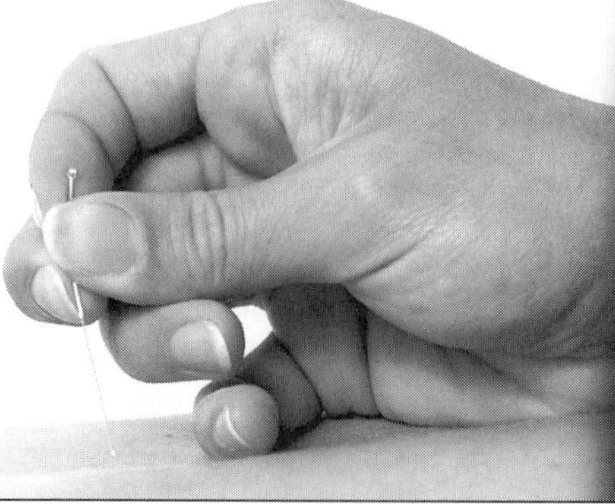

swelling or limited movement. Degeneration of cartilage and bone can cause arthritis at the base of the thumb. Everyday wear and tear is the most common factor. Other contributors may be heredity and a previous injury, such as dislocation of your thumb.

Diagnosis

A physical examination and X-rays often can indicate the severity of the problem.

Treatment

Simply avoiding or modifying the aggravating activities may cause the swelling and pain to subside. Applying ice also may help. Medical supply stores carry splints that wrap and stabilize your thumb joint to reduce pain and stress on the joint. For a custom-fitted splint, see a physical or occupational therapist.

Ask your doctor or a therapist about tools and utensils specially designed for people with arthritis, such as special scissors that close automatically and tools and utensils with large, padded handles that make them easier to grip.

Medication

To relieve pain in the joint, your doctor may recommend an over-the-counter pain reliever such as acetaminophen (Tylenol, others), aspirin or ibuprofen (Advil, Motrin, others). Or your doctor may prescribe a prescription pain relief medication.

Surgery

If the pain is severe or limits mobility of your thumb, your doctor may recommend surgery. If the joint surfaces are severely damaged, a surgeon may replace the joint with an artificial joint.

Recovery typically takes several months. Although you won't end up with a normal thumb, most people who have the surgery are pleased with the improvement in pain and joint strength and stability.

Baker's Cyst

Any condition that causes inflammation of the knee joint can cause the membrane lining of the joint (synovium) to produce excess lubricating (synovial) fluid. The fluid can accumulate in the popliteal bursa behind the knee, resulting in the development of a painless cyst called a Baker's cyst. Other names for the condition include popliteal bursitis or synovial cyst of the popliteal space.

Often, no treatment is needed. If the cyst is large and causes a lot of pain, your doctor may remove (aspirate) excess fluid from the knee joint with a needle. Sometimes, a doctor will inject a steroid medication, such as cortisone, into the knee to reduce the volume of fluid being produced.

If the cyst is related to an injury, such as a cartilage tear, you may need surgery to repair the torn cartilage.

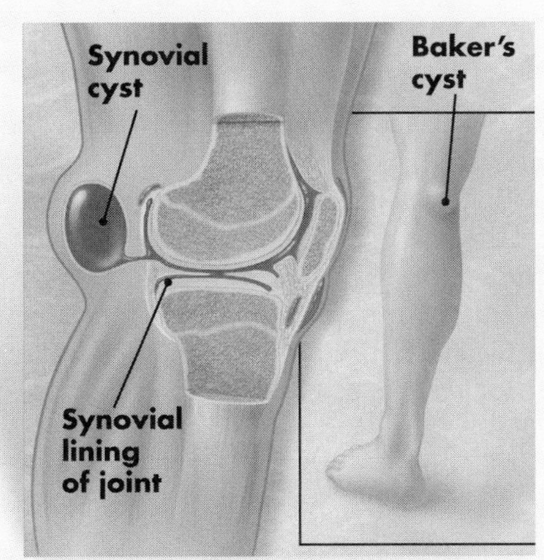

Rheumatoid arthritis

Signs and symptoms

- Pain and swelling in the joints of the feet, wrists and hands
- Pain and swelling in symmetric joints, such as both feet
- Diffuse aching or stiffness
- Redness and warmth over the joints
- Fatigue and malaise
- Appetite and weight changes
- Anemia
- Lumps under the skin

Unlike the more common osteoarthritis, rheumatoid arthritis isn't the result of joint wear and tear. Rather, it's an autoimmune disease in which your body's immune system attacks healthy tissues, specifically the thin synovial lining of the joints and some internal organs.

Inflammation in affected joints causes pain, stiffness, warmth, redness and swelling. The inflamed synovium often proliferates, invading and damaging bone and cartilage and disrupting the stability of joints. Inflammatory cells release enzymes that digest bone and cartilage and cause further damage.

Researchers suspect that certain viruses may trigger rheumatoid arthritis in some people who have an inherited susceptibility to the disease. Many people with the disease have a genetic marker called HLA-DR4. Other genes are thought to influence the development of rheumatoid arthritis, as well.

Unlike osteoarthritis, which affects only the musculoskeletal system, rheumatoid arthritis is a systemic disease. In some people, it affects several organs, such as the heart, lungs, skin and eyes. It also tends to affect multiple joints, resulting in diffuse stiffness and aching.

Rheumatoid arthritis tends to be symmetric, affecting, for example, both ankles or both wrists. It may also produce small lumps under the skin (rheumatoid nodules) near the elbows, on the fingers, on the feet, along the Achilles tendons or on the buttocks. The lumps range in size from that of a pea to that of a walnut. Usually, the lumps aren't painful and present no physical problems.

Rheumatoid arthritis can lead to deformity in the fingers. The hand may lose strength and be painful during flares of the disease.

Rheumatoid arthritis can strike at any age, but most often it develops between ages 20 and 50. A variant of rheumatoid arthritis called juvenile rheumatoid arthritis occurs at a younger age (see page 1004). Roughly three times as many women as men have rheumatoid arthritis.

Diagnosis

If your doctor suspects that you have rheumatoid arthritis, he or she will look for characteristic features of the disease, such as whether you have joint involvement on both sides of your body. X-rays and laboratory tests can help establish the diagnosis, but no single test can confirm or exclude the condition.

A special blood test that determines the erythrocyte sedimentation rate can indicate the presence of inflammation and differentiate rheumatoid arthritis from some other conditions. Another blood test measures the level of an autoantibody called rheumatoid factor (RF). About 80 percent of people with rheumatoid arthritis test positive for RF. RF doesn't

Joint Replacement

Every year, about a half million people in the United States have joint replacement surgery to regain physical function and eliminate pain in their joints caused by a joint disorder such as osteoarthritis or rheumatoid arthritis.

A surgical procedure called arthroplasty, which literally means "reforming the joint," may be the best remedy for a damaged hip or knee joint.

Replacement arthroplasty involves replacement of joint surfaces with plastic and metal implants (prostheses). Cement is used to fasten the implants to the bone. Some prostheses are made from material that enables bone to grow into it.

The hip and knee joints are the most commonly replaced. In a hip arthroplasty, a ball on a stem replaces the top of the thighbone (femur). A polyethylene cup replaces the socket of the hip. The results are often remarkable: People who were unable to walk before their hip or knee surgery are able to do so afterward.

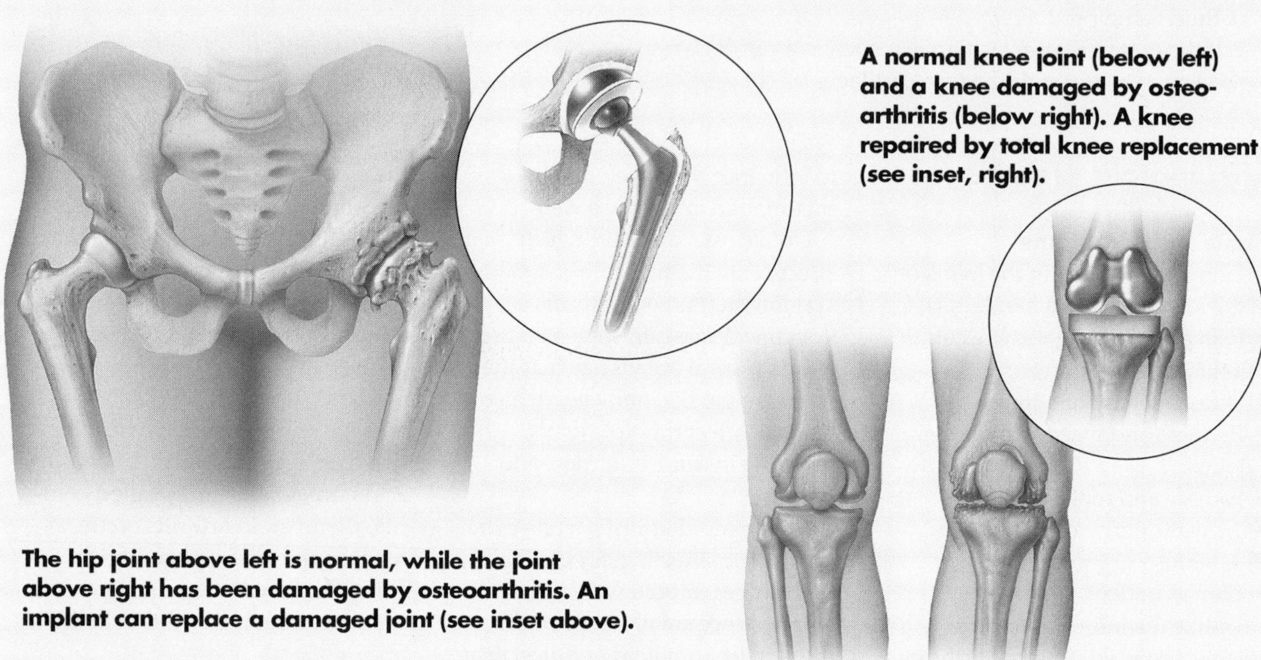

A normal knee joint (below left) and a knee damaged by osteoarthritis (below right). A knee repaired by total knee replacement (see inset, right).

The hip joint above left is normal, while the joint above right has been damaged by osteoarthritis. An implant can replace a damaged joint (see inset above).

PREVENTION TIP

There's some evidence that omega-3 fatty acids found in certain fish, such as salmon, trout and herring, may help reduce joint inflammation when consumed in sufficient quantities. Omega-3 fatty acids are also found in flaxseed and in over-the-counter supplements. It's generally best to get omega-3s from a healthy diet rather than from supplements.

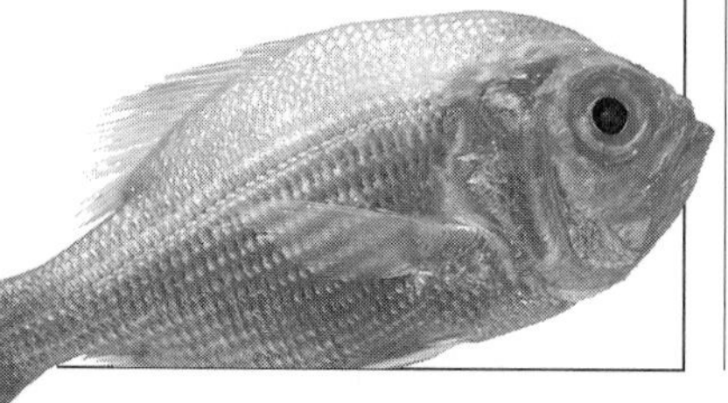

confirm the diagnosis, however, because it sometimes is present in healthy people or in those with unrelated diseases, such as tuberculosis or chronic liver disease.

As the disease advances, X-rays help monitor its progression.

How serious is rheumatoid arthritis?

Rheumatoid arthritis can be the most debilitating form of arthritis. The disease can damage the cartilage, bones, tendons and ligaments of affected joints. People with rheumatoid arthritis often have joint deformity, which leads to loss of mobility. Some people also experience sweats and fever along with loss of strength in muscles attached to affected joints.

For most people, the condition is long-lasting (chronic). Inflammation may fluctuate in severity but generally persists. In mild cases, periods of increased disease activity, called flare-ups or flares, alternate with periods of relative remission, during which symptoms such as swelling, pain, difficulty sleeping and weakness fade or disappear. For others, the disease is continuously active and progresses over time. Only 1 in 10 people with the disease have a single episode followed by long-lasting remission.

It's difficult to predict initially how severe the disease will be in any one person. People who have continuous symptoms for 4 or 5 years are likely to have a lifetime of problems with the disease.

Although the long-term durability of joint prostheses remains a concern, evidence to date suggests that replacement parts last for many years with moderate use. New developments and technologies are becoming available that provide the possibility of dramatically lowering joint-surface wear, which may further increase durability. These new technologies include metal-on-metal and ceramic-on-ceramic surfaces and a new class of polyethylenes (plastics). The goal is to eliminate friction, which may cause an artificial joint to shed particles that can irritate and destroy bone.

Other new technologies involve the way joint implants are affixed to the bone. Cement can loosen over time. Soft tissues attach themselves to some new materials, such as tantalum, which gives it an advantage over some other materials.

Prostheses can also replace ankles, elbows, shoulders, fingers, wrists and hands. Wrist and hand joint replacements are less common because the joints are small and complex and they rely heavily on soft tissue for proper function.

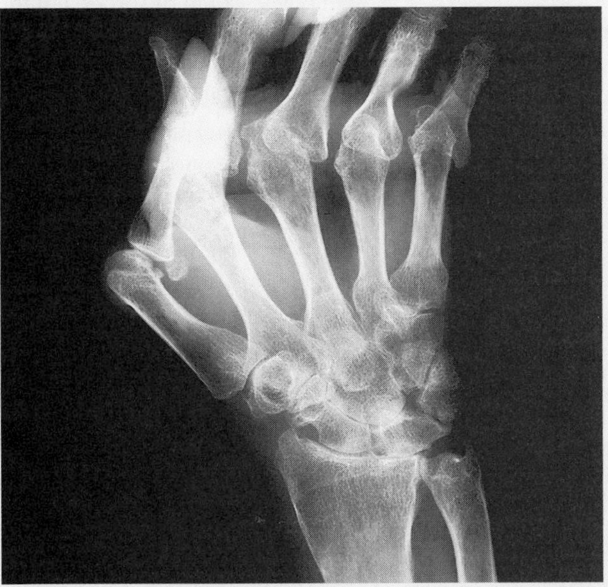

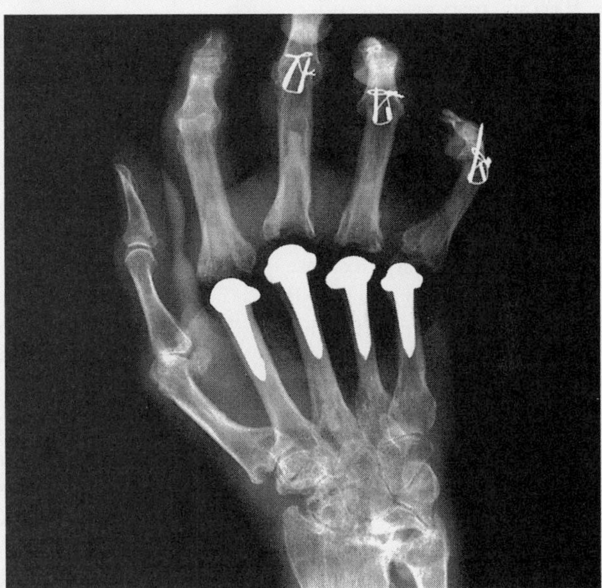

These X-rays show the deforming effects of rheumatoid arthritis on a hand (left) and the same hand following joint replacement surgery (right).

Most people are able to live long, productive and nearly normal lives despite the disease. However, proper and prompt medical care is essential for dealing effectively with the condition.

Treatment

Highly effective drug treatments are available for rheumatoid arthritis. It's important to diagnose the disease early because delay in starting treatment may reduce its effectiveness. Current treatments focus on relieving pain, reducing inflammation, stopping or slowing joint damage, helping people with the disease function as normally as possible and preventing associated medical problems, such as heart or lung disease.

Medication

Medications for treating rheumatoid arthritis fall into two categories: those used to relieve symptoms and those used to control the disease.

- Nonsteroidal anti-inflammatory drugs (NSAIDs), including ibuprofen (Advil, Motrin), naproxen (Aleve, Naprosyn) and others, are basic to treating the pain and inflammation of rheumatoid arthritis. If you're sensitive to NSAIDs, your doctor may prescribe derivatives of aspirin called nonacetylated salicylates (magnesium trisilicate, salsalate). Another alternative is COX-2 inhibitors, such as rofecoxib (Vioxx), celecoxib (Celebrex) and valdecoxib (Bextra). COX-2 inhibitors are NSAIDs that may be easier on the stomach. Acetaminophen (Tylenol, others) may be used for pain relief, but it doesn't reduce inflammation.
- Corticosteroid medications, such as prednisone, are very effective for relieving pain and inflammation but not for controlling disease progression. They should be used with caution and in the smallest effective dosage because of numerous and potentially serious side effects (see page 998).
- Disease-modifying medications may help reduce symptoms and slow joint damage. These include hydroxychloroquine (Plaquenil and other antimalarial drugs), sulfasalazine (Azulfidine),

minocycline (Minocin, Dynacin), methotrexate (Rheumatrex), leflunomide (Arava), azathioprine (Imuran), cyclosporine (Neoral), cyclophosphamide (Cytoxan), penicillamine (Cuprimine, Depen) and gold therapy (Ridaura). Each of these drugs can cause serious side effects, so you and your doctor need to weigh the risks and the benefits.
- Biologic response modifiers, such as etanercept (Enbrel) and infliximab (Remicade), block the action of tumor necrosis factor, a chemical that plays an important role in inflammation and tissue damage. Another biologic response modifier, called anakinra (Kineret), decreases inflammation by blocking the chemical called interleukin-1. These medications can be very effective, but because they block immune responses, a possible side effect is serious infection.

Rest and exercise

Another key component in managing rheumatoid arthritis is to establish the optimal balance between rest and exercise. The preservation of function in affected joints requires muscle-building and range-of-motion exercises, but you also need sufficient rest.

Because of the ebb-and-flow nature of the disease, strategies used during flares and periods of remission differ. Intense disease activity during a flare puts you at risk of joint damage, so your doctor may advise a combination of rest, pain reduction strategies and gentle activity. During flares, refrain from exercises that strain your affected joints, but don't stop moving. During periods of remission, exercise and carry on activities as tolerated. It's important to recognize your limits and avoid undue fatigue.

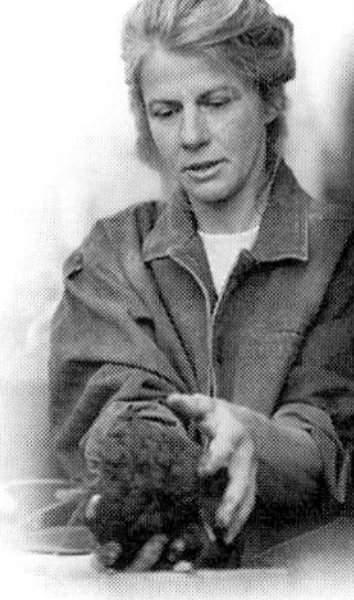

Surgery

The surgical removal of inflamed synovium (synovectomy) may be recommended if the arthritis isn't responding adequately to medications or if joint function is impaired. Depending on the type of joint, the procedure may be done with traditional surgery (open synovectomy) or with an arthroscope. For severely eroded joints, joint replacement may be the best solution.

Juvenile rheumatoid arthritis

Signs and symptoms

- Swelling and stiffness in the joints
- Fever
- A rash
- Fatigue and irritability
- Inflammation of the eye

Juvenile rheumatoid arthritis resembles rheumatoid arthritis in some ways but differs in others. Differences include the age of onset — juvenile rheumatoid arthritis affects children and can even begin in infancy — and the long-term nature of the ailment.

Juvenile rheumatoid arthritis actually includes three distinct forms of childhood arthritis: pauciarticular, polyarticular and systemic onset (Still's disease). Fifty percent of children with the disease have the pauciarticular type, 40 percent have the polyarticular type and 10 percent have the systemic type.

Each form has its own distinguishing characteristics. The pauciarticular variety usually affects four or fewer joints in an asymmetrical fashion. For instance, if the right knee is affected, the left knee probably isn't. Polyarticular juvenile rheumatoid arthritis affects more than four joints, usually in a symmetric pattern. It's more aggressive and frequently causes chronic joint problems.

The systemic type affects many body systems in addition to the joints, including the heart, liver, spleen and lymph nodes. It may also cause fever, chills, rash and anemia.

The cause of juvenile rheumatoid arthritis is unknown. Most likely several factors are involved, including genetics. A virus or bacterium may trigger the disease in children with a genetic predisposition.

Juvenile rheumatoid arthritis most often begins during the toddler or early teenage years. Certain types and subtypes are more prevalent in one sex than the other, but in general the disease affects more girls than boys.

About half of the children with short-term (acute) juvenile rheumatoid arthritis recover completely, and half develop the long-lasting (chronic) form.

Diagnosis

Diagnosing the disorder generally involves a thorough physical examination and laboratory tests to measure inflammation and to detect autoantibodies — these are antibodies that attack the body's own cells.

Children with juvenile rheumatoid arthritis should have a special eye examination with a slit lamp because of the high risk of a potentially serious eye condition called uveitis (see page 643).

How serious is juvenile rheumatoid arthritis?

As with adult rheumatoid arthritis, juvenile rheumatoid arthritis puts the person who has it at risk of permanent joint damage. In addition, a growing child with the disease may experience abnormal bone growth. For example, the disease may accelerate growth in one leg bone but not in the other. Another risk is that a child will instinctively refrain from moving an affected joint to avoid pain. This can result in weakened and contracted muscles and even a joint deformity over time.

Treatment

In general, treatment of juvenile rheumatoid arthritis resembles that for adult rheumatoid arthritis, although many of the drugs used to treat adults aren't approved for use in children.

Medication

A doctor may prescribe ibuprofen (Advil, Motrin), naproxen (Aleve, Anaprox), aspirin or other anti-inflammatory drugs. If the disease is progressive, disease-modifying antirheumatic drugs, such as methotrexate (Rheumatrex), gold therapy (Ridaura) or the newer biologic agent etanercept (Enbrel), may be used.

Corticosteroid medications, such as prednisone, are usually used only in children with internal organ involvement or eye inflammation because of the drug's potential to stunt growth when given in high doses.

Other therapies

Range-of-motion exercises and splints may be recommended to prevent loss of motion and deformity. There's a delicate balance between maintaining some semblance of normal activity and getting sufficient rest to avoid fatigue and excessive stress on affected joints. During periods of severe disease activity, bed rest or tutoring at home may be necessary, but it's important for psychological and physical reasons to avoid isolating children from all of their normal routines.

Surgery

If a child sustains severe joint damage, reconstructive procedures or joint replacement may be required. In general, though, it's advisable to wait until the child has stopped growing.

Other types of inflammatory arthritis

The most common form or inflammatory arthritis is rheumatoid arthritis. Other types may take one of several forms, each with somewhat different manifestations. These forms of arthritis have genetic factors. Each of them has characteristic gene markers that indicate a genetic predisposition to the disease.

A tissue-typing test can detect the presence of the marker. Having a certain gene marker doesn't mean you'll get one of these conditions, only that you're predisposed to it, which increases your risk. Why one of these disorders develops in one person and not another remains a mystery.

Psoriatic arthritis

People with the skin condition psoriasis may develop psoriatic arthritis. Signs and symptoms include:

- Pain, swelling and decreased mobility in one or more joints, often the small joints of the hands and feet, but possibly in larger joints and the spine
- Swelling of fingers or toes that gives them a sausage-like appearance
- Pitting and discoloration of the nails, which may separate from the nail beds
- Eye inflammation

Psoriasis is a common skin disease in which areas of the skin become inflamed and reddish in color (see page 1176). The skin over the elbows and knees often becomes scaly. The fingernails may become pitted and discolored. Psoriatic arthritis develops in about 1 in 10 people with psoriasis. More women than men have psoriatic arthritis, which typically strikes people in their 20s, 30s and 40s.

For most people, the effects of psoriatic arthritis are relatively minor, with some pain and discomfort in affected joints but little effect on overall health. In some, however, it can cause severe deformity and disability if left untreated.

Treatment

First-line medications for the disease include nonsteroidal anti-inflammatory drugs (NSAIDs), such as ibuprofen (Advil, Motrin, others) or aspirin. For persistent symptoms, your doctor may prescribe other drugs, such as the disease-modifying drugs methotrexate (Rheumatrex) or sulfasalazine (Azulfidine) or tumor necrosis factor (TNF) blockers, such as etanercept (Enbrel) and infliximab (Remicade).

Other treatments include range-of-motion exercises, application of heat to relax muscles around painful joints and relaxation exercises.

Reiter's syndrome

Some people inherit a susceptibility to this form of arthritis, which is often precipitated by an infection including those transmitted by sexual contact. Ingestion of contaminated food or water also can bring on the disease. Signs and symptoms include:

- Pain in joints, usually in the lower extremities, and in the heels
- Inflammation of the urethra or intestine
- Painful inflammation of the eye
- A rash

Reiter's syndrome usually appears in stages. Usually, inflammation of the urethra or intestine comes first. Some time later, joint pain occurs, most often in the finger, toe, ankle, hip and knee joints. Skin lesions similar to those of psoriasis also may appear, as well as a painful eye inflammation called conjunctivitis.

Reiter's syndrome may appear once or episodically. Attacks tend to last a few weeks or months. Inflammation associated with a sudden, severe attack can produce tenderness and pain and may lead to permanent joint damage.

Treatment

Treatment generally includes nonsteroidal anti-inflammatory drugs (NSAIDs) to relieve pain and inflammation. For more severe symptoms, other medications may be prescribed.

Ankylosing spondylitis

This form of arthritis predominantly affects the spinal joints.

However, peripheral joints of the arms and legs and the tendons and ligaments where they attach to bones also may be affected. Signs and symptoms include:

- Pain and stiffness in the spine and perhaps other joints
- In advanced stages, a stiff, inflexible spine

People with this disorder have the same genetic marker found in people with Reiter's syndrome. Males are affected more often than females, with onset generally before age 40. The condition may be associated with inflammatory bowel disease.

Typically, ankylosing spondylitis begins with soreness in the spine. As the disease progresses, the affected bones begin to fuse together, rendering the joints immobile and causing a stiff, inflexible spine (bamboo spine). Some people develop a peripheral arthritis resembling rheumatoid arthritis.

In most cases, ankylosing spondylitis is mild, so it may go undiagnosed for decades. However, once joints fuse, treatment won't help restore mobility.

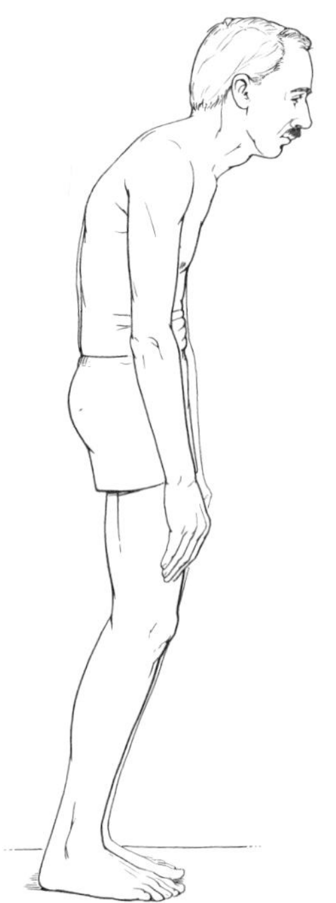

Ankylosing spondylitis can lead to a stiff, inflexible spine.

Treatment

Nonsteroidal anti-inflammatory drugs (NSAIDs), such as ibuprofen (Motrin, Advil, others) and naproxen (Aleve, Anaprox, others) may relieve the chronic pain and stiffness.

Other drugs used to treat this condition include disease-modifying antirheumatic drugs, such as sulfasalazine (Azulfidine) and methotrexate (Rheumatrex), and occasionally corticosteroids. Newer medications, such as the tumor necrosis factor (TNF) blockers etanercept (Enbrel) and infliximab (Remicade), are reported to be effective in treating this condition.

Physical therapy and exercise are essential components of treatment. Try to remain as active as possible. Range-of-motion and stretching exercises can help maintain flexibility in joints and preserve good posture.

If you smoke, try to quit because the condition affects mobility of the rib cage and may hamper your breathing ability.

Arthritis of inflammatory bowel disease

People with inflammatory bowel disease (ulcerative colitis and Crohn's disease) may develop a characteristic form of arthritis. Signs and symptoms include:

- Pain and swelling in peripheral joints, especially knees, ankles and feet
- Pain and stiffness in the spine

Joint pain and swelling — often in the large and small joints of the legs — occurs in approximately 1 in 10 people with ulcerative colitis and in 1 in 5 people with Crohn's disease. The pain and stiffness in the spine is similar to that brought on by ankylosing spondylitis.

Treatment

Symptoms are generally treated with anti-inflammatory drugs. Control or cure of the inflammatory bowel disorder is the long-term solution.

Palindromic rheumatism

Also called palindromic rheumatoid arthritis, this disease is a rare type of inflammatory arthritis. Signs and symptoms include:

- Recurrent attacks of painful swelling, usually of one or two joints and surrounding tissues
- Attacks that start abruptly and last several hours to a few days
- Unpredictable frequency of attacks, from every few days to every few months

The term *palindromic* means "to come and go." Attacks of palindromic rheumatism can recur for many years. The disease affects

Rheumatic Fever

The management of rheumatic fever is one of modern medicine's success stories. It was once the cause of serious heart problems in many children. The advent of prompt antibiotic treatment of streptococcal infections, however, markedly reduced its incidence.

A common manifestation of the illness is a form of arthritis. It characteristically occurs several weeks after a streptococcal infection, usually of the throat (strep throat). Your joints may become swollen, reddened and painful to move. Typically, your joints are affected in a migratory manner — first, one joint is painful for a time, and then the pain improves and occurs in another joint.

The arthritis of rheumatic fever isn't due to joint infection. Rather it's a hypersensitivity reaction in the joints associated with a previous strep infection. In general, the treatment is the same as that for rheumatic fever, although your doctor may remove fluid from swollen joints with a needle to reduce the discomfort.

? Question and Answer

What's pseudogout?

Pseudogout is similar to gout, but it involves the deposit of crystals of a calcium salt rather than uric acid in joints. Affected joints are more likely to be knees, wrists and ankles than those of the foot. Pseudogout strikes women and men with roughly equal frequency, but the age at onset is late, typically 70 years.

Doctors usually treat pseudogout with anti-inflammatory medications, although colchicine, used for centuries to treat gout, may be effective.

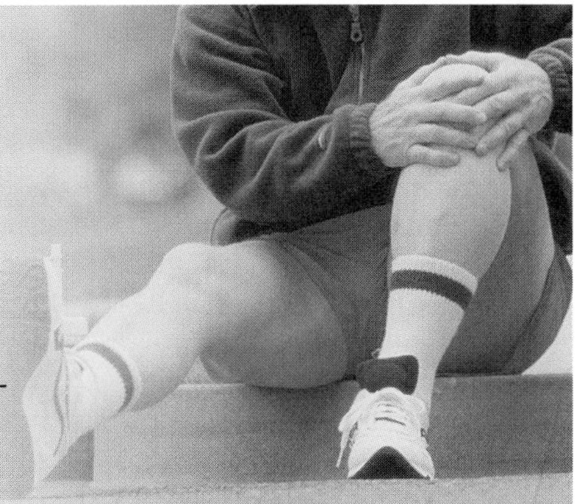

both men and women, typically between the ages of 20 and 50. Palindromic rheumatism usually doesn't cause joint damage, but people with the disease are at higher risk of developing rheumatoid arthritis.

Treatment
Some doctors recommend nonsteroidal anti-inflammatory drugs (NSAIDs) to relieve symptoms, but their benefit isn't clear. Corticosteroids usually aren't beneficial. Colchicine, an anti-inflammatory medication used to treat gout, and gold therapy may prevent attacks.

Infectious arthritis

Signs and symptoms

- Pain and stiffness in one joint, typically a knee, shoulder, hip, ankle, elbow, finger or wrist
- Warmth and redness in surrounding tissues
- Chills and fever
- Weakness

Bacteria, viruses, fungi or other infectious agents can cause a joint infection. Typically, the infecting agent enters the body and spreads to the joint via the bloodstream. In some instances, an open wound or puncture provides direct access to the joint. Unlike other joint disorders, infectious arthritis can affect anyone, anytime, regardless of age, sex or race.

Types

Here's a look at some representative types of infectious arthritis.

Lyme disease
Named for the town in Connecticut where it was first observed, Lyme disease is contracted from a tick bite.

Usually, a disk-shaped rash will develop around the bite, and other signs and symptoms may follow, including fever, chills, sore throat, fatigue and nausea. Some weeks later, you may develop stiffness and pain in your joints.

Gonococcal infection
Roughly one-third of individuals who contract gonorrhea, a sexually transmitted bacterial disease, experience pain in several joints. A rash also may develop. This type of infectious arthritis occurs 10 times more frequently in women than in men.

Staphylococcal infection
When a boil or other infection releases staphylococcal bacteria into your bloodstream, the infection can spread to a knee or other joint. The pain is usually intense and sudden.

Tuberculous infection
A small number of people with tuberculosis have arthritis caused by the bacterium that causes tuberculosis (*Mycobacterium tuberculosis*). Nontuberculosis mycobacteria may also cause infectious arthritis.

Viral infections
Arthritis symptoms may occur in people who have hepatitis B, hepatitis C, human parvovirus B19, German measles (rubella), mumps and other diseases caused by viruses.

In general, the arthritis resolves as the infection clears or, with viral infections such as hepatitis C, with successful treatment of the underlying disease.

Diagnosis

If your doctor suspects a form of infectious arthritis, he or she may perform a biopsy, removing fluid from an affected joint with a needle for laboratory analysis. Your doctor may also order blood tests.

How serious is infectious arthritis?

In most cases, early diagnosis and treatment of a joint infection result in rapid and complete recovery.

Treatment

Because of the risk of permanent damage to the bone or cartilage, a joint infection needs to be treated promptly. Hospitalization may be necessary.

Unless the cause of the infection is viral, your doctor will likely prescribe an antibiotic. Your doctor may use a needle to drain the infected joint, or a surgeon may open the joint surgically to remove infected and damaged tissues. After the infection has resolved, you may need reconstructive surgery if your joint has been seriously damaged.

During recuperation from an infection, the joint may be immobilized with a splint. Physical therapy may be necessary to regain strength and mobility in the affected joint.

Gout

Signs and symptoms

- Sudden, severe pain in a single joint, often at the base of your big toe
- Swelling, redness and warmth of tissues surrounding the joint

One of humankind's oldest known diseases, gout has been recognized for more than 2,000 years. It's caused by too much uric acid, a substance your body naturally forms from proteins called purines. When you have gout, your body either produces too much uric acid or excretes too little in the urine. In 90 percent of individuals with gout, the problem is underexcretion.

Uric acid typically dissolves in your blood and passes through your kidneys into your urine. In people with gout, the excess uric acid can build up and form sharp crystals, which deposit in a joint and surrounding tissue, causing pain, inflammation and swelling. Gout typically affects the joint of the big toe, but it can strike other joints in the feet, as well as the ankles, knees and, occasionally, the hands and elbows. Not everyone with excess uric acid develops gout symptoms.

Other factors that may contribute to gout are eating foods high in purines — organ meats, anchovies, herring and mackerel — drinking alcohol, being overweight, having high blood cholesterol or diabetes and taking certain medications. For instance, taking a thiazide diuretic for high blood pressure may interfere with your kidneys' ability to remove uric acid from the body.

Daily low-dose aspirin also can raise uric acid levels in the blood by decreasing excretion. The stress of an injury such as a bone fracture or a surgical procedure may provoke an attack of gout.

An episode of acute gout develops in a matter of hours. A joint suddenly becomes intensely painful, and the area around it becomes hot, red and swollen. The joint will remain very painful for several days. The discomfort generally subsides gradually over the next 1 to 2 weeks.

Ninety percent of people with gout are men older than age 40. One in four have a family history of the ailment. Women become increasingly susceptible after menopause.

Gout has a reputation as an illness that's caused by excessive consumption of food and drink. Although that may contribute to the problem, gout can strike at any time and for no apparent reason.

Diagnosis

To confirm the diagnosis and rule out infection as the cause, your doctor may withdraw fluid from the affected joint to look for crystals of uric acid within the white blood cells. He or she may also order blood tests to check levels of uric acid. However, blood tests can be misleading because the levels may be nearly normal during an acute attack of gout. In addition, many people with high levels of uric acid never experience gout.

A long-term accumulation of uric acid may produce lumps (tophi) just beneath the skin. The most common sites are the cartilage of the ear, elbows and Achilles tendons. Infrequently, kidney stones develop from accumulation of uric acid.

How serious is gout?

After an attack of gout has run its course — generally a matter of days and no more than a few weeks — the affected joint usually returns to normal. You may never have another attack, or you may have them several times a year. If you don't receive proper treatment, the condition can permanently damage affected joints, and uric acid deposits may cause kidney problems, including the development of kidney stones.

Treatment

An acute attack of gout is generally treated with nonsteroidal anti-inflammatory drugs (NSAIDs) and followed up with other medication to prevent a recurrence. Lifestyle changes also may help prevent a recurrence.

Medication

NSAIDs, such as ibuprofen (Advil, Motrin), naproxen (Aleve, Naprosyn) and others, are the treatment of choice for an acute gout attack. The medication colchicine has been used for centuries to relieve the pain and swelling of an acute episode. But it's more likely to cause gastrointestinal upset and toxicity than NSAIDs. Another treatment option is cortisone, either in pill form or as an injection into the affected joint.

Once the attack is under control, your doctor may advise preventive treatment to keep uric acid levels down and prevent recurrence. This usually involves taking medication such as allopurinol (Aloprim, Zyloprim) for months or years.

Self-care

Although doctors no longer consider food and drink the main cause of gout, lifestyle changes can help. If you have gout, limit or avoid alcohol, maintain a healthy weight and avoid foods that are high in purines, including sardines, anchovies and organ meats. Don't try fad diets. Diets that involve rapid weight reduction may provoke an acute attack.

If you're taking a medication such as allopurinol to prevent future attacks of gout, don't abruptly discontinue the drug because this may provoke an acute attack of gout. In addition, if you start taking allopurinol during an acute attack of gout, you may worsen and prolong the attack.

Bursitis

Signs and symptoms

- Pain around a joint
- Stiffness and difficulty moving the joint
- Warmth over the joint

- Swelling and skin redness
- Increasing pain, redness or warmth over the joint, along with fever and chills

Your body houses more than 150 bursae, tiny sacs that help lubricate and cushion pressure points between your bones and the fibrous tissues of the muscles and tendons. Bursae facilitate movement by limiting friction.

Repetitive movements or pressure may cause inflammation in a bursa, a condition known as bursitis. For instance, if you spend a lot of time kneeling, such as when you garden, the pressure could cause a bursa in front of your kneecap to become inflamed. Swinging a racket or golf club or throwing a ball repeatedly can affect a bursa in your shoulder.

Although you can usually trace bursitis to overuse or pressure, in some cases, there is no obvious cause.

Diagnosis

Your doctor may be able to identify tenderness in a localized area. If it appears that something else may be causing the discomfort, your doctor may want an X-ray of the affected area. If bursitis is the cause, X-ray images are usually normal.

How serious is bursitis?

Bursitis often improves on its own with simple self-care remedies. With proper care, you might prevent bursitis from recurring. However, if the pain is disabling or doesn't subside after a week, see your doctor. Sometimes a bursa becomes infected, especially those near the knee or elbow. If you develop increasing pain, redness or warmth over the joint, along with fever and chills, seek medical care promptly.

Treatment

Bursitis usually disappears within 2 weeks, given reasonable care of the painful joint. Physical therapy may be useful to decrease pain and restore motion and strength as the pain subsides. Physical therapy may also prevent recurrences.

Medication

Acetaminophen or nonsteroidal anti-inflammatory drugs (NSAIDs), such as aspirin or ibuprofen (Advil, Motrin, others), may help relieve the discomfort. In some cases, a doctor may inject a corticosteroid drug into the affected bursa. If a bursa becomes infected, your doctor may drain the infected fluid and prescribe an antibiotic.

Self-care

Apply ice for 5 to 10 minutes at a time several times a day to reduce swelling. Use ice for the first 2 days or until the swelling has significantly subsided. After the swelling has improved, you can use heat to relieve pain and stiffness.

Doing gentle stretches can help maintain or restore your range of motion. But until the pain and swelling subside, avoid strenuous activities that stress the joint. Keep pressure off the area of the bursa until the swelling goes down. Depending on which joint is affected, you might want to use an elastic bandage, sling or soft foam pad.

Surgery

When bursitis occurs repeatedly in the same location, your doctor might suggest that the affected bursa be removed surgically. This procedure is done infrequently.

Prevention

With proper care, you may be able to keep bursitis from recurring or reduce the severity of the signs and symptoms if it does. Warm up before physical activity and stretch afterward. Strengthening exercise can help keep your muscles strong.

When doing repetitive tasks, take frequent breaks. Avoid standing or sitting for excessively long periods. Protect your joints by sitting in well-supported, cushioned chairs or using foam kneeling pads.

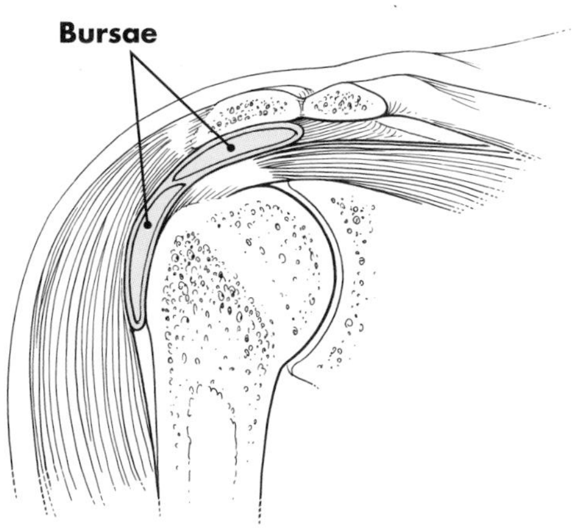

Bursae

Bursae serve as cushions between bones and fibrous tissue. Overuse of a joint can lead to bursitis, an inflammation of a bursa.

Frozen shoulder

Signs and symptoms

- Aching or burning pain in your shoulder
- Limited shoulder motion
- Pain in your upper arm or, possibly, your neck
- Often, shoulder pain that worsens at night

As its name suggests, frozen shoulder is characterized by stiffness in the shoulder joint, along with pain. Also known as adhesive capsulitis, the condition most often affects only one shoulder.

Your shoulder is a ball-and-socket joint. The round end of your upper arm bone (humerus) fits into a shallow groove on your shoulder blade (scapula). Tough connective tissue, called the shoulder capsule,

Rotator Cuff Injuries and Exercises

Your shoulder joint has the greatest range of motion of any joint in your body, thanks largely to your rotator cuff, which is made up of four muscles and their attached tendons. The muscles connect your upper arm bone (humerus) with your shoulder blade. They also help hold the ball of your upper arm firmly in your shoulder joint socket.

A rotator cuff injury is a painful strain or tear in the tendons and muscles surrounding your shoulder joint, often caused by falling, lifting and repetitive overhead arm activities, such as throwing a ball or placing items on a shelf above your head. As you age, your risk of rotator cuff injury increases.

The symptoms of rotator cuff injury may resemble those of frozen shoulder, although the range of motion restrictions are not as severe. If you're unable to use your arm or your pain is severe or persistent, see your doctor as soon as possible.

For a minor shoulder injury, resting your shoulder, applying ice and heat and taking an over-the-counter pain reliever may be sufficient. After a day or two, do gentle exercises to keep your shoulder muscles limber. For a more severe injury, your doctor may give you a corticosteroid injection in your shoulder joint to relieve pain and inflammation. If you have a large tear in your rotator cuff, you may need surgery to repair the tear.

In addition, you may need shoulder exercises. Your doctor or a physical therapist will give you specific exercises designed to help heal your injury, improve flexibility of your shoulder and provide balanced shoulder muscle strength. Physical therapy may last from 3 weeks to several months.

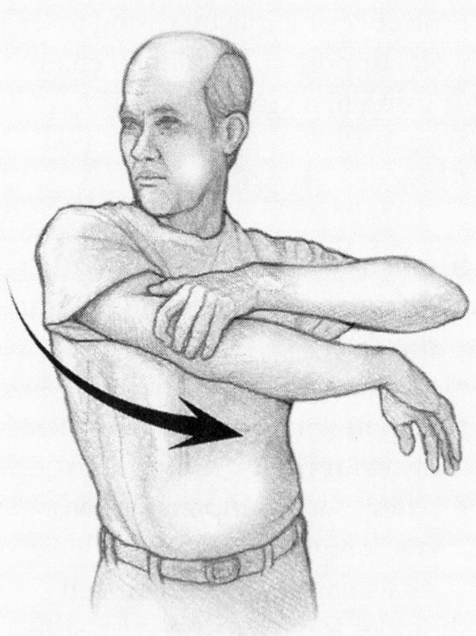

Gently pull your arm across your body so you feel the back of your shoulder stretch. Hold for 30 seconds. Repeat two to three times. Switch arms and repeat.

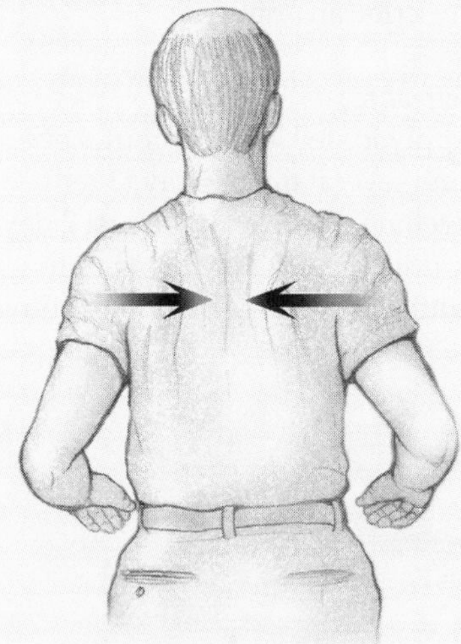

With your arms bent forward at the elbows, pull your elbows back to squeeze your shoulder blades closer together. Hold for 10 seconds. Repeat three to five times.

surrounds the joint and allows movement. With frozen shoulder, the shoulder capsule becomes inflamed and stiff, causing pain and loss of movement.

Frozen shoulder typically develops slowly and in three stages: painful, freezing and thawing. During the painful stage, which can last from 2 to 9 months, you feel pain with shoulder movement. The pain often worsens at night.

Motion, particularly extending your arm to the side or putting on a coat, may produce or increase pain. Sometimes, people hold the affected arm close to their body and avoid moving it. Ligaments and other tissues around the joint tend to stiffen. This is the freezing stage. Try to use your involved shoulder for activities of daily living as much as your pain and range-of-motion limitations will allow.

Pain may diminish during the freezing stage, which can last from 4 to 12 months, but your shoulder's range of motion gradually decreases by perhaps as much as 50 percent to 75 percent. Movement can cause pain. During the thawing stage, which can last from 1 to 3 ½ years, the condition may begin to improve.

No one knows what causes frozen shoulder, but it can occur after a shoulder injury or prolonged immobilization of your shoulder, such as following surgery or after a fracture of your arm. Twenty percent of people with diabetes develop the condition, which raises the possibility that frozen shoulder may have an autoimmune component, meaning that your own immune system may attack the shoulder capsule, causing the inflammation.

More women than men get frozen shoulder, most often between the ages of 40 and 65.

Diagnosis

The primary means of diagnosing frozen shoulder is by physical examination. Your doctor may ask you to raise and lower your arm to the front, side and back of your body. He or she may also move your arm to determine your passive range of motion of the shoulder joint and press on parts of your shoulder to check for tender areas.

Your doctor may order an X-ray of your shoulder and possibly a magnetic resonance imaging (MRI) scan to exclude other structural problems.

How serious is frozen shoulder?

In some cases, mobility can decrease to the point where it's difficult if not impossible to perform many everyday tasks, such as combing your hair, putting on your coat or brushing your teeth. Usually, though, the condition improves on its own over time, and most people regain nearly full range of motion and strength in the shoulder.

Treatment

Most often, treatment for frozen shoulder involves gently and gradually stretching your shoulder to restore range of motion. Stretching may not alleviate the problem, but it may help restore enough flexibility for you to resume everyday activities. Icing the shoulder also may be helpful.

Medication

Acetaminophen (Tylenol, others) and nonsteroidal anti-inflammatory drugs (NSAIDs), such as ibuprofen (Advil, Motrin, others) and naproxen (Aleve, Naprosyn, others), may help relieve the pain. Or your doctor may prescribe a COX-2 inhibitor, such as celecoxib (Celebrex), rofecoxib (Vioxx) and valdecoxib (Bextra).

If pain and inflammation persist, a corticosteroid injection into the joint may be helpful. Newer treatment options include injecting fluid into the shoulder joint to expand the shoulder capsule and break up adhesions. However, the long-term results of this treatment aren't yet clear.

Physical therapy

Once the pain begins to subside, your doctor may refer you to a physical therapist who can help you with exercises to stretch tissue and help preserve a range of motion that permits you to perform everyday activities.

In rare cases of severe stiffness, your doctor may gently manipulate your shoulder while you're under general anesthetic.

Frozen shoulder usually takes a year or two to resolve. Your tendency will be to keep your shoulder as still as possible because of the pain and stiffness when you move your arm. But restoring and maintaining range of motion is critical.

Move your shoulder joint through its available range four times a day to avoid further stiffening. If necessary, ask a friend to help you gently move your arm.

Once the pain improves, exercise your arm daily. Flexibility and strengthening exercises, such as swimming and lifting weights, may help. A physical therapist can guide you in appropriate exercises at each stage of this condition.

Prevention

When your shoulder is sore from overuse or tendinitis, you may be able to avoid the freezing stage by regularly moving your shoulder through range-of-motion exercises.

Immunologic Rheumatic Diseases

Immunologic rheumatic diseases are sometimes called connective tissue diseases or collagen vascular disorders. They result from alterations in your body's immune system. Common to all of them is inflammation of unknown cause that can affect almost all tissues of the body.

Lupus

Signs and symptoms

- Joint pain, swelling and redness that come and go, most often in fingers and wrists
- A rash, especially across the nose and cheeks
- Localized chest pain that increases with moving, coughing or taking a deep breath
- Sunlight sensitivity that produces a rash, fever and tiredness following minimal sun exposure
- Sores inside the mouth or nose
- Fatigue and weakness
- Fever
- Weight loss
- Raynaud's disease

Lupus is a chronic disease in which an individual's immune system attacks healthy tissues, typically the joints. This causes inflammation, pain, stiffness and occasional redness in the joints. It may also produce a rash across the nose and cheeks. Both the joint discomfort and the rash tend to be episodic, with alternating periods of remission and flares.

Systemic lupus erythematosus, the most common form, affects about 70 percent of individuals who have the disease. *Systemic* means that several body systems may be affected. The disease may affect your skin, kidneys, nervous system, lungs and heart. About half the people with systemic lupus erythematosus have major internal organ involvement. For the other half, skin and joints are primarily affected.

Other types of lupus include discoid and cutaneous lupus, which may be limited to the skin, and drug-induced lupus. Drug-induced lupus is the least common form, and it can develop in people who are using several prescription medications. Typically, the symptoms clear up once the drugs are stopped.

Lupus most often develops in females between the ages of 15 and 45 years, but it can occur in younger children and older adults.

Approximately 10 times as many women as men have lupus, and it's more common in blacks than in whites. Lupus sometimes appears for the first time during pregnancy, usually with little or no effect on the unborn child. Some people may inherit a genetic predisposition to lupus.

Diagnosis

Your doctor may order laboratory studies, such as an antinuclear antibody (ANA) test and other antibody tests. A positive ANA test may suggest lupus, but because healthy individuals also can have a positive ANA test, this test alone can't confirm the disease. Your doctor may do other blood tests to check immune function. You may also have urine tests because lupus can affect kidney function. A chest X-ray or echocardiogram can help determine if the disease is affecting the lining around your heart.

How serious is lupus?

For many people with lupus, the disease doesn't cause serious problems. For others, it's a major illness that needs to be managed carefully to prevent or treat serious complications, especially kidney and heart disease, as well as complications of treatment. Typically, lupus is a lifelong ailment that comes and goes.

Treatment

The treatment of lupus depends on its severity and the forms it assumes.

Medication

Nonsteroidal anti-inflammatory drugs (NSAIDs), such as ibuprofen (Advil, Motrin, others) and aspirin, may help control pain and inflammation associated with lupus. Another option is COX-2 inhibitors, such as rofecoxib (Vioxx), celecoxib (Celebrex) and valdecoxib (Bextra). These prescription medications provide options if your current pain reliever causes side effects, such as gastrointestinal pain and bleeding.

Sometimes, a doctor may prescribe a corticosteroid medication, such as prednisone, to control inflammation. Other medications for lupus include the antimalarial drug hydroxychloroquine (Plaquenil) and immunosuppressant medications such as azathio-

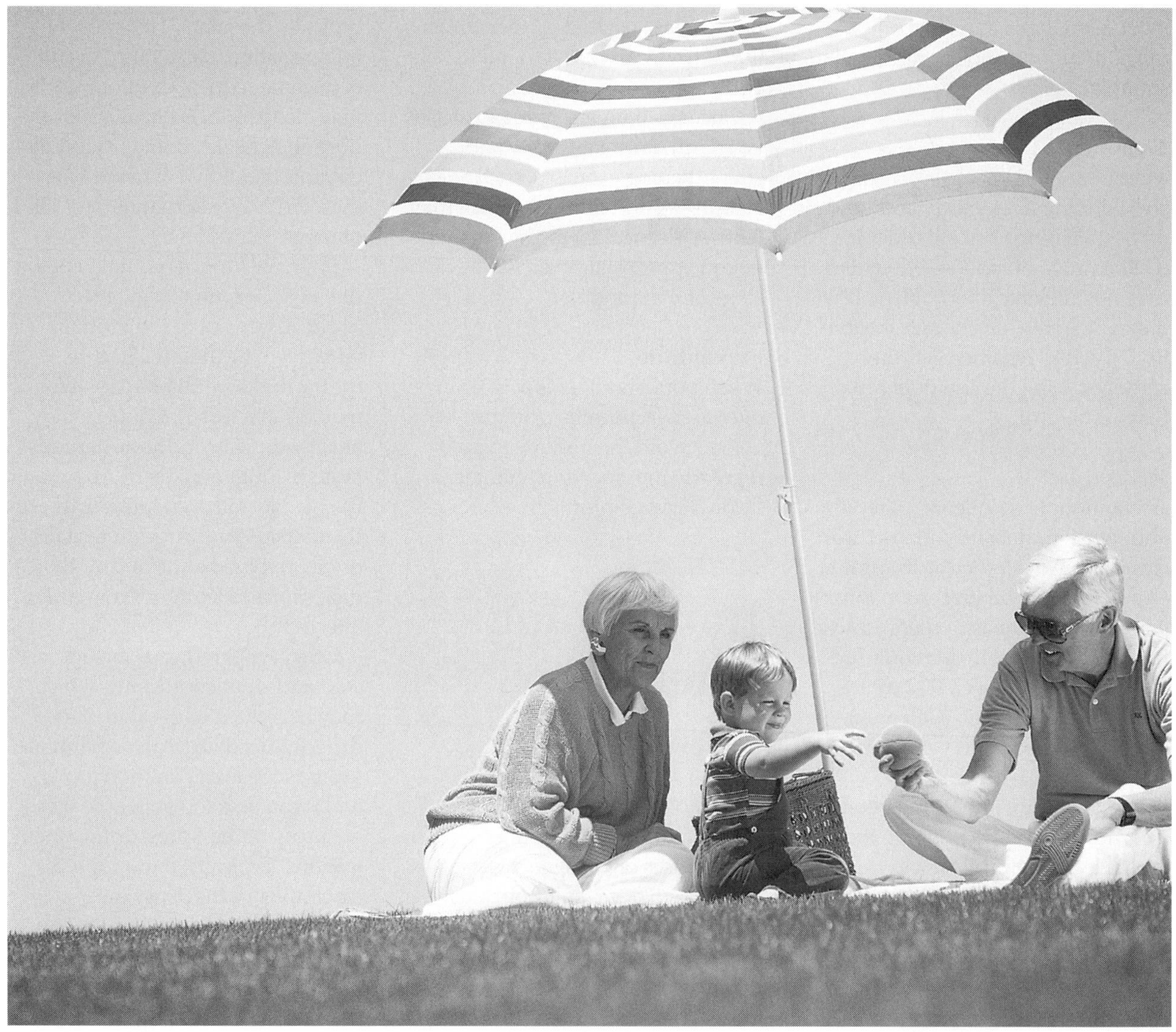

Ultraviolet rays from the sun can aggravate lupus. Avoid prolonged exposure to sunlight and use a sunscreen.

prine (Imuran), cyclophosphamide (Cytoxan) and mycophenolate mofetil (CellCept).

Because of long-term risks associated with lupus and its treatment, your doctor will carefully monitor the status of the disease and the medications you use to treat it.

Exercise
As with other conditions that affect muscles and joints, management of lupus includes daily activity to prevent muscle weakness and ease joint stiffness. You may not feel up to exercising during flares, but even then you should do gentle range-of-motion exercises such as stretching. A physical therapist can design an exercise program to suit your physical condition.

Other therapies
Your doctor may recommend that you wear sunscreen and that you limit exposure to the ultraviolet rays in sunlight and avoid tanning beds. Sunlight and ultraviolet light from the beds may help trigger the autoimmune flares of lupus. As with any chronic disease, sometimes the illness can lead to depression, which may require treatment.

Scleroderma

Signs and symptoms

- A thickening and tightening of the skin, especially on your arms, face or hands
- Change in skin color
- Puffy hands and feet, particularly in the morning
- Joint pain and stiffness
- Skin that appears shiny
- Numbness, pain or color changes in your fingers, toes, cheeks, nose or ears
- Swallowing and digestive problems
- Heart, lung or kidney problems
- Fatigue

Scleroderma, which means "hard skin," is a rare autoimmune disease that leads to an overproduction of the protein collagen. The condition causes thickening, hardening and tightness of the affected tissues. Affected skin takes on a shiny appearance. Another name for the disease is progressive systemic sclerosis.

There are several types of scleroderma. Those that are limited and

Vasculitis

Vasculitis is a general term used to describe an inflammation of the blood vessels, usually the arteries. The inflammation damages the wall of the blood vessel and may impair circulation to part of the body. Signs and symptoms of vasculitis depend on the part of the body that's affected. General symptoms may include fever, muscle weakness, loss of appetite and fatigue. If a particular organ is involved, such as the intestines, vasculitis may cause more specific symptoms, such as abdominal pain.

Vasculitis is often associated with autoimmune disorders and is therefore treated by rheumatologists. A doctor may confirm a diagnosis of vasculitis by blood tests, an X-ray of blood vessels (angiography), or biopsy of an affected blood vessel, in which a tissue sample is removed for laboratory study.

Treatment of vasculitis depends on the type, location and severity of the problem. It often includes anti-inflammatory medications such as corticosteroids and immunosuppressant drugs.

Different types of vasculitis may include:

Polyarteritis

This serious disorder involves an inflammation of many arteries. Inflammation can result in obstruction of the vessels, reducing the supply of blood to the affected area. The skin, intestines, kidneys and heart are at greatest risk.

Typical symptoms include weight loss, fever, weakness and fatigue. If the intestines are involved, you may have abdominal pain and bloody diarrhea.

Middle-aged men are most likely to suffer from polyarteritis, although there's also a juvenile form of the illness. In the past, this disease often was fatal. Today, with proper treatment, many people with polyarteritis can lead normal lives.

Allergic granulomatous angiitis

Also called Churg-Strauss syndrome, this ailment also may affect multiple organ systems, but it generally includes the lungs. People affected by this type of vasculitis often have asthma.

Hypersensitivity vasculitis

This form of vasculitis is the result of exposure to a drug or foreign substance. It usually involves the small blood vessels of the skin.

Granulomatous arteritis

This disorder occurs almost exclusively in people older than age 50, and it affects women more often than men. Also called cranial, temporal or giant cell arteritis, this condition involves medium-sized arteries, especially those in the head. The condition is characterized by headache and a tender, thickened artery that can be felt at the side of the head. It's often associated with polymyalgia rheumatica.

Malaise, fatigue, loss of appetite, weight loss, fever and night sweats are common accompanying symptoms. Occasionally, chewing fatigues the jaw and vision problems develop. Left untreated, it can lead to partial or total blindness.

diffuse are defined by the amount of skin affected by the disease. Overlap syndromes have features of scleroderma and other connective tissue diseases, such as systemic lupus erythematosus, polymyositis and rheumatoid arthritis. Localized scleroderma includes morphea and linear scleroderma.

Raynaud's disease, a condition in which poor blood flow to the extremities causes the skin color to change to a dead white pallor, then to blue and finally to a reddish color, occurs more commonly in scleroderma than in any of the other connective tissue diseases. Emotional stress or exposure to cold may bring on the symptoms of Raynaud's disease (see page 792).

Most people with scleroderma develop the disease between the ages of 35 and 55, although it can occur in children and older adults. Women are about four times as likely as men to get scleroderma.

Diagnosis

Because it's rare and can resemble other immune system diseases, scleroderma can be difficult to diagnose. A diagnosis typically is based on medical history, physical examination and laboratory tests. Your doctor may perform a biopsy, in which a tissue sample is removed for laboratory study. You may also have blood tests and tests to check the status of your heart, lungs and gastrointestinal tract.

How serious is scleroderma?

Limited scleroderma may stop progressing on its own, although in rare instances the hands may be damaged permanently.

Diffuse scleroderma can severely affect internal organs and may result in high blood pressure, heart disease, lung impairments, kidney failure and intestinal tract problems that can lead to malnutrition. When there's severe internal organ involvement, the life expectancy may be shortened, especially if the heart or lung is involved.

Treatment

There's no cure for scleroderma, but a number of medications may help control it. Localized scleroderma may disappear or stop progressing without treatment. With systemic scleroderma, treatment generally involves medications to help protect internal organs and attempt to halt progression of the disease.

Medication

Medications used to treat the disease include nonsteroidal anti-inflammatory drugs (NSAIDs) and low doses of corticosteroids to ease pain and reduce stiffness and inflammation. Your doctor may prescribe a blood vessel dilator if you have Raynaud's disease, high blood pressure medication to control high blood pressure, acid blockers or pantoprazole (Protonix) for heartburn or gastroesophageal reflux disease (GERD), and antibiotics for intestinal problems. Certain types of antihypertensive drugs called angiotensin-converting enzyme (ACE) inhibitors may have a protective effect on the kidneys.

Self-care

Exercise is important to overall health and because it may limit stiffening of skin tissues and increase blood flow to the tissues. Your doctor may refer you to a physical or occupational therapist. If you smoke, quitting is important because nicotine causes blood vessels to constrict.

Using a paraffin bath — in which you dip your hands into warm, melted paraffin — can help maintain finger flexibility. Also be sure to wear mittens for protection when you're outside in cold temperatures or even when you reach into a freezer. Dress in layers for warmth. If you have heartburn, avoid eating 3 to 4 hours before bedtime.

Sjogren's syndrome

Signs and symptoms

- Dry eyes with a feeling of sandiness or grittiness
- Dry mouth
- Fatigue
- Difficulty chewing or swallowing
- A dry nose, throat and lungs
- Muscle and joint pain

Sjogren's syndrome is an autoimmune disorder in which the immune system attacks glands that produce moisture. It causes dryness of moist mucous membranes, primarily in the eyes and mouth. Your eyes may feel as if foreign bodies have lodged in them, and you may have difficulty chewing or swallowing. It may cause vaginal dryness in women. It may also cause problems with other parts of the body, including muscles, joints, lungs, kidneys and stomach.

A primary form of the condition occurs alone, but the secondary form occurs with disorders that affect the joints and muscles, such as rheumatoid arthritis or other ailments, such as lupus, scleroderma or polymyositis. Most people who have Sjogren's syndrome are middle-aged women.

Diagnosis

When making a diagnosis, your doctor will consider your symptoms, combined with blood tests and an eye exam. He or she may also order an inner lip biopsy, in which a tissue sample is removed for analysis, and salivary gland tests to determine if inflammation is damaging the salivary glands.

How serious is Sjogren's syndrome?

Sjogren's syndrome can seriously affect your quality of life, including your ability to work and to participate in day-to-day activities.

Treatment

Therapy is aimed at symptom relief. Besides taking medications, you may find it helpful to use skin moisturizers, drink plenty of fluids, use artificial saliva and get regular dental care, because reduced saliva can cause cavities.

Preservative-free artificial tears and eye ointments may help relieve the discomfort in your eyes. You can relieve your dry mouth by sucking on sugar-free lemon drops or other hard candies to stimulate the production of saliva and by sipping beverages, preferably water, throughout the day.

Medication

Your doctor will review the medications you're taking to be sure that they're not aggravating your dryness. He or she may prescribe medications, such as pilocarpine (Salagen) or cevimeline (Evoxac) to stimulate the production of saliva.

Your doctor may also prescribe corticosteroids or an immunosuppressant drug such as Cytoxan if your case is severe and it involves kidney, lung or neurologic problems.

Polymyalgia rheumatica

Signs and symptoms

- Pain and stiffness in the muscles, usually in the neck, shoulders, and hips, particularly in the morning
- Fatigue
- Lack of appetite leading to weight loss
- Anemia
- A general feeling of illness
- Sometimes, a slight fever

The phrase *polymyalgia rheumatica* is from the Greek words that mean "pain in many muscles." Polymyalgia rheumatica typically causes pain and stiffness around the neck, shoulders and hips due to an inflammation of the joints and surrounding tissues. Most of the inflammation occurs in the hip and shoulder joints, but inflammation may occur elsewhere in the body, as well. Anemia often accompanies the disease.

Polymyalgia rheumatica usually affects adults older than age 50 and is more common in whites than in other races. It affects women more often than men. The cause is unknown, but researchers suspect that genetic and environmental factors are involved.

Diagnosis

Information about the onset of pain and recent changes in your health are important in making a diagnosis.

In polymyalgia rheumatica, the pain usually strikes suddenly and may involve most muscles, although the neck and shoulders frequently are the most painful. The discomfort is likely to be worse in the morning, but it may occur at night too. No specific tests can confirm the diagnosis, but X-ray or laboratory tests may be done to eliminate other possible causes.

With polymyalgia rheumatica, your erythrocyte sedimentation rate and C-reactive protein levels are usually elevated, indicating the presence of inflammation.

How serious is polymyalgia rheumatica?

The typical disease course is about 1 to 2 years, after which it usually disappears. However, it can recur.

Polymyalgia rheumatica may be associated with a disease called giant cell arteritis (temporal or cranial arteritis), a condition that causes inflammation and tenderness in the arteries just under the scalp near the temples. If you have polymyalgia rheumatica and develop vision problems, scalp tenderness or headaches, call your doctor promptly.

Treatment

Medication and exercise may ease symptoms.

Medication

Corticosteroids often produce improvement within just a few days. You may have to take a corticosteroid until the disease runs its course. Because the medications can cause side effects, your doctor will want to give you the smallest dosage possible to control the symptoms (see page 998). For a mild case, nonsteroidal anti-inflammatory drugs (NSAIDs) may provide adequate relief of symptoms without the need for corticosteroids.

Exercise

Exercise is essential to help maintain your energy and muscle strength. It can also help prevent weight gain, a possible side effect of taking corticosteroids. Your doctor may refer you to a physical therapist for suggestions on the types of exercises that will work best for you.

Polymyositis and dermatomyositis

Signs and symptoms

- Muscle weakness
- Pain and swelling in the small joints
- Reddish patches of skin on the face, knuckles, elbows, knees or ankles

Polymyositis is a disorder in which the muscles become inflamed, resulting in damage to muscle fibers. When a particular skin inflammation accompanies the muscle inflammation, the disorder is called dermatomyositis.

Adults between the ages of 30 and 60 are most likely to have these disorders, but they can occur at any age. Children between ages 5 and 15 may develop dermatomyositis. Women are about twice as likely as men to have polymyositis or dermatomyositis.

Diagnosis

Your doctor will likely take a medical history and perform a physical examination, focusing on your skin and testing your muscle strength. Your doctor may also order a series of blood tests to determine the presence of certain muscle enzymes. A test called electromyography can measure the electrical activity in your muscles. In addition, a biopsy, in which a tissue sample is removed for laboratory study, may be conducted on affected muscles.

How serious are polymyositis and dermatomyositis?

Signs and symptoms of dermatomyositis and polymyositis may persist for many months or even years. A particular danger is the potential effect on the muscles of the throat, which can make swallowing difficult. Lung problems also may occur, including weakness of the muscles that help you breathe.

Treatment

The primary treatment of polymyositis and dermatomyositis is immunosuppressant medication. The corticosteroid prednisone is commonly used. Other medications that a doctor may prescribe include methotrexate (Rheumatrex), azathioprine (Imuran) or intravenous immunoglobulin.

Once the medication begins to take effect and the inflammation improves, your doctor may recommend an exercise program to prevent muscle wasting (atrophy) and stiffness. ■

CHAPTER **32** PART V

Endocrine System

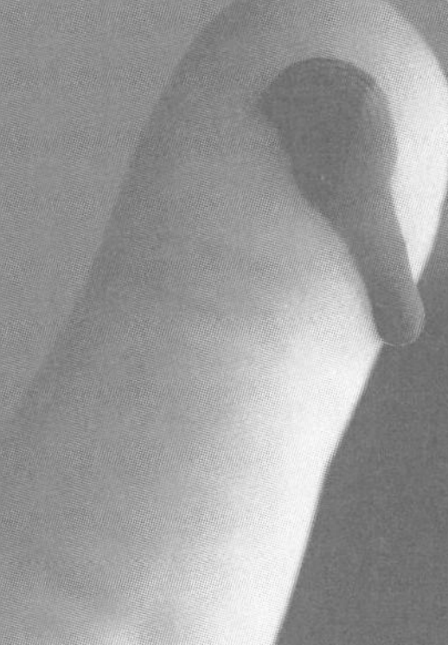

Your body's endocrine system consists of several glands that function as your body's control mechanism. Along with your nervous system, your endocrine glands coordinate how your body responds to usual and unusual events.

Endocrine glands produce hormones, the key component of the system. A hormone is a chemical messenger. Different endocrine glands secrete different types of hormones. Most of these are released into the bloodstream so that they can deliver instructions to various organs and tissues.

Although hormones circulate throughout the body, each hormone influences specific organs or tissues, so it regulates only certain body processes. The pancreas, for example, secretes the hormone insulin, which enables the body to regulate the amount of sugar in the bloodstream.

In response to physical or emotional stress, the adrenal glands secrete adrenaline (epinephrine), which can produce a sudden and remarkable burst of energy. Similarly, the pituitary, thyroid, parathyroid and sex glands each influence particular body functions. Some hormones, including many produced by the pituitary gland, control the activity of other glands. Virtually every system in your body is directly or indirectly influenced by hormones.

Occasionally, the endocrine system malfunctions. Because the system is so complex, a malfunction can lead to a wide range of problems. For example, in diabetes, the most common endocrine disorder, if the pancreas doesn't secrete enough insulin, excess sugar (glucose) stays in the blood. And if a child's pituitary gland malfunctions, he or she may experience growth problems.

A doctor whose special area of expertise is the endocrine system is called an endocrinologist. In the following pages, hormonal problems that endocrinologists commonly encounter are discussed.

Because hormones affect many tissues and organs throughout the body, an endocrinologist may also have expertise in areas that aren't commonly thought of as related to the endocrine system, such as bone development and blood pressure disorders.

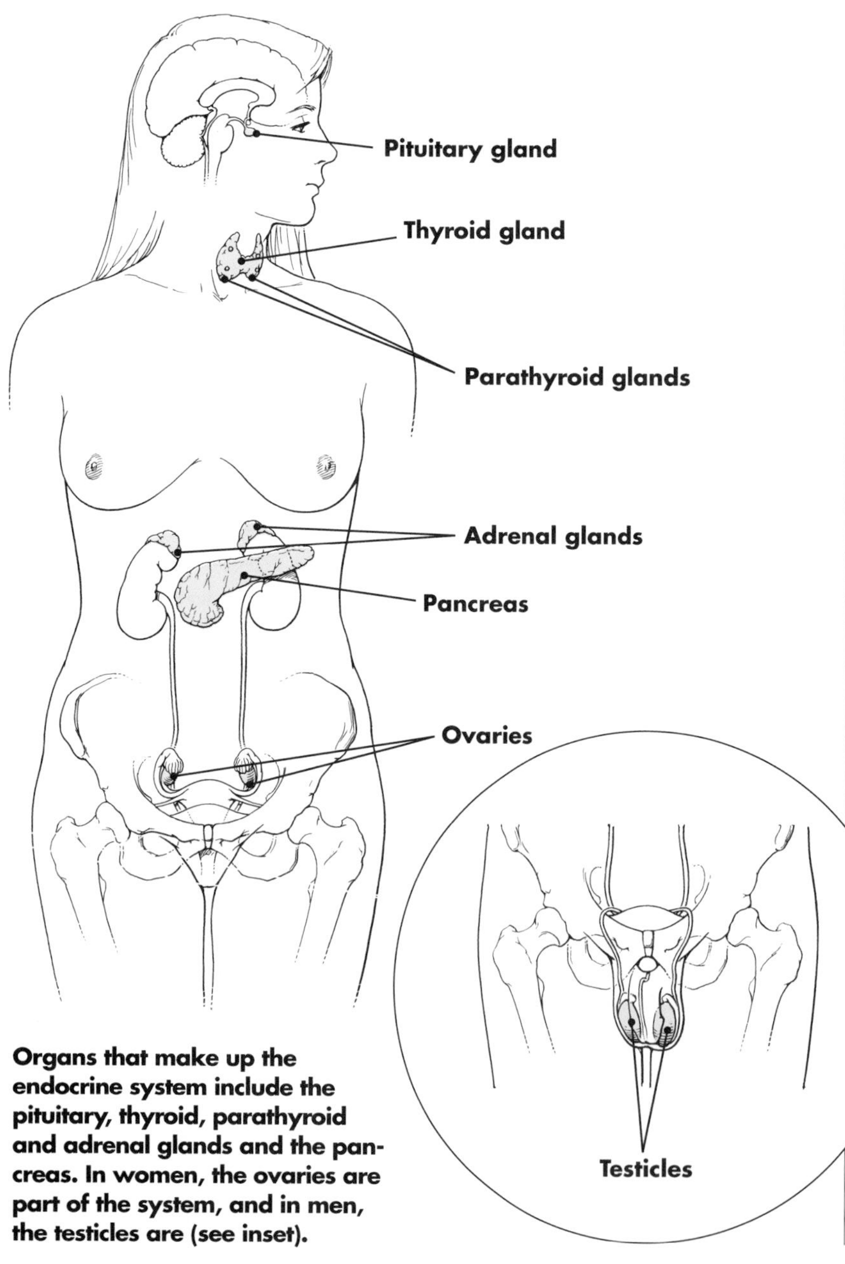

Organs that make up the endocrine system include the pituitary, thyroid, parathyroid and adrenal glands and the pancreas. In women, the ovaries are part of the system, and in men, the testicles are (see inset).

Diabetes

The medical term for diabetes is *diabetes mellitus.* The origins of the term are Latin, referring to the sweetness, or honey (mellitus), that passes through to the urine as a result of the condition.

Another, much less common form of diabetes is diabetes insipidus. It involves a different hormone that's secreted from the pituitary gland and influences the kidneys' conservation of water (see page 1036).

Diabetes mellitus, or diabetes, has become one of the most common diseases in the United States, largely due to the aging of the American population and the increasing number of people who are overweight. More than

16 million Americans, including more children and teenagers than ever before, have diabetes.

What is diabetes?

Diabetes refers to an excess amount of sugar (glucose) in your blood. The condition is often related to a malfunction of the pancreas.

Located behind your stomach, the pancreas is a long, thin organ roughly the length of your hand. It plays an important part in the digestive process, producing enzymes essential for breaking down (metabolizing) the food you eat.

The other key role of the pancreas might best be described as fuel control. The pancreas regulates your body's use of blood sugar, which provides energy for all of your cells, fueling your brain and other organs and tissues.

When your pancreas is functioning normally, the sugar concentration in your blood changes within a narrow, set range in response to a wide variety of factors, including meals, exercise, stressful situations and infections. But sometimes this precisely balanced system of control fails.

Instead of the majority of sugar being transported into your cells, significant amounts remain in your bloodstream. This excess sugar often is more than the kidneys can handle, and sugar may spill into the urine, where it can be detected by urinalysis.

Following an overnight fast, most people have blood sugar levels between 70 and 110 milligrams of glucose per deciliter of blood (mg/dL). This concentration range — equal to about 1 teaspoon of sugar in a gallon of water — is considered normal.

If your blood sugar is consistently 126 mg/dL or higher after fasting, you have diabetes. If your blood sugar measures between 111 and 125 mg/dL, you have impaired fasting glucose, which is commonly referred to as borderline diabetes or prediabetes.

Normal Metabolism

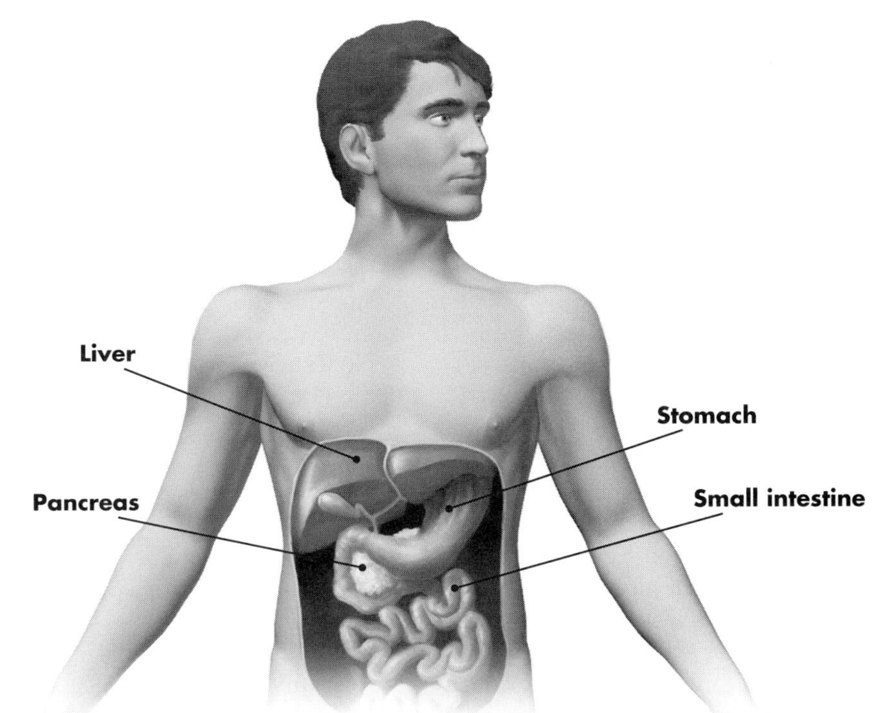

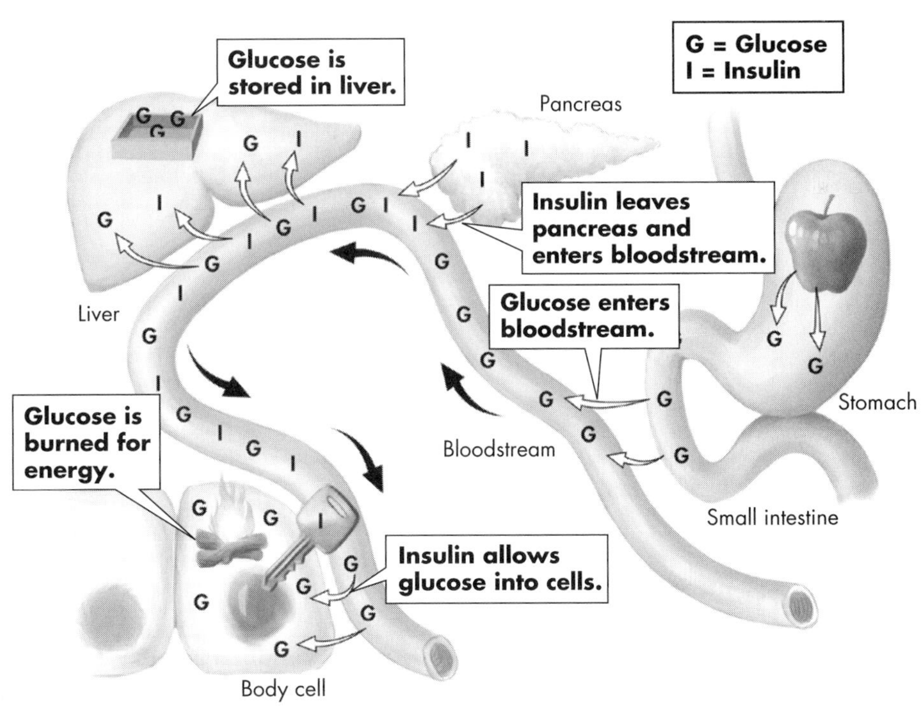

Sugar (glucose) from the food you eat provides energy to fuel your body. Insulin, released by your pancreas, escorts glucose to individual cells, where it's needed for energy, and to your liver, where extra sugar is stored.

Causes

Excess sugar may accumulate in your blood for a variety of reasons:

Insulin
Diabetes occurs when the pancreas is unable to produce enough of the hormone insulin or when body cells become unresponsive (resistant) to insulin's effects.

Normally, when you eat, sugar is absorbed into your bloodstream from food particles in your small intestine. Cells that make up your muscles and organs rely on sugar for energy. But sugar can't enter the cells without the help of insulin.

At the same time sugar is entering your bloodstream, your pancreas is releasing insulin into your blood. The insulin circulates with the sugar and acts like a key, unlocking microscopic doors so that sugar can enter your cells. This lowers the amount of sugar in your blood. Without insulin, sugar remains in your blood and can't get into the cells where it's needed.

Liver
Your liver acts as a blood sugar storage and manufacturing center. When the level of insulin in your blood is high, such as after a meal, your liver stores extra sugar in case your cells need it later. When insulin levels are low, such as when you haven't eaten in a while, the pancreas releases a hormone called glucagon, which converts sugar stored in your liver (glycogen) into glucose and releases it into your bloodstream. This helps keep your blood sugar within a narrow and safe range.

Other hormones
In addition to insulin and glucagon, several other hormones can affect your blood sugar level. In certain circumstances, hormones such as adrenaline (epinephrine) and cortisol counteract the effects of insulin, preventing sugar from entering your cells. The hormones may also encourage your liver to release its stored sugar, even if the sugar isn't needed.

Types

People often think of diabetes as one disease. But excess sugar can accumulate in your blood for various reasons, reflecting different types of diabetes.

Type 1
Type 1 diabetes develops when your pancreas makes little or no insulin. Without insulin circulating in your bloodstream, sugar can't get into your cells, so it remains in your blood.

Type 1 diabetes used to be called insulin-dependent or juvenile diabetes. *Insulin-dependent* means that you need to administer insulin medication daily to make up for the insulin that your body doesn't produce. The term *juvenile diabetes* was used because this form of diabetes most often develops in children and teenagers. The names *insulin-dependent diabetes* and *juvenile diabetes* are used less often today because they're not entirely accurate. Use of insulin isn't limited

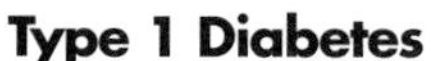

Type 1 Diabetes

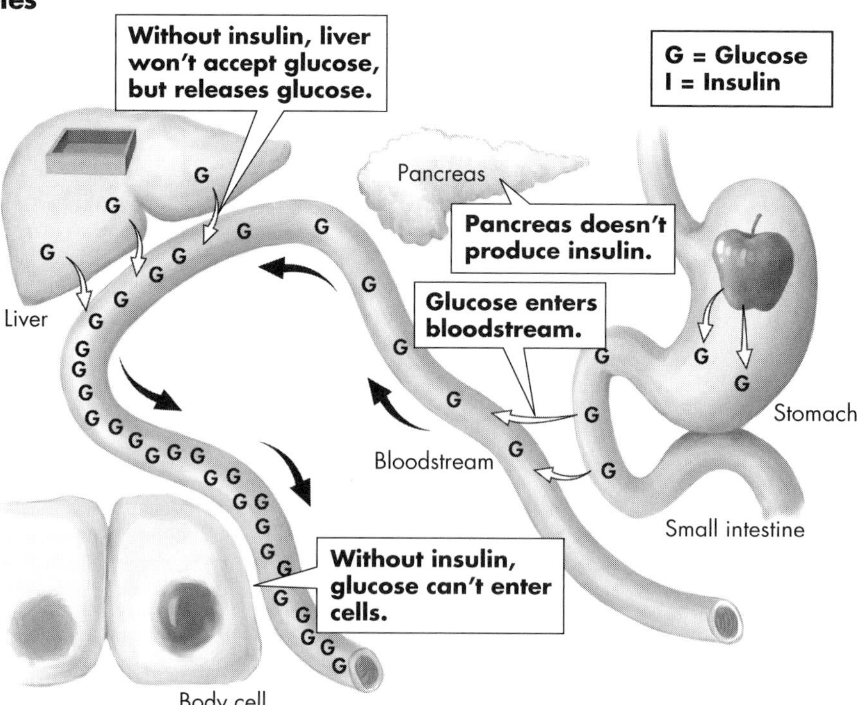

In type 1 diabetes, your pancreas produces little if any insulin. Without insulin to escort sugar (glucose) from the food you eat into your cells, sugar remains in your bloodstream.

only to people with type 1 diabetes. People with other forms of the disease may also need insulin. In addition, although less common, adults as well as juveniles can develop type 1 diabetes.

Type 1 diabetes is an autoimmune disease, meaning that your own immune system is the culprit. Similar to how it attacks invading viruses and bacteria, your body's infection-fighting system may attack your pancreas, zeroing in on the beta cells that produce insulin. Researchers aren't certain why this happens, but they believe that genetic factors, diet and exposure to certain viruses may be involved.

Between 5 percent and 10 percent of people with diabetes have type 1. Although the disease can smolder and remain undetected for several years, it usually comes on quickly, commonly following an illness.

Type 2

Type 2 diabetes is by far the most common form — 90 percent to 95 percent of people over age 20 with diabetes have type 2. Like type 1 diabetes, type 2 used to be called by a couple of other names: noninsulin-dependent diabetes and adult-onset diabetes. These names reflect that many people with type 2 diabetes don't need insulin shots and that the disease usually develops in adults. But as with type 1, the alternative names aren't entirely accurate.

Children and teenagers, as well as adults, can develop type 2 diabetes. In fact, the incidence of type 2 diabetes in young people is increasing. In addition, some people with type 2 diabetes need insulin to control their blood sugar.

Unlike type 1 diabetes, type 2 isn't an autoimmune disease. In type 2, your pancreas makes at least some insulin, but one or two other problems develop:

- Your pancreas doesn't make enough insulin.
- Your muscle and tissue cells become resistant to insulin.

When your cells develop a resistance to insulin, they refuse to accept it as the key that unlocks the door for sugar. As a result, sugar accumulates in your bloodstream. Exactly why the cells become insulin resistant is uncertain, although excess weight and fatty tissue seem to be important factors. Most people with type 2 diabetes are overweight.

It's unclear why excess weight is associated with increased risk of type 2 diabetes. However, scientists have identified a protein, which they call resistin, that's produced by fat cells and appears to induce insulin resistance.

Some people with type 2 diabetes can keep their blood sugar in a healthy range and control the disease by keeping their weight down, eating a healthy diet, exercising and, in some cases, taking oral medication.

Other people need more insulin than their pancreas can supply. Like people with type 1 diabetes, these individuals need insulin replacement medication to control their blood sugar.

Type 2 Diabetes

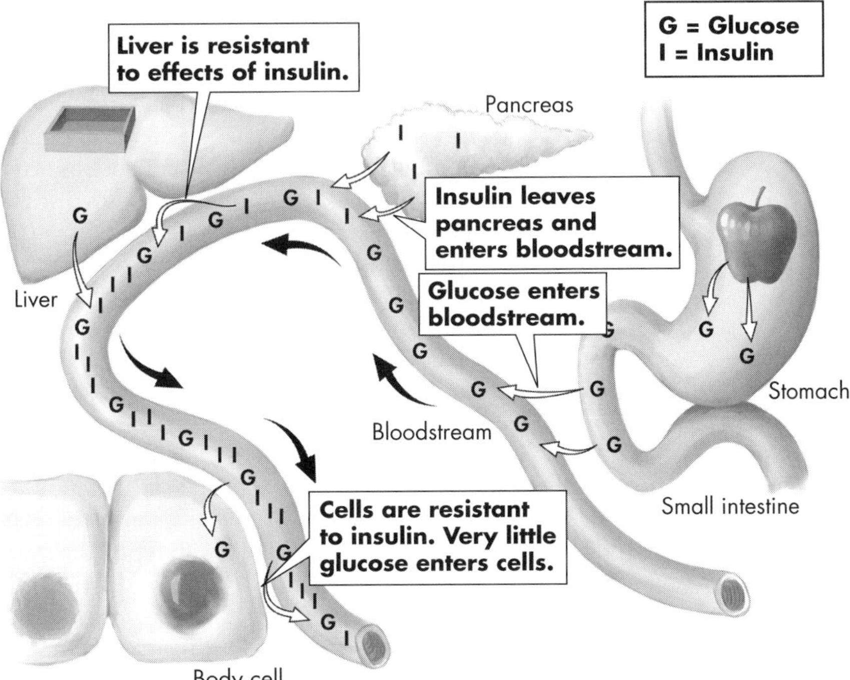

In type 2 diabetes, your pancreas produces insulin, but your cells don't respond to insulin's effects, causing excess sugar (glucose) to remain in your bloodstream after you eat.

Are You at Risk?

Researchers don't fully understand why some people develop diabetes and others don't. However, they've identified a number of factors that increase your risk:

Impaired fasting glucose or impaired glucose tolerance
If blood sugar (glucose) testing shows that you have prediabetes or borderline diabetes, you're at high risk of developing diabetes.

A family history of diabetes
Your chance of developing either type 1 or type 2 diabetes increases if you have a parent, brother or sister with the disease.

Excess weight
Being overweight significantly increases your risk of getting diabetes. The majority of people with type 2 diabetes are overweight. The more fatty tissue you have, the more resistant your muscle and other tissue cells become to your own insulin, especially if your excess weight is concentrated around your abdomen.

Inactivity
The less active you are, the greater your risk.

Age
Your risk of type 2 diabetes increases with age.

Race or ethnicity
Though it's not clear why, people of certain races or ethnic groups are more likely to develop type 2 diabetes than are others. You're at higher risk if you're Hispanic, black, Asian-American, American Indian or Pacific Islander.

In women, a history of gestational diabetes
More than half the women who experience gestational diabetes develop type 2 diabetes later in life. Women who give birth to at least one baby weighing 9 pounds or more also are at increased risk.

Polycystic ovary syndrome
Polycystic ovary syndrome (PCOS) is due to a common form of hormonal imbalance in women. It's associated with an increased risk of type 2 diabetes. Research suggests a link between PCOS and insulin. Many women with PCOS have high blood insulin levels and are less sensitive to the effects of insulin than other people are.

High blood pressure or abnormal blood fats
Because the underlying processes that put someone at risk of developing diabetes also increase the risk of high blood pressure and abnormal blood fat (lipid) levels, anyone affected by these should be screened for diabetes.

When your blood pressure is measured, it's written like a fraction. Your pressure is considered high if your systolic blood pressure (upper number) is consistently 140 millimeters of mercury (mm Hg) or higher or your diastolic blood pressure (lower number) is consistently 90 mm Hg or higher or both. If diabetes is diagnosed in someone with high blood pressure, the goal for blood pressure often is 130/80 mm Hg or less.

Undesirable levels of blood fats — cholesterol and triglycerides — are indicated if your total cholesterol is 240 or above, your low-density lipoprotein (LDL or "bad") cholesterol is 160 or above, your high-density lipoprotein (HDL or "good") cholesterol is below 40, or your triglyceride level is 200 or higher. Desirable levels are much lower if you have diabetes.

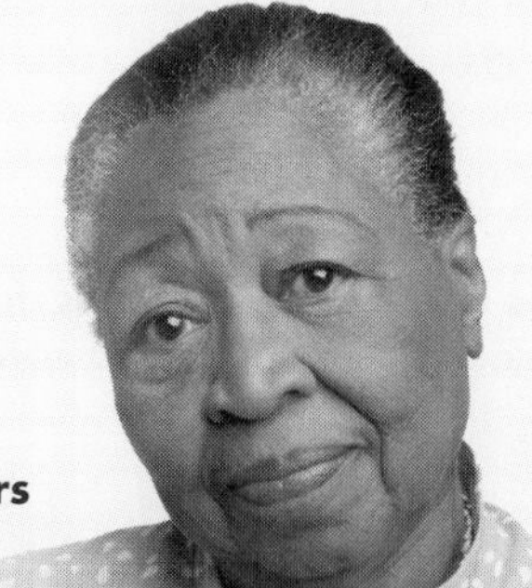

Gestational
Gestational diabetes develops in pregnant women. This can happen temporarily when hormones secreted during pregnancy increase your body's resistance to insulin. About 2 percent to 5 percent of pregnant women develop gestational diabetes, typically during the second half of pregnancy.

Gestational diabetes often can be treated with diet alone and usually goes away after the baby is born. But more than half the women who experience gestational diabetes develop type 2 diabetes later. Type 1 diabetes also may begin during pregnancy, but this is less common.

Most pregnant women are screened for gestational diabetes to detect the condition early. If you develop this form of the disease, controlling your blood sugar level through the remainder of your pregnancy can reduce risk of complications for you and your baby.

Other
Approximately 1 percent to 2 percent of the people with diabetes can trace the cause to illnesses or medications that interfere with the production of insulin or its action. These include:

- Inflammation of the pancreas (pancreatitis)
- Adrenal or pituitary gland disorders, such as acromegaly or Cushing's disease
- Removal of the pancreas
- Corticosteroid medications
- Malnutrition
- Infection

Signs and symptoms

Often, diabetes develops gradually and causes few, if any, signs or symptoms. This is most common with type 2 diabetes. Other times, signs and symptoms can develop rather suddenly. These include:

- Increased thirst
- A frequent need to urinate
- Hunger
- A flu-like feeling, including weakness and fatigue

- Unexplained weight loss
- Blurred vision
- Irritability
- Slow healing of cuts and bruises
- Tingling or numbness in your hands or feet
- Red, swollen and tender gums
- Recurring infections of the gums, skin, vagina or bladder

Two classic symptoms that most people with diabetes experience are increased thirst and a frequent need to urinate. When the level of sugar in your blood is high, the kidneys can't reabsorb all of the filtered sugar. The circulating sugar carries water with it, which is drawn from your tissues. As a result, you're dehydrated and feel thirsty.

To replenish the fluids being drawn out, you're almost constantly drinking water and other beverages. This water-intensive filtering process leads to more frequent urination.

Diagnosis

Often, people are shocked to learn that they have diabetes because they didn't notice any symptoms. Many people with type 2 diabetes first learn they have diabetes when blood tests are done for another condition or as part of a routine physical examination. Type 1 diabetes tends to come on more suddenly, with noticeable signs and symptoms.

Sometimes, a doctor may test specifically for diabetes if he or she suspects, based on your symptoms and risk factors, that you have the disease. Individuals at high risk of developing diabetes should be tested beginning at age 30.

To determine if you have diabetes, your fasting blood sugar level will be measured. The amount of sugar in anyone's blood naturally fluctuates, but within a narrow range. Following an overnight fast, most people have blood sugar levels between 70 and 110 milligrams of glucose per deciliter of blood (mg/dL). This concentration range is considered normal.

Methods of measuring blood sugar include:

Finger-prick screening

Finger-prick screening tests are fast, easy and inexpensive. Many health fairs offer them for free.

A drop of blood is collected from a tiny prick in your fingertip and placed on a chemically treated strip that's inserted into a small machine that displays your blood sugar level. If the result is 126 mg/dL or above, see your doctor for a more formal diagnostic test.

Random blood sugar test

A random blood sugar test is part of routine blood work done without prior fasting during a physical examination, when blood is drawn for a variety of laboratory tests. If the results are above 200 mg/dL, your doctor may want to do a fasting blood sugar test another day.

Fasting blood sugar test

Your blood sugar level typically is highest after a meal and lowest after an overnight fast. The preferred way to test your blood sugar is after you've fasted overnight, or for at least 8 hours. Blood is drawn from a vein, and its glucose content is measured at a laboratory.

If your blood sugar measures 126 mg/dL or higher, your doctor may repeat the test. If your blood sugar is very high, a second test may not be necessary to reach a diagnosis. When a second test is ordered, if the results are again 126 mg/dL or higher, you'll likely receive a diagnosis of diabetes.

Glucose tolerance test

The glucose tolerance test is used less often today because other tests are less expensive and easier to administer. A glucose tolerance test involves drinking about 8 ounces of a sweet liquid following an overnight fast. Your blood sugar is measured before you drink the liquid and every hour for a 3-hour period afterward. If you have diabetes, this test will show that your

PREVENTION TIP

People with diabetes who take insulin or oral medications need to learn to recognize symptoms of low blood sugar (hypoglycemia) and know how to deal with them. Low blood sugar can occur any time or place. Take the following steps in case you have a low blood sugar reaction:

- Carry with you at all times a concentrated source of sugar, such as hard candy or glucose tablets. This type of sugar can lead to a predictable rise in blood sugar. Other types of candy can raise blood sugar excessively.
- If you take insulin, keep a glucagon emergency kit with or near you at all times. This kit includes glucagon and a syringe. The shot is easy to administer, and the medication starts to act in 5 minutes. This kit requires a prescription.
- Educate your family and friends about what to do if they notice that you're having a low blood sugar reaction. Be sure they know how to recognize and treat low blood sugar. Teach your children how to call 911 for emergency assistance if needed. Teach adult family members how to inject glucagon.
- Wear a medical alert necklace or bracelet or carry a card that identifies you as a person with diabetes. If you become confused or lose consciousness, your medical identification will make it easier for medical personnel to make a correct diagnosis and treat you.

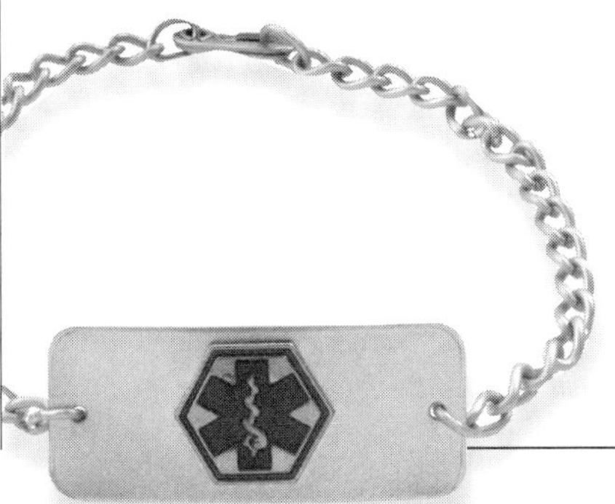

blood sugar rises higher than expected. Doctors sometimes use a modification of this test to check pregnant women for gestational diabetes.

Complications of Diabetes

Excessive sugar (glucose) in your blood threatens many major organs, including your heart, nerves, eyes and kidneys. You might not feel the effects right away, but you may eventually if you don't take steps to manage and control your disease.

Researchers continue to make progress in understanding what triggers complications of diabetes and how to manage or prevent them. If you keep your blood sugar level close to normal, you can dramatically reduce your risk of complications.

Short-term complications

Diabetes can produce both short- and long-term complications. Short-term complications are medical emergencies requiring immediate attention. These include low blood sugar (hypoglycemia), high blood sugar (diabetic hyperosmolar syndrome) and excessive blood acids (ketoacidosis).

Low blood sugar

Low blood sugar — a level below 60 milligrams of glucose per deciliter of blood (mg/dL) — results from too much insulin and too little sugar in your blood. Not enough glucose enters individual cells, which become starved for energy.

Sometimes, overtreatment of diabetes with medication can cause low blood sugar (hypoglycemia). This is most common among people taking insulin. It can also occur in people taking oral medications that enhance the release or action of insulin.

Your blood sugar level can drop for many reasons. Among people with diabetes, some common reasons include skipping a meal, exercising longer or more vigorously than usual or not adjusting your medication to accommodate changes in your blood sugar.

Signs and symptoms

Hypoglycemia symptoms vary from one person to another. Common early symptoms and signs include:

- Weakness
- Sweating, often a cold sweat
- Shakiness
- A fast heartbeat
- Visual disturbances, such as blurred vision
- Hunger
- Nervousness
- A tingling sensation in your hands and feet
- Irritability
- Nausea

If your blood sugar continues to drop, headache and difficulty walking may follow. In addition, you may behave unusually, appearing confused and sometimes stubborn or uncooperative.

As the condition worsens, you may seem intoxicated and feel drowsy and very confused. Your speech may be slurred. In extreme cases, unconsciousness and seizures may occur, particularly in children.

Treatment

Low blood sugar is a serious condition. But if it's recognized early, it can usually be treated easily.

When symptoms appear, stop all activity — bring the car to a halt, turn off the lawn mower, stop running — and eat or drink something that will raise your blood sugar level quickly. This might be hard candy (about five Life Savers), a regular (not sugar-free) soft drink, a half cup of fruit juice or glucose tablets, which are nonprescription sugar pills made especially for treating low blood sugar. Glucose is also sold in squeeze tubes, allowing you to squirt the contents into your mouth.

Your blood sugar level should rise within 10 or 15 minutes. If the signs and symptoms continue after 15 minutes, repeat the treatment. If they still don't go away, contact your doctor.

If you lose consciousness or are unable to swallow, placing food in the mouth is no longer safe. Blood sugar must be raised by injection. One option is injecting glucagon under your skin.

Glucagon is a fast-acting hormone that stimulates the release of sugar into your blood. Help your close friends and family members become familiar with this medication, including where you keep it and how to give you a shot of it in case of an emergency.

Another option is administering glucose in the form of dextrose directly into the bloodstream. This requires emergency medical personnel.

If you ever find someone unconscious, whether or not they have diabetes, call for emergency medical assistance.

High blood sugar

Sometimes, blood sugar can reach such a high level — 600 mg/dL or higher — that your cells can't absorb it all and sugar passes into your urine. This triggers a filtering process that draws tremendous amounts of fluid from your body and leads to dehydration.

Extremely high blood sugar (diabetic hyperosmolar syndrome) is most common in people with type 2 diabetes, especially those who don't monitor their blood sugar or are unaware they have diabetes. It can also occur in people with diabetes who are taking high-dose steroids or drugs that increase urination.

Older people with type 2 diabetes who also have another illness and who don't drink enough water may develop a very high level of sugar in the blood. High blood sugar may be brought on by an

Care of Your Feet

If you have diabetes, you're at increased risk of foot problems. When the network of nerves in your feet is damaged, you lose some of your ability to sense pain. You can cut your foot or develop a blister without realizing it.

Diabetes can also narrow your arteries, reducing blood flow to your feet. With less blood to nourish tissues, sores don't heal as well.

When you have diabetes, cuts, blisters, corns, calluses and other conditions that are nothing more than minor irritations to someone without diabetes can become serious medical problems. Infections and ulcers can result. In severe cases, amputation of the foot or leg may be required. Proper foot care can help you minimize this risk.

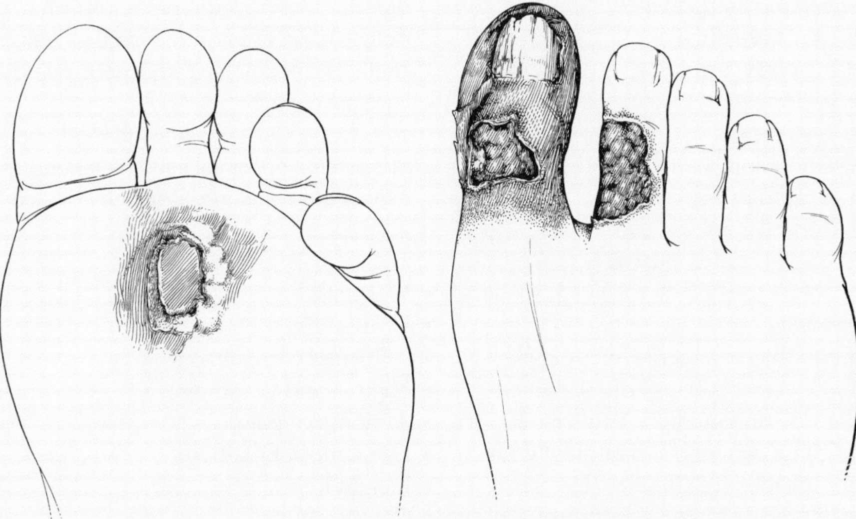

Over a period of years, diabetes can result in damage to nerves and blood vessels in your feet and other extremities. Minor wounds may lead to development of open sores (left). In some instances, the deterioration of blood vessels can severely limit blood flow, leading to gangrene (right).

Check your feet every day

Every day, examine your feet carefully, including the tops, bottoms, areas between the toes and toenails. Use a small mirror if you have difficulty seeing the bottoms of your feet.

Look for cuts and scrapes, cracks, calluses, bruises, corns, swelling, redness or other changes that may not be painful but could become more serious.

Keep your feet clean and dry

Wash your feet carefully every day, using lukewarm water and mild soap or a cleanser recommended by your doctor. To avoid burning your feet, test the water temperature with a thermometer — it should be no warmer than 90 F. Or test the water by touching a dampened washcloth to a sensitive area of your body, such as your face or wrist.

Dry your skin by blotting or patting it. Dry carefully between your toes to prevent fungal infection. Use a moisturizer regularly.

Wear clean, dry socks

Wear socks that pull (wick) sweat away from your skin. Avoid socks that are tight enough to reduce circulation or that cause your feet to sweat excessively.

Trim your toenails properly

Don't use scissors or rounded clippers on your toenails because they can cause injury to the nails and surrounding skin. Cut your toenails straight across and not too short. They should be even with the end of your toe. File rough edges so they won't cut the adjacent toe.

Use foot products cautiously

Don't use a file or scissors on calluses, corns or bunions, and don't use chemicals such as wart removers on your own. See your regular doctor or a podiatrist for treatment of warts, calluses and other problems.

Always wear shoes

Wear comfortable, safe shoes at all times to protect your feet from injury. Around the house, wear sturdy slippers. Avoid tight shoes.

Exercise carefully

Exercise increases circulation and helps maintain the health of your feet. In selecting your physical activities, however, consider the risk of injury to your feet and avoid extremes of hot and cold. When your feet or legs become tired, sit down and elevate them for a few minutes.

See your doctor if a problem develops

Consult your doctor promptly if you notice any areas of soreness or if a wound isn't healing, appears to be getting bigger or looks as if it may be infected. Your doctor also should inspect your feet at your regularly scheduled visits. He or she may recommend that you see a podiatrist, a doctor who specializes in foot care.

infection, illness, stress or drinking excessive amounts of alcohol.

Signs and symptoms
- Excessive thirst
- Increased urination
- Weakness
- Leg cramps
- Confusion
- A rapid pulse
- Convulsions
- Loss of consciousness

Treatment
If your blood sugar level is persistently above 300 mg/dL, seek medical care immediately. You'll likely be given emergency treatment with intravenous (IV) fluids to restore water to your tissues and short-acting insulin to help your cells absorb sugar. Without prompt treatment, the condition can be fatal.

Increased blood acids
Increased blood acids (diabetic ketoacidosis) is an acute complication of diabetes. It occurs when your muscle cells become so starved for energy that your body takes emergency measures and breaks down fat, a process that forms acids known as ketones. Increased amounts of ketones in your blood make it more acidic.

Diabetic ketoacidosis is most common among people with type 1 diabetes and usually occurs because of insufficient insulin. This can happen when you miss or skip some of your insulin shots, are under extreme stress or have an acute illness or injury.

Signs and symptoms
Many of the signs and symptoms of diabetic ketoacidosis can be confused with those of the flu. These include:
- Increased urination and an unquenchable thirst that develops over several hours, which occurs more quickly in a child
- Loss of appetite
- A sweet, fruity smell on your breath that may be confused with the smell of alcohol
- Weakness
- Drowsiness
- A flushed complexion
- Nausea and vomiting
- Abdominal pain
- Deep, rapid breathing
- Weight loss
- Confusion

At an advanced stage, you may lose consciousness.

Treatment
Diabetic ketoacidosis demands immediate treatment because death can result. If you feel sick, check your urine for ketones. Also check for ketones if you're feeling especially stressed or whenever your blood sugar is persistently above 240 mg/dL. You can buy a ketone test kit at a drugstore or pharmacy and do the test at home. If the test results indicate a high ketone level, call your doctor.

Ketoacidosis requires emergency medical treatment, which involves replenishing lost fluids through intravenous (IV) lines. Insulin can be combined with IV fluids.

Gradually, your blood sugar level is brought down to normal. Your blood sugar and fluid status will be closely monitored. With prompt treatment, recovery from ketoacidosis is usually rapid and complete.

Long-term complications

Long-term (chronic) effects of diabetes develop slowly and generally with few early symptoms. Long-term complications involve damage to large and small blood vessels, resulting in a variety of health problems. Studies show that tight blood sugar control — keeping your blood sugar within a normal or near-normal range — can dramatically reduce your risk of long-term complications.

Nerve damage
Nerve damage (neuropathy) is a common long-term complication of diabetes. An intricate network of nerves runs throughout your body, connecting your brain to your muscles, skin and other organs. High blood sugar levels can damage these delicate nerves, affecting their ability to send messages.

Your feet and legs, and sometimes your hands and arms, might tingle, burn or feel numb, a condition called peripheral neuropathy. Over time you may lose all sense of feeling in the affected areas, leaving you more vulnerable to injury and infection.

Diabetes can also reduce blood flow to your feet. This, along with nerve damage, can lead to development of an open sore (ulcer) and possibly to gangrene. Practice good foot care to help avoid developing an infection.

Damage to nerves that control your muscles may leave you with an unsteady gait. Damage to nerves that control autonomic functions can increase your heart rate and perspiration. Such damage can also lead to problems with bladder control and diarrhea. In men it can lead to impotence.

An uncommon nerve-related problem is Charcot's joint. In this condition, the small bones of the arch of your foot gradually disintegrate, and your feet become

PREVENTION TIP

The American Diabetes Association recommends that most people over age 30 who have diabetes take an aspirin every day. Studies show that daily aspirin use can reduce their risk of heart attack by up to 60 percent. The recommended dose is one baby or adult tablet (81 to 325 milligrams) a day.

It's best to take aspirin with food and to take coated tablets that dissolve in your small intestine instead of your stomach. Regular aspirin use can cause stomach irritation, bleeding or an ulcer.

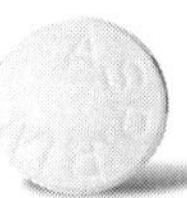

swollen, deformed and very flat. Although this condition causes little pain, it can be crippling.

Kidney disease

Kidney disease eventually affects more than 30 percent of people with type 1 diabetes and 10 percent of those with type 2. Either type of diabetes can impair your kidneys' ability to filter wastes from your body. The longer you have diabetes, the greater your risk of kidney damage.

In its early stages, kidney disease produces few symptoms. A rise in blood pressure can be one of the first signs. Generally, signs and symptoms emerge only after extensive damage. These may include swelling of the ankles, feet and hands, shortness of breath, confusion or difficulty concentrating, poor appetite, nausea, fatigue and itchy and dry skin.

If you have diabetes, your doctor will likely periodically examine your urine for protein to check for kidney damage. Keeping your blood sugar levels and blood pressure under control will prevent or reduce kidney damage.

Angiotensin-converting enzyme (ACE) inhibitors — medications used to treat cardiovascular problems — can help slow progression of diabetic kidney damage.

Eye disease

Diabetic eye disease includes diabetic retinopathy (see page 657). Tiny blood vessels at the back of your eye (retina) can be damaged by high blood sugar, causing a range of effects, from mild vision problems to blindness.

Nearly everyone with type 1 diabetes and more than 6 of 10 people with type 2 diabetes develop some form of eye damage by the time they've had the disease for 20 years. If you have diabetes, you're also at increased risk of developing cataracts (see page 648) and glaucoma (see page 644).

Early eye disease often produces no symptoms until it's well advanced. For this reason, schedule yearly eye examinations with an eye specialist to identify and treat problems before permanent damage occurs.

Cardiovascular disease

Diabetes dramatically increases your risk of developing one of many cardiovascular problems, including chest pain (angina), heart attack, stroke, high blood pressure and narrowing of your arteries (atherosclerosis).

Diabetes can damage your major arteries as well as your body's small blood vessels. The damage makes it easier for fatty deposits (plaques) to form in the arteries, a condition called atherosclerosis. Atherosclerosis that develops in blood vessels that supply oxygen and nutrients to the heart is called coronary artery disease.

Diabetes also increases pressure in your arteries and reduces blood circulation. High blood pressure can damage blood vessels, tissues and organs. People with diabetes are at particular risk of silent heart attacks, which don't cause typical symptoms.

You can reduce your risk of heart and blood vessel disease by not smoking, controlling high blood pressure, limiting fat and calories in your diet, getting more exercise, and losing weight if you're overweight.

To decrease the risk of heart and blood vessel disease and kidney disease, people with diabetes should have blood pressure readings of no higher than 130/80 millimeters of mercury (mm Hg). Your doctor may prescribe medications to help you control abnormal levels of blood fats.

Occasionally, people with diabetes get pain in their calves (claudication) while walking or climbing stairs. The pain eases when the activity is stopped. See your doctor if you experience such discomfort. It may be a sign of circulatory problems in the vessels that supply blood to your legs.

Increased risk of infection

High blood sugar impairs the ability of your immune system cells to fight off invading germs and bacteria, putting you at higher risk of infection. High blood sugar can also damage nerves that might alert you to a potential infection. The mouth, gums, lungs, skin, feet, bladder and genital area are common infection sites.

Fever is common with many infections. Other signs and symptoms vary depending on the location of the infection. If your gums are infected, you may experience red, bleeding gums. A bladder infection typically causes frequent urination and a burning sensation while urinating. A vaginal infection commonly causes discharge and itching.

Self-care

If you have diabetes, you can do a great deal to remain healthy and reduce your risk of developing complications of the disease. In addition to keeping your blood sugar in control and seeing your doctor regularly to monitor your diabetes, take the following self-care measures:

- Have a yearly physical in addition to your regular checkups to monitor your diabetes.
- Get a yearly eye exam.
- See your dentist regularly.
- Keep up-to-date on your vaccinations, especially those for the flu (influenza) and pneumonia.
- If you're a smoker, quit. Smoking is especially hazardous for people with diabetes and significantly adds to their risk of heart disease and stroke.
- Take proper care of your feet.
- Monitor your blood pressure and take steps to control high blood pressure through diet, exercise and medications, if needed. Your goal is 130/80 mm Hg or less.
- Manage stress. Stress and depression can make it more difficult to take care of yourself and your diabetes. Excessive or prolonged

stress may also increase production of hormones that block the effects of insulin, causing your blood sugar to rise. Stress relaxation techniques or counseling may be helpful.

Treating Diabetes

When it comes to managing diabetes, your health, to a great extent, is in your hands. A number of health care professionals may be involved in your medical care, yet your role is crucial.

The single most important thing that you can do to feel your best and prevent complications is to control your blood sugar level on a daily basis. Only you can do that. The keys to managing diabetes are:

- Monitoring your blood sugar
- Eating a healthy diet
- Staying active
- Maintaining a healthy weight
- Using medications appropriately, as prescribed
- Having regular checkups

Blood sugar monitoring

To control your blood sugar, you need to keep track of your blood sugar level. You want it to stay within a desirable range that's not too high or too low. Your doctor will help you determine your blood sugar goals.

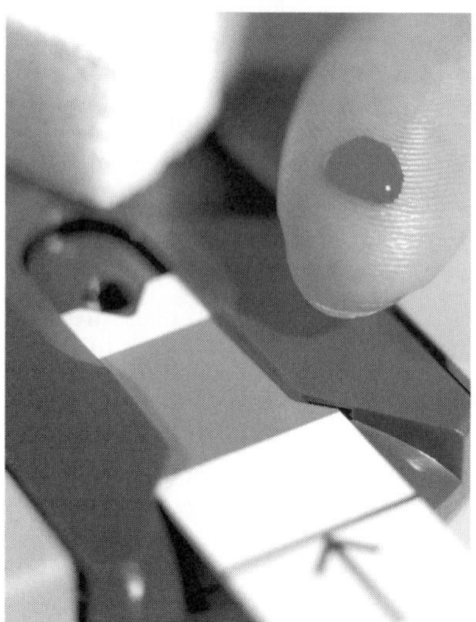

Testing your blood sugar on a regular basis is the only way to know whether you're achieving those goals and if your treatment is working. If you take insulin, test your blood sugar frequently. Testing is normally done before meals and at bedtime, times when glucose levels should be relatively normal. If you don't take insulin, you may not need to check your blood sugar as often.

Testing your blood sugar is a quick and easy process that usually takes only a couple of minutes. The tools include:

- *A lancet.* A small needle is used to prick the skin on a finger to draw a drop of blood. Spring-loaded lancets generally are less painful.
- *A test strip.* A drop of blood is placed on a chemically treated strip that's inserted into a blood glucose monitor.
- *A blood glucose monitor.* This is a small device that measures and displays glucose levels. Monitors come in many forms.

After your blood test, record the results in a logbook. Note the date and time of testing, test results, type and dosage of medication you're taking, any episodes of low blood sugar and any circumstances that may have affected the levels, such as unusual stress or excitement, illness, travel or an especially large meal. This information can help you and your doctor track how various factors affect your blood sugar.

Diet

Healthy eating is a key part of managing diabetes. However, that doesn't mean that you have to start buying specialized foods or follow a highly detailed and boring diet plan. For most people with diabetes, a healthy diet simply translates into variety and moderation. That means eating more of certain foods, such as fruits, vegetables and grains, which are high in nutrients and low in fat and calories — and less of others, such as animal products and sweets. It's the same eating plan recommended for all Americans.

? Question and Answer

What's the ideal blood sugar level?

Ideally, everyone should aim to keep his or her blood sugar in the normal range of 70 to 110 milligrams of glucose per deciliter of blood (mg/dL). However, that's not realistic for many people with diabetes. Instead, your goal may be to achieve near-normal levels, often referred to as target ranges.

Target ranges differ depending on a variety of factors, including your age and overall health. Among younger adults who don't have complications, a typical target range before meals is 80 to 120 mg/dL, and after meals, below 180 mg/dL. Others may have a different target range. For older adults with complications, the goal before meals might be 100 to 140 mg/dL, and after meals, less than 200 mg/dL.

Healthy eating basics

Depending on your blood sugar level, whether you need to lose weight and if you have other health problems, you need to tailor your diet to your own personal needs. But even though the details may differ, the basics remain the same. Each day eat a variety of foods to achieve the right balance of three key nutrients — carbohydrates, protein and fat.

- *Carbohydrates.* Carbohydrates include starches (bread, cereal, rice, pasta, beans and certain vegetables, such as corn, potatoes and squash), fruits, milk products and nonstarchy vegetables.

Carbohydrates: Sugar and Starch

Carbohydrates are classified as either simple carbohydrates (sugar) or complex carbohydrates (starch). During digestion, your body breaks down complex carbohydrates into simple sugars. Sweets, milk, fruit and some vegetables contain simple sugars. Grain products and certain vegetables contain complex carbohydrates.

It's best to eat a mixture of complex and simple carbohydrates. The advantage of complex carbohydrates is that it takes your body longer to break them down into sugar. This means that sugar enters your bloodstream at a steadier rate. Include in your carbohydrate mix foods that are high in fiber. The more fiber a food contains, the more slowly it's digested and the more slowly your blood sugar (glucose) level rises.

For years, people with diabetes were told to avoid candy, cookies and other sugary foods because it was assumed that they would raise blood sugar faster and higher than complex carbohydrates would. But studies have shown that this isn't true. All carbohydrates, including table sugar, affect blood glucose about the same way. Sweets don't produce an exaggerated rise in blood sugar, provided they're eaten with your meal and counted as a carbohydrate source.

The most important thing about carbohydrates is not so much what type you eat but how much. If you eat more carbohydrates than usual, you may not have enough insulin available to transport the excess sugar into your cells, causing an increase in your blood sugar level. One way you can help control your blood sugar is by eating the same amount of carbohydrates at similar times each day.

Although sugar isn't forbidden, it's still best to limit sweets. Candy, soda pop, cookies and other sugary foods have little nutritional value. They're empty calories that can easily lead to weight gain.

Consume about half your daily calories from carbohydrates.

- *Protein.* Foods high in protein include meat, poultry, eggs, cheese, fish, legumes and peanut butter. Most people should consume 10 percent to 20 percent of their daily calories from protein, or about two to three servings a day.

  When planning your meals, select proteins that are lower in fat, such as plant products, fish, poultry without skin, lean meats and low-fat or fat-free cheese. Limit or avoid fatty meats, eggs and high-fat cheeses.
- *Fats.* Fats are found in meat, poultry, fish, cheese, butter, margarine, oils, salad dressing, whole milk and many desserts and snack foods. Limit total fat consumption to 30 percent or less of your daily calories and saturated fat to less than 10 percent of your daily calories.

  Saturated fat, which is found in animal products such as meat, cream and butter, raises blood cholesterol, and high blood cholesterol is a risk factor for heart disease. If you need to lose weight or have high cholesterol, consuming less than 7 percent of your calories from saturated fat is healthier.

Planning meals

The first step in meal planning is to establish a routine of eating meals and snacks at regular times every day. Some people can keep their blood sugar in good control simply by eating three regular meals a day and avoiding too many sweets. Others need to follow a more deliberate plan, eating only the recommended number of servings from each food group, based on their individual calorie needs.

You may find it helpful to talk with a registered dietitian about meal planning. A dietitian can provide you with a variety of tools to help you establish an eating plan that fits your health goals and concerns, food tastes, family or cultural traditions and lifestyle.

Whether or not you work with a dietitian, aim for consistency in your eating habits. Every day try to eat about the same amount at the same time, with the same proportion of carbohydrates, protein and fats. This can help keep your blood sugar at a consistent level.

Some people use tools such as exchange lists or carbohydrate counting. Exchange lists are part of a system of grouping foods by food group and serving size. Carbohydrate counting is a way to calculate meal-related insulin doses based on the carbohydrate content of meals. Talk to your doctor or dietitian if you're interested in learning about these tools.

Physical activity

Being physically active on a regular basis is another key element in treating diabetes. It takes special effort to incorporate physical activity into a daily routine — but physical activity brings with it a bounty of health benefits. Even a moderate amount of exercise can improve control of diabetes.

Improves blood sugar control

As muscles contract and relax during exercise, they use sugar for energy. To meet this energy need, sugar is removed from your blood during and after exercise. This lowers your blood sugar level. In addition, exercise reduces blood sugar by increasing your sensitivity to insulin: your body requires less insulin to escort sugar into your cells.

Along with a healthy eating plan, regular exercise can reduce your need for medication that lowers your blood sugar level. Some people manage their diabetes through just diet and exercise.

Reduces risk of heart disease
Exercise is good for your heart and blood vessels. It improves the flow of blood through small blood vessels and increases your heart's pumping efficiency.

In combination with a healthy diet, exercise helps lower high blood pressure and it improves blood cholesterol levels.

Controls your weight
Physical activity helps you lose weight and maintain a healthy weight. Regular exercise takes off pounds by burning calories and increasing your metabolism. Exercise can also reduce resistance to insulin that commonly occurs from being overweight.

Your doctor can help you establish guidelines for how frequently and how vigorously you should exercise. Chapter 4, "Keeping Active," discusses how to develop a fitness program to meet your needs.

Because physical activity usually lowers your blood sugar level, you want to be alert to symptoms of low blood sugar when exercising (see page 1024). Make sure your blood sugar isn't too low or too high before you start. If you're going to be active for a long period, especially if you take insulin, take a break and check your blood sugar while you're exercising.

Weight control

Being overweight is by far the greatest risk factor for type 2 diabetes — about 90 percent of people with newly diagnosed type 2 diabetes are overweight. By contrast, most people with type 1 are at or below their ideal weight.

Why is weight so important? Fat alters how your cells respond to insulin. It causes them to become more resistant to insulin's effects, reducing the amount of sugar the hormone is able to transport from your blood to your cells.

You can reverse this process by losing weight. As you take off pounds, your cells become more responsive to insulin. For some people with type 2 diabetes, losing weight is all that's necessary to control their diabetes and return their blood sugar to normal.

The amount of weight loss doesn't have to be extreme to result in health benefits. A modest loss of 10 to 20 pounds, or 5 percent to 10 percent of your weight, can lower your blood sugar level, as well as reduce your blood pressure and blood cholesterol levels.

Exercise and Diabetes

To avoid problems with low or high blood sugar during or after physical activity, especially if you take insulin, follow these guidelines:

- Check your blood sugar approximately 30 minutes before you exercise and then again right before you start. This will help you determine if your blood sugar level is stable, rising or dropping. If your blood sugar level is under 100 mg/dL, eat a carbohydrate-containing snack to avoid having low blood sugar while you exercise. If your blood sugar level is more than 300 mg/dL, don't exercise. Exercise can raise your blood sugar further.
- If you have type 1 diabetes and your blood sugar level before exercising is 250 mg/dL or higher, test your urine for ketones (see page 1026). If the result indicates a moderate or high ketone level, don't exercise.
- Check your blood sugar during and after exercise. This is especially important when you're trying a new activity or sport or if you're increasing the intensity or duration of your activity. If you exercise for more than an hour, especially if you have type 1 diabetes, stop and test your blood sugar every 30 minutes. If it starts to fall, have a snack. Until you have a good idea of how your body reacts to exercise, check your blood sugar frequently after your activity. Hypoglycemia can occur hours after exercise.
- If you start to experience symptoms of low blood sugar while exercising, stop immediately and — if possible — test your blood sugar. If you have symptoms, treat yourself for low blood sugar even if you don't have your testing equipment with you. If your test is low, eat something with sugar.
- If you take insulin, adjust your dose for planned exercise. Avoid exercise within 3 hours after injecting short-acting insulin due to the potential risk of low blood sugar. Ask your doctor when would be the best time to exercise and follow the precautions listed above.
- People with type 1 diabetes who exercise for more than an hour or do strenuous activities may benefit from eating a snack before or while exercising. For most people with type 2 diabetes, a snack before exercise generally isn't necessary.

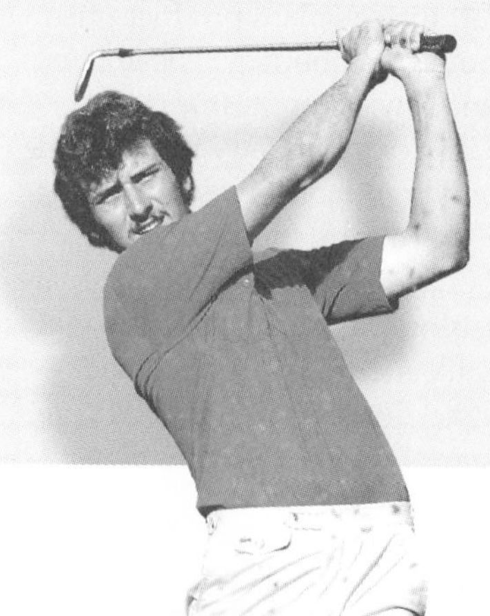

As many who've tried to lose weight know, it can be very difficult. But with a positive attitude and the right advice, it's a challenge that you can meet. To determine if you're overweight and to learn about weight management strategies, see Chapter 3, "Controlling Your Weight."

Medication

Depending on the type and severity of your diabetes, your doctor may prescribe an oral medication or insulin. All people with type 1 diabetes need to take insulin. Most people with type 2 diabetes eventually need to take a medication that lowers blood sugar — either insulin or an oral medication.

Insulin

Insulin is administered by injection with a syringe or insulin pen, or through constant infusion with an insulin pump. Insulin isn't available in pill form because its chemical structure is destroyed during digestion, making the hormone ineffective by the time it gets to your bloodstream.

Many types of insulin are available. They differ in the time it takes for them to begin working and in their duration. Short-acting insulin works quickly but only for a short time. Intermediate-acting insulin starts working later but lasts longer. Long-acting insulin takes several hours to work, but its peak action — the time when it has the greatest effect — lasts longer than other forms of insulin.

The type and dosage of insulin you take depend on your specific needs. Some people take more than one type of insulin. For example, some people mix short-acting and intermediate-acting insulin.

For many people, the best blood sugar control is achieved by taking one dose of long-acting insulin a day along with an injection of short-acting insulin before each meal. Your doctor will help you decide which approach best suits your needs.

Injections

The most common way to receive insulin is by using a syringe or an insulin pen. These methods deliver insulin underneath the skin, where it's absorbed into the bloodstream.

Insulin pens offer a convenient, more accurate and discreet means of taking insulin. The device looks like a pen with a cartridge, but the cartridge is filled with insulin rather than ink. A fine-point needle, much like the one on a syringe, is on the tip of the pen. You turn a dial on the pen to select the desired dose, insert the needle under your skin and click down on a button to deliver the insulin under the skin.

Insulin jet injectors are another way to deliver insulin. They use high-pressure air to send a fine spray of insulin under your skin. This can be a painful way to take insulin, and it's not as accurate as other methods. Jet injectors may be an option for people who can't use needles.

PREVENTION TIP

Occasionally — especially when you first use insulin — you may notice redness and slight swelling at the injection site. If the skin irritation lasts more than 2 to 3 weeks or causes discomfort, talk to your doctor. To minimize pain from injections:

- Make sure the insulin is at room temperature.
- Be sure no air bubbles are in the syringe.
- Relax your muscles in the area of the injection.
- Penetrate the skin quickly with the needle.
- Don't change the direction of the needle during the injection.

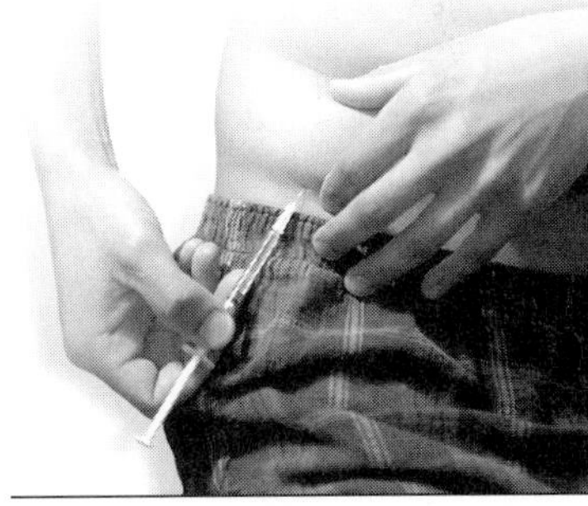

Pumps

An insulin pump is a small device filled with insulin that you wear outside your body. A small, flexible tube connects the insulin supply to a catheter inserted under the skin of

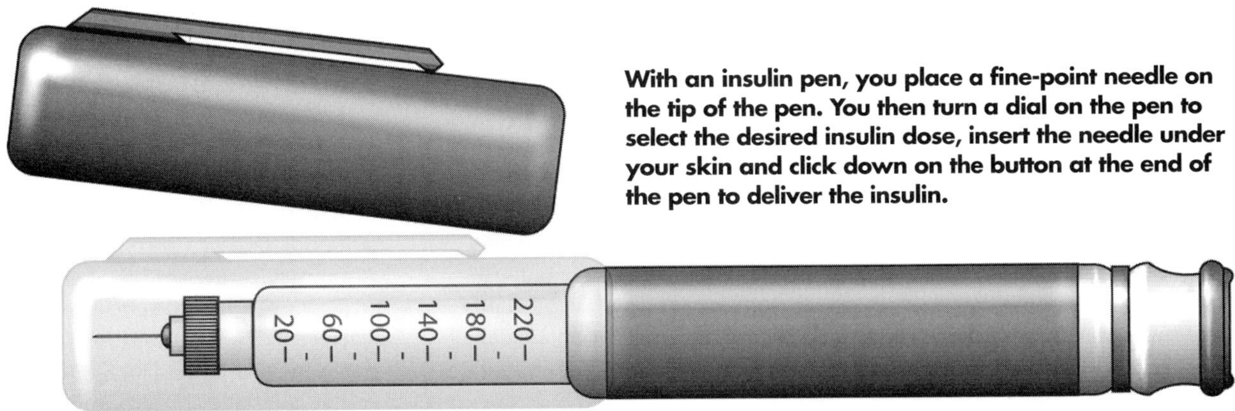

With an insulin pen, you place a fine-point needle on the tip of the pen. You then turn a dial on the pen to select the desired insulin dose, insert the needle under your skin and click down on the button at the end of the pen to deliver the insulin.

your abdomen. The pump dispenses the desired amount of insulin through the catheter and into your body, based on the information programmed into its microprocessor.

The main advantages of an insulin pump are flexibility and a better match of insulin needs and delivery. People who use a pump often are able to achieve normal or near-normal blood sugar levels, and say it provides them with a more flexible lifestyle. Before you can use an insulin pump, you must go through a short training program on how to use it and be committed to obtaining frequent blood sugar measurements throughout the day.

It's essential to have a clear understanding of the relationship between insulin, food and activity so that you can program the pump to accommodate changing situations. Results depend on the person controlling the pump.

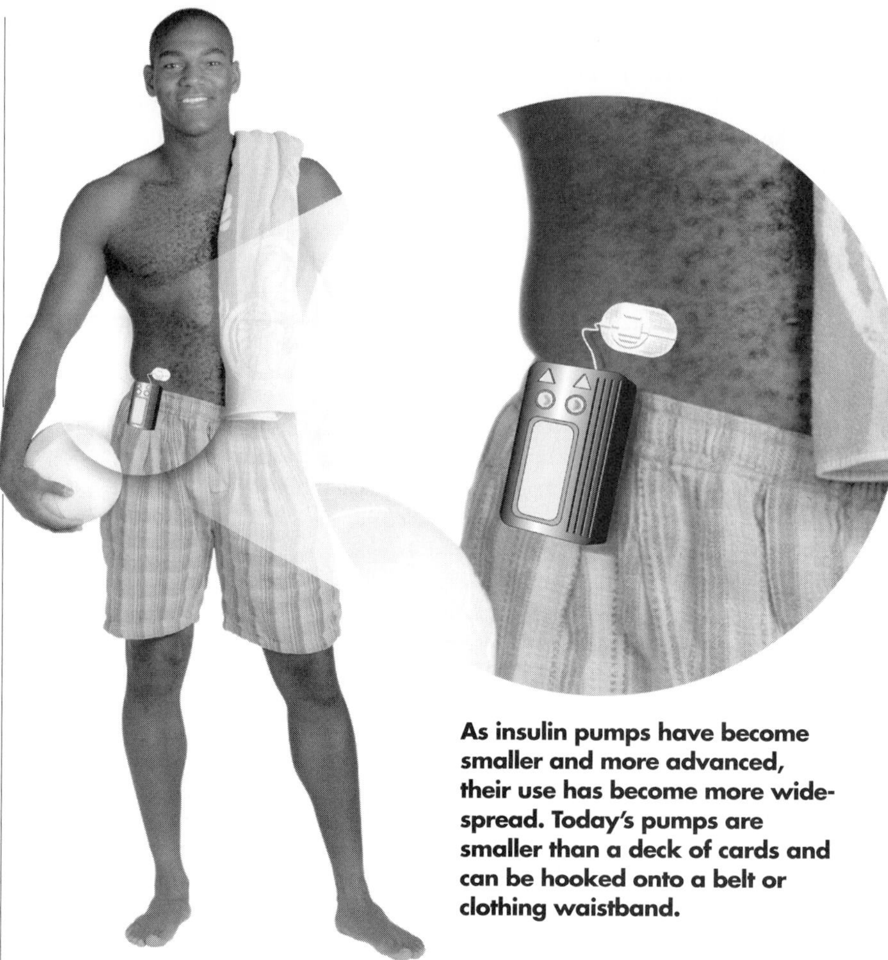

As insulin pumps have become smaller and more advanced, their use has become more widespread. Today's pumps are smaller than a deck of cards and can be hooked onto a belt or clothing waistband.

Oral medications

A variety of oral medications are available for treating type 2 diabetes. In addition to insulin, five types of oral medications are available. Each has its own method for lowering blood sugar.

To effectively control your blood sugar, you may need a combination of more than one oral medication or an oral medication plus insulin. Your doctor can determine if you need medication and which type. Let your doctor know if you're taking other medications or using alcohol while taking diabetes drugs so that he or she can alert you to the possibility of drug interactions.

Sulfonylureas

Sulfonylureas have been used for decades. They work by stimulating the pancreas to produce more insulin. To benefit from the medication, your pancreas must be able to produce some insulin on its own.

Sulfonylureas include:

- Chlorpropamide (Diabinese)
- Glimepiride (Amaryl)
- Glipizide (Glucotrol)
- Glyburide (DiaBeta, Glynase PresTab, Micronase)
- Tolazamide (Ronase, Tolinase)
- Tolbutamide (Orinase)

Possible side effects of these medications include low blood sugar, especially during the first 4 months of therapy. If you have impaired liver or kidney function, your doctor may not prescribe a sulfonylurea drug. Newer versions of sulfonylureas may be used safely in people with kidney impairment.

Meglitinides

Meglitinides cause a rapid but short-term release of insulin by your pancreas. These medications are taken with meals and begin working shortly thereafter, when your blood sugar level is highest. Repaglinide (Prandin) is presently the only such medication available. Low blood sugar is a possible side effect.

Biguanides

Biguanides improve your body's response to insulin by decreasing insulin resistance. They enhance the ability of tissues to take up glucose and reduce the amount of glucose released by the liver.

Biguanides are associated with less weight gain than other diabetes medications, and generally are prescribed to people with type 2 diabetes who are overweight. Metformin (Glucophage) is the only such medication available.

Possible side effects include an unpleasant metallic taste in your mouth, loss of appetite, nausea or vomiting, abdominal bloating, discomfort or pain, gas or diarrhea and a rash. When combined with another diabetes medication, metformin may cause low blood sugar. A rare but serious side effect is lactic acidosis due to a buildup of lactic acid in your body. This is more likely if you have kidney disease or severe heart disease, if you drink alcohol daily or excessively, or if you take the medication cimetidine (Tagamet). People with impaired kidney function generally shouldn't take metformin.

Alpha-glucosidase inhibitors

Alpha-glucosidase inhibitors delay digestion of carbohydrates, slowing the rise in blood sugar after eating. These drugs are taken with each meal and typically are prescribed if your blood sugar reaches its highest levels right after eating. Alpha-glucosidase inhibitors include the medications acarbose (Precose) and miglitol (Glyset).

Possible side effects include abdominal bloating or discomfort, gas and diarrhea. When taken with another diabetes medication, risk of low blood sugar is increased.

People with certain medical conditions — including irritable bowel syndrome, ulcerative colitis and Crohn's disease — or a chronic malabsorption disorder such as celiac disease shouldn't take these drugs.

Thiazolidinediones

Thiazolidinediones reduce resistance to insulin. They're generally best absorbed when taken with a meal. They include the medications pioglitazone (Actos) and rosiglitazone (Avandia).

Possible side effects include swelling, weight gain and fatigue. A rare but serious side effect is liver injury. Therefore, it's important to have your liver checked through blood tests every 2 months during the first year of treatment and to be aware of the signs and symptoms of liver damage.

If you're taking birth control pills, thiazolidinediones may make them less effective. In addition, you shouldn't take thiazolidinediones if you have congestive heart failure.

Transplantation

Medication and lifestyle changes can effectively control diabetes, but a common question remains: What about a cure?

Presently, there is no cure for diabetes. Researchers continue to explore therapies that they hope will one day bring about a cure. One area of study that receives a lot of attention is transplantation. Since the late 1970s, doctors have performed pancreas transplants to halt or reverse complications of diabetes, and the procedure has met with some success. Researchers are also experimenting with transplanting islet cells — the cells in the pancreas that produce insulin.

Pancreas transplantation

In the United States, more than 900 pancreas transplants are done each year, usually in conjunction with or following a kidney transplant. Kidney failure is one of the most common complications of diabetes. A kidney transplant can restore a number of crucial functions. Receiving a new pancreas at the same time doesn't jeopardize — and may actually improve — kidney survival. Unlike kidney transplants, in which a living person donates a kidney, a pancreas used for transplantation usually comes from a person who has just died.

After a successful pancreas transplant, many people with diabetes no longer need to use insulin or measure their blood sugar as frequently. They're no longer at risk of the dangers presented by widely fluctuating blood sugar levels.

However, transplantation isn't always successful. In addition to the risks inherent in any major surgery, the body can reject the new organ days or years after the transplant.

Because the immune system treats the new organ as a foreign invader and tries to destroy it, transplant recipients generally need to take immunosuppressant medications the rest of their life to prevent organ rejection. Such medications carry significant health risks.

Islet cell transplantation

A human pancreas contains about 1 million islets, which make up about 2 percent of the gland. Beta cells within these small islets produce insulin. In people with type 1 diabetes, their immune system has attacked and destroyed their islet cells, so their pancreas is unable to produce insulin.

Researchers have studied different methods of transplanting islet cells. Although the procedure has been fraught with problems, recent studies have shown promise. Improved techniques and new immunosuppressant medications are leading to more successful outcomes.

One of the main advantages of islet cell transplantation is that it's less risky than pancreas transplantation. Because it's still considered experimental, however, the procedure isn't covered by medical insurance. Additional studies are underway to learn more about the long-term effects of islet cell transplantation and complications from immunosuppressant medications.

Regular checkups

Another important part of diabetes treatment is staying in regular contact with your health care team and making sure that you receive appropriate tests to evaluate how well you're controlling your blood sugar. Regular checkups give your doctor an opportunity to look for early evidence of diabetes complications.

Many potential complications show up in simple blood and urine tests and examinations performed in your doctor's office. The checkups also give you a chance to review your successes and difficulties in meeting your blood sugar goals.

How often you see your doctor and other health care professionals depends on what's happening with your health. In general, if you're feeling good and keeping your blood sugar within the range that you and your doctor have agreed on, you probably need to see your doctor at least once every 3 months.

If you're having trouble keeping your blood sugar levels in the target range or you're changing medication, you may need to contact a member of your health care team weekly or even more often.

During a checkup, you may receive one or more of these tests:

Glycated hemoglobin test

A glycated hemoglobin test measures hemoglobin A-1C, which indicates how well you've controlled your blood sugar over the past 2 to 3 months. It can alert you to potential problems. If you take insulin, you'll probably have this test three or four times a year. If you have type 2 diabetes and your blood sugar is under good control, you may not need the test that often.

Lipids test

A lipids test measures the level of fats (lipids) in your blood. After a meal, your body digests fat in the food you eat and releases it into your bloodstream in two forms: cholesterol and triglycerides.

People with diabetes should have this test at least once a year. A rising level of certain blood fats can alert your doctor to an increased risk of blood vessel damage. You may need to take medication to lower your cholesterol or triglyceride levels.

Serum creatinine test

The serum creatinine test is a blood test that can warn of kidney problems. It measures the level of creatinine in your blood. Creatinine is a chemical waste product that's produced when you use your muscles.

If the kidneys aren't functioning properly, they aren't able to remove as much creatinine from your blood. People with diabetes should have this test at least once a year.

Urine microalbumin test

A urine microalbumin test assesses the health of your kidneys. When your kidneys are functioning normally, they filter out blood waste products pumped through them. The waste is excreted in your urine, and protein and other helpful substances remain in the bloodstream.

When your kidneys become damaged, waste products remain in your blood, and protein (albumin) leaks into your urine. A urine microalbumin test screens for protein leakage into your urine. You should have the test every year if you have type 2 diabetes or if you've had type 1 diabetes for more than 5 years and you're past puberty.

Other Pancreatic Disorders

Diabetes is the most common disorder of the pancreas. Less commonly, the organ may become inflamed (pancreatitis) or develop tumors that may be noncancerous (benign) or cancerous (malignant). Because the pancreas produces digestive enzymes as well as hormones, pancreatic disorders can cause both digestive and metabolism-related symptoms.

Islet cell tumors

Rarely, tumors may arise from islet cells in the pancreas that secrete the hormones insulin and glucagon. These tumors often release excessive amounts of the hormones, resulting in serious metabolic effects.

Types

There are different types of islet cell tumors, each named after the hormone that it produces.

Insulinoma

An islet cell tumor that produces insulin is called an insulinoma. It causes periods of low blood sugar (hypoglycemia). Signs and symptoms may include episodes of weakness, sweating, a fast heartbeat and confusion. They're relieved by eating food.

Symptoms tend to develop gradually over several months to a year. A diagnosis is usually made when your blood tests, obtained during a fast, show very low blood sugar associated with a high insulin level. This fasting test is generally performed in a hospital setting. If the results are positive, the insulinoma is located with imaging tests and then surgically removed.

Gastrinoma

A second type of hormone-producing tumor is a gastrinoma. Although most gastrinomas develop in the upper portion of your small intestine (duodenum), they also may occur in the pancreas. Gastrin is a hormone that stimulates the stomach to secrete acid and digestive juices. A tumor that overproduces gastrin will cause severe ulcer symptoms that respond poorly to standard ulcer treatments.

Signs and symptoms associated with a gastrinoma include watery diarrhea and stomach pain that's relieved temporarily by food and antacids but grows more severe over weeks or months. Generally, gastrinoma is diagnosed when blood tests show excessive gastrin. The condition associated with this type of tumor is called Zollinger-Ellison syndrome.

Glucagonoma

A third type of tumor that arises in the pancreas secretes glucagon and is called a glucagonoma. Signs and symptoms associated with a glucagonoma include a rash on various areas of the body, a sore tongue, weight loss and an elevated blood sugar level.

A rash is important in diagnosing glucagonoma. Your doctor may conduct blood tests to determine if your blood sugar (glucose) concentration is abnormally high.

Others
Other hormone-producing tumors are extremely rare. They have a wide range of manifestations, including watery diarrhea — even while fasting — weight loss and a low blood potassium level. If you experience severe watery diarrhea accompanied by fatigue and weight loss over a period of several weeks, your doctor may want to do stool, blood and radiologic tests to rule out those rare conditions.

Treatment
Like other tumors, pancreatic tumors often can be treated successfully if diagnosed promptly. Surgical removal of the affected tissues is usually the key component of treatment. Some of these tumors may be cancerous (malignant).

Pancreatic cancer

Although cancer of the pancreas accounts for only about 2 percent of all cancers in the United States, it's the fourth leading cause of cancer death. The reason it's so deadly is that the cancer typically produces no symptoms until it's advanced and incurable. Because the pancreas is located deep in your abdomen behind other organs, your doctor usually can't detect a lump by feeling the area.

The cancer may grow undetected for years and in later stages may affect normal metabolism. For more information on pancreatic cancer, including risk factors and treatment, see page 902.

Pancreatitis

Inflammation of the pancreas (pancreatitis) disrupts the normal functions of the organ. Pancreatitis can result in a variety of signs and symptoms, including abdominal pain, nausea, bloating and weight loss.

The condition can occur for various reasons, and in some cases the cause is unknown. The two most common causes of the disease are gallstones and excessive use of alcohol. For more information on pancreatitis, see page 900.

Pituitary Gland Disorders

Located at the base of the brain, behind the nasal passages, the pituitary gland is roughly the size and shape of a hazelnut. Despite its diminutive size, it's the most important endocrine gland. It serves as a control center for your body's long-term growth, day-to-day functioning and reproductive capabilities.

The pituitary gland consists of two parts, the front (anterior) lobe and the rear (posterior) lobe. The anterior lobe produces six distinct hormones, including prolactin to stimulate the production of breast milk and growth hormone to regulate your body's physical growth and use of fuel.

The other four hormones influence other glands of the endocrine system, stimulating activities in the thyroid gland, ovaries, testicles and adrenal glands.

The posterior lobe is responsible for the release of two hormones, oxytocin and antidiuretic hormone. Oxytocin prompts uterine contractions during childbirth and stimulates the breasts to release milk during breast-feeding. Antidiuretic hormone acts on the kidneys to control urine output.

Most problems with the pituitary gland are caused by pituitary tumors, which can be classified as either functioning or nonfunctioning. Functioning tumors release excess amounts of one of the normal pituitary hormones. In contrast, nonfunctioning tumors don't produce excessive hormone amounts.

Both types of tumors can cause problems simply because their increased size exerts pressure on neighboring vital tissues. For example, the nerves that control eye movement and vision lie close to the pituitary gland and can be affected by a pituitary tumor. Although the vast majority of pituitary tumors aren't cancerous and don't spread, they can lead to significant problems.

Acromegaly

Signs and symptoms
- Gradual enlargement of hands, feet, jaw and forehead
- Widely spaced teeth
- A large tongue
- Excessive perspiration
- Sleep apnea
- Carpal tunnel syndrome
- Pressure on surrounding structures, resulting in symptoms such as headaches or visual disturbances
- Hypopituitarism

Acromegaly is a disorder involving excessive growth of the forehead, jaw, hands and feet. It usually results from overproduction of growth hormone from a pituitary tumor in an adult. Acromegaly most commonly affects middle-aged adults. In children, a tumor that produces excess growth hormone causes a condition called gigantism, characterized by significantly accelerated growth and increased height.

Excess growth hormone can cause growth of the bones and internal organs. Other possible effects are high blood pressure, diabetes, colon polyps, arthritis and loss of vision. If acromegaly is untreated, the heart may become enlarged, leading to heart failure. These changes occur gradually, usually over several years, and often aren't apparent to the person with the disorder or to his or her family.

Diagnosis
The presence of certain physical features may suggest acromegaly. Your doctor may ask if you've had an increase in glove, shoe or hat size and whether your older rings

still fit. In addition, with acromegaly, blood tests show excessive amounts of growth hormone and insulin-like growth factor-I (IGF-I).

To confirm the diagnosis, it may be necessary to measure growth hormone after you've ingested glucose. A test of your vision may be done because an enlarged pituitary can press on the nerves that control vision, producing a defect in your visual field.

A computerized tomography (CT) scan or magnetic resonance imaging (MRI) of the head is frequently used to detect a tumor within the pituitary gland. Very rarely, a tumor located outside the pituitary can cause this syndrome.

Treatment

Surgery to remove the tumor is the most common treatment for acromegaly. Many times, it's not possible to remove the entire tumor. In this situation, radiation therapy or medications may be used. Radiation destroys the tumor and in turn stops production of growth hormone. Medications decrease growth hormone production but don't destroy the tumor.

Focused radiation — Gamma Knife or stereotactic radiosurgery — is often used. This procedure delivers a high dose of radiation to the tumor while minimizing the amount of radiation to surrounding normal tissues.

An injectable medication that decreases the production of growth hormone from the tumor may be used. A small number of people with acromegaly respond to oral medications. A promising new medication that blocks the effect of growth hormone is being tested.

If the pituitary gland is damaged by the tumor or during the course of treatment, hormone replacement therapy will be necessary. This involves taking medications that perform similar actions to those hormones the pituitary gland is no longer able to produce.

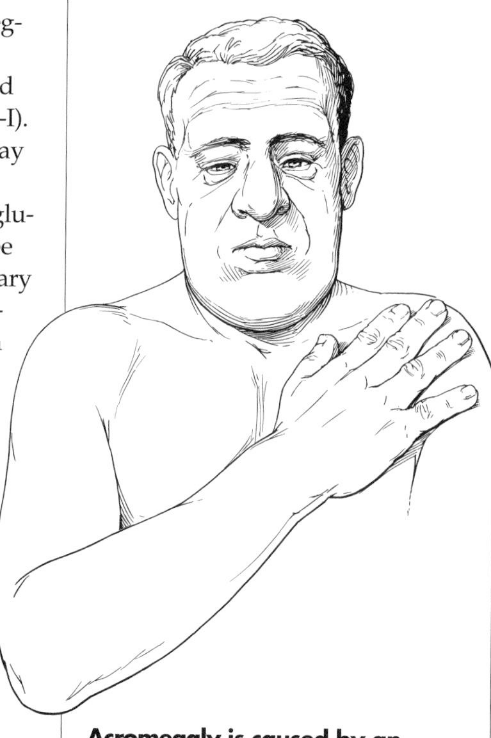

Acromegaly is caused by an excess of growth hormone in adulthood. The condition may result in enlargement of the hands, feet, jaw and forehead.

Diabetes insipidus

Signs and symptoms

- Excessive thirst
- Increased urination

Emergency signs and symptoms

- Dehydration, physical collapse and low blood pressure

Despite the similarities in symptoms and name, diabetes insipidus shouldn't be confused with diabetes mellitus. Diabetes mellitus, most commonly called just diabetes, stems from a deficiency of or resistance to the hormone insulin. Diabetes insipidus results from a deficiency of or resistance to antidiuretic hormone (ADH).

When the disorder results from a deficiency of ADH, it's called central diabetes insipidus. When it results from resistance to ADH, it's termed nephrogenic diabetes insipidus. The release of ADH is controlled by the pituitary gland.

A shortage of antidiuretic hormone or action can disturb the water balance in your body. Rather than reabsorbing enough water to maintain proper fluid levels, your kidneys simply pass the water out.

The cause of diabetes insipidus is unknown in about half the people who have it, although a pituitary disorder may become evident several years after symptoms begin.

Identifiable causes of central diabetes insipidus include damage to the pituitary gland from a head injury, surgery for a pituitary tumor and some inflammatory conditions. Identifiable causes of nephrogenic diabetes insipidus include certain medications and some types of kidney disease.

Diagnosis

The key sign of diabetes insipidus is the large volume of urine that's excreted — 5 quarts to 20 quarts within 24 hours isn't uncommon. Dehydration that results from increased urination causes insatiable thirst and, sometimes, dry skin.

If your doctor suspects that you have diabetes insipidus, he or she may conduct a water deprivation test, in which you consume no fluid for several hours. Urine produced during that time is analyzed. If you have normal amounts of antidiuretic hormone, the volume of urine will decrease. If you have diabetes insipidus, you'll eliminate substantial volumes of water. Your doctor may also conduct blood tests to determine the water and salt balance in your blood.

Treatment

Treatment focuses on determining the cause of diabetes insipidus, eliminating the cause, if possible, and controlling symptoms.

Diet

If you have nephrogenic diabetes, your doctor may advise that you limit consumption of salt because reducing sodium may help alleviate symptoms.

Medication

For central diabetes insipidus, you may be given an antidiuretic hormone, available by prescription. It can be taken in pill form, as a nasal spray or by injection. Hormone therapy usually is lifelong. However, if the disease resulted from an injury to the head or surgery, the pituitary may regain its normal function over a few months to a year. In such instances, hormone medication can be discontinued.

For nephrogenic diabetes insipidus, a thiazide diuretic drug may be prescribed. Although diuretics ordinarily are used to increase urination, thiazides have been effective for treating nephrogenic diabetes insipidus.

Surgery

If a tumor in your pituitary gland is the cause of the disorder, surgery or radiation therapy may be appropriate treatment.

Hypopituitarism

Signs and symptoms

- Lightheadedness
- Intolerance to cold
- Constipation
- Excessive thirst
- Fine wrinkling of the skin adjacent to the eyes and mouth
- Fatigue and low ambition
- Decreased appetite and, sometimes, weight loss

In children

- Slowed growth and sexual development
- Low blood sugar (hypoglycemia)

In women

- Irregular or absent menstrual periods
- Infertility
- An inability to lactate after childbirth

In men

- Decreased sexual interest
- Erectile dysfunction
- Loss of facial or body hair

Emergency signs and symptoms

- Fever
- A decrease in blood pressure

Hypopituitarism is a disorder in which your pituitary gland doesn't produce enough of one or more of the pituitary hormones. The name is derived in part from the Greek prefix *hypo*, which means "under." Some people inherit a tendency toward hypopituitarism. Others acquire the ailment for unknown reasons. In many instances, the cause is identifiable.

The condition may be associated with a tumor or inflammation of the pituitary gland, or it can develop after a serious head injury. Some women experience hypopituitarism after childbirth because the gland, which normally increases in size during pregnancy, grows so large that the body is unable to provide it with the oxygen and other nutrients it needs. As a result, some or all of the pituitary tissue dies. This form of hypopituitarism is called Sheehan's syndrome.

Because the pituitary gland also produces hormones that activate other glands, underproduction of those hormones can result in symptoms of other endocrine disorders.

If the hormone that controls adrenal function is impaired, your body won't be able to respond normally to physical stresses such as injury or infections. This can be life-threatening. Underactive thyroid (hypothyroidism) also may occur. Individuals with underactive thyroid may have a higher risk of developing cardiovascular and respiratory disease.

Diagnosis

Hypopituitarism in a child results in dwarfism. The key sign is abnormally slow growth. This condition is rare — very few children who are shorter than average have such a hormone insufficiency.

If hypopituitarism is suspected, your doctor may order tests to measure hormone concentrations in your blood and urine. Subsequent testing may involve administering other hormones or medications to stimulate the pituitary gland to produce its hormones, which are then measured.

If test results indicate a shortage of pituitary hormones, further tests may be performed to try to determine the underlying cause.

Treatment

If a cause for hypopituitarism is identified, specific treatment may improve the hormone levels. If not, various hormone replacement therapies will be necessary, depending on the degree of deficiency of each hormone. In children, injections of synthetic growth hormone can stimulate growth. Growth hormone replacement restores normal body proportions of fat and muscle and can improve fatigue that occurs with hypopituitarism.

Estrogen replacement for girls and testosterone replacement for boys may be required for sexual development. Adults also may need sex hormone replacement or specific fertility treatments. Adrenal hormones such as prednisone or hydrocortisone may need to be taken daily, with higher doses during times of illness.

People who require hormone replacement should wear a medical alert bracelet or necklace identifying their medical condition.

Nonfunctioning pituitary tumors

Signs and symptoms

- Loss of side (peripheral) vision
- Double vision
- Drooping of an eyelid
- Headache
- Excessive thirst and urination
- Fatigue and lightheadedness
- Intolerance to cold
- Constipation

In women

- Irregular or absent menstrual periods
- Infertility
- Discharge from the breasts

In men

- Decreased sexual interest
- Erectile dysfunction
- Decreased body hair

In children

- Slowed growth and development

Several types of nonfunctioning tumors — those that don't produce excessive amounts of a particular hormone — also can develop in the pituitary gland. Two of the most common are a pituitary adenoma and a craniopharyngioma.

Nonfunctioning tumors cause symptoms by pressing on the tissues surrounding the gland rather than by producing excess hormones. The pituitary's own normal function also can be affected, leading to deficiencies of the thyroid, adrenal, growth, water balance or sex hormones.

In some instances, these tumors cause few, if any, problems. In others, they cause hormone deficiencies or serious and life-threatening pressure on the brain. Symptoms generally progress gradually, but in rare cases they occur suddenly.

Diagnosis

A computerized tomography (CT) scan or magnetic resonance imaging (MRI) can confirm the presence of a nonfunctioning tumor. Many such tumors are found on scans performed for an unrelated condition. Your blood and urine may be tested for an excess or deficiency of certain hormones.

Treatment

If treatment is necessary, the tumor is usually removed surgically. Ra-

Hormone Supplements and Aging

Because hormone levels generally decline with age, some scientists speculate that hormones may play a role in the aging process. This has led some anti-aging enthusiasts and product manufacturers to promote the use of hormone supplements as a way to set back your body's clock.

If only it were that simple. Aging is an intricate, complex process that involves many body functions and tissues. When evaluating claims about hormone supplements, some old advice remains wise — if it sounds too good to be true, it probably is. Despite tempting claims, no hormone product has been proved to prevent or reverse aging. In addition, some may have dangerous side effects.

Here's a look at some hormone supplements that are touted as anti-aging therapies:

Human growth hormone

Growth hormone, produced in the pituitary gland, fuels growth and development during childhood and adolescence. In youths and adults who have a documented deficiency of the hormone, injections of the hormone are beneficial.

Proponents of human growth hormone (HGH) supplements for healthy adults say the hormone burns fat, builds muscle and renews energy. No evidence, however, shows that taking HGH results in health or lifestyle benefits for normal, aging adults. Moreover, possible side effects include fluid retention, joint pain, diabetes, high blood pressure and colon polyps.

DHEA

Dehydroepiandrosterone (DHEA) is a precursor hormone that's converted by the body into other hormones, including the sex hormones estrogen and testosterone. Normally, DHEA levels in your body peak during early adulthood and then gradually decline. Levels are quite low in older adults.

DHEA is sold over-the-counter as a dietary supplement and is advertised as a product that can slow aging, increase muscle and bone strength, burn fat, improve cognition, strengthen the immune system and protect against many chronic diseases. None of these claims has been proved. More troubling, DHEA may have harmful side effects. Even when taken for a short time, it may cause liver damage. Other potential problems include menstrual irregularities and unwanted facial hair in women, promotion of prostate cancer in men and an increased risk of heart disease.

Melatonin

Melatonin is a hormone that helps regulate your body's schedule for sleeping and waking. Claims that melatonin can slow or reverse aging, fight cancer and enhance sexuality remain unproved. Supplements on the market typically contain many times the amount of melatonin produced by your body. If taken improperly, melatonin can actually disrupt your sleep cycle.

Testosterone

In general, levels of the male sex hormone testosterone decline over time, although the rate of decline varies greatly among individual men. Anti-aging advocates say that increasing your level of testosterone by taking prescription supplements will improve your energy, well-being, complexion and sex drive. Such claims also remain unproved.

In high doses, testosterone can cause prostate problems, aggravate sleep apnea, stimulate excessive blood production and elevate cholesterol levels. However, in men whose testosterone level is low due to testicular disease or a pituitary problem, treatment with testosterone can be beneficial.

Estrogen

One type of hormone therapy that has been shown to have benefits for normal aging in women is hormone replacement therapy (HRT). It can help prevent osteoporosis, improve vaginal lubrication and maintain or improve skin elasticity. However, the data also point to possible risks, including increased risk of breast cancer. Therefore, it's important to weigh the risks and benefits of the therapy with your doctor. For more information, see page 1082.

diation therapy may be required if the tumor can't be adequately removed. Hormone deficiencies are generally treated with the appropriate hormone replacements.

Prolactinoma

Signs and symptoms

In women

- Irregular or absent menstrual periods
- Milky discharge from the breasts

In men

- Erectile dysfunction, decreased sexual interest and body hair
- Enlarged breasts

In both

- Hypopituitarism
- Pressure on surrounding tissues or structures
- Infertility

Prolactinoma is a condition in which a pituitary tumor overproduces the hormone prolactin. The tumor may range in size from microscopic to several centimeters in diameter. The major effect of increased prolactin is a decrease in normal levels of sex hormones: estrogen in women and testosterone in men. Although such deficiencies aren't life-threatening, they can lead to long-term complications, such as osteoporosis, and may cause infertility and sexual dysfunction.

High prolactin levels can also result from causes other than a prolactinoma, including several medications.

Diagnosis

Your doctor will likely take a careful medical history and conduct a physical examination to exclude other causes of high prolactin. Blood tests will measure your level of prolactin and other hormones. A computerized tomography (CT) scan or magnetic resonance imaging (MRI) of the pituitary gland can often identify a tumor.

Treatment

Oral medications can often decrease the production of prolactin and eliminate symptoms. Medications also may shrink the tumor. However, long-term treatment with medications is needed. Surgery offers the chance of a cure with small tumors and also may be necessary to relieve pressure on the nerves controlling vision.

Thyroid Disorders

Shaped like a bow tie or butterfly, your thyroid gland is located at the base of your throat, just below your Adam's apple. The gland wraps around your windpipe (trachea). A crossbar of tissue (isthmus) connects its two lobes.

Although the thyroid gland weighs less than an ounce, it has an enormous effect on your health. It helps set the rate at which your body functions, regulating all aspects of your metabolism, from how fast your heart beats to how quickly you burn calories. In response to direction from the pituitary gland, the thyroid gland secretes the hormone thyroxine. The more thyroxine that's circulating in your bloodstream, the greater the speed at which chemical activities occur in your body. The thyroid gland also produces calcitonin, a hormone that helps control the calcium level in your blood.

As long as your thyroid gland produces the right amount of thyroxine, your metabolism functions normally. But sometimes the gland produces and releases too much or not enough of this hormone, upsetting the delicate balance of chemical reactions in your body. Disorders of the thyroid gland generally fall into two categories, one involving its function and the other involving its structure. The thyroid can have both functional and structural abnormalities, which may or may not be related to each other.

Overproduction of thyroxine causes hyperthyroidism (overactive thyroid disease). The opposite condition — underproduction of thyroid hormone — causes hypothyroidism (underactive thyroid disease). Hyperthyroidism and hypothyroidism are functional disorders because they involve problems with the gland's functioning. Both disorders have various underlying causes. Goiter, an enlargement of the thyroid, is an example of a structural abnormality.

Hyperthyroidism

Signs and symptoms

- Weight loss despite increased appetite
- A rapid or irregular heartbeat or pounding of the heart
- Nervousness and irritability
- Sweating
- Swelling at the base of the neck (goiter)
- More frequent bowel movements, sometimes diarrhea
- Fatigue and muscle weakness
- Increased sensitivity to heat
- In women, changes in menstrual patterns
- Difficulty sleeping

Emergency signs and symptoms

- Fever
- A very rapid pulse
- Agitation and delirium

Hyperthyroidism (overactive thyroid disease) occurs when the thyroid gland produces or releases too much of the hormone thyroxine. Excessive thyroxine accelerates your body's metabolism.

Women are more likely to have hyperthyroidism than are men. Although it can occur at any age, it's most common in young or middle-aged adults.

Several different disease processes can cause your thyroid to release too much thyroid hormone. The most common underlying cause is an autoimmune disorder called Graves' disease. Other causes include inflammation of the thyroid gland (thyroiditis) and some lumps or nodules in the gland.

Hyperthyroidism can have serious consequences if untreated.

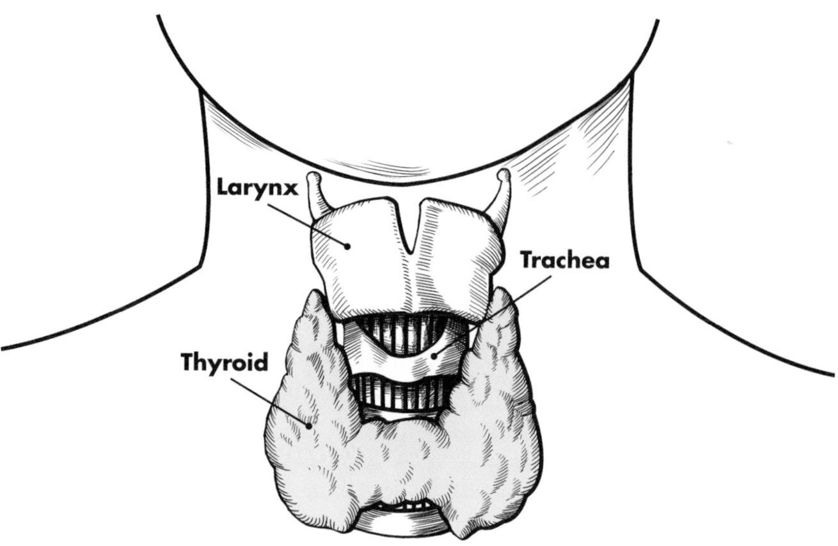

The thyroid gland consists of two lobes. It's located at the base of the throat.

Complications include heart problems, such as a rapid heart rate, an irregular heartbeat (atrial fibrillation) or congestive heart failure. Untreated hyperthyroidism can cause loss of bone mass (osteoporosis). If you have overactive thyroid disease, you're also at risk of thyrotoxic crisis. This is a sudden intensification of signs and symptoms that leads to fever and even delirium. It requires urgent medical attention.

Common manifestations of the speeded-up metabolism of hyperthyroidism include an increase in appetite, feeling warm while others may be cool or comfortable, and hands that tremble. Your heart may pound forcibly at a rapid rate and occasionally develop an irregular rhythm. Sleep difficulties are common. Your thyroid gland may be enlarged, but often so slightly that it isn't noticeable. If hyperthyroidism is due to Graves' disease, your eyeballs may protrude and become dry, and your skin may feel moist and sweaty.

Diagnosis

Hyperthyroidism is generally diagnosed based on a medical history, physical examination and blood tests. During the exam, your doctor may try to detect a slight tremor in your fingers when they're extended. You may be asked questions about any changes in your bowel movements or sensitivity to temperature. Your doctor may ask you to swallow while he or she examines your thyroid, as this makes it easier to feel.

Blood tests can detect an increase in thyroxine concentration. They may also show low or no amounts of thyroid-stimulating hormone, which is produced by the pituitary gland and is suppressed when too much thyroid hormone is circulating. These results may indicate hyperthyroidism. However, tests results only indicate that the thyroid is overactive — they don't identify the cause.

Your doctor may use a radioactive iodine uptake test to help establish the diagnosis and to aid in planning your treatment. In this test, you're given a small amount of radioactive iodine that you take orally. Over time, the iodine collects in your thyroid gland, where it's absorbed and used to manufacture thyroxine. You may be checked after 2, 6 or 24 hours — or sometimes all three — to determine how much iodine your thyroid has absorbed.

A high uptake of radioactive iodine indicates that your thyroid gland is producing too much thyroxine, as occurs with Graves' disease and hyperfunctioning thyroid nodules. If the uptake is low, thyroiditis is more likely the cause. In this inflammatory condition of the thyroid, iodine uptake is blocked, but stored thyroid hormone in the gland is released excessively.

Your doctor may also obtain a picture of your thyroid gland (thyroid scan) to help determine the cause and possible treatment.

Treatment

Treatment for hyperthyroidism depends on its underlying cause, your physical condition, your age and the severity of the disorder. Treatments include:

Radioactive iodine

Radioactive iodine is the most common treatment for hyperthyroidism. Taken as a single dose in liquid or capsule form, radioactive iodine is absorbed by the thyroid gland. The irradiation harmlessly and painlessly destroys thyroid tissue, causing the gland to shrink and slow its production of thyroid hormone.

The dose of radioactive iodine depends on the size of the thyroid gland and the findings on the uptake test. The elevated levels of thyroxine gradually decline over 2 to 3 months. Some people may require a second dose of radioactive iodine.

More than 80 percent of people who take radioactive iodine for hyperthyroidism are cured. However, because this treatment causes thyroid activity to slow considerably, it can result in the opposite condition — too little production of the thyroid hormone thyroxine. Many people need to take oral thyroxine every day to replace thyroxine that's no longer being produced.

Antithyroid medications

Another treatment involves taking antithyroid medications — methimazole (Tapazole) and propylthiouracil — in tablet form. These medications gradually reduce

PREVENTION TIP

Hyperthyroidism (overactive thyroid disease) during pregnancy increases the risk of miscarriage, so it's best to avoid getting pregnant until your hyperthyroidism is treated. If you've been treated with radioactive iodine, avoid getting pregnant for at least 6 months afterward. If hyperthyroidism occurs or recurs during pregnancy, you'll be given the lowest possible dose of an antithyroid drug. Radioactive iodine isn't used if you're pregnant or breast-feeding.

symptoms of hyperthyroidism by preventing the gland from producing excess amounts of hormones.

Within 6 to 8 weeks after the therapy is started, the symptoms of hyperthyroidism often disappear. Treatment, however, is long-term and may cause adverse liver or bone marrow effects. For some people, 1 to 2 years of antithyroid medications clear up the problem permanently, but many experience a relapse.

Beta blockers
A class of drugs called beta adrenergic blockers, or beta blockers, commonly used to treat coronary artery disease and high blood pressure, also block the action of thyroid hormone in your body. Beta blockers can decrease your hand tremor and heart rate and make you feel more comfortable within hours, but they don't change the high levels of thyroxine in your blood.

A beta blocker such as propranolol (Inderal), atenolol (Tenormin), metoprolol (Lopressor, Toprol) or nadolol (Corgard) may be prescribed to reduce symptoms of hyperthyroidism until another treatment takes effect, or it may be used in combination with another type of treatment.

Surgery
If medications aren't able to treat the problem, you may be a candidate for thyroid surgery. During a procedure called thyroidectomy, your doctor removes part or most of the thyroid gland, reducing or stopping hormone production. If all of the gland is removed, you'll need to take medication daily to replace the hormones normally produced by the gland.

Self-care
If you've lost a great deal of weight or are experiencing muscle wasting, work with your doctor or a dietitian to plan an appropriate diet. With successful treatment, nearly everyone regains weight. It's also important to get enough calcium every day to help prevent osteoporosis. Aim for a total of 1,500 milligrams daily, either from the food you eat, calcium supplements or both.

Hypothyroidism

Signs and symptoms

- Fatigue and sluggishness
- A slow heart rate
- Increased sensitivity to cold
- Unexplained weight gain
- Constipation
- Dry skin and hair
- Heavy menstrual periods
- Depression
- A hoarse voice
- A puffy face
- An elevated blood cholesterol level

Hypothyroidism (underactive thyroid disease) is a condition in which the thyroid gland fails to produce and release adequate levels of the hormone thyroxine. This disease slows your body's metabolic activities.

Because thyroid hormones have such a significant effect on growth, development and daily functioning, a deficiency can lead to a wide variety of health problems. Children with the condition may experience developmental disabilities. Adults may experience a slowing of physical and mental functioning and even heart disease. In addition, an underactive thyroid can increase cholesterol levels and blood pressure.

Signs and symptoms of hypothyroidism vary widely, depending on the severity of the hormone deficiency. In adults, the condition usually develops slowly over months or even years. As your metabolism continues to decrease, symptoms become more obvious.

Often, the first symptoms are constant fatigue with muscle aches and an inability to stay warm in cool or cold temperatures. You may become constipated, and your skin may dry out and lose its luster. Your voice may become hoarse. Some people also gain weight, usually in the range of 10 to 20 pounds.

Advanced hypothyroidism is called myxedema. It can develop if hypothyroidism goes unrecognized for several years. Symptoms of myxedema may include drowsiness, intense intolerance of cold and low body temperature, followed by profound lethargy and finally unconsciousness. Myxedema coma may be triggered by infection, use of sedatives, surgery or another stress on your body.

Hypothyroidism can occur in either sex and at any age. Middle-aged women are most commonly affected, and older adults are most likely to remain undiagnosed. The condition has various causes.

The thyroid gland may be destroyed by an autoimmune disorder, in which your own immune system attacks the gland. Hypothyroidism can result from an inflammation of the gland or from a failure of your pituitary gland to produce thyroid-stimulating hormone. This hormone signals your thyroid gland to produce thyroxine.

In addition, treatment for excess production of thyroid hormones (hyperthyroidism) can result in hypothyroidism. Some women develop hypothyroidism before or

Are You at Risk?

Hypothyroidism occurs mainly in women age 40 or older, and the risk of developing the disorder increases with age. However, it can affect either sex, from infants to older adults.

You're at increased risk of hypothyroidism if you:

- Have a close relative, such as a parent or grandparent, with an autoimmune disease
- Have diabetes or an autoimmune disease and are or have been pregnant
- Have been treated with radioactive iodine or antithyroid medications
- Have had thyroid surgery
- Have been treated with radiation for cancer of the head or neck

after pregnancy. In rare instances, infants are born with a defective thyroid gland or no thyroid gland.

Diagnosis

Because hypothyroidism is more prevalent in older women, some doctors recommend that women age 60 and older be screened for the disorder during routine physical examinations. Some doctors also test pregnant women for hypothyroidism.

Your doctor may also test for an underactive thyroid if you're feeling increasingly tired or sluggish, have dry skin, constipation and a hoarse voice or have had previous thyroid problems.

The most effective way to diagnose hypothyroidism is with blood tests that measure levels of thyroid-stimulating hormone (TSH) and thyroxine. Low levels of thyroxine and high levels of TSH suggest hypothyroidism.

Treatment

Treatment for an underactive thyroid involves use of the synthetic thyroid hormone levothyroxine (Levothroid, Levoxyl). You must take the hormone daily. This oral medication restores adequate hormone levels.

After you start treatment, symptoms such as fatigue should start to subside, although all of your symptoms may not improve for several months. The medication may gradually lower your cholesterol level and reverse any weight gain caused by the disease.

Treatment with levothyroxine is usually lifelong and must be followed with periodic blood tests because your body's thyroid hormone requirement may change slightly over time.

Other thyroid disorders

The following thyroid conditions may lead to hyperthyroidism or hypothyroidism, or pose similar signs and symptoms. Appropriate testing can determine the cause of the problem and the best form of treatment.

Graves' disease

Graves' disease is an autoimmune disorder named for Robert Graves, the Irish doctor who first described it. The process that triggers the disease involves your body's immune system. The immune system produces proteins called antibodies to inactivate and destroy foreign invaders such as bacteria and viruses. In the case of Graves' disease, something causes your immune system to produce an antibody that imitates the action of thyroid-stimulating hormone (TSH) and stimulates your thyroid gland.

Women are about seven times more likely to have Graves' disease than are men. Researchers suspect that for some people, a stressful life event, such as divorce or the death of a loved one, may trigger the disease by affecting antibody production of the immune system. But many people who develop the disease have no identifiable stress in their life.

Graves' disease is the most common cause of hyperthyroidism. Immune system abnormalities that stimulate excess hormone production may also cause an uncommon condition called Graves' ophthalmopathy. In this disorder, the eyeballs protrude beyond their protective orbit because tissues and muscles behind the eyes swell and cause the eyeballs to move forward (see page 659). Your eyes may also be red and irritated. Some people experience double vision. A small number of people with Graves' disease develop reddening and swelling of the skin, often on their shins and the top of their feet.

Treatment

No treatment exists that can stop your immune system from producing the antibodies that cause Graves' disease, but medication can control the symptoms by decreasing the production of thyroxine. Treatment for Graves' ophthalmopathy is discussed on page 660.

Screening in Infants

All states in the United States require that newborns be screened with routine blood tests for hypothyroidism. That's because in an infant, untreated hypothyroidism can result in serious problems with physical and mental development. If the condition is diagnosed within the first few months of life, the chances of normal development are excellent.

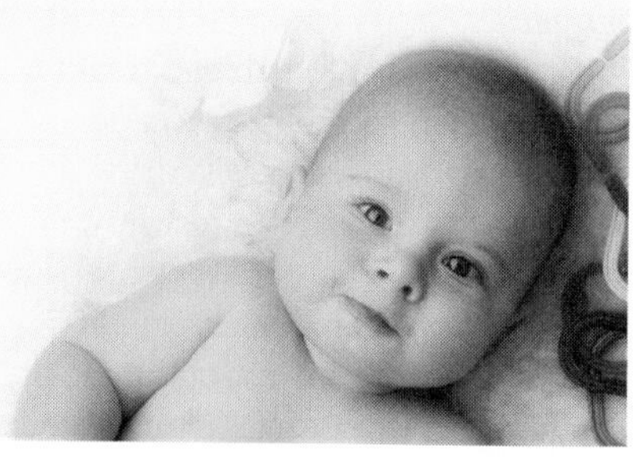

Goiter

Goiter is a general term for an enlarged thyroid gland. The word comes from the Latin for "throat." The enlargement may be a small, localized lump or a swelling of both lobes of the thyroid gland. A goiter is usually painless.

An enlarged thyroid gland can produce normal, low or excessive amounts of hormones. In rare instances, in which the enlarged gland grows around the windpipe, the enlargement can interfere with swallowing or breathing.

Thyroid enlargement has many causes. In the past, the most common cause of goiter was a shortage of iodine in the diet. Goiter is now rare in the United States because table salt is supplemented with iodine, and the food supply is generally rich in iodine. In some parts of the world that lack dietary iodine, goiters are still common.

Other causes of goiter include:

Simple enlargement

A soft, widespread enlargement of the thyroid gland is called simple goiter. Although infrequent, it's most common during pregnancy or adolescence. Other times, the cause is unknown, although there may be a genetic component in some instances.

Thyroiditis

Thyroiditis is an inflammation of the thyroid gland, which can cause it to enlarge. The gland may become rubbery, or it may be tender and cause pain when swallowing. Chronic lymphocytic thyroiditis, also called Hashimoto's thyroiditis, is the most common cause of thyroid enlargement in the United States. It results from an autoimmune disorder.

Graves' disease

Graves' disease causes an overactive thyroid. It usually produces a slight but generalized enlargement of the thyroid, although the gland can become quite large.

Thyroid nodules

Nodules or lumps in the thyroid gland may cause enlargement of one or both lobes. A nodule needs to be evaluated to determine if it's cancerous. Rarely, a nodule partially blocks your windpipe (trachea), causing breathing difficulties that may resemble asthma.

If your goiter isn't causing any problems, treatment may not be necessary. If the gland becomes large enough to be of cosmetic concern, medication can be taken to decrease its size. If the enlargement interferes with eating or breathing, medication may be prescribed or all or part of the gland may be removed.

If the gland contains nodules or bumps, diagnostic tests will likely be performed to make sure the growths aren't cancerous (malignant). In case of cancer, removal of all or a portion of the gland may be necessary.

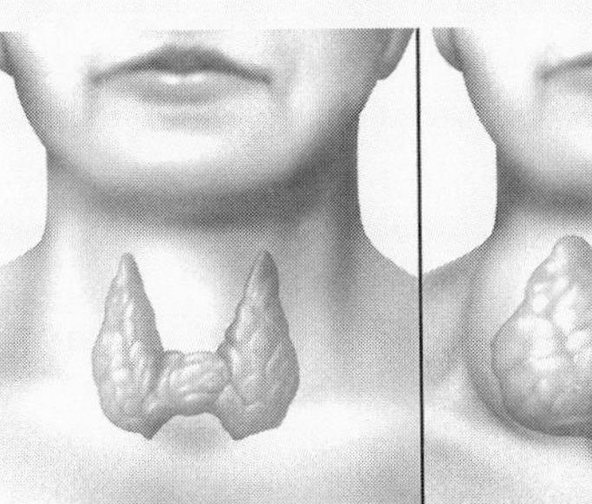
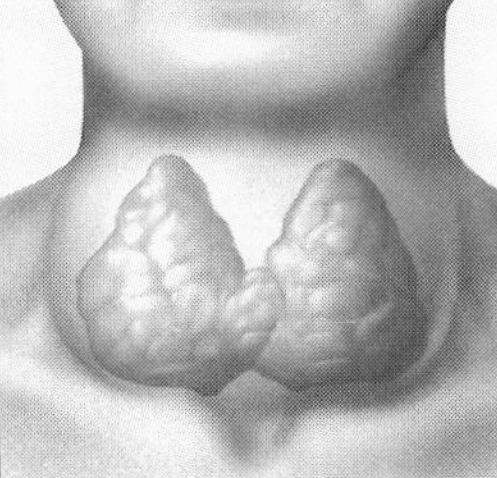

Normal thyroid **Enlarged thyroid**

Thyroiditis

Thyroiditis, an inflammation of the thyroid gland, can cause enlargement of the gland. There are several types of thyroiditis.

The most common is chronic lymphocytic thyroiditis, also called Hashimoto's thyroiditis. It's an autoimmune disease in which the immune system creates antibodies that damage the thyroid gland, causing underproduction of thyroid hormone. This disease is most common in older women and tends to run in families.

Thyroiditis after pregnancy is called postpartum thyroiditis. It's a painless inflammation of the thyroid gland that occurs in about 6 percent of women approximately 4 to 12 months after childbirth.

A short period of hyperthyroidism may occur, but thyroid function usually returns to normal after a few months. Some women, though, experience significant or long-term hypothyroidism. These women generally require treatment with thyroid hormone replacement medication.

Another less common condition is subacute granulomatous thyroiditis. This condition, which is probably caused by a virus, begins more suddenly than Hashimoto's thyroiditis and causes the thyroid gland to become painful and enlarged. Either hyperthyroidism or hypothyroidism may occur temporarily. This type of thyroiditis usually goes away by itself within a few months.

Treatment

If you have discomfort or swelling around your thyroid gland or symptoms of hyperthyroidism or hypothyroidism, your doctor may examine your thyroid gland and request blood tests to measure hormone levels and antibodies.

Most people with Hashimoto's thyroiditis must take thyroid hormone replacement medication for the rest of their lives. In other forms of thyroiditis, the thyroid gland generally returns to normal in a few months.

Aspirin or other nonsteroidal anti-inflammatory drugs can relieve the pain and inflammation of subacute thyroiditis. In more severe cases, a doctor may prescribe corticosteroid medications.

Thyroid nodules

A thyroid nodule is a lump within the thyroid gland. You may have several or only one. Thyroid nodules are relatively common and rarely cancerous (malignant).

One noncancerous (benign) type of nodule is an adenoma, in which a portion of the thyroid walls itself off from the rest of the gland. It forms a lump, often half an inch or more in diameter, which you can feel and sometimes see.

Most thyroid adenomas produce little or no thyroid hormone, but occasionally an adenoma manufactures an excessive amount of the hormone, a condition called hyperfunctioning thyroid nodule causing hyperthyroidism.

Treatment

Most thyroid nodules are discovered during a routine physical examination. To determine what type of nodule it is and if it's cancerous, a doctor may do an ultrasound test to get an image of the lump. He or she may also do a biopsy, a procedure in which a thin needle is used to take a sample of the tissue (fine needle aspiration) for examination. Typically, you'll also have a blood test to check the level of thyroid hormones.

Often, a nodule requires no specific treatment, as most don't produce symptoms. Adenomas that produce excessive thyroid hormone are treated with radioactive iodine, which destroys the nodule, or with surgery.

Cancerous nodules require surgical removal of the thyroid gland. If your thyroid gland is removed, you'll need to take thyroid hormone replacement medication for the rest of your life.

Thyroid cancer

Cancer of the thyroid is rare, making up less than 1 percent of all cancers. There are four main types of thyroid cancer, based on what the cancer cells look like under a microscope. The two most common types are papillary and follicular. The papillary type tends to spread to the lymph nodes in the neck. The follicular type may spread to your lungs and other more distant parts of your body. Most thyroid cancers grow slowly.

In an unusual form of thyroid cancer called medullary cancer, the cancer cells secrete the hormone calcitonin. The progress of this cancer can be followed by measuring calcitonin in blood. Medullary cancer frequently occurs in members of the same family. Medullary thyroid cancer is also associated with a rare hereditary disorder called multiple endocrine neoplasia (MEN) type 2 (see page 1054).

Cancer of the thyroid is more common in women than in men. You're at increased risk of developing thyroid cancer if you've been exposed to large amounts of radiation, if you've had radiation treatment to your head or neck or if someone in your family has had medullary thyroid cancer or pheochromocytomas, rare tumors that arise from cells in the core (medulla) of the adrenal gland.

Treatment

If a thyroid lump is malignant, the tumor and all or part of the gland will likely be surgically removed. Because thyroid cancer may spread to nearby lymph nodes, these may be removed as well.

Under certain circumstances, radioactive iodine is given to supplement surgical treatment. It destroys thyroid tissue that can't be removed by surgery. The thyroid gland and tumor absorb the radioactive iodine, which can destroy thyroid tissue and cancer without affecting the rest of the body.

If your thyroid gland is removed, your body can no longer make thyroid hormone, so you'll have to take thyroid hormone tablets daily to replace those no longer being produced. Thyroid hormone also may stop the growth of any remaining cancer cells. It does this by suppressing the release of thyroid-stimulating hormone.

If you have medullary thyroid cancer, ask your doctor about genetic counseling and testing. Family members can be tested to see if they carry the genetic defect that causes inherited forms of the cancer. Thyroid surgery can prevent cancer in carriers who have not yet developed cancer.

Parathyroid Gland Disorders

The parathyroid glands are located on the four corners of the thyroid gland, which lies at the front and base of your neck. The parathyroid glands are very small — each is about the size of a grain of rice — and they secrete parathyroid hormone. When too much of this hormone is produced, the resulting disorder is called hyperparathyroidism. When too little of the hormone is released, the condition is called hypoparathyroidism.

The parathyroid glands maintain the level of calcium in your blood within very narrow limits by secreting more or less hormone. Increased hormone secretion by one or more of the parathyroid glands raises the calcium level in your blood by increasing the release of calcium from your bones — the storage area for calcium in your body — and by increasing the amount absorbed in your small intestine. Vitamin D also is necessary for regulating the amount of calcium in your blood.

Hyperparathyroidism

Signs and symptoms

- Kidney stones
- Osteoporosis
- Fatigue
- Frequent urination and increased thirst
- Abdominal pain, indigestion or ulcer symptoms

When one or more of the parathyroid glands produce an excess of parathyroid hormone, hyperparathyroidism results. When excess parathyroid hormone circulates in your body, the calcium level in your blood becomes elevated, and the concentration of phosphorus is lowered.

Phosphorus, like calcium, is a mineral essential to your body's functioning and is of particular importance to the development and health of your bones and teeth.

Most of the time, the cause of hyperparathyroidism is a noncancerous (benign) tumor in one of the parathyroid glands. In some instances, all four of the glands become enlarged and overproduce the hormone. Cancer of the parathyroid glands is very rare.

Women are about twice as likely to have hyperparathyroidism as men are. The condition is associated with multiple endocrine neoplasia (MEN) type 1, which is a rare hereditary disorder.

Hyperparathyroidism may be symptomless at first, unless there's pain from kidney stones. Symptoms may not appear for many years.

Diagnosis

About half the people with hyperparathyroidism have no symptoms. Often the diagnosis is made when an abnormally high calcium level is discovered by a routine blood test for some other reason.

Low amounts of phosphorus in the blood also indicate that you might have the disorder. Direct measurement of the amount of parathyroid hormone in the blood helps confirm the diagnosis.

Your doctor may order an ultrasound examination or other imaging scans of the thyroid region to look for tumors in the parathyroid glands.

Treatment

For some people with hyperparathyroidism, no treatment is necessary. Your doctor may simply monitor your condition. He or she may periodically order image tests of your kidneys, because of increased risk of kidney stones, and measure your bone mineral density to assess the status of your bones, which are at risk of thinning if you have this disorder.

If your blood calcium level is very high or there's evidence of bone thinning or kidney stones, you may need treatment. Treatment involves surgical removal of the tumor or the glands that are overproducing parathyroid hormone. Special scans can accurately locate the tumor, which allows a surgeon to remove it during minimally invasive surgery.

Hypoparathyroidism

Signs and symptoms

- Muscle spasms or tingling, especially in your hands, feet, face and throat
- Breathing difficulties
- Dry skin
- Yeast infections
- In children, vomiting, convulsions and headache

When the parathyroid glands produce too little of their hormone, the disorder that results is called hypoparathyroidism. Hypoparathyroidism is far less common than hyperparathyroidism.

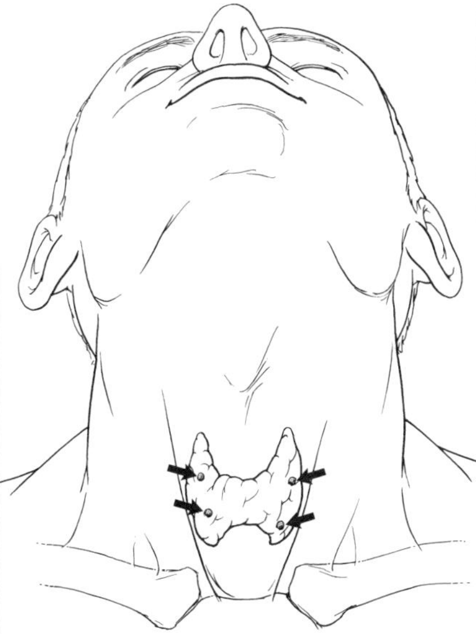

Located on your thyroid gland, the tiny parathyroid glands (arrows) produce a hormone that controls the level of calcium in your blood.

Without sufficient quantities of parathyroid hormone circulating in your body, the amount of calcium in your blood falls below normal levels, and the amount of phosphorus rises. A low blood calcium concentration can produce various problems, particularly muscle spasms and cramps.

Muscle spasms associated with hypoparathyroidism can be uncomfortable or painful, and breathing difficulties can result from spasms of the muscles controlling your vocal cords. If the amount of calcium in your blood has been low for many years, cataracts and convulsions can occur.

There are two types of hypoparathyroidism. One type is called spontaneous hypoparathyroidism. Its cause is unknown, but the condition may be associated with susceptibility to yeast infections and failure of the ovaries or adrenal glands. Children are affected more often than adults. The second type results when the parathyroid glands are removed or damaged during neck surgery.

Diagnosis

The key findings in hypoparathyroidism are an abnormally low level of calcium in the blood (hypocalcemia), an abnormally high concentration of phosphorus, and an inappropriately low level of parathyroid hormone.

Treatment

To treat the condition, your doctor may prescribe vitamin D and calcium supplements. If muscle spasms are especially severe, you may be given an intravenous (IV) injection of calcium to provide immediate, temporary relief.

You will likely need to take calcium and vitamin D supplements for the remainder of your life in amounts considerably larger than those typically required for ordinary nutrition.

In addition, because levels of calcium in your blood must be monitored, your doctor will establish a schedule of regular blood tests. These tests are important to make sure you maintain normal levels of calcium in your blood.

Adrenal Gland Disorders

Your adrenal glands are located on top of your kidneys. Each gland is about the size of the end of your thumb and is shaped like a boomerang. The adrenal gland consists of two portions: the inner core, called the medulla, and the outer layer, called the cortex.

The medulla produces hormones called catecholamines. The most important of these are adrenaline (epinephrine) and noradrenaline (norepinephrine). Physical and emotional stresses usually trigger their release. When secreted into the bloodstream, catecholamines increase your heart rate and blood pressure and affect several other body functions.

The cortex produces hormones called corticosteroids. An area of your brain called the hypothalamus and the pituitary gland control the production of these hormones.

There are three groups of corticosteroids:

Sex hormones

Sex hormones include male androgens and female estrogens, which affect sexual development and reproduction. Sex hormones also are produced in larger amounts in the testicles and ovaries.

Glucocorticoids

The cortisol family of hormones (glucocorticoids) influence the conversion of starchy foods into glycogen, a stored form of blood sugar. One important glucocorticoid is cortisol, which has many functions. Among other tasks, it helps regulate the immune system, helps maintain proper blood pressure and blood volume and helps your body deal with physical stress.

Mineralocorticoids

Mineralocorticoids are corticosteroids that control the body's content of the minerals sodium and potassium. Aldosterone is the main member of this group.

Unlike other corticosteroids — which are controlled by the pituitary gland hormone adrenocorticotropic hormone (ACTH) — aldosterone is mainly controlled by the hormone renin. Renin is produced by the kidneys.

Adrenal gland hormones affect virtually every system in your body to some degree. Their effects are complex, and some of their actions overlap. When problems occur in this intricate system, serious diseases and disorders can develop.

Addison's disease

Signs and symptoms

- Weakness and lethargy
- Weight loss and decreased appetite
- Darkening of the skin
- Lightheadedness when standing
- Abdominal pains accompanied by diarrhea, nausea and vomiting
- Decreased sexual interest
- Joint and muscle aches
- Persistent fever
- Salt craving

Emergency signs and symptoms

- Severe diarrhea and vomiting
- Dehydration
- Shock
- Loss of consciousness

Addison's disease is named for Thomas Addison, the 19th-century English physician who first identified it. The disease occurs when the outer portion (cortex) of the adrenal gland fails to produce enough steroid hormones.

Addison's disease most commonly results from an autoimmune disorder, a condition in which the body's own immune system attacks itself. Other causes include infections of the adrenal glands, spread of cancer to the adrenal glands or bleeding into the glands. The disorder can occur at any age, including infancy, and occurs equally in males and females.

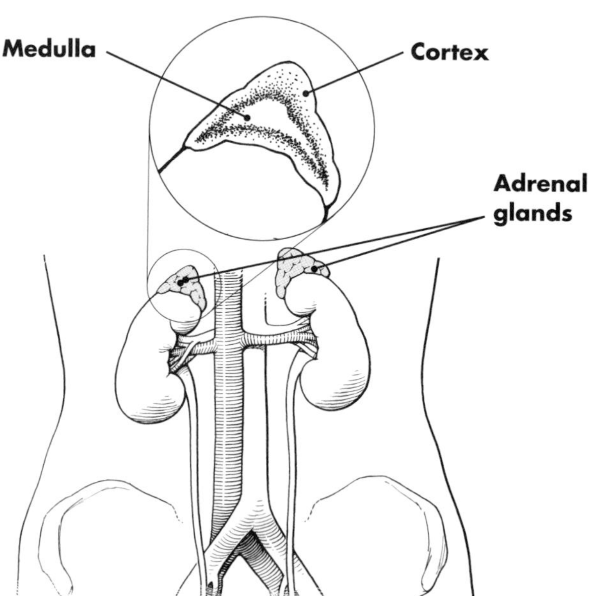

The adrenal glands are located on the top of the kidneys. They produce corticosteroid and catecholamine hormones. Catecholamines include adrenaline and noradrenaline.

Signs and symptoms of Addison's disease usually develop slowly, perhaps over several months, but they may appear suddenly. In acute adrenal failure (addisonian crisis), signs and symptoms generally include severe diarrhea, vomiting, dehydration, shock and loss of consciousness.

Diagnosis

If your doctor thinks that you may have Addison's disease, he or she will likely request blood and urine tests to measure the amounts of corticosteroid hormones. To confirm the diagnosis, your doctor may measure your body's response to an adrenal-stimulating hormone, adrenocorticotropic hormone (ACTH), which is produced by the pituitary gland. In this procedure, you receive an injection of synthetic ACTH, and the output of hormones from your adrenal cortex is measured. If your adrenal glands are damaged, the response is blunted or nonexistent.

Treatment

Hospitalization is essential for treatment of acute adrenal failure, which may be provoked by physical stress, infection, injury, vomiting, diarrhea or the use of diuretic medications. Adrenal failure is a life-threatening condition that requires prompt medical care, including intravenous (IV) salt solutions and steroid hormones. Treatment for Addison's disease can alleviate symptoms and allow you to live a normal life.

Medication

Because your body isn't producing sufficient steroid hormones, your doctor may prescribe one or more hormone medications to treat the deficiency. These replacement hormones may include hydrocortisone or prednisone to replace cortisol.

A second drug, fludrocortisone, is used to replace aldosterone. Aldosterone controls your body's sodium and potassium needs and keeps your blood pressure normal.

You take the hormones in daily dosages that mimic the amount your body would normally produce, thereby minimizing side effects. If you're facing a stressful situation, such as an operation, infection or illness, your doctor may prescribe a temporary increase in your dosage. If you don't take the hormones as directed, you may be at risk of acute adrenal failure.

Carrying a medical alert card and wearing an alert bracelet at all times is critical if you're taking steroid medications for Addison's disease. When you're traveling, it's also wise to carry an emergency kit that includes a needle, syringe and injectable form of corticosteroid medications.

Supplemental sodium

A low-salt diet can provoke symptoms of acute adrenal failure. If you have Addison's disease, it's important that you consume adequate amounts of sodium daily.

Congenital adrenal hyperplasia

Signs and symptoms

- In male infants, enlargement of the penis
- In female infants, enlargement of the clitoris
- Acute adrenal failure (occasionally)
- High blood pressure (rarely)
- Accelerated growth in early childhood that stops early, resulting in short stature

This condition is the most common adrenal gland disorder in infants and children. It's the result of a genetic abnormality that leads to an enzyme deficiency, which in turn causes the adrenal glands to produce an abnormal pattern of steroid hormones. Some women have only a partial or mild deficiency of the enzyme. They develop normally in childhood but as young adults may have problems with abnormal hairiness (hirsutism), menstrual irregularities or infertility.

Diagnosis

When congenital adrenal hyperplasia is suspected, the doctor may conduct blood and urine tests to measure the levels of hormones produced by the adrenal gland.

Treatment

Once this disorder has been diagnosed, it can usually be treated with medication. For most people, treatment consists of oral corticosteroid medication on a daily basis. Some people have both adrenal glands removed, allowing for treatment with lower doses of corticosteroids.

The main long-term risk is potential side effects from the medication, so the doctor will closely monitor skeletal and other growth patterns in young people.

Cushing's syndrome

Signs and symptoms

- Thinning of the skin with easy bruising, slow healing and stretch marks
- Obesity concentrated in trunk
- A hump between the shoulders (buffalo hump)
- Rounding of the face and fullness of the neck
- Muscle weakness and wasting
- Fatigue
- A flushed face
- Osteoporosis
- Diabetes
- High blood pressure
- Swelling
- In men, erectile dysfunction
- In women, absence of menstrual periods
- Excess hair growth
- Depression

Cushing's syndrome is sometimes referred to as hypercortisolism. It occurs when excess cortisol circulates in the bloodstream. The syndrome is named for Harvey Cushing, an early 20th-century American surgeon who first described the disorder.

Extended use of steroid medications to treat another ailment can cause Cushing's syndrome. In addition, the syndrome can result from

Discovery of Adrenal Tumors

Most adrenal gland tumors are discovered incidentally during imaging studies conducted for another reason. For example, you might see your doctor because of abdominal pain. An ultrasound or computerized tomography (CT) scan of the abdomen is performed, and your doctor discovers a mass on one of your adrenal glands. Typically, this tumor is small and has nothing to do with whatever is causing your symptoms.

An adrenal tumor found in this way is sometimes called an adrenal incidentaloma — meaning it's discovered incidentally in the absence of symptoms of adrenal disease. In the last 20 years, development of more sensitive imaging equipment has greatly increased discovery of such tumors.

Once an adrenal tumor is found, the next step is to determine if it's cancerous. A CT scan or magnetic resonance imaging (MRI) of the mass may be ordered to check for characteristics such as size and density that can help in determining whether the tumor is cancerous (malignant). Most adrenal gland tumors are noncancerous (benign). If the tumor looks benign, your doctor probably will monitor it at regular intervals to check for any changes in size. Surgery may be recommended for large or growing tumors.

Your doctor will also want to find out if the tumor is overproducing hormones. You may need to undergo urine and blood tests to check for abnormally high or low hormone and electrolyte concentrations. Electrolytes are salts in your blood that are regulated by hormones.

overproduction of cortisol by the adrenal glands.

A tumor on an adrenal gland, enlargement of both glands or a lung or other tumor that produces a hormone that stimulates the adrenal glands can cause this overproduction. When caused by a tumor in the pituitary gland, the form is called Cushing's disease. This affects women five times more frequently than men.

If you have Cushing's syndrome, you're at increased risk of heart attack or stroke because the disorder can accelerate buildup of fatty deposits (plaques) in your arteries (atherosclerosis). Thinning of your bones (osteoporosis) and bone fractures also are common, as is impaired ability to resist or fight infections. Left untreated, Cushing's syndrome can be fatal.

Diagnosis

A round, red face and extra fatty tissue above the collarbone and between the shoulder blades are physical clues to Cushing's syndrome. Frequent or even spontaneous bruising on the arms and legs is another common sign.

Cushing's syndrome is generally determined by measuring hormone levels in your blood and urine, often before and after taking a synthetic hormone. Magnetic resonance imaging (MRI) or a computerized tomography (CT) scan of the pituitary or adrenal glands or lungs can help determine if a tumor is present. Direct blood sampling from the veins draining the pituitary gland also may be necessary.

Treatment

Treatment depends on the cause of the excess cortisol. If your signs and symptoms are due to taking steroid medications, treatment consists of stopping their use or decreasing the dosage. Sudden discontinuation of steroid treatment can aggravate the underlying disease, such as asthma or arthritis. Your doctor will likely recommend a gradual reduction in the dosage of steroids.

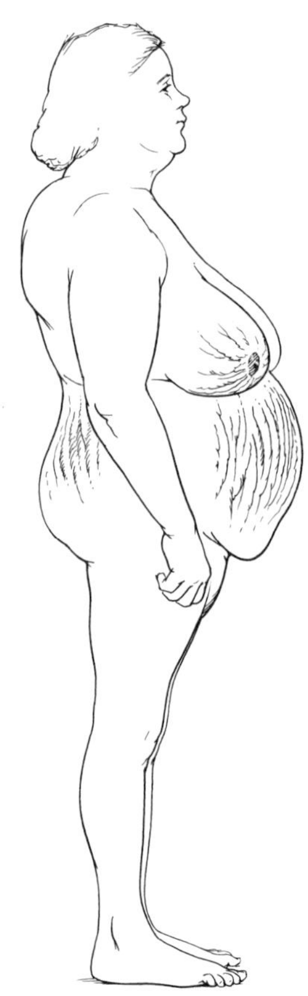

If Cushing's syndrome is untreated, it can cause an individual's face to become very round, abdominal obesity, the back to develop a characteristic hump and skin to develop pink or purple stretch marks.

In some cases, another drug may be used in place of the steroid originally prescribed. For as long as a year after steroid medication is stopped, physical stress from an injury, infection or surgery may result in a dangerous insufficiency of adrenal hormones, requiring emergency treatment.

For Cushing's syndrome that's caused by a tumor in the pituitary gland, adrenal gland or lung, removal of the tumor is usually the best treatment. Surgical techniques continue to evolve. Newer techniques require smaller incisions, result in shorter hospital stays and generally produce less pain and other complications. Successful removal of a tumor is likely to result in a full recovery, although long-term hormone replacement therapy may be required.

Hirsutism

In some women, hair may begin to grow on the face, chest, abdomen and other locations where typically only men have hair. Such excessive hair growth, called hirsutism, may stem from use of drugs such as phenytoin (Dilantin), used to treat some seizure disorders, and from some medications used to control high blood pressure. Certain disorders of the adrenal glands and ovaries also can cause hirsutism.

If a doctor can't find an explanation for the abnormal hair growth, the condition is referred to as idiopathic hirsutism — hairiness of unknown cause. Women with idiopathic hirsutism may have a slight increase in sensitivity to, or production of, androgen hormones. These are male sex hormones that are also normally produced by women. The condition poses no health risk but is often a matter of cosmetic concern.

No oral medication has been approved specifically for treating abnormal hair growth, but several drugs may be effective for suppressing androgen levels and controlling hirsutism. These include corticosteroids, the diuretic spironolactone, and oral contraceptives that contain the hormones estrogen and progestin. A prescription cream (eflornithine) applied twice daily may slow the growth of facial hair.

Keep in mind, however, that these are potent drugs with possible side effects. In addition, they don't work for everyone and may take several months to produce an effect. Other methods to control unwanted hair, such as laser hair removal, may be preferable.

If surgery isn't possible or successful, treatment may include radiation and medications to block adrenal hormone production. If treatment renders the adrenal glands incapable of providing the hormones your body requires, you'll need oral medications to replace the missing hormones.

Pheochromocytoma

Signs and symptoms

- High blood pressure
- Excessive sweating
- Increased heart rate or the sensation of a pounding heart
- Headache
- A pale complexion

Pheochromocytoma is a rare tumor in the core (medulla) of the adrenal gland that can produce large amounts of the hormones adrenaline (epinephrine) and noradrenaline (norepinephrine). People with a rare inherited disorder called multiple endocrine neoplasia (MEN) type 2 often develop pheochromocytomas. The high blood pressure may be constant or come in episodes associated with sweating, headache, pale skin and a fast or pounding heartbeat.

About 10 percent of pheochromocytomas are cancerous (malignant). The tumors may be associated with malignant tumors in other endocrine glands, such as the thyroid (medullary thyroid cancer). Pheochromocytomas can be life-threatening if untreated. They can release dangerously high levels of adrenaline into the bloodstream after an injury or during surgery.

Diagnosis

Blood or urine tests that reveal elevated levels of epinephrine and norepinephrine or their breakdown products (metanephrines) strongly suggest pheochromocytoma. Additional testing to detect a tumor may include a computerized tomography (CT) scan, magnetic resonance imaging (MRI) or a radioisotope scan.

This type of scan involves injecting a radioactive substance. You wait for the substance to travel to and become concentrated in the designated organ — in this case the adrenal glands. A camera that detects gamma rays given off by the radioactive substance is then positioned near your body. Areas of disease generally give off abnormal amounts of radiation.

Treatment

Surgical removal of the entire gland is the usual treatment, and in most cases the signs and symptoms disappear. Before surgery, your doctor will prescribe medications to block the effects of the adrenal hormones and control blood pressure.

Primary aldosteronism

Signs and symptoms

- High blood pressure
- Muscle weakness or cramps
- Occasionally, increased urination and thirst

Primary aldosteronism is a syndrome characterized by excess production of the hormone aldosterone from the outer portion (cortex) of the adrenal gland. The condition causes your body to retain too much sodium and water and to lose potassium, resulting in high blood pressure and low blood potassium levels.

Overproduction of aldosterone may result from a noncancerous (benign) tumor in an adrenal gland (aldosterone-producing adenoma) or overactivity of both adrenal glands (idiopathic hyperaldosteronism). Very rare causes include an inherited form of the disease and cancerous (malignant) adrenal tumors.

Diagnosis

A combination of high blood pressure and low blood potassium may be clues to the condition. Further blood and urine tests indicating excess aldosterone can confirm the diagnosis. A computerized tomography (CT) scan of the adrenal glands and, sometimes, direct blood sampling of the veins that drain the glands are done to help determine the underlying cause.

Treatment

The main concerns of this condition are the problems that can arise from increased blood pressure. Very low potassium levels also may cause muscle weakness, cramps, fatigue and serious heart problems.

If a tumor is found in one adrenal gland, surgery to remove the gland usually improves blood pressure and normalizes hormone and potassium levels. Some individuals may continue to need medication for high blood pressure. For idiopathic hyperaldosteronism, your doctor may recommend a medication that blocks the effects of aldosterone. Medication may also be an alternative to surgery for disease caused by a tumor.

Others

Rarely, adrenal tumors can produce sex hormones of the opposite sex. Men may experience erectile dysfunction or breast enlargement. Women may experience abnormal hair growth, menstrual irregularities and deepening of the voice.

Cancers of the adrenal cortex are very rare but usually aggressive. They can overproduce any of the adrenal hormones. Some, however, don't produce hormones.

Several other conditions can cause enlargement of the adrenal glands, including fatty tumors, infections and the spread of cancer from another location in the body (metastasis).

Sex Gland Disorders

The sex glands are the testicles (testes) in men and the ovaries in women. These organs, also known as gonads, produce sperm and eggs, respectively. They also produce hormones that control secondary sexual characteristics, such as facial hair and breasts, that determine the differences between men and women. Sex hormones play an important role in the reproductive process.

Both men and women produce male sex hormones (androgens) and female sex hormones (estrogen and progesterone), but androgens predominate in men and estrogen and progesterone are dominant in women. Disorders of the sex glands may result in various health disorders involving the secondary sexual characteristics.

Male sex gland disorders

Testosterone is the most important of the male sex hormones (androgens). During fetal development, testosterone is needed to form male genital organs. During puberty, it's required for the development of masculine physical characteristics, and in adult men, the hormone maintains muscle mass and strength, fat distribution, bone mass, sperm production, sex drive and potency.

Deficiencies or imbalances in testosterone and other sex hormones can affect sexual development, sexual characteristics and fertility.

Abnormal puberty

In boys, normal puberty begins between ages 9 and 14, often around age 12. The milestones of puberty for boys include:

- Enlargement of the testicles and penis
- Appearance of pubic and armpit hair
- Deepening of the voice
- Accelerated growth
- Increase in muscle mass
- Facial hair

Disorders of puberty may include delayed puberty, premature (precocious) puberty and incomplete or absent puberty. Delayed puberty is the most common problem. In most children, delayed puberty is just a variation of the normal process, and no specific cause is found. In these instances, puberty just occurs late, and the child becomes a normal adult. Both early and late puberty can run in families.

Sometimes, abnormal puberty is due to a medical condition. Delayed puberty may result from conditions such as hypopituitarism, genetic abnormalities, hypogonadism and some long-term illnesses, such as asthma and kidney disease. Puberty may also be delayed in children who are involved in extensive athletic training or excessive exercise, who have an eating disorder, who are malnourished or who've had chemotherapy or radiation.

Typically, precocious puberty is caused by the abnormally early onset of the hypothalamus and pituitary changes that start puberty. The reasons for this early onset — which can occur several years earlier than usual — are usually unknown. But it can also be caused by tumors of the brain, testicles or adrenal glands.

Additional causes include congenital adrenal hyperplasia (see page 1047) or severe hypothyroidism. Precocious puberty can result in shorter adult height.

Boys whose penis and testicles haven't completely developed 5 years after the start of development, or who haven't experienced any testicular development by age 14, may be experiencing late puberty. On the other hand, puberty may be early if a young boy has an increase in testicle size and penis length before age 9.

Diagnosis

To evaluate the possible cause of abnormal puberty, take your child in for a physical exam. The doctor might order some tests, including:

- Hormone levels in the blood
- An X-ray of the wrist to see if bone growth is normal
- A computerized tomography (CT) scan or magnetic resonance imaging (MRI) of the head to look for a tumor or brain injury
- Genetic studies

Treatment

Treatment depends on the cause. Sometimes, a cause can't be found, even after several tests. Hormone replacement may be given to start development of secondary sex characteristics. Hormone treatments are also available for certain types of premature puberty.

Sometimes, children experiencing abnormal puberty need help dealing with issues related to being either less or more sexually developed than their peers. Psychological counseling may be helpful. If you think that your child could benefit from counseling, talk to your doctor.

Gynecomastia

Gynecomastia is the term for male breast enlargement. It's common during puberty. As many as two-thirds of boys experience breast tenderness and enlargement during this time. Gynecomastia occurs as a result of changes in hormones — an imbalance in the ratio of estrogen to testosterone that can normally occur at puberty or as part of aging.

It's normal for newborn boys to have enlarged breast tissue due to exposure to maternal estrogen. This typically disappears soon after birth. In adult males, the most common cause of gynecomastia is hypogonadism. It may also occur as a result of using alcohol, some medications and some illicit drugs, including marijuana, amphetamines and heroin. Chronic liver disease, hyperthyroidism and rare endocrine tumors can cause breast enlargement, as can breast cancer, which occurs very rarely in men.

Some men and boys have fat on their chests that makes it look as if they have breasts. This isn't the same thing as gynecomastia.

Treatment

Whether you need treatment for gynecomastia depends on your age and what the doctor learns from your medical history and exam. In teenagers, breast enlargement usually goes away on its own in 2 or 3 years, and no treatment is necessary. Younger boys and adult men with gynecomastia usually should be evaluated to find out what's causing the problem.

Treatment is necessary if the breast enlargement is caused by a disease or tumor. In men with testosterone deficiency, hormone replacement can produce a dramatic improvement. Rarely, surgery may be necessary to remove the extra breast tissue. If there's concern that it could be cancer, you may have a mammogram and a small sample of tissue may be removed (biopsied) for laboratory analysis.

Hypogonadism

Male hypogonadism, sometimes referred to as testosterone deficiency, results from an inability of the testicles to produce testosterone, sperm or both. Hypogonadism can develop at any age, even before birth. Approximately 1 in 500 men and boys are affected.

The two basic types of male hypogonadism are primary testicular failure, caused by an abnormality in the testicles, and secondary testicular failure, which stems from a problem in the hypothalamus or pituitary gland. In secondary testicular failure, the testicles are normal, but they function improperly due to lack of stimulation by pituitary hormones.

Both forms of male hypogonadism can have many causes. It's important to establish the precise cause so that appropriate treatment can be prescribed. Common causes of primary male hypogonadism include:

- Klinefelter's syndrome, a congenital abnormality of the sex chromosomes
- Undescended testicles
- Too much iron in the blood
- Injury to the testicles
- Mumps infection
- Prior hernia surgery
- Cancer treatment using chemotherapy or radiation

Causes of secondary hypogonadism include:

- Kallmann's syndrome, a hypothalamic disorder
- Pituitary tumors
- Other pituitary disorders
- Medications, including some psychiatric drugs
- Normal aging

The effects of male hypogonadism are determined primarily by the stage of life when it occurs. During fetal development, hypogonadism may affect development of the external genitalia, leading to a condition called ambiguous genitalia, in which the sex of the newborn isn't clear from external examination.

When hypogonadism occurs during puberty, it may slow growth and impair development of many secondary sex characteristics. A boy with this condition may not develop increased muscle mass, a deepened voice and body hair. The penis and testicles may not grow. Changes in skeletal development can lead to unusually long arms and legs, disproportionate to body height.

In adult males, hypogonadism can cause erectile dysfunction and infertility. It may also lead to a decrease in facial and body hair growth, thinning of the skin, development of breast tissue (gynecomastia) and loss of bone mass. In addition, mental and emotional changes, such as mood swings, irritability, decreased sex drive and depression, can accompany hypogonadism.

Diagnosis

Early diagnosis and treatment can help boys prevent delayed puberty and can protect adult men against osteoporosis and other risks of untreated hypogonadism.

A diagnosis of hypogonadism is based on symptoms and the results of blood tests that measure testosterone levels. Additional studies may be done to determine the cause. These may include hormone testing, semen analysis, pituitary imaging, genetic studies and testicular biopsy.

Treatment
Treatment depends on the cause. Testosterone replacement therapy given by injection, patch or gel is effective to restore normal testosterone levels. In boys, it can stimulate puberty. No effective treatment exists to restore sperm production if you have primary hypogonadism. If a pituitary problem is the cause, pituitary hormones may stimulate sperm production and restore fertility. A pituitary tumor may require surgical removal, medication or hormone replacement.

Female sex gland disorders

In females, sex hormones work together in an intricate pattern to make the reproductive cycle function smoothly. The major female sex hormones are estrogen and progesterone, which are produced mainly by the ovaries during the reproductive years.

Besides helping control ovulation, conception and pregnancy, estrogen maintains bone strength and helps regulate cholesterol. Progesterone works with estrogen to prepare a woman's body for conception and pregnancy and helps regulate her menstrual cycle.

Problems with production and release of sex hormones can affect sexual development, sexual characteristics and fertility.

Abnormal puberty

In girls, puberty normally begins between ages 8 and 14. Some researchers suggest that normal puberty may begin earlier — as young as age 6 or 7. In girls, milestones of puberty include:

- Development of breast buds
- Appearance of pubic and armpit hair
- Menstruation

Abnormal puberty may include delayed puberty, premature (precocious) puberty and incomplete or absent puberty. Delayed puberty is the most common problem. In most children, delayed puberty is just a variation of the normal process, and no specific cause is found. In these instances, puberty occurs late, but the child becomes a normal adult. Both early and late puberty can run in families.

Sometimes, abnormal puberty is due to a medical condition. Delayed puberty may be caused by hypopituitarism, genetic abnormalities, hypogonadism and some long-term illnesses, such as asthma and kidney disease. Puberty may also be delayed in children who are involved in extensive athletic training or excessive exercise, who have an eating disorder, who are malnourished or who've had chemotherapy or radiation.

Typically, precocious puberty is caused by the abnormally early onset of the hypothalamus and pituitary changes that start puberty. The reasons for this early onset — which can occur several years earlier than usual — are often unknown. Precocious puberty can also be caused by tumors of the brain or adrenal glands, or severe hypothyroidism. A potential long-term consequence of premature puberty is shorter height.

A girl may be experiencing early puberty if she develops breasts and pubic hair before age 8. Puberty may be delayed if a girl hasn't developed breast tissue by age 14 or hasn't had a menstrual period within 5 years of the first appearance of breast tissue.

Diagnosis
To evaluate the possible cause of abnormal puberty, a doctor will perform a physical examination and may order some tests. These include:

- Blood tests to check hormone levels
- An X-ray of the wrist to see if bone growth is normal
- A computerized tomography (CT) scan or magnetic resonance imaging (MRI) of the head to look for a tumor or brain injury
- Ultrasound of the ovaries
- Genetic studies

Treatment
Treatment depends on what's causing the problems. Sometimes the cause can't be found. Hormone replacement treatment may initiate the development of secondary sex characteristics. It also may be used for certain types of premature puberty.

Some children need help dealing with issues related to being either less or more sexually developed than their peers. Psychological counseling may be helpful. If you think your child could benefit from counseling, talk to your doctor.

Hypogonadism

Female hypogonadism occurs when the ovaries produce inadequate quantities of sex hormones. Primary hypogonadism originates from an abnormality in the ovaries, and secondary hypogonadism stems from a problem in the hypothalamus or pituitary gland. In secondary hypogonadism, the ovaries function improperly due to lack of stimulation by pituitary hormones.

Primary hypogonadism may be caused by Turner's syndrome, a congenital abnormality of the sex chromosomes, by other genetic disorders or by an autoimmune disease that causes ovarian failure. Causes of secondary hypogonadism include hypopituitarism, disorders involving the hypothalamus, polycystic ovary syndrome, severe stress, anorexia nervosa and excessive exercise. Many times, no clear cause can be found.

Except in Turner's syndrome, symptoms of female hypogonadism usually aren't apparent until puberty. In premenopausal women, signs and symptoms include:

- Irregular or absent menstrual periods
- Infertility
- Decreased vaginal secretions
- Decreased sex drive
- A decrease in breast size

Left untreated, females with hypogonadism are at increased risk of developing osteoporosis.

Diagnosis
A diagnosis of hypogonadism is based on symptoms and the results of blood tests that measure estrogen and other sex hormone levels. Other studies may include chromosomal (genetic) testing, an MRI of the pituitary gland and an ultrasound scan of the ovaries.

Treatment
Treatment depends on the cause. Hormone replacement with estrogen and progesterone can help women maintain secondary sexual characteristics and restore a normal menstrual cycle. To treat infertility, medications that stimulate ovulation may be used.

If a pituitary problem is the cause, pituitary hormones may be prescribed. A pituitary tumor may require surgical removal, medication or hormone replacement.

Virilization
Normally, a woman's ovaries and adrenal glands secrete some male hormones (androgens) such as testosterone. Virilization is a rare condition in which excess androgens circulate in your body, most often because your ovaries or adrenal glands are overproducing these hormones. Excess androgens may also come from taking androgen hormones, such as dehydroepiandrosterone (DHEA).

An excess of male hormones in a woman leads to development of masculine physical characteristics such as excessive hair growth, increased muscle bulk, deepening of the voice, and irregular menstrual periods. Hair growth similar to a man's (hirsutism) may be the first manifestation of virilization, but the two disorders aren't the same. Virilization is much less common than hirsutism and may be associated with a serious underlying condition, such as an ovarian or adrenal gland tumor.

Diagnosis
If you have signs of virilization, seek prompt medical attention because a cancerous (malignant) tumor is possible. Your doctor will likely perform a physical exam and request blood tests to measure the levels of male hormones. You may also have an ultrasound of your ovaries or a CT scan or MRI of the adrenal glands to detect the presence of a tumor or identify polycystic ovaries.

Treatment
Once the underlying cause of the condition is identified, treatment may include surgery to remove a tumor or medication to reduce androgen production.

Endocrine Syndromes

Some disorders of the endocrine system affect more than one gland. As a result, an individual may have symptoms of several endocrine problems.

Two main groups of disorders affect multiple endocrine glands. In polyglandular autoimmune syndromes (PGA), several endocrine glands become underactive and produce lower than normal amounts of hormones. In multiple endocrine neoplasia (MEN) syndromes, tumors develop in more than one of the endocrine glands.

Polyglandular autoimmune syndromes and MEN syndromes are inherited. Some of these conditions are associated with a particular genetic defect. For that reason, family members of a person with an endocrine syndrome are usually screened for a possible genetic defect or to detect signs of a disorder before serious problems appear.

Polyglandular autoimmune syndromes

Polyglandular autoimmune (PGA) syndromes cause several endocrine glands to underproduce hormones. A person with such a syndrome has an inherited tendency to develop antibodies that react to cells in the endocrine glands. An autoimmune reaction can cause inflammation of endocrine glands and, eventually, progressive destruction of the glands. As the glands are destroyed, they stop producing hormones, leading to various disorders.

Types
There are two PGA syndromes — type 1 and type 2:

PGA 1
Type 1 is a rare inherited disorder that usually develops in early childhood and is equally prevalent among girls and boys. Frequent yeast infections in childhood are often the first sign of the syndrome. The two other most common features are an underactive parathyroid gland (hypoparathyroidism) and underactive adrenal glands. These problems may not develop until middle age. People with PGA 1 may also have hypogonadism, hepatitis, gallstones, difficulty in absorbing food, loss of pigmentation and type 1 diabetes.

PGA 2
Type 2 is more common. It also runs in families, and is seen more often in women than in men. The first manifestations usually appear around age 30. In this disorder, the adrenal glands are underactive, and the thyroid gland may be underactive or overactive. A person with PGA 2 may have Addison's disease, Graves' disease or autoimmune (Hashimoto's) thyroiditis, type 1 diabetes, hypogonadism, myasthenia gravis and celiac disease. Unlike PGA 1, type 2 doesn't involve recurrent yeast infections or hypoparathyroidism.

Treatment
Treatment depends on the type you have and your symptoms. If you have a hormone deficiency, you may need to take hormone replacement therapy. This may include thyroid hormone, corticosteroids

and insulin. Screening tests often can detect problems before serious signs and symptoms develop.

Multiple endocrine neoplasia syndromes

Multiple endocrine neoplasia (MEN) syndromes are rare inherited diseases in which tumors develop in several endocrine glands. The syndromes are generally inherited, but there's variability, even within the same family, of which glands will develop tumors. The tumors may appear as early as infancy or as late as age 70. They may be noncancerous (benign) or cancerous (malignant). Signs and symptoms result mostly from production of excess hormones.

Types

There are two main types of MEN, based on which glands develop tumors.

MEN 1

People with MEN type 1 (MEN 1) have tumors of the parathyroid gland, the islet cells of the pancreas, the pituitary gland or all three. This type involves a genetic abnormality on chromosome 11.

MEN 2

MEN type 2 has two subtypes, MEN 2A and MEN 2B. Both are associated with genetic defects on chromosome 10 and include a rare type of thyroid cancer (medullary thyroid cancer) and adrenal gland tumors called pheochromocytomas. Parathyroid tumors can occur in MEN 2A but are rarely seen in MEN 2B.

Individuals with MEN 2 typically have long limbs and loose joints, as well as growths or nodules around the nerves (ganglioneuromas) that may be noticeable on the eyes, lips and tongue. The nodules are also found in the gastrointestinal tract.

Treatment

Doctors generally treat each tumor individually, either by removing it or by correcting the hormone imbalance. Sometimes one surgery doesn't resolve the problem. Some people need multiple surgical procedures on two or more endocrine glands during their lifetime.

As soon as someone receives a diagnosis of MEN 2B — even in infancy — a doctor will likely recommend removing the thyroid gland, since medullary thyroid cancer is particularly aggressive in this disease. Removal of the thyroid before there is any apparent disease in the gland is also often recommended in a person with type 2A.

If you receive a diagnosis of MEN, screening of your immediate blood relatives is very important. Early detection and treatment can be life-saving. Genetic testing and blood and urine tests to measure hormone levels can detect early stages of the tumors. When detected early, these tumors have a much greater chance of being removed with a favorable outcome.

Obesity

It's common to hear people attribute their weight gain or being overweight to "low metabolism," heredity or a medical problem.

Actually, obesity doesn't have just one cause. Being overweight stems from a complex interaction of several factors. Genes and metabolism do play a role in your weight, but in most cases, the amount you weigh is determined by your diet and physical activity. Consuming too many calories, leading an inactive lifestyle or a combination of both leads to obesity.

Genetics

A family history of obesity increases your chance of becoming obese by about 30 percent. Your genes affect the rate at which your body accumulates fat and where that fat is stored. By influencing the amount of body fat and fat distribution, genes can make you more susceptible to gaining weight.

Researchers have identified several genes known to contribute to obesity. In most cases, multiple genes — rather than a single "fat gene" — interact in complex ways to cause obesity. These mechanisms aren't fully understood. A few rare inherited diseases, such as Prader-Willi syndrome and Cohen syndrome, are known to cause obesity.

For common forms of obesity, it's clear that environmental factors exert an enormous influence. It's easy to eat too much in a society where large portions of high-fat foods are the norm and many people get little daily physical activity.

Metabolic and endocrine disorders

Some people have a naturally high metabolic thermostat — they tend to burn more calories than average even when they're asleep. Other individuals need fewer calories for the same physical activity. A low metabolic rate is rarely a cause of obesity, however.

In fact, most overweight people have a higher metabolic rate and burn more calories at rest than do lean people of the same height. However, when some obese people lose weight, they burn fewer calories at rest, making it hard to keep the weight off.

Some endocrine disorders can cause weight gain. However, less than 5 percent of all cases of obesity can be traced to a metabolic disorder or hormonal imbalance. Endocrine disorders that may lead to obesity include:

- Cushing's syndrome
- Hypothyroidism
- Insulinoma
- Tumors, injury or inflammation of the hypothalamus
- Polycystic ovary syndrome

For information on how to lose weight, see Chapter 3, "Controlling Your Weight." ■

CHAPTER 33 PART V

Female Reproductive System

The primary biological function of the female reproductive system is the creation of offspring. But the sex organs also play a crucial role in a woman's overall health and well-being. Maintaining good reproductive health is important. Doing so involves having regular checkups and tests. Understanding how the female reproductive system functions also can help you understand natural changes that take place during a woman's life.

Female Reproductive Organs

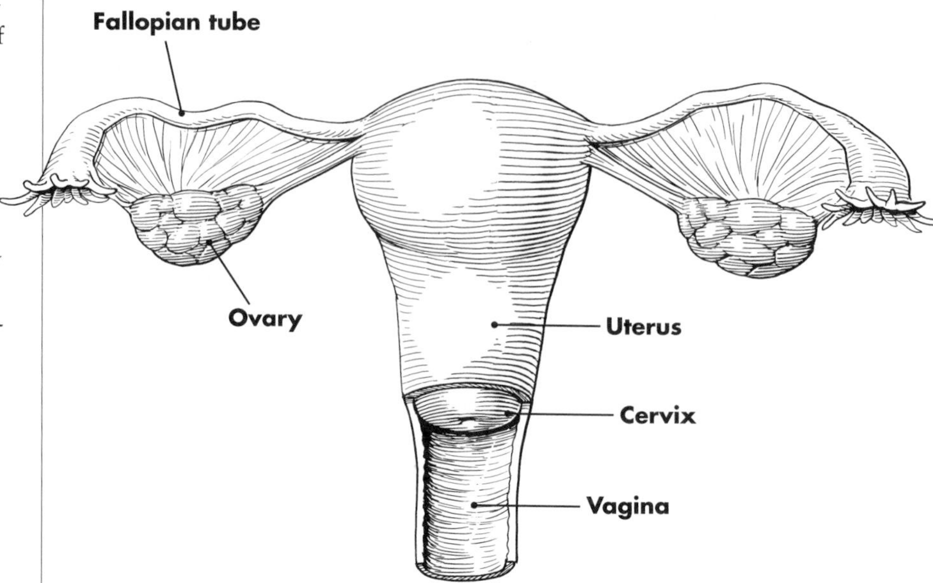

Reproductive Organs

The female reproductive system is made up of the organs associated with childbearing. These organs include the two ovaries, the fallopian tubes, the uterus and the external genitalia.

Ovaries

The ovaries are situated in the lower part of a woman's pelvis, about 4 or 5 inches below the waist. Before birth, a female fetus contains hundreds of thousands of eggs (ova), many of which disappear before birth. By the time a baby girl is born, her ovaries are stocked with all the eggs she'll need. Beginning in puberty, the ovaries regularly release an egg into the fallopian tubes in a process called ovulation. The ovaries also produce the female sex hormones estrogen and progesterone, which are important in the development and maintenance of feminine physical characteristics.

The ovaries constantly change in size during the reproductive years, the normal range varying from the size of an almond to the size of a walnut.

Fallopian tubes

Between each ovary and the uterus lies a thin, 4- or 5-inch-long passageway called a fallopian tube. Each tube is no wider than a needle. Fertilization takes place within a fallopian tube when a sperm penetrates an egg that has been released from one of the ovaries. The fertilized egg then travels down the tube and into the uterus.

Uterus

The uterus is a pear-shaped organ, about $2\frac{1}{2}$ inches long in a nonpregnant woman. The walls of the uterus are thick and made up primarily of powerful muscles.

When a fertilized egg reaches the uterus, it implants itself within the uterine wall and begins to develop into a baby. If the egg isn't fertilized, it degenerates and the lining of the uterus is shed during menstruation.

The narrow neck of the uterus (cervix) also has thick walls. Ordinarily, the opening of the cervix is very small — big enough for menstrual fluids to pass through but not large enough that you could accidentally thrust a tampon, for example, into it. During labor, the cervical opening expands (dilates) to allow passage of the baby, and the muscles of the uterine wall contract to push the baby out.

The cervix extends into the vagina, a muscular tube about 5 inches long. Most of the time, the walls of the vagina touch, but they can expand to accommodate something as small as a tampon or as large as a full-term baby. Cells in the vaginal walls secrete lubricants. In girls, the hymen — a thin membrane — partly blocks the opening of the vaginal canal. It often remains intact until first sexual intercourse. In rare cases, a doctor has to make an incision in the hymen before a girl can menstruate.

External genitals

The female external genitals — the mons pubis, the labia, the clitoris and the opening (vestibule) of your vagina — are called the vulva. The mons pubis is the pad of fatty tissue at the base of the abdomen that becomes covered with hair at puberty. The labia are double folds of tissue that extend downward on either side of your vagina — the outer folds are the labia majora and the inner folds are the labia minora. *Labia* is the Latin word for "lips."

Where the labia meet near the front of the body, they cover a small protrusion, which is the tip of the clitoris. During sexual arousal, the clitoris, like the male penis, becomes erect. Bartholin's glands, which empty into the vestibule of

Successful Reproduction

During sexual intercourse — when a man inserts his erect penis into a woman's vagina and ejaculates sperm-saturated semen — the vagina is flooded with millions of sperm swimming in all directions in search of an egg to fertilize. Most sperm die within the vagina and never even reach the woman's cervical canal, the opening between the vagina and the uterus. Of those that make it to the 1-inch cervical canal, most never make it any farther.

Only a few sperm reach the uterus and successfully make the journey midway down one of the fallopian tubes where an egg is located, provided it's the time of the month when the woman has released an egg from an ovary (ovulated). When a sperm finds and penetrates an egg, fertilization has occurred and a pregnancy has begun. The sperm that fertilizes an egg has overcome enormous odds.

To result in pregnancy, sexual intercourse usually must take place within the 72 hours before an egg (ovum) enters a fallopian tube. Some of these sperm are stored in the woman's cervical mucus and released over time into the uterus and fallopian tubes. If some of these sperm stay viable for up to a few hours after an egg is released from an ovary, one of them may find and fertilize the egg. The best chance of becoming pregnant is just before the release of an egg (ovulation). Ovulation usually occurs once every menstrual cycle, about 14 days before the start of a woman's next period.

Even perfect timing, though, doesn't guarantee a pregnancy. At best, in fact, couples have only about a 30 percent chance of achieving pregnancy in any one cycle. To become pregnant through sexual intercourse requires both a healthy female reproductive system and a healthy male reproductive system.

In a woman, an irregular ovulation pattern can make fertilization of an egg more difficult. The fallopian tubes must be open and receptive to the egg and sperm. Women whose tubes contain scar tissue from a previous infection or surgery may not be able to get pregnant without surgery or reproductive assistance.

Even cervical mucus must have just the right characteristics to allow sperm entry. Mucus that's too thick or acidic can prevent fertilization. Acidic mucus can make the vagina hostile to sperm, which thrive in alkaline surroundings.

As for the man, he must produce not only an adequate number of sperm but sperm that are active and healthy (see Chapter 34, "Male Reproductive System").

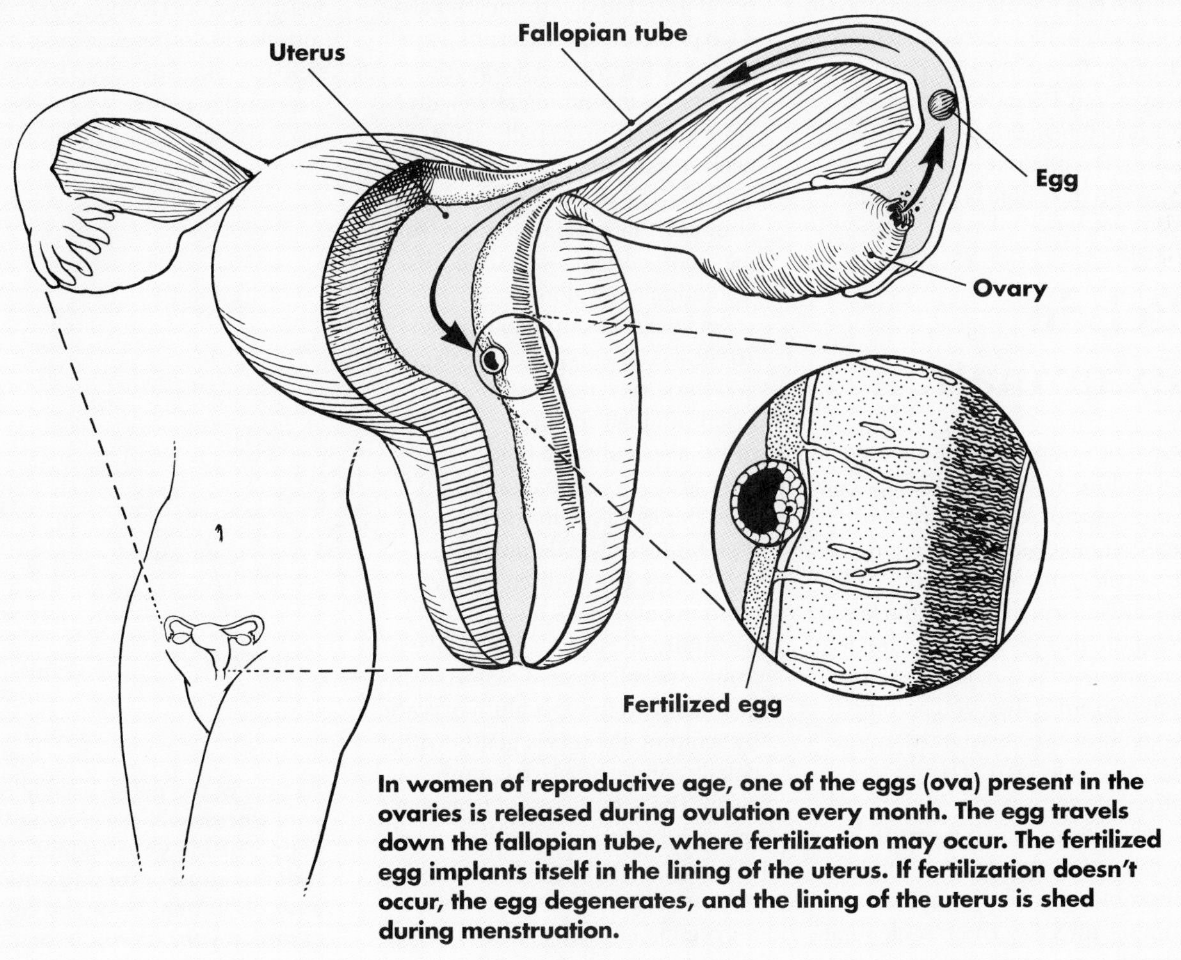

In women of reproductive age, one of the eggs (ova) present in the ovaries is released during ovulation every month. The egg travels down the fallopian tube, where fertilization may occur. The fertilized egg implants itself in the lining of the uterus. If fertilization doesn't occur, the egg degenerates, and the lining of the uterus is shed during menstruation.

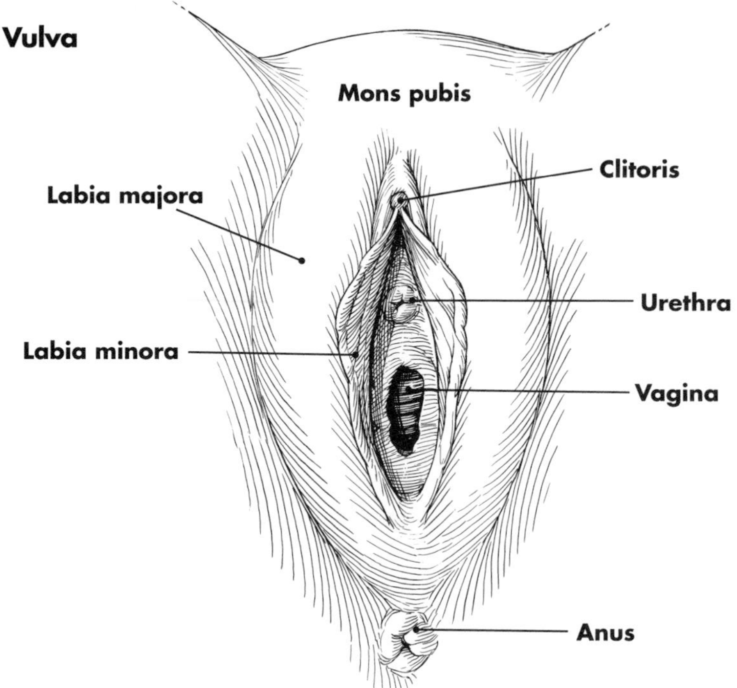

the vagina, secrete substances that lubricate the vaginal opening.

The smaller opening between the clitoris and vagina is the entrance to the urethra. Not involved in reproduction, the urethra is a passageway, about $1\frac{1}{2}$ inches long, that leads to the bladder, which stores urine. The bladder is situated between the pubic bone and uterus.

Pelvic Examination

A pelvic examination is a simple procedure that can be done by your family doctor, a gynecologist or another health care professional. A gynecologist is a doctor trained to treat disorders that affect the female reproductive system. It's extremely important to begin having regular pelvic exams when you become sexually active. A pelvic examination is usually part of a routine physical examination.

Pelvic exams are important because they can detect a number of problems, including cysts, tumors, infection and muscle weakness that can cause the uterus or vagina to sag. If you have a suspicious discharge, your doctor can obtain a sample of material that can be analyzed to determine the cause.

To perform a pelvic exam, your doctor will have you lie on your back on an examining table with your knees bent. Usually, your heels rest in metal supports called stirrups. The doctor first examines your external genitals to make sure they look normal — no sores, discoloration or swelling.

An internal examination is next. To see the inner walls of the vagina and the cervix, the doctor inserts an instrument called a speculum to hold the vaginal walls apart and then shines a light inside to look for lesions, inflammation, signs of abnormal discharge or anything else that's unusual. Generally, the next step is to take a sample of cells from the cervix. This is done, with the speculum in place, by scraping the cervix gently with a small spatula, brush or cotton swab. The sample is sent to a laboratory for a Pap test, which is used to screen for cancer of the cervix.

Your doctor can't see your internal organs, such as your uterus and ovaries, but can examine them by touch (palpation) after removing the speculum. To do this, your doctor inserts two lubricated, gloved fingers into your vagina. By pressing down on your abdomen with the other hand while maneuvering the fingers inside your vagina, he or she can locate your uterus, ovaries and other organs, judge their size and confirm that they're in their proper positions. By exploring the contours of these organs, your doctor sometimes can detect tumors or cysts.

To palpate the same organs from a different angle, and to examine your rectum, your doctor may also insert a finger into your rectum and manipulate that finger, together with a finger in your vagina.

As your doctor palpates your internal organs, you may feel somewhat uncomfortable. However, the experience shouldn't be painful. If you do experience pain or tenderness, say so immediately. You'll feel less discomfort if you can relax the muscles in your pelvic area. It often helps to take slow, deep breaths.

A routine gynecological checkup also often includes a medical his-

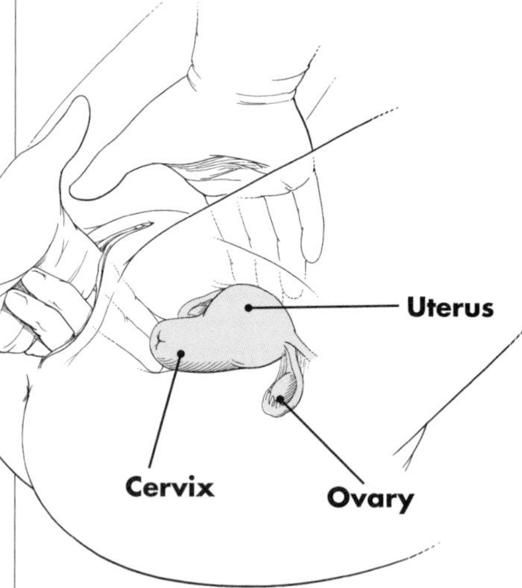

As part of the pelvic examination, your doctor will insert two gloved fingers inside your vagina. While simultaneously pressing down on your abdomen, he or she can examine your uterus, ovaries and other organs.

tory and an examination of your breasts. If you've begun menstruating, your doctor will want to know the date of your last menstrual period. You'll likely be asked about past pregnancies and their outcomes and about what form of birth control you're using, if any. You may be weighed and have your blood pressure measured, and you may be asked for urine and blood samples to be analyzed in the laboratory.

The American College of Obstetricians and Gynecologists recommends that you have an initial pelvic examination at age 18, or earlier if you're sexually active.

Menstrual Cycle

From puberty through menopause, most women cycle through a complex monthly process of hormonal fluctuations and bodily changes. Designed to enable them to bear children, the process most often ends in the shedding of the uterine lining known as menstruation.

Puberty and menarche

At birth, your ovaries contain all the eggs (ova) they'll ever have. However, the eggs remain almost dormant until stimulated by a surge of pituitary hormones. That happens at puberty, which begins when a girl is about 8 years old. At that time, a few eggs each month begin to enlarge and to develop additional layers of outer cells. The cells form a capsule (follicle) around the egg, and they begin to produce the hormone estrogen.

During childhood, a girl's body produces estrogen in very small quantities, but at puberty her estrogen level increases about 20-fold. Meanwhile, the ovaries themselves grow larger as the eggs develop, and other internal reproductive organs also grow and mature.

External signs of change appear during puberty, as well. A girl's breasts begin to bud as estrogen induces the development of milk ducts. One breast may start to grow before the other, and the two may develop at different rates, but they usually end up approximately the same size. Next, the girl develops pubic hair and, later, underarm hair. She experiences a growth spurt, and as her hips and breasts become more rounded, she begins to look more like a woman.

Approximately 2 years after a girl's breasts begin to bud, she reaches menarche — that is, she menstruates for the first time. Menarche marks the beginning of her reproductive life, just as menopause — the cessation of ovarian functioning — marks the end of it.

In addition, during puberty a girl's pituitary gland begins to secrete increasing amounts of two key hormones: follicle-stimulating hormone (FSH) and luteinizing hormone (LH). As a result of FSH secretion, fluid develops within some of the follicles that surround the eggs. Some grow larger and bulge, while others shrivel and die. Every month after puberty, one — or sometimes two — of these fluid-filled follicles reaches full development.

A surge of LH stimulates the follicle to release an egg, which then bursts through the surface of the ovary into the pelvic cavity where it's picked up by the fallopian tube. This process is called ovulation, which generally occurs at the midpoint of the menstrual cycle. In any

Seeing a Gynecologist

Gynecology is the branch of medicine concerned with the health and study of the female organs of reproduction. The term originates from the Greek words *gyne*, meaning "woman" and *logos*, meaning "study." Gynecologists are medical doctors trained to treat disorders affecting female reproductive organs. You might consult a gynecologist for any of the following:

- Menstrual problems
- Breast problems
- Advice on birth control, abortion or sexual problems
- Treatment of infertility or sexually transmitted diseases (STDs)
- Difficulties during menopause
- Cancer that develops in any of your reproductive organs

Because gynecologists are also trained as obstetricians, many also see women through pregnancy and childbirth. Many women choose a gynecologist as their primary care doctor during their reproductive years. Family physicians, internists and some nurse practitioners also can provide routine gynecological care.

Another alternative is a certified nurse midwife, a nurse who has had specialized training in obstetrics and gynecology. Certified nurse midwives may deliver babies under some circumstances and provide well-woman care, including routine breast examinations and pelvic examinations with Pap tests. They should always work with at least one doctor who's available for consultations and in emergencies.

To find a gynecologist, you can ask another doctor to recommend one, call a local medical clinic or hospital for suggestions or ask women friends for a recommendation.

During your first visit to a gynecologist, you'll be looking for answers to important questions: Is the doctor willing to take time to explain things in language you can understand? Are you comfortable with this person? If you're not, you may want to consult other gynecologists before making a final choice.

given cycle, ovulation usually occurs from only one ovary.

Males have no counterpart to menarche, which marks a dramatic change in a female's biologic status. A girl's attitude toward menstruation and her feelings about what it means to be a woman may be influenced by the way her family and friends respond to her first menses.

Menarche typically happens after age 9 and before age 16. On average, American girls begin menstruating at 13 years, which is younger than the age at which previous generations of American women began. For the past 100 years, the average age at menarche in the United States has been dropping at the rate of 3 or 4 months every decade. Medical experts attribute the change to better nourishment.

Apparently, before hormonal changes can begin, a girl must reach a critical body weight — around 106 pounds — or she must be at that weight and also have a specific amount of body fat and body water. At any rate, girls who are overweight usually have their first menstrual period earlier than those who aren't. Very athletic girls, or those who are malnourished or have a chronic, debilitating disease generally begin menstruating later.

If a girl's breasts begin to bud before she's 8 years old or if she has her first period before age 9, consult her doctor. This rare condition is called precocious puberty. It has several possible causes, but it's usually treatable. It's also a good idea to consult a doctor if a girl has no breast development by age 14 or if she hasn't begun to menstruate by the time she's 16 years old, especially if she's concerned about her development.

For the first few years after menarche, it's normal for a girl's menstrual cycle to be irregular and for her to skip a period at times. Her ovaries probably aren't yet releasing an ovum every month. However, young women need to be aware that they can become pregnant even before their first period, because the first egg may be released before menstruation begins.

In medical terms, puberty ends only after menstruation is established and is regular.

Normal menstrual cycle

Your menstrual cycle begins on the first day of flow of one menstrual period and ends on the first day of flow of the next. The release of an egg — a single cell barely visible to the naked eye — occurs approximately in the middle of the normal menstrual cycle.

Each month, as you menstruate, several follicles begin to develop in one of your ovaries, getting your next cycle under way. After a week or so, one follicle begins to outgrow the others, which shrink to normal size. Meanwhile, your ovaries secrete more estrogen, much of it produced by the outer cells of that single, dominant follicle. The estrogen acts on the lining of the uterus (endometrium), causing it to grow and thicken.

A day or two before ovulation, estrogen levels peak. They then start to decrease, and the dominant follicle begins to produce tiny amounts of the hormone progesterone. The follicle swells, ruptures and releases its egg, while the other follicles that were in the race for ovulation disappear. Other bodily changes include a slight increase in body temperature and a change in secretions from the glands in your cervix.

After its release from the follicle, the egg is picked up by one of the fallopian tubes and begins a journey to your uterus that generally takes about 6 days. While the egg is in transit, a sperm may fertilize it if you've recently had sexual intercourse. Fertilization generally takes place within a few hours after ovulation, before the egg has traveled more than a third of the way down the tube.

Even as the egg travels toward your uterus, its empty follicle in your ovary changes. Once again, it enlarges rapidly — at this stage it's called the corpus luteum — and begins to secrete large quantities of progesterone and estrogen. Under the impact of these hormones, your endometrium begins to function. Its glands secrete substances and release nutrients, and its blood supply and number of tiny blood vessels in the tissue increase. By the end of your menstrual cycle, the uterine lining has doubled in thickness, and large amounts of nutrients have been stored there, ready to nourish a fertilized egg.

If you become pregnant — meaning that a fertilized egg has become implanted in your endometrium — the hormones secreted by the corpus luteum will help to sustain the pregnancy. If you don't become pregnant, the egg disintegrates or leaves your body in vaginal secretions, usually before menstruation begins.

About 2 weeks after ovulation, the corpus luteum begins to shrink, and levels of estrogen and progesterone decrease. Your uterus starts to shed its lining, and menstrual bleeding (menses) begins.

Menstrual flow contains blood, vaginal and cervical secretions and tissue sloughed from the lining of your uterus. By the fourth or fifth day of your period, the endometrium has become thin, and the process of rebuilding it has already begun.

On average, a menstrual cycle is 28 days long, although cycles normally range anywhere from 23 to 35 days. If your cycle doesn't fall within this range, it may not be a problem. However, extremely long or extremely short cycles are sometimes associated with infertility. On average, menstrual bleeding lasts 4 to 5 days, but periods as short as 2 days or as long as 7 aren't unusual.

At times, your period may become temporarily irregular for no obvious reason. You may skip a period or have one that's much longer, shorter or heavier than usual. Sometimes this change simply reflects your age. Menstrual cycles are apt to last longer both at menarche and as you approach menopause. At other times, stress may play a role.

Preventing Pregnancy

Thanks to several effective contraceptive methods, women can choose whether they want to become pregnant and when. Some birth control methods rely primarily on actions taken by the man (see page 1107). Others rely on the actions of the woman. The following methods depend primarily on the woman.

Natural family planning

Natural family planning encompasses several methods that rely on a woman's menstrual cycle to determine what days may be safe for intercourse. They're variations of the so-called rhythm method.

Each of the approaches in natural family planning involves a conscientious awareness of when you can become pregnant, which is but a brief span in the middle of each menstrual cycle — from about 72 hours before ovulation to about 24 hours after ovulation. The key is to determine when these days occur in your cycle and to avoid having intercourse at that time.

Highly motivated couples can use natural family planning effectively. In population-based studies, natural family planning has a failure rate of about 20 percent. Predicting ovulation is difficult because a woman's cycle may vary from month to month. If you decide to try natural family planning, keep records for several months to establish a pattern for your menstrual cycle.

There are four ways to calculate the time of ovulation: the temperature method, the calendar method, the cervical mucus inspection method and the mucothermal

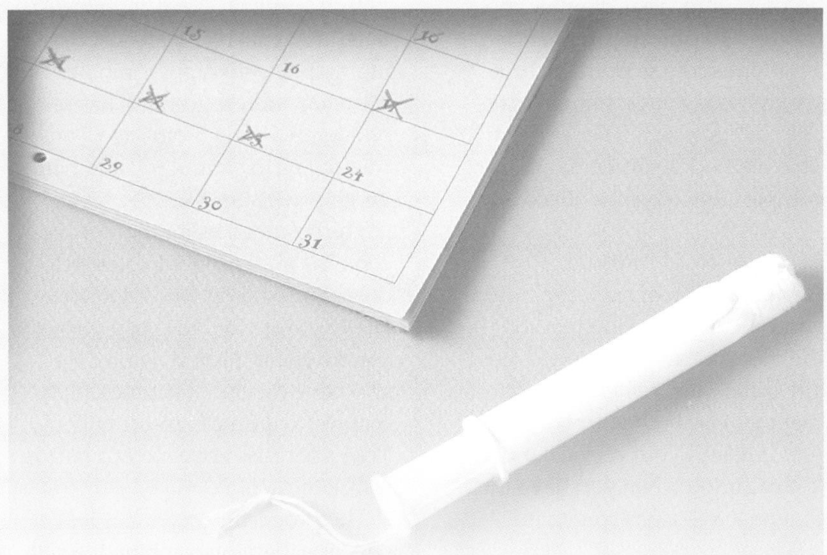

Menstrual Products

Years ago, women who were menstruating used cloths to catch their menstrual flow, rinsing them out and reusing them. Today, commercially made sanitary napkins are available, as are tampons and menstrual sponges that women insert into the vagina to absorb menstrual fluids. Menstrual sponges are rarely used today.

Napkins and tampons are often labeled regular or super. These terms refer to the product's ability to absorb, rather than to its physical size. Because there are no common standards and one brand's "regular" may be as absorbent as another brand's "super," you'll have to find out by trial and error what works best for you.

Change the tampon every few hours, and use a pad instead of a tampon at night. One reason for such precautions is toxic shock syndrome, a rare but potentially dangerous disorder that's associated most often with tampons and occasionally with extended use of contraceptive sponges, especially among women younger than age 30.

In the early 1980s, there was a small epidemic of toxic shock syndrome, for the most part involving young, menstruating women who had been using a particular brand of superabsorbent tampons. Researchers reported that the syndrome appeared to be caused by toxins produced by a type of bacteria called *Staphylococcus aureus.*

Some researchers theorized that when the women left superabsorbent tampons in place for a long time, the tampons became a breeding ground for these bacteria. Others suggested that the fibers in the tampons scratched the surface of the vagina, making it possible for the bacteria or their toxins to enter the bloodstream.

The brand of tampons associated with the original epidemic was taken off the market. Since then, the number of cases of toxic shock syndrome has declined, even though most tampons today contain some superabsorbent fiber. Still, it's a good idea to change your tampon every few hours.

If you use a napkin or tampon that's scented or deodorized, your vagina or vulva may begin to itch or become irritated during your period. Some women are allergic to the chemicals used in these products. Menstrual fluid is actually odorless until it comes into contact with bacteria and air. In general, if you bathe regularly and change napkins or tampons often, you won't have a problem with odor.

method. Effective natural family planning requires using all of these techniques.

Temperature method

Most women have a slight rise in body temperature just after ovulation. To detect a temperature change, take and record your temperature every day when you wake up. You'll need to use a basal thermometer — a special thermometer designed to detect the postovulatory rise in temperature. Basal thermometers are available in most pharmacies. This technique can be helpful in recognizing patterns, but since temperatures change only after ovulation, it's not effective alone.

Calendar method

To use this method, you need to keep a record of your cycles for a year. Then take the number of days in your shortest cycle and subtract 18 (18 is used because it equals 14 days from ovulation to the first day of your period plus 4 days for the average life span of a sperm). Subtract 10 from the number of days in your longest cycle (10 equals 14 days from ovulation to the first day of your period minus 1 day for the life span of an egg and minus 3 more days for a margin of error). The results of your calculations are the first and last days of your cycle during which you can become pregnant.

For example, if your shortest cycle is 24 days and the longest is 35 days, then the time during which you can become pregnant is between 24 days minus 18 days (the 6th day) and 35 days minus 10 days (the 25th day). So, potentially, you could become pregnant from the 6th through the 25th days of each cycle.

This method requires that menstrual cycles be very regular, and it demands long periods of abstinence.

Cervical mucus inspection method

About 4 days before the release of an egg, your vaginal mucus becomes thin, clear, runnier and profuse. To prevent pregnancy, avoid intercourse from the time such mucus appears until 4 days after it becomes thicker and drier. This method is somewhat more complex, but it can be effective.

Mucothermal method

A combination of the temperature and mucus inspection methods — the mucothermal method — generally is the most reliable natural method. Use both your basal temperature and your cervical mucus to determine when you have the potential to become pregnant.

Birth control pills

One of every four American women younger than age 45 use birth control pills. And about 1 in 100 of these women become pregnant each year.

Today's birth control pills are very different from the original formulation because manufacturers have reduced the dose of female hormones. When oral contraceptives contained high levels of estrogen, they carried a significant risk of blood clots. You still face some risk of blood clots if you take the newer, lower-dose pills, but the danger is slight. Smoking greatly increases the risk of side effects from birth control pills. Smokers older than age 35 shouldn't use birth control pills.

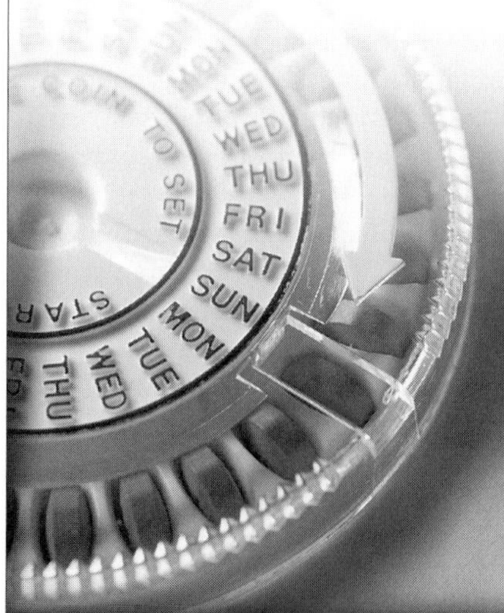

Two families of oral contraceptives are available. The most commonly prescribed pill combines estrogen and progestin. It has only one-tenth as much estrogen as the original birth control pill and half as much progestin.

The so-called minipill, which contains only progestin, is also low dose. For women who are breast-feeding and want to take a birth control pill to protect against another pregnancy, doctors often will prescribe a progestin-only pill. That's because estrogen can reduce milk production.

The progestin-only pill is less effective than the combination pill, but when combined with breast-feeding — which suppresses ovulation — this pill is often adequate. Breast-feeding alone reduces, but doesn't eliminate, the possibility of getting pregnant.

Once a baby can eat cereal, or if the baby takes a combination of breast milk and formula, a doctor may prescribe the combination progestin and estrogen pill. The baby still can get adequate nutrition even if estrogen decreases the mother's milk supply, and ovulation is no longer suppressed by breast-feeding.

How they work

Birth control pills prevent the hypothalamus, the hormone control center in the brain, from instructing the pituitary gland to mobilize follicle-stimulating hormone and luteinizing hormone. With these hormones suppressed, you don't release an egg (ovulate).

In addition, the pill prevents the cervical mucus from becoming watery, as it normally does during ovulation. Instead, the mucus remains scant throughout your cycle, making it difficult for sperm to reach the fallopian tubes.

The pill doesn't keep you from menstruating, but the flow generally isn't as heavy and doesn't last as many days as normal menstruation. In some women, the flow may be so light they wonder whether they're having a period. Most women on the pill don't experience cramps before and during menses.

Getting started

To start on the pill, you need a prescription and instructions from your doctor. A common method is to begin taking the pill on the first Sunday after the start of your period. Most brands today contain 28 pills, 21 with hormones and 7 with inactive ingredients. You take a pill every day so as not to interrupt the pattern. You start a new package the day after you finish the previous one. About 3 days after you take the last active pill, your period will start.

With another method you receive a pack with only 21 active pills. You take one a day, stop for 7 days, then start a new pack.

Don't worry if you don't menstruate. If you have a 28-pill pack, just keep taking the pills. If you have a 21-pill pack, simply begin your new pills 1 week after you finish the previous pack. If you miss a second period, consult your doctor but don't stop taking your pills.

Oral contraceptives aren't recommended for some women. You shouldn't take the combination pill if you have a history of a stroke, blood clots, severe diabetes or breast or uterine cancer, or if you have active liver disease or sickle cell disease. Risks associated with oral contraceptives increase with smoking, and studies show that the risks may increase slightly with age.

Side effects

Although effective and easy to use, birth control pills may have side effects, most of which are minor. They include nausea, breast tenderness, fluid retention, depression, decreased libido and nervousness. In addition, you may gain weight, either because of water retention or because the pill has increased your appetite, causing you to eat more.

You may also have spotting or bleeding between periods, or you may not menstruate at all, especially when you first start to take the pill. There are dozens of birth control pills on the market, and often your doctor can eliminate these problems by prescribing a different brand.

Some women menstruate regularly while they're taking the pill but stop having periods after they discontinue using it. This effect is almost always temporary.

Because there's still a small risk that the pill will cause serious side effects, watch for danger signs if you're taking it. If you have pain or swelling in your legs or severe headaches, contact your doctor.

The most serious side effect is a tendency to develop blood clots in your veins, which can be fatal if they dislodge and travel to your lungs. The incidence of blood clots is slightly higher in women who take the pill than in those who don't.

In addition, roughly 5 percent of women who use oral contraceptives develop some increase in blood pressure after about 5 years. In most cases, their blood pressure returns to normal if they stop taking the pill.

The combination pill doesn't appear to increase the incidence of cancer in the reproductive organs. In fact, there's good evidence that oral contraceptives may decrease the risk of ovarian and endometrial (uterine) cancers. In addition, the pill is beneficial for reducing the risks of ovarian and breast cysts, anemia that results from excessive menstrual flow and the incidence of rheumatoid arthritis and pelvic infections.

Drug interactions

Before you start a new medication, remember to tell your doctor that you're taking the pill. It may interact with other drugs, such as some anticonvulsants and antibiotics.

PREVENTION TIP

To lessen the chance of forgetting to take your birth control pills, get in the habit of taking the pill at the same time every day. This will also help to keep the level of hormones in your blood constant.

Contraceptive implants

Contraceptive implants are similar in action to mini birth control pills. The implants contain a hormone that keeps cervical mucus thick and impedes fertilization. Your doctor can implant these small, match-sized hormone sticks under the skin on the inside of your upper arm. They last for 5 years, and during that time there's no need to remember to do anything.

Contraceptive implants cause spotting and irregularity in your menstrual cycle, which limits their use. They may also adversely affect blood sugar (glucose) control if you have diabetes.

This method is somewhat expensive initially, but effective. Fewer

Hormonal Vaginal Ring

The first hormonal vaginal contraceptive ring approved by the Food and Drug Administration is called NuvaRing. The product consists of a flexible, transparent vaginal ring containing a combination of estrogen and progestin hormones, similar to the active ingredients in some oral contraceptives. After you insert the ring into the vagina, it releases a continuous low dose of the hormones. You wear the ring for 3 weeks and then remove it for 1 week, during which time you have your menstrual period. Following your period, you insert a new ring.

than 5 in 100 women who use the implants become pregnant in a year. If you opt for implants, take care to select a doctor well trained and experienced in placing and removing them.

Intrauterine devices

Intrauterine devices (IUDs) are about 95 percent to 99 percent effective for preventing pregnancy. An IUD is a small piece of plastic inserted into your uterus by your doctor, usually during your menstrual period when the cervix is more open. The device has a small string hanging from it. The string makes it easy for a doctor to remove the device. In addition, the wearer can check for the string with her finger to make sure the IUD remains in place. IUDs prevent pregnancy in several ways, but primarily they keep sperm from reaching an egg in the fallopian tubes.

Common side effects are increased bleeding during your period and increased menstrual pain. IUDs may also cause irregular menstrual bleeding. Sometimes the IUD can be expelled during a menstrual period, so it's important that you periodically check to make sure the device is still in place. The most serious side effects of IUDs are pelvic infection and tubal (ectopic) pregnancy. Although rare, sterility can result from severe pelvic infection.

A new IUD, called Mirena, contains progestin. It's similar to getting a shot of the medication Depo-Provera except that it delivers the hormone directly to your uterus. Unlike other IUDs, rather than increasing blood flow during your period, Mirena decreases it.

Barrier methods

Barrier methods of contraception block the sperm from getting to the egg. There are physical barriers, such as the diaphragm and cervical cap, and chemical barriers (spermicides) that come in the form of creams, gels, foams and suppositories. You can enhance the 80 percent to 90 percent effectiveness of these methods by combining a physical barrier with a spermicide.

Diaphragm

The diaphragm is an effective barrier method for women when it's used consistently and correctly. Developed more than 100 years ago, the diaphragm is a rubber disk that you insert into your vagina to cover your cervix. The device needs to be fitted by a doctor. Proper fit is essential because the diaphragm must cover the entire cervical opening to be effective. If you gain or lose a large amount of weight or deliver a baby, you may require a diaphragm of a different size.

Before intercourse, insert your diaphragm with about a teaspoon of spermicidal cream or jelly spread around the edge and in the center of the device. After intercourse, wait at least 6 hours to remove the diaphragm. Always use spermicide with a diaphragm. If you have intercourse again within the 6 hours, you must apply more spermicide without removing the diaphragm. Try not to leave it in place for more than 24 hours.

Clean your diaphragm with soap and water. Periodically check for holes or thinning of the rubber. If you find either, you need a new diaphragm.

Side effects with a diaphragm are rare as long as you're not allergic to the spermicide or latex. The most common complaint among women who use a diaphragm is having to interrupt sex to insert it.

Cervical cap

The cervical cap is a plastic cap designed to fit snugly over the cervix. It's similar to the diaphragm

Birth Control Shots and Patches

A medroxyprogesterone (Depo-Provera) shot contains the synthetic hormone progestin, similar to a contraceptive implant. To maintain protection against pregnancy, you need to have a shot in the arm or buttock every 3 months.

This method is safe immediately after childbirth and during breast-feeding. You may experience irregular monthly periods and spotting, and chances are good that you'll stop having periods entirely after 6 months. There's a slightly higher rate of pregnancy among women who weigh more than 160 pounds. If you exceed this weight, your doctor may need to adjust the amount of medication you receive. This is true of implants, as well.

Another birth control method, called Lunelle, is a monthly shot that acts like birth control pills. This combination estrogen-progestin shot offers the advantage of convenience. It's designed for women who have trouble remembering to take their pills every day. It has the same risks as birth control pills but is potentially more effective.

A birth control patch also is available. The patch emits the same hormones as the pill. You apply a new patch to a slightly different spot on your lower abdomen, buttocks or upper body — but not on your breasts — once a week. The patch carries the same potential risks as the pill, including nausea and breast tenderness and, rarely, blood clots and stroke, particularly if you smoke. Women who weigh more than 198 pounds may not be able to get a high enough contraceptive dose from the patch.

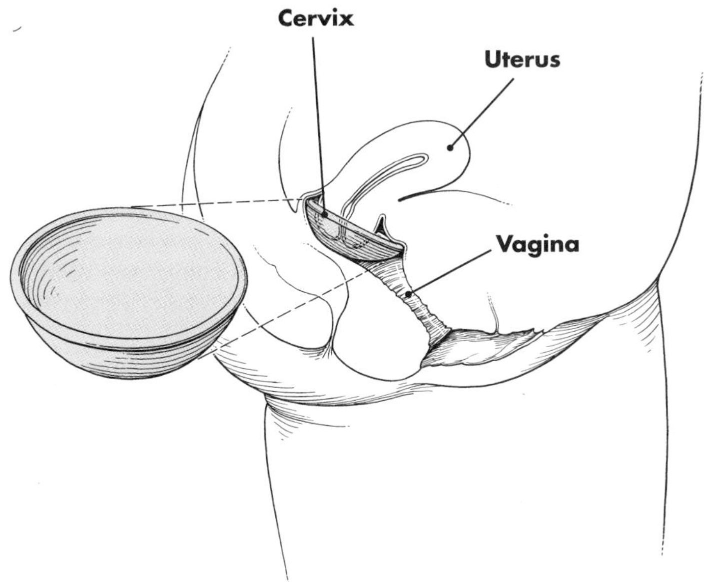

The contraceptive device known as a diaphragm is a rubber disk that's inserted into the vagina to cover the cervix, the opening to the uterus.

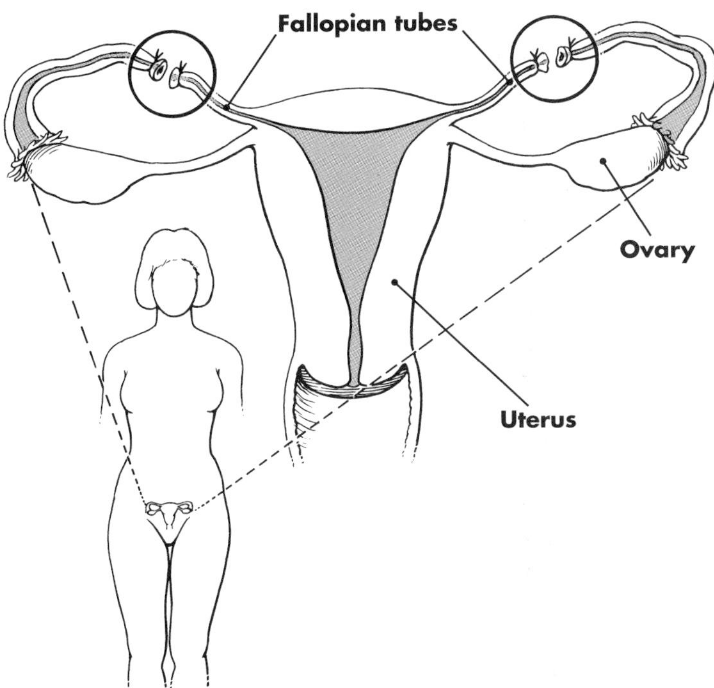

In a tubal ligation, the most common surgical procedure to sterilize a female, the path normally taken by eggs (ova) is interrupted by cutting and sealing off the fallopian tubes.

in that a doctor must fit it. Unlike the diaphragm, however, the cap is difficult for many women to insert because it needs to be placed deep within the vagina. As a result, women are tempted to leave the cap in for extended periods. That can cause problems because the cap can become a breeding ground for bacteria.

The cervical cap is about 85 percent effective for preventing pregnancy, a rate comparable to that of the diaphragm.

Female condom

The female condom, which is a type of condom worn by the woman, comes in several forms. Many are made of thicker latex than typical male condoms. All extend to the outside of the vagina, and several have a diaphragm-like end that fits over the cervix. Insertion methods vary. The breakage rate is generally less than half that of male condoms.

Tubal ligation

Tubal ligation works by keeping the egg and the sperm from meeting. To perform a tubal ligation — the most common method of female sterilization — a surgeon cuts and seals off the fallopian tubes so that eggs (ova) can't travel down the tubes and sperm can't move up. Tubal ligation failure rates appear to be higher than previously reported. Failures up to 5 percent over multiple years have been seen in some studies.

A hysterectomy — the removal of the uterus — isn't recommended for the sole purpose of sterilization. A hysterectomy should only be done if a woman has another medical condition that warrants it.

Many women opt to be sterilized immediately or shortly after giving birth. This is an opportune time for a tubal ligation because the woman is already in the hospital. The abdominal wall is relaxed and the top of the uterus is near the navel, the entry point of operation, which makes direct access to the tubes easy. Short-term anesthesia is necessary, but the procedure doesn't lengthen a postpartum hospital stay. If the abdomen is already open for a Caesarean delivery, a doctor can perform a tubal ligation in a matter of minutes.

For a woman who has recently had a vaginal delivery, a common method for performing a tubal ligation is minilaparotomy. The doctor makes a small incision below the navel through which he or she raises a "knuckle" of each tube, ties the base, cuts the tube, then ties the two separated ends. A laparoscope is most often used for sterilizations done weeks or months after delivery. It isn't used for procedures performed soon after delivery because of the size of the uterus.

A laparoscope is a thin instrument that's inserted through a small incision below the navel after the abdomen has been inflated with gas. The instrument has a viewing scope through which a doctor can see the reproductive organs. Using operating instruments through either the same incision or a second one, the doctor locates the tubes and either cauterizes them or attaches plastic clips or rings to them.

As with any operation, tubal ligation carries risk. About 1 in 1,000 women develop a complication from the procedure. These include reactions to the anesthetic, pelvic infection, injury to blood vessels in the abdomen and bowel or bladder injuries.

After a tubal ligation, you may require mild pain medication for your sore abdomen. You may also experience dizziness, fatigue, nausea and bloating. Within 8 hours, most women can walk around, eat a regular diet and care for their infants. Most women go home the same day and resume their normal schedules within a few days.

If you're pregnant and considering sterilization, discuss options with your doctor. Some doctors perform the tubal ligation immediately after childbirth, while others prefer to wait 3 to 6 months. Before doctors perform tubal ligations, they often recommend that the parents wait to be sure their last child is healthy. If there's a problem, the parents may decide they want another child. Tubal ligation can be done in a hospital or an outpatient surgical center at a later date.

When considering sterilization, you and your partner may also want to discuss the possibility of a vasectomy rather than a tubal ligation. Vasectomies involve making a small cut in the man's scrotum, then cutting and tying or clipping the vas deferens, the two tubes that carry sperm from the testicles. Vasectomies are safer, less complicated and cheaper than tubal ligations. They may also be more effective, with a failure rate of less than 1 percent.

Reversing a Tubal Ligation

Some women who've been sterilized later decide they want to become pregnant. An operation can be done to reverse tubal ligation. Sixty percent to 80 percent of women who have it are eventually able to conceive. However, the risk of tubal (ectopic) pregnancy increases. For these reasons, doctors stress that before you undergo sterilization, be very sure you won't want to become pregnant.

Another possibility for women who want to conceive after tubal ligation is in vitro fertilization, a procedure in which mature eggs are removed from the ovary, fertilized with the partner's sperm in a laboratory and implanted into her uterus. This procedure is more common today than tubal reversal surgery.

Infertility

At least 10 percent to 15 percent of couples experience infertility. Fortunately, many cases of infertility can be solved.

Problems of infertility may include problems with the sperm, the egg or difficulties encountered in their union. Abnormal function of the fallopian tubes or uterus, infections, immunologic and other factors may cause infertility. Infertility problems can also result from sexual dysfunction.

To doctors, the term *infertility* usually means the inability to achieve pregnancy after 1 year of frequent sexual intercourse without using contraception. Infertility often can be overcome, but for many couples pregnancy may not occur for more than a year after starting treatment.

Note that infertility is not the same thing as sterility, which means the inability to conceive a child under any circumstances. With infertility, conceiving a child may be possible.

In about 30 percent of cases, the man is the infertile partner. The woman is infertile about 40 percent of the time. In the remaining cases, both partners contribute to infertility, or the cause can't be determined.

Being infertile doesn't make a man any less a man or a woman any less a woman. Infertility doesn't mean anyone is incomplete or defective. It has nothing to do with attractiveness or sexual prowess. Moreover, it's not a comment on a couple's relationship.

Medically speaking, infertility is simply the existence of some obstacle in the long and exceedingly complex chain of events that leads to pregnancy. Infertility can be frustrating and disappointing and a source of great sorrow for couples experiencing it.

Evaluation

If you and your partner are unable to achieve conception within a reasonable time, seek help. A gynecologist, urologist or family doctor can determine if there's a fertility problem that may require the services of an infertility specialist.

Before deciding to undergo infertility testing, be aware that the process requires commitment. The doctor will need to know your sexual habits and may make recommendations about how to change those habits. Tests and periods of trial and error may extend over several months, and, in some cases, may include operations or uncomfortable procedures. Evaluation is expensive and may not be covered by your medical insurance. Finally, there's no guarantee, even after all the tests and procedures, that you'll be able to conceive. However, if you're determined to try to have your own child, infertility evaluation is the route to take, and it often results in a successful pregnancy.

Male tests

For a man to be fertile, his testicles must produce enough sperm, the sperm must be able to reach the seminal vesicles, and the sperm must be ejaculated effectively into the woman's vagina. Male fertility tests attempt to determine if any of these steps are impeded.

A doctor will likely begin with a medical history, including illnesses and disabilities, medications and sexual habits. You may then have a physical examination, including examination of your genitals.

The doctor will likely ask for a specimen of ejaculated semen. You provide the sample by masturbating and ejaculating the semen into a clean container. You may need to provide more than one specimen during the fertility testing process.

A laboratory analysis of the semen notes its quantity and color as well as the number of sperm and the presence of infections or blood. Laboratory analysis also determines the concentration of sperm present in the ejaculate, their shape and their activity (motility).

You may be asked to take other tests, such as a blood test to determine your level of testosterone or other hormones.

Female tests

For a woman to be fertile, her ovaries must release healthy eggs regularly, and her reproductive tract must allow the eggs and sperm unobstructed passage for a possible union in the fallopian tubes. Your doctor will likely start with a medical history, followed by a general physical examination, including a gynecological examination. He or she may also ask you questions about medications you take, your menstrual cycle and your sexual habits.

The following tests are used to determine the possible causes of female infertility. Not everyone needs to undergo all, or even many, of the tests before the cause is found. Your doctor will discuss the tests with you and, with your agreement, determine which ones to use and in what order. In up to 20 percent of infertile women, despite careful testing, no cause can be found.

Blood tests

You may be asked for a blood sample to test for levels of hormones involved in successful ovulation and, sometimes, to look for infections. After receiving the results of one or more of these tests, your doctor will know if ovulation occurs and whether sperm can survive in your reproductive tract. If the tests reveal no problems, additional information may be needed.

Biopsy

An endometrial biopsy can help determine if ovulation occurs and whether the lining of the uterus is hormonally prepared for pregnancy. In this test, a doctor takes a small sample of tissue from the uterine lining shortly before the onset of your menstrual period.

Ultrasound

A doctor may use ultrasound to examine the pelvic area and look for abnormalities in your ovaries and uterus.

Hysterosalpingography

This procedure may be used to evaluate the condition of the uterus as well as the fallopian tubes. After a contrast fluid is injected into the uterus, an X-ray determines if the fluid travels out of the uterus and up the fallopian tubes. This test often can locate blockages or find other problems.

Hysteroscopy

Hysteroscopy is a procedure in which your doctor uses a small instrument to examine the interior of your cervix and uterus for irregularities that might lead to infertility. This test may be done under general anesthesia. It's not effective in studying the fallopian tubes.

Surgery

Sometimes, a doctor will perform a minimally invasive operation — in either a hospital or outpatient surgical center — with local or general anesthesia. During the procedure, a doctor inserts a thin, illuminated viewing device (laparoscope) into your abdomen and pelvis to examine your fallopian tubes, ovaries and uterus.

Causes of infertility most commonly identified with laparoscopy are fallopian tube or ovarian adhesions or endometriosis, a condition in which uterine tissues escape the uterus and implant themselves on other reproductive organs. Through the laparoscope, a doctor can spot blockages or scarring of the fallopian tubes and uterus, which may prevent fertilization.

Causes

Rarely, the cause of infertility is a sexual one. For example, an impotent man might be fertile if he could achieve an erection sufficient for intercourse. Similarly, premature ejaculation — ejaculation that takes place before the penis is far enough into the vagina — greatly lessens the chances of a sperm meeting up with the egg.

Most of the time, the cause isn't sexual dysfunction but a problem with fertility.

Female causes

In women, the failure to release an egg each menstrual cycle (anovulation) is responsible for infertility in up to 15 percent of cases. It can result from various factors. If a woman doesn't menstruate, there may be a problem with the way her uterus or ovaries developed. However, even a woman who has normal periods can have impaired ovulation.

Hyperprolactinemia, a condition in which the blood contains an excess amount of the hormone prolactin, can prevent ovulation. The hypothalamus in the brain produces hormones that normally stimulate a woman's pituitary gland, which in turn triggers the release of an egg. If the hypothalamus doesn't secrete the hormones, no egg is released.

Polycystic ovary syndrome also may result in infertility. With this condition, a woman's body produces an excess of male hormones. The ovaries may become large and studded with cysts. Most women who experience this condition never establish a normal menstrual rhythm. Some never start menstruating. Additional causes of anovulation include chronic debilitating diseases such as uncontrolled diabetes and thyroid disease.

If ovulation is normal, the problem lies elsewhere. Up to one-third of the time, abnormalities of the fallopian tubes are the problem, or contribute to it. Damage from infection in the fallopian tubes can block passage of an egg. In a condition called endometriosis, some of the tissue that lines the uterus and is shed each month during the menstrual cycle is present in the abdomen somewhere outside the uterus. This tissue can interfere with fertility.

Sometimes after ovulation, the egg passes successfully through the fallopian tubes, only to encounter other problems. Many processes under hormonal control, from cervical mucus production to proliferation of the lining of the uterus, may fail in their functions.

Sometimes the cause of infertility stems from the uterus. An irregular-shaped uterus or tumors in the uterine cavity can cause problems. Surgical correction may or may not restore fertility. Problems of the cervix that can cause infertility include cervical narrowing (stenosis) or problems with the cervical mucus that damage the sperm or impede its passage.

Male causes

The prime cause of infertility in a man is impaired sperm production. Azoospermia, the absence of sperm in the semen, generally is due to a disorder of the testicles or, rarely, a blockage in the passageways leading from the testicles. With oligospermia, sperm are present in the semen but not in enough quantity to readily fertilize an egg.

One potential cause of male infertility is a varicocele, a condition in which varicose veins surrounding the testicles prevent normal cooling of the testicles. An increase in testicular temperature impairs sperm production. Other problems with the testicles also may be responsible for infertility.

A blood test often can identify hormonal disorders that may be the underlying cause of testicular problems. Sexually transmitted diseases (STDs) or other infections can block the passageways through which sperm travel, or they can injure or kill sperm, causing infertility. Mumps and some other infections sometimes cause an inflammation of one or both testicles (orchitis) that can permanently impair or prevent sperm production in the affected testicle. Injuries also can affect sperm production.

Some men have a condition called retrograde ejaculation, in which they produce sperm normally but ejaculate into the bladder rather than out the penis. This is most frequently seen in men with diabetes.

Male and female causes

Immunologic factors may cause infertility. A few women produce antibodies that kill sperm before one can penetrate an egg. Similarly, some men produce antibodies that are meant to fight an infection but inadvertently attack sperm instead. Clearing up an infection may eradicate this problem.

In men as well as women, numerous diseases that can affect the genitourinary tract can cause infertility. These include sexually transmitted diseases (STDs). Pelvic inflammatory disease commonly is caused by sexually transmitted diseases such as gonorrhea, chlamydia and vaginitis and, less commonly, by tuberculosis and anaerobic streptococcal infection. In women with pelvic inflammatory disease, aggressive treatment with antibiotics can clear up the infection and re-establish fertility. Even with treatment, pelvic inflammatory disease may result in tubal obstruction (occlusion) and infertility.

Treatment

Treatments for infertility are numerous, and recent developments have increased the number of once infertile couples who can achieve pregnancy. The method that may work best for you depends on the cause of your infertility. Some causes of infertility can't be corrected. However, even in those cases, various means of insemination or embryo transfer may be possible so that a woman can still become pregnant.

Restoring fertility

Sperm survive in the female reproductive tract for up to 72 hours, and an egg can be fertilized for a few hours after its release. Therefore, by having intercourse every 2 to 3 days at midcycle, couples can effectively eliminate faulty timing as a factor contributing to infertility. Sexual problems, such as impotence or premature ejaculation, also can be treated to improve fertility.

When the source of infertility is the man's sperm, restoring or initiating fertility is sometimes possible. For example, surgically correcting varicocele appears to restore fertility in some cases. Some problems with the testicles, prostate gland, seminal vesicles and urethra also may be corrected.

When sperm production is impaired because of damage to the sperm-producing cells of the testicle, drug treatment has proven to be of little benefit. In extremely rare instances, when a pituitary gland problem impairs sperm production, the use of human chorionic gonadotropin or human pituitary gonadotropin to replace pituitary hormones has been helpful. When infections hamper sperm production, resolving the infection may restore fertility. This is particularly true of sexually transmitted diseases, for which both partners must be treated.

For a woman, treatment also depends on the results of her examination and tests. Treating any infection or underlying illness is the first step. If the fertility problem is related to failure to release an egg (anovulation), a doctor can attempt to bring about ovulation by administering substances that promote ovulation, such as clomiphene citrate, human gonadotropins or gonadotropin-releasing hormones with or without human chorionic gonadotropin.

Surgery sometimes is used to correct blockages or other problems in the fallopian tubes. Microsurgical techniques make such delicate operations possible. Surgical repair offers a chance of pregnancy. Today, however, assisted reproductive technology is often used instead of an operation.

Although birth control pills can be effective in treating endometriosis and relieving its pain, they're not useful in treating infertility caused by endometriosis. If you have endometriosis, your doctor may attempt to treat it during laparoscopic surgery. Restoring fertility may also require superovulation therapy. If neither treatment works, in vitro fertilization may be considered.

Assisted reproductive technology

Assisted reproductive technology (ART) refers to medical procedures that enable many couples to have children when fertility can't be restored. In vitro fertilization is the most commonly used ART technique. It involves retrieving mature eggs from the woman, fertilizing them with sperm in a petri dish in a laboratory and implanting the fertilized eggs in the uterus 2 days later.

You begin in vitro fertilization by taking fertility drugs to stimulate your ovaries to produce more eggs than usual. About 1 week before your period — before your hormones start the process of egg stimulation — you may receive an injection of a medication that reduces the hormones that promote the development of eggs in the ovaries. After about 10 days, a vaginal ultrasound and blood test determine if the drug has reduced egg development. If not, you may continue the drug therapy for another week or two.

When the function of the ovaries has been temporarily stopped, you'll receive hormone injections for about 7 days to stimulate the development of ovarian follicles, fluid-filled sacs in which the eggs mature. More blood tests and a vaginal ultrasound exam determine follicle growth. It's important to monitor follicle growth to be able to retrieve mature eggs.

After the ovaries have been stimulated appropriately, you'll receive an injection of another hormone, human chorionic gonadotropin (HCG), to help the eggs mature and to trigger ovulation. Eggs are retrieved 34 to 38 hours after the HCG injection, or shortly before egg release would normally occur.

It usually takes 20 to 50 minutes to retrieve the eggs. You receive medication through an intravenous (IV) line to help keep you comfortable and relaxed throughout the procedure. Using transvaginal ultrasound, your doctor guides a needle through the vagina to an ovary. In general, eggs are recovered from about 80 percent of the mature follicles seen on ultrasound.

After being removed from the follicles, the fluid that contains the eggs is taken immediately to a laboratory, where the eggs are immersed in a special solution and placed in an incubator. How long the eggs remain in the incubator depends on their maturity. When mature, the eggs are mixed with sperm (inseminated). Typically about 80 percent of the eggs are

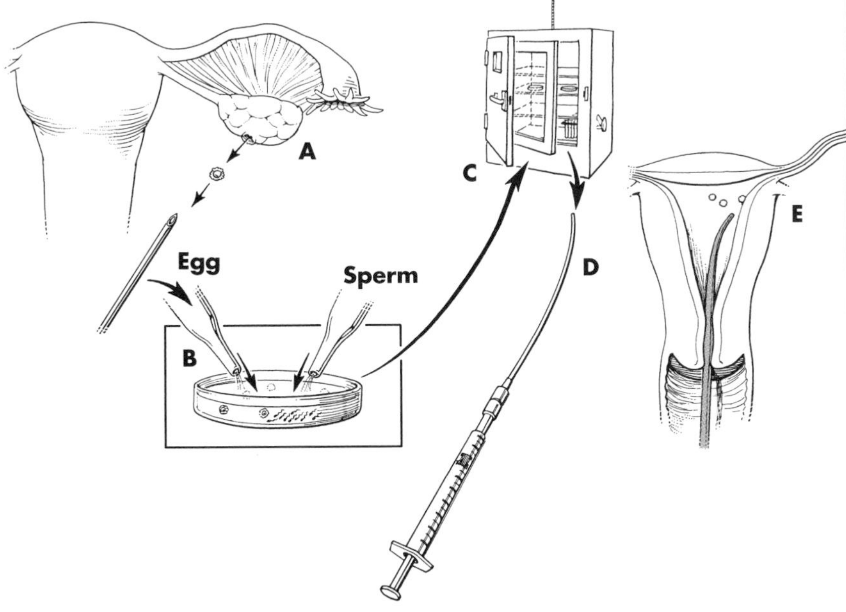

During in vitro fertilization: (A) A doctor uses a needle to remove eggs (ova) from the ovary. (B) The eggs and sperm from a donor are combined in a petri dish and (C) placed in an incubator. (D) After fertilization, the ova are retrieved by means of a cannula and (E) transferred to the uterus.

successfully fertilized, provided there's no male factor contributing to the infertility.

Some of the embryos are transferred to your uterus 2 days after fertilization is confirmed. Embryo transfer is a brief procedure in which your doctor threads a soft, flexible catheter (cannula) through your cervix into your uterus. Usually two or three embryos are transferred. Extra embryos can be cryopreserved (frozen) so that you don't have to repeat the ovarian stimulation and retrieval process. If conception doesn't occur following the embryo transfer or if you want more children, the frozen embryos may be used at a later date. You'll have a pregnancy test, usually 2 weeks after the procedure.

The national success rate for in vitro fertilization — the percentage of ART cycles started that resulted in a live birth — is approximately 25 percent. In vitro fertilization is generally the treatment of choice when both fallopian tubes are blocked. It's also used widely for a number of other infertility conditions, including endometriosis, unexplained infertility, cervical factor infertility, male factor infertility and ovulation disorders.

ART works best when the woman has a healthy uterus, responds well to fertility drugs and ovulates naturally. The success rate is lower in women older than age 40 and women with untreated conditions of the uterus, such as scar tissue, fibroids and polyps. The success rate is also lower in men with low sperm counts, low sperm motility or abnormal sperm function.

Among other forms of ART that aren't used as often is zygote intrafallopian transfer. In this procedure, a fertilized egg (zygote) is placed into a fallopian tube the day after removal. With gamete intrafallopian transfer, unfertilized eggs and sperm are placed into a fallopian tube, where the egg is fertilized. Another technique is called intracytoplasmic sperm injection. It involves a microscopic technique in

Factors to Consider

Determining the cause of infertility and treating it can be demanding for both the couple and the doctor. It requires energy and commitment for what may be a prolonged period.

Personal attitudes

It's important for a man and woman considering fertility therapy to take into account their attitudes about the process. Just because something is possible doesn't mean that it should be done. Attitudes toward conception vary greatly. Some couples believe that if sexual intercourse doesn't produce a child, they should accept the situation and not take further steps toward possible pregnancy. Conversely, other couples are so eager to have their own biological child that they believe no procedure is too much, no therapy too complicated and no expense or hardship too great.

Most couples find themselves somewhere between these two positions. Doctors who specialize in fertility problems are often prepared to discuss these issues with you. They can help you to examine your attitudes and to keep your expectations realistic. Even though medical science has provided many new techniques, they all have limitations, and none is 100 percent successful.

Ethical considerations

When fertilization is only possible through medical intervention, some couples believe that taking advantage of the latest technology crosses a line. It raises questions and ethical considerations for them.

A significant issue for many people is using donor sperm or donor eggs from someone other than their own partner. Using sperm or eggs from a stranger raises many questions: Does the donor have any rights concerning the child? Might future court decisions award donors visitation rights?

Other ethical considerations concern issues of selective reduction in the number of embryos in case of a multiple pregnancy.

In the end, only you and your partner can decide how far you should go and whether you can deal with issues that may arise. The time to consider your ethical positions on fertility therapy is before you embark upon these treatments.

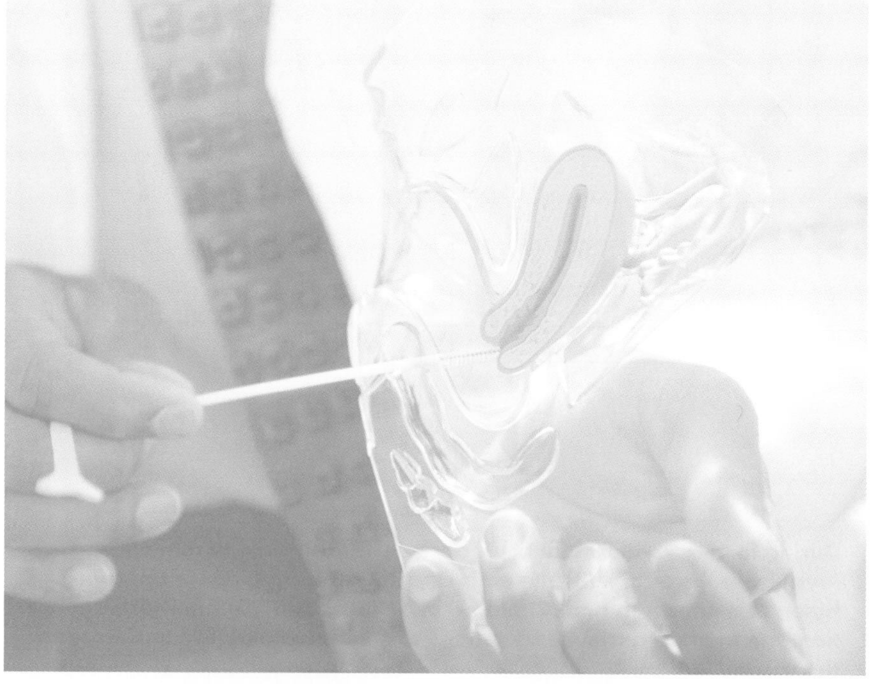

which a single sperm is injected into an egg to achieve fertilization. Fertilization rates are higher than those achieved with standard insemination. This procedure is especially helpful for couples who've failed to achieve fertilization with standard techniques and for men with low sperm concentrations.

Additional aides to ART include electroejaculation, which uses an electric stimulus to bring about ejaculation to obtain semen. This procedure can be used in men with spinal cord injuries who can't otherwise achieve ejaculation. Aspiration techniques include removing sperm from parts of the male reproductive tract such as the epididymis, vas deferens or testicle.

The risks associated with ART involve the medications and procedures used to remove the eggs. These risks include hemorrhage, infection, damage to adjacent organs and overstimulation of ovaries, which causes ovarian enlargement and abdominal discomfort. The greatest risk is an increased chance of a multiple pregnancy.

Sexual Dysfunction

Different women respond differently to sexual stimulation, but generally, women go through a four-stage sexual response cycle:

- *Desire.* Wanting to have sex
- *Arousal.* Physical changes, such as lubrication of your vagina and swelling of your clitoris and labia, that prepare your body for sex
- *Orgasm.* Contraction of the vaginal muscles that causes pleasure
- *Resolution.* Your body's return to its pre-sex state

For women, sexual response is complex. It often has as much to do with a woman's feelings for her partner as it does with the sexual stimuli. Beyond having a sex drive, many women are sexual because they want to get closer or communicate their affection to their partner.

Sexual dysfunction simply implies problems or obstacles encountered in one or more of the stages of sexual response. Both men and women can experience problems, and most people experience sexual difficulties at some point in their lives. In fact, results from a national survey of people ages 18 to 59 indicate that sexual dysfunction is common — 43 percent of women and 31 percent of men reported having sexual problems.

Many instances of sexual dysfunction are due to a lack of basic sex education. It's important to understand your anatomy and your body's normal physiologic response to sexual stimulation. It can be hard for you to achieve orgasm if you've never had one, don't know what it feels like or what stimulation your body requires to get there. Also, many people are unaware that it often takes a woman longer to become sexually aroused than it does a man.

A common problem for women is fatigue and the various stressors and demands on them as they try to meet myriad needs and fill multiple roles, such as worker, wife, mother and caretaker of aging parents. Among men, factors that can lead to sexual dysfunction include high blood pressure, certain medications, chronic diseases such as diabetes and substance abuse. More recent findings indicate that women have many of these same risk factors.

Sexual dysfunction in women is generally divided into four categories: hypoactive sexual desire, sexual arousal disorder, orgasmic disorder and sexual pain disorder. Keep in mind that these are categories, not causes. The categories have many commonalties. Hormonal changes, such as those experienced during pregnancy or menopause, can affect sexual response. So can breaches in your relationship with, or negative feelings toward, your partner. Emotional problems, such as anxiety or depression, can contribute to any of the sexual disorders. So can a history of sexual abuse. Conversely, sexual dysfunction can affect your self-esteem or that of your partner, your relationships and your quality of life.

Hypoactive sexual desire

Signs and symptoms

- Diminished or absent sexual desire, including recurrent or long-lasting lack of sexual thoughts and fantasies
- Insufficient sexual desire to sustain interest in sexual activity
- Distress over the lack of desire

Possibly the most common type of sexual disorder among women, hypoactive sexual desire means a woman has poor libido, or lack of sex drive. She doesn't think about or fantasize about sex. You may even be having sex and experiencing orgasm, but lack desire. This condition is considered a sexual disorder only if the woman is distressed by it.

On average, men desire sexual relations more often than women. Your partner's wanting sex more frequently than you do doesn't necessarily mean that you have a desire problem. Instead, it suggests a disparity between the two of you. In such cases, counseling might help. It can lead to compromise and better understanding between the two of you.

Hypoactive sexual desire doesn't mean there's anything psychologically or interpersonally wrong. Almost every woman experiences it at some point in her life. It's common after giving birth, when many new mothers are fatigued and focusing their energy on their baby. There's not much left over for sex.

Hypoactive sexual desire generally is transient. Diminished or absent desire that persists, however, can cause distress, create problems for a woman's self-image and damage the sexual life of both partners.

Sexual arousal disorder

Signs and symptoms

- Loss of arousal during desired sexual activity
- Vaginal dryness during sexual intercourse, despite sufficient sexual stimulation during foreplay
- Sometimes, painful intercourse
- Distress over the lack of arousal

With sexual arousal disorder, your desire for sex is intact, but you're unable to maintain your arousal during intercourse. Your body won't cooperate. It doesn't produce enough lubrication or sensation to sustain your arousal.

As with other sexual problems, an occasional lack of arousal doesn't mean you have a disorder. It's only considered dysfunctional if it persists and causes you distress. A lack of sexual response when your partner doesn't provide sufficient stimulation or foreplay isn't a disorder. It's a normal reaction to inadequate sexual stimulation.

Many things can affect sexual arousal. Physical causes include radiation therapy to the pelvis, certain medications or underlying peripheral vascular disease that decreases blood flow to the genitals.

Orgasmic disorder

Signs and symptoms

- An inability to reach orgasm during sex after sufficient stimulation
- Delay in reaching orgasm despite sufficient stimulation
- Distress over the lack of orgasm

Although most women are biologically able to have an orgasm, some women never attain orgasm, some attain orgasm only sometimes, and others have orgasm every time they have intercourse. A change in your normal pattern that causes you distress and leads to dissatisfaction with sexual activity warrants evaluation.

Orgasmic disorder is defined as persistent or recurrent difficulty or delay in achieving orgasm after sufficient sexual stimulation and arousal. If the situation doesn't distress you, it's not considered a disorder. When a woman who has never experienced an orgasm receives this diagnosis, it's termed primary orgasmic disorder. In a woman who has previously achieved orgasm but no longer can, it's called secondary orgasmic disorder.

Orgasmic disorder is closely related to sexual arousal disorder. In general, if you don't experience pleasurable sensations from sexual activity, you won't have an orgasm. In some cases of orgasmic disorder, a woman does experience orgasm, but has to work unreasonably hard or long to attain it.

Female sexual response is complex, involving sexual desire and sexual stimulation. Understanding how your body responds to sexual stimulation, knowing what gives you pleasure and communicating your sexual needs to a responsive partner is important for achieving orgasm.

A large percentage of women — estimates range from one-third to two-thirds of all women — require stimulation of the clitoris to reach orgasm. Don't assume that you have orgasmic disorder until your partner or you have tried direct stimulation of the clitoris before, during or after intercourse and you find you still can't attain orgasm.

Another common cause of this condition is a class of antidepressants known as selective serotonin reuptake inhibitors (SSRIs). These include fluoxetine (Prozac), paroxetine (Paxil), sertraline (Zoloft) and citalopram (Celexa). Other physical causes include spinal cord injury, other neurologic disorders or trauma. Nonphysical causes can include sexual inhibition, fear of losing control or other distractions that affect your ability to focus on pleasurable sexual sensations.

Sexual pain disorder

Signs and symptoms

- General pain during sexual stimulation without intercourse
- Pain upon penile entry into the vagina
- Distress over the pain

With sexual pain disorder, women find sexual stimulation without intercourse causes them pain or they have pain upon entry of the penis. Some have recurrent or persistent genital pain associated with sexual intercourse (dyspareunia) or painful, involuntary spasms of the muscles that surround the entrance to the vagina (vaginismus).

Several physical ailments affecting the genital area can be responsible for dyspareunia, including hormonal changes, poor vaginal lubrication, vaginitis, endometriosis and reactions to devices or substances used for contraception. The absence of sufficient vaginal lubrication can cause painful intercourse. Following menopause, the mucosol lining of the vagina generally becomes thinner and drier, and

Vaginismus

A rare cause of painful intercourse is vaginismus. If you have vaginismus, the natural lubrication of your vagina isn't activated when you're sexually aroused. At the same time, the muscles surrounding the entrance to the vagina contract, making intercourse difficult, if not impossible.

The cause of vaginismus may be psychological, perhaps as a response to a traumatic sexual experience. If you have vaginismus, consult a doctor or therapist trained in treating sexual disorders.

Treatment often combines counseling with progressive vaginal enlargement (dilation). You begin by inserting a small tube into your vagina. Once you can tolerate that without pain, you insert progressively larger sizes until you can insert a penis-sized dilator without pain. This technique usually requires ongoing counseling, as well.

previously pleasurable intercourse may become painful.

Psychological trauma, such as rape or sexual molestation, can be a cause of sexual pain disorder. With vaginismus, vaginal muscle spasms often are a conditioned response to painful penetration, or they can be the result of emotional trauma.

Seeking help

If your sexual disorder causes you distress, you may want to seek help. Sexual disorders are common, and there's no reason to be embarrassed. Doctors are becoming more sensitive to sexual problems. Look for a doctor who shows interest and starts to ask questions in an effort to help.

An understanding doctor can help determine the cause of your disorder and suggest treatment. He or she can check for and treat underlying causes. Your doctor may also ask about your relationship with your partner, your physical and emotional condition, your medical history, any medications you're taking, as well as questions about sexual desire and whether you've experienced sexual abuse.

The seriousness of sexual disorders lies more in the distress they cause or their effect on your relationship with your partner than in the dysfunction itself.

Treatment

If you have an underlying illness that may be causing your dysfunction, your doctor will likely take steps to treat it. He or she may also alter or eliminate medications you take to determine if they may be affecting your sexual responsiveness.

Vaginal lubricants can help alleviate pain during intercourse. If you're postmenopausal your doctor may recommend estrogen — oral, vaginal cream or a patch — to counteract vaginal drying and thinning brought on by menopause.

If you have orgasmic disorder, your doctor may suggest a set of simple exercises (Kegel exercises, see page 1089) that can help you develop the muscles in the outer third of the vagina that are involved in pleasurable sensations. These same muscles also help control the flow of urine.

In some cases, counseling may help you and your partner. It may include suggestions to increase your sexual pleasure. If there's an underlying problem in your relationship with your partner, counseling may help you work through it.

Menstrual Disorders

Your menstrual cycle is regulated by hormones that are ultimately controlled by your hypothalamus, an area at the base of your brain that acts as a kind of regulator for your whole reproductive system. Your hypothalamus interacts with your pituitary gland, some of whose hormones regulate the hormone action of your ovaries. It's primarily the ovarian hormones that affect the uterus.

Given the complexity of this system and that both physical and mental stress can affect the hypothalamus, it's remarkable that women's menstrual cycles are as regular as they are. Sometimes, though, irregularities in the cycle can occur. Various factors can cause menstrual disorders.

Absence of periods

Signs and symptoms

- No menstruation by age 16
- A 3-month absence of menstruation in women who aren't pregnant or menopausal

Failure to menstruate is called amenorrhea. If you've never menstruated, the condition is called primary amenorrhea.

If you reach the age of 16 without menstruating, chances are you're developing normally but later than most girls. Being very athletic or quite thin can delay menarche. However, there's a small possibility that you have a hormonal abnormality that causes the absence of periods (amenorrhea). Consult a doctor, especially if other sexual changes are also delayed, such as in development of breasts and pubic hair.

If you've been menstruating for years and you miss three or more periods, you have secondary amenorrhea. There are several possible explanations for this. The most obvious is pregnancy. Other reasons for missed periods include a condition called polycystic ovary syndrome (see page 1074), losing a lot of weight over a short period, exercising a lot, being under stress, obesity or use of medication that suppresses menses as a side effect. Oral contraceptives also may cause absence of periods, especially during the first few months of use. If this occurs, it's important to keep taking the pills.

If you just stopped use of oral contraceptives, you may not have a period for several months. Breastfeeding also can delay menstruation. If you're reaching the age of menopause, skipping periods is a normal part of that process.

Secondary amenorrhea due to such causes is quite common. More serious problems, such as tumors or disorders of the pituitary gland, also can cause amenorrhea, but they're rare. Failure to resume menstruation after childbirth, particularly if you can't produce breast milk (lactate), may mean that the pituitary gland failed either partly or completely at the time of delivery, a rare condition called postpartum pituitary necrosis (Sheehan's syndrome).

If you've been menstruating regularly and your period is more than 2 weeks late, you may want to perform a home pregnancy test or see your health care provider to find out whether you're pregnant. However, if you're sure you couldn't be pregnant and you have no other symptoms, there's no harm in waiting 3 months before consulting a doctor. Keep in mind, though, that you could still become pregnant even though you're not menstruating. Continue contraceptive practices until you've gone a year without a period.

Diagnosis

Whether you have primary or secondary amenorrhea, your doctor may do a pelvic examination to determine if your vaginal walls seem moist and otherwise normal. He or she may examine your cervical mucus, looking for signs that your ovaries are producing normal amounts of estrogen.

Another way to determine your estrogen status is to take progesterone for a few days and wait to see if it induces vaginal bleeding. Bleeding indicates that estrogen isn't the problem. If you don't bleed despite taking progesterone, then your ovaries are probably secreting little or no estrogen. Blood tests and X-rays can help your doctor determine the cause.

How serious is absence of periods?

Amenorrhea often indicates that something isn't working properly and should be treated. If you're not menstruating, you may find it difficult to become pregnant. Amenorrhea can be the result of conditions that could cause you problems later in life. If you're producing estrogen but not having periods, you could be at a greater long-term risk of endometrial (uterine) cancer.

Treatment

Treatment depends on the underlying cause. Your doctor may prescribe oral contraceptives or hormone replacement therapy to induce regular periods. If an underlying disorder is to blame for either primary or secondary amenorrhea, your doctor will likely prescribe appropriate treatment to correct the problem.

Primary amenorrhea

Signs and symptoms

- No menstruation by age 16
- Undeveloped breasts and pubic hair
- Abnormal-looking genitals

Failure to begin menstruating at puberty can be the first sign of a chromosomal abnormality that causes some girls to be born without all the usual internal or external organs of their sex. Sometimes the problem is noticeable at birth. Other times, the problem doesn't become evident until puberty, when a girl may or may not develop breasts and pubic hair, depending on the nature of her genetic problem.

One-third of girls who fail to menstruate have incompletely developed ovaries (gonadal dysgenesis). Several types of gonadal dysgenesis occur, but the most common is Turner's syndrome, which occurs in 1 of every 2,500 female newborns. A teenage girl with Turner's syndrome is very short, and her body appears childlike. Her breasts don't develop, and she has little or no pubic or underarm hair. Her internal reproductive organs are also childlike, and her ovaries are simply streaks of fiber (streak gonads) with no follicles or ova.

In another condition, a girl develops breasts but little or no pubic or underarm hair. Her genitals appear to be normal, but her vagina is short and she has no cervix, uterus, ovaries or fallopian tubes. Some girls with this condition have no vagina. In place of the female organs, gonadal tissue is present somewhere in the abdominal cavity, and the risk of cancer of that tissue is increased. The tissue is usually removed.

Diagnosis

When girls reach their late teens without menstruating, most often the cause is simply late development. However, a doctor may check for congenital problems by doing a pelvic examination and possibly ordering blood tests to measure and evaluate circulating hormones. If there's an abnormality, chromosome studies can help pinpoint which chromosomes are involved.

A doctor can also learn more about the status of the girl's ovaries by prescribing a course of the female sex hormone progesterone. If the ovaries are producing estrogen, progesterone will induce bleeding from the uterus. This bleeding also implies that the uterus has a lining (endometrium) that can be stimulated.

How serious is primary amenorrhea?

Without surgery to remove the gonadal tissue, the child is at increased risk of cancer. The condition can also cause emotional difficulties.

Treatment

In some cases of primary amenorrhea, the ovarian tissue is so underdeveloped that treatment with female sex hormones is needed to help the girl develop breasts and other female secondary sex characteristics. Pregnancy generally isn't possible without donor eggs.

Polycystic ovary syndrome

Signs and symptoms

- Unpredictable menstrual periods or a failure to menstruate
- Infertility
- An unusual amount of facial and body hair
- High blood sugar

Polycystic ovary syndrome (PCOS) is the most common hormonal disorder among women of reproductive age in the United States, affecting an estimated 4 percent to 12 percent. Most women with PCOS never establish a normal menstrual rhythm in their teens and eventually stop menstruating altogether. Some never start. Menses generally occur without cramping, and women with this disorder rarely ovulate.

With PCOS a women's body produces an excess of male hormones (androgens), which may lead to excess facial hair and acne. Women with this condition may also be overweight.

The name of the condition comes from the appearance of the ovaries in some women with the disorder. They're large and studded with numerous (poly) cysts. These cysts are follicles, fluid-filled sacs that contain immature eggs. This condition may cause infertility but is usually treatable.

Doctors don't know the cause of PCOS, but research suggests a link to insulin, the hormone produced in the pancreas that facilitates transport of sugar (glucose) from blood to individual cells. Usually, the condition is lifelong and requires close supervision and management to prevent endometrial cancer.

Diagnosis

During a pelvic examination, your doctor may detect an enlargement of both ovaries. Blood tests may reveal a typical pattern of hormones present in abnormal amounts. Your doctor may request an ultrasound exam to check the thickness of the lining of your uterus or an endometrial biopsy, in which a tissue sample is removed for laboratory study, to detect any precancerous conditions.

How serious is polycystic ovary syndrome?

Women with PCOS are at increased risk of diabetes, high blood pressure, abnormal blood fats and coronary artery disease. Because PCOS disrupts the reproductive cycle and exposes the uterus to a constant supply of estrogen — due to the lack of ovulation — women with PCOS are at increased risk of abnormal uterine bleeding and uterine cancer.

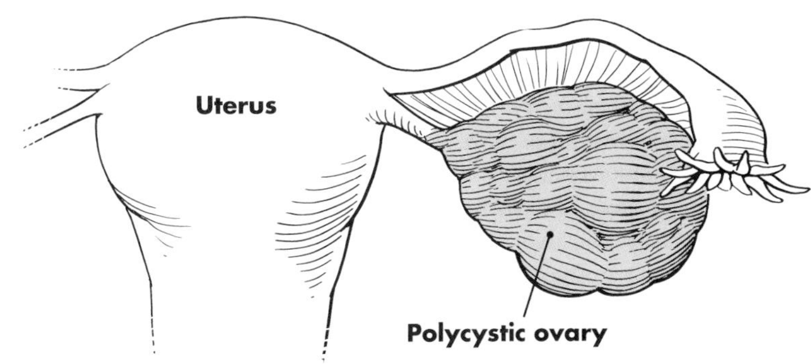

Polycystic ovary syndrome is a disorder involving irregular menstrual periods and occasionally an excess of facial and body hair. The ovaries develop multiple cysts and fail to release eggs.

Treatment

Overweight women with PCOS have more severe signs and symptoms. Weight loss can reduce both insulin and androgen levels. If you don't want to become pregnant, your doctor may prescribe birth control pills or long-acting progestins such as medroxyprogesterone to suppress ovulation and forestall development of possible precancerous changes in the lining of your uterus. Your doctor may add a medication, such as spironolactone (Aldactone), to counter the effects of excess androgen.

Researchers are evaluating the use of metformin (Glucophage), an oral medication for type 2 diabetes (formerly called adult-onset or non-insulin-dependent diabetes) to treat PCOS. Metformin inhibits the production and release of glucose from the liver, thus requiring less insulin to transport blood sugar into cells.

If you want to conceive, you may be given a fertility drug to induce ovulation. About half of the women with PCOS who take a fertility drug become pregnant. If, despite medication, you fail to conceive, in rare cases a procedure may be performed on the wall of your ovary that may improve your chances of conception.

Premenstrual syndrome

Signs and symptoms

- Bloating, fluid retention, abdominal swelling, swollen hands and feet and weight gain
- Breast soreness
- Clumsiness
- Fatigue
- Headache
- Gastrointestinal upset, including nausea, vomiting, diarrhea and constipation
- Skin and respiratory problems
- Mood swings, difficulty concentrating and lethargy
- Irritability, anxiety, anger and tension

Premenstrual syndrome (PMS) is a predictable pattern of physical and emotional changes that occur just before menstruation. For 2 percent to 5 percent of women, PMS is a significant problem. Many others experience the condition to only a mild degree. The symptoms can develop any time after the midpoint in your menstrual cycle, and they generally disappear soon after your period starts. PMS symptoms tend to wax and wane from month to month, and they are more apt to trouble women in their 20s and 30s.

No one really knows what causes PMS. It's undoubtedly related to cyclic changes in hormone levels because symptoms disappear during pregnancy and after menopause. Stress can aggravate the problem, but it's not the sole cause. Occasionally, some women with severe PMS may have undiagnosed depression, though depression alone doesn't explain all of the symptoms of PMS. Caution should be used in blaming PMS for mood abnormalities.

Diagnosis

A doctor will attribute a particular symptom to PMS only if it's part of a predictable premenstrual pattern. To determine if there's a pattern, your doctor may ask you to keep a record of your symptoms over several menstrual cycles. On a calendar or in a diary, you record all of your symptoms, the day you first noticed them and the day they disappeared. Note, too, the day your period began.

How serious is premenstrual syndrome?

PMS can be hard to tolerate, but it's not associated with any underlying disease process. PMS often disappears on its own before menopause. If you find your PMS symptoms hard to live with, there are potential treatments.

Treatment

Your doctor usually can offer relief from some of the symptoms of PMS and help ease your discomfort.

Medication

None of the medications used to treat PMS help all women. But individual reactions to the drugs differ, and each helps some women.

For severe PMS, a class of antidepressants known as selective serotonin reuptake inhibitors (SSRIs) has become the initial drug of choice. The most studied drug is fluoxetine (Prozac), but others, such as paroxetine (Paxil) and sertraline (Zoloft), also may be effective.

A diuretic, sometimes called a water pill, may reduce premenstrual water retention and bloating, although some studies show no benefit from its use, and this treatment can have serious side effects. Oral contraceptives also have been effective in treating some women's PMS symptoms.

Nutrition and exercise

By avoiding salt for a few days before your period, you can help reduce bloating and fluid retention. If you avoid caffeine, you may feel less irritable and tense and have less breast soreness. Many women say that regular exercise helps provide an emotional lift.

Women who have only mild PMS sometimes find that simply recording their symptoms for a few months is all the help they need. Once it's clear that their problems are predictable and short-lived, they find their PMS easier to tolerate.

Mittelschmerz

Signs and symptoms

- Pain in the lower abdomen at the time of ovulation
- Slight vaginal bleeding accompanying the pain

Mittelschmerz is a German word meaning "middle pain." The condition occurs at the midpoint in the menstrual cycle, about the time of ovulation. Typically, the pain is a dull ache that lasts anywhere from a few minutes to a few hours. It may be accompanied by minimal bleeding.

When an ovarian follicle ruptures and releases an egg, fluid from the follicle escapes into your abdominal cavity and may cause irritation. Stretching the ovary with a developing egg also may be painful. The rapid drop in estrogen that occurs at the time of ovulation may cause bleeding.

The timing and location of the pain usually serve to identify mittelschmerz. On rare occasions, the pain is severe enough to resemble that of appendicitis.

Treatment

Treatment varies depending on how often you experience mittelschmerz and how painful it is. You can take a mild analgesic such as acetaminophen, aspirin or ibuprofen to ease the pain. If it's severe and occurs most months, your doctor may recommend that you take birth control pills to prevent ovulation.

Painful periods

Signs and symptoms

- Pain in the lower abdomen during menstruation, possibly extending to the hips, lower back or thighs

More than half of all women have mild abdominal cramps on the first day or two of their periods. However, 10 percent experience such severe menstrual pain (dysmenorrhea) that they can't manage their normal routine without taking medication.

If the pain isn't a symptom of an underlying gynecological disorder, but is instead an exaggeration of normal menstrual processes, the problem is called primary dysmenorrhea. The prefix *dys* means "difficult," *men* signifies "month," and *rhoia* means "a flow." Medical experts believe that production of prostaglandins, substances that make the uterus contract, cause primary dysmenorrhea.

When a gynecological disorder causes painful menstruation, it's known as secondary dysmenorrhea. In general, there's likely to be a secondary cause when the pain lasts longer than the first 1 to 3 days of the menstrual period. The underlying cause could be fibroids, adenomyosis, endometriosis, pelvic inflammatory disease or an ovarian cyst or tumor.

Diagnosis

Your doctor's first concern is to check for the underlying disorders that cause secondary dysmenorrhea. You'll likely have a pelvic examination and perhaps blood tests and a urinalysis. Your doctor may also order diagnostic tests, such as ultrasound, to get images of your pelvic organs.

How serious are painful periods?

Primary dysmenorrhea can be extremely painful, but it's not harmful. More common during adolescence, it's likely to ease or disappear by the time you're in your mid-20s or after you've had your first baby. Secondary dysmenorrhea is more serious, but most of the disorders that underlie it are treatable.

Treatment

Treatment depends on the type of dysmenorrhea you have. For primary dysmenorrhea, your doctor may prescribe a nonsteroidal anti-inflammatory drug (NSAID) such as ibuprofen (Advil, Motrin, others) or naproxen (Aleve, Naprosyn, others) to help relieve the pain. These medications, which block prostaglandin formation, work for about 80 percent of the women who take them. Oral contraceptives consistently relieve the discomfort. For secondary dysmenorrhea, treatment is generally focused on curing or managing the underlying cause.

Dysfunctional uterine bleeding

Signs and Symptoms

- Vaginal bleeding that occurs at irregular intervals
- Vaginal bleeding that's unpredictable in amount or duration

The menstrual cycle varies from woman to woman, but menstrual flow generally occurs about every 28 days, lasts 4 to 5 days and produces a blood loss of 60 to 250 milliliters (4 tablespoons to about a cup).

Dysfunctional uterine bleeding refers to irregular bleeding that's not caused by an anatomic abnormality. Common and usually painless, it occurs most often in girls who have just begun to menstruate, in women approaching menopause or as a consequence of stress or illness. In most cases, the uterine lining grows too thick because the ovaries aren't producing hormones normally.

Dysfunctional uterine bleeding can take a number of forms, including heavy periods (menorrhagia), infrequent periods (oligomenorrhea), abnormally frequent periods (polymenorrhea) and irregular, heavy periods (metrorrhagia).

When it's not due to life stage or stress, dysfunctional uterine bleeding is most commonly due to anovulation associated with polycystic ovary syndrome. Less frequently, the problem is an estrogen-producing ovarian tumor or abnormal estrogen metabolism due to liver disease.

Rarely, a woman who's not nearing menopause begins to menstruate infrequently and develops acne and an unusual amount of hair on her face and body. In this case, the problem may be an excess of androgen, produced either by her adrenal glands or by an ovarian tumor.

Diagnosis

Your doctor will most likely ask you about your medical history and menstrual cycles and do a pelvic examination to make sure the source of the bleeding is your uterus and not your bladder, vagina or cervix. Your doctor may also try to determine if a tubal (ectopic) pregnancy or an early miscarriage could be the cause of your bleeding. Associated symptoms that are cause for concern are excessive facial hair, breast discharge, thyroid problems or abnormal blood clotting.

Your doctor may recommend a dilatation and curettage (D and C) to determine the cause of bleeding. In this minor surgical procedure, your doctor dilates your cervix and scrapes the lining of your uterus with a thin, spoon-shaped instrument (curette). Samples of the lining are sent to a laboratory to check for cancer.

Sports and Menses

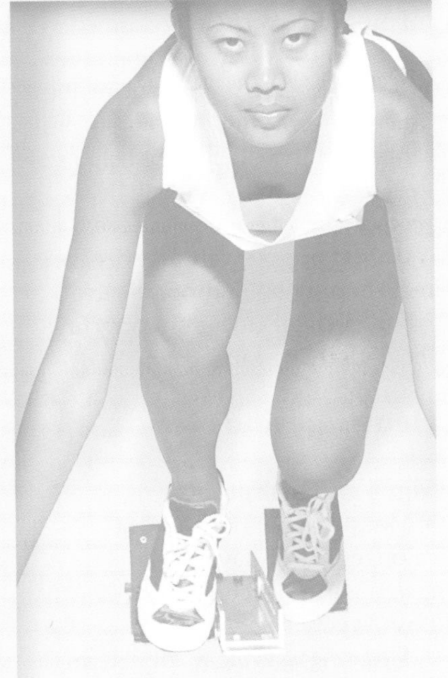

Female dancers, runners and females involved in vigorous sports frequently find that they skip menstrual periods or stop menstruating (amenorrhea). This is more likely to happen if you're young, especially if your menstrual cycle tends to be irregular. In fact, some teenagers who train heavily for an athletic event reach their late teens before they start menstruating.

Medical experts believe that several factors are involved, including stress and perhaps the ratio of fat cells to other cells in your body. In either case, you stop menstruating because your ovaries don't produce hormones in the cyclic manner that causes the uterine lining to thicken and then shed.

Reducing your exercise schedule or gaining weight may cause you to begin menstruating again. If that doesn't work, or if you don't want to exercise less or gain weight, your doctor may suggest hormone therapy, often in the form of oral contraceptives. There's a good reason for this. If you're not producing normal amounts of estrogen, you are more susceptible to osteoporosis, which makes fractures more likely in later years.

Keep in mind that spontaneous recovery is common, and you could ovulate at any time and be at risk of pregnancy, so don't forget about birth control.

How serious is dysfunctional uterine bleeding?

If you're bleeding in a pattern outside of what's normal for your periods, see your doctor. Dysfunctional uterine bleeding usually requires treatment. If you menstruate infrequently and can't achieve a desired pregnancy, you may need to see a fertility specialist. Women with chronic bleeding are sometimes infertile.

Treatment

Treatment depends on the cause of the condition. Once the cause is defined, oral contraceptives can be very useful in promoting regular menstrual cycles. If the bleeding is heavy, you may require hospitalization, bed rest and injections of estrogen or progesterone. If you've become anemic, you may need iron supplements. In rare cases, a surgical procedure may be performed to try to control heavy bleeding.

If your ovaries are producing too little estrogen, your doctor may prescribe hormone therapy to help prevent osteoporosis. Estrogen helps protect against bone loss. If the cause of your problem is excessive male hormones (androgens), treatment will likely focus on correcting the underlying cause.

Heavy periods

Signs and symptoms

- Menstrual periods that last longer than 7 days
- Periods in which bleeding is unusually heavy

Menorrhagia is the medical term for heavy periods. The disorder also is known as hypermenorrhea.

Heavy periods are common, especially in young women who aren't ovulating regularly and in women approaching menopause. However, any woman at any time in her reproductive years may experience heavy menstrual bleeding. Some women have heavy periods almost every cycle.

Approximately 30 percent of women complain of heavy menstrual bleeding, but only 10 percent experience blood loss severe enough to be defined as menorrhagia. Often, heavy periods reflect some spontaneous disturbance of the hormone cycle. They can also be the result of fibroids, a pelvic infection, certain medications, such as anticoagulants, or endometriosis. Some intrauterine devices used for birth control also can cause menorrhagia.

If you bleed heavily later than your expected period, you could be having a miscarriage. If the miscarriage is incomplete, you may need to have a dilatation and curettage (D and C) or a suction procedure.

You probably don't need medical attention if you have a single heavy period. If the bleeding doesn't stop or slow significantly within 24 hours, call your doctor. If you have several heavy periods, see a doctor to make sure that you're not developing iron deficiency anemia, a condition that results from the loss of blood.

Diagnosis

Your doctor will likely do a pelvic examination to check for abnormalities of your uterus. Your doctor may also do a Pap test and a biopsy of your uterine lining (endometrium).

In addition, you may have other tests, such as an ultrasound exam or a dilatation and curettage procedure to try to identify the cause of the heavy bleeding. Your doctor may request a blood test to make sure you're not anemic.

How serious are heavy periods?

Menorrhagia is inconvenient, and it can be distressing. However, most of the time it doesn't indicate a serious underlying disorder. You have to be sure you aren't becoming anemic.

Treatment

Treatment may depend on your age and the condition of your uterus.

Medication

If you're young and your uterus is normal, your doctor may prescribe birth control pills to reduce the bleeding. Nonsteroidal anti-inflammatory drugs (NSAIDs), such as ibuprofen (Advil, Motrin, others) or naproxen (Aleve, Naprosyn, others), also may decrease the amount of blood flow, as can other hormonal treatments. If you're anemic, you may need iron tablets.

Surgery

If other treatments fail, your doctor may recommend a hysterectomy or a procedure called endometrial ablation.

Postmenopausal bleeding

Signs and symptoms

- Vaginal bleeding a year or more after your last menstrual period
- Occasional bleeding after intercourse

Vaginal bleeding after menopause has a number of possible explanations. It may stem from a vaginal infection or vaginal atrophy, in which the walls of your vagina become thinner and more fragile. Bleeding due to vaginal atrophy commonly occurs after sexual intercourse. Hormone replacement therapy can cause bleeding. Vaginal bleeding following menopause can also be an early symptom of uterine cancer.

Diagnosis

See your doctor if you experience vaginal bleeding following menopause. Your doctor will likely perform a pelvic examination. The first concern will be to establish the source and cause of the bleeding.

This may involve a Pap test, a vaginal ultrasound exam or other diagnostic procedures. If any of the tests are abnormal, the next step may be a hysteroscopy or a uterine dilatation and curettage (D and C) to further evaluate the source of bleeding.

Sometimes, exhaustive study fails to reveal the cause of postmenopausal bleeding. However, even if a cause isn't found, if the

Endometrial Ablation

Newer surgical procedures may make hysterectomy unnecessary for some women with heavy menstrual periods. The procedures are typically done in outpatient settings, and you usually can return to full activity within 48 hours. However, you're only eligible for these procedures if you have no desire to become pregnant because a pregnancy can't progress normally after the uterine lining (endometrium) has been surgically removed or destroyed.

The surgical alternatives involve removing or destroying (ablating) the uterine lining. The most common techniques are standard ablation, roller-ball diathermy and thermal balloon ablation. Other types of ablation are being developed, as well.

You may be a candidate for one of the newer treatments if:

- You often need to change your pad or tampon more than every hour
- You develop iron deficiency anemia as a result of your blood loss
- Excessive bleeding interferes with your normal activities
- Hormonal or other treatments fail
- The cause of your bleeding is noncancerous (benign)
- You wish to avoid hysterectomy

Be aware that up to 25 percent of women who undergo ablation still may need a later hysterectomy to control bleeding or for other reasons.

Hysteroscopic ablation

Using a scope to see inside your uterus, a surgeon treats the uterine lining with a laser beam or electric current. Possible complications include uterine perforation and fluid imbalance, a result of absorbing excessive fluid during the procedure.

Thermal balloon ablation

This procedure uses a fluid-filled balloon that's inflated inside the uterus. After a probe inside the balloon heats the fluid, the balloon is left in place for about 8 minutes. The heat destroys cells in the uterine lining, and the lining eventually sloughs off. The whole procedure takes about 30 minutes. Most balloons used are latex-free, so women with latex allergies can be treated. This procedure is less likely to cause uterine rupture than hysteroscopic techniques.

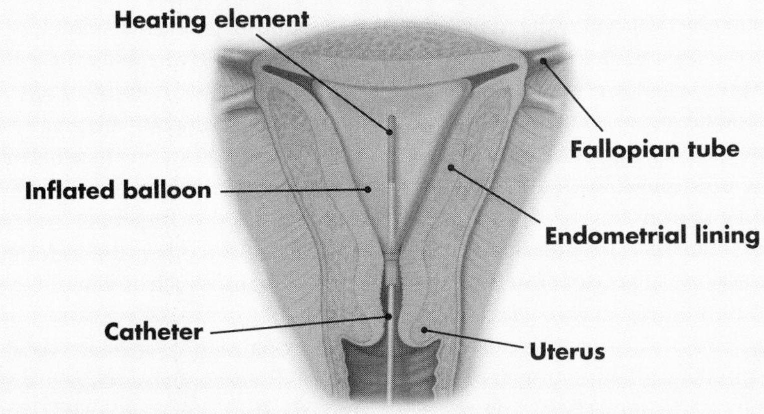

A doctor inserts a fluid-filled thermal balloon and inflates it. A heated probe inside the balloon heats the fluid. The balloon is left in place for about 8 minutes. The heat destroys cells in the uterine lining.

bleeding recurs, you should be re-examined.

How serious is postmenopausal bleeding?

In most instances, postmenopausal bleeding isn't serious, but it's the most common symptom of endometrial (uterine) cancer. Early diagnosis and treatment offer the best chances for a cure.

Treatment

Treatment depends on the underlying disorder. Vaginal infections are generally treated with antibiotics. If the tissue lining your vagina has become fragile, your doctor may prescribe estrogen, either systemically or just in the vagina. Estrogen helps protect against thinning of vaginal tissue. If the bleeding is a result of a cancer, surgery and other treatments may be necessary.

Menopause

Signs and symptoms

- Cessation of periods
- Hot flashes, a sudden reddening of the face and neck associated with a feeling of warmth
- Thinning of vaginal tissues and decreased lubrication, which can cause painful intercourse
- Insomnia

Menopause is a stage of life, not a medical condition. In the simplest terms, it's a transition from the time when you menstruate and can bear children to the time when you no longer menstruate and can no longer become pregnant. It happens when your ovaries no longer contain eggs and no longer produce enough estrogen to adequately stimulate the lining of your uterus and vagina.

Menopause comes naturally to most women between the ages of 45 and 55. Once you reach midlife, you'll suspect you're approaching menopause when your periods become irregular. You may menstruate more or less often, you may skip periods, or your periods may become shorter or longer and heavier.

An estimated one-third of women experience no menstrual irregularities prior to menopause. They simply stop menstruating. For most women, menopause is a gradual process that takes anywhere from several months to several years as the ovaries produce less and less estrogen. You still may produce some estrogen elsewhere in your body, but the total amount available decreases dramatically at menopause. When your estrogen level is so low that it can no longer stimulate your uterine lining (endometrium) to proliferate and grow, you've reached menopause.

Literally, menopause occurs when you menstruate for the last time. Clinical menopause occurs when you have had no menses for 12 months. Perimenopause is the 5- to 10-year period that begins when you first experience menstrual irregularities and lasts until your body has adjusted completely to hormonal changes.

Although girls in this country are reaching menarche at younger ages than girls in previous generations, the onset of menopause has stayed relatively constant. Although it's not unheard of for a woman to be menstruating in her mid-50s, the median age at the last menstruation is 50 to 51 years. Because a woman's life expectancy may be almost 80 years, she has almost a third of her life left to live following menopause.

Common changes

Menopause is associated with a number of signs and symptoms such as hot flashes (hot flushes) and vaginal changes. Hot flashes happen when blood vessels dilate. Some women experience only mild flashes. Other women's flashes cause extreme discomfort. Women in the latter group may wake up drenched with perspiration many times each night (night sweats). During the day, they may feel conspicuous and embarrassed when flashes strike as they feel their faces heat up and they begin to perspire. It helps to remember that most of the time the flashes produce only a slight change in skin color, so others don't usually notice.

All women experience gradual vaginal changes with menopause. Thinning vaginal tissues and less lubrication may make intercourse painful. Vaginal changes and thinning of tissues in the urinary tract may cause increased susceptibility to both vaginal and urinary infections.

Osteoporosis, a disorder in which your bones become porous and brittle, can become a serious problem. It's most common in postmenopausal women. Other diseases, such as coronary artery disease and breast cancer, are more prevalent after menopause.

Many women develop sleep problems during menopause, and a small percentage develop emotional difficulties. However, the connection between emotional difficulties and menopause is hard to prove or disprove, because midlife is often a difficult time for both women and men, especially if children leave home, spouses and friends become ill and elderly parents die. Any of these changes can trigger the mood disorders that are sometimes attributed to menopause.

Menopause can also affect your physical and mental health in positive ways. For instance, if you have migraines or endometriosis, the symptoms often diminish or disappear after menopause. Fibroids usually shrink. In addition, you no longer need to worry about becoming pregnant.

Seeing a doctor

Menopausal problems aren't life-threatening and are generally self-limited. If you do nothing about them, they'll generally go away on their own within a few months or a few years. You may want to see a doctor, though, to get relief from hot flashes and other discomforts of menopause, such as vaginal dryness.

Menopause does increase your risk of diseases such as osteoporosis and coronary artery disease. Therefore, it's a good idea to talk with your doctor about steps you can take to reduce your risk of these common diseases.

Hormone Abnormalities and Menstruation

A complex cascade of hormones governs the menstrual cycle. The hypothalamus in your brain sends chemicals called releasing factors to your pituitary gland. Your pituitary then releases pituitary hormones (gonadotropins) that travel through your bloodstream to your ovaries. These hormones cause ovarian follicles to produce estrogen and progesterone. Estrogen and progesterone prepare your uterus for a possible pregnancy. At any stage in this process, things can go wrong.

Many hormone-related disorders can cause menstrual irregularity. The hypothalamus may be affected by illness, stress or drugs. More rarely, your hypothalamus develops a disorder such as a tumor or infection, which can affect menstruation.

If the hypothalamus fails to stimulate the pituitary gland, estrogen production and menstruation will cease. Sometimes, the pituitary gland produces too much of the hormone prolactin. Prolactin stimulates milk production when a woman is breast-feeding. Released in excess at other times, it can prevent ovulation and menstruation.

Treatment

Although ovarian function can't be preserved, signs and symptoms of menopause can often be treated with medication. Lifestyle habits also help prevent or control symptoms of menopause.

Lifestyle

A well-balanced diet, regular exercise and avoidance of triggers may help you ease through this stage of life with fewer or less severe symptoms.

Diet
Eating a nutritious diet that's low in saturated fat and cholesterol and maintaining a healthy weight may reduce hot flashes and reduce your risk of developing coronary artery disease.

To help reduce your risk of osteoporosis, eat a diet rich in calcium, especially while you're young. Calcium is found in dairy products and green vegetables. Women under age 50 should have 1,000 milligrams (mg) of calcium daily, and those over age 50 should have 1,200 to 1,500 mg daily.

Exercise
Weight-bearing exercise, such as walking or lifting weights, can slow bone loss. Exercise also contributes to an overall feeling of well-being that can make coping with menopausal symptoms easier.

Triggers
To reduce hot flashes and night sweats, identify your hot flash triggers and try to manage or avoid them. Triggers may include stress, warm temperatures, spicy foods, caffeine and hot drinks.

Medication

Hormone replacement therapy (HRT) has been used to relieve the symptoms of menopause or to reduce the risk of conditions associated with decreased estrogen levels (see page 1082). Because of concerns about risks associated with HRT, other medications may also be used to treat specific symptoms.

Menopausal signs and symptoms
Signs and symptoms commonly associated with menopause, such as hot flashes, night sweats, vaginal dryness and mood swings, may be treated with the following medications:

- *Antidepressants.* Some antidepressant medications can help reduce hot flashes and night sweats. Venlafaxine (Effexor) is the one most widely used and has been found to be effective against hot flashes for women who can't take estrogen. Other antidepressants, such as fluoxetine (Prozac) and paroxetine (Paxil) may also help reduce hot flashes for some women. Antidepressants may also be beneficial in controlling mood swings that can develop during menopause.
- *Supplements.* Vitamin E and the herb black cohosh may have some effect in reducing hot flashes. Although black cohosh may have some estrogen-like effect, it's unknown if it also has estrogen-like risks. Its safety and effects beyond 6 months have not been studied. The Food and Drug Administration can't regulate supplements closely, so there's no guarantee of safety, purity and quality control.
- *Oral contraceptives.* Oral contraceptives may be an option during the years just preceding menopause (perimenopausal years). They can help regulate irregular bleeding, decrease heavy periods and reduce hot flashes, night sweats and vaginal dryness. There are risks associated with these medications, including blood clots and high blood pressure.
- *Topical estrogen.* Estrogen tablets, creams or slow-release rings that are applied to or inserted into the vagina may be used to relieve vaginal dryness, painful intercourse and bothersome urinary symptoms that may develop after menopause. Vaginal tissues absorb the estrogen, and the rest of the body is largely unaffected.
- *Lubricants.* A water-based lubricant, such as Astroglide or liquid K-Y, may be helpful during intercourse. The over-the-counter lubricant Replens may help moisturize and increase the elasticity of vaginal tissues if used on a regular basis. In addition, regular sexual stimulation increases blood flow and may help keep tissues supple.

Osteoporosis
You may be able to slow or prevent the development of this bone-thinning disease with:

- *Bisphosphonates.* The drugs alendronate (Fosamax) and risedronate (Actonel) help prevent bone loss and reduce your risk of fractures as effectively as or more effectively than hormone therapy. Concerns include gastrointestinal symptoms and rarely, risk of esophageal ulcers, especially if you take them incorrectly or you've had a previous acid reflux problems.
- *Selective estrogen receptor modulators (SERMs).* The drug raloxifene (Evista) falls into this category. SERMs provide estrogen-like benefits for bone density and blood fats, and they reduce the risk of spinal fractures. Unlike HRT, SERMs don't stimulate breast and uterine tissue, so they don't cause uterine bleeding or increase breast tenderness. SERMs do carry the same risk of causing blood clots as HRT. They also often make hot flashes worse.
- *Calcitonin.* Calcitonin is a hormone produced in your thyroid gland that helps maintain bone density and prevent fractures. However, calcitonin supplementation appears to be less beneficial than other osteoporosis treatments and may not prevent fractures in bones other than your spine. The medication is usually administered as a nasal spray. It's typically prescribed to

people who can't take bisphosphonates or other osteoporosis treatments. The main side effect is occasional nasal irritation.

Coronary artery disease

In addition to lifestyle changes, several medications may help prevent narrowing of your coronary arteries. They include:

- *Statins.* The cholesterol medications atorvastatin (Lipitor), fluvastatin (Lescol), lovastatin (Mevacor), pravastatin (Pravachol) and simvastatin (Zocor) are much more effective at treating high cholesterol and reducing coronary artery disease than is estrogen.
- *Others.* Other medications that may reduce cholesterol levels include bile acid sequestrants, nicotinic acid and fibric acids (see page 737).

Breast cancer

For women at high risk of breast cancer, doctors may prescribe:

- *Tamoxifen.* Tamoxifen (Nolvadex) is a synthetic hormone that's been used for 20 years to treat breast cancer. It's also approved for use in reducing the risk of breast cancer for women at increased risk.

  In addition, tamoxifen may improve bone density in women who are postmenopausal. However, it tends to cause hot flashes and carries the same risk of blood clots as HRT and raloxifene. It can also increase your risk of uterine cancer.

Hormone replacement therapy

Hormone replacement therapy (HRT) partially replenishes the hormones that diminish with menopause. It does so by providing a low dose of the hormone estrogen, often in combination with a progestin — a natural or synthetic form of the hormone progesterone.

HRT is most commonly used for controlling menopausal symptoms, such as hot flashes (hot flushes) and vaginal dryness. It may also be prescribed for long-term protection against medical conditions that can occur following menopause, such as osteoporosis. However, despite its long-term use, HRT's benefits and risks aren't fully known. One large study indicates that the therapy may carry more risks than once thought. It found that the risk of breast cancer, heart attacks, stroke and serious blood clots was slightly higher in women taking a particular combination of estrogen and progestin (Prempro) than in women taking a placebo.

It's important to weigh the benefits and disadvantages of hormone replacement therapy with your doctor. The decision about whether to use HRT should be made jointly on the basis of these discussions.

Forms of HRT

If you decide to take HRT, the type of therapy your doctor recommends depends in part on whether you've had your uterus surgically removed, a procedure called hysterectomy.

- *If you haven't had a hysterectomy.* If you still have your uterus, you'll likely be advised to take progestin along with estrogen. Estrogen stimulates growth of your uterine (endometrial) lining, which, if left unchecked, could become cancerous. Progestin balances estrogen's effect on the uterus. If you take progestin with estrogen, your risk of developing endometrial (uterine) cancer is not increased.
- *If you've had a hysterectomy.* If your uterus has been removed, estrogen is given alone, without progestin. Because you no longer have a uterus, you don't have to worry about the increased risk of endometrial cancer.

Estrogen is most commonly taken as a pill. It's also available in the form of a patch, cream, tablet or vaginal ring. Progestin also comes in pill form. It can be taken separately or as a combination pill that includes both estrogen and progestin. Progestin is also sold in the form of a patch or gel.

Both estrogens and progestins come in natural and synthetic forms. Natural isn't necessarily better than synthetic. Each form can affect your body in a different way.

You generally take HRT according to one of two schedules:

- *Cyclic.* A cyclic method provides estrogen daily and progestin 10 to 14 days of the month. This usually leads to predictable, monthly vaginal bleeding, at least in the early years of HRT use.
- *Continuous.* A continuous method provides low doses of estrogen and progestin daily and, though it doesn't cause monthly bleeding, may result in irregular spotting, particularly in the first year of use.

HRT is also prescribed in a number of dosing strengths. Moderate- to low-dose regimens may be as effective as higher-dose regimens in reducing symptoms and can still help prevent osteoporosis. While low-dose estrogen helps prevent osteoporosis, it's not as effective as regular-dose estrogen. Some women need to take higher doses of estrogen for a period of time to relieve hot flashes. This dose can be tapered over time.

Risks and benefits

If you're considering HRT, understand the risks and benefits of the therapy. The accompanying chart lists some of the known, probable and possible benefits and risks. In addition, each form of HRT has its own pros and cons.

Pills

Taken by mouth, estrogen enters your body through your intestines, where it's absorbed and passed on to the liver before it makes its way to your circulatory system. Avoid the pill form if you have a history of liver and gallbladder problems and you haven't had your gallbladder removed. Estrogen may worsen symptoms and may cause gallstones.

Oral estrogen can also increase your risk of blood clots. In addition, it may increase levels of certain blood fats (triglycerides). High triglyceride levels increase your risk of cardiovascular disease. At the same time, oral estrogen may help lower low-density lipoprotein (LDL or "bad") cholesterol and increase high-density lipoprotein (HDL or "good") cholesterol.

One specific type of oral combination HRT — prescribed as a single pill (Prempro) — was shown in a recent large study to slightly increase your risk of heart problems, stroke, blood clots and breast cancer. This risk may also apply to oral combination HRT that includes estrogen plus medroxyprogesterone acetate (Provera, Cycrin, others).

Hormone Replacement Therapy Risks and Benefits

These are known, probable and possible risks and benefits of hormone replacement therapy (HRT) in general. Talk with your doctor about how these factors might pertain to you.

	Known*	Probable**	Possible †
Short-term benefits	• Reduces frequency or severity of hot flashes • Reduces vaginal and urinary tract symptoms • Improves sleep in women bothered by nighttime hot flashes	Not applicable	• May help maintain skin tone • May decrease depression and mood swings • May improve sleep, even in women not experiencing hot flashes
Long-term benefits	• Slows bone loss • Can raise high-density lipoprotein (HDL or "good") cholesterol and lower low-density lipoprotein (LDL or "bad") cholesterol	• Reduces bone fractures • May decrease risk of colorectal cancer	• May protect against Alzheimer's disease • May improve memory and mental function • May protect against macular degeneration, an eye disease
Short-term risks	• Blood clotting • Irregular vaginal bleeding • Fluid retention • Breast tenderness • Headache • Nausea	• May slightly increase risk of heart disease, including heart attack	Not applicable
Long-term risks	• Blood clotting • Irregular vaginal bleeding • Gallbladder disease • Oral estrogen can cause triglyceride levels to rise • If taken without progestin, increases risk of endometrial (uterine) cancer	• May slightly increase risk of heart disease, including heart attack, and stroke • May slightly increase risk of breast cancer, particularly if used for many years — risk may be higher with use of progestin	Not applicable

*Based on multiple, conclusive studies that are broadly accepted.
**Based on at least one large study. Additional studies are ongoing.
†Theoretical, or based on small studies or case reports.

Patches

Applying an estrogen patch to your abdomen one or two times a week delivers estrogen directly through your skin into your blood. This method initially bypasses your liver, reducing the aggravating effect that oral estrogen can have on liver and gallbladder problems. Plus it won't increase triglyceride levels.

The patch is comparable to oral estrogen in relieving menopausal symptoms and preventing osteoporosis. If a progestin is needed, you can take it orally or use a combination estrogen-progestin patch. The patch sometimes irritates your skin, and some women have difficulty keeping it attached to the skin. Newer patches have been changed to reduce these problems.

Vaginal creams, tablets and rings

Hormone creams, tablets and rings applied vaginally are useful in treating menopausal symptoms such as vaginal dryness, urinary changes and painful intercourse. Because estrogen applied this way is only minimally absorbed into your bloodstream, it won't protect against osteoporosis or improve cholesterol levels.

You usually apply a hormone cream vaginally, on a regular basis, with an applicator that resembles those used to treat yeast infections. A vaginal estrogen ring is inserted into the upper third of your vagina, where it remains and releases a constant dose of estrogen for up to 90 days. You replace it with another ring at 3-month intervals. With vaginal tablets, you insert them into the vagina twice a week.

Vaginal and Vulvar Disorders

Your vagina is the passageway that connects your uterus to your external genitals. Its walls are lined with strong muscles. Most of the time your vagina is so narrow that the walls touch, but it can expand dramatically. The neck of your uterus, the cervix, extends into your vagina at the upper end.

In girls, the outer end of the vagina is partially blocked by a thin membrane called the hymen. In very rare cases, the hymen may close off the vagina altogether. The membrane is sometimes semicircular and covers just part of your vaginal opening, or it may be circular with a central opening.

The area of the external genitals is called the vulva. It includes the lip-like folds of tissue — labia majora and labia minora — that shield your vagina and urethra.

Just below the mons pubis, where the labia come together, is the clitoris, a small organ that becomes distended during sexual arousal. Your urethra, which opens just below your clitoris, leads to your bladder, where urine is stored. Below your urethra is your vaginal opening. Glands located in the vulva and vagina lubricate this area during sexual arousal.

Developmental disorders

Signs and symptoms

- Undersized or absent vagina, or a very short vagina and no cervix
- Genitals in a female that resemble male genitals

At conception, the embryo acquires either male (XY) or female (XX) chromosomes. For the next 40 days, males and females are indistinguishable. After that time, if the fetus has a Y chromosome, testicles begin to develop. In the absence of a Y chromosome and the presence of two X chromosomes, ovaries develop. These organs secrete male or female hormones, respectively, that cause the fetus to develop either a male or a female urogenital tract.

Sometimes, a female is born with sexually ambiguous genitals. She may have an unusually large clitoris, or the labia majora may be partially fused together and resemble a scrotum. The most common cause for ambiguous genitals is congenital adrenal hyperplasia, sometimes called pseudohermaphroditism. In such cases, the body doesn't produce enough of certain enzymes at a crucial time in fetal development. The internal organs of a female born with this condition are usually normal.

Early surgery can alter the genitals, if necessary. If the genital ambiguity is due to congenital adrenal hyperplasia, a potentially fatal complication (addisonian crisis) could develop unless your doctor is on the alert to prevent it.

Diagnosis

A doctor will do a physical examination and, because developmental disorders occasionally run in families, may take a family history. Laboratory tests on blood or skin cells can establish if a chromosomal problem caused the condition. Laboratory tests can also identify hormonal problems.

How serious are developmental disorders?

Girls with congenital adrenal hyperplasia have normal internal organs. Given surgical correction of abnormalities in the vulva and proper medication, they may be able to have children.

Treatment

Depending on the cause of the disorder, treatment may involve medication or surgery or both. For congenital adrenal hyperplasia, doctors often prescribe corticosteroids to prevent a buildup of undesirable hormones. For girls born without a normal vagina, surgeons can create an artificial one, which allows sexual activity.

Vulvitis

Signs and symptoms

- Swelling of the vulva, with redness and itching
- Blisters that may ooze or crust over

- White or thickened areas of the vulva

Vulvitis is an inflammation of your external genitals (vulva). It can be caused by a reaction to a vaginal spray, to the detergent with which you wash your underwear or to a medication. Or it could stem from excess moisture or a bacterial, viral or fungal infection.

Diagnosis

Your doctor will likely do a pelvic examination and order blood tests, a urinalysis and other laboratory tests. If there's a possibility you have a sexually transmitted disease (STD), he or she may test for that. If the inflammation persists, you may need a biopsy to make sure there's no malignancy.

Treatment

Treatment varies depending on the cause of the problem. Usually, medication is prescribed. To help reduce symptoms and prevent a recurrence, keep the area clean and dry and wear loose, absorbent clothing and cotton underpants. If the vulvitis consistently develops after you use a spray or deodorant, stop using the product. The vulvitis may be a reaction to what you're using. An allergic reaction usually takes several days to develop.

Vulvar dystrophy

Signs and symptoms

- Dry, reddened areas in the vulva
- Itching in the affected area
- White or thickened areas of the vulva
- Papery or shiny skin around the vulva and anus
- A shrinking of the labia minora and vaginal opening

Dystrophy is a kind of degeneration of tissue. The word is derived from the Greek words for poor nutrition. Vulvar dystrophy usually occurs in women who are past menopause. It can cause patchy white and thickened areas of the vulva (hypertropic vulvar dystrophy) or thin, whitish skin around the vulva and anus (lichen sclerosus).

Diagnosis

To make sure that you don't have cancer, your doctor may remove a small piece of tissue for microscopic analysis (biopsy). He or she may also check for signs of an underlying infection. Vulvar dystrophy generally isn't life-threatening.

Treatment

Treatment depends on the source of the problem. Your doctor may prescribe a topical steroid cream, such as clobetasol propionate, to relieve symptoms, including itching. It's important to have periodic examinations to determine whether precancerous changes have developed.

Vulvodynia

Signs and symptoms

- Burning or stinging, irritation, itching of the vulva
- Stabbing pain in the vulvar area
- Rawness in the vulvar area

Vulvodynia means "painful vulva." Your vulva is the area around the opening to your vagina. It consists of the labia, the clitoris and the opening of your vagina.

The pain of vulvodynia may be constant or intermittent, localized or widespread and can last for months or even years. It can also vanish as suddenly as it started. In a type of vulvodynia known as vulvar vestibulitis, you may experience pain only when there's pressure on the area surrounding the entrance to your vagina, such as from a bicycle seat or tight jeans.

Diagnosis

Vulvodynia can be difficult to diagnose because it may have no visible signs, and the pain may come and go. The discomfort can be serious enough to interfere with your lifestyle, but the condition itself isn't life-threatening.

Treatment

Treatments for vulvodynia focus on relieving symptoms. Tricyclic antidepressant medications, such as amitriptyline (Elavil), sometimes help lessen the pain. Applying cool compresses to your genital area also may help improve your symptoms.

Vaginal Hygiene

Normally, your vagina is self-cleansing. Your vaginal walls produce their own fluid, which carries away dead cells and organisms as it flows downward. This healthy discharge is either clear or milky, becoming yellowish when it dries. It's somewhat slippery and has a mild, not unpleasant odor. It increases in amount at about the time you ovulate and during sexual arousal. If you have a vaginal discharge that's a different color or has a strong smell, you may have a vaginal infection and should see a doctor.

Washing your genitals once a day with a mild soap and water is sufficient. Douches and feminine hygiene sprays are unnecessary, and at times they can be harmful. Some commercial douches contain irritating chemicals. Douching can change the normally acidic vaginal environment that discourages the growth of yeast and other organisms that can cause infections.

Bacteria and fungi that cause vaginal infections tend to thrive in warm, moist conditions. For that reason, it's a good idea to wear cotton underpants or synthetic underpants with a cotton lining and to avoid tight pantyhose. Tight, nylon underpants and pantyhose trap heat and moisture in the genital area. Sleeping without underpants — except, perhaps, during your period — can be helpful.

One last point: Always wipe from front to back to avoid contaminating your vagina with bacteria from a bowel movement.

Genital warts

Signs and symptoms

- Tiny pink or white nodules in your genital area

Genital warts (venereal warts or condyloma acuminata) are caused by the human papillomavirus. You can get them from direct sexual contact with someone who has them. The incubation period is 1 to 6 months. In women, these warts can grow on the vulva, the walls of the vagina, the cervix or around the anus. In men, they may be found on the shaft of the penis, the scrotum or the anus. They can also develop on the mouth or in the throat of a person who has had oral sex with an infected person.

Diagnosis

A doctor usually can diagnose genital warts by their appearance. However, because you can acquire other sexually transmitted infections, such as chlamydia or the human immunodeficiency virus (HIV), from the same sexual exposure that caused the warts, you may need to be tested for other infections. Sometimes, a doctor will do a biopsy, in which a tissue sample is removed for laboratory study, to rule out cancer.

How serious are genital warts?

By themselves, genital warts are mainly a nuisance because they have a tendency to recur. However, they've also been associated with cancers of the cervix and rectum. The human papillomavirus that causes the warts may cause cancer in those tissues. If you've had genital warts, be sure to have a Pap test annually.

Treatment

How genital warts are treated depends on their size and location. Sometimes, medical treatment can take care of the virus that causes genital warts as well. If the underlying virus isn't completely eliminated, however, the warts may reappear even after treatment.

Medication

Medications are available that can be applied directly to the skin. These topical treatments include imiquimod (Aldara), podofilox (Condylox), trichloroacetic acid (TCA) or 5 percent 5-fluorouracil cream. Don't use over-the-counter wart removers. They aren't intended for use in the genital area.

Other therapies

Warts may also be removed with laser surgery or by freezing with liquid nitrogen (cryosurgery) or burning (electrocautery). Sometimes, surgery is necessary to remove large warts or those that don't respond to treatment.

Bartholin's abscess

Signs and symptoms

- A hot, tender, swollen lump in the labia majora

Bartholin's glands, named for Danish anatomist Casper Bartholin, are situated at the entrance to your vagina, one on each side. A gland or the duct on its surface can become infected. At first, the infection may ooze pus. If the opening to the gland becomes blocked, an abscess results.

Diagnosis

Your doctor will do a pelvic examination, examine the lump and possibly order laboratory tests to check for sexually transmitted diseases (STDs). The abscess itself generally requires surgical treatment. Sometimes, a chronic Bartholin's cyst forms afterward and may need to be removed surgically.

Treatment

Treatment generally involves draining the abscess.

Pubic lice

Signs and symptoms

- Grayish insects the size of a pinhead in pubic hair
- Tiny white particles —the eggs of the lice — clinging to the hair
- Severe itching in the pubic area

You can catch pubic lice by having intercourse with someone who has them or, rarely, from clothing or bedding. They can cause intense itching and a slight rash. Pubic lice are often called crabs because they hang on with crab-like claws. This problem is also known as pediculosis pubis.

Treatment

Prescription and over-the-counter medications can kill the lice. To keep from becoming reinfested, dry-clean the clothing you've worn and the sheets, blankets and towels you've used, or wash them in very hot water.

Put the rest of your clothes, towels and bedding away for 2 weeks where they won't come into contact with people. During that time, the louse eggs (nits) will hatch, and the lice will die of starvation. Treat infested mattresses the same way.

Vaginitis

Signs and symptoms

- Unusual vaginal discharge
- Itching and irritation in the vaginal area
- Pain during intercourse
- An unpleasant odor from the vaginal area
- Pain in the lower abdomen

PREVENTION TIP

To reduce your chances of getting genital warts or other sexually transmitted diseases (STDs), you need to practice safe sex. Aside from abstinence, having a monogamous partner who has no sexually transmitted diseases is the surest way to protect yourself. Using condoms is the next best thing. However, condoms aren't foolproof against disease.

Vaginitis is an inflammation of your vagina, usually caused by an infection. A vaginal infection can be sexually transmitted, though most vaginal infections aren't the result of a sexually transmitted disease (STD). Ask your doctor if your sexual partner needs treatment too.

Most vaginal infections are common and treatable, but those resulting from an STD may be more serious. It's possible to have an infection but no symptoms.

Common types

The three common causes of vaginitis are trichomoniasis, yeast infections (candida) and bacterial vaginosis.

Trichomoniasis

This type of infection is caused by a parasite. You may have no symptoms, or you may develop a smelly, greenish-yellow, sometimes frothy discharge. Most of the time, trichomoniasis is contracted through intercourse.

Yeast infection

The main symptom of a yeast infection is itchiness in the vaginal area, but you may also have a white discharge that resembles cottage cheese. You're more likely to develop a yeast infection if you're pregnant or if you're taking antibiotics, corticosteroid medications or birth control pills.

Bacterial vaginosis

This type of vaginitis may result from several bacteria and is very common. Symptoms include a white or grayish, fishy-smelling vaginal discharge.

Diagnosis

Your doctor will take a medical history and do a pelvic examination. He or she may take a sample of the discharge to identify the organism responsible. Vaginitis is common and, because it tends to recur, can be annoying.

Treatment

Treatment depends on the type of vaginitis you have. Doctors usually treat trichomoniasis with vaginal or oral metronidazole (MetroGel) and yeast infections with antifungal creams, suppositories or pills (Diflucan). For bacterial vaginosis your doctor may prescribe oral metronidazole (Flagyl) or clindamycin (Cleocin).

Atrophic vaginitis

Signs and symptoms

- Soreness, burning, or itching in your vagina
- Bleeding after intercourse
- Painful intercourse
- Thin, watery vaginal discharge

Atrophic vaginitis is an inflammation of the vagina caused by thinning (degeneration) of vaginal tissue. This condition is most likely to develop after menopause, although it can occur during breast-feeding. In both situations, estrogen production is decreased, and the walls of the vagina may become drier, thinner, less elastic and more prone to bleeding.

Diagnosis

A pelvic examination may be all that's necessary to diagnose the problem, although your doctor may order some tests if it appears that you have a vaginal infection. Atrophic vaginitis isn't serious, but it can interfere with sexual intercourse and therefore may require treatment.

Treatment

In breast-feeding women, the problem is temporary. If you're past menopause, it's not.

Your doctor may prescribe hormone replacement therapy or you can apply estrogen directly to your vagina as a cream, ring or tablet. If the primary problem is painful intercourse, using a water-soluble lubricant also may help.

Vaginal cysts

Signs and symptoms

- Small swellings in the walls of your vagina
- A lump that bulges out of your vaginal opening

Several types of noncancerous (benign) cysts can develop in your vagina. The most common are inclusion cysts and Gartner's cysts. Inclusion cysts are caused by trauma, such as an operation or childbirth. Gartner's cysts are remains of a duct that serves a purpose during fetal development and then disappears. Sometimes, a Gartner's cyst enlarges enough to poke through your vaginal opening.

Vaginal Pain

When vaginal pain occurs during intercourse, it's called dyspareunia. A frequent cause is atrophic vaginitis. The symptoms are vaginal soreness or persistent or recurrent pain during intercourse. Sometimes your vagina may simply be irritated by a feminine hygiene spray or contraceptive cream or jelly.

Rarely, dyspareunia can result from bladder problems such as cystitis or urethritis. If intercourse causes deep internal pain, you may have endometriosis, or you could have some other disorder of your cervix, uterus, fallopian tubes, ovaries or pelvic floor.

If you're breast-feeding or you're past menopause, your vaginal lining may have thinned because you're producing less estrogen. Some women also have a problem called vaginismus — involuntary contractions of muscles at the opening to the vagina.

To determine the causes of vaginal pain, your doctor will likely do a pelvic examination and may order imaging tests. Treatment depends on what's causing your pain.

Diagnosis
A doctor can identify most cysts during a pelvic examination. A cyst generally isn't a problem unless it's so large that it interferes with intercourse.

Treatment
If it's not bothering you, you may elect to ignore a vaginal cyst. If a cyst causes discomfort, a doctor can remove it surgically.

Loss of pelvic support

Signs and symptoms
- A bulge in the walls of your vagina
- A feeling of fullness and discomfort when you bear down, sometimes with backache
- Difficulty defecating
- Urinary incontinence when you laugh or cough
- Pelvic pressure when lifting or when you stand for a long time

Your pelvic floor consists of a sheet of muscles and ligaments that support the organs — such as your bladder, uterus, colon and small intestine — that fill the pelvic cavity. These muscles also help close off your urethra where it leaves your bladder.

The muscles can become stretched or slack as a result of childbirth or aging or because of a hereditary weakness. When that happens, some of your internal organs may sink lower in your body (prolapse). Prolapse is more likely to develop in older women and in those who've given birth to several children.

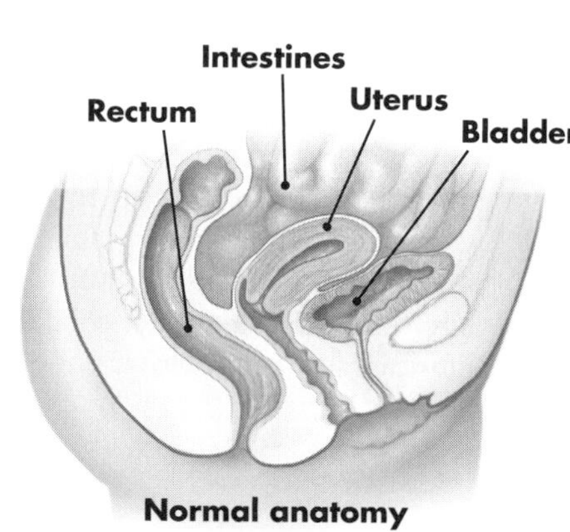

Normal anatomy

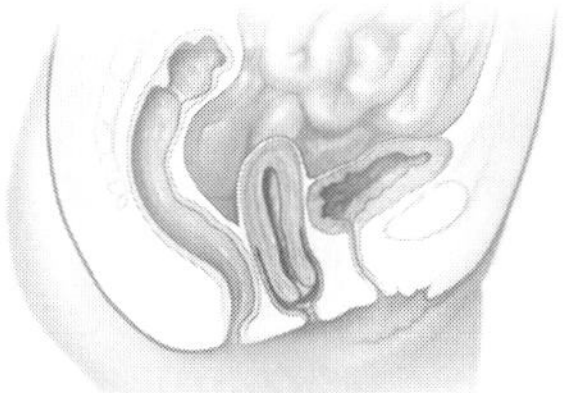
Uterine prolapse involves the uterus

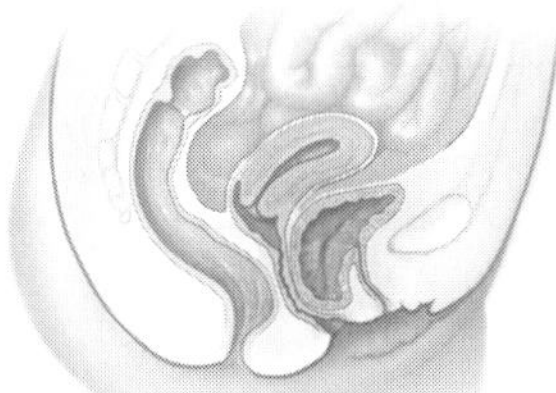
Cystocele involves the bladder

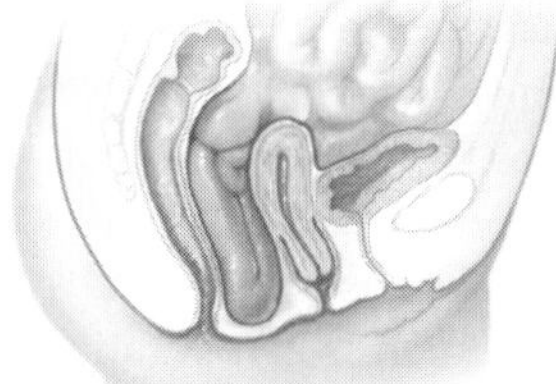
Enterocele involves the intestines

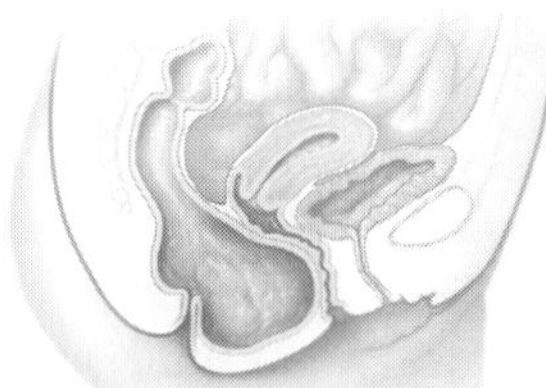
Rectocele involves the rectum

One or more female pelvic organs may be affected by pelvic floor muscle weakness. This weakness can cause prolapse of the uterus (uterine prolapse), bladder (cystocele), intestines (enterocele) or lower rectum (rectocele).

Sometimes, weakened pelvic muscles allow your uterus to drop downward into your vagina. In extreme cases, your cervix may actually protrude from your vaginal opening. When either your bladder or your urethra prolapses, they produce a bulge in the front wall of your vagina. A bulge in the back wall may mean that either your small intestine or your lower rectum has prolapsed. When that happens, bowel movements may become difficult.

Diagnosis
Telltale bulges in your vaginal wall usually make prolapses easy to diagnose during a pelvic examination. Minor prolapses are common, especially in older women. They're probably not serious if they don't cause too much discomfort. Serious cases may require treatment.

Treatment
Depending on the severity of the prolapse, self-care measures may provide the relief you need. Bladder and urethral prolapse can cause incontinence or repeated urinary tract infections. Surgical repair may be the best solution. A prolapsed lower rectum doesn't generally require an operation unless the bulge is large or there's difficulty with bowel movements. Any time a bulge is severe enough to extend outside the vaginal opening, treatment is in order.

Self-care
Sometimes, simple exercises called Kegel exercises are the only treatment you need. If you're overweight, losing weight may also improve your symptoms. Eating high-fiber foods also helps by allowing you to have bowel movements without straining.

Devices
If self-help measures aren't beneficial and an operation would be risky, your doctor can fit you with a vaginal pessary, a rubber device that fits around your cervix and

helps to prop up prolapsed organs. You'll have to remove it regularly to clean it.

Surgery
Surgery might include a vaginal repair, in which a surgeon elevates your prolapsed organ or organs back into place and tightens the muscles and ligaments of your pelvic floor. Another option is removal of the uterus (hysterectomy) with repair of any remaining prolapsed organs.

Your doctor may also consider collagen injections to treat incontinence caused by the prolapse. Collagen is a protein found in skin that thins with estrogen loss.

Kegel Exercises

Your pelvic floor muscles — those that surround your anus and vagina — are called the pubococcygeal muscles. In the 1950s, a physician by the name of A.M. Kegel developed an exercise regimen that may be helpful in strengthening these muscles:

- *Find the right muscles.* This is very important. Imagine that you're trying to stop urinating. When you use the correct muscles, you'll have a pulling feeling.
- *Pull in the pelvic muscles.* Hold them for a count of three and then relax for a count of three. Work up to 10 to 15 repetitions at a time.
- *Repeat the exercise at least three times a day.* You can exercise the muscles most anytime — while lying down, sitting in your car or standing in your kitchen. Using different positions makes the muscles strongest.

As the tone in your pubococcygeal muscles gradually improves, you'll likely have better pelvic support. Be patient. You may not feel the improvement for 3 to 6 weeks. As a bonus, many women find that they're also more responsive sexually.

During a collagen injection, the protein is injected through a cystoscope into the lining of your urethra. Collagen is a naturally occurring skin protein. Estrogen loss causes it to thin, so injecting it into the urethral lining adds bulk to the tissues of your urethra, helping to close the gap that allowed urine to leak.

Cervical, Uterine and Fallopian Tube Disorders

Your uterus (womb) is the organ that shelters the fetus when you're pregnant. The uterus is shaped like an upside-down pear. The narrower end, the cervix, extends into the vagina.

The fallopian tubes are connected to the uterus, one on each side of its broad top. Each tube extends from the interior of your uterus to a location close to each ovary. Once a month, one of the ovaries releases an egg that travels down a fallopian tube to the uterus.

Developmental disorders

Signs and symptoms

- Failure to begin menstruating at puberty
- An inability to conceive or to carry a pregnancy to term

Because of genetic problems or because something goes wrong during fetal development, some women are born with abnormalities of the cervix, uterus or fallopian tubes. These can range from a near-total absence of female reproductive organs to minor abnormalities that make it difficult to conceive or carry a pregnancy to term.

For instance, in a female fetus, an internal duct called the mullerian duct normally develops into fallopian tubes, a uterus and the upper portion of the vagina. If something interferes with this process, the baby may be born without a uterus or with one that's very short. This condition is known as mullerian agenesis.

Because most of these abnormalities are internal, if the child has a vaginal opening, there may be no indication of the problem until she reaches puberty and fails to menstruate.

Diagnosis

If your doctor suspects a developmental disorder, he or she may order a type of X-ray called a hysterosalpingogram. Because soft tissues can't be seen on an X-ray, this procedure uses a special dye that registers on the film. The dye is injected into your uterine cavity and travels up your fallopian tubes and into your abdominal cavity, where your body absorbs it. While the dye is spreading, a radiologist takes a series of X-rays.

Other diagnostic procedures may include ultrasound and magnetic resonance imaging (MRI). In some cases, laparoscopic surgery may be performed to get a direct view of the internal organs.

How serious are developmental disorders?

Although generally not life-threatening, these disorders can be emotionally difficult. Girls who have mullerian agenesis are infertile.

Treatment

Treatment varies depending upon the abnormality and its cause. Surgery can sometimes correct a cervix that's unable to sustain a pregnancy to term and fix certain structural problems of the uterus.

Cervical polyps

Signs and symptoms

- Bleeding after intercourse, between periods or after menopause
- Watery, bloody discharge from your vagina

Cervical polyps are growths, rather like grapes, that generally protrude from the mouth of your cervix. You may have one polyp or a cluster. They're common, often occurring during pregnancy because of hormonal changes.

Diagnosis
A doctor can often detect cervical polyps during a pelvic examination. He or she may remove the growth for laboratory testing.

How serious are cervical polyps?
They're almost never cancerous. A small polyp may produce no symptoms and may not be detected until your doctor finds it during a routine pelvic examination. Large polyps can cause bleeding, so you may want to have them removed.

Treatment
Your doctor may remove a single polyp in a brief office procedure. If you have many large polyps, you may need an operation, although this is rarely necessary.

Cervicitis

Signs and symptoms
- Vaginal discharge that's grayish or yellow
- Pain during intercourse
- Bleeding after intercourse

Cervicitis is an inflammation of your cervix. Most often, there are no symptoms and the condition is discovered as a result of a Pap test or a biopsy done for another condition. Common sexually transmitted diseases (STDs), as well as exposure to certain bacteria, can cause cervicitis.

Diagnosis
Your doctor will likely take samples of cervical secretion with a swab to be analyzed in a laboratory.

Treatment
If the cause of the inflammation is an STD, both you and your sexual partner may require treatment. You may not need treatment if you have only a minor inflammation that isn't caused by an STD.

Nabothian cyst

Signs and symptoms
- A fluid-filled lump on your cervix that you're not likely to feel

A nabothian cyst is named for German anatomist Martin Naboth. It forms when a mucus gland on your cervix becomes obstructed. This is most common in adolescence or after childbirth. A doctor generally can diagnose a nabothian cyst during a routine pelvic examination.

Treatment
The condition rarely requires treatment. If necessary, a doctor can remove the cyst by cauterizing it or through application of extreme cold (cryosurgery).

Cervical dysplasia

Cervical dysplasia is an abnormality of the cells at the surface of the cervix. This condition isn't cancer, but it may indicate an area that could become cancerous.

Cervical dysplasia is detected by means of a Pap test. The condition can occur at any age once sexual intercourse has begun. It's strongly linked to a virus called the human papillomavirus. Dysplasia is more likely to occur in someone who began sexual intercourse as a teenager or has had several sexual partners.

Diagnosis
If your Pap test reveals dysplasia, you may need further diagnostic testing, including an additional Pap test or a colposcopy. A colposcope is an instrument equipped with a magnifying lens and a light. A doctor uses it to examine the cervix. If your doctor spots an abnormality, he or she may remove a tissue sample (biopsy) to send for laboratory analysis to confirm the dysplasia and its severity.

Depending on the results of your tests, your doctor may recommend treatment or monitoring of the condition.

How serious is cervical dysplasia?
Left untreated, the condition could lead to cancer. Benign cell abnormalities sometimes disappear.

Treatment
Doctors may treat cervical dysplasia with a variety of procedures:
- *Observation.* This involves a period of time to see if the body will "clear" the problem on its own.
- *LEEP.* During this procedure, known as loop electrosurgical excision procedure (LEEP), a doctor removes abnormal tissue using a thin wire loop and a carefully controlled electric current.
- *Cryocautery.* Cryocautery involves freezing the cervix to destroy abnormal tissue.
- *Laser surgery.* During laser surgery, a high-energy beam of light burns away (vaporizes) the abnormal tissue. There's little or no damage to surrounding tissue, and the area heals quickly.
- *Conization.* For deeper or more worrisome dysplasias, a portion of the cervix is removed.

Fibroids

Signs and symptoms
- Heavy or prolonged menstrual periods
- Pain or pressure in your lower abdomen or lower back

Emergency signs and symptoms
- Sudden sharp pain low in your abdomen

A fibroid is a noncancerous (benign) tumor that develops within your uterine wall or is attached to it. Also called leiomyomas, myomas or fibromyomas, fibroids are extremely common. About 20 percent to 40 percent of women older than age 40 have them.

Rather than a single fibroid, you're more likely to have several. They can be as small as a pea or larger than a grapefruit. They often cause no symptoms. Normally, fibroids grow slowly, but they may respond to increased levels of hormones, which allows them to enlarge rapidly during pregnancy. After menopause, these tumors usually shrink and often disappear completely.

Diagnosis

A doctor often detects fibroids during a pelvic examination. If there's any question about what they are, your doctor will likely order a diagnostic test such as a computerized tomography (CT) scan or ultrasonography. During another procedure called hysteroscopy, a small scope is inserted into the uterus, allowing your doctor to look for fibroids.

How serious are fibroids?

Fibroids very rarely become cancerous, and most cause few problems. Nevertheless, if you have fibroids, schedule regular checkups to make sure they don't grow too large.

Fibroids can cause your menstrual periods to become very heavy, which could result in iron deficiency anemia. They can also make conception difficult, and they can cause miscarriage or interfere with delivery. Sometimes, a fibroid attached to your uterine wall becomes twisted, cutting off its blood supply. If that happens, then you may feel a sudden, sharp pain in your lower abdomen. This situation requires emergency surgery to remove the fibroid.

Treatment

If your fibroids don't cause symptoms, your doctor may suggest a wait-and-see approach. You may need regular follow-up visits and, possibly, ultrasound exams to monitor the size of the fibroids.

If you do develop symptoms, your doctor may recommend medication or surgery.

Medication

Oral contraceptives may help control regular bleeding. The hormonal treatment danazol (Danocrine) also may be useful to control excessive menstrual flow. However, these therapies don't control fibroid growth. Medications known as gonadotropin-releasing hormone (Gn-RH) agonists (Lupron, Viadur) may help shrink fibroids by reducing the amount of estrogen in your body. This form of drug therapy isn't a long-term solution, but it may be used as a preparation for surgery.

Unfortunately, Gn-RH agonists cause all of the symptoms of menopause, including hot flashes, mood swings, headaches, vaginal dryness and bone loss. If you need prolonged treatment, your doctor may use other medications to reduce menopausal symptoms.

Surgery

Sometimes you may need surgery to remove a fibroid. One option is myomectomy, a procedure in which only the fibroids are removed and your uterus is left intact. This is an important option if you're considering having children. Following myomectomy, fibroids return in about 10 percent of cases.

If you have symptoms and you're not planning to have children, your doctor may recommend removal of your uterus (hysterectomy). Hysterectomy has a lower rate of complications than myomectomy and is a permanent solution for fibroids.

Another procedure called uterine fibroid embolization may be an option for some women who want to avoid surgery. It's designed to shrink fibroids by cutting off the blood supply that feeds them. A doctor guides a thin tube (catheter) through an artery in your leg to those arteries in your uterus that nourish the fibroids. The doctor inserts tiny particles of plastic or gelatin through the catheter to block blood flow inside the fibroids, causing the fibroids to shrink over time.

The long-term effects of uterine fibroid embolization require more research. The procedure's effect on future pregnancies and chances of recurrence of the fibroids are unclear.

Endometrial polyps

Signs and symptoms

- Spotting between menstrual periods
- Pelvic cramps
- Heavy or prolonged periods

Endometrial polyps are small, soft growths in the lining of your uterus (endometrium). You may have one or a cluster of them.

Bleeding is the most common symptom. Sometimes the polyps produce no symptoms. However, they may protrude into your vagina, causing cramps as they impinge on the opening of your cervix. If protruding polyps become twisted and lose their blood supply, they can become infected.

Diagnosis

Sometimes the growths can be detected by ultrasound. Most often a procedure called hysteroscopy is used. A small scope is inserted into the uterus to look for polyps. At the same time, instruments can be inserted into the scope to remove the growths.

Treatment

The polyps may be removed by hysteroscopy or a procedure called dilatation and curettage (D and C), a minor operation in which your doctor scrapes the lining of your uterus. After removal, your doctor will likely have the polyps analyzed to be sure they're not cancerous (malignant). On occasion, the polyps may recur.

Endometrial hyperplasia

Signs and symptoms

- Bleeding between menstrual periods
- Heavy or prolonged menstrual periods

Simple endometrial hyperplasia occurs when the uterine lining (endometrium) grows too thick as a result of estrogen stimulation. Women with irregular menstrual cycles who don't ovulate are most apt to have this problem. It must be distinguished from a condition called complex hyperplasia, which can lead to endometrial (uterine) cancer.

Diagnosis

If your doctor suspects endometrial hyperplasia, he or she will likely do an endometrial biopsy to remove a small sample of your endometrium for laboratory analysis. This may be done with a procedure called hysteroscopy, in which a small scope with attached instruments is inserted into the uterus or a procedure called dilatation and curettage (D and C), in which tissue is scraped from your uterine lining.

How serious is endometrial hyperplasia?

Simple endometrial hyperplasia isn't serious. It may indicate a hormone imbalance, which should be corrected. Complex endometrial hyperplasia may be a precursor to endometrial cancer.

Treatment

Treatment is fairly simple as long as a tissue analysis reveals no precancerous cells. Taking birth control pills or progesterone medications for a few months will often correct the problem. If a biopsy indicates the presence of precancerous cells, you may be advised to have a hysterectomy.

Hydatidiform mole

Signs and symptoms

- During pregnancy, uterine growth that's too rapid
- Vaginal bleeding
- Severe nausea and vomiting
- No fetal movement
- Passage of grape-like tissue from your vagina
- High blood pressure

A rare noncancerous (benign) growth called hydatidiform mole sometimes develops at the beginning of pregnancy from tissue surrounding the fertilized egg that would normally produce a placenta. Because of this condition, the fetus never forms.

The tumor grows quickly and can become large. Although more than 80 percent of such moles are benign, 15 percent develop into a condition called invasive mole. This mole, though still benign, reaches so deeply into your uterine wall that it can cause a hemorrhage and other serious problems. A choriocarcinoma, a fast-growing cancerous (malignant) tumor that soon spreads to other parts of the body, follows 2 percent to 3 percent of hydatidiform moles. Hydatidiform mole, invasive mole and choriocarcinoma are all gestational trophoblastic diseases.

Hydatidiform moles are more common in older women. One occurs in about every 2,000 pregnancies in the United States, and the prevalence is higher in other parts of the world.

Diagnosis

The condition is most often detected during an ultrasound exam. Because hydatidiform moles produce quantities of human chorionic gonadotropin, a hormone that can be detected in blood or urine, your doctor may order a blood test to check for the condition.

How serious is a hydatidiform mole?

A noninvasive mole can be removed, and invasive moles and malignant tumors are treatable if caught early. Even for choriocarcinoma, the overall cure rate is 75 percent to 85 percent.

Treatment

A noninvasive mole can be removed surgically. If it's invasive or malignant, it may require chemotherapy.

Surgery

Your doctor may remove the mole in a procedure called dilatation and curettage (D and C), in which tissue is scraped from your uterine lining. Afterward, he or she will likely monitor your levels of human chorionic gonadotropin, which should return to normal. If they don't, you may have developed an invasive mole or choriocarcinoma. Rarely, a doctor will recommend a hysterectomy.

Chemotherapy

For both invasive moles and choriocarcinoma, chemotherapy is the treatment of choice. Pregnancy is possible after these diseases, but there's a risk of recurrence.

Endometriosis

Signs and symptoms

- Painful periods, sometimes with pain before and several days after the start of your period
- Heavy periods
- Pain during intercourse
- Infertility
- Pain when straining to have a bowel movement

Endometriosis occurs when bits of the tissue that lines your uterus (endometrium) become implanted on pelvic organs. Some experts believe the implants are a result of menstrual flow that backs up into the fallopian tubes and spills into the pelvic cavity, but that may be just one factor. Most often, the implants develop on the outside of the ovaries, fallopian tubes or the uterus or its supporting ligaments.

These cells cause bleeding as menstruation begins. Because the implants are embedded within other tissue, there's nowhere for the blood to go. Blood irritates the surrounding tissue, which may lead to the development of cysts. The cysts, in turn, may form a scar that binds organs together (adhesion). Scars and adhesions on your ovaries or fallopian tubes can prevent pregnancy.

Experts estimate that 10 percent to 15 percent of American women of childbearing age have endometriosis. Most have no symptoms and require no treatment, but for some, endometriosis is a progressive disease that becomes more painful and debilitating with time. The condition, which may run in families, usually occurs between the ages of 25 and 40 and is more common in women who haven't had children.

Menopause cures endometriosis. Very rarely, hormone replacement therapy may reactivate it.

Diagnosis

A doctor may be able to feel nodules of endometriosis during a pelvic examination, but a surgical procedure called laparoscopy can confirm the diagnosis. A laparoscope is a slim instrument equipped with a light. It's inserted into your abdomen through a small incision. Your doctor looks through the scope to examine your pelvic organs. Laparoscopy may be done with either local or general anesthesia, often on an outpatient basis.

How serious is endometriosis?

Endometrial implants aren't cancerous (malignant), but they're frequently associated with infertility. Although the symptoms may wax and wane, they often get worse with time.

Treatment

Treatment focuses on relieving symptoms and, if you want to have a child, making it possible for you to conceive and carry the pregnancy to term. Although there's no one treatment option that works for everyone, most women who seek help for endometriosis find some, if not complete, relief from their symptoms.

Finding a doctor with whom you feel comfortable is crucial in managing and treating endometriosis.

Medication

Your doctor may recommend that you take over-the-counter pain relievers to help ease painful menstrual cramps. However, if you find that you're taking more than the recommended dosage, it may be a sign that you need to try another treatment approach to manage your symptoms.

Hormone medications are very effective at reducing or eliminating the pain of endometriosis. That's because the rise and fall of hormones during a woman's menstrual cycle causes endometrial implants to thicken, break down and bleed. Hormone therapies used to treat endometriosis include:

- *Birth control pills.* Birth control pills help control hormones responsible for the buildup of endometrial tissue each month. Taking the pill long-term can reduce or eliminate the pain of endometriosis. Most women also experience lighter and shorter menstrual flow when taking the pill. Women over the age of 35 who smoke are generally advised not to take the pill because of a risk of blood clots.
- *Gonadotropin-releasing hormone (Gn-RH) agonists and antagonists.* These drugs block the production of ovarian-stimulating hormones. This prevents menstruation, which helps shrink endometrial implants. Gn-RH agonists and antagonists can force endometriosis into remission during the time of treatment and sometimes for months or years afterward.
- *Danazol.* Danazol (Danocrine) blocks the production of ovarian-stimulating hormones, preventing menstruation and the symptoms of endometriosis. Danazol may not be the first choice because it can cause annoying side effects, such as acne and facial hair.
- *Medroxyprogesterone.* This injectable drug sold under the brand name Depo-Provera is effective at halting menstruation and the growth of endometrial implants, relieving symptoms of endometriosis. Its side effects include weight gain and depressed mood.

Surgery

Although hormone therapies are effective at relieving or eliminating symptoms of endometriosis, they prevent pregnancy. If you have endometriosis and are trying to become pregnant, surgery to remove implants may increase your chances of success. If you have severe pain from endometriosis, you may also benefit from surgery:

- *Conservative surgery.* Conservative surgery refers to removal of endometrial growths, scar tissue and adhesions without removing reproductive organs. The procedure may be accomplished

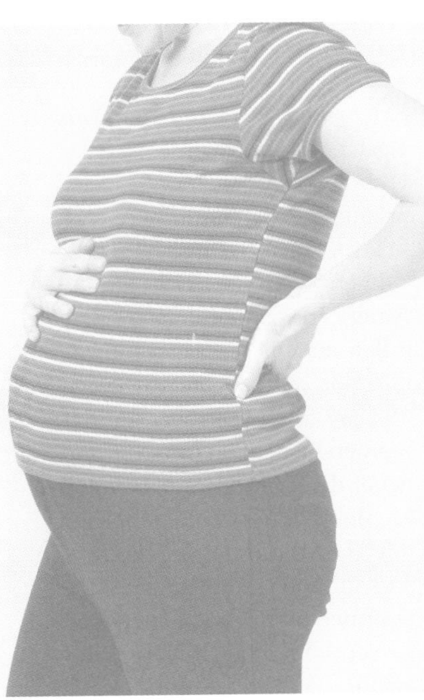

Endometriosis and Pregnancy

If you have early-stage endometriosis, your doctor may suggest that you try to become pregnant as soon as it's appropriate if you want to have children. It may become more difficult to conceive later on. During pregnancy, endometriosis implants generally shrink and the symptoms may disappear. However, endometriosis increases your risk of having an ectopic pregnancy, in which the fertilized egg implants itself outside of your uterus.

laparoscopically or through traditional abdominal surgery. In laparoscopic surgery, a slender viewing instrument (laparoscope) is inserted through a small incision near your bellybutton. The laparoscope is equipped with a laser, a cautery — an instrument that destroys tissue with heat — or small surgical instruments.

If surgery is ineffective at improving fertility, other procedures, such as in vitro fertilization techniques, may help.

- *Hysterectomy.* In severe cases of endometriosis, surgery to remove some or all of a woman's reproductive organs (hysterectomy) may be the best treatment. But this type of surgery is typically considered a last resort, especially for women still in their reproductive years.

Self-care

If pain persists or it takes awhile for you and your doctor to find a treatment that works, you can try measures at home to relieve your discomfort. Warm baths and a heating pad can help relax pelvic muscles, reducing cramping and pain.

Regular exercise may help reduce the symptoms of premenstrual syndrome and take the edge off endometriosis symptoms. Some women find that giving up or cutting back on caffeine, sugar and alcoholic beverages helps their symptoms.

Adenomyosis

Signs and symptoms

- Menstrual cramps that last throughout a period and worsen as you grow older
- Prolonged, excessive menstrual bleeding

In adenomyosis, some of the endometrial tissue that lines your uterus begins to grow within its muscular walls. This is most likely to happen late in your childbearing years and after you've had children. Many women with adenomyosis have no symptoms.

Diagnosis

During a pelvic examination, your doctor may discover that your uterus is enlarged and tender. This along with prolonged painful cramps and excessive menstrual bleeding suggests adenomyosis. Ultrasound and magnetic resonance imaging (MRI) may be helpful in making a diagnosis. Although it can be painful, the condition is generally harmless.

Treatment

Adenomyosis usually resolves after menopause, so treatment may depend on how close you are to that stage of life. If you're nearing menopause, your doctor may prescribe painkillers and suggest no other treatment. If your pain is severe or menopause is years away, your doctor may suggest a hysterectomy.

Pelvic inflammatory disease

Signs and symptoms

- Severe pain in your lower abdomen
- Mild, recurrent pain in your lower abdomen, perhaps with backache and irregular menstrual periods
- Infertility
- Pain during intercourse
- Irregular bleeding
- Vaginal discharge

Emergency signs and symptoms

- Severe pain low in your abdomen
- Nausea and vomiting
- Temperature above 102 F

Every year, about 1 million American women develop pelvic inflammatory disease (PID), an infection of the pelvic organs that can cause scarring. Some women have no symptoms and are never diagnosed, some develop a low-level, long-lasting (chronic) infection and others have a severe and sudden (acute) attack. After treatment about 15 percent to 25 percent of women develop PID again.

Usually, you acquire the organisms responsible for pelvic inflammatory disease through sexual intercourse. PID develops in almost 15 percent of women with gonorrhea. Chlamydia is an even more frequent cause.

If your partner uses a condom, you're somewhat protected from PID. If you have PID, your sexual partner should seek treatment too, even if he has no symptoms. If he is infected, he may reinfect you.

Diagnosis

During a pelvic examination, your doctor may take samples from your vagina and cervix for laboratory analysis to determine what organism is causing the infection. Blood tests are also helpful. If there's any question about the diagnosis or about how widespread the infection is, your doctor may do a surgical procedure known as laparoscopy. It involves inserting a thin, lighted instrument through a small incision in your abdomen and viewing your pelvic organs.

How serious is pelvic inflammatory disease?

Without treatment, PID can be serious. An abscess may develop on your fallopian tubes or ovaries, creating an emergency if it perforates. Your tubes or ovaries may be damaged or scarred, causing infertility. PID can also lead to peritonitis, an inflammation of the membrane that lines your abdominal cavity. Peritonitis is always serious and needs intensive treatment with antibiotics. In rare cases, bacteria may invade your bloodstream, leading to blood poisoning (septicemia) and infection in your joints.

Long-term consequences of PID include chronic pelvic pain and tubal (ectopic) pregnancy, in which the fetus grows outside your uterus, usually in one of your fallopian tubes.

Treatment

Treatment may consist of medication, rest and possibly surgery.

Medication
Your doctor may prescribe a combination of an antibiotic and a pain reliever.

Rest
Your doctor may recommend bed rest. You may even be hospitalized for a short time if you have a severe case or if your condition fails to respond quickly to medication.

Surgery
Surgery is rarely necessary. However, if an abscess ruptures or threatens to rupture, it may require drainage or removal. Removal may mean that a fallopian tube or an ovary or both also be removed. Occasionally, total hysterectomy is necessary.

Pelvic Pain

Any time you have pain in your pelvic region that lasts longer than a few hours, recurs or is accompanied by fever or vaginal bleeding, see your doctor. He or she will want to know if your pain is new or if it's a condition that's been with you for a while (chronic). If it's chronic, your doctor will want to know if it comes and goes (is episodic) or is continuous.

Your doctor may also ask other questions about your pain, such as if it's associated with your menstrual periods, is related to bowel or bladder habits or occurs with intercourse or physical activity.

Chronic pelvic pain

Signs and symptoms

- Persistent pain in your pelvic region
- Painful intercourse and bowel movements

Chronic pelvic pain can take many forms: It can be steady or intermittent. It can be a dull ache, a sharp pain, cramping or an overall feeling of pressure or heaviness deep in your abdomen. The pain may be worse when you sit or stand and better when you lie down.

Determining the cause can be difficult, if not impossible. Possible causes of chronic pelvic pain include:

- Endometriosis (see page 1092)
- Adenomyosis (see page 1094)
- Pelvic inflammatory disease (see page 1094)
- Spasms of the pelvic floor muscles
- Pelvic congestion syndrome resulting from varicose-type veins around the ovaries that cause pooling of blood
- A piece of ovary left after hysterectomy (ovarian remnant) that develops tiny, painful cysts
- Fibroids (see page 1090)

Studies show that women who are depressed or under excessive stress or who have been sexually or physically abused are more likely to experience chronic pelvic pain. That may be because emotional distress can worsen pain, possibly by causing you to tense your pelvic floor muscles or by causing chemical changes that affect your ability to cope with pain.

Diagnosis

Diagnosis may require a pelvic exam and various tests to try to identify the cause of the pain. It may also involve pain mapping, in which your doctor uses a smaller version of a laparoscope (microlaparoscope) to see inside your pelvic area. You remain awake but sedated while your doctor touches different areas and notes which ones cause pain.

How serious is chronic pelvic pain?

Typically, chronic pelvic pain is a debilitating, long-term condition that often results in the loss of reproductive function. However, it's almost never caused by a life-threatening condition.

Treatment

Treatment depends on the cause, but it often requires a multidisciplinary approach. Medical professionals from several specialties may be consulted or involved in your care.

Medication
Antibiotics may be prescribed to treat pelvic inflammatory disease (PID), and hormones to suppress ovulation may be used to treat endometriosis and pelvic adhesions. If psychological factors are contributing to your condition, your doctor may prescribe an antidepressant, which may lessen the pain and improve your mood so that you're better able to cope with your pain.

Self-care
Stress management and relaxation techniques, such as meditating, listening to music and practicing yoga, may help with forms of chronic pelvic pain. Working with a physical therapist, you can learn how to relax and stretch your pelvic floor muscles if those muscles are causing the pain.

Devices
An ultrasound device inserted into your vagina can apply soothing heat to your pelvic floor muscles and help relieve spasms.

Surgery
Surgery — sometimes a hysterectomy — may be used to treat endometriosis. PID and fibroids also may require a hysterectomy. Surgery may also be necessary to remove ovarian remnants.

Ovarian Disorders

Each of your two ovaries is about the size of an almond. The ovaries are situated in your abdomen, above and to the side of your uterus and about 4 to 5 inches below your waist. At birth, a female has roughly 1 million eggs (ova) stored in her ovaries, each egg housed in its own follicle. Every month, from the time of puberty until menopause, one ovum grows until rupture of its follicle releases it. The ovum moves through your fallopian tube into your uterus.

Your ovaries also produce the female sex hormones estrogen and progesterone, which regulate your menstrual cycle. During the first half of the cycle, your ovaries secrete estrogen. The outer cells of the single follicle where the ovum is growing manufacture most of it. Estrogen causes your uterine lining to thicken in preparation for receiving a fertilized egg.

Just before ovulation, the same follicle begins to produce tiny amounts of progesterone. After the egg is released, the follicle — at this stage it's called the corpus luteum — expands rapidly and steps up production of both progesterone and estrogen.

These hormones act together to complete the development of your uterine lining. If pregnancy occurs, hormones secreted by the corpus luteum help to sustain the pregnancy. Otherwise, the corpus luteum begins to shrink, and levels of estrogen and progesterone decrease. As a result, your uterus sheds its lining, resulting in menstruation.

Ovarian cysts and noncancerous tumors

Signs and symptoms

- A dull ache, pressure or fullness in your abdomen
- Pain during intercourse
- Delayed, irregular or painful menstrual periods
- Abrupt onset of sharp pain in your lower abdomen

Emergency signs and symptoms

- Sudden, severe abdominal pain and perhaps vomiting

A cyst is a sac filled with fluid. Most ovarian cysts are harmless and disappear of their own accord. Often, they're noncancerous (benign) and don't cause symptoms. Other types of cysts warrant attention. Your doctor may find one or more cysts during a routine pelvic examination. Cysts that develop after menopause are somewhat more likely to be an indicator of ovarian cancer.

In women who haven't gone through menopause, the ovaries normally grow cyst-like structures called follicles each month. Follicles are little "chemical factories" that produce the hormones estrogen and progesterone and release an egg (ovum) when you ovulate.

Sometimes, a normal monthly follicle just keeps growing. When that happens, it becomes what's known as a functional cyst. This means it started during the normal function of your menstrual cycle. There are two types of functional cysts:

- *Follicular cyst.* Ovulation initiates a complex chain reaction. The follicle holding your egg takes its cue from your brain's pituitary gland via a surge in the level of a hormone called luteinizing hormone (LH). When everything goes according to plan, your egg is released and begins its journey down the fallopian tube in search of fertilization. A follicular cyst begins when LH doesn't surge, and the chain reaction doesn't start. The result is a follicle that doesn't rupture or release its egg. Instead it grows and grows until it becomes a cyst. Follicular cysts are usually harmless, rarely cause pain and often disappear on their own within two or three menstrual cycles.
- *Corpus luteum cyst.* If LH does surge and your egg is released, another chain of events starts. The follicle then responds to LH by producing large quantities of estrogen and progesterone in preparation for conception. This changes the follicle. At this stage it's called the corpus luteum. However, sometimes after the egg's release, its escape hole seals off and tissues accumulate inside, causing the corpus luteum to expand into a cyst. Although this cyst usually disappears on its own in a few weeks, it can grow to almost 4 inches in diameter and has the potential to bleed into itself or twist the ovary, causing pelvic or abdominal pain. If it fills with blood, the cyst may rupture, causing internal bleeding and sudden, sharp pain.

A tumor is a solid lump. Benign tumors don't invade neighboring tissue or spread to other parts of the body. Cancerous (malignant) tumors may do both.

However, if a benign tumor or ovarian cyst is large, it can cause abdominal discomfort. In some cases, it may interfere with your production of ovarian hormones and result in irregular bleeding from your vagina or an increase in body hair. If a large tumor or cyst presses on your bladder, you may need to urinate more frequently because your bladder's capacity is diminished.

If a tumor or cyst becomes twisted, you may experience spas-

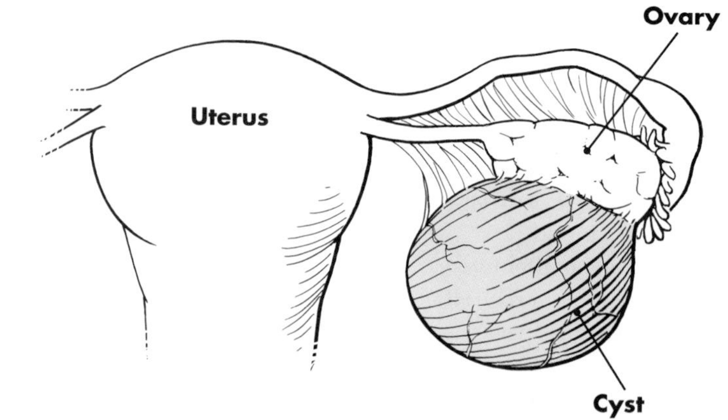

An ovarian cyst may be detected during a routine pelvic examination.

modic pain. Sudden or sharp pain may mean a cyst has ruptured. If you have severe abdominal pain, fever and vomiting, or if you have symptoms of shock, such as cold, clammy skin and rapid breathing, seek immediate medical help.

Diagnosis

If during a pelvic examination your doctor detects something that feels like an ovarian cyst or tumor, he or she may order an ultrasound examination or another imaging procedure to confirm the diagnosis. Your doctor may also perform laparoscopic surgery, in which a slim, lighted instrument is inserted into your abdomen to examine your ovaries.

Treatment

Most ovarian cysts go away without treatment. Watchful waiting, including regular monitoring with ultrasound, is a treatment option if a cyst is fluid-filled and less than 2 inches in diameter. Your doctor will likely recommend that you get follow-up pelvic ultrasounds at periodic intervals to see if the cyst has changed in size.

If you have a functional cyst that's large and causes considerable symptoms, your doctor may recommend birth control pills to help shrink it. Taking birth control pills may also reduce the chance that your cyst will grow.

Your doctor may suggest removal of a cyst or benign tumor if it's large, solid, filled with debris, growing or if it persists through two or three menstrual cycles. Cysts that are irregularly shaped, cause pain or other symptoms and can be found on both ovaries also may be removed.

If a cyst is cancerous, your doctor may advise a hysterectomy to remove both ovaries and your uterus. After menopause the risk of ovarian cancer increases. As a result, doctors more commonly recommend surgery when a cystic mass develops on the ovaries after menopause.

Cancers of the Reproductive Tract

Cancer can develop in the fallopian tubes, uterus, ovaries, cervix, vagina and vulva. The chance of a successful outcome depends on which organ is involved and how early the cancer is diagnosed.

Endometrial cancer

Signs and symptoms

- Vaginal bleeding after menopause
- Before menopause, heavy periods or bleeding between periods
- A pink, watery discharge from your vagina

Endometrial (uterine) cancer starts in the endometrium, the lining of your uterus. It's one of the most common cancers in American women. It's also one of the most curable, if it's detected early. It most often occurs after menopause, in women between the ages of 50 and 70.

Obesity predisposes you to endometrial cancer. Postmenopausal women who are overweight are at especially high risk of uterine cancer because fat cells make estrogen, but their ovaries are no longer making progesterone to balance it out. Obesity can also make treatment more difficult. Hormone replacement therapy (HRT) was once a risk factor as well. Current HRT uses lower doses of estrogen combined with progestin. Appropriate use poses no increase in the risk of endometrial cancer.

In addition to those who are obese, women at higher risk for endometrial cancer include those who have never given birth, those who experience menopause later in life than most women and those with a history of infertility or irregular periods. The medication tamoxifen, which has been used to lower the risk of breast cancer in some women, also increases the risk of endometrial cancer, as does estrogen taken without progestin, for menopausal symptoms.

Use of birth control pills decreases the risk of endometrial cancer.

Diagnosis

The first symptom of endometrial cancer is vaginal bleeding. If you have abnormal bleeding, your doctor will likely do an endometrial biopsy. This involves removing a small piece of tissue from your uterine lining for laboratory analysis. This procedure may be done in your doctor's office and usually doesn't require anesthesia. If enough tissue can't be obtained during a biopsy or the biopsy suggests cancer, your doctor will most likely want to perform a dilatation and curettage (D and C). In this procedure, which requires you to be in an operating room under anesthesia, tissue is scraped from the lining of your inner uterus and examined under a microscope for cancer cells.

Your doctor may also recommend a transvaginal ultrasound to help rule out other conditions. In this painless procedure, a wand-like device (transducer) is inserted into the vagina. The transducer uses sound waves to create a video image of your uterus. This test helps your doctor look for abnormalities in your uterine lining. Sometimes, saline water is inserted into your uterus via a thin tube (catheter) before the test is done. The saline water enhances the image, making any abnormalities of the uterine lining more visible on video.

If cancer of the endometrium is found, you'll likely be referred to a gynecological oncologist — a doctor who specializes in treating cancers involving the female reproductive system. More tests will be done to evaluate the extent of the disease.

How serious is endometrial cancer?

Because this type of cancer causes abnormal vaginal bleeding, it's likely to be discovered at an early

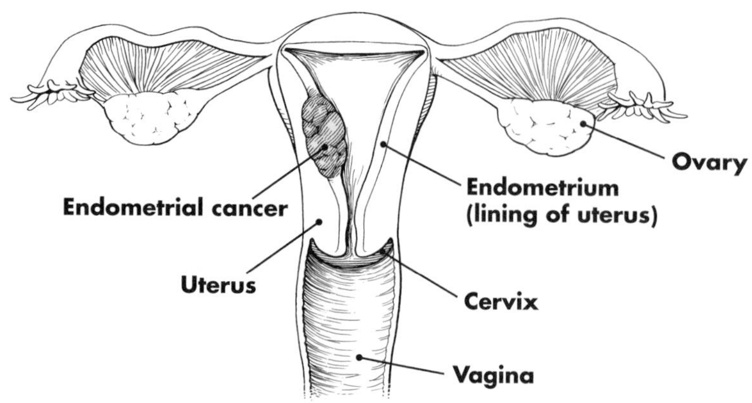

Endometrial (uterine) cancer develops in the lining of your uterus (endometrium). Treatment is usually very successful if the cancer is diagnosed early.

stage, when it's still localized. Therefore, treatment is successful in many cases. Rarely, the tumor is a faster-growing, deadlier type, and results aren't as good.

Treatment

Depending on how aggressive the cancer is and whether it has spread, treatment may require just one or a combination of therapies.

Surgery

Surgery is the most common treatment for endometrial cancer. Most doctors recommend either the surgical removal of the uterus alone (hysterectomy), or, more often, the surgical removal of the uterus, fallopian tubes and ovaries (complete hysterectomy). Lymph nodes in the area also may be removed during surgery. Lymph nodes are small, bean-shaped structures found throughout the body that produce and store infection-fighting cells but may also contain cancer cells.

If you have an aggressive form of endometrial cancer or the cancer has spread to other parts of the body, additional treatments may be required.

Radiation

Radiation therapy is the use of high-dose X-rays to kill cancer cells. If your doctor believes you're at high risk of cancer recurrence, he or she may suggest that you have radiation therapy after a hysterectomy. Your doctor may also recommend radiation therapy if the cancerous tumor is fast-growing or invades deeply into the muscle of the uterus or involves blood vessels. Rarely is radiation used before or instead of surgery.

Hormone therapy

If the cancer has spread to other parts of your body, synthetic progestin, a form of the hormone progesterone, may stop it from growing. The progestin used in treating endometrial cancer is given in different doses than the progestin used in hormone replacement therapy for menopausal women. Some other medications may be used as well. Treatment with progestin may be an option for women with early endometrial cancer who want to have children and, therefore, don't want to have a hysterectomy. However, this approach is new and not without risk that the cancer will return.

Chemotherapy

Chemotherapy is the use of drugs to kill cancer cells. In some cases, your doctor may recommend chemotherapy for endometrial cancer. Chemotherapy may be taken by pill or administered intravenously. These drugs enter the bloodstream and then travel through the body, killing cancer cells.

Cervical cancer

Signs and symptoms

- Bleeding from your vagina after intercourse, between periods or after menopause
- Bloody discharge from your vagina
- In advanced stages, a dull backache

Cancer of the cervix is one of the most common cancers that affect a woman's reproductive organs. Various strains of the human papillomavirus (HPV), a sexually transmitted infection, are responsible for at least 95 percent of cases of cervical cancer.

When exposed to HPV, the immune system response in most women prevents the virus from doing harm. In a small group of women, however, the virus survives for years before it eventually converts cells on the surface of the cervix into cancer cells. Cervical cancer is most likely to occur between the ages of 30 and 55.

Thanks largely to Pap test screening, the death rate from cervical cancer has decreased significantly over the last 40 years. Still, every year an estimated 12,900 women in the United States find out that they have invasive cervical cancer, and approximately 4,400 die of the disease.

Diagnosis

This type of cancer is generally detected with a Pap test. If the test results come back abnormal, your doctor may also perform a colposcopy exam and biopsy. A colposcope is an instrument with a magnifying lens that permits a close look at the cervix. A biopsy is a procedure in which your doctor removes specimens of tissue from your cervix for microscopic study to determine if the tissue is cancerous (malignant).

How serious is cervical cancer?

Cervical cancer is serious, especially if it has spread. For about 3 percent of American women who

Hysterectomy

A hysterectomy is the removal of your uterus. A hysterectomy is most often performed for the following reasons:

- Endometrial (uterine) cancer
- Severe endometriosis or fibroids
- Severe, uncontrollable bleeding
- Protrusion of the uterus from the vagina (uterine prolapse)

Hysterectomies aren't all alike. A supracervical hysterectomy leaves your cervix in place. In a total hysterectomy, the entire uterus, including the cervix, is removed. A complete hysterectomy with bilateral salpingo-oophorectomy is removal of your uterus, cervix, fallopian tubes and both ovaries. A radical hysterectomy, usually performed for cancer of the cervix, extends even further to include the removal of the upper part of your vagina and some pelvic lymph nodes.

In performing a hysterectomy, the surgeon most often makes an incision in the lower abdomen, either horizontally just above the pubic hairline or vertically from the navel to the hairline. Recovery generally takes about 6 weeks. Sometimes, for noncancerous (benign) disease, a surgeon will perform a vaginal hysterectomy, done without an abdominal incision. Some surgeons use a laparoscope to help accomplish a vaginal hysterectomy. Recovery may be easier and faster than that following a traditional vaginal hysterectomy. Either operation takes 1 to 2 hours and is performed using general anesthesia.

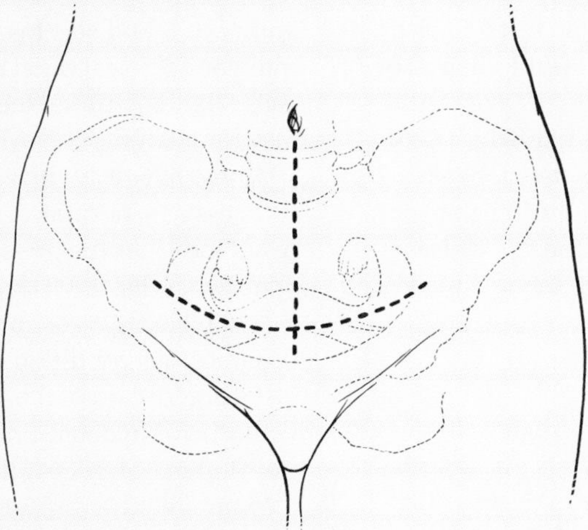

In performing an abdominal hysterectomy, your surgeon may elect either a horizontal or vertical incision.

In case of a large ovarian or uterine tumor, a surgeon will usually use the abdominal approach. For uterine prolapse, the vaginal approach often is preferred.

Some surgeons routinely advise removal of the ovaries in women older than 40 to prevent ovarian cancer, but this is a controversial issue. On one hand, ovarian cancer is deadly, with a cure rate of only 10 percent to 20 percent, and is usually prevented by removing the ovaries. On the other hand, cancer of the ovaries is uncommon.

Possible complications of a hysterectomy include pelvic infections, kidney and bladder infections and hemorrhage. After you get home, you'll have to forgo intercourse and lifting heavy objects for a time. For 6 to 8 weeks, you can't engage in active sports.

die of cancer, invasive cancer of the cervix is the cause.

Treatment

Determining if and how extensively the cancer has spread is called staging. The stage of your cancer is the key to determining how extensive your treatment should be. Whatever treatment you receive, you'll need regular checkups and tests for at least 5 years after you've completed it.

Surgery

For invasive cancer that's confined to the uterus and upper vagina, your doctor will likely recommend a radical hysterectomy. In this procedure, a surgeon removes the uterus (including the cervix), upper vagina, some surrounding tissue and lymph nodes and the fallopian tubes but may leave one or both ovaries in place if you're a young woman. You may have radiation therapy afterward.

Radiation

Most cervical cancers that have spread to neighboring structures are treated with radiation. Radiation treatment often involves both external beam radiation delivered by a machine and internal radiation. To administer internal radiation, a surgeon implants radioactive material in your uterus or in the upper part of your vagina and leaves it there for several days while you remain in the hospital. The implantation is done under general anesthesia.

Radiation may cause some distressing side effects. These include diarrhea, rectal bleeding and fatigue. For a few months afterward, you may have trouble retaining urine. Radiation treatments will disrupt your menstrual cycle and may cause symptoms of menopause, including hot flashes. Radiation therapy also can cause some narrowing and shortening of the vagina.

Chemotherapy

Using drugs to kill cancer may enhance the effects of radiation.

Tumors tend to shrink rapidly with aggressive chemotherapy, but the drugs can be toxic to people with cervical cancer. Chemotherapy has been shown to improve survival rates in women with more advanced forms of cervical cancer and is often used in conjunction with radiation therapy.

Ovarian cancer

Signs and symptoms

- In early stages, generally none
- Vague abdominal discomfort and mild indigestion
- In later stages, a swollen abdomen and lower abdominal pain

Ovarian cancer often is deadly. In its early stages, it produces few noticeable signs or symptoms and may be discovered during a routine pelvic examination. If undetected, it eventually causes signs and symptoms, and the tumor may produce fluid that causes your abdomen to swell. Seventy percent to 80 percent of the time, the disease has advanced by the time you receive a diagnosis. That's because there's no acceptable, cost-effective, accurate screening test for this disease.

Ovarian cancer typically develops after menopause. You're somewhat more likely to get cancer of the ovaries if you've never been pregnant or you had trouble conceiving. Conversely, you're less likely to get it if you've had several children or have taken birth control pills. Either way, an annual pelvic examination is important because early diagnosis and treatment give you the best chance for long-term survival.

Diagnosis

If a pelvic examination reveals a growth on an ovary, your doctor will likely order an ultrasound, magnetic resonance imaging (MRI) or a computerized tomography (CT) scan to evaluate it. Three out of four ovarian tumors are noncancerous (benign).

How serious is ovarian cancer?

When detected early, the 5-year survival rate is 60 percent to 80 percent. However, the survival rate is only 30 percent to 40 percent overall because this type of cancer is seldom found early enough. Nevertheless, with aggressive surgery and chemotherapy, more

Pap Test

Since the early 1940s, the death rate of women with cervical cancer has decreased by 70 percent, largely because so many women have Pap test screening. Although not infallible, this test detects 95 percent of cervical cancers and, more importantly, detects precancerous conditions that are virtually 100 percent curable. Occasionally, a Pap test will also detect evidence of endometrial or ovarian cancer.

The Pap test is named for G.N. Papanicolaou, its developer. It's typically performed during a pelvic examination. At most, it causes slight discomfort. Using a wooden spatula or brush, your doctor gently samples the surface of your cervix to gather cells and also inserts a brush into your cervical canal to sample its cells. The cells are sent to a laboratory for analysis.

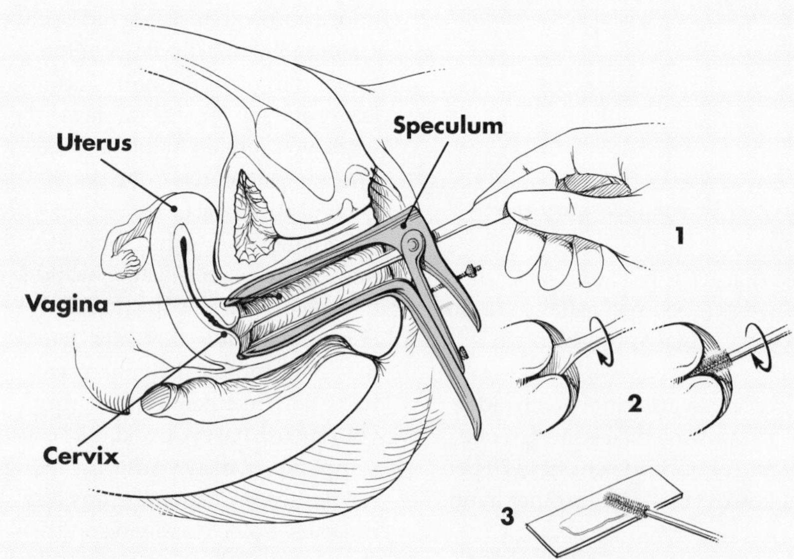

With a speculum in place, your doctor rotates a spatula and then a brush to remove a sample of cells (1 and 2). The cells are smeared onto a glass slide for examination under a microscope (3).

A negative result means your cervical tissue is normal. A positive result indicates the presence of abnormal cells, but it doesn't prove that you have cancer or dysplasia, a precancerous condition. A pathologist's description of the cells can aid your doctor in determining the next step. Often, further evaluation is recommended.

You should have your first Pap test at age 18, or earlier if you start having intercourse. A second and third Pap test should occur at 1-year intervals. If three Pap tests have normal results, and you're at low risk, your doctor may suggest that you can have less frequent exams.

If you're in a high-risk group, continue to be tested annually. Women at highest risk are those who began having intercourse before age 18 and who've had multiple sex partners, a sexually transmitted disease or a previous abnormal Pap test.

women with advanced ovarian cancer are surviving longer.

Treatment
Your doctor may advise a combination of surgery and chemotherapy to treat the cancer.

Surgery
In a young woman who wants to have children and whose tumor is discovered early, a surgeon may remove only the involved ovary and its fallopian tube. However, the most common type of ovarian cancer requires removal of both ovaries, as well as your uterus, fallopian tubes, nearby lymph glands and a fold of tissue known as the omentum. In addition, your doctor will likely take many samples of tissue and fluid from your abdomen to examine for cancer cells.

Chemotherapy
Ovarian cancer is generally treated with a combination of several medications. After chemotherapy, a tumor usually shrinks. However, it often begins to grow again. Your doctor may use a different combination of drugs in the second course of chemotherapy.

Radiation
In rare instances, radiation therapy is used to inhibit tumor growth.

Vaginal cancer

Signs and symptoms
- Watery discharge from your vagina
- Bleeding after intercourse or a pelvic examination
- Pain during intercourse
- A frequent or urgent need to urinate
- Painful bowel movements

Vaginal cancer is extremely rare. Of all the cancers that can develop in a woman's reproductive organs, only about 1 percent is cancer of the vagina. This type of cancer is most likely to occur in women between the ages of 45 and 65, and 95 percent of these cancers are slow-growing squamous cell tumors. They often extend to your bladder or rectum, causing painful defecation or a frequent, urgent need to urinate.

Diagnosis
You may receive a diagnosis of this cancer after you develop signs and symptoms and your doctor performs an examination of the vagina. Abnormal tissue may be removed for examination (biopsy).

How serious are vaginal cancers?
They're rare but they can be deadly, especially if not detected and treated early.

Treatment
Surgery, possibly followed by radiation therapy, is the main treatment for vaginal cancers. The extent of the operation generally depends on where the cancer is located, how far it extends and your age.

Vulvar cancer

Signs and symptoms
- A small, hard, lump that may itch in the skin of the vulva
- An ulcer on the vulva with raised edges that may bleed or seep fluid

Cancer of the vulva is rare. It accounts for just 3 percent to 4 percent of all tumors of the female reproductive organs. It's more common after menopause.

Diagnosis
Because women often don't seek care for complaints such as itching, diagnosis is sometimes delayed. To diagnose a suspicious lump in your vulva, your doctor will remove a tiny piece of tissue for laboratory analysis.

How serious is vulvar cancer?
With effective treatment, there's a good chance of full recovery.

Treatment
Typically, a vulvectomy is necessary. In this procedure, a surgeon removes the tumor, surrounding skin and perhaps lymph nodes in your groin. The type of cancer and size of the tumor determine how much tissue must be removed. Radiation therapy also may be recommended.

Sexual Crises

Physical abuse and rape are crises in which the victims are usually — but not always — women. These conditions are serious and require prompt intervention and treatment.

Physical abuse

Physical abuse involves physical damage inflicted by someone you know, such as a spouse, companion, significant other or relative. It typically occurs at home. Rape is a particular form of physical abuse.

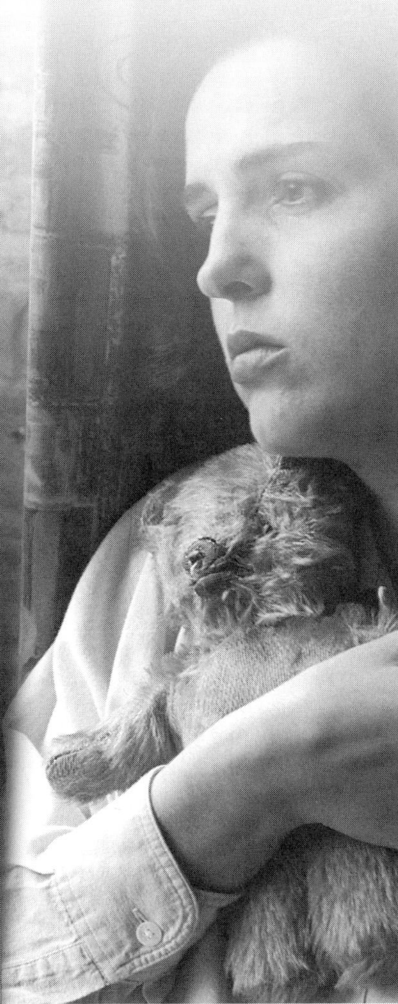

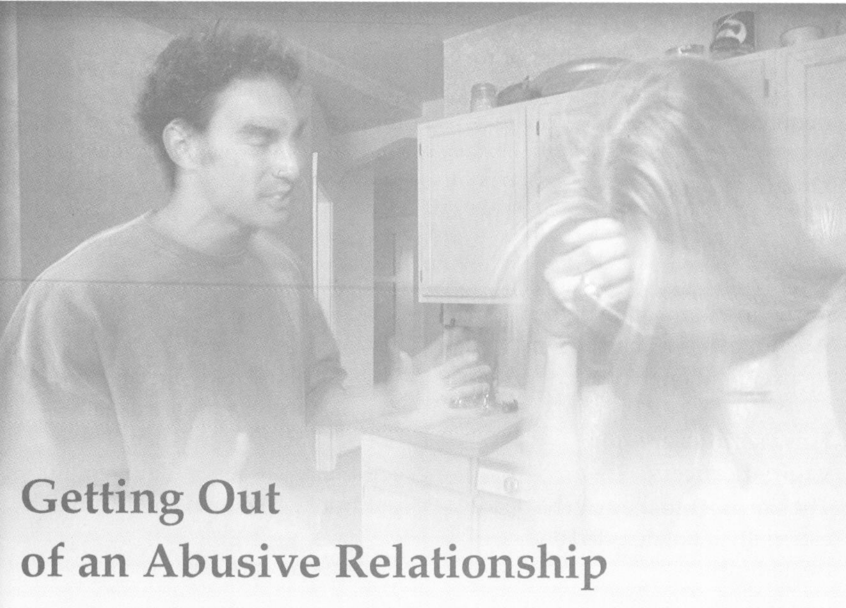

Getting Out of an Abusive Relationship

Abuse can include battering and physical assault, sexual assault and psychological abuse, in which you may be verbally forced into doing degrading or humiliating things.

If you've already experienced family violence, sexual assault or incest or physical abuse from a partner, you have a higher risk of being in another abusive relationship. The following are signs that you're involved in an unhealthy relationship:

- Your partner frightens you with threats of violence or by throwing things when angry.
- Your partner says it's your fault that he or she hits you.
- Your partner promises that it won't happen again, but it does.

What should you do?

If you're in an abusive relationship:

- Confide in someone you trust so that you can contact the person in case you need to leave suddenly.
- Ensure your safety. In case you need to leave quickly, pack a suitcase and leave it with a friend or neighbor. Keep important documents handy so that you can take them with you. Know where to go and how you'll get there at any time of day.

Signs of impending danger

You may be in danger if any of the following are true:

- Your partner talks about using or has access to a weapon, especially a gun.
- Your partner extends the threats to children, other family members or pets.
- Your partner sexually assaults you.
- Your partner shows little guilt and remorse after a violent episode.

If you recognize these or other signs of impending danger, get away.

If you can't avoid an attack

- Call the police.
- Call your doctor or go to an emergency department if you're hurt, even if you think your injuries are minor. Keep a copy of the medical records so that you can file charges.

There are people who can and will help you face difficult decisions regarding your future. Seek them out.

Some cultures once held that a man had the right to beat his wife. In fact, the "rule of thumb" refers to the size of the stick a man could use to beat his wife — no wider than his thumb. This attitude is no longer acceptable in most cultures, but remnants of it remain.

The clearest dividing line between what's acceptable and unacceptable is mutual enjoyment. When something hurts, you avoid it or stop it. If a partner forces you to participate in some activity that hurts you, that's physical abuse. It's not OK for your spouse or anyone else to threaten, beat or rape you. If you're a victim, you're entitled to help and protection.

Deliberate infliction of harm to another, regardless of whether sexual activity is involved, is a crime. In addition to contacting law enforcement authorities, see your doctor or go to a hospital emergency department for treatment of injuries. Medical personnel or law enforcement authorities can refer you to a shelter or to people who can provide counseling and intervention.

Abuse can cause severe physical injuries and death. Even minor injuries that accumulate over time can be debilitating. The emotional and psychological damage inflicted by abuse can be just as devastating as the physical damage. A psychotherapist, counselor or social worker often can be helpful.

Rape

Lack of consent differentiates rape from acceptable sexual activity. Rape is sexual activity that's forced upon you, sometimes by violence or threats of violence and sometimes by deception. Although it takes the form of sex, rape is an act of aggression fueled by hostility and anger.

People of all ages, from infancy through old age, can be rape victims. About half of the instances of rape occur in the victim's home. The rapist can be a stranger, but in about half of cases the victim knows the rapist. Often the rapist is a member of the victim's extended family. Some women are raped by their husbands. Rape can be both psychologically and physically devastating.

There are techniques you can use to avoid becoming a rape victim. When a potential rapist attacks a woman, how to resist — or whether to resist — depends on the individual and the circumstances. One technique is to stall for time, in the hope that someone will come along and help. Some women have avoided rape by saying they have a sexually transmitted disease (STD). Other possibilities include using self-defense techniques, such as screaming, breaking a window or kicking the attacker in the testicles to disable him long enough for you to escape.

However, if you think you'll be harmed if you resist, or if resistance fails, then it may be best to submit. It's preferable to being killed or seriously injured. Rape is still a crime whether you resist or submit.

In case of a rape, seek immediate medical care from your regular doctor or at an emergency department. Don't bathe or douche before you're examined. Semen, blood or other materials from the rapist could be used as evidence.

The doctor who examines you can treat any injuries you sustained and provide psychological support. He or she will also obtain evidence that can be used to prosecute the rapist. In most cases, physical damage, such as wounds and scratches, will heal.

If there's a possibility of pregnancy as a result of the rape, your doctor may give you something called the morning-after pill, one of several oral contraceptives that may prevent pregnancy. You may also receive medications to reduce the risk of developing an STD. It's likely you'll need to be tested for human immunodeficiency virus. You'll likely need to return in several weeks for a follow-up examination.

The emotional and psychological consequences are often harder to

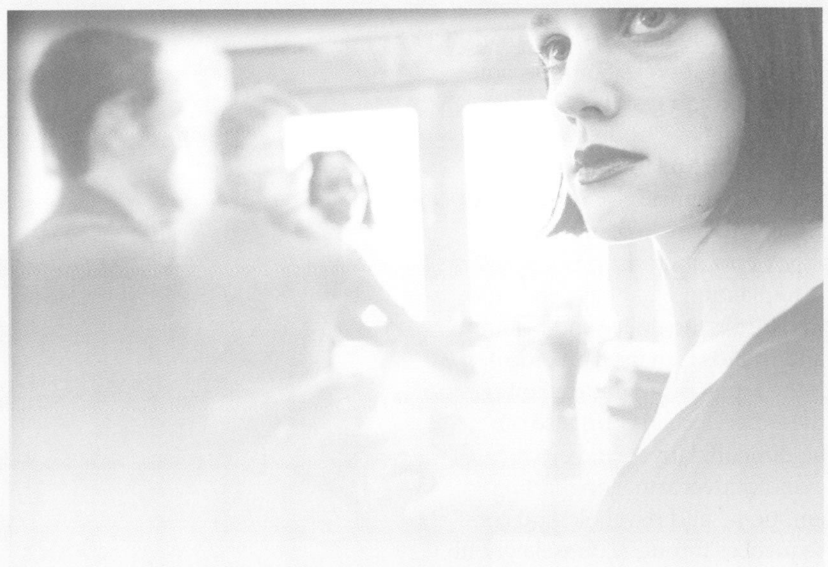

Rape Prevention Tips

You can't always prevent rape, but you can take steps to reduce your risks. Here are some techniques that might help:

Set sexual limits
How friendly is too friendly? This is a judgment call — one that you must make whenever you're alone with a man. Always remember that you have the right to establish limits and that it's OK to change those limits as required by the circumstances. When it comes to sexual intercourse, you should never feel you've lost control.

Communicate
Make your limits known to the other person.

Know yourself
Pay attention to your emotions. Don't let circumstances override your good judgment. If it seems as though you're being pressured, then you *are* being pressured, and it's time to say goodbye.

Be observant
Sometimes you can anticipate circumstances that could lead to rape. For example, avoid eye contact with an individual who stares at you. If someone sits or stands too close to you, move. If an individual blocks your way, walk confidently in another direction, avoiding eye contact. Avoid people who speak or act as though they know you intimately when they don't.

Assert yourself
If someone grabs or pushes you or disregards your negative response to any physical or verbal act, tell the individual, in a firm tone of voice, to bug off. The language may seem unrefined or rude, but in circumstances such as this you may need to be uncharacteristically direct. Remember that it's OK to become angry. It's also important to react quickly with your negative response. If assertiveness is a problem for you, you might consider an assertiveness training course. Avoid being alone with people you don't know well.

deal with. Some women become unreasonably fearful, rather than rationally cautious. Some become depressed as a result of the rape. They may have trouble with existing or future relationships with men. Sometimes, women wrongly assume they're to blame for the rape or for not resisting effectively.

Explaining what happened to the doctor, the police and to family and friends is in itself an ordeal. If the rapist is caught, recounting the experience in court also can be difficult. However, you can avoid or overcome long-lasting emotional and psychological consequences through counseling with someone who's trained to help rape victims. ■

CHAPTER 34 PART V

Male Reproductive System

The main biological function of the male reproductive system is to produce sperm cells and transport them to the female reproductive system. Unlike a woman, whose reproductive ability usually comes to a halt in midlife, a man is capable of reproducing well into old age. Once a male reaches sexual maturity, he produces sperm constantly.

Each time a man ejaculates, millions of microscopic sperm are propelled in the semen. Whether one sperm finds its way to an egg (ovum) and fertilizes it depends on several factors, including how well the man's reproductive system is functioning, whether he's engaging in sexual intercourse with a woman at the time of ejaculation and whether that woman has recently released an egg from her ovaries (ovulated).

As with females, there's some overlap in function between the reproductive and urinary systems, with some organs being used in each. The link is so close in men that a genital disorder often causes urinary symptoms, and vice versa.

Reproductive Organs

The male reproductive organs include the penis, testicles, sac of skin that holds the testicles (scrotum), tubes through which semen passes (epididymides and vasa deferentia), prostate gland and seminal vesicles.

The penis has a sexual function and a urinary function. Urine and ejaculated semen both leave the body by way of the urethra, which runs through the length of the penis. The two can't, however, use this pathway at the same time because right before ejaculation, a valve closes off the path of urine from the bladder.

The penis is made up of soft, spongy tissues. But when a man is sexually aroused, these tissues become engorged with blood, causing an erection. The penis becomes firm and gets longer and wider. With sufficient stimulation, the man ejaculates, sending semen through the urethra and out the opening in the head (glans) of the penis.

Male Genital Organs

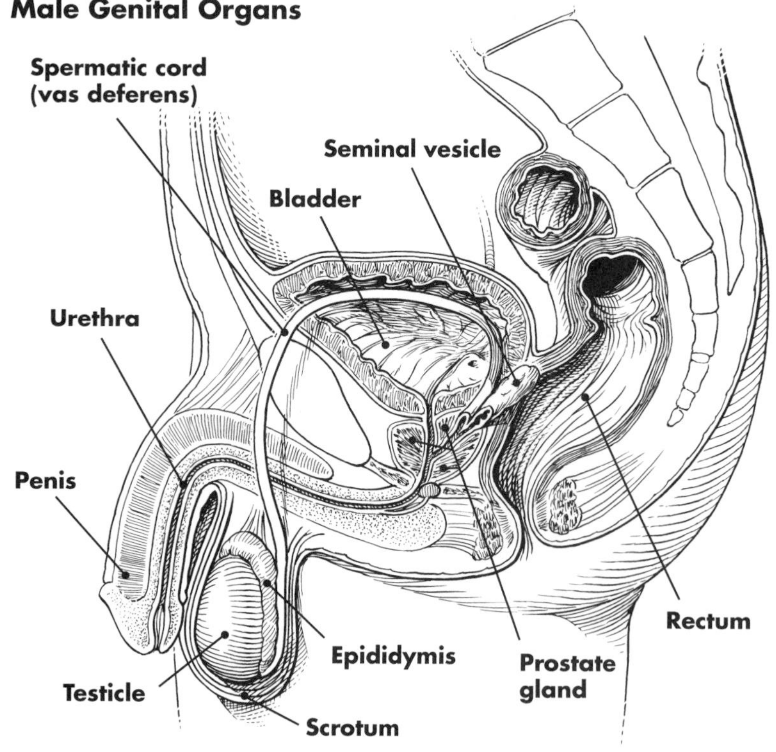

Semen is the ejaculated fluid that contains sperm. It's produced by the prostate gland and seminal vesicles. The amount of semen produced depends to some extent on the amount of time between ejaculations. The average amount of semen ejaculated varies from $^1/_2$ to $1^1/_2$ teaspoons. This white, sticky fluid helps the sperm survive inside the vagina. The average ejaculation contains about 100 million sperm.

Sperm are produced in the testicles, two oval-shaped organs about 2 inches long. They're contained in a pouch of skin, called the scrotum, which hangs below the abdomen and behind the penis. Each testicle contains a tightly packed mass of coiled tubes in which sperm are produced.

A human sperm is made up of a head — which contains the genetic material of the cell — a body and a tail. Sperm are microscopically small. It would take about 600 of them lined up end to end to measure an inch.

When a boy reaches puberty, his testicles begin to produce sperm cells. This process continues throughout his life. In addition to producing sperm cells, the testicles secrete the male hormone testosterone. Other hormones — chemical messengers — are produced in other parts of the body.

Testosterone plays an important role in the development and maintenance of masculine physical characteristics, such as facial hair, greater muscle mass and strength and a deeper voice. It also influences body shape, sex drive and the ability to have an erection.

Inside the testicles are the cells that make sperm. These cells are extremely sensitive to temperature. Sperm production only takes place at a temperature that's lower than the normal temperature within the rest of the body. That's why the testicles are located outside the abdominal cavity.

The scrotal sac acts as a highly efficient thermostat, maintaining the temperature of the testicles about 6 degrees below the normal internal body temperature. When a man is cold, muscles in the scrotum contract to raise the testicles closer to the body to maintain adequate heat. When he's hot, the scrotum becomes larger and flaccid to expose more area for heat loss. Tight-fitting underwear can hold the testicles too close to the body, and the increased heat can reduce the number of sperm produced.

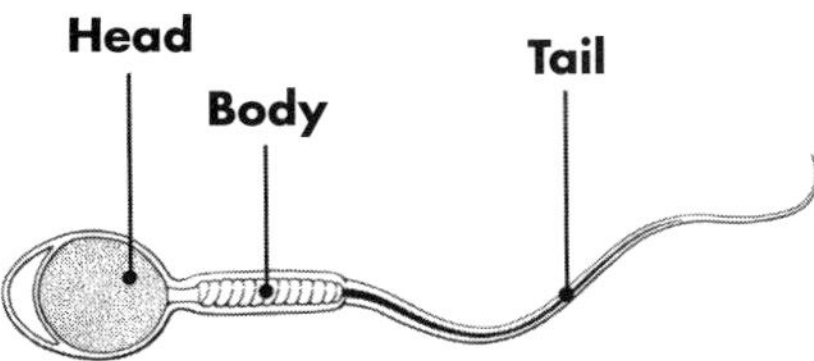

About 1/600 of an inch long, a human sperm is made up of a head — which contains the nucleus, or center, of the cell — a body and a tail to propel it.

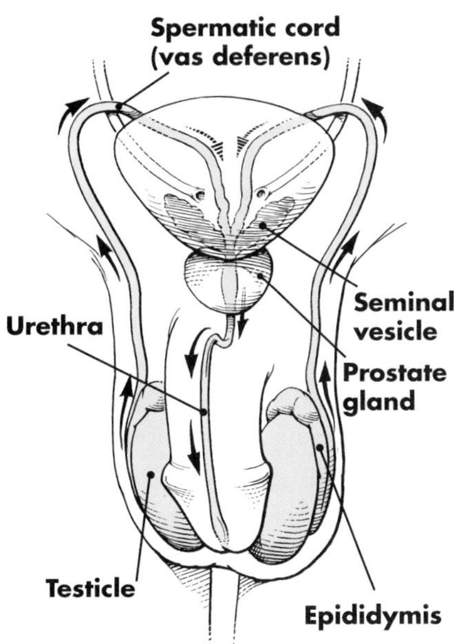

From the testicle, sperm move by contractions through the epididymis and vas deferens. Fluids are added by the seminal vesicle and prostate gland. Semen is a combination of these fluids and sperm. Following sufficient sexual stimulation, a man ejaculates, sending semen through the urethra inside the penis and out the opening in the head of the penis.

After being produced in a testicle, sperm travel to the epididymis, where they continue to ripen. The epididymis is a long, coiled tube. A man has two of these organs, one attached to the top of each testicle. When sperm are ready, they're propelled by contractions out of these tubes and into the vasa deferentia.

The vasa deferentia are the body's warehouses for sperm as well as the conduits that carry sperm from the scrotum to the urethra. They're each about 18 inches long and run from the upper scrotum into the urethra at the base of the prostate. Millions of sperm enter the vasa deferentia every day.

The prostate gland surrounds the urethra. The prostate gland and seminal vesicles produce fluids that mix with sperm before ejaculation to make semen. After the semen is ejaculated from a man's penis into a woman's vagina, sperm cells search for a woman's egg to fertilize. The tail on the sperm whips to propel it. A sperm can travel an inch in 4 to 16 minutes in the vagina, depending on if the female's cervical mucus is watery or thick. For pregnancy to occur, one sperm must penetrate an egg.

Preventing Pregnancy

Throughout history, men and women have tried — and not always successfully — to prevent pregnancy.

More than 1,500 years ago, a collection of Jewish writings known as the Talmud recommended that couples drink a beverage derived from roots to prevent pregnancy. Some American Indians brewed a special tea for those who wished to avoid conception.

And as early as the 1500s, Arabs were inserting into the vagina of female camels a crude version of today's intrauterine device in an effort to prevent an unwanted increase in the number of animals in the herd.

Today, many couples in the United States use some form of birth control (contraception). Some contraceptive methods depend on the actions of the woman. Three depend primarily on the actions of the man — condoms, withdrawing the penis from the vagina before ejaculation *(coitus interruptus)* and vasectomy.

The Reproductive Process

The first step in reproduction is sexual arousal, which is regulated by a combination of psychological factors, sex hormones and physical stimulation. When a man is sexually stimulated, he gets an erection. During sexual intercourse he inserts his erect penis into a woman's vagina, and sexual excitement intensifies to the point of orgasm. It's usually during orgasm that ejaculation occurs. Muscles that surround the prostate gland and the seminal vesicles go through a series of involuntary contractions that suddenly propel the sperm-saturated semen through the urethra. This fluid traverses the length of the penis and is released into the vagina.

The vagina is flooded with millions of sperm swimming in all directions in search of an egg to fertilize. Most sperm die within the vagina and never even reach the woman's cervical canal — the opening between the vagina and uterus. Of those that make it to the 1-inch cervical canal, most never make it any farther. Only a few sperm reach the uterus and successfully make the journey midway down one of the fallopian tubes, where an egg is located if it's the time of the month when the woman has released an egg from an ovary (ovulated). When a sperm finds and penetrates an egg, fertilization has occurred and a pregnancy has begun. The sperm that fertilizes an egg has overcome enormous odds.

Condoms

About 10 percent to 15 percent of all couples practicing birth control use condoms. A condom is a thin sheath, usually made of latex (rubber), that's placed over the man's erect penis just before sexual intercourse. When the man ejaculates, the semen remains inside the condom and doesn't enter the vagina.

When used correctly, condoms are about 96 percent effective in preventing pregnancy. An added benefit is that condoms, if used properly, can help to protect against the spread of sexually transmitted diseases (STDs).

One reason condoms are so popular is that they're easy to buy. Condoms are available without a prescription in many stores. You can also buy them from vending machines in some restrooms. They come with or without a lubricant, are packaged in small or large quantities and are available in several sizes.

They also come in various materials, including plastic and lambskin. Latex condoms offer the best protection from leakage and sexually transmitted diseases. Packaged condoms are good for at least 2 to 5 years if they're kept in a cool, dry environment.

The proper use of a condom
If you decide to use a condom, make sure that as you unroll it onto the penis, you leave room at the tip for semen to collect. If you're uncircumcised, also make sure to pull back the foreskin before you put on the condom.

After intercourse, withdraw the penis from the vagina while holding the base of the condom so that the condom doesn't come off before your penis is out of the vagina. Then remove the condom and dispose of it.

Condom accidents can occur during intercourse, usually as a result of the condom breaking. The chance of such an accident can be reduced by:

- Allowing extra room at the condom's tip for semen to collect.
- Applying a water-based lubricant such as K-Y jelly on the condom after you've put it on, especially if your partner's vagina seems dry. An oil-based lubricant such as petroleum jelly or baby oil may weaken the latex material.

The most common complaint about condoms is that they dull sensation for the man, which can diminish his sexual pleasure. Some couples also complain that spontaneity is lost because they have to stop their lovemaking to put on the condom. Others think that putting on a condom enhances lovemaking, especially when the woman places it on the man during foreplay.

Using a condom with a spermicide gives you added protection against pregnancy. A spermicide is a sperm-killing cream that's inserted into the vagina before intercourse or used as a lubricant on the condom.

Withdrawal before ejaculation

Coitus interruptus means withdrawing the penis from the vagina before ejaculation. It's probably the oldest method of birth control — and one of the least effective. Its ineffectiveness is one reason that fewer than 3 percent of adults in the United States use it as their main form of contraception. Throughout the world, however, *coitus interruptus* is used more than any other kind of contraception.

Although some couples have used *coitus interruptus* effectively, the overall failure rate is high, and most doctors don't recommend it. Aside from being frustrating for both partners, *coitus interruptus* requires that the man maintain stringent control. Even with excellent control and no ejaculation into the vagina, often small discharges of semen are released into the vagina, which can cause pregnancy.

Vasectomy

When couples make the decision not to have any more children — or not to have any children — they often consider sterilization. Either the man or the woman may be sterilized. The procedure in men is called vasectomy. Compared with female sterilization (tubal ligation), a vasectomy is less physically traumatic, less expensive and usually involves less time away from work.

A vasectomy is a relatively simple operation that can be done in an outpatient surgical setting. The procedure involves cutting and sealing the vasa deferentia, the two tubes that carry sperm from the testicles to the urethra. The procedure in no way interferes with your ability to maintain an erection or reach orgasm. Nor does it block the production of male hormones or of sperm in the testicles. The only change is that the transport of sperm has been interrupted, preventing it from mixing with semen.

After a vasectomy, you continue to ejaculate about the same amount of semen because sperm account for only a tiny part of the ejaculate. Sperm continue to be produced, but at a slower rate. The sperm are broken down and reabsorbed in the epididymis and a portion of the vas deferens.

A Male Birth Control Pill?

Researchers have been talking for years about developing a male birth control pill. In fact, some hormonal treatments have been tested that do render a man temporarily infertile. Unfortunately, they also take away his sex drive and ability to maintain an erection. Research continues, but so far a male birth control pill still isn't available.

How it's done

Before a vasectomy, you're given an injection of local anesthetic behind the scrotum to numb the area. After your doctor locates the vasa deferentia, two small cuts are made in the skin of the scrotum. Each vas deferens is pulled through one of the openings until it forms a loop.

Approximately a half inch is cut out of each tube and removed. The ends of each are closed by stitches, cauterization or both and placed back into the scrotum. The incisions are then closed with stitches.

The procedure takes about 20 to 40 minutes, after which you may be asked to stay for a short period of observation. After a vasectomy, refrain from any strenuous activity for at least 2 days.

If your work doesn't involve physical labor, you may be able to return to your job as soon as you feel able to. The stitches will most likely be the type that dissolves in 7 to 10 days.

You may notice some swelling, bruising and minor discomfort in your scrotum for several weeks. If the pain becomes severe or if you develop a fever, call your doctor. This may indicate an infection.

The failure rate for a vasectomy is less than 1 percent. But keep in mind that your vasectomy isn't an instant guarantee against pregnancy. That's because afterward you'll still have some sperm stored above the point where the vasa deferentia were severed.

In most men, the semen becomes sperm-free after 8 to 10 ejaculations following the vasectomy. Your doctor will want to test your ejaculate for sperm a few weeks after the procedure. Until your doctor has determined that your ejaculate doesn't contain sperm, continue to use contraception.

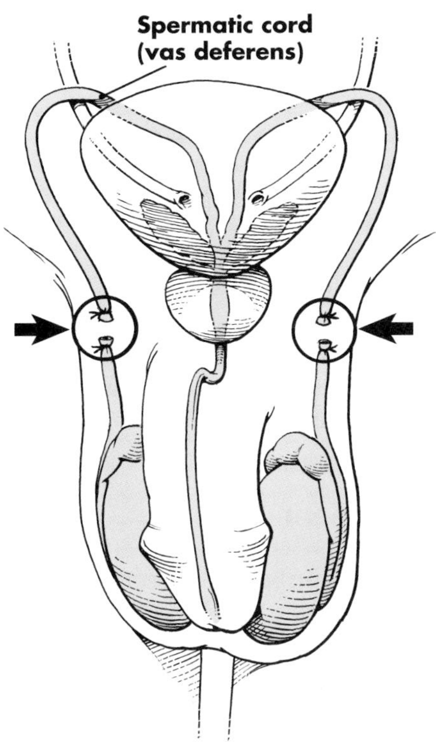

In a vasectomy, the doctor severs and seals the spermatic cords (vasa deferentia), closing off the sperm's only paths to the outside.

Reversing a Vasectomy

A vasectomy is done for permanent sterilization, but it might be reversible. Perhaps your circumstances have changed — for example, you've remarried after being widowed or divorced, and you and your spouse want a child.

It's usually possible to reattach the previously cut ends of the vasa deferentia. Unlike a vasectomy, a vasovasostomy, as the procedure is called, requires the skill of a surgeon trained to operate using a microscope. And the surgery isn't something that can be performed in a few minutes during an office visit. It takes 1 to 2 hours and is relatively expensive.

About 80 percent to 90 percent of men who have their vasectomies reversed do ejaculate semen-containing sperm. But only 30 percent to 40 percent are able to father children after the reversal. The reason for this discrepancy may be that as a result of the vasectomy many men develop antibodies that attack and damage their sperm — a kind of natural spermicide.

Consult your family doctor or a urologist — a specialist who treats urinary and male genital problems — for referral to a surgeon experienced in this procedure.

Infertility

Doctors generally use the term *infertility* to describe the inability of a couple to conceive after 1 year of frequent sexual intercourse without using contraception. Infertility isn't the same as sterility, which means the inability to conceive a child under any circumstances. With infertility, the possibility of conceiving a child has by no means been ruled out.

Infertility is a common problem. Fortunately, major advances in treating it have been made in recent decades, and infertility can often be overcome. It can be caused by problems with the sperm or egg or by difficulties in their union.

Ten percent to 15 percent of couples are infertile. Of such couples, the man is the infertile partner in about 30 percent of cases and contributes to the infertility problem in an additional 20 percent of cases. In both men and women, various factors can account for infertility.

Inadequate sperm

Forty percent of infertile couples have more than one cause of their infertility. Because of this, your doctor may begin a comprehensive infertility examination of both partners. The most common diagnostic test for men is semen analysis. Other tests may involve determining the man's level of testosterone and other hormones.

For a man to be fertile, his testicles must produce enough sperm, the sperm must be able to reach the seminal vesicles, and the sperm must be ejaculated effectively into the woman's vagina. Male infertility tests attempt to determine if any of these steps are impeded.

The first step of your fertility evaluation is a general physical examination. This includes examination of the genitals and questions about your medical history, illnesses or disabilities, medications and sexual habits. Your doctor may ask you for a specimen of ejaculated semen. To obtain this you masturbate or interrupt intercourse, and ejaculate semen into a clean container.

The fresh semen is analyzed in a laboratory. Technicians evaluate its quantity and color and search for evidence of infection or blood.

Principally, however, they analyze the sperm, determining the concentration of sperm present in the ejaculate, their shape and their activity (motility). Sperm disorders include:

Azoospermia
Azoospermia is the complete absence of sperm in the semen, generally due to a disorder of the testicles or a blockage in the passage leading from the testicles.

Oligospermia
Oligospermia is a condition in which sperm are present in the semen but not in enough quantity to readily fertilize an egg.

Other causes

Sometimes the problem isn't really one of infertility but a more general sexual problem. For example, you may be fertile but impotent — unable to obtain an erection sufficient to have intercourse.

Premature ejaculation — ejaculation during foreplay or before the penis is very far into the vagina — also greatly reduces the chances of a sperm meeting an egg. In some men, sperm production is perfectly normal, but the sperm are ejaculated backward into the bladder rather than out the penis, a condition called retrograde ejaculation (see page 1115).

Another cause of male infertility is varicocele, a swelling of the scrotum caused by enlarged (varicose) veins surrounding the testicle. The enlarged veins may prevent normal cooling of the testicles, which impairs sperm production.

Several other problems with the testicles also can be responsible for infertility. Sexually transmitted diseases (STDs) or other infections also can block the passageways through which sperm travel, or they can injure or destroy sperm. Mumps and other infections sometimes can cause an inflammation of one or both testicles that can permanently impair or prevent sperm production in the affected testicle.

In addition, some men produce antibodies that are meant to fight infection but inadvertently attack sperm instead. Injuries to the genitals also can affect the production of sperm.

Treatment

Infertility can be treated in many ways. The type of treatment your doctor recommends will depend on what's causing the infertility. Recent developments in therapy have increased the number of once infertile couples who can achieve pregnancy. Some causes of infertility can't be corrected, but even then, various means of insemination may be possible so that the woman can still become pregnant.

When the source of infertility is the man's sperm — or a lack of sperm — restoring or initiating fertility is sometimes possible. For example, varicocele can be corrected surgically. Problems with the testicles, prostate gland, seminal vesicles and urethra also may be successfully treated.

In extremely rare instances, sperm production is impaired because of a pituitary gland problem. For this condition the hormones human chorionic gonadotropin and human pituitary gonadotropin have been helpful. When infections hamper sperm production, block the transport of sperm or kill sperm, treatment of the infection may restore fertility.

Loss of Sexual Desire

Men can experience various physical problems that make it difficult to have sexual intercourse. But what if the urge to have sex goes away?

It's unusual for a man to have no sexual desire at all. But it's common for men to experience reduced desire. With increasing age most men experience somewhat diminished sexual desire, although this can vary greatly from one man to another.

The first cause to consider is a physical ailment. Illnesses that cause persistent pain, weakness or fatigue tend to reduce your sexual desire. So do emotional problems such as depression or difficulty dealing with stress. Medications taken to combat these disorders also can reduce sexual desire. When this happens your doctor can usually find substitute medications.

Lack of enthusiasm from you or for your sexual partner also can lead to dampened desire. In addition, you may experience a loss of desire because you don't tell your partner what arouses you or what stops your arousal. Or, your timing may be off. For example, you want to have intercourse when you or your partner is tired.

Loss of desire often can be cured. If you experience a continuing loss of sexual desire, don't assume that this is the natural course of events. Seek help from your doctor to search for the cause. You may benefit from counseling, changes in medication or other forms of therapy.

This is particularly true for sexually transmitted diseases.

For men with low sperm concentrations, a technique called intracytoplasmic sperm injection might be used. It involves a microscopic technique (micromanipulation) in which a single sperm is injected directly into an egg to achieve fertilization. Fertilization rates are comparable to those achieved with standard in vitro fertilization (see page 1069).

Sexual Dysfunction

Sexual dysfunction refers to problems encountered during sexual intercourse that may be experienced by either the man or woman. For men, the most common problems are erection abnormalities and premature ejaculation.

The solution to sexual problems in either partner requires understanding and cooperation from both partners. One of the first steps in solving sexual problems in men is understanding the male sexual sequence and how it can be interrupted. The sequence involves:

- Stimulation
- Erection
- Orgasm with ejaculation
- Loss of erection

For men, the ability to function sexually depends on psychological, hormonal, neurologic and vascular factors. That's because the ability to have an erection is controlled by both the nervous system and vascular system, and sexual arousal is governed by a variety of hormones and psychological factors. If a man's hormone levels are low or if he is under a lot of emotional stress, he may lose interest in sex.

Ejaculation is controlled by the nervous system. The normal loss of an erection after sex is controlled by the neurologic and vascular systems. Some neurologic disorders and diseases of the urinary and reproductive systems directly interfere with sexual performance. Many other chronic diseases, such as diabetes and cancer, can impede a man's ability to perform sexually because of their debilitating effect on overall health. Diabetes can also damage nerves that control an erection. The use of alcohol or some other drugs also may impair sexual function.

The good news is that effective treatments are available for most of the common causes of male sexual dysfunction.

Impotence

Impotence is a persistent inability to obtain an erection or to keep it long enough for sexual intercourse. The term comes from the Latin word *impotentia*, which means "lack of strength."

Diminished sexual desire or even the loss of sexual desire isn't the same as impotence. Impotence refers to the inability to use the penis for sexual activity even when desire and opportunity are present.

It's important to realize that an occasional episode of impotence happens to most men. It's perfectly normal and nothing to worry about. When it becomes a persistent problem, impotence can hurt a man's self-image as well as his sex life. Impotence affects about 30 million American men — mostly older men. Nearly 20 percent of impotent men are in their 60s and 70s, and more than 70 percent are age 80 or above. Impotence is by no means an inevitable consequence of aging, and treatment in older men is often as effective as it is in younger men.

The biology of an erection

To deal with impotence, it's important to understand how an erection occurs. The penis has two cylindrical, sponge-like structures that run along its length. When a man is sexually aroused, nerve impulses cause blood flow to the cylinders to increase to about seven times the normal amount. This sudden influx of blood expands the sponge-like structures and enlarges, straightens and stiffens the penis, producing an erection. Continued sexual arousal maintains the higher rate of blood flow and closes the valves that would allow blood to drain from the penis, which maintains the erection.

After ejaculation, or when the sexual excitement passes, the excess blood drains out of the spongy tissue, and the penis returns to its nonerect size and shape.

Three important steps are necessary to produce the erection. The

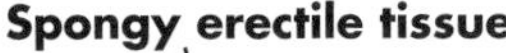

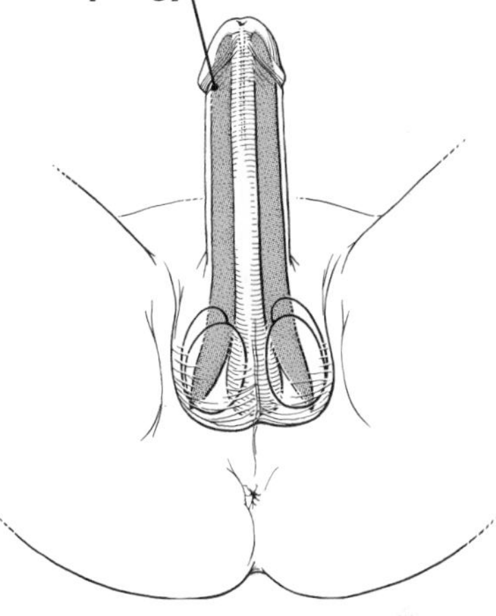

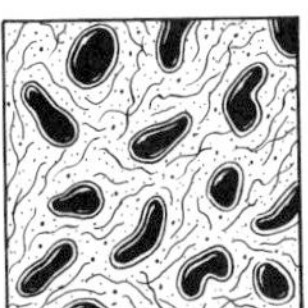

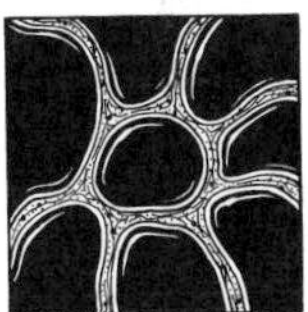

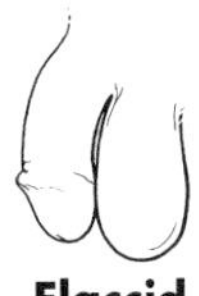

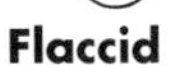

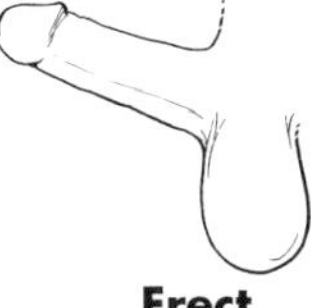

When a man is sexually aroused, two cylindrical, sponge-like erectile structures become engorged with blood. Veins that normally drain blood from the penis clamp down, keeping extra blood in the penis and maintaining the erection. After orgasm the excess blood drains from the spongy tissue, leaving the penis flaccid.

first is sexual arousal, which can come from the senses of sight, touch, hearing, taste and smell and from thoughts. The second step is communication of the sexual arousal from nerves in the brain to nerves in the penis.

The third step is a relaxing action of the blood vessels that supply the penis, allowing more blood to flow into the cylinders. This produces an erection because exit valves of the veins in the penis close, trapping the blood. If something affects any of these steps, impotence can result.

Causes

Some causes of impotence aren't physical. The most common nonphysical cause is stress or anxiety. If you can't relax and focus on the sexual situation, or if you're overwhelmed or confused by life circumstances, it's difficult for the three-stage erection process to take place. This happens to almost every man at some time.

Impotence is also an occasional side effect of psychological disorders such as depression. Other contributing factors include negative feelings toward the sexual partner, or expressed by the sexual partner, such as resentment, hostility or lack of interest.

The important thing is not to assume that an episode of impotence means that you have a permanent problem and that you should expect it to happen again. The best thing to do if you experience an episode of impotence is to treat it as something that happens once in a while to all men, and to expect a more successful experience at another time. Impotence isn't reflective of your self-worth or masculinity.

Conditions that account for most cases of impotence include:

- Diabetes-related nerve damage
- Vascular disorders, such as blocked arteries to the penis or leaking valves in penile veins
- Some prescription medicines
- Surgery in the pelvic area, such as for prostate cancer
- A spinal cord injury
- Multiple sclerosis
- Hormone disorders
- Alcoholism and other forms of drug abuse

Physical and nonphysical causes can work together to trigger impotence. For example, a minor physical problem that slows sexual response might cause anxiety about attaining an erection, and the anxiety worsens the impotence.

Diagnosis

If you experience recurring episodes of impotence, consult your doctor. If your doctor suspects a nonphysical cause, he or she may ask if you get erections in other circumstances, such as during masturbation or while you're asleep. Most men experience many erections — without remembering them — during sleep. Testing for nocturnal erection can be done in many ways. One way is to wrap a special perforated tape around the penis before sleeping. If the tape is separated in the morning, your penis was erect at some point during the night. Tests like this can help determine the cause of your impotence by, for example, ruling out physical problems such as vascular disorders.

If your doctor suspects a physical cause, you may need to undergo further testing. An ultrasound procedure that measures blood flow to the penis is often used. A more complicated procedure called angiography can help determine if there's blood vessel blockage in the penis. This is a special type of X-ray study using a die injection to enhance the image. Neurologic tests evaluate communication problems from the brain. Your doctor may also want to measure hormone levels in your blood. If he or she suspects a prescription drug may be responsible for your impotence, you may be prescribed a different medication.

Treatment

The type of treatment your doctor recommends will depend on the cause of your impotence. There are a variety of options.

Psychological therapy

If the cause of your impotence isn't physical, your doctor may suggest that you visit a psychiatrist, psychologist or sex therapist, either alone or with your partner. These medical specialists can help you address problems such as stress and anxiety.

Medication

Sildenafil (Viagra), an oral medication for men taken about an hour before sexual intercourse, has become a common treatment for many impotent men. Unlike most other treatments for impotence, Viagra produces a natural erection instead of an artificial one, such as the kinds that results from implants. One Viagra tablet is often effective for about 4 hours, and this medication shouldn't be used more than once a day. Many men are able to maintain an erection even after multiple orgasms. However, Viagra, isn't the best choice for all men.

Among men whose impotence is related to hormone deficiencies, synthetic hormones can sometimes help. Hormones usually aren't prescribed unless your doctor has documented that your hormone levels are low and the cause of the low levels is well established. Men with a history of prostate cancer normally aren't given hormone shots or pills because male sex hormones can make cancer cells grow faster.

Another medication for men that's used to treat impotence is called alprostadil (Caverject, Edex, others). It's delivered as either a suppository or an injection. The suppository method involves inserting the suppository — about half the size of a grain of rice — into the urethra through the tip of your penis. This medication increases blood flow in the penis, causing an erection. A rubber ring placed around the base of your penis before the suppository is inserted helps trap the blood and maintain an erection.

Alprostadil can also be self-injected into the base of your penis with a fine needle. It generally takes 5 to 20 minutes for the drug to work, producing an erection that lasts about an hour.

You need to be careful to insert the needle along the side of your penis and not at the top or bottom. At the top are arteries, veins and nerves, and at the bottom is the urethra, the tube through which semen and urine pass. If you hit either area, you won't get an erection, and you'll need to wait at least 24 hours before you can use the medication again.

Candidates for alprostadil treatment undergo a test dose of the medication in their doctor's office and are taught how to use it on their own.

The Dangers of Viagra

Rarely has a new drug been greeted with as much fanfare as the impotence medication sildenafil (Viagra). Even so, this medication does have potential serious side effects, and it needs to be used with caution.

The Food and Drug Administration reports that since Viagra's introduction in April 1998, more than 100 men have died shortly after taking the medication. Most deaths were due to cardiovascular disease.

Viagra shouldn't be taken with nitrate medications, such as the heart drug nitroglycerin. And the drug isn't recommended for people in whom sexual activity could trigger a cardiac event and in potentially high-risk groups in whom the drug hasn't been studied. This includes people who've had a heart attack, stroke or life-threatening arrhythmia in the past 6 months, as well as people with unstable angina, low or high blood pressure or an eye condition called retinitis pigmentosa. For some people with heart disease, exercise testing may help determine if Viagra can be safely used.

It's wise to be cautious. Before taking Viagra make sure you discuss with your doctor its potential benefits and its side effects.

A vacuum device

A vacuum device is a method of impotence treatment that uses vacuum pressure to draw blood into the penis. It's made up of a plastic tube and hand pump.

You place the tube over your penis and use the pump to draw the air out of the plastic tube. As you do this, blood is drawn into the tissue of your penis, producing an erection. You then slip off the elastic ring mounted on the base of the tube and pull it onto the base of your penis. The ring traps the blood inside your penis, allowing you to keep your erection once the vacuum tube is removed.

You should remove the ring within 30 minutes to restore normal blood flow to your penis. If you don't, you could damage tissue in your penis.

Some men find the elastic ring uncomfortable and believe that it looks unnatural. In addition, your penis may feel cold because there's no blood circulation. However, a vacuum device is effective in more than 90 percent of men who try it, it doesn't require surgery or use of medication, and it's reasonably priced.

Surgery

Among men with insufficient blood flow to the penis due to vascular problems, surgery might be performed in rare instances to increase circulation to the penis. Surgery might also be performed to implant a penile prosthesis. Various types of penile implants are available, ranging from semirigid rods to inflatable devices.

Semirigid, bendable rods are the easiest implant to use and the least likely to malfunction. Two firm, flexible rods made of wires and covered with silicone or polyurethane are placed inside your penis. They give you a permanent erection. You bend your penis down toward your body to hide the erection and bend it up to have sexual intercourse.

Inflatable implants work more naturally than semirigid rods because instead of having a permanent

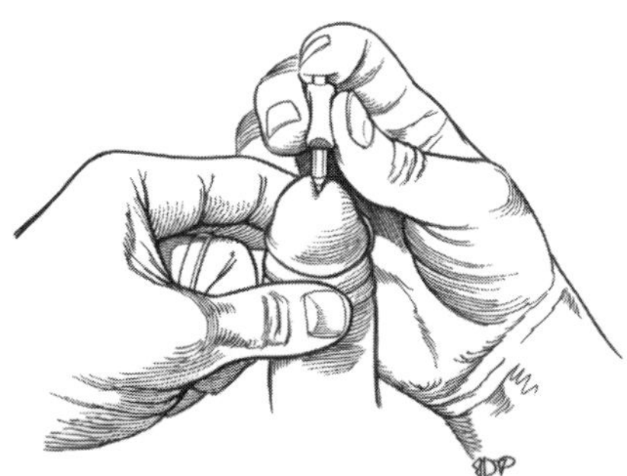

One therapy for impotence involves inserting a tiny suppository into the tip of your penis to help relax muscle tissue and increase blood flow to the penis.

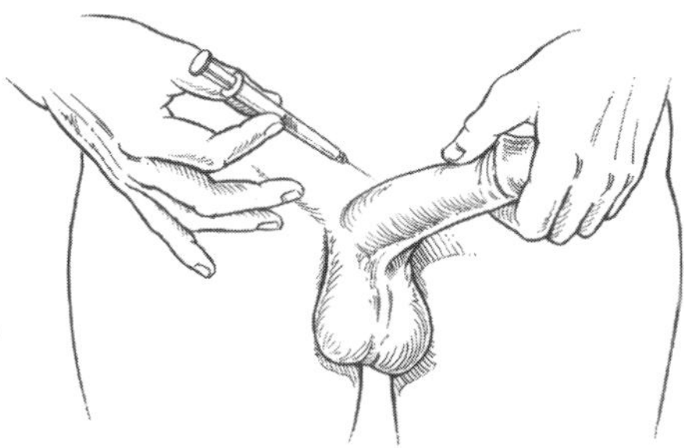

Self-injection therapy involves injecting medication directly into a specific area of the penis to increase blood flow and cause an erection.

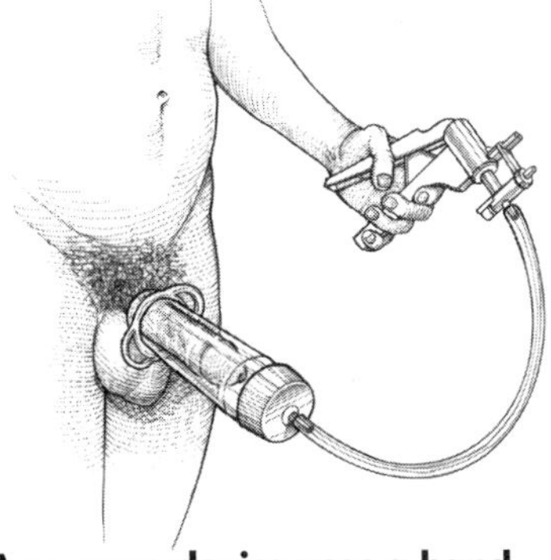

A vacuum device uses a hand pump to draw blood into the penis, creating an erection. An elastic ring placed at the base of the penis keeps it erect.

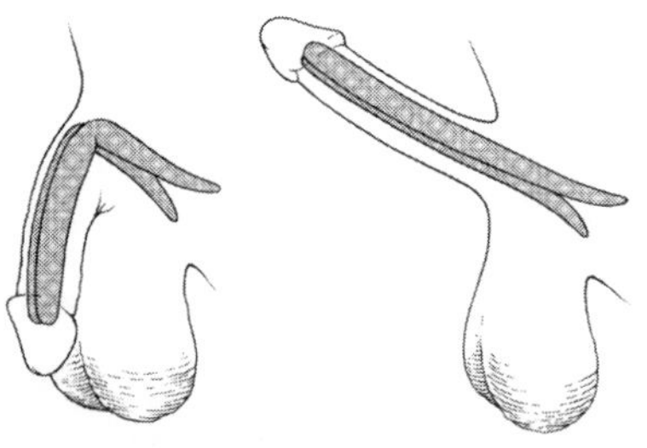

With semirigid implants, the penis is always erect. To hide the erection, the implanted rods are bent down.

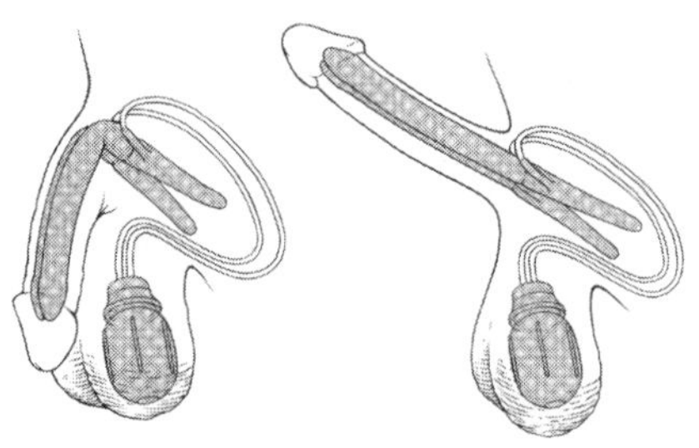

With some inflatable implants, you squeeze a pump, causing fluid from a reservoir to fill inflatable cylinders in the penis and produce an erection. When an erection isn't wanted, the fluid is directed back to the reservoir.

erection, you produce an erection only when you want one. Two hollow, inflatable cylinders are placed into your penis. The cylinders are attached to a reservoir in either your scrotum or your lower abdomen. In some devices these cylinders are connected to a tiny pump in your scrotum.

To produce an erection, you squeeze the pump or a device at the head of the penis and fluid from the reservoir fills the cylinders. This device gives you the most natural erection of any implant, but it's more likely than most other implants to suffer mechanical failure.

Peyronie's disease

Peyronie's disease involves a curvature of the penis during an erection, which can be painful. The name comes from the French physician who first described the disorder.

Peyronie's disease occurs most often between the ages of 40 and 60 and can make sexual intercourse difficult or impossible. The disease is caused by scar tissue that forms inside the penis for unknown reasons. Sometimes, this tissue calcifies into hard lumps known as plaques. The scar tissue and plaques are dense and firm and won't allow the adjacent part of the penis to fill with blood during an erection. This causes the penis to curve toward the side of the scar tissue.

Peyronie's disease isn't related to any infection, tumor, contagious disease or sexual practice. Some researchers speculate that the problem might begin with mild trauma to the penis that results from it being hit or bent abnormally, especially during sexual intercourse. The trauma can cause small tears in penile tissue or ruptured blood vessels. The condition might also stem from wear and tear of the lining of the penile cylinders.

How serious is Peyronie's disease?

The symptoms of Peyronie's disease are often mild. In about three of four men with this problem, the disease goes away on its own. But this may take several years.

Treatment

Researchers have been testing vitamin E and injections of substances such as steroids, collagenase and verapamil as a means of breaking down the scar tissue and plaques. In severe cases, surgery may be an option. The following four methods are commonly used:

- Tissue on the side of the penis opposite the scar tissue and plaques is removed or pinched, countering the bending effect.
- The scar tissue and plaques are removed, and a patch of skin or artificial material is used to replace it.
- The scar tissue and plaques are cut to allow straightening, and the incision is covered with grafted material.
- A penile prosthesis is implanted to straighten and increase the rigidity of the penis.

Priapism

Priapism is a condition in which you have a sustained, often painful, erection that occurs without sexual stimulation. The term *priapism* comes from the Latin name for a male fertility god in ancient mythology, Priapus. The condition occurs most often as a reaction to medication used to create erections in impotent men, but it may also occur as a result of a spinal cord disorder, leukemia, sickle cell anemia or inflammation of the urethra.

In priapism the penile shaft is firm, but the head of the penis is soft. The penis becomes filled with blood as during a normal erection, but the blood doesn't drain out, and the erection doesn't go away as it normally should after sexual stimulation ceases.

How serious is priapism?

If an erection continues for more than 4 hours, blood trapped inside the penis becomes thick because of oxygen loss. This can damage penile tissue.

If you have a painful erection that doesn't go away, seek medical help. Prompt treatment is necessary to preserve the ability of your penis to have a normal erection. Your doctor may examine the penis and perform tests to determine the underlying cause of your condition.

Treatment

Should you experience a prolonged erection, placing a towel-covered ice pack over the penis usually stops the erection. Taking an over-the-counter decongestant that causes your blood vessels to shrink also may relieve the condition. If these methods don't help and the erection continues for more than 4 hours, call your doctor or go to an emergency department. Blood may be withdrawn from the penis using a needle.

If the erection recurs, other medications, such as adrenaline (epinephrine) can be used to constrict the blood vessels. In rare cases, a surgical procedure to allow blood to drain from the penis may be necessary. The longer you wait before seeking treatment, the greater the risk that damage may be done to the penile tissue.

Premature ejaculation

Premature ejaculation refers to ejaculation that occurs during foreplay with a sexual partner or before the penis is inserted very far during intercourse. The only thing wrong with premature ejaculation is its timing — which is too soon, before either partner has had an opportunity to enjoy the sex act fully. In rare cases, merely touching a partner is enough to bring about ejaculation.

Premature ejaculation is a common sexual problem, especially in young men. The cause is rarely physical, and treatment that involves the partner's help is almost always successful.

Although premature ejaculation isn't serious, untreated it can have a detrimental effect on the sex life of both your partner and you — your partner doesn't have time to attain orgasm, and you experience orgasm but after so little sexual activity as to deprive you of much of the pleasure involved.

On occasion, some men become so frustrated at premature ejaculations that they eventually become impotent. Such anxiety is unnecessary because effective treatment is often available.

Treatment

Premature ejaculation can be treated with the squeeze technique. This method works as follows: Begin sexual activity as usual, including stimulation of the penis, until you feel almost ready to ejaculate. Then have your partner squeeze the end of the penis, at the point where the head (glans) joins the shaft, and maintain the squeeze for several seconds, until the urge to ejaculate passes.

After the squeeze is released, wait for about half a minute, then go back to foreplay. You may notice that squeezing the penis causes it to become less erect, but when sexual stimulation is resumed, it soon regains full erection.

If you again feel you're about to ejaculate, have your partner repeat the squeeze process. By repeating this as many times as necessary, you can reach the point of entering your partner without ejaculating. After a few practice sessions, the feeling of knowing how to delay ejaculation will most likely become a habit that no longer requires the squeeze technique, and you'll continue through successful intercourse. Some men, however, need medication to help delay ejaculation.

Retrograde ejaculation

In retrograde ejaculation, little or no semen is ejaculated out from the penis during a sexual climax. Retrograde ejaculation is a fairly unusual phenomenon in which the semen travels backward into the bladder during ejaculation instead of emerging from the end of the penis. The word *retrograde* refers to the backward direction of the semen. Retrograde ejaculation is harmless. Semen that enters the bladder is simply expelled during urination. Retrograde ejaculation does, however, prevent fertility if no semen exits the penis. And it diminishes fertility if a decreased quantity of semen emerges.

You can tell you have retrograde ejaculation by observing the urine that you void. If retrograde ejaculation has occurred, your urine will look cloudy because of the semen in it.

Various conditions can cause retrograde ejaculation, including prostate or urethral surgery and some medications used to treat high blood pressure or mood swings. The condition occurs most commonly in men who have diabetes-related nerve damage.

Treatment

If retrograde ejaculation stems from medication you're taking, switching to a different medication may solve the problem. Retrograde ejaculation may also be corrected by certain prescription drugs such as ephedrine or adrenaline (epinephrine). Infertility due to retrograde ejaculation sometimes can be reversed through artificial insemination. The sperm is retrieved from the bladder by way of a catheter immediately after ejaculation.

Blood in Semen

Blood in semen (hemospermia) alarms most men but is seldom something to worry about.

The color of semen in men with this condition ranges from pink to red. If you or your partner notices blood in your ejaculated semen but you have no other symptoms, you probably don't have a physical disorder. But to make sure, visit your doctor and have a thorough examination of your genital area, including your prostate gland and testicles. If your doctor doesn't find anything, further tests usually aren't helpful in revealing the cause.

The source of blood in semen isn't clear. It probably comes from vessels lining the seminal vesicles and may be the result of harmless inflammation.

Testicular and Scrotal Disorders

The testicles play two main roles. They produce sperm for reproduction, and they make hormones, such as testosterone, to generate and maintain masculine features.

The location of the testicles within the scrotum keeps them at a temperature slightly lower than inside your abdominal cavity — a requirement for healthy sperm production. This relatively exposed location makes the testicles vulnerable to injury. But it also makes them easy to examine for early detection of potentially life-threatening conditions, such as cancer.

Sharp or sudden pain in your testicles can be a symptom of a serious medical condition, such as infection or testicular torsion. See a doctor if the pain doesn't go away in 10 or 15 minutes or if it subsides and then returns.

Testicular torsion

Signs and symptoms

- Sudden, severe pain in one testicle
- Elevation of one testicle within the scrotum
- Swelling of a testicle
- Nausea and vomiting
- Faintness
- Fever

Each testicle is suspended in the scrotum on a spermatic cord that contains the vas deferens and blood vessels supplying the testicle. In a condition called testicular torsion, the testicle twists on its spermatic cord, closing off the blood supply to the testicle. Testicular torsion may occur without any apparent cause, even during sleep. At other times it happens after strenuous physical activity. Testicular torsion is uncommon and can occur at any age.

Diagnosis

To distinguish testicular torsion from other conditions affecting the testicles, your doctor may order an ultrasound examination of the testicle. Or you may need surgery to confirm the diagnosis and correct the torsion.

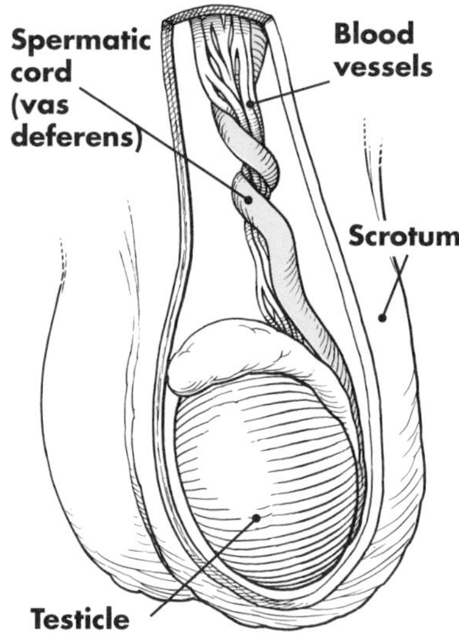

In testicular torsion, the testicle twists on its spermatic cord, cutting off the blood supply and producing sudden, severe pain.

How serious is testicular torsion?

If a testicular torsion isn't corrected within a few hours — often by an operation — the testicle can be permanently damaged from a lack of blood supply and may even have to be removed. Severe pain in a testicle for no apparent reason or after strenuous physical activity requires prompt medical attention.

Treatment

Surgery to correct testicular torsion may be avoided, at least temporarily, if your doctor is able to manipulate the twisted testicle back to its normal position. But even then, you may need an operation later to secure the testicle in its normal position to prevent a recurrence. During surgery the surgeon returns the testicle to its normal position and anchors it in place. The other testicle also may be anchored to prevent possible torsion of that testicle.

Testicular Injury

Because the testicles are located outside the abdomen, they're vulnerable to injury. Pain caused by striking the testicles is often severe.

Fortunately most injuries are minor. The sponginess of testicular tissues and the flexibility of their location generally enable them to absorb considerable shock without permanent harm.

If your testicles have been injured by a blunt object or in a fall and the pain and swelling of the scrotum go away within about an hour, there's probably no serious damage. If the scrotum remains swollen or is bruised or if the pain persists, seek prompt medical care. Untreated testicular injury can have serious complications, such as infertility or the loss of a testicle. If the scrotum has been penetrated by a sharp object, seek emergency care.

The same precautions apply to male babies and children. Persistent pain, swelling or bruising signal the need to see a doctor promptly. A young male can become infertile from an untreated testicular injury even though he hasn't reached sexual maturity.

Testicular failure

Signs and symptoms

- Infertility
- A lack of sex drive
- A delay of puberty or of the development of masculine characteristics

The term *testicular failure* refers to the inability of the testicles to produce sperm or, in some cases, male hormones. This condition may stem from chromosome abnormalities present before birth, problems involving sexual maturation or damage to normally developed testicles from disease, drugs or injury.

Diagnosis

Testicular failure is one of many possible causes of infertility. To find out if a couple's infertility is caused by testicular failure, your doctor will likely interview and examine both sexual partners and perform blood, urine and semen tests.

In cases of slowed or absent sexual maturation of the testicles, the diagnosis may be revealed by the history gathered during the interview. In addition, it may emerge after a physical examination and other tests.

How serious is testicular failure?

Testicular failure isn't life-threatening. But it can produce infertility, lack of sex drive or delayed sexual maturation.

Treatment

If you have testicular failure, administering male hormones can often help restore your normal sex drive or continue normal sexual development. But it usually can't produce fertility.

Epididymitis

Signs and symptoms

- Pain in the scrotum, generally severe, which develops gradually over several hours or days
- Pain generally limited to one testicle
- Fever
- Swelling of a testicle
- Pain during urination

At the top and rear of each testicle is a coiled tube called the epididymis, which transports sperm to the vas deferens. Epididymitis is inflammation of this tube.

The swollen area will feel hot and sausage-shaped to the touch. Bacteria can cause epididymitis, but often the cause is unknown.

Diagnosis

Your doctor may take a urine sample and a sample of prostate gland secretions in an attempt to identify an infecting organism.

How serious is epididymitis?

Epididymitis usually is an acute ailment — that is, one that comes on suddenly — that can be corrected with medication and without permanent damage. Occasionally, chronic — that is, long-lasting — epididymitis develops. Surgical treatment is rarely necessary with chronic epididymitis.

Treatment

If bacteria are the culprits, antibiotics are prescribed to treat the infection. Additional treatment may include bed rest, application of ice packs to the scrotum, elevation of the scrotum and over-the-counter anti-inflammatory medication. Because your sex partner may be infected with the same bacteria, treatment of your partner may be recommended as well.

Scrotal masses

Signs and symptoms

- A lump or swelling in the scrotum
- Local pain or tenderness

A lump in the scrotum can stem from any number of problems, including a tumor, physical injury, a cyst, infection or inguinal hernia. The tumors may be noncancerous (benign) or cancerous (malignant). A tumor growing inside a testicle is most often cancerous. Those located elsewhere in the scrotum are generally noncancerous.

A common type of painless, benign cyst is a spermatic cyst (spermatocele). It's located in the epididymis, near the top of a testicle. Other benign sources of scrotal swelling include hydroceles, hematoceles and varicocele. A hydrocele is a collection of watery fluid. A hematocele is a pocket of blood caused by physical injury.

Varicocele is a swelling in the scrotum caused by enlarged (varicose) veins. With an inguinal hernia, a section of intestine can sometimes drop into the scrotum and appear as a scrotal mass.

Diagnosis

Every scrotal mass should be evaluated by a doctor. Tests such as an ultrasound examination help to distinguish the many harmless causes of scrotal masses from serious tumors. Sometimes holding a light next to the scrotum can aid in diagnosis. If the light shines through, the mass is probably not cancerous but something less serious, such as a hydrocele. A mass within the testicle usually must be removed surgically before an accurate diagnosis can be made.

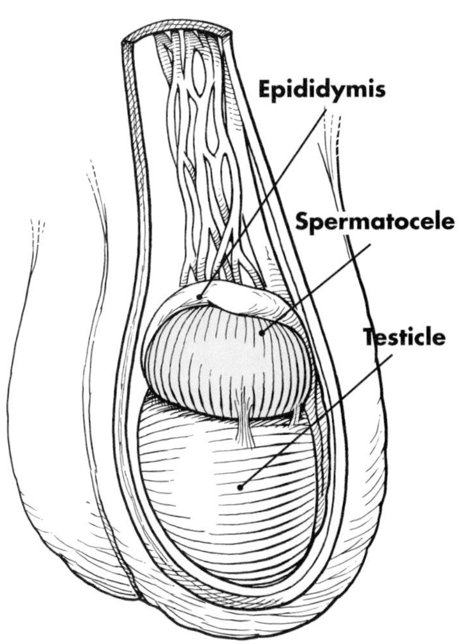

A painless, noncancerous, fluid-filled enlargement above the testicle is called a spermatic cyst (spermatocele).

How serious are scrotal masses?

Cancerous tumors are serious and can be fatal. For more on testicular cancer, see page 1119.

Treatment

Many scrotal masses don't require any treatment unless they cause discomfort. Some problems require surgery. Testicular cancer requires surgical removal of the entire testicle and possibly additional treatment as well. Inguinal hernias also generally require surgical repair (see page 894).

Hydrocele

Signs and symptoms

- Soft, usually painless, swelling in the scrotum

The term *hydrocele* comes from the Greek terms *hydro* for "water" and *cele* for "tumor" or "cavity." A testicular hydrocele is a collection of watery fluid in the sheath around the testicle. Normally, this sheath contains a tiny amount of fluid. An excessive amount, which produces the hydrocele, develops either because your genital area produces too much fluid or because it doesn't absorb enough fluid.

Hydroceles are a common cause of scrotal swelling and may occur on one or both testicles. Hydroceles can occur at any age but are most common in young boys and older men.

Diagnosis

To help differentiate a hydrocele from a tumor or another source of swelling, your doctor will feel the swollen area and may hold a light to the scrotum. If the swelling is a hydrocele, the light will shine through it. An ultrasound examination also may be done.

How serious are hydroceles?

Hydroceles aren't serious. Treatment usually isn't required unless the scrotum is so swollen that it's uncomfortable.

Treatment

If discomfort persists, your doctor may draw off hydrocele fluid with a needle and syringe. This procedure is simple, but because the fluid usually will accumulate again, it provides only temporary relief. Another disadvantage is that needle aspiration is potentially hazardous because it can cause an infection. A more common option is surgery.

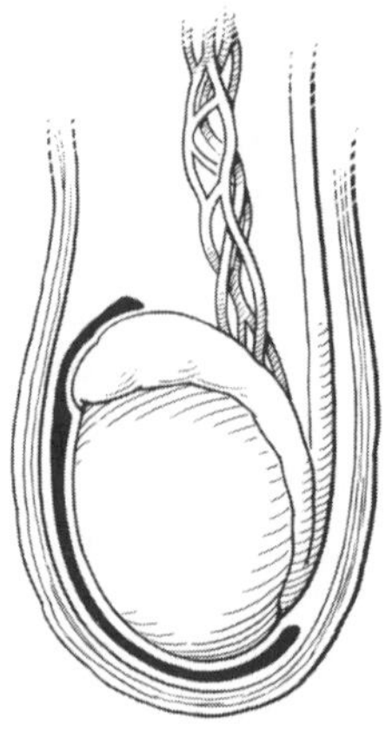
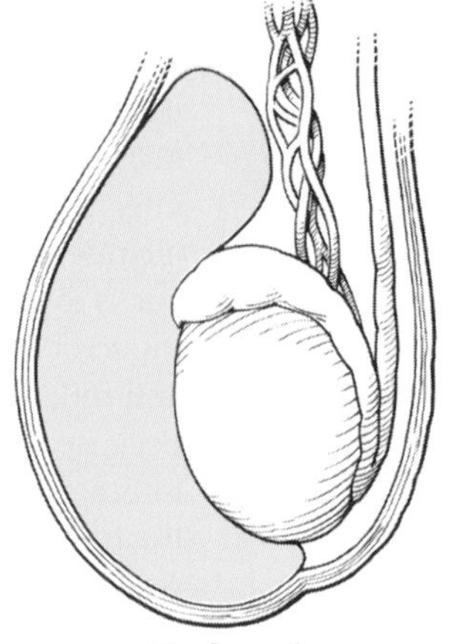
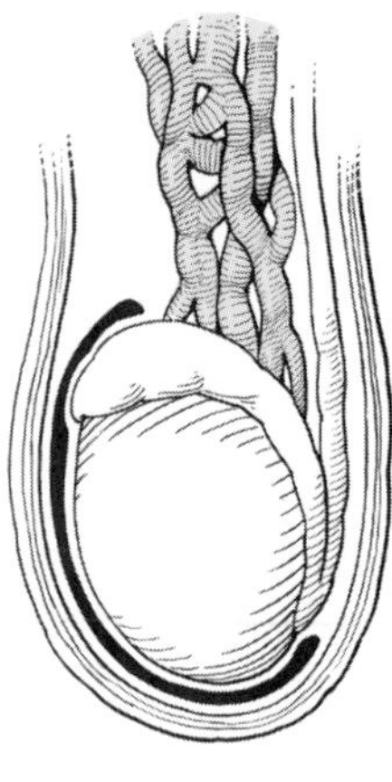

Normal testicle **Hydrocele** **Varicocele**

A hydrocele (middle) is a harmless but abnormal accumulation of watery fluid within the scrotum. It usually requires no treatment. Varicocele (right) is a swelling in the scrotum due to enlarged (varicose) veins. This condition may require treatment to prevent infertility.

Varicocele

Signs and symptoms

- Painless swelling in the scrotum, usually on the left side
- An area of the scrotum that feels like a bag of worms — a sensation that may nearly disappear when you lie down

Varicocele is a swelling in the scrotum caused by enlarged (varicose) veins. Due to a problem with tiny valves inside the veins, blood backs up in the veins that lead from the testicles.

Diagnosis

Your doctor will examine the swollen scrotum and may hold a light to the swollen area. If the problem is varicocele, light won't shine through the blood in the veins. An ultrasound examination also may be done.

How serious is varicocele?

Varicocele itself isn't a serious disorder, but backed-up blood in the testicles can contribute to infertility by increasing the temperature in the scrotum.

Treatment

Unless varicocele is associated with infertility or causes pain, treatment is rarely necessary. When infertility occurs, surgery to tie off the enlarged veins may be necessary. Another treatment involves making a tiny incision that requires no stitches and inserting a tiny blocking object directly into a vein to cut off excessive flow of blood.

Orchitis

Signs and symptoms

- Pain in a testicle
- Swelling, generally on one side of the scrotum only
- A heavy feeling in the scrotum

Orchitis is an inflammation of the testicle, usually due to a bacterial infection or the mumps virus. Orchitis may also develop if you have an infection of the prostate gland or epididymis.

Diagnosis

Your doctor will probably examine your scrotum. Because symptoms of orchitis are similar to those of epididymitis and other conditions affecting the testicles, your doctor may take a urine sample and perform other tests to identify associated infections.

How serious is orchitis?

Orchitis can permanently damage one or both testicles, possibly resulting in infertility or reduced testicular size.

Treatment

Orchitis caused by a bacterial infection is treated with antibiotics. Orchitis associated with mumps or other viral infections is usually treated with rest and medication to relieve pain and reduce the inflammation.

Undescended testicle

Before birth the testicles develop inside the male infant's abdomen. Usually, the testicles move into their permanent place in the scrotum about a month before birth. A small percentage of male infants are born with one or both testicles undescended. In most of these babies, the testicles descend into the scrotum during the first few months of life, without any medical intervention. In some cases surgery may be necessary.

Diagnosis

Your doctor can confirm the absence of or the stunted development of a testicle by feeling the scrotum. Other tests may be required before determining the appropriate action for correcting the condition.

How serious is an undescended testicle?

Before age 2, an undescended testicle isn't serious. In infants, the condition often corrects itself or can be corrected with surgery. But after age 2, the condition can lead to a nonfunctional testicle.

A testicle that remains undescended by age 2 might not produce sperm later in life, though if the other testicle functions normally, it will produce enough sperm to maintain fertility. An undescended testicle — even one that has been corrected naturally or surgically — is more vulnerable to cancer than is a normal testicle.

Treatment

Hormones may help induce an undescended testicle to descend into the scrotum. For testicles that don't descend early in life or in response to hormones, surgery is required to prevent loss of function of the testicle and to decrease the risk of testicular cancer. The best age for surgery is 12 to 18 months.

Testicular Self-Examination

Cancer of the testicles is a potential killer. But if detected early, it can usually be treated successfully. A simple self-examination that takes only 1 or 2 minutes can detect a growth in the testicles in its early stages. Like the breast self-examination for women, self-examination of the testicles is important. Because cancer of the testicles often occurs in younger men, monthly self-examination of the testicles should begin in the teen years.

Perform the examination after a warm shower or bath, when the skin of the scrotum is loose and relaxed. Examine one testicle at a time. Grasp the testicle and roll it gently between your thumb and forefinger. As you do so, feel for any lump on the surface of the testicle. Also notice if the testicle is enlarged, hardened or, if you've done a self-exam before, somehow different than it was during your last examination. If you feel a lump on a testicle or any change in the testicle, you don't necessarily have cancer. However, do see your doctor about it as soon as possible.

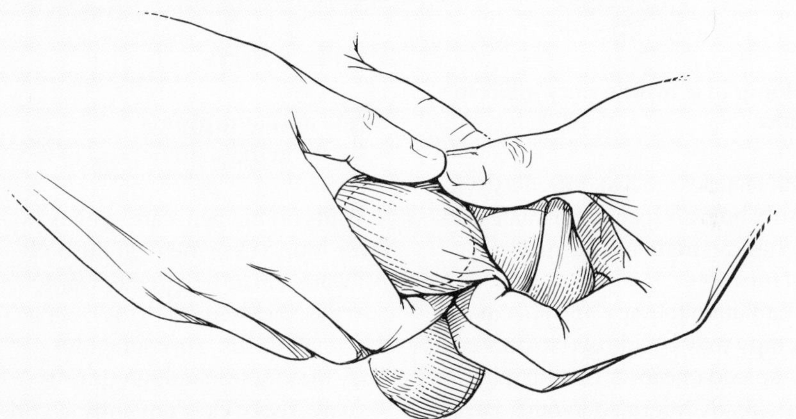

Grasp and roll the testicle between your thumb and forefinger, feeling for lumps, swelling, hardness or other changes.

Testicular cancer

Signs and symptoms

- A lump in a testicle
- Swelling of a testicle
- A heavy feeling in a testicle

Cancer of a testicle often begins in the cells that produce sperm. In the early stages, it has no symptoms. The first noticeable sign is often a hard lump in a testicle. Most men discover the lump themselves during a self-examination.

Generally, testicular cancer affects only one testicle. It's more common among men ages 15 to 35, and it's more common in white men than in black men. If one or both testicles are undescended at birth, the risk of cancer in either testicle later in life is increased. If it's detected and treated early, testicular cancer often can be cured.

Diagnosis

A self-examination can often detect the presence of a growth or tumor within the scrotum. An ultrasound examination may be performed to help in the diagnosis. A tumor in the testicle is almost always cancerous, but other conditions affecting the testicles and scrotum can produce a lump that feels quite similar.

How serious is testicular cancer?

The most common type of testicular cancer, seminoma, can be cured in nearly all cases if it's discovered and treated early. When all types of testicular cancers are considered, including cancers discovered at a late stage, about 90 percent of men with this condition will live for 5 years or more after treatment.

Treatment

Surgical removal of a cancerous testicle is necessary. Blood tests, X-rays and other tests may be necessary to determine if the cancer has spread to other parts of the body.

Removing a testicle doesn't cause any loss of virility because the remaining healthy testicle can maintain the body's normal sexual and hormone-producing functions. If

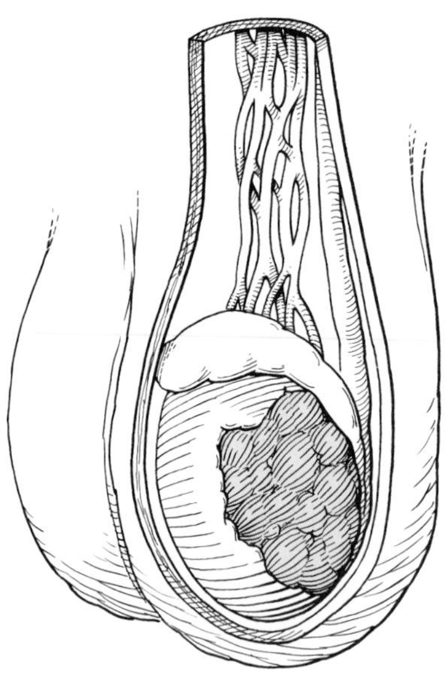

A lump in a testicle may indicate cancer.

both testicles are lost, infertility will result, but replacement of male hormones can maintain normal sexual function.

Radiation therapy and chemotherapy may be advised to prevent the spread of cancer or treat it if it has already migrated to other parts of the body. Even with cancer that has spread, chemotherapy can be very effective in destroying the cancer. For more information on radiation and chemotherapy, see Chapter 19, "Cancer."

Penile Disorders

The penis is both a sexual organ and urinary tract organ. Infections and other conditions can sometimes interfere with its functions, causing a variety of signs and symptoms including pain, irritation and skin lesions.

Penile warts

Signs and symptoms

- Warts on the shaft or head of the penis

Warts on the penis are similar to those found elsewhere on the body. All warts, including penile warts, are caused by viruses. This means that penile warts are contagious. They may be transmitted during sexual activity. Consequently, if you have penile warts, both you and your sexual partner may require treatment.

Diagnosis

Penile warts are diagnosed on the basis of their appearance. Sometimes, however, a growth on the penis that looks like a wart may instead be a symptom of another sexually transmitted disease or even a cancerous tumor. Warts that aren't visible may become visible when they're dabbed with vinegar (acetic acid), showing up as a white patch. Your doctor may use this procedure on you if your sex partner has physical changes suggesting that the virus has been transmitted.

How serious are penile warts?

Penile warts should be treated because they can spread to a sexual partner and can also proliferate on your penis. Women are at increased risk of cervical cancer when exposed to the virus that causes penile warts.

Treatment

Your doctor may prescribe a preparation that's applied to the warts to remove them. Don't use over-the-counter wart products because they're designed for skin that's less sensitive than the skin of the penis. Other possible treatments include laser surgery, freezing the warts or destroying the warts with electrical current. These procedures may require local or general anesthesia.

Balanitis

Signs and symptoms

- Irritation and redness of the head of the penis

Balanitis is an inflammation of the head of the penis. It's a fairly common genital problem, especially in uncircumcised males whose foreskin is narrowed so that it can't be easily pulled back for cleaning.

Balanitis has many causes, including yeast or bacterial infection, reaction to contraceptive creams, and irritation from clothing that rubs against the penis or from chemicals used in the cleaning or manufacturing of clothing. Men with diabetes

Sexually Transmitted Diseases

Sexually transmitted diseases (STDs) are diseases that are passed on by contact with an infected person through vaginal intercourse, anal intercourse or oral sexual activity. In the case of human immunodeficiency virus (HIV) and AIDS, possible additional routes of transmission include infected semen and blood and needles shared for illegal intravenous (IV) drug use.

Symptoms of sexually transmitted diseases may not develop immediately, and the course and consequences of the diseases vary. For more information on STDs, see Chapter 20, "Infectious Diseases."

Proper use of a condom during sexual activity offers protection against acquiring or passing along a sexually transmitted disease. But condoms don't provide foolproof protection. You can avoid STDs by being abstinent or by engaging in sexual activity only with a noninfected partner. AIDS and HIV can also be avoided by not sharing needles used for inappropriate use of drugs.

are especially prone to balanitis, although it's unclear why.

Diagnosis
If you have an inflammation of the penis that doesn't go away in a day or two, see your doctor or a urologist — a specialist who treats urinary and male genital problems. The doctor will examine your penis and may perform some tests to help establish the cause of the inflammation.

Treatment
Antibiotics or antifungal agents are used to cure bacterial or yeast infections. In an uncircumcised man whose foreskin doesn't easily retract, circumcision may be necessary to cure balanitis and prevent its recurrence.

Prevention
The best way to prevent balanitis is by using good penile hygiene. Wash your penis and scrotum daily with soap and water.

Phimosis

Phimosis is a condition in which the uncircumcised foreskin covers the penis so tightly around its head that the foreskin can't be pulled back to expose and clean it. Sometimes this condition can interfere with urination and sexual activity.

Phimosis is fairly common in newborn boys. The foreskin normally loosens up in time, without treatment. In older boys and men, the foreskin may shrink or tighten because of an inflammation. Sometimes this requires circumcision.

Paraphimosis

Paraphimosis occurs when tight foreskin of an uncircumcised penis is pulled back and can't be returned over the head of the penis. This can cause painful swelling at the tip of the penis. If you experience severe swelling in the end of the penis, seek emergency medical help.

Penile Hygiene

Wash your penis and scrotum the same way you wash other parts of your body — with soap and water every day. If your penis is uncircumcised, pull back the foreskin and clean the head of the penis beneath it. These basic hygienic practices will help keep the genitals clean and free from minor infections.

Simply washing your penis won't keep you from getting a sexually transmitted disease. Seek medical attention as soon as possible if you notice signs of disease, such as sores or growths.

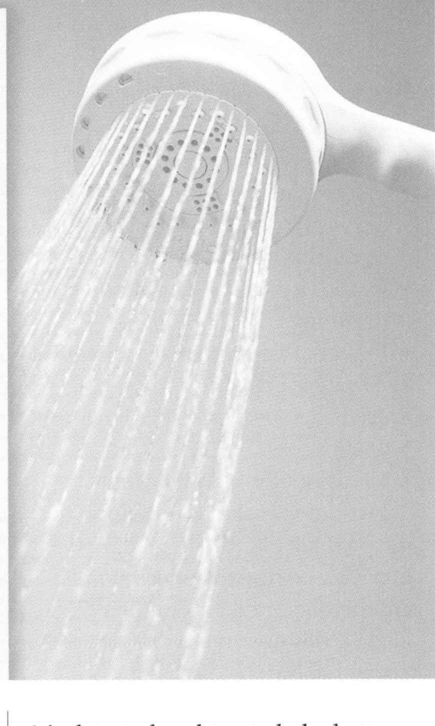

Surgical treatment by circumcision or partial circumcision may be necessary to release the foreskin. If treatment is prompt, permanent damage to the penis generally can be prevented.

Cancer of the penis

Signs and symptoms
- A painless ulcer, nodule or wart-like bump on the penis

Cancer of the penis is rare. When it occurs it's almost always in uncircumcised males. In its early stages, small, painless growths occur on the penis, usually near its tip. Without surgical removal and examination of the tissue by a pathologist, these growths may be indistinguishable from penile warts. As the cancerous (malignant) growth progresses, you may experience pain and bleeding.

Diagnosis
Through examination, testing and possible surgical removal of the growth, your doctor can determine if it's malignant. If it is, more tests can determine if the cancer has spread to other parts of your body.

How serious is cancer of the penis?
Like any other cancer, penile cancer can be life-threatening. The earlier it's detected and treated, the better your chances of recovery.

Treatment
Removal of the malignant growth, and possibly of portions of the penis surrounding the growth, will likely be necessary. Often, enough of the penis can be left to allow for sexual activity and normal urination. Radiation therapy and chemotherapy may be used to prevent or control the spread of the disease to other parts of the body. For more information on radiation and chemotherapy, see Chapter 19, "Cancer."

Prostate Gland Disorders

The prostate is a walnut-sized gland located in the pelvic area, just below the outlet of the bladder. Present only in males, it surrounds the urethra, the tube that carries urine from your bladder to the tip of your penis. The prostate gland plays an important role in the reproductive process, producing the majority of the fluid that blends with sperm to create semen. The prostate gland tends to become a health concern as men age.

Prostatitis

Signs and symptoms

- Pain in the lower back and in the area between the rectum and the scrotum (perineum)
- Pain or a burning sensation while urinating
- Frequent and difficult urination
- An urgent need to urinate
- A sudden moderate to high fever
- Chills
- Occasionally, blood in urine

Prostatitis is an inflammation of the prostate gland. The inflammation may be due to an infection or another factor that's irritating the gland. Although many things are unclear about the disease, an accurate diagnosis is crucial to successfully treating it. Prostatitis occurs in at least three forms:

Acute bacterial prostatitis
Acute bacterial prostatitis is the most severe form of the disease. It results from an infection in the prostate gland that produces severe and often sudden symptoms. Bacteria found in the urinary tract or large intestine are often responsible for this type of infection.

Chronic bacterial prostatitis
Chronic bacterial prostatitis also results from a bacterial infection. Unlike acute bacterial prostatitis, its symptoms typically develop more slowly, and they're often less severe. The cause of the infection usually isn't clear. It may result from bacteria in your urinary tract, a bladder infection or a blood infection. The infection may also follow trauma to your urinary tract or insertion of an instrument such as a catheter or cystoscope.

Chronic nonbacterial prostatitis
Chronic nonbacterial prostatitis is the most common form of prostatitis. Unfortunately, it's also the most difficult to diagnose and treat. Symptoms of chronic nonbacterial prostatitis tend to be similar to those of chronic bacterial prostatitis, but one distinguishing factor separates the two: With nonbacterial prostatitis there's no evidence of bacteria in your urine or in fluid from the prostate gland, but white blood cells identified in urine specimens may signal the presence of inflammation.

The main reason this type of prostatitis is so difficult to diagnose and treat is that its cause is unknown. Possible causes include a reduction in the frequency of sexual intercourse, anxiety or stress, heavy lifting, occupations that subject the gland to a great deal of vibration, or an infectious agent that current techniques can't detect.

Diagnosis
Prostatitis is generally diagnosed by feeling the prostate gland. To do this your doctor inserts a gloved finger into your rectum and feels the outside wall of the gland. An inflamed prostate usually feels enlarged and tender. You may also

Are You at Risk?

There's no simple formula to tell precisely who will encounter prostate problems. However, the following factors — some controllable, some not — can increase your risk:

Uncontrollable risk factors

Factors in life that you can't control include the following:

Your age
The older you get, the greater your risk of developing prostate problems. More than half the men older than age 50, and 80 percent of men in their 70s, experience prostate enlargement. In addition, 8 out of 10 men with diagnosed prostate cancer are older than age 65.

Your racial or ethnic group
For reasons unclear to researchers, black men are more likely to develop prostate cancer than are men of any other group. The risk for Hispanic and American Indian men is lower than it is for whites or blacks.

Your family history
Some diseases, including prostate cancer, can run in the family. Studies show that if your father or brother had prostate cancer, your risk of the disease is about double what it would be normally.

Controllable risk factors

Factors in life that you can control include the following:

Your environment
Studies suggest that your risk of prostate cancer can be influenced by where you spend much of your time. Higher death rates from prostate cancer can be found in certain blue-collar workers — such as farmers, mechanics, welders and industrial employees — than in men in other occupations.

Your diet
Eating fatty foods may increase your risk of prostate cancer. One study showed that men who ate high-fat diets were nearly twice as likely to have prostate cancer as men who ate less fat. On the other hand, some foods, such as soy products and certain vegetables and fruits, seem to lower your risk.

need to provide urine and semen samples to be tested for bacteria that may be causing the infection. To effectively treat this disorder, it's important to determine the cause, when possible.

How serious is prostatitis?

Left untreated, acute bacterial prostatitis can cause serious problems, including an inability to urinate. Chronic prostatitis tends to be more frustrating and debilitating. Without treatment, chronic bacterial prostatitis can lead to serious infection.

Treatment

Antibiotics are used to treat bacterial prostatitis. Sometimes a catheter is needed temporarily to drain the bladder. Warm sitz baths may provide relief from the symptoms. So may dietary changes and the use of anti-inflammatory medicine.

Prostatitis vs. Painful Prostate

Sometimes men who see a doctor for what appears to be prostatitis may actually have a condition called painful prostate (prostatodynia, or prostatalgia). Men with this condition often refer to their symptoms as pain "down there," meaning anywhere in the genital (perineal) area. Symptoms typically mimic those of chronic nonbacterial prostatitis. The difference is that with prostatodynia, urine and prostate fluid samples show no evidence of infection or inflammation. Bacteria or white blood cells aren't detectable in the samples.

Rather than being a problem with your prostate gland, prostatodynia may instead stem from your pelvic floor muscles. When you're under stress, you may not completely relax the pelvic floor muscles supporting your bladder and urethra, causing urination difficulties. Many men with prostatodynia tend to be hard-driven, tense and stressed. Prostatodynia also seems to occur more frequently among marathon runners, bicyclists, weightlifters and truck drivers.

Treatment for prostatodynia is similar in many ways to treatment for chronic nonbacterial prostatitis. Your doctor may also recommend physical therapy to help you relax your pelvic floor muscles and stress management to help you prevent and cope with stress.

Benign prostatic hyperplasia

Signs and symptoms

- A frequent, sometimes urgent, need to urinate
- Difficulty in starting the urine stream
- Decreased force of the urine stream
- An inability to sleep through the night without getting up to urinate
- Dribbling at the end of urination

Emergency signs and symptoms

- An inability to urinate

The prostate gland tends to enlarge with age. Enlargement usually begins around age 50. In some men it may not occur until their 70s or 80s.

Noncancerous enlargement of the prostate is called benign prostatic hyperplasia (BPH). The word *benign* distinguishes this condition from prostate cancer. *Hyperplasia* means an increase in size.

Four of every five men experience benign enlargement of the prostate by age 80. It's estimated that 25 percent to 30 percent of men in the United States will need some type of treatment for BPH symptoms during their lifetime.

Symptoms vary in severity from slight to severe. At first the symptoms tend to be only annoying. As the prostate continues to grow, they gradually worsen.

Diagnosis

Your doctor may ask you about your prostate symptoms to determine the seriousness of your problem. He or she will likely also examine your prostate gland by inserting a gloved finger into your rectum and feeling the size and firmness of the gland. You might also be given a test to determine the strength of your urine flow and a prostate-specific antigen (PSA) blood test. The PSA test assesses the possibility that cancer of the prostate is contributing to your symptoms. Your bladder may be examined with a cystoscope.

How serious is BPH?

BPH isn't life-threatening unless symptoms become severe, making it difficult or impossible to urinate. Retention of urine increases your risk of developing urinary tract infections, which may damage your kidneys.

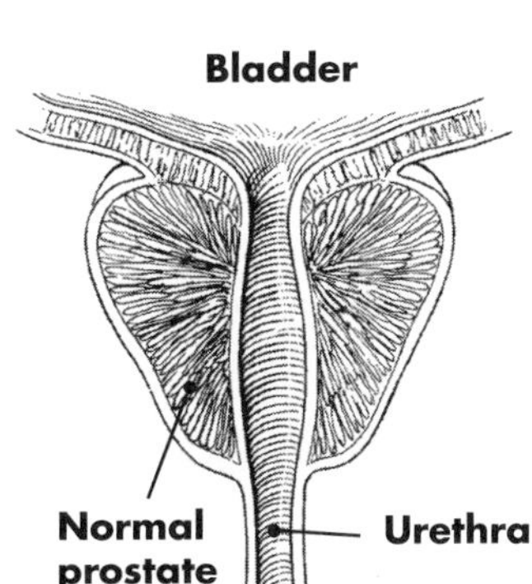

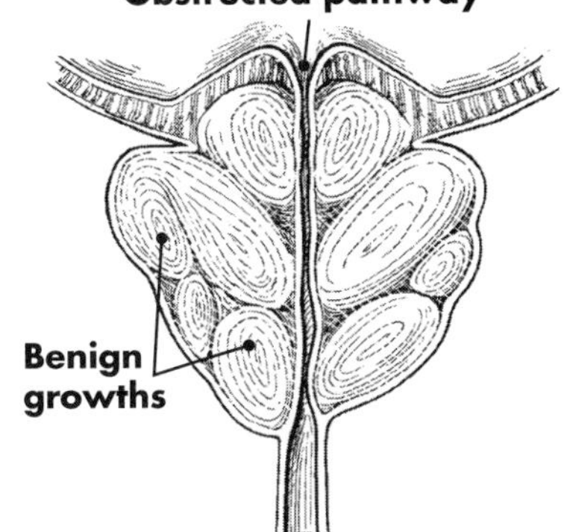

The urethra, the tube that drains the bladder, is surrounded by the prostate gland. Benign prostatic hyperplasia (BPH) results when tissues in the center of the prostate gland enlarge and press on the urethra, affecting normal urine flow.

Treatment

Treatment for BPH depends on its severity and your preference of options. Possible options include:

Watchful waiting

If your symptoms are mild and you're not bothered by them, you and your doctor may decide that watchful waiting is appropriate. Your doctor should periodically evaluate your symptoms to see if they stay the same or worsen.

Medication

Medication may control moderate symptoms of BPH. Medication is also an option for men with mild symptoms who find them annoying or who don't care for watchful waiting. Medications called alpha blockers (Cardura, Flomax, others) improve the flow of urine by relaxing muscles in the area of the prostate gland. These are usually the most effective drugs to relieve the symptoms. Another type of drug, finasteride (Proscar), shrinks the prostate gland by suppressing certain hormones that stimulate prostate growth.

Surgery

Surgical treatment that removes part of the prostate gland can reduce pressure on the urethra. The most common surgical procedure is transurethral resection of the prostate (TURP), which is performed without an incision (see color illustration on page 425).

During this procedure the surgeon inserts an instrument called a resectoscope into the urethra and uses small cutting tools to remove excess prostate tissue. TURP is effective and relieves symptoms quickly. Most men experience a strong urine flow within a few days. If the prostate gland is excessively large, the surgeon may have to perform surgery through an incision in your abdomen.

After prostate surgery it's common for semen to enter the bladder during ejaculation (retrograde ejaculation) rather than being ejaculated through the penis. There's no harm in this, and the semen is eventually voided with the urine. However, retrograde ejaculation can cause infertility because no semen reaches the vagina. In rare cases, TURP can lead to impotence or the inability to control urination.

Other options

Several less invasive techniques also may be used to destroy prostate tissue. Microwave therapy uses computer-controlled heat in the form of microwave energy to destroy the central part of the enlarged gland. Another treatment involves using radio waves to heat and destroy prostate tissue. The radio waves are transmitted through needles inserted into the prostate gland. Electrical therapy uses a metal instrument that emits a high-frequency electrical current to cut and vaporize excess tissue. Laser therapy produces concentrated light that heats and destroys the tissue.

COMPLEMENTARY MEDICINE

Many herbal products are marketed to relieve common prostate problems. One that shows some promise in treating benign prostatic hyperplasia (BPH) is saw palmetto (Serenoa repens).

No one is sure how saw palmetto works. One theory is that it prevents the hormone testosterone from breaking down into another form associated with prostate tissue growth.

Saw palmetto is slow-acting. Most men who see an improvement in their urinary symptoms do so within 1 to 3 months. If after 3 months you haven't noticed any benefit from the product, then it may not work for you. Possible effects from long-term use are unknown.

One drawback of this herb is that it may suppress prostate-specific antigen (PSA) levels in your blood. This action can interfere with the effectiveness of the PSA test to screen for prostate cancer. If you take saw palmetto, it's important to tell your doctor before having a PSA test.

Prostate cancer

Signs and symptoms

- Sometimes none
- A sudden need to urinate
- Difficulty starting your urine flow
- Pain during urination
- A weak urine flow and dribbling
- Starting and stopping of your urine flow
- A sensation that your bladder isn't empty after voiding
- Frequent urination at night
- Blood in your urine
- Painful ejaculation
- Pain in the lower back, hips or upper thighs
- Loss of weight and appetite

Prostate cancer is the most common cancer in American men. As you age your risk of prostate cancer increases. It's estimated that by age 50, up to one in four men have cancerous cells in the prostate gland. By age 80 this increases to one in two. The average age at diagnosis of prostate cancer is 72.

Prostate cancer is the second leading cause of cancer deaths in American men — not because it's so deadly but because it's so common. You're more likely to die *with* prostate cancer than you are to die *of* it. Typically, prostate cancer grows slowly and remains confined to the prostate gland, where it doesn't cause any serious harm. But not all cancers act the same. Some forms of prostate cancer can be extremely aggressive and quickly spread to other parts of the body.

It isn't known what causes prostate cancer and why some types of prostate cancer behave differently than others. Research suggests a combination of factors

Screening for Prostate Cancer

A prostate checkup usually includes a digital rectal exam. Many doctors recommend that men age 40 and older have a yearly digital rectal exam. For this exam you're asked to bend over — perhaps leaning on an examination table — while your doctor gently inserts a lubricated, gloved finger into your rectum. Because the prostate gland is located just in front of the rectum, your doctor can feel the gland for lumps or hard spots in the part of the gland where 70 percent of cancerous tumors develop.

Another component of a prostate checkup is the prostate-specific antigen (PSA) blood test. PSA is naturally produced by your prostate gland to help liquefy semen. A small amount of it, however, enters your bloodstream and circulates in your blood. If a higher than normal level of PSA is detected in your blood, it could indicate prostate inflammation, enlargement or cancer.

Using the PSA test as a screening tool for prostate cancer is controversial. It isn't always able to distinguish between cancer and other diseases. As a result, some men who don't have cancer undergo additional tests — such as a needle biopsy to remove tissue samples from the gland — to rule out cancer.

Some doctors feel that because prostate cancer is generally so slow in developing, the PSA test leads to some men undergoing unnecessary surgery or radiation to treat a form of cancer that might not have caused any health problems if left alone. Other doctors strongly support regular use of the test because it's the best tool currently available for detecting prostate cancer in its early stages, and it's especially beneficial for younger men with treatable cancers.

Many urologists — specialists who treat urinary and male genital problems — recommend an annual PSA test beginning at age 50, unless you're at high risk of the disease, in which case they suggest that you begin getting an annual test sooner. Beyond age 75 a yearly PSA test may no longer be necessary. Men who develop prostate cancer late in life generally die of causes other than their cancer.

may play a role, including family history, race, ethnicity, hormones, diet and environment.

Diagnosis

A digital rectal examination and the prostate-specific antigen (PSA) test are usually the first steps in diagnosing prostate cancer. If the results of one or both tests are abnormal and your doctor suspects cancer, he or she may recommend an ultrasound examination and an ultrasound-guided needle biopsy to retrieve part of the tissue for examination. During an ultrasound examination of your prostate gland, a small, lubricated probe that emits sound waves is inserted into your rectum. The reflections from the sound waves are converted into a video picture. Because cancerous tissue is thicker and denser than healthy tissue, it often reflects the sound waves differently.

To determine if a tumor is cancerous, a biopsy may be done. A biopsy involves removing a small sample of tissue for microscopic examination. For a prostate biopsy, the tissue may be taken by inserting a biopsy needle into the prostate gland through the area between the anus and the scrotum. More often, though, the needle is directed alongside the ultrasound probe and inserted through the wall of the rectum. Sections of tissue may be taken from various areas of your prostate. If a sample proves cancerous (malignant), more tests may be performed to determine if the cancer has spread to other parts of the body and to plan treatment.

How serious is prostate cancer?

Prostate cancer is the second leading cause of cancer deaths in American men, following lung cancer. But if found early — when the cancer is confined to the prostate gland — prostate cancer often can be cured. It's after the cancer has spread to nearby organs that treating the disease becomes more difficult, but not impossible.

Treatment

Prostate cancer can be treated in a number of ways. Your doctor might even recommend a combination of treatments, such as surgery followed by radiation or hormone therapy. Which treatment you and your doctor choose will depend on several factors — including how

Mayo Clinic's PSA Standards

Mayo Clinic urologists — specialists who treat urinary and male genital problems — use the following age-adjusted scale to determine whether the prostate-specific antigen (PSA) level in your blood is within a normal range.

Age	Normal PSA range*
40	0 to 2.0 ng/mL
50	0 to 2.8 ng/mL
60	0 to 3.8 ng/mL
70	0 to 5.3 ng/mL

*Upper limits increase almost every year as you age. For example, the upper limit for a 45-year-old is 2.4 ng/mL. Measurements are in nanograms per milliliter (ng/mL), based on the test used at Mayo Clinic.

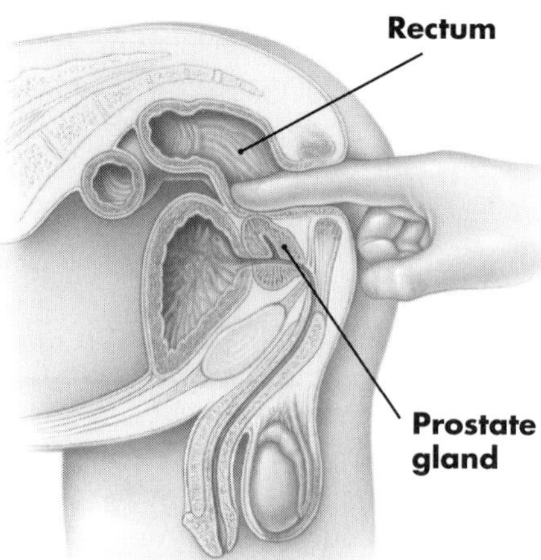

During a digital rectal exam, your doctor inserts a gloved, lubricated finger into your rectum and feels the back wall of the prostate gland for enlargement, tenderness, lumps or hard spots.

fast the cancer is growing, whether it has spread, your age and your overall health. The most common treatments for prostate cancer are:

Watchful waiting
Because blood tests can detect prostate cancer at a very early stage, many men prefer this treatment option. It involves follow-up PSA tests and digital rectal exams to check for new signs or symptoms. You may also need to have occasional biopsies. But watchful waiting isn't the best approach for all men, and it can allow cancer that's at a highly treatable stage to grow and spread.

If you're healthy and in your 40s, 50s, 60s or even 70s, your doctor probably won't recommend this approach. The younger you are, the longer the cancer has to grow. Even a small, slow-growing cancer might eventually reach the point when it needs additional treatment. The cancer cells could also suddenly become aggressive and spread so much that a cure becomes difficult or impossible.

If the cancer is small and slow-growing and you're in your 70s or older, or in poor health, watchful waiting might be a good option. Chances are you'll live 10 more years without treatment — and without the cancer spreading or causing you problems.

Surgery
The most effective way to treat cancer confined to the prostate gland is to remove the gland. This type of surgery is called a radical prostatectomy. Research indicates that this type of surgery cures prostate cancer in about 70 percent of men who have it. This surgery has better long-term results than other therapies, especially in men with a life expectancy of 10 years or more.

During a radical prostatectomy, surgeons use special techniques to totally remove the prostate gland while sparing muscles and attached nerve bundles that control urination and sexual function (see color illustration on page 425).

This surgery wasn't always so successful at retaining urinary and sexual function and sometimes resulted in impotence or incontinence. A decade ago only 1 in 10 men with prostate cancer chose this option. Now, because of refinements in surgical technique, one in four men with prostate cancer choose surgery. The surgery may be performed one of two ways: retropubic or perineal.

- *Retropubic.* In retropubic surgery the gland is removed through a lower abdominal incision that typically runs from just below the navel to an inch above the base of the penis. This is the most common approach to prostate removal for two reasons: The surgeon can use the same incision to remove adjacent lymph nodes, which are tested to see if the cancer has spread, and the procedure gives the surgeon better access to the prostate, making it easier to save the nerve bundles that control erection.
- *Perineal.* With perineal prostate surgery, an incision is made between the anus and the scrotum. There's generally less bleeding with perineal surgery, and heavier men tend to recover

Question and Answer

Should I get a second opinion before deciding how to treat my prostate cancer?

It depends. If you feel confident in your doctor, understand what the options are and are comfortable with your treatment plan, you may not need a second opinion. But if you have some concerns about your diagnosis, you don't feel confident in your doctor or you don't feel comfortable with the treatment recommended, then it might be a good idea to get another opinion.

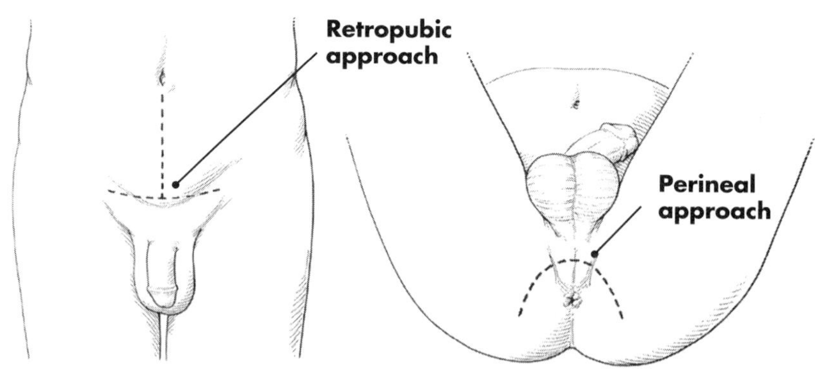

With retropubic surgery, the prostate gland is removed through an incision in the lower abdomen. Perineal surgery involves removing the gland through an incision between the anus and the scrotal sac.

sooner than they would with retropubic surgery. Unfortunately, this approach makes it a bit more difficult for your surgeon to locate and protect the nerve bundles attached to the prostate. It also doesn't allow the surgeon to remove nearby lymph nodes. That's why this surgery is less commonly used.

Radiation

Radiation treatment uses high-powered X-rays or other radiation to destroy cancer cells. It's generally the preferred treatment if you're older or in poor health and might have a hard time withstanding surgery. It may also be the preferred option if the cancerous tumor is located in a part of the prostate gland that makes surgery more difficult. For cancer confined to the prostate, radiation is often as effective as surgery for up to 10 years.

Radiation is also used to treat cancer that's spread outside your prostate. It can destroy cancerous cells, shrink tumors and relieve painful symptoms. Two forms of radiation therapy for prostate cancer are external beam and radioactive seed implants.

- *External beam.* External beam radiation is delivered by beams from a large machine that's placed over your body. Unfortunately, these external beams do more than destroy cancerous cells. They can also damage healthy tissue in the same area. That's why the first step in radiation therapy is to map out the areas in your body to receive radiation to find the best angles to direct the beams.

  Treatments are generally given 5 days a week for about 6 or 7 weeks. Each treatment takes about 15 minutes, but much of this is preparation time. The actual length of time that you receive radiation is only about 1 minute. New forms of external beam therapy are being tested that cause less damage to surrounding tissue.

? Questions to Ask Your Doctor

To help determine the best form of prostate cancer treatment for you, ask your doctor these questions:

1. What options are available to me?
2. How fast will the cancer grow if it's left untreated?
3. Do you think the cancer can be cured with treatment? If so, what are the chances?
4. Which treatment do you recommend, and why?
5. How many times have you performed this procedure? (The more often, the better.)
6. How soon will we know if the treatment has worked?
7. What are my risks of lasting side effects, such as impotence or incontinence?
8. How soon will I be able to return to work?
9. Will I have to restrict any activities?
10. If the treatment doesn't work, do I still have other options?

- *Radioactive seed implants.* An alternative method of radiation uses ultrasound-guided needles to inject rice-sized radioactive seeds into your prostate gland. These seeds deliver double the dose of radiation of external beams with less damage to healthy tissue. Because this technique is relatively new, its long-term effects are unknown, but early results are encouraging. Of men with cancer limited to the prostate, radioactive seeds control cancer growth for 5 years in 90 percent of cases.

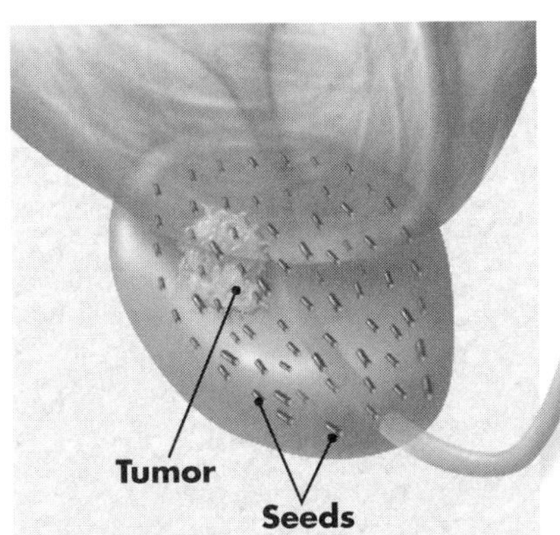

Rice-sized radioactive seeds are inserted into the prostate gland. The seeds emit radiation designed to destroy the cancer.

Cryotherapy

Another way to kill prostate cancer is to freeze the prostate. Cryotherapy involves inserting five to seven thin metal rods — each about 6 inches long — through the area between your scrotum and anus (perineum) and into the prostate. An ultrasound probe in the rectum helps your doctor position the rods. Once the rod tips are in place, liquid nitrogen is released into the rods, where it circulates and lowers the temperature. As the tissue around the rods freezes, the formation and expansion of ice crystals within the cancerous cells cause them to rupture and die. To keep the urethra from freezing along with your prostate, a catheter is placed inside the urethra and filled with a warming solution.

Short-term results of this therapy are encouraging, but the long-term survival rates appear lower than those of surgery or radiation, and its side effects can be quite severe. In addition, the procedure doesn't always kill all of the cancer cells.

Hormone therapy

Male sex hormones make cancer cells in the prostate gland grow

trait were more likely to survive malaria epidemics. Sickled red blood cells interfere with the growth of the parasite that causes malaria.

Over time, the survivors migrated and had children. In some cases, carriers of the gene married each other, and some of their children inherited two copies of the mutated gene. Today, sickle cell anemia affects millions of people worldwide. It's particularly common among people with ancestors from Africa, Spain, the Mediterranean region, the Middle East and India. In the United States, it most commonly affects blacks and Hispanics.

Diagnosis

People who have sickle cell anemia usually receive the diagnosis as newborns. Sickle cell anemia is detected by various blood tests. The diagnosis is confirmed by hemoglobin electrophoresis, a laboratory procedure that can isolate and identify hemoglobin S.

How serious is sickle cell anemia?

There's no known cure for sickle cell anemia, a potentially fatal disease. However, treatments can relieve symptoms and prolong life. Many people with sickle cell anemia lead fairly normal lives and enjoy reasonably good health into their 40s and beyond.

Serious complications of the disease include:

Stroke

A stroke can occur if sickled red blood cells block blood flow to an area of the brain. Stroke is one of the most serious complications of the disease. Roughly 10 percent of children with sickle cell anemia suffer a stroke. The risk is highest between the ages of 2 and 5.

Signs and symptoms of stroke include seizure, weakness or numbness of the arms and legs, sudden speech difficulties and loss of consciousness. A baby or child with any of these signs and symptoms should receive prompt medical care. A stroke can be fatal.

Acute chest syndrome

Acute chest syndrome is a life-threatening complication of sickle cell anemia caused by a lung infection or trapped sickled blood cells in the lung. Similar to pneumonia, it causes chest pain, cough, fever and difficulty breathing. It requires emergency treatment with antibiotics, blood transfusions and drugs that open up lung airways. Recurrent attacks can damage the lungs.

Organ damage

Sickled red blood cells can block blood flow through blood vessels, depriving an organ of blood and oxygen. Chronic deprivation of oxygen-rich blood can damage nerves and organs, including the kidneys, liver and spleen.

Blindness

Tiny blood vessels in the eye may become plugged with sickle cells. Over time, this can damage the retina, the portion of the eye that processes visual images, and lead to blindness.

Other conditions

Sickle cell anemia can lead to leg ulcers, caused by sickled red cells obstructing blood vessels that nourish the skin. When red blood cells are destroyed, a substance called bilirubin is produced, which can cause yellowing of the skin and eyes (jaundice) and lead to gallstones.

Men with sickle cell anemia may experience painful and prolonged erections when sickled red blood cells prevent blood flow out of an erect penis (priapism). Over time, priapism can damage the penis and lead to impotence.

Treatment

Although there's no cure for sickle cell anemia, your doctor can do a great deal to help you or your child live with the disease. In addition, treatments are continually improving. People with sickle cell anemia may benefit from treatment by specialists at a hospital or a sickle cell anemia clinic. Regular visits to the doctor are important.

Medication

Medications used to treat sickle cell anemia include:

- *Antibiotics.* Starting at 2 to 3 months of age and continuing until age 5 or 6, a child with sickle cell anemia usually needs to take regular doses of an antibiotic, typically oral penicillin.

  Penicillin helps prevent infections such as pneumonia, which can be life-threatening to an infant or child with sickle cell anemia. Antibiotics may also help adults with sickle cell anemia prevent or treat infections.
- *Pain-relieving medications.* To relieve pain during a sickling attack, your doctor may advise over-the-counter pain relievers and application of warm heat to the affected area. Sometimes, stronger prescription pain medications are necessary.
- *Hydroxyurea.* This prescription drug, usually used to treat leukemia, has been shown to reduce the number of painful sickling crises and reduce the need for blood transfusions. Hydroxyurea (Hydrea, Droxia) appears to stimulate production of fetal hemoglobin, a type of hemoglobin found in newborns, which helps prevent sickling of red blood cells.

  The Food and Drug Administration has approved hydroxyurea for treating sickle cell anemia in adults. Studies are under way to determine the proper dosage for children. The long-term effects of hydroxyurea are unknown. People taking it need frequent blood tests because the drug can cause a dangerous drop in blood cell counts. Taking hydroxyurea with a medication called erythropoietin, a hormone

PREVENTION TIP

Taking steps to prevent sickling is critical for anyone with sickle cell anemia. Good nutrition, adequate rest and protection against infections all are important in maintaining good health.

To help stay healthy, people with sickle cell anemia can:

- *Take folic acid supplements daily.* Bone marrow needs folic acid to make new red blood cells.
- *Drink plenty of water.* Staying hydrated helps keep your blood diluted. With more diluted blood, the chance of sickling is less.
- *Avoid temperature extremes.* Both high and low temperatures can trigger sickling.
- *Avoid stress.* Stress also can trigger sickling.
- *Get vaccinated.* Infants and children need regular childhood vaccinations, and it's recommended that children and adults have a yearly flu (influenza) shot and be immunized against pneumococcal pneumonia.

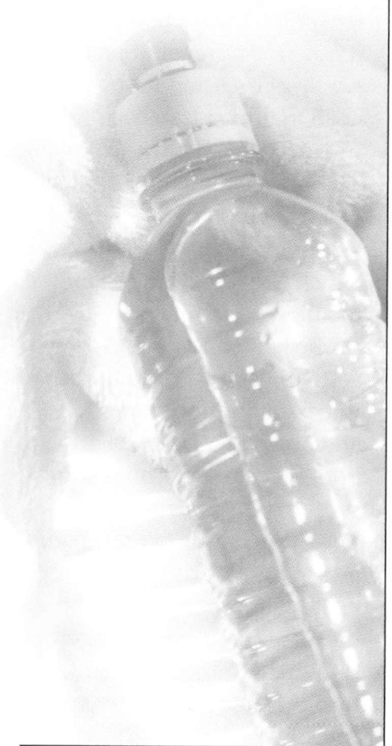

that stimulates the bone marrow to make red blood cells, may increase the effectiveness of hydroxyurea and allow for lower doses of the medication.

- *Folic acid.* Your doctor may prescribe a daily oral supplement of folic acid because the disease increases your body's need for this vitamin.

Blood transfusions

Blood transfusions can increase the number of normal red blood cells in circulation to relieve anemia. In children with sickle cell anemia at high risk of stroke, periodic blood transfusions can cut the risk of a first or second stroke by up to 90 percent.

Supplemental oxygen

You may be given oxygen through a breathing mask during a sickling crisis or with acute chest syndrome to add oxygen to your blood and help you breathe easier.

Stem cell transplantation

Rarely, sickle cell anemia can be successfully treated with a stem cell transplant (see page 1162). This treatment tends to be more successful in children. Adults with sickle cell anemia have a higher rate of transplant rejection and other complications.

Experimental treatments

In the past 30 years, scientists have gained new insights into the symptoms and causes of sickle cell anemia that have led to newer treatments.

Researchers are studying:

- *Gene therapy.* Researchers are exploring whether inserting a corrected gene to control production of hemoglobin into the bone marrow of people with sickle cell anemia will result in the production of normal hemoglobin.

  Scientists are also exploring the possibility of turning off the defective gene while reactivating another gene responsible for the production of fetal hemoglobin, which would prevent sickling.
- *Butyrate.* This fatty acid, widely used as a food additive, increases the level of fetal hemoglobin in blood.
- *Clotrimazole.* This over-the-counter medication, which is used to treat fungal infections, may prevent a loss of water from red blood cells that can contribute to sickling.
- *Nitric oxide.* This gas, used by anesthesiologists to put patients to sleep, may also prevent red blood cells from sickling, and may even promote the unsickling of sickled cells. It's also being studied as a treatment for acute chest syndrome.

Treating complications

Most complications of sickle cell anemia are treated as they occur. Treatment may include antibiotics, blood transfusions, pain relief medications and, possibly, surgery to correct vision problems, remove a damaged spleen or treat other complications.

Prevention

If you know that sickle cell anemia runs in your family, genetic counseling may help you prevent passing it on to your children. If both you and your spouse carry the trait, the risk is one out of four that your child will have sickle cell anemia.

Sickle cell anemia can be detected in an unborn baby. By sampling some of the fluid around the baby in the mother's womb (amniotic fluid) or some of the placenta, doctors can tell if the fetus has sickle cell anemia or carries the sickle cell gene.

In vitro fertilization can improve the chances that parents who both carry the sickle cell gene will have a child with normal hemoglobin. In the procedure, eggs are taken from the mother, and sperm is taken from the father.

In a laboratory, the eggs are fertilized with the sperm. The fertilized eggs are then tested for presence of the sickle cell gene. Fertilized eggs

Rare Hemoglobin Diseases

Rare hemoglobin diseases, called hemoglobinopathies, result from variant forms of hemoglobin. Over 400 variants have been identified. These abnormal hemoglobins tend to be less efficient at transporting oxygen to tissue cells.

One example is hemoglobin SC disease. People with this disease have inherited the sickle cell trait (hemoglobin S) from one parent and another variant (hemoglobin C) from the other parent. Their life span is slightly decreased, and they experience persistent mild-to-moderate anemia. Individuals with hemoglobin SC can have attacks of pain similar to those experienced by people with sickle cell anemia.

that are free of the sickle cell gene are implanted into the mother for normal development. However, this procedure is new and not always successful.

Hemolytic anemias

Signs and symptoms

- Fatigue
- Pale skin
- Breathlessness
- A faster and more noticeable heartbeat, particularly on exertion
- Yellowing of the skin
- Dark urine
- Pressure or fullness under the left ribs from an enlarged spleen

Emergency signs and symptoms

- The sudden onset of pain in the upper abdomen

Hemolytic anemias refer to those anemias in which red blood cells are broken down (hemolyzed) faster than the bone marrow can produce new ones to replace them. The word *hemolytic* comes from Greek roots meaning "destruction of blood."

Hemolytic anemias can be inherited or acquired. Inherited hemolytic anemias generally result from abnormalities in the red blood cell membrane or from red blood cell enzyme deficiencies. In one inherited type, called spherocytosis, red blood cells are small, round and fragile. Another inherited type, called glucose-6-phosphate dehydrogenase deficiency, results from an enzyme deficiency.

Acquired forms may result from medications taken for other conditions, such as infections or high blood pressure. Hemolytic anemia may also develop from an immune response in which your immune system attacks your own red blood cells.

Diagnosis

If your doctor thinks that you may have a hemolytic anemia, he or she will likely have your blood examined to count the number of young red blood cells (reticulocytes) and to see if the cells are deformed. The number of young red cells is increased in hemolytic anemia. Your doctor may examine your upper abdomen to see if your spleen or liver is enlarged.

How serious is hemolytic anemia?

Some forms of hemolytic anemia are hard to treat, but these types of anemia are seldom fatal.

Treatment

When hemolytic anemia is caused by a medication, stopping use of that medication often improves or eliminates the condition.

Medication

For hemolytic anemia caused by an immune response, medications are often prescribed to treat the condition. Corticosteroid medications, such as prednisone, are often helpful in preventing the destruction of red blood cells (hemolysis).

Surgery

If the condition has caused an enlarged spleen, the spleen may need to be removed. The spleen filters out and stores defective red blood cells, and certain hemolytic anemias can cause it to become enlarged with damaged red blood cells.

Other anemias

In addition to the more common types of anemias, other, more rare forms exist. Some uncommon anemias include:

Glucose-6-phosphate dehydrogenase deficiency

This type of anemia is the result of an inherited defect in an enzyme, glucose-6-phosphate dehydrogenase, in red blood cells. Like hemolytic anemia, this disorder causes the premature breakdown of red blood cells. It occurs commonly in people of Mediterranean and African ancestry.

Symptoms range from mild to severe, depending on which form of defective gene is present. Symptoms tend to be less severe in people of African ancestry than in those of Mediterranean ancestry.

The gene for the glucose-6-phosphate dehydrogenase enzyme is carried on the X chromosome. Like the blood disorder hemophilia, this disease almost always affects boys and men — who have only one X chromosome — rather than girls and women — who have two X chromosomes. If you have two X chromosomes, then you're likely to have one without the defect.

Thalassemia

Thalassemia is a disease that has two forms. Both are based on inherited defects in hemoglobin. In alpha-thalassemia, not enough of the portion of hemoglobin called alpha-globin is produced. In beta-thalassemia, beta-globin is lacking.

Alpha-thalassemia occurs most often in people of Southeast Asian descent. Beta-thalassemia, also

Enlarged Lymph Nodes

Lymph nodes are distributed throughout the body, in the neck, armpits, chest, abdomen and groin. They serve an immune function similar to that of the spleen, filtering out foreign substances (antigens) from lymph fluids.

Enlarged lymph nodes (lymphadenopathy) commonly occur with infections. They're due to an increase in certain white blood cells (lymphocytes) needed to fight the infection. Other causes of lymph node enlargement include autoimmune disorders, such as lupus, and certain cancers, such as leukemias and lymphomas. If cancer is suspected, a lymph node biopsy may be analyzed for cancerous cells. When cancer is the cause of lymph node enlargement, the nodes typically aren't painful. In other conditions, they may be.

called Cooley's anemia or Mediterranean anemia, is common in the Mediterranean region.

The thalassemia genes are recessive, so you have to inherit them from both parents to get the disease. If you have only one defective gene, you carry the trait but have no symptoms. Thalassemia frequently causes severe chronic anemia with poor growth, an enlarged spleen and, sometimes, heart failure.

Without treatment, death occurs in early childhood. There's no cure, but therapy can often prolong life into the 20s or 30s. Treatment involves repeated transfusions of red blood cells. These cells carry a great deal of iron, which can overload the body's vital organs. To lessen this effect, medication may be given that causes extra iron to be excreted in the urine. Stem cell transplantation is another possible treatment. Genetic counseling can help individuals avoid passing the disorder on to their children.

A milder form of thalassemia, called thalassemia minor or thalassemia trait, is common. This disorder produces blood cells that look like those present in iron deficient blood, but they produce no symptoms. By itself, the disorder doesn't cause problems.

Anemia of chronic disease

Some chronic diseases interfere with the production of red blood cells, resulting in chronic anemia. Kidney failure is one example. Your kidneys produce a hormone called erythropoietin, which stimulates your bone marrow to produce red blood cells. A shortage of erythropoietin can result in a shortage of red blood cells. The bone marrow of some people with rheumatoid arthritis doesn't use erythropoietin efficiently, resulting in anemia. A shortage of erythropoietin can also be caused by chemotherapy.

Other chronic diseases associated with anemia include AIDS, cancer, chronic liver disease, acute and chronic infections and certain ulcers.

Anemia of chronic disease is curable only if the underlying disorder causing it can be cured or improved with treatment. If you have severe anemia of chronic disease, treatment consists of red blood cell transfusions and, in some cases, erythropoietin injections.

Aplastic anemia

Aplastic means "failure in development." This form of anemia is caused by a drastic decrease in the bone marrow's production of all types of blood cells, including white blood cells that fight germs and platelets that help blood clot. This condition puts you at risk of infections and uncontrolled bleeding.

This uncommon and life-threatening illness can be inherited — Fanconi's anemia — or triggered by a serious infection such as hepatitis, a bone marrow disorder such as leukemia, high-dose radiation, chemotherapy, exposure to toxic chemicals or use of certain medications. It results from damage to your bone marrow.

Aplastic anemia can come on suddenly and last only a short while, or it can persist. Without treatment, it may progress and become fatal.

Treatment generally begins with eliminating the cause, if it's known. For example, aplastic anemia caused by radiation, chemotherapy or other drug treatment usually improves once the treatment is stopped.

Your doctor will try to protect you from infections and will likely aggressively treat any that do occur with antibiotics. Other treatment options include transfusions of red blood cells and platelets and, if your case is severe and a suitable donor is available, stem cell transplantation.

Occasionally, aplastic anemia is due to an autoimmune disorder that causes your immune system to damage bone marrow. To prevent this, doctors sometimes prescribe medications that suppress the immune system. However, these medications make you more susceptible to infections.

Sideroblastic anemia

Sideroblasts are young red blood cells that contain excess iron. Sideroblastic anemias are rare disorders in which the red blood cells contain a high concentration of iron and hemoglobin production is defective.

Treatment depends on the cause. You can acquire this anemia as a result of certain medications or exposure to toxins, such as ethanol and lead. When the offending agent is removed, the anemia may disappear. Sideroblastic anemia is also associated with certain cancers, such as leukemia, lymphoma and myeloma, and with inflammatory diseases, such as rheumatoid arthritis. As the underlying condition is treated, the anemia may improve.

There's also an inherited form of sideroblastic anemia. In some cases, no cause can be identified. For these forms, blood transfusions may be needed, along with a medication to remove extra iron via your urine.

Leukemias

Leukemias are cancers of the body's blood-forming tissues. Leukemia generally begins with one or a few white blood cells that have a lost or damaged DNA sequence.

These abnormal cells remain immature in what's known as blast form, but they maintain the ability to multiply, causing the formation of excessive numbers of abnormal white blood cells. These abnormal cells reach high concentrations in bone marrow, the lymphatic system and bloodstream and begin to interfere with the functions of vital organs.

Normal white blood cells are potent infection fighters. Leukemia interferes with this ability. The abnormal white blood cells decrease production of normal white blood cells, impairing your ability to fight off infection.

Abnormal white blood cell production that takes control of the bone marrow interferes with the production of red blood cells and platelets in the bone marrow.

A deficiency in red blood cells means that your body's organs don't receive enough oxygen. A shortage of platelets makes the blood-clotting process less effective, leaving your body more vulnerable to bleeding and bruising.

Many people perceive leukemia as a disease of childhood, but this form of cancer affects about 10 times as many adults as children. In the United States, new cases of leukemia number more than 30,000 annually.

Risk factors

Experts aren't sure what causes abnormal cells to develop and multiply, but they've identified certain factors that place you at increased risk of leukemia:

- *Age.* The risk of genetic mutations increases with age. More than half the people who develop leukemia are older than age 60.
- *Cancer therapy.* People who've had certain types of chemotherapy and radiation therapy for other cancers have a slightly elevated risk of developing leukemia.
- *Genetics.* At least part of the risk of leukemia may be inherited. Some genetic disorders, such as Down syndrome, are associated with an increased risk.
- *Environmental hazards.* Smoking, exposure to intense radiation and long-term exposure to benzene, a chemical found in unleaded gasoline, may mutate genes. These hazards are linked to greater risk.

Types

Leukemias are classified depending on the type of white blood cell affected.

Myelogenous leukemia is a cancer of the granulocytes, a type of white blood cell formed in the bone marrow. Lymphocytic leukemia involves the lymphocytes, a type of white blood cell produced in the lymph system and bone marrow.

Types of leukemia are further divided according to how quickly they progress. In acute leukemia, leukemia cells multiply rapidly, and the disease worsens in weeks or months (see the color illustration on page 429).

Acute leukemia requires aggressive, immediate treatment. In chronic leukemia, abnormal blood cells replicate or accumulate more slowly and can function normally for a period of time. As a result, chronic leukemia worsens gradually and may not require immediate

Treating Leukemia

Various medications and other therapies are used to treat leukemia. The form of treatment your doctor recommends is based on a number of factors, including the type of leukemia you have.

- *Chemotherapy.* Chemotherapy, which uses chemical agents to kill cancer cells, is the major form of treatment for leukemia. Depending on the type of leukemia that you have, you may receive a single chemical agent or a combination of agents. Rapidly multiplying cells are often more sensitive to the effects of chemotherapy. For this reason, acute leukemia is usually quite responsive to chemotherapy.
- *Radiation.* Radiation therapy uses X-rays or other high-energy rays to damage leukemic cells and stop their growth.
- *Stem cell transplantation.* Chemotherapy or radiation therapy destroys your body's bone marrow, affecting its ability to produce healthy new blood cells. Your doctor may use a stem cell transplant to repopulate your blood with healthy cells (see page 1162).
- *Interferon-alfa.* Interferon is an antiviral agent that works to stop the spread of leukemic cells and helps bolster your immune system.
- *Cell-specific antibodies.* Antibodies that can destroy leukemic cells can be removed from your body and their number greatly increased in a laboratory. This larger number of antibodies then can be put back in your body to help destroy more cancer cells.
- *Retinoic acid.* One of the problems associated with leukemia is that the abnormal white blood cells produced don't mature as normal cells do. They multiply, but they don't mature and die off. All-trans-retinoic acid (ATRA) causes leukemic cells to mature and die.

Superficial Bleeding

Petechiae are round, pinpoint-sized spots caused by superficial bleeding into the skin. The spots aren't raised and initially are red but turn bluish-purple with time. Petechiae commonly appear on the lower legs but may appear over the whole body. A petechial rash isn't a disease but a sign of an underlying blood problem.

A common cause of petechiae is a marked decrease in the number of platelets in the blood. Platelets play an important role in controlling bleeding. A low platelet count (thrombocytopenia) can have many causes, including:

- Bone marrow disorders, such as leukemia
- Autoimmune diseases, such as lupus or rheumatoid arthritis
- Viral infections, such as mononucleosis and German measles (rubella)
- Drug reactions

Petechiae usually go away upon successful treatment of the underlying problem. Because of the seriousness of some causes of petechiae, it's important to determine the cause. If you develop a petechial rash, see your doctor promptly.

treatment. Chronic leukemia sometimes progresses to acute leukemia. Both acute and chronic forms occur somewhat more frequently in men than in women.

Chronic myelogenous leukemia

Signs and symptoms

- Symptoms of anemia
- Bone pain
- Fever and infections
- Night sweats
- Weight loss
- Pressure or fullness under the left ribs from an enlarged spleen
- Bleeding and bruising
- In some cases, none

Emergency signs and symptoms

- Fever with a temperature of 101 F or more
- Severe bleeding
- Sudden appearance of small red marks on the skin

Chronic myelogenous leukemia (CML) results from production of cancerous versions of granulocytes. Granulocytes are a type of white blood cell formed in the bone marrow.

This type of leukemia may also be called myeloid, myelocytic or granulocytic. The disorder tends to occur in middle-aged people.

Diagnosis

Often, people receive a diagnosis of the disease before symptoms develop, when routine blood tests reveal abnormal results.

Further tests are used to determine if you have chronic myelogenous leukemia. These include a complete blood count, a differential count of the various types of white blood cells, and measurement of an enzyme called leukocyte alkaline phosphatase. The bone marrow also may be examined.

The presence of an abnormal chromosome — known as the Philadelphia chromosome — also is helpful in making a diagnosis. This abnormality is found in 96 percent of people with chronic myelogenous leukemia.

Molecular genetic techniques can often identify the genetic abnormality in chronic myelogenous leukemia, even in individuals who don't have the Philadelphia chromosome.

How serious is chronic myelogenous leukemia?

Chronic myelogenous leukemia is a progressive disease. In most people with the disorder, an acute phase, called a blast crisis or blastic phase, develops within 3 to 5 years.

The blast phase is characterized by a high concentration of immature white blood cells (blasts) in the blood and by red pinpoints (petechiae) on the skin that result from bleeding due to lack of platelets. A blast crisis is a form of acute leukemia that's particularly resistant to treatment and may be fatal.

Treatment

The drug treatment of choice for chronic myelogenous leukemia is the oral medication imatinib mesylate (Gleevec), which stops the growth of abnormal white blood cells. Imatinib mesylate can be used to treat both the chronic phase and the blastic phase. The medication blocks a specific enzyme that's a key factor in the disease. Remission rates are high, especially in the chronic phase of the disease.

Another option for the chronic phase is allogeneic stem cell transplantation. Allogeneic stem cell transplantation is used in people younger than age 65, and it's the only proven curative treatment.

The choice between therapy with imatinib mesylate and allogeneic stem cell transplantation is made after taking into consideration various factors, including your age and preference. The best initial treatment for chronic myelogenous leukemia will evolve as more long-term results with imatinib mesylate become available.

Other options for therapy include hydroxyurea and chemotherapy combined with interferon. Interferon is an antiviral agent that works to stop the spread of leukemic cells and helps bolster the immune system. With the advent of imatinib mesylate, the role for these approaches as initial therapy has lessened.

If your spleen is extremely enlarged, it may be removed surgically (splenectomy). This doesn't appear to increase the duration of survival and is usually done only to decrease pain and reduce the risk of a ruptured spleen.

Acute myelogenous leukemia

Signs and symptoms

- Fatigue, weakness and general malaise
- Fever
- Bruising, small red marks on the skin or a rash
- Weight loss
- Overgrowth of the gums
- Blurred vision or loss of vision
- Headache
- Seizures
- Swollen lymph nodes
- Pressure or fullness under the left ribs from an enlarged spleen
- In some cases, none

Emergency signs and symptoms

- Bleeding from the digestive tract
- An altered state of consciousness
- An inability to talk or move an extremity
- Fever, with bacterial infection in the blood

Acute myelogenous leukemia causes overproduction of immature white blood cells known as blasts. Normally, these cells develop into granulocytes, but in this disease they remain immature. This form of acute leukemia is also referred to as nonlymphocytic, myeloid, monocytic, myelogenic or myelocytic leukemia. Acute myelogenous leukemia is the most common type of acute leukemia in adults. In most cases, its cause is unknown.

Diagnosis

Diagnosis of acute myelogenous leukemia is generally based on the results of a complete blood count, a differential count of the various types of white blood cells and examination of bone marrow. Your doctor may also look for certain chromosome abnormalities that can help establish the diagnosis or indicate how your body may respond to the disease. In some cases, spinal fluid is taken for analysis.

How serious is acute myelogenous leukemia?

The course of acute myelogenous leukemia can be extremely rapid. Without treatment, death can occur within weeks. Treatment with combinations of certain chemotherapy medications can produce remission in 30 percent to 75 percent of people.

Younger individuals generally respond better to treatment than do older adults. However, recurrences develop in the majority of people who enter remission. When given further treatment, approximately 30 percent to 40 percent of individuals experience prolonged remission.

Treatment

Standard treatment generally involves combinations of different chemotherapy medications. Antibiotics can treat or prevent bacterial infections, which can frequently occur in people with this disease. Autologous or allogeneic stem cell transplantation (see page 1162) may be performed during an initial remission, in relapse or during a second remission.

Acute lymphocytic leukemia

Signs and symptoms

- Abnormal bruising, including small hemorrhages into the skin
- Bleeding from mucous membranes
- Fatigue, weakness and general malaise
- Fever
- Paleness
- Enlarged liver, spleen or lymph nodes
- Bone pain

Acute lymphocytic leukemia is a form of cancer that causes overproduction of immature blood cells (lymphoblasts, or blasts for short) that, under normal circumstances, would eventually develop into lymphocytes.

The disorder is also known as acute lymphoblastic leukemia. Although it occurs in both adults and children, it's sometimes referred to as childhood leukemia because it's the most common leukemia among children.

Diagnosis

The symptoms of acute lymphocytic leukemia may appear suddenly or develop over weeks or months. Your doctor will likely perform blood tests, including a complete blood count (see page 1131) with a differential count of the various types of white blood cells. If the results of these tests suggest acute lymphocytic leukemia, a sample of your bone marrow will likely be examined to see if it contains a high concentration of blasts.

In many medical centers, further tests are often performed to determine what subtypes of lymphoblasts are present. These and other tests help characterize the disease and indicate the best treatment.

How serious is acute lymphocytic leukemia?

Without treatment, bleeding and infection can lead to death within months. Before current treatments were developed, this was the inevitable outcome of the disease. Fortunately, one of medicine's great success stories is the treatment of this leukemia in children.

The younger an individual is and the lower his or her white blood cell count at the time the disease is diagnosed, the better the chances of a cure. With a combination of chemotherapy, up to 80 percent of children are in complete remission 5 years after detection of the disease. The prognosis isn't as good for older children and adults. About 40 percent achieve long-term survival. The outcome also depends on the particular type of lymphoblast that's present.

Treatment

Treatment of acute lymphocytic leukemia has two phases. The first, called induction therapy, is intended to kill as many leukemia cells as possible, leading to no signs or symptoms of disease (remission). The second phase, called continuation therapy, takes place during remission. The goal is to kill any remaining leukemia cells.

Induction therapy
With induction therapy, an attempt is made to achieve remission, usually by administering chemotherapy. Using combinations of medications maximizes the effect of the treatment. A chemotherapeutic drug such as methotrexate may also be injected into spinal fluid (central nervous system prophylaxis).

In adults, radiation therapy to the brain is often used in addition to methotrexate for central nervous system prophylaxis. Radiation therapy to the brain may also be used if cancer cells have already invaded the brain.

Chemotherapy drugs can cause side effects, interfering with the normal functions of the bone marrow, the immune system and other organs. In addition, some drugs temporarily slow a child's growth. The child usually catches up following treatment.

Consolidation and maintenance therapy
Once remission has been achieved, further chemotherapy is usually administered as consolidation therapy to kill lingering cancer cells. If lingering cancer cells aren't destroyed, they can cause a relapse later on. Finally, maintenance treatment involving lower-dose chemotherapy is given for 2 to 3 years.

Stem cell transplantation
Doctors may recommend stem cell transplantation for people who've had a relapse, are at high risk of relapse or fail to achieve a complete remission with induction therapy.

Lymphocytosis

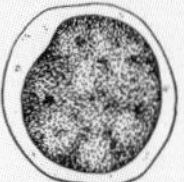

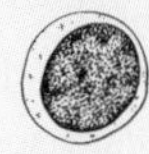

Lymphocytosis is the term for an increase in the percentage of lymphocytes — a type of white blood cell — in your blood. The condition generally causes no symptoms and may be discovered during a routine blood test performed for some other purpose.

Your bone marrow produces lymphocytes in great quantities. These white blood cells play an important role in your immune system response, defending against infection.

A marked increase in lymphocytes commonly occurs in response to a viral infection, but it may also be due to chronic lymphocytic leukemia. Sometimes, the percentage of lymphocytes increases because of a decrease in the number of other white blood cells. Doctors refer to this as relative lymphocytosis.

Chronic lymphocytic leukemia

Signs and symptoms

- Swollen lymph nodes
- Fatigue, weakness and general malaise
- Infection
- Fever
- Weight loss
- Night sweats
- Pressure under the left ribs from an enlarged spleen
- Bone pain
- In many cases, none

Chronic lymphocytic leukemia is a cancer of the bone marrow that causes a slow increase in the number of white blood cells known as lymphocytes (see the color illustration on page 429). It's the most common leukemia in the Western world. It most often occurs in men and people older than age 50. The disease can run in families.

Diagnosis
The onset of chronic lymphocytic leukemia tends to be insidious, with symptoms developing gradually. Most cases are detected by routine blood tests performed on people without symptoms. Your doctor may then conduct further tests to establish what subtypes of lymphocytes are affected. Results of these tests can help predict how rapidly or slowly the disorder will advance, and they'll help you and your doctor determine how to proceed with treatment.

How serious is chronic lymphocytic leukemia?
The course of chronic lymphocytic leukemia varies widely. Because the lymphocytes are mature and functional, people with this disorder may survive for many years without treatment. In some people, the disorder progresses more rapidly, requiring earlier treatment.

Treatment
Current treatment guidelines recommend no treatment if the only abnormality is an increased lymphocyte count or if the only evidence of disease is swollen lymph nodes. Your doctor may want to keep track of your condition with periodic blood tests.

Treatment of more advanced disease involves the use of chemotherapy. Following initial treatment, many people with advanced chronic lymphocytic leukemia feel well for years without further treatment.

Medication
If anemia or the bleeding disorder thrombocytopenia accompany chronic lymphocytic leukemia, treatment is generally necessary. Three classes of chemotherapy medications are used to treat chronic lymphocytic leukemia. These include alkylating agents such as chlorambucil (Leukeran), antimetabolites such as fludarabine (Fludara) and monoclonal antibodies such as rituximab (Rituxan). Sometimes, chemotherapy includes corticosteroid medications such as prednisone.

Surgery
Rarely, removal of the spleen (splenectomy) is necessary. This is

generally done if the spleen has become huge or if it's causing problems, such as immune complications that interfere with drug treatment.

Hairy cell leukemia

Signs and symptoms

- Fatigue, weakness and general malaise
- Infection
- Fever
- Pressure under the left ribs from an enlarged spleen

Hairy cell leukemia is characterized by an enlarged spleen and cancer cells covered by hair-like villi (hairy cells).

The disease affects the lymphocytes, a type of white blood cell. The cancerous cells generally collect in the spleen, causing it to swell. The cause of this rare form of leukemia is unknown. It primarily affects men.

Diagnosis

Hairy cell leukemia is generally diagnosed based on results from blood tests and a bone marrow sample.

How serious is hairy cell leukemia?

Hairy cell leukemia is a progressive disease that can be fatal if not treated. Since the 1980s, this disease has been treatable with medications, and many people are able to live a normal life span.

Treatment

Cladribine (Leustatin) — also known as 2-chlorodeoxyadenosine and 2-CdA — is used to treat hairy cell leukemia. It's given intravenously over 7 days. The medication destroys both the cancerous cells that are dividing and those at rest. Interferon may also be used. Other medications are available or are under development.

Lymphomas

Lymphomas are cancers of the lymphatic system, the disease-fighting network spread throughout your body. The lymph system includes the lymph nodes, which are located throughout the body and are connected by small vessels called lymphatics. The tonsils, adenoids, spleen, thymus and bone marrow also are part of the lymphatic system.

Often, the first symptom of lymphoma is enlargement of lymph nodes with no other obvious symptoms. However, lymphomas may also occur outside the lymph nodes in virtually any part of the body.

Hodgkin's disease

Signs and symptoms

- Painless enlargement of lymph nodes in the neck, armpits or groin

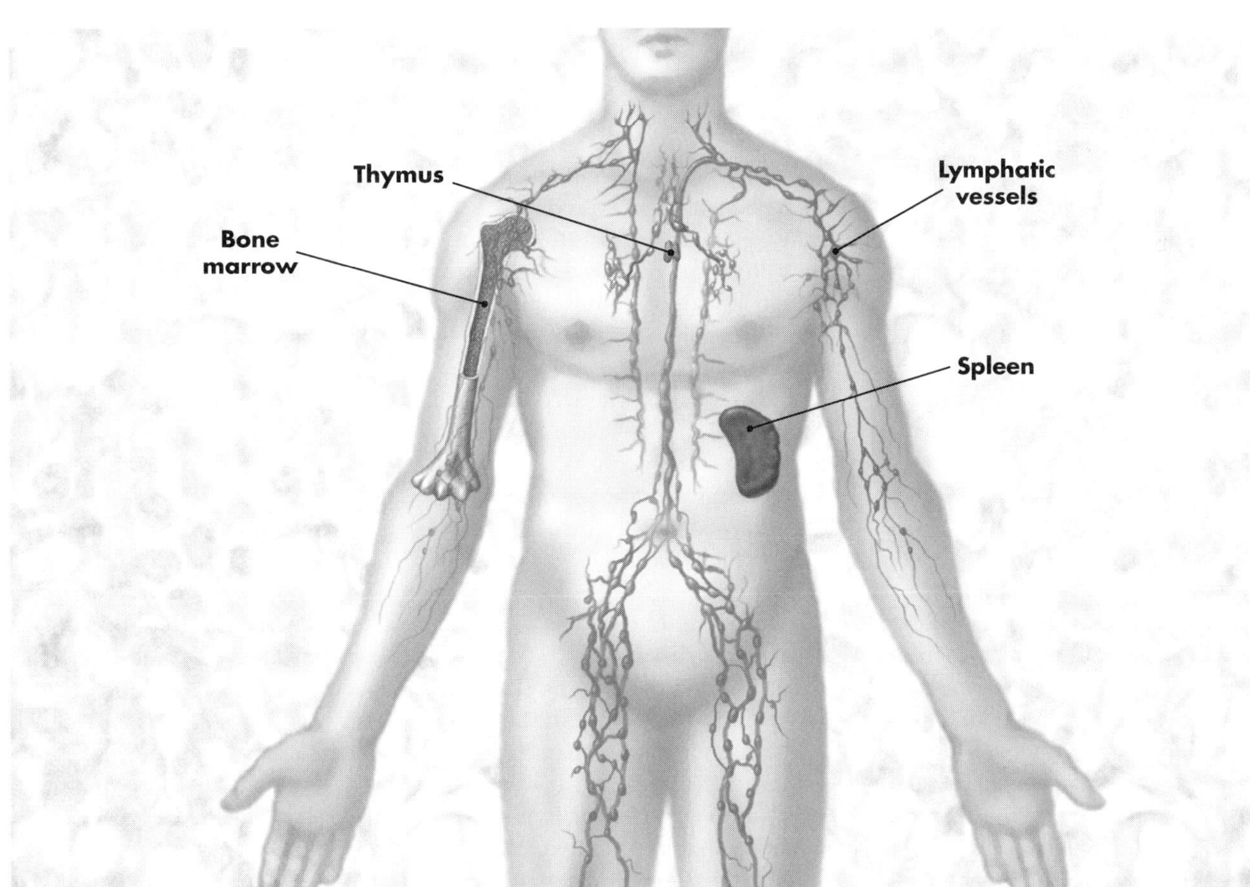

Your lymphatic system is a complex network of thin-walled vessels. It includes the spleen, thymus, bone marrow, lymphatic vessels and, not shown here, the tonsils and adenoids.

- Fatigue
- Fever and chills
- Night sweats
- Weight loss and loss of appetite
- Severe itching

Emergency signs and symptoms

- Sudden onset of high fever from any cause
- Loss of bladder or bowel control
- Numbness or loss of strength in the arms and legs

Hodgkin's disease (Hodgkin's lymphoma) is named after the 19th-century English doctor Thomas Hodgkin who first described it in 1832. It's an uncommon cancer of the lymphatic system with several characteristics that distinguish it from other lymphomas.

In Hodgkin's disease, cells in the lymphatic system grow abnormally and may spread beyond the lymphatic system. As the disease progresses, it compromises your body's ability to prevent or fight infection, and signs and symptoms begin to appear.

Many signs and symptoms of the disease are similar to those of influenza, such as fever, fatigue and night sweats. Eventually, cancerous tumors develop. Hodgkin's disease most often affects people between the ages of 15 and 24 and people older than age 55.

Hodgkin's disease is far less common than non-Hodgkin's lymphoma. In 2001, about 7,400 new cases of Hodgkin's disease caused about 1,300 deaths in the United States. During the same year, about 56,200 new cases of non-Hodgkin's lymphoma caused about 26,300 deaths.

Causes

Hodgkin's disease causes the development of abnormal B cells, which originate in bone marrow and are an important component of the immune system response. B cells normally work with T cells, derived from the thymus, to fight infection. T cells kill foreign invaders directly. B cells become plasma cells, which produce antibodies that neutralize foreign invaders.

In most cases of Hodgkin's disease, B cells develop into large, abnormal cells called Reed cells. Instead of undergoing the normal life-and-death cycle of cells, Reed cells continue to live and to produce more cancerous (malignant) B cells. What causes these changes is unknown. In about 50 percent of the individuals with Hodgkin's disease, the Epstein-Barr virus is contained in malignant cells. Whether this is the cause of the disease isn't known.

Diagnosis

Diagnosis of Hodgkin's disease usually involves a medical history, thorough physical examination, a chest X-ray and blood and urine tests. A lymph node biopsy, in which lymph node tissue is removed and studied for the presence of the patterns typical of Hodgkin's disease, may confirm the diagnosis. Sometimes, only a portion of the node is removed for examination under a microscope, which allows the doctor to use the remainder of the node as a marker to evaluate the response to treatment.

If you receive a diagnosis of Hodgkin's disease, your doctor may conduct more tests to find out how advanced the cancer is and to determine how best to treat it. This process is called staging and may involve a bone marrow biopsy (see page 1132), a computerized tomography (CT) scan of your abdomen and chest and other tests, such as a gallium scan. In rare cases, surgery is performed to determine the extent of the disease.

How serious is Hodgkin's disease?

When Hodgkin's disease is detected and treated early, the 5-year survival rate is higher than 90 percent. Fifty years ago, the disease was almost always fatal. Even for people with the most advanced stage of the disease, 80 percent are free of disease 5 years after treatment.

Many individuals who die within 15 years following treatment do so because of complications of the treatment, such as secondary cancers or heart failure, rather than of the disease itself. The challenge for researchers is to decrease the long-term complications of treatment without reducing its effectiveness.

Treatment

Your treatment depends on several criteria, including the type and stage of the disease, the number and regions of lymph nodes affected, your age and your overall health status. Treatment options include:

Radiation

When the disease is limited to one or two areas, radiation therapy is often used in combination with chemotherapy. Radiation is applied to the affected nodes following 2 to 4 months of chemotherapy. Occasionally, individuals may be treated with radiation therapy alone.

If you have a relapse following radiation therapy — usually within 2 years after conclusion of radiation treatment — then chemotherapy may be recommended.

Chemotherapy

When the disease progresses and involves more lymph nodes or other organs, chemotherapy is often the preferred treatment. Chemotherapy uses specific drug preparations to kill cancer cells.

Currently, the greatest concerns about using chemotherapy for Hodgkin's disease are long-term side effects and complications, which include heart, kidney and liver damage and development of secondary cancers, such as leukemia. Drug regimens have been developed that substantially diminish the likelihood of such long-range, life-threatening complications in people who receive multiple courses of chemotherapy and radiation therapy.

The two most common drug regimens are MOPP and ABVD. Both are combinations of four chemotherapy drugs.

MOPP stands for mechlorethamine, vincristine (Oncovin), procarbazine and prednisone. This used to be the basic regimen, but it's very toxic, and serious side effects often appear several years after treatment.

ABVD stands for doxorubicin (Adriamycin), bleomycin, vinblastine and dacarbazine. This is a newer regimen with less severe side effects, and it's now the preferred treatment. Doctors still occasionally use MOPP because ABVD may cause heart failure in some people.

Stem cell transplantation

If the disease recurs following an initial chemotherapy-induced remission, an autologous stem cell transplant (see page 1162) may be considered.

Non-Hodgkin's lymphoma

Signs and symptoms

- Painless enlargement of lymph nodes in the neck, armpit or groin areas
- Fatigue
- Fever or chills
- Night sweats
- Weight loss

Emergency signs and symptoms

- Sudden onset of unexplained high fever
- Mental confusion
- Drowsiness
- Involuntary loss of urine or stool
- Numbness or loss of strength in the arms and legs

Non-Hodgkin's lymphomas are a group of cancers (malignancies) that develop from white blood cells (lymphocytes) in your lymphatic system, often at different locations in your body. These tumors are classified according to their cell type as seen under a microscope. They're also grouped into two broad categories by the level of activity of the cancerous cells: indolent and aggressive.

Normally, lymphocytes go through a predictable life cycle. Old lymphocytes die, and your body creates new ones to replace them. But in non-Hodgkin's lymphoma, your body produces abnormal lymphocytes that continue to divide and grow without control. This oversupply of lymphocytes crowds into your lymph nodes, causing them to swell. There are more than 20 different types of non-Hodgkin's lymphoma.

Non-Hodgkin's lymphoma accounts for about 5 percent of all new cancers in the United States. The disease is more than seven times more common than the other common form of lymphoma — Hodgkin's disease.

Non-Hodgkin's lymphoma occurs more frequently among people who have received organ transplants, because their immune systems are inhibited by immunosuppressant therapy. Individuals with AIDS are at higher risk of developing this disorder. The disease usually occurs in people between the ages of 45 and 70.

Non-Hodgkin's lymphoma has been one of the most rapidly increasing types of cancer in the United States since the 1970s. The good news is that during the 1990s, the rate of increase began to slow.

Causes

Doctors don't know what causes non-Hodgkin's lymphoma. Researchers believe that activation of certain genes may be associated with some cancers that develop in B lymphocytes. Lymphocytes occur either as B cells, those that originate in bone marrow, or T cells, which derive from the thymus gland. About 85 percent of non-Hodgkin's lymphomas occur in B cells, and the rest in T cells.

Non-Hodgkin's lymphoma typically involves cancer in your lymph nodes, but the disease can spread to other parts of your lymphatic system. This includes the lymphatic vessels, tonsils, adenoids, spleen, thymus and bone marrow. Occasionally, non-Hodgkin's lymphoma involves organs outside the lymphatic system.

Diagnosis

Your doctor may use these procedures to help diagnose non-Hodgkin's lymphoma:

- *Physical examination.* Your doctor may examine not only your swollen lymph nodes but also other lymph nodes to determine their size and consistency.
- *Blood and urine tests.* Much of the time, having swollen lymph nodes means you're fighting an infection. Blood and urine tests may help your doctor rule out an infection or other disease, or they may help identify the particular type of non-Hodgkin's lymphoma you have.
- *Imaging techniques.* An X-ray or computerized tomography (CT) scan of your chest, neck, abdomen and pelvis may detect the presence and size of tumors.
- *Lymph node biopsy.* Taking a sample of lymph node tissue for examination in the laboratory may reveal whether you have non-Hodgkin's lymphoma and, if so, which type.
- *Bone marrow biopsy.* To find out if the disease has spread, your doctor may request a biopsy of your bone marrow (see page 1132).

How serious is non-Hodgkin's lymphoma?

Indolent non-Hodgkin's lymphoma isn't curable, but it's typically very responsive to initial therapy. The survival rate for people with non-Hodgkin's lymphoma is good. If you have this disease but have no symptoms, your doctor may recommend observation only.

In contrast, aggressive non-Hodgkin's lymphomas require aggressive treatments in an attempt to produce a complete remission. Sixty percent to 80 percent of affected individuals enter a complete remission with chemotherapy.

Treatment

Treatment decisions depend on the type and stage of your lymphoma, your age and your overall condition. A combination of chemotherapy medications is often used.

Newer treatments include antibody and vaccine therapies. Rituximab (Rituxan) is a monoclonal antibody that responds to a special antigen found on lymphoma cells. The Food and Drug Administration (FDA) also recently approved the medication ibritumomab tiuxetan (Zevalin), which consists of a monoclonal antibody joined to a radioactive isotope, as part of a treatment regimen for one type of low-grade non-Hodgkin's lymphoma.

Both Rituxan and Zevalin are designed to help your immune system target and destroy cancer cells. Zevalin produces serious side effects, including reduced blood cell counts, and the FDA has approved its use only for people who've had no success with other treatments.

Radiation

For some types of non-Hodgkin's lymphoma, high doses of radiation are used to kill cancerous cells and shrink tumors. Sometimes, radiation is used along with chemotherapy to treat specific sites, such as the brain.

Stem cell transplantation

An autologous stem cell transplant (see page 1162) is primarily used if the cancer relapses following initial, successful treatment.

Bleeding Disorders

Bleeding disorders result from a disruption in the complex process by which blood clots form. The clotting process (coagulation) involves blood platelets as well as plasma proteins involved in coagulation (clotting factors).

The process begins when platelets stick to a blood vessel at the site of an injury. An intricate cascade of enzyme reactions occurs to produce a web-like protein network that encircles the platelets and holds them in place (platelet phase) to form a clot (coagulation phase). In this cascade, each clotting factor is transformed, in turn, from an inactive to an active form. Specialized laboratories can study the coagulation mechanism in an affected person's blood to pinpoint the place in the cascade at which the fault lies.

Problems with clotting factors cause bleeding disorders such as hemophilia, von Willebrand's disease and disseminated intravascular coagulation. Bleeding disorders based on clotting factor problems tend to cause bleeding in deep tissues and joints, although excessive bruising, severe nosebleeds and other types of bleeding can occur as well.

When platelets are too few (thrombocytopenia) or fail to function, one result is reddish-purple pinpoint hemorrhages seen in the skin (petechiae).

Hemophilia

Signs and symptoms

- Many large or deep bruises
- Joint pain and swelling caused by bleeding
- Blood in urine or stool
- Prolonged bleeding from cuts or injuries or after surgery or tooth extraction

Emergency signs and symptoms

- Bleeding into the head, neck or digestive tract
- Sudden pain, swelling and warmth of large joints — such as the knees, elbows, hips or shoulders — and of arm or leg muscles
- Excessive bleeding from a minor injury, especially if you have a severe form of hemophilia

Hemophilia includes several inherited disorders characterized by a deficiency of selected clotting factors in your body's blood-clotting system. At least 10 clotting factors are involved in the clotting process. Three of these factors are involved in hemophilia, leading to three types of disease: hemophilia A, B and C.

The most common type of hemophilia is hemophilia A (classical hemophilia), in which there isn't enough of clotting factor VIII. Hemophilia B (Christmas disease), in which factor IX is lacking, makes up most of the remaining cases. Hemophilia C, better known as factor XI deficiency, is rare, with only about 200 known cases in the United States since it was identified in 1953. In total, about 17,000 Americans have hemophilia.

Both the A and B forms of the disorder have also been called the royal disease because hemophilia was inherited by descendants of England's Queen Victoria and introduced into the royal houses of Spain, Germany and Russia. Although hemophilia is one of the most commonly inherited bleeding disorders, it's still uncommon.

Hemophilia A and B occur almost always in males. Generally, hemophilia A and B are passed from mother to son through one of the mother's genes. Men can't pass along the gene that causes hemophilia to their sons.

Everyone has two sex chromosomes, one from each parent. Females inherit an X chromosome from their mother and an X chromosome from their father. Males inherit an X chromosome from their mother and a Y chromosome from their father. The gene that causes hemophilia A or B is located on the X chromosome. Most women who have the defective gene that causes hemophilia are simply carriers. They carry the hemophilia trait but exhibit no signs or symptoms of hemophilia. It's also possible for hemophilia A or B to occur through spontaneous mutation of a gene.

Factor XI deficiency (hemophilia C) can occur in boys and girls. It's milder than hemophilia A or B. The defective gene that causes factor XI

PREVENTION TIP

Physical therapy and daily physical activity can help joints damaged by hemophilia function better. Swimming, bicycle riding and walking can build up your muscles to help protect your joints. Regular physical activity may help you avoid surgery to replace a severely damaged joint. But don't engage in contact sports. Contact sports carry a high risk of injury and bleeding.

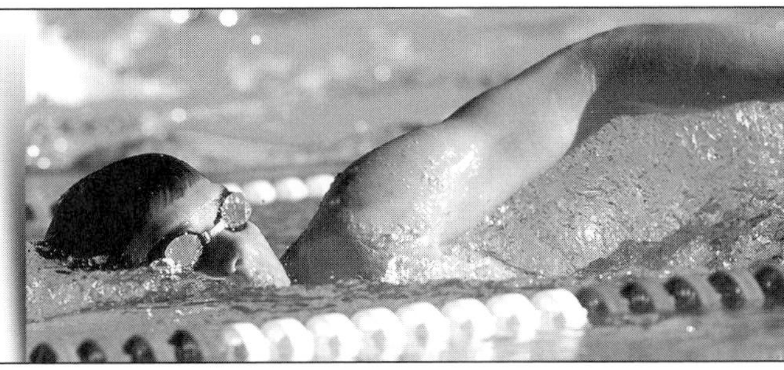

deficiency can be passed on to children by mothers and fathers by an inheritance pattern that differs from that of hemophilia A and B.

The major problem for people with hemophilia isn't superficial, external cuts, which can be easily treated with pressure and a bandage, but is uncontrolled internal bleeding. The severity of bleeding varies from person to person. The more severe forms of hemophilia typically become apparent early in life. Excessive bleeding happens often and even spontaneously without any apparent cause.

In its mild forms, hemophilia may not become apparent until later in life, and troublesome bleeding episodes may happen only after surgery, tooth extraction or major injury. Newborns often show no signs of hemophilia because of their limited mobility. But as your baby begins to move around, falling and bumping into things, bruising may develop beneath the skin. Most of the time, these bumps and bruises aren't serious and don't require medical treatment.

Diagnosis

The diagnosis of hemophilia may be established in several ways. For people with a family history of the disease, it's possible to test the fetus to determine if the child is affected. Analysis of a blood sample from either a child or an adult can show a deficiency of a clotting factor.

Prolonged bleeding following circumcision may be the first indication that a baby boy has hemophilia. On occasion, in boys who aren't circumcised, easy bruising when the child becomes more mobile between ages 9 and 18 months may lead to the diagnosis. Sometimes, mild hemophilia isn't diagnosed until a person has surgery and excessive bleeding results.

How serious is hemophilia?

Hemophilia is a lifelong disease. But with medication, replacement of deficient clotting factors and proper self-care, most people with hemophilia can lead active, productive lives.

Depending on the severity of the hemophilia, it may be necessary to take extra care to minimize bleeding as a result of physical activity or surgical or dental procedures. Sometimes, the disorder becomes more difficult to control due to the development of antibodies to the clotting factor used in the treatment.

Without treatment, recurrent bleeding into the joints can cause chronic pain and weakness and may even destroy the joint. Bleeding into muscle and soft tissue may put pressure on nerves, producing pain, stiffness and numbness.

Without adequate treatment, permanent nerve damage and muscle wasting eventually may occur. If bleeding occurs in your head, neck or digestive system, the condition is considered extremely serious. It's important to treat such episodes promptly.

If you're considering having children and either have hemophilia or think that you may carry the trait, prenatal testing and genetic counseling can help you learn if you could pass the disorder on to your children.

Treatment

Treatment varies with the severity of the disorder. If you have mild hemophilia A, a bleeding episode may be treated with slow injection into a vein of the medication desmopressin (DDAVP). This drug helps stop bleeding by stimulating the release of factor VIII and making blood vessels contract. Occasionally, desmopressin (Stimate) is given by nasal inhalation.

If you have hemophilia B or more severe hemophilia A, bleeding episodes may stop only after an infusion of clotting factors derived from donated human blood or genetically engineered products called recombinant clotting factors. For factor XI deficiency, plasma infusions are used to stop bleeding episodes.

Infusion of a clotting factor two or three times a week may help prevent bleeds in hemophilia A and B. This approach may be a way to reduce time spent in the hospital and away from home, work or school and to limit side effects such as damage to joints. Your doctor may train you to do your own infusions of desmopressin or of clotting factor at home, work or school.

Wear a medical alert bracelet so that emergency medical personnel will be alerted to your condition and the type of clotting factor that's best for you. Don't use medications that might worsen bleeding, such as aspirin.

If you experience a small cut or scrape, using pressure and a bandage will usually take care of the bleeding. For small areas of bleeding beneath the skin, use an ice pack.

Surgery
When recurrent internal bleeding destroys a joint, your doctor may recommend replacing the joint with an artificial joint.

Von Willebrand's disease

Signs and symptoms

- Bleeding from the gums or nose
- Excessive and prolonged menstrual bleeding
- Easy bruising, often noticeable on parts of the body that typically aren't injured during normal activity — such as the thighs, upper arms, back, abdomen, chest, hands and feet
- Blood in the stool, characterized by a black or tarry appearance, or blood in urine

This chronic bleeding disorder is caused by a defect in a clotting factor called von Willebrand's factor. In many cases, there's also a deficiency of clotting factor VIII. Ordinarily, these two factors combine to form the active substance (complex) needed to cause platelets to gather at the site of blood vessel injury. In von Willebrand's disease, both platelet aggregation and clot formation are impaired.

The disease is named for the Finnish doctor who described it in 1926. It's also referred to as pseudohemophilia or vascular hemophilia.

Von Willebrand's disease is the most common hereditary bleeding disorder. It affects 1 percent of the U.S. population, men and women equally. In the majority of cases, it's a mild disorder, called type 1. Type 2 produces mild to moderate symptoms. Type 3, which is rare, is the most severe.

Before adolescence, a key sign is nosebleeds that may be severe enough to require a visit to your doctor or the emergency department. In women, the menstrual flow is heavy and prolonged, sometimes lasting weeks. Many women assume this is normal, and the disease goes undiagnosed.

Other signs and symptoms are marked bruising, blood in the urine or stool, bleeding gums, and bleeding during and after surgery or tooth extraction. Some people also experience persistent gastrointestinal or urinary tract bleeding.

Diagnosis

Specialized blood tests are needed to diagnose the disease. Tests include bleeding time, platelet function, the level of active von Willebrand's factor and, in some cases, tests for factor VIII.

Treatment

Type 1 is treated with the medication desmopressin in a nasal spray form (Stimate), typically taken before surgery or menstruation. The medication stimulates release of von Willebrand's factor and factor VIII from blood vessel walls.

Types 2 and 3 require more complicated treatments. Transfusion of plasma or cryoprecipitate may be used. Cryoprecipitate is a clotting factor concentrate derived from donated human blood.

If you have von Willebrand's disease, avoid medications that might worsen bleeding, such as aspirin and other nonsteroidal anti-inflammatory drugs (NSAIDs), which interfere with clotting. Also avoid antihistamines, because they can affect platelet functioning.

The only way to prevent this inherited disorder is by genetic counseling of prospective parents who have it. If you're found to have von Willebrand's disease, it's possible that your brothers, sisters or children also might have it. And they may want to seek appropriate testing and counseling.

Disseminated intravascular coagulation

Signs and symptoms

- Bleeding from many sites in the body
- In some cases, none

Emergency signs and symptoms

- Severe bleeding, especially with trauma or at surgical incision sites

Disseminated intravascular coagulation is a nonhereditary bleeding disorder that results paradoxically from excessive coagulation. It occurs when activated clotting factors are present throughout the bloodstream instead of being limited to sites of injury. These factors can cause blood to clot (coagulate) in small blood vessels all over the body.

Because so much of the body's supply of clotting factors and platelets is used up by this inappropriate coagulation, not enough is available for the formation of clots at injury sites. The body also reacts by stepping up the system that dissolves clots, promoting generalized bleeding.

Although it's seen only rarely, the disorder almost always occurs as a complication of a serious underlying disease, including infection and malignancy, or following trauma or surgery.

Diagnosis

If your doctor suspects that you have disseminated intravascular coagulation, he or she will likely request a variety of tests to establish the diagnosis.

How serious is disseminated intravascular coagulation?

The severity of this disorder varies. When disseminated intravascular coagulation occurs with cancer or some other disorder, it may be chronic. In such instances, you may not experience spontaneous bleeding and the condition might be detected by blood tests done for other reasons.

More often, the disorder is acute, causing severe bleeding from multiple sites, such as surgical incisions. Clots may form in the legs, or a stroke may occur. Rarely, it's serious enough to cause gangrene in the fingers, genitals or nose.

The conditions that cause the disorder tend to be life-threatening, but if they're successfully treated, disseminated intravascular coagulation will often stop.

Treatment

The only really effective approach is to treat the underlying condition. Transfusion of various blood products also may be necessary to replace the clotting factors depleted by the widespread coagulation. Treatment with heparin, a medication that prevents clotting, may be necessary if there's evidence of clotting or if there's continued bleeding despite blood product transfusions.

Thrombocytopenia

Signs and symptoms

- Easy or excessive bruising
- A reddish-purple skin rash, usually on the lower legs
- Prolonged bleeding from cuts
- Spontaneous bleeding from your gums or nose
- Blood in urine or stools
- Heavy menstrual flow
- Bleeding during surgery

Emergency signs and symptoms

- Serious or widespread bleeding, including bleeding in the brain and digestive system

Your bone marrow makes new platelets daily. Each platelet lives only about 10 days. At any given time, you should have 150,000 to 450,000 platelets per cubic millimeter of circulating blood. Thrombocytopenia means a shortage of platelets in blood. The condition is often asymptomatic but may be associated with bleeding.

Causes of thrombocytopenia include:

- Reduced production of platelets by bone marrow
- Early destruction of platelets by the immune system
- Trapping of platelets in the spleen, which filters blood

Sometimes, mild thrombocytopenia is a temporary problem that's self-correcting. A routine blood test may show that your platelet count is low even though you haven't been experiencing symptoms. Other more serious forms of the condition require treatment.

One form that requires treatment is idiopathic thrombocytopenic purpura (ITP). This condition results when the immune system malfunctions and antibodies attack healthy platelets. It may be related to an autoimmune disease, follow a recent infection or result from certain medications. ITP occurs most often in children and young adults but can occur in people of any age. It generally affects more women than men.

Thrombotic thrombocytopenic purpura (TTP) is a rare, life-threatening condition that causes a sudden, sharp drop in platelets. The drop occurs when platelets are drawn into small blood clots that suddenly form throughout the body. The clots can put you at risk of stroke-like symptoms. A few anticlotting medications have been linked to the condition.

Thrombocytopenia may also be caused by a number of disorders, such as systemic lupus erythematosus, lymphoma, chronic lymphocytic leukemia, sarcoidosis, ovarian cancer and viral infections. It can be caused by an overwhelming infection following a transfusion or use of certain medications. Medications that can cause thrombocytopenia include heparin, quinidine, sulfonamides, procainamide, rifampin and most chemotherapy drugs.

Diagnosis

To detect thrombocytopenia, your doctor will obtain a platelet count and examine your blood under a microscope. Your doctor may order special blood tests and a bone marrow examination to determine the cause.

How serious is thrombocytopenia?

The seriousness of thrombocytopenia depends on its cause. Thrombocytopenia may occasionally resolve without any treatment, particularly in children. In these cases, the bone marrow may make up for the shortened life span of platelets by producing large numbers of new ones until the initiating cause subsides. Young platelets are especially active in clotting, so even though the total concentration of platelets is low, you might experience no bleeding problems and need no special treatment.

ITP in adults is often chronic. It may vary in severity over time, and it can even recur after an apparently complete remission. Fortunately, the most serious complications, such as bleeding into the brain and digestive tract, occur only rarely.

Treatment

Sometimes, treatment isn't necessary. If the cause of thrombocytopenia is apparent, treating the underlying condition or stopping use of the offending medication may be sufficient.

Medication

In rare situations, a doctor may use thrombopoietin, a hormone that stimulates platelet production.

For idiopathic thrombocytopenic purpura, treatment may include medications that suppress or otherwise alter the immune system, such as a corticosteroid or intravenous immunoglobulin therapy.

Surgery

Sometimes, the spleen is removed (splenectomy) to relieve symptoms or to help cure chronic ITP that doesn't respond to corticosteroids. The spleen destroys platelets that are attacked by antibodies.

Blood transfusion

For severe bleeding, lost blood is replaced with transfusions of packed red blood cells. Platelet concentrates are given to treat severe thrombocytopenia, particularly those related to cancer or chemotherapy.

Thrombosis

Thrombosis occurs when a blood clot forms in a vein or artery. A blood clot that remains in a vein is called a thrombus, and the condition is called venous thrombosis. Sometimes, clots that remain localized don't cause symptoms, but often they cause localized pain and swelling. Some people have a tendency to develop blood clots spontaneously, a condition called thrombophilia, or hypercoagulable state.

A blood clot is made up of a plug of platelets, colorless blood cells that repair injured blood vessels, enmeshed in a network of red blood cells and a protein called fibrin. Clots are the end result of a complex process that helps stop bleeding after you've been injured. Sometimes, though, clots form for no purpose.

Most of these unwanted clots originate in a vein in your leg or pelvis. The affected vein may be near the surface of your skin (superficial thrombosis) or deep within a muscle (deep vein thrombosis).

Clots in superficial veins rarely present a serious problem and often clear on their own. But clots in deep veins may detach and travel in the blood to another part of your body. A clot that travels to another part of your body is called an embolus. A clot can migrate to your lungs, causing a pulmonary embolism, or to the brain, causing a stroke.

Risk factors

Factors that increase your risk of deep vein thrombosis may be inherited or acquired.

Inherited risk factors

Inherited risk factors include deficiencies in natural anticlotting substances (anticoagulants) and high levels of clotting factors (procoagulants) in blood.

- *Activated protein C resistance.* Factor V is a protein that's important for formation of blood clots (a procoagulant protein). In order to control its clotting activity, a protein called protein C normally breaks it down. When factor V resists this breakdown or protein C is inactivated, the condition is called activated protein C resistance or factor V Leiden. The condition is due to a genetic defect in coagulation factor V.

  Up to 7 percent of whites have this abnormality, making it the most common inherited risk factor for deep vein thrombosis in this group. Of individuals who experience the condition, 20 percent have protein C resistance.
- *Deficiencies of anticoagulant proteins.* Inherited deficiencies in two natural proteins called protein C and S and antithrombin, which prevent blood from clotting, can increase risk of deep vein thrombosis. Together, they account for less than 10 percent of people with the condition.
- *Prothrombin gene abnormality.* This inherited condition is found in up to 6 percent of individuals with deep vein thrombosis. It's also present in up to 2 percent of whites without the condition.

People with deep vein thrombosis are treated with anticoagulant medications to prevent blood from clotting. How long the medications are used depends on which inherited abnormality you have.

Acquired risk factors

Medical conditions and lifestyle factors that can increase the risk of a venous thrombosis include:

- *Certain types of cancer.* Pancreatic, ovarian and lung cancers, in particular, are known to increase levels of clotting factors. Some studies indicate that menopausal women with a history of breast cancer taking tamoxifen also have an increased risk.
- *Estrogen use.* The female hormone estrogen found in birth control pills and hormone replacement therapy may increase clotting factors in the blood, especially when the medications are combined with tobacco use.
- *Pregnancy.* Women are at increased risk during pregnancy and the period immediately following delivery, possibly due to extra pressure on veins in the legs and pelvis. A blood clot traveling to a lung artery (pulmonary embolism) is the most frequent cause of maternal death associated with childbirth. Many women who have pregnancy-related venous thromboembolism also have an inherited clotting disorder.
- *Long periods of inactivity.* Inactivity during prolonged bed rest or a long plane or car trip can decrease blood flow, causing pooling of blood in leg veins and increasing the risk of clotting. Cramped airline seats with little legroom likely have contributed to an increase in deep vein thrombosis — so much so that it has been referred to as economy class syndrome. In addition, people who are immobilized after surgery, a heart attack or serious injury are more likely to develop blood clots than individuals who are able to get up and walk around. The highest incidence of pulmonary embolism occurs among patients in hospitals.
- *Certain medical conditions.* People with cardiovascular disease associated with localized clot formation, such as heart attack or stroke, are more likely to develop blood clots in their veins.
- *Injury to veins.* This may occur during certain surgical procedures, especially hip surgery or knee replacement. It may also result from leg or pelvic fractures. Finally, a direct traumatic injury to the leg may injure the veins and cause a subsequent clot.
- *Being overweight.* Researchers aren't certain why excess body weight increases risk of blood clots. One theory is that increased levels of estrogen stored in fatty tissue may contribute to blood clots in some women.
- *Antiphospholipid-antibody syndrome.* The presence of anticardiolipin antibodies predisposes you to venous or arterial blood clots. The clots can occur for no appar-

ent reason or in association with diseases like systemic lupus erythematosus. In addition to increased risk of blood clots, antiphospholipid-antibody syndrome is associated with obstetrical complications, stroke and other blood disorders, such as autoimmune breakdown of red blood cells or platelets.

Combined risk factors

Inherited risk factors for venous thrombosis are prevalent among the general population. Yet only some people with these abnormalities develop blood clots in their veins. The combination of an inherited risk factor and an acquired risk factor, such as vein damage from surgery, may increase your overall risk of venous thrombosis.

If you have a family history of excessive clot formation, you may want to talk to your doctor about preventive measures to take during high-risk situations, such as orthopedic surgery or travel. Certain inherited and acquired risk factors for venous thrombosis also can lead to problems during pregnancy, such as premature labor, fetal growth retardation or recurrent spontaneous abortions.

Tests are available to diagnose some genetic conditions that cause excessive clot formation, but the pros and cons of such testing must be weighed carefully. Although testing might give you a greater awareness of your risk, it could lead to difficulty obtaining health and life insurance.

Treatment

People with venous thrombosis are generally treated with anticoagulants (blood thinners) such as warfarin (Coumadin) or heparin to help stop clot formation.

The exact duration of the treatment depends on your particular situation. If you have a chronic disorder that puts you at high risk of recurrent clot formation and pulmonary embolism, you may need to stay on these medications for the rest of your life. In general, though, you only take the medication for a limited time, usually 3 to 6 months, for deep blood clot treatment.

As with all medications, the benefits of anticoagulants in preventing clots needs to be weighed against the risks. Anticoagulants increase your risk of bleeding complications. Many of these complications are minor, such as bleeding from your gums, but some bleeding may be severe and life-threatening.

People taking warfarin need periodic blood tests to check whether their dosage is appropriate: too high a dose can lead to bleeding, and too low a dose isn't effective in preventing clot formation.

During anticoagulant therapy, avoid use of aspirin and other nonsteroidal anti-inflammatory drugs (NSAIDs), such as ibuprofen (Advil, Motrin, others). These medications also affect your platelets' ability to form clots, and when combined with warfarin or heparin, may increase your risk of bleeding.

Because more than 100 other medications, including over-the-counter medications, and herbs can interact with anticoagulants, tell your doctor about all of the medications you're taking, even nonprescription medications and supplements.

Transfusions and Transplants

A variety of treatments are used to treat blood disorders. Two of the most common forms of treatment are blood transfusions and stem cell transplants.

Blood transfusions

Blood transfusions are often a necessary component of treatment for people with certain blood disorders. Blood transfusions increase the blood's ability to transport oxygen, boost immunity and speed clotting time. Transfusions are also used to replace lost blood after an accident or surgery. More than 4 million Americans receive blood transfusions each year.

During a blood transfusion, either whole blood (blood cells plus plasma) or a component of blood is infused into your bloodstream. The blood used in a transfusion is compatible with your blood type and enters your bloodstream through an intravenous (IV) line.

Types

Various components of blood may be transfused. These include packed red blood cells, fresh-frozen plasma, cryoprecipitate, coagulation factor concentrate, granulocytes (a type of white blood cell) and platelets.

When donated blood stored as collected is infused, this is known as whole blood transfusion. The type of transfusion given usually depends on the condition being treated.

Red blood cells

If you're deficient in red blood cells but not in the other components of blood, a transfusion of packed red blood cells is often best. This provides only the red blood cells that you need, without extra blood volume from other blood components. Too much blood circulating in your blood vessels can cause complications such as congestive heart failure.

Transfusions of red blood cells are often used to treat various types of anemia. Red blood cells may also be infused during an acute crisis of inherited anemias such as sickle cell disease, thalassemia or glucose-6-phosphate dehydrogenase deficiency.

Red blood cells can be kept in storage in a liquid form for a maximum of 6 weeks. Frozen red blood cells may be stored for up to 10 years.

Autologous Transfusions

The safest blood for you to receive is your own. Your immune system won't consider your blood foreign, and you can't give yourself any infections that you don't already have. Transfusing one's own blood, known as autologous transfusion, is becoming more popular.

In an emergency, you may have to rely on transfusions from random donors unless you're at a medical center that can salvage blood otherwise lost during surgery. However, if your doctor is planning elective surgery, ask if you can donate your own blood ahead of time. Usually, you give it over a period of a few weeks in advance of your operation. Your blood will be stored and used, if necessary, to replace blood that you lose during the operation.

It may cost more to receive your own blood than to get a random donor transfusion. The reason is the extra work involved in specially labeling your own blood, storing it separately and delivering it to you at the right time. However, many people consider the added expense to be worth it. If, for some reason, you can't donate your own blood, a blood bank will select a donor whose blood shouldn't cause an adverse reaction.

During surgery, it's possible to recover the blood a patient loses during an operation and return it to that patient. In this procedure, known as intraoperative autologous transfusion, surgeons salvage blood cells from the wound while they're operating. The cells are washed free of debris from the wound and then returned to the patient.

Because there will always be situations in which using your own blood is impossible, the increase in autologous transfusions doesn't eliminate the need for blood donors.

Fresh-frozen plasma

Fresh-frozen plasma is used to treat clotting disorders, including mild forms of hemophilia and von Willebrand's disease, as well as serious burns. This blood product can be stored frozen for 1 year.

Cryoprecipitate

People who are missing certain blood-clotting factors sometimes receive cryoprecipitate, a component of plasma containing certain blood-clotting factors. It's used to treat hemophilia, von Willebrand's disease and other clotting disorders.

Coagulation factor concentrate

Coagulation factor concentrates are freeze-dried preparations of specific clotting factors from plasma. Before being transfused, the concentrate must be reconstituted. It's used to treat certain disorders, such as hemophilia.

Granulocytes

Transfusions of granulocytes may be used to treat severe neonatal sepsis, a widespread infection in the body. However, these transfusions are rarely needed today because of the availability of antibiotics. Granulocytes can be stored for only a few hours.

Platelets

Platelet transfusions are used to control bleeding in people who have conditions with certain blood abnormalities. Among people who have undergone chemotherapy or radiation to treat diseases such as leukemia, lymphoma or thrombocytopenia, production of platelets may be suppressed. These individuals are sometimes given transfusions of platelets. Platelets can be stored for only about 5 days before they become inactive.

Blood groups

When a transfusion is necessary, not just any blood will do. Your blood type dictates the type of blood you can receive.

Blood groups were discovered around 1900, when it was observed that blood collected for transfusions was compatible in some recipients but not in others. It was determined that each person spontaneously forms antibodies against specific proteins (antigens) that his or her own red blood cells lack. If you receive blood that contains proteins different from those in your own blood, your antibodies attack the cells in the transfused blood that carry them.

Blood groups are based on the proteins (antigens), carried on your red blood cells. Like other physical characteristics, the specific antigens in your blood are determined by genes inherited from your parents.

There are four major blood groups: A, B, AB and O. Each of these is divided into two rhesus (Rh) types, positive and negative. The most common blood group in the United States is O positive, followed by A positive, B positive, O negative, A negative, AB positive, B negative and AB negative.

If your blood group is A, your red blood cells are coated with A antigens, and your plasma develops antibodies against B. If your blood group is B, you have B antigens and your plasma develops antibodies against A. Type AB blood has both A and B antigens, and type O has neither.

In most cases, blood that's the exact same type as yours must be used in a transfusion. For example, if you have A positive blood, you must receive A positive blood. However, type O negative can be used in emergencies for all of the blood types.

If your blood is Rh-negative, your red blood cells don't carry an antigen called the rhesus (Rh) factor. If it's Rh-positive, they do.

Women may develop anti-Rh antibodies after exposure to Rh-positive blood at the time of their first pregnancy. If exposed again to Rh-positive blood, serious complications and even death could result. To avoid risks, Rh-typing is done

Blood Safety

Which is safer? Getting in your car and driving to the grocery store or receiving a blood transfusion? A blood transfusion is far safer.

Emergence of the AIDS epidemic prompted significant changes in the way blood is donated, tested and transfused. As a result, the nation's blood supply is safer than at any time in the past.

- *Blood banks are carefully regulated.* All blood banks in this country are federally regulated by the Food and Drug Administration (FDA).
- *Potential donors are carefully screened.* Donors must fill out a written medical history that includes direct questions about behaviors that may lead to a higher risk of transmitting blood-borne infection. They're also interviewed by a trained health care professional who reinforces the importance of a safe blood supply and risk factors that compromise that goal.
- *All donated blood is thoroughly tested.* A highly sensitive test for human immunodeficiency virus (HIV) is used to screen all donated blood. Screening tests also are done to check for hepatitis viruses, human T-lymphotropic viruses and syphilis.

Researchers also continue to investigate methods for sterilizing various blood components. Certain techniques are in clinical trials but have yet to receive FDA approval.

Donating Blood

Individuals 18 years of age or older and who weigh at least 110 pounds are eligible to donate blood. However, having certain communicable diseases may preclude you from giving blood. These include hepatitis and the human immunodeficiency virus (HIV). In addition, don't donate blood if you think that you may have an infection. Instead, see your doctor.

When you agree to give blood, trained staff will take a small sample of your blood to check if it contains adequate hemoglobin, the oxygen-carrying component of your blood. They'll also ask you some questions about your health and check your heart rate, blood pressure and temperature. If your health is good and your hemoglobin concentration is normal, staff will draw a pint of blood from a vein in your arm.

Giving blood is quick and generally causes little, if any, pain. It's also safe. New, sterile, disposable equipment is used for each donor. Therefore, there's no risk of contracting a blood-borne disease by donating blood.

The average volume of blood in the body is 10 to 12 pints in men and 8 to 9 pints in women. The usual amount of blood taken during donation is 1 pint. If you're a healthy adult, you can spare this amount without affecting your well-being. Within a few hours, your body will have replaced the fluid you've lost. Your red blood cells will have returned to their usual numbers well before you're eligible to give blood again in about 8 weeks.

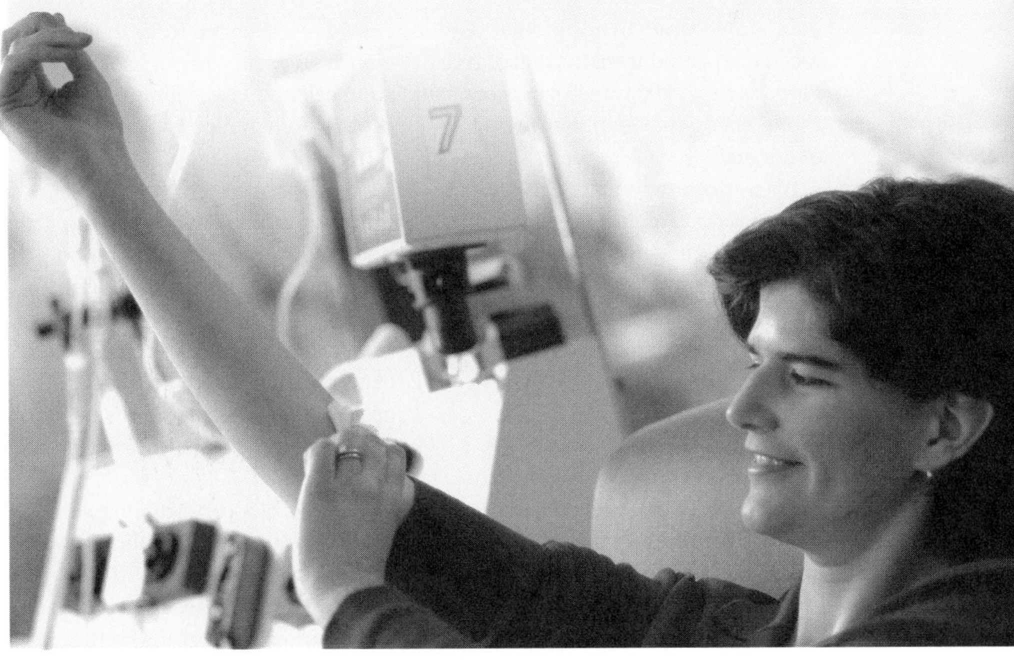

routinely before transfusions, and blood of the same Rh type is used for transfusions.

Many other minor blood subgroups also occur that can become important in circumstances such as multiple transfusions or organ transplantation.

Risks

Blood transfusions are generally safe, but risks exist. They include:

Antibody reactions

Before you receive a blood transfusion, a blood bank typically mixes a sample of the donor's blood with yours to check compatibility — a process called crossmatching. Despite these precautions, it's possible that you may carry antibodies against the donor's red blood cells, white blood cells or platelets. This can lead to an immune reaction, which can cause a variety of signs and symptoms, including shaking, chills, fever, hives, wheezing and shortness of breath, chest pain, low back pain, pink urine, nausea and pain along the vein that received the transfusion. Shock, kidney failure or intravascular coagulation rarely ensue but may cause death.

Your risk of having such an immune reaction is increased if you've received multiple blood transfusions in the past. Exposure to blood antigens from multiple donors may lead to antibodies against obscure blood groups.

Communicable diseases
Although the risk of contracting a communicable disease from a blood transfusion is remote, it's always a possibility. All blood donors are screened, and donated blood is tested for viruses such as the human immunodeficiency virus (HIV), hepatitis and human T-lymphotropic virus. Methods to sterilize blood components have been developed and are being tested in clinical trials. These methods may further improve safety in the future.

Other reactions
Other adverse reactions to transfusions are possible. For instance, if you have heart trouble, you may have difficulty handling an increase in blood volume. In addition, if you receive repeated transfusions of red blood cells — 200 transfusions or more — you may experience iron overload.

It's important to realize that most people who receive a transfusion have no adverse reactions or infections as a result. If you need a transfusion, don't let unfounded or exaggerated fears keep you from accepting it.

Future products
Researchers at many medical centers are working to develop synthetic substitutes for blood. There are several reasons for this effort.

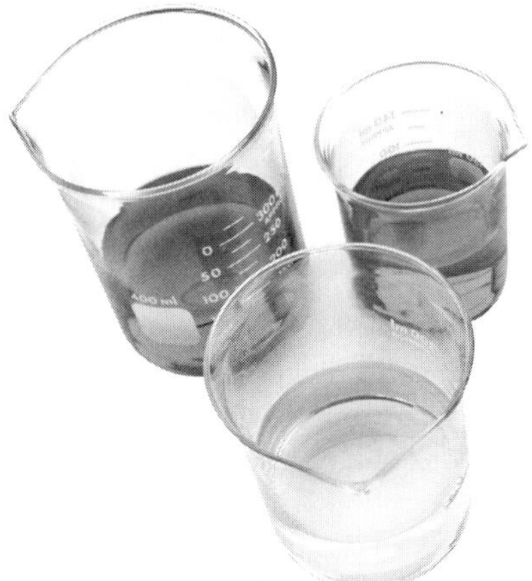

Synthetic substitutes could help to prevent transfusion complications, such as infection and immunologic reactions, and overcome shortages of donated blood. The substances are still experimental. In addition, although they're designed to carry oxygen, they can't perform other important functions of the blood.

Stem cell transplantation

Transplanting stem cells offers hope to people with certain blood and bone marrow disorders, including aplastic anemia, leukemia, lymphoma and multiple myeloma.

Stem cells produce all the different types of cells and tissues that make up your body. When a stem cell divides, one of the resulting cells becomes specialized — it creates certain types of cells in your body, such as blood, heart or brain cells. The other cell from that division is an exact copy of the original stem cell and is available for future division when repair is needed.

Transplanting blood-producing stem cells harvested from bone marrow or blood can allow the body to replenish healthy blood cells when existing cells are damaged, either due to disease or use of medication to destroy disease. For example, high doses of chemotherapy or radiation treatments used to kill cancer cells also destroy stem cells.

Healthy blood-producing stem cells generate the 200 billion new oxygen-carrying red blood cells required by your body each day, as well as infection-fighting white blood cells and platelets that help stop bleeding. Blood-producing stem cells can be harvested from the bone marrow or blood, either from a donor or from the individual in need of them.

When treating blood disorders, bone marrow has traditionally been used as the source of blood-producing stem cells. This sponge-like material found inside certain bones produces most stem cells. After treatments such as chemotherapy and radiation to treat cancer, bone marrow is transplanted into the individual receiving treatment. Bone marrow transplants have been performed successfully for more than 30 years.

Currently, stem cell transplants commonly use blood rather than bone marrow as the source of the stem cells. In the early 1980s, researchers discovered that stem cells circulate in the bloodstream. These cells are called peripheral blood stem cells. They're rather scarce in the bloodstream, but their numbers can be increased by medications that encourage bone marrow to release stem cells.

Use of peripheral blood stem cells instead of bone marrow makes transplants safer, particularly for older adults. This type of transplant procedure is called peripheral blood stem cell transplantation.

Types
A stem cell transplant may be performed in a variety of manners:

Syngeneic
In a syngeneic transplant, the donor is the identical twin of the stem cell recipient. Identical twins have the same genetic makeup, so the recipient isn't at risk of a severe reaction to the transplant. However, few people have identical twins.

Allogeneic
In this type of transplant, the donor is, preferably, a sibling or parent of the recipient. In order to establish the compatibility of the potential donor's stem cells, a test for human lymphocyte antigens (HLA test) is done to determine if there's an HLA match.

This test examines six proteins found on the surface of the white blood cells and most other cells. The odds of an HLA donor match are about 25 percent with two siblings in a family, but they increase to about 75 percent with six siblings.

If no relative is found with an HLA match, an unrelated donor is selected on the basis of that person's HLA results being identical or nearly identical to the recipient's. A National Bone Marrow Registry has been set up to help locate HLA-matched bone marrow donors.

Autologous

An autologous transplant is often used in individuals with cancer. In an autologous stem cell transplant, stem cells are collected from the person with cancer and stored for later transplant. After the individual receives treatment with high doses of chemotherapy or radiation that can destroy stem cells, the stored cells are transplanted back into the individual. Because the person's own cells are used, there's no risk of rejection.

The procedure

The first step in the transplantation process is the collection (harvest) of stem cells. The procedure used depends on whether blood or bone marrow is chosen as the source of the cells. If blood is chosen, growth factor injections are administered with or without chemotherapy in an attempt to release (mobilize) stem cells from the bone marrow into the bloodstream.

Blood tests are then done to determine if sufficient stem cells have been mobilized. The cells are then collected from a vein — much like when donating blood — but using an apheresis machine. This machine separates the blood into its various components, and only those parts that are needed are saved. The other parts are returned into the body.

When bone marrow is selected as the source of the cells, the person is put under general anesthesia and marrow is removed from a pelvic bone. This involves making small cuts in the skin over the pelvic bone and inserting a large needle to draw marrow from the bone. The process takes about an hour.

The next step typically is administration of chemotherapy with or without radiation therapy to kill the cancer cells. This is followed by preparation of the recipient's bone marrow to accept the transplanted stem cells. Finally, the collected stem cells are injected into the recipient's veins. The cells travel in the bloodstream until they reach bone marrow, where, in about 2 to 3 weeks, they produce new cells.

In syngeneic and allogeneic stem cell transplantation, the stem cells generally are removed from the donor and injected into the recipient on the same day. In autologous transplantation, the stem cells are removed and frozen. These cells can remain frozen for months to years — until the individual has completed treatment.

Diseases when transplantation is used

The best results from allogeneic and syngeneic transplantation have been obtained in cases of severe aplastic anemia, chronic granulocytic leukemia and acute nonlymphocytic leukemia. Clinical trials are evaluating use of stem cell transplantation for treating acute nonlymphocytic leukemia in remission, acute lymphocytic leukemia in remission, lymphoma in remission and neuroblastoma in remission.

In autologous transplantation, the best results have been obtained in treating Hodgkin's disease and non-Hodgkin's lymphoma. Studies suggest that those whose disease is responsive to chemotherapy or who achieve complete remission following use of chemotherapy after a relapse are the best candidates for this procedure. The role of stem cell transplants in breast cancer, ovarian cancer and other solid tumors isn't well established.

Risks

The major cause of toxicity and death in stem cell transplantation is graft-versus-host disease (GVHD). This complication occurs when the transplanted white blood cells from the donor marrow (graft) attack the marrow recipient's (host's) own cells because they perceive the host's cells as foreign.

GVHD can affect the skin, liver, gastrointestinal tract and lungs of the transplant recipient. It's the major complication in allogeneic transplantation, but it isn't a problem in syngeneic or autologous transplantation.

The mortality rate among recipients of an allogeneic transplant ranges from about 10 percent to 40

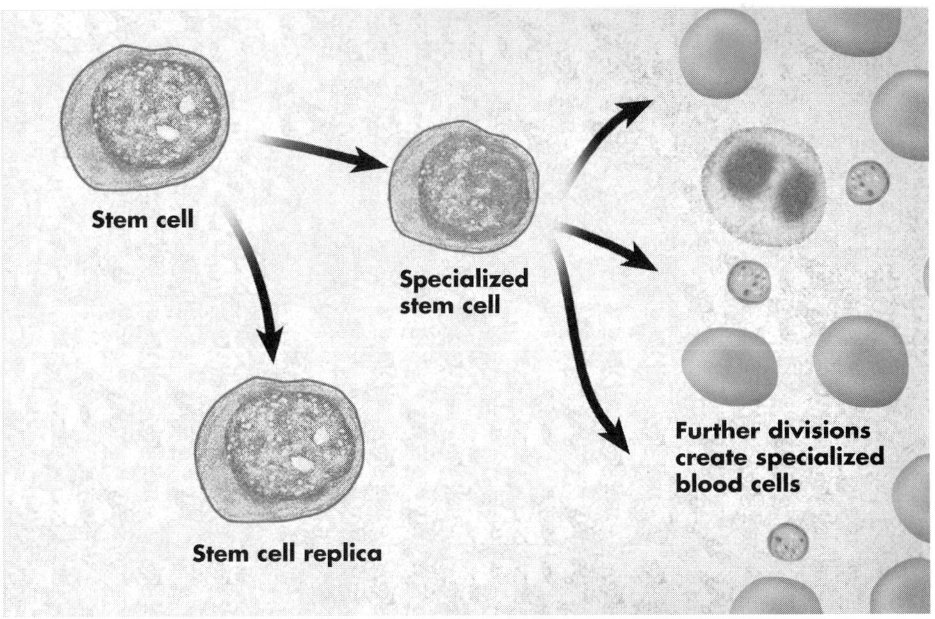

When a stem cell divides, it creates a stem cell that's specialized — one that can create cells, such as blood cells, that perform specific functions. It also creates an exact replica of itself.

percent in the first 100 days after the procedure, primarily from infection or GVHD. Another major problem is pneumonia, which can result from an infection or other complications.

Among people receiving an autologous stem cell transplant, the mortality rate in the first 100 days after the procedure ranges from less than 5 percent to 15 percent.

Clinical trials are being conducted to determine methods to prevent graft-versus-host disease and to otherwise increase the safety and effectiveness of stem cell transplants. ■

CHAPTER **36** PART V

Skin, Hair and Nails

Your skin is a unique and remarkable organ. The 2 square yards of skin that cover the average adult constitute approximately 15 percent of the body's total weight. Each square inch of your skin contains millions of cells and many specialized nerve endings for sensing heat, cold and pain. In addition, skin contains oil glands, hair follicles and sweat glands. An intricate network of blood vessels nourishes this complex structure.

Your skin serves many purposes. For one, it's your body's first line of defense against the environment around you. It helps protect you from injury, infection and harmful substances. By its texture, temperature, color and clarity, your skin gives information about your general health.

Your skin also serves as your body's heat regulator. Blood vessels in your skin dilate or constrict according to your body's temperature. When you're hot, you sweat and the evaporation of the sweat on your skin lowers your body's temperature. When your body is chilled, these blood vessels become narrowed, and your skin becomes pale and cold. This constriction decreases the flow of blood through your skin, reducing heat loss and conserving heat for other organs of your body.

Your sweat glands also excrete waste products, such as urea. However, this is a minor pathway of waste disposal compared with your kidneys' production of urine.

Your skin plays a major role in your sense of touch. Sensory nerves send signals to your brain about hazards. Another group of specialized nerve endings in your skin can arouse your nerve and endocrine systems to sexual excitement.

Your nails and your hair serve important functions too. Your nails, which are a product of your skin cells, help you pick up and handle objects and provide signs of your general health. Each individual hair on your body grows from its own follicle located in your skin. Your hair helps protect your scalp from excessive sun exposure and your head from trauma.

Over your lifetime, you may develop problems with your skin, hair and nails. Most of these conditions are best treated by a skin specialist, called a dermatologist.

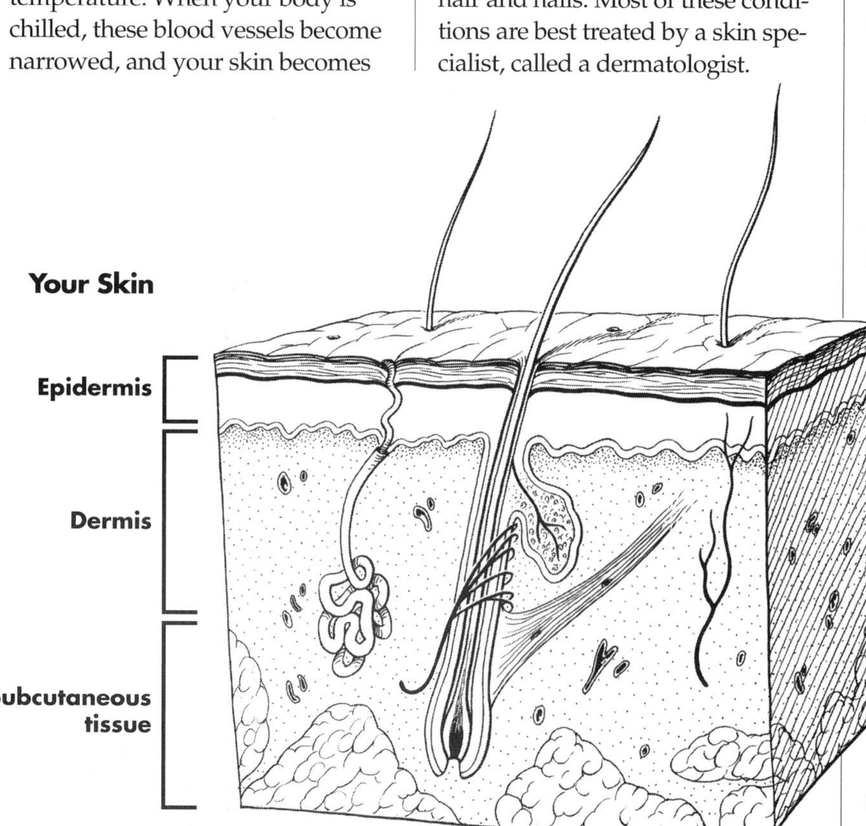

The Basics

Your skin, hair and nails are interrelated. Your nails, hair and outer layer of skin (epidermis) are each composed of the protein keratin. But each of these three body parts has its own unique characteristics.

Your skin

Your skin is composed of three layers — the epidermis, the dermis and the subcutaneous tissue. Your skin averages only a tenth of an inch in thickness, ranging from very thin on your eyelids and the inner folds of your elbows to very thick on the palms of your hands and soles of your feet. Housed in your skin are sweat glands, oil glands and hair follicles.

Epidermis

Your skin's outer layer, the epidermis, is as thin as a pencil line. It provides a protective layer of skin cells that you continuously shed. Squamous cells lie just below the outer surface. Basal cells, which produce new skin cells, are at the bottom of the epidermis.

It takes approximately 1 month for new skin cells to move from the basal cells to the outer surface. As the cells move away from their source of nourishment, they become smaller and flatter, changing into a lifeless protein called keratin. They remain on the surface only briefly as a protective cover and then flake off as a result of washing and friction. Thus, the skin is a dynamic organ that's constantly replenished.

Cells that manufacture skin constitute about 95 percent of your epidermis. The remaining cells produce a black pigment, called melanin.

Melanin provides the coloring of your skin and helps protect it from ultraviolet light. People of all races are born with the same number of pigment cells (melanocytes). The rate at which melanin granules are formed in these cells and their concentration in the epidermis are inherited characteristics and major factors in skin color differences.

Dermis

Just below the epidermis is the dermis, which makes up 90 percent of the bulk of your skin. It's a dense bed of strong, white fibers (collagen) and yellow, elastic fibers (elastin) through which blood vessels, muscle cells, nerve fibers, lymph channels, hair follicles and glands are interspersed.

The dermis gives strength and elasticity to your skin. As you age, the dermis layer becomes thinner and your skin more transparent. This accounts for the prominence of blood vessels in the skin of older adults.

Subcutaneous tissue

The deepest layer of skin is the subcutaneous tissue, through which blood vessels and nerves run. This layer, composed primarily of fat, insulates and protects your inner organs and helps keep your skin resilient. The roots of your oil and sweat glands are located here. Subcutaneous tissue also thins with aging.

Oil glands

Oil glands (sebaceous glands) are distributed throughout your skin but are most concentrated in your scalp, face, midchest and genitals. They're each attached to a hair follicle and secrete an oily substance (sebum) that rises through the follicle to the surface of the skin. The oily sebum — made up of fatty acids, cholesterol, various hydrocarbons, unsaturated alcohols and waxes — lubricates and protects your skin.

Sweat glands

You have two types of sweat glands. The eccrine glands are distributed throughout your body, with the richest supply in your palms, soles, scalp and underarms. The apocrine glands are specialized sweat glands that secrete sweat in times of stress or emotion. In the ear, they form a portion of the earwax. They're most abundant under your arms and around your nipples and genitals.

Your hair

The human being is a hairy animal. Only your lips, palms and soles are truly hairless. Each hair grows from a single, live follicle that has its roots in the subcutaneous tissue of your skin.

Oil from an oil gland next to the hair follicle provides gloss and, to some degree, waterproofing for the hair. Your hair follicles are nourished by minerals, proteins, vitamins, fats and carbohydrates brought to them by tiny blood vessels (capillaries).

Like the surface of your epidermis, hair is made up of the dead protein keratin and also contains melanin. Just as the pigment cells determine your skin color, the number of melanin granules in your hair determines its color.

Your fingernails and toenails

Your fingernails and toenails also are products of your epidermis and are composed of the protein keratin. Each nail grows outward from a nail root (matrix) that extends into a skin nail fold.

Contrary to common belief, the structure of your nails isn't related to the structure of your bones. You can't strengthen brittle fingernails or toenails by taking extra calcium or gelatin.

Your fingernails normally grow at the rate of an eighth of an inch a month, approximately two to three times faster than your toenails. Nail growth slows in old age. Sudden or significant changes in the appearance of your nails can be an early sign of illness.

Hair Follicle

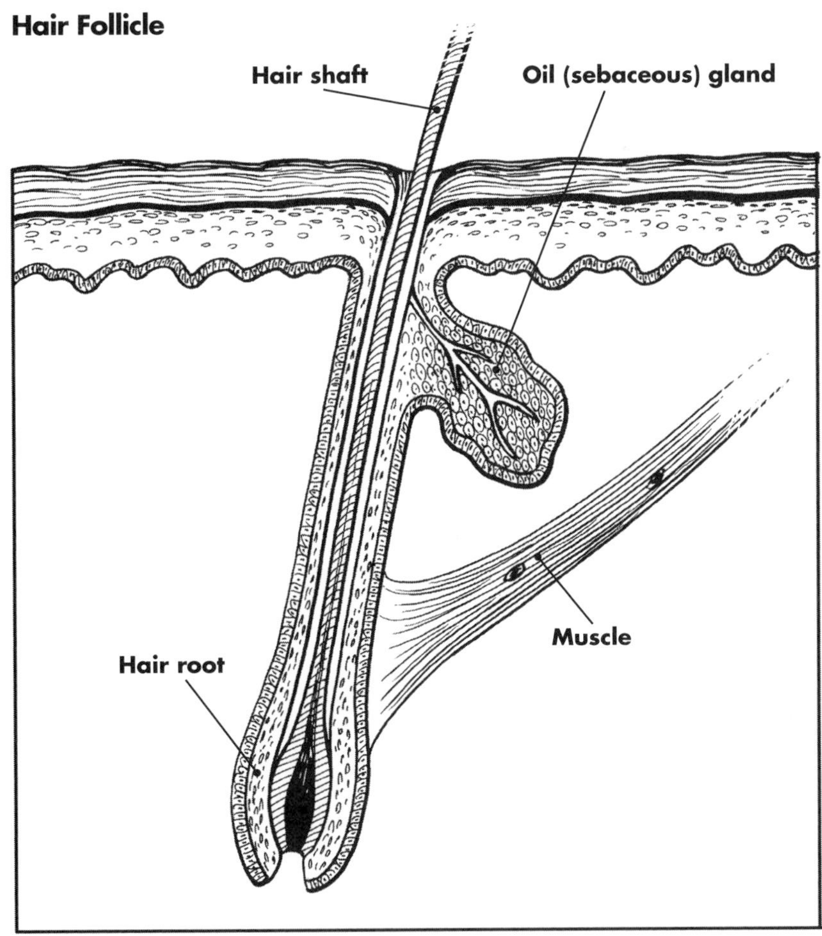

Your Fingernail

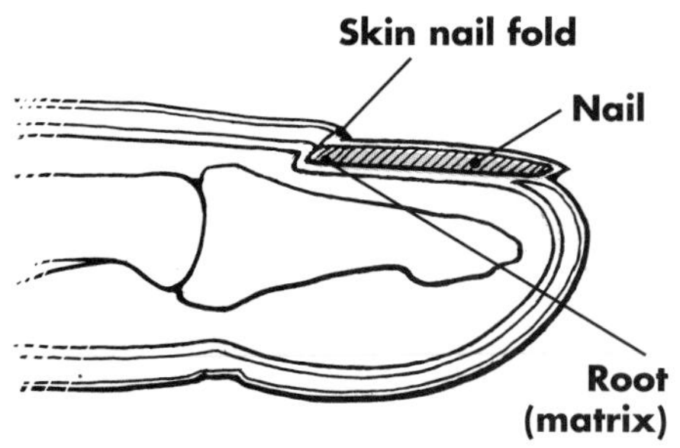

Proper Skin Care

Your skin isn't the baby-soft body glove you were born with. With age, your skin normally becomes thinner and finely wrinkled. Oil-producing (sebaceous) glands become less active, and your skin becomes drier. The number of blood vessels in your skin decreases, and your dermis can get thinner and more fragile, so you lose your youthful color and glow.

In addition, with aging your skin replaces old cells more slowly, and cells repair themselves less effectively. This can result in slower turnover of surface skin and slower healing of damaged skin.

Good self-care habits can help delay the natural aging process and prevent many skin problems. The single most important goal is to protect your skin from ultraviolet light. Follow these tips to keep your skin healthy. The benefits of good skin care will become increasingly apparent as you grow older.

Avoid the sun

Regardless of your skin color or your age, avoiding exposure to ultraviolet rays from the sun and tanning beds can help prevent unnecessary aging as well as later skin cancer.

Dark skin can tolerate more sun than fair skin. However, any skin can become blotchy, leathery and wrinkled from long-term overexposure to the sun. Avoiding the sun — particularly during peak hours — wearing protective clothing, applying sunscreen and lubricating or moisturizing your skin daily can help protect it from the sun's harmful effects.

Don't smoke

Nicotine in tobacco smoke constricts blood vessels that nourish your skin. Over time, smoking can cause your skin to become pale and sallow. It can also cause deep wrinkles to develop around your lips and slow your skin's ability to heal.

Use appropriate cosmetics

If you use cosmetics, be sure to match them to your skin type: If you have dry skin, use makeup with a heavier, creamier base. If you have skin that's oily or acne prone, use a water-based product that's labeled noncomedogenic, which means that it's less likely to clog the small openings in your skin (pores). Preferably, choose a brand of foundation, lipstick and eyeliner that's nonallergenic. Look for a moisturizer that's fragrance-free and has the least amount of preservatives. If you know that you're allergic to any of the ingredients in a product, avoid it.

Cleanse gently

Proper cleansing is another important strategy in protecting your skin. The best procedures and cleansing ingredients vary according to the type of skin you have — oily, dry, balanced or a combination.

If you wear eye makeup, remove it first using cotton balls to avoid damaging the delicate tissue around your eyes. When washing your face, use tepid, never hot, water and a washcloth or sponge to remove dead cells. Use a mild soap for your face and skin. A mild superfatted variety of soap, such as Dove or Basis, may be better if your facial skin is dry. You may need to clean oily skin two or three times each day.

What's Your Skin Color?

Skin color is defined by the degree to which you tan or burn when exposed to the sun. Your skin color affects your risk of skin cancer and photoaging, a term that describes damage from ultraviolet rays to the skin, including wrinkles, pigmentation and roughness.

The Fitzpatrick Classification of Skin Type divides skin into the following six categories:

1. Always burns, never tans (pale, white skin)
2. Always burns easily, tans minimally (white skin)
3. Burns moderately, tans uniformly (light brown skin)
4. Burns minimally, always tans well (moderate brown skin)
5. Rarely burns, tans profusely (dark brown skin)
6. Never burns (deeply pigmented dark brown to black skin)

Type 1 people typically have pale, white skin, red or blond hair, blue or green eyes and Celtic (Irish, Scottish, Welsh or Breton) ancestry. People with this skin type have the greatest risk of sun-induced skin problems, including skin cancer and photoaging. Type 2 and 3 people have more pigmented shades of white skin and have a moderate to strong risk of sun-induced skin problems. Type 4 and 5 people have olive to medium brown skin color and have moderate to low risk of sun-induced skin problems. Type 6 people have dark brown to black skin color. Their risk of skin problems related to sun exposure is minimal.

Because no one is completely immune from sun damage and skin cancer, dermatologists recommend using a broad-spectrum sunscreen with a sun protection factor (SPF) of 15 or higher for all skin types.

Bathing can dry your skin. Especially during dry weather, follow the antidrying bathing basics found on page 1178.

Shave gently

Shaving can irritate thin, dry or photoaged skin. If you shave with a blade razor, always use a sharp blade.

Men can soften their beard before shaving by applying a warm washcloth for a few seconds and use plenty of shaving cream. Pass the blade over your beard only once, in the direction of hair growth. If you reverse the stroke to obtain a close shave, you can cause a skin irritation called razor burn. Using an electric razor too vigorously also can irritate your skin. You can buy various preparations to prevent skin irritation caused by an electric razor.

Women who shave or use hair remover also need to avoid skin irritation. If you're using a hair remover for the first time, determine whether the product is irritating to your skin by applying the preparation to a small area.

What's Your Skin Type?

The skin of your face is generally the best guide in classifying skin type. Examine your skin closely, especially the pores.

Oily skin

Oily skin is caused by overactivity of the oil-producing (sebaceous) glands. Oily skin has large pores. People with oily skin tend to develop acne, and they're less likely to develop wrinkles as early in life as people with dry skin are. Most people with oily skin also have oily hair.

Dry skin

Dry skin can be caused by underactivity of the sebaceous glands, environmental conditions or normal aging. Dry skin is usually more easily irritated. It's often associated with dry hair and small pores. People with dry skin tend not to develop acne. As they age, their skin tends to become drier and more wrinkled than that of people with oily skin.

Balanced skin

Balanced skin is neither oily nor dry. It's smooth with fine texture and few problems. It has a tendency to become dry as a result of environmental factors and aging.

Combination skin

Combination skin consists of oily regions — often on the forehead and around the nose — and regions that are balanced or dry.

Skin Disorders

Your skin is surprisingly resistant to a wide variety of insults, but it's still susceptible to various problems. The skin disorders that follow aren't life-threatening or contagious, but they can cause acute discomfort or make you upset about your appearance. Your symptoms may disappear in a week, may require surgery or may call for a long-term treatment program.

The term *dermatitis*, which is used interchangeably with the term *eczema*, simply means an inflammation of the skin. Generally, dermatitis involves swollen, reddened and itchy skin. It has many causes.

Contact dermatitis

Signs and symptoms

- Redness and itching
- Blisters and weeping from the involved skin in severe cases
- Skin changes limited to the area of contact with the causative agent

Contact dermatitis (see the color illustration on page 432) results from direct contact with an irritant or allergen. Common irritants include laundry soap, skin soap and cleaning products. Possible allergens include rubber, metals, jewelry, perfume, cosmetics and plants such as poison ivy. If you're sensitive to an allergen, just brief exposure to a small amount of allergen can cause dermatitis.

In contact dermatitis, only the areas of skin contacted by the offending substance react. The area with the greatest exposure reacts most severely.

Diagnosis

If your dermatologist suspects your skin problem is the result of an allergic reaction, he or she may test your skin by applying small amounts of different substances and examining the site for allergic reactions 48, 72 and 96 hours later. This assessment, called patch testing, determines if you have allergic contact dermatitis, which is caused by an immune system reaction. Relatively few people have such a response. In allergic contact dermatitis, the allergen might be something that you had been in contact with for years without trouble until now.

Substances such as acids, solvents, strong soaps and detergents are usually irritants rather than allergens. When an irritant causes a skin reaction, the condition is known as irritant contact dermatitis. Some substances are both allergens and irritants.

Some hard-to-identify causes of contact dermatitis include ingredients in:

- Medicinal lotions, such as antihistamines, antibiotics or antiseptics
- Plants, ranging from trumpet creeper to mangoes
- Rubber
- Metals, such as nickel
- Dyes
- Cosmetics
- Chemicals used in manufacturing, such as those used in the production of shoes or clothing

Some substances cause dermatitis only when they contact skin exposed to sunlight (see page 1183). Typical examples include shaving lotions, sunscreens, ointments containing sulfa drugs, some perfumes and coal-tar products. Other causes of contact dermatitis may be airborne, such as ragweed pollen and insecticide spray.

Treatment

Treatment of contact dermatitis consists primarily of identifying the offending agent and avoiding it. Sometimes, hydrocortisone-containing creams or slightly astringent wet dressings may help relieve redness and itching. A slightly astringent dressing can be made by wetting a dressing with a solution of 1 ounce white vinegar to 16 to 32 ounces water.

Neurodermatitis

Signs and symptoms

- Itching, aggravated by nervous tension
- Small patches of thickened, leathery skin
- Scratch marks (excoriations)

Neurodermatitis is a common skin disorder, sometimes referred to as lichen simplex chronicus, that consists of small, flat growths (plaques) of various sizes, generally 1 to 10 inches in diameter. The growths have definite margins that have become thickened and leather-like (lichenified).

Neurodermatitis can occur when something such as a tight garment rubs or scratches your skin. This irritation may lead you to rub or scratch your skin repeatedly. Common locations for the disorder include the ankles, waist, outer forearm or arm and the back of your neck.

Generalized neurodermatitis is a similar condition, but it tends to involve more of the body. The affected skin tends to be less leathery. Long-standing neurodermatitis may lead to brownish pigmentation. This condition is often associated with nervous tension and anxiety.

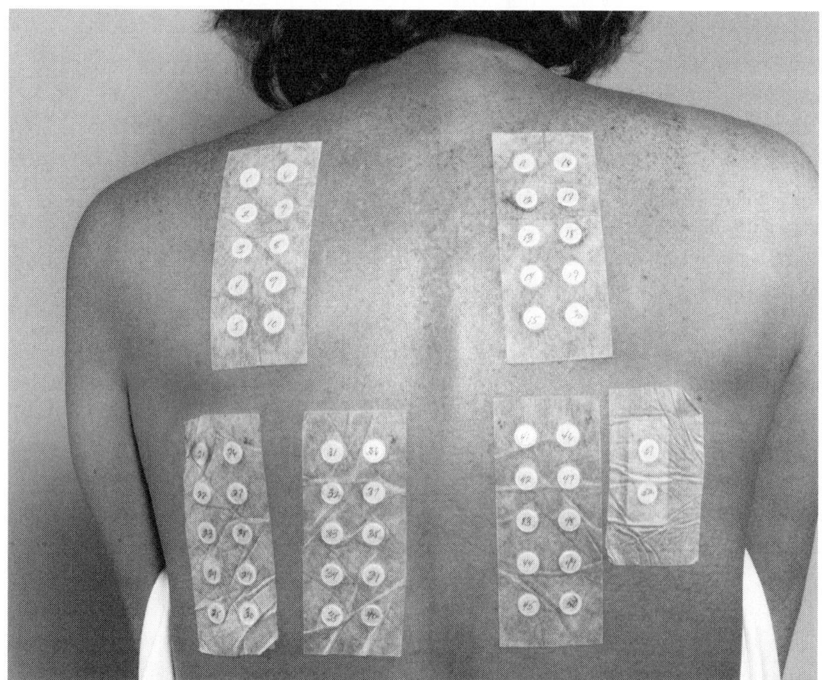

Patch testing can be helpful in determining if you're allergic to a specific substance. Small amounts of different substances are placed on your skin under an adhesive coating.

Treatment

The primary treatment for these skin problems is to stop the scratching. Scratching makes the skin itch more, creating a vicious cycle. If you have trouble ignoring the itchy area, try placing a dressing over it that's difficult to remove.

Antihistamines or anti-anxiety medications (anxiolytics) may help you stop the scratching, but your doctor will want to monitor your use of anxiolytics because they can be addictive.

Your doctor may recommend over-the-counter hydrocortisone-containing lotions to decrease the itching and inflammation. If the inflammation is more severe, your doctor may prescribe a stronger cortisone preparation. In addition, the thickened plaques may be thinned by applying tar or salicylic-acid-containing ointments, which have a soothing and peeling effect.

Eczema

Signs and symptoms

- Thickened, fissured skin, most often in the folds of the elbows or

- backs of the knees and on the face, neck, hands and feet
- A rash
- Itching

Eczema (atopic dermatitis) is an itchy inflammation of the skin (see the color illustration on page 436) that's often accompanied by asthma and allergies such as hay fever (allergic rhinitis). Frequently, it runs in families in which other family members have asthma or hay fever. The condition can cause extreme itching and great frustration.

Eczema is common. In the United States, it affects about 10 percent of infants and 3 percent of all Americans. When it occurs in infants, it's called infantile eczema. This condition typically begins in infancy and may vary in severity during childhood and adolescence. It tends to become less of a problem in adulthood, unless it's caused by allergens or irritants in the workplace.

In infants, the condition often involves an oozing, crusting rash, mainly on the face and scalp, but it can occur anywhere. The condition typically improves before age 2, and treatment can help relieve the itching until then. After infancy, the rash becomes dryer and tends to be red to brownish-gray in color. The skin may be scaly or thickened. The intense itching may continue.

In teens and young adults, the patches typically occur on the hands and feet but can occur anywhere, including the bends of the elbows, backs of the knees, ankles, wrists, face, neck and upper chest.

Treatment

Although eczema is related to allergies, eliminating allergens is rarely helpful in treating the condition. Occasionally, items that trap dust — such as feather pillows, down comforters, mattresses, carpeting and drapes — can worsen the condition. Allergy shots usually aren't successful in treating eczema and might even make the condition worse.

Avoid clothing that's rough, tight, scratchy or made from wool. Rapid changes of temperature, sweating and stress also can worsen the condition. Avoid direct contact with wool products, such as rugs, bedding and clothes, as well as harsh soaps and detergents.

Treatment often consists of applying hydrocortisone-containing lotions or nonsteroidal creams to the affected areas. Tacrolimus (Protopic) and pimecrolimus (Elidel) are nonsteroidal creams that help suppress itching, redness and inflammation. Both are approved for short-term or long-term intermittent treatment, generally when other treatments don't work or aren't well tolerated. Tacrolimus and pimecrolimus are more commonly used for mild to moderate eczema.

If your skin cracks open, your doctor may prescribe mildly astringent wet dressings to prevent infection. If itching is severe, oral antihistamines may help. Diphenhydramine (Benadryl, Sominex) has substantial sedative action and may be helpful at bedtime.

Stasis dermatitis

Signs and symptoms

- Thickening of the skin at your ankles and shins
- Discolored — reddish or brownish — skin
- Itching
- Varicose veins

Varicose veins and other circulatory conditions in which the return of fluids to the heart is reduced can cause an increase of fluid in tissues beneath the skin (edema). Such areas may be poorly nourished and become fragile.

Because your ankles are the lowest part of the body and have less supportive tissue, they're often the site of edema. The overlying skin may inflame, itch and discolor. In severe situations, open ulcers that are hard to heal may develop in the skin around the ankles. This condition is called stasis dermatitis (see the color illustration on page 432).

Although initially the skin may become thin, it later becomes irregularly thickened, perhaps in response to the itching and excessive scratching.

Treatment

Treatment of stasis dermatitis consists of correcting the condition that causes fluid to accumulate in your ankles. In case of varicose veins, surgery or other therapies, such as vein sclerosis, may be recommended.

Other options for controlling edema include frequently elevating your legs above the level of your heart. The mainstay of treatment, however, is the use of elastic support stockings that help prevent fluid from accumulating in the ankles by exerting graduated pressure over the ankles and lower legs.

Mildly astringent dressings may be used to soften the thickened, yet fragile, skin and to control infection. Low-potency topical corticosteroids also might be helpful.

Seborrheic dermatitis

Signs and symptoms

- Greasy-appearing, scaling, itching areas in your scalp, at the sides of your nose, between your eyebrows, behind your ears or over your breastbone
- Stubborn, itchy dandruff

Seborrheic dermatitis (see the color illustration on page 432) is characterized by greasy scaling and a somewhat reddened appearance of the skin. It's predominantly found in the scalp and in the folds at the sides of the lower portions of the nose, above the bridge of the nose and over the breastbone. It also occurs beneath the breasts, in the folds of skin in the genital regions and around the navel (umbilicus) in obese people.

Seborrheic dermatitis can cause stubborn, itchy dandruff. It also may appear as cradle cap — crusty, scaly skin on your baby's scalp. Cradle cap usually doesn't appear in children older than 1 year.

Some people are born with an inherited tendency to seborrheic

Infant Skin Conditions

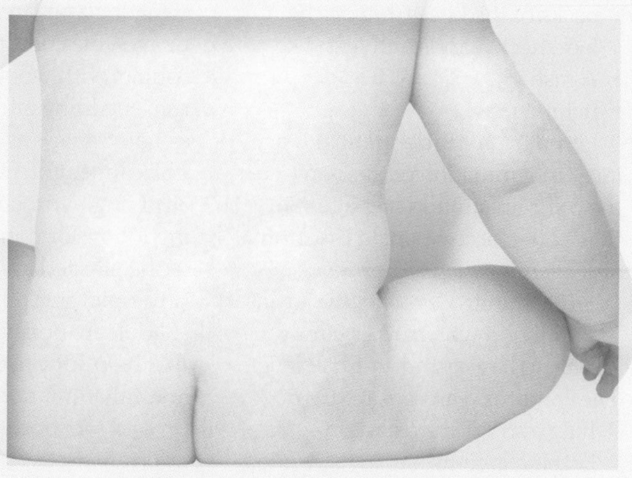

Many parents expect their newborn baby's skin to be flawless. The blemish-free babies in magazine ads may have raised your expectations, but most babies — even those who will someday be in ads — have rashes or blemishes in the early weeks. Most of the time, infant skin conditions are easily treated.

Common infant skin conditions include:

- *Cradle cap.* This crusty skin on the baby's scalp is also called seborrheic dermatitis. Shampooing your baby's hair once a week can help. If cradle cap persists, your baby's doctor may suggest a medicated lotion or another treatment.
- *Diaper rash.* This redness of the skin is caused by moisture, chafing of diapers and the acid in urine or stool. Frequent diaper changes may prevent the rash, but most newborns have diaper rash periodically because their skin is tender. If your child has diaper rash, change your child's diaper frequently, taking care to dry his or her bottom thoroughly, and use a protective cream or ointment. If the rash is mild, you may not need to use the cream or ointment. Check with your baby's doctor if the rash persists.
- *Erythema toxicum.* This is a blotchy, red rash, sometimes with yellowish centers. Most newborns have this rash, typically on the face and torso. It generally disappears without treatment.
- *Heat rash.* In hot, humid weather, your baby may develop tiny, pink bumps on the skin — usually on the back of the neck and upper back. This condition may also be a result of your baby's being wrapped too warmly. The rash usually disappears without treatment, though giving your child cool rinses and dressing him or her in lighter clothing can help.
- *Infant acne.* Infant (newborn) acne may occur within the first 6 to 8 weeks. Whiteheads appear on the face, neck, upper chest or back. This, too, is temporary and doesn't mean that the child will have future skin problems. Treat the condition by gently washing your baby with water daily and with mild soap and water weekly.
- *Infantile eczema.* Infantile eczema (atopic dermatitis) is a rough, red, patchy rash usually associated with extremely dry, sensitive skin. It tends to appear on the cheeks and forehead. Avoid temperature extremes. Most babies with eczema do better in a mild climate with moderate humidity because sweating seems to aggravate the rash. Avoid wool clothing and don't lay the baby on wool carpeting. Keep baths to a minimum and use bath oil to lubricate the dry skin.
- *Milia.* Milia are tiny, white spots on the nose and cheeks. More than half of all newborns have these little spots, which eventually disappear and don't require treatment.
- *Neonatal pimples.* About 20 percent of babies have pimples at birth or in the first 1 or 2 months after birth. Periodic cleaning with mild soap and water is usually adequate. Neonatal pimples don't indicate that your child will have skin blemishes later in life.
- *Peeling, dry skin.* Dry skin on the feet and hands is common in the first 2 weeks and will respond to over-the-counter lotions such as Nivea and Lubriderm.
- *Yeast infection.* This is a persistent, bright red rash in the diaper region, with surrounding lesions, that usually follows a diaper rash. Yeast infections are caused by a fungal organism *(Candida albicans)* that flourishes in a warm, moist environment. If your baby has such a yeast infection, an antifungal cream will help. In addition, frequent diaper changes and airing of the bottom promote dryness.

Although rashes are common and most often treatable at home, have your baby examined if you notice a rash that's purple, crusty, weepy or blistering.

Birthmarks are also common among babies. They include:

- *Cafe au lait spots.* As the name implies, these permanent birthmarks are the color of coffee with cream, occurring most commonly on the baby's torso, arms and legs.
- *Mongolian spots.* This is the traditional term, but you may hear them called blue-gray macule of infancy. These large, blue-gray birthmarks sometimes resemble bruises. They're more common in dark-skinned babies, appearing on the lower back and, less commonly, on the buttocks and legs. They usually disappear later in childhood.
- *Salmon patches.* Sometimes affectionately called stork bites or angel kisses, these reddish or pink patches often occur above the hairline at the back of the neck, on the eyelids or between the baby's eyes. These marks are caused by collections of tiny blood vessels (capillaries) close to the skin. They fade within a child's first 2 years but may not completely go away.

For more on infant skin conditions, see page 167.

dermatitis and will never completely get rid of it, although treatment can help keep it under control. It may occur during times of stress or in people who have neurologic conditions such as Parkinson's disease.

In folds of skin that are kept moist by contact with other skin, for example, beneath your breasts or around your genitals, secondary yeast infections may complicate the condition. You may be more susceptible to these infections if you're taking antibiotics.

Treatment

For dandruff, treatment consists of frequent shampooing of your scalp, followed by careful rinsing. Your doctor may recommend that you shampoo alternately with a regular shampoo and a medicated shampoo, such as Nizoral A-D, which contains ketoconazole and is available over-the-counter or by prescription.

Application of hydrocortisone-containing creams or solutions or ketoconazole cream (Nizoral) may soothe your skin. You may also need treatment for a secondary infection.

Overtreatment dermatitis

Signs and symptoms

- Redness and sensitivity of the skin in areas treated for another skin disorder

Overtreatment dermatitis is the result of overtreatment of a skin condition. Dermatologists often see people who have inflammation of the skin that has persisted for several weeks or months and worsened, despite frequent application of several ointments or other treatments. The inflammation resulting from the excessive treatment obscures the underlying disease, which may or may not still be present. Typically, there's no way that the underlying disorder can be identified.

Treatment

In this situation, your doctor may recommend that you discontinue all treatment other than the most soothing measures for a week or two. This can be hard to accept. Assessing the problem is possible only after all medications are withdrawn. Meanwhile, the problem may improve considerably — or even disappear.

Dandruff

Everyone has some degree of scaling of the skin on their scalp because of the normal process of shedding your outer layer of skin cells. If the flaking becomes obvious on your hair and clothing, it's commonly called dandruff. New studies suggest that a yeast-like organism may cause dandruff. The *Malassezia ovalis* fungus causes irritation and increased sloughing of the top layer of skin cells on your scalp.

If your dandruff persists or you have large flakes together with redness or scaling around your nose, ears or chest, you may have a more severe form of dandruff or perhaps even psoriasis of the scalp. If you have questions about the seriousness of your condition, consult your doctor or a dermatologist.

Treatment

Several over-the-counter products are available to treat dandruff. Try them, along with the following suggestions, to see if they improve your dandruff:

- Shampoo regularly. Start with a mild, nonmedicated shampoo. Gently massage your scalp to loosen flakes. Rinse thoroughly.
- Use medicated shampoo (Head & Shoulders, Selsun Blue) for stubborn cases. Look for shampoos containing pyrithione zinc, salicylic acid, coal tar or selenium sulfide. If necessary to control flaking, use a dandruff shampoo each time you shampoo. Rotating different types of shampoo may help. For mild dandruff, alternate dandruff shampoo with your regular shampoo.
- Consider trying the antifungal shampoo Nizoral A-D to kill dandruff-causing fungi that may live on your scalp. Nizoral A-D is available both over-the-counter or by prescription.
- If you use tar-based shampoos, use them carefully. They can leave a brownish stain on light-colored or gray hair and make your scalp more sensitive to sunlight.
- Use a conditioner regularly.

If dandruff persists or your scalp becomes irritated or severely itchy, you may need a prescription shampoo. Dandruff isn't contagious and is rarely serious, but your skin may be more susceptible to infection. If your dandruff persists, you may have another skin condition. See your doctor.

Acne

Signs and symptoms

- Blackheads or whiteheads on the face, neck, shoulders or back
- Pimples ("zits")
- Cysts

Acne, a skin disorder characterized by pimples due to clogged pores, is a common frustration for teens. In fact, it affects four of every five people between the ages of 12 and 24. But it can affect people of all ages. An estimated one in five adults between 25 and 44 experience acne, and nearly half of all adult women experience mild to moderate acne.

Acne occurs when the hair follicles of your skin become plugged. Each follicle contains oil-producing (sebaceous) glands that secrete a fatty oil (sebum) to lubricate your hair and skin. When your body produces sebum and dead cells faster than they can exit from the pore, the two solidify as a soft, white plug. This plug may close the pore, causing the follicle wall to bulge, thus creating a whitehead. If the pore stays open, the top surface of the plug may darken, causing a blackhead.

A pimple is inflammation that develops when a whitehead ruptures a hair follicle wall below the skin surface. After the rupture, solidified sebum, dead cells and bacteria invade your skin. Ruptures deep within your skin form boil-like lesions called cystic acne (see the color illustration on page 435).

In some situations, the sebaceous gland continues to secrete material that doesn't rupture through the skin. Instead, a flattened, pliable lump forms under the skin. This is called a sebaceous cyst (wen). Sometimes, the lumps can be an inch or more in diameter. Generally, there's no discoloration or pain unless the cyst becomes infected.

Acne is most prevalent in adolescence because hormonal changes stimulate the sebaceous glands to increase sebum production during these years. Acne related to hormonal changes is also common in:

- Women and adolescent girls 2 to 7 days before their periods
- Pregnant women
- People under stress
- People using certain medications, including corticosteroids

Other risk factors for acne include:

- Exposing your skin directly to greasy or oily substances
- Having a family history of acne
- Using sports equipment or wearing clothing that rubs against your skin
- Being Caucasian

Application of oil or grease to your skin can aggravate acne. This includes use of oil-based makeup, suntan oil or hairdressing solutions, as well as oils from machinery or cooking. Acne isn't caused by dirt. In fact, scrubbing the skin too hard or cleansing with harsh soaps or chemicals can cause irritation, which may make acne worse.

Diagnosis

Acne usually is easy to diagnose. Pimple-like pustules alone, with no blackheads or whiteheads, may be another skin disease or a reaction to medications such as corticosteroids.

How serious is acne?

For many people, acne is an ongoing (chronic) problem from puberty through early adulthood. It eventually clears up in most cases, but you may want to seek treatment from a dermatologist for persistent pimples or inflamed cysts to avoid scarring or other damage to your skin.

In addition, the condition can affect self-esteem, confidence, personality and social life. These potential problems are also legitimate reasons to treat acne. Medical treatment usually provides visible improvement within a few months.

Sudden onset of severe acne in a mature adult may signal an underlying disease, such as a tumor that affects certain hormone production. This requires prompt medical attention.

Treatment

Don't pick or squeeze blemishes. Picking or squeezing can cause infection or scarring. Most acne will clear up without this kind of intervention. If aggressive treatment is needed, see your doctor or dermatologist.

Acne treatments work by reducing oil production, speeding up skin cell turnover, controlling bacterial infection or doing all three. With most prescription acne treatments, you may not see results for 6 to 8 weeks, and your skin is likely to get worse before it gets better. Most oral prescription medications for acne shouldn't be used during pregnancy, especially during early stages or while you're nursing.

Treatment for acne may include one or more of the following:

Lotions

Acne lotions dry up oil, kill bacteria and promote sloughing of dead skin cells. Over-the-counter lotions are generally mild and contain benzoyl peroxide, sulfur, resorcinol or salicylic acid as the active ingredient. These products can be helpful for mild acne.

If your acne doesn't respond to such treatments, you may want to see your primary care doctor or dermatologist to get a stronger prescription lotion. Retinoic acid, also called tretinoin (Avita, Retin-A), and adapalene (Differin) are topical prescription products derived from vitamin A. They work at the level of the pore to prevent plug formation.

A number of topical antibiotics also are available. They work by killing excess skin bacteria. Often, a combination of such products is required to achieve optimal results.

Antibiotics

For moderate to severe acne, oral antibiotics such as tetracycline may be needed to reduce bacteria and fight inflammation. You may need to take these antibiotics for months and in combination with topical products.

Some antibiotics may interfere with the effectiveness of oral contraceptives, and some shouldn't be used during pregnancy.

Isotretinoin

For deep cysts, antibiotics may not be enough. Isotretinoin (Accutane) is a powerful medication available for cystic acne, scarring acne or acne that doesn't respond to other treatments. This medicine is reserved for the most severe forms of acne. Accutane is very effective, but people who take it require close monitoring by a dermatologist because of the possibility of severe side effects, including depression, bone or joint pain, vision problems, rectal bleeding and severe stomach pain.

In addition, severe birth defects are likely to occur if Accutane is taken during pregnancy. Accutane should not be taken by women who may become pregnant either intentionally or unintentionally. Strict guidelines and safety measures exist for the use of Accutane in women of reproductive potential, and the drug should be prescribed only by doctors familiar with these guidelines.

Oral contraceptives
Oral contraceptives, which include norgestimate (Ortho-Cyclen, Tri-Cyclen) and ethinyl estradiol (Demulen, Ovral), have been shown to improve acne in women. Some antibiotics may interfere with the birth control effectiveness of oral contraceptives.

Cosmetic procedures
Cosmetic surgery may diminish scars left by acne. Procedures include chemical peel, dermabrasion and laser resurfacing (see page 1213). However, if your skin tends to form scar tissue (keloids), these procedures can make your complexion worse.

? Question and Answer

Does diet affect acne?

Contrary to what many people think, foods have little effect on acne. Neither chocolate nor greasy foods like french fries are likely to cause or aggravate acne. However, if certain foods seem to make your acne worse, it may be best to avoid them. Discuss this with your doctor.

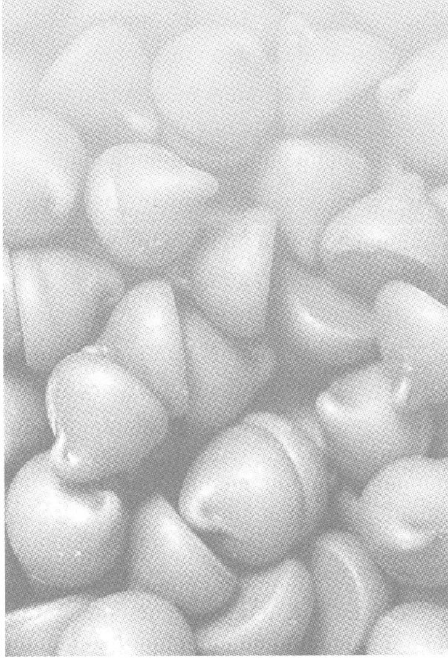

Rosacea

Signs and symptoms

- Red facial areas
- A tendency to flush or blush easily
- Visible small blood vessels on nose and cheeks (telangiectasia)
- Small red bumps or pustules on the nose, cheeks, forehead and chin
- Inflammation of the cheeks, nose, forehead and chin
- A burning or gritty sensation in the eyes (ocular rosacea)
- A red, bulbous nose (rhinophyma)

Rosacea is an inflammatory skin condition often resulting in redness of the face (see the color illustration on page 435). Its characteristics — a red nose, flushed cheeks and small red, pus-filled bumps (pustules) — are frequently mistaken for acne. Rosacea is also sometimes referred to as adult acne or acne rosacea, but in reality it has little to do with the pimples and blackheads that commonly afflict teenagers.

The condition may be progressive, meaning it tends to get worse over time. But in most people it's cyclic. It may be active for a time, lessen in intensity, then be followed by a flare-up.

Besides acne, rosacea can also be mistaken for other skin problems, such as a skin allergy. Once diagnosed, it's highly treatable.

Rosacea affects mostly fair-skinned adults between the ages of 30 and 60. About 13 million Americans have this skin condition. Although rosacea is more common in women, men are more likely to have the severe form, with a bright red, bulbous nose (rhinophyma). Rosacea isn't life-threatening, but it can affect appearance — and self-esteem.

Common progression

Rosacea may begin as a simple tendency to flush or blush easily, then progress to a persistent redness in the central portion of your face, particularly the nose. This redness results from the dilation of blood vessels close to the skin's surface.

As symptoms worsen, vascular rosacea may develop — small blood vessels on your nose and cheeks swell and become visible (telangiectasia). Your skin may become overly dry and sensitive. However, rosacea may also be accompanied by oily skin, as well as dandruff.

Small red bumps may appear and persist, spreading across your nose, cheeks, forehead and chin. This is sometimes known as inflammatory rosacea. In severe and rare cases, the oil glands (sebaceous glands) in the nose and sometimes the cheeks become enlarged, resulting in a buildup of tissue on and around the nose (rhinophyma).

More than half the people with rosacea experience ocular rosacea at times. They may feel a burning and gritty sensation in the eyes, and the eyelids may be inflamed or appear scaly.

The cause of rosacea is unknown, but researchers believe it's likely due to a combination of genetic and environmental factors. One thing is certain — rosacea isn't caused by alcoholism. Although alcohol consumption does lead to flushing of the skin and may worsen rosacea, people who don't consume alcohol may still experience severe signs and symptoms.

A number of factors can aggravate rosacea or make it worse by increasing blood flow to the surface of the skin. Some of these include:

- Hot foods or beverages
- Spicy foods
- Alcohol
- Caffeine withdrawal (caffeine itself isn't a factor)
- Temperature extremes
- Sunlight
- Stress, anger or embarrassment
- Strenuous exercise
- Hot baths, saunas
- Corticosteroids, as well as drugs that dilate blood vessels
- Skin care products that contain ingredients such as acids, alcohol and other irritants

Diagnosis

If you experience persistent redness in your face, see your doctor or a dermatologist. Because of the progressive nature of rosacea, an early diagnosis is important.

Treatment

Although there's no cure for rosacea, effective treatment can relieve its signs and symptoms. Most often this requires a combination of prescription treatments and self-care measures. Treatment is most effective if started early.

Prescription treatment usually involves antibiotics that you apply directly to your skin (topical) or that you take orally. In many cases, dermatologists initially prescribe both oral and topical antibiotics to lessen symptoms, followed by long-term use of a topical antibiotic alone to maintain remission.

Ocular rosacea might be treated with oral antibiotics. Laser surgery may reduce visible blood vessels and improve a red, bulbous nose (rhinophyma).

In addition, your doctor may recommend certain moisturizers, soaps, sunscreens and other products to improve your skin. If your rosacea is brought on by hot flashes, you might ask your doctor about estrogen to control them.

Medication

A common topical antibiotic prescribed is metronidazole. This medication comes in a cream, lotion or gel form. Other topical antibiotics include sulfacetamide, erythromycin and clindamycin. Topical treatment with a preparation containing sulfur and salicylic acid also may be helpful.

Some of the most common oral antibiotics prescribed include tetracycline, minocycline, doxycycline and erythromycin. Oral antibiotics tend to work faster than topical ones and are most effective in treating the pustules of rosacea.

Isotretinoin (Accutane) is a powerful medication sometimes used for more severe cases of rosacea. Usually prescribed for cystic acne, it works to inhibit the production of oil by sebaceous glands. Isotretinoin must be used cautiously. It can have significant side effects and is known to cause severe birth defects if taken during pregnancy.

The duration of your treatment will depend on the type and severity of your symptoms, but typically you'll notice an improvement within 1 to 2 months. Because symptoms may recur if medications are stopped, long-term regular treatment is often necessary.

Surgery

Enlarged blood vessels, some redness and changes due to rhinophyma often become permanent. In these cases, surgical methods, such as laser surgery and electrosurgery, may be used to reduce the visibility of blood vessels, remove tissue buildup around the nose and generally improve appearance.

Self-care

Along with your doctor, you can play an active part in your treatment. One of the most important things that you can do is to minimize your exposure to anything that causes a flare-up.

Because everyone is different, it's important to find out what factors affect you and avoid them. Keeping a running list might help. Here are other suggestions for preventing flare-ups:

- Protect your face from the sun by wearing a broad-brimmed hat or using sunscreen with a sun protection factor (SPF) of 15 or higher.
- Protect your face in the winter with a scarf or ski mask.
- Avoid irritating your facial skin by rubbing or touching it too much.
- Avoid facial products that contain alcohol or other skin irritants.
- When using a moisturizer with a topical medication, apply the moisturizer after the medication has dried.
- Use products that are labeled noncomedogenic to avoid clogging your pores.
- Stay cool on hot days.
- Try to avoid stressful situations.
- If you wear makeup, try green-tinted prefoundation creams. They may counter skin redness.

Psoriasis

Signs and symptoms

- Dry, red patches of skin covered with silvery scales
- Small scaling spots (most commonly seen in children)
- Swollen and stiff joints

Emergency signs and symptoms

- Reddening and scaling affecting the entire skin

Psoriasis, a common skin disease, affects the life cycle of skin cells. Normally, it takes about a month for new cells to move from the lowest skin layer, where they're produced, to the outermost layer, where they die and scale off in tiny flakes. With psoriasis, the entire cycle takes only days. As a result, cells accumulate rapidly, forming thick patches with scales.

Psoriasis (see the color illustration on page 432) is a persistent, long-lasting (chronic) disease. It affects about 5.5 million Americans. Psoriasis can occur suddenly at any age, but the onset is usually gradual and begins between ages 15 and 35.

The inflammation can be frustrating if you have it, causing unsightly patches of skin, discomfort and even pain. The attacks can range from a few spots of dandruff-like scaling to large areas with major eruptions. Psoriasis most commonly affects the elbows, knees, trunk and scalp. Pits or ridges may develop in the nails. The eruptions take various forms, including pustules, cracking skin, itching or minor bleeding. Psoriasis isn't contagious.

Arthritis accompanies psoriasis in about 1 in 10 people. For most of these individuals, the effects of psoriatic arthritis are minor. It produces some pain in affected joints but has little effect on overall health. Less commonly, the joint symptoms can lead to significant disability, similar to that sometimes experienced by people with rheumatoid arthritis.

Causes

In psoriasis, skin cells reproduce rapidly, forming a thickened, less coherent superficial layer. This usually doesn't stop unless treatment interrupts the cycle.

Factors that may trigger psoriasis include:

- A systemic infection such as strep throat
- An immune system response to disease
- Injury to the skin
- Reaction to a medication or vaccine
- Stress
- Excessive alcohol consumption
- Environmental factors, such as exposure to the sun or to chemicals such as disinfectants and paint thinners

Doctors believe psoriasis is an inherited disease influenced by many factors. But researchers haven't yet identified the precise gene or genes responsible for it.

Diagnosis

A diagnosis of psoriasis usually is based on a physical inspection. Your doctor may need to obtain a skin sample (biopsy) for microscopic analysis to rule out other disorders or a fungal infection.

How serious is psoriasis?

Psoriasis ranges from mild and short term (acute) to severe and chronic. The disease can't be cured, but treatments are usually effective. If almost all of your skin is affected, you may require prompt treatment. Acute secondary infections also can start during any flare-up.

Treatment

One reason psoriasis is so difficult to control is its wide variation in type, severity and response to treatment. Because each case of psoriasis is unique, your doctor will tailor a treatment specifically to you. The goal of treatment is to restore order to the growth and maturation of your skin cells. In mild cases, over-the-counter coal-tar soaps, shampoos, cleansers or ointments used together with bath oils often will suffice.

Other treatment approaches include:

Creams and ointments

Calcipotriene (Dovonex) is a prescription ointment that contains a derivative of vitamin D. Calcipotriene controls the overproduction of skin cells. It's a useful treatment for mild to moderate psoriasis. Another option is a topical retinoid medication, such as tazarotene (Tazorac). Your doctor may also prescribe a corticosteroid or a coal-tar preparation.

If you have patches of psoriasis on your scalp, they may require a phenol and sodium chloride (salt) lotion or a stronger tar preparation in addition to a daily tar shampoo. Topical calcipotriene or corticosteroid lotions or solutions also may be prescribed.

Oral medication

Acitretin (Soriatane) may help reduce excess growth of skin cells in cases of severe psoriasis. Extreme care must be used when taking this drug because it can produce side effects such as eye and lip inflammation, hair loss and sun sensitivity, as well as birth defects if taken during pregnancy.

Other oral medications include methotrexate, which blocks the growth of skin cells in psoriasis, and cyclosporine, which suppresses your immune system. These drugs can also cause serious side effects, including liver and kidney toxicity, and are usually reserved for the most severe cases of psoriasis.

Phototherapy

Psoralen plus ultraviolet A (PUVA), a combination of light-sensitizing medications (psoralens) and ultraviolet A (UVA) light, is effective in suppressing the growth of skin cells in severe psoriasis. Long-term use of PUVA — 250 treatments or more — may increase the risk of skin cancer, including melanoma, a potentially deadly form of skin cancer.

Exposure to moderate sunlight, while being careful to avoid sunburn, as well as the application of coal tar combined with ultraviolet B radiation (Goeckerman treatment) also are effective treatments.

A newer form of phototherapy treatment called narrow-band ultraviolet B (NB-UVB) may be as effective as PUVA and not require oral medications before each treatment. It may not carry as high a potential for skin cancer as PUVA.

Topical treatments and phototherapy are often combined to increase their effectiveness. Doctors sometimes use phototherapy and oral medications in rotation or simultaneously in lower dosages to minimize side effects.

Self-care

You can take a number of steps to control your psoriasis:

- Eat a nutritionally balanced diet, get adequate rest and exercise regularly.
- Maintain a healthy weight. Psoriasis often occurs in skin creases or folds.
- Avoid scratching, rubbing or picking at patches of psoriasis.
- Bathe daily to soak off the scales. Avoid hot water or harsh soap.
- Keep your skin moist. Pat rather than rub dry after bathing, apply a heavy, water-in-oil moisturizing cream immediately after bathing while your skin is still moist, avoid creams or lotions containing alcohol, use a humidifier and keep room temperatures cool.
- Use soaps, shampoos, cleansers or ointments containing coal tar or salicylic acid.
- Expose your skin to moderate sunlight, but avoid sunburn.
- Apply an over-the-counter cortisone cream, 0.5 percent or 1 percent, for a few weeks when symptoms are especially bad.

Lichen planus

Signs and symptoms

- A rash that appears as raised, flat areas that may vary in color from violet to pink to red
- A rash that typically appears on the arms and legs but sometimes involves the scalp or the mucous membranes that line the mouth, nose, vagina and anus
- Itching
- Soreness or a burning sensation involving the mucous membranes

Lichen planus is a rare, persistent, itchy rash characterized by shiny, reddish purple spots on the skin and gray-white ones in the mouth. Most commonly, lichen planus appears in midlife, between the ages of 45 and 60. The initial attack may persist for weeks or months, and recurrences can continue over many years. Oral symptoms often consist of a dry mouth and a metallic taste or blunted taste sensation, or burning in the mouth. They may appear before the rash and be the only evidence of the disease.

The cause of this disorder usually can't be determined. In some cases, it may represent a reaction to medication or stress. Some cases have been linked to infections, such as hepatitis.

How serious is lichen planus?

Lichen planus of the skin is generally noncancerous (benign). It may clear up with treatment but can persist for months to years.

People with long-term lesions of the mucous membranes are at greater risk of squamous cell carcinoma — a form of skin cancer. In these cases, a doctor may advise regular examinations to monitor any changes in the lesions. It's also important to stop any tobacco use, which raises your risk of squamous cell carcinoma.

Diagnosis

A diagnosis of lichen planus is generally made by inspection or laboratory examination of a tissue sample (biopsy).

Treatment

Treatment usually focuses on relieving the itching and may include:

- An ointment or cream containing a corticosteroid medication
- Phototherapy with ultraviolet light
- Oral corticosteroid medications, in severe cases
- Immune-modulating therapy, in severe cases

Pityriasis rosea

Signs and symptoms

- A mild, itchy rash, ranging from pink to tan
- A rash that starts as one large spot on an arm, a leg or the trunk

Pityriasis rosea is a skin condition that causes a fine, scaly rash ranging in color from pink to tan. The itchy rash may start as one large spot, called a herald patch, on an arm, a leg or your trunk. After several days, the rash may spread to other parts of the body. The rash may peel.

The cause of pityriasis rosea isn't clear. It may be due to a viral infection. Pityriasis rosea usually affects children and young adults. The rash may last for 3 to 12 weeks. It rarely recurs.

Treatment

There's no specific treatment for pityriasis rosea. The rash usually disappears without treatment. Exposure to sunlight may help reduce the rash — but avoid sun-

Bathing Basics

Follow these tips to minimize the drying effects of bathing on your skin:

1. Bathe less frequently. Two or three times a week is often enough for most people. Limit yourself to 15 minutes, and use warm, rather than hot, water.
2. Choose mild superfatted soaps such as Basis or Dove, which dry skin less. Add Aveeno oatmeal powder or bath oils to your bath water. Soap substitutes in bar, gel and liquid forms are less drying than deodorant and antibacterial soaps. Use soap only on your face, underarms, genital areas, hands and feet. Use clear water elsewhere.
3. After bathing, brush your skin rapidly with the palms of your hands or gently pat your skin with a towel.
4. Apply an oil or cream to your skin immediately after drying. Use a heavy, water-in-oil moisturizer, not a light "disappearing" cream that contains mostly water. Avoid creams or lotions containing alcohol. Pay special attention to your legs, arms, back and the sides of your body.

burn. You may relieve the itching by applying a moisturizing cream or an over-the-counter hydrocortisone cream.

Dry skin

Signs and symptoms

- Itching
- Flaking, scaly skin

Dry, itchy skin, also known as asteatosis, is a common problem, especially in older adults. Cold air and low humidity can be especially tough on your skin.

The season for dry weather depends on where you live. Minnesotans experience winter itch, while Arizonans suffer from summer itch.

Symptoms of dry skin result from the loss of natural moisture and oil from the skin. Your skin may become cracked. Round patches of irritated skin may develop, resembling ringworm. The most common sites are the lower legs, upper arms, sides (flanks) and thighs.

Treatment

To help decrease the dryness that causes asteatosis, bathe less frequently during the dry season and moisturize your skin daily with a lubricating cream or oil. In addition, use a humidifier and keep room temperatures cool. If your symptoms persist, apply an over-the-counter hydrocortisone cream to your skin. For a severe rash with itching, your doctor may prescribe a stronger corticosteroid preparation to lessen the itching. If you have generalized, persistent itching, consult your doctor. This may be a symptom of other disorders.

Ichthyosis

Signs and symptoms

- Severely dry, scaly skin starting in early childhood

Ichthyosis is a group of inherited skin disorders that affects more than 1 million Americans. *Ichthy* is taken from the Greek root for "fish" and refers to the dry, scaly appearance of skin associated with the disease. Ichthyosis occurs when the skin's natural shedding process is too slow or the production of skin cells is too fast.

Most cases of ichthyosis are mild, but some can be severe. The disorder occasionally is seen at birth, but often appears between ages 1 and 4. Sometimes it disappears entirely for most of the adult years, only to return in later years. The rash tends to be most predominant on the elbows, knees and hands. It usually worsens in the winter. Ichthyosis may be associated with eczema (see page 1170).

Treatment

There's no known cure for ichthyosis, so the goal of treatment is to manage symptoms by moisturizing the skin. The simplest treatment may consist of petroleum jelly applied to the affected areas, sometimes with a plastic wrap to keep the petroleum jelly from staining clothes or furniture. Twice daily applications of a lactic acid, urea or other creams also may help.

In severe cases, your doctor might prescribe retinoids — medications derived from vitamin A. They reduce the proliferation of skin cells. Side effects from the medication may include eye and lip inflammation, bone spurs and hair loss, as well as birth defects if taken during pregnancy.

Itching

The medical term for itching is *pruritus.* No matter what you call it, itching can be a miserable, distressing condition.

Causes

Although the most common cause of itching is dry skin, itching occurs in a variety of diseases or disorders. It can on occasion indicate a systemic condition such as liver or kidney disease and some blood disorders. Itching may also result when larvae of the hookworm family of parasites penetrate your skin. This includes swimmers' itch, eruption caused by the larvae of cat and dog hookworm and ground itch caused by the true hookworm.

Many other skin disorders also can have itching as a major symptom, including insect bites, dermatitis, hives and skin parasites, such as scabies. Some medications, such as aspirin and codeine-related pain relievers, can cause itching, which may or may not be accompanied by a rash.

Emotional stress can contribute to or increase the sensation of itching, no matter what the underlying cause may be. If emotional factors are the primary cause, the condition is known as psychogenic itching.

Treatment

Antihistamines may relieve itching due to hives, certain drug rashes and some forms of dermatitis. Most antihistamines also have a mild sedative effect and may help you sleep. Creams or ointments containing hydrocortisone, menthol, camphor and other medications may help control the itch of insect bites and dermatitis.

For dry skin associated with aging, moisturizing the skin is key. For severe itching from dry skin, use Aveeno, a form of oatmeal soap, in your bath water.

You can get much the same effect from an oatmeal bath or a starch-and-soda bath. For an oatmeal bath, tie a handful of oatmeal into a piece of cotton cloth. Boil it just as you would cook the oatmeal. Then use this "oatmeal sponge" while you bathe in a tub half full of lukewarm water. To prepare a starch-and-soda bath, add half of a 16-ounce box of baking soda and one 16-ounce box of laundry starch to a tub half full of lukewarm water. Mix well and bathe without using soap.

Hives

Signs and symptoms

- Raised, red, often itchy welts of various sizes that appear and disappear at random on the surface of the skin
- The development of welts where the skin is scratched (dermatographism)

Hives is common. Typically, the condition appears as a reaction to internal or external allergens. A rare form of hives, called angioedema, can be life-threatening. Therefore, it's important to avoid substances that trigger hives, if possible. For a detailed discussion of hives and angioedema, see page 542.

Treatment

When hives occur, the typical treatment is with an antihistamine. For more severe cases, other drugs may be used, such as an injection of adrenaline (epinephrine). Occasionally, hives is treated with a prescription corticosteroid medication.

Pigmentary changes

Signs and symptoms

- Slowly growing white patches of skin
- Dark brown patches of skin

Skin color is the result of the melanin pigment created by certain cells (melanocytes) in skin. Occasionally, something happens to this mechanism.

Chloasma

When an area of skin produces too much melanin and becomes darker, it's called chloasma (see the color illustration on page 433). Chloasma patches are most common on the face. They seldom spread far. In women, they're often associated with pregnancy or use of birth control pills, but both men and women can get them for no known reason.

Vitiligo

When no melanin is produced, the involved patch of skin becomes white. When a white patch grows, it may be due to a skin disorder called vitiligo (see the color illustration on page 433). Although vitiligo can start at any age, it often first appears between the ages of 20 and 30. The white patches may begin on the face above the eyes or on the neck, armpits, genitalia, hands or knees. They're often symmetric and can spread over the entire body. Heredity is often a factor.

Sometimes, vitiligo results from the destruction of melanin-producing cells by the immune system. Some people with vitiligo also have associated immune-related disorders, such as thyroid problems or pernicious anemia.

How serious are pigmentary changes?

Neither vitiligo nor chloasma is life-threatening. Cosmetics or skin dyes often are used to hide the patches. Because vitiligo patches sunburn easily, you'll need to use skin protection — clothing, sunscreen, sun avoidance or all three.

Treatment

Repigmentation and depigmentation treatments are used to restore uniform skin color. Phototherapy is perhaps the best therapy to date.

Repigmentation of vitiligo patches is done with psoralen ultraviolet A (PUVA) therapy, which combines light-sensitizing medications (psoralens) and ultraviolet A (UVA) light. This technique has been used for several decades.

In recent years, narrow-band ultraviolet B (NB-UVB) has also been used with success. Both therapies are administered under the direction of a dermatologist.

Long-term use of PUVA may increase your risk of skin cancer. Proper dosing and supervision is required to limit these risks. Mild cases of vitiligo may respond to topical corticosteroid preparations or to the newer topical medications pimecrolimus (Elidel) or tacrolimus (Protopic).

A cream containing retinoic acid (Avita, Retin-A) applied nightly may help to lighten the dark patches of chloasma. Bleaching creams also may be helpful. These are available by prescription and contain a low concentration of hydroquinone. Sun protection is a must to avoid rapid repigmentation of chloasma.

Drug rashes

Signs and symptoms

- Skin changes, including redness, hives, blisters and bleeding into the skin
- Itching

Drug rashes are a result of an allergic reaction to either an over-the-counter medication or one prescribed by your doctor. If a rash develops while you're taking any kind of drug, the medication may be the cause.

Drug reactions can involve more than an itch or rash. Signs and symptoms of a drug reaction may be extremely varied. In addition to the rash, you might experience fever, seizures, nausea, vomiting, diarrhea, heartbeat irregularities, difficulty breathing, asthma or decreased urine flow. In addition, laboratory tests may demonstrate an effect on your hemoglobin value or white blood cell count.

Fever is often the earliest sign of a drug reaction. Fortunately, rashes usually appear early during the course of a drug reaction and warn you that you may be experiencing a drug reaction. If you take one or more medications, a persistent rash is a warning to seek medical advice.

Treatment

If your rash is caused by a medication, the signs and symptoms will usually improve when you stop taking the drug. If the drug is a prescription medication, consult your doctor before discontinuing its use.

If your rash is itchy, oatmeal baths or wet dressings may soothe it (see page 1179). Topical hydrocortisone cream also may help. Antihistamines sometimes relieve the itch and diminish the rash of certain types of drug rashes.

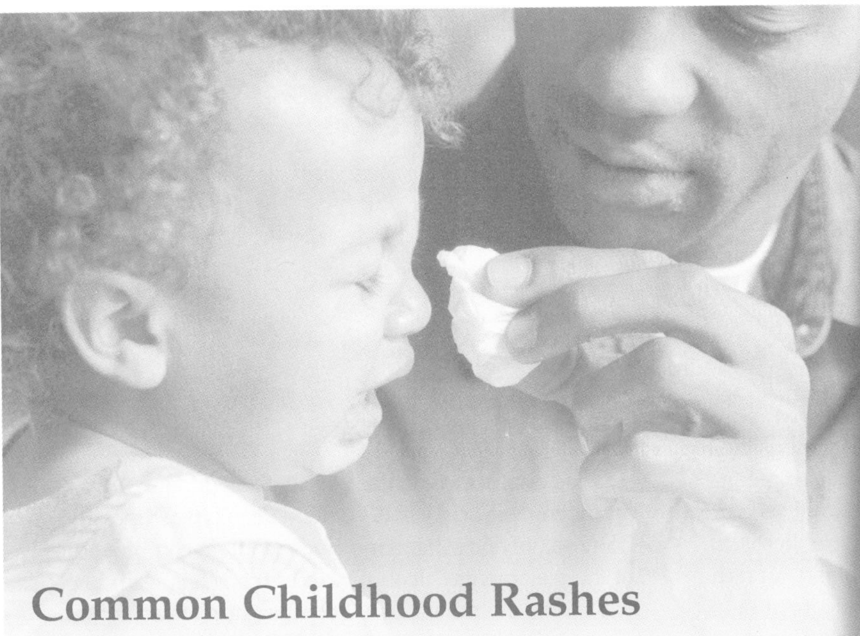

Common Childhood Rashes

Sometimes it can be difficult to determine the cause of a rash. Here are four childhood illnesses that commonly cause a rash:

Chickenpox

Chickenpox (varicella) causes itchy, red spots on the face or chest that spread to the arms and legs. These spots quickly fill with a clear fluid to form blisters that rupture and turn crusty. New spots generally continue appearing over 4 to 5 days. Fever, runny nose or cough often accompanies chickenpox, which is contagious until the rash crusts.

Seek medical help if the rash involves the eyes or is accompanied by a cough or shortness of breath. In addition, seek medical help if chickenpox develops twice in the same person or occurs after immunization.

Fifth disease

With fifth disease, bright red, raised patches appear on both cheeks, giving a slapped-cheek appearance. During the next few days, a pink, lacy, slightly raised rash may also develop on the arms, trunk, thighs and buttocks. The rash may come and go for up to 3 weeks. Some children develop a slight fever and other mild, cold-like symptoms.

Measles

Measles (rubeola) typically begins with a fever, often as high as 104 to 105 F, a cough, sneezing, a sore throat and inflamed, watery eyes. A rash appears 2 to 4 days later. It often begins as fine, red spots on the face and spreads to the trunk, arms and legs. Spots may become larger and usually last about a week. Small, white spots may appear on the inside lining of the cheek.

See a doctor if you suspect that your child may have the measles. It may lead to uncommon but potentially serious complications, such as pneumonia, encephalitis or a bacterial infection.

Roseola

Roseola often begins with a high fever lasting about 3 days. When it subsides, a rash appears on the trunk and neck and lasts a few hours to a few days. The virus most often affects children between ages 6 months and 3 years. See a doctor if the rash lasts longer than 3 days.

Sunburn

Signs and symptoms

- Red, tender, swollen skin
- Water blisters
- Peeling skin

Emergency signs and symptoms

- Fever and chills
- Nausea
- Delirium

Sunburn is the result of the skin's overexposure to ultraviolet (UV) radiation from the sun or tanning beds. Congestion in the capillaries that supply blood to your skin causes the swollen, red skin of a sunburn.

Sunburn is thought to play a role in the dramatic increase in malignant melanoma, the most lethal form of skin cancer. A history of painful, blistering sunburns, especially in childhood, increases your risk of developing melanoma later in life (see page 1200). Intense, brief exposure to the sun is also a hazard. Whatever your age, there's no such thing as a healthy tan.

The UV content of sunlight varies. It's greater at higher elevations because it isn't filtered out by clouds or haze. Cold air doesn't reduce UV radiation from the sun. Reflected UV light from snow, sand, water and other surfaces can burn as severely as direct sunlight. The darker your skin, the less these rays penetrate because they're absorbed by the melanin pigment.

Mild sunburn or exposure to sun may stimulate your skin to produce extra melanin as protection against further ultraviolet penetration. More melanin means a deeper tan, if the additional pigment is distributed evenly. Otherwise, it forms freckles, liver spots or discolored splotches. Melanin production and dispersal are under genetic control. There's nothing you can do to change your tanning capacity.

Your skin, eye and hair color are good predictors of how much sun you can tolerate before you suffer a sunburn (see page 1168). You're most likely to sunburn without tanning if you have fair skin, blue or

Protecting Your Skin From the Sun

It's the first warm, sunny day after a long winter. You step outside for a deep breath of fresh air, close your eyes and turn your face to the sun. The soothing warmth of the sun on your skin feels so good. You imagine the look of a nice suntan, but what you may be getting instead are wrinkles and liver spots.

Despite the still-prevalent image of a tan being healthy, excessive exposure to the sun is responsible for much of the skin damage associated with aging. It's a lifelong process, as over time your skin slowly accumulates the damaging effects of the sun.

Accumulated exposure to the ultraviolet (UV) radiation in sunlight and tanning beds causes your skin to age prematurely and leads to wrinkles and skin discoloration. Much of the damage is merely cosmetic, but some effects can be deadly. Excessive sun exposure is the leading cause of skin cancer, by far the most common form of cancer diagnosed today. Almost half of all Americans who reach age 65 will have at least one skin cancer.

Sun sense

Armed with adequate sunscreen and protective clothing, you can — at any age — prevent damage to your skin.

Avoidance

When possible, avoid overexposure to the sun by planning outdoor activities for early morning or late afternoon. UV radiation is most intense from 10 a.m. to 2 p.m.

Tanning beds also damage skin. They emit ultraviolet A (UVA) rays, which are often touted as less dangerous than ultraviolet B (UVB) rays. But UVA light penetrates even deeper into your skin, causes precancerous skin lesions and increases your risk of skin cancer.

Proper clothing

If you expect to be exposed to sunlight for lengthy periods, protect yourself. Wear a hat, select shirts with long sleeves and avoid shorts. Several clothing manufacturers (MasqueRays, Solumbra) market items designed to provide protection from the sun while you're outdoors.

Sunscreen

Use a premium-quality sunscreen lotion whenever you're outdoors for sustained periods. A sunscreen can protect you from burning and allow some tanning. Avoid lotions touted as tan accelerators, such as coconut oil, cocoa butter or baby oil. These products don't make you tan faster, and they provide very little protection from UV radiation.

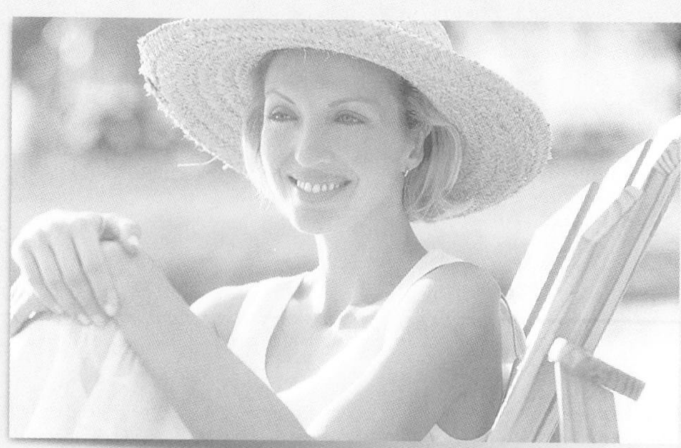

Good sunscreens contain derivatives of para-aminobenzoic acid (PABA), cinoxate, oxybenzone, homosalate or avobenzone. Some contain combinations of these elements. Alcohol-based sunscreens seem to penetrate deeper and are less likely to aggravate acne. Some sunscreens also contain physical blockers such as zinc oxide or titanium dioxide, which provide even better protection and are more resistant to water and perspiration.

Sunscreens are rated by their sun protection factor (SPF) in a range from 2 to 45, with 45 offering the most protection. These numbers mainly relate to the ability of the sunscreen to block UVB, not UVA. It's best to use a sunscreen with an SPF rating of at least 15 that blocks both UVA and UVB rays.

Apply it at least half an hour before exposure. Reapply your sunscreen frequently because protection diminishes as the sunscreen evaporates. Swimming and perspiration can wash it away as well.

Also be sure to use a sunscreen for winter sun exposure. The greatest hazard in winter months is on cloudy days after a fresh snow, especially at higher altitudes, where UV radiation is greater.

The delicate skin around your eyes, nose and lips needs extra protection. Some people prefer to use a sunblock, such as zinc oxide or titanium dioxide, which stops all radiation from reaching the skin. Many people use a special lip sunscreen with an SPF rating of 15 or higher.

Sun sensitizers

Certain medications and skin products may make you more sensitive to the sun, including some antibiotics and antihistamines. Be especially careful to avoid the sun and tanning beds when using these substances. Avoid perfumes and after-shave lotion before sun exposure because such preparations may produce discolored patches on your skin.

Cleansing

After sun exposure, bathe or shower away perspiration, salt, pool chemicals and sunscreen products. Then apply a lubricant to your skin.

green eyes and blond or red hair. Resistance to sunburn and easy tanning are most likely if you have dark brown eyes, brown or black hair and brown or black skin.

Diagnosis

Symptoms of sunburn don't appear until a few hours after exposure, but then the pain, redness and occasional blistering of sunburned skin are unmistakable.

How serious is sunburn?

The effect of sunburn is like that of any burn, although its development is relatively slow rather than rapid, as from a heat burn. If the sunburn is severe, skin cells die and blisters form. The skin then heals in a period of 1 to 2 weeks. During the healing process, skin damaged by sunburn may peel off in patches.

Damage to your skin cells from recurrent sunburn is cumulative, and continued overexposure to UV radiation produces long-term effects. These can include skin discolorations, actinic keratosis and skin cancer. Ninety percent of all skin cancer is due to such irreversible skin damage.

Treatment

Treat your sunburn with cool tap water compresses and, if severe, hydrocortisone cream several times daily. Soaking in cool tub water with or without oatmeal may help. Leave water blisters intact to speed healing. If they break open on their own, remove the skin fragments and apply an antibacterial ointment on the open areas to help prevent infections. Keep the wounds clean.

For a severe sunburn, contact your doctor before signs and symptoms fully develop. Your doctor may prescribe an oral corticosteroid to decrease the reaction.

Photosensitivity

Signs and symptoms

- Redness
- A rash
- Blistering or swelling

Photosensitivity is a heightened reaction of skin to ultraviolet (UV) rays from the sun or tanning beds, usually after consuming certain medications or touching certain substances or plants. When skin products cause a sunlight allergic reaction, the condition is called photocontact dermatitis.

Medications that sometimes can cause photosensitive reactions include:

- Antibiotics
- Anticonvulsants
- Antidepressants
- Antihistamines
- Birth control pills
- Chemotherapy medications
- Diuretics
- High blood pressure medications
- Nonsteroidal anti-inflammatory drugs (NSAIDs)
- Oral diabetes medications
- Topical antiseptic creams
- Tranquilizers

Some substances and plants can cause photosensitivity when they come in contact with your skin. These include:

- Artificial sweeteners (cyclamates)
- Perfumes containing bergamot, sandalwood, lavender or citron oils
- After-shave lotions
- Antibacterial deodorant soaps
- Detergents
- Medicated cosmetics
- Skin-bleaching creams
- Shampoos or soaps with coal-tar ingredients
- Sunscreens with para-aminobenzoic acid (PABA)
- Certain fruits and plants, such as limes, parsley, celery, parsnips, carrots and figs

Types

The two categories of photosensitive reactions are photoallergic and phototoxic.

Photoallergic

A photoallergic reaction is a result of changes in your immune system. When this occurs, your skin reacts each time it's exposed to sunlight after exposure to or contact with a particular sensitizing drug, chemical or plant.

Your skin becomes red, although not necessarily sunburned, and develops a bumpy rash, similar to that caused by poison ivy. Discolored patches, blisters or swelling also can occur. Symptoms can extend to areas not exposed to the light. Once your body becomes sensitized to a certain substance, you can react to it, and chemically similar substances, again and again.

Phototoxic

A phototoxic reaction looks and feels like an exaggerated sunburn with inflammation, redness, blisters and the characteristic discomfort. You may have this reaction any time a sufficient amount of the sensitizing chemical is present in your body or on your skin and you're exposed to the activating wavelength of light.

Treatment

A photosensitive reaction usually disappears within a week after you take steps to protect your skin from UV exposure and avoid the sensitizing substance.

If you've had a photoallergic reaction, it's especially important to wear protective clothing and use a broad spectrum sunscreen that blocks both ultraviolet A and ultraviolet B rays when you're outdoors.

For a severe reaction, your doctor may prescribe a corticosteroid ointment or cream or hydroxychloroquine tablets to help suppress photoallergic reactions.

Solar elastosis

Signs and symptoms

- Loose, sagging or wrinkled skin
- Dry, tough, leathery skin

Excessive exposure to sunlight over many years damages collagen and elastin fibers that help support skin. This can lead to loose, sagging, tough and wrinkled skin that can look 15 to 20 years older than normal.

Care for Wrinkled Skin

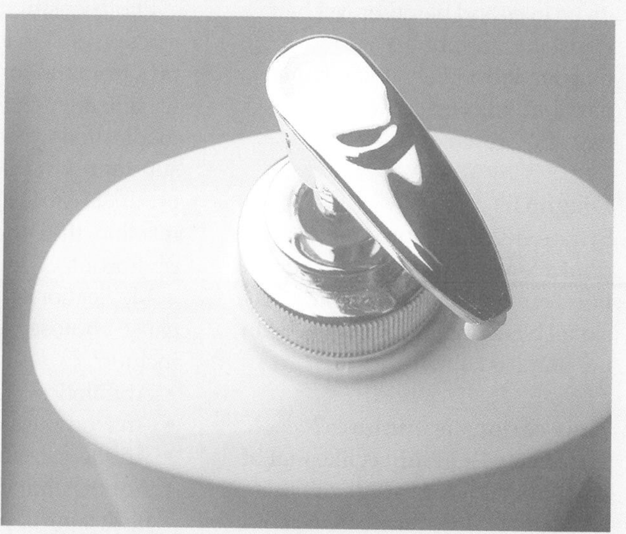

Wrinkling is a natural part of aging. As you grow older, your skin gets thinner, drier, less elastic and more wrinkled. And it tends to lose its youthful color and glow.

Dryness is a result of decreased oil production within your skin. Deterioration in the connective tissues (elastin and collagen) in your dermal layer causes sagging, wrinkling and thinning. Finally, as your blood supply slows, your rosy glow begins to fade.

Although aging of your skin is inevitable, it can be slowed by consistently using sunscreen whenever you're outdoors and by not smoking. Overexposure to sun and cigarette smoking accelerate skin wrinkling dramatically.

Over-the-counter products

Although sunscreen is the most important product for preventing wrinkles, regular use of a moisturizer can help keep skin healthy. When choosing a moisturizer, avoid products that contain propylene glycol or sorbitol. Although propylene glycol holds moisture in the skin, it also repels it, prohibiting any benefit.

Many over-the-counter products promise to diminish fine lines, but choosing from among the myriad products on the shelf can be difficult. The American Academy of Dermatology recommends looking for products that contain tretinoin (such as retinoid creams) or alpha-hydroxy acid. Another ingredient to look for is furfuryladenine (Kinerase, Kinetin), a newer agent that helps retain water in the skin.

It's stronger prescription skin creams, not over-the-counter products, that have been found truly effective. The dab of an alpha-hydroxy acid, for example, in over-the-counter moisturizers and facial treatments may not make much difference in your skin.

Prescription creams

If you're serious about reducing wrinkles, see a dermatologist about using prescription tretinoin or alpha-hydroxy acids. Prescription products contain a much higher concentration of these effective ingredients than do over-the-counter products.

Tretinoin

Retin-A and Avita are prescription creams containing tretinoin (retinoic acid), a synthetic derivative of vitamin A. They're not miracle drugs, but they have been shown to improve fine wrinkling, roughness and pigment changes in mildly to moderately affected skin. Also used for treating acne, retinoic acid sloughs off the outer layers of the skin, exposes the skin underneath and causes collagen to re-accumulate, which thickens the skin fibers that preserve moisture.

You apply the cream nightly to your face, neck, upper chest and hands. Possible side effects include increased sensitivity, dryness, redness and excessive peeling. If you experience side effects, less-frequent applications — perhaps three times a week — may be appropriate. You must avoid sun exposure while using these medications. Talk with your doctor about how to prevent sunburn. Skin treated with retinoic acid shouldn't come into contact with dyes, hair removal wax or perfume.

Alpha-hydroxy acids

Alpha-hydroxy acids (AHAs) are less irritating than retinoic acid but don't penetrate as deeply. In one clinical trial, more than 70 percent of those treated with AHAs (either lactic acid or glycolic acid) reported improvement in the appearance of their skin.

Botulinum toxin

Another way dermatologists and plastic surgeons smooth wrinkles is by injecting them with botulinum toxin, a poison that temporarily paralyzes skin muscles. Frown lines and crow's-feet partially result from repetitively contracting muscles. Botulinum toxin weakens the pull of these muscles, causing the skin to flatten out and appear smoother and less wrinkled.

The procedure has been shown to be generally safe. The only worry is that the injection can migrate to a different area of the face. If that happens, it can cause temporary facial weakness or drooping. You're usually told not to rub the area after injection to prevent migration of the toxin. The effects of the treatment are temporary and may need to be repeated every few months.

Cosmetic procedures

Other options for reducing wrinkles include resurfacing techniques, soft-tissue fillers and face-lifts (see page 1213).

Your skin is composed of two types of connective tissue. One type is a strong, white fiber (collagen). The other is an elastic, yellow fiber (elastin). Ultraviolet radiation penetrates skin and can damage these tissues. Orderly structural arrangement of skin cells and connective tissues deteriorates, and abnormal cell growth begins.

Each exposure to ultraviolet light causes slight but irreversible changes, so the damage within your skin accumulates over the years. Signs and symptoms of solar elastosis appear gradually as the skin loses its resilience, flexibility and water-holding capacity.

If you sunburn easily and tan poorly, you're most susceptible to solar elastosis. The condition usually occurs in fair-skinned, blue- or green-eyed people with blond or red hair who are frequently exposed to intense sunlight without protection. The risk is highest for sunbathers, farmers, sailors and others who are often outdoors. Those who live in regions with intense sunlight are more at risk. Such areas include higher elevations and the Western plains.

Diagnosis

You can see the effects of solar elastosis by comparing your protected skin to overexposed skin. Your dermatologist can establish the diagnosis by examination.

How serious is solar elastosis?

No medical treatment can reverse the damage or rejuvenate your skin. If your skin has been damaged enough to cause solar elastosis, your risk of acquiring skin cancer is increased. See your doctor whenever you have a new growth or a change in an existing growth such as a mole.

Treatment

To prevent further damage, avoid sunlight whenever you can. If you can't, protect your skin with sunscreen and proper clothing.

Your dermatologist may recommend lubricating creams to reduce dryness and soften your skin. Facial massages and masks can make your face feel better for a while by toning muscles and stimulating blood circulation.

Senile skin

Signs and symptoms

- Skin discolorations, including liver spots, freckles and red, yellow, gray or brown blotches
- Skin texture changes, including coarse wrinkles, sagging folds, sallowness, roughness, excessive dryness or leathery toughness
- Skin growths, including scaly patches

The effects of aging on skin are generally gradual. However, signs of aging may appear more quickly and at a younger age if you're susceptible to sun damage and your skin has had considerable sun exposure.

Treatment

Senile skin is irreversible. For more information on common conditions related to aging, see liver spots (page 1196), solar elastosis (page 1183) and actinic keratosis (page 1196).

Xanthelasma and xanthoma

Signs and symptoms

- Soft, fatty, yellowish bumps beneath the surface of your skin

Both xanthelasma and xanthoma are yellowish bumps that appear beneath the skin and have sharply defined margins. The bumps can be removed, but they may reappear.

Xanthelasmas

Xanthelasmas are flat and appear in the skin above your eyelids near your nose. They don't hurt, and they may be harmless. However, they're often associated with high levels of fat (lipids) in the blood (hyperlipidemia), so you'll probably want to have your blood tested for increased concentrations of cholesterol and triglycerides.

Xanthomas

Xanthomas are a symptom of an underlying metabolic disorder that increases the fat (lipid) concentration in the blood. Xanthomas can appear anywhere on your body but most commonly occur over joints or tendons. With certain disorders, they tend to appear where your skin receives persistent pressure,

Spider Veins

Spider veins really have nothing to do with spiders, although the pattern of bluish veins seen through your skin may look a bit like a spider. Spider veins result when blood vessels close to the skin's surface widen (dilate). Spider veins are most common on the legs and face. They're not dangerous, but if associated with varicose veins, they can on occasion cause your legs to ache after extended time on your feet.

The cause of spider veins is unknown and nothing can be done to prevent them from appearing. Unlike varicose veins, spider veins are primarily painful to your vanity. For some people, wearing a skirt or shorts is no longer an option because of worries about the appearance of the purple-blue veins on their legs.

Treatment

The easiest course is to ignore the veins. They're a common, mild and medically insignificant variety of varicose veins. If the unsightly blood vessels concern you or, more importantly, if they prevent you from taking part in activities you would otherwise enjoy, ask your doctor about treating them with sclerotherapy, laser surgery or other options (see page 791).

such as on your knees, elbows, hands, feet or buttocks. The bumps are flat and can vary from less than 1 inch to more than 3 inches across.

In addition to hyperlipidemia, xanthomas may also be associated with diabetes, primary biliary cirrhosis, some cancers and several inherited metabolic disorders.

Corns and calluses

Signs and symptoms

- Thickened, hardened layers of skin or raised bumps of hardened skin on your hands and feet

Corns often appear as raised bumps of hardened skin less than 1/4 inch long. Calluses vary in size and shape. Corns and calluses are your skin's attempt to protect itself. Although they can be unsightly, treatment generally is necessary only if they cause discomfort. For most people, eliminating the source of friction or pressure helps corns and calluses disappear.

Treatment

In most cases, you can treat your corn or callous on your own at home. If it becomes painful or inflamed, contact your doctor. Try the following self-care tips:

- Wear properly fitted shoes with adequate toe room. Have your shoe shop stretch your shoes at any point that rubs or pinches. Place pads under your heels if your shoes rub. Try over-the-counter remedies to cushion or soften the corn while wearing shoes.
- Wear padded gloves when using hand tools or try padding your tool handles with cloth tape or covers.
- Rub your skin with a pumice stone or a washcloth during or after bathing to gradually thin some of the thickened skin. Do not do this method if you have diabetes or poor circulation.
- Try over-the-counter corn dissolvers containing salicylic acid.
- Don't cut or shave corns or calluses with a sharp instrument.

Perspiration Disorders

Sitting in the heat of the sun, working out at the gym, giving a presentation at work — all of these things can make you sweat. It's natural to sweat under these conditions. In fact, when you exercise strenuously, are exposed to heat or are under extreme emotional stress, you may lose several quarts of fluid in perspiration.

Sometimes the complex mechanism of perspiration goes awry, resulting in either excessive perspiration (hyperhidrosis) or little or no perspiration (anhidrosis). Excessive sweating can be embarrassing and may sometimes signal a more serious health problem. Anhidrosis is potentially life-threatening.

For most people, sweating is simply a minor nuisance. The odor that sometimes occurs when you sweat is probably more upsetting. Although perspiration is basically odorless, it can take on an unpleasant smell when it comes into contact with bacteria on your skin. Americans spend close to $750 million a year on antiperspirants and deodorants.

But how much you sweat and even the way your sweat smells can be influenced by your mood, certain foods and beverages, some drugs and medical conditions and even your hormones. Because it's almost impossible to define normal sweating, try to learn what's normal for you. That will help you pinpoint any unusual changes.

Anhidrosis

Signs and symptoms

- Lack of perspiration in hot weather and when exercising

Many people worry about excessive sweating. But some people sweat very little or not at all — a condition that can be potentially life-threatening. Factors that may affect your ability to perspire normally include:

- Certain drugs, including some antipsychotic medications
- Hypohidrotic ectodermal dysplasia, a rare disorder in which children are born without sweat glands or with underdeveloped sweat glands
- Autonomic neuropathy, a disorder of nerves
- Infections of the sweat glands
- Burns

Prickly Heat Rash

To some of us, hot weather means the arrival of prickly heat rash. The condition is characterized by a rash of pinhead-sized bumps surrounded by a zone of red skin. Prickly heat rash itches intensely. Often, there's an accompanying prickling, stinging sensation. Typically, it occurs on the neck, upper chest, groin and armpits. The medical name for the most common variety of prickly heat is *miliaria rubra*.

Excessive perspiration produces prickly heat because the moisture damages cells on the surface of your skin. These damaged cells form a barrier that blocks the free flow of sweat out to the surface of your skin. Instead, the sweat accumulates beneath your skin.

The best treatment for prickly heat rash is prevention. Avoid situations that lead to excessive perspiration. If you already have a prickly heat rash, keep the affected area cool and dry, and the problem will likely clear up spontaneously within a few days.

An air-conditioned environment can be helpful. In addition, avoid antiperspirants, lotions, insect repellents or powders if you're still perspiring. After your skin is cool and dry, use a calamine-type lotion to help relieve the symptoms.

- Dehydration
- Heatstroke
- Diabetes, which can cause autonomic neuropathy

How serious is anhidrosis?
When you stop sweating or don't perspire enough to cool your body, the results can be serious or even fatal. Complications of too little perspiration include heat exhaustion and heatstroke. The main sign of heatstroke is a high temperature — generally greater than 104 F — with hot, dry skin and confusion. Early signs and symptoms may include abnormal irritability, headache and nausea. Coma can result from unrecognized and untreated heat exhaustion.

Treatment
Treating anhidrosis involves treating the underlying condition, if possible. In some instances, this may mean changing medications. It's also important to take steps to prevent heat exhaustion, heatstroke and dehydration.

Hyperhidrosis

Signs and symptoms
- Abnormally excessive and bothersome perspiration during exercise or in hot weather
- Excessive and bothersome perspiration on your face, underarms, palms and the soles of your feet that's triggered by nervousness, anxiety or stress

You have two types of sweat glands in your skin: eccrine glands and apocrine glands. Eccrine glands occur over most of your body and open directly onto the surface of your skin. Apocrine glands develop in association with hair follicles on your scalp, underarms, nipples and genitals.

You have between 2 million and 5 million eccrine sweat glands. When your body temperature rises, your autonomic nervous system stimulates these glands to secrete fluid onto the surface of your skin, where it cools your body by evaporation. This fluid (perspiration) is composed of water, salt (sodium chloride) and trace amounts of other electrolytes — substances that help regulate the balance of fluids in your body.

Apocrine glands, on the other hand, secrete a fatty sweat directly into the tubule of the gland. When you're under emotional stress, the wall of the tubule contracts, and the sweat is pushed to the surface of your skin where bacteria begin breaking it down. Most often, it's the bacterial breakdown of apocrine sweat that causes the strong odor.

Some people simply sweat more than others for no apparent reason. But certain factors may make you sweat heavily. These include:
- Certain foods and beverages, including caffeine, alcohol and spicy foods
- Certain drugs, including some antipsychotic medications, morphine, certain painkillers and excess doses of the thyroid hormone thyroxine
- Fever
- Menopause
- Low blood sugar (hypoglycemia)
- Hyperthyroidism (overactive thyroid)
- A heart attack
- Tuberculosis
- Malaria

Complications
Common skin disorders associated with excessive sweating include:
- Fungal nail infections
- Athlete's foot and jock itch
- Bacterial infections and warts

Diagnosis
See your doctor if you suddenly begin to sweat more than usual or experience night sweats for no apparent reason. Infections, thyroid gland problems, menopause and certain types of cancer, such as leukemia and lymphoma, can produce unusual sweating patterns.

A cold sweat is usually your body's response to a serious illness, anxiety or severe pain. Seek immediate medical attention for a cold sweat if you have signs of lightheadedness or chest and stomach pains. Also talk to your doctor if you notice a change in body odor. This can be a sign of certain medical conditions. A fruity smell, for example, may be a sign of diabetes, while an ammonia-like smell could indicate liver disease.

In addition, a rare condition known as fish-odor syndrome (trimethylaminuria) causes an odor similar to rotting fish. People with fish-odor syndrome have a defective gene that prevents them from metabolizing trimethylamine (TMA) — a natural byproduct in the digestion of foods such as saltwater fish, eggs and liver.

Treatment
For some people who sweat excessively, the answer may be simple: an over-the-counter antiperspirant used on the hands and feet as well as the underarms. Antiperspirants work by inhibiting the action of your sweat ducts with aluminum salts, thereby reducing the amount of perspiration that reaches your skin. Deodorants, which can eliminate odor but not perspiration, turn your skin acidic, which makes it less attractive to bacteria. Although you may have heard stories linking antiperspirants and breast cancer, there's no evidence of such a link.

Continued use of antiperspirants can cause irritation or even contact dermatitis — red, swollen, itchy skin. In fact, antiperspirants are the cosmetic product most associated with skin irritation.

If over-the-counter products aren't strong enough, your doctor may suggest a prescription antiperspirant. For more severe problems with sweating, your doctor may recommend other treatments, including:

Iontophoresis
Iontophoresis is a procedure in which a dermatologist uses a battery-powered device to deliver a low current of electricity to the affected area. The instrument

introduces ions into the skin, which prevent the sweat glands from working. Although iontophoresis is painless and quite safe, it may be no more effective than a topical antiperspirant.

Botulinum toxin injections
Botulinum toxin is the same product that helps smooth facial wrinkles by paralyzing certain muscles. Researchers have discovered that botulinum toxin (Botox) injections are also an effective way to treat severe hyperhidrosis. The Botox blocks the nerves that control the sweat glands. It's used mainly in the armpits.

Careful application is required, as in some situations it can cause muscle atrophy. This procedure isn't a cure-all. It may take several injections to achieve the desired results, the treatment can be painful and the results only last about 4 months.

Surgery
In rare cases, surgery may be an option. If excess sweating occurs just in your armpits, removing the sweat glands there may help. This can be done surgically or through liposuction.

If excess sweating occurs on your hands, one possible treatment is to cut the nerves that carry messages from the sympathetic nerves to the sweat glands. The surgery, which generally requires only a day in the hospital and produces minimal scarring, typically doesn't reduce sweating of the underarms, feet or body, but it can permanently stop sweating on the hands. As a side effect of surgery, increased sweating can occur elsewhere on your body.

Self-care
You can do a number of things on your own to reduce sweating and body odor. The following suggestions may help:

- *Bathe daily.* This helps keep the number of bacteria on your skin in check.
- *Dry your feet thoroughly after you bathe.* Microorganisms thrive in the damp spaces between your toes. Use over-the-counter foot powders to help absorb sweat.
- *Apply antiperspirants nightly.* At bedtime, apply antiperspirants to sweaty palms or soles of the feet. Try perfume-free antiperspirants.
- *Choose shoes and socks made of natural materials.* Shoes made of natural materials, such as leather, can help prevent sweaty feet by allowing your feet to breathe. In addition, wear the right socks. Cotton and wool socks help keep your feet dry because they absorb moisture. When you're active, moisture-wicking athletic socks are a good choice.
- *Change your socks often.* Change your socks or hose once or twice a day, drying your feet thoroughly each time. Women who wear pantyhose may want to try those with cotton soles.
- *Rotate your shoes.* Shoes won't completely dry overnight, so if you have trouble with sweaty feet, try not to wear the same pair 2 days in a row.
- *Air your feet.* Go barefoot when you can or at least slip out of your shoes now and then.
- *Choose natural-fiber clothing.* Wear natural fabrics, such as cotton, wool and silk, that allow your skin to breathe. When you exercise, you might prefer high-tech fabrics that wick moisture away from your skin, such as CoolMax or Driline.
- *Try relaxation techniques.* Consider relaxation techniques such as yoga, meditation or biofeedback. These may help you learn to control the stress that can trigger perspiration.

Skin Infections

Because your skin is your first line of defense, it often must deal with attacks from bacteria, viruses, fungi and insects. Skin infections range from localized, superficial infections to widespread, life-threatening infections. The signs and symptoms depend on where the infection develops and the organism causing it.

Impetigo

Signs and symptoms

- Itchy, red sores with yellow or gray crusts, on the face, legs or arms

Impetigo is a fairly common superficial skin infection caused by bacteria — staphylococci (staph), streptococci (strep) or both. It may occur on normal skin, but the bacteria usually invade through a crack, abrasion, insect bite or an area of dry or inflamed skin.

The infection starts as a red sore that blisters briefly and then oozes during the next few days to form a sticky crust (see the color illustration on page 436). The sore tends to grow and is contagious through contact with bacteria in the blister's fluid. Physical contact — including scratching — can spread the infection to other parts of the body or even to other people.

An ulcerating form of impetigo (ecthyma) appears as itchy, thick, brown-black crusts ringed by red skin. In rare instances, the bacteria may infect the bloodstream and, in children, lead to kidney disease. The incidence of impetigo is highest among children with poor hygiene. In adults, it appears mostly as a complication of an underlying skin problem.

Diagnosis
A diagnosis of impetigo may be made after examination of the skin and a lab analysis of the bacteria causing your infection.

Treatment
Topical medications are often effective for limited and minor infections. It may also help to apply a diluted vinegar compress. To make this type of compress, fold a clean cloth and moisten it with a solution

of one ounce white vinegar to 16 to 32 ounces water. For more extensive infections, your doctor may prescribe an oral antibiotic.

Wash the area several times each day with antibacterial soap or cleanser to soften the crusts, and then gently remove them. To avoid spreading the infection, don't share towels, clothing and razors. Avoid skin contact until the condition clears. The sores heal slowly, but the rate of successful treatment is very high.

Folliculitis

Signs and symptoms

- Small, white-headed pimples around the hair follicles

Folliculitis is a superficial infection of the hair follicles (see the color illustration on page 438). This type of infection is common and is usually caused by staphylococci (staph) bacteria, yeast or fungi.

It can occur anywhere on your skin as a result of clothing friction, hair follicle blockage or injury. For example, shaving your neck or underarms can produce a rash that becomes long-lasting (chronic) unless treated.

Barber's itch is a bacterial infection of the hair follicles in the bearded area, especially the upper lip near the nose. Itching may occur a day or two before the pinhead-sized pustules erupt. Shaving is a major aggravating factor.

A similar eruption due to a fungal infection is called tinea barbae. This requires antifungal treatment. Pseudofolliculitis barbae occurs primarily in black men when the hair of the beard curls into the hair follicle or adjacent skin and forms a small, curled-up mass within the follicle, causing a persistent (chronic) infection.

Treatment

For mild folliculitis, a topical antibiotic alone may treat the condition. For more extensive folliculitis, oral antibiotics may be necessary. You might find some relief by applying a washcloth or compress moistened by warm water. If you have folliculitis of the beard, use a new razor blade each time you shave to avoid reinfection from a contaminated razor. Pseudofolliculitis barbae may respond to treatment only if the infected person doesn't shave.

Boils and carbuncles

Signs and symptoms

- A swollen, tender nodule on your skin, usually pink or red, that often eventually drains pus
- A spreading area of swelling, redness and pain in the skin
- Fever
- Exhaustion

A boil (furuncle) is a local infection in one or more hair follicles and is usually caused by staphylococci (staph) bacteria. When multiple boils appear anywhere on the body, the condition is called furunculosis. In contrast, a carbuncle is a cluster of boils that forms a connected area of infection under the skin. Contact with other parts of the body and other people can easily spread these infections.

Sometimes a boil will go away after the initial stage of itching or mild pain. More often, it grows rapidly over a few days. As pus collects within the lesion, pressure and pain increase. It comes to a head with a white or yellow center in the nodule and then bursts, drains and heals. It may recur later near the same site and go through the same cycle.

Boils are common, and most people get one at some time during their lifetime. A boil can occur anywhere on your skin but is most likely to appear on your face, neck, armpits, buttocks or thighs. Poor health, clothing that binds or chafes and disorders such as acne, dermatitis, diabetes and anemia can increase your risk of infection.

Carbuncles commonly appear on the upper back and on the nape of your neck. They're less common than boils. Men are more prone to have them than are women. Carbuncles develop slowly and may not reach your skin's surface to drain on their own.

Diagnosis

A boil or carbuncle can usually be identified by a visual inspection of the affected area. A culture of the pus may be necessary to determine the specific bacteria that caused the infection. Further tests of your blood and urine may be necessary if your doctor suspects an underlying associated disorder.

How serious are boils and carbuncles?

A boil usually will burst within 2 weeks. Any carbuncle or boil that persists longer might spread the infection to your bloodstream. Internal staph infections, which can be life-threatening, often start as skin infections.

A boil or carbuncle on or near your nose, cheeks, forehead or spine can spread rapidly to become a brain abscess or spinal abscess. Prompt medical treatment can help prevent these serious complications.

A boil or carbuncle can produce permanent scarring. The frequent occurrence of boils may indicate an underlying disorder that needs medical attention.

Treatment

To avoid spreading the infection and to minimize discomfort, follow these self-care measures:

- For about 30 minutes every few hours, apply a washcloth or compress moistened with warm salt water. Doing so may help the boil burst and drain much sooner. To prepare warm salt water, add 1 teaspoon of salt to 1 quart of boiling water and let it cool. Prevent the drained matter from contacting other skin areas.
- Gently wash the sore twice a day with antibacterial soap. Cover the sore with a bandage to prevent the infection from spreading.
- Apply an over-the-counter antibiotic ointment.

- Never squeeze or lance a boil because you might spread the infection.
- Launder towels, compresses and clothing that have touched the infected area.

Contact your doctor if the infection is located over your spine or on your face, if it worsens rapidly, causes severe pain, hasn't disappeared within 2 weeks or is accompanied by fever or reddish lines radiating from the boil. In some cases, antibiotics or surgical drainage may be necessary to clear your infection.

Erysipelas and cellulitis

Signs and symptoms

- Painful area of hot, red, swollen skin, sometimes accompanied by red streaks

Cellulitis is an acute inflammation of the connective tissue of your skin that results from a bacterial or fungal infection. It may appear gradually over a couple of days or rapidly over a few hours. It begins as a localized area of red, painful, warm skin, and it may be accompanied by fever and swelling (see the color illustration on page 438).

This infection occurs when bacteria or fungi enter your body through a break in the skin, such as from dermatitis, a fungal infection or a skin injury. People with chronic leg or foot swelling, immune deficits or circulatory deficiencies, such as those related to diabetes, are more prone to developing cellulitis.

Erysipelas is a severe form of cellulitis caused by streptococci (strep) bacteria, in which the infected area is shiny and sharply defined. It's characterized by high fever and recurrences. Gangrene is a rare complication of these infections.

Treatment

After an examination, your doctor may prescribe an antibiotic. This treatment usually stops the infection within a week. Elevating the infected area and applying hot, moist compresses to the site also may help. If the infection spreads, you may require intravenous antibiotics and possibly surgery to control the infection.

Lymphadenitis and lymphangitis

Signs and symptoms

Lymphangitis

- Swollen areas of skin, sometimes with redness and pain
- Throbbing pain in the area of the wound
- Malaise
- Fever, sweating and chills
- Loss of appetite

Emergency signs and symptoms

- A red streak running from the site of the infection up the extremity, or running to the armpit or groin

Lymphadenitis

- Enlarged lymph nodes, such as in the neck, armpits and groin
- Tender or painful lymph nodes
- A smooth, irregular, soft or rubbery feel to the lymph nodes, which indicates an abscess may have formed
- Reddened, hot skin over the lymph nodes

Lymphadenitis is an inflammation of lymph nodes caused by infection from bacteria, viruses, fungi or other microorganisms. Areas where you can easily feel lymph nodes, especially if they're enlarged, are the groin, armpits and neck. Lymphangitis is a similar infection of the lymphatic channels. Both may be associated with pus-filled abscesses and cellulitis.

Lymphangitis often occurs following an acute infection of the skin, such as cellulitis, or an abscess in the skin or soft tissues. It causes a throbbing pain, malaise, fever and loss of appetite. If you develop a red streak running from the site of the infection up the extremity or to the armpit or groin, immediate treatment is essential. The infection can spread rapidly to the bloodstream and may be fatal if untreated.

Lymphadenitis causes enlargement of the lymph nodes, which may be tender or painful. It often results from cellulitis or a bacterial infection by streptococci (strep) or staphylococci (staph), but it can result from any bacterial, fungal, viral or other infection. Sometimes an abscess occurs.

Diagnosis

Diagnostic tests may include blood cultures, a white blood cell count and a lymph node culture or biopsy.

Treatment

Treatment varies, depending on the source of the infection. Antibiotic treatment, begun immediately, usually brings the disease under control in a few days with a complete

PREVENTION TIP

To prevent wound infections, follow these basic self-care measures:

- Keep skin wounds clean.
- Apply an antibiotic cream or ointment. If a rash develops, stop using the ointment and talk to your doctor or pharmacist. Ingredients in such ointments can cause a mild rash in some people.
- Cover the area with a bandage to help keep it clean and keep harmful bacteria out. Repeatedly drain covered blisters until a scab forms.
- Change the bandage daily or whenever it becomes wet or dirty.

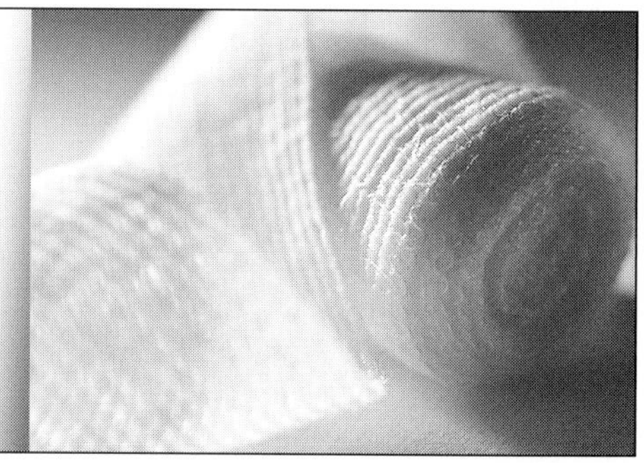

recovery. Aspirin can help relieve the pain, inflammation and swelling. Abscesses may need to be surgically drained.

Cold sores

Signs and symptoms

- Small, fluid-filled blisters on a raised, red, painful area of skin, usually located on the lips but sometimes on your nostrils, cheeks or fingers
- Pain or tingling, often preceding the blisters by 1 to 2 days

The scenario is all too familiar: You feel a tingling on your lip and a small, hard spot that you can't see. Sure enough, in a day or two, a red blister appears on your lip (see the color illustration on page 440). It's another cold sore, probably happening at a bad time, and there's no way to hide it or make it go away quickly.

Cold sores — also called fever blisters — affect millions of Americans, perhaps more than half the population.

Cold sores are quite different from canker sores, a condition people sometimes associate them with. Cold sores are caused by a form of the herpes simplex virus, and they're contagious. Canker sores, which aren't contagious, are ulcers that occur in soft tissues inside the mouth. Although it's unusual, cold sores may appear on the gums or the roof of your mouth (hard palate). Cold sores usually appear on your lip, but occasionally they occur on your nostrils, cheeks or fingers.

Certain strains of the herpes virus cause cold sores. Herpes simplex virus type 1 usually causes cold sores. Herpes simplex virus type 2 is usually responsible for genital herpes. However, either form of the virus can cause sores in the facial area or on the genitals.

You get cold sores from another person who has an active lesion. Shared eating utensils, razors and towels may spread this infection. The greatest risk of infection is from the time the blisters appear until they've completely dried and crusted over. Cold sores seem to run in families. You may have a greater tendency to get cold sores if an immediate family member also experiences cold sores. This may be due to the contagious aspect of cold sores, but it's more likely due to genetic susceptibility.

Symptoms of your first cold sore may start as long as 20 days after exposure to the virus and may last for 7 to 10 days. The blisters form, break and ooze. A yellow crust forms and finally sloughs off to uncover pinkish, healing skin. The virus then reverts to a latent form within your nerve cells.

The herpes virus may emerge again as an active infection on or near the original site causing another cold sore. You may experience an itch or heightened sensitivity at the site preceding each attack. Recurrences are generally milder than the initial infection and may be triggered by menstruation, sun

Blister Basics

Blisters develop when pressure or friction causes fluid to accumulate between the layers of your skin. If you feel a hot spot developing, stop what you're doing and cover the affected area with an adhesive bandage. A blister is a common minor injury.

Don't puncture a blister unless it's painful or prevents you from walking or using one of your hands. Cover a small blister with an adhesive bandage and cover a large one with a porous, plastic-coated gauze pad that absorbs moisture and allows the wound to breathe.

If you must open the blister, first wash your hands and the blister area with soap and warm water. Swab the blister with iodine or 70 percent alcohol. Then puncture the blister at several points along the base with a sterile needle. Drain the fluid, but leave the overlying skin intact. Apply antibiotic ointment to the site and cover it with a gauze pad. After a few days, use a tweezers to lift any dead skin and a scissors to cut it away. Reapply ointment and gauze and check for signs of infection (redness or pus). See a doctor if the blister appears to be infected.

PREVENTION TIP

The virus that causes cold sores can spread as long as the blisters have moist secretions — even after the blisters crust over. The following list includes prevention tips for people who want to guard against a cold sore and for those who already have one but want to avoid spreading it to other parts of their body or to other people:

If you have a cold sore:
- Avoid kissing and intimate skin contact with people.
- Don't share food or beverages with others.
- Wash your hands carefully before touching another person.
- Be careful about touching other parts of your body. Your eyes and genital area are particularly susceptible to spread of the virus.

If you don't have a cold sore:
- Avoid kissing and intimate skin contact with people who have a cold sore.
- Don't share food or beverages with people who have a cold sore.
- Use sunblock on your lips and face before prolonged exposure to the sun — during both the winter and summer.

exposure, stress or any illness accompanied by a fever.

Diagnosis
Your doctor can diagnose cold sores by physical examination. A culture or smear of material from your sore can confirm the presence of herpes simplex virus but is rarely necessary.

How serious are cold sores?
Cold sores are common and rarely cause problems other than discomfort and cosmetic bother. Treatment often can relieve some of the discomfort. However, the infection can cause some potentially serious complications.

If you have a cold sore, avoid contact with infants, anyone who has eczema (atopic dermatitis) and individuals with a suppressed immune system, such as people with cancer or AIDS or those who have received an organ transplant. The herpes virus can be a life-threatening condition for these individuals.

Treatment
For most adults and especially children, cold sores generally clear up without treatment in 7 to 10 days. In the meantime, the following may provide relief:

- Apply rubbing alcohol or diluted white vinegar to help dry up the sore.
- Try over-the-counter anesthetics containing benzocaine (Anbesol, Orajel). They can provide comfort, but they don't speed healing.
- Apply ice to the blisters to ease the pain.
- Take a pain reliever if the sore is still painful after it has dried up and anesthetics and ice aren't helpful.
- Avoid squeezing, pinching or picking at any blister.

If you experience frequent or severe bouts with cold sores, your doctor may prescribe an antiviral medication. Commonly used antivirals include acyclovir (Zovirax), available in both pill and ointment forms, the oral drugs famciclovir (Famvir) and valacyclovir (Valtrex), and the ointment penciclovir (Denavir). Medication may shorten the duration of cold sores, but it won't prevent recurrences.

Shingles

Signs and symptoms
- Pain, burning, tingling or itching in a localized area
- A red rash characterized by small, fluid-filled blisters
- Fever
- Headache

The same virus that causes chickenpox (varicella) causes shingles (herpes zoster). After you've had chickenpox, the virus may remain dormant within your nerve cells. It can re-emerge years later as shingles, a localized infection.

Symptoms generally occur in a sequence as the virus reactivates. The initial sensation is pain, burning, tingling or itching as the virus proliferates along a peripheral nerve that spreads outward from your spinal cord. Shingles affects only the area of your body served by that nerve. A rash of small, fluid-filled blisters appears 2 or 3 days later, after the virus reaches the nerve endings in your skin (see the color illustration on page 438).

Over the next 3 to 5 days, the rash reaches its maximum extent. It may appear as a rectangular strip or belt (*zoster* is Latin for "belt") on one side of your body running from your spine to your breastbone. Or it may appear over an extremity, such as an arm, or on one side of your face or head. The blisters dry up in a few days, forming crusts that fall off 2 or 3 weeks after your initial symptoms.

Shingles is more common in adults than in children. About one in five adults experience shingles, usually after age 50. You can develop shingles more than once, although that's uncommon.

Because your immune system protects you from a new invasion by the virus that causes chickenpox, you can't get shingles from someone else if you've already had chickenpox. However, shingles is contagious for anyone who hasn't had chickenpox and can be debilitating for those with a weakened immune system.

If you have blisters, avoid physical contact with the following individuals. Once your blisters scab over, there's less chance of you spreading the infection to another person.

- Anyone who has never had chickenpox
- Pregnant women, because the infection is dangerous to fetuses
- Newborns, because their immune systems are still forming
- People who are immune compromised, such as those with cancer or AIDS or those who have had an organ transplant

Diagnosis
A diagnosis of shingles is generally made based on your symptoms and the characteristic appearance of the rash. A diagnosis can't be made in absence of the rash.

How serious is shingles?
Shingles normally isn't a serious condition and usually resolves in 2 to 3 weeks. However, some people may have continuing pain for months or even years along the peripheral nerve involved. This painful condition is called postherpetic neuralgia. It occurs more often in people who've had shingles after age 70. Most often, though, postherpetic neuralgia clears up in less than a year, even in people older than age 70.

Shingles damages nerve fibers. The ability of your nerves to send messages from your skin becomes confused and exaggerated. People with postherpetic neuralgia often say they have multiple types of pain, sometimes at the same time.

When shingles affects a major nerve in your face, such as the trigeminal nerve, the rash can occur on your face, inside of your mouth or in or near an eye. Any pain or rash in or near your eye requires prompt medical attention by an ophthalmologist. An eye infection can lead to permanent vision damage.

Treatment

Early treatment of shingles is important. Prompt intervention can shorten the duration of infection and possibly decrease your risk of persistent pain due to neuralgia.

See your doctor as soon as symptoms occur, especially if you're older than age 60. Be sure to see an ophthalmologist if the pain or rash occurs near your eyes or on your nose because the cornea could become involved. You'll need special treatment to avoid visual complications.

Medication

Your doctor will probably take a three-pronged approach to your treatment:

- High doses of an antiviral drug to reduce the duration and severity of symptoms.
- An anti-inflammatory drug to ease inflammation.
- Pain relievers to control pain. For relief of severe pain, narcotics (opioids) may be needed.

Self-care

Your doctor may also recommend that you take these self-care steps:

- Wash the blisters twice a day with regular soap and water, but don't bandage them.
- To help relieve the pain, apply to the blisters cool, wet compresses of water or water mixed with white vinegar — 1 ounce vinegar to 32 ounces water. Do this one to three times a day.
- Soak in a tub of lukewarm water, with or without an oat-bath additive (Aveeno).
- Apply a soothing calamine-type lotion.

Molluscum contagiosum

Signs and symptoms

- Tiny, pearl-like papules on the skin with a core of white, cheesy matter

Molluscum contagiosum is a relatively common viral infection of the skin. Each small, globular papule characteristically has a small indentation or dot on its summit (see the color illustration on page 436).

In children, nodules usually appear on the face, trunk or limbs. In adults, common sites for the nodules are the genitals, abdomen and inner thighs. The infection is contagious by contact.

In adults, it's often spread through sexual contact. Adults with reduced immunity sometimes experience multiple molluscum lesions on the face.

The firm nodules are often painless and disappear within a year. If the nodules and surrounding skin are injured, local spreading can occur.

Treatment

Left untreated, more lesions may occur as the virus sheds from lesions to normal skin. Your doctor can remove the nodules by freezing them, surgical scraping or squeezing out the core matter.

Fungal infections

Signs and symptoms

- Itching, stinging or burning skin
- Cracking and peeling skin
- Extremely dry skin with small, white scales
- Itchy, red or grayish, scaly patches on the scalp
- Itchy, red, scaly, slightly raised rings
- Moist, well-marked, reddened patches rimmed with small, red bumps
- Reddened areas with white patches inside

Fungal skin infections are caused by microscopic fungal organisms that become parasites on your skin. Your body hosts a great variety of microorganisms including mold-like and yeast-like fungi. Some serve useful purposes and cause no problems. Others can proliferate as infectious colonies.

Athlete's foot, jock itch and ringworm

Mold-like fungi (dermatophytes) cause athlete's foot and jock itch as well as ringworm of the skin or scalp. These fungi live on dead tissues of your hair, nails and the outer layer of your skin. Poor hygiene, continuously moist skin and minor skin or nail injuries increase your susceptibility to infection by these fungi.

The primary symptoms of jock itch and athlete's foot are itching and a rash. Jock itch affects the groin and anal areas. Athlete's foot can affect the soles of the feet, the palms and between the toes and fingers.

Ringworm most often affects children. The characteristic rings may be irregular. They start on the scalp but can expand beyond it. The ring grows outward as the infection spreads and the central area becomes less actively infected (see the color illustration on page 436). This type of infection is very contagious and can be passed from shared hats, combs, brushes and barber tools. It's also possible to be infected with ringworm from pets or domestic animals.

Candida albicans

A persistent, bright red rash in the diaper region may indicate a yeast infection caused by *Candida albicans,* which flourishes in a warm, moist environment. Other candida infections include oral thrush and rubbing or chafing infections, which can occur in the folds of skin of overweight people.

Conditions and diseases that can increase your susceptibility to a candida infection include pregnancy, obesity, diabetes, cancer, AIDS, human immunodeficiency virus (HIV) and use of certain medications, such as antibiotics and corticosteroids.

Tinea versicolor

Tinea versicolor is a type of yeast infection that appears as a tissue-thin coating of fungus on your skin (see the color illustration on page 438). The only symptoms are patches of discolored skin that slowly grow. Tinea versicolor is common among teenagers and young adults.

Diagnosis

Your doctor may only need to examine your skin to make the diagnosis of a fungal skin infection. Other times, he or she may need to obtain material from the lesion for laboratory analysis.

How serious are fungal infections?

Fungal infections are rarely life-threatening. They can range from mild to severe and often persist or recur. Treatment is generally successful, but in some cases it may include long-term medication use and continued measures to prevent recurrence.

Rarely, a skin infection by candida yeast can spread through your bloodstream to internal organs. Although some people blame candida infections for a wide variety of symptoms, including chronic fatigue syndrome, evidence for this is lacking.

Treatment

The appropriate treatment depends on the type of fungal infection.

Athlete's foot, jock itch and ringworm
For athlete's foot, ringworm and jock itch, apply an over-the-counter antifungal ointment, lotion, powder or spray. Most infections respond well to these topical agents.

Your doctor may prescribe an oral antifungal medication if the infection is persistent (chronic) or severe. Side effects from oral antifungal medications can be severe and include gastrointestinal upset, rash and liver failure. They may also interfere with the effects of certain medications, including warfarin (Coumadin). In May 2001, the Food and Drug Administration issued a public health advisory regarding two antifungal medications, itraconazole (Sporanox) and terbinafine (Lamisil), because of concerns they may cause congestive heart failure. This medication-induced effect stopped when use of the drug was discontinued. The warning doesn't apply to cream and solution forms of Lamisil, which are applied topically.

Candida infections
Diaper rash and chafing can be treated using an antifungal cream and by keeping the affected area clean and dry. Frequent diaper changes will help promote dryness. For other candida infections that are severe or persistent, your doctor may prescribe an oral antifungal medication. It's important that your doctor supervise this treatment because long-term use of this type of drug can have serious side effects.

Tinea versicolor
For tinea versicolor, frequent showering can help. In addition, apply topical agents such as selenium sulfide (Selsun, Exsel) or antifungal creams such as ciclopirox (Loprox).

Insect bites

Signs and symptoms

- Itchy, red bumps
- A red, painful, ulcerating sore
- Local numbness or a pins-and-needles sensation

PREVENTION TIP

Preventing jock itch and athlete's foot requires good personal hygiene. Follow these suggestions:

Jock itch

- Keep the affected area clean and dry.
- Avoid clothes that chafe.
- If you use athletic supporters, launder them frequently.
- Shower and change clothes after exercise.

Athlete's foot

- Keep your feet dry, especially between the toes.
- Wear socks that are made of natural material, such as cotton or wool.
- Change socks and stockings regularly — twice a day if your feet sweat a lot.
- Wear light, well-ventilated shoes made of natural, not synthetic, materials.
- Alternate the pairs of shoes that you wear so that they can dry between wearings.
- Wear waterproof sandals or shower shoes in communal showers, pools, fitness centers and other public areas.
- Use an antifungal foot powder or spray daily.
- Don't borrow shoes.

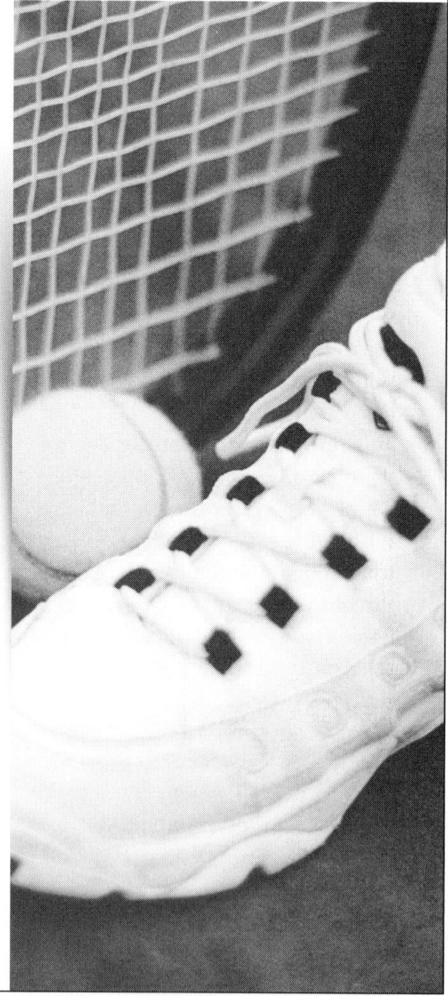

Emergency signs and symptoms
- A swollen face
- Widespread numbness
- Muscle cramping
- Difficulty breathing
- Headache
- Nausea
- Fever
- Coma

The injection of venom or other agents into your skin causes the symptoms from insect bites. Most often the reaction is local and temporary, but the venom can affect your entire body if you're hypersensitive to the venom or if it's exceptionally potent.

The bite of a black widow spider feels like a pinprick. Some people aren't aware they've been bitten. At first, they may experience only slight swelling and faint red marks in the area of the bite. Within a few hours, intense pain and stiffness begin.

Other symptoms may include chills, fever, nausea and severe abdominal pain. Generally, the pain lessens after a few hours but may return over the next 2 to 3 days.

Bites by the brown recluse and other spiders cause a mild stinging followed by local redness and intense pain within 8 hours. A fluid-filled bump forms at the site and then sloughs off, sometimes leaving a large, deep, growing ulcer. Symptoms can vary from a mild fever and rash to nausea and listlessness.

Most ant bites cause only local redness and swelling. Fire ants, however, can produce many small, fluid-filled bumps that ulcerate like spider bites. Other biting insects inject chemicals as they feed on you. These insects include mosquitoes, fleas, flies, bedbugs and chiggers.

Stings by bees, wasps and hornets inject venom that causes immediate pain and rapidly enlarging red bumps. A few hours after a sting, the pain generally subsides, and the affected area turns itchy.

Diagnosis

Sometimes you can recognize an insect bite or sting easily because you feel the sting when it happens. At other times, bites just seem to appear. If you have a severe reaction, knowing what bit you will help your doctor determine the treatment.

How serious are insect bites?

Symptoms from a typical bite or sting generally last a few hours or days. However, if you're allergic to bee stings or if you receive multiple stings, you may experience a life-threatening reaction called anaphylactic shock (see page 545). This requires emergency treatment.

Approximately 1 in 250 Americans are allergic to bee stings. These stings cause more deaths than do snakebites. Poisonous spider bites are rarely fatal. However, small children and older adults are especially vulnerable to the effects of spider bites.

Treatment

Mild insect bites may be treated by applying ice cubes to the affected area to decrease pain. In addition, applying over-the-counter hydrocortisone cream or calamine-type lotion may help relieve itching or inflammation.

For a more severe reaction, your doctor may prescribe a corticosteroid cream.

An individual who's allergic to the venom of a particular insect, such as a bee or hornet, may require an immediate injection of adrenaline (epinephrine) if stung. A doctor can prescribe an emergency medical kit to keep handy that includes emergency medication. If faintness, listlessness or shortness of breath occurs, seek emergency medical care immediately.

If you're bitten by a black widow spider, you may need to be hospitalized. Treatment may include hot soaks, injections of antivenin and intravenous infusion of calcium gluconate to relieve cramps.

Treatment for a brown recluse spider bite often involves corticosteroid injections and surgical removal of the ulcer.

Portuguese man-of-war stings

Signs and symptoms
- Stinging and pain
- Red, hive-like lesions in a line
- Shortness of breath
- Nausea and stomach cramps
- Emotional upset

The Portuguese man-of-war is a jelly-like marine animal that has no backbone (invertebrate). It's easy to recognize on account of the highly characteristic blue or red bell-shaped body that floats at the surface of the water and ranges from less than 1 inch to more than a foot in diameter.

A cluster of tentacles hangs beneath the body of the man-of-war. Most are short and frilly, but one or more can be many feet long. These long fishing tentacles are responsible for the stings.

If you touch one of these tentacles, it will whip around the contact area and inject a toxic venom into your skin. Because the venom (a neurotoxin) remains potent long after the man-of-war is dead, wading in shallow water or walking along the beach can be hazardous. The tentacles discharge their venom for long periods, even after they're separated from the main body of the man-of-war. The venom is carried into the victim by tiny barbs on the tentacles.

Diagnosis

Common symptoms range from mild prickling to severe burning and numbness. A red line develops on the area of the skin exposed to the tentacles. Sometimes a line of welts or blisters develops.

How serious are Portuguese man-of-war stings?

Death from Portuguese man-of-war stings is unusual, but the stings can be painful. Severe stings can lead to muscle cramping, fainting, coughing, vomiting and difficulty breathing. In rare cases, a potentially fatal reaction called anaphylactic shock (see page 545) may occur.

Treatment

Here are practical tips for coping with Portuguese man-of-war stings:

- *Get out of the water.* The pain and cramps can be disabling and cause you to drown.
- *Deactivate the stinging.* Sprinkle the affected area with vinegar, salt, sugar or even dry sand. This often offers quick relief.
- *Cleanse the wound.* Approximately 15 minutes after deactivating the wound, gently wash the area with seawater. Don't use fresh water and don't rub the skin because either action could trigger discharge of more venom.
- *Remove the stinging tentacles.* Apply a paste made of seawater and sand, baking soda, talcum powder or flour. Scrape the residue with a knife or other suitable object, such as a clamshell. It's best to wear gloves or use a towel while removing the residue.
- *Apply medication.* Use a nonprescription hydrocortisone cream to relieve redness and swelling. A local anesthetic ointment, such as those containing benzocaine, can help relieve pain, and a calamine-type lotion reduces itching.

If you have a significant reaction to a sting, see a doctor.

Prevention

Extra clothing, particularly a wet suit or body stocking, is your best protection from Portuguese man-of-wars if you're swimming in waters where they live. In addition, wear sneakers or plastic beach shoes while walking along the beach. And watch where you step.

Noncancerous Skin Tumors

Noncancerous (benign) skin tumors are common and usually harmless. As you grow older, you're likely to have a number of them. With the exception of actinic keratoses and certain moles, benign tumors don't require removal unless they're irritating or cosmetically displeasing. As a precaution, however, consult your doctor about any new growth or changes in old growths.

Actinic keratoses

Signs and symptoms

- Gritty, scaly, pale-gray to dark-pink patches on the face, scalp and back of hands

Actinic keratoses (solar keratoses) occur mostly in fair-skinned people with sun-damaged skin. Initially, the keratoses are flat and scaly. Later, they have a hard, wart-like surface (see the color illustration on page 433). Their sandpaper-like surface is more easily felt than seen. Actinic keratoses are considered noncancerous (benign) tumors, but they may represent precancerous changes in your skin.

Treatment

Medical attention is needed for an actinic keratosis because left untreated it may develop into squamous cell skin cancer. Your doctor can remove it by freezing it with liquid nitrogen or by using topical medication, electrical burning or surgery. A sample of the tissue may be examined for signs of cancer.

Cherry angiomas

Signs and symptoms

- A small, smooth, cherry red spot on the skin

Cherry angiomas are noncancerous (benign) skin tumors of unknown origin that appear most frequently after age 40. They can occur almost anywhere on your skin but most commonly are found on the torso. Cherry angiomas range from pinhead size to 1/4 inch across (see the color illustration on page 433). Large angiomas can bleed profusely when they're injured.

Treatment

A cherry angioma is painless and harmless, but you may want it removed for cosmetic reasons. Your doctor can remove it easily by freezing the angioma with liquid nitrogen, using laser treatment or destroying it by a minor electrosurgical procedure.

Keloids

Signs and symptoms

- Flesh- or lighter-colored nodular or ridged growths over scars on the skin

A keloid is an overproduction of scar tissue. It's sometimes called hypertrophic scarring.

A keloid occurs at the site of a skin injury resulting from, for example, an operation, a vaccination, severe acne, a burn or even a minor scratch. It's fairly common on black skin and much less common on white skin.

A keloid is harmless, but it may be tender, itchy or disfiguring. Some keloids stop growing or even disappear without treatment.

Treatment

Surgical removal of a keloid often causes further scarring unless it's followed by X-ray treatment or injection of steroids at the site. Small keloids may be removed by freezing them with liquid nitrogen.

Liver spots

Signs and symptoms

- Flat spots of increased pigmentation — usually brown, black or gray — on your face or the backs of your hands

Liver spots (senile lentigines) are harmless flat patches of increased pigmentation that range from freckle-sized to a few inches across. These flat, gray, brown or black spots affect more than 90 percent of fair-skinned people over age 50.

Liver spots are most common on areas most exposed to the sun — your face and the backs of your hands (see the color illustration on page 433). They tend to darken with sun exposure. Despite the name, they're unrelated to the liver.

How serious are liver spots?

True liver spots hardly ever become cancerous, although they can look like some cancerous growths. In rare circumstances they may turn into lentigo maligna, a slow-growing, nonaggressive form of skin cancer.

Treatment

For cosmetic reasons, liver spots can be lightened with skin-bleaching products or removed by freezing or laser therapy. You can help prevent new spots by avoiding the sun and using sunscreen.

Moles

Signs and symptoms

- Flesh-colored, brown, blue or black spots on the skin

Nearly everyone has moles. These noncancerous (benign) tumors are nests of pigment cells. They may be smooth, contain hairs, and become raised or wrinkled (see the color illustrations on page 434). New moles may appear up until age 40, but most appear by age 20. Some moles disappear with advancing age.

Moles are usually harmless, but they can become cancerous (see page 1203). Consult your doctor if a mole changes in color or size or if it develops itching, pain, bleeding or inflammation. Certain moles — such as those that are irregular in shape and are located around or under your nails or near your genitals — should be monitored by a doctor for evidence of melanoma. Some moles have a higher-than-average risk of becoming cancerous. They include:

- *Large moles present at birth.* Large moles that are present at birth are called congenital nevi and may increase your risk of malignant melanoma, a form of skin cancer. Moles that are more than 8 inches in diameter pose the greatest risk. Any mole that has been present since birth and is the size of a credit card or larger should be examined by a doctor.
- *Moles that run in families.* Moles that are larger than average — about the diameter of a pencil eraser — and irregular in shape are known as atypical or dysplastic nevi. These moles tend to be hereditary and usually have dark brown centers and lighter, uneven borders. Overall, they may look red or tan. If you have dysplastic nevi, you have a greater risk of developing malignant melanoma.
- *Numerous moles.* If you have many moles larger than 6 millimeters across — about the diameter of a pencil eraser — you may be at greater risk of developing melanoma.

Other important factors that increase your risk of melanoma include family history, a history of severe sunburns and a fair complexion with reddish hair and blue eyes. Not all melanomas arise from pre-existing nevi.

Diagnosis

If your doctor suspects that a mole may be cancerous, he or she may take a sample of the tissue to be examined (biopsied) under a microscope.

Treatment

If your doctor finds that your mole is cancerous, the entire mole and a margin around it will be removed. Usually, a mole that has been removed won't reappear. If it does, see your doctor promptly.

Most moles don't require treatment, but if you want one removed for cosmetic reasons, it can be done in several ways. Your doctor may use a method known as shave

Monitor That Mole

Moles have no known purpose, and no one knows why they develop. Most moles are harmless, but you do need to monitor them for changes that may signal melanoma, a serious form of skin cancer.

The best way to catch potential problems at an early stage is to become familiar with the location and pattern of your moles. Remember to check areas that aren't exposed to sunlight, including your scalp, armpits, feet (between the toes) and genital area.

Examine your skin carefully on a regular basis. If necessary, use a hand-held mirror along with a wall mirror to scan hard-to-see places like your back. If your moles are larger than average — about the diameter of a pencil eraser — and irregular in shape, you're at greater risk of developing malignant melanoma and may want to consider having a dermatologist check your moles on a regular basis.

When checking your moles to determine if they may be cancerous, follow the A-B-C-D guide from the American Academy of Dermatology (see page 1203). Watch for irregular borders, changes in color and an increasing diameter. Other factors to watch for include:

- *Height.* Noncancerous (benign) moles tend to be flat or dome shaped. Be wary of moles that are partially flat and partially elevated.
- *Texture.* Scales, shedding of skin, oozing or mild bleeding can signal melanoma. So can hardening or softening of the colored area.
- *Sensation.* Is there itching, tenderness or pain?
- *Nearby skin.* Pay attention to swelling, redness or other coloring that spreads into skin near the pigmented area.

excision in which the area around the mole is numbed and the mole is removed close to the skin. Moles may also be removed with a small incision or punch biopsy technique. The procedure is usually performed in a doctor's or dermatologist's office and takes only a short time.

Seborrheic keratoses

Signs and symptoms

- Brown, black or pale growths on the face, chest, shoulders and back that look waxy, as if they were dripped on the skin by a candle

Seborrheic keratoses are noncancerous (benign) skin tumors of unknown origin that commonly appear after age 40. The oval growths have a waxy, wart-like, scaly, slightly elevated surface and range from 1/3 to 1 inch or more across (see the color illustration on page 433). Their color varies from pale yellow to dark brown or black, and they have a pasted-on appearance. Occasionally, they appear singly but most often are multiple.

Treatment

A seborrheic keratosis is normally painless and requires no treatment unless it itches, irritates or detracts from your appearance. This type of growth is never deeply rooted, so removal is simple and nonscarring. Your doctor can remove it with a simple surgical procedure or freeze it off with liquid nitrogen. Sometimes it recurs.

Skin tags

Signs and symptoms

- Small tags of skin on your neck, armpits, upper trunk and body folds

Skin tags (acrochordons) are tiny, noncancerous (benign) tumors of unknown origin that protrude from your skin on a narrow stalk (see the color illustration on page 434). They're soft and normally skin-colored but may appear darker. Skin tags are common, especially after middle life. They're usually painless but can become irritated by friction with clothing.

Treatment

Treatment of a skin tag is unnecessary unless it's bothersome. Your doctor can remove it by freezing it with liquid nitrogen, cutting it off or burning it off with electricity.

Warts

Signs and symptoms

- Small, fleshy, grainy bumps that may be skin-colored, white, pink or tan

Warts are skin growths caused by the human papillomavirus (HPV), which stimulates the rapid growth of cells on the outer layer of your skin. More than 50 types of warts occur and can affect any part of your body, most often the hands and feet. Warts may disappear in a few weeks, or they may last a long time.

Types

The two kinds of warts most often seen by doctors are common warts and plantar warts.

Common warts

Common warts appear as skin growths near the fingernails but can also appear on any part of the hand (see the color illustration on page 434). Young adults and children appear to be affected most often. Common warts are typically painless.

Plantar warts

Plantar warts appear on the feet and may appear to have tiny black dots in them. The dots are small, clotted blood vessels. Plantar warts can be painful because they press inward when you stand on them.

Causes

You can acquire warts through direct contact with an infected person or surface, such as a shower floor. Warts usually spread through breaks in your skin.

Each person's immune system responds differently, meaning that not everyone who comes in contact with HPV will develop warts. Generally, the incubation period — the time from when you're initially infected until warts appear — is about 3 months, but the virus can lie dormant for years. Because warts are more common in children, some experts believe that adults may develop an immunity to HPV.

How serious are warts?

Common warts and plantar warts aren't usually a serious health concern, and many disappear on their own within 2 years. But they may be bothersome, requiring medical treatment to remove them. Warts may also recur after treatment and become a persistent problem.

Warts that don't occur in your genital areas are neither a sign of cancer nor a precursor to it. Because warts shed HPV, new warts can appear nearby. There's also a potential to infect others, such as family members who might share bathing facilities.

Warts that occur on the sexual organs are called genital warts and are considered a sexually transmitted disease. They can be a serious health concern because they may increase the risk of cervical cancer in women. Various strains of HPV are responsible for at least 95 percent of cases of cervical cancer. In addition, a pregnant women infected with HPV can pass on the virus to a newborn during childbirth.

Treatment

For warts that aren't located on your genitals, home treatment may be possible. Don't try to treat genital warts with over-the-counter medications, which are not intended for use in the moist tissues of the genital areas. Doing so can cause pain and soreness in the treated areas. See your doctor if warts occur on your genitals.

Over-the-counter wart medications are available at drug, discount

Laser Surgery

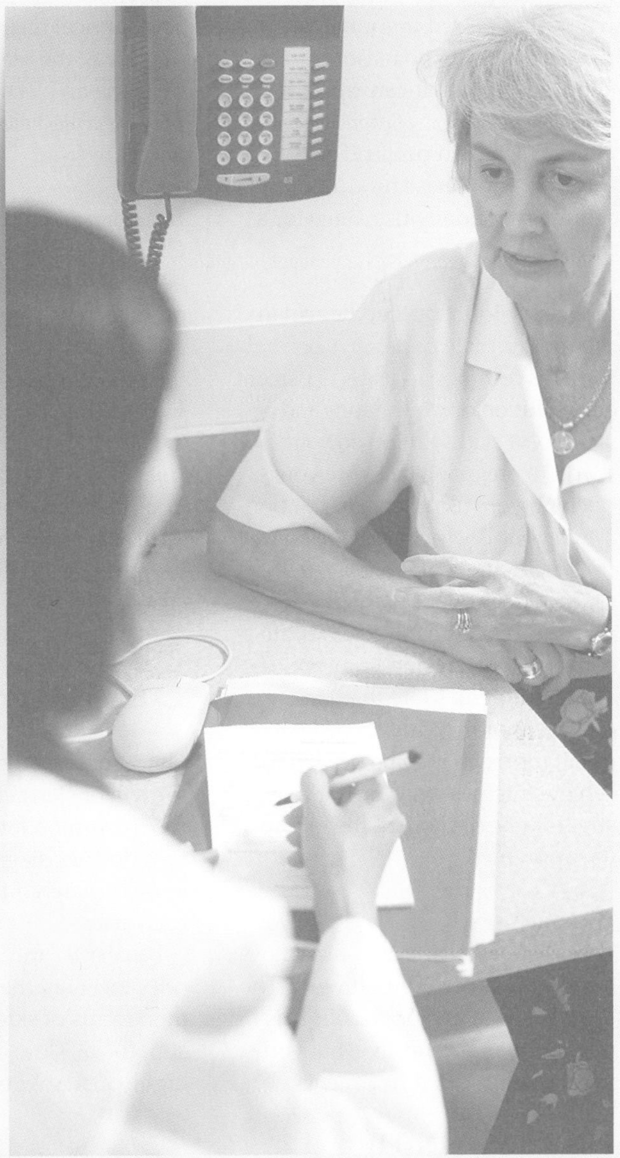

Laser beams are strong enough to cut through diamonds, yet they can be gentle enough to sculpt your skin. In the medical world, these scalpels of light are helpful in many procedures. But as high-tech as these magic wands are, they can't zap away every problem. They may be the right tool for some procedures but not the best choice for others.

In addition, as with any operation, the success of laser surgery depends largely on the surgeon's skill and on whether the procedure is appropriate for you.

Intense light

The word *laser* stands for light amplification by stimulated emission of radiation. Laser beams are strong beams of light produced by electrically stimulating a particular material. A solid, liquid or gas is used. Generally, lasers are named for the substances that produce them and vary from carbon dioxide and argon to ruby.

The combination of light intensity and the ability to focus it on a small area gives lasers their unique role in medicine. Lasers can be used to:

- Cut or destroy tissue that's abnormal or diseased
- Shrink or destroy tumors or lesions
- Burn off or vaporize tissue
- Sculpt tissue
- Seal blood vessels

Basically, what lasers do is vaporize tissue. A scalpel cuts tissue with a blade. Lasers cut tissue by destroying (vaporizing) the cells.

Distinct advantages

Lasers haven't replaced scalpels, but they do help doctors perform some procedures more effectively than with traditional methods. Lasers cause minimal bleeding, providing surgeons a clear view of the area of surgery. Because of their precision, lasers allow doctors to work on small and hard-to-reach parts of the body. Doctors can also vary how deeply the laser penetrates tissue by adjusting the light's intensity.

In addition, laser surgery may pose less risk of infection and scarring. In some cases, laser surgery is faster than traditional surgery, shortening recovery time. Some laser surgeries are performed under a local anesthetic in a doctor's office. Others require general anesthesia and hospitalization.

Versatile tool

Laser surgery is used in many dermatological procedures. They can be used to remove or lighten:

- Birthmarks such as port-wine stains
- Fine wrinkles
- Pigmentation disorders, such as freckles and liver spots
- Spider veins
- Noncancerous (benign) skin growths
- Some skin cancers
- Warts
- Unwanted hair
- Tattoos

Precautions

Despite what some advertisements might suggest, lasers aren't magical, fix-all tools. Risks associated with using a laser are similar to those of using a more conventional procedure. They include pain, infection and, rarely, scarring. Imprecisely aimed lasers can burn or destroy healthy tissue. Although lasers can remove marks on skin, they can also change skin pigmentation and, therefore, coloring.

and grocery stores. Unless you have an impaired immune system, there's generally no reason you shouldn't try a self-care approach. Look for products containing salicylic acid, which peels off the infected skin. These products require twice daily use, often for a few weeks.

One caution about over-the-counter products is that the acid in them can irritate or damage normal skin. It's common to use a 17 percent acid solution on your hands and a 40 percent acid solution on your feet. If you're pregnant, talk with your doctor before using an acid solution.

See your doctor if, despite home treatment, the warts persist or spread. Warts, especially plantar warts, can be difficult to eradicate completely. New ones may appear after treatment. More than one treatment or more than one treatment approach may be needed to achieve success. Your doctor may suggest one or more of the following approaches:

Freezing
Your doctor may destroy a wart by freezing it with liquid nitrogen. The dead tissue later sloughs off. This method may be effective, but you may need repeated treatments.

Minor surgery
The surgical method involves cutting away the wart or destroying it by using an electric needle in a process called electrodesiccation and curettage.

Laser surgery
One type of laser emits a narrow beam of intense light that cuts away or vaporizes growths. Another type of laser emits a beam that vaporizes the blood vessels supplying the wart so that the wart dies.

Injection
Your doctor may inject medications such as interferon alfa or bleomycin into the wart to kill the HPV virus.

PREVENTION TIP

To reduce the risk of spreading or contracting warts:

- Avoid brushing, clipping, combing or shaving over areas where you have a wart.
- Don't walk barefoot in public areas, such as pools and locker rooms. Wear shoes or sandals in these public places.
- Avoid using the same file or nail clipper on nails with warts as you use on healthy nails.
- Don't pick at warts. Picking may spread the virus. If you have a child with a wart, consider covering his or her wart with an adhesive bandage to discourage picking.

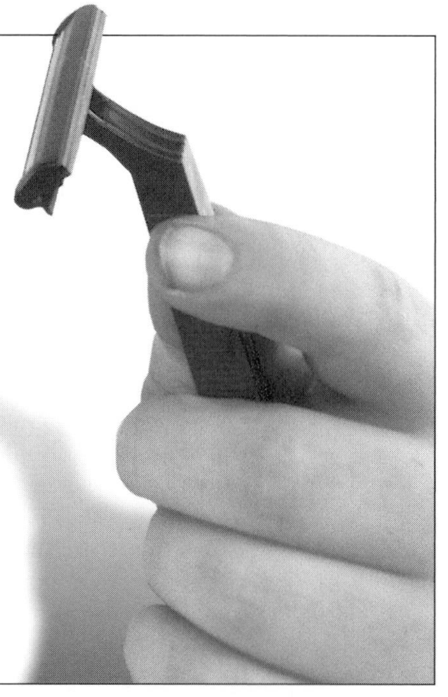

Skin Cancer

Skin cancer — the abnormal growth of skin cells — is by far the most common form of cancer. In fact, doctors diagnose skin cancer in approximately 1 million Americans each year.

Basal cell cancer and squamous cell cancer are the two most common forms of skin cancer. Both are superficial, slow growing and highly treatable, especially if found early. Melanoma is a more serious form of skin cancer. It can affect deeper layers of the skin and has the greatest potential to spread to other tissues in the body.

Skin cancer is on the rise. Fair-skinned people who live in areas with a lot of sunlight are at greatest risk. But anyone can develop skin cancer, which is most commonly caused by overexposure to ultraviolet (UV) radiation. Nearly half of all Americans will develop a cancerous skin lesion at least once by the age of 65. The good news is that nearly 90 percent of skin cancers are preventable. If caught early, most are also highly curable.

It's important to protect your skin from UV radiation and to check your skin regularly for signs of cancer. Left undetected or untreated, skin cancer can be damaging and even deadly. Skin cancer claims nearly 10,000 lives a year in the United States.

Risk factors

Generally, your risk of developing skin cancer increases with age. But skin cancer isn't limited to middle-aged and older people. People in their 20s and 30s can develop skin cancer. Half of all melanomas occur in people under the age of 50.

Although overexposure to UV radiation is the most common cause of skin cancer, several factors may increase your risk of developing skin cancer:

Fair skin
Having less pigment (melanin) in your skin provides less protection from damaging UV radiation from the sun or tanning beds. If you have blond or red hair, light-colored eyes and you freckle or sunburn easily, you're 20 to 30 times more likely to develop skin cancer in your lifetime than is a person who doesn't have these traits.

A history of sunburns
Sunburn is the result of overexposure to the sun's UV radiation.

Every time you sunburn your skin, you increase your risk of developing skin cancer. People who've had one or more severe, blistering sunburns as a child or teenager are at increased risk of skin cancer as an adult. Sunburns in adulthood also are a risk factor.

Excessive sun exposure
Individuals who spend considerable time in the sun, including those who tan, may develop skin cancer. This is especially true if the skin is unprotected by sunscreen or clothing.

Sunny or high-altitude climates
People who live in sunny, warm climates are exposed to more sunlight than are people who live in colder climates. In the United States, for example, skin cancer is much more prevalent in Arizona than it is in Minnesota.

In addition, people who live at higher elevations are exposed to more UV radiation than are people who live at lower elevations.

Moles
People who have multiple moles called dysplastic nevi are at increased risk of skin cancer (see page 1197).

Precancerous skin lesions
Having skin lesions known as actinic keratoses can increase your risk of developing skin cancer (see page 1196).

Genetics
Chronic sun exposure doesn't explain melanomas or other skin cancers that develop on skin not exposed to sunlight, such as the soles of the feet. Genetics seem to play a role. If your parent or a brother or sister has had skin cancer, you may be at higher risk of the disease.

Personal history of skin cancer
If you develop skin cancer once, you're at risk of developing it again.

A weakened immune system
People with impaired immune systems are at greater risk of many diseases, including skin cancer. This may include individuals who've undergone an organ transplant, people receiving cancer treatment or individuals with human immunodeficiency virus (HIV) or AIDS.

Fragile skin
Skin that has been burned or injured from disease is more susceptible to sun damage and skin cancer. Certain psoriasis treatments also can increase the risk of skin cancer.

Exposure to environmental hazards
Exposure to environmental chemicals, including some herbicides, may increase the risk of skin cancer.

Detection and diagnosis

A skin change is the most common warning sign of skin cancer. You may notice the appearance of a small growth or a sore that bleeds, crusts over, heals and then reopens. The first sign of melanoma may be a change in an existing mole or the development of a new, suspicious-looking mole.

Skin cancer develops mainly on areas of skin that are exposed to a lot of sun — the scalp, face, lips, ears, neck, chest, arms and hands. But skin cancer can also develop on unexposed areas, such as the palms, the spaces between toes and the genital area. A cancerous skin lesion can appear suddenly, or it can develop slowly.

Check your skin regularly and report changes to your doctor. Examine your skin at least every 3 months for the development of new skin growths or changes in existing moles, freckles, bumps and birthmarks. With the help of mirrors, check your face, neck, ears and scalp. Examine your chest and trunk and the tops and undersides of your arms and hands. Examine the front and back of your legs, your feet, including the soles and between your toes, your genital area and between your buttocks.

Although skin cancers don't all look the same, they all involve a change in the skin's appearance in a localized area. If you notice any change in your skin, consult your doctor right away. Don't wait for the area to start hurting because skin cancer seldom causes pain.

If your doctor suspects skin cancer after a visual inspection of your skin, he or she may want to take a small sample of your skin (biopsy) for analysis in a laboratory to confirm the diagnosis. A biopsy can usually be performed in a doctor's office after administering a local anesthetic.

Doctors generally divide skin cancer into two stages: local, affecting only the skin, or metastatic, spreading beyond the skin. Because superficial skin cancers such as basal cell cancer or squamous cell cancer rarely spread, a biopsy often is the only test needed to determine the cancer stage.

In cases where a growth is very large or has existed for a while, your doctor may check your lymph nodes in the area. You may also need additional tests, such as special X-rays, to determine whether the cancer has spread to other parts of the body. Knowing the stage of a skin cancer helps your doctor plan the best treatment.

Basal cell cancer

Signs and symptoms
- A pearly or waxy bump on the face, ear or neck
- A flat, flesh-colored or brown scar-like lesion on the chest or back

Basal cell cancer is a common form of skin cancer. Approximately 1 million diagnoses are made every year in the United States.

When basal cells in your epidermis become cancerous, they form a pearl-like or waxy bump or a flat lesion. The lesion may ulcerate after a few months, slowly enlarge and never heal completely (see the color illustration on page 434).

Basal cell skin cancers usually occur on unprotected areas of skin. The primary cause of this type of skin cancer is repeated overexposure to ultraviolet radiation from the sun, or from tanning beds or sunlamps.

Basal cell cancer most commonly occurs after age 40. The cancer generally remains a local growth and only rarely spreads to other parts of the body. However, lack of medical attention can allow the growth to invade nearby tissues and underlying structures, including your nerves, bones or brain.

Treatment
In order to make a diagnosis of basal cell cancer, your doctor will need a sample of the lump or lesion to be examined in a laboratory (biopsied). Treatment depends on the cancer's size, depth and location and may include scraping and cauterization of the cancer, freezing

Skin Cancer Treatments

The appropriate treatment for skin cancer depends on the size, type, depth and location of a lump or lesion. Most treatments use a local anesthetic and can be performed in an outpatient setting.

Standard therapies

Methods used to treat skin cancer include:

Freezing
To prevent skin cancer, a doctor may destroy precancerous skin lesions that increase the risk of skin cancer, such as actinic keratoses, by freezing them with liquid nitrogen (cryosurgery). This procedure may also be used on some small, early skin cancers. The dead tissue later sloughs off. The treatment may leave a small, white scar. You may need a repeat treatment to remove the growth completely.

Laser therapy
Laser therapy involves a precise, intense beam of light that vaporizes growths, generally with little damage to surrounding tissue and with minimal bleeding, swelling and scarring. A doctor may use this therapy to treat superficial skin cancers or precancerous growths on lips.

Excisional surgery
Excisional surgery may be appropriate for any type of skin cancer. A doctor cuts out (excises) the cancerous tissue and a margin of healthy skin around it. A wide excision — removing extra normal skin around the tumor — may be best for melanoma. To minimize or avoid scarring, especially on the face, skin reconstruction may be needed.

Mohs' micrographic surgery
Mohs' micrographic surgery is a technique used for larger, recurring or difficult-to-treat skin cancers, which may include both basal cell and squamous cell types. A doctor removes the skin growth layer by layer, examining each layer under the microscope, until no abnormal cells remain. Mohs' surgery is the treatment of choice to remove skin cancer without taking an excessive amount of surrounding healthy skin.

Curettage and electrodesiccation
With this procedure, a doctor scrapes away layers of cancer cells using a circular blade (curette). An electric needle destroys any remaining cancer cells. This simple, quick procedure is common in treating small or thin basal cell cancers. It leaves a small, flat, white scar.

Radiation therapy
If surgery isn't an option, your doctor may recommend daily radiation treatments, usually for 1 to 4 weeks, to destroy basal cell and squamous cell skin cancers.

Chemotherapy
In chemotherapy, drugs are used to kill cancer cells. With skin cancer, chemotherapy can be delivered topically by applying to the skin creams or lotions containing anticancer agents. This treatment is useful for cancers limited to the top layer of the skin. Chemotherapy drugs can also be taken by mouth (orally) or given intravenously to treat skin cancer that has spread to other parts of the body.

Experimental therapies

Other treatments for skin cancer that are currently under study include:

Photodynamic therapy
Photodynamic therapy destroys skin cancer cells with a combination of intense light and medications that make cancer cells sensitive to light.

Biological therapy
The medications interferon and interleukin-2 are under study as a treatment for melanoma. These biological therapy (immunotherapy) drugs stimulate the body's own immune system to fight the cancer. Although these drugs showed promise initially, later studies had somewhat disappointing results.

Limb perfusion
Limb perfusion is an experimental method of administering chemotherapy. The procedure is being studied for use when melanoma involves only an arm or leg. In limb perfusion, the flow of blood to and from the limb is stopped temporarily with a tourniquet. Chemotherapy drugs are then given intravenously into the limb. This allows for the cancer to be treated with higher doses of chemotherapy.

(cryosurgery), radiation, surgical excision or a series of microscopically controlled shaved excisions, called Mohs' surgery (see page 1202).

Because many skin cancers are on the face, a surgeon may also perform a reconstructive procedure, such as a skin graft, if necessary.

With early treatment, basal cell cancer has a cure rate of more than 95 percent. You'll need to diligently practice good sun protection techniques to avoid further growths. Avoid the midday sun, wear protective clothing and use sunscreen on exposed skin. In addition, have regular medical examinations.

Squamous cell cancer

Signs and symptoms

- A firm, red nodule on the face, lip, ear, neck, hand or arm
- A flat lesion with a scaly, crusted surface on the face, ear, neck, hand or arm

Squamous cell cancer is a cancerous (malignant) tumor that arises from the midportion of the epidermal layer of the skin. In the United States, about 200,000 diagnoses of this type of skin cancer are made each year.

Squamous cell cancer is more aggressive than basal cell cancer. It can spread (metastasize) to other locations, including lymph nodes or internal organs.

The tumor initially is painless, although pain may develop if it ulcerates and never completely heals (see the color illustration on page 434). It may begin in normal skin, in a burn or scar or at a site of chronic inflammation. Squamous cell cancer also may originate from precancerous skin tumors such as actinic keratoses (see page 1196).

Ultraviolet radiation is usually the main cause of this type of cancer, but genetic predisposition may be a contributing factor. Fair-skinned, blue-eyed, blond or red-haired people are the most vulnerable. The onset of squamous cell cancer most commonly occurs after age 50.

Treatment

Treatment depends on the cancer's size, depth, location and evidence of spread (metastasis). The tumor and the skin around it will likely be removed through surgery. In some cases, radiation may be necessary. Some individuals also need a skin graft to replace excised skin. For cancers that recur after surgical removal, the Mohs' procedure may be necessary (see page 1202), followed by a reconstructive procedure.

With early treatment, the cure rate for squamous cell cancer is approximately 95 percent. Persistent use of high-protection sunscreens and other sun protection techniques can help minimize further development of skin lesions. Be sure to follow up with regular medical examinations to detect possible recurrence.

Melanoma

Signs and symptoms

- A mole that changes in color, size or consistency
- A mole that bleeds or has new hair growth
- A small lesion with an irregular border
- Red, white, blue or blue-black spots on your trunk or limbs
- Shiny, firm, dome-shaped bumps anywhere on the skin
- Dark lesions on the palms, soles of the feet, tips of the fingers and toes or mucous membranes
- A large brownish spot with darker speckles

Melanoma is the most deadly skin cancer. It's less common than basal and squamous cell cancers, but incidence is on the rise, with the number of new cases of melanoma doubling in the past 20 years alone. About 1 in 75 Americans will develop melanoma in their lifetime. Men who receive a diagnosis of this disease have a higher mortality rate than do women with this disease.

Melanoma typically arises painlessly from cells that produce the skin's pigment (melanin). Approximately 70 percent of melanomas

The ABCDs of Melanoma

Melanoma is often curable if you find it early. Follow this self-examination guide, adapted from the American Academy of Dermatology's A-B-C-D guide, to determine if an unusual mole or suspicious spot on your skin may be melanoma.

A is for asymmetry
Symmetrical round or oval growths are usually noncancerous (benign). Look for irregular shapes where one half is a different shape than the other half.

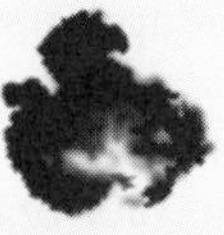

B is for border
Growths with irregular, notched scalloped or vaguely defined borders need to be checked out.

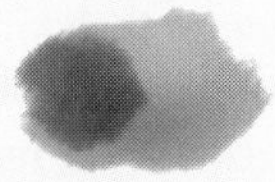

C is for color
Look for growths that have many colors or an uneven distribution of color. Often, growths that are the same color all over are benign.

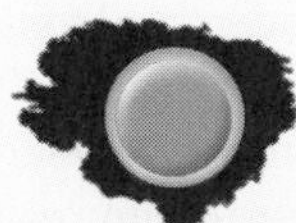

D is for diameter
Have your doctor check any growths that are larger than 6 millimeters, about the diameter of a pencil eraser.

appear on normal skin and 30 percent arise from an existing mole that undergoes changes in color or size or that becomes painful, itches, bleeds or swells (see the color illustration on page 434).

The cancer first spreads to the surrounding skin and is highly curable at this phase. If not treated, the tumor begins to spread downward into other areas of the skin or to lymph nodes or internal organs. Ultraviolet radiation is the chief cause of melanoma. Certain moles also tend to transform into melanoma. Other risk factors include your skin type, a history of sunburns, your health status and genetics.

Melanomas are divided into four types:

- *Superficial spreading melanoma.* Superficial spreading melanoma accounts for 70 percent of melanoma cases and strikes at any age. It appears as a small lesion with an irregular border. The color of the lesion may be red, white, blue or blue-black. It can occur anywhere on the body but most commonly appears on the trunk or limbs.
- *Nodular melanoma.* Nodular melanoma is the most aggressive type of melanoma. It appears as a shiny, firm, dome-shaped bump anywhere on the skin. It's usually black, but it can be blue, gray, white, brown, tan, red or the color of your skin. It may ulcerate and fail to heal completely. Nodular melanomas account for 10 percent to 15 percent of melanoma cases.
- *Acral-lentiginous melanoma.* Acral-lentiginous melanoma appears as dark lesions on the palms, soles, tips of fingers and toes or the mucous membranes. It accounts for 10 percent of melanoma cases and is more common in non-Caucasians.
- *Lentigo maligna melanoma.* Lentigo maligna melanoma appears as a large, brownish spot with darker speckles on skin that has been overexposed to the sun, such as that on the face, ears, arms and upper trunk. It accounts for about 5 percent of melanoma cases. It frequently afflicts older adults and is associated with senile skin (see page 1185). A noncancerous (benign) brownish spot may appear several years before turning cancerous.

Diagnosis

Your doctor may suspect a melanoma from visual inspection. To confirm the diagnosis, he or she will take a sample of skin tissue to be examined in a laboratory (biopsied). If your doctor thinks that the melanoma may spread to other locations, he or she may order further testing, including a complete physical examination with a chest X-ray and computerized tomography (CT) scan. A procedure to determine if the cancer has entered the lymph system may be performed.

How serious is melanoma?

Prompt treatment in the early stages of the disease leads to successful treatment in 85 percent of people with melanoma. When the tumor has grown downward or spread to the lymph nodes or other organs, the 5-year survival rate is approximately 30 percent.

Treatment

The usual treatment for melanoma is surgical removal of the tumor along with a wide margin of normal skin (see page 1202). Sometimes, nearby lymph nodes are removed. This may be followed by a skin graft at the site of the operation. If the cancer has spread to other organs, additional treatment may include chemotherapy or radiation therapy.

Long-term management of melanoma includes periodic medical examinations for evidence of recurring cancer.

Kaposi's sarcoma

Signs and symptoms

- Red to purple nodules anywhere on the skin
- Dark blue or purple-brown nodules on the toe or leg
- Swelling of the legs, groin or skin around the eyes

Kaposi's sarcoma is a cancer that starts in connective tissues, such as the dermis — the layer of skin just beneath the surface layer — cartilage, bone, fat, muscle, blood vessels or fibrous tissue. It typically appears as a nodule on the skin or the mucous membranes. Early lesions are red to purple and resemble a birthmark, and older lesions become brown to black, tend to be flatter and occur with scarring of the skin.

The disease can cause blockage of lymph nodes or lymph vessels, leading to painful swelling (lymphedema) that usually affects the legs, groin or the skin around the eyes. Kaposi's sarcoma is sometimes associated with other cancers, including leukemia or lymphoma, as well as immune deficiency disorders, including human immunodeficiency virus (HIV) and AIDS.

The disease appears in two forms: aggressive and indolent. The aggressive form occurs both internally and externally. It's now occurring with greater frequency because of its association with HIV and AIDS. Before AIDS, Kaposi's sarcoma was a rare disease that appeared primarily in older Italian and Jewish men.

The indolent form, which is generally marked by darker tumors, is caused by blood vessel involvement. It can spread to the hands and arms or produce fungus-like growths or both. This cancer may penetrate underlying tissue and invade bone, lymph nodes and internal organs.

Treatment

Treatment for Kaposi's sarcoma may include local procedures such as freezing therapy (cryotherapy) or surgery, radiation, chemotherapy or therapies that affect the immune system. Elastic support hose may provide some relief by reducing swelling.

Hair

Your hair is composed of keratin, the same protein that makes up nails and the outer layer of your skin. The part of the hair that rises out of your skin is the hair shaft. An average head has about 100,000 of them. Below your skin is the hair root, enclosed by a sac-like structure called the hair follicle. Tiny blood vessels at the base of the follicle provide nourishment to your hair. Nearby oil-producing glands keep your hair shiny and somewhat waterproof.

Each hair shaft consists of three layers. The outermost layer (cuticle) is thin and colorless. The middle layer (cortex) is the thickest. It determines your hair color and whether your hair is straight or curly. Your hair color results from melanin from your pigment cells. Blond hair has few melanin granules in the cortex layer, and dark hair has many. The innermost layer (medulla) is nearly colorless and doesn't extend all the way to the tip of the hair shaft. Light reflected from the medulla creates sheen and the variations in color tone.

Like skin cells, hair grows and is shed regularly. In most people, about 90 percent of the hair on the scalp is in a 4- to 5-year growth stage at any given time. The other 10 percent is in a 2- to 3-month resting phase, after which it's shed. Most people lose 50 to 100 hairs a day. This hair is usually replaced by new hair, which grows at a rate of approximately ½ inch each month. When the rate of shedding exceeds the rate of regrowth, hair loss results. The new hair may be thinner than the hair shed, or it may not come back, leading to baldness.

Hair loss

It may have started with a few extra hairs in the sink or in your comb, but now you can't look in the mirror without seeing more of your uncovered scalp. Anyone can experience hair loss — men, women and children. Hair loss — thinning of your hair or excessive loss of hair from your scalp (baldness) — can be the result of genetics, use of certain medications or an underlying medical condition.

The medical term for hair loss is *alopecia.* The most common type is known as androgenetic alopecia, or pattern baldness. It's generally permanent and usually can be chalked up to heredity. About 95 percent of baldness is due to family history. Heredity also affects the age at which you begin to lose hair, as well as the speed, pattern and extent of your loss.

Alopecia is influenced by hormones called androgens, major determining factors for hair distribution in both sexes. Hair loss can also occur any time your hair's delicate growth cycle is upset. Diet, medications, hormones, pregnancy, improper hair care, poor nutrition, underlying diseases and other factors can cause too many follicles to rest at once, producing bald patches or diffuse thinning.

Sudden hair loss in a defined area is usually due to a condition called alopecia areata. This fairly rare condition is usually temporary and can involve hair loss on the scalp or the body. Its specific cause is unknown.

No matter what causes hair loss, the results can be traumatic. That may be why hair-growth schemes are among the most common medical scams. Many products marketed to reverse baldness avoid regulation by the Food and Drug Administration (FDA) because they aren't considered drugs. FDA-approved medications and surgical procedures are available to treat baldness. Before pursuing any of these options, talk with your doctor about the cause of your hair loss and the best possible treatments.

Female-pattern baldness

Signs and symptoms

- General thinning of hair all over the head
- Loss of hair on the crown of your head or at the hairline

Hair loss in women is generally less prominent than hair loss in men. Instead of baldness, women generally experience thinning of their hair, a condition called female-pattern baldness (androgenetic alopecia). This type of hair loss accounts for 99 percent of hair loss in women. It's normal for a woman's hair to thin out gradually as she grows older. Some women have as much hair at age 80 as they did at 18, but this is unusual.

The distribution of your hair is largely controlled by your endocrine system through a group of hormones known as androgens. Major changes in androgen production can have a significant effect on your hair. For example, you may find that during or after menopause, the hair on your head is thinner and your facial hair is more coarse. Genetic factors also play a large role.

Poor nutrition, pregnancy, internal or scalp disorders, hair damage and medications can cause hair loss in women. When some substance or condition causes a temporary condition, you may experience temporary hair loss (see page 1206).

Diagnosis

Doctors generally diagnose female-pattern baldness by ruling out other causes for the hair loss.

Treatment

A dermatologist can advise you on various methods that might stop the hair loss or stimulate new hair growth, including medication (see page 1207). You may also want to seek the advice of a hair care expert in choosing a new hairstyle or perhaps a hairpiece.

Male-pattern baldness

Signs and symptoms

- A receding hairline
- Moderate to extensive loss of hair, especially on the rear crown of your head

Male-pattern baldness (androgenetic alopecia) usually begins with thinning at your hairline, followed by the appearance of a thinned or bald spot on the crown of your head. You also may find your hair is finer and doesn't grow as long as it once did. This type of hair loss accounts for 99 percent of hair loss in men. Unlike hair loss resulting from disease or other nonhereditary factors, hair loss due to male-pattern baldness is permanent.

Your hair grows in a continuous cycle. In male-pattern baldness, the rate of growth shortens and more roots fail to produce new hair at the end of each growth cycle.

Treatment

Although there's no known cure for male-pattern baldness, treatment is possible with hair transplants, scalp reduction surgery, flap surgery or medication. These approaches can be costly. In addition, medications aren't always effective, and their lifelong benefits haven't been established.

If you choose not to undertake medical treatment for your baldness or if you don't respond to treatment, you may want to check with a hair care expert about wearing a hairpiece or changing your hairstyle.

Some people think that on some men shorter hair minimizes the contrast produced by male-pattern baldness and creates a distinguished image. However, a hairpiece can be used to cover either permanent or temporary hair loss. Quality, natural-looking hairpieces are available.

Temporary, sudden hair loss

Signs and symptoms

- Small bald patches on the scalp
- Overall thinning of hair on the scalp
- Loss of scalp, eyebrow and eyelash hair
- Complete loss of hair over the body

Temporary, sudden hair loss most commonly is due to alopecia areata, a condition that occurs in 2 percent of the population. Alopecia areata starts abruptly with one or more circular bald patches, up to 3 inches across, that may overlap.

Causes

Alopecia areata is classified as an autoimmune disease, but its exact cause is unknown. In fact, people who develop this type of baldness are generally in good health. A family history of alopecia areata makes you more likely to develop it.

Unlike female-pattern baldness or male-pattern baldness (androgenetic alopecia), the hair will generally grow back, but it may take several years. Other causes of temporary hair loss include:

- *Disease.* Diabetes, lupus and thyroid disorders, as well as some eating disorders, can cause hair loss. Lichen planus of the scalp is associated with hair loss.
- *Poor nutrition.* If you don't receive adequate protein or iron in your diet or are poorly nourished in other ways, you can experience hair loss. Fad diets and crash diets also can result in poor nutrition.
- *Medications.* Certain drugs used to treat gout, arthritis, depression, heart problems and high blood pressure may cause hair loss in some people. For some women, taking birth control pills or going off of birth control pills may result in hair loss.
- *Medical treatments.* If you're undergoing chemotherapy or radiation therapy, you may experience temporary hair loss. After your treatment is complete, your hair should begin to regrow.
- *Recent high fever, severe infection or surgery.* You may notice that you have less hair 4 weeks to 3 months following an illness or surgery. Sometimes illness or surgery causes hair to shift rapidly into a resting phase, resulting in less new hair growth. A normal amount of hair typically will appear after the growth phase resumes. The medical term for this condition is *telogen effluvium.*
- *Childbirth.* Many women experience an increase in hair loss several months after delivering a baby. This usually corrects itself.
- *Infancy.* Newborn babies often lose hair during the first few months of life. This baby hair is eventually replaced by more permanent hair. It's also common for babies from 3 to 6 months of age to lose a patch of hair on the back of their heads from rubbing against mattresses, playpens and car seats. Hair will grow back once a baby begins to spend more time sitting up.
- *Hair treatments.* Overuse or incorrect use of chemicals used for dying, tinting, bleaching, straightening or perming can cause hair to become damaged and break off. Excessive hairstyling or hairstyles that pull your hair too tightly also can cause some hair loss.
- *Scalp infection.* Infections such as ringworm (see page 1193) can invade the scalp and cause changes on the skin's surface, which can lead to hair loss. Once the infection is treated, hair generally returns.

Diagnosis

A complete medical history and examination can help in a diagnosis. Tests may be necessary if the cause of your hair loss isn't readily apparent.

Treatment

Treatment depends on the cause. If an underlying condition is found, efforts will be made to cure or control that condition. In some cases, you may have to let time take its course.

Hirsutism

Signs and symptoms

- Growth of hair in unwanted locations, such as on the face in women

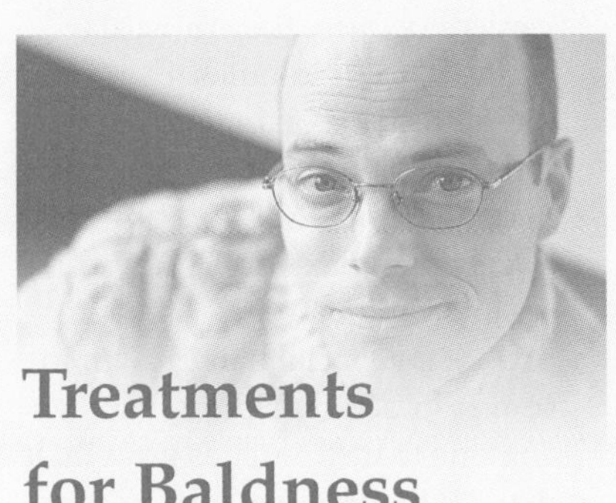

Treatments for Baldness

Baldness typically can't be cured, but a variety of treatments are available to help promote hair growth or hide hair loss.

Medications

The effectiveness of medications depends on the cause of hair loss, the extent of the loss and your response to the drugs. Generally, treatment is less effective for more extensive hair loss. Medications approved by the Food and Drug Administration for treatment of hair loss include:

Minoxidil

Available over-the-counter, minoxidil (Apo-Gain, Rogaine) is a liquid that you rub into your scalp twice daily to help regrow hair and prevent further hair loss. About 25 percent of men and 20 percent of women experience some hair regrowth with regular strength minoxidil. A nonprescription extra-strength version of minoxidil is approved for use by men only.

When using this medication, your new hair often grows in thinner and lighter in color but in enough quantity to hide bald spots. New hair stops growing soon after you discontinue use of minoxidil. If you don't experience significant results within 6 months, your doctor may recommend that you discontinue using it. Side effects of minoxidil use can include dryness and scalp irritation.

Finasteride

Finasteride (Propecia) is the only approved treatment for male-pattern baldness that comes in pill form. Like minoxidil, results may take several months. If you don't experience results within 12 months, your doctor may recommend that you discontinue using it.

Finasteride is a prescription medication that works by inhibiting the conversion of testosterone into dihydrotestosterone (DHT), a hormone that shrinks hair follicles and is a significant factor in male-pattern hair loss. In clinical trials, more than 80 percent of men taking finasteride experienced a slowing of hair loss, and more than 60 percent showed some new hair growth. Rare side effects include diminished sex drive and sexual function. As with minoxidil, benefits stop if usage is discontinued.

Finasteride hasn't been shown effective for women. In fact, it poses significant danger to women of childbearing age. Pregnant women shouldn't even handle crushed or broken finasteride tablets because absorption of the drug may cause serious birth defects in male fetuses. No side effects have been observed in women as a consequence of their partner's use of finasteride.

Cortisone

If you experience sudden hair loss (alopecia areata), injections of cortisone into the scalp may help stimulate the hair follicles to grow new hair. Treatment may be repeated. For extensive hair loss due to alopecia areata, oral cortisone medication is sometimes prescribed.

Anthralin

Available as a prescription cream or ointment, anthralin (Drithocreme, Dritho-Scalp) is a synthetic, tarry substance that you apply to your scalp and wash off daily. It's typically used to treat psoriasis, but doctors sometimes prescribe it to treat other skin conditions. Anthralin creates mild irritation of the skin, which may stimulate new hair growth for mild cases of sudden hair loss.

Surgery

Surgical treatments for hair loss are generally expensive and aren't covered under most insurance plans because they're cosmetic. They can be painful and carry a slight risk of infection. A very small percentage of people experience persistent (chronic) head pain afterward. The following techniques are most often used in people with pattern baldness.

Hair transplants

During a hair transplant, a dermatologist or surgeon takes tiny grafts of skin from the back or side of your scalp and implants them into the bald sections. Using micrografts (minigrafts) containing only one or two hairs takes longer, but this approach can result in a more natural-looking hairline. Several surgeries may be needed. The transplanted hair may fall out within the first few weeks, but it grows back about 3 months later. Additional transplants may be needed as the bald area becomes larger with age.

Scalp reduction

As its name implies, scalp reduction means decreasing the area of bald skin on your head. Your scalp and skull may seem to have a snug fit, but the skin can be stretched enough for some of it to be surgically removed. The areas with hair are pulled more closely together, decreasing the area of baldness.

Flap surgery

Doctors can fold hair-bearing skin over an area of bald skin. The surgeon makes cuts in a section of hair near the balding area, creating a flap of skin with hair, and then rotates the flap into the balding section.

Flap or scalp reduction surgery can be combined with hair transplantation to fashion a natural-looking hairline. Flap or scalp reduction surgery might also be used in combination with medications.

There's a paradox about hair. People generally regard an ample and healthy head of it as beautiful. But the presence of hair in other locations may be considered anything but beautiful. On women, for example, hair on the cheeks, upper lip, underarms or legs is considered by many women and men to be unattractive.

Amounts of facial and body hair vary greatly from one person to another. Many women develop considerable amounts of body and facial hair during puberty. In some cases, even faint mustaches appear. The normal secretion of androgen hormones produces many changes in a young girl's body, including hair growth in the pubic and armpit regions.

In women, the amount of facial and body hair usually increases slowly with age, even past menopause. Similarly, men may develop considerably more body hair as they age.

Too much hair is called hirsutism. How much is too much is largely a matter of personal perception. Part of the solution to a cosmetic problem of excessive hair is the simple acceptance that the amount you have is right for you. On the other hand, if you have a sudden increase in hair — for example, over a period of a few months — consult your doctor. This type of hair growth may have a medical cause, such as a tumor of the ovary or adrenal gland or a side effect of a medication.

Treatment

If you feel that you have too much facial or body hair and would like to get rid of it, you have several treatment options.

- *Plucking.* This is the most common cosmetic method, if your problem is a few scattered hairs. Wash the area first and dab on a little alcohol with a cotton ball to help prevent an infection in the hair follicle. Use good tweezers to remove the hair by pulling it out in the direction it's growing. Plucking is a temporary solution. The hair will likely grow back.
- *Shaving.* This popular but temporary method can be irritating to your skin if you do it haphazardly. Women commonly shave their underarms and lower legs, but shaving is also safe for facial hair. Similar to plucking, shaving doesn't make your hair grow faster or become darker or coarser.
- *Wax removal.* This method is popular among American women for removing hair on the eyebrows, upper lip, chin and legs. Waxing can be painful and may irritate your skin. Seek the services of a trained cosmetician. First, the cosmetician applies melted wax to the area, then, after it cools and sets, quickly strips it off in the direction of the hair growth. The results last longer than other temporary methods because the hair is pulled out below your skin's surface. New hairs generally appear after a month. As with plucking, infection of the hair follicles may occur.
- *Abrasive agents.* The use of pumice and other abrasive agents is the oldest method of hair removal. The process is slow and tedious, and the vigorous rubbing can irritate your skin. You may find it useful for scattered hairs, but it's not practical for large areas.
- *Bleaching.* Bleaching is useful for large areas, such as forearms or thighs, to make unwanted hair less conspicuous. Use a product specially designed for this purpose and follow the directions. Be sure to do a test on a small area to check for possible irritation before applying the product over a large area.
- *Depilatories.* Chemical agents called depilatories dissolve hair protein. You can buy them in foam, cream or lotion form. Follow the directions and test the product on a small area of your skin for possible irritation. Some women find depilatories inconvenient because they must stay on for 10 to 15 minutes. Don't use these products on injured or inflamed skin.
- *Eflornithine hydrochloride.*This relatively new prescription topical cream (Vaniqa) reduces the rate of excessive facial hair growth in some women by blocking an enzyme that stimulates growth. It may take up to 2 months to work. The possible side effects include stinging, tingling, ingrown hairs and acne.
- *Electrolysis.* Electrolysis is the most permanent method of hair removal. An electrologist inserts a very fine needle into each hair follicle, and a burst of electric current is delivered through the needle to destroy the hair root. The hair grows back about 30 percent of the time. Infections, scarring or discoloration around the follicle may occur. It's wise to have the electrologist do a few hairs and observe the results before embarking on an extensive program of hair removal. You may need several sessions because the maximum removal rate is about 100 hairs a visit. Electrolysis treatment can be long, tedious and expensive, but it might be a permanent solution to unwanted hair.
- *Lasers.* Lasers use light energy produced by a special type of laser to destroy hair follicles. Although tedious and expensive, this technique has been gaining in popularity as an option for semipermanent or permanent hair removal. Multiple treatments are required.

The idea for laser hair removal surfaced in 1992 when a laser physicist accidentally zapped his arm, which at the time was covered with carbon residue, and some of his arm hair fell off. The Food and Drug Administration (FDA) approved the use of lasers for hair removal in 1995. The first laser to win FDA approval worked by coating your skin with a black carbon solution that attracts the laser light,

Caring for Your Hair

Healthy, lustrous hair is a sought-after symbol of beauty as evidenced by the millions of dollars spent on hair care products each year. Use the following tips to help keep your hair healthy:

Handle your hair gently

Wet hair is especially fragile because it might become stretched. When possible, allow your hair to air-dry. A natural-bristle brush is preferable to a synthetic one because the synthetic material may cut your hair. Brush your hair gently from your scalp to disperse scalp oil over your hair. If you prefer a comb, use a wide-toothed comb to avoid injury to your hair. If you must use a blow-dryer, use it on a low setting and leave your hair slightly damp.

Shampoo your hair as needed

The amount of washing that your hair needs depends on your hair type, the weather, your physical activities and perhaps even your occupation. Daily shampooing won't damage your hair if you do it gently.

Buy shampoos tailored to your hair type — oily, dry or normal. Protein shampoos don't penetrate your hair, but they do coat it, temporarily giving your hair more bulk. A protein shampoo acts as a shampoo and conditioner in one. Permanent-waved, straightened or dyed hair needs a low-pH shampoo. Follow your shampoo with a cream rinse or conditioner. These products lubricate your hair between washings and help minimize damage from brushing or combing.

Choose a hair-healthy style

Certain hairstyles and treatments can cause breakage or root damage. Avoid excessively tight braiding, buns or ponytails and don't roll your hair too tightly in curlers. Curling is safest if you twist your hair into pin curls overnight. For safe curling of fine hair, wind slightly dampened hair around sponge rollers and let it air-dry. Use of excessively hot rollers or curling irons may damage even coarse hair. Use these devices cautiously. Teasing and back-combing should be done gently or not at all.

A styling gel or mousse can give your hair more body or thickness. These products don't necessarily damage your hair, but they might make it extra dry, especially at the ends. Permanent waving (a perm) is safe for healthy hair, but you may find that it results in increased dryness and splitting. Straightening and permanent waving use the same chemical methods to change the properties of hair strands. The initial (waving) solution dissolves a chemical linkage in the hair. After the hair is arranged in its new, curly configuration, application of the second solution, the neutralizer, restores the linkage. Like other aggressive cosmetic treatments, permanent waving can be damaging when done to excess.

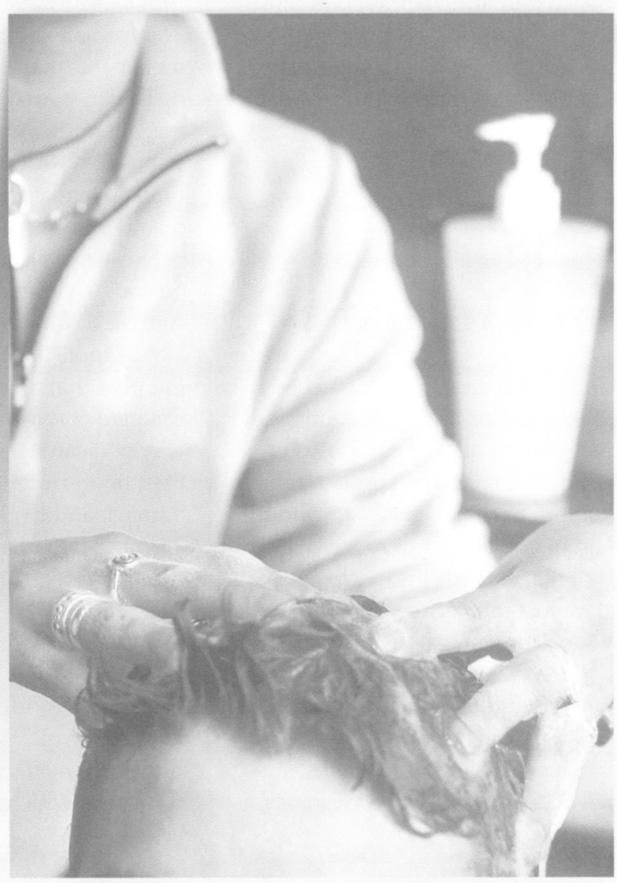

Be careful with coloring

Hair bleaches chemically alter the melanin granule in the middle layer of each hair strand. Despite careful treatment, persistent bleaching eventually damages even healthy, strong hair shafts, but it doesn't injure the roots from which future hair growth takes place.

Hair dyes work more like paint by covering hair strands with color or by mixing with the melanin granules without altering them. Dyes come in temporary form, which eventually wash out, and semipermanent and permanent forms, which penetrate your hair.

Avoid chemical and sun damage

Too much exposure to sun, wind and swimming pool chemicals will dry out your hair and cause it to knot.

Eat a balanced diet

The quality of your hair reflects, in part, the adequacy of your diet. Contrary to what you may have heard or read, consuming extra protein or amino acid preparations won't promote hair growth. However, crash diets and eating disorders such as anorexia nervosa can damage hair dramatically.

which damages hair follicles. Since that time, significant improvements have been made in the multiple laser systems that are now available to reduce hair.

Fingernails and Toenails

Cells at the base of your nail beds produce your fingernails and toenails. Your nails are composed of laminated layers of a protein called keratin. Each nail grows toward the end of your finger or toe from a nail root that extends into a groove of skin. Just in front of your nail root is your cuticle skin, which is attached to the nail surface and helps protect new keratin cells that slowly emerge from below.

Your nails may give the first signal of an illness. They occasionally provide clues for diagnosis as well as information about your age and diet. In addition, your fingernails assist you with the tasks of daily living, although you may not be conscious of how much you use them until an injury, infection or other disorder limits your use of them.

Healthy nails are smooth, without ridges or grooves. They're uniform in color and consistency and free of spots or discoloration. Remember that no nail care product can give you healthy nails. The only way you can help your nails to look their best is to protect them from damage and irritants such as chemicals and detergents and clean and trim them regularly.

Paronychia

Signs and symptoms

- A red, swollen, painful area on the skin next to a nail
- Blisters, which may ooze pus

Signs and symptoms of a severe infection

- A raised cuticle
- A detached nail
- Nail distortion or discoloration
- Red lines along your skin

Paronychia is a superficial infection of the skin around the nail. The most common cause of paronychia is either staphylococci (staph) bacteria or yeast. The infection is usually the result of an injury, such as biting off a hangnail, or is caused by manipulating or pushing back the cuticle.

Bacterial paronychia is usually a sudden and painful infection. Superficial pus-filled blisters may appear. Pressing the affected area can produce oozing pus.

Another form of paronychia is caused by fungal infections and is common among people with diabetes and individuals who have their hands in water for long periods of time. Fungal infections develop slowly but tend to persist. Sometimes, both bacteria and fungi are present.

A severe (acute) infection, which usually affects fingers, can extend around your nail and cuticle to invade beneath them. Your cuticle becomes raised. The nail may become detached. Nail distortion or discoloration might occur. Red lines along your skin are a signal that bacteria have entered your bloodstream. If this occurs, see your doctor. The diagnosis may require a culture to determine which type of microorganism is causing your paronychia.

Treatment

Soaking the affected area in warm water will help decrease inflammation of the tissues. Topical application of an antibacterial agent will help fight a bacterial infection. If a fungal infection is present, you might try a 1 percent solution of gentian violet, an antifungal medication that's available over-the-counter. Or try soaking in a dilute vinegar solution of 1 ounce white vinegar to 16 ounces water.

Ingrown Toenails

Ingrown toenails usually occur on the big toe. They form when the edge of your nail curls and grows into the soft underlying tissue. Ingrown toenails are caused by:

- Improper cutting of nails
- Faster nail growth at the edge than at the center
- Pressure from poorly fitting shoes

If you experience severe discomfort, pus or redness that seems to be spreading from the side of the toe, seek medical attention. Your doctor may need to remove the ingrown portion of the nail and prescribe antibiotics.

You can do several things to prevent and treat ingrown toenails at home. Follow these self-care tips:

- Trim your toenails straight across and not too short.
- Wear socks and shoes that fit properly and don't place excessive pressure on your toes.
- Wear open-toe shoes or sandals, if appropriate.

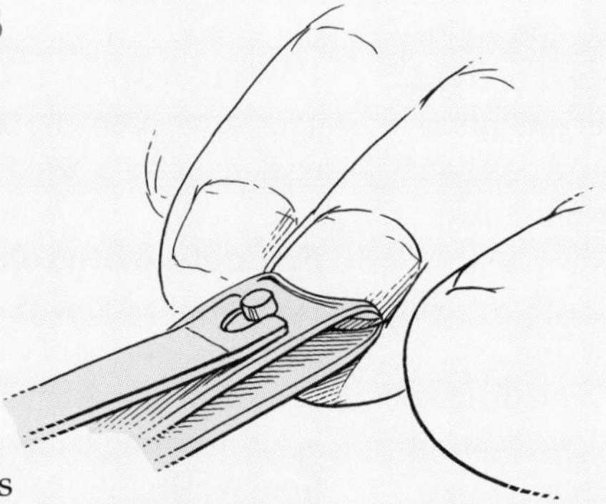

To avoid ingrown toenails, cut your nails straight across and not too short.

- Soak your feet in warm salt water — 1 tablespoon of salt per quart of water — for 30 minutes four times a day to reduce swelling and relieve tenderness.
- After soaking, put tiny bits of sterile cotton under the ingrown edge. This will help the nail eventually grow above the skin edge. Change the cotton daily until the pain and redness subside.
- Apply an antibiotic ointment to the tender area.

Fungal infection

Signs and symptoms

- Thickened, lusterless fingernails or toenails
- Nail discoloration, usually yellow or brown
- Crumbling nail edges
- A detached nail

Fungus spores may attach themselves to the dense bed of keratin cells that make up your nails. These microscopic plants can digest the keratin and live within it. The resulting infection, called onychomycosis, can persist indefinitely.

When infected by a fungus, your nails may become thickened, detached and shed (see the color illustration on page 438). There's usually an accumulation of keratinous debris beneath the free edge of an infected nail. You may feel some pain in the nail and detect a slight odor. In some cases, the nail is destroyed.

You can contract fungal infections in several ways, including walking barefoot in public places or as a complication of athlete's foot or paronychia. People with decreased blood circulation or diabetes are more prone to infection. Your risk of fungal infection of a toenail is greater if your feet perspire heavily and if you wear socks and shoes that hinder ventilation and don't absorb perspiration. Fingernail fungal infections often result from overexposure to water and detergents. Moisture caught under artificial nails also can encourage fungal growth.

Fungal infections are more common among older adults. After age 40, nails grow more slowly and begin to thicken, making them more susceptible to infection. Once a fungal nail infection begins, it can persist indefinitely if not treated. See your doctor at the first sign of infection. Fungal nail infections usually begin as a tiny white or yellow spot on your nail.

Diagnosis

Your doctor's diagnostic tests may include scraping up some of the debris beneath the nail edge for microscopic examination to identify the fungus. Presence of a fungus rules out other diseases of the nails.

Treatment

Fungal nail infections can be difficult to treat, and repeated infections are common. If you have a fungal infection, your doctor may prescribe an oral antifungal medication. These drugs, which are effective most of the time, include itraconazole (Sporanox), fluconazole (Diflucan) and terbinafine (Lamisil). These drugs help a new, infection-free nail grow out while the older, infected portion of your nail is slowly replaced. Although these drugs can usually eliminate an infection in 4 to 12 months, recurrent infections are possible.

These oral medications, however, may cause side effects ranging from skin rashes to liver damage. Itraconazole and fluconazole also can cause adverse interactions with other drugs, including some anticoagulant and allergy medications. In May 2001, the Food and Drug Administration issued a public health advisory regarding itraconazole and terbinafine over concerns that they may cause congestive heart failure. The warning doesn't apply to the cream and solution forms of Lamisil, which are applied topically. Before you and your doctor decide to use oral therapy, consider the possible side effects.

Over-the-counter antifungal nail creams may help soften your nail and keep a fungal infection from spreading while a new nail grows. Other antifungal creams or lotions are available by prescription.

Another option is a topical antifungal lacquer. You paint the lacquer onto infected nails and surrounding skin once daily. After 7 days, you remove the painted-on layers and start with a fresh application. Daily use for up to 1 year or longer has been shown to help clear up some fungal nail infections.

If your nail infection is severe or extremely painful, your doctor may suggest removing your nail. A new nail will usually grow in its place.

PREVENTION TIP

To help prevent a fungal nail infection:

- Keep your nails dry and clean. Dry your feet, including between your toes, thoroughly after bathing.
- If your feet sweat excessively, change your socks often. Take your shoes off occasionally during the day and after exercise. Alternate closed-toe shoes with open-toe shoes.
- Use an antifungal spray or powder on your feet and inside your shoes.
- Wear rubber gloves to protect your hands from overexposure to water. Between uses, turn rubber gloves inside-out to dry.
- Don't pick at or trim the skin around your nails. This may give germs a route into your skin and nails.
- Avoid walking barefoot around public pools, showers and locker rooms.
- Choose a reputable manicure and pedicure salon that sterilizes its instruments. And avoid using nail polish and artificial nails, which may trap unwanted moisture and make the condition worse.
- Wash your hands after touching an infected nail. Fungal nail infections can spread from nail to nail if you're not careful.

Care of your nails

Perhaps the single most important element in taking care of your nails is to avoid abusing them. Don't use them as tools and don't bite them or pick your cuticles. Lubricate your nails and cuticles with lotion as you do for your skin — rub in the lotion. Even a minor cut alongside your nail can allow bacteria or fungi to enter and cause an infection. Because your nails grow slowly, an injured nail retains signs of its injury for several months.

Weekly fingernail trimming is important because nails that are smooth and cared for are less likely to become damaged. Use sharp manicure scissors or clippers to trim your fingernails and use an emery board. Bevel the edges with the fine side of the emery board. Trim your toenails straight across and not too short.

You need to do this only about once a month because toenails grow more slowly than fingernails. They also tend to be thicker, especially on your big toe, so the best time for a trim is after bathing when your nails are softer.

If you have a hangnail, don't attempt to pull it off. Pulling almost always rips into living tissue. Instead, clip it off neatly, leaving a slight angle outward. This may help prevent recurrence. Using hand lotion regularly can help prevent hangnails.

Be fashion wise

Some women treat their nails as accessories, going to great lengths to keep them looking lovely. However, what looks good isn't always good for your nails. Although fashion encourages trimmed cuticles, avoid this practice. It can create a point of entry for bacteria and fungi and thus promote infection. Artificial nails can produce reactions beneath your nails.

Some nail products can be hard on your nails. Cuticle removers are corrosive alkali-based products that destroy these naturally protective bands. Some nail strengtheners can discolor or break your nails. Polish removers dry and weaken your nails.

Despite advertising claims, most polishes are chemically similar. They make your nails stronger only in the sense that the polish itself coats and thus protects the nail. If you polish your nails, apply several thin coats instead of one heavy one.

Nail Discoloration or Deformity

Your nails can tell you a lot about your general health. Take a look at your fingernails. Are they strong and healthy looking? Or do you see ridges or areas of unusual color or shape?

Many less-than-desirable nail conditions can be avoided through proper nail care, but some conditions may be indications of an illness that requires attention.

Some nail conditions are harmless. These include vertical ridges, which tend to worsen as you age. A minor injury can cause nail discoloration. The black spot under your thumbnail after a hammer blow is blood. White, cloud-like marks on the tips of your nails are the result of minor trauma.

Overexposure to strong soaps or chemicals can cause splitting, peeling or brittleness, and tight or ill-fitting shoes can cause ingrown or thickened toenails.

Other nail conditions may indicate disease, so remove your nail polish when you see your doctor. Here are some conditions that might require medical attention:

Separation of a nail from its bed

Separation of a nail from its bed (onycholysis) may be associated with injury, psoriasis, drug reactions, fungal disease or a reaction to nail hardeners or acrylic nails.

Yellow nail syndrome

Swelling in the hands or a respiratory condition, such as chronic bronchitis, can cause one or more of your nails to turn yellow or green. The condition is associated with very slow nail growth — your nails may need clipping only once every several months.

Pitting

Small depressions in the nail are common in people with psoriasis or nail injuries.

Terry's nails

Terry's nails is a condition in which your nails look opaque, but the tips each have a dark band. This may be a sign of serious illness, such as cancer, congestive heart failure or diabetes, or it may just be a sign of aging.

Clubbing

Nails that curve around the fingertips or toes, along with broadening of the fingers or toes, may be a sign of lack of oxygen. It's associated with a number of diseases, including heart disease and emphysema.

Beau's lines

Beau's lines are indentations that run across the nail. They can appear when growth at the nail bed is interrupted by severe illness, such as a heart attack or pneumonia, or by high fever.

Mees' lines

Mees' lines are caused by arsenic poisoning. They're white lines that run across the nail.

Spoon nails

Spoon nails — soft nails that look scooped out — may be a sign of iron deficiency anemia. The depression is usually large enough to hold a drop of liquid.

It's not unusual for your nails to be affected during an illness and to recover afterward. Damage can be repaired only by the slow process of new growth, about 1/8 inch a month for fingernails and 1/24 inch for toenails. After your underlying disorder is under control or cured, your nails will gradually return to normal. But report any new changes in color or markings to your doctor.

Keep them tough

Here are some tips to toughen or protect weak fingernails:

- Keep your nails short, square-shaped and slightly rounded on top.
- Apply a nail hardener, but avoid products containing toluene sulfonamide formaldehyde or formaldehyde, which can cause itchiness, redness or irritation of the skin.
- Apply a moisturizer each time you wash your hands. At bedtime, moisturize your nails and cuticles and wear cotton gloves.
- Wear cotton-lined rubber gloves when exposing your hands to water or household chemicals. Between uses, turn rubber gloves inside-out to dry to prevent microorganisms from growing inside them.
- Don't use nail polish remover more than twice a month. Instead, touch up the polish. When you do need a remover, avoid those that contain acetone, which may dry nails.
- Trim brittle nails after a bath or a 15-minute hand-soak in bath oil. Then apply a moisturizer.
- Repair splits or tears with nail glue or clear polish.
- Avoid dietary practices that supposedly strengthen nails. They won't work. Unless you're deficient in protein, which is uncommon among people in the United States, adding protein to your diet won't strengthen your nails. Similarly, soaking your nails in gelatin won't help.

Cosmetic Procedures

As you grow older, you'll no doubt see the effects of time and aging when you look in the mirror. You may be perfectly happy to proudly wear evidence of your life's ups and downs. But if you find these signs distressful and have money to spend, consider cosmetic procedures, which can markedly diminish many signs of aging. You can meet with a dermatologist or plastic surgeon to discuss the limitations, benefits, risks and side effects of available procedures.

Keep in mind that cosmetic procedures usually aren't covered by health insurance, and they may have to be repeated to maintain benefits.

Common cosmetic concerns

Cosmetic procedures are used to treat a number of skin-related conditions. Some of the most common cosmetic concerns include:

Aging and sun-exposed skin

Skin resurfacing techniques, such as chemical peels, dermabrasion or laser resurfacing, can help get rid of wrinkles, sags and bags, as well as scars resulting from acne. Other procedures to reduce wrinkles include soft tissue fillers and facelifts.

Varicose and spider veins

Some women are so embarrassed by varicose or spider veins that they refuse to wear shorts and skirts. Several options are available to get rid of these unwanted veins.

Fat

Liposuction may be an option for men or women who aren't happy with the shape of their thighs or who want to get rid of those love handles that never seem to disappear.

Selecting a surgeon

No cosmetic procedure is without risks. That's why it's crucial to find the right doctor if you're considering cosmetic surgery. Be sure the person is properly trained and board certified in a specialty dealing with cosmetic surgery: a plastic surgeon, dermatologic surgeon or an ear-nose-and-throat (ENT) surgeon. If you're considering laser surgery, make sure the doctor has experience working with lasers.

When talking to a surgeon about a particular procedure, ask the following questions:

- Are there other treatments that might work just as well or better for me?
- Am I a good candidate for this procedure? Why or why not?
- Are you experienced in these procedures, and what results have your patients had? However, don't expect to see the results of surgery performed on other people. Their results may not be what you can expect, and a doctor showing them to you would violate patient confidentiality rules.
- What results can I expect?
- What are the possible complications?
- How will you monitor my progress after surgery? What follow-up care will you provide?
- What percentage of people require touch-up surgery, and who is responsible for the cost?

Skin resurfacing techniques

Skin resurfacing techniques can be used to reduce fine wrinkles, scars such as those left by acne and pigmentation problems such as liver spots. This is done by removing the outer layer of skin (epidermis) to let smoother, younger-looking skin grow back in its place.

Resurfacing techniques include:

Chemical peel

With a chemical peel, your doctor applies an acid that burns the outer layer of your skin, which peels off, causing new, smoother skin to regenerate. Your skin will develop a scab for about 7 to 10 days and will be pink for about 3 months.

Risks

Even with a successfully completed procedure, you may be left with small scars. If the procedure isn't done correctly or if you develop an infection, you may have severe scarring. Your skin will be permanently lighter, without sun-protecting pigmentation. This makes you more susceptible to sunburn and to developing skin cancer. In people with dark skin, chemical peels can cause blotchy skin.

Dermabrasion
Fine wrinkles, liver spots and scars can be sanded down with a small, rotating wheel. Scabbing and swelling generally last 7 to 10 days. Complete healing takes longer. Dermabrasion has largely been replaced by laser resurfacing.

Risks
If you tend to get cold sores (fever blisters), they can flare up after the procedure. Exposure to the sun may cause a bad burn that can permanently discolor your skin. Dermabrasion isn't recommended for people with dark skin because it can cause blotchiness.

Laser resurfacing
Laser resurfacing is a procedure in which the doctor uses an intense, pulsating beam of light to vaporize the outer layer of skin (epidermis). At a lower power, the laser can shrink individual wrinkles. When the underlying skin (dermis) eventually heals, it's tighter and smoother than it was before.

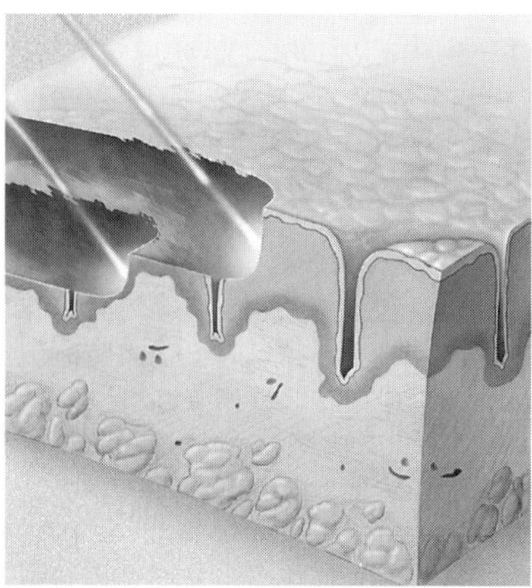

With laser resurfacing, an intense, pulsating beam of light vaporizes outer skin tissues. Underlying skin eventually heals more tightly and smoothly.

For the first 48 to 72 hours after surgery, your face is bright red, sore, oozing and itchy. Some people react less severely than others. Your skin grows back in about a week. In 2 weeks, your swelling is mostly down, but it will take at least 3 to 4 months for all of the redness to go away. It's especially important to use sunscreen liberally after the procedure.

The new generation of lasers give surgeons more control over how much skin is vaporized compared with older types of lasers and traditional resurfacing methods. The latest lasers, when used correctly, produce less scarring and pigment changes, create less discomfort and require a shorter recovery time than older lasers.

Risks
The scarring rate is about 1 percent, similar to dermabrasion and chemical peels. Hyperpigmentation usually can be controlled by pretreating the skin with bleaching cream for 2 weeks before and 3 weeks after the procedure. Laser resurfacing works best on individuals with medium-colored skin.

Electrosurgical resurfacing
Another technique, not widely used, is electrosurgical resurfacing, which uses microelectrical frequency (coblation) to remove skin tissue. The procedure delivers electrical energy rather than heat or chemicals used in some other resurfacing techniques.

Risks
Your skin will be swollen and red for the first couple of days after you have the procedure done. Within a week it should be only moderately pink, and after 2 weeks the redness should be gone. The healing time is usually no more than a month. Unlike other resurfacing techniques, electrosurgical resurfacing can be used on individuals with darker skin.

Soft tissue fillers

Collagen from cattle or fat from your thigh or abdomen can be injected into wrinkles on your face. The injected collagen plumps up your skin, smoothing out the wrinkles and filling in furrows, such as those around your nose and mouth and between your eyebrows. The collagen gradually degrades over several months but it may trigger your body to produce new collagen. To maintain the effect, you may need to have the procedure repeated every few months.

Risks
Some people are allergic to collagen from cattle, so prior testing is necessary.

Face-lift

A face-lift requires more extensive surgery to remove drooping skin and jowls and smooth out wrinkles. It involves removing excess skin and fat, tightening the underlying muscle and connective tissue, and doing it all without leaving prominent, visible traces. Each operation varies, depending on what your surgeon thinks is appropriate for you.

Not everyone is a good candidate for a face-lift. You have the best chance of good results if your skin still has some elasticity, if you have a strong and well-defined bone structure and if you're not overweight. Most people who have a facelift are between ages 40 and 70, but if you're in your 70s or even 80s, you can still have good results.

Surgeons can also perform eyelid surgery to correct droopy eyelids, a procedure called blepharoplasty. This can be done alone or at the same time as a face-lift.

Typically, your surgeon makes incisions that start inside your hairline at your temples and extend downward in front of your ears, then around behind your ear lobes and into your lower scalp. A small incision under your chin may also be necessary if the tissue of your neck needs tightening too. Your surgeon separates your skin from the fat and muscle that lie underneath. Fat from around your neck and chin may be trimmed or suctioned away.

Your surgeon may tighten the underlying tissue (submuscular aponeurotic system) that lifts your jowls, tightens your neck and elevates your cheeks. Your skin is then pulled back and the excess trimmed off. This two-layer face-lift technique is an improvement over earlier procedures in which only the skin was tightened, but it's not necessary for all people.

Finally, your surgeon closes your incisions with stitches. Metal clips may be used on your scalp. Your surgeon may temporarily insert a small, thin tube under your skin behind your ear to allow drainage of any fluid that accumulates there. He or she will also apply a dressing to help reduce bruising and swelling.

Following surgery

With all that pulling, tugging, suctioning and snipping, your face is bound to look and feel like it has been pummeled. Although it's elective and cosmetic, a face-lift is no walk in the park. The first time you look in the mirror, expect to see a pale, puffy and bruised face staring back at you.

Levels of discomfort vary, but usually can be managed with pain medication. You need to keep your head elevated and as still as possible for a couple of days after surgery to help minimize swelling. Sleeping in this position can be uncomfortable. If you had a drainage tube inserted, it's usually removed 1 or 2 days after surgery. Dressings are removed several days after that.

Parts of your face may feel numb for a few weeks or even months. This is normal and eventually disappears, although some tingling sensations may persist for a while longer. Scars take longer to fade, but because they're hidden in hairlines, behind the ears and in natural folds, they're barely noticeable.

Risks

Although complications are uncommon, when they occur they can be serious. They include:

- *Hematoma.* This is a collection of blood under the skin. The excess blood can be removed by your surgeon. Small hematomas may resolve on their own.
- *Weakness of your facial muscles.* This is usually temporary, but until the nerves heal, parts of your face may not move normally.
- *Poor healing.* Smokers are more likely to be affected by poor healing, because substances in cigarettes constrict the small blood vessels of the skin.
- *Infection.* Incisions can become infected.

Liposuction

The concept behind liposuction seems almost too good to be true: Unwanted fat deposits can simply be sucked away with a tiny vacuum. However, the problem isn't that easy to fix.

Liposuction is a serious surgical procedure that involves a potentially painful recovery. Although rare, the surgery also can cause serious complications. A decision about whether to undergo liposuction should be considered very carefully.

A popular choice

Instant fat reduction holds great appeal to many, making liposuction one of the most common cosmetic procedures performed in the United States. According to the American Society of Plastic Surgeons, more than 350,000 liposuction procedures were performed in the United States in 2000.

The areas most commonly treated are the outer thighs and abdomen in women and the flanks or love handles in men. Liposuction can also remove unwanted fat from your hips, buttocks, knees, upper arms, chin, cheeks, neck and other areas.

Liposuction is most effective for removing localized fat deposits in parts of your body that don't respond to dieting or exercising. After the procedure, it's important to continue with an exercise and weight management program for best results.

Liposuction techniques

Two basic techniques are used in liposuction: tumescent, developed

Vein surgery

Eighty million Americans, mostly women, are bothered by varicose veins or spider veins, a mild variation of varicose veins. Varicose veins are gnarled, enlarged veins close to your skin. The name *varicose* comes from the Latin root varix, which means "twisted." Any vein may become varicose, but the most commonly affected areas are the legs and ankles. Spider veins result when small veins close to the skin's surface dilate. They're most common on the legs and face.

For many people, varicose veins and spider veins are simply a cosmetic concern. For other people, they can cause aching pain and discomfort. Sometimes varicose veins lead to more serious problems such as leg ulcers.

Self-care measures — such as exercising, losing weight, not wearing tight clothes, elevating your legs and avoiding long periods of standing or sitting — can ease the pain and prevent varicose veins from getting worse. If your varicose veins don't respond to self-help or if they're more severe, your doctor may advise surgery — including removal of the enlarged vein or another type of procedure to seal off the vein. For information on treatment of varicose and spider veins, see page 791.

by dermatologic surgeons, and ultrasonic, developed by plastic surgeons. Both techniques share core surgical elements. In fact, even if ultrasound is used, it will be followed by tumescent liposuction. Whether you use tumescent or ultrasonic liposuction depends on a number of individual factors that your surgeon will discuss with you.

Some new devices have been developed that liquefy fat when applied externally — so-called noninvasive liposuction. However, their effectiveness has not been established.

Tumescent liposuction

In tumescent liposuction, your surgeon pre-injects your fat deposits with a saltwater solution containing the hormone adrenaline (epinephrine). The solution might also contain a local anesthetic.

Your surgeon will decide whether to use additional anesthetics — local, regional or general — or use only the saltwater solution with a local anesthetic. The decision on what type of anesthetic to administer is based largely on the amount of fat to be suctioned and whether ultrasound will be used.

To begin the procedure, a surgeon typically makes one or more small incisions near the area to be suctioned. Whenever possible, the incisions will be placed within the natural folds or contour lines of your skin so that they aren't highly noticeable.

A slim, hollow tube called a cannula is then inserted into your skin through the incision so that its tip penetrates the underlying fat. After the cannula is connected by flexible tubing to a suction pump, your surgeon moves the cannula back and forth through the fat. The fat is then vacuumed into the tube. Minimal bleeding, bruising and swelling result from tumescent liposuction.

Ultrasonic liposuction

Ultrasound-assisted liposuction (UAL) is a two-step technique that uses the energy from sound waves to liquefy fat deposits before they're suctioned. In UAL, your surgeon inserts a small, heated probe that produces vibrations at frequencies above what your ear can hear (ultrasonic). This energy causes your fat cells to rupture, releasing their oily contents. These oily contents are then suctioned out using the tumescent technique.

Potential advantages to UAL include the ability to remove fat in difficult areas, such as the upper abdomen, the flanks, the back and the male chest. However, UAL is associated with significantly greater complications than tumescent liposuction, such as more pain, swelling, skin burns and other complications.

Following surgery

Recovery from liposuction can be uncomfortable, but most people are back to their normal routine within 3 to 10 days. During the first few weeks, most people experience varying degrees of pain, burning, swelling and temporary areas of numbness.

Pain medications can offer some relief, and special compression garments can reduce swelling. You may be advised to refrain from strenuous physical activity other than walking for about a week after the procedure.

Although your new body contour usually begins to emerge in the first couple of weeks, some swelling may remain for several months. Major weight gain or loss after liposuction can produce unwanted skin surface irregularities.

Many people assume that because liposuction removes fat cells, it's impossible to regain weight in the treated areas. However, remaining fat cells may grow larger, especially if you abandon exercise and a healthy diet. This means problem spots can return. It's more likely, though, that weight gain following liposuction will be distributed to other parts of your body instead of settling entirely back into old problem areas.

Risks

Liposuction isn't without risks. In general, the larger the volume of fat removed, the higher the potential for complications. Some surgeons will suction a greater amount of fat at one time and complete the job in one procedure, whereas others will suction smaller volumes over the course of multiple procedures. Ask your surgeon which course he or she follows.

People with certain medical conditions, such as diabetes, heart disease, lung disease and poor circulation, as well as individuals who smoke or are subject to blood clots, are at increased risk of complications from liposuction, just as they are for any surgical procedure.

Rare but serious complications include blood clots, which can migrate to the lungs and cause death, infection and allergic reactions. In addition, the combination of liposuction, general anesthesia and having other cosmetic procedures — for example a face-lift — at the same time has been associated with increased risks. ■

CHAPTER 37 PART V

Mental Illness

Mental illness is mysterious and confusing to many people. Is a stretch of sleepless nights the result of depression? Are your worries normal, or do you have an anxiety disorder?

Part of the challenge is that there's no clear dividing line between mental health and mental illness. A recent report by the U.S. Surgeon General views mental health and mental illness as points on a continuum. To some extent, any definition of mental health reflects culture and circumstances. Different cultures have different ways of coping with stress and adversity. Behavior that's considered abnormal in one culture may be perfectly acceptable in another.

In general, mental health refers to normal mental functioning that allows a person to be productive, develop fulfilling relationships, adapt to change and cope with adversity. Mental illness refers to changes in thinking, mood or behavior that cause distress and interfere with a person's ability to function in a variety of ways. A person with a mental illness has trouble — to a lesser or greater degree — with daily activities, family responsibilities, relationships, work or school.

Like other illnesses, mental disorders range in severity from mild to severe. The signs can be as subtle as increased irritability or as obvious as staying in bed all day. Some mental disorders last a short time and gradually improve. Others are lifelong, requiring on-going treatment.

A Common Problem

Mental illnesses are common. A study by the World Health Organization, the World Bank and Harvard University found that mental illness is second only to cardiovascular disease in causing disability and premature death in developed countries. In the United States, about 18.5 percent of the adult population — more than 37 million people — experiences a mental disorder in any given year.

Mental illness can take a great toll on your quality of life, and that of those who care about you — family, friends, employers and co-workers. Many people with unrecognized, untreated or inadequately treated mental illness endure lives that are sapped of vitality or undermined by tension and conflict.

Fortunately, most mental illnesses are treatable. Many people can recover, and others with more long-term (chronic) disorders can learn to manage their symptoms, much as people learn to manage and live with diabetes or arthritis. A growing body of research is helping to identify effective therapies and new medications that cause fewer or less severe side effects.

Despite such significant advances, too many people don't recognize or acknowledge mental illness, and many don't receive care until a crisis occurs. The misconception that mental disorders aren't true illnesses and the fear of appearing emotionally weak make many people reluctant to seek help for emotional distress. Unfortunately, despite growing awareness of mental illness, a societal stigma is still attached to mental disorders.

Mental illnesses don't involve lack of willpower and self-discipline. As with cancer and heart disease, they arise from a mixture of influences — the complex interplay of heredity, biology and environmental factors.

Life Issues and Mental Illness

Following years of research on brain function and human behavior, scientists are ending the artificial split between illnesses of the mind and of the body. Mental disorders are now recognized as illnesses with a biologic basis that are often influenced by psychological and social stress. Even in the womb, experience shapes brain development, influencing the types and amounts of chemicals that convey messages throughout the nervous system. Changes in these pathways may even set the stage for some mental disorders.

Although many mental illnesses have a strong biologic or genetic basis, that's not the entire story. Many factors can play a role in the development of mental disorders. A disorder can occur as a manifestation of another illness, as a reaction to a medication or to drug or alcohol abuse, or as a result of a stressful or emotionally difficult life experience.

One person may have mental illness due to nature — a specific genetic defect that alters brain circuitry. Another may have mental illness caused by nurture — one or more environmental factors that alter natural brain chemistry. Mental illness is often thought to be a complex interaction of both nature and nurture.

Risk factors

Some of the factors that can contribute to mental illness are as follows:

Genetics

Hereditary traits are conveyed through individual genes, which carry instructions that direct the formation and guide the function of every structure of the human body. Some genes are actively expressed throughout an individual's life, and others lie dormant unless stimulated.

Genetic factors play a role in many human diseases. An inherited susceptibility to a disease occurs when one or more genes fail to give correct instructions for the manufacturing or functioning of cells. This failure may make you more vulnerable to disease. Genes can also influence the severity or progression of a disease.

It's unlikely that a single genetic abnormality can cause mental illness, but a composite of genetic abnormalities may increase susceptibility to some mental illnesses. Genetic factors alone probably aren't enough to trigger the illness. Other factors also come into play.

Sex and stress hormones are among the substances produced by the body that may play a role. External factors, such as stress or drug or alcohol abuse, may activate a genetic susceptibility to mental illness.

If someone in your family has or had a mental illness, such as depression, it doesn't necessarily mean that you'll develop it too. But a family history of mental illness does increase your risk.

Stress and grief

Stressful life events can unmask vulnerability to mental illness. For example, if you have a major crisis in your life, such as a divorce or the death of a loved one, you may become sad and depressed. Even after your life situation has improved, these symptoms may persist. Stress or grief can trigger an illness that needs professional treatment.

The death of a loved one is a common trigger of mental disorders. Grief is a normal and necessary response to such a loss, but grief that's especially severe or lasts longer than a year may be complicated by a mental disorder, such as depression.

Stress can result from many other situations, such as relationship or work troubles, major life changes and illness.

Past experiences

People who have experienced deeply upsetting events — for example, childhood abuse or wartime combat — are at higher risk of developing mental disorders such as depression and post-traumatic stress disorder.

Any form of abuse during childhood — sexual, physical or emotional — can make a person more vulnerable to mental disorders. Other aspects of family environment that may contribute to mental disorders include a high level of conflict between parents, family violence, substance abuse or loss of a parent due to death.

The connection between past traumas and mental illness is partly related to the way the human body responds to danger and stress. When confronted with real or perceived danger, your body gears up to face the challenge (fight) or to move out of harm's way (flight). This fight-or-flight response results from the release of hormones that cause your body to shift into overdrive. Severe or ongoing stressful experiences trigger stress responses in your brain circuits, and hormonal systems may become chronically hyperactive.

In addition, children who don't acquire good coping skills when growing up may be less able to cope when they're faced with a stressful situation during adulthood. Consequently, they may be more adversely affected by stress than is a person with better coping skills.

Substance abuse

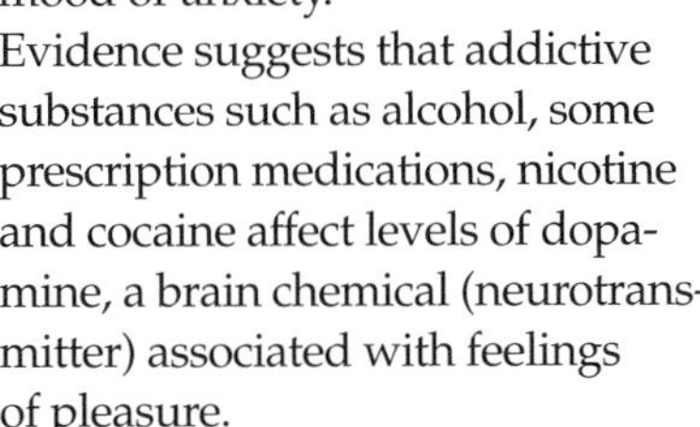

Approximately 30 percent to 60 percent of people with substance abuse problems also experience a disorder of mood or anxiety. Evidence suggests that addictive substances such as alcohol, some prescription medications, nicotine and cocaine affect levels of dopamine, a brain chemical (neurotransmitter) associated with feelings of pleasure.

Addictive substances are thought to create an oversupply of dopamine, which influences emotion and motivation.

Other medical conditions

Other physical illnesses and medical conditions may trigger a mental illness. For example, some hormone-related diseases, such as an underactive thyroid (hypothyroidism), have a direct link to the development of depression. Medical conditions such as stroke, cancer, Alzheimer's disease, Parkinson's disease, obstructive sleep apnea, epilepsy and chronic pain also are associated with an increased risk of depression.

Children and mental illness

Despite its image as a carefree time of life, childhood is far from easy. Many children and adolescents experience emotional difficulties as they deal with a wide range of issues — self-control, learning to socialize with peers, separation from parents, and so on. Adolescence is a time of tumultuous physical and emotional changes, including increasingly intense self-awareness and developing sexuality, which often make for a traumatic and rocky road from being a dependent child to becoming a young adult.

For some children and adolescents, these normal developmental struggles are compounded by a mental illness. Some of the disorders that may develop during childhood or adolescence are depression, anxiety disorders, eating disorders and substance abuse. Depression and anxiety disorders, in particular, are common among children and teens. Less commonly, bipolar disorder and schizophrenia may first appear during the teenage years. In addition to these mental conditions, a number of disorders involving learning and development are typically first diagnosed during childhood or adolescence.

When children and teenagers have untreated mental illness, their family relationships can suffer, their social development may be affected, they may do poorly in

Is Your Child at Risk?

The American Psychiatric Association lists the following warning signs of possible mental illness in children:

- Frequent crying
- Frequent requests or hints for help
- Constant anxiety, worry or preoccupation
- Fears or phobias that are unreasonable or interfere with normal activities
- An inability to concentrate on schoolwork and other age-appropriate tasks
- A decline in school performance that doesn't improve
- A loss of interest in playing
- Isolation from other children
- Fighting with other children
- Low self-esteem and little self-confidence
- Setting fires

If your child is experiencing any of these signs or symptoms, it may be appropriate to consult your child's pediatrician, your family doctor or a mental health professional.

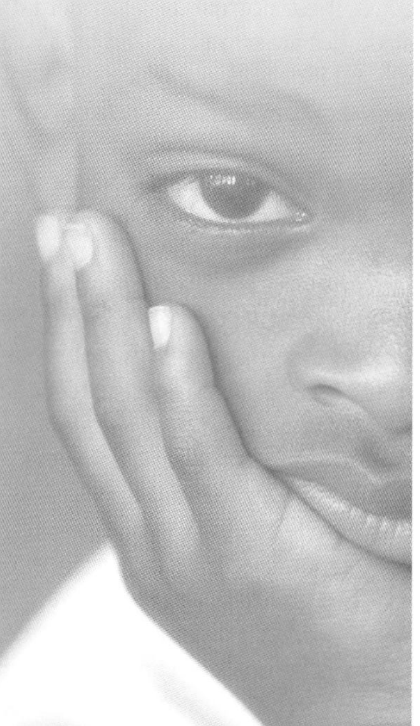

school, they may abuse alcohol or drugs, and they may be at risk of suicide. Suicide is the third leading cause of death for 15- to 24-year-olds and the sixth leading cause of death for 5- to 15-year-olds. These rates have tripled since 1960.

Prompt identification and treatment of mental disorders in children and teenagers can reduce the severity and duration of illness and the risk of complications. During the last two decades, health care professionals have improved efforts to better understand, recognize and treat mental illness in children and adolescents.

In response to the increasing rate of depression in children and teens, more efforts are being made to recognize and treat depression in this age group. Studies show that early treatment of mild to moderate depression may help prevent severe depression and related disorders, such as substance abuse and eating disorders. For children and teens at high risk of mental illness due to family history, short-term, family-based educational intervention seems to help reduce the risk of a first episode of illness.

For more information about specific conditions in children and adolescents, see Chapter 13, "Preschool to Preteen Years," and Chapter 14, "Teenage Years."

Older adults and mental illness

Just as young people struggle to adjust to the changes that occur in their lives, so too do older adults. The aging process may bring a number of physical and mental changes that can contribute to mental illness, especially depression. Increased health problems, a change in normal routine, financial stress, loss of independence or mobility and the death of family and friends can increase the risk of depression. More than 6 million adults age 65 and older experience depression, but many don't receive treatment.

Depression can occur with illnesses that are more common later in life, such as Alzheimer's disease, Parkinson's disease, stroke, heart disease and cancer. Because signs and symptoms of these diseases may overlap with those of depression, depression is often underdiagnosed in people with these health conditions. Some medications may trigger depression and anxiety.

Undiagnosed and untreated mental illness in older adults can diminish their quality of life. It can lead to decreased physical functioning and an increased reliance on others. Depression may even be associated with an increased risk of early death among people with certain forms of heart disease. Fortunately, treatment for depression is generally as effective in older adults as it is in younger people.

Depression

Many people say that they're "depressed" when they feel sad, lonely, down or dejected. But the medical diagnosis of depression implies more than a fleeting bad mood or period of stress. True depression — what medical professionals generally refer to as depressive illness — is different from normal sadness or despair.

In contrast to the blues, a period of several days when you seem to be feeling down, depression continues for a longer time. In its most common form, depressive illness lasts at least 2 weeks, and often much longer. It exhibits specific symptoms related to mood, behavior, thinking and outlook. It impairs your ability to function on a daily basis and requires treatment with medications or psychotherapy or both.

For centuries, people viewed depression as a sign of mental weakness. "It's all in your head" was a common phrase heard by people experiencing depression. Following years of research, though, doctors came to recognize depression as a medical disorder. People with depression may have abnormally low levels of certain brain chemicals (neurotransmitters) and slowed cellular activity in areas of the brain that control mood, appetite, sleep and other functions. Brain imaging studies have shown changes in brain activity during depression.

Many factors play a role in bringing about these chemical changes. Development of depression may be related to the genes you inherit from your parents. It may stem from medical conditions, such as diseases of the thyroid and adrenal glands or changes in the production of sex hormones. Physical and emotional stress, especially if it's severe or persistent, also can produce changes in brain activity, that can trigger depression.

Depression is one of the most common medical problems in the United States. It affects approximately 18 million American adults at any given time and can strike anyone, regardless of age, race, nationality, occupation, income level or sex. However, women have significantly higher rates of depression than do men.

A person's first episode of depression typically occurs between the ages of 25 and 44. But the illness also affects children, teenagers and older adults.

Depression can occur by itself, or it can be a complication of another illness. It may occur as a reaction to a medication. It may occur after childbirth or as a result of alcohol or drug abuse. It can be a response to stress from a job change, loss of a loved one or another difficult event. Sometimes it just happens, with no apparent trigger but is likely due to decreased amounts of neurotransmitters in the brain.

Signs and symptoms

The hallmark symptom of depression is a depressed mood. You may feel sad, helpless and hopeless. Your self-esteem and self-confidence may plummet, and you may feel guilty or worthless. Some people, however, experience depression without feeling depressed.

Depression can affect more than just your mood. It can also cause physical changes and changes in thinking and behavior. It can disrupt your sleeping and eating patterns and reduce your sexual drive. It affects how you think about things, making your thoughts more negative and pessimistic and hampering your ability to concentrate or make a decision. It impacts how you act. You may be more irritable, withdrawn or ambivalent.

Depression often goes unnoticed and untreated. Health care providers may fail to associate physical symptoms such as fatigue, headaches, pain and insomnia with depression. And individuals who are depressed often deny or minimize their symptoms, or rationalize them as reactions to stress.

Depression is characterized by several of the following signs and symptoms:

- Persistent sadness
- Irritability
- Feelings of anxiety
- Loss of interest or pleasure in life
- Neglect of personal responsibilities or personal care
- Changes in eating habits or a weight loss or gain
- Changes in sleeping patterns, including early awakening, sleeping too much or having trouble falling asleep or staying asleep
- Fatigue and loss of energy
- Decreased concentration, attention and memory
- Extreme mood changes
- Feelings of helplessness, hopelessness, worthlessness or guilt
- Continuous negative thinking or pessimism
- Physical symptoms, such as headache, digestive problems and chronic pain, that don't respond to treatment
- Increased alcohol or drug use
- Thoughts of death or suicide

Brain Communication

Brain cells communicate by sending messages along a complex system of nerve bundles that connect different regions of the brain. The ends of brain cells contain chemical messengers, called neurotransmitters, that serve as communication links between nerve cells (neurons). It's thought that neurotransmitters play a key role in depression and other mental disorders.

Nerve cells release neurotransmitters into a small gap (synapse) between a sending nerve cell and a receiving nerve cell (see the color illustration on page 414). The neurotransmitter binds to a receptor on the receiving nerve cell. During the transfer of information, electric signals from the sending nerve cell are changed into chemical signals that communicate the message to the receiving nerve cell. When the transfer is complete, the receiving cell changes the chemical signals back to electric signals. Communication from one cell to another occurs very rapidly.

People who are depressed may have lower levels of certain neurotransmitters, such as serotonin and norepinephrine, in the synapse between nerve cells compared with people who aren't depressed. Antidepressant medications increase the amount and activity of neurotransmitters in the synapse. This allows nerve cells in the treated individual to get messages in a way similar to that of people who aren't depressed.

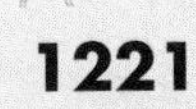

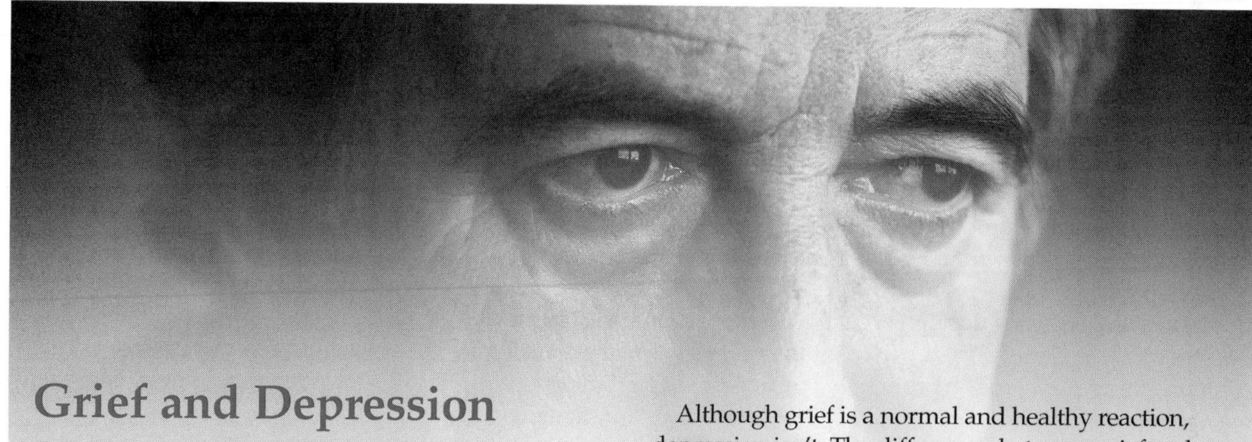

Grief and Depression

Grief is the emotional and physical response to a significant loss, such as the death of a loved one, the end of a relationship, a move to a new town, a change in health or the death of a pet. Grieving is a process of coming to terms with the loss and letting go. It takes a long time, and it's hard work. Grieving is a private journey that's different for everyone.

In many ways, grief and depression are similar. They share many signs and symptoms, including feelings of sadness, lack of interest in usually pleasurable activities, problems with sleeping and eating, irritability, sexual difficulties and difficulty concentrating. Other symptoms you may experience if you're grieving are a sense of confusion or disorientation, headaches or other physical complaints, anger, resentment or bitterness and withdrawal from social activities.

Although grief is a normal and healthy reaction, depression isn't. The differences between grief and depression are in how long the feelings last and to what extent your daily activities are impaired. Depression can complicate grief in two ways: It can produce short-term symptoms that are more severe than those typically associated with grief, and it can cause symptoms of grief to be more intense and to persist longer than normal.

There's no specific treatment for grief, other than time. The grief process can take a year or more. During this time it's important to surround yourself with people who are supportive. If your grief is severe or lasts longer, it may be complicated by depression. Studies suggest that another difference between grief and depression is self-denigration. People who are depressed often have feelings of worthlessness, but people who are grieving usually don't have such feelings.

Signs and symptoms may come on suddenly, or they may develop slowly over months and years. They may vary according to the type of depression an individual has.

Types

Depression can take many forms, differentiated by the symptoms and circumstances associated with each and the duration and severity of symptoms. Often, though, different types of depression have no clear-cut distinctions, and they share many characteristics. People may have more than one type of depression.

Major depression

Major depression is the most common form of the illness. It's characterized by a mood change that lasts more than 2 weeks and includes one or both of the primary signs of depression — overwhelming feelings of sadness or grief and loss of interest in usually enjoyable activities. People with major depression also experience at least four of the following signs and symptoms regularly, if not daily:

- Sleep disturbance
- Slowed or restless movement
- Fatigue or loss of energy
- Low self-esteem or inappropriate guilt
- Feelings of worthlessness, helplessness or hopelessness
- Impaired thinking or concentration
- Loss of sexual desire
- Significant weight loss or gain
- Recurrent thoughts of death or suicide

You may experience major depression only once, or it may return. After your first bout of major depression, you have more than a 50 percent chance of having it again, and the odds of recurrence increase with each episode.

If not treated, episodes of major depression typically last from 6 to 18 months. Early treatment may keep depression from becoming more severe, and continuing treatment can keep it from coming back.

Dysthymia

Dysthymia is a long-lasting form of mild depression that's characterized by a persistently gloomy outlook. The term originates from the Greeks, who thought that the thymus gland was the root of all emotions. *Dys* means "bad," and *thymia* means "a condition of the mind."

Dysthymia generally lasts for at least 2 years and sometimes more than 5 years. Periods of dysthymia may alternate with brief intervals of feeling normal. The condition can interfere with work and social life. Many people with dysthymia become socially withdrawn and less productive. Individuals with dysthymia also have a greater risk of developing major depression.

Signs and symptoms of dysthymia are like those of major depression but not as intense, and you may not experience as many of them. They may include:

- Difficulty concentrating or making decisions
- Social withdrawal
- Irritability
- Restlessness or sluggishness
- Problems sleeping
- Weight gain or loss

Some people with dysthymia first experience feelings of depression in childhood or adolescence. Others develop dysthymia later in life, often following a medical illness.

Adjustment disorder

An adjustment disorder occurs when your response to a stressful situation causes signs and symptoms of depression that aren't strong enough to meet the criteria for major depression.

For example, if your marriage falls apart, your business fails or you receive a diagnosis of cancer, it's normal to feel tense, sad, overwhelmed or angry. Eventually, most people come to terms with the consequences of such stresses. But people with an adjustment disorder don't. Often times, an adjustment disorder precedes major depression.

Adjustment disorders can affect anybody. They often occur at a time in your life when you are particularly vulnerable — for instance, when you move away from your parents or at the end of a fulfilling career. Some people develop an adjustment disorder in response to a single event. For others the condition stems from a combination of stressful events.

Postpartum Depression

Many women experience temporary feelings of sadness following childbirth. These so-called baby blues tend to gradually diminish and usually don't require treatment. Some women, though, experience a major form of depression following childbirth called postpartum depression. Compared with the baby blues, the signs and symptoms of this type of depression are more severe and persistent. An episode of postpartum depression increases the likelihood that you'll have recurrent bouts of depression, either after subsequent births or at other times.

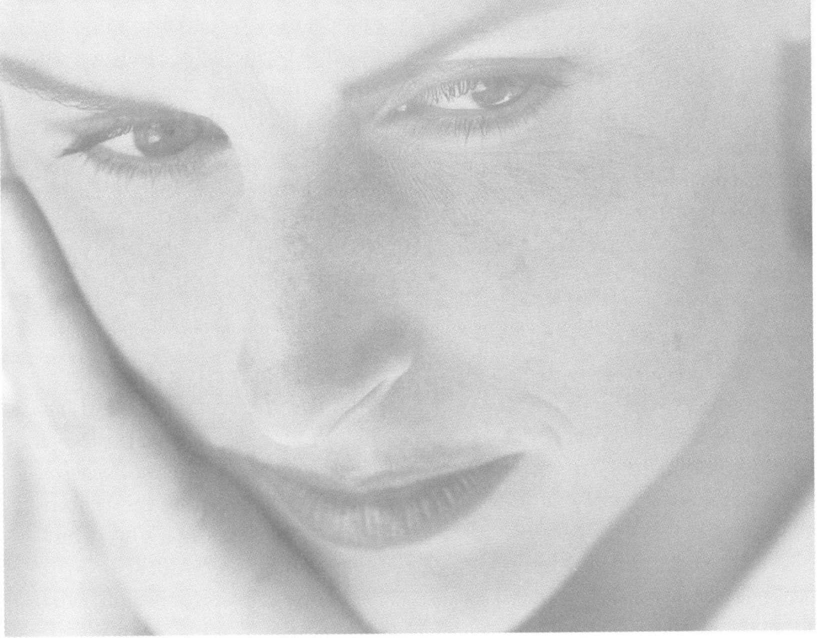

Bipolar disorder

Some people have bipolar disorder, recurring cycles of depression and euphoria (mania). This illness, with emotions at both extremes (poles), is also known as manic depression or manic-depressive disorder.

Bipolar disorder isn't as common as major depression or dysthymia. The illness typically emerges in adolescence or young adulthood and continues intermittently throughout life. It often runs in families. Both men and women are equally at risk.

During a manic phase, you feel unstoppable. You might spend money recklessly or make unwise decisions. Your grandiose ideas may result in anything from a bad business decision to promiscuous behavior. Some people have bursts of increased creativity and productivity during a manic phase.

Signs and symptoms of mania include:

- Abnormal or excessive elation
- Markedly increased energy
- A decreased need for sleep
- Unusual irritability
- Unrealistic beliefs in one's abilities and powers
- Increased talkativeness
- Racing thoughts
- Poor judgment
- Increased sexual desire
- Provocative, intrusive or aggressive social behavior
- Abuse of alcohol or other substances

Your euphoria might not be obvious to those who don't know you well, but friends and loved ones may come to recognize it as typical of the manic phase. Your speech and thoughts seem to run at high speed. Your speech may become so laden with puns, jokes and plays on

Depression and Other Mental Illnesses

Depression often accompanies other mental illnesses, most commonly anxiety disorders, eating disorders and substance abuse. For example, up to 50 percent of individuals who are depressed experience anxiety, and 50 percent to 75 percent of people with an eating disorder have a history of depression.

Of people who abuse alcohol, about 30 percent meet the criteria for depression. Experts speculate that some people who abuse alcohol or drugs may be trying to self-medicate or "normalize" their neurotransmitters in an attempt to feel better. But even moderate amounts of alcohol or other substances can cause or increase the severity of depression.

The intermingling and intensity of symptoms in combined mental disorders can present challenges and obstacles to diagnosis and treatment. The only way to untangle the interdependence of combined disorders is to recognize and treat both conditions. One way you can help yourself is to be honest and forthcoming when you discuss your symptoms with your doctor or a mental health professional. This can help greatly in recognizing combined disorders and determining the best treatment approach.

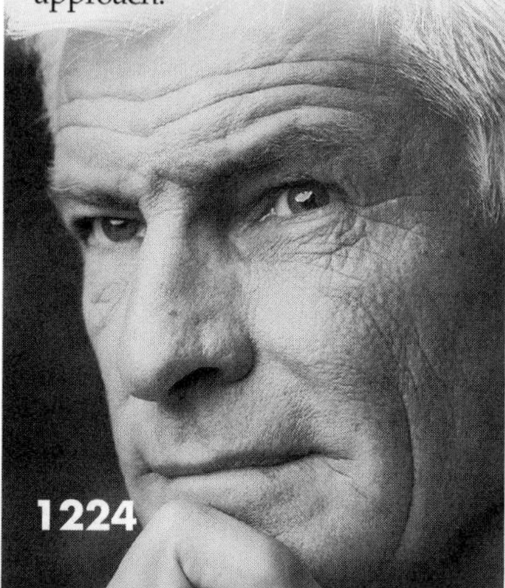

words that after a while it makes little sense.

Signs and symptoms of bipolar disorder tend to become more severe over time. You may start out with episodes of depression, mania or a mixture of both moods, separated by periods with no symptoms. Over time, episodes of mania and depression become more frequent, with shorter normal periods. Severe depression or elation may be accompanied by psychosis, including hallucinations and delusions.

The different forms of bipolar disorder are classified by their severity and symptom patterns. As with other forms of depression, it's critical to get treatment early to prevent the illness from progressing and to decrease the risk of suicide.

Seasonal affective disorder

Seasonal affective disorder (SAD) is the term for depressive periods that are related to a change of season. This disorder is more than cabin fever — most people with cabin fever don't have SAD.

No one knows for certain what causes SAD. Some researchers believe that a lack of daylight disrupts your circadian rhythms, which regulate your body's internal clock. SAD is more common in places where daylight hours are seasonally limited. People with SAD usually notice mood changes starting in late fall, with improvement in spring. But some people experience summer depression.

SAD usually begins in adolescence or young adulthood and is more common among women than among men. You may have the condition if you've experienced depression and related symptoms during at least two consecutive winters, followed by nondepressed periods in the spring and summer.

Individuals with SAD generally sleep a great deal in the winter, crave carbohydrates and gain weight, become irritable and low on energy, experience headaches and stress and have crying spells.

Treatment

Once you suspect or recognize depression in yourself, it's crucial that you seek treatment. Untreated depression can raise your risk of a number of other health conditions. Studies show that even mild depression may be associated with poor physical and social functioning, increased risk of future depression and suicide attempts.

With appropriate treatment, approximately 8 out of 10 people with depression improve and return to their usual, productive lives. From medications to psychotherapy, many options are available for treating depression, and each can play an important role. Just as the cause of depression may be a complex interplay of factors, so too finding the most effective treatment for your illness can be a complex process that takes time and professional guidance.

Medication

Antidepressant medications are often the first line of treatment for depression (see page 1241). Antidepressants can relieve symptoms, generally with few side effects. Many types are available. If one type doesn't work for you, another may.

The initial goal of treatment is to relieve signs and symptoms. After beginning to take an antidepressant, you may not notice a change for 2 weeks or longer. It's important not to feel discouraged and to keep taking the medication even if at first it seems to be having no effect. Once your signs and symptoms have eased, use of medication (maintenance treatment) typically continues for 4 to 12 months to prevent a relapse. Even though you may feel fine, it's important to keep taking your medication as prescribed. If you've had recurrent episodes of depression, your doctor may recommend that you continue taking medication longer — perhaps for years. Episodes of depression recur in 80 percent to 90

Light Therapy for SAD

Light therapy, or phototherapy, is a common treatment for seasonal affective disorder (SAD). The therapy consists of exposure to intense light under specified conditions. The lighting system most often used is a box that you set on a table or desktop. The box contains a set of special fluorescent bulbs with a diffusing screen to help block out ultraviolet rays, which can cause cataracts and skin problems.

Treatment involves sitting near the light box with the lights on and your eyes open. You shouldn't look directly at the light, but you want your head and body oriented so that the light can enter your eyes. Researchers believe that when bright light enters your eyes, it has antidepressant-like effects, causing changes in brain chemical activity in certain areas of the brain.

Light therapy improves symptoms in about three out of four people with SAD. Many people begin to feel better in a few days, but symptoms often reappear if therapy is stopped. It's important that light therapy be monitored by a health care professional.

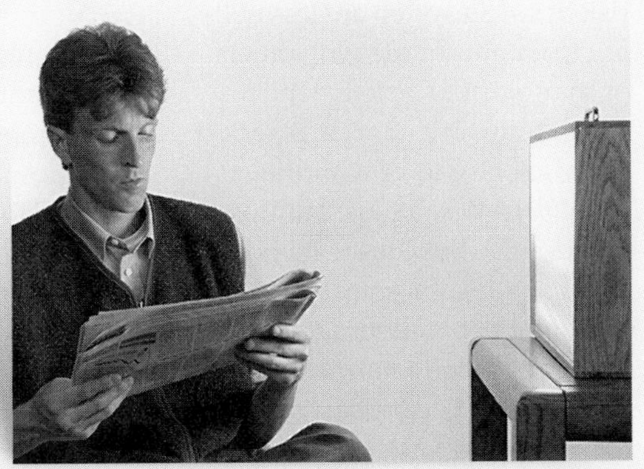

Phototherapy for seasonal affective disorder involves sitting near a bright light for a specified period each day. You shouldn't stare at the light, but you want the light to enter your eyes.

percent of people who have had one episode. The longer you stay on medication, the less likely it is that depression will recur.

Depending on the type of depression you have, your doctor may recommend a second medication in addition to an antidepressant. Mood stabilizers are used to treat bipolar disorder. If your depression is accompanied by a condition such as anxiety, your doctor may recommend an anti-anxiety medication. Often, the most effective treatment is a combination of medication and psychotherapy.

Psychotherapy

Psychotherapy, also known as talk therapy, may be combined with medication. Psychotherapy involves help from a mental health professional through a combination of talking and listening. Psychotherapy can help you understand the source of your feelings and find better ways of coping with problems and conflicts.

When you're acutely depressed, psychotherapy can provide support during the time needed for your medication to take effect. As symptoms improve, psychotherapy can help you understand why the depression occurred and what you can do to prevent a recurrence.

Several different types of psychotherapy are used to treat depression. Cognitive-behavioral therapy (CBT), for example, has been shown to be very effective in treating depression. For more information on CBT and other therapies, including interpersonal therapy, group therapy and family therapy, see page 1243.

Electroconvulsive therapy

Electroconvulsive therapy (ECT) is one of the most dramatically effective treatments for severe depression. Unlike antidepressants, ECT works quickly, often within a few days.

No one knows for certain how ECT helps treat depression. Researchers theorize that when administered on a regular basis for a short period of time, ECT produces chemical changes in the brain that build upon one another, somehow reducing depression. The procedure is effective in about 80 percent of people who complete the course of treatment. For more information on ECT, see page 1246.

Depression and suicide

More than 30,000 Americans commit suicide each year, and an estimated 10 to 20 times that number attempt to kill themselves. About 90 percent of people who commit suicide have one or more mental illnesses, most commonly depression. The more severe the depression — especially if it's untreated or inadequately treated — the greater the suicide risk.

Several warning signs indicate that someone may be at risk of suicide. Many of the warning signs are also features of depression, and it can be difficult to determine if they represent suicidal intentions or are symptoms of depression.

If you or someone you know displays any of the following warning signs of potential suicide, seek professional help as soon as possible:

- *Suicidal threats.* Sometimes, an individual will tell others outright that he or she is thinking of committing suicide. The person may say things like, "I wish I'd never been born," "I'd be better off dead," or "You'll be better off when I'm gone." The common assumption that people who threaten suicide don't do it isn't true.

- *Withdrawing from others.* People at risk of suicide often are less willing to communicate with others or may want to be left alone. Trouble at work or poor grades can also be signs of withdrawal.
- *Moodiness.* We all have our ups and downs. But drastic mood swings — an emotional high one day and deep discouragement the next — aren't normal.
- *Difficulty with a personal crisis.* A major life crisis, such as a divorce, a lost job or the death of a loved one, can be difficult for anyone to manage. Among people who are depressed, such a crisis can push them over the edge, triggering a suicide attempt.
- *Personality changes.* Before someone commits suicide, he or she may exhibit marked changes in personality and routines, such as eating or sleeping patterns. For example, an individual who's shy may become the life of the party, or an outgoing person may become withdrawn. You might notice a change in his or her energy level or attitude toward personal appearance.
- *Displays of risky behavior.* Uncharacteristically dangerous activities, such as high-speed driving, unsafe sex or drug abuse, may be signs of a desire to die.
- *Giving away possessions.* Sometimes, a person who is considering suicide may begin to give away cherished belongings, believing they won't be needed any longer.

Unfortunately, some people being treated for depression kill themselves 2 to 3 months into their recovery.

If someone has been struggling with depression for months or years, this may be the first time he or she sees the problems the depression has caused or has the energy to act on suicidal feelings. The person may not yet have overcome the hopelessness and negative thinking that commonly accompany depression.

Anxiety Disorders

Everyone has moments of anxiety, worry and fear. It's normal to feel your stomach churn if you have a disagreement with your boss. It's normal to experience a wave of concern if your partner or child is late getting home. Feeling anxious about the future after a terrorist attack or during a war is a normal reaction.

A moderate amount of anxiety is essential for human survival. It helps you respond appropriately to real danger, and it may help motivate you to excel at work and at home. But when worries or fears center on events that are unlikely to occur and when they consume your life and dictate your actions, you've moved beyond reasonable levels of anxiety. You may not even know what's causing your distress, or the source of your anxiety may seem minor compared with the intensity of your reaction. This type of anxiety can be a symptom of or a form of mental illness. Persistent anxiety that affects your daily life is termed an anxiety disorder.

Anxiety disorders are some of the most common mental disorders, affecting about 12 million Americans each year. About twice as many women as men are affected. Some personality types are more prone to anxiety disorders, and they tend to run in families.

Anxiety may be associated with another medical illness, such as a thyroid condition or cardiovascular disease. Anxiety disorders frequently occur in combination with depression. About half of all depressed people experience anxiety. When their depression is treated, their anxiety often improves as well.

The stress response

Scientists are beginning to map circuits and structures of the nervous system that are prominent in mental disorders such as anxiety. They believe that the amygdala, an almond-shaped structure in the temporal lobe of the brain, may transmit emotions and sensations that typify anxiety. The amygdala picks up and processes signals from areas of the brain that sense danger.

Evidence suggests that, like a dispatcher in a taxi company, the amygdala sends signals to parts of the nervous system that perceive fear and prompt the stress (fight-or-flight) response. Nerve cells (neurons) in the amygdala and other regions of the brain secrete a hormone known as corticotropin-releasing factor. CRF turns on a cascade of other hormones that can cause your heart to pound, breathing to quicken, sweat to increase, mouth to go dry, blood pressure to rise and muscles to tense. You may also experience nausea or diarrhea.

When anxiety gets out of control, this response can occur almost continuously. It can also occur during periods of calm. Why this happens isn't fully understood. One theory is that an anxiety disorder may develop after you experience one or more fearful events that trigger the fight-or-flight response. The deeply etched memory of the event may prime you to become hypervigilant and to overreact to everyday situations.

Signs and symptoms

Signs and symptoms vary depending on the type of anxiety disorder you have. Physical signs and symptoms triggered by the stress response are common in many anxiety disorders. These include:

- Muscle tension
- A rapid heartbeat
- Rapid breathing or the feeling that you're unable to get enough air
- Tremors
- Gastrointestinal distress, such as diarrhea
- Sweating
- Dry mouth
- Dizziness

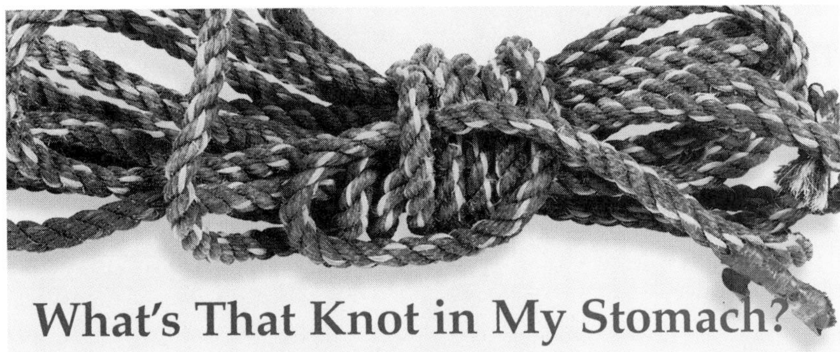

What's That Knot in My Stomach?

Stress or anxiety can bring on not only a tension headache but also tension in your gut. Muscles in the wall of your stomach and intestines may suddenly contract, giving you the feeling of a knot, much like a muscle cramp in your leg.

This may cause discomfort or pain, but it isn't serious. As your anxiety lessens, the feeling usually goes away. If the knot is persistent or intense or if you also have nausea, vomiting, diarrhea or difficulty swallowing, see your doctor. These symptoms could indicate some other problem.

- Restlessness or an inability to relax
- Irritability or impatience
- Problems sleeping
- Difficulty concentrating

Your signs and symptoms may become long term (chronic) and progressively worse if you don't receive appropriate help. Treatment for an anxiety disorder can be highly effective at calming you or eliminating many of your signs and symptoms.

Types

Anxiety may accompany depression, or it may develop as a separate disorder:

Generalized anxiety disorder

One of the most common anxiety disorders is generalized anxiety disorder. You feel anxious most of the time, usually without a readily identifiable cause. You may be plagued by a sense of self-doubt and indecisiveness and have a nagging feeling that something bad is about to happen. You worry about your kids, your job, your health, for no apparent reason. You may feel tense all of the time, making it difficult for you to function at home or at work.

If you have this condition, you may have trouble sleeping and wake up feeling wired. You may experience fatigue, exhaustion, muscle tension, irritability, chest pain, a lump in your throat, fast breathing, stomachache, diarrhea, headaches, dry mouth or sweaty palms.

Generalized anxiety disorder can begin at any age and continue throughout your life. In children and adolescents with the disorder, their worries often center on their performance at school or in sports. In older adults generalized anxiety often coincides with depression.

Adjustment disorder with anxiety

An adjustment disorder with anxiety occurs when your response to a stressful situation causes signs and symptoms of anxiety, such as nervousness, worry or jitteriness. The stressor may be a single event, such as the end of a romantic relationship, or multiple events. Most people eventually come to terms with the consequences of such stress, but people with an adjustment disorder don't.

Adjustment disorders can affect anybody. They often occur at a time in your life when you're more vulnerable — when you move away from your parents or at the end of your career, for instance.

Panic disorder

A panic disorder typically includes feelings of terror that strike suddenly and repeatedly with no warning and often for no reason. During a panic attack your heart may race, you may sweat or hyperventilate, and you may feel weak, faint or dizzy. The physical symptoms are so intense that you may think you're dying or losing your mind. Symptoms can mimic a heart attack. You may have chest pain, shortness of breath or a feeling that you're being smothered. You may experience a sense of unreality or of losing control.

Attacks can occur at home or in public, and they can even awaken you from a deep sleep. An attack typically lasts only a few minutes but may go on for up to 10 minutes or longer. You may feel fatigued and worn out after it subsides.

Because the attacks are unpredictable, people with panic disorder often develop intense anxiety or lingering worry about the possibility of having another attack at any time. About half the people with panic disorder develop agoraphobia, a condition in which you become afraid to leave your home. In addition, about half the people who experience panic attacks experience at least one episode of depression.

Between 10 percent and 20 percent of Americans experience a panic attack at some time in their life, but a much smaller number of people have true panic disorder. People with panic disorder experience four or more panic attacks a month, or their fear of having an attack limits their daily activities. Panic disorder tends to run in families.

Without treatment, panic disorder can become debilitating and destructive. Fear of recurrent attacks can cause you to adopt avoidance behavior, such as

A Perfectionist or an Obsessive-Compulsive?

There's a difference between being a perfectionist and having obsessive-compulsive disorder. Perhaps you get all of your work done a week ahead of schedule, your hair is never out of place, and the floors in your house are so clean that you could eat off them. That doesn't mean you have obsessive-compulsive disorder. Instead, you may belong to the large group of people who hold themselves to a very high standard in all that they do. This behavior can build self-esteem and success. In contrast, behaviors associated with obsessive-compulsive disorder interfere with normal functioning.

However, sometimes the distinction isn't so clear. You may feel that your perfectionism isn't extreme, but family members disagree. They may claim that your behavior is excessive. In such cases, it may be useful to get an evaluation from a mental health professional.

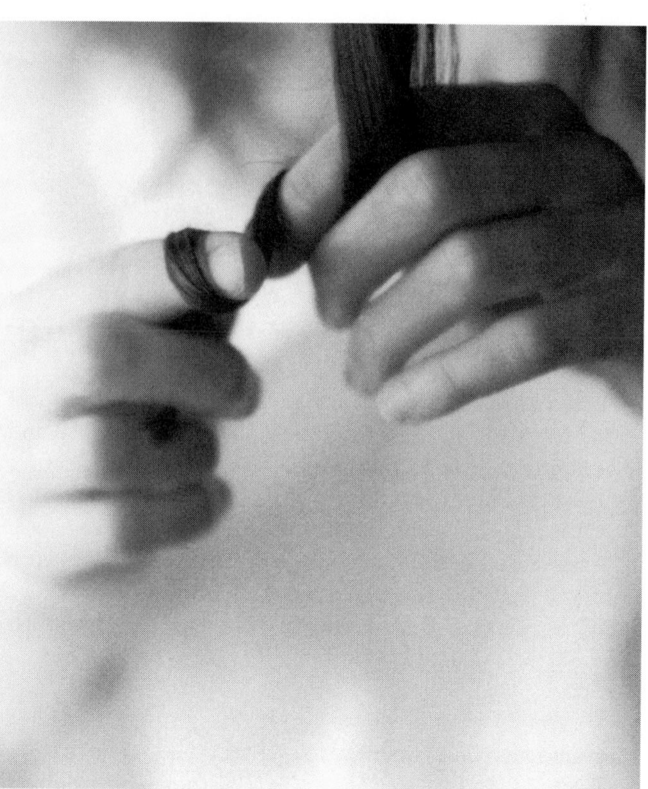

refusing to go shopping or to leave the house by yourself.

In children, panic attacks can interfere with normal development, disrupting their social life and schoolwork. Children and teenagers may refuse to go to school or to leave the house.

Phobias

A phobia is a persistent, irrational fear of an object or a situation. You may be afraid of enclosed spaces, bridges, heights, flying or creatures such as snakes or spiders. Even though you understand that your fear is excessive or unwarranted, you try to avoid the object of your phobia at all costs.

It's normal to feel some discomfort about certain objects or situations. But if your fears become irrational and uncontrollable and your avoidance of the feared object affects your social interactions and daily activities, you may have a phobia.

Fears of animals and other objects are common in childhood but usually pass. Such fears aren't categorized as phobias unless they impair the child's functioning — for example, if the child refuses to go to school for fear of encountering a dog on the street.

When exposed to the feared object or situation, a person with a phobia becomes panicky and has signs and symptoms similar to those experienced with panic disorder. Just anticipating an encounter with the feared object may provoke feelings of intense anxiety, so you go out of your way to avoid what you fear.

Children may express their anxiety by crying, tantrums, freezing or clinging. Phobias usually first occur in childhood or early adolescence. Evidence suggests that certain types of phobias may run in families.

Social anxiety disorder

Everyone feels nervous from time to time. Going on a first date or giving a speech often prompts a queasy stomach. But for some people, normal nervousness mushrooms into extreme fear. Everyday activities such as starting a conversation, eating with others or attending a party become impossible. This condition is known as social anxiety disorder or social phobia.

You may receive a diagnosis of social anxiety disorder if your fears significantly interfere with your day-to-day life or cause significant distress. You may become anxious when you're around people you don't know, or you may fear a particular situation, such as talking in front of others.

Common, everyday experiences such as using a public restroom or telephone, returning items to a store, writing in front of others, making eye contact or ordering food in a restaurant can cause severe anxiety.

People with social anxiety disorder experience signs and symptoms of anxiety — sweating, blushing, tremors, gastrointestinal discomfort, muscle tension, a racing heart, confusion — in the feared social situations.

The disorder typically starts in the teenage years or after a stressful or humiliating experience. It can vary in intensity over the course of a person's life but generally is lifelong. Like other anxiety disorders, it appears to have a hereditary component.

If shyness interferes greatly with your life and causes emotional distress, you may want to see a doctor or mental health professional who specializes in anxiety disorders.

Obsessive-compulsive disorder
A person with obsessive-compulsive disorder may perform the same rituals over and over again to the point that the behaviors dominate his or her life. If you have this disorder, you may feel that you must eat the same lunch every day and eat the food in the same order. You may wipe off the doorknobs in your home each time someone touches them. You may leave home only to return several times to make sure you turned off the coffeepot or locked the door.

Individuals with this disorder experience obsessions or compulsions or both. Obsessions are recurrent, persistent, unwanted ideas, thoughts or impulses that you experience involuntarily and that appear to be senseless. They commonly intrude when you're trying to think of or do other things. Common obsessions include:

- Fear of dirt or contamination
- Concern with order, symmetry and exactness
- Constantly thinking about certain sounds, images, words or numbers
- Fear of harming a family member or friend
- Fear of thinking thoughts you consider evil or sinful
- Worry about making a mistake

Compulsions are repetitive behaviors that you're driven to perform regularly to combat your obsessions. Typical compulsions include:

- Excessive hand washing
- Checking repeatedly that doors are locked and appliances are turned off
- Arranging items in a precise order
- Counting over and over to a certain number
- Touching certain objects several times

If you have obsessive-compulsive disorder, you may do everything in a meticulous, precise, orderly fashion. If the compulsive need isn't fulfilled, you may experience overwhelming anxiety. When you perform these rituals, you may feel some relief from anxiety, but not for long. Your discomfort soon returns, and you feel compelled to repeat the behaviors.

You realize that your repetitive thoughts and behaviors are irrational and senseless, but you can't free yourself from them. You may be able to control the unwanted behaviors for a while, but your resistance may weaken after months or years of struggle. Eventually, your rituals may take up more of your time, making it difficult to lead a normal life.

Obsessive-compulsive disorder generally begins in late adolescence or young adulthood, and it may be accompanied by depression. Shame and embarrassment may keep you from seeking treatment. Even if your rituals are deeply ingrained, treatment can help.

Post-traumatic stress disorder
As the name implies, post-traumatic stress disorder is a form of anxiety disorder triggered by a traumatic experience that you lived through or witnessed.

The disorder may affect survivors of sexual assault, physical abuse, war, torture, natural disasters, automobile accidents, airplane crashes, hostage situations or death camps. It can also affect rescue workers at an airplane crash or mass shooting or someone who witnessed a traumatic accident. Whatever the trauma, the person has lived through a period in which he or she was faced with intense fear, a sense of helplessness and loss of control.

Relatively few people involved in a traumatic event experience post-traumatic stress disorder. Very young and very old people who experience major traumas seem to be especially susceptible to post-traumatic stress, probably because young children have inadequately developed coping mechanisms and older adults may have fewer social supports.

Post-traumatic stress disorder shares many of the same signs and symptoms of depression. The major difference is that with post-traumatic stress disorder, you

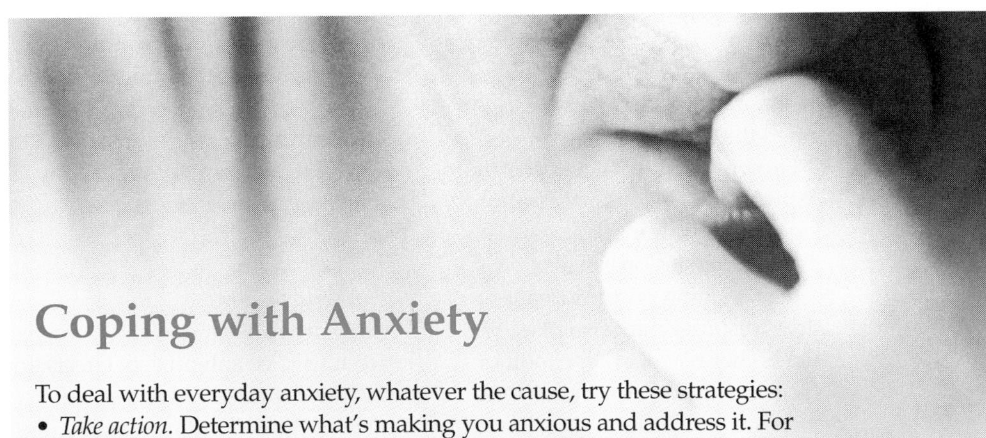

Coping with Anxiety

To deal with everyday anxiety, whatever the cause, try these strategies:

- *Take action.* Determine what's making you anxious and address it. For example, if you're worried about finances, draw up a budget.
- *Let it go.* Try not to dwell on past concerns. Change what you can and let the rest take its course.
- *Break the cycle.* When you feel anxious, take a brisk walk or delve into a hobby.
- *Take care of yourself.* Get enough rest, eat a balanced diet, exercise and take time to relax. Avoid caffeine and nicotine, which can worsen anxiety. Don't turn to alcohol or unprescribed drugs.
- *Talk to someone.* Share your problems with a friend or counselor who can help you gain perspective.

continue to have prominent memories and intrusive thoughts of the event or events that initially triggered the disorder.

Growing evidence indicates that depression develops after prolonged post-traumatic stress disorder, but depression can also precede it. Having post-traumatic stress disorder may also place you at a higher risk of other conditions such as drug abuse, alcohol abuse and eating disorders.

Signs and symptoms of post-traumatic stress disorder typically appear within 3 months of the traumatic event. In some instances, they may not occur until years later and may include:

- Flashbacks, disturbing dreams and hallucinations
- Distress at anniversaries of the traumatic event or events
- Efforts to avoid thoughts, feelings and activities associated with the trauma
- A sense of detachment or estrangement from others and an inability to feel love
- Markedly diminished interest or participation in activities that once were an important source of satisfaction
- In young children, delayed development or regression in areas such as toilet training and language
- A sense of hopelessness about the future
- Increased emotional or physical arousal, which may include at least two of the following: trouble sleeping, anger, difficulty concentrating, an exaggerated startle response to noise, increased blood pressure, a rapid heart rate, rapid breathing, muscle tension, nausea and diarrhea

Treatment

Treatment for an anxiety disorder depends on the type of disorder you have. With treatment most people with anxiety disorders are able to resume everyday activities. For the most effective results, your doctor may recommend a combination of medication and psychotherapy.

Medications

Several types of medications may relieve signs and symptoms of anxiety:

Antidepressants

Many drugs used to treat depression also have anti-anxiety effects. In fact, antidepressants are the treatment of choice for some anxiety disorders. Examples of antidepressant drugs used to treat anxiety include fluoxetine (Prozac), paroxetine (Paxil) and imipramine (Tofranil). For more on these medications, see page 1241.

Anti-anxiety medications

Anti-anxiety medications include a class of tranquilizing drugs called benzodiazepines, as well as the medication buspirone (BuSpar). See page 1242 for more information.

Beta blockers

Beta blockers are often used to treat cardiovascular conditions. They may help anxiety disorders by blocking the stimulating effects of the hormone adrenaline (epinephrine). Adrenaline causes many of the signs and symptoms associated with anxiety, including a pounding heart and increased heart rate and blood pressure.

Psychotherapy

Types of psychotherapy that are especially effective in treating anxiety disorders are cognitive-behavioral therapy, relaxation therapy and desensitization and exposure therapy. These therapies are discussed on page 1243.

Addictive Behaviors

The word *addiction* tends to bring to mind drugs. But you can be addicted to many substances and practices, from alcohol to nicotine to gambling to spending time online. The main characteristic of addictive behavior is that you feel a compelling need to engage in the activity or to use the addictive substance.

Addictive behaviors commonly occur in combination with other mental illnesses. Studies indicate that more than half the people who abuse alcohol or drugs have another mental illness or have experienced one in the past.

About 20 percent of people who abuse drugs and 30 percent of those who abuse alcohol have depression. Researchers aren't sure why these rates are so high, but it may have to do with the way addictive substances act on brain chemicals (neurotransmitters) that affect mood.

Alcohol addiction

Alcoholism and alcohol abuse cause major social, economic and public health problems in the United States. According to the National Council on Alcoholism and Drug Dependence, about 14 million Americans abuse alcohol. Each year more than 100,000 Americans die of alcohol-related causes.

You may begin to become dependent on alcohol after discovering that having a few drinks helps to relieve stress from family problems, difficulties at work or social isolation. Despite occasional hangovers and the fact that relief from life's stresses is only temporary, you gradually fall into the pattern of drinking alcohol whenever you feel tense.

Unfortunately, the more an alcohol-dependent person drinks, the less tension he or she can tolerate without using alcohol.

The actual number of drinks you have is not the critical issue. The diagnosis of alcohol dependency is made when you have difficulty getting through the day without regular alcohol consumption.

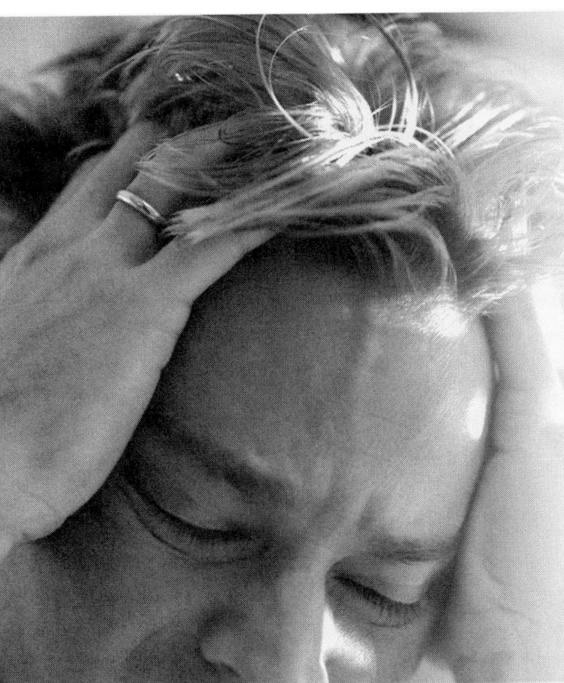

Alcohol Intoxication

The form of alcohol in the beverages people drink is ethyl alcohol (ethanol), a colorless liquid that, in its pure form, has a burning taste. Ethanol is produced by the fermentation of sugars in grains and fruits such as barley and grapes.

The intoxicating effects of alcohol relate to the concentration of alcohol in the blood. For example, if you're not a regular drinker and your blood alcohol concentration is more than 100 milligrams of alcohol per deciliter of blood (100 mg/dL), you may be quite intoxicated and have difficulty speaking, thinking and moving around. Most states define legal intoxication as a blood alcohol concentration of at least 70 to 100 mg/dL — .07 percent to .10 percent.

Your response to alcohol is affected by how much food you've eaten and how recently you ate before drinking. Size, body fat and tolerance to the effects of alcohol also play significant roles. Women generally have a higher blood alcohol concentration per drink than men do because they tend to be smaller, resulting in the alcohol being less diluted in their bodies. In addition, they may metabolize alcohol more slowly than men do.

Alcohol addiction — physical dependence on alcohol — occurs gradually as drinking alcohol alters the balance of some brain chemicals, causing a strong desire for more alcohol. These chemicals include:

- Gamma aminobutyric acid (GABA), which inhibits impulsiveness
- Glutamate, which stimulates the nervous system
- Norepinephrine, which is released in response to stress
- Dopamine, serotonin and opioid peptides, which can produce pleasurable feelings

Excessive, long-term drinking can deplete or increase the levels of some of these chemicals, causing the body to crave alcohol to restore good feelings or to avoid negative feelings. Other factors that can lead to excessive drinking contribute to the addiction process. These include:

- *Genetics.* Your genetic makeup doesn't cause alcoholism but may make you more susceptible to it.
- *Emotional state.* High levels of stress or anxiety, depression or other emotional pain can lead some people to drink alcohol to reduce or eliminate the turmoil.
- *Psychological factors.* Having friends or a close partner who drinks regularly, but who may not abuse alcohol, could lead to excessive drinking on your part. It may be difficult for you to not join in the drinking behavior.
- *Social and cultural factors.* The glamorous way that drinking alcohol is portrayed in advertising and in the entertainment media commonly sends the message that it's both common and OK to drink excessively.

For more information on alcohol addiction and treatment, see Chapter 6, "Addressing Risky Behaviors."

Drug addiction

Drug addiction involves compulsively seeking to use a substance — legal or illicit — regardless of social, psychological and physical consequences of its use. Certain drugs, such as narcotics and cocaine, are more addicting than other drugs.

The range of drugs to which you can become addicted is wide. They include illicit drugs such as marijuana, amphetamines, cocaine, Ecstasy and heroin as well as prescription drugs, including pain relievers such as morphine and codeine, sedatives, tranquilizers and stimulants such as methylphenidate (Concerta, Ritalin). Everyday substances such as glue, paint and solvents can also be used in an addictive manner.

Most people use prescription medications as directed, but prescription drug abuse appears to be on the rise in the United States. It's thought to be the most common form of drug abuse among older adults. A dramatic increase in the use of prescription drugs for nonmedical purposes among teenagers and young adults has been seen.

Dependence on drugs is destructive because of its long-term physical effects, its disruptive effect on family and work and the risks associated with sudden withdrawal. Illegal drugs are hazardous not only by their nature but also because of the risk of contamination with toxic or infectious substances and the risk of serious legal and social consequences.

Drug use or abuse crosses the line to drug addiction when you feel you need the drug to function and you increase the amount you take. Various factors, such as your personality, your genetic makeup and peer pressure affect your risk of becoming addicted to a drug.

Addiction appears to occur when repeated use of a drug alters reward

Types of Chemical Dependency

The three forms of chemical dependency are:

Increased tolerance
As your body becomes accustomed to a drug, the drug can lose its effectiveness. To receive the same degree of relief, you need to take increasing amounts of the drug.

Physical dependence
When you're physically dependent on a drug, you experience signs and symptoms of physical withdrawal when use of the drug is abruptly stopped or its dosage is substantially reduced. To control your pain, you rely on your medication at regular intervals.

Addiction
Addiction involves both physical and psychological dependence on a drug. This is possible with prescription medications as well as alcohol and illicit drugs. You become fixated or obsessed with a drug, and lose control over its use.

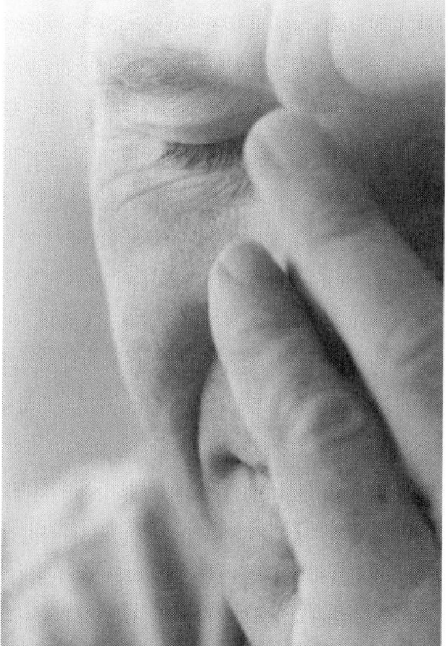

pathways in the brain. The drug changes the process by which nerve cells (neurons) in the brain use chemicals (neurotransmitters) to communicate. The changes vary with the type of drug being used.

For more information on drug abuse and treatment, see Chapter 6, "Addressing Risky Behaviors."

Nicotine addiction

Nicotine, one of the key ingredients in tobacco, can be as addictive as cocaine. Nicotine increases the amount of the brain chemical dopamine, which makes you feel good. Getting that dopamine boost is part of the addiction process.

Addiction to nicotine alters your mood. When you try to stop smoking, you may develop withdrawal symptoms — irritability, a depressed mood, insomnia, restlessness, anxiety and a decreased ability to concentrate. Indications that you may be addicted to nicotine include:

- An inability to quit smoking despite a desire to stop
- Withdrawal symptoms if you stop smoking
- Smoking to avoid withdrawal symptoms
- Using up your supply of cigarettes or other nicotine-containing products faster than you expected
- Forgoing an activity because it takes place in an area where smoking is prohibited
- Continuing to smoke or use any nicotine-containing product despite having medical problems related to tobacco use

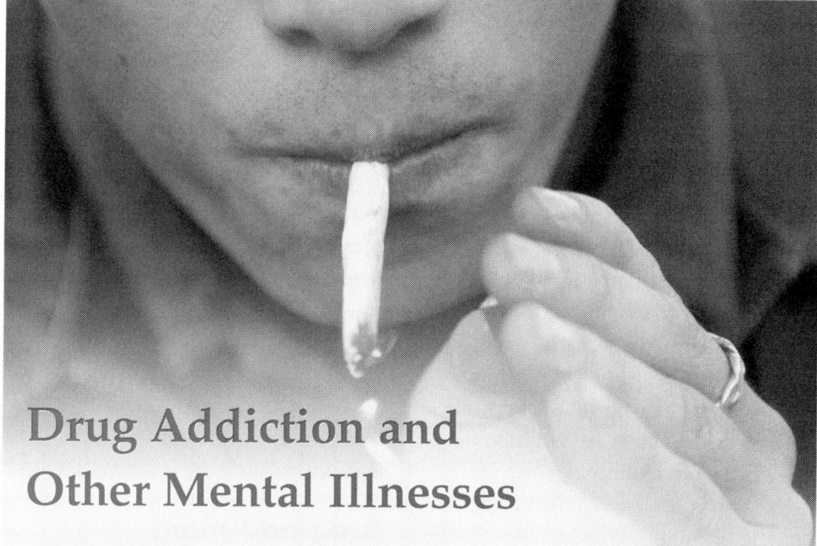

Drug Addiction and Other Mental Illnesses

Drug addiction may be associated with symptoms of another mental illness, such as depression or schizophrenia. For successful recovery, it's critical that you receive an accurate diagnosis of and treatment for all relevant disorders.

It can be difficult to determine whether drug abuse is causing symptoms of mental illness or if the mental illness is prompting the drug abuse. Either way, drug abuse can worsen the symptoms of other mental illnesses and complicate treatment.

If symptoms of mental illness are caused by substance abuse, they usually diminish within weeks after the person stops taking the substance. But it may take 4 to 6 months for the effects of a drug to resolve. Sometimes, the effects never fully disappear. People who have taken LSD, for example, may experience flashbacks for the rest of their life. Ecstasy is another drug that may cause long-term mental effects.

It's helpful to work with a professional who has expertise in treating both chemical dependence and mental illness.

Although more than 80 percent of individuals who smoke say they want to stop — and 35 percent try each year — less than 5 percent are successful in quitting without help.

For more information on nicotine addiction and treatment, see Chapter 6, "Addressing Risky Behaviors."

Compulsive gambling

Most people who gamble don't have a mental health problem. But a minority — an estimated 1 percent to 2 percent of the general population — become compulsive gamblers. People in this group lose control of their betting, often with serious consequences. Compulsive gambling often goes hand in hand with excessive alcohol use.

Signs and symptoms

Indications that you or someone you know may be a compulsive gambler include:

- Being preoccupied with gambling — reliving past gambling experiences, planning the next venture or thinking of ways to get money to gamble
- Gambling habitually, often with increasing amounts of money to achieve the desired excitement
- Trying repeatedly but unsuccessfully to cut back or stop gambling
- Feeling restless or irritable when attempting to cut down or stop gambling
- Neglecting other interests, such as family or work
- Keeping losses secret
- Lying to others about the extent of gambling involvement
- Continuing to gamble until the place closes or there's no money left
- Chasing losses — after losing money, returning the next day to get even
- Relying on others to provide money to relieve a desperate financial situation
- Having jeopardized or lost a significant relationship, job or career because of gambling
- Resorting to unlawful activities to finance gambling

Treatment

Treatment for compulsive gambling is similar to that for other forms of addiction. It involves education, psychotherapy and support groups such as Gamblers Anonymous, a 12-step program patterned after Alcoholics Anonymous.

Medications to augment the process of recovery are being investigated. Some of the drugs being considered are those that have been helpful in treating conditions such as alcoholism, obsessive-compulsive disorder and depression.

Eating Disorders

Eating disorders are characterized by a preoccupation with weight that results in severe disturbances in eating behavior. In general, eating disorders, like other forms of mental illness, often involve a complex interplay of medical, psychological and social factors.

It's not easy to distinguish between an eating disorder and the whims and fads of adolescence. Most teenage girls, and some boys, go on diets to lose weight and then stop dieting after 2 or 3 weeks. Binge eating and dieting aren't uncommon among teenage girls. These behaviors also occur, though not as frequently, among teenage boys.

General indications of an eating disorder include:

- Not wanting to eat meals with the family
- Frequent, lengthy visits to the bathroom during or just after meals — especially if running water is used to obscure the sound of induced vomiting
- Skipping meals
- Excessive exercise or preoccupation with weight, shape and body image
- Wanting to be alone
- Weight loss

Types

The three main eating disorders are anorexia nervosa, bulimia nervosa and binge-eating disorder.

Anorexia nervosa

People with anorexia nervosa have a distorted body image and view themselves as fat even when they're underweight. They go to great lengths to keep a low body weight. They eat very little, often to the point of starvation, and may compulsively exercise. Individuals with anorexia nervosa are likely to be perfectionists.

Teenage girls and young women account for about 90 percent of cases of anorexia nervosa. The disorder occurs infrequently in adult women and males.

Left untreated, anorexia nervosa may result in serious medical complications or death. Signs and symptoms of anorexia nervosa include the following:

- Resistance to maintaining a healthy body weight
- An irrational fear of gaining weight
- An unrealistic view of body shape and size
- Among women, infrequent menstrual periods or a cessation of menstruation

Bulimia nervosa

Bulimia nervosa involves eating large amounts of food within a short period (bingeing) and then purging the food by vomiting or using enemas, laxatives or diuretics. Many people with this disorder also exercise compulsively. Between the bingeing and purging episodes, people with bulimia nervosa usually restrict how much they eat.

Teenage girls and young women account for about 90 percent of cases of bulimia nervosa. Individuals with the disorder are more likely to act compulsively, and similar to individuals affected by

Are You at Risk?

The following factors increase your risk of developing an eating disorder:

- *Sex.* Teenage girls and young women are more likely to develop eating disorders than are teenage boys and young men.
- *Age.* Although eating disorders can occur in midlife, they're most common among people in their teens and 20s.
- *Family influences.* People who feel less secure in their families — whose parents and siblings may be overly critical — are at higher risk.
- *Heredity.* Eating disorders are more common in people who have close family members with eating disorders.
- *Emotional disorders.* People with depression, anxiety disorders and obsessive-compulsive disorder are more likely to have an eating disorder.
- *Athletics.* People who participate in some athletic activities may be at greater risk of developing an eating disorder. Young women in sports such as gymnastics, ballet and figure skating are at particular risk of developing anorexia nervosa.

anorexia nervosa, they tend to be preoccupied with weight and body image. Feelings of disgust or shame related to the illness can trigger further bulimic episodes, leading to the development of a vicious cycle. Excessive purging causes changes in body chemistry and may produce serious medical complications or death.

Binge-eating disorder

Binge eating involves a loss of control over eating behavior and the consumption of excessive amounts of food within a short time. The disorder is defined as having binge-eating episodes at least 2 days a week for at least 6 months. Unlike the bingeing associated with bulimia nervosa, the eating episodes in binge-eating disorder aren't followed by purging or excessive exercise.

As with other eating disorders, people with binge-eating disorder are usually preoccupied with weight and food. They often have high personal standards. The disorder is most common in adult, overweight women.

Causes

Doctors aren't certain of the exact causes of eating disorders. It appears that a variety of factors are involved, including genetics, family and culture. In some instances, abnormal biologic systems in the brain that govern mood and appetite may contribute to an eating disorder.

Part of the explanation may lie in advertising messages that emphasize excessive thinness as attractive. In an effort to be as thin as some actors and models, many people try to achieve and maintain a weight that's not healthy for them.

For some young people, the media message of thinness contributes to a distorted body image. A bright, high-achieving 14-year-old who's rational in every other way may begin skipping meals, denying herself the fuel that her body needs to develop normally. She gets thinner but still believes she's fat. Eventually, she may become so undernourished that she needs hospital care.

Complications

People with anorexia nervosa have a greater variety of health complications and a greater risk of death than do people with other eating disorders. However, any eating disorder can result in serious health problems. Possible complications include:

- *Heart disease.* Anorexia nervosa and bulimia nervosa can cause irregular heart rhythms. Heart complications are a common cause of death for people with anorexia.
- *Hormonal changes.* Changes in sex hormones and thyroid hormones can cause absence of menstruation (amenorrhea), infertility, bone loss and retarded growth.
- *Imbalance of minerals and electrolytes.* Your body needs adequate levels of minerals, particularly calcium and potassium, to maintain normal function of organs. Disruption of your body's fluid and mineral content can create an electrolyte imbalance that can be life-threatening.
- *Nerve damage.* Anorexia nervosa may cause brain and nerve damage, seizures and loss of feeling in hands and feet.
- *Blood disorders.* Lack of nutrition can deplete your body's vitamin B-12, causing anemia.
- *Digestive problems.* Anorexia nervosa can cause constipation and bloating. Vomiting and purging may cause irritation of the walls of your esophagus and rectum.
- *Teeth and gum disease.* Gastric acid in your mouth from induced vomiting can damage your teeth and gums.
- *Drug dependence.* Over-the-counter drugs used during purge

cycles may lead to drug dependence. These include laxatives, diuretics, appetite suppressants and ipecac syrup, a drug that induces vomiting.

- *Weight gain.* People with binge-eating disorder often are overweight, which raises the risk of diabetes, heart disease and other conditions.
- *Lowered self-esteem.* Binge eaters may feel self-loathing, shame or disgust about their eating pattern, leading to poor self-esteem.

Treatment

Treatment of eating disorders may include nutrition education, psychotherapy and medications. In severe cases of anorexia, hospitalization may be necessary to rehydrate your body and restore electrolyte balance.

Nutrition education

Your doctor or nutritionist may discuss with you the importance of a healthy diet and help establish a routine for eating meals.

Psychotherapy

Individual counseling with a mental health professional may help identify emotional problems or stressful life events that contribute to the eating disorder. Family counseling can help address feelings of guilt and anxiety within a family that may have led to a child's eating disorder. For more information about psychotherapy, see page 1243.

Medication

Doctors sometimes treat bulimia with antidepressant medications, in addition to psychotherapy. Antidepressants generally aren't effective for people with anorexia nervosa. If an eating disorder is accompanied by depression and anxiety — and many are — antidepressant medications will benefit those conditions as well. More detailed information about antidepressants is provided on page 1241.

Personality Disorders

Personality disorders stem from inflexible and problematic patterns of perceiving, relating to and thinking about yourself and the world. If you have a personality disorder, your inner experiences and outward behavior are consistently different from what's usual or expected in your culture. The disorder likely interferes with your interactions with family or other people at work or play.

You may have long-standing difficulties in your marriage, employment and friendships. Other people in your life may be more distressed by your thoughts and behaviors than you are.

Of the many different types of personality disorders, the most common is borderline personality disorder, which may affect up to 3 percent of the U.S. population. This disorder is characterized by disappointing and unstable relationships, fear of abandonment, intense anger and feelings of emptiness.

Personality disorders typically emerge during adolescence or young adulthood. Borderline personality disorder and antisocial personality disorder may become less evident or diminish with age.

Before making a diagnosis of a personality disorder, your doctor must rule out other conditions that can mimic a personality disorder.

Types

Personality disorders are generally classified into three groups, based on their major characteristics:

- Antisocial, borderline, histrionic and narcissistic disorders
- Paranoid, schizoid and schizotypal disorders
- Avoidant, dependent and obsessive-compulsive personality disorders

Antisocial, borderline, histrionic and narcissistic personality disorders

People with these personality disorders often appear dramatic, emotional or erratic. Antisocial personality disorder is diagnosed more frequently in men, and borderline and histrionic personality disorders are more common in women.

Antisocial personality disorder

People with antisocial personality disorder — sometimes termed sociopaths — show a lack of concern for societal rules and expectations and repeatedly violate the rights of others. Before age 15, these individuals often display a pattern of lying, trouble with the law, truancy, delinquency and substance abuse. As adults, people with this disorder often commit crimes, fail to live up to their employment, financial or parenting responsibilities and are reckless in personal behavior. They're generally unable to sustain long-term relationships, frequently abuse alcohol or drugs and are aggressive and irritable.

Borderline personality disorder

People with borderline personality disorder have disturbed thinking and are frequently in a state of emotional turmoil. They're calm and rational at times but may explode into inappropriate anger or rage at perceived rejection or criticism. Individuals with this disorder are often terrified of being alone, yet repel people with their erratic behavior. These individuals tend to be exceedingly demanding and to see others in black-and-white terms as all good or all bad. They may gamble excessively, spend money irresponsibly, binge eat and abuse addictive substances.

Histrionic personality disorder

Histrionic personality disorder is a pattern of excessive emotionality and attention seeking. Often lively and overly dramatic, people with this disorder continually demand to be the center of attention and the life of the party. The disorder usually leads to stormy and ungratifying interpersonal relationships.

Narcissistic personality disorder
The narcissistic person has an inflated sense of his or her own uniqueness, importance and gifts. When rejected, he or she displays excessive anger or shame and has trouble viewing others realistically, characterizing them as perfect or worthless.

Paranoid, schizoid and schizotypal personality disorders
People with these disorders often appear odd or eccentric.

Paranoid personality disorder
Paranoid personality disorder is a pattern of distrust and suspiciousness — an ongoing sense that others are "out to get you." People with this disorder spend a great deal of energy looking for hidden, sinister meanings behind others' behavior and are easily offended. They show a limited range of emotions and may appear cold and humorless. They often become hostile.

Schizoid personality disorder
Individuals with schizoid personality disorder appear to have little need for other people and are usually loners. They generally lack close friendships and remain aloof from everyone they encounter.

Schizotypal personality disorder
Schizotypal personality disorder is similar in many ways to schizophrenia, but symptoms — including odd ways of thinking, perceiving the world and speaking — aren't pervasive or strong enough to warrant a diagnosis of schizophrenia.

Avoidant, dependent and obsessive-compulsive personality disorders
Individuals with these disorders often appear anxious or fearful.

Avoidant personality disorder
People with avoidant personality disorder are preoccupied with their own perceived shortcomings and consequently fear rejection. This causes them to withdraw from others. Despite their lack of close ties, they often wish for intimacy.

Dependent personality disorder
People with dependent personality disorder generally prefer to have others make decisions for them — simple daily choices as well as major life decisions. They tend to view themselves as inadequate and generally avoid taking responsibility. They willingly subordinate their own desires and needs to those of others. This disorder is diagnosed more often in women than in men.

Obsessive-compulsive personality disorder
Obsessive-compulsive personality disorder isn't the same as obsessive-compulsive disorder (see page 1229). Individuals with obsessive-compulsive personality disorder tend to be preoccupied with detail, rules and procedures. They often insist that things be done a specific way. These individuals place a higher value on work and possessions than on interpersonal relationships. They often have difficulty expressing warm feelings toward others and are sometimes perceived as being aloof, cold or indifferent.

Treatment

Treatment for personality disorders can be effective in reducing or eliminating many of the most troubling symptoms, but it requires that the individual acknowledge his or her difficulties and commit to the hard work needed to overcome them. With treatment, people with personality disorders can feel good about themselves, sustain loving relationships and enjoy meaningful careers. However, treatment can be difficult and may be needed for years.

Treatment generally consists of psychotherapy. There may be a role for medications, including antidepressants, antipsychotic drugs or anti-anxiety drugs. These are discussed on page 1241.

People who have the best chance for successful recovery are generally those who seek treatment for themselves and who find a therapist experienced in personality disorders. Success depends on sticking to the treatment and taking personal responsibility for one's thoughts and actions.

Psychotic Disorders

Over the years, the word *psychotic* has been used in several different ways, and it still has no universally accepted definition. People sometimes use the term in everyday speech to mean insane or dangerous. The American Psychiatric Association defines psychotic as referring to the presence of certain signs and symptoms — hallucinations, delusions and, to a lesser extent, bizarre speech or behavior.

Psychosis refers to an impairment of thinking in which your interpretation of reality is severely abnormal. Although psychosis is often associated with other mental illnesses, psychotic symptoms may also result from physical illnesses, including some infections, cancer, nervous system disorders, thyroid disorders and immune system disorders. Psychotic signs and symptoms can also be a complication of Parkinson's disease, Alzheimer's disease and other dementias. Psychosis may also represent a distinct type of mental disorder that can occur by itself.

Signs and symptoms

The two hallmark symptoms of psychotic disorders are hallucinations and delusions.

Hallucinations

Hallucinations occur when you sense things that don't exist. A common hallucination is hearing voices. A person experiencing hallucinations may carry on a conversation with voices that no one else can hear. Or the individual may perceive voices telling him or her what to do.

Delusions

Delusions are firmly held personal beliefs that have no basis in reality. For example, individuals with paranoid schizophrenia hold irrational beliefs that others are persecuting them or conspiring against them. For instance, a delusional person may believe that the television is directing his or her behavior or that Martians are controlling his or her thoughts.

Types

Three types of psychotic disorders are schizophrenia, brief psychotic disorder and substance-induced psychotic disorder.

Schizophrenia

Schizophrenia is the most common type of psychotic disorder. It affects approximately 1 percent of the population worldwide, including more than 2 million Americans. This disorder is often long term (chronic) and debilitating. It commonly causes delusions and hallucinations that result in unusual behavior and strained relationships.

An individual with schizophrenia may withdraw from people and activities. Schizophrenia generally causes progressive deterioration in a person's ability to function in various roles, especially in a job and personal relationships.

Schizophrenia is rare in children. In men, the disease typically emerges in the teens or 20s. In women, onset typically is in the 20s or early 30s. Schizophrenia may exist alone or in combination with other psychiatric conditions.

Signs and symptoms

Schizophrenia may be diagnosed in a person if he or she displays or experiences two or more of the following:

- Delusions
- Prominent hallucinations for much of the day
- Incoherence
- Lack of emotions or inappropriate display of emotions
- Trouble functioning at work, interacting in social settings and managing personal hygiene
- Continuous and progressive signs and symptoms lasting at least 6 months

Signs and symptoms of schizophrenia may vary greatly. People with this disorder may behave differently at different times. They may become extremely agitated and distressed. Or they may fall into a trance-like, immobile, unresponsive (catatonic) state. Other times they may behave normally.

Early on in the course of the disease, an individual and his or her family may not see a need for treatment. A person with schizophrenia may experience gradual deterioration of function and become less sociable.

Signs and symptoms may include a lack of expression, inappropriate expression of emotions, such as laughing while describing terrifying images, and a change in speech, such as speaking in a dull monotone. In addition, conversation may jump from one idea to a completely unrelated one, or the person may chatter away yet fail to convey any information. He or she may play with language and make up new words.

Treatment

By its nature, schizophrenia isn't an illness for which people are likely to seek treatment on their own. To someone with schizophrenia, the delusions and hallucinations are real, so he or she sees no need for medical help. If you're a family member or friend of someone who's exhibiting possible signs of schizophrenia, you may need to arrange for a medical evaluation for that person.

There's often no cure for schizophrenia, but by working closely with mental health professionals,

Schizophrenia: What It Is and Isn't

People hold many misconceptions about schizophrenia and its relation to other mental illnesses.

- Schizophrenia isn't the same as having a split or multiple personality. Multiple personality disorder is a separate, rare condition.
- Although some people with schizophrenia become violent, most don't. Many withdraw into themselves rather than interact with others.
- Not everyone who is paranoid or distrustful has schizophrenia. People who have paranoid personality disorder are suspicious or distrustful of others, but this disorder doesn't include other features of schizophrenia.
- Not everyone who hears voices is schizophrenic. Some people with severe depression may hear voices. Hearing voices may also occur as a result of a serious medical illness or from side effects of medication.

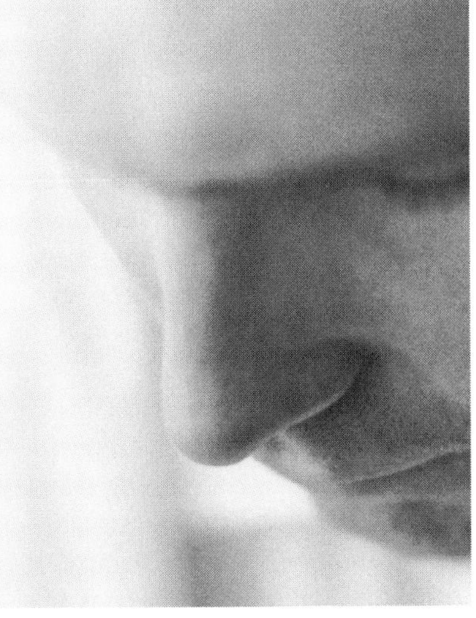

many people can successfully manage the condition — especially when they receive an early diagnosis. Newer medications have greatly helped to make this sometimes-devastating disorder more manageable than ever before.

- *Antipsychotic medications.* Antipsychotic medications are the cornerstone of treatment. Newer antipsychotics provide more effective management of a wider range of symptoms and have resulted in greater independence and a higher quality of life for many people with schizophrenia. They include the medications clozapine (Clozaril), risperidone (Risperdal), olanzapine (Zyprexa), quetiapine (Seroquel) and ziprasidone (Geodon).

  In addition, these medications cause fewer side effects than earlier antipsychotic drugs. For example, there's a lower incidence of tardive dyskinesia, a condition that causes involuntary movements of the mouth, lips, tongue and other parts of the body.

  In general, the goal of treatment with antipsychotic medication is to control signs and symptoms at the lowest effective dosage. The appropriate medication and dosage vary widely from one individual to another. Even with the best care, an individual can experience relapses, but medications may reduce the frequency of relapses.

  Noncompliance with medication schedules remains a difficult problem. Some people with schizophrenia ignore or forget to follow treatment recommendations or deny that anything is wrong with them. For more on antipsychotic medications, see page 1243.
- *Psychotherapy.* An individual with schizophrenia may benefit from psychotherapy by learning ways to cope with stressful thoughts and situations. Psychotherapy may also help reduce the risk of a relapse. In addition, a therapist can help an individual with schizophrenia follow his or her recommended schedule of medications.

  Family members may benefit from therapy that provides support and education. Studies show that people with schizophrenia have a better chance of improving if their family members understand the illness, recognize stressful situations that might trigger a relapse and help the person follow through with recommended treatment.

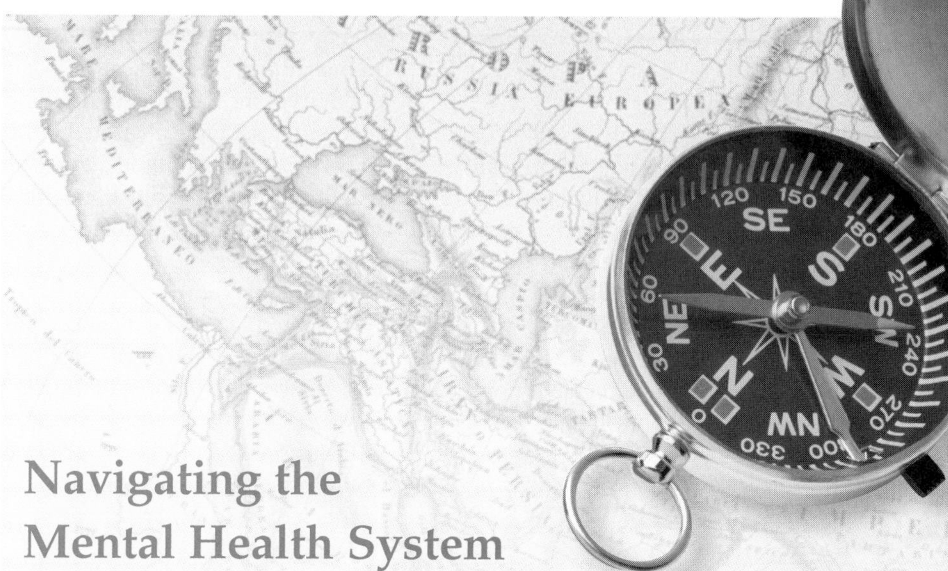

Navigating the Mental Health System

According to the U.S. Surgeon General, each year about 15 percent of adults and 20 percent of children and adolescents in the United States use mental health services.

Because services are spread across many professions and agencies, deciding where or how to get help may be a challenge. The following overview of resources may help you find the help that's best for you:

Primary care doctor

Your primary care doctor may be able to help determine the nature of your problem and the type of help best suited to your circumstances. If your symptoms are mild, he or she may provide the treatment. Or your primary care doctor may refer you to a psychiatrist, psychologist or other mental health professional.

Hospitals and medical schools

A hospital in your area may be staffed with mental health professionals. The psychiatry department of the medical school in your area may provide treatment or referrals.

Advocacy groups

Local branches of organizations such as the National Alliance for the Mentally Ill (NAMI) often supply contact information. NAMI distributes brochures, books and videos about mental illness and offers advice on talking to mental health professionals.

Professional societies

Local or state branches of professional organizations such as the American Psychiatric Association or the American Psychological Association can help you find local mental health providers.

For more information on psychotherapy, see page 1243.

- *Rehabilitation.* Training in social and vocational skills necessary for independent living is an important part of recovery. With the help of a therapist, an individual can learn social skills such as good hygiene and skills for appropriate communications. People with schizophrenia who participate in vocational training and job placement programs experience greater improvement than do those who don't.

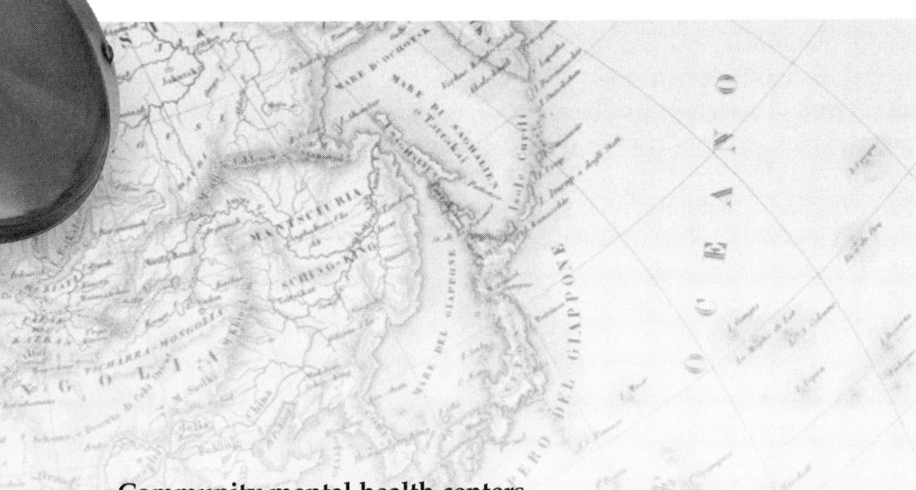

Community mental health centers

Community mental health centers were established on a national scale in the 1960s in an effort to allow individuals with severe mental illness to move from psychiatric hospitals into local neighborhoods. Today, these centers help people with mild and severe illness. Services include psychotherapy, management of medication, crisis intervention and substance abuse treatment.

Insurance companies

Often third-party payers have lists of health care workers, but they may include only — and pay only for services performed by — mental health professionals within their own network.

Employee assistance programs

Many employers provide referrals to workers for problems that can affect work performance, such as substance abuse, family and relationship problems and mental and emotional difficulties.

Hot lines and help lines

Many communities have telephone lines that provide referrals for mental health problems. Check the telephone directory.

Social service organizations

Agencies such as the United Way can supply information about community resources, including mental health providers.

Clergy

Religious leaders often are a source of comfort and advice. A clergy member at your place of worship may be able to provide assistance.

School districts

Your child's teachers, school principal, counselor or school nurse may be a good resource.

Brief psychotic disorder

Brief psychotic disorder involves the sudden onset of at least one type of psychotic sign or symptom — delusions, hallucinations, speech that makes no sense or wanders, or disturbed or catatonic behavior. The disturbance lasts for at least a day but less than a month, and the individual eventually returns to his or her previous level of functioning.

The signs and symptoms often appear after an extremely stressful event, such as military combat or the loss of a loved one. A person with this disorder may experience overwhelming confusion or a rapid fluctuation of emotions.

Behavior and dress may be bizarre, and the individual may adopt peculiar postures and scream or become mute. Speech may sound foolish, often involving the repetition of nonsense phrases. Disorientation and memory impairment may occur. After the symptoms subside, the individual may continue to feel a loss of self-esteem or be mildly depressed for a while.

Treatment may include antipsychotic medications (see page 1243) and psychotherapy (see page 1243).

Substance-induced psychotic disorder

Substance-induced psychotic disorder is a psychosis caused by the use of certain drugs, particularly hallucinogens or amphetamines, by a drug overdose or by drug or alcohol withdrawal.

Overdoses of cocaine, amphetamines, over-the-counter sleeping pills and antihistamines, antidepressants and medications used for Parkinson's disease can cause psychotic symptoms. A psychotic reaction following use of hallucinogenic drugs such as LSD or phencyclidine (PCP or angel dust) and occasionally marijuana or hashish is often referred to as a bad trip. Signs and symptoms may include anxiety or panic as well as delusions and hallucinations.

Treatment generally addresses the drug addiction and may involve antipsychotic drugs and psychotherapy.

Medically Unexplained Disorders

The common features of some mental disorders include physical signs and symptoms that seem to indicate a medical problem but that can't be fully explained by a medical condition.

Signs and symptoms associated with medically unexplained disorders (somatoform disorders) may begin at a time of crisis in your life and clear up when the situation improves or when you learn to better adapt. The signs and symptoms often resemble those that normally accompany stress or emotional upset, but in somatoform disorders they're more intense and last for a sustained period.

Types

Disorders that may cause medically unexplained signs and symptoms include:

Somatization disorder

Somatization refers to the conversion of mental experiences or states into bodily symptoms. Individuals with this disorder may have many physical complaints over a period of several years. When investigated by a doctor, the complaints have no evident physical basis.

Signs and symptoms

- Pain, such as back pain, headache, joint pain and chest pain
- Gastrointestinal problems, such as nausea, vomiting and diarrhea
- Sexual problems, such as a lack of interest in sex and erectile dysfunction
- Neurologic problems, such as numbness and tingling

The signs and symptoms usually begin in adolescence, and the disorder is more common in females.

Pain disorder

Pain disorder involves long-term (chronic) pain without physical findings that explain its cause or intensity. This disorder isn't the same as chronic pain that does have a physical basis, such as that associated with arthritis.

Pain disorder usually begins between ages 30 and 50. It typically appears suddenly and worsens over a few weeks or months. The disorder is diagnosed almost twice as frequently in females as in males.

People with this disorder may quit work, go from one doctor to the next, use too many pain relievers and assume the role of an invalid. The disorder can lead to depression.

Conversion disorder

Signs and symptoms of this disorder tend to be sensory related and involve motor functioning. Sensory symptoms may include the loss of touch or pain sensation, double vision, blindness and deafness. Signs and symptoms related to motor function may include impaired coordination or balance, paralysis, difficulty swallowing or loss of voice. You may also experience seizures or convulsions.

Results of neurologic and other tests reveal no abnormalities. However, psychological factors, such as stress, generally are believed to trigger or worsen signs and symptoms of this disorder. It usually appears in adolescence or early adulthood.

Hypochondriasis

Hypochondriasis is a preoccupation with the fear of developing a serious disease — or the belief that you have one. You interpret physical signs or sensations as evidence of serious physical illness. An unwarranted fear of disease continues even after a doctor finds no serious physical disorder following a thorough examination.

You may interpret a change in heart rate, perspiration or gastrointestinal pain as evidence of serious disease. Or you may become preoccupied with a specific organ — for example, worrying that you have heart disease.

Often, someone with hypochondriasis is overdemanding of doctors and unappreciative of their attempts to help. Unlike Munchausen syndrome (factitious disorder) — in which an individual fabricates a physical illness or self-inflicts an injury to gain attention — people with hypochondriasis genuinely believe they're physically ill.

Treatment

Your doctor may conduct a thorough examination to search for possible physical causes for your symptoms. When a cause can't be found — and no other mental illness such as depression or anxiety is believed to be present — treatment generally focuses on helping you live with the condition so that you're not unduly affected or limited. It may include psychotherapy and, possibly, antidepressant medications. Antidepressants help treat depression that may accompany a medically unexplained disorder. They may also help control pain and improve sleep.

Common Treatments

Mental illness may seem like an unbearable burden, but in reality most forms are treatable. Three general approaches to treating mental illnesses are medication, psychotherapy and other medical therapies, which include electroconvulsive therapy (ECT). Frequently, a combination of approaches is most effective.

PREVENTION TIP

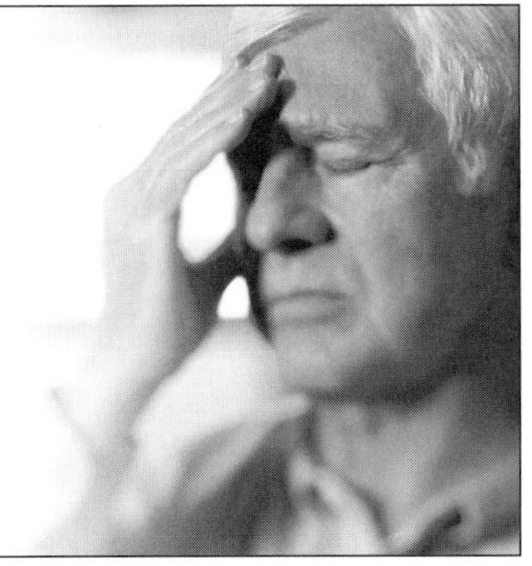

A rare but potentially life-threatening side effect of selective serotonin reuptake inhibitors (SSRIs) is serotonin syndrome. Signs and symptoms include confusion, hallucinations, fluctuations in blood pressure and heart rhythm, fever, seizures and possibly coma.

Serotonin syndrome most often develops when an SSRI interacts with other antidepressants, usually a monoamine oxidase inhibitor. But it can also occur when an SSRI is taken with other medications that influence serotonin. For this reason you shouldn't take an SSRI with St. John's wort, which is a nonprescription herbal supplement that affects serotonin activity. It's also important to always inform your doctors of all of the medications — prescription and nonprescription — that you take.

Treatment for any mental illness must be tailored to the individual. No single treatment regimen will work for everyone. Although most treatment occurs in an outpatient setting, some people receive care in a hospital or residential setting, such as a halfway house.

Medication

The evolution of mental health care over the past 50 years has been fueled by the discovery of new medications and new uses for long-available medications. In 1949, doctors discovered that a compound of the element lithium could relieve symptoms of intense elation (mania).

In the following year, chlorpromazine (Thorazine) was found to ease hallucinations and other manifestations of psychosis. Similar medications followed and eventually led to many people with severe mental illness being able to move from large, state-run psychiatric hospitals to community settings.

In the last 20 years, the development of newer antidepressant and mood-stabilizing medications has revolutionized treatment of illnesses such as depression and anxiety.

Antidepressants

Scientists don't know exactly how these medications improve symptoms, and the mechanism may be different in different people. It is known, though, that antidepressants influence the activity of certain brain chemicals (neurotransmitters) that help nerve cells (neurons) in the brain send and receive messages.

All antidepressants are about equally effective, with a 60 percent to 80 percent chance of improving symptoms. Doctors can't predict which medication will or won't be effective for any given person. You may have to try more than one type to find the drug that works the best for you.

An important point to remember about antidepressants is that they usually don't work immediately. The medication may begin to work within 2 weeks, but it may take up to 8 weeks before you realize its full effects.

Types of antidepressants include:

Selective serotonin reuptake inhibitors

This group of antidepressants influences the activity of the neurotransmitter serotonin. Serotonin is thought to play a crucial role in depression and other mood disorders.

Selective serotonin reuptake inhibitors (SSRIs) include citalopram (Celexa), escitalopram (Lexapro), fluvoxamine (Luvox), fluoxetine (Prozac), paroxetine (Paxil) and sertraline (Zoloft). These newer medications aren't necessarily more effective than earlier antidepressants, but they're safer to use and produce milder, more tolerable side effects.

If you take an SSRI for depression, it's often effective in improving your mood and eliminating other signs and symptoms of depression. If you take an SSRI for an anxiety disorder, the medication may help you become less tense and anxious.

Side effects of SSRIs include gastrointestinal problems, which often decrease or disappear over time. SSRIs may reduce sexual desire or prevent orgasm. In men, they can cause inability to achieve an erection.

Tricyclic antidepressants

These older antidepressants have been used since the 1950s. Tricyclic antidepressants include the medications amitriptyline (Elavil), clomipramine (Anafranil), desipramine (Norpramin), imipramine (Tofranil), nortriptyline (Aventyl, Pamelor), protriptyline (Vivactil) and trimipramine (Surmontil).

Tricyclic antidepressants can cause more bothersome side effects than newer antidepressants, but many people tolerate them well. Side effects may include dry mouth, blurred vision, dizziness, drowsiness, weight gain, constipation and difficulty urinating. Tricyclics may trigger or worsen certain medical conditions, including an enlarged prostate, some forms of glaucoma and some types of heart disease.

Monoamine oxidase inhibitors

Because they can cause serious side effects and because so many alternative medications are available, monoamine oxidase inhibitors (MAOIs) are used infrequently today.

MAOIs include the medications phenelzine (Nardil) and tranylcypromine (Parnate). Food and drug interactions are a serious concern with MAOIs.

Others

Several other types of antidepressants are available that work in a variety of ways. Unlike SSRIs — which affect mainly the brain chemical serotonin — these medications affect other brain chemicals, including norepinephrine and dopamine. Some of the medications affect several neurotransmitters.

These other antidepressants include trazodone (Desyrel), nefazodone (Serzone), venlafaxine (Effexor), bupropion (Wellbutrin), maprotiline (Ludiomil) and mirtazapine (Remeron).

Some people who take venlafaxine experience an increase in blood pressure. Bupropion is less likely to cause an increase in blood pressure or other side effects associated with antidepressants, such as sexual problems or weight gain. However, the medication can increase your risk of seizures and therefore isn't recommended for people with a history of seizures.

Trazodone is more likely than other antidepressants to cause drowsiness. It's commonly used in low doses to help treat sleep problems.

Mood stabilizers

Mood stabilizers are taken for bipolar disorder. The two main types of mood stabilizers are lithium and anticonvulsants. Lithium curbs mania, helps prevent extreme mood swings and, in some people, can ease sadness. It's sold by prescription under the brand names Eskalith and Lithobid and as the generic drug lithium carbonate.

If you take lithium, your doctor will measure lithium levels in your blood to adjust the dose. He or she will also need to know what other medications you take, including over-the-counter medications, to avoid drug interactions. The most common side effects of lithium are nausea, diarrhea, fatigue, confusion and trembling hands.

Divalproex (Depakote) and carbamazepine (Carbatrol, Tegretol) are prescribed primarily for seizure disorders, but they're also used to treat bipolar disorder. It's uncertain exactly how these anticonvulsant drugs help the disorder. An anticonvulsant may be taken in combination with lithium.

Side effects of valproic acid include drowsiness, increased appetite, weight gain and digestive problems. Carbamazepine may cause drowsiness, dizziness, confusion, headaches, nausea, a skin rash and a lowered white blood cell count. Both medications can cause liver problems in some people.

Anti-anxiety medications

Anti-anxiety medications are used to treat various disorders, including anxiety disorders and phobias. Sedatives called benzodiazepines ease anxiety — often within 30 to 90 minutes. But these drugs can be habit forming if taken for more than a few weeks. For this reason, doctors usually prescribe them only for a short time to help you get through a particularly anxious period.

The most commonly prescribed sedatives to control anxiety include alprazolam (Xanax), chlordiazepoxide (Librium), clonazepam (Klonopin), diazepam (Valium) and lorazepam (Ativan). These medications may cause dizziness, drowsiness, imbalance and reduced muscle coordination. Higher doses and long-term use can cause memory problems. You shouldn't drive, use alcohol or operate heavy machinery while using them.

When discontinuing use of a sedative, it's important to reduce the dose gradually over several days or weeks, with the advice of your doctor. This can help prevent withdrawal symptoms, such as nausea, loss of appetite, irritability, insomnia, headaches, dizziness and trembling.

Another medication prescribed for anxiety is buspirone (BuSpar). It influences the activity of serotonin but in a different way than SSRI antidepressants do. Buspirone often doesn't work as well if you've taken benzodiazepines in the past. A common side effect of buspirone is a brief feeling of lightheadedness shortly after taking the medicine. Less common side effects include headaches, nausea, nervousness and insomnia.

? Question and Answer

Since I started taking an antidepressant, I've developed sexual difficulties. Is there anything I can do?

Selective serotonin reuptake inhibitors (SSRIs) are among the medications most frequently prescribed for treating depression and anxiety, but these drugs can cause sexual side effects, such as delayed ejaculation, inability to achieve orgasm and loss of interest in sex. Men and women experience sexual side effects in similar numbers. People who are affected usually experience problems within weeks of starting the medication or after increasing the dosage.

Sometimes, the problem improves over time or if your doctor reduces your dosage. Switching to a drug in a different class of antidepressant, such as bupropion (Wellbutrin), mirtazapine (Remeron) or nefazodone (Serzone), also may help. In addition, certain medications may counter the side effects of SSRIs.

Talk with your doctor about possible ways to overcome sexual difficulties associated with your medication.

Use of Stimulants

When an individual is severely depressed, a doctor may prescribe both a stimulant and an antidepressant. Stimulants include methylphenidate (Ritalin, Concerta) and dextroamphetamine and amphetamine (Adderall). They help boost your mood and energy level during the time before an antidepressant becomes fully effective. Typically, after a few weeks you stop taking the stimulant and remain on the antidepressant.

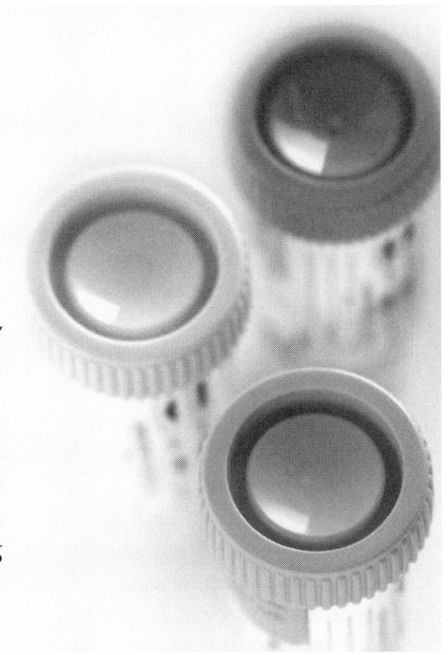

Antipsychotic medications
Available since the 1950s, antipsychotic medications are typically prescribed to treat symptoms of psychosis, including hallucinations and delusions. Some of the more commonly used medications include haloperidol (Haldol), olanzapine (Zyprexa), quetiapine (Seroquel), risperidone (Risperdal), thioridazine (Mellaril), trifluoperazine (Stelazine) and ziprasidone (Geodon).

Antipsychotics block the effects of the neurotransmitter dopamine, which is associated with psychosis. The medications are often effective but may cause side effects, including weight gain, dry mouth, blurred vision, constipation, drowsiness and increased tendency to sunburn (photosensitivity).

Psychotherapy

Long before medical treatments were developed for mental illness, some people found comfort from emotional distress by "unburdening the soul" — discussing their problems and fears. During difficult times it's natural to turn to a friend, family member, doctor or member of the clergy. Talking with someone you trust in order to relieve distress and receive advice still remains an integral part of treatment for mental illness. Today, these discussions often take place with a licensed mental health professional.

The term *psychotherapy* is most often used to describe this component of treatment. It refers to receiving help from a mental health professional through a combination of talking and listening. *Talk therapy* is another common term for this practice.

Depending on how severe your disorder is and the type of psychotherapy you receive, your treatment may last just a few sessions or it may continue for several months or longer. In general, the more severe or complicated the disorder, the longer the time needed to treat it.

Over the long term, psychotherapy can provide many benefits. It can help you understand yourself better, equip you with problem-solving skills, provide you with more effective ways of dealing with life events and help you handle powerful emotions.

However, the therapy can be successful only when both you and your therapist are dedicated to achieving a successful outcome. It's important during therapy sessions to be honest, face up to some possibly painful truths, deal with uncomfortable feelings and be open to new insights and ways of coping. In turn, the therapist will listen carefully, interpret and help guide you toward more healthy behaviors. The process involves mutual trust, respect and confidentiality.

Much as a variety of medications are used to treat mental illness, so too are different forms of psychotherapy used.

Cognitive-behavioral therapy
Cognitive-behavioral therapy, also called cognitive therapy, examines distortions in thinking that lead to psychological problems. It's the most studied therapy and is highly effective in treating mental illness. Brain imaging research shows that cognitive therapy can produce changes in brain activity in regions associated with depression.

This type of therapy is based on the foundation that you are what you think. You identify — with your therapist's help — distorted thoughts and beliefs that trigger psychological stress, fears or depression. You learn to replace negative thoughts with more positive, realistic perceptions, and you learn ways you can view and cope with life events differently.

The treatment emphasizes learning to develop a sense of mastery and control of your thoughts and feelings. Cognitive therapy is generally a short-term treatment.

Interpersonal therapy
Interpersonal therapy focuses on relationships as the key to understanding and overcoming signs and symptoms of mental illness. The goal is to improve your relationship and communication skills and boost your self-esteem. Interpersonal therapy typically explores four major areas: unresolved grief, conflicts with others, transitions from one social or occupational goal to another and difficulties with interpersonal or people skills.

Like cognitive-behavioral therapy, interpersonal therapy is usually short term. It can help improve

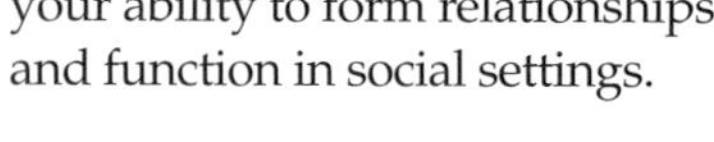
your ability to form relationships and function in social settings.

Desensitization and exposure therapy

Desensitization and exposure therapy is a behavioral therapy that's especially helpful for treating phobias, post-traumatic stress disorder and obsessive-compulsive disorder.

Treatment focuses on changing your response to a particular object or situation. For example, repeated exposure to a feared object or obsession may help you conquer your fear. You gradually increase your exposure to more anxiety-provoking thoughts and situations while learning how to remain calm. Eventually, your fear and anxiety diminish so that you no longer need to avoid certain situations and thoughts.

Psychodynamic psychotherapies

Psychodynamic psychotherapies are intended to help people understand and change behaviors or interactions that have become outdated, ineffective or destructive. Using concepts related to unconscious mental processes, these therapies evolved from principles developed by Sigmund Freud.

Psychodynamic psychotherapies generally take longer than 6 months and may continue for several years. Individuals most likely to benefit from long-term therapy are those who have more than one mental disorder or who have persistently painful or costly patterns of behavior, such as fear of commitment or difficulty maintaining good relationships with others.

Group therapy

Group therapy involves a group of unrelated people and one or more mental health professionals who help facilitate the therapy sessions. It isn't the same as a support group, which may be led by peers or laypersons rather than professionals. The group may be formed on the

COMPLEMENTARY MEDICINE

According to one study, more than one in three people with severe depression or anxiety use some form of complementary or alternative care to treat their illness. This includes herbal and dietary supplements sold without a prescription. Some of the more popular supplements marketed or taken for treatment of depression include:

St. John's wort

An herbal preparation from the plant *Hypericum perforatum,* St. John's wort has long been used in folk medicine and is widely used in Europe to treat anxiety, depression and sleep disorders. In the United States it's sold in the form of tablets or a tea.

Some studies have suggested that St. John's wort may work as well as a prescription antidepressant for mild to moderate depression. But a large clinical trial found it ineffective for treatment of major depression.

Adverse reactions to this herbal preparation can include dry mouth, dizziness, digestive problems, fatigue, confusion and sensitivity to sunlight. St. John's wort can interfere with the effectiveness of certain prescription medications, including antidepressants and drugs used to treat human immunodeficiency virus (HIV) infection and AIDS.

SAM-e

S-adenosyl-methionine (SAM-e) is a chemical substance that's available in Europe as a prescription drug for the treatment of depression. In the United States it's sold as an over-the-counter supplement. SAM-e is found in human cells and plays a role in many body functions. In supplement form it's thought to increase levels of serotonin and dopamine, though this has not been confirmed in larger studies. Taken in large quantities, SAM-e can be harmful.

Omega-3 fatty acids

Omega-3 fatty acids, a kind of nutrient found in fish oils and certain plants, are being investigated as a possible mood stabilizer for people with bipolar disorder. Fish oil capsules containing omega-3 fatty acids are sold in many stores. The capsules are high in fat and calories and may produce gastrointestinal problems. A better way to get more of these fatty acids is simply to eat more cold-water fish, such as salmon, mackerel and herring.

5-HTP

One of the raw materials that your body needs to make the neurotransmitter serotonin is a chemical called 5-hydroxytryptophan (5-HTP). It's prescribed in Europe to treat depression and is available over-the-counter in the United States. Although it's possible that 5-HTP may help some individuals with depression, more research on safety and effectiveness is needed before it can be recommended.

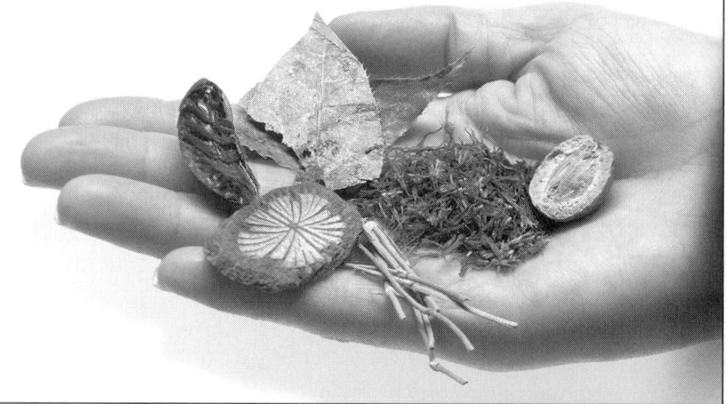

Mental Health Professionals

Professionals who provide mental health care include:

Psychiatrists

A psychiatrist is a medical doctor who has had at least 4 years of specialty training after earning a doctor of medicine (M.D.) degree. Psychiatrists must be licensed to practice medicine in the state in which they work and most are certified by the American Board of Psychiatry and Neurology. Psychiatrists are qualified to carry out many aspects of treatment, including prescribing medication.

Psychologists

A psychologist usually has a doctoral degree (Ph.D., Ed.D. or Psy.D.) in psychology or counseling, although some states allow providers with master's degrees (M.A. or M.S.) to practice under the supervision of a practitioner with a doctorate. A period of supervised training is required after completion of the doctorate. All states license psychologists, who may also be certified by the American Board of Professional Psychology.

Psychologists use testing and other methods to help evaluate and treat individuals with psychological problems. They use various forms of psychotherapy, but in most states they can't prescribe medications.

Social workers

Clinical social workers must have a master's degree in social work and be licensed or certified by the state in which they practice. Many states also require continuing education.

To be designated a licensed clinical social worker (L.C.S.W.) or licensed independent clinical social worker (L.I.C.S.W), candidates usually undergo supervised training in psychotherapy. A clinical social worker may work for a social service agency, in a private practice or as part of a hospital- or clinic-based multidisciplinary treatment team that includes a psychiatrist, a psychologist, nurses and recreational and vocational therapists. Social workers can't prescribe medicines.

Psychiatric nurses

A psychiatric nurse has a degree in nursing, is licensed as a registered nurse (R.N.) and has additional experience in psychiatry. A clinical nurse specialist (C.N.S.) has a bachelor's degree in nursing, is licensed as an R.N. and holds a master's degree in psychiatric and mental health nursing or a related field. The clinical nurse specialist can provide psychotherapy and in some states may prescribe psychiatric medications. Nurse practitioners (N.P.s) also work in psychiatry. They have advanced training in physical assessment, physiology, pharmacology and physical diagnosis, and they may prescribe medications.

Others

Other types of mental health professionals include couples and family therapists and pastoral counselors. Couples and family therapists may be psychiatrists, psychologists, social workers or nurses, or they may have other training. They diagnose and treat mental illness within the context of relationships. Those who are members of the American Association for Marriage and Family Therapy have at least a master's degree and 2 years of supervised practice with couples and families.

A pastoral counselor is a member of the clergy who integrates religious concepts with training in the behavioral sciences, according to the American Association of Pastoral Counselors (AAPC). Licensure isn't required, but counselors can seek certification with the AAPC.

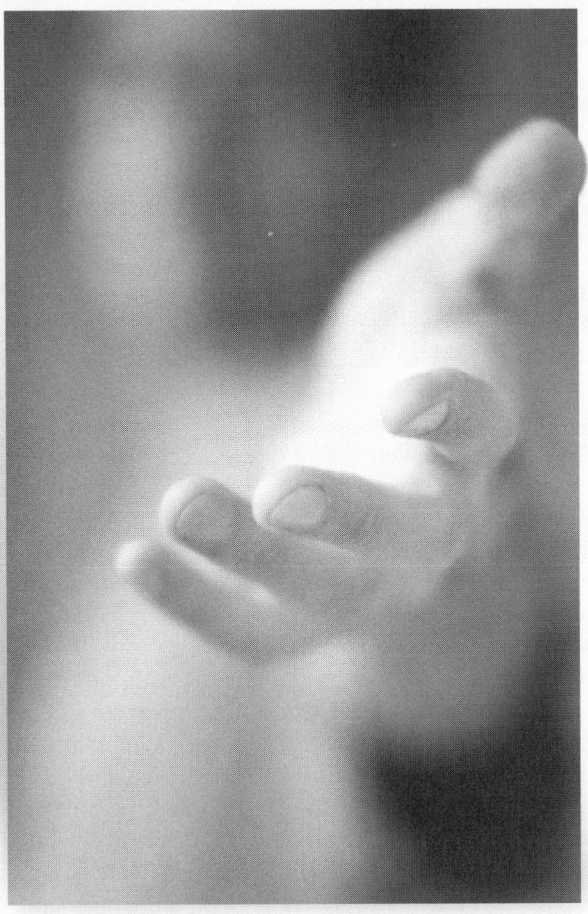

basis of diagnosis, gender, age or other characteristics.

Group therapy strives toward many of the same goals as individual therapy but relies in part on advice, feedback and support from group participants. This type of therapy can be useful in treating social phobia, eating disorders and addictions to drugs, alcohol and gambling.

Couples and family therapy

Couples and family therapy can be useful in helping spouses, partners and families work together to deal with the emotional turmoil and stress that mental illness can cause. Instead of focusing on the individual, couples and family therapy focuses on the interaction between the couple or family members.

Electroconvulsive therapy

Sometimes, medication and psychotherapy aren't effective in treating mental illnesses. Or, based on a person's health status, they may not be appropriate. For some illnesses, such as depression, another option is electroconvulsive therapy (ECT). Study after study indicates that ECT is a safe, effective and efficient treatment.

How it works

During this procedure a doctor places small electrodes, each about the size of a silver dollar, on your head. While the electrodes are being positioned, you're given intravenous (IV) injections of a short-acting anesthetic to make you go to sleep and a muscle relaxant to prevent strong muscle contractions that can occur during the procedure. Then a doctor presses a button on the ECT machine that causes a small electric current to pass through your brain, producing a seizure that usually lasts 30 to 60 seconds. Following the seizure you're taken to a recovery room, where a nurse monitors you while the effects of the anesthesia and muscle relaxant wear off. The total duration of anesthesia is about 10 minutes, followed by 30 to 45 minutes in the recovery room.

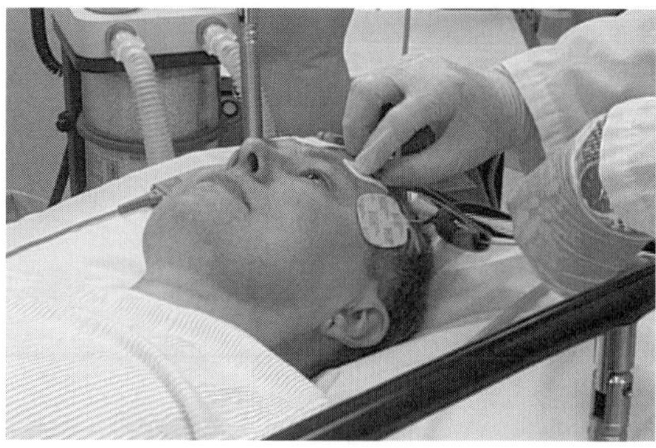

During electroconvulsive therapy (ECT), a doctor places small pads with attached wires (electrodes) on your scalp. The electrodes are connected to the ECT machine. Pads that measure brain activity are also placed on your scalp.

It's not known for certain how ECT helps mental illness. It is known, however, that many chemical aspects of brain functioning are altered during and after seizure activity.

Doctors consider ECT one of the most effective treatments for major depression and some other types of severe mental illness. Unlike antidepressant medications or psychotherapy, which can take weeks to show an effect, ECT often begins to work within a few days, although a series of treatments is often necessary. In people who complete the course of treatment, ECT is effective in approximately 80 percent of cases.

Following a successful course of ECT treatment, some form of ongoing treatment is important to prevent a relapse. Ongoing treatment may include medication or maintenance ECT.

Side effects

A major side effect of ECT is memory impairment. Immediately following an ECT treatment, you're likely to experience a period of confusion. You may not know where you are or why you're there. This period generally lasts from a few minutes to several hours and may get longer with each successive treatment. Occasionally, the confusion may last several days. After the course of treatment is over, the confusion gradually clears up. New memories that may have formed during your treatment may be lost.

In rare instances, people have trouble remembering life events going back several years. Sometimes, these long-term memories return after the ECT treatments are done. Other times they remain permanently forgotten.

After an ECT treatment, you may experience nausea, headache, muscle ache or jaw pain. These minor side effects are common and can be treated with medications. They may be distressing, but they're not serious.

Self-care

After professional treatment brings your mental disorder under control and helps you feel better, you still have to cope on a day-to-day basis. Life inevitably presents challenges and frustrations. In addition to the help you get from a mental health professional, it's up to you to look for ways to enhance your overall well-being. Adopting healthy habits can help you recover from a mental illness and reduce your risk of a recurrence. These healthy living strategies are grounded in the importance of taking good care of your whole being:

Keep active

Research shows that regular exercise can help manage mild to moderate depression, anxiety and possibly other psychiatric disorders. One study, for example, found that individuals with depression who exercised for 20 to 60 minutes three times a week experienced noticeable improvements in their mental health. Exercise stimulates the production of endorphins, brain

Future Directions

Researchers continue to study new treatments for mental illness that are more effective or cause fewer side effects than current methods. Two treatments being investigated for depression include transcranial magnetic stimulation and vagal nerve stimulation.

Transcranial magnetic stimulation

In some ways, transcranial magnetic stimulation (TMS) is similar to electroconvulsive therapy (ECT). With TMS, electric current passes through a wire coil inside a hand-held device. The electric current creates a strong magnetic pulse that passes through your scalp and skull to stimulate nerve cells in the brain.

TMS doesn't require anesthesia and doesn't intentionally cause a seizure. On occasion, a seizure may occur. Another advantage of TMS is that it doesn't cause memory difficulties such as those associated with ECT.

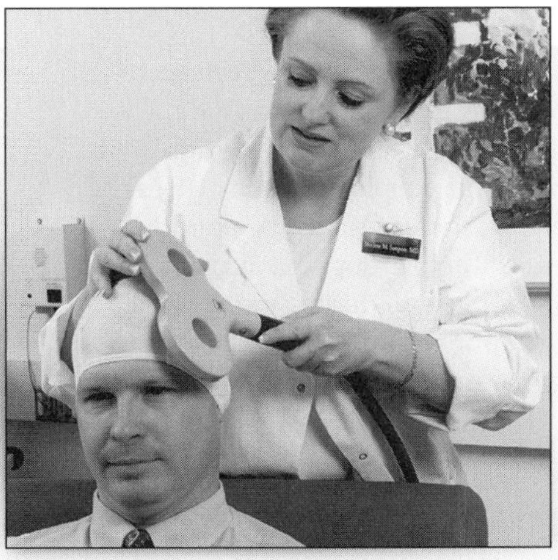

During transcranial magnetic stimulation, a device that emits a strong magnetic pulse is held to your scalp. The magnetic energy passes through your skull and stimulates nerve cells in your brain.

Vagal nerve stimulation

Vagal nerve stimulation (VNS) was originally developed to treat seizure disorders that continued despite use of medication. Researchers began to study its use in treating depression after they noted that people who received VNS to treat seizures experienced an improvement in mood.

VNS requires surgery, during which a small electric pulse generator similar to a cardiac pacemaker is permanently placed in the upper-left side of your chest. Tiny wires are routed under your skin and up to your neck, where they're wrapped around the vagus nerve. The vagus nerve connects your brainstem with organs in your chest and abdomen. The generator is programmed to deliver tiny electric pulses to the vagus nerve every few minutes.

As with so many other treatments, no one knows for certain how VNS improves depression.

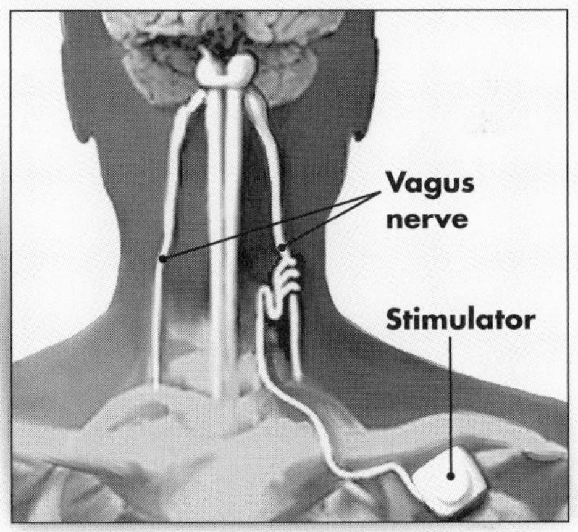

A vagal nerve stimulator delivers tiny, intermittent electric pulses to the vagus nerve.

chemicals that produce feelings of satisfaction and wellness. Exercise also provides many other health benefits and generally improves quality of life.

Eat well

A balanced diet can improve the way you feel on many levels. Both your body and your brain need good nutrition to function efficiently.

Get adequate sleep

Sleep refreshes you. It improves your attitude and gives you energy for physical activity and coping with stress.

Control stress and practice relaxation techniques

Relaxation helps produce a physical and mental state of calm that's the opposite of the fight-or-flight response triggered by stress. Leisure and recreational activities also may help reduce stress.

See Chapter 5, "Managing Stress," for information on relaxation techniques and managing stress.

Get involved

A strong social network is an important component of overall health, including your mental health.

Good friends and a supportive family can provide a sense of purpose or meaning, encouragement and feedback, and they can lend a hand when you need help.

Attend to your spiritual needs

Spiritual practices — whether they involve meditation, religious services, nature or something else — have a beneficial effect on health. Your spirituality can help you live more fully despite your symptoms.

Consider a support group

Self-help organizations can be potent allies for many people who are coping with mental illness or who care about someone with such an illness. These groups include Alcoholics Anonymous and similar groups for people with other types of addictions. In many communities, self-help groups are available for people with depression, anxiety, schizophrenia and other mental illnesses. ■

CHAPTER **38** PART V

Sleep Disorders

Sleep is a basic necessity, as fundamental to your health and well-being as fresh air, clean water and nutritious food. Humans spend about one-third of their life in the state of unconsciousness known as sleep. But sleep is more than just a timeout from daily life or a passive retreat. It's an active state that renews mental and physical health. After a good night's sleep, you wake up feeling refreshed, alert and ready to tackle the day's tasks. As Shakespeare wrote, untroubled sleep is "sore labor's bath, balm of hurt minds ... chief nourisher in life's feast."

When you don't get enough sleep, you may feel less alert and less vigorous and, perhaps, more confused, irritable and fatigued. Lack of sleep affects not only your energy level but also your mental and social functioning. It can make it more difficult for you to concentrate, and you may be impatient with others, less interactive in your relationships and less productive at work. Insufficient sleep also can be downright dangerous. According to the National Highway Traffic Safety Administration, more than 100,000 crashes each year are due to drivers falling asleep at the wheel.

So how much sleep is enough? The amount needed each night varies from person to person. The average is $7\frac{1}{2}$ to 8 hours of sleep a night, but some people feel fine with only 4 to 6 hours while others need 8 to 9 hours. More important than counting hours is assessing how you feel during the day. If you feel alert, are functioning well and aren't tired, even when you sit down and relax for a few minutes, you're probably getting enough sleep.

Unfortunately, many Americans don't get the sleep they need for optimum health, safety and performance. More than 100 million Americans of all ages have occasional sleep problems. For many people, a hectic lifestyle and increased work demands put time at a premium, and sleep often takes a back seat.

Various sleep disorders also deprive people of their needed slumber. Insomnia, characterized by difficulty falling or staying asleep, is the most common sleep problem. Insomnia and other sleep disorders are discussed in this chapter, along with normal sleeping patterns. Fortunately, most sleep difficulties are treatable, and addressing them often leads to a better night's sleep.

Sleep Stages and Patterns

While you're sleeping, many things are happening within your body. Sleep is a dynamic process, and not all sleep is the same. By measuring brain waves, sleep researchers have identified several stages of sleep that recur in fairly regular cycles throughout the night.

Are You Getting Enough Sleep?

Many people think they're getting adequate sleep but really aren't. You may not be getting the right amount and quality of sleep if:

- You routinely ignore your alarm clock or snatch a few extra minutes to snooze before getting up.
- You look forward to catching up on your sleep on the weekends.
- You have to fight to stay awake during long meetings, in overheated rooms or after a heavy meal.
- You're irritable with co-workers, family and friends.
- You have difficulty concentrating or remembering.
- It takes you longer than 30 minutes to fall asleep at night.
- You wake repeatedly throughout the night.
- You wake up groggy and not refreshed.
- Your spouse or partner complains about your snoring or fitful sleeping.

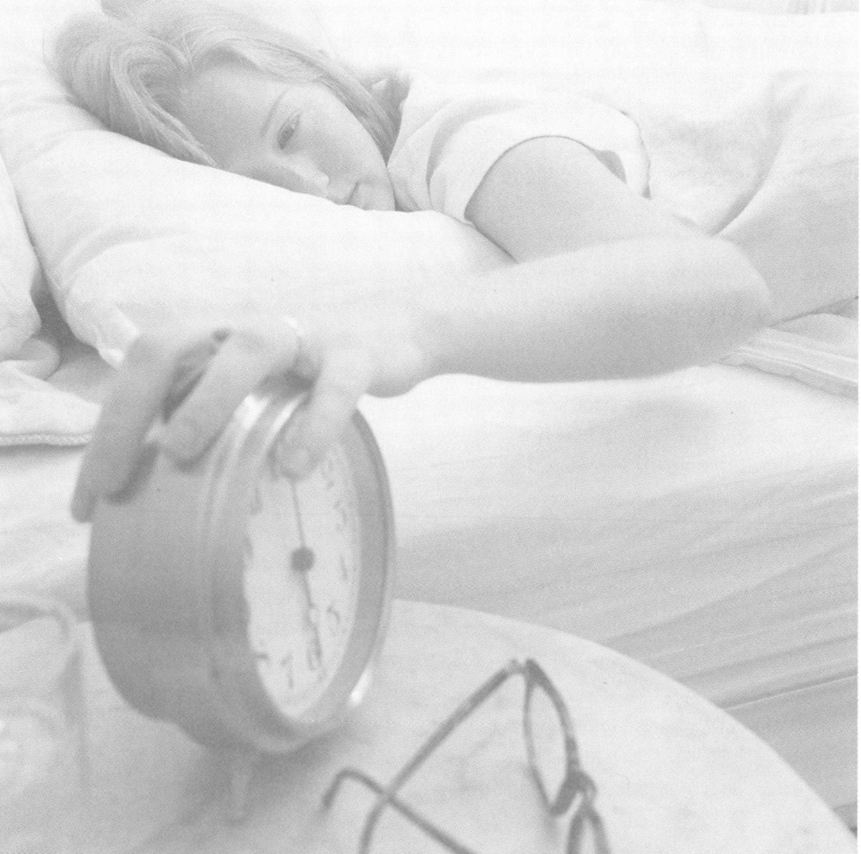

Sleep types and stages

The two types of sleep are non-rapid eye movement (NREM) and rapid eye movement (REM).

NREM sleep

Your nightly journey begins as you pass into stage 1 of NREM sleep, a light sleep. During NREM sleep, your brain activity and body functions slow. This type of sleep has three other stages: Stage 2 is the one in which we spend the most time. During this stage, your brain waves become larger, with bursts of electrical activity. Stages 3 and 4, called deep sleep, are the most restful. In these stages, brain waves are large and slow, and you're more difficult to awaken.

REM sleep

REM sleep, or dream sleep, occurs about 1½ to 2 hours after you fall asleep. During REM sleep, your eyes move rapidly behind your closed lids, hence the name. This is a period of increased activity during which you dream and your body functions speed up.

During REM sleep, your brain waves show faster electrical activity at lower amplitude than at other sleep stages, a pattern that's similar to the brain waves of wakefulness. This suggests that you do more thinking, in the form of dreaming, in this state than in the other sleep stages. People awakened during REM sleep may recall vivid dreams.

Your brain requires increased amounts of oxygen, increasing your blood flow, during REM sleep. Even though some body functions speed up, most of your muscles are paralyzed — probably to keep you from acting out your dreams.

Sleep Cycles

Throughout the night, you continuously move from one stage or type of sleep to another in cycles that can last from 70 to 90 minutes each. Early REM periods are very short, usually 5 to 10 minutes long. You may experience several longer REM periods as the night progresses. Because REM sleep is more active, people often feel that sleep during the second half of the night is much shallower than that of the first half.

Your Natural Sleep Cycle

Typically, you have four to six sleep cycles a night. Each cycle lasts 70 to 90 minutes. At the end of each cycle, you are nearly awake.

Light sleep
Body movement decreases. Spontaneous awakening may occur.

Intermediate sleep
Most of the night is spent in this stage. Helps refresh body.

Deep sleep
Difficult to arouse. Most restorative stage, lasting 30-40 minutes in first few cycles, less in later cycles.

REM (rapid eye movement)
Dreaming occurs. Heart rate increases. Lasts about 10 minutes in first cycle, 20-30 minutes in later cycles.

Sleep patterns

Your sleep patterns and needs are regulated by a biological clock in your brain. The natural pattern of waking and sleeping that occurs within a 24-hour day is called the circadian rhythm. The word *circadian* comes from two Latin words, *circa* for "around" and *dia* for "day." Circadian rhythms guide not only your wake and sleep cycle but also your metabolism and your body temperature.

This internal clock usually makes you sleepy at night and ready to wake up in the morning. Most people's clocks run on a cycle of about 24 hours, but individual clocks vary. Some people are morning people and find that they have more energy and are more alert in the morning. Others, commonly referred to as night owls, are more alert late in the day. However, almost everyone needs to sleep between midnight and dawn. Many people are also somewhat sleepy in the middle of the day, which is what makes an afternoon nap so appealing.

When your natural circadian rhythm is upset, sleep can become difficult. This can happen if you spend prolonged periods in bed, you're in an area with little natural light for an extended period, you go to bed or wake at random times, or you experience a few nights of insomnia. Crossing several time zones during air travel can interrupt your circadian rhythm, causing jet lag. People who change work shifts often experience sleep difficulties. Temperature, metabolism and your mood also can affect your sleep pattern.

Changing sleep patterns with age

Sleep patterns vary according to age. During the first few weeks of life, most babies spend at least half their time sleeping. When they're born, infants seem unaware of the difference between night and day, but eventually they establish their own circadian rhythm, adapting their habits to fit a 24-hour day.

Babies spend about half their sleep time in rapid eye movement sleep, compared with about 20 percent for adults. Infants sometimes fall into REM sleep immediately, but adults must pass through other sleep stages first. Scientists believe that REM sleep activates the learning areas of the brain.

As children grow, their sleeping habits become more organized. Frequent, unpredictable periods of sleep give way to about 11 hours of sleep at night, often in addition to a nap during the day. By about age 5, most children stop napping, and the number of hours of sleep they need gradually decreases. Although 8 hours of sleep a night is often sufficient for younger children, many adolescents need a bit more — 8½

Sleep and Aging

Some people have more trouble sleeping as they get older. In a study of more than 9,000 people age 65 and older, over half reported at least one long-term sleep problem. Older adults often have trouble falling asleep at night, or they may wake up very early in the morning and not be able to go back to sleep.

Many factors conspire to make it more difficult to get a good night's sleep with age. These include:

Changes in sleep-wake pattern
Around your 60s or 70s, your circadian rhythm typically changes. Older adults often get sleepy earlier in the evening and wake up earlier in the morning.

Lifestyle changes
You may be less physically or socially active. Activity helps promote good sleep. You may have more free time and, as a result, drink more caffeine or alcohol or take a daily nap. These things can interfere with nighttime sleep.

Medical conditions and life changes
Chronic pain from conditions such as arthritis or back problems can disrupt sleep. Other illnesses that can interfere with your sleep include osteoporosis, heartburn, Parkinson's disease, dementia, Alzheimer's disease and lung disease.

Older men often develop noncancerous enlargement of the prostate gland (benign prostatic hyperplasia, or BPH). This can lead to more frequent urination at night. In women, hot flashes associated with menopause can disrupt sleep.

Mental health issues
Depression, stress and bereavement are common in older adults as they cope with life changes such as physical limitations, loss of loved ones and leaving their home. These conditions often cause sleep difficulties.

Medications
Many medications have stimulating effects and can cause sleep difficulties. Medications that can interfere with sleep include some antidepressants, decongestants, bronchodilators, corticosteroids and high blood pressure medications.

Sleep disorders
Several sleep disorders become more common with age. These include sleep apnea, restless legs syndrome, periodic limb movement disorder and rapid eye movement (REM) sleep behavior disorder.

Despite all of these changes, however, poor sleep isn't inevitable with age. You can do many things to improve the quality of your sleep. For example, daily exercise or more exposure to sunlight can help reinforce your sleep-wake cycle.

Women and Sleep

Menstruation, pregnancy and menopause all can affect how well women sleep. That's because changing levels of the female sex hormones estrogen and progesterone affect sleep.

During your menstrual cycle, the hormone progesterone rises after ovulation and may cause you to feel more sleepy or tired. Progesterone levels peak around days 19 to 21 of the cycle and then begin to fall. During this low point, you may find it more difficult to fall asleep. During the week before menstruation, some women who experience premenstrual syndrome (PMS) commonly report insomnia and daytime sleepiness.

Sleep disturbances during pregnancy also are common, especially as the pregnancy progresses. During the first trimester, daytime sleepiness may occur as a result of high progesterone levels. In the last trimester of pregnancy, physical discomfort, leg cramps, heartburn and an increased need to urinate may disturb sleep. Some pregnant women develop restless legs syndrome, which

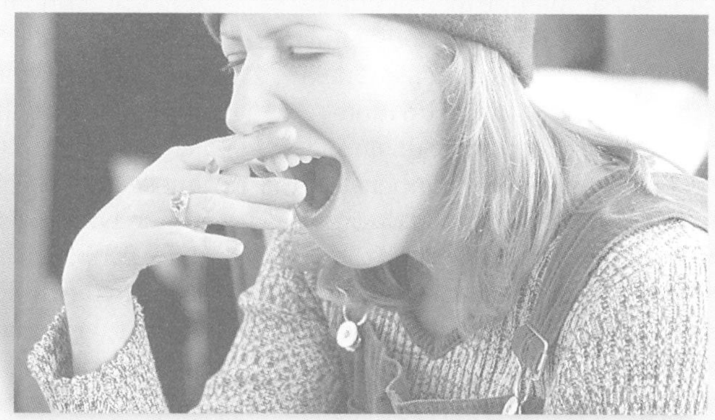

usually ends after the baby is born. Sleep often continues to be interrupted after delivery because of the necessity to tend to the baby's needs during the night.

Women report the most sleep problems during menopause. Changing and decreasing levels of estrogen can cause symptoms that can disrupt sleep, such as hot flashes. Snoring is more common and more severe in postmenopausal women.

Sleep apnea is less common in women than in men, but it does occur and often goes undiagnosed.

to 9 hours each night. During adolescence, the biological clock also changes. Teens start to stay up later and have a harder time waking up early. Studies suggest that this change is due to a delay in the secretion of melatonin, a hormone that induces sleepiness and helps set a person's circadian rhythm.

Sleep needs generally remain constant throughout adulthood. Despite the popular notion that you need less sleep as you age, the amount of sleep your body and brain require changes little. However, sleep patterns change with age.

Between the ages of 50 and 60, sleep may become less restful. You may spend more time in light sleep — stages 1 and 2 of NREM sleep — and less time in the deep sleep stages — stages 3 and 4 of NREM sleep. You not only get less restorative sleep but also sleep more lightly and awaken more easily. Frequent awakenings during the night may make you feel sleepier the next day.

Insomnia

Insomnia is the most common sleep disorder. It's defined as an inability to get enough sleep, to the point where your daytime functioning is affected. Almost everyone has occasional sleepless nights, perhaps due to stress, heartburn or drinking too much caffeine or alcohol. Insomnia differs in that it occurs on a regular or frequent basis.

Signs and symptoms

- Difficulty falling asleep at night
- Frequent awakenings during the night
- Waking up too early in the morning
- Daytime fatigue or sleepiness
- Daytime irritability

About one-third of all people experience insomnia at some point. Symptoms of insomnia include difficulty falling asleep, waking up often during the night, waking up early in the morning and being unable to get back to sleep. Insomnia can be temporary or chronic.

Consequences

For most people, a night or two of poor sleep, or even a night of no sleep, isn't that bad. Lost sleep may sap your motivation and make it difficult to concentrate, but as long as you get back to a normal sleep schedule within a few days, you'll experience no lasting consequences. One good night of sleep after a few poor ones usually is enough to catch up.

However, chronically losing sleep can result in sleep debt, which can lead to serious consequences. Sleep debt is cumulative, and even small nightly sleep losses can add up to affect daytime function. Possible consequences include increased accidents and poor performance on the job or in school.

Long-term sleep deprivation can affect your physical and mental health. Sleep helps bolster your immune system so that you can fight off viruses and bacteria. After a few nights of absolutely no sleep, some people begin hallucinating.

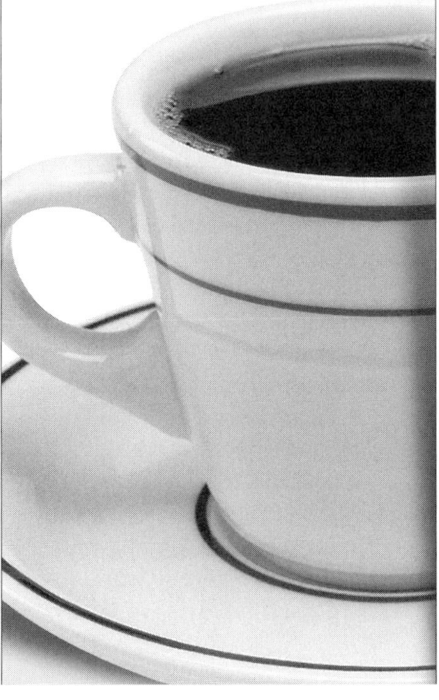

Causes

The causes of insomnia are many and varied. They include:

Stress and anxiety
Concerns about work, school, health or family can keep your mind too active and unable to relax for sleep. Excessive boredom, such as during a long illness, also can create stress and keep you awake. Everyday anxieties as well as severe anxiety disorders may keep your mind too alert to sleep.

Depression
People who are depressed often either sleep too much or have trouble falling asleep. This may be due to chemical imbalances in the brain or because anxiety that can accompany depression prevents relaxation.

Environment or work changes
Long-distance air travel or having to work a late or early shift can disrupt your body's circadian rhythms.

Age
Insomnia becomes more prevalent with age.

Stimulants and medications
Drinking coffee, tea or colas can trigger insomnia. If you're especially sensitive to caffeine, even a cup or two during the day can keep you awake at night.

Smoking also can contribute to insomnia. Nicotine is an addictive stimulant that can keep you awake. In addition, smokers experience withdrawal symptoms at night, making it harder both to fall asleep at night and to wake up in the morning.

Some prescription medications, including steroids, some high blood pressure medications and antidepressants, can interfere with sleep. Many over-the-counter medications, including some brands of aspirin, decongestants and weight-loss products, contain caffeine and other stimulants. Antihistamines may initially make you groggy, but they can worsen urinary problems, causing you to get up more often during the night.

Sleep medications
Doctors generally recommend using sleeping pills only for up to 4 weeks. Sleeping pills often become less effective over time.

Alcohol
Although a drink or two of an alcoholic beverage seems to help some people relax enough to fall asleep, even moderate amounts of alcohol can distort normal sleeping patterns. Alcohol may help you get to sleep, but it also frequently wakes you up in the middle of the night.

Learned insomnia
After a few nights of poor sleep, you may start worrying about sleep. The more you worry, the less you sleep. You may come to associate being in your bedroom with being awake. Most people with this condition sleep better when they're away from their usual sleep environment or when they're not trying to sleep, such as when they're watching television.

Medical conditions and life changes
Diseases or disorders that cause pain, such as arthritis, fibromyalgia or a nerve disorder (neuropathy), can interfere with sleep. Allergies, thyroid problems and menopause also can affect your sleep.

Eating too much too late
Eating too much before bedtime may cause you to feel physically uncomfortable while lying down, making it difficult to sleep. After eating, many people experience heartburn, a reflux of food from the stomach into the esophagus. This uncomfortable feeling may keep you awake.

Poor sleep environment
A bed partner's snoring, a barking dog and an overheated room are just a few of the environmental conditions that can make it difficult to get to sleep.

Diagnosis

If you're more tired than usual, you haven't been able to sleep well for more than a month and you have fitful sleep, you may have insomnia. See your doctor. Your doctor may ask you questions about your sleep patterns, such as how long you've experienced troublesome symptoms and whether they occur every night. He or she may also ask about your mood, your work schedule, whether you snore, how well you function during the day and if you take any medications or have other health disorders. You might be asked to complete a questionnaire to determine your level of daytime sleepiness.

Your doctor may have you keep a sleep diary for a couple of weeks, with observations about when you went to bed, when you got up, how long it took to fall asleep, how much you think you slept during the night and how restful you felt the next morning. He or she may also suggest that you spend a night at a sleep disorders center where your sleep can be monitored and studied.

> **? Question and Answer**
>
> **I work the night shift and have trouble sleeping during the day. Is there anything I can do?**
>
> Keep your bedroom as quiet and dark as possible and stick to a sleep schedule. If possible, remain "shifted" on the days that you're not working, that is, follow the same sleep-wake pattern as you would on a workday.
>
> Avoid using sleeping pills to improve your sleep. They can be addictive and can actually worsen sleep problems. Using caffeine to keep awake while you're working also may make it more difficult to sleep once you get home. If it's daylight when you're on your way home from work, try wearing sunglasses to prevent confusing your internal clock.
>
> For many shift workers, sleep is particularly elusive. Shift work forces you to try to sleep when activities around you and your own biological rhythms signal you to remain awake — and vice versa.
>
> Some people's sleep problems are a result of frequent changes in their work shifts. If possible, remain on a specific shift, such as the night shift, instead of rotating between day, evening and night shifts.

Treatment

Insomnia is usually temporary. If self-help measures don't work, your doctor may recommend other approaches.

Behavioral and cognitive therapy
Behavioral and cognitive therapy can educate you about sleep and help you try to adjust your sleep behaviors. Behavioral and cognitive therapy may include:

Relaxation training
Relaxation training, in which you learn different relaxation techniques, can be helpful if you're having trouble sleeping because of stress or anxiety.

Stimulus control
Stimulus control trains you to associate your bedroom with sleep. You may be asked to limit activities in your bedroom to sleep and sex, to go to bed only when you're sleepy and to leave the bedroom if you don't fall asleep quickly.

Sleep restriction
Your doctor may ask you to reduce the time you spend in bed to as few as 5 hours a night, then gradually increase the time until the desired quality and duration of sleep are achieved. The idea is to reduce the amount of time spent in bed without sleeping. Nine out of 10 people with insomnia stay in bed longer than necessary.

Medication

To help you sleep, your doctor may recommend medications, often as a short-term treatment until other therapies begin to work.

Prescription sleeping pills
You may take a prescription sleep aid for a couple of weeks until you have less stress in your life or until you notice benefits from lifestyle changes or use of behavioral or cognitive therapies. When your sleep seems to be improving, your doctor will gradually lower the dose of the medication. Sleeping pills aren't recommended for long-term use because they can lead to dependence and other unwanted side effects.

Benzodiazepines are older forms of sleeping pills. They include

Tips for Better Sleep

Sleeping patterns are highly individual, and techniques that help one person sleep better may not help someone else. The first thing to consider when suffering from insomnia is whether simple changes in your bedtime routine may help you sleep. Here are some ways to improve your sleep:

- *Stick to a sleep schedule.* Go to bed and get up at about the same time every day, including on weekends.
- *Establish and follow a bedtime ritual.* In the evening, slow the pace of your activities.
- *Limit your time in bed to no more than 8 hours.* Contrary to what you may have thought, spending too much time in bed usually disrupts sleep in the middle of the night.
- *Don't eat or drink a lot before bed.* A light snack may help you sleep, but avoid heavy meals and fluids or foods that stimulate stomach acid production, which could cause heartburn. Drink less liquid before bedtime so that you won't have to go to the bathroom as often.
- *Avoid or limit naps.* Regular daytime naps may contribute to insomnia. If you can't get by without one, keep it to less than 30 minutes.
- *Schedule worry time.* If worries keep you awake, attempt to deal with them before bedtime. Set aside a worry time during the day. Make a list of problems and identify possible solutions.
- *Avoid or limit caffeine, nicotine and alcohol.* Don't drink caffeinated coffee, tea, cocoa or cola after lunchtime. Don't smoke before bedtime because nicotine can cause shallow sleeping and sleeplessness.
- *Don't watch the clock.* If a bedside clock keeps you awake at night, put it in a dresser drawer or under the bed.
- *Exercise and stay active.* Aim for 30 minutes of moderate exercise most days of the week. Physical activity enhances deep, refreshing sleep. But avoid exercising too close to bedtime. Afternoon exercise seems to have the most positive effect on sleep.
- *Find ways to relax.* Taking a warm bath or drinking a cup of warm milk may help. Try relaxation exercises.

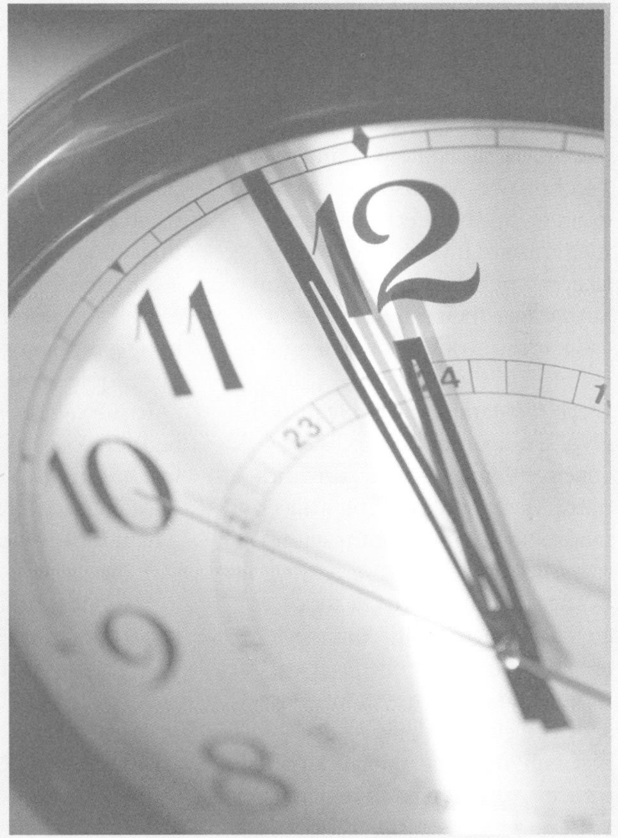

- *Create a comfortable sleep environment.* Keep your sleeping environment quiet, dark and comfortably cool. Make sure your bed is comfortable.
- *Don't rely on sleeping pills.* If you do take a sleep medication for a few days, reduce the dosage gradually when you want to discontinue using it.
- *Check your medications.* Ask your doctor if your prescription medications may be contributing to your insomnia. Check the label of over-the-counter products to see if they contain caffeine or other stimulants, such as ephedrine or pseudoephedrine.
- *If sleep doesn't come naturally, get up.* Read a book, listen to music or watch television until you feel drowsy. Then go to your bedroom to fall asleep. But don't change your rising time in the morning. It's important to keep a firm time for going to bed and arising.

medications such as flurazepam (Dalmane) and estazolam (ProSom), which slow down your central nervous system. After 4 to 6 months of use, they not only lose their effectiveness but also disturb your sleeping pattern and contribute to insomnia.

Although the newer sleeping pills zolpidem (Ambien) and zaleplon (Sonata) are less habit-forming than the previous ones, they're still not recommended for long-term use.

Your doctor may caution you against taking sleeping pills if you drink alcohol or have to operate machinery soon after waking up. Alcohol, which is also a sedative, exaggerates the effects of sleep medications. If you're over age 65, sleeping pills may not be appropriate because their sedating effects can increase your risk of falling.

Over-the-counter sleeping pills
Over-the-counter sleep pills are less effective than prescription medications. Many nonprescription sleep medications contain antihistamines to induce drowsiness.

These products are OK for occasional sleepless nights, but they, too, often lose their effectiveness the more you take them. Many nonprescription sleeping pills contain diphenhydramine, which can cause difficulty urinating and may make you feel drowsy during the daytime.

Antidepressants
Treating depression can help improve sleep, but most antidepressants don't improve sleep right away, and some can even interfere with sleep.

Your doctor may prescribe a low dose of a sedating antidepressant, such as trazodone (Desyrel), nortriptyline (Aventyl, Pamelor) or amitriptyline (Elavil, Endep), to help you sleep. Sedating antidepressants taken in low doses aren't habit-forming and can be taken for a longer period than other sleep medications.

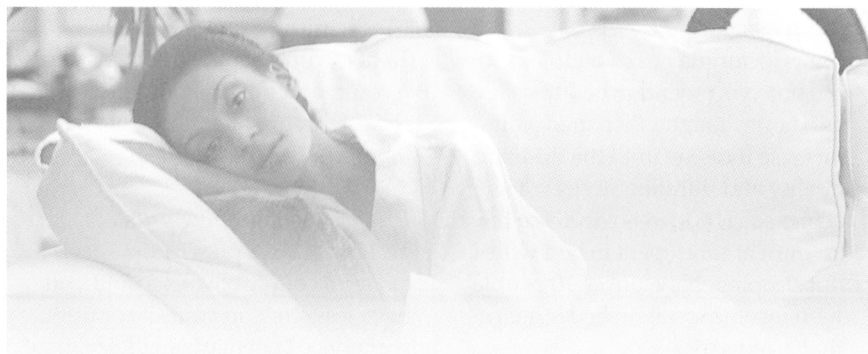

To Nap or Not to Nap?

It's midafternoon and your eyelids are getting heavy. You try to ignore the feeling, but you have to fight to stay awake. Should you follow the irresistible urge to snooze, or will that keep you from sleeping well at night?

It depends. If you're not getting enough sleep, napping may or may not help. The best solution is to try to go to bed earlier. If that's not possible, a daytime nap may give you the boost you need, helping you feel more energized and alert. For people who have insomnia, however, a daytime nap may make sleeping at night more difficult.

An urge for a midday nap is built into your body's biological clock. Usually between 1 p.m. and 4 p.m., you experience a slight drop in your body temperature, indicating nap time. Most Americans ignore the urge, but people of many other cultures incorporate it into their lifestyle.

To discover how naps affect your energy level and the quality of your nighttime sleep, do an experiment. Take a daily nap for a week. The next week, don't nap. Every morning, rank your sleep quality on a 10-point scale. Every evening, rate your day on a similar scale. After 2 weeks, judge whether naps work for you.

If you do nap, keep it short — limit it to 20 or 30 minutes late in the morning or in the midafternoon. And don't rely on naps to keep you going. Try to get enough sleep to avoid building a sleep deficit.

COMPLEMENTARY MEDICINE

Melatonin is an over-the-counter supplement that's marketed to prevent jet lag and help overcome insomnia, among other things. Melatonin is a hormone that occurs naturally in the human body and helps establish your sleep-wake rhythm. The supplements sold in stores are a synthetic or animal form of the hormone.

Some studies indicate that melatonin may help a small number of individuals who have a deficiency of the hormone. However, only about 5 percent of people who've taken melatonin say it helped them.

In addition to melatonin, the herbal supplement valerian has been shown to be effective as a sleep aid in a small number of studies. Valerian may help some people fall asleep more quickly and improve sleep quality. Some people find drinking chamomile tea helpful.

To determine if these remedies work for you, you'll need to experiment. Try each one for 2 weeks and rate your sleep on a scale of 1 to 10 every morning. Then don't take it for 2 weeks and rate your sleep daily.

Keep in mind that herbal products are less regulated than are medications. Therefore, you need to be careful. Ask your doctor if he or she thinks any of these alternative products may be helpful.

Obstructive Sleep Apnea

Obstructive sleep apnea is a potentially serious disorder in which your airway is repeatedly obstructed while you sleep. Often, your breathing stops altogether, but sometimes it may be only partially restricted. In addition, you may repeatedly awaken due to your own snoring.

Signs and symptoms

- Excessive daytime sleepiness
- Usually, loud snoring
- Observed episodes of breathing stoppage during sleep
- Morning headache
- Elevated blood pressure

If you have sleep apnea, you'll usually snore loudly. The snoring may be followed by a pause and then a deep gasp or snort. In the daytime, you're likely to be very sleepy, especially after lunch or while driving, reading or otherwise being inactive. You may wake up in the morning with a headache and feel mentally dull or disoriented, with a sense that your sleep wasn't refreshing. Other symptoms include irritability, impotence, decreased sex drive and dry mouth.

During sleep, the muscles in the back of your throat (pharynx) relax. These muscles normally keep your airway open, and they support structures in your mouth and throat, such as the small, teardrop-shaped tissue at the back of your throat (uvula), the soft palate, your tonsils and your tongue.

In sleep apnea, the muscles collapse on themselves and obstruct airflow. Obstruction of airflow lowers the level of oxygen in your blood. After 10 to 30 seconds or more of insufficient exchange of air, your brain senses the decrease in oxygen and rouses you to a lighter level of sleep or brief wakefulness. The muscles then regain their normal tone (tenseness), the obstruction is relieved, and you resume breathing, possibly with a snort.

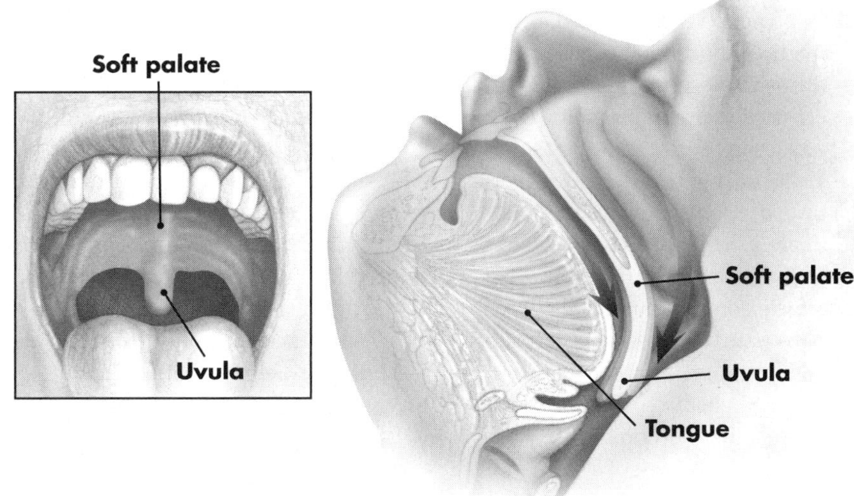

In obstructive sleep apnea, the muscles that normally keep your airway open relax and sag during sleep, causing your tongue, tonsils, soft palate or uvula to repeatedly block your breathing.

This pattern can repeat itself 10 or more times an hour, all night long. You may not be aware of these momentary interruptions of your sleep. In fact, many people with sleep apnea think they sleep well. But the repetitive obstructions prevent you from ever reaching the deep, restorative phases of sleep, causing you to feel sleepy when you're awake.

Another, less common type of sleep apnea is central sleep apnea. In this disorder, the brain fails to send proper signals to the muscles that control breathing. The airway stays open, but the diaphragm and chest muscles stop working, resulting in an interruption in breathing. The level of carbon dioxide in the blood rises, which may cause you to wake up. People with central sleep apnea are more likely to remember waking up than are people with obstructive sleep apnea.

Sleep apnea is most common in middle-aged, overweight men, although women, young people and people who aren't overweight also may have it. After menopause, women who aren't taking hormone replacement therapy generally develop sleep apnea at about the same rate as men.

Are You at Risk?

Certain factors may put you more at risk of having obstructive sleep apnea. They include:

- *Excess weight, especially around the neck.* A fat or thick neck tends to narrow the airway in your throat.
- *Enlarged tonsils or adenoids.* They can narrow your airway.
- *Being male.* Men are more likely than women to suffer from sleep apnea.
- *Being age 40 or older.* Most sleep apnea occurs in people between the ages of 40 and 70.
- *A family history of sleep apnea.* The disorder runs in families.
- *Use of alcohol, sedatives and tranquilizers.* They relax the throat muscles.
- *Race.* Obstructive sleep apnea is more common in black Americans.

Dangers

Sleep apnea is considered a serious medical condition because sudden drops in blood oxygen levels strain the cardiovascular system. The pauses in breathing (apneas) force your heart to pump harder every time it's deprived of oxygen. Untreated sleep apnea is associated with an increased risk of heart attack, coronary artery disease, stroke and congestive heart failure.

In addition, almost half the people with obstructive sleep apnea have high blood pressure, which also raises the risk of stroke and heart failure. One study found that obstructive sleep apnea can damage the layer of cells that line the blood vessels. These cells help regulate blood pressure. Treating sleep apnea usually reduces elevated blood pressure.

The repeated awakenings associated with sleep apnea make normal, restorative sleep impossible. They can also keep a roommate or bed partner from sleeping well. People with sleep apnea may have difficulty concentrating and may find themselves falling asleep at work, while watching television or even when driving. People with sleep apnea are three to five times more likely to have motor vehicle accidents than are people without the disorder.

Diagnosis

Occasional pauses in breathing are common and are no cause for alarm. Reasons to see your doctor include:

- Having more than a few pauses in breathing during a night's sleep
- Snoring loudly enough to disturb another person's sleep
- Excessive daytime drowsiness, which may cause you to fall asleep while you're working, watching television or driving

Your doctor may ask you and your bed partner questions about your snoring, any pauses in breathing and other sleep behaviors. Excess weight or high blood pressure also suggest the possibility of sleep apnea.

Your doctor may refer you to a sleep disorders clinic for a sleep evaluation to confirm the diagnosis. A sleep evaluation usually involves an overnight stay at the facility during which staff monitor your breathing and other body functions during sleep.

In a test called polysomnography, sensors (electrodes) are placed at various locations on your body and are attached to equipment that monitors your heart, lung and brain activity, breathing patterns, arm and leg movements and blood oxygen levels. Because treatments for sleep disorders differ, it's important to get an accurate diagnosis and determine exactly what's causing your sleeping problem.

Treatment

Sleep apnea rarely goes away on its own, but it can be treated. If you have mild sleep apnea, your doctor may recommend treatment with self-care measures such as losing weight and avoiding sleeping on your back. For most people with moderate to severe sleep apnea, the best treatment is nasal continuous positive airway pressure (CPAP). For some people, surgery may be necessary.

Self-care

A number of self-care steps are used to treat obstructive sleep apnea or to keep it from getting worse. These include:

- *Losing excess weight.* Even small reductions in weight can produce major improvements in sleep apnea.
- *Sleeping on your side or stomach.* Sleeping on your back can cause your tongue and soft palate to rest against the back of your throat and block your airway. To help stop yourself from sleeping on your back, you might try sewing a pocket or an athletic stocking on the back of your pajamas and placing a tennis ball inside.
- *Avoiding alcohol and certain medications.* Alcohol, tranquilizers and sleeping pills relax the muscles in the back of the throat, interfering with your breathing.

CPAP

With CPAP, you place a mask over your nose. The mask is connected to a small machine that gently blows air into the mask. The pressure is just enough to keep your upper airway passages open, preventing apnea and snoring. This form of treatment is extremely effective. It can eliminate snoring, dramatically improve the quality of your sleep, eliminate excessive daytime sleepiness and lower your blood pressure. In some individuals, a full mask, which covers both the nose and mouth, is recommended.

The drawback is that CPAP isn't a permanent cure — when you stop using the machine, sleep apnea returns. In addition, some people won't use the machine. They don't like the feel of the mask, or they're self-conscious about wearing it.

Oral devices

Your doctor may recommend a dental device designed to open your throat by bringing your jaw forward or holding your tongue forward. You wear the device at night. It may relieve snoring and mild sleep apnea.

Surgery

If you can't tolerate a CPAP machine and don't benefit from other treatments, your doctor may recommend surgery to increase the size of your airway.

The most common type of surgery used to treat snoring and sleep apnea has the tongue-twisting name of uvulopalatopharyngoplasty (UPPP). During this procedure, tissue from the back of your mouth and top of your throat is removed. Tonsils and adenoids are

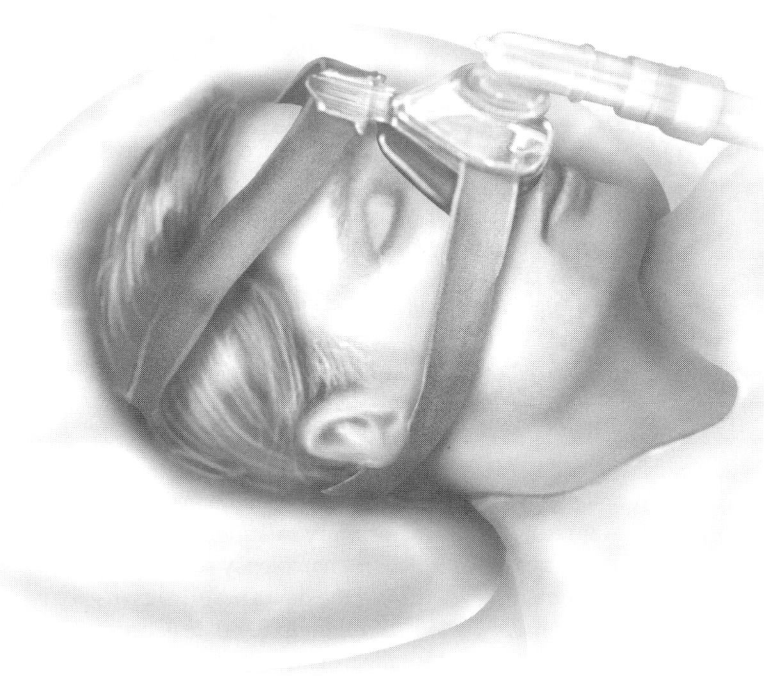

A nasal continuous positive airway pressure (CPAP) device delivers just enough air pressure to keep your upper airway passages open, preventing apnea and snoring.

usually removed as well. UPPP can decrease or eliminate snoring, but it's effective in treating sleep apnea only about 50 percent of the time.

Another surgical procedure is laser-assisted uvulopalatoplasty (LAUP), in which a laser is used to remove tissue from the back of your throat. This method, like UPPP, has been effective in reducing snoring but has shown minimal success in treating obstructive sleep apnea, so it generally isn't recommended.

If your jaw or nasal structures are contributing to a blocked airway, your doctor may recommend surgery to remove polyps, straighten a deviated septum, remove enlarged tonsils or adenoids, or move the jaw and tongue forward.

Another form of surgery, a tracheotomy, may rarely be necessary if other treatments have failed and you have severe, life-threatening sleep apnea. In this procedure, an opening is made in the windpipe (trachea). During the day, the opening is kept covered, but at night it's uncovered to allow air to pass in and out of the lungs, bypassing the blocked air passage in your throat.

Narcolepsy

Narcolepsy is an abnormal tendency to sleep during the day. The term comes from the Greek word *narke,* meaning "stupor." This sleep disorder is a neurologic problem involving sleep-wake mechanisms in the brain and abnormalities of rapid eye movement (REM) sleep.

Signs and symptoms

- Excessive daytime sleepiness
- Sudden loss of muscle tone (cataplexy)
- A feeling of paralysis when going to sleep or waking up
- Dream-like hallucinations

People with narcolepsy may at any time begin to feel drowsy and instantly enter REM sleep, without first passing through the non-rapid eye movement (NREM) sleep

Snoring

Snoring is very common. It affects about 50 percent of men and 30 percent of women — most age 50 or older. It occurs when air flows past relaxed tissues in your throat, causing the tissues to vibrate. We hear this vibration as snoring.

If snoring is disturbing your sleep, you may have sleep apnea, and a sleep study may be necessary. Even if your snoring isn't associated with sleep apnea, it can be disruptive to your partner's sleep. And research has shown that snoring may disrupt your sleep as well — even though you may not realize it — making you sleepy during the day. Evidence suggests that loud, frequent snoring even without obstructive sleep apnea may lead to high blood pressure.

Treatment of snoring is much the same as treatment of sleep apnea. Losing weight, sleeping on your side, treating nasal congestion or obstruction and avoiding alcohol and sedating medications may help. Nasal strips help many people increase the area of their nasal passages, enhancing their breathing.

In addition to traditional uvulopalatopharyngoplasty (UPPP), laser-assisted uvulopalatoplasty (LAUP) and somnoplasty are used at some medical centers to treat snoring. During somnoplasty, high-frequency sound waves heat throat tissue and shrink part of the tongue and soft palate. In LAUP, the surgeon uses a laser to remove the uvula and a small portion of the soft palate. These treatments aren't advised for occasional or light snoring, but may be an option if your snoring is frequent, loud and disruptive. The long-term effectiveness of either of these procedures isn't known.

stages. Researchers believe that genetics, brain chemicals called neurotransmitters and some sort of trigger, such as a virus, all play a role in causing narcolepsy.

As many as 200,000 Americans have the disorder, but only about 50,000 have received a diagnosis, according to the National Institutes of Health. Narcolepsy is often mistaken for depression, lack of sleep or other conditions that may cause daytime sleepiness. Men are affected slightly more often than women. The first symptoms usually appear in the teens or early 20s.

The primary symptom of narcolepsy is an overwhelming drowsiness and uncontrollable need to sleep during the day. These sleep attacks often occur after lunch and during sedentary or boring situations, but they may also happen during active times — for example, while you're driving a car or having a conversation. Extreme sleepiness may cause low sex drive or impotence. People with narcolepsy may even fall asleep during sexual intercourse.

Cataplexy is the second most common symptom. This loss of muscle tone can cause a range of physical changes, from slurred speech to total physical collapse, lasting for a few seconds to a few minutes. Cataplexy is often triggered by strong emotions, such as laughter, anger, embarrassment, excitement, surprise or joy.

Some people with narcolepsy experience sleep paralysis, a temporary inability to move or talk while falling asleep or waking. People often feel awake or half awake during this paralysis, which may last from a few seconds to a few minutes.

Hallucinations can take place if you fall quickly into REM sleep. Because you may be semi-awake when you begin dreaming, you interpret the dreams as reality, and they may be particularly vivid and frightening.

Other signs and symptoms include memory difficulties, restless nighttime sleep and occasional automatic behavior when you perform routine tasks without awareness or memory of doing them.

Diagnosis

Your doctor may make a preliminary diagnosis of narcolepsy based on your experience of both excessive daytime sleepiness and cataplexy — the hallmark symptoms of the disorder. You may be referred to a sleep specialist for additional studies and evaluation.

Methods of diagnosing narcolepsy and determining its severity include polysomnogram tests taken while you're asleep to measure brain waves, body movements and nerve and muscle functions. A multiple sleep latency test measures how long it takes for you to fall asleep during the day. You may be asked to take four or five naps, each 2 hours apart. Sleep specialists will observe your sleep patterns.

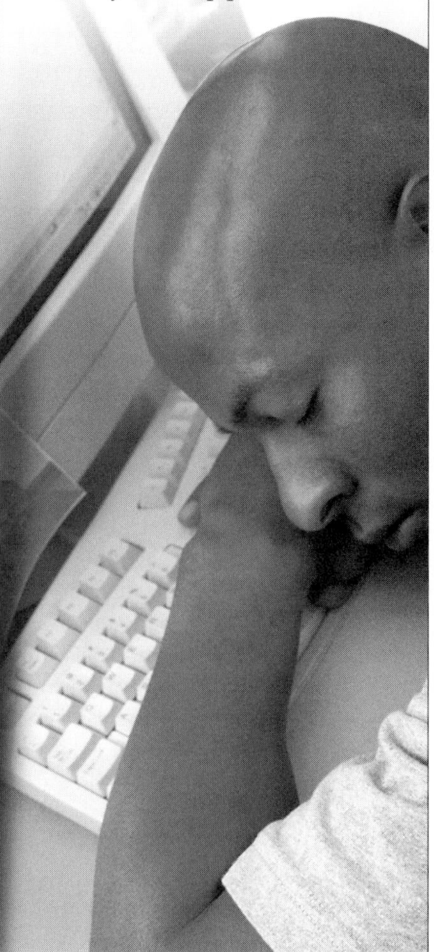

Treatment

A combination of medications and lifestyle adjustments are generally used to manage narcolepsy. The goal is to enhance your alertness during critical times of the day, such as at work and school and while driving.

Medication

Medical treatment of narcolepsy includes the following medications:

Stimulants

Medications that stimulate the central nervous system have long been the primary treatment to help people with narcolepsy stay awake during the day. These drugs include methylphenidate (Concerta, Ritalin), dextroamphetamine (Dexedrine) and pemoline (Cylert).

Although these medications improve symptoms in many people, they may cause side effects and can be addictive.

Modafinil

The medication modafinil (Provigil) also improves alertness in people with narcolepsy. Although how it works isn't clearly understood, it differs from traditional stimulants. Researchers are trying to determine if modafinil is as effective as the central nervous system stimulants. Results so far show that it's less addictive and has fewer side effects.

Antidepressants

Doctors often prescribe antidepressant medications, which suppress REM sleep, to help alleviate the symptoms of cataplexy, hallucinations and sleep paralysis. These medications affect levels of neurotransmitters, brain chemicals that may play a role in narcolepsy.

Antidepressants used to treat narcolepsy include tricyclic antidepressants, such as protriptyline (Vivactil) and imipramine (Tofranil), as well as selective serotonin reuptake inhibitors (SSRIs), such as fluoxetine (Prozac, Sarafem) and paroxetine (Paxil).

Self-care

Lifestyle modifications are important in managing the symptoms of narcolepsy. Self-care measures include:

- Going to sleep and waking up at the same time every day, including weekends
- Allowing plenty of time for sleep at night
- Scheduling several 10- to 15-minute naps each day
- Stopping for naps and exercise breaks whenever you feel drowsy
- Drinking moderate amounts of coffee, tea or cola drinks to help you stay awake during the day and avoiding caffeine and nicotine in the evening
- Eating light meals during the day and avoiding a heavy meal just before an important activity
- Working with your doctor to establish a medication schedule that ensures the greatest likelihood of wakefulness when you drive
- Telling your employer, co-workers or teachers about your condition and working together to find ways to accommodate your needs — including napping during the day, breaking up monotonous tasks, tape-recording meetings or class periods and taking brisk walks at various points throughout the day

Having narcolepsy can be a challenge to your personal and professional life. Others may perceive you as lazy, lethargic or rude. Narcolepsy can affect intimate relationships because of sexual dysfunction and emotional difficulties. Support groups and counseling can help people with narcolepsy and their loved ones cope with the disorder. Ask your doctor to help you locate a support group or a qualified counselor in your area.

Sleep Centers

Many hospitals and medical centers operate sleep clinics to diagnose sleep disorders. These centers are accredited by the American Academy of Sleep Medicine. About 250 sleep centers are accredited nationwide.

If you have a sleep problem, you may be referred to a sleep center. During your first visit, a sleep history will likely be assembled based on questions about your sleep and daytime habits. Family members also may be asked to provide information about your sleep habits.

After the initial consultation, you may spend a night at the center so that your sleep can be monitored by a team of specialists. Before you go to sleep, dime-sized sensors (electrodes) are placed on your head and body to record a variety of bodily activities during the night, including brain wave patterns, breathing and heart rate, muscle activity and eye and body movements. This monitoring, called a polysomnogram, isn't painful. Other tests may be conducted.

The results of these studies often allow sleep disorder specialists to identify your condition so that it can be treated appropriately.

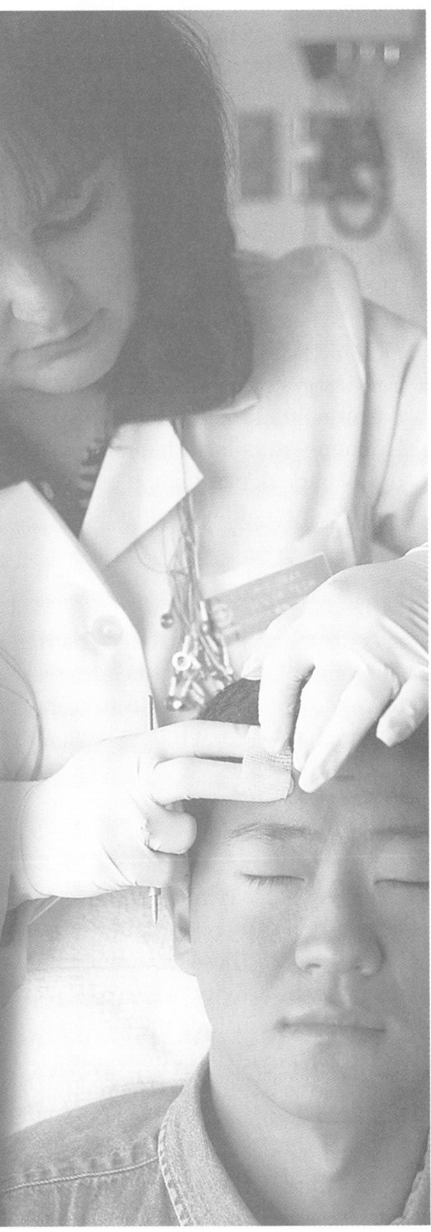

Restless Legs Syndrome

Restless legs syndrome (RLS) is a condition in which your legs feel increasingly uncomfortable until you move them. People typically describe the sensations associated with this condition as creeping, crawling, jittery, tingling, burning or aching — like insects crawling inside your legs. The feelings are unpleasant but not painful. To combat the sensations, people stretch or jiggle their legs, pace the floor or exercise. These activities relieve the symptoms only briefly.

Signs and symptoms

- Unpleasant creeping sensations deep inside the calves and occasionally in the feet, thighs or arms while awake, especially while sitting or lying down
- An irresistible urge to move the legs
- Temporary relief of the sensations by moving the legs
- Symptoms are worst during the early night and better during the day

The creepy-crawly sensation associated with this condition commonly begins shortly after you go to bed. As a result, many people with restless legs syndrome find it difficult to get to sleep or stay asleep, resulting in daytime sleepiness.

The disorder isn't dangerous, but it can be intensely uncomfortable and disruptive to sleep. Many people with RLS also experience involuntary leg twitches and jerks during sleep, called periodic limb movements of sleep.

Researchers estimate that RLS affects as many as 12 million Americans, although the condition is thought to be underdiagnosed. The disorder may start in childhood and is sometimes confused with growing pains, but it's most common in middle-aged and older individuals.

The cause of RLS is unknown, but approximately half those who have it have a family history of the disorder. Some people with RLS have anemia or iron deficiency. Chronic diseases such as kidney failure, diabetes and Parkinson's disease are associated with RLS. Some pregnant women develop restless legs syndrome, especially in their last trimester. For most, symptoms disappear within a month after delivery.

Diagnosis

Your doctor may diagnose RLS by evaluating your symptoms and asking questions about your sleep habits. Blood tests may be done to check your iron levels and look for other conditions, such as anemia or diabetes.

If an underlying condition such as kidney failure or peripheral neuropathy is causing your symptoms, treating that condition often alleviates many of the symptoms. In people who are iron deficient, iron replacement may relieve symptoms. But iron should only be taken under your doctor's supervision after a blood test has confirmed an iron deficiency, because iron overload can be harmful to your health.

Treatment

For people with mild to moderate symptoms of RLS, lifestyle changes can often reduce or eliminate symptoms. If they don't help, a prescription medication may be helpful.

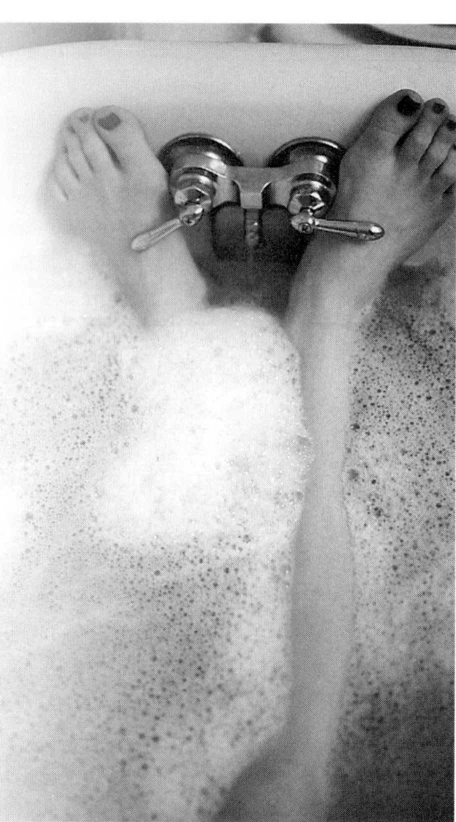

Self-care

These steps may help prevent or ease bothersome symptoms:

- *Take a pain reliever.* Taking an over-the-counter pain reliever such as ibuprofen (Advil, Motrin, others) when symptoms begin may relieve the sensations.
- *Try baths and massages.* Taking warm baths and massaging your legs before bed can relax your muscles.
- *Exercise.* Moderate, regular exercise may relieve symptoms of RLS, but overdoing it at the gym or working out too late in the evening may intensify symptoms.
- *Avoid caffeine, alcohol and tobacco.* These substances may aggravate or trigger symptoms in people who are predisposed to develop RLS.

Medication

The most commonly used medications to treat RLS are dopaminergics, medications developed to treat Parkinson's disease. They reduce the amount of motion in your legs. Dopaminergics include pramipexole (Mirapex), pergolide (Permax), and a combination of carbidopa and levodopa (Sinemet).

Sleep medications, particularly benzodiazepines such as clonazepam (Klonopin) and diazepam (Valium), may be prescribed to help you obtain more restful sleep, although they don't fully alleviate leg sensations.

For more severe symptoms, narcotics such as codeine may be used to induce relaxation, but they can be addicting if taken for a long time. Medications for epilepsy may also be prescribed. These medications decrease the activity of nerve cells in your legs and include the medications gabapentin (Neurontin) and lamotrigine (Lamictal). The high blood pressure medication clonidine (Catapres) is used occasionally. It may diminish the activity of your muscles and nerves.

Periodic Limb Movement Disorder

Periodic limb movement disorder (PLMD), formerly called nocturnal myoclonus, may occur independently or accompany restless legs syndrome, sleep apnea or other sleep disorders. In this condition, your legs twitch or jerk during sleep.

Signs and symptoms

- Twitches, jerks or kicks of the legs or upward flexing of the feet during sleep
- Daytime sleepiness

The involuntary movements typical of this disorder last 1 to 3 seconds and are spaced 10 to 60 seconds apart. The movements aren't harmful, but they can wake you from sleep and disturb your bed partner. Many people with PLMD experience no symptoms, but their bed partners are aware of the leg movements because they may be the ones getting kicked at night.

Some people with the condition feel sleepy during the day because the leg movements disrupt their sleep.

PLMD occurs in about 5 percent of people between the ages of 30 and 50 and in 30 percent to 45 percent of people over age 65. Men and women are equally affected. As with restless legs syndrome, iron deficiency anemia and kidney failure increase the risk of developing this condition.

Diagnosis

Your doctor may diagnose PLMD based on your symptoms. However, an overnight evaluation at a sleep clinic may be necessary to rule out other possible sleep disorders that also can cause restless sleep, such as restless legs syndrome and sleep apnea.

Treatment

The significance of periodic limb movement must be decided on an individual basis. Avoiding caffeine, nicotine and alcohol may be beneficial in limiting the disorder.

Medications may be needed to provide relief in some cases. Your doctor may recommend a low dose of a medication used to treat Parkinson's disease, such as pramipexole (Mirapex), pergolide (Permax) or a combination of carbidopa and levodopa (Sinemet).

Your doctor may measure the amount of iron in your body and suggest iron supplements if you have iron deficiency.

Other Sleep Disorders

Among the other types of sleep disorders are conditions that involve unusual physical behaviors, such as walking during sleep. These types of disorders are called parasomnias. Another sleep-related problem is teeth grinding (bruxism).

Nightmares and night terrors

Signs and symptoms

Nightmares

- Unpleasant or frightening dreams that take place during rapid eye movement (REM) sleep

Night terrors

- Arousal from sleep often accompanied by screaming or crying, usually with no memory of a frightening dream

A nightmare is a scary dream from which you may awaken in fright. When they recur, nightmares may suggest a psychological disturbance or stress brought on by a difficult life situation. However, most people have nightmares from time to time throughout life.

Night terrors are most common in children between the ages of 2 and 6. They're infrequent after that. During deep, non-rapid eye movement sleep (NREM), the child may wake up screaming, terrified and unable to explain what happened. He or she can't be comforted or fully awakened.

Although the terror may last for several minutes, the child usually doesn't remember the episode the next morning. Unless awakened, the child typically returns to peaceful sleep.

Night terrors are often more distressing for parents than the child. The best response to your child's night terror is usually to just let it run its course without waking the child.

Night terrors usually happen during the first third of the night, while nightmares tend to occur near morning. Individuals generally don't remember night terrors, but you may recall a nightmare vividly.

Night terrors seem to run in families. In adults, they can worsen with the use of alcohol. Emotional stress also can make them more likely to occur. Adults who frequently have nightmares or night terrors usually are experiencing considerable conflict and stress during their waking hours.

Treatment

Children usually outgrow night terrors. In adults, there's no specific treatment for night terrors, but a psychiatrist or psychologist may help resolve stress and emotional conflicts that may be triggering the episodes. You may also consider seeing a psychiatrist or psychologist if you have frequent nightmares.

Sleepwalking

Signs and symptoms

- Walking or doing other activities during sleep
- Eyes are open
- Blank or dazed facial expression
- Confusion or disorientation if awakened

Sleepwalking involves not only walking but also other activities performed during sleep, such as rearranging furniture, dressing or undressing and even getting into a car and driving, although this is rare. However, young children, who often sit up in bed and appear to be awake, rarely leave the bed and actually walk.

Sleepwalking usually occurs during the first third of the night and typically lasts a few minutes to a half-hour. The sleepwalker's eyes are open. He or she will have a blank or dazed facial expression and will be confused or disoriented if awakened. Many people believe that sleepwalkers don't get hurt during their travels. This is a misconception. Sleepwalkers commonly are injured by tripping or losing their balance.

Sleepwalking is most frequent between the ages of 6 and 12. Fatigue and prior sleep loss probably increase sleepwalking in children. Sleepwalking in adults may be associated with personality disorders as well as anxiety and stress. Sleepwalking also tends to run in families.

Treatment

There's no specific treatment for sleepwalking. To prevent injury, it's a good idea to make your bedroom and house safe for the sleepwalker. Avoid leaving small objects, electrical cords and furniture in the middle of rooms. Block the top of staircases with gates and lock outside doors.

Sometimes, a doctor will prescribe short-acting sleeping pills. Psychotherapy and relaxation training may improve the problem. Avoiding alcohol and other central nervous system depressants also might help.

REM sleep behavior disorder

Signs and symptoms

- Excessive physical movements while dreaming — such as thrashing, flailing, punching, kicking, falling or leaping from bed
- Daytime sleepiness

Most people experience a type of paralysis as they begin dreaming in the rapid eye movement (REM) phase of sleep. Usually this paralysis keeps you from acting out your dreams.

In REM sleep behavior disorder, this paralysis is incomplete or missing. It may get weaker with age. As a result, dramatic, often violent behaviors occur during REM sleep, usually accompanied by vivid, striking dreams.

People with this disorder may thrash about in bed, sometimes falling or leaping out of bed. They may yell, punch or kick. Injuries to themselves or their bed partner are common.

These episodes may occur once every few weeks or months or up to several times a night. Most people with the disorder say their dreams have become more vivid, action packed and violent over the years. Some people feel sleepy during the day as a result of the disruption of their sleep at night.

The disorder is most common in older men. It's often associated with a neurologic disorder such as Parkinson's disease, dementia or multiple system atrophy. REM sleep behavior disorder may be the first manifestation of these conditions, so be sure to inform your doctor of your symptoms.

Treatment

The first step is to make your sleep environment safer by removing dangerous objects from the bedroom and moving furniture away from the bed. Some people even place their mattress on the floor. Your bed partner may need to move to a separate bed.

If your symptoms are mild, medication may not be necessary. For people with moderate to severe symptoms, the sleep medication clonazepam (Klonopin) is effective.

Teeth grinding

Signs and symptoms

- Grinding, gnashing or clenching of the teeth during sleep
- The tips of teeth worn down, flattened or chipped
- Worn tooth enamel
- Increased tooth sensitivity
- Jaw pain or tightness in the jaw muscles
- Popping, clicking or locking of jaw joint
- Dull morning headache
- Earache due to jaw muscle contractions
- Chronic facial pain

Teeth grinding (bruxism) is a condition in which you grind, gnash or clench your teeth during sleep. About 15 percent of people are affected.

Bruxism can be mild and occasional or frequent and violent. It usually occurs in the early part of the night and may disturb your bed partner. Some people grind (brux) so loudly that they can't duplicate the sound while awake.

Severe bruxism can damage your teeth and cause tension headaches, facial pain and temporomandibular disorders. Temporomandibular disorders occur in the temporomandibular joint (TMJ) located just in front of your ear.

Sometimes, bruxism is caused by a problem in the way your upper and lower teeth fit together when your jaws are closed. Psychological factors also may be involved.

People with bruxism are often tense or anxious. Bruxism can be an uncommon side effect of some psychiatric medications, including antidepressants such as sertraline (Zoloft), paroxetine (Paxil) and fluoxetine (Prozac).

Treatment

Treatment for bruxism varies, depending on the cause. If it's stress related, your doctor may recommend strategies to help you relax and may recommend that you see a psychiatrist or psychologist. Muscle relaxation medications or the medication botulinum toxin (Botox) may help relax your jaw. Cutting back on caffeine and alcohol also may help. Bruxism is often made worse by alcohol.

If your bruxism is related to dental problems, your dentist may treat it by adjusting your bite pattern to correct any misalignment. Wearing a mouth guard or bite plate can prevent tooth damage from bruxism.

If you develop bruxism as a side effect of antidepressant medication, your doctor may change your medication or prescribe another medication to counteract the bruxism. ■

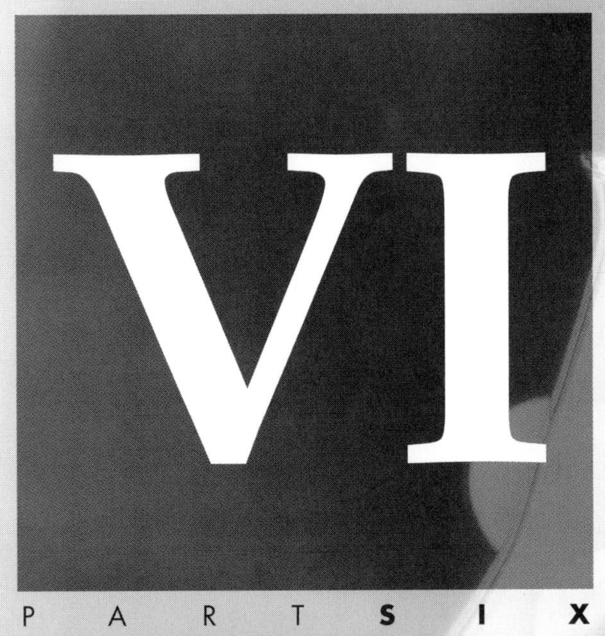

PART SIX

Tests and Treatments

CHAPTER 39 PART VI

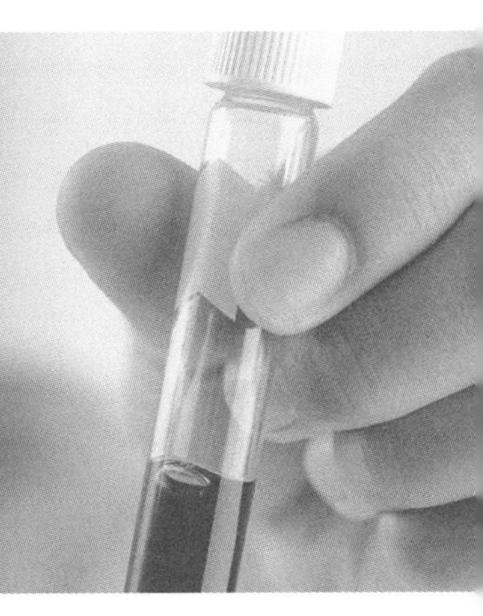

Diagnostic Tests

When you see a doctor for a general physical examination or because you aren't feeling well, he or she may order a variety of tests to help assess your health. Diagnostic tests are common tools used to identify diseases and disorders, monitor chronic illnesses or decide on the most appropriate treatment plan.

There are many diagnostic tests. The types of tests that your doctor recommends will depend on the information needed. Sometimes, several tests are necessary before a diagnosis can be made or a treatment plan determined.

Blood Tests

Your blood contains many components that provide important information about your health. Tests that identify the composition and chemical makeup of your blood are frequently used to evaluate your overall health and help diagnose many diseases.

The drawing of a blood sample usually takes only a few seconds. Blood can be drawn from various sites. For tests that require only a drop or two, the blood is often taken from a fingertip. If more blood is needed, the blood is generally drawn from a vein in your forearm with a needle (venipuncture). In some instances, blood may be taken from a vein in a foot or hand or from an artery in a wrist or the groin.

There are literally hundreds of blood tests. Those most commonly performed on blood samples include complete blood counts, blood-clotting tests, blood chemistry tests, blood lipid tests, blood tests for inflammation, blood hormone tests, tumor marker tests and blood gases measurements.

Complete blood count

A complete blood count (CBC) is a common blood test that's often part of a general physical examination. Laboratory instruments determine the number of white and red cells and platelets in a cubic milliliter of blood. Platelets are colorless, round or oval disks in blood that play a vital role in blood clotting. A CBC also measures the size of red blood cells, the proportion of blood made up of red blood cells and the hemoglobin level in the red blood cells. Hemoglobin is the oxygen-carrying substance that gives red blood cells their color. The results of a CBC may signal the presence of a wide variety of conditions.

Red blood cells

A lower-than-normal level of red blood cells or a low hemoglobin level can indicate anemia, a condition often characterized by paleness and fatigue. The size of the cells also can suggest the cause. In iron deficiency anemia, red blood cells are pale and smaller than normal. Anemia caused by a vitamin B-12 deficiency produces red blood cells that are larger than normal.

White blood cells

A slightly to moderately increased number of white blood cells is often related to an infection or inflammation of body tissues. A marked increase in white blood cell count may be due to a bone marrow disorder, such as leukemia. Conversely, a lower-than-normal level of white blood cells is often associated with an immune disorder. Medications such as chemotherapy to treat cancer commonly reduce the white blood cell count.

Platelets

A lower-than-normal level of blood platelets in a blood sample may be associated with a bleeding disorder.

Blood-clotting tests

Blood-clotting (coagulation) tests measure the time it takes for a sample of blood to clot after substances that encourage clotting are added to it. The tests are typically performed if signs or symptoms suggest that your blood may be clotting more slowly than normal or your blood has a tendency to clot too easily.

Inherited bleeding disorders can cause blood to clot more slowly than normal. The tendency for blood to clot too easily may be associated with unprovoked blood clots in the legs (deep vein thrombosis) or lungs (pulmonary emboli). If you have a liver disorder, you may need routine clotting tests because the liver makes the chemicals in blood that enhance clotting. People on blood-thinning (anticoagulant) medications require regular testing to monitor the effects of the medication.

Blood chemistry tests

As blood circulates through your body, it carries with it a variety of substances released by cells in your organs and tissues. When organs and tissues aren't functioning normally, certain substances in blood may increase or decrease. Blood chemistry tests help diagnose disease by measuring levels of such substances in your blood.

Sugar measurements

A higher-than-normal level of sugar (glucose) in blood is commonly an indication of diabetes. For sugar to pass from blood into tissue cells, it needs to team up with the hormone insulin. If your pancreas fails to produce adequate levels of insulin or if insulin receptors in your body don't use insulin effectively, excess sugar accumulates in your blood.

Bone mineral measurements

Higher-than-normal levels of calcium in blood can indicate disorders such as an overactive parathyroid gland or a bone tumor, conditions that cause extra amounts of bone minerals to be released into blood.

Kidney tests

Blood tests to evaluate kidney function measure the levels of dissolved salts (electrolytes) and certain waste products. When levels of these substances are outside their normal range, your kidneys may not be working optimally. Two of the most frequently measured waste products are blood urea nitrogen (BUN) and creatinine.

Liver tests

Blood tests are a common method of determining liver health. When liver cells are damaged, enzymes normally found inside the cells will leak into blood. Your blood may also contain higher-than-normal amounts of waste products, such as bilirubin, because these substances aren't being removed by your liver as they would be normally. In addition, your blood may contain abnormal amounts of certain proteins made in the liver.

Muscle damage tests

When muscle is damaged, an enzyme called creatine kinase can leak from the damaged muscle into blood. Increased levels of this enzyme in blood can signal many possible disorders, from a simple muscle tear to muscular dystrophy.

A particular form of creatine kinase occurs only in the heart muscle. An increased level of this form of the enzyme is often an indication of a heart attack. Another substance released into blood immediately following a heart attack is a protein called troponin. Generally, the higher the level of troponin in your blood, the greater is the damage to the heart muscle.

Blood lipid tests

Blood lipid tests measure the levels of the fatty substances (lipids), such as cholesterol and triglycerides, in blood. A high level of many of these substances increases the risk that they'll form fatty deposits (plaques) in arteries, narrowing the arteries and increasing your risk of a heart attack or stroke.

In addition to the total amount of cholesterol, blood cholesterol tests can also measure specific types of

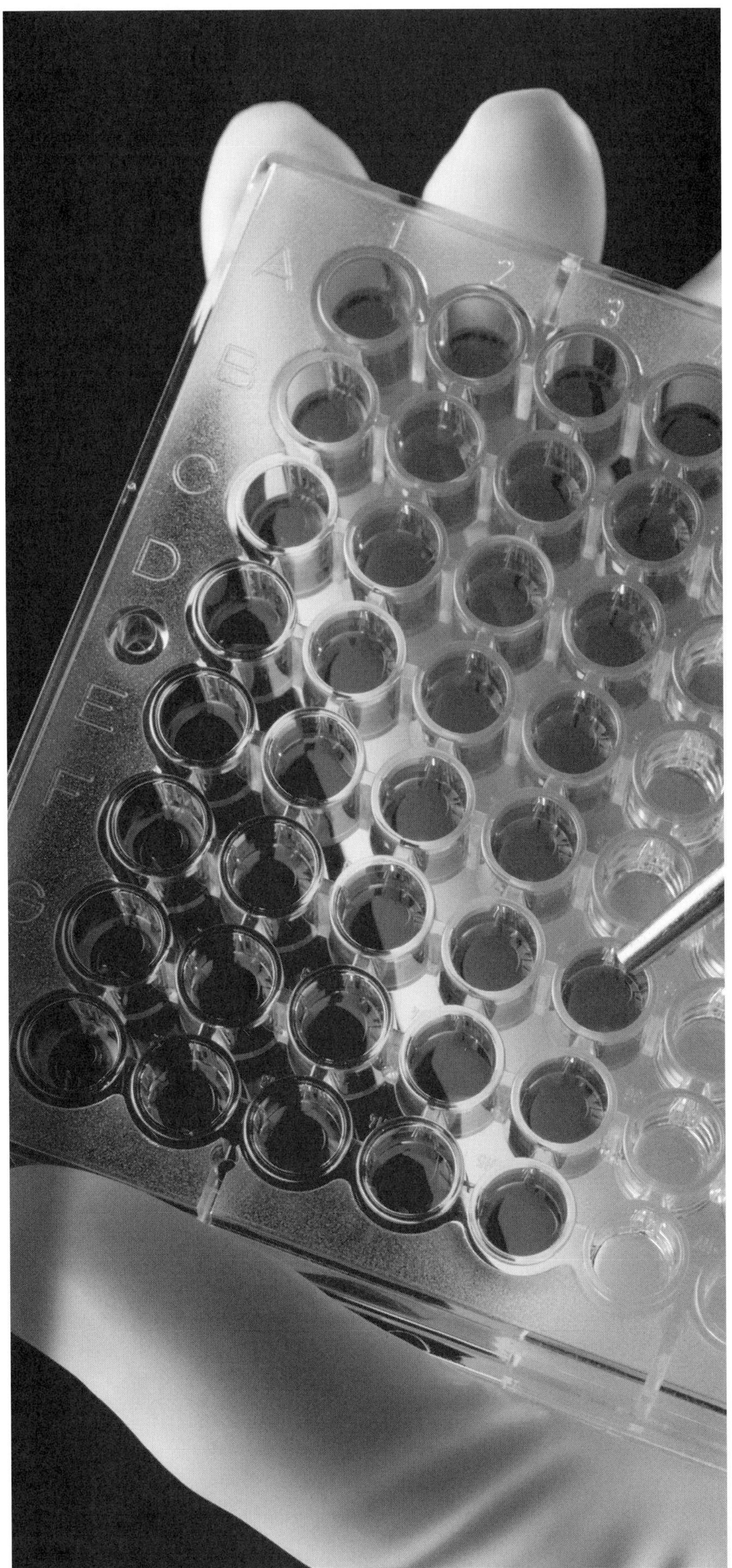

cholesterol: high-density lipoprotein (HDL) cholesterol and low-density lipoprotein (LDL) cholesterol. LDL cholesterol, the "bad" cholesterol, is a risk factor for formation of plaques (atherosclerosis). HDL cholesterol, the "good" cholesterol, seems to have a protective effect against cardiovascular disease.

Blood tests for inflammation

When tissues in your body become inflamed, they produce higher-than-normal amounts of certain proteins, called inflammatory proteins. If your doctor suspects that you may have an infection or inflammatory disorder, he or she may have your blood tested to see if it contains higher-than-normal levels of these proteins. The same tests are also used to monitor the progression of certain inflammatory diseases, such as rheumatoid arthritis.

One of the more specific indicators of inflammation is a protein called C-reactive protein. Its levels quickly rise and fall in association with development and treatment of inflammation. Another blood test commonly used to help identify inflammatory disorders is called the erythrocyte sedimentation rate (sed rate). It measures the speed at which red blood cells sink to the bottom of a glass tube. Generally, when inflammation is present, red blood cells clump together and settle more rapidly than normal, causing the sed rate to increase.

Blood hormone tests

Blood hormone tests measure the levels of specific hormones produced by the glands that make up the endocrine system: pituitary gland, thyroid and parathyroid glands, adrenal glands, ovaries in women and testes in men. An abnormal level of a certain hormone may mean that a particular gland isn't functioning properly. A common reason to have a hormone test is to confirm pregnancy. Hormone tests are also used to help investigate thyroid disorders, infertility, abnormal growth or early or delayed puberty.

Tumor marker tests

Some cancers produce certain substances that can be detected in blood. These substances, called tumor markers, are often present in healthy individuals in small amounts. With the development of certain cancers, their levels may increase. One of the better-known tumor markers is prostate specific antigen (PSA), sometimes associated with prostate cancer.

Blood gases measurement

Measuring the levels of oxygen and carbon dioxide in blood is helpful in diagnosing and monitoring lung disorders. Reduced oxygen and increased carbon dioxide levels can be a warning that your lungs aren't functioning properly.

One way to measure the level of gases in blood is to take a sample of blood from an artery, generally one in a wrist. Blood is drawn from an artery instead of a vein because the blood sample must contain freshly oxygenated blood. A more common method for measuring blood gases is with a small device called a pulse oximeter, which attaches to the end of a finger. The device indirectly measures blood oxygen levels by shining a light through soft tissues containing tiny arteries.

Urine and Stool Tests

Like your blood, your urine contains many chemicals and waste products. Abnormal levels of certain hormones, proteins, minerals or salts in your urine — or the presence of substances not normally found in urine, such as blood — can guide doctors and others in diagnosis and medical care. Blood in stool also can be a warning of a possible medical condition.

Urinalysis

A urinalysis is a common medical test and may be included in a comprehensive physical examination. For this test you provide a small sample of your urine, and it's taken to a laboratory for analysis. Other tests require careful timing or collection of the urine under sterile conditions.

Some urine tests can be performed at home using home test kits. For example, home pregnancy kits allow women to test their own urine to determine if they may be pregnant. The tests are designed to detect a hormone called human chorionic gonadotropin (HCG), which is produced by a developing placenta.

24-hour urine collection

A 24-hour urine collection test requires that you collect and store all of your urine in a large plastic jug for 24 hours. The stored urine is then taken to your doctor's office where it's sent to a laboratory and analyzed. This type of test is performed when a simple urine sample isn't adequate in determining the presence or severity of certain diseases.

An example is the urine microalbumin test used to help assess kidney status in people with diabetes. It measures the amount of a protein called albumin that leaks from your kidneys into your urine when your kidneys aren't functioning properly.

Fecal occult blood test

A fecal occult blood test detects small amounts of blood contained in a sample of stool. Nonvisible (occult) blood in stool may be due to a gastrointestinal disorder that can cause bleeding in the digestive tract, such as polyps, colorectal cancer, gastritis or an ulcer.

For this test, you generally provide a small stool sample. In a laboratory, some of the sample is placed on a special piece of paper and a chemical is added to it. If a color change occurs, blood may be present in the sample. Further tests are then necessary to confirm the presence of blood and look for a cause.

Microbiologic Tests

Microorganisms such as bacteria, viruses and fungi can lead to illness. If a doctor suspects that an illness may be due to the presence of a microorganism, he or she may request a sample of tissue or fluid from your body to be examined under a microscope.

Because samples often contain few organisms, the organisms may be grown (cultured) to increase their numbers and make them easier to detect. Before viewing, most tissue or fluid samples are treated with stains to aid in the identification of microorganisms. Different types of microorganisms can be recognized by their size, shape and how they react with certain stains. Microorganisms can also be tested for possible resistance to antibiotics. This can help determine the best medication to treat the infection.

Examples of tissue and fluid cultures include throat culture, urine culture, blood culture, cerebrospinal fluid analysis, synovial fluid analysis and tests for antigens and antibodies.

Throat culture

A throat culture is most often done when a doctor notices redness or pus on your tonsils or the tissues in the back of your throat. To determine if a virus or bacterium may be causing the inflammation or infection, a sterile swap is rubbed over the red tissues to obtain a sample of the secretions. The swab is sent to a laboratory where it's cultured and analyzed. Swab contents are placed on a growth medium to see if any contents in the medium grow.

One of the most common reasons for a throat culture is to diagnose strep throat, an infection of throat tissues by the streptococcus bacterium. For some time, a rapid test has been available that gives an initial result within 1 hour, but it misses up to 30 percent of strep cases, requiring the need for a throat culture to confirm the results. Mayo Clinic recently developed a new diagnostic test that provides a final, confirmed result in about 8 hours, compared to 1 to 2 days with a traditional throat culture.

Urine culture

A urine culture is used to identify inflammation or infection of the urinary tract. You provide a sample of urine, which is taken to a laboratory where it's analyzed for bacteria or other microorganisms. Increased levels of white blood cells in urine also may indicate infection or inflammation.

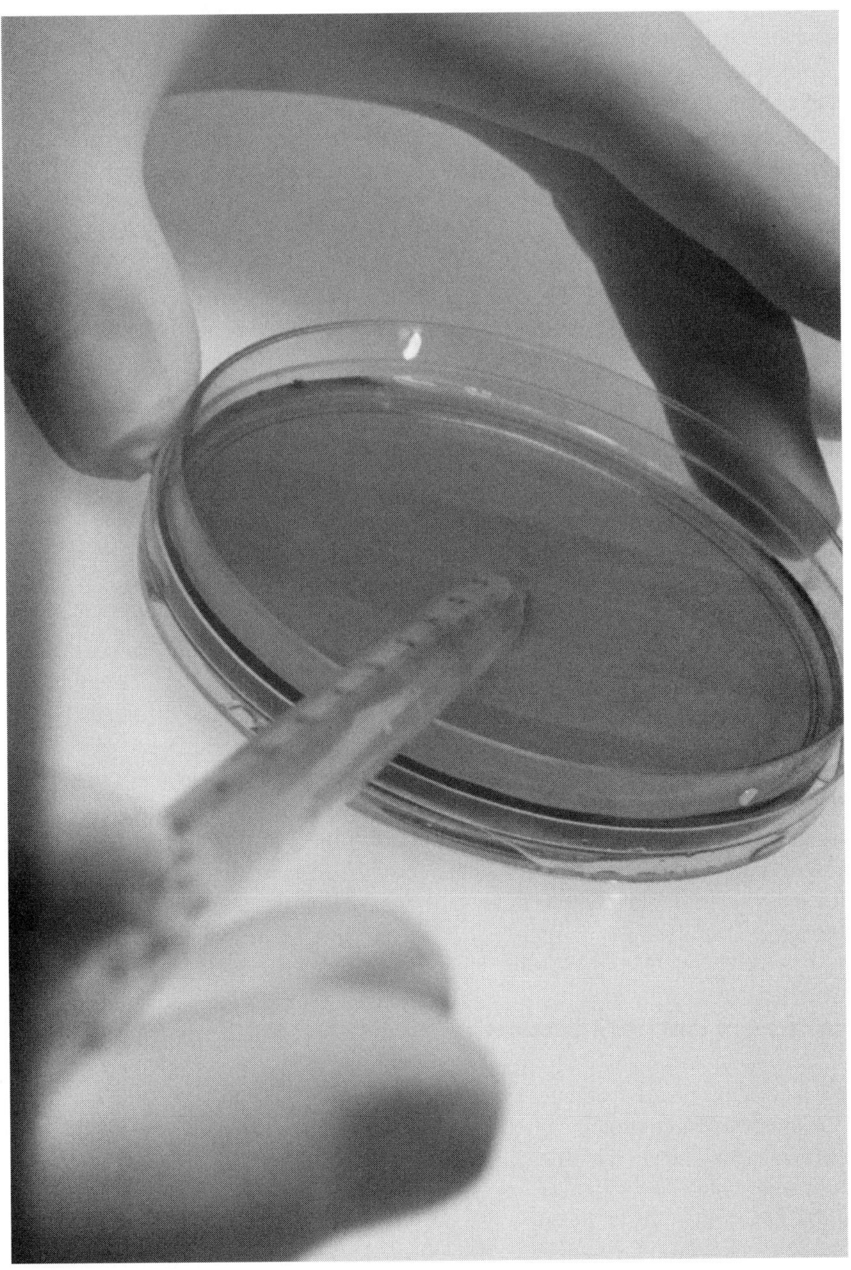

Blood culture

A blood culture can detect a possible bloodstream or heart valve infection. A sample of blood is taken from your arm and examined for evidence of bacteria, viruses or other organisms.

Cerebrospinal fluid analysis

For a cerebrospinal fluid test, a small amount of fluid is removed from your spinal canal for analysis. The fluid is removed by inserting a needle in the lower part of your spine (lumbar puncture). This process is also known as a spinal tap.

Analysis of cerebrospinal fluid can help confirm the diagnoses of infections such as meningitis and syphilis and other infections of the central nervous system. It can also help to identify multiple sclerosis, spinal tumors and bleeding into cerebrospinal fluid.

Synovial fluid analysis

Synovial fluid is the lubricating fluid that's secreted by the membranes that line your joints, called the synovial membranes. Infection of these membranes can be detected by examination of the synovial fluid. To identify joint infection, a doctor inserts a thin needle into the joint and draws out fluid for analysis. In addition to identifying infection, this test may also analyze the fluid for other conditions that can cause joint inflammation. Gout or pseudogout is associated with joint pain and inflammation due to crystals that form in the fluid. These crystals can be detected under a microscope.

Tests for antigens and antibodies

All microorganisms that enter the human body have proteins on their surface, called antigens. When your immune system detects these foreign invaders, it produces substances called antibodies that attach to particular antigens and help to destroy them. Every microorganism carries unique antigens, so the antibodies produced by your immune system also are unique.

One way doctors can quickly and accurately identify a possible source of infection is to test your blood or another body fluid for a certain antigen or antibody. These tests are useful when a rapid diagnosis is needed or when there aren't enough microorganisms in tissue or fluid samples to be visible under a microscope.

Cell and Tissue Tests

Body tissues are made up of cells with unique characteristics. Some diseases, such as cancer, cause cells to appear abnormal under a microscope. With other diseases, such as inflammatory disorders, certain tissues may contain normal cells that shouldn't be present in the tissue.

Cell tests

The most common use of cell tests (cytology) is to screen for cancer. The tests can detect precancerous or cancerous cells before signs or symptoms of the cancer develop. The cells used for testing are collected in different ways. They may be scraped off of tissue surfaces, as in a Pap test where cells are removed from the surface of the cervix, they may be taken from body fluids, or they may be gathered by inserting a needle into an area of tissue and removing cells.

Before they're examined under a microscope, the cells are generally treated with a preservative and stained to make them easier to identify.

Tissue tests

Tissue tests, more commonly called biopsies, differ from cell tests in that a sample of tissue, not just individual cells, is taken from a particular organ or body area. The tissue may be gathered with a needle, through an incision or with a device called an endoscope, which is threaded into your upper or lower digestive tract. Once removed, the tissue is treated with chemicals and sliced into very thin sections. The sections are placed onto glass slides, stained to make the tissue easier to see and then examined under a microscope.

Biopsies are used to confirm or rule out a variety of diseases. They're commonly used in the diagnosis of cancer. They're also used to identify conditions such as cirrhosis of the liver, in which excess fibrous tissue forms in the organ. Biopsies can also help doctors distinguish between diseases that share similar signs and symptoms, such as the inflammatory bowel diseases ulcerative colitis and Crohn's disease.

Imaging Tests

Imaging tests provide detailed images of structures within your body to help detect the presence and extent of disease. They can also help determine how well some organs are functioning. As imaging techniques have improved, the need for exploratory surgery to detect and identify illnesses has declined.

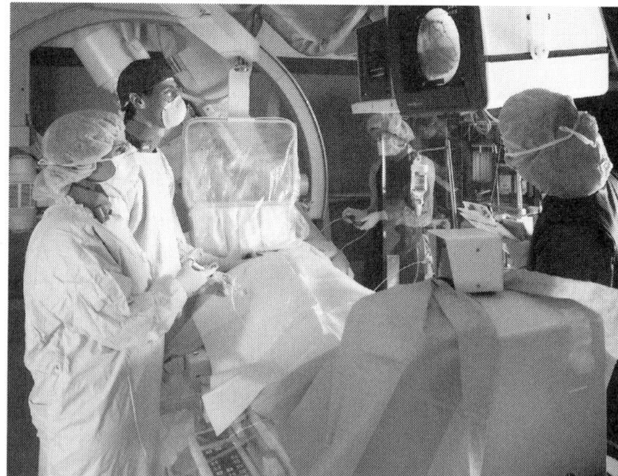

Coronary angiography is performed in a catheterization laboratory, under the guidance of the catheterization team.

X-rays

Since its invention in 1895, the X-ray machine has been an integral part of medicine. During an X-ray, electromagnetic radiation passes through your body onto film or a screen. Dense structures, such as bone, absorb the most radiation and appear white on the film or screen. Less dense tissues, such as your lungs and intestines, absorb less radiation and are contrasted in black and shades of gray. To make less dense structures more visible, you may be injected with, or asked to swallow, a contrast material before an X-ray examination. The contrast material absorbs radiation in the same manner as do dense tissues.

X-rays are most often used to view:

Bones

One of the most common reasons that an X-ray is taken is to detect a fractured bone. Electromagnetic radiation isn't absorbed where the bone is fractured, making the extent and location of most breaks visible on an X-ray image.

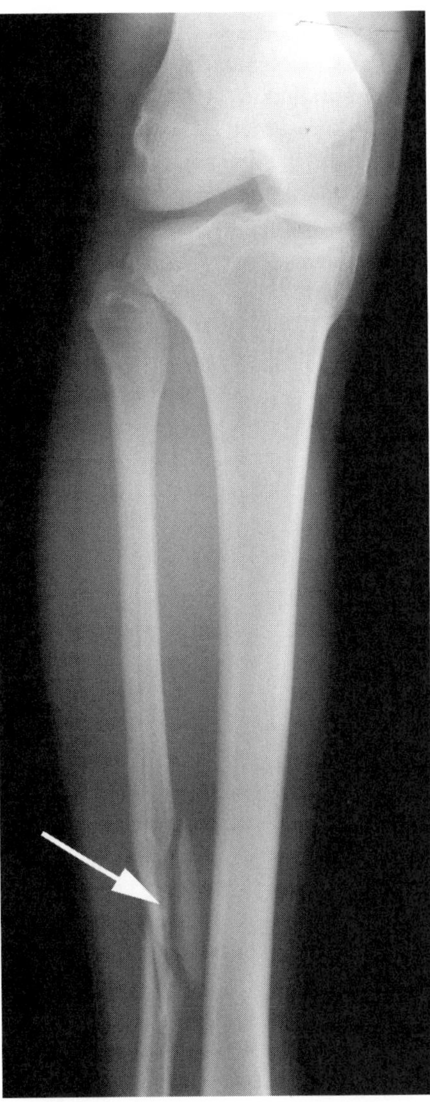

This X-ray shows a fractured bone (fibula) in a leg (see arrow).

Chest

A chest X-ray is another commonly performed procedure. A chest X-ray can supply information about your heart, lungs and chest wall, including your ribs. In a normal chest X-ray, the ribs are visible, the heart is outlined, and the lungs appear black because they contain air.

A chest X-ray can identify conditions such as a broken rib, an enlarged heart, pneumonia, a collapsed lung or a lung tumor. In the case of pneumonia, for example, instead of appearing black, portions of one or both lungs may appear white.

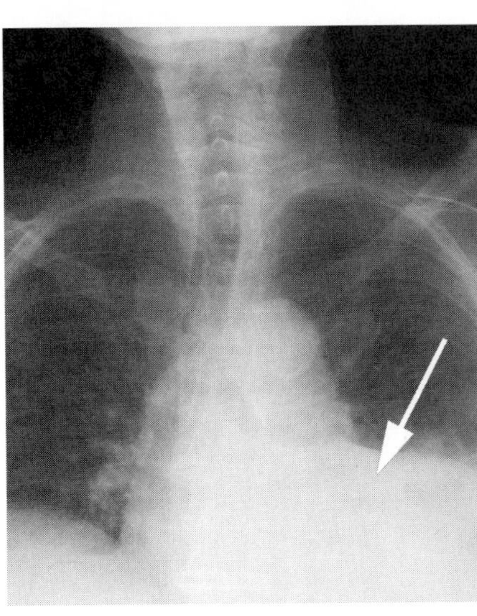

This chest X-ray shows a collection of fluid (pleural effusion) on the left side.

Breast

The medical term for X-ray imaging of a woman's breast is *mammography*. The procedure is done to detect early breast cancer. As X-rays pass through breast tissue, denser tissues in the breast absorb more radiation, making them visible on X-ray film. The presence of dense tissues could be an indication of cancer. For more information, see page 839.

Digestive tract

X-ray examinations of the digestive tract are commonly referred to as barium X-rays because they usually involve use of the contrast material barium. Barium is a liquid, metallic alkaline material that temporarily coats the lining of your digestive tract, making the lining show up more clearly on X-ray films.

Depending on whether your upper or lower digestive tract is being examined, you may either swallow a fluid containing barium, or the barium may be delivered into your colon by a tube inserted through your rectum (barium enema). X-rays of the digestive tract can identify many problems, such as ulcers, cancerous (malignant) and noncancerous (benign) tumors and blockage (obstruction) in the digestive tract.

Blood vessels

X-ray imaging of blood vessels is commonly referred to as angiography or arteriography. During the procedure, contrast material is injected into a blood vessel by way of a tiny, long, flexible tube (catheter) that's threaded into a vessel. As the solution travels through blood vessels, X-ray images are taken of the vessels. The X-rays can indicate if blood is flowing normally or is being interrupted or slowed by a blockage in a vessel.

When contrast material is injected into arteries that supply blood to the heart muscle (coronary arteries), the procedure is called coronary angiography (see page 753). Coronary angiography is most commonly used to identify narrowing or blockage of a coronary artery due to formation of plaques (atherosclerosis) or clots. When the contrast material is injected into a major artery leading to the brain, the procedure is referred to as cerebral arteriography or cerebral angiography.

These tests are used to detect abnormalities in the neck or brain such as a blood clot, a blood vessel tear or an aneurysm. They're performed less frequently now than in past years due to the development of magnetic resonance imaging (MRI) and magnetic resonance angiography (MRA).

Urinary tract

During a procedure called intravenous pyelography, contrast material is injected into a vein. It circulates in the bloodstream and is concentrated in the kidneys, where the contrast material is excreted in urine. As the dye passes through the urinary tract, it outlines the tract, making it more visible on an X-ray.

This test is most often done to look for obstructions in the urinary tract caused by stones or tumors or to check for kidney or urinary tract abnormalities, such as tumors. For more information on this test, see page 918.

Bile and pancreatic ducts

X-ray examination of the bile and pancreatic ducts can help identify gallstones, narrowings (strictures), cancer or other abnormalities. A contrast medium is injected into the ducts through a long tube (endoscope) that's inserted into the digestive tract and threaded through the tract until it reaches the bile or

Barium X-rays

Barium X-rays involve the use of the contrast material barium to examine the upper or lower gastrointestinal tract. When swallowed, barium outlines the upper digestive tract, allowing a doctor to check for abnormalities such as an ulcer, tumor and tract narrowing (stricture). It also allows visualization of motion abnormalities of the esophagus, stomach and small intestine.

To examine the lower gastrointestinal tract, barium may be inserted into the rectum and colon using an enema. A barium enema permits visualization of the lining of your rectum, colon and often a portion of the small intestine. The test can aid in the diagnosis of diseases such as colorectal polyps, colorectal cancer, Crohn's disease and ulcerative colitis.

Preparation

Before the examination you generally need to fast overnight. For the ingestion of barium, you'll be asked to drink a chalky liquid that may be flavored to make it more pleasant tasting.

If you're having a barium enema, you'll probably be given a laxative the night before to prepare your colon. You may also need a cleansing enema an hour or two before the procedure. With a barium enema, barium is infused into your rectum. Although you'll feel the urge to expel it, it's important that you hold the barium until the examination is completed.

The procedure

After the barium mixture coats and fills in the hollows of your digestive tract, X-rays are taken that reveal a clear silhouette of the shape and condition of these organs.

Normal Stomach

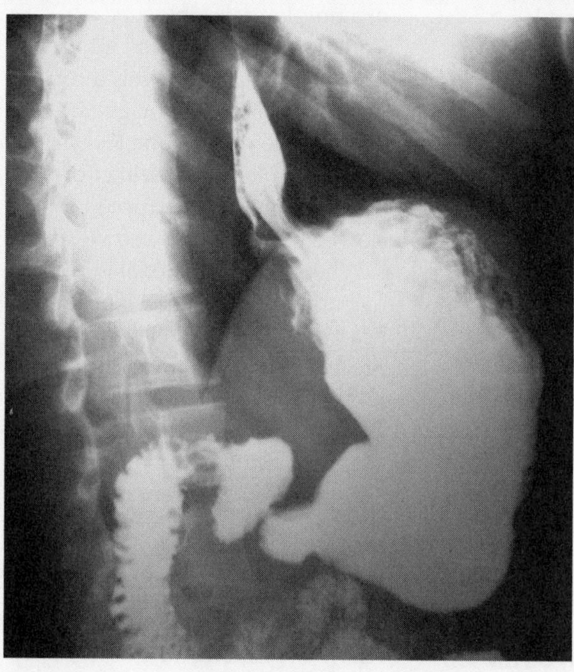

Stomach Cancer (see arrow)

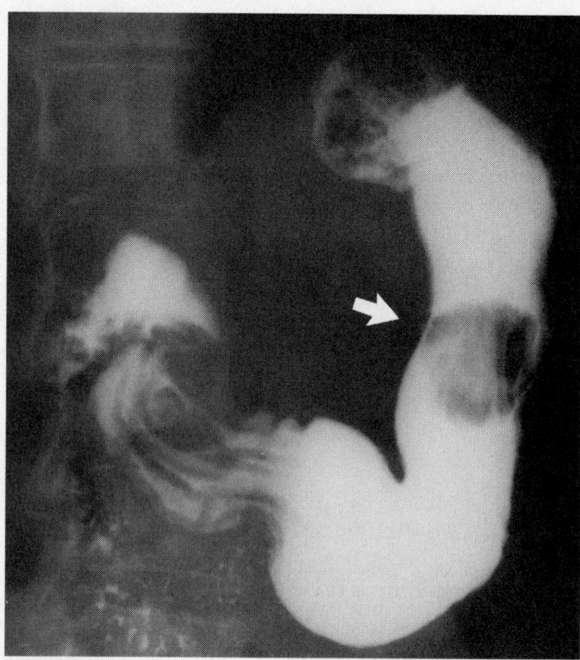

Question and Answer

What does catheterization mean?

Catheterization refers to any procedure in which a catheter — a long, flexible tube — is inserted into the body.

Sometimes the term *angiography* is used synonymously with the phrase *catheterization of the heart and blood vessels* (cardiac catheterization). Angiography refers to injection of a contrast material through a catheter so that the heart and blood vessels can be seen on an X-ray. Some cardiac catheters also have miniature devices at the tips that can measure blood oxygen, blood flow and pressures within blood vessels. In addition, some catheters are equipped to take a sample of tissue (biopsy) from a blood vessel or the heart or to treat disease.

Catheters are also used in other situations. For example, urinary catheters are used to drain urine from the bladder when an individual isn't able to go to the bathroom.

A fluoroscope is also used to visualize passage of the barium. This device uses a fluorescent screen to convert the X-ray image into visible light. The fluoroscope is also capable of providing a conventional X-ray film at any point during the procedure.

For an even clearer picture of the stomach, you might be asked to take a powder or pill that releases gas into your stomach. The gas will expand (dilate) your stomach to provide a more detailed picture of the organ.

During a barium examination of the colon, the doctor may place you in various positions and push down on (palpate) your abdomen as the barium flows through your colon. He or she will attempt to force the barium into the small intestine. At times, the radiologist may instill some air into your colon to obtain better delineation of fine features of its lining. This is particularly effective in detecting very small polyps and intestinal changes associated with ulcerative colitis or Crohn's disease.

Side effects

The barium is expelled in the stool and generally causes few ill effects. It can lead to temporary constipation. Therefore, a laxative is commonly advised after a barium test of the small intestine. A barium enema has been known to occasionally aggravate ulcerative colitis or, rarely, lead to perforation of the colon.

You should be able to eat a normal diet immediately after the examination, and you'll probably be advised to drink plenty of liquids during the remainder of the day. For several days after the test, your stool may be light pink or white as you eliminate the remaining barium from your gastrointestinal tract.

Normal Colon

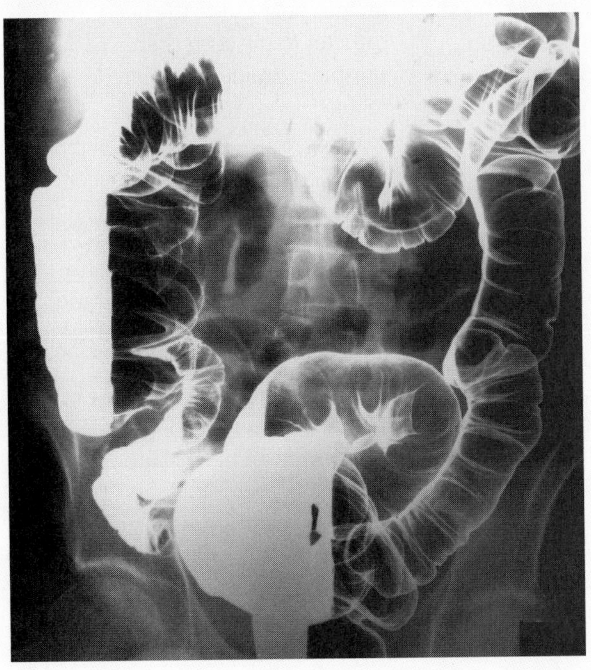

Colon Cancer (see arrow)

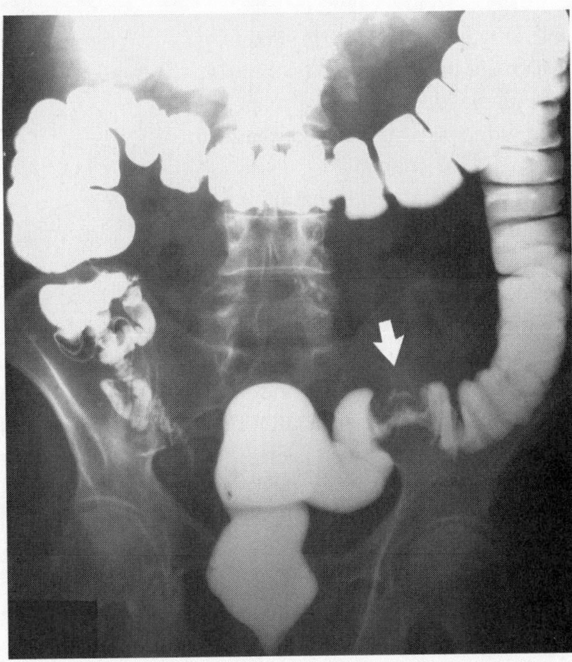

pancreatic duct. This procedure is called endoscopic retrograde cholangiopancreatography (ERCP). For more information, see page 897.

Ultrasound scans

Ultrasound scanning, also known as ultrasonography or sonography, uses very high-frequency sound waves to produce images of the inside of the human body. Ultrasound operates similarly to sonar devices on submarines or fish finders on fishing boats.

A device called a transducer converts electric current into high-frequency sound waves that are inaudible to the human ear. The transducer is usually a hand-held device that's placed on the skin surface over the area of your body to be examined. Sometimes, it's attached to a probe that's inserted into a natural opening, such as your esophagus, rectum or vagina.

Once the transducer is in place, sound waves are emitted from the device. The sound waves pass through body tissues — more readily through soft tissues and fluid and less readily through dense tissues. The waves are reflected to a receiver located within the transducer. The receiver converts the sound waves into electric signals, which are processed by a computer and displayed as moving images on a video screen. Selected images are saved for analysis.

An ultrasound examination is usually performed by a technician trained in ultrasound imaging (sonographer), and the images are analyzed by a doctor, generally a radiologist or an obstetrician.

Ultrasound is very safe and causes relatively little discomfort. Because of this, its role has expanded considerably since its development. Ultrasound may be used to examine:

A fetus

Ultrasound is routinely used in pregnancy to view the developing fetus and check for uterine disorders (see page 263).

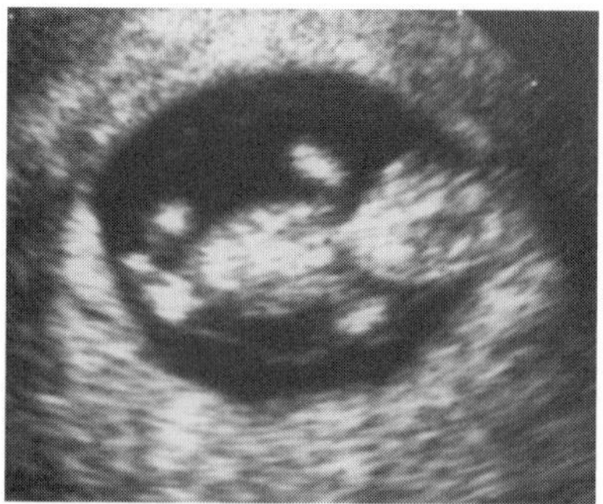

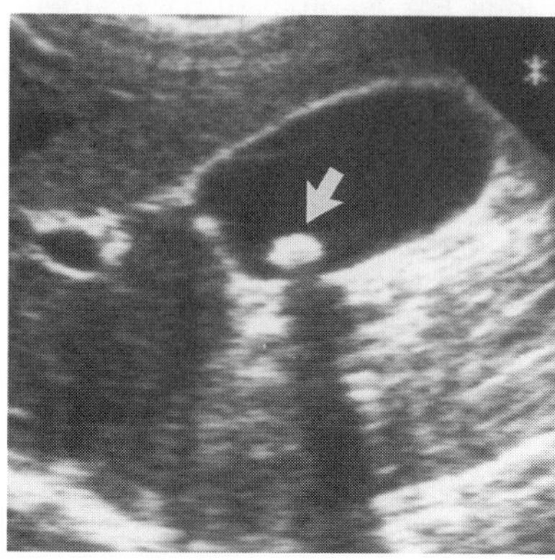

The ultrasound scan on top shows a fetus in the uterus. The scan on the bottom reveals a gallstone (see arrow).

Heart

Ultrasonography allows doctors to detect heart valve defects by watching the flow of blood through the chambers of the heart. It's also used to determine the thickness of the walls of the heart and to measure the heart's pumping function (ejection fraction). For more information on this procedure, called echocardiography, see page 776.

Blood vessels

A specific type of ultrasound, called Doppler ultrasound, allows doctors to monitor blood flow through arteries and veins. Doppler ultrasound uses short pulses of ultrasound to determine the speed and direction of blood flow. Blood flowing away from the probe appears one color on the screen, and blood flowing toward it appears another. This type of ultrasound is most often used to identify blood clots and damaged valves within veins.

Internal organs

Ultrasound is often used to identify possible disorders of the kidneys, spleen, prostate gland, testicles, thyroid, uterus and ovaries. Ultrasound can also help identify disorders of the esophagus, stomach, gallbladder, liver, biliary ducts, pancreas and rectum.

In addition to assessing the health of internal organs, ultrasound guidance may be used in some invasive procedures, such as a biopsy, drainage of an infection or treatment of a cancerous mass. Ultrasound images help guide the needle or catheter to the correct area to be sampled, drained or treated.

Endoscopic Ultrasound

Endoscopic ultrasound is similar to upper gastrointestinal endoscopy, a procedure in which a thin, flexible instrument with an attached camera (endoscope) is inserted into the digestive tract to view the interior of the tract. With endoscopic ultrasound, an ultrasound probe is also attached to the endoscope.

The ultrasound probe is used to view internal organs and structures that are adjacent to the stomach and intestines. These include the liver, pancreas, gallbladder and bile ducts. Endoscopic ultrasound can help diagnose gallstones, as well as identify tumors located in the pancreas, liver and bile ducts. Miniature cutting tools located in the endoscope allow tissue samples to be taken from an abnormality, such as a tumor.

Endoscopic ultrasound may provide clearer images and help obtain tissue samples. Preparation for the procedure, as well as the procedure itself, is similar to that of an endoscopy.

Computerized tomography scans

Computerized tomography (CT) uses X-ray images in conjunction with a computer to produce images of your body. As you lie on a table, the part of the CT scanner that resembles an enormous doughnut rotates around you. As the machine is rotating, it emits a series of thin X-ray beams that pass through your body at different angles. A computer compiles the images into two-dimensional "slices" of your organs. These slices are called tomograms.

The advantage of computerized tomography is that it provides much greater detail than an ordinary X-ray. An ordinary X-ray can show only a few levels of density: bone, soft tissues and air. A CT scan can identify hundreds of levels of density, making organs that are difficult or impossible to see on an ordinary X-ray, such as lymph nodes and the liver, more visible. CT scans are often used to examine the head, chest, abdomen and pelvis for tumors, inflammation of tissues, bleeding within large organs and organ enlargement. CT scans may also be used during biopsy procedures, to monitor blood flow (CT angiography) and to treat cancerous masses.

Magnetic resonance imaging

Magnetic resonance imaging (MRI) uses magnetic fields and radio waves to generate images. You're placed on a motorized bed that's moved into the tunnel (cylinder) of the scanner. The scanner houses a powerful magnet that surrounds the cylinder.

When atoms in your body are exposed to a very strong magnetic field, they line up parallel to one another. Radio waves from a radiofrequency magnet briefly knock the atoms out of their parallel alignment. As they realign, the atoms emit tiny signals, which are picked up and passed on to a

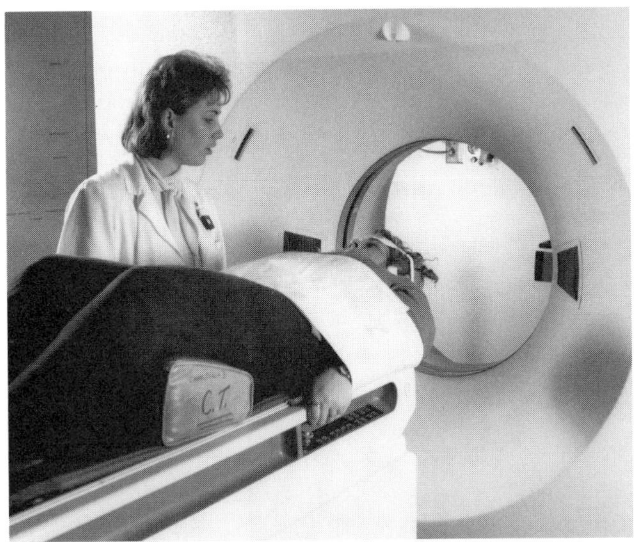

A person entering a computerized tomography (CT) scanner.

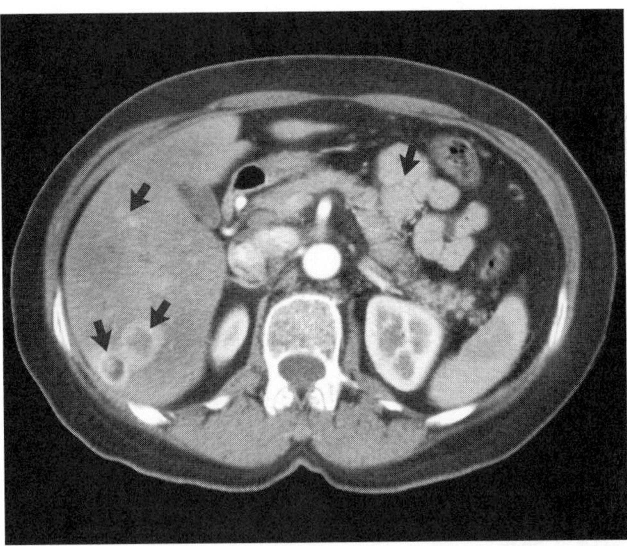

A CT scan reveals tumors in the pancreas and liver (see arrows).

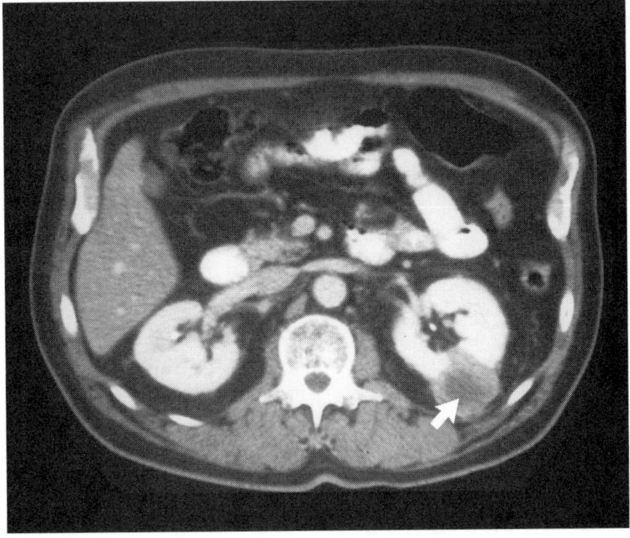

A CT scan shows a kidney tumor (see arrow).

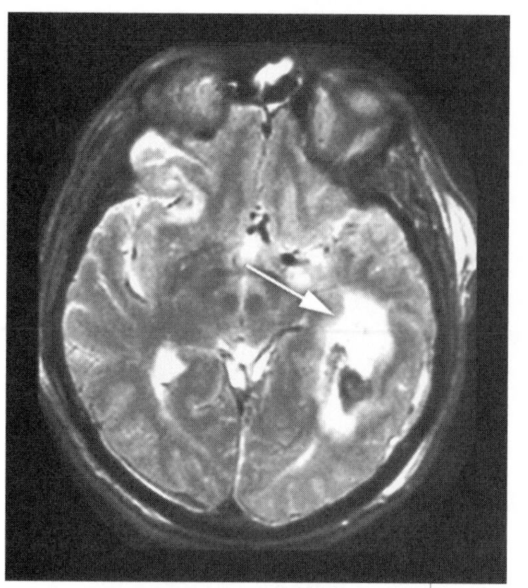

The arrow on this magnetic resonance image (MRI) points to an area of bleeding in the brain (brain hemorrhage).

computer. The computer then converts these signals into an image.

Magnetic resonance imaging is particularly useful for imaging areas of the brain because it produces detailed images of the brain's white and gray matter. It's also often used to image the spinal cord and help diagnose disorders such as multiple sclerosis. MRI also is used

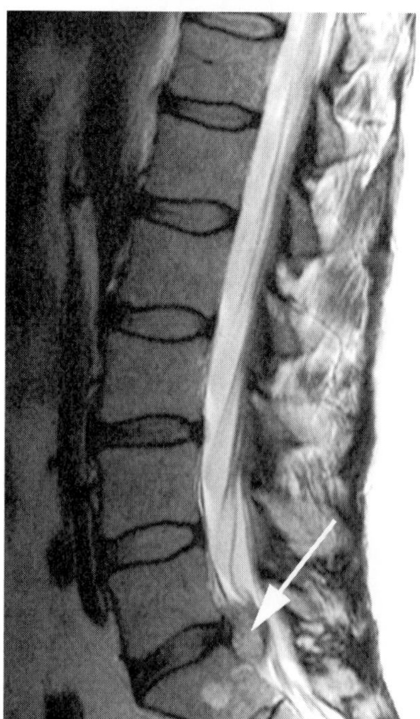

An MRI reveals compression of the spinal canal from a herniated disk (see arrow).

to diagnose disorders affecting many internal organs.

The procedure is painless and has the advantage of not exposing you to radiation. However, it can trigger feelings of claustrophobia in some people. The tunnel of the scanner into which you're placed is not much wider than your body. For individuals who are claustrophobic, sedation or, occasionally, general anesthesia may be used.

A form of magnetic resonance imaging called magnetic resonance angiography (MRA) is used to examine arteries in the neck and brain and the rest of the body. It doesn't require the use of a catheter, as does angiography. It's also less costly, and the recovery time is considerably shorter.

However, an MRA can't always match the clarity of images produced by conventional arteriography. Thus, cerebral arteriography is needed to detect very small abnormalities, such as a small brain aneurysm. Specialized MRI procedures may also be used to evaluate the heart, bones, joints and muscles.

Radionuclide scans

Radionuclide (nuclear) scanning involves the use of a tiny amount of a radioactive substance (radionuclide) that's generally injected into the bloodstream. A radionuclide gives off minute amounts of energy (radiation) in the form of gamma rays. These rays are detected by a device called a gamma camera. Information from the camera is processed by a computer and converted into images.

Different tissues take up different radionuclides, and therefore the radioactive substance used during the procedure depends on the organ a doctor wants to investigate.

Radionuclide scans portray parts of the body as images of varying intensity. Areas of high uptake of radionuclide are called hot spots.

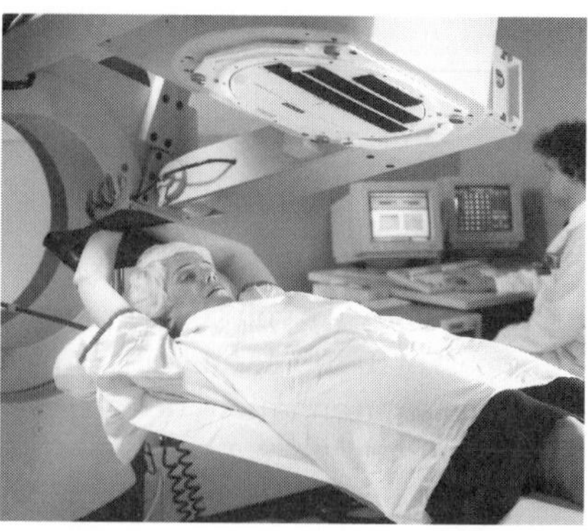

A radionuclide (nuclear) scan is obtained by a special camera that detects radiation given off by a radioactive substance put into the body. During the scanning the camera moves while you remain still.

Areas of less intense color, which indicate a low uptake of radionuclide, are called cold spots.

Radionuclide scans are generally used to assess how an organ or tissue is functioning. They're used to detect abnormal levels of activity in organs such as the thyroid gland, kidneys and bone. Radionuclide scans are also used to evaluate the circulation of blood through the lungs and the size and function of the heart. Sometimes, a radionuclide scan is used in conjunction with exercise testing (a stress test) to assess function of the heart muscle during exercise. Radionuclide scans may also be used to detect tumors or inflammation. In addition, these scans may be used to evaluate the passage of food through the digestive tract.

Positron emission tomography scans

Positron emission tomography (PET) is a special form of radionuclide scanning. Unlike other scanning techniques, PET scans don't produce clear structural images of organs. Instead, they're used to provide information about chemical activity within certain tissues or organs.

PET uses radioactive substances (radionuclides) that emit particles called positrons. The radiation that these particles generate is detected by a PET scanner. The number of positrons emitted by an organ or area of tissue indicates how much of the radioactive substance the organ or tissue has taken up and, therefore, how chemically active it is.

PET is used mostly to study the brain and the heart. PET scans may be of help in locating the origin of epileptic activity associated with seizures and in investigating brain function in certain mental health disorders, such as depression. In the heart, PET can identify areas of the heart receiving decreased blood flow. PET is also used to detect abnormal masses in the body that may be cancerous.

Single-photon emission computerized tomography scans

Single-photon emission computerized tomography (SPECT) is another specialized form of radionuclide scanning. It's similar to PET scanning. SPECT scans are used most often to assess heart and brain function.

Endoscopic Tests

A direct view of certain organs and tissues is often the best way to determine if an organ is healthy or affected by disease. Structures that are easily accessible, such as your ears, are examined using simple viewing instruments. Many structures located deeper inside your body can be examined using fiber-optic instruments called endoscopes.

Endoscopic devices contain a lens and a fiber-optic lighting system that allow your doctor to view organs and tissues that make up the gastrointestinal tract and the airways of the lungs. A channel within the endoscope also permits the passage of instruments that allow your doctor to take samples of tissue (biopsy), remove fluid and perform certain treatments.

Upper gastrointestinal endoscopy

Upper gastrointestinal endoscopy (esophagogastroduodenoscopy) provides your doctor a direct view of the upper part of your digestive tract. An endoscope can be inserted through your mouth and threaded into your esophagus, stomach and the first part of the small intestine (duodenum).

Before the tube is inserted, a local anesthetic may be sprayed into your mouth and throat to dull the gag reflex that can result from the pressure of the tube on the back of your tongue and throat. You may also be given an intravenous (IV) sedative to relax you. You may feel some mild discomfort or fullness as the tube is inserted or if air is introduced to allow better visibility.

Endoscopy is useful in the diagnosis and treatment of many upper gastrointestinal diseases and disorders. During the procedure, your doctor may do one or more of the following:

- Look for and inspect inflamed tissue, ulcers and growths
- Take tissue samples (biopsy)
- Remove foreign objects or noncancerous growths (polyps)
- Stretch (dilate) the esophagus if it's narrowed by scar tissue
- Identify and treat bleeding lesions

Certain chronic conditions of the upper gastrointestinal tract, such as Barrett's esophagus, may predispose an individual to the development of cancer. In such cases, regular endoscopic examinations may be helpful to screen for early signs of cancer.

Bronchoscopy

Bronchoscopy allows for the direct examination of air passageways. During this procedure, an endoscope is inserted into your mouth, threaded through the larynx and into lung bronchial tubes. This procedure may be performed to look for abnormal growths, damage to lung tissues or foreign objects in lung airways. For more information, see page 819.

Colonoscopy

Colonoscopy involves the examination of the large intestine (colon) with an endoscope. Colonoscopy is the most accurate method of examining your colon for polyps or cancer. In people known to be at increased risk of these conditions, periodic colonoscopy may be very useful.

Other common uses include:

- Removing polyps and taking tissue samples (biopsies)

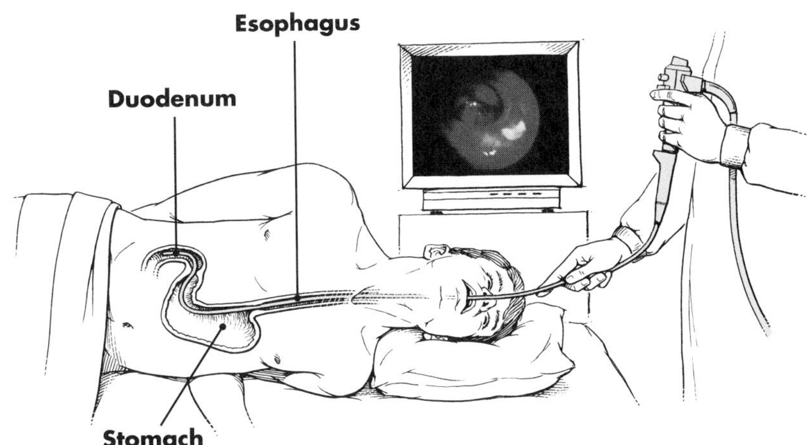

An endoscope provides a direct view of the upper gastrointestinal tract: esophagus, stomach and upper part of the small intestine (duodenum). Images from inside the gastrointestinal tract appear on a monitor screen.

- Searching for a cause of chronic or acute bleeding and treating bleeding sites
- Identifying pouches (diverticula) and obstructions
- Stretching narrowed areas
- Differentiating the causes of inflammatory bowel disease
- Identifying a cause of chronic diarrhea

The night before the test you'll likely be given a liquid solution and a laxative to cleanse the colon for better viewing. Just before to the examination, you may receive medication to partially sedate you and help you to relax.

During the procedure you lie on your left side, and air is introduced into your colon to inflate it and allow better viewing of the interior walls. You may feel some abdominal cramping or pressure during the exam, which should end when the endoscope is removed.

Sigmoidoscopy

Sigmoidoscopy is similar to colonoscopy, except that during

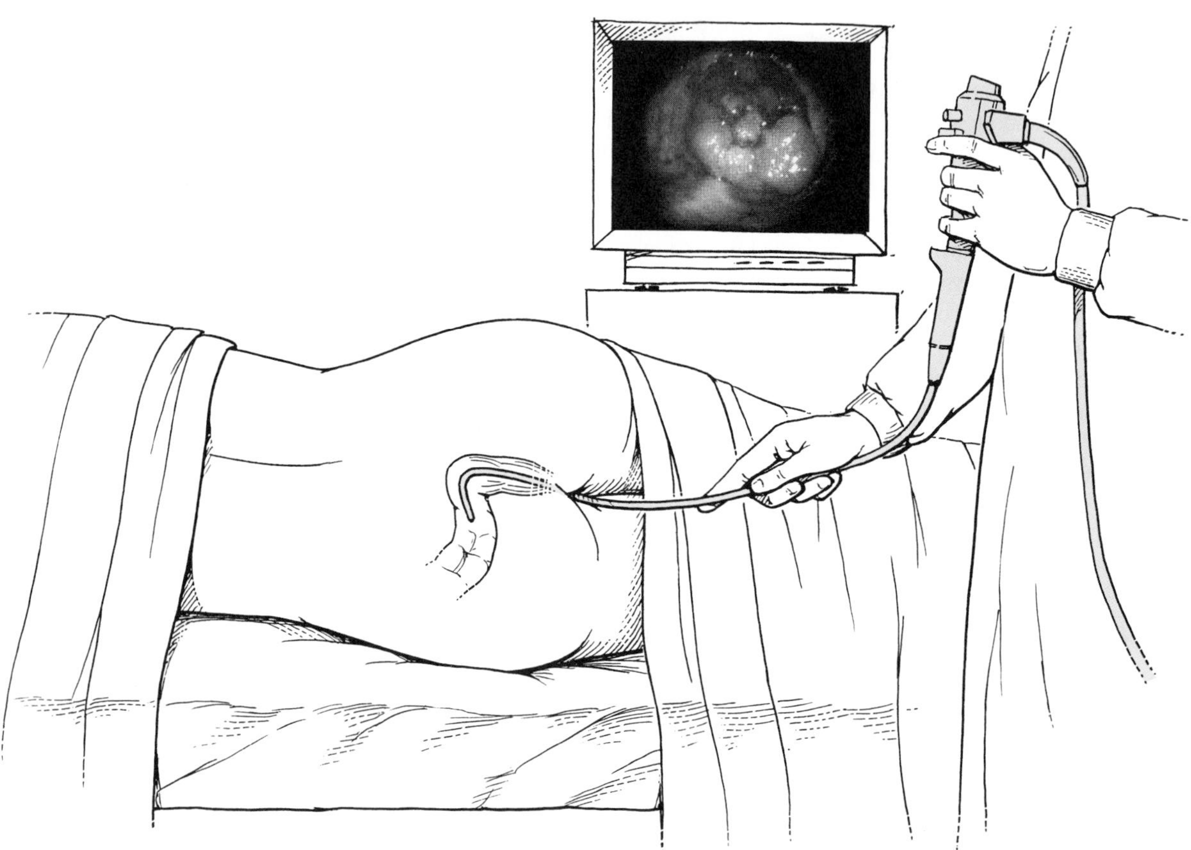

During a sigmoidoscopy examination, a doctor uses a flexible, lighted fiber-optic tube (sigmoidoscope) to examine the rectum and sigmoid colon. The image on the screen shows colon cancer.

Virtual Colonoscopy

Computerized tomographic (CT) colography is a new, noninvasive technique for examining the large intestine (colon). Commonly referred to as virtual colonoscopy, this diagnostic procedure provides two- and three-dimensional pictures of your colon and rectum without having to use an endoscope or sedation.

Before the scan you're given laxatives, and perhaps an enema, to clear your colon. Your colon is filled with air by inserting a small catheter tip just inside the rectum. Pictures are then taken of the entire colon with a CT scanner. A scan of the entire colon generally takes less than 10 minutes.

CT colography is more comfortable and faster than traditional colonoscopy. Research studies are now comparing its effectiveness to traditional colonoscopy. CT colography can identify most polyps that are larger than half an inch. However, if suspicious areas are found, you'll still need traditional colonoscopy to get a better view of the area, perform biopsies or remove polyps. Researchers are also studying whether CT colography can be done successfully without prior bowel preparation.

this procedure a doctor examines just your rectum and the lower portion of your large intestine (sigmoid colon), not the entire colon. Sigmoidoscopy is performed in the same manner as colonoscopy, except that you usually aren't sedated.

Sigmoidoscopy may be used to find the cause of diarrhea, constipation or bleeding or to look for polyps or cancer.

Cystoscopy

Cystoscopy involves insertion of an endoscope into the urethra and bladder, allowing for examination of these organs. Cystoscopy may be used to look for bladder stones, bladder cancer or the cause of recurring urinary tract infections. In men, the procedure can help assess the degree of urethral constriction caused by an enlarged prostate gland (benign prostatic hyperplasia, or BPH). For more information, see page 934.

Arthroscopy

Arthroscopy is an endoscopic examination of a joint, most commonly the knee. A tiny incision is made in the skin on one side of the joint, and an endoscope is inserted through the incision. Arthroscopy is often used to diagnose damaged cartilage or ligaments in the knee. For more information, see page 964.

Tests That Monitor Electric Impulses

The human body continuously generates and transmits electric impulses. This activity occurs primarily in your brain, heart, muscles and nerves. If a doctor suspects that a disease or disorder may be related to an abnormal electric pattern or a disruption in a nerve pathway, he or she may have you undergo a test to measure electric impulses within a certain organ or nerve.

Electrocardiography

Electrocardiography (ECG) measures the pattern of electric impulses generated by your heart. During the test — which takes only a couple of minutes — approximately 12 to 15 adhesive electrode patches are attached to your skin, generally at your chest, arms and legs. The electrodes detect electric impulses generated by your heart and transmit the information to an electrocardiograph. This machine records information from the electrodes, which is displayed on a monitor or graph paper in the form of waves.

By interpreting the wave patterns, a doctor usually can tell if you've recently had a heart attack or are presently experiencing one. An electrocardiogram can also help identify the extent of damage from a heart attack and detect irregular heart rhythms and enlarged heart muscle. For more information, see page 751.

Cardiac stress test

Many different types of cardiac stress tests are used (for more information see page 752). A common type is the treadmill test. It's similar to electrocardiography (ECG), but unlike ECG it's performed while you're exercising. For this test, you typically walk on a treadmill while electrodes attached to your chest and back record your heart's response to increased exertion. ECG recordings are taken before, during and after you exercise.

Cardiac stress testing is used most often to identify inadequate blood circulation to the heart muscle and heart rhythm abnormalities that are more likely to occur during exercise.

Electroencephalography

Electroencephalography (EEG) measures electric activity produced

Electrophysiologic Testing

Sometimes, an electrocardiogram and other related tests are inconclusive, particularly in individuals who have experienced unexplained dizziness, fainting spells or abnormal heart rhythms. In these situations, electrophysiology (EP) tests may be done in a controlled hospital setting to find out where the problem is and what can be done to fix or control it.

EP testing is done in a special laboratory that has equipment for recording the heart's electric signals and for electrically stimulating the heart when needed. Electrode catheters are inserted through blood vessels, usually veins, into the heart chambers, most commonly the right atrium and ventricle. These catheters sense electric impulses in various regions of the heart and measure how the heart conducts impulses from one area to another. By determining where and when impulses occur, a doctor can map the electric system of your heart.

The electrodes can also pace the heart with a small electric current that's similar to a pacemaker electrode. Pacing the heart can help in the mapping procedure. It may also be used to trigger abnormal heart rhythms. Observing the rhythm problem may enable your doctor to determine the cause.

During the test, various medications can be given to see if they can correct the problem. Doctors may also check to see how well the problem responds to use of a pacemaker. Catheter ablation also may be done at the time of EP testing. This procedure uses radiofrequency energy to destroy specific heart muscle cells responsible for the rhythm disturbance.

by the brain. Similar to an ECG, this test gathers information through small, adhesive patches containing electrodes that are attached to your forehead and scalp. Electric impulses from your brain are sent to an electroencephalography machine, which displays the impulses on a monitor or graph paper in the form of waves. This test is used most often to diagnose and manage seizure disorders and to assess sleep patterns.

Electromyography

Electromyography (EMG) measures tiny electric discharges produced within muscles. During the procedure a needle-thin electrode is gently inserted into each muscle to be studied. A fine wire attached to the needle is connected at the other end to an electronic instrument that detects electric current in the muscle. Patterns of electric activity are recorded when the muscle is at rest and as the muscle is tightened and relaxed. These patterns are monitored on a screen and may be recorded for further analysis. Electromyography is used to help diagnose muscle or nerve disorders, such as muscular dystrophy and amyotrophic lateral sclerosis (ALS).

Nerve conduction study

A nerve conduction study is a variation of electromyography that measures the speed at which nerves transmit electric signals. Another name for this test is electroneurography.

To prepare you for a nerve conduction study, two adhesive electrodes are placed directly over the nerve to be studied at different locations along its path. Electrodes may also be placed over a muscle connected to the nerve. A small instrument with metal prongs applies a mild shock to the nerve. The electric signal moves down the nerve, passing under the electrodes.

By comparing the recording of the signal at each electrode site and calculating the time it takes to travel between them, your doctor can determine the speed of conduction along the nerve. The nature of the signal from the nerve or muscle also helps to determine if nerve or muscle fibers have been damaged by disease or trauma. Nerve conduction tests are often used to diagnose peripheral nerve disorders, such as carpal tunnel syndrome.

Other Tests

Additional tests may be used to diagnose a disease or disorder. For a digestive problem, these may include an esophageal muscle test or an ambulatory acid probe test.

Esophageal muscle test

An esophageal muscle test (esophageal motility study or esophageal manometry) is most often performed when a person has a swallowing difficulty thought to result from abnormal contraction of the muscles of the esophagus.

An esophageal muscle test records movement and pressures in the esophagus. A tube is passed through your mouth or nose into your esophagus. There it performs continuous recordings of pressures in the esophagus over a period of 10 to 15 minutes. These recordings demonstrate the strength and coordination of those muscles used to propel food into the stomach. They can also evaluate function of the lower esophageal sphincter.

Ambulatory acid probe test

An ambulatory acid probe test can help determine if you have acid reflux, a condition in which stomach acid regurgitates into your esophagus. The test uses an acid-measuring (pH) probe to identify when, and for how long, stomach acid regurgitates into your esophagus.

While you're sitting, a nurse or technician may spray your throat with a numbing medication before a catheter is threaded through your nose or, less frequently, your mouth and into your esophagus. The probe is positioned just above the muscular valve (lower esophageal sphincter) between your esophagus and stomach. A second probe may be placed in your upper esophagus. The catheter doesn't interfere with your breathing, and most people experience little or no discomfort.

Connected to the other end of the catheter is a small computer that you wear around your waist or shoulder during the test. It records acid measurements. Knowing the frequency and duration of acid reflux can help your doctor determine how best to treat the problem. ■

CHAPTER 40 PART VI

Medications Guide

Medications can be a marvel. When used properly they may soothe minor aches and pains, downshift a rapidly progressing disease into slow motion, improve your quality of life or mean the difference between life and death.

But almost anything with the power to heal also carries the power to harm if used incorrectly. And many Americans *do* use medications incorrectly. In one study, researchers found numerous problems with use of both prescription and over-the-counter drugs. These problems included taking a different dose than recommended, not taking a medication or taking an inappropriate medication.

As helpful as medications can be, they can also be dangerous and even deadly if used inappropriately. This chapter will help you understand:

- How medications work
- Why two people can be affected by the same medication in different ways
- How to take your medications safely and avoid harmful interactions with other drugs or certain foods
- The potential advantages and drawbacks of cheaper generic drugs and brand-name medications
- How to make sure you're taking the right medications at the right time

At the end of the chapter, you'll find an overview of many common medications.

How Medications Work

Given the wide variety of medications and the different forms in which you can take them — tablets, capsules, lozenges, syrups, suppositories, suspensions, elixirs, creams, ointments, pastes, sprays, patches, inhalers, drops and injections — it's impossible to sum up exactly how they work in a sentence or two. In general, the most common medications are in pill form and are absorbed into your bloodstream through the lining of your gastrointestinal tract. Once in the bloodstream, the medication is carried to your liver, your body's chemical processing center. Some medications aren't affected by the liver, but many are. The liver converts some medications into a chemically active form. These active chemicals are then distributed throughout your body, including the site where the medication is needed. The kidneys inactivate medications so that they can be excreted.

Means of delivery

The most common methods of administering medications are as follows:

- Swallowed as a liquid, tablet or capsule
- Chewed and swallowed
- Placed under the tongue
- Sprayed into the mouth or nose
- Injected into a vein or muscle
- Dropped into or applied to an eye
- Dropped into an ear
- Placed in the rectum
- Placed in the vagina
- Applied to the skin

Oral medications

Swallowing a tablet or capsule and drinking a liquid are the most com-

Not Everyone Responds the Same

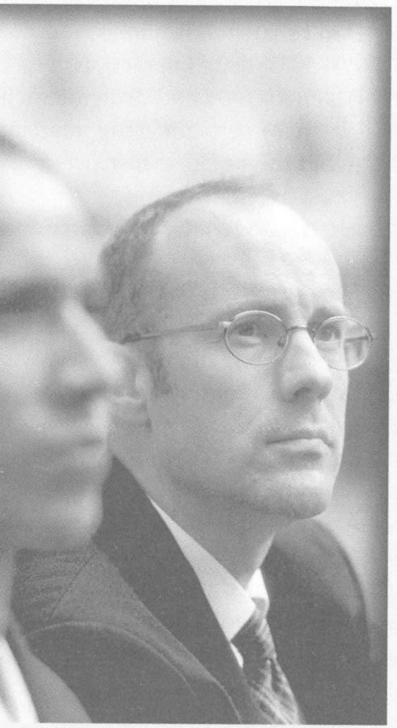

Medications don't affect everyone the same way. That's because no two people are alike. Differences in your makeup may cause you to react to a medication differently than someone else does. What works for you could actually harm someone else, and vice versa. Allergies, age, gender, race, weight, genetic differences and the general status of your health can affect your reaction to a drug.

Newborns, for example, aren't just smaller versions of adults. Their immature organs don't process drugs in the same way as adult organs do. So even small doses of an adult medication can produce an entirely different — and potentially lethal — chain of chemical reactions.

At the other end of the age scale, older adults tend not to process medication as efficiently as they did earlier in life. As people age, their kidneys and liver often become less effective in breaking down and removing drugs from the body.

Women may require smaller doses of some medications because they generally have more body fat than men do. Fat contains less water than does muscle. That means in women, medications aren't as diluted by body fluids as they are in men.

mon methods of taking medication. They're convenient, noninvasive, painless and inexpensive methods of getting medication into your body.

When swallowed, the medication travels down your esophagus to your stomach and eventually reaches your small intestine, where it's absorbed into your bloodstream and distributed throughout your body. Sometimes, though, a tablet or capsule may stick to the inner lining of your esophagus. If it dissolves there — instead of inside your stomach or intestines — it may cause irritation, possibly even vomiting or chest pains.

Here are some ways to help your medications make it to their destination:

- Before swallowing a pill, sip a little water to lubricate your esophagus.
- Swallow the pill with a mouthful of water.
- Drink the rest of the water to wash the medication down. Drink at least half of an 8-ounce glass of water to help flush the pill into your stomach.
- Don't lie down when taking the pill. Stand up or sit up straight.
- Stay upright for at least a minute or two after you swallow the pill.

If you have trouble swallowing pills, ask your doctor or pharmacist if the drug is available in liquid form. Another option is to take the pill with a soft, bulky food, such as a banana. The food will pass down your esophagus, carrying the pill with it. You can also try taking the pill with applesauce, perhaps crushing it if necessary. But check with your doctor first because crushing a pill can disrupt the timed release of some medications and damage the protective coating.

Metered-dose inhalers

A variety of inhalers are available, but basically they fall into two categories — metered-dose and dry powder. To use a metered-dose inhaler, shake the inhaler vigorously five or six times immediately before using it. Remove the cap from the mouthpiece. If the cap wasn't on while you were carrying the inhaler, check the mouthpiece for dirt and foreign objects before using it. If the inhaler hasn't been used for several days, do a test spray into the air.

If your inhaler doesn't have a spacer built into it, attach a spacer to the nozzle end. A spacer is a 4- to 8-inch length of tubing that helps get more of the medication deep into your lungs. Without a spacer, medication is deposited in the back of your throat, which can lead to harmful side effects. You can buy a spacer or make your own out of a cardboard, plastic or paper tube.

Hold your head erect and sit up straight or stand. Breathe in and out normally once, then stop for a moment. Don't try to push all of the air from your lungs. Close your mouth around the end of the spacer. Squeeze the inhaler once as you breathe in slowly. Keep inhaling even after finishing the squeeze. Continue inhaling for 5 to 7 seconds. This process mixes the medication with the incoming air and pulls it into your lungs slowly.

After inhaling, remove the spacer from your mouth and hold your breath for 10 seconds. Then slowly exhale through your nose. Wait 1 minute before taking your next inhalation. If you've been directed to take two doses at a time, breathe normally four or five times and repeat the process just described, beginning with shaking the inhaler. When you're done, gargle or brush your teeth and spit out the water.

Nasal sprays

Shake the sprayer gently. Tilt your head back. Close one nostril by pressing a finger against it. Insert the sprayer tip about a half-inch into your other nostril, with the tip pointing toward the inside corner of the eye above that nostril. Squeeze the sprayer and sniff at the same time. Repeat these steps with the opposite nostril. Try not to blow your nose for a couple of minutes to allow time for the medication to be absorbed into the blood vessels in your nose. Clean the sprayer tip with warm water and dry it. Put the cap over the tip to keep it clean.

Nose drops

Lie down or sit with your head tilted back. Check the tip of the dropper to be sure it's not chipped or cracked. Breathing through your mouth, place the prescribed number of drops in each nostril. Try not to touch the sides of your nasal openings with the dropper, which would contaminate the dropper and the rest of the nose drops when you put it back in the container. Remain reclining or seated with your head tilted for several minutes to give the medication time to spread within your nasal cavity.

Eye ointments

Always wash your hands before applying an eye ointment. Next, lie down or sit or stand with your head tilted back. Draw the lower eyelid down, look upward and place approximately a half-inch bead of the ointment along the inside margin of your eyelid. Don't touch your eye or eyelid with the tube because doing so can contaminate the medication in the tube. Close your eye and roll it around to distribute the ointment across the surface of the eye. With a tissue, gently remove any excess ointment from your eyelashes.

Eyedrops

Wash your hands, tilt your head back, draw the lower eyelid down and look upward. Place the drops in the pocket formed between your lower eyelid and eye. Avoid putting drops directly on the cornea and don't touch the dropper to your eye. This could contaminate the rest of the eyedrops. Close your eye and use a tissue to gently remove any excess solution from your eyelashes or eyelid.

Eardrops

Tilt your head so that the affected ear is angled up. Straighten the ear canal to receive the medication by drawing your earlobe down and back. Then deliver the prescribed number of drops into your ear. Try to avoid touching your ear canal with the dropper to prevent it from becoming contaminated. Keep your head tilted for a few minutes to allow the medication to drain deep into the ear.

Rectal suppositories

Before inserting a rectal suppository, put on latex gloves. To make the suppository easier to insert, coat it with a lubricant such as petroleum jelly.

Lie on your side and insert the suppository, pointed end first, as far as possible into the rectum. Push the bottom of the suppository sideways to be sure that some portion of it touches the bowel wall. If you have trouble keeping the suppository inside the rectum, you may not have inserted it far enough. You may also find it helpful to hold your buttocks together for a short while after inserting the suppository.

Vaginal medications

Most vaginal medications, such as those for yeast infections, come in the form of creams, gels, foams and suppositories. Wash your hands before and after applying the medication. Spread the vaginal lips and insert the medication as directed, typically a few inches inside the vagina. Don't insert a tampon afterward because it will absorb some of the medication. Wearing a panty liner will help protect your clothes from medication that may leak out.

Topical medications

Creams, gels, ointments and sprays that you put directly on your skin can deliver medication directly to the site that needs it. Wash your hands before and after applying the medication. With creams, gels and ointments, apply the prescribed amount onto the center of the affected area and spread it out into a thin layer. With sprays, shake the can and hold the nozzle at least 6 inches from the skin, unless otherwise directed.

As with other forms of medications, more isn't better. In fact, an overdose of some topical medications, such as the steroid hydrocortisone, can affect others parts of your body and cause serious side effects.

Skin patches

One of the newest ways to deliver medication is through a patch worn on your skin. Patches can be filled with many medications, from fentanyl, which helps control severe pain, to estrogen, which helps reduce symptoms of menopause. Patches release a steady flow of medication until it's exhausted.

Your doctor will tell you where to place the patch on your body and when to change it. This information is also available in the instructions that come with the medication. To help avoid skin irritations, rotate where you place the patches. If you still experience a skin irritation, tell your doctor. Don't cut the patches unless your doctor directs you to do so. In addition, follow your doctor's advice about how to discard a patch. Generally, it's best to fold it in half, with the medicated side facing in.

PREVENTION TIP

For most women, douching is unnecessary and actually can be harmful, as some commercial douches contain irritating chemicals. Douches can also change your vagina's normal acidic environment. This acidity resists the growth of yeast and other organisms that can cause infections.

Safety

To make sure your medication works as it's supposed to, take it as instructed. To ensure your safety, take the following steps:

Read the instructions

Before taking any new medication, read the label and any accompanying information to learn all you can about it. If you have unanswered questions, check with your pharmacist or doctor. For example, the label may contain directions about usage or information about side effects that you didn't know or weren't told about.

The label on the container of a prescription medication should bear your first and last name, the name of the person who prescribed it, the pharmacy address and telephone number, the prescription number, the date of dispensing and directions for use. Some states may have additional requirements. An expiration date may be given.

All of this information is important in identifying your medications and using them properly. Don't remove the label from a container and always keep a medication in its original container.

Don't share medications

Medication that calms your throbbing headache may not help a friend or relative in the same way. In fact, the medication could cause a life-threatening allergic reaction or other complications. Allergies, age, gender, race, weight, genetic factors and the general status of your health all can affect your reaction to medication.

Even if someone uses the same type of prescription medication as you, his or her prescription may be

Some Common Drug Interactions

Here are some examples of drugs that don't mix. Many others that aren't listed here can cause interactions. It's important to talk with your doctor or pharmacist before taking any new medication.

Type of medication	Possible risk of interaction if you:
Antacids	• Take any prescription drugs • Have kidney disease
Antinausea medications*	• Take sedatives or tranquilizers • Have a breathing problem, such as emphysema, asthma or bronchitis • Have glaucoma • Have difficulty urinating due to an enlarged prostate gland
Antihistamines*	• Take sedatives or tranquilizers • Take a prescription drug for high blood pressure or depression • Have a breathing problem, such as emphysema, asthma or bronchitis • Have glaucoma • Have difficulty urinating due to an enlarged prostate gland
Inhalers (bronchodilators)	• Have heart disease, high blood pressure, thyroid disease or diabetes • Have difficulty urinating due to an enlarged prostate gland • Take prescription drugs for asthma or have ever been hospitalized for asthma
Cough and cold medications	• Take any prescription drugs • Have high blood pressure, diabetes or heart, thyroid, kidney or liver disease • Have a breathing problem, such as emphysema, asthma or bronchitis • Have glaucoma • Take sedatives or tranquilizers • Have difficulty urinating due to an enlarged prostate gland
Laxatives	• Have kidney disease • Have stomach pain, nausea or vomiting
Decongestants	• Have heart disease, high blood pressure, thyroid disease or diabetes • Have difficulty urinating due to an enlarged prostate gland
Sleep medications*	• Take prescription sedatives or tranquilizers • Have a breathing problem, such as emphysema, asthma or bronchitis • Have glaucoma • Have difficulty urinating due to an enlarged prostate gland
Pain relievers (acetaminophen,* ibuprofen** or naproxen**)	• Drink three or more alcoholic beverages a day • Have kidney or liver disease • Take prescription drugs
Aspirin**	• Drink three or more alcoholic beverages a day • Take anticoagulant medications (blood thinners) • Have kidney or liver problems • Have asthma or high blood pressure

*Avoid alcohol when using these products.
**Check with your doctor first if you have stomach problems.

Source: Food and Drug Administration, 2001

Mixing Alcohol and Medication

Alcohol can change how some medications work. If you drink alcohol while you're on medication, you're putting yourself at risk of illness, injury and death. Because alcohol is sedating, this danger is especially true of drugs that tend to make you sleepy, such as many antihistamines and medications used to treat anxiety, depression and muscle spasms. You could end up with two sedatives instead of one — an overdose.

Individuals who drink moderate to excessive amounts of alcohol on a regular basis (chronic drinkers) and who take acetaminophen (Tylenol, others) — even at the standard dose — are at increased risk of liver damage. In addition, ibuprofen (Advil, Motrin, others) and naproxen (Aleve, Naprosyn, others), like alcohol, can irritate your stomach. When taken with alcohol, they can cause stomach ulceration and bleeding. Consuming excessive amounts of alcohol while taking the anticoagulant drug warfarin (Coumadin) may enhance its effect, increasing your risk of life-threatening hemorrhages.

If you take medication regularly and wonder if it's OK to have an occasional alcoholic drink, ask your doctor.

? Question and Answer

What should I do if I forget to take my medication?

Try to take your medication on schedule. But if you're an hour or two late and you're not scheduled to take the medication again for several more hours, it's usually best to go ahead and take it right away. If, however, you're more than several hours late and are getting close to your next scheduled dose, wait until the next time you're scheduled to take the drug.

If you miss a dose, don't take a double dose the next time.

of a different strength or a different preparation. The pills may look the same, and the labels may appear to match, but that doesn't mean your medication is safe for that person.

In determining what's best for you, your doctor takes into consideration what other medications you're taking, your health, your age and any drug allergies or sensitivities that you may have. Keeping these factors in mind, your doctor decides the appropriate medication, the appropriate dose and the duration of treatment.

Watch for drug interactions

If you take more than one medication, you need to watch out for potentially dangerous interactions. Two or more drugs taken together may produce an interaction that makes you feel worse instead of better. Work with your doctor and pharmacist to make sure your medications don't clash.

Drug interactions become an increasing problem as you age because older adults tend to take more medications than younger people do. Take the following precautions to prevent such adverse drug reactions from both prescription and over-the-counter drugs:

- Bring a list of all of the medications you're taking and their dosages — or a bag with all of your medication containers — when you have your checkup. Make sure to include nonprescription medications, including herbal supplements.
- Have all of your prescriptions filled at the same pharmacy, if possible. Having a pharmacist who can help you keep track of your medications and explain their proper use may prevent an adverse reaction.
- Talk to your doctor or pharmacist about possible drug interactions before taking any nonprescription medication.

Signs of drug interactions

During a checkup your doctor might notice signs of a possible drug interaction, such as an abnormal heart rhythm or changes in the results of your laboratory tests. But you may spot signs of potential problems even sooner.

If you experience any of the following symptoms after you start a new medication, contact your doctor right away:

- A tendency to bruise more easily than usual
- Skin rashes
- Persistent diarrhea
- Persistent constipation
- Continuing heartburn
- Dizziness
- Confusion
- Persistent nausea and vomiting
- A fever
- Extreme fatigue

Watch for food and drug interactions

When you mix certain foods and drugs, you can end up with different results than if you had taken them separately. In most cases, the interaction reduces the absorption of the drug. But in some cases, it blocks the breakdown of the drug, causing increases in drug concentration, possibly producing excessive blood levels of the drug.

Like many people, you might enjoy grapefruit or grapefruit juice at breakfast. But if you also take prescription drugs at breakfast, the combination could result in a higher blood level of the medication than intended.

Researchers first discovered an interaction between grapefruit juice and felodipine (Plendil), a drug used to treat cardiovascular disease. Later studies revealed that grapefruit juice alters the effects of many other medications as well. Among juices made from citrus fruits, grapefruit juice is unique. Chemicals in this juice interfere with certain enzymes in your liver that break down many prescription drugs. This can result in higher blood levels of the drug than your doctor intended.

Avoid taking any medications when you're eating grapefruit or drinking grapefruit juice, unless you have approval from your doctor or pharmacist.

Here are some other effects of combining certain foods and drugs:

- Eating excessive amounts of leafy vegetables, liver and other foods that contain vitamin K can promote blood clotting, reducing the effects of anticoagulant medications.
- The antibiotic tetracycline may not be fully absorbed if taken with dairy products.
- Antidepressants called monoamine oxidase inhibitors (MAOIs) can cause dangerously high blood pressure if taken with foods containing tyramine. Tyramine is found in aged cheeses, aged meats, sauerkraut and some alcoholic beverages.

Watch for herb and drug interactions

Although herbal supplements are considered natural, many contain active ingredients that don't safely mix with prescription or over-the-counter medications. Therefore, it's important to inform your doctor of any herbal supplements you take.

Here are 10 commonly used herbs and the prescription and over-the-counter drugs you shouldn't mix them with:

Feverfew, garlic, ginger, ginkgo
These herbs may augment the anticoagulant effect of the following drugs and may cause spontaneous and excessive bleeding:

- Aspirin (Bayer, Bufferin, others)
- Ticlopidine (Ticlid)
- Clopidogrel (Plavix)
- Dipyridamole (Persantine)
- Warfarin (Coumadin)

St. John's wort
St. John's wort has been shown to increase the body's breakdown of the following drugs. Many other medications may also be affected.

- Antidepressants
- Indinavir (Crixivan)
- Digoxin (Lanoxicaps, Lanoxin)
- Theophylline (Elixophyllin, Uniphyl)
- Cyclosporine (Neoral, Sandimmune)

The combination of St. John's wort and some antidepressants may cause an excess of serotonin (serotonin syndrome). Typical symptoms include headache, stomach upset and restlessness.

Ephedra
Ephedra by itself has been shown to increase risk of heart attack, stroke, seizure or death. Combined with the following drugs, the risk is increased even further:

- Decongestants
- Stimulants
- Heart drugs
- Antidepressants
- Medications containing caffeine

Ginseng
Avoid mixing ginseng with:

- Warfarin (Coumadin)
- Phenelzine (Nardil)
- Digoxin (Lanoxicaps, Lanoxin)

PREVENTION TIP

Take these precautions to guard against food and drug interactions:

- Follow instructions from your doctor or pharmacist on how and when to take your medications.
- Don't take medications at the same time that you take vitamin or mineral supplements. Some supplements, especially calcium, can bind with many medications and impair their absorption.
- If you're instructed to take a drug on an empty stomach, take it at least 1 hour before or 2 hours after eating.
- Don't stir your medication into food. Acid or minerals in some foods may alter the drug's ingredients.
- Don't mix medications into hot beverages. Heat can change or destroy some drug ingredients.

Taken with warfarin, ginseng can increase the risk of bleeding. Used with phenelzine, it may cause headache, trembling and mania. Used with digoxin, it may interfere with the drug's intended action.

Kava
Combined with the following drugs, kava can produce deep sedation and even coma:

- Sedatives
- Sleeping pills
- Antipsychotics
- Alcohol
- Drugs used to treat anxiety or Parkinson's disease

Echinacea
Echinacea can be toxic to the liver and shouldn't be combined with other drugs that can cause liver damage. Because this herb stimulates the immune system, it can also interfere with the effects of some immunosuppressants. Avoid mixing echinacea with:

- Anabolic steroids
- Methotrexate
- Amiodarone (Cordarone, Pacerone)
- Ketoconazole (Nizoral)
- Cyclosporine (Neoral, Sandimmune)

Cayenne
Cayenne may increase the absorption and impact of the following drugs:

- Angiotensin-converting enzyme (ACE) inhibitors, used for heart failure, high blood pressure, kidney disease
- Theophylline, an asthma medication

Cayenne may also increase the likelihood of developing a cough when it's taken with an ACE inhibitor.

Avoid the sun, if so instructed

Some medications can make your skin more sensitive to ultraviolet rays in sunlight. If you take such a medication, even slight sun exposure can result in skin redness, itching, swelling and blisters. This is known as a photosensitivity reaction, or photoreaction.

Medications that can produce this reaction include:

- Nonsteroidal anti-inflammatory drugs (NSAIDs), such as ibuprofen (Advil, Motrin, others) or naproxen (Aleve, Naprosyn, others)
- Some birth control pills
- Some antibiotics, such as tetracycline, sulfa drugs or quinolones
- Antinausea medications
- The high blood pressure medication hydrochlorothiazide (Esidrix, Hydrodiuril, Microzide, others)
- Tricyclic antidepressants
- Phenothiazines, taken for nausea and some psychological disorders
- Some chemotherapy drugs
- Some diabetes medications, such as glyburide (DiaBeta, Glynase, Micronase)
- The heart drug amiodarone (Cordarone, Pacerone)
- Tretinoin, used in prescription antiwrinkle creams and acne medications
- The acne medication isotretinoin (Accutane)

Anyone can have a photoreaction to a medication. Some reactions are mild, and others are quite severe. If the combination of sun and your medication seems to be causing a photoreaction, ask your doctor for advice on how to protect against future reactions.

Over-the-Counter vs. Prescription Medications

Over-the-counter, or nonprescription, medications can be purchased without a prescription. Innumerable over-the-counter medications, including aspirin, cough syrups and laxatives, are sold in drugstores, groceries, discount stores and convenience stores.

Prescription medications can be purchased only from a licensed pharmacy and with a written prescription from your doctor. These include an array of drugs from antibiotics to painkillers.

Some medications are available both over-the-counter and by prescription. Generally, the over-the-counter version contains a reduced strength of the medication. Often, an over-the-counter product contains about half the amount of the drug as its prescription counterpart.

Even nonprescription medications can cause side effects and be dangerous if misused. Follow the same safety precautions for over-the-counter products as you do with prescription medications.

Name Brand vs. Generic Drugs

When a new drug is developed, the pharmaceutical company that developed it generally gets 20-year patent rights to it — meaning that during this time, the developer is the only company that can sell the drug. This allows the pharmaceutical company to recoup money spent in research and in continuing clinical trials.

Extensions and new patents on the drug are sometimes granted, but once a patent expires, other pharmaceutical companies are free to produce and sell their own version of the drug. This generic form of a drug must meet the same Food and Drug Administration (FDA) standards established for the original drug.

Because companies that produce generic drugs don't incur the large expenses in research and development, they can offer the drug at a much lower price — often 30 percent to 50 percent less than the brand-name drug.

Generics get their name from the fact that when a drug is discovered or produced in a laboratory, it's first given a generic name that's designated by a committee of drug experts and approved by governmental agencies. This name identifies the drug as unique and it distinguishes the drug from all others. The generic name is nonproprietary, meaning it's not owned by anyone.

When the drug receives approval for sale to the public, it's usually given another name (brand name) by the original manufacturer. Other pharmaceutical companies that decide to produce their own version of the drug after the patent expires often market the drug under its generic name, or under another brand name. In either case, it's usually cheaper than the original brand.

Common Myths About Generics

You've taken the brand-name medication for years. Now your pharmacist says you have a choice — a generic drug is available too. Is what you've heard about generics true?

Myth: Generic drugs aren't as strong as brand-name drugs, nor as safe.
Fact: Generics are required by the Food and Drug Administration (FDA) to have the same quality, strength, purity and stability as their brand-name counterparts. And because generics have the same active ingredients, generics have the same risk and benefit as their brand-name counterparts.

Myth: Generic drugs don't act as quickly in the body.
Fact: A generic drug must deliver the same amount of active ingredient in the same amount of time as the original brand-name drug.

Myth: Generic drugs have more side effects.
Fact: The FDA monitors reports of adverse drug reactions and has found no marked difference in the incidence of side effects.

Myth: Generics are often made in substandard facilities.
Fact: The FDA conducts thousands of inspections each year to ensure that the manufacturing facilities of both brand-name and generic drugs meet government standards. In fact, about half of all generics are produced by brand-name firms that make copies of their own or other brand-name drugs.

Generics are available for about half of all drugs now on the market. Aside from the name, price and inactive ingredients — such as dyes, fillers and coatings — there's typically little difference between a generic drug and a brand-name drug. The FDA found that on average generic and brand-name drugs have the same clinical effect. Some generics, however, may be slightly less effective — which is why you should check with your doctor before making the switch to a generic medication.

Even slight differences between generics and their brand-name counterparts are important when it comes to certain medications, which are sometimes called narrow therapeutic index (NTI) drugs. With these drugs, the difference between the dosage that you need and a dosage that can harm you is very small. These include medications for:

- Epilepsy, such as phenytoin (Dilantin)
- Heart rhythm regulation, such as digoxin (Lanoxicaps, Lanoxin)
- Lung disease, such as theophylline (Elixophyllin, Uniphyl)
- Thyroid disorders, such as levothyroxine (Levoxyl, Synthroid)
- Anticoagulation, such as warfarin (Coumadin)

Changing from one brand of NTI drug to another should be done only in close consultation with your doctor. As for the effectiveness of over-the-counter generics, check with your pharmacist.

If your doctor is prescribing a medication, ask if a generic is available at a lower cost and if it would be OK to use it. Pharmacists may substitute lower priced generics — and sometimes are required to do so by certain health plans — unless you disapprove or your doctor has specifically directed otherwise.

Managing Your Medications

One of the most important steps you can take to get the most from your medications is to take an active role in your health care. Medical professionals will work with you, but ultimately you have to take responsibility for your own health.

Work with your doctor

An important key to successfully managing your medications is to make sure that both you and your doctor know:

- What medications you're taking
- Why you're taking them
- How you're taking them

Review the medications you're taking
Find out the exact name of each medication — both the generic name and the brand name. Record this in a personal record that you update at least once a year, or whenever you change a medication. Next to each listed drug, identify which doctor prescribed it.

Ask why you're taking each medication
Some people take so many medications that they find it hard to remember why they're taking some of them. Keep tabs on how each medication fits into your treatment plan.

Make sure you're taking each medication correctly
That means reviewing the dosages, the time of day you take the drugs and how you take them — on an empty stomach or with food.

Use only one pharmacy

A pharmacist is an important member of your health care team. In addition to performing traditional services, such as dispensing medications, your pharmacist can help you understand your medications and how to take them safely and effectively. Because a pharmacist can play a vital role in protecting and improving your health, find a pharmacy that you feel comfortable with and that has staff willing to assist you with your questions and concerns.

Other issues to consider include:
- Are you able to talk to a pharmacist without other people hearing you?
- Can a pharmacist be reached in case of an emergency?
- Does the pharmacy accept your health maintenance organization (HMO) or third-party payment plan?

If you change to a new pharmacy that doesn't have access to your medication records, it's important that you inform the pharmacists there, as fully as possible, about your medical history and the medications you're taking.

A pharmacist can also help you with information on the price of your medications. Many medications are available from more than one pharmaceutical company. They may have equal effects but different costs.

Your insurance company, HMO or other third-party payment group may reimburse you for only some of these medications or for only part of their costs. A pharmacist can often help you determine which medications are covered by your medical payment plan and which cost less.

Develop a routine

Make use of reminders, if you need to, to make sure that you take your medication at the right time:

Pillbox reminders
Once a week or once a day, fill each compartment with the pills that you need to take. Some boxes have separate compartments for doses needed at different times of the day. Ask your pharmacist or doctor if it's OK to use a pillbox container for your medications. Some pills, such as nitroglycerin, should be kept in their original container.

Medication containers with alarms
Use a medication container that has a cap with a small clock in it. This clock can be set to sound an alarm or flash a small light when it's time to take your medication.

Reminder watches
You can buy a special watch with an alarm that you can program as a medication reminder. Such watches may be available at your pharmacy or a medical supply store.

Charts and calendars
Develop a chart or calendar that lists your medication schedule. Keep it near your medications. Each time you take a drug, check it off the list.

Ordering Drugs by Mail

People order medications by mail instead of purchasing them from a local pharmacy for two main reasons:
- *Convenience.* You don't have to go farther than your mailbox to get them.
- *Money.* Mail-order drugs may be cheaper.

A big disadvantage of using mail-order services is that you don't have a local pharmacist who knows you, keeps a list of your medications, checks to make sure there are no drug interaction problems and can personally tell you about warnings and special instructions.

Another disadvantage is time lag. It can take several weeks to get drugs by mail. However, your doctor may be willing to write two prescriptions — one for the mail-order medication and a second, smaller prescription that you can fill at your local pharmacy and have on hand until the mail-order medication arrives.

Your Home Medicine Cabinet

Having a designated area for medications that you take regularly can help you keep them organized, easy to find and out of the reach of children.

Location
Many bathrooms have built-in medicine cabinets. But bathing and showering areas aren't always the best locations for storing drugs. Consider the following tips:
- Don't store your medications in humid places. Heat, moisture and direct light can change a medication's strength. For these reasons, don't leave your medication on a windowsill or in a car.
- Store your medications in a dark, dry, cool place.
- Keep liquid medications from freezing.
- Don't store medication in the refrigerator unless directed to do so.

Safety
Regardless of where you keep your medications, they should be out of the reach of children. Even if visits from youngsters are rare, take precautions. Cabinet and dresser drawer locks are a good idea for keeping toddlers away from medications inside. Child-resistant caps provide a second line of defense.

Common Medications

The purpose of this section is to provide some basic information about commonly used medications in the hope that the information may help answer some of your questions. Following is a list of some of the most frequently used medications and their functions. The medications are listed in alphabetical order. We've included products available by prescription as well as some that are sold without a prescription. Most of the listed medications are taken orally. Others are administered by injection, applied topically, inhaled, given intravenously or taken as drops. When side effects are listed for a group of medications, they're generally common to several of the listed drugs but may not apply to every one of them.

The availability of medications is subject to change. New medications are continuously being developed, and some brand name medications may be discontinued. For additional information regarding a particular medication, talk with your doctor or pharmacist.

Acne medications

Anti-infectives

Generic and common brand names

- Azelaic acid (Azelex, Finevin)
- Benzoyl peroxide (Benzac, Brevoxyl, Clearasil)
- Clindamycin (Cleocin T)
- Demeclocycline (Declomycin)
- Doxycycline (Doryx, Vibramycin)
- Erythromycin (Erygel, Staticin, others)
- Metronidazole (MetroGel, Noritate)
- Minocycline (Minocin)
- Tetracycline (Achromycin V, Sumycin)

Action

Stop growth and reproduction of certain microorganisms that cause infection.

Common uses

To treat acne. Some of these antibiotics also are used to treat other infections, such as traveler's diarrhea, gum infections, Lyme disease and some sexually transmitted diseases (STDs).

Common side effects

Rash, itching, stomach pain, diarrhea, sore throat and increased skin sensitivity to light

Note

Antacids, calcium and dairy products can reduce absorption of these medications. Some of the medications can cause birth defects if taken while pregnant. In children under age 8, the medications may cause permanent discoloration of teeth.

Retinoids

Generic and common brand names

- Adapalene (Differin)
- Isotretinoin (Accutane)
- Tazarotene (Tazorac)
- Tretinoin (Avita, Retin-A)

Action

Help inhibit oil gland function.

Common uses

To treat acne.

Common side effects

Dry, irritated skin, burning sensation and increased skin sensitivity to sunlight.

Note

Retinoids can cause birth defects if used during pregnancy.

Salicylic acid

Common brand names

- Clearasil
- Oxy Balance
- Stri-Dex

Action

Promotes shedding of dead skin cells.

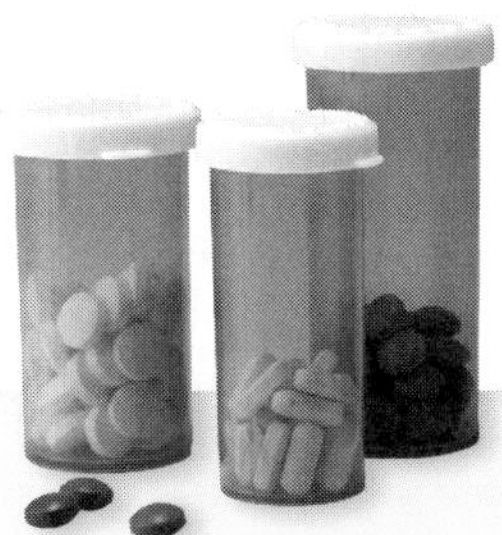

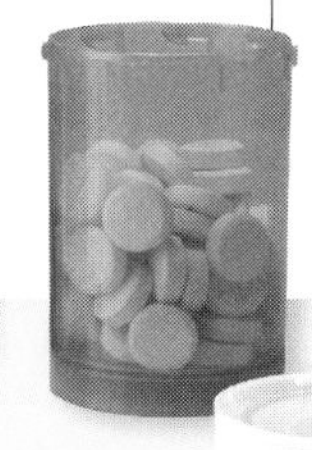

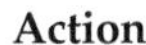

It's easy to absentmindedly leave medication on a kitchen counter or bedside table where a toddler may find the bright colors irresistible. So don't get in the habit of leaving the drugs out. If you have medication that must be refrigerated, put it on a high shelf so that young children can't reach it, or in a place where it's not visible.

Cleaning

Periodically go through your medicine cabinet. Get rid of unused, outdated prescription drugs. Medication deteriorates over time — even sooner than the printed expiration date if it hasn't been stored properly. If the expiration date isn't listed, the general rule is to discard the medication 1 year after it has been dispensed.

If you develop the same health problem you had several years ago, don't take leftover medication.

Keep medications in their original containers — otherwise you or members of your family may get confused about what drug is what and when it expires. If the label gets separated from its container and you're not sure what's in the container, discard the medication or call your pharmacist, who may be able to identify the medication according to the unique imprint codes each drug is required to have.

Common uses
To treat many skin disorders, including acne.

Common side effects
Skin irritation and stinging.

Note
Wash your hands after applying this medication.

Allergy medications

Antihistamines

Generic and common brand names
- Brompheniramine and pseudoephedrine (Bromfed, Bromfenex)
- Cetirizine (Zyrtec)
- Chlorpheniramine (Chlor-Trimeton)
- Clemastine (Tavist)
- Desloratadine (Clarinex)
- Dimenhydrinate (Dramamine)
- Diphenhydramine (Benadryl Allergy Relief)
- Fexofenadine (Allegra)
- Loratadine (Claritin)

Action
Prevent histamine from binding to its receptors, thereby preventing runny nose, itchy and watery eyes and sneezing due to an allergy.

Common uses
To treat allergies. Diphenhydramine and dimenhydrinate are also used to treat motion sickness and sleep disorders.

Common side effects
Some antihistamines cause drowsiness. Others may also cause dry mouth, nervousness, weakness and occasional headache.

Note
Avoid alcohol while taking antihistamines that cause drowsiness. Don't eat grapefruit or drink grapefruit juice while taking fexofenadine or loratadine. Doing so could lead to toxic blood levels of the medicine. Antihistamines can cause excitement in children.

Corticosteroids (nasal sprays)

Generic and common brand names
- Beclomethasone (Beconase, Vancenase)
- Budesonide (Rhinocort)
- Flunisolide (Nasalide)
- Fluticasone (Flonase)
- Mometasone (Nasonex)
- Triamcinolone (Nasacort)

Action
Reduce inflammation by slowing the reaction of individual cells to substances that trigger inflammation.

Common uses
To relieve symptoms of seasonal or year-round allergies and to prevent regrowth of nasal polyps following surgery to remove them.

Common side effects
Nasal stinging, sore throat, nosebleed, nausea and headache.

Note
Relief of symptoms may come in a day, or it may take a couple of weeks before the full effects of the medication become noticeable.

Mast cell stabilizers

Generic and common brand names
- Cromolyn sodium (Nasalcrom)

Action
Act on specific cells called mast cells, preventing them from releasing histamine and other substances that cause allergic reactions.

Common uses
To treat mild to moderate nasal allergies and asthma.

Common side effects
Burning, stinging or irritation of nasal membranes, flushing and increased sneezing.

Note
It may take a couple of weeks before the full effects of the medication become noticeable.

Alzheimer's disease medications

Cholinesterase inhibitors

Generic and common brand names
- Donepezil (Aricept)
- Galantamine (Reminyl)
- Rivastigmine (Exelon)

Action
Slow the breakdown of the brain chemical acetylcholine. Loss of acetylcholine is thought to be associated with Alzheimer's disease.

Common uses
To treat symptoms of mild to moderate Alzheimer's disease, such as memory loss, concentration and initiative.

Common side effects
Diarrhea, loss of appetite, muscle cramps, nausea, trouble sleeping, unusual tiredness or weakness and, uncommonly, heart rhythm changes.

Note
This medicine won't cure Alzheimer's disease or stop it from getting worse, but it may improve the ability to think.

Anemia medications

Erythropoietin

Generic and common brand names
- Darbepoetin alfa (Aranesp)
- Epoetin alfa (Epogen, Procrit)

Action
Stimulates your bone marrow to make red blood cells. Erythropoietin is a synthetic version of the natural hormone erythropoietin.

Common uses
To treat individuals with a chronically reduced number of red blood cells, such as individuals with kidney (renal) failure.

Common side effects
Chest pain, shortness of breath, headache, increased blood pressure, swelling and weight gain.

Note
Tell your doctor about all of your allergies, including allergies to foods, preservatives and dyes. This information can provide a clue about possible allergic reactions to the medication.

Folic acid

Action
Increases the folate (vitamin B-9) content in your body.

Common uses
To treat macrocytic anemia and other disorders associated with decreased folate levels. Also taken to reduce risk of birth defects in early pregnancy and decrease the risk of coronary artery disease in some people.

Common side effects
Generally doesn't cause side effects.

Note
Folic acid shouldn't be taken if you have pernicious anemia without also treating the vitamin B-12 deficiency.

Iron

Generic and common brand names
- Ferrous fumarate (Femiron)
- Ferrous sulfate (Feratab)

Action
Increases the iron content in your body. Iron is needed to produce hemoglobin in red blood cells, and hemoglobin is a key to maintaining good health and energy.

Common uses
To treat iron deficiency anemia.

Common side effects
Generally doesn't cause side effects. In some instances, may cause upset stomach, chest or throat pain and charcoal-colored stools.

Note
Too much iron can cause a condition called hemochromatosis. Talk with your doctor to make sure you're getting the right amount.

Vitamin B-12

Action
Increases the vitamin B-12 content in your body.

Common uses
To treat pernicious anemia and other disorders due to decreased levels of vitamin B-12.

Common side effects
Generally doesn't cause side effects. Injectable form may cause irritation at the injection site.

Note
Some strict vegetarians need vitamin B-12 supplements because they don't get enough of the vitamin in their daily diet.

Asthma medications

Beta agonists

Generic and common brand names
- Albuterol (Proventil, Ventolin)
- Bitolterol (Tornalate)
- Epinephrine (Adrenalin Chloride, Primatene Mist, others)
- Formoterol (Foradil)
- Levalbuterol (Xopenex)
- Metaproterenol (Alupent)
- Pirbuterol (Maxair)
- Salmeterol (Serevent)
- Terbutaline (Brethine)

Action
Relax muscles in the bronchial tubes, increasing the size of the airways.

Common uses
To prevent and treat spasms in airways (bronchospasms).

Common side effects
Shaking, nervousness, dizziness, headache, rapid heart rate and nausea.

Note
Don't take salmeterol or formoterol for asthma emergencies because they're slow-acting inhalants.

Corticosteroids

Generic and common brand names
- Beclomethasone (Qvar, Vanceril)
- Budesonide (Pulmicort)
- Flunisolide (AeroBid)
- Fluticasone (Flovent)
- Prednisolone (Pediapred, Prelone)
- Prednisone (Deltasone, Sterapred, others)
- Triamcinolone (Azmacort)

Action
Reduce inflammation and swelling of airways. Corticosteroid inhalers are slow acting and must be used on a regular basis. Oral medications (prednisone, prednisolone) generally are prescribed only for severe attacks of asthma.

Common uses
To prevent flares of asthma or relieve severe symptoms and to reduce inflammation associated with allergies, rheumatoid arthritis and certain skin disorders

Common side effects
Inhaled corticosteroids may cause sore throat, dry mouth, hoarseness and yeast infection of the mouth and throat. Oral corticosteroids may cause increased appetite, water retention, weight gain and difficulty sleeping. Long-term side effects of oral corticosteroids include glaucoma, cataracts, osteoporosis, muscle weakness and adrenal insufficiency. Adrenal insufficiency is the reduced ability of the adrenal glands to produce

increased amounts of corticosteroids in response to severe stress, including surgical trauma.

Note
Rinse your mouth after each use of a corticosteroid inhaler, to prevent yeast infection. Don't suddenly stop taking oral corticosteroids. Their use needs to be tapered.

Fluticasone and salmeterol

Brand name
- Advair Diskus

Action
A combination medication. Fluticasone is a corticosteroid that reduces airway inflammation and swelling. Salmeterol opens up lung airways.

Common uses
To control symptoms of asthma and improve lung function.

Common side effects
Throat dryness, hoarseness, runny nose, sneezing, a high-pitched noise when breathing, voice changes, trouble swallowing and body aches.

Note
Don't take this medication to relieve an asthma attack that has already started.

Leukotriene blockers

Generic and common brand names
- Montelukast (Singulair)
- Zafirlukast (Accolate)
- Zileuton (Zyflo)

Action
Keep airways open by blocking action or formation of chemicals called leukotrienes.

Common uses
For prevention and long-term treatment of asthma.

Common side effects
Headache and, less commonly, rash, fatigue, dizziness and nausea.

Note
Montelukast should be taken in the evening, and zafirlukast should be taken on an empty stomach.

Mast cell stabilizers

Generic and common brand names
- Cromolyn sodium (Intal)
- Nedocromil sodium (Tilade)

Action
Block the release of histamine and other mast cell chemicals that cause swelling and narrowing of bronchial tubes.

Common uses
To treat mild to moderate asthma and to prevent exercise-induced bronchospasms.

Common side effects
Sore throat, cough, hoarseness, sneezing and bad taste from the aerosol spray.

Note
A few swallows of water can lessen sore throat and hoarseness. Don't use these medications in emergency situations.

Methylxanthines

Generic and common brand names
- Theophylline (Elixophyllin, Uniphyl)

Action
Increase the chemical cyclic AMP that relaxes bronchial muscles, relieving bronchospasms and increasing lung capacity.

Common uses
To relieve shortness of breath and wheezing associated with asthma.

Common side effects
Nervousness, rapid heart rate, insomnia and increased urination.

Note
A test that measures the amount of theophylline in your blood can help determine the right dose for you.

Blood pressure medications

Alpha blockers

Generic and common brand names
- Doxazosin (Cardura)
- Prazosin (Minipress)
- Terazosin (Hytrin)

Action
Block the central nervous system from stimulating muscles that constrict smaller arteries and raise blood pressure.

Common uses
To treat high blood pressure and symptoms caused by benign enlargement of the prostate gland.

Common side effects
Dizziness, headache, rapidly pounding heart, nausea and weakness.

Note
Standing up slowly after lying or sitting will help reduce dizziness.

Angiotensin-converting enzyme (ACE) inhibitors

Generic and common brand names
- Benazepril (Lotensin)
- Captopril (Capoten)
- Enalapril (Vasotec)
- Fosinopril (Monopril)
- Lisinopril (Prinivil, Zestril)
- Moexipril (Univasc)
- Quinapril (Accupril)
- Ramipril (Altace)
- Trandolapril (Mavik)

Action
Block production of a substance called angiotensin II, which narrows your blood vessels and causes you to retain salt and fluids, increasing blood pressure. These medications also enhance the action of a compound called bradykinin, which opens blood vessels.

Common uses
To treat high blood pressure. Some ACE inhibitors are also used to

treat congestive heart failure or kidney disease and to prevent recurrent heart attacks and strokes. These medications also help prevent or reduce complications of diabetes.

Common side effects
Dry cough, swelling of the face, rash, altered sense of taste, reduced appetite, dizziness, sunlight sensitivity and increased potassium in blood.

Note
Notify your doctor immediately if you notice swelling in your face or lips. Don't take these medications if you're pregnant or plan to become pregnant. The drugs can cause serious birth defects.

Angiotensin II receptor blockers

Generic and common brand names
- Candesartan (Atacand)
- Eprosartan (Teveten)
- Irbesartan (Avapro)
- Losartan (Cozaar)
- Telmisartan (Micardis)
- Valsartan (Diovan)

Action
Prevent angiotensin II from binding to tissues, inhibiting blood vessel narrowing and retention of salt and fluids.

Common uses
To treat high blood pressure, kidney failure and congestive heart failure, and to prevent stroke.

Common side effects
Dizziness, nasal congestion, musculoskeletal pain, indigestion, coughing and insomnia.

Note
These medications have less of a tendency to cause coughing compared with ACE inhibitors. Don't take these drugs if you're pregnant or planning to become pregnant because they can cause birth defects.

Beta blockers

Generic and common brand names
- Acebutolol (Sectral)
- Atenolol (Tenormin)
- Betaxolol (Kerlone)
- Bisoprolol (Zebeta)
- Carteolol (Cartrol)
- Carvedilol (Coreg)
- Metoprolol (Lopressor, Toprol)
- Nadolol (Corgard)
- Penbutolol (Levatol)
- Pindolol (Visken)
- Propranolol (Inderal)

Action
Interfere with the response of certain nerve impulses in parts of the body, decreasing the heart's need for blood and oxygen and thereby reducing its workload.

Common uses
To treat high blood pressure. Some beta blockers are also used to treat heart attacks, angina and anxiety and to prevent heart attacks, heart failure and migraine.

Common side effects
Fatigue, a reduced capacity for strenuous physical activities, cold hands, trouble sleeping, impotence and loss of sex drive.

Note
These drugs may aggravate asthma and diabetes.

Calcium channel blockers

Generic and common brand names
- Amlodipine (Norvasc)
- Diltiazem (Cardizem, Dilacor XR, Tiazac)
- Felodipine (Plendil)
- Isradipine (DynaCirc)
- Nicardipine (Cardene)
- Nifedipine (Adalat, Procardia)
- Nisoldipine (Sular)
- Verapamil (Calan, Isoptin, others)

Action
Prevent calcium from flowing through channels in muscle cells. When calcium enters the cell, it causes muscle cells in arteries to contract, narrowing the arteries and increasing blood pressure.

Common uses
To treat high blood pressure. Some calcium channel blockers are also used to treat chest pain (angina) and kidney failure and to prevent repeat heart attacks.

Common side effects
Constipation, headache, rapid heartbeat, rash and swelling in the feet and lower legs.

Note
Don't eat grapefruit or drink grapefruit juice while on these medications. A substance in the juice reduces your liver's ability to eliminate the medications from your body, potentially allowing them to accumulate to toxic levels.

Central-acting agents

Generic and common brand names
- Clonidine (Catapres)
- Guanabenz (Wytensin)
- Guanadrel (Hylorel)
- Guanfacine (Tenex)
- Methyldopa (Aldomet)

Action
Prevent your brain from sending signals to your nervous system to speed up your heart rate and narrow your blood vessels.

Common uses
To treat high blood pressure.

Common side effects
Extreme fatigue, drowsiness, impotence, dry mouth, headache, weight gain and impaired thinking and psychological problems, including depression.

Note
Abruptly stopping some of these drugs can cause your blood pressure to rise to dangerously high levels very quickly.

Diuretics

Generic and common brand names
Loop diuretics
- Bumetanide (Bumex)
- Furosemide (Lasix)
- Torsemide (Demadex)

Potassium-sparing diuretics
- Amiloride (Midamor)
- Eplerenone (Inspra)
- Spironalactone (Aldactone)
- Triamterene (Dyrenium)

Thiazide diuretics
- Chlorothiazide (Diuril)
- Chlorthalidone (Hygroton, Thalitone)
- Hydrochlorothiazide (Hydrodiuril, Microzide, others)
- Indapamide (Lozol)
- Methyclothiazide (Aquatensen, Enduron)
- Metolazone (Mykrox, Zaroxolyn)

Action
Cause your kidneys to excrete more sodium than usual. The sodium takes with it water from your blood. Less blood volume reduces blood pressure. Each class of diuretics works on a different part of your kidney.

Common uses
To treat high blood pressure and reduce swelling caused by accumulation of fluid (edema).

Common side effects
Frequent urination, dehydration, weakness and dizziness when standing.

Note
Reducing sodium and getting ample potassium in your diet will help the drugs work more effectively. Thiazide and loop diuretics can decrease potassium in your body. Therefore, use of these medications may require potassium supplementation.

Cholesterol and triglyceride medications

Bile acid sequestrants

Generic and common brand names
- Cholestyramine (Questran)
- Colesevelam (Welchol)
- Colestipol (Colestid)

Action
Lower cholesterol in your blood by binding with bile acids in your small intestine, tying up the acids and forcing your liver to make more. Bile acids are made from cholesterol.

Common uses
To reduce elevated cholesterol levels.

Common side effects
Bloating, abdominal fullness, constipation, gas, stomach upset and headache.

Note
To avoid drug interactions, inform your doctor of all other medications you take. Don't take bile acid sequestrants within 1 to 2 hours of taking other medicines.

Fibric acid

Generic and common brand names
- Fenofibrate (Tricor)
- Gemfibrozil (Lopid)

Action
Alters the synthesis of blood fats, lowering triglycerides and raising high-density lipoprotein (HDL or "good") cholesterol. Also lowers total cholesterol levels.

Common uses
To lower triglyceride levels in people with too much of this type of blood fat. Also to raise HDL cholesterol levels and reduce total cholesterol levels.

Common side effects
Abdominal pain, nausea, diarrhea, headache and muscle pain.

Note
Contact your doctor promptly if you experience unexplained muscle pain, tenderness or weakness.

Nicotinic acid (niacin)

Brand names
- Niaspan
- Slo-Niacin

Action
Lowers triglyceride levels in blood and raises levels of high-density lipoprotein (HDL or "good") cholesterol.

Common uses
To manage triglycerides and cholesterol in people with elevated levels.

Common side effects
Flushing, dizziness, headache, nausea, vomiting, dry skin and itching.

Note
Talk to your doctor before taking over-the-counter niacin supplements because they can interact with other medications. These medications can occasionally cause drug-induced hepatitis (liver inflammation).

Statins

Generic and common brand names
- Atorvastatin (Lipitor)
- Fluvastatin (Lescol)
- Lovastatin (Mevacor)
- Pravastatin (Pravachol)
- Simvastatin (Zocor)

Action
Decrease cholesterol synthesis and improve removal of low-density lipoprotein (LDL or "bad") cholesterol from blood.

Common uses
To lower total blood cholesterol level in individuals whose levels are abnormal. To increase high-density lipoprotein (HDL or "good") cholesterol in blood and lower total cholesterol.

Common side effects
Muscle pain, headache, nausea, diarrhea and gas.

Note
These medications can cause drug-induced hepatitis (liver inflammation). Therefore, it's important to have periodic blood tests to check liver enzyme levels.

Cold medications

Cough suppressants (antitussives)

Generic and common brand names
- Benzonatate (Tessalon)
- Dextromethorphan (Robitussin)
- Guaifenesin and codeine (Guiatuss AC, Robitussin AC, others)

Action
Relieve coughs by acting directly on the lungs and breathing passages, and perhaps on the cough center in your brain. Or, thin mucus in your lungs to help your lungs clear it out.

Common uses
To treat coughs caused by colds, flu (influenza) or other illnesses.

Common side effects
Drowsiness, weakness, dryness in nose, mouth and throat, constipation, dizziness, nausea and headache.

Note
If your cough lingers for more than a week, consult your doctor. Drink lots of fluids, especially if you're taking an expectorant, such as guaifenesin.

Decongestants

Generic and common brand names
- Oxymetazoline (Afrin, Dristan, others)
- Phenylephrine (Alconefrin, Neo-Synephrine, others)
- Pseudoephedrine (Dimetapp, Sudafed, Triaminic, others)
- Xylometazoline (Inspire, Otrivin, others)

Action
Narrow blood vessels in your nose and sinuses and decrease congestion.

Common uses
To relieve nasal congestion caused by cold, flu (influenza), allergies or sinus infection. These medications may be combined with an antihistamine to further relieve symptoms.

Common side effects
Nervousness, restlessness, anxiety, trouble sleeping and increased heart rate.

Note
If you regularly take a decongestant nasal spray for more than 3 days, you may experience rebound congestion.

Diabetes medications

Alpha-glucosidase inhibitors

Generic and common brand names
- Acarbose (Precose)
- Miglitol (Glyset)

Action
Block action of enzymes in your digestive tract that break down carbohydrates into sugar, delaying the digestion of carbohydrates. Sugar is absorbed into your bloodstream more slowly.

Common uses
To reduce blood sugar (glucose) in people with type 2 diabetes.

Common side effects
Abdominal bloating, gas and diarrhea.

Note
Starting with a low dose and gradually increasing it usually minimizes side effects.

Biguanides

Generic and common brand names
- Metformin (Glucophage)

Action
Reduce the amount of sugar your liver releases into blood and the amount the intestine absorbs. Also, increase insulin sensitivity.

Common uses
To control blood sugar (glucose) in people with type 2 diabetes.

Common side effects
Altered sense of taste, such as a metallic taste, nausea, vomiting or loss of appetite, abdominal discomfort, gas, diarrhea and skin rash.

Note
Metformin can cause a serious condition called lactic acidosis. Lactic acidosis is more likely to occur in people with heart failure, kidney or liver problems or who use alcohol excessively. Risk of the condition also increases with certain medical procedures, such as surgery or X-ray procedures that require use of a contrast dye. Your doctor may ask you to stop taking the drug prior to a medical procedure.

Insulin

Generic and common brand names
- Insulin zinc suspension — Lente (Humulin L, Novolin L, others)
- Insulin zinc suspension, extended — Ultralente (Humulin U)
- Isophane insulin suspension (Humulin N, Novolin N, others)
- Isophane insulin suspension with regular insulin injection (Humulin 50/50, Humulin 70/30, Novolin 70/30)
- Regular insulin (Humulin R, Novolin R, others)

Action
Transports sugar from your bloodstream into individual cells, where it's used as a source of energy.

Common uses
To treat type 1 diabetes and type 2 diabetes.

Common side effects
Low blood sugar and redness and irritation at the injection sites.

Note
Rotate the injection sites to prevent skin side effects.

Insulin analogues

Generic and common brand names
- Insulin aspart (NovoLog)
- Insulin glargine (Lantus)
- Insulin lispro (Humalog)

Action
Transport sugar from your bloodstream into individual cells, where it's used as a source of energy. The onset and duration of these newer types of insulin more closely resemble those of natural insulin.

Common uses
To treat type 1 diabetes and type 2 diabetes.

Common side effects
Low blood sugar, weight gain and irritation at the injection sites.

Note
Insulin lispro and insulin aspart are rapid-acting. Take them just before you eat. Insulin glargine is long-acting.

Meglitinides

Common brand names
- Repaglinide (Prandin)

Action
Cause a rapid, short-lived release of insulin by the pancreas.

Common uses
To reduce blood sugar levels in people with type 2 diabetes.

Common side effects
Low blood sugar, headache, drowsiness, nausea and rash.

Note
Let your doctor know if the medication makes you feel lightheaded, nervous or tired. Your dosage may need adjusting.

Nateglinide

Brand name
- Starlix

Action
Causes a rapid, short-lived release of insulin by the pancreas.

Common uses
To reduce blood sugar (glucose) levels in people with type 2 diabetes.

Common side effects
Low blood sugar, cough, runny or stuffy nose and sore throat.

Note
Don't take other medications unless you have discussed their use with your doctor.

Sulfonylureas

Generic and common brand names
- Chlorpropamide (Diabinese)
- Glimepiride (Amaryl)
- Glipizide (Glucotrol)
- Glyburide (DiaBeta, Glynase, Micronase)
- Tolazamide (Tolinase)
- Tolbutamide (Orinase)

Action
Stimulate beta cells in your pancreas to produce and release more insulin.

Common uses
To reduce blood sugar (glucose) levels in people with type 2 diabetes.

Common side effects
Low blood sugar, dizziness, upset stomach and loss of appetite.

Note
Your risk of low blood sugar levels is greatest the first few months after starting to use the medication.

Thiazolidinediones

Generic and common brand names
- Pioglitazone (Actos)
- Rosiglitazone (Avandia)

Action
Make body tissues more receptive to insulin and increase glucose disposal by the liver.

Common uses
To reduce blood sugar (glucose) levels in people with type 2 diabetes.

Common side effects
Weight gain, fatigue, nausea, abdominal pain, loss of appetite, dark urine and yellowing of the skin and eyes (jaundice).

Note
A rare but serious side effect of thiazolidinediones is liver injury. Have your liver enzymes checked every 2 months during the first year of use of the medication.

Ear medications

Antibiotic and steroid combinations

Generic and common brand names
- Acetic acid and hydrocortisone (Acetasol HC, VoSol HC)
- Ciprofloxacin and hydrocortisone (Cipro HC)
- Neomycin, polymyxin B and hydrocortisone (Cortisporin, Pediotic, others)

Action
Destroy bacteria that cause ear infections and reduce swelling and inflammation.

Common uses
To treat infections of the outer ear canal.

Common side effects
Skin irritation and slight stinging in the ear canal.

Note
To keep the medicine germ-free, don't touch the eardropper to any surface, including the ear canal.

Antibiotics

Generic and common brand names
- Acetic acid and aluminum acetate
- Chloramphenicol (Chloromycetin)
- Neomycin combinations (Coly-Mycin, Cortisporin, others)

Action
Destroy some bacteria that cause external ear infection.

Common uses
To treat infections of the outer ear canal.

Common side effects
Skin irritation or burning or stinging in the ear.

Note
To keep the medicine germ-free, don't touch the eardropper to any surface, including the ear canal.

Pain relievers

Generic and common brand names
- Antipyrine and benzocaine (Allergen, Auralgan, others)

Action
Relieve pain and swelling.

Common uses
To treat symptoms associated with an ear infection. An antibiotic is necessary to treat the infection itself.

Common side effects
Skin irritation or burning or stinging in the ear.

Note
To keep the medicine germ-free, don't touch the eardropper to any surface, including the ear canal.

Eye medications

Alpha-adrenergic agents

Generic and common brand names
- Apraclonidine (Iopidine)
- Brimonidine (Alphagan)

Action
Reduce the production of aqueous humor, which lowers pressure in the eye.

Common uses
To treat glaucoma and other conditions associated with elevated pressure inside the eye.

Common side effects
Red, itchy and teary eyes.

Note
These medications can cause dizziness and drowsiness in some people.

Anti-infectives

Generic and common brand names
- Chloramphenicol (Chloromycetin, Chloroptic, others)
- Ciprofloxacin (Ciloxin)
- Erythromycin (Ilotycin)
- Gentamicin (Garamycin, Genoptic)
- Levofloxacin (Levaquin)
- Neomycin, bacitracin, polymyxin B (Neosporin)
- Norfloxacin (Chibroxin)
- Ofloxacin (Ocuflox)
- Sulfacetamide sodium (Bleph-10)
- Sulfisoxazole (Gantrisin)
- Tobramycin (Tobrex, Tobi)

Action
Kill bacteria that cause eye infections.

Common uses
To treat eye infections, such as conjunctivitis.

Common side effects
Itching, burning eyes and blurred vision.

Note
To avoid contaminating the medicine, wash your hands before using it and don't touch the applicator tip to your hands or eye.

Artificial tears

Generic and common brand names
- Carboxymethylcellulose (Celluvisc, Refresh Plus)
- Hydroxypropyl methylcellulose (Artificial Tears, Goniosol, others)

Action
Lubricate dry eyes with fluid chemically similar to natural tears.

Common uses
To relieve dryness and irritation caused by reduced tear flow.

Common side effects
Eye irritation, blurred vision and matting or stickiness of eyelashes.

Note
To keep the medicine as germ-free as possible, don't touch the applicator tip to your hands or eye.

Beta blockers

Generic and common brand names
- Betaxolol (Betoptic)
- Carteolol (Ocupress)
- Levobunolol (Betagan)
- Metipranolol (Optipranolol)
- Timolol (Betimol, Timoptic)

Action
Reduce the production of aqueous humor, which lowers pressure in your eye.

Common uses
To treat glaucoma and other conditions associated with elevated pressure inside the eye.

Common side effects
Stinging of the eye.

Note
For a short time after using the medication, your vision may be blurred.

Carbonic anhydrase inhibitors

Generic and common brand names
- Acetazolamide (Diamox)
- Brinzolamide (Azopt)
- Dichlorphenamide (Daranide)
- Dorzolamide (Trusopt)
- Methazolamide (Neptazane)

Action
Reduce the secretion of fluid inside the front of the eyeball (aqueous humor), lowering pressure inside the eye.

Common uses
To treat glaucoma and other conditions associated with elevated pressure inside the eye.

Common side effects
Burning in the eyes, blurred vision and a bitter taste. Oral medications can cause a tingling sensation in the fingers and toes, rash, fatigue and stomach upset.

Note
Take oral medication with meals to reduce stomach upset. With eyedrops, don't touch the eyedropper to the eye.

Mast cell stabilizers

Generic and common brand names
- Cromolyn sodium (Crolom, Opticrom)
- Nedocromil (Alocril)

Action
Act on certain inflammatory cells (mast cells) to prevent them from releasing substances that cause itching eyes.

Common uses
To treat eye symptoms associated with allergies.

Common side effects
Blurry vision, change in color vision, difficulty seeing at night, increased sensitivity to sunlight and eyelid swelling.

Note
Don't wear contact lenses when your eyes are itching and irritated.

Mydriatics

Generic and common brand names
- Atropine (Isopto Atropine)
- Homatropine (Isopto Homatropine)
- Scopolamine (Isopto Hyoscine)

Action
Reduce inflammation and relax muscles in the eye, enlarging the pupil.

Common uses
To treat uveitis, an inflammation of the iris and the muscles that control focusing, and to open (dilate) the pupil for eye examinations.

Common side effects
Increased eye sensitivity to light and blurred vision.

Note
After use of the medication, wear sunglasses to protect your eyes from the light.

Prostaglandin analogues and prostamides

Generic and common brand names
- Bimatoprost (Lumigan)
- Latanoprost (Xalatan)
- Travoprost (Travatan)

Action
Increase the outflow of fluid inside the front of the eyeball (aqueous humor), reducing pressure inside the eye.

Common uses
To treat glaucoma and other conditions associated with elevated pressure inside the eye.

Common side effects
Red and itchy eye, blurry vision, darkening of the iris and eyelid skin and increased sensitivity to light.

Note
Bimatoprost and lantanoprost can cause your iris to darken and your eyelashes to become thicker and darker. These changes may be permanent.

Vasoconstrictors

Generic and common brand names
- Naphazoline (Vasoclear, Vasocon)
- Tetrahydrozoline (Murine Plus, Visine)

Action
Constrict the blood vessels of the eye, reducing redness.

Common uses
To relieve redness due to minor irritations of the eye, such as those caused by allergies, dust, smoke and wind.

Common side effects
Stinging of the eyes, dizziness, headache, blurry vision, eye sensitivity to light and watery eyes.

Note
Don't use these medications for more than 3 days at time, and don't use them if you have glaucoma.

Gastrointestinal medications

Acid blockers (histamine blockers)

Generic and common brand names
- Cimetidine (Tagamet)
- Famotidine (Pepcid)
- Nizatidine (Axid)
- Ranitidine (Zantac)

Action
Interfere with the ability of the chemical histamine to stimulate your stomach to release acid.

Common uses
To treat or prevent gastrointestinal disorders, such as gastroesophageal reflux disease (GERD) and ulcers.

Common side effects
Headache, bowel changes, dizziness and drowsiness.

Note
Some of these medications shouldn't be taken with other medications because of the risk of a drug interaction.

Antacids

Generic and common brand names
- Aluminum hydroxide (Alternagel)
- Calcium carbonate (Rolaids, Tums)
- Magaldrate (Riopan)
- Magnesium hydroxide (Milk of Magnesia)
- Products with multiple acid-absorbing chemicals (Gaviscon, Maalox, others)

Action
Neutralize stomach acid.

Common uses
To treat mild heartburn.

Common side effects
Constipation or diarrhea.

Note
If you take some antacids with certain medications, they may reduce the absorption of those medications.

Aminosalicylates

Generic and common brand names
- Balsalazide (Colazal)
- Mesalamine (Asacol, Pentasa, Rowasa)
- Olsalazine (Dipentum)
- Sulfasalazine (Azulfidine)

Action
Reduce inflammation in the small and large intestines by blocking production of certain inflammatory substances.

Common uses
To treat intestinal inflammations, such as ulcerative colitis and Crohn's disease.

Common side effects
Loss of appetite, nausea, vomiting, skin rashes and headache.

Note
Some of these medications come in capsule form. Others are administered as an enema or suppository.

Antidiarrheals

Generic and common brand names
- Attapulgite (Kaopectate)
- Bismuth subsalicylate (Pepto-Bismol)
- Loperamide (Imodium)

Action
Some decrease intestinal secretions, others absorb intestinal secretions, and still others decrease contraction of your intestinal muscles, reducing cramping and diarrhea.

Common uses
To treat diarrhea. Bismuth subsalicylate also helps relieve nausea.

Common side effects
Constipation, temporary stool darkening (with bismuth subsalicylate) and drowsiness.

Note
Don't take bismuth subsalicylate if you're allergic to aspirin.

Antispasmodics

Generic and common brand names
- Dicyclomine (Bentyl, Quentyl)
- Hyoscyamine (Levsin, Levsinex)

Action
Relax intestinal muscles and relieve spasm.

Common uses
To relieve cramps and spasms of the stomach, small intestine and colon.

Common side effects
Headache, dizziness, dry mouth, increased heart rate, constipation and urine retention.

Note
Older adults may experience some confusion or agitation from this type of medication. It can also aggravate glaucoma.

Interferons

Generic and common brand names
- Interferon alfa-2a (Roferon-A)
- Interferon alfa-2b (Intron A)
- Interferon alfacon-1 (Infergen)

Action
Interfere with the growth and replication of the attacking virus.

Common uses
To treat chronic hepatitis. Interferon alfa-2a and interferon alfa-2b are also used to treat certain cancers. Other interferons are used to treat multiple sclerosis and some types of cancer.

Common side effects
Flu-like symptoms, fatigue, depression and reduced white blood cell and platelet counts.

Note
Side effects are more common in older adults.

Laxatives and stool softeners

Generic and common brand names
- Bisacodyl (Correctol, Dulcolax, Fleet, others)*
- Docusate (DSS)
- Methylcellulose (Citrucel)
- Psyllium (Fiberall, Metamucil, others)
- Senna (Senokot)*

*stimulants

Action
Some of these products soften stool by helping fat and liquids mix with the stool or by providing bulk to help the stool pass more easily. Others stimulate bowel muscles to contract and move the stool out. Still others, such as mineral oils, lubricate the stool so that it passes more easily.

Common uses
To treat constipation and to prepare the intestinal tract for certain tests or surgery.

Common side effects
Abdominal cramps, nausea and vomiting

Note
Ask your doctor for advice before taking a laxative. Even some nonprescription laxatives may be harmful. Long-term use of stimulant laxatives may lead to dependency and severe constipation.

Motility agents

Generic and common brand names
- Metoclopramide (Reglan)

Action
Increase the speed of stomach emptying by stimulating muscle contractions.

Common uses
To treat stomach acid reflux and delayed stomach emptying (gastroparesis).

Common side effects
Drowsiness, fatigue, restlessness and, occasionally, breast tenderness and swelling, headache and diarrhea.

Note
This medicine adds to the sedating effects of alcohol and other drugs that depress the central nervous system.

Proton pump inhibitors

Generic and common brand names
- Esomeprazole (Nexium)
- Lansoprazole (Prevacid)
- Omeprazole (Prilosec)
- Pantoprazole (Protonix)
- Rabeprazole (Aciphex)

Action
Block acid secretion by inhibiting an enzyme system in your stomach lining called the proton pump.

Common uses
To treat gastroesophageal reflux disease (GERD) and ulcers.

Common side effects
Abdominal pain, diarrhea, headache and nausea.

Note
These medications are most effective when taken on an empty stomach before meals.

Ulcer-protective agents

Generic and common brand names
- Misoprostol (Cytotec)
- Sucralfate (Carafate)

Action
Misoprostol protects the stomach lining by stimulating mucus and bicarbonate production, forming an alkaline barrier or coating over the lining. Sucralfate coats an ulcer, providing a barrier against stomach acid.

Common uses
To prevent or treat peptic ulcers.

Common side effects
Diarrhea, stomach pain, indigestion and gas. Constipation is the most frequent complaint with sucralfate.

Note
Don't take antacids 30 minutes before or after taking sucralfate. They may keep the medication from working properly. Misoprostol can cause birth defects if taken during pregnancy.

Heart medications

Angiotensin-converting enzyme (ACE) inhibitors

Generic and common brand names
- Benazepril (Lotensin)
- Captopril (Capoten)
- Enalapril (Vasotec)
- Fosinopril (Monopril)
- Lisinopril (Prinivil, Zestril)
- Moexipril (Univasc)
- Quinapril (Accupril)
- Ramipril (Altace)
- Trandolapril (Mavik)

Action
Block production of angiotensin II, which constricts blood vessels, causing retention of salt and fluids and formation of fibrous tissue (fibrosis).

Common uses
To treat congestive heart failure, high blood pressure and kidney disease and to prevent recurrent heart attacks and strokes. These medications help prevent or reduce complications of diabetes.

Common side effects
Dry cough, swelling of the face, rash, altered sense of taste, reduced appetite, dizziness, sunlight sensitivity and increased potassium in the blood.

Note
Notify your doctor immediately if you notice swelling in your face or lips. Don't take these medications if you're pregnant or plan to become pregnant. The drugs can cause serious birth defects.

Anti-arrhythmics

Generic and common brand names
- Amiodarone (Cordarone, Pacerone)
- Disopyramide (Norpace)
- Dofetilide (Tikosyn)
- Flecainide (Tambocor)
- Mexiletine (Mexitil)
- Procainamide (Procanbid, Pronestyl, others)
- Propafenone (Rythmol)
- Quinidine (Cardioquin, Quinidex, others)
- Toncainide (Tonocard)

Action
Delay electric impulses through the nerves and muscle of the heart, helping to restore and maintain normal heart rate and rhythm.

Common uses
To correct irregular or rapid heartbeats (arrhythmias).

Common side effects
Dry mouth, constipation, dizziness, blurred vision and reduced urination.

Note
Amiodarone can be associated with thyroid and lung dysfunction, therefore, it's important to see a doctor regularly if taking this medication.

Anticoagulants (injected)

Generic and common brand names
- Dalteparin (Fragmin)
- Danaparoid (Orgaran)
- Enoxaparin (Lovenox)
- Heparin

Action
Prevent the activation of clotting factors, proteins that are essential for normal blood clotting. Injected anticoagulants work more quickly than oral anticoagulants.

Common uses
To treat circulatory disorders such as deep vein thrombosis. Also commonly used after surgeries or during hospitalizatin to prevent blood clotting.

Common side effects
Easy bruising and bleeding and irritation at the injection site.

Note
Low molecular weight heparin (dalteparin, danaparoid, enoxaparin) may be prescribed on an outpatient basis for certain individuals who have blood clots in the leg (deep vein thrombosis) and are capable of giving themselves daily injections of the drug.

Anticoagulants (oral)

Generic and common brand names
- Warfarin (Coumadin)

Action
Decrease the formation of clotting factors, proteins that are essential for normal blood clotting. Often referred to as blood thinners, though they don't actually thin the blood.

Common uses
To reduce risk of heart attack and stroke in people with artificial heart valves, irregular heart rhythms and blood-clotting disorders.

Common side effects
Easy bruising, bleeding, rashes and diarrhea.

Note
Check with your doctor before taking other medications to avoid harmful interactions. Dosage may need to be adjusted depending on the amount of vitamin K in your diet. Watch for bruising and bleeding.

Antiplatelet drugs

Generic and common brand names
- Aspirin (Bayer, Bufferin, others)
- Clopidogrel (Plavix)
- Dipyridamole (Persantine)

Action
Reduce blood clotting by inhibiting the ability of platelets to cross-link, forming blood clots.

Common uses
To help prevent blood clots, reducing your risk of heart attack and stroke.

Common side effects
Prolonged bleeding after an injury, stomach irritation, abdominal cramps, diarrhea and dizziness.

Note
Talk with your doctor or pharmacist before you take any nonprescription medicine.

Beta blockers

Generic and common brand names
- Acebutolol (Sectral)
- Atenolol (Tenormin)
- Carvedilol (Coreg)
- Metoprolol (Lopressor, Toprol)
- Nadolol (Corgard)
- Propranolol (Inderal)

Action
Block beta adrenergic receptors in certain parts of the body, decreasing the heart's need for blood and oxygen and reducing its workload.

Common uses
To treat high blood pressure, chest pain (angina), some arrhythmias and congestive heart failure and to prevent a repeat heart attack or stroke.

Common side effects
Fatigue, a reduced capacity for strenuous physical activities, cold hands, trouble sleeping, impotence, loss of sex drive, shortness of breath and wheezing.

Note
These medications can cause worsening of symptoms in people with asthma.

Calcium channel blockers

Generic and common brand names
- Amlodipine (Norvasc)
- Diltiazem (Cardizem, Dilacor XR, Tiazac)
- Nicardipine (Cardene)
- Nifedipine (Adalat, Procardia)
- Verapamil (Calan, Isoptin, others)

Action
Prevent calcium from flowing through channels in muscle cells. When calcium enters muscle cells in arteries, it causes the arteries to contract, narrowing them and increasing blood pressure.

Common uses
To treat high blood pressure, arrhythmias, chest pain (angina), coronary artery spasm and kidney

failure. Sometimes used to prevent a repeat heart attack.

Common side effects
Constipation, headache, rapid heartbeat, rash, swelling in the feet and lower legs.

Note
Don't eat grapefruit or drink grapefruit juice while on these medications. A substance in the juice reduces your liver's ability to break down these medications, allowing the drugs to potentially accumulate to toxic levels.

Digitalis

Generic and common brand names
- Digoxin (Lanoxicaps, Lanoxin)

Action
Increases the force of your heart muscle contractions and delays electric impulses through the nerves and muscle of your heart.

Common uses
To improve heart strength and efficiency in people with congestive heart failure and to control heart rate and rhythm, improving blood circulation and reducing swelling (edema).

Common side effects
Anxiety, blurred vision, confusion, dizziness, depression, headache, nausea, gastrointestinal discomfort and loss of appetite.

Note
It's important that this medication be taken exactly as recommended by your doctor. Stopping its use suddenly can cause a serious change in heart function.

Diuretics

Generic and common brand names
Loop diuretics
- Bumetanide (Bumex)
- Furosemide (Lasix)
- Torsemide (Demadex)

Potassium-sparing diuretics
- Amiloride (Midamor)
- Eplerenone (Inspra)
- Spironalactone (Aldactone)
- Triamterene (Dyrenium)

Thiazide diuretics
- Chlorothiazide (Diuril)
- Chlorthalidone (Hygroton, Thalitone)
- Hydrochlorothiazide (Hydrodiuril, Microzide, others)
- Indapamide (Lozol)
- Methyclothiazide (Aquatensen, Enduron)
- Metolazone (Mykrox, Zaroxolyn)

Action
Cause your kidneys to excrete more sodium than usual, taking with it water from your blood. Less blood volume can lower blood pressure. Each class of diuretics works on different parts of your kidneys.

Common uses
To treat high blood pressure and reduce accumulation of fluid (edema) associated with congestive heart failure.

Common side effects
Increased urination, weakness, dizziness while standing, thirst and dehydration.

Note
Reducing sodium and making sure that you have ample potassium in your diet will help the drugs work more effectively. Thiazide and loop diuretics can decrease potassium in your body, so you may need potassium supplementation.

Nitrates

Generic and common brand names
- Isosorbide dinitrate (Isordil, Sorbitrate, others)
- Isosorbide mononitrate (Imdur, Ismo)
- Sublingual nitroglycerin (Nitrogard, Nitrostat, others)

Action
Dilate your blood vessels, increasing blood and oxygen to your heart and reducing your heart's workload. Also dilate the veins, reducing the return of blood to the heart.

Common uses
To treat chest pain (angina) and to prevent angina attacks.

Common side effects
Headache, blurred vision, dry mouth, lightheadedness, skin flushing and rash.

Note
Keep sublingual nitroglycerin in the original bottle and put that bottle in a container or location that protects it from sunlight. Replace every 3 to 6 months to ensure a fresh supply. When taking sublingual nitrates, always be seated and don't attempt to drive or operate dangerous equipment because fainting is possible. Call for emergency help if your symptoms persist after two doses of sublingual nitroglycerin or if they last longer than 20 minutes.

HIV and AIDS medications

HIV protease inhibitors

Generic and common brand names
- Amprenavir (Agenerase)
- Indinavir (Crixivan)
- Nelfinavir (Viracept)
- Ritonavir (Norvir)
- Ritonavir and lopinavir (Kaletra)
- Saquinavir (Fortovase, Invirase)

Action
Block the HIV enzyme (protease) to keep the virus from maturing.

Common uses
To treat HIV infection.

Common side effects
Nausea, abdominal pain, diarrhea, headache and rash.

Note
It's critical that you take doses precisely as scheduled.

Non-nucleoside reverse transcriptase inhibitors

Generic and common brand names
- Delavirdine (Rescriptor)
- Efavirenz (Sustiva)
- Nevirapine (Viramune)

Action
Interrupt an early stage of HIV replication, reducing the severity and extent of HIV infection.

Common uses
To treat HIV infection.

Common side effects
Rash, itching, headache, fatigue, dizziness, insomnia and liver inflammation.

Note
To get the full effect from the medication, it's important that you take doses precisely as scheduled.

Nucleoside reverse transcriptase inhibitors

Generic and common brand names
- Abacavir (Ziagen)
- Abacavir, lamivudine and zidovudine (Trizivir)
- Didanosine (Videx)
- Lamivudine (Epivir)
- Stavudine (Zerit)
- Tenofovir (Viread)
- Zalcitabine (Hivid)
- Zidovudine (Retrovir)
- Zidovudine and lamivudine (Combivir)

Action
Interrupt an early stage of HIV replication to limit the severity and extent of HIV infection.

Common uses
To treat HIV infection. Lamivudine is also used to treat hepatitis B infection.

Common side effects
Stomach pain, diarrhea, nausea, vomiting, headache, dizziness, rash, itching, dry mouth and altered sense of taste.

Note
To get the maximum benefit from the medication, it's critical that you take doses precisely as scheduled.

Impotence medications

Alprostadil

Common brand names
- Caverject
- Muse

Action
Relaxes smooth muscle tissue in the penis, increasing blood flow to the penis.

Common uses
To induce and help maintain erections in men with erectile dysfunction.

Common side effects
Penile pain and a prolonged erection. Caverject may cause bruising at the injection site, and Muse may cause burning with urination.

Note
Both medications require manual dexterity for their appropriate use.

Sildenafil

Brand name
- Viagra

Action
Delay the action of an enzyme called phosphodiesterase, which works on the penis.

Common uses
To help maintain erections in men with erectile dysfunction.

Common side effects
Flushing, nasal congestion, headache, stomach upset and a blue-green haze to vision.

Note
This medication shouldn't be taken by men who take nitroglycerine-types of medication or who have significant coronary artery disease.

Medications that prevent blood clotting

Antiplatelet drugs

Generic and common brand names
- Aspirin (Bayer, Bufferin, others)
- Clopidogrel (Plavix)
- Dipyridamole (Persantine)

Action
Reduce blood clotting by blocking the activation and accumulation of blood platelets, which help form blood clots.

Common uses
To help prevent blood clots, reducing your risk of heart attack and stroke.

Common side effects
Prolonged bleeding after an injury, stomach irritation, abdominal cramps, diarrhea and dizziness.

Note
Talk with your doctor or a pharmacist before you take any non-prescription medicine.

Injected anticoagulants

Generic and common brand names
- Dalteparin (Fragmin)
- Danaparoid (Orgaran)
- Enoxaparin (Lovenox)
- Heparin

Action
Prevent the activation of clotting factors, proteins that are essential for normal blood clotting. Injected anticoagulants work more quickly than oral anticoagulants.

Common uses
To treat circulatory disorders such as deep vein thrombosis. Also used after surgeries or during hospitalization to prevent blood clotting.

Common side effects
Easy bruising and bleeding and irritation at the injection site.

Note
Low molecular weight heparin (dalteparin, danaparoid, enoxaparin) may be prescribed on an outpatient basis for certain individuals who have blood clots in the leg (deep vein thrombosis) and are capable of giving themselves daily injections of the drug.

Oral anticoagulants

Generic and common brand names
- Warfarin (Coumadin)

Action
Decrease the formation of clotting factors, proteins that are essential for normal blood clotting. Often referred to as blood thinners, though they don't actually thin the blood.

Common uses
To reduce risk of heart attack and stroke in people with artificial heart valves, irregular heart rhythms and blood-clotting disorders.

Common side effects
Easy bruising, bleeding, rashes and diarrhea.

Note
Check with your doctor before taking other medications to avoid harmful interactions. Dosage may need to be adjusted depending on the amount of vitamin K in your diet. Watch for bruising and bleeding.

Medications that relieve inflammation

Corticosteroids

Inhalers
See *Asthma medications*

Nasal sprays
See *Allergy medications*

Oral corticosteroids

Generic and common brand names
- Betamethasone (Celestone)
- Cortisone
- Dexamethasone (Decadron)
- Hydrocortisone (Cortef, Hydrocortone)
- Methylprednisolone (Medrol)
- Prednisolone (Pediapred)
- Prednisone (Deltasone, Sterapred, others)
- Triamcinolone (Aristocort)

Action
Decrease the inflammatory process by blocking the natural defensive function of white blood cells.

Common uses
To treat a wide variety of allergic and inflammatory conditions, such as asthma, skin disorders and arthritis.

Common side effects
Increased appetite, water retention, weight gain, elevated blood sugar (glucose), difficulty sleeping, muscle weakness and mild euphoria.

Note
After prolonged use of one of these medications, sudden withdrawal from it can be dangerous. You need to be gradually weaned from the drug.

Topical corticosteroids

Generic and common brand names
- Alclometasone (Aclovate)
- Betamethasone (Diprolene)
- Desonide (DesOwen)
- Fluocinonide (Lidex)
- Halobetasol (Ultravate)
- Hydrocortisone (Cortizone-10, Hytone)
- Mometasone (Elocon)
- Triamcinolone (Aristocort, Kenalog)

Action
Reduce inflammation by slowing the reaction of cells to substances that trigger inflammation.

Common uses
To treat skin disorders, such as eczema, which cause inflammation and itching.

Common side effects
Thinning of the skin and increased susceptibility to bruising with long-term use.

Note
Apply a thin film sparingly. Avoid putting the medication in sensitive areas, such as your eyes, mucous membranes, groin and armpits.

COX-2 inhibitors

Generic and common brand names
- Celecoxib (Celebrex)
- Rofecoxib (Vioxx)
- Valdecoxib (Bextra)

Action
Inhibit an enzyme in your body called cyclooxygenase-2 (COX-2). This enzyme makes hormone-like substances called prostaglandins, which are involved in the development of inflammation and pain.

Common uses
To treat pain caused by inflammation, such as that of arthritis.

Common side effects
Diarrhea, indigestion, nausea and headache.

Note
These medications may be less damaging to the stomach than are aspirin and other NSAIDs.

Nonsteroidal anti-inflammatory drugs (NSAIDs)

Generic and common brand names
- Diclofenac sodium (Voltaren)
- Etodolac (Lodine)
- Fenoprofen (Nalfon)
- Flurbiprofen (Ansaid)
- Ibuprofen (Advil, Motrin, others)
- Indomethacin (Indocin)
- Ketoprofen (Orudis)
- Ketorolac tromethamine (Toradol)

- Meloxicam (Mobic)
- Nabumetone (Relafen)
- Naproxen (Aleve, Naprosyn, others)
- Oxaprozin (Daypro)
- Piroxicam (Feldene)
- Sulindac (Clinoril)

Action
Relieve pain by blocking an enzyme in your body called cyclooxygenase-2 (COX-2). This enzyme makes substances called prostaglandins, which are involved in the development of inflammation and pain.

Common uses
To treat pain caused by inflammation and swelling, such as arthritis and tendinitis.

Common side effects
Nausea, stomach pain, stomach bleeding and ulcers.

Note
Many nonprescription pain relievers contain NSAIDs. Talk with your doctor or pharmacist to make sure you aren't double dosing.

Salicylates

Common brand names
- Aspirin (Bayer, Bufferin, others)
- Choline salicylate (Arthropan)
- Diflunisal (Dolobid)
- Magnesium salicylate (Doan's pills, Mobidin, others)
- Salsalate (Disalcid)

Action
Inhibit the synthesis of prostaglandins, chemicals in the body that produce inflammation. Specific types of NSAIDs.

Common uses
To treat mild pain caused by inflammation, such as with arthritis, and to control fever. Aspirin helps prevent blood clots, reducing the risk of heart attack and stroke.

Common side effects
Stomach irritation, prolonged bleeding after an injury, skin rash and ringing in the ears.

Note
Intestinal tract irritation and bleeding can occur if aspirin is taken regularly. Alcohol use with aspirin increases the risk of intestinal problems.

Medications that suppress the immune system

Corticosteroids

Generic and common brand names
- Dexamethasone (Decadron)
- Hydrocortisone (Cortef, Hydrocortone)
- Methylprednisolone (Medrol)
- Prednisolone (Pediapred)
- Prednisone (Deltasone, Sterapred)
- Triamcinolone (Aristocort)

Action
Modify the body's immune response in multiple ways, including blocking certain white blood cells (lymphocytes) from multiplying, which prevents them from attacking elements that they consider to be foreign invaders.

Common uses
To suppress your immune system in order to keep your body from

Aspirin's Wide Range of Uses

Aspirin is a powerful medication with a wide range of uses, yet it's often taken for granted as a mere fever reducer, headache tamer or arthritis soother.

Aspirin also helps to prevent heart attack and stroke. According to the American Heart Association, chewing an aspirin at the first sign of a heart attack, such as chest pain, could save 5,000 to 10,000 lives each year. Because aspirin makes your blood less likely to clot, it lowers your risk of an obstructed coronary artery. Chewing the aspirin gets the medicine into your bloodstream faster.

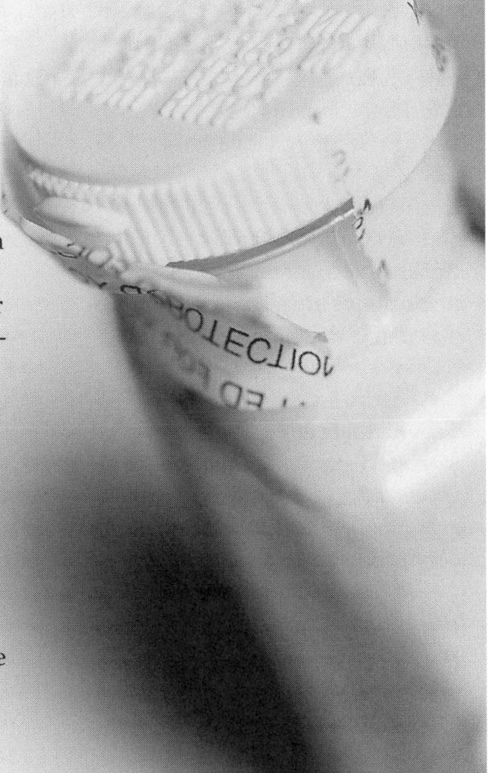

What is aspirin?
Aspirin is acetylsalicylic acid. This natural substance comes from the bark of willow trees. Aspirin is referred to in medical terms as an analgesic (pain reliever) and a nonsteroidal anti-inflammatory drug (NSAID).

Side effects
With its many benefits, aspirin also carries some potentially serious side effects: stomach irritation, gastrointestinal bleeding and urinary tract bleeding. In children it can cause Reye's syndrome. If you take aspirin regularly, talk to your doctor about ways to reduce its side effects.

rejecting a newly transplanted organ. Also used for allergic and inflammatory conditions.

Common side effects
Increased appetite, water retention, weight gain, elevated blood sugar, difficulty sleeping and muscle weakness.

Note
These medications can make you more susceptible to viral, bacterial and fungal infections. When taking them, protect yourself by washing your hands frequently and thoroughly and avoiding contact with people who are sick.

Immunosuppressants

Generic and common brand names
- Azathioprine (Imuran)
- Basiliximab (Simulect)
- Cyclosporine (Neoral, Sandimmune)
- Daclizumab (Zenapax)
- Mycophenolate (CellCept)
- Sirolimus (Rapamune)
- Tacrolimus (Prograf)

Action
Block certain white blood cells (lymphocytes) from being activated, preventing them from attacking elements that they consider to be foreign invaders.

Common uses
To keep your body from rejecting a transplanted organ. Some of these medications are also used to treat severe rheumatoid arthritis and psoriasis.

Common side effects
Increased susceptibility to infections, shaking, excessive hair growth, increased blood pressure, confusion and seizures.

Note
When you're using this type of medication, your body is less able to resist infections, so see your doctor immediately if you become ill.

Medications to treat infection (antimicrobials)

Antibiotics

Aminoglycosides

Generic and common brand names
- Amikacin (Amikin)
- Gentamicin (Garamycin)
- Kanamycin (Kantrex)
- Neomycin

Action
Bind with the bacteria's microscopic building blocks (ribosomes), interfering with the bacteria's growth process and thereby eliminating bacterial cells.

Common uses
To treat many bacterial infections, including skin, eye and intestinal infections.

Common side effects
Topical medications and eardrops may cause skin irritation. Side effects of intravenous (IV) and oral drugs include loss of appetite, nausea, vomiting, hearing problems (tinnitus), clumsiness or unsteadiness and dizziness.

Note
Serious side effects of IV and oral drugs are more likely among older adults and children.

Cephalosporins

Generic and common brand names
- Cefaclor (Ceclor)
- Cefadroxil (Duricef)
- Cefdinir (Omnicef)
- Cefixime (Suprax)
- Cefpodoxime (Vantin)
- Cefprozil (Cefzil)
- Ceftibuten (Cedax)
- Cefuroxime (Ceftin)
- Cephalexin (Keflex)
- Loracarbef (Lorabid)

Action
Kill certain bacteria by interfering with each cell's ability to produce protective cell walls as they grow.

Common uses
To treat many bacterial infections, especially of the skin, soft tissues and respiratory tract.

Common side effects
Nausea, abdominal pain, diarrhea and rash.

Note
Inform your doctor of any drug allergies, especially to penicillin, before taking these drugs. People with serious allergic reactions to penicillin also may be allergic to these medications.

Fluoroquinolones

Generic and common brand names
- Ciprofloxacin (Cipro)
- Gatifloxacin (Tequin)
- Levofloxacin (Levaquin)
- Moxifloxacin (Avelox)
- Norfloxacin (Noroxin)
- Ofloxacin (Floxin)

Action
Block bacterial DNA enzyme needed for reproduction and repair, stopping growth of the bacteria.

Common uses
To treat bacterial infections that tend to be resistant to commonly used antibiotics. Infections that may be treated effectively with these medications include those affecting the urinary tract, prostate, sinuses and lungs, as well as gonorrhea and chlamydial infections and complicated skin, soft tissue and bone infections.

Common side effects
Nausea, diarrhea, abdominal pain, headache and rash.

Note
Don't take aluminum- or magnesium-containing antacids or the drug sucralfate (Carafate) at the same time you take this medication. These drugs can interfere with absorption of fluoroquinolones.

Macrolides and ketolides

Generic and common brand names
- Azithromycin (Zithromax)
- Clarithromycin (Biaxin)
- Erythromycin (Erygel, Erythrocin, others)
- Telithromycin (Ketek)

Action
Interfere with bacteria's formation of essential proteins, preventing growth and multiplication of cells.

Common uses
To treat bacterial infections, such as strep throat, pneumonia, Legionnaires' disease and some sexually transmitted diseases (STDs). Azithromycin and clarithromycin are effective against certain bacterial infections in people with AIDS.

Common side effects
Nausea, vomiting, diarrhea, abdominal pain and headache.

Note
People with severe liver disease may have an increased risk of side effects. Erythromycin and clarithromycin can cause significant drug interactions. Discuss this with your doctor.

Metronidazole

Common brand names
- Flagyl
- MetroCream
- MetroGel

Action
Destroys bacteria or protozoa causing an infection.

Common uses
To treat certain sexually transmitted diseases (STDs) and some gastrointestinal infections.

Common side effects
Oral preparations may cause diarrhea, lightheadedness, headache, nausea and abdominal pain. Gels or creams may cause itching or vaginal discharge.

Note
If you experience stomach upset with an oral form of this medication, try taking it at mealtime. Refrain from using alcohol while taking oral metronidazole.

Penicillins

Generic and common brand names
- Amoxicillin (Amoxil, Trimox)
- Amoxicillin and clavulanate (Augmentin)
- Ampicillin (Omnipen, Principen)
- Bacampicillin (Spectrobid)
- Carbenicillin (Geocillin)
- Cloxacillin
- Dicloxacillin (Dynapen)
- Nafcillin (Unipen)
- Oxacillin
- Penicillin V (Veetids)

Action
Kill many bacteria by interfering with cells' ability to produce protective cell walls as they grow.

Common uses
To treat many bacterial infections, including those of the skin and soft tissues and upper and lower respiratory tract (strep throat, ear infections, pneumonia and sinusitis).

Common side effects
Nausea, diarrhea, abdominal pain and vomiting.

Note
Don't take any of these drugs if you've had an allergic reaction to any kind of penicillin.

Sulfonamides

Generic and common brand names
- Silver sulfadiazine (Silvadene)
- Sulfamethoxazole
- Sulfisoxazole
- Trimethoprim and sulfamethoxazole (Bactrim, Septra)

Action
Stop growth and reproduction of microorganisms by interfering with formation of folate, an essential nutrient for these organisms.

Common uses
To treat urinary tract infections, sinusitis, ear infections and, in some individuals, respiratory infections.

Common side effects
Rashes, itching, headache, dizziness and ringing in the ears.

Note
Some of these drugs may increase your sensitivity to sunlight and may produce allergic reactions.

Tetracycline

Generic and common brand names
- Doxycycline (Doryx, Vibramycin, others)
- Minocycline (Minocin)
- Tetracycline (Achromycin V, Sumycin)

Action
Interfere with production of proteins needed for replication of certain microorganisms.

Common uses
To treat a variety of infections, such as respiratory tract infections, skin infections, chlamydial infections and tick-borne diseases. Doxycycline may be prescribed to travelers to prevent malaria.

Common side effects
Rash, itching, abdominal pain, diarrhea, sore throat and increased sensitivity to sunlight.

Note
Antacids, calcium and dairy products can decrease absorption of tetracyclines. Medications can cause birth defects if taken during pregnancy. In children under age 8, the medications can cause permanent discoloration of teeth.

Antifungals

Generic and common brand names
- Flucytosine (Ancobon)
- Fluconazole (Diflucan)
- Griseofulvin (Fulvicin, Grisactin, others)

- Itraconazole (Sporanox)
- Ketoconazole (Nizoral)
- Nystatin (Mycostatin)
- Terbinafine (Lamisil)

Action
Kill fungi by damaging cell walls and blocking enzymes necessary for growth and reproduction.

Common uses
To treat serious fungal infections as well as fungal nail disease and yeast infections.

Common side effects
Oral medications may cause nausea, headache, diarrhea and rash.

Note
Mothers who are breast-feeding shouldn't use an antifungal drug because it'll show up in breast milk. For treatment of nail infections, you may need to take the medication for months. Some antifungals, especially itraconazole and terbinafine, can cause liver damage.

Antivirals

Generic and common brand names
- Acyclovir (Zovirax)
- Amantadine (Symmetrel)
- Famciclovir (Famvir)
- Ganciclovir (Cytovene)
- Oseltamivir (Tamiflu)
- Penciclovir (Denavir)
- Ribavirin (Virazole)
- Rimantadine (Flumadine)
- Valacyclovir (Valtrex)
- Valganciclovir (Valcyte)
- Zanamivir (Relenza)

Action
Block viruses from entering cells and inhibit viruses from replicating.

Common uses
To treat infections caused by certain viruses, such as chickenpox (varicella), shingles, flu (influenza), herpes and cytomegalovirus.

Common side effects
Nausea, vomiting, diarrhea, dizziness and weakness.

Note
Older adults taking amantidine may experience confusion and agitation.

Medications to treat mental illness

Antipsychotics

Generic and common brand names
- Chlorpromazine (Thorazine)
- Clozapine (Clozaril)
- Fluphenazine (Prolixin)
- Haloperidol (Haldol)
- Molindone (Moban)
- Olanzapine (Zyprexa)
- Perphenazine (Trilafon)
- Prochlorperazine (Compazine)
- Quetiapine (Seroquel)
- Risperidone (Risperdal)
- Thioridazine (Mellaril)
- Thiothixene (Navane)
- Trifluoperazine (Stelazine)
- Ziprasidone (Geodon)

Action
Block the effects of the brain chemical dopamine, which is associated with psychosis.

Common uses
To treat psychotic mental illnesses, such as schizophrenia, some forms of manic-depressive illness and severe depression with psychosis.

Common side effects
Weight gain, dry mouth, blurred vision, constipation, drowsiness and increased tendency to sunburn.

Note
Clozapine requires strict monitoring due to potentially dangerous side effects.

Benzodiazepines

Generic and common brand names
- Alprazolam (Xanax)
- Chlordiazepoxide (Librium)
- Clonazepam (Klonopin)
- Diazepam (Valium)
- Lorazepam (Ativan)

Action
Slow down (sedate) the central nervous system by increasing the activity of the neurotransmitter gamma aminobutyric (GABA).

Common uses
To treat anxiety. Some benzodiazepines may be taken for short periods to help promote sleep.

Common side effects
Drowsiness, dizziness, imbalance and reduced muscle coordination.

Note
Prolonged use can lead to dependence on the medication. Alcohol can magnify the sedating effects of the medication.

Beta blockers

Generic and common brand names
- Propranolol (Inderal)

Action
Reduce the effect of the hormone adrenaline.

Common uses
To treat high blood pressure and some heart-related disorders and to control anxiety.

Common side effects
Fatigue, cold hands, trouble sleeping, impotence and loss of sex drive.

Note
The medication may aggravate asthma and diabetes.

Monoamine oxidase inhibitors

Generic and common brand names
- Phenelzine (Nardil)
- Tranylcypromine (Parnate)

Action
Block the action of enzymes inside nerve cells that break down the brain chemicals norepinephrine and serotonin.

Common uses
To treat depression.

Common side effects
Headache, increased blood pressure and increased heart rate.

Note
Food and drug interactions are a serious concern. Foods that contain a high level of the amino acid tyramine, such as cheese and wine, can interact with monoamine oxidase inhibitors to cause a severe increase in blood pressure.

Mood stabilizers

Generic and common brand names
- Lithium (Eskalith, Lithobid)

Action
Produce brain chemical changes that help curb mania, ease sadness and prevent extreme mood changes.

Common uses
To treat bipolar disorder.

Common side effects
Nausea, diarrhea, fatigue, confusion and trembling of the hands.

Note
Certain medications can increase lithium levels in the bloodstream. They include nonsteroidal anti-inflammatory drugs (NSAIDs) and some high blood pressure medications.

Selective serotonin reuptake inhibitors (SSRIs)

Generic and common brand names
- Citalopram (Celexa)
- Escitalopram (Lexapro)
- Fluoxetine (Prozac)
- Fluvoxamine (Luvox)
- Paroxetine (Paxil)
- Sertraline (Zoloft)

Action
Increase levels of the brain chemical serotonin.

Common uses
To treat depression, anxiety and obsessive-compulsive disorder.

Common side effects
Diarrhea, nausea, headache, drowsiness, insomnia, dry mouth, decreased libido, inability to reach orgasm, impotence, sweating, tremor and decreased appetite.

Note
May take 2 to 3 weeks for the medication to begin working, possibly longer in those with obsessive-compulsive disorder.

Tricyclic and tetracyclic antidepressants

Generic and common brand names
- Amitriptyline (Elavil)
- Clomipramine (Anafranil)
- Desipramine (Norpramin)
- Doxepin (Sinequan)
- Imipramine (Tofranil)
- Maprotiline
- Mirtazapine (Remeron)
- Nortriptyline (Aventyl, Pamelor)
- Protriptyline (Vivactil)
- Trimipramine (Surmontil)

Action
Increase levels of the brain chemicals noradrenaline and serotonin, among multiple other actions.

Common uses
To treat depression. Some medications are used to treat anxiety and obsessive-compulsive disorder.

Common side effects
Drowsiness, dry mouth, dizziness, blurred vision, weight gain, nausea, constipation and difficulty urinating.

Note
May take 2 to 3 weeks for the medication to begin working.

Others

Generic and common brand names
- Bupropion (Wellbutrin)
- Nefazodone (Serzone)
- Trazodone (Desyrel)
- Venlafaxine (Effexor)

Action
Increase the levels of several brain chemicals in which low levels are thought to be associated with depression.

Common uses
To treat depression. Bupropion is also used in smoking cessation therapy (Zyban).

Common side effects
Headache, insomnia, drowsiness, dizziness, diarrhea, constipation, nausea, dry mouth and weight gain or loss.

Note
It may take 2 to 3 weeks for the medication to begin working.

Migraine medications

Antiseizure medications

Generic and common brand names
- Divalproex (Depakote)

Action
Affect the actions of nerve fibers and brain transmitters.

Common uses
To treat seizures and to prevent migraines.

Common side effects
Nausea and vomiting, heartburn, diarrhea, hair loss, fatigue, dizziness and unsteadiness.

Note
It may take 2 to 3 weeks before you begin to notice benefits from these drugs. Maximal benefits may not be evident for 2 to 3 months.

Beta blockers

Generic and common brand names
- Atenolol (Tenormin)
- Metoprolol (Lopressor, Toprol)
- Nadolol (Corgard)
- Propranolol (Inderal)

Action
Unclear how their action prevents migraines.

Common uses
To treat high blood pressure and other cardiovascular conditions and to prevent migraines.

Common side effects
Fatigue, cold hands, trouble sleeping, impotence and loss of sex drive.

Note
These medications will slow your heart rate.

Ergot derivatives

Generic and common brand names
- Dihydroergotamine (D.H.E. 45)
- Ergotamine (Ergomar)
- Methysergide (Sansert)

Action
Interact with serotonin receptors and, possibly, constrict blood vessels in the outer area of your brain and scalp.

Common uses
To relieve migraine symptoms and to help prevent cluster headaches.

Common side effects
Cold hands and feet, tingling in and mild numbness of hands and feet, drowsiness, dizziness, confusion and nausea.

Note
Methysergide is a preventive agent and not intended for treatment of an acute migraine. Alcohol counteracts the effects of these medications.

Gabapentin

Brand name
- Neurontin

Action
Unclear.

Common uses
To treat seizures and certain types of pain, including migraine.

Common side effects
Sedation, fatigue, dizziness and weight gain.

Note
You may not experience maximal benefits of these drugs for 2 to 3 months.

Tricyclic antidepressants

Generic and common brand names
- Amitriptyline (Elavil)
- Doxepin (Sinequan)
- Nortriptyline (Aventyl, Pamelor)
- Protriptyline (Vivactil)

Action
Unclear. May modify brain chemicals that play a role in headaches.

Common uses
To prevent migraines and tension-type headaches.

Common side effects
Sedation, weight gain, dry mouth and lightheadedness.

Note
It may take several weeks before you begin to notice the benefits of these medications.

Triptans

Generic and common brand names
- Almotriptan (Axert)
- Frovatriptan (Frova)
- Naratriptan (Amerge)
- Rizatriptan (Maxalt)
- Sumatriptan (Imitrex)
- Zolmitriptan (Zomig)

Action
Mimic the brain chemical serotonin to deactivate nerves and decrease swollen blood vessels.

Common uses
To relieve migraine symptoms.

Common side effects
Nausea, dizziness, muscle weakness, sensation of chest and neck pressure, thirst, frequent urination, altered sense of taste, changes in blood pressure and fatigue.

Note
These medications are used only to treat, not prevent, migraines. They are not recommended for individuals with significant heart disease.

Muscle relaxants

Generic and common brand names
- Baclofen (Lioresal)
- Carisoprodol (Soma)
- Chlorzoxazone (Parafon Forte)
- Cyclobenzaprine (Flexeril)
- Metaxalone (Skelaxin)
- Methocarbamol (Robaxin)
- Orphenadrine (Norflex)
- Tizanidine (Zanaflex)

Action
Act on your central nervous system, causing your muscles to relax.

Common uses
To relieve the pain and discomfort caused by muscle cramping and spasm.

Common side effects
Clouded thinking, drowsiness, fatigue and dizziness.

Note
Alcohol dramatically increases the side effects of these medications.

Osteoporosis medications

Bisphosphonates

Generic and common brand names
- Alendronate (Fosamax)
- Etidronate (Didronel)
- Pamidronate (Aredia)
- Risedronate (Actonel)
- Zoledronic acid (Zometa)

Action
Help preserve bone mass by preventing excess breakdown of bone.

Common uses
To prevent or treat osteoporosis and to treat Paget's disease of bone.

Common side effects
Nausea, abdominal pain, irritation of the esophagus and difficulty swallowing.

Note
Take oral bisphosphonates with a full glass of water to protect against irritation of the esophagus. Take your dose 30 minutes before eating or drinking any beverage other than water. Don't lie down for 30 minutes after taking the drug.

Calcitonin

Brand name
- Miacalcin

Action
Helps maintain bone density and prevent bone loss. Available as a nasal spray for treatment of osteoporosis.

Common uses
To treat osteoporosis, Paget's disease and too much calcium in the blood (hypercalcemia).

Common side effects
Can cause nasal irritation.

Note
Blow your nose gently before using the spray and don't inhale while spraying.

Calcium supplements

Generic and common brand names
- Calcium carbonate (Caltrate, Os-Cal, others)
- Calcium citrate (Citracal)
- Calcium glubionate (Calcionate)

Action
Help maintain bone density and prevent bone loss.

Common uses
To treat or prevent osteoporosis and other conditions resulting from reduced calcium levels. These products are available without a prescription.

Common side effects
Constipation and headache.

Note
Chewable calcium tablets and calcium powders and solutions may be more easily absorbed than hard, compressed calcium tablets. Calcium is absorbed better when taken with food.

Hormone replacement therapy

Generic and common brand names
- Conjugated estrogens (Premarin)
- Esterified estrogens (Estratab)
- Estradiol (Estrace, Estraderm)
- Estropipate (Ogen)

Action
Mimics actions of naturally produced female estrogen hormones. Estrogens prevent the excess breakdown of bone that occurs after menopause.

Common uses
To help prevent osteoporosis in postmenopausal women and to reduce symptoms of menopause.

Common side effects
Fluid retention, weight gain, breast pain, swelling of feet and lower legs, abnormal menstrual bleeding.

Note
Women in menopause who are on hormone replacement therapy but haven't had a hysterectomy should take a progestin along with estrogen to prevent endometrial cancer.

Pain relievers

Acetaminophen

Brand name
- Tylenol

Action
Blocks the effects of pyrogens, which are natural fever inducers, along with substances that lead to pain.

Common uses
To reduce fever and relieve pain.

Common side effects
Side effects are extremely rare. Excessive doses can cause liver damage.

Note
If you regularly combine even usual amounts of acetaminophen with alcohol, your chances for liver damage are increased.

COX-2 inhibitors

Generic and common brand names
- Celecoxib (Celebrex)
- Rofecoxib (Vioxx)
- Valdecoxib (Bextra)

Action
Relieve pain by blocking an enzyme called cyclooxygenase-2 (COX-2), which stimulates production of substances (prostaglandins) involved in pain and inflammation.

Common uses
To treat pain from inflammation.

Common side effects
Rash, dizziness and stomach irritation.

Note
These medications are thought to be less irritating to the stomach than are standard NSAIDs.

Narcotics (opiates and opioids)

Generic and common brand names
- Butorphanol (Stadol)
- Codeine
- Fentanyl (Actiq, Duragesic)
- Hydrocodone and acetaminophen (Lortab, Vicodin, others)
- Hydromorphone (Dilaudid)
- Levorphanol (Levo-Dromoran)
- Meperidine (Demerol)
- Methadone (Dolophine)
- Morphine (MS Contin, Roxanol, others)
- Oxycodone (OxyContin, Roxicodone)
- Propoxyphene (Darvon)

Action
Decrease the brain's perception of pain.

Common uses
To relieve severe pain caused by serious illness, a severe injury or surgery.

Common side effects
Nausea, constipation, sedation and unclear thinking.

Note
Don't take the medication with alcohol because both act as depressants. Some people can become addicted to these narcotics if they're taken for a lengthy period.

Nonsteroidal anti-inflammatory drugs (NSAIDs)

Generic and common brand names
- Aspirin (Bayer, Bufferin, others)
- Diclofenac sodium (Voltaren XR)
- Etodolac (Lodine)
- Fenoprofen
- Flurbiprofen (Ansaid)
- Ibuprofen (Advil, Motrin, others)
- Indomethacin (Indocin)
- Ketoprofen (Orudis)
- Ketorolac tromethamine (Toradol)
- Meloxicam (Mobic)
- Nabumetone (Relafen)
- Naproxen (Aleve, Naprosyn, others)
- Oxaprozin (Daypro)
- Piroxicam (Feldene)
- Sulindac (Clinoril)

Action
Relieve pain by blocking an enzyme called cyclooxygenase-2 (COX-2), which stimulates production of substances called prostaglandins, which are involved in inflammation and pain. Reduce fever by affecting the part of your brain that controls body temperature.

Common uses
To relieve pain from inflammation and swelling and to reduce fever. Aspirin is also taken to inhibit formation of blood clots.

Common side effects
Nausea, stomach pain, stomach bleeding and ulcers.

Note
Many nonprescription pain relievers contain NSAIDs. Talk with your doctor or pharmacist to make sure you aren't double dosing. Risk of side effects increases with age, especially among women.

Tramadol

Brand name
- Ultram

Action
Interferes with the transmission of pain signals and triggers the release of the brain chemicals noradrenaline and serotonin, both of which help reduce pain.

Common uses
To relieve moderate pain from illness or following surgery.

Common side effects
Dizziness, sedation, headache, nausea and constipation.

Note
Although a narcotic, tramadol is a weak one and less addicting than the others.

Parkinson's disease medications

Amantadine

Brand name
- Symmetrel

Action
Causes complex actions within the brain, including increasing the release of the brain chemical dopamine. Blocks some actions of another brain chemical called glutamate. These actions are thought to be beneficial in the treatment of Parkinson's disease.

Common uses
To treat the flu (influenza) and Parkinson's disease. It helps control involuntary movements (dyskinesias) caused by another Parkinson's drug, levodopa.

Common side effects
Red or purple skin discoloration of the legs, often accompanied by swelling. This isn't worrisome medically.

Note
Common side effects resolve if the drug is reduced or discontinued.

Anticholinergics

Generic and common brand names
- Benztropine (Cogentin)
- Biperiden (Akineton)
- Procyclidine (Kemadrin)
- Trihexyphenidyl (Artane)

Action
Block the action of the brain chemical acetylcholine.

Common uses
To treat Parkinson's disease. But these drugs are only mildly beneficial and the benefits are often offset by side effects.

Common side effects
Reduced memory, blurred vision, dry mouth, constipation and reduced urination.

Note
These medications may make you sweat less, causing your body temperature to increase. Take care to avoid becoming overheated during hot weather and exercise.

COMT inhibitors

Generic and common brand names
- Entacapone (Comtan)
- Tolcapone (Tasmar)

Action
Prolong the effect of the medication levodopa by blocking an enzyme that breaks down levodopa.

Common uses
To treat Parkinson's disease in conjunction with the use of levodopa.

Common side effects
Diarrhea. These drugs also worsen side effects that may occur with levodopa use.

Note
Tolcapone can cause serious liver damage.

Dopamine agonists

Generic and common brand names
- Bromocriptine (Parlodel)
- Pergolide (Permax)
- Pramipexole (Mirapex)
- Ropinirole (Requip)

Action
Mimic the action of the brain chemical dopamine.

Common uses
To treat Parkinson's disease.

Common side effects
Confusion, dizziness, fainting due to low blood pressure, drowsiness, hallucinations and involuntary body movements.

Note
If you're taking one of these medications, make sure you know how your body reacts to it before driving or operating equipment.

Levodopa and carbidopa

Generic and common brand names
- Levodopa (Larodopa)
- Levodopa and carbidopa (Sinemet)

Action
Increase amounts of the brain chemical dopamine. Levodopa is a natural substance that the brain transforms into dopamine. Carbidopa, used in combination with levodopa, helps reduce nausea and enhances levodopa's potency.

Common uses
To treat Parkinson's disease. It's the most potent and effective treatment for the disease.

Common side effects
Involuntary movements (dyskinesias), low blood pressure when standing, nausea and hallucinations.

Note
For people taking levodopa alone, vitamin B-6 may reduce the effects of the medication. Don't take vitamins containing B-6. Foods that contain B-6 include bananas, egg yolks, lima beans, meats and white-grain cereals.

Selegiline

Brand name
- Eldepryl

Action
Inhibits the enzyme that breaks down dopamine in the brain.

Common uses
To treat Parkinson's disease.

Common side effects
Unusual body movements, mood changes and dry mouth.

Note
Sugarless candy, gum or a saliva substitute may help with dry mouth.

Prostate medications

Alpha blockers

Generic and common brand names
- Doxazosin (Cardura)
- Tamsulosin (Flomax)
- Terazosin (Hytrin)

Action
Relax certain smooth muscles in the urinary tract, making it easier to urinate.

Common uses
To treat high blood pressure and noncancerous (benign) enlargement of the prostate gland.

Common side effects
Nasal stuffiness, dizziness, headache, rapidly pounding heart, nausea, weakness, fatigue and ankle swelling.

Note
To minimize side effects, take the medicine before bedtime.

Anti-androgens

Generic and common brand names
- Bicalutamide (Casodex)
- Flutamide (Eulexin)
- Nilutamide (Nilandron)

Action
Stop production of most, but not all, male sex hormones that nourish the prostate gland and cancerous tumors of the prostate.

Common uses
To treat prostate cancer.

Common side effects
In men, reduced or eliminated sex drive and impotence. Hot flashes, enlarged and sensitive breasts, weight gain, reduced muscle and bone mass, nausea, diarrhea and fatigue.

Note
Nilutamide may temporarily change the way your eyes react to light. You may not be able to see well for several minutes after going from bright light to darkness or vice versa.

Conversion blockers

Generic and common brand name
- Finasteride (Proscar)

Action
Shrink prostate gland tissue by inhibiting conversion of testosterone to dihydrotestosterone.

Common uses
To treat noncancerous (benign) enlargement of the prostate gland. A weaker version of this medicine (Propecia) is used to prevent male-pattern baldness.

Common side effects
Impotence, decreased sex drive and reduced semen release during ejaculation.

Note
It generally takes 6 months to a year for the treatment to produce its full effect.

Gonadotropin-releasing hormone agonists

Generic and common brand names
- Goserelin (Zoladex)
- Leuprolide (Lupron)

Action
Decrease estrogen and testosterone in the blood.

Common uses
To treat a number of medical problems including prostate cancer in men and, in women, breast cancer and endometriosis.

Common side effects
Hot flashes, constipation and, in men, an inability to achieve or maintain an erection.

Note
In rare instances, these medications can cause chest pain. See a doctor immediately if this occurs.

Seizure medications

Generic and common brand names
- Acetazolamide (Diamox)
- Carbamazepine (Carbatrol, Tegretol)
- Clonazepam (Klonopin)
- Divalproex (Depakote)
- Ethosuaximide (Zarontin)
- Ethotoin (Peganone)
- Felbamate (Felbatol)
- Fosphenytoin (Cerebyx)
- Gabapentin (Neurontin)
- Lamotrigine (Lamictal)
- Levetiracetam (Keppra)
- Methsuximide (Celontin)
- Oxcarbazepine (Trileptal)
- Phenytoin (Dilantin, Phenytek)
- Primidone (Mysoline)
- Topiramate (Topamax)
- Valproate (Depacon)
- Valproic acid (Depakene)
- Zonisamide (Zonegran)

Action
Reduce excessive electric activity in the brain, reducing or preventing seizures. The mechanism by which the medications reduce electric activity varies.

Common uses
To treat seizures and related disorders. Divalproex and gabapentin may be used to treat migraines. Carbamazepine, gabapentin and oxcarbazepine may be prescribed for trigeminal neuralgia and painful peripheral neuropathy.

Common side effects
Drowsiness, dizziness, nausea, impaired coordination and memory.

Note
It may take 2 to 3 weeks before you can see benefits of the medication.

Sex hormones

Androgens

Generic and common brand names
- Danazol (Danocrine)
- Fluoxymesterone (Halotestin)
- Methyltestosterone (Android, Testred, others)
- Testosterone (AndroGel, Delatestryl, others)

Action
Mimic the action of natural male sex hormones (androgens).

Common uses
To provide additional male sex hormones when a male is unable to produce enough (hypogonadism). Also used to treat hereditary angioedema and certain types of breast cancer in females.

Common side effects
Oily skin and acne. In men, may enlarge the prostate gland. In women, may decrease breast size, increase facial and body hair and produce a lowered voice.

Note
Tell your doctor about any other medications you're taking, including nonprescription drugs.

Estrogens

Generic and common brand names
- Chlorotrianisene
- Conjugated estrogens (Premarin)
- Esterified estrogens (Estratab)
- Estradiol (Estrace, Estraderm, others)
- Estropipate (Ogen)
- Ethinyl estradiol (Estinyl)

Action
Mimic the action of the natural female sex hormone estrogen.

Common uses
To provide additional estrogen when your body isn't able to produce enough. Used in women to treat hot flashes and vaginal dryness and to prevent osteoporosis.

Common side effects
Fluid retention, weight gain, breast pain and swelling of the feet and lower legs. In women, an altered menstrual pattern and bleeding in the middle of the menstrual cycle.

Note
Discuss the benefits and risks of estrogen hormones with your doctor. Women in menopause who are on hormone replacement therapy but have not had a hysterectomy need to take a progestin along with estrogen to prevent endometrial cancer.

Progestins

Generic and common brand names
- Medroxyprogesterone (Amen, Provera, others)
- Megestrol (Megace)
- Norethindrone (Aygestin, Micronor)
- Progesterone (Prometrium)

Action
Mimic the action of the natural female sex hormone progesterone.

Common uses
To regulate the menstrual cycle, help maintain an existing pregnancy or treat endometriosis or abnormal uterine bleeding. Some progestins are used to treat cancers of the breast, kidney and uterus.

Common side effects
Fluid retention, weight gain and changes in vaginal bleeding.

Note
These medications can worsen symptoms among people bothered by migraines.

Smoking cessation medications

Generic and common brand names
- Bupropion (Zyban)
- Nicotine gum (Nicorette)
- Nicotine inhaler (Nicotrol)
- Nicotine nasal spray (Nicotrol)
- Nicotine transdermal system patch (Habitrol, Nicoderm CQ, others)

Action
Deliver controlled amounts of nicotine to your brain via your bloodstream. Bupropion is thought to raise the level of the brain chemical dopamine, the same chemical affected by nicotine.

Common uses
To reduce the symptoms of nicotine withdrawal.

Common side effects
Bupropion may cause agitation and anxiety. Nicotine gum may irritate oral membranes. An inhaler may irritate the throat. A nasal spray may cause nasal irritation, a runny nose and watery eyes. A transdermal patch may cause a local skin irritation.

Note
If not used as directed, nicotine replacement products can cause a nicotine overdose. Follow the directions carefully. Individuals with seizure disorders shouldn't take bupropion.

Stimulants

Generic and common brand names
- Dextroamphetamine and amphetamine (Adderall)
- Methamphetamine
- Methylphenidate (Concerta, Ritalin)
- Pemoline (Cylert)

Action
Stimulate cells in the brain and spinal cord (central nervous system), increasing alertness and concentration.

Common uses
To treat narcolepsy and attention-deficit/hyperactivity (ADHD) disorder.

PREVENTION TIP

Take these precautions to guard against food and drug interactions:
- Follow instructions from your doctor or pharmacist on how and when to take your medications.
- Don't take medications at the same time that you take vitamin or mineral supplements. Some supplements, especially calcium, can bind with many medications and impair their absorption.
- If you're instructed to take a drug on an empty stomach, take it at least 1 hour before or 2 hours after eating.
- Don't stir your medication into food. Acid or minerals in some foods may alter the drug's ingredients.
- Don't mix medications into hot beverages. Heat can change or destroy some drug ingredients.

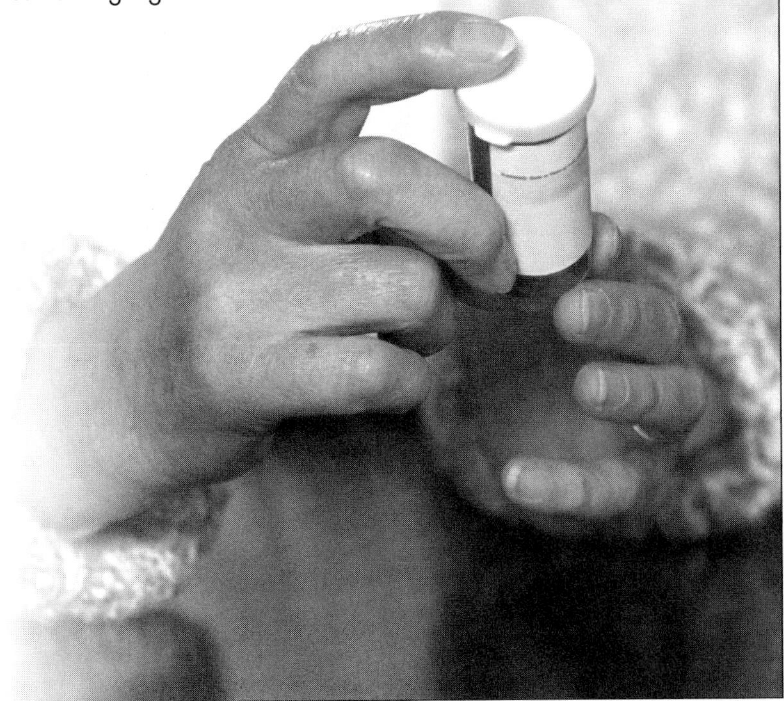

Common side effects
Nervousness, sleeping problems, increased heart rate and appetite loss.

Note
When taking one of these medications, avoid caffeine, which is also a stimulant.

Thyroid medications

Hyperthyroidism medications

Generic and common brand names
- Methimazole (Tapazole)
- Propylthiouracil, or PTU

Action
Interfere with iodine, required to produce thyroid hormone.

Common uses
To treat an overproductive thyroid gland (hyperthyroidism) by preventing it from producing excessive amounts of thyroid hormone.

Common side effects
Rash, itching, nausea, vomiting and abdominal pain.

Note
It may take several days or weeks for these medications to work. Rarely, they can impair blood cell production or cause liver inflammation.

Hypothyroidism medications

Generic and common brand names
- Levothyroxine (Levothroid, Synthroid, others)
- Liothyronine (Cytomel)
- Liotrix (Thyrolar, others)
- Thyroid (Armour Thyroid)

Action
Increase thyroid hormone in the bloodstream.

Common uses
To restore thyroid hormone levels to normal if the thyroid gland doesn't produce enough. Also used for thyroid hormone replacement after removal or destruction of the thyroid gland.

Common side effects
Generally, none.

Note
Treatment is generally lifelong. Blood tests can confirm the appropriate dose. ■

CHAPTER 41 PART VI

Surgery

For many people, an operation is a frightening prospect. Taking an active role in your care and making sure that you understand the process can help relieve your anxieties. Knowing what's going on helps reduce the fear factor in most situations.

Presurgical Evaluation

Before you have an operation, your doctor or surgeon reviews your medical history and looks for any medical conditions, reactions or allergies that may affect the outcome. As much as possible, existing medical problems are corrected before an operation.

In most instances, an anesthesiologist also visits you before your operation. The purpose of this visit is to detect any conditions that might affect your reaction to anesthesia. The anesthesiologist reviews any pertinent medical problems and asks you if you've had any adverse reactions to anesthesia in the past.

Be sure to inform the doctors of all medications that you're taking, even seemingly insignificant over-the-counter medications and supplements. These are easy items to overlook because they're used so commonly, but they can have a significant effect on your recovery.

As part of your presurgical evaluation, you may undergo laboratory tests, particularly if you're older than 40 or have other medical problems. These tests may include an electrocardiogram (ECG) to evaluate your heart and a chest X-ray. You may also have blood tests.

Anesthesia

Anesthesia is the loss of sensitivity to pain brought about by various drugs (anesthetics). Anesthesia is used during many medical procedures, including surgery. Anesthesia specialists, including physician anesthesiologists and certified registered nurse anesthetists, administer anesthetics.

The type of anesthesia you receive during surgery depends on the procedure being performed and your physical and emotional status.

For most surgeries, it's important that you avoid solid foods for at least 8 to 10 hours before you receive an anesthetic. This precaution helps to prevent you from breathing in (aspirating) stomach contents into your lungs during or after the surgery.

You may also be given instructions as to when to stop drinking liquids before the procedure. In most situations, you should take your usual medications, with sips of water, the morning of your surgery.

Types of anesthesia include:

Conscious sedation

Conscious sedation or intravenous (IV) sedation is used to relax you and make you feel sleepy, though you remain conscious. This type of anesthesia is used for procedures such as colonoscopy, an exam of your colon and rectum. It generally includes intravenous administration of pain medication and a mild sedative to minimize any discomfort.

Local anesthesia

Local anesthesia is used to block pain in a part of your body, allowing you to remain fully alert. Typically, a local anesthetic is used for procedures such as dental work, skin biopsies or stitching up a cut. Sometimes, a local anesthetic is used for a more extensive procedure in people for whom general or regional anesthesia is inadvisable.

For local anesthesia, an anesthetic is injected at or near the site of the procedure. The injection numbs the area to pain and any other sensation. For a more extensive procedure, you may have a catheter inserted into one of your veins — usually in an arm — so that you can receive fluids intravenously. This catheter provides access for giving sedatives and other medications, if needed.

Local anesthetics are generally of short duration. They come in different forms, including injections, sprays and ointments. Only rarely do they cause an allergic reaction.

Regional anesthesia

Regional anesthesia is used to block sensation in a particular region of your body. As with local anesthesia, you remain conscious during regional anesthesia. Sometimes, a

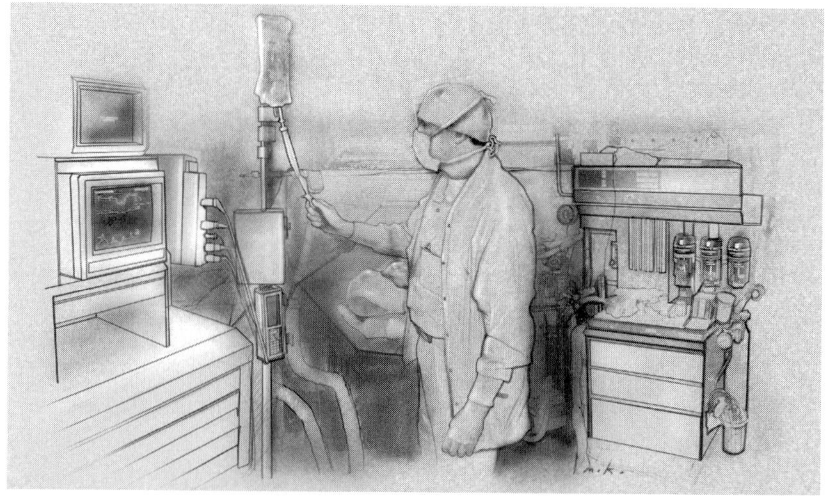

Anesthesia specialists today have sophisticated monitors to help track a patient's condition during surgery. That's one of the reasons deaths from anesthesia have dropped 25-fold in the last decade.

sedative also is administered intravenously before the procedure to relax you. The sedative may make you feel sleepy, although you remain conscious.

The anesthetic is injected around a single nerve or network of nerves that serve the area involved in the surgical procedure. You receive the injection, which generally is painless, while lying on your side or sitting. Spinal, epidural and caudal anesthesia involve injecting an anesthetic near the spinal cord. This eliminates pain in the lower half of the body. These forms of anesthesia are often used for pelvic operations and leg and hip surgery. Epidural anesthesia is often used during childbirth.

Side effects, which may include nausea and vomiting, breathing difficulties, lightheadedness or headache, are infrequent and are usually easy to manage. Afterward, you may have some minor discomfort at the site of the injection.

Regional anesthesia may also be used in an arm or another part of the body. This type is commonly referred to as a regional nerve block. An anesthesia specialist places a small needle into the area through which a major nerve passes. Often, you'll feel a sensation similar to a mild electric shock. This tells the specialist that the needle is in the correct place. He or she then injects a local anesthetic drug so that the intended area of your body becomes numb and immobile.

The main advantage of regional anesthesia is that it's useful for more extensive procedures than those that require only local anesthesia, but it affects only the region of your body needing it. It has little effect on other areas, such as your heart, lungs and brain. Regional anesthesia may also be used to provide pain relief after an operation.

General anesthesia

General anesthesia is used for more extensive procedures that require you to be unconscious. The medications used in general anesthesia are given intravenously or by inhalation through a mask. The drugs circulate in your bloodstream to all areas of your body, including your brain. They act as hypnotics, painkillers and muscle relaxants, and they block the memory of the surgery. Your age, condition and the type of surgery you're having determine the type of drug or drugs you receive.

Because general anesthetics affect all areas of your body, such as the heart and lungs, effects from the medications are more common. However, most are temporary and easily managed by medical personnel. To prevent problems, your blood pressure, heart rate and rhythm, breathing and temperature are continuously monitored throughout the procedure.

At the end of surgery requiring general anesthesia, the anesthesiologist reverses the effects of the anesthetic drugs. As you regain consciousness, you'll be carefully monitored by medical personnel skilled in postoperative recovery. If you experience pain, let your doctor or nurse know so that you can be given something to control the pain. Tolerating excess pain after surgery gains nothing and can actually be detrimental.

Side effects from general anesthesia after an operation include nausea, vomiting and muscle aches. These are usually of brief duration and can be treated. More serious complications, such as heart attack, kidney damage and stroke, are extremely rare. Proper screening and treatment of any serious medical illnesses in advance of the procedure, as well as careful monitoring of your vital signs during the operation, reduce such risks.

The Operation

Often, you're brought to the operating room on a rolling table and transferred to and appropriately positioned on the operating table. Then various monitoring devices are attached to your body, and anesthesia is administered.

Medical personnel may shave and disinfect the area involved in your surgery. Or, this preparation may be done before you come to the operating room. During the operation, the surgical team may rotate or tilt the operating table to provide the best access to the surgery site.

Great care is taken to avoid infection during the procedure. All instruments and supplies are sterile, and the medical team wears sterile gowns, gloves and surgical masks.

During surgery, your vital signs are carefully monitored. Intravenous (IV) access to a vein can be used to maintain normal levels of water in your body and to serve as an avenue for giving drugs, as necessary, during your operation.

Types of surgery

Years ago, the only way to perform surgery was to make a large incision in the skin at the site of the procedure. This is generally known as traditional surgery or open surgery. Traditional surgery is still performed for many types of procedures in which a doctor needs adequate room to reach the organ needing repair or removal.

Increasingly, more surgeries are performed through a less invasive technique called endoscopic surgery. Endoscopic surgery relies on use of a sophisticated device called an endoscope — a pencil-thin tube with its own lighting system and miniature video camera. It allows a surgeon to see inside your body without making a large incision.

To perform endoscopic surgery, a surgeon inserts the endoscope through an incision less than an inch long. While viewing the procedure on a video screen, the surgeon operates with miniature instruments inserted through one or more other small incisions.

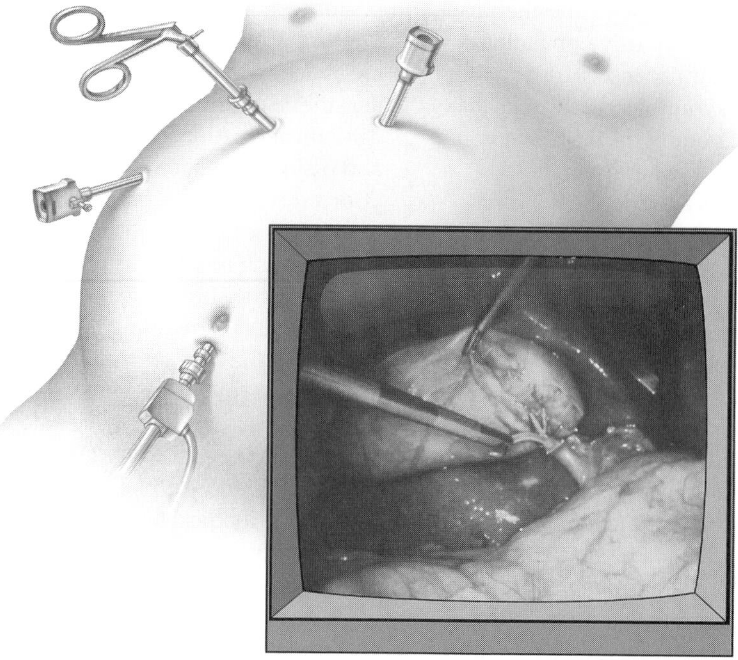

This illustration shows removal of the gallbladder with laparoscopic surgery. During the procedure, several small incisions are made in the abdomen and tiny tube-like instruments called endoscopes are inserted into the incisions. A camera and television monitor give the surgeon a clear view of the internal organs.

The specific area of your body treated determines the type of endoscopic surgery performed. For example, arthroscopy refers to joint surgery performed with an endoscope, and laparoscopic surgery refers to abdominal procedures performed with an endoscope.

The advantages of endoscopic surgery over traditional surgery generally include a speedier recovery, a shorter hospital stay, fewer complications and less expense.

Outpatient surgery

Outpatient surgery, ambulatory surgery, same-day surgery — these are all terms for the same concept. You come to the surgical facility, have the operation and leave all on the same day. Given the high cost of staying overnight at a hospital and increasing pressure to keep costs down, outpatient surgery has become increasingly common.

Outpatient surgery may be performed at an outpatient clinic within a hospital or at a separate, free-standing facility. The advantage of being located within a hospital is that it's easier to deal with major complications if they arise.

Before the surgery, you receive a presurgical evaluation. When you arrive for your surgery, a doctor or nurse tells you what to expect. If you haven't already done so, let your doctor or nurse know of any illnesses that you have and medications that you take.

If you receive regional or general anesthesia, you may not be able to drive yourself home after the surgery. Have a family member or friend provide transportation for you.

How long you remain in the hospital after the operation depends on several factors, including whether your pain is under control and whether you can drink fluids, walk and urinate.

Postoperative recovery

After your operation, you'll likely be taken to a recovery room where you'll stay until the anesthetic wears off and your vital signs are stable. Specially trained personnel will monitor your breathing and pain control.

Following some major operations, such as neurologic or cardiac procedures, you may be moved to an intensive care unit (ICU). This area has sophisticated monitoring equipment, mechanical devices to assist breathing and resuscitation equipment.

In the days immediately following surgery, you may experience:

- *Delirium.* It's common to feel confused and to have trouble remembering events surrounding your surgery. General anesthesia combined with the stress of surgery can have this effect.
- *Nausea and vomiting.* Nausea and vomiting may be caused by pain or a side effect of medication.
- *Digestive difficulties.* Some surgeries can cause your gastrointestinal system to stop functioning normally for a brief period. You may have difficulty eating and drinking in the first few days following surgery.

While you're in the hospital, staff will likely encourage you to do deep-breathing exercises and to sit up and walk. These steps are important to your recovery and to reduce your risk of complications, such as pneumonia and blood clots.

Besides providing for your care, a nurse or other medical personnel will educate you on any procedures you must follow while in the hospital or when you return home. After dismissal, you'll probably need to come back to the hospital or your doctor's office for a follow-up examination.

Recovering from surgery may require dedication, discipline and physical exertion. Although you'll receive coaching in the early stages of your recovery, it's up to you to motivate yourself after you leave the hospital. ■

CHAPTER **42** PART VI

Pain Management

Physical pain is a part of life. You see evidence of this in drugstores, their shelves stacked high with pain relievers. And, chances are, you feel the evidence, at least from time to time.

There are times when pain is beneficial. Perhaps you've grabbed a hot iron skillet with a bare hand or stubbed your toe on a dresser. Like a blaring alarm, pain screams its urgent warning that something is wrong and that you need to tend to the problem.

But other pain — the day-after-day ache of arthritis or the constant throbbing of a headache — serves no useful purpose. You already know that something is wrong, and you're doing everything that you can to treat the problem. Relentless pain like this can be overwhelming.

Pain is also unique. Two people injured in much the same way may experience radically different levels of discomfort and react quite differently. Each individual's pain tolerance is the result of a variety of factors, including his or her biological, psychological and cultural makeup.

Strategies on how best to manage pain continue to evolve. For acute pain, such as that following surgery or an accident, medication can often alleviate the pain while the injury heals. For persistent pain — commonly called chronic pain — medication alone isn't always adequate or the best form of treatment. A comprehensive approach that includes exercise, relaxation techniques and behavior changes may improve pain control.

People today are living longer, but often with disease that causes pain. Successful approaches for managing pain are important.

How You Feel Pain

Understanding how your body feels pain can help you appreciate how unique your pain experiences are. It can also help you better understand why chronic pain is often difficult to treat.

Pain basically results from a series of electrical and chemical exchanges involving three major components: your peripheral nerves, spinal cord and brain.

Peripheral nerves

Your peripheral nerves encompass a network of nerve fibers that branch throughout your body, all the way down to your fingers and toes. Attached to some of these sensory fibers are special nerve endings that detect an unpleasant stimulus, such as a cut, burn or painful pressure. These nerve endings are called nociceptors, from a Latin word meaning "to injure."

You have millions of nociceptors in your skin, bones, joints and muscles and in the protective membranes around your internal organs. You can't feel pain in your internal organs themselves. Nociceptors are concentrated in areas more prone to injury, such as your fingers and toes. That's why a splinter in your finger hurts more than one in your thigh or shoulder.

There may be as many as 1,300 nociceptors in just 1 square inch of skin. Muscles, protected beneath your skin, have fewer nerve endings. And organ membranes, protected by skin, muscle and bone, have fewer still.

Some nociceptors sense sharp blows, others heat. One type senses pressure, temperature and chemical changes. Nociceptors can also detect inflammation caused by injury, disease and infection.

When nociceptors detect a harmful stimulus, they relay the pain messages — in the form of electrical impulses along a peripheral sensory nerve — to your spinal cord and brain. The speed by which the messages travel can vary, even if they're related to the same stimulus. For example, if you hit your finger with a hammer, you first feel a fast, sharp pain and then, more slowly, an aching.

Spinal cord

When pain messages reach your spinal cord, they're adjusted (modulated) within a network of neural connections. Depending on the circumstances, this modulation may either decrease or increase the rate at which the signals are relayed to the brain.

For severe pain that's linked to an immediate danger, such as when you touch a hot stove, the messages take an express route to your brain. Nerve cells in your spinal cord also respond to these urgent warnings by triggering into action other parts of the nervous system, such as your

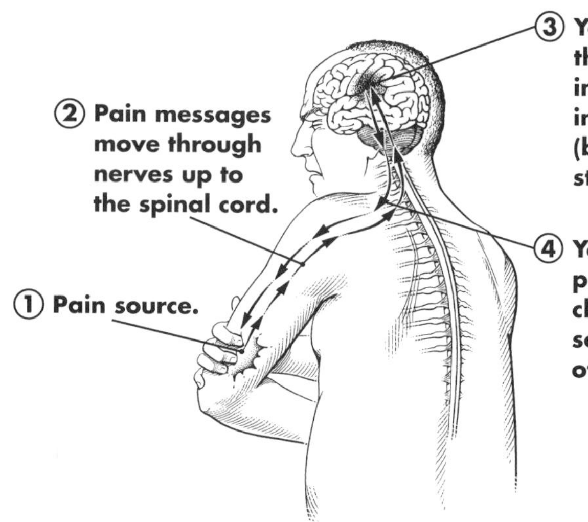

motor nerves. Motor nerves can signal your muscles to contract and pull your hand away from the burner. Weaker pain signals, though, such as from a scratch, may not even be passed on to the brain.

Within your spinal cord, the messages can change in other ways. Other sensations may overpower and diminish the pain messages. This happens when you massage or apply pressure to the injured area. The result is that the warnings sent by your peripheral nerves are downgraded to a lower intensity.

Change also occurs when nerve cells in your spinal cord release chemicals that amplify or subdue the messages. This affects the speed at which these messages travel to your brain.

Brain

When pain messages reach your brain, they arrive at the thalamus, a sorting and switching station located deep inside your brain. The thalamus quickly forwards them simultaneously to both the thinking part of your brain, called the cerebral cortex, and to your brain's limbic center.

The limbic center produces the emotions that often accompany pain, such as anxiety, fear and frustration. It's at this point that you actually begin to feel pain.

Your cerebral cortex reacts to the pain messages by locating the source of the injury, assessing the damage and determining a course of action, such as ordering you to take pressure off your foot if you've sprained your ankle.

The cerebral cortex relays additional key messages. For instance, if you've cut your finger, the cerebral cortex signals your autonomic nervous system — the system that controls your blood flow — to send additional blood and nutrients to the injury site to help repair the damage. And it dispatches the release of pain-suppressing chemicals and sends stop-pain messages to the spinal cord.

Pain response

When pain messages reach your brain, two components determine how you respond to the pain: the physical sensation and your personal makeup.

Physical sensation

Pain comes in many forms: sharp, jabbing, throbbing, burning, stinging, tingling, nagging, dull and aching. Sharp and jabbing pain generally produces greater discomfort than does dull, aching pain. It's also more likely to make you anxious or fearful.

Pain also varies from mild to severe. Severe pain grabs your attention more quickly, and it generally produces a greater physical and emotional response than does mild pain. Severe pain can incapacitate you, making it difficult or impossible to sit or stand.

The location of your pain also can affect your response to it. A headache that interferes with your ability to work or concentrate may be more bothersome, and therefore receive a stronger response, than arthritic pain in your knee or a cut to your finger.

Personal makeup

Your emotional and psychological state, memory of past painful experiences, upbringing and attitude also affect how you interpret pain messages and tolerate pain. For example, a minor sensation that would barely register as pain, such as a dentist's probe, can actually produce exaggerated pain for someone who has never been to the dentist but has heard horror stories of what it's like.

But your emotions can also work in your favor by reducing even major pain messages. This was illustrated in a pain study that compared formerly wounded war veterans with men in the general population. Men in both groups had the same kind of surgery. The combat veterans, however, required less pain medication than the others did, perhaps because they thought that the pain from surgery was minor compared with what they had experienced in battle.

Athletes also can condition themselves to endure pain that would incapacitate others. In addition, if you're brought up in a home or culture that teaches "Grin and bear it," "No pain, no gain" or "Bite the bullet," you may experience less discomfort than do people who focus on their pain or are more prone to complain.

Acute vs. Chronic Pain

The two main types of pain are acute and chronic. Acute pain is usually short term and useful because it alerts you to a physical problem that you need to address. Chronic pain is long term, and instead of being helpful, it's often debilitating.

Acute pain

You probably already know about acute pain from firsthand experience. Acute pain is triggered by tissue damage. It's the type of pain that generally accompanies an injury or surgery. When you have acute pain, you usually know exactly where it hurts. In fact, the word *acute* comes from the Latin word for "needle," referring to a sharp pain.

Pain might be mild and last just a moment, such as from a pinch. Or it might be severe and last for weeks or months, such as from a burn, pulled muscle or broken bone. Examples of acute pain include a toothache from a cavity, a burning elbow from a scrape and a sore throat from having your tonsils removed.

Some acute pain, though, is more difficult to link to its cause. For example, your left arm may hurt when you're having a heart attack, or you may have generalized abdominal pain when you have acute appendicitis.

When you have acute pain, doctors can generally figure out what the problem is and fix it. The goal of treatment is to manage the pain over the short term until healing occurs — when the cavity is filled, the skins grows back or the incision heals.

Chronic pain

Chronic pain is pain that hangs on even after the injury has healed, seemingly unaffected by the passing of time. Chronic pain can also result from progressive injury that doesn't heal, such as from arthritis and some cancers. This is reflected in the word itself: *chronic*, like *chronology*, comes from the Greek word for "time."

Like acute pain, chronic pain can span the full range of sensations and intensity. It can be dull or sharp, and it can tingle, jolt or burn. The pain may remain constant, or it can come and go, such as a headache that suddenly develops without warning.

Sometimes, the cause of chronic pain can't be determined. There may not be any evidence of disease or damage to body tissues that doctors can link to the pain. Other times, doctors are able to identify the cause.

Often, chronic pain results from one of the following three broad types of injury:

Joint and bone injury

Chronic conditions such as osteoarthritis, rheumatoid arthritis, degenerative disk disease and spinal stenosis are common causes of chronic bone and joint pain. Osteoporosis, a common, chronic bone disorder among women older than 45, causes porous and weak bones. It can result in increased risk of fractures, which can be painful, especially compression fractures of the vertebrae.

Tissue injury

Damage to tendons or muscles is another common cause of chronic pain. Conditions such as tendinitis or fibromyalgia can produce persistent aching.

Nerve injury

Occasionally, chronic pain may stem from an accident, infection or surgery that damages a peripheral or spinal nerve. The damaged nerve continues to cause pain even after the original injury has seemingly healed. This type of nerve pain is called neuropathic pain. Neuropathic pain can also result from diseases that damage nerves, such as diabetes or shingles (herpes zoster).

Once damaged, the nerve may send pain messages that are unwarranted. For example, an increased blood sugar level from diabetes can damage the small nerves in your hands and feet, leaving you with a painful burning sensation in your fingers and toes.

Mystery shrouds many of the reasons why injured nerves sometimes misfire and send wrong messages. However, when a nerve cell is damaged, the ends of surviving fibers can sprout a tangle of unorganized nerve fibers (neuroma). This bundle of nerve tissue may start sending warnings of injuries that don't exist. Damaged nerves may actually be more sensitive to external stimuli, or they may send signals spontaneously in the absence of painful stimuli.

The chronic pain challenge

Acute pain tends to be easier to treat than chronic pain. It often responds well to medication, and with time — a few days to a few weeks — it begins to subside.

Chronic pain can be difficult to treat. For some types of chronic pain, medication or injections are beneficial. But these measures don't always work, or their effects are short-lived. Infrequently, surgery may cure or reduce the pain.

When pain can't be controlled, treatment often centers on ways to live with the pain, reducing its intensity and its effect on daily life. Learning to cope with chronic pain has a lot to do with attitude and lifestyle. People who can approach their condition with a positive attitude and a willingness to change their lifestyle to prevent or reduce pain triggers are often the most successful in coping with pain.

Methods for Treating Pain

When it comes to controlling pain, the first thing most people think of is medication. That's understandable. Medication is the most common method for treating pain. But it's not the only method. A variety of methods can be used to relieve pain, or to reduce its sting:

- Medications, ranging from aspirin to narcotics
- Mechanical therapies, such as ice, heat and massage
- Invasive therapies, including injections
- Behavior therapies, beginning with exercise and stress management

Often, a combination of therapies provides the best approach for managing pain and reducing unwanted side effects.

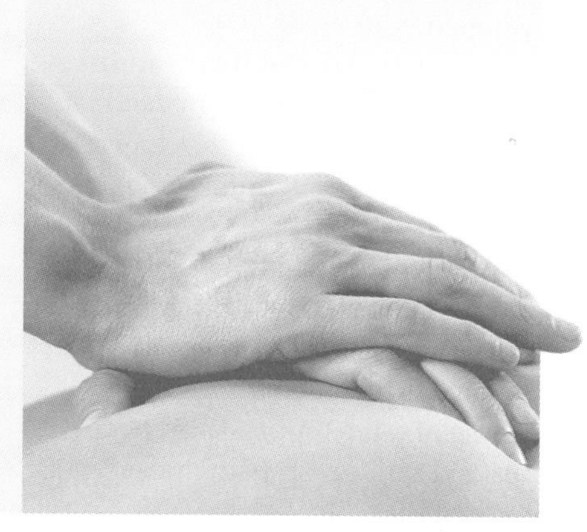

Pain Medications

Pain relievers (analgesics) are the most widely used medication for controlling pain. They control pain by interfering with the development of pain messages, their frequency, their path or how they're interpreted. Many types of over-the-counter and prescription pain relievers are available.

Acetaminophen

Acetaminophen is most effective for minor to moderate pain that isn't accompanied by inflammation. Acetaminophen doesn't interfere with the enzyme in your body that serves as a catalyst for inflammation. But this drug is often effective at controlling other types of pain.

Over-the-counter generic products are available. Brands of pain medication with acetaminophen include:

- Anacin Aspirin Free
- Aspirin Free Excedrin
- Anacin-3
- Tylenol

When taken occasionally and as recommended, acetaminophen is generally safe. But if you take more of the medication than recommended on the product label, it could lead to liver damage. Alcohol appears to enhance this risk.

Acetaminophen is sometimes combined with a narcotic to provide stronger pain relief. This form of the drug is available only by prescription. It's generally effective, but it can become habit-forming if taken regularly for a long period.

Nonsteroidal anti-inflammatory drugs

Nonsteroidal anti-inflammatory drugs, or NSAIDs, are most effective for mild to moderate pain that's accompanied by swelling and inflammation. These drugs relieve pain by inhibiting production of pain-intensifying chemicals activated by tissue damage.

NSAIDs are especially helpful for arthritis and pain resulting from muscle sprains, strains, back and neck injuries or cramps.

Over-the-counter NSAIDs include:

- Aspirin (Bayer, Bufferin, others)
- Ibuprofen (Advil, Motrin, others)
- Ketoprofen (Orudis)
- Naproxen (Aleve)

NSAIDs available by prescription include:

- Diclofenac sodium (Voltaren XR)
- Etodolac (Lodine)
- Fenoprofen
- Flurbiprofen (Ansaid)
- Indomethacin (Indocin)
- Ketorolac (Toradol)
- Meloxicam (Mobic)
- Nabumetone (Relafen)
- Naproxen (Naprelan, Naprosyn)
- Oxaprozin (Daypro)
- Piroxicam (Feldene)
- Sulindac (Clinoril)

When taken occasionally and as directed, NSAIDs are usually safe. But if you take them regularly for months or years, or if you take more than the recommended dosage, NSAIDs might cause nausea, stomach pain, stomach bleeding and ulcers.

Large doses of NSAIDs can also lead to kidney problems, fluid retention and heart failure. Risk of these conditions increases with age, especially among women. If you regularly take NSAIDs, talk to your doctor about monitoring potential side effects.

NSAIDs can also have a ceiling effect — a limit on how much pain they can control. Beyond a certain dosage, they don't provide additional pain relief benefits. If you have moderate to severe pain, an NSAID may not be able to relieve your pain.

COX-2 inhibitors

COX-2 inhibitors are a newer type of NSAID designed to relieve pain with fewer side effects than traditional NSAIDs.

NSAIDs relieve pain by inhibiting enzymes in your body called cyclooxygenase (COX). These enzymes make hormone-like substances called prostaglandins, which are involved in the development of pain and inflammation.

Traditional NSAIDs work against two versions of cyclooxygenase present in your body: COX-1 and COX-2. However, there's evidence that suppressing COX-1 can cause stomach and bleeding problems because COX-1 is the enzyme that protects your stomach lining and allows platelets to form blood clots.

COX-2 inhibitors primarily suppress COX-2 enzymes. Because they don't affect COX-1 as much, the drugs are considered less harmful to your digestive system. However, COX-2 inhibitors don't protect against blood clots, like aspirin and other NSAIDs do — an important point for people with cardiovascular disease.

Examples of prescription COX-2 inhibitors include:

- Celecoxib (Celebrex)
- Rofecoxib (Vioxx)
- Valdecoxib (Bextra)

In studies of COX-2 inhibitors, participants reported a 30 percent to 70 percent reduction in pain without common side effects associated with traditional NSAIDs. COX-2 inhibitors are usually more expensive than traditional NSAIDs. Possible side effects include diarrhea, indigestion, gas, nausea and headache. Long-term effects of COX-2 inhibitors are unknown.

Tricyclic antidepressants

Some medications developed to manage other conditions, such as depression or seizures, are also used to treat chronic pain. One such group of medications is tricyclic antidepressants. Although tricyclic antidepressants aren't analgesics, they can be very effective in reducing some forms of pain. The medications interfere with certain chemical processes in your brain that cause you to feel pain.

When Is It Addiction?

Chemical dependency can manifest itself in three ways: increased tolerance, physical dependence and addiction. People often lump all three forms under the term *addiction*, but addiction has a very specific meaning. Although addiction poses serious health risks, the other two forms of dependency aren't necessarily "bad."

Increased tolerance
As your body becomes accustomed to a drug, the medication can lose its effectiveness. To receive the same degree of relief, you may have to take higher doses. Don't increase your dosage unless you're under the supervision of a doctor and he or she recommends that you do so.

Physical dependence
To control your pain, you rely on receiving your medication at regular intervals. When use of the drug is abruptly stopped or its dosage substantially reduced, you experience physical withdrawal symptoms. Withdrawal can be avoided by tapering the medication dosage gradually. If you take narcotic medications regularly, ask your doctor for guidance before decreasing the dosage.

Addiction
Addiction involves both physical and psychological dependence on a drug. You can develop this dependence with a prescription medication, nicotine, alcohol and illegal drugs, such as marijuana and cocaine. In cases of psychological dependence, you crave the psychological effects of the medication, leading to loss of control over its use. You take the drug even though it isn't helping you, and, in fact, the habit leads to harm — professionally, socially and psychologically.

Tricyclic antidepressants include:
- Amitriptyline (Elavil)
- Clomipramine (Anafranil)
- Desipramine (Norpramin)
- Doxepin (Sinequan)
- Imipramine (Tofranil)
- Nortriptyline (Aventyl, Pamelor)
- Protriptyline (Vivactil)
- Trimipramine (Surmontil)

Unlike narcotics, tricyclic antidepressants don't lead to dependency or addiction. They can, however, make you drowsy, so it's generally recommended that you take the medication at bedtime.

In addition, the drugs may cause dry mouth, constipation, weight gain and difficulty with urination. To reduce or prevent these symptoms, your doctor will likely start you off at a low dose and slowly increase the amount of the drug you take. Most people are able to take tricyclic antidepressants with only mild side effects.

Antiseizure medications

Developed mainly to reduce or control epileptic seizures, antiseizure medications also may help control the stabbing, shooting or jabbing pain that can accompany nerve damage. The drugs seem to work by slowing or preventing damaged nerves from sending uncontrolled pain signals.

Antiseizure medications used for chronic pain include:
- Carbamazepine (Carbatrol, Tegretol)
- Gabapentin (Neurontin)
- Lamotrigine (Lamictal)
- Phenytoin (Dilantin, Phenytek)
- Topiramate (Topamax)

Although these medications can cause dizziness, nausea and constipation, most people who take them are bothered only minimally by these side effects. More severe but less common side effects include blood, heart and liver disorders.

To reduce your risk of side effects, your doctor may start you on a small amount of the drug and gradually increase the dose over a period of several weeks — possibly monitoring you with blood tests during that time.

Narcotics

Some narcotics are natural compounds derived from opium. Others are synthetic medications that work in a similar fashion. These potent painkillers, known as opioids and opiates, interfere with the transmission of pain signals and are taken most often to relieve pain from a severe injury, surgery, cancer or a terminal illness.

Narcotics include the following — those marked with an asterisk are multi-ingredient:
- Butorphanol (Stadol)
- Codeine (aspirin with codeine, acetaminophen with codeine)
- Fentanyl (Actiq, Duragesic)
- Hydrocodone (Lorcet*, Lortab*, Vicodin*, others)
- Hydromorphone (Dilaudid)
- Levorphanol (Levo-Dromoran)
- Meperidine (Demerol)
- Methadone (Dolophine)
- Morphine (MS Contin, Roxanol)
- Oxycodone (OxyContin, Percocet*, Roxicet*, Tylox*, others)
- Propoxyphene (Darvon, Darvocet*)

Short-term use of narcotics generally causes only minor side effects, such as nausea, constipation, sedation and unclear thinking. When taken for several weeks to months, these side effects can become more bothersome. A narcotic drug can lose its effectiveness as your body develops a tolerance to it.

The biggest concern with narcotics is the risk of addiction. Narcotics can become habit-forming, and that's why doctors have tended to limit their use to acute pain. In recent years, however, some difference of opinion has arisen regarding the use of these medications. More doctors have begun prescribing narcotics for some forms of chronic pain, in response to studies that suggest the risk of addiction is less than once thought.

Several studies indicate that most people who regularly take a narcotic over a long period of time become physically dependent on the drug and experience some minor withdrawal symptoms if they abruptly stop using it. But only a small percentage of people actually abuse the medication or become addicted to it. Although addiction is a serious problem, physical dependence itself may not result in serious problems, provided the medication is taken as directed.

Nonetheless, the potential risks associated with long-term use of narcotics still make it difficult to justify the use of narcotics for many forms of chronic pain.

Tramadol

Tramadol (Ultram) is a prescription pain medication that works in two ways. It interferes with the transmission of pain signals, like a narcotic, and it triggers release of the brain neurotransmitters norepinephrine and serotonin, which help reduce pain.

Tramadol is used mainly to relieve moderate to severe acute pain. Its use for chronic pain hasn't been as well studied. In a few studies in which the drug was prescribed for chronic pain, some people experienced significant pain relief and others had none.

Because it's a weak narcotic, risk of physical dependence and addiction is low. Side effects from tramadol can include dizziness, sedation, headache, nausea and constipation. Possible long-term effects from the drug are unknown.

Mechanical Therapies

Methods that try to relieve pain by targeting muscles and connective tissues involved in an injury are called mechanical therapies. They include cold therapy, heat therapy, exercise, massage, chiropractic care, ultrasound therapy and transcutaneous electronic nerve stimulation (TENS).

Cold

Ice decreases pain by numbing the affected area. It works best for muscle spasms, swelling and joint pain. When the cold area warms up, extra blood rushes back to the area of the injury, speeding the healing.

Ice massage

To give yourself an ice massage, gently rub a piece of ice over the affected area for 5 to 7 minutes, until it becomes slightly numb. Watch for color changes in your skin. If you notice your skin losing its underlying red tone, stop immediately because it could indicate the onset of frostbite. If your skin becomes more than slightly numb during the ice massage, end the treatment.

Cold packs

To use a cold pack, place a damp towel over the painful area. Then put a cold pack — such as a small bag of frozen peas — on the towel and cover it with dry towels for

Pain-Relieving Creams

Some pain relievers come in the form of a cream or gel. The medication is absorbed through your skin. Pain relief creams and gels can occasionally help relieve pain and inflammation just below your skin, such as pain from arthritis or nerve damage or pain near a surgical incision.

EMLA

EMLA is a prescription pain-relieving cream made from two topical anesthetics: lidocaine and prilocaine. Your skin becomes numb within an hour after application, and the benefits of the cream are greatest 2 to 3 hours following application. EMLA is commonly used — especially on children — to reduce pain before a shot, drawing blood, inserting an intravenous line or treating a wart.

Capsaicin

Capsaicin (Dolorac, Zostrix) is a topical nonprescription cream made from the seeds of hot chili peppers. It's thought to work by depleting nerve cells of a chemical involved in transmitting pain messages. You rub the cream on your skin three or four times a day. It usually takes 1 to 2 weeks before its effects become noticeable. Maximum effects are often achieved after 3 to 4 weeks.

Capsaicin is most effective for temporary relief of arthritic pain in joints close to the skin, such as your fingers, knees and elbows. It's also used to help relieve skin sensitivity from shingles, pain resulting from nerve damage, pain that follows a mastectomy and chronic pain near healed surgical scars.

Methyl creams

Nonprescription multi-ingredient medications such as ArthriCare, Ben-Gay and Icy Hot use heat or cold to cover up the pain. These creams may relieve occasional, mild muscle aches, but they're not effective for most forms of chronic pain.

Aspirin-like creams

Nonprescription trolamine creams such as Aspercreme, Sportscreme and Myoflex Creme contain a chemical that's similar to aspirin. The Food and Drug Administration describes these creams as safe but not necessarily effective for pain relief.

insulation. Don't leave the pack on the area for more than 20 minutes at a time. Check your skin regularly for loss of underlying redness, a clue that frostbite is beginning.

Heat

Heat increases blood flow and nutrients to painful muscles and joints. This helps the healing process and can improve flexibility.

Hot packs

To treat your pain with a hot pack, place several towels over the painful area. Lay a hot pack on top. Cover the pack with more towels for insulation. Add or remove towels between your skin and the pack to vary the heat. Check your skin every 15 minutes. If you see red and white blotches, stop the treatment at once to prevent a burn.

Heating pads

To treat your pain with an electric heating pad, first place a towel over the painful area. Then put the pad on top. Limit your use of a heating pad to 30 minutes at a time. Check occasionally for red and white blotches — signs that you've made the area too hot.

Heat lamps

A heat lamp produces infrared rays that warm your skin, which in turn increases blood circulation. Use a 250-watt reflector heat bulb. Position the lamp 18 to 20 inches from your skin. To decrease the heat intensity, move the lamp farther away. Apply heat to the sore area for no longer than 30 minutes. If you think you might fall asleep while under the lamp, use an alarm clock or timer.

Baths and hot tubs

A 15-minute hot bath can be just as effective as a hot tub in relieving muscle and joint pain. Don't get the water too hot. You don't want to burn yourself. If you have a hot tub, limit its use to no more than 30 minutes at a time.

Looking for a Helping Hand?

For help with designing and getting started on your physical activity program, contact one of these professionals:

A physical therapist
Most hospitals and clinics have physical therapists on staff. A physical therapist is trained in the use of exercise to achieve physical fitness. He or she can help you select the most appropriate exercises based on the location of your pain and show you how to do them properly.

An occupational therapist
Occupational therapists also are available in most hospitals and clinics. An occupational therapist can teach you how to do daily activities in ways that can reduce stress on your joints.

A certified exercise therapist
Many health clubs have employees who are trained in exercise therapy. If you belong to a health club — or are thinking of joining one — make an appointment to meet with a certified exercise therapist for help with developing an exercise plan.

Exercise

A common misconception is that exercise increases pain. Actually, exercise can help reduce it. During physical activity, your body releases chemicals — endorphins and enkephalins — that block pain signals from reaching your brain. These chemicals also help alleviate anxiety and depression, conditions that can make your pain more difficult to control.

A regular exercise program that includes flexibility, aerobic and strengthening exercises can help improve your fitness and control pain. Regular exercise can also:

- Increase your energy and improve sleep
- Promote weight loss, reducing stress on your joints
- Increase bone mass, reducing your risk of injury

It's important to play it safe when it comes to exercise. Here are some precautions to observe:

- If you've recently suffered an injury or haven't exercised in the past, consult a doctor before beginning an exercise program.
- Get advice on choosing the exercises best for you.

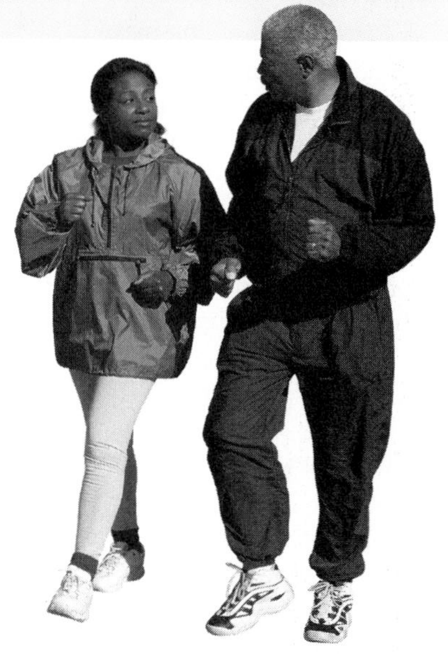

- Be careful not to overdo it. Start out slowly, and gradually increase the time and pace of your exercise.

To help you get and stay active, see Chapter 4, "Keeping Active."

Massage

Massage is one of the oldest methods of therapy that's still practiced. It involves use of different manipulative techniques to move your body's muscles and soft tissues.

A massage therapist primarily uses his or her hands to manipulate muscles and tissues. However, the therapist sometimes may use his or her forearms, elbows or feet.

Massage therapy is based on the belief that when muscles are overworked, waste products accumulate in them, causing soreness and stiffness. The therapy aims to improve circulation in the muscles, increasing the flow of nutrients and removing waste products.

Massage can relax your muscles, improve the range of motion in your joints and increase production of your body's natural painkillers. It may also help relieve stress and anxiety. Avoid massage if you have open sores, acute inflammation or circulatory problems.

Chiropractic

Chiropractic care is based on the belief that certain illnesses and conditions, including pain, result from impairment of your nervous system due to problems with your joints and especially your spine. To relieve or eliminate negative effects on your nerves, chiropractors manipulate associated joints. They typically do this by slightly stretching or adjusting the joints.

There are two types of chiropractors. Those who depend solely on traditional chiropractic practices are often referred to as straight practitioners. Chiropractors who combine standard chiropractic care techniques with other therapies, such as exercise, acupuncture or dietary and herbal supplements, are known as mixers.

The effectiveness of some chiropractic therapies is controversial. Back pain is the most common reason people see a chiropractor, and studies indicate that for some types of low back pain, especially acute pain, chiropractic therapy may be effective.

Ultrasound

Ultrasound can do more than allow doctors to see inside your body. Physical therapists use ultrasound to treat painful injuries and to speed the healing process. Ultrasound acts as a deep-heating tool, warming tissue below the surface of the skin.

The heating effects — which you can't feel — are especially helpful in treating injured muscles, tendons and ligaments. They can also help relieve the pain associated with these injuries. In addition, the sound pulses may be used to help "push" a topical anti-inflammatory cream deep into damaged tissues.

Transcutaneous electronic nerve stimulation

Transcutaneous electronic nerve stimulation (TENS) is a treatment prescribed by a doctor. It's intended to relieve pain by preventing pain signals from reaching your brain. TENS is safe and usually painless.

With TENS, small electrodes are placed on your skin near the area of your pain. The electrodes are attached to a small portable stimulator that you wear.

The battery-powered stimulator delivers tiny electric impulses through the electrodes to nearby nerve pathways. You turn the TENS unit on and off as needed to control pain.

Exactly how the impulses relieve pain is uncertain. One theory is that TENS blocks the transmission of pain signals during modulation at the spinal cord. Another theory is that TENS stimulates production of endorphins, your body's natural painkillers.

TENS generally works best for acute pain associated with a pinched nerve. It's less successful for chronic pain, although some people receive benefit from it. Most often, the therapy is used in conjunction with other treatments, including exercise.

A related and newer procedure under study, called percutaneous electronic nerve stimulation (PENS), uses acupuncture-like needles, instead of electrodes placed on the skin, to transmit electric current to your nerves.

Invasive Therapies

Invasive therapies range from simple injections to surgical implants. For some types of pain, the most effective approach is to treat the pain locally, near the pain site. Invasive therapy can also be an option when medications or mechanical approaches don't produce satisfactory results.

Injections

An injection (a shot) is most effective for nerve, joint or muscle pain that's confined to a specific location. The injections may include an anesthetic to control the pain, a steroid to reduce inflammation or a combination of the two.

The benefit of injections is that the medication works primarily on the painful area and doesn't spread throughout your body. This reduces potential side effects from the drug. The disadvantage of injections is that many times their effects are only temporary. In addition, there's a limit as to how often you can receive an injection, depending on the injection site and the type of medication used.

The two classes of injections are diagnostic and therapeutic. Diagnostic injections are used to test where the pain is coming from. Therapeutic injections are used to help provide long-term relief of symptoms. Sometimes the two are combined.

Injections generally aren't a cure, but they can help some people through an initial period of intense pain or a severe flare-up. The three general types of pain management injections are joint, soft-tissue and nerve block.

Joint injection

If you're experiencing inflammation and pain caused by bone rubbing against bone, your doctor may recommend an injection near or

Question and Answer

What's the difference between a pain clinic and a pain center?

Usually, a pain clinic offers a more narrow range of services than does a pain center.

A pain clinic is typically a facility with one or more doctors who specialize in the treatment of one or several painful conditions. For example, the doctors may specialize in the treatment of back pain or headache pain.

A pain center is generally composed of a multidisciplinary group of doctors who specialize in the comprehensive treatment of pain. Their collective expertise allows for the management of a wide variety of pain problems. Frequently, a pain center does research and participates in the training of pain specialists.

A pain center or clinic is similar to many things in life — you get from it only what you put into it. If you're unwilling to learn new pain-coping skills and you have a negative attitude, the program may be of little help. But if you have a positive attitude and realistic expectations, you can come away with a better understanding of your pain and what you can do to manage it.

into the affected joint. The joint is generally injected with a preparation of a local anesthetic to numb the area and then a medication. The two main types of medication used for joint injections are corticosteroids and hyaluronic acid.

Corticosteroids
Corticosteroids suppress inflammation. They often begin working in 3 to 4 days and may offer some pain relief for 4 to 6 months. When used for many months to years, they tend to become less effective.

Hyaluronic acid
Hyaluronic acid — hyaluronate (Hyalgan, Supartz) and hylan G-F 20 (Synvisc) — is used to treat osteoarthritis of the knee and may eventually be used for other joints. Hyaluronic acid is a substance found in normal joint fluid, which acts as a lubricant. Hyaluronate and hylan G-F 20 help relieve pain by substituting for hyaluronic acid. Often, a local anesthetic is administered first, to relieve pain from the injections. Relief may last from 6 to 12 months.

Soft-tissue injection

When a specific body part, such as a muscle or a cushioning sac near a joint (bursa), is inflamed or painful, an injection can be given directly into the surrounding soft tissue.

Trigger point injection
Trigger points are areas where your muscles and nearby tissues underneath your skin are sensitive to touch or movement. These areas are generally in the upper and lower back muscles. A trigger point (field block) injection — usually a preparation of a local anesthetic and a corticosteroid — is used to treat such an area. Depending on the medication used, a trigger point injection can reduce pain in a muscle, reduce inflammation, relax a muscle or increase movement.

Bursa injection
Bursae are tiny, fluid-containing sacs that lubricate and cushion pressure points between your bones and the tendons or muscles near your joints. They help you move without pain. When a bursa becomes inflamed (bursitis), movement or pressure may cause pain. Bursitis most often affects a shoulder, elbow or hip joint. A corticosteroid injection can be given to reduce inflammation in the bursa.

Nerve block injection

A nerve block procedure involves injecting an anesthetic around a nerve's fibers, preventing pain messages from traveling along that nerve pathway to your brain. Nerve blocks are used most often to relieve pain for a short period until other therapies or medications can take effect. They're also used to provide regional anesthesia for surgery or to control labor pain.

There are three main types of nerve blocks:

Peripheral
With a peripheral nerve block, an anesthetic is injected at a specific location, such as an ankle, to reduce feeling and pain in that area.

Spinal
Spinal nerve blocks are most often used for pain that affects a broader area, such as your lower back or a leg. An anesthetic is injected near the spinal cord at the base of your spine to reduce pain all the way down the path of the nerve to your toes. These techniques include spinal (intrathecal) and epidural injections.

Sympathetic
Some forms of chronic pain, such as complex regional pain syndrome, may result from abnormally increased activity of your sympathetic nervous system. Your sympathetic nerves, part of your autonomic nervous system, control circulation and perspiration. To prevent messages produced by your sympathetic nerves from reaching the affected area of the body, an anesthetic may be injected near the sympathetic nerves. These injections are done in the neck for pain in the arms and in the low back for pain in the legs.

Spinal cord stimulation

A spinal cord stimulator is a small device that's surgically implanted, usually in your lower abdomen. It's wired to your spinal cord to deliver electric pulses that block pain messages to your brain. The device is battery powered, much like a pacemaker, and is controlled by an external programming unit that turns the stimulator on and off and adjusts the level of the electric pulse. Some people who use this device say the pulse causes a tingling sensation.

Spinal cord stimulation is usually used only after other treatments have failed. However, studies indicate that it can provide substantial pain relief. The procedure is used for a variety of pain, including back pain not relieved by surgery and pain from nerve injury.

Pain pumps

For some people with excruciating pain that isn't helped by other measures, one option to control the pain is a pain pump. The small device is surgically implanted in the lower abdomen, where it provides a steady injection of medication — typically a narcotic — to the spinal cord. Sometimes, the medication is a combination of drugs, such as a narcotic, muscle relaxant and local anesthetic.

Pain pumps are used most often to control pain associated with severe nerve damage or a terminal illness. Most people who receive a pain pump continue to experience pain, but the medication dulls the pain enough to make it tolerable.

Behavior Therapy

The goal of behavior therapy is to identify and modify personal pain triggers and reactions and to adjust your lifestyle to better manage your pain.

Simple things, such as how you organize your day, can have a significant effect on your ability to manage your pain. If you overdo it to meet a deadline at work or overcommit yourself so that you're running from one activity to the next, fatigue sets in and your pain increases. The opposite — avoiding all activities and lying around the house — isn't any better. The isolation can cause you to focus only on your pain. Behavior therapy is about finding a healthy balance of work, socialization, recreation and relaxation.

Time management

For many people an important step to balancing their day is learning to use time more efficiently. Juggling work, household tasks and social activities can consume large amounts of your day. Procrastination, perfectionism or overcommitting yourself can make time management even more difficult.

Try these strategies for using your time more wisely:

Plan
Schedule your day so that you have time for the things you must do and those you want to do. Write down all of your activities in a daily planner. Then frequently refer to your planner to make sure you stay on track.

You might also place a central calendar near your telephone to mark down all events and appointments so that they don't come as a surprise and to avoid becoming overcommitted.

Identify
Notice when you waste time and avoid these time wasters. If you can't avoid them, try to make them productive. For example, while waiting for a doctor's appointment or during your daily train commute, listen to a relaxation tape or balance your checkbook.

Prioritize
If you're involved in too many activities that are competing for your time, decide which are the most important and let go of the rest. Your health needs should come before the wants of others. The consequences of not taking care of yourself likely can be increased pain and fatigue.

Delegate
On days when you have more to do than you can comfortably handle, seek help from others. Have your spouse, son or daughter do the laundry or prepare dinner.

Evaluate
Think about your day. Do you have realistic expectations regarding the number of tasks that you can complete in a day?

Educate
Discuss your time needs with those who rely on you the most. If family members, friends or co-workers make unreasonable demands on your time, explain to them that you need to pace yourself.

Organizational skills

Becoming more organized can save you time so that you can incorporate more activities into your day. Organization also helps conserve energy by eliminating wasted steps and unnecessary motions.

Think before you act
Before you begin a task, gather all of the items you need or make a list of what needs to be done. For example, keep all of your cleaning supplies in one container to avoid multiple trips up and down the stairs. Before you run errands, list all of the things you need to do to avoid a second trip later on.

Keep items accessible
Organize your work areas at home and at your job so that items you use frequently are close at hand. This can save you unnecessary bending or reaching.

Reduce clutter
Searching for items takes both time and energy. Organize your counters,

Cancer Pain

In the United States, about 9 million people live with cancer — nearly 1 in 30 people. Although not all people with cancer experience pain, at least one-third do. Cancer pain can't always be eliminated, but it frequently can be controlled to lessen its impact on normal daily activities.

Treatment of cancer pain

Cancer-related pain can be treated in many different ways. The ideal method is to remove the source of the pain, for example, through surgery, chemotherapy, radiation or some other form of treatment. If that can't be done, the next option might be pain medication.

The type of medication prescribed for cancer pain depends on the severity of the pain. Sometimes, a simple analgesic such as acetaminophen (Tylenol, others) or a nonsteroidal anti-inflammatory drug (aspirin, ibuprofen, others) is helpful. Other times a stronger pain reliever is needed. This may include a weak narcotic, such as codeine, or a strong narcotic, such as morphine. To provide more consistent pain control, narcotics are often prescribed in a sustained-release formulation. You take the long-acting medication on a scheduled, regular basis. Your doctor may also prescribe a shorter-acting narcotic for intermittent use to control breakthrough pain. If swallowing pills is difficult, narcotics can be given in patch form, where they're absorbed through the skin. Other routes of delivery include transmucosal (lollipop), inhaled, intravenous, subcutaneous, spinal and rectal.

For some types of cancer, such as pancreatic cancer, a nerve block may effectively control the pain. During this procedure a doctor injects medication into the major nerves around the affected area to destroy the nerves and prevent them from sending pain signals to the brain.

Undertreatment of cancer pain

Unfortunately, cancer pain often isn't adequately controlled. One reason has to do with doctors' knowledge of pain and their ability to evaluate and treat pain. Some doctors and other health care professionals may not specifically ask about pain, which should be a normal part of every cancer checkup.

A second factor is reluctance on the part of the person with cancer. Some people fear that pain means that their cancer is getting worse, or they worry that their doctor may think of them as weak if they complain of pain. Many people feel they're supposed to have pain with cancer and that they should be able to deal with it on their own. This simply isn't true.

Another factor is fear of addiction. People with cancer worry that they may become addicted to narcotics used to control cancer pain. But the risk of addiction for people who take pain medications appropriately is low. The problem is estimated to occur in only about 1 in 10,000 people with cancer.

Some people worry that taking medications, such as morphine, may shorten their life. If the medication is dosed properly, it shouldn't shorten life or cause other severe side effects. Many people taking morphine still remain active.

A team approach

Inform your doctor if you're experiencing pain, and work together on a pain management plan. Set a main goal, such as keeping the pain at a level with which you're comfortable. If you aren't achieving that goal, keep working with your doctor. You might also ask to consult a pain specialist. Many medical facilities, especially major medical centers, have pain centers or pain clinics in which medical personnel are trained in a variety of pain management techniques.

cabinets, closets and drawers so that you can easily find what you need.

Moderation skills

Moderation involves how much, how long or how fast you do things to avoid overdoing or underdoing your day. Moderation helps you avoid large swings in your pain level so that at the end of each task, your pain is near the same level as when you began. To practice moderation:

Break apart lengthy tasks

Lengthy activities often sap your energy and may increase your pain. Instead of spending all day planting your garden, spend 1 or 2 hours a day in the garden for 3 or 4 days. Spread out a 10-hour car trip to visit friends or relatives over 2 days.

Alternate activities

Mix activities that require a lot of effort with those that require little energy. After vacuuming one room of the house, sit down and read or pay some bills. Then do a load of laundry. Note times of the day when you have the most energy and the least pain. Plan your priority tasks during these times.

Rest periodically

How often you should take a break depends on the activity. You may find that you can do some activities, such as word processing, for 30 minutes to an hour before you need a break. More strenuous tasks, such as mowing the lawn, may require a break every 10 to 20 minutes.

Pace yourself

Instead of rushing to complete a task, work at a comfortable speed — a pace at which you feel like you're exerting yourself but not overdoing it. You expend twice as much energy when you work at a fast pace than you do at a moderate one. It may take you a little longer to get the job done, but in the end you'll feel better.

Stress management

Pain and stress go hand in hand. When you're in pain, you're less able to handle everyday stressors. Common hassles turn into major obstacles. Stress also causes you to do things that intensify your pain, such as tense your muscles, grit your teeth and stiffen your shoulders. In short, pain causes stress, and stress intensifies pain.

The first step in breaking this pain-stress cycle is to realize that stress is your response to an event, not the event itself. It's something you can control. That's why events that are stressful for some people aren't for others.

For example, your morning commute may leave you anxious and tense because you use it as worry time. A co-worker, however, finds the same commute relaxing. She enjoys her time alone, perhaps listening to music or a book on tape.

Understanding that you have control over your stress helps you develop positive strategies for dealing with it. For information on stress management techniques, see Chapter 5, "Managing Stress."

Treatment for depression and anxiety

As many as half of people with chronic pain experience mild to severe depression and anxiety. It's natural to feel down, frustrated or anxious when the pain first develops or for short periods afterward.

Your pain itself may cause signs or symptoms associated with depression, such as slowed movements or loss of energy. But if your symptoms linger for several months or they become severe, you may be experiencing depression or anxiety.

Depression and anxiety are complex conditions that can make your pain worse. That's because it's difficult to separate your mood from the intensity of your pain. People who are depressed or anxious often report stronger, longer-lasting and more severe pain than do people who aren't depressed. They're less able to tolerate pain.

Depression and anxiety should be treated. With appropriate treatment most people begin to show improvement, usually in a matter of weeks. For information on these conditions, see Chapter 37, "Mental Illness."

Common Chronic Conditions

Chronic pain can strike just about any part of your body, from your head to your toes, from your skin to your well-protected internal organs. Arthritis pain, back pain and headache are the most common types of chronic pain. But chronic pain can occur in many forms and for many reasons.

Your pain may be related to an existing illness or stem from an accident or injury. Perhaps your pain is linked to a condition that doctors don't fully understand. Or maybe it has no apparent cause.

This section briefly reviews some of the more common types of chronic pain.

Bone and joint disorders

There are many painful disorders of the bones and joints, but the most common is arthritis. The word *arthritis* means "joint inflammation." Although people often talk about arthritis as one disease, it's not. It takes many forms. Some forms appear gradually. Others appear suddenly and then disappear, only to return again later.

The disease can strike any joint in your body and may be triggered by various causes, including an injury, lack of physical activity, natural wear on your joints and genetic disease. The two most common forms of arthritis are osteoarthritis and rheumatoid arthritis.

Osteoarthritis

Osteoarthritis affects close to 20 million Americans. This common condition results when cartilage that cushions the ends of bones in your joints starts to deteriorate. If the cartilage wears down completely, you may be left with bone rubbing against bone, irritating the joint and producing pain.

Your body tries to repair the damage, but often the repairs are unsuccessful, even resulting in growth of new bone along the sides of existing bone. The new bone may produce bony lumps, most

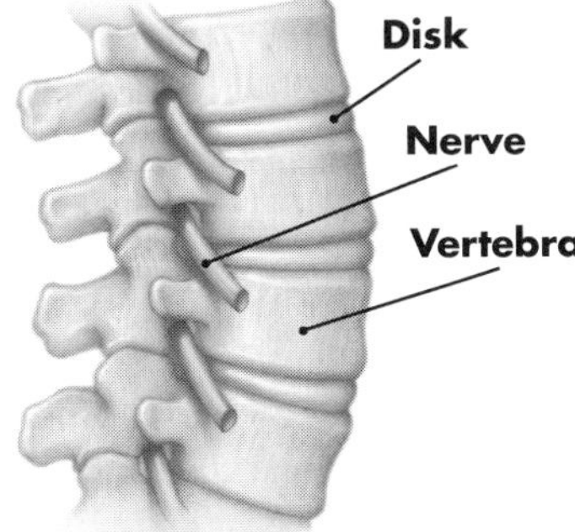

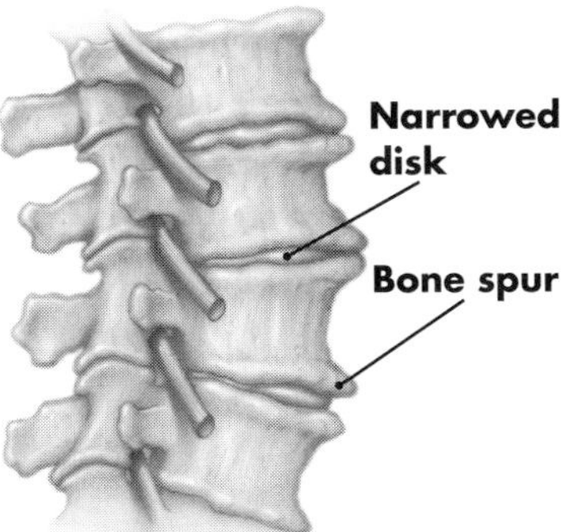

In a normal spine, your vertebrae are cushioned by elastic structures called disks, which help to keep the spine flexible. When you have osteoarthritis in the spine, the disks narrow, leading to bony lumps along the sides of vertebrae. Pain and stiffness may occur where bone surfaces rub together.

noticeably in your hands and feet, and especially at the middle joints or ends of your fingers and toes. These lumps, some of which are called spurs, may or may not produce pain and tenderness.

Osteoarthritis can develop anywhere in your body, but it tends to be most common in your hands and feet and in major joints in your neck, back, knees and hips. Initially, arthritis pain may be minor and hurt only when you use the affected joint. But in time, the pain can intensify and occur even when you're not using the joint.

Although there's no known cure for osteoarthritis, in recent years treatments to reduce pain and maintain joint movement have improved. Pain management generally includes a combination of medication, self-care and physical therapy, including daily exercise.

Medications include both topical medications, such as creams and gels that temporarily relieve the pain, and oral medications, such as nonsteroidal anti-inflammatory drugs (NSAIDs), including COX-2 inhibitors. Over-the-counter medications may be sufficient for mild osteoarthritis. For moderate to severe disease, you may need a stronger, prescription medication.

The dietary supplements glucosamine and chondroitin sulfate are popular alternative treatments for osteoarthritis, but so far, research hasn't confirmed that the supplements can actually prevent cartilage loss. However, several smaller studies suggest that for some people, the two supplements can relieve arthritis pain as effectively as NSAIDs can. No significant side effects are known to be associated with the supplements, but they may raise blood sugar levels, which may be a concern for people who have diabetes.

Rheumatoid arthritis

Unlike osteoarthritis, rheumatoid arthritis is thought to stem from an immune system disorder that causes your immune system to inappropriately attack the lining of your joints, just as it appropriately attacks invading viruses or bacteria.

White blood cells designed to destroy viruses and bacteria move into joint tissues, producing inflammation and pain. Swelling of the tissues triggers the release of natural chemicals that eventually dissolve cartilage and damage tendons and ligaments in the joint. Gradually, the joint becomes deformed. Rheumatoid arthritis most often affects joints in your wrists, hands, feet and ankles.

Anti-inflammatory drugs can often help ease pain associated with rheumatoid arthritis. Over-the-counter medications may be sufficient for mild pain. For moderate to severe disease, you may need a stronger, prescription medication.

Connective tissue disorders

Your muscles help you move. Each skeletal muscle is attached to bones by fibrous bands called tendons. Muscles and tendons work with other soft tissues, such as cartilage in your joints, to enable you to run, walk or climb stairs. Damage to connective tissues can make movement painful. Common connective tissue disorders include low back pain, bursitis, tendinitis and fibromyalgia.

Low back pain

Back pain ranks second only to headaches as the most frequent type of pain. Four of five adults, at some time in life, experience a bout of back pain that causes them to see a doctor.

Most back pain occurs in your lower back (lumbar area), which bears most of your weight. Muscle strain is a common cause of low back pain. It can occur if you lift something too heavy, twist too sharply or stand on your feet too many hours. Muscle spasm may also occur. Spasm is your back's response to injury. It's designed to immobilize you and prevent further damage. Any movement of the injured muscles can set off a wave of stabbing pains.

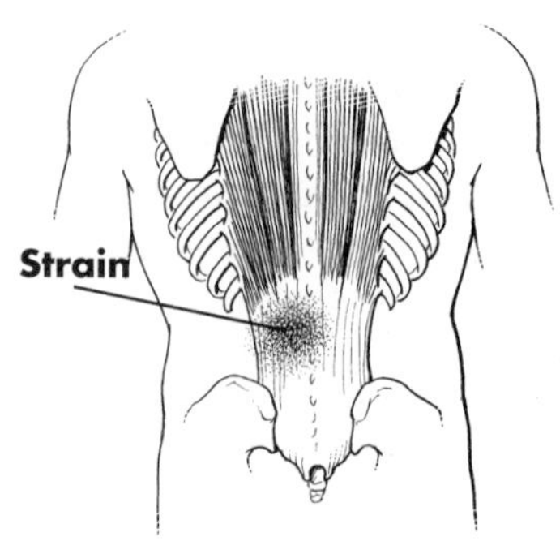

Your lower back, a pivot point for turning at your waist, is vulnerable to muscle strains.

The good news is that about 90 percent of muscle strains heal within 4 weeks, usually much sooner. The remaining 10 percent take longer. In some cases, the pain becomes chronic and never goes away.

Treatment typically includes rest, anti-inflammatory medicines such as nonsteroidal anti-inflammatory drugs (NSAIDs), exercise and heat and cold therapy. If these measures don't work, other options may include ultrasound or transcutaneous electronic nerve stimulation (TENS).

Bursitis

You have more than 150 bursae in your body. These tiny, fluid-containing sacs lubricate and cushion pressure points between your bones and the tendons and muscles near your joints. They help you move without pain. But when they become inflamed — often through overuse or an injury such as a hard bump — movement or pressure is painful.

Most often bursitis affects the shoulder, elbow or hip joint. It can also affect your knee, heel and even the base of your big toe. With proper treatment, bursitis pain usually goes away within a week or so, but return flare-ups are common.

An injection of a steroid into the bursa may help relieve the inflammation. Often an anesthetic is included to relieve pain. Other options include a nonsteroidal anti-inflammatory drug (NSAID), such as a COX-2 inhibitor, to help relieve pain and inflammation. Heat and cold therapy may help. And an elastic bandage, sling or soft pad can help protect the joint until the swelling goes down.

Tendinitis

Tendinitis is inflammation or irritation of a tendon — a thick, fibrous cord that attaches muscles to bone. The most common cause of tendinitis is injury or overuse during work or play. The condition generally causes tenderness and stiffness near a joint that's aggravated by movement. Most often, tendinitis develops in a shoulder, elbow (tennis elbow) or knee.

If tendinitis is severe and causes a rupture of a tendon, you may need surgical repair. In many cases, though, rest and medications to reduce pain and inflammation may be the only treatment you need. Sometimes, a doctor may inject a steroid into tissue around the tendon to relieve the inflammation.

Fibromyalgia

Fibromyalgia is a disorder that targets your muscles, tendons and ligaments. It differs from arthritis in that the pain is in nearby tissues instead of the joints themselves. Also unlike arthritis, it doesn't cause inflammation — just pain.

The main symptom of fibromyalgia is aching all over. The pain may be a deep ache or a burning sensation. Symptoms of fibromyalgia may flare and subside, but they usually don't disappear completely.

In general, fibromyalgia is treated with a combination of medications to reduce pain and improve sleep. The emphasis is on minimizing symptoms and improving general health. Medications often include over-the-counter or prescription pain relievers. Antidepressants may be prescribed to help promote sleep and relieve pain. Medications are often combined with behavior therapies, including stress management and daily exercise.

Nerve disorders

Pain from nerve damage or disorders can be among the most difficult to treat. Your body's intricate network of nerves is what controls the pain messages sent to your brain. When nerves don't work properly, they can cause a variety of symptoms that can be difficult to control.

Diabetic neuropathy

High blood sugar characteristic of diabetes can be associated with damage to delicate peripheral nerves in your feet and hands. About 6 of 10 people with diabetes experience this kind of nerve damage, which can be painful and disabling. Most commonly, nerves in the feet are affected, and less often, nerves in the fingers. Peripheral neuropathy may produce a tingling sensation, numbness, pain or a combination of all these.

Medications that tend to provide the greatest relief of nerve pain include antiseizure or antidepressant medications. Another treatment option is the nonprescription cream capsaicin (Dolorac, Zostrix) made from hot chili pepper extract. When you rub it over the painful area, the extract helps block pain sensations. However, it can take 1 to 4 weeks for the cream to become effective. Other therapies that may be beneficial include acupuncture, biofeedback and relaxation techniques.

Shingles and pain after shingles

Shingles (herpes zoster) can result in acute pain and also in persistent nerve pain known as postherpetic neuralgia.

Shingles is the re-emergence of the virus that caused an earlier case of chickenpox. The virus reactivates after lying dormant for years within your nerve cells. When it reactivates, the virus typically causes pain or tingling in a limited area, usually on part of one side of your body or face. As the virus travels along a nerve that spreads outward from your spine or face, this pain or tingling can continue for several days or longer. Subsequently, a rash with small blisters typically appears.

Most people with shingles have pain requiring treatment with pain relievers, even prescription narcotics. Antiviral medications, such as acyclovir (Zovirax) and famciclovir (Famvir), can hasten healing of skin lesions and reduce the severity of some complications caused by shingles.

If pain persists after the rash heals, it's known as postherpetic neuralgia. This chronic pain results from damage to nerve fibers from the shingles infection. Postherpetic neuralgia can be treated with tricyclic antidepressants and antiseizure drugs, among other medications. Some people are helped most by these drugs, which help suppress pain messages from damaged nerves.

Other steps that may reduce the pain include applying an analgesic cream, such as capsaicin (Dolorac, Zostrix), and placing a wet, cool compress over the blisters.

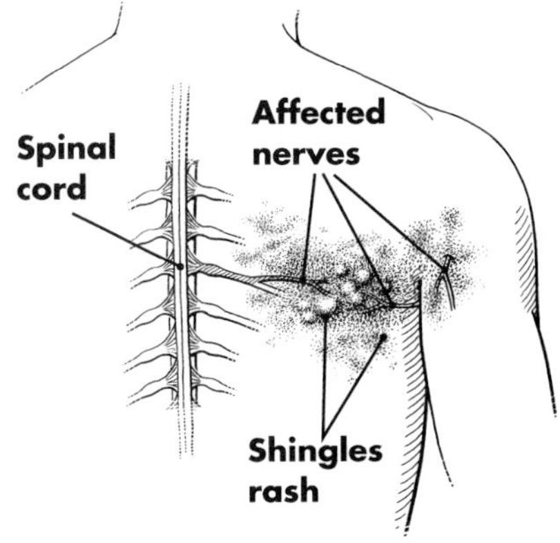

Shingles (herpes zoster) is a rash associated with an inflammation of nerves beneath the skin. Damage to the nerves may produce pain even after the rash has healed (postherpetic neuralgia).

Sciatica

Sciatica is named for the sciatic nerves, one of which extends down the back of each leg from your buttock to your heel. Nerve inflammation or compression of a nerve root in your lower back can cause sciatica. You may feel the pain radiating from your back through your buttock to your lower leg. Tingling, numbness or muscle weakness also can occur.

Usually, the pain goes away on its own. However, severe nerve compression can cause progressive muscle weakness and continued pain. Your doctor may recommend hot and cold compresses to relieve inflammation around the nerve. An anti-inflammatory medication, such as a nonsteroidal anti-inflammatory drug (NSAID), also may help reduce swelling and pain.

If these don't work, other mechanical or behavior therapies may be beneficial. An injection of a corticosteroid near the spinal column also may be used. Back surgery to relieve pressure on the nerve is generally a last resort.

With this kind of pain, as with other kinds, a combination of medication, physical therapy and behavior therapy can usually allow you to live a normal life. ■

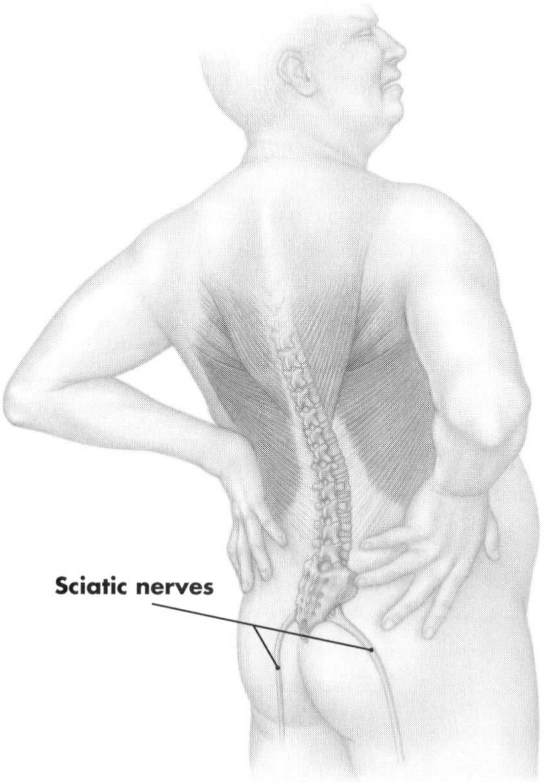

Nerve irritation in your lower back can cause sciatica — pain radiating from your back through your buttock to your lower leg.

PREVENTION TIP

Sciatica can stem from many factors, but one common cause is sitting for prolonged periods. To help minimize the symptoms of sciatica caused by sitting:

- Use chairs with firm support and sit back in your chair. This helps to avoid concentrated pressure on the sciatic nerve, which runs from your lower back to your foot.
- Avoid crossing your legs. Plant your feet on the floor or on a footrest.
- Take frequent breaks. Walk around at least once every hour.
- Get regular exercise to strengthen your back muscles and improve your posture.
- Adjust your car seat so that your legs are bent at the knees and hips. Use a lumbar support or a rolled-up towel to support your lower back.
- Don't carry a wallet in your back pocket because sitting on a wallet can put pressure on the sciatic nerve.

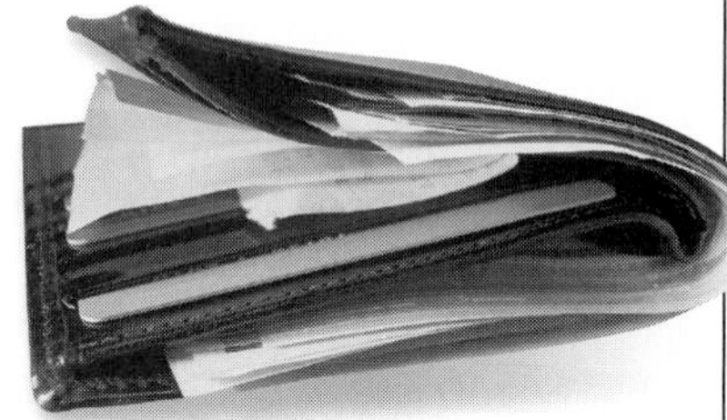

Pain of Unknown Cause

Sometimes, chronic pain develops for no apparent reason. Despite repeated tests, your doctor isn't able to link it to an identifiable physical cause or condition. This doesn't mean that the pain doesn't exist. It simply means that your pain may be associated with factors that are difficult to diagnose.

Your health is affected by the interaction of your mind and body. Among some people, psychological issues can play a major role in chronic pain. For example, people who've endured sexual or physical abuse appear to be at greater risk of developing some types of chronic pain. It's unknown whether the pain is the result of physical injuries or if it stems from emotional scars or stress. It may be due to a combination of factors.

CHAPTER **43** PART VI

Complementary and Alternative Medicine

As people seek to play a greater role in their health, more and more are turning to techniques outside the mainstream of conventional medical practice — what's known collectively as complementary and alternative medicine. Perhaps you've already experimented with such techniques. Maybe you've meditated to reduce stress or tried acupuncture to relieve pain.

The National Center for Complementary and Alternative Medicine (NCCAM), a division of the National Institutes of Health (NIH), defines complementary and alternative medicine as treatments and health care practices that aren't taught widely in medical schools, not generally used in hospitals and usually not covered by medical insurance. These include a broad range of healing philosophies, approaches and therapies. Some examples might be practicing tai chi — in addition to taking medication — to treat anxiety or using an herbal preparation instead of traditional chemotherapy or radiation to treat cancer.

Often, the emphasis of complementary and alternative medicine is on a holistic approach that considers physical, mental, emotional and spiritual aspects of health. Prevention — preventing health problems rather than treating them after they've developed — also is stressed. Some alternative and complementary therapies are consistent with conventional Western medicine and are becoming part of mainstream practice. Others aren't accepted in conventional practice.

Many alternative and complementary practices aren't new. In fact, some, such as acupuncture, have been around for thousands of years. Others change with the times because they fall out of favor, prove to be dangerous or become accepted as mainstream medicine. Digitalis, originally considered an alternative medication, is now used routinely by doctors in treating cardiovascular disease.

Changing Times

According to a study published in the *Journal of the American Medical Association*, between 1990 and 1997 Americans visited alternative and complementary practitioners more frequently than they did primary care physicians, even though many complementary and alternative services weren't covered by medical insurance.

Why? For one thing, people are trying to take more control over their own health. For another, many consider complementary treatments as natural. The treatments are also largely noninvasive and readily accessible. In addition, many nontraditional therapies focus on the whole person, attending to the physical, mental, emotional and spiritual well-being of each individual. This holistic approach is appealing to some who see conventional medicine as being too disease oriented instead of person oriented.

Greater interest in complementary and alternative practices isn't limited to those seeking treatment. Many doctors have been highly skeptical of alternative and complementary treatments, but today an increasing number of doctors in the United States either use some type of unconventional treatment or refer their patients to others who do. At the least, doctors are more knowledgeable about unconventional treatments than they were in the past.

The option to pick and choose among nontraditional treatments makes the complicated world of health care even more so. Take a careful look at your options and don't believe everything that you hear or read about complementary and alternative treatments. You may find something that works for you, but some practices can do more harm than good.

When deciding on any unconventional treatment — or conventional, for that matter — you need to consider its safety and effectiveness. According to the NCCAM, safety means that the benefits of a treatment outweigh its risks. A safe practice is one that does no harm when used as intended. Effectiveness is the likelihood that the treatment will be of benefit when used appropriately.

Where to Find Information

Complementary and alternative medicine is a fast-changing field. You can find considerable information about these practices in medical libraries, public libraries, bookstores and on the Internet. Unfortunately, you'll also encounter a lot of misinformation, particularly on the Internet.

When you're looking for information online, the best way to find reliable information is to stick with health Web sites associated with major medical centers, reputable national organizations, universities or the federal government. One example of a good online resource is the Web site of the National Center for Complementary and Alternative Medicine (see page 1385). From there, you can link to organizations such as the National Institutes of Health and the National Library of Medicine.

Another online resource is the Health On the Net Foundation (HON). This foundation, created in 1995, is a not-for-profit organization designed to guide nonmedical Internet users and medical practitioners to useful and reliable online medical and health information (see page 1383). HON also provides leadership in setting ethical standards for Web site developers.

If you don't have Internet access, check with your public library. Many libraries make computers with Internet connections available for public use.

Apply the 3 *D*'s

You can find thousands of Web sites devoted to health. The material ranges from solid research to outright quackery. To evaluate the quality of the information you find, apply the three *D*'s.

Dates
Search for the most recent information you can find. Reputable Web sites include a date for each article posted and indicate whether and when the article has been updated.

Documentation
Check for the source of information. Notice whether articles refer to published medical research. Look for a board of qualified professionals who review content before it's published. Be wary of commercial sites or personal testimonials that push a single point of view or hype miracle cures.

Double-checking
Visit several health sites and compare information. Before you follow any medical advice, check with your doctor.

What to Watch For

People who do exhaustive research before deciding on a new car or appliance often don't approach health care in the same way. Cliche or not, knowledge is power. If you're considering a complementary or alternative treatment, find out all you can about it. In the interest of protecting your health and your wallet, evaluate the benefits and risks — especially the risks. "Natural" doesn't mean harmless.

The difference between complementary or alternative practices and conventional medicine is scientific evidence of safety and effectiveness. For that, doctors rely on research and they would advise you to do the same.

Ask your doctor for information on research results to help you make an informed decision about any treatment you're considering. Or, dig up the information on your own, keeping in mind that not all research meets the same exacting standards for credibility. It's important for you to understand the quality of the studies you're reading.

Pay attention to the terms

Various terms are used to describe different types of research. For example:

- Clinical studies involve research on people, rather than animals. Clinical studies are usually preceded by studies that demonstrate the safety and effectiveness of the treatment in animals.
- In randomized, controlled trials, participants are usually divided into two or more groups. One group receives the treatment under investigation. Another is a control group — the people in this group receive standard treatment, no treatment or an inactive substance called a placebo. Participants are assigned randomly to these groups to help prevent bias and ensure that the groups are similar in makeup.
- In double-blind studies, neither the researchers nor the human subjects know who receives the active treatment and who gets the placebo.
- Prospective studies are forward looking. Researchers establish criteria for study participants to follow and then measure or describe the results. Information from these studies is usually more reliable than retrospective studies. Retrospective studies involve looking at past data — for example, asking participants to recall information — which leaves more room for bias and errors in interpretation.
- Peer-reviewed medical journals, such as the *Journal of the American Medical Association* and the *New England Journal of Medicine,* publish only articles that have been reviewed by independent medical experts.

Rely on the best studies

Now that you know the terms, here's what to look for: prospective, double-blind studies that have been controlled, randomized and published in peer-reviewed journals. They're considered the gold standard of medical research. If they involve large numbers of people (several hundred or more) who have been studied over several years, then they gain even more credibility.

In addition, doctors like studies that are replicated by different investigators who end up with similar results.

Common Categories

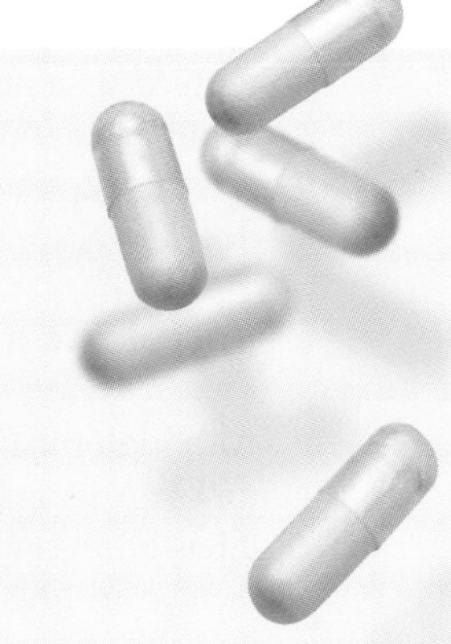

Hundreds of complementary and alternative therapies are available. Most can be classified into the following five major groups:

- Herbal preparations
- Manipulation and touch
- Mind-body interventions
- Natural energy restoration
- Alternative systems

To date, little research involving complementary and alternative treatments meets these rigorous standards. For the majority of unconventional treatments, you'll find mostly anecdotal reports from practitioners and people who have undergone the treatments, inconclusive data and opinion — from opponents as well as proponents.

Herbal Preparations

The Food and Drug Administration (FDA) classifies herbal supplements, along with vitamins and minerals, as dietary supplements. Used for centuries for healing, herbs such as St. John's wort and echinacea have evolved from folk remedies into a multibillion-dollar industry in the United States.

An estimated 60 million Americans use herbal supplements. Because herbs are derived from plants, many people consider them "natural" and therefore assume they're safe. That's not necessarily so. Research has identified a number of herbal substances, such as ephedra, that can cause harmful, even deadly, effects. In addition, the effectiveness of most herbal preparations hasn't been established, and the relative lack of regulation of the products means that you don't know what you're getting when you purchase them.

Unlike prescription drugs, most herbal preparations aren't standardized to provide consumers with consistent products. Only with standard manufacturing practices can the safest and most effective doses be assured.

Regulation

Although the FDA is responsible for overseeing herbal supplements, it has little control over their manufacture. In 1993, the agency proposed a regulation that would require companies to prove the claims they made for their products. Implementing the regulation would have required the companies to conduct adequate studies on every product. Herbal manufacturers and concerned consumers mounted an effective campaign to block the FDA from limiting access to herbs and dietary supplements. Congress responded by passing the Dietary Supplement Health and Education Act (DSHEA) of 1994. This act limits the FDA's control over products labeled as dietary supplements.

As a result, herbal products are not subjected to the same rigorous standards as over-the-counter and prescription drugs. Therefore, the contents of one package of ginkgo, for example, can vary considerably from another. Herbal products can also be sold with no proof of effectiveness or safety, and manufacturers can make certain claims about their herbal products based on their own review and interpretation of studies — without FDA review. That's why herbal supplement labels are required to carry a disclaimer: "This statement has not been evaluated by the Food and Drug Administration. This product is not intended to diagnose, treat, cure or prevent any disease." However, FDA can pull a product off the market once it has been proved dangerous.

Of all the unconventional treatments, herbal preparations may present the greatest potential for serious harm.

Safety

If you decide to use an herbal preparation, exercise as much caution as you would with any prescription or over-the-counter medication.

Read the label

The quality and strength of an herbal preparation can vary greatly by brand. Look for the letters *USP* (United States Pharmacopeia) or *NF* (National Formulary), which indicate the supplements meet certain standards of quality. Some companies voluntarily follow standards set for drugs — you'll know them by the words "Good Manufacturing Practices" on their packages. Look for those.

Follow directions

Don't exceed recommended dosages. In addition, some herbs can be harmful if taken for too long a time. Get advice from your doctor and other reputable resources.

Tell your doctor what you're taking

Most people don't tell their doctors they take herbal remedies, because they think their doctors will disapprove, they think it doesn't matter, or the doctors don't ask. Tell your doctor what you're taking. Some herbs can interfere with the action of prescription or over-the-counter drugs or have other harmful effects. In addition, if you're taking an herbal preparation to treat a symptom, that symptom might also mean that you have an underlying medical condition that requires treatment by your doctor.

Keep track of what you take

Keep a record of what you take, the dosage and how it makes you feel. Note any side effects, such as drowsiness, sleeplessness, headache or nausea.

Check where it's manufactured

In general, herbs prepared and packaged in Europe are better regulated and standardized than those manufactured elsewhere. Some herbal supplements manufactured in China, India and other countries have contained toxic ingredients — including lead, mercury and arsenic — and prescription drugs, such as prednisone.

Buy single-herb products

Make sure the label on the product states how much of the herb each dose contains. Mixed-herb products often contain less of each herb than the amount found in single-herb products.

Avoid herbs considered harmful

Herbs the FDA has determined to be harmful include belladonna, scotch broom, comfrey, lobelia and pennyroyal. Goldenseal and ephedra also are controversial herbs that can cause serious side effects. And kava, an herb used to treat anxiety, reportedly has been associated with liver damage in some people. There may be other harmful herbs. Overdoses of any of these herbs can be fatal.

Avoid herbs if you're pregnant or breast-feeding

Herbal preparations may harm your baby or cause you to miscarry. Avoid them if you're pregnant or breast-feeding.

10 popular herbs

People take herbs for a host of reasons. Here's a look at some of the most popular ones, what they claim to do and what the research says about them.

Black cohosh *(Cimicifuga racemosa)*

With some effects similar to the female hormone estrogen, black cohosh is used to relieve menstrual cramps, painful periods and menopausal symptoms, such as hot flashes, anxiety and depression. A number of clinical studies indicate that black cohosh is effective, but more long-term studies are needed.

Echinacea *(Echinacea purpurea, Echinacea pallida)*

Derived from the purple coneflower, echinacea typically is used to prevent colds and flu. Studies show that although it may shorten the duration of colds and flu, it probably doesn't keep you from getting them.

Some researchers have raised concerns about the potential of this herb to be toxic to the liver. Don't take it for more than 8 weeks at a time. Echinacea affects your immune system, so some medical professionals advise against its use if you have diabetes, an autoimmune disease such as multiple sclerosis, lupus or rheumatoid arthritis, or impaired immunity from a condition such as cancer or human immunodeficiency virus (HIV).

Feverfew *(Tanacetum parthenium)*

The leaves of the feverfew plant are used to prevent migraines. Studies indicate that the herb's active ingredient, parthenolide, may reduce the frequency and severity of migraines. Don't take feverfew if you're pregnant because it may cause a miscarriage.

Garlic *(Allium sativum)*

Some people believe that garlic can lower cholesterol and blood pressure and keep blood clots from forming.

Garlic is supposedly more effective if eaten raw and in large amounts — five or more cloves a day. But eating that much can irritate your stomach, not to mention affect your breath and body odor. Garlic supplements may be effective if they contain the active ingredient allicin. Because garlic can have blood-thinning properties, don't use it if you're taking anticlotting drugs such as warfarin (Coumadin). And before combining garlic with a daily dose of aspirin, talk to your doctor.

Ginger *(Zingiber officinale)*

The root of the ginger plant is used to relieve nausea and indigestion. Studies show it may be effective for preventing nausea associated with motion sickness and anesthesia. However, if you take ginger regularly and need surgery, stop taking it 2 to 3 weeks before the date of your surgery because it may increase your risk of bleeding.

Ginger isn't recommended for treatment of morning sickness. In addition, if you have gallstones, check with your doctor before using ginger because it increases the production of digestive juices and bile.

Too Good to Be True?

The Food and Drug Administration and the National Council Against Health Fraud recommend that you watch for the following claims or practices, which can be warning signs of potentially fraudulent products or treatments:

- The advertisements or promotional materials include words such as *breakthrough, magical* or *new discovery*. If the product were in fact a cure, then it would be widely reported in the media, and your doctor would recommend it.
- Promotional materials include pseudomedical jargon such as *detoxify, purify* or *energize*. Such claims are difficult to define and measure.
- The manufacturer claims that the product can treat a wide range of symptoms or cure or prevent a number of diseases. No single product can do that.
- The product is supposedly backed by scientific studies, but the references aren't provided or they're limited or out-of-date.
- The product promotion mentions no negative effects, only benefits.
- The manufacturer of the product accuses the government or medical profession of suppressing important information about the product's health benefits. There's no reason for the government or medical profession to withhold information that could help people.

Ginkgo *(Ginkgo biloba)*
Ginkgo is used to increase blood flow to the brain in an effort to ease symptoms such as short-term memory loss, dizziness, ringing in the ears and headache. It's also taken to treat activity-related leg pain caused by poor circulation in the legs (claudication). Evidence shows that ginkgo has a mild positive effect on claudication and on memory, and it's being studied to determine whether it can slow the progression of Alzheimer's disease. But more research on the herb is needed. Don't use ginkgo if you're taking anti-clotting medication or a thiazide diuretic.

Ginseng *(Panax ginseng, Panax quinquefolius)*
Some people use ginseng to boost energy, increase sexual stamina, reduce stress and counter the effects of aging. No scientific evidence indicates that it does these things, but it may improve your overall sense of well-being. Don't use it for more than 3 months or exceed the recommended maximum dose. Don't use ginseng if you have an estrogen-related disease, such as breast cancer. In addition, don't use it if you have uncontrolled high blood pressure.

Kava *(Piper methysticum)*
Some people use kava to relieve anxiety and insomnia. In late 2001 — following reports from Europe of liver problems in some people who used kava — the FDA began investigating the risks of kava. Until the FDA knows more, don't start taking kava or products that contain it. If you already use kava, contact your doctor for advice. You shouldn't take kava if you have a history of liver problems, you're depressed or if you take antidepressants or prescription sedatives.

St. John's wort *(Hypericum perforatum)*
Most widely prescribed in Germany, St. John's wort is used to treat mild to moderate depression. Some studies suggest that St. John's wort may work as well as some antidepressant drugs for mild depression, and with fewer side effects. It hasn't been shown to be effective in treating major depression. A major concern is that the herb can dangerously alter the effects of a number of prescription drugs, including other antidepressants, digoxin, warfarin and cyclosporine. Until more is known, a good rule of thumb is to not mix St. John's wort with any medication without discussing it in advance with your doctor.

Saw palmetto *(Serenoa repens)*
Some research indicates that saw palmetto may improve urine flow and bladder emptying in men with noncancerous enlargement of the prostate gland (benign prostatic hyperplasia). Studies are inconclusive as to whether saw palmetto can affect results in the prostate-specific antigen (PSA) blood test used to screen for prostate cancer.

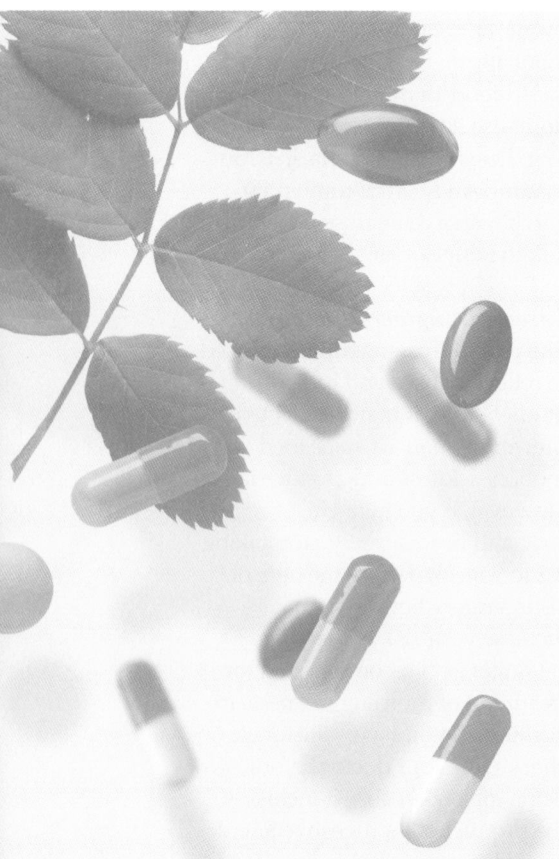

Avoiding Dangerous Interactions

Herbal supplements contain ingredients that may not be taken safely with prescription or over-the-counter medications. Certain medical problems also may increase your risk of adverse effects from taking herbal products.

Talk to your doctor before taking any herbal products, especially if you're pregnant or nursing or if you regularly take prescription or over-the-counter medications. Also talk to your doctor if you have any of the following conditions:

- High blood pressure
- A history of stroke
- Blood-clotting problems
- Thyroid problems
- Diabetes
- Cardiovascular disease
- Epilepsy
- Parkinson's disease
- Glaucoma
- An enlarged prostate gland
- Human immunodeficiency virus (HIV), AIDS or other diseases of the immune system
- Depression or other psychiatric problems

Some herbal supplements also can be dangerous when combined with anesthesia. If you're having surgery, tell your doctor about any medications, including herbal supplements, that you're taking. Stop taking herbal supplements at least 2 to 3 weeks before surgery to allow them to clear from your body. If this isn't possible, then bring the herbal product in its original container to the hospital so that the anesthesiologist knows what you're taking.

Manipulation and Touch

If you've ever had a massage, not to mention a hug from a friend or loved one, then you know how comforting human touch can be. Touch and manipulation of body tissues are at the core of several complementary and alternative treatments.

Chiropractic treatment

You may be surprised to learn that chiropractic treatment is considered complementary or alternative. There are more than 45,000 chiropractors in the United States. One-third of all Americans visit chiropractors, making these practitioners second only to doctors as primary care providers.

In the early days of chiropractic treatment, practitioners claimed that misaligned vertebrae were the source of all disease and that the cure depended on spinal adjustments. According to chiropractic theory, misaligned vertebrae can restrict your spine's range of motion, which affects nerves that radiate from your spine. The organs affected by those nerves then can malfunction or become diseased. Chiropractic adjustments aim to realign your vertebrae, increase range of motion, free nerve pathways and restore health.

Many of today's chiropractors use a hands-on type of adjustment known as spinal manipulative therapy to treat back pain. Studies show that within 4 to 6 weeks of the onset of acute, uncomplicated back pain, manipulation can improve function and decrease pain, possibly as well as other treatments. In fact, the Agency for Healthcare Research and Quality has concluded that spinal manipulation may provide temporary relief from acute low back pain. After 6 weeks of symptoms, however, there's no evidence to support continuing spinal manipulation. There's also no evidence to suggest that spinal manipulation is useful for anything other than back pain.

Chiropractors sometimes work with medical doctors. Although chiropractors can't prescribe medication or perform surgery, they may use some standard medical procedures. Their services may be covered by medical insurance, so check with your insurance firm.

Osteopathic medicine

Doctors of osteopathy (D.O.s) receive training similar to that of medical doctors (M.D.s), including attending medical schools, completing residencies and passing specialty certification exams. Like M.D.s, they can prescribe medicine and perform surgery. And they also specialize in all areas of medicine, such as pediatrics or radiology.

There is, however, one difference in the training osteopaths undergo: Some of it centers on manipulation to address joint and spinal problems. They may perform manipulations to release pressure in your joints, align your muscles and joints and improve the flow of body fluids. The treatment you receive at the hands of an osteopath may not be noticeably different from the treatment you receive from a conventional doctor. Not all osteopaths use spinal manipulation in their practice, or they may use it only occasionally.

Massage

Massage involves manipulation of your body's soft tissues — your skin, muscles and tendons. The type of manipulation — including its rhythm, intensity, rate and direction — varies with the type of massage, from the traditional kneading and rubbing in Swedish massage to the use of pressure at acupuncture points in shiatsu massage.

Often used as part of physical therapy, sports medicine and nursing care, massage can relieve muscle tension, reduce stress and help you feel better as you undergo medical treatment for various illnesses. But you don't have to be ill to benefit from massage. Healthy people use it as a means of relieving stress relief and relaxation.

A massage should feel good or cause little discomfort. If it hurts, immediately inform the person who's performing it. Avoid massage in areas where you have open wounds, skin infections, phlebitis, weakened bones or inflamed joints. If you've been injured, consult your doctor before getting a massage.

Mind-Body Interventions

Your mind and body are inextricably linked, so your thoughts and emotions affect your body. That's the premise behind mind-body interventions.

Traditional medicine has long concentrated on the biology of the body and brain. But that's changing. Over the past few decades, researchers and doctors have focused more attention on the effects the mind has on the body, particularly for diseases that appear to be brought on or exacerbated by stress, such as cancer, heart disease and asthma.

Practitioners of mind-body therapies believe that negative thoughts and feelings may produce bodily symptoms. They use a number of relaxation techniques aimed at calming the mind.

Biofeedback

Biofeedback is a procedure in which a trained therapist uses monitoring instruments to help teach you how to control certain bodily responses that can affect your health, such as your heart rate, muscle tension and blood pressure.

The therapist applies electrodes and other sensors to various parts of your body. The electrodes attach to devices that monitor your responses and provide you with auditory or visual feedback. For example, patterns on a monitor might indicate your brain wave activity.

With the feedback, you can learn to produce positive changes that indicate relaxation. For instance, when you're under stress, your blood vessels constrict, which can worsen conditions such as migraines. Thermal biofeedback uses an instrument that measures your skin temperature. By concentrating on raising your skin temperature, you can ease the constriction.

Therapists often combine biofeedback with other relaxation techniques to further calm you. Performed in physical therapy clinics, medical centers and hospitals, biofeedback is used for a variety of conditions, including anxiety, high blood pressure, asthma, irritable bowel syndrome, chronic pain, migraines and tension type headaches.

Hypnosis

Hypnosis is a technique that induces a state of deep relaxation while keeping your mind alert and open to suggestion. No one knows for sure how it works, but experts believe it alters your brain wave patterns in much the same way as do other relaxation techniques.

About 80 percent of adults can be hypnotized. Whether hypnosis can work for you depends on the expertise of the practitioner and your desire to cooperate. If you're using hypnosis to give up a bad habit, such as smoking or taking drugs, then you need to be strongly motivated to change for it to help.

Hypnosis has been used in place of anesthesia during some surgery, childbirth and dental procedures. It's more commonly used to help manage pain, such as headache or postoperative pain, or to control asthma attacks or relieve performance anxiety, such as the fear of speaking in front of an audience.

Some psychiatrists and psychologists practice hypnosis, as do professional hypnotists. But the field is poorly regulated. Before you put yourself in the hands of a hypnotist, get a recommendation from someone you know and trust.

Yoga

Yoga is an ancient practice that aims to induce physical, mental and spiritual well-being through a combination of postures (asanas), breathing techniques and meditation. This practice is increasingly popular among people seeking relaxation, a spiritual path or improvements in flexibility, coordination, balance, strength and endurance.

The National Center for Complementary and Alternative Medicine (NCCAM) says that yoga may ease arthritis, help people stop smoking and improve some of the symptoms of carpal tunnel syndrome. According to the NCCAM, other benefits of yoga, when practiced regularly, may include reduced anxiety, slowed breathing, lowered blood pressure, altered brain waves and more efficient heart blood flow. Many yoga enthusiasts claim that yoga can treat specific mental and physical disorders, but there aren't enough randomized, controlled studies to support the claims.

At the very least, yoga can relax you, and some forms may improve your physical conditioning. If you find an experienced instructor who adapts postures to your levels of flexibility, yoga is likely to help you and unlikely to be harmful. But yoga isn't easy. It requires discipline and concentration.

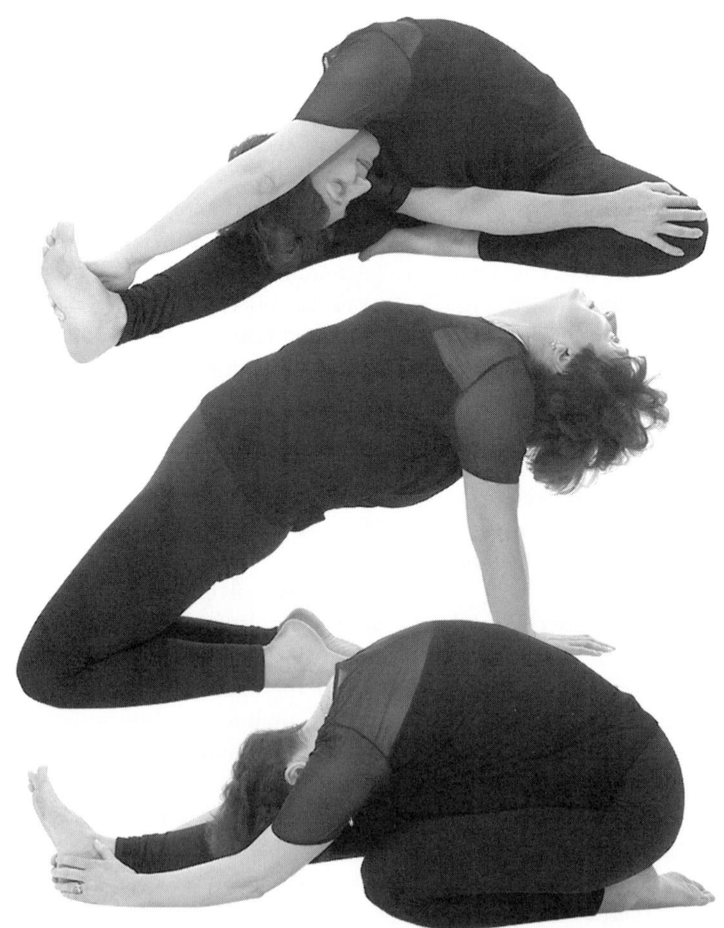

With continued practice, you can use yoga to help improve flexibility, coordination, posture, balance, strength and endurance.

Meditation

Spending time each day trying to quiet your mind with meditation can help you relax, slow your breathing and heart rate and decrease muscle tension.

Meditation can lessen your body's response to the chemicals it produces when you're stressed, such as adrenaline, which can raise your blood pressure and make your blood more likely to clot — both risk factors for heart disease. With continued practice you may reach a point where meditation can help reduce your blood pressure.

Meditation helps you enter a deeply restful state. The ensuing relaxation may help you manage pain and reduce stress and anxiety that can trigger or worsen an illness.

During meditation you sit still and make an effort to focus on a single thing, such as a particular word. When your thoughts wander, as they inevitably do, you bring your focus back to where it was.

A related practice is guided imagery, in which someone's voice, whether taped or live, directs you through a visualization exercise.

Once you reach a state of deep relaxation, most likely through meditation, you conjure up a visual image of whatever the person directing the exercise suggests. Perhaps it's a peaceful place, such as a garden or on a sandy beach, where you feel calm and safe. If you have an illness, you may be asked to visualize healthy cells attacking the disease.

Brain studies of people undergoing guided imagery sessions show that visualizing or imaging something stimulates the same parts of your brain that are stimulated during the actual experience. If sitting by the ocean relaxes you, you may achieve the same level of relaxation by visualizing yourself sitting by the ocean.

Finding a Yoga Class and Teacher

If you decide to give yoga a try, your best bet is to learn in a class. But first you have to pick the style that's right for you, from gentle to power styles. Basic hatha yoga is a gentle form that combines breathing techniques with a series of postures, called asanas.

Here's a rundown of variations of hatha yoga:

- Iyengar yoga, developed by an influential teacher from India, emphasizes mental clarity and precision in doing the asanas.
- Svaroopa yoga uses postures that focus on the spine and hips. If you turn to yoga primarily for stress relief and relaxation, you may find this form of yoga appealing.
- Ashtanga and vinyasa yoga — often advertised as power yoga — teach asanas connected in a flowing, coordinated series combined with deep, rhythmic breathing. Power yoga offers an aerobic benefit.
- Bikram yoga is a system of 26 poses performed in the same sequence every time. Classes are held in a heated room, even when it's warm outside, for the purpose of promoting greater flexibility.
- Kripalu yoga emphasizes release of tension and trust in your body wisdom (intuition).

Yoga classes are generally easy to find in larger cities. Check with local health clubs, YMCAs, YWCAs, churches and community education centers. There's no certification for yoga instructors, so look for one with a serious interest in yoga who has studied and practiced for years. Observe the class before you sign up.

How to Meditate

You don't have to twist your legs into a pretzel or spend your life at an ashram to learn to meditate. All you need to do is find a quiet place where you won't be disturbed. Sit or lie in a comfortable position and determine a focus for your mind. Here are a few to consider:

- *Focus on your breath.* Breathe in and out through your nose and pay attention to some aspect of your breathing, such as the pause between breaths or the sensation of air leaving your nostrils.
- *Focus on a word, phrase or prayer.* In Transcendental Meditation you mentally repeat a mantra, usually a Sanskrit word or sound assigned by your instructor. But you can choose your own mantra, such as the word *peace*, or you can count from one to four over and over. You can also coordinate your mantra with your breathing.
- *Focus on the moment.* This is also known as mindfulness meditation. You become aware of sensations, sounds and thoughts. You simply notice them and let them go. Or you may notice the sensations in your body — stomach growling or thigh cramping.

Many people meditate with their eyes closed. Others prefer to keep their eyes partially open with a soft focus. It doesn't matter whether you lie down or sit on the floor, a chair, a meditation cushion or a bench, as long as you're comfortable. But keep your spine straight and don't get so comfortable that you fall asleep.

Start with 5-minute meditation sessions once or twice a day and work up to 20-minutes sessions.

Natural Energy Restoration

Natural energy techniques are based on the idea that the energy that flows through your body, or the field of energy that supposedly surrounds your body, can be disturbed or blocked and needs to be restored. Although many of the mind-body practices are based on the same premise, these energy-based techniques differ greatly from one another.

Acupuncture

A component of Chinese traditional medicine, acupuncture has existed for at least 2,500 years. The Eastern philosophy behind it is that health depends on a vital energy called chi, or qi (pronounced chee), that flows through your body along 14 pathways called meridians. According to this ancient theory, if your chi is out of balance, you develop pain and disease. Inserting needles into specific points along the meridians unblocks the energy flow and restores your body's healthy balance.

A consensus statement on acupuncture by the National Institutes of Health (NIH) acknowledges a lack of well-designed and controlled research and research comparing acupuncture with a placebo or sham acupuncture, in which needles are inserted randomly in the body. Still, acupuncture is one of the most researched and accepted nontraditional medical practices.

In addition, the consensus statement says that studies indicate acupuncture may help provide relief from pain after dental surgery and from nausea and vomiting

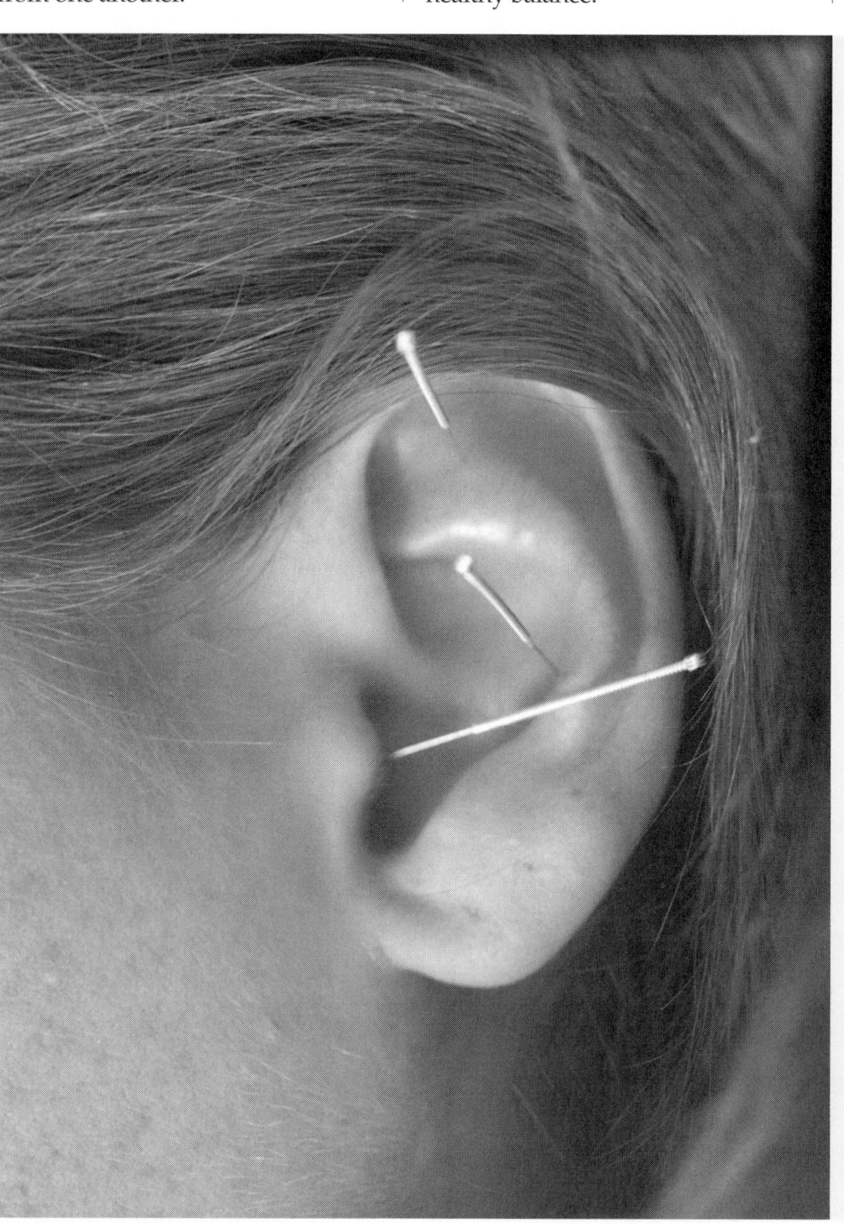

There should be little or no pain from the insertion of the needles. Some people even find it relaxing.

Acupuncture Tips

If you seek acupuncture, here's what you can expect:

- From 1 to 20 or more hair-thin needles are inserted under your skin.
- Some may go in as deep as 3 inches, depending on where they're placed in your body and what the treatment is for. Others are placed superficially.
- The needles usually are left in for 15 to 30 minutes.
- You should feel little or no pain from insertion. Significant pain is a sign that the procedure is being done improperly.
- Once inserted, the needles may be moved gently by hand or stimulated with an electrical current or heat.
- You'll probably have several sessions. You may not get relief from the first one, but if nothing's happening after six or eight sessions, then acupuncture probably isn't for you.
- If you feel some relief, give it a chance to work. It could take months to alleviate your pain.

from chemotherapy, anesthesia and pregnancy. According to the panel that released the consensus statement, acupuncture may be useful as adjunctive therapy in helping to control the pain of menstrual cramps, tennis elbow, fibromyalgia, low back pain, osteoarthritis, headache and other conditions that involve chronic pain. Mayo Clinic pain specialists have used acupuncture in some pain treatment since 1974. According to the NIH panel, study findings indicate that acupuncture may work, in part, by releasing natural painkillers and other chemicals in the central nervous system.

Adverse side effects from acupuncture are rare, but they do occur. They include transmission of hepatitis B from needles that aren't properly sterilized, possible lung puncture, tissue or nerve damage, or a needle breaking off under the skin. Most adverse effects are the result of the practitioner's lack of medical knowledge, unhygienic practices or inadequate training. That's why it's so important to find an experienced practitioner.

Tai chi

Developed as a martial art in China more than 1,000 years ago, tai chi is based on a series of slow, flowing movements that resemble a dance. It's designed to foster the free flow of energy (chi) that practitioners believe is necessary for good health.

Today's practitioners use tai chi to gain emotional and physical balance, reduce stress and strengthen muscles and joints. Because it can help you feel both alert and tranquil, some people use it as a form of moving meditation.

Tai chi comprises hundreds of combinations of continuous movements that require concentration, balance and grace. When combined with deep, rhythmic breathing, these movements can increase your circulation, relax your mind and body and ease chronic pain. Practicing tai chi has also been shown to improve balance, reducing the risk of falling.

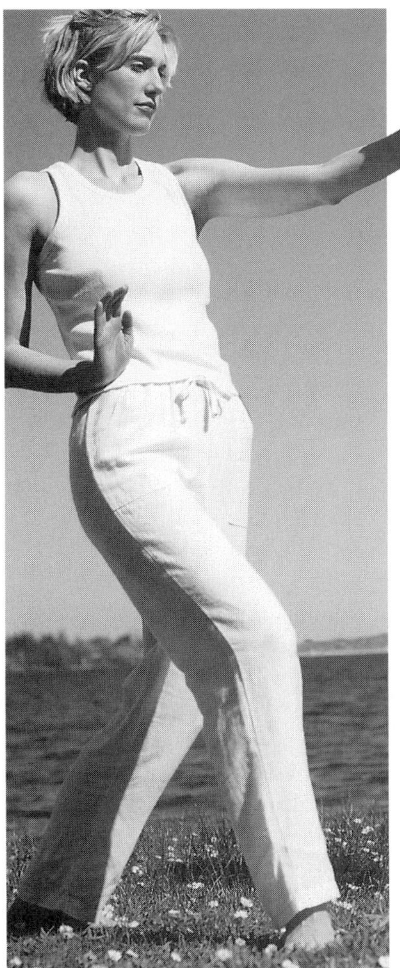

Literally hundreds of combinations of movements are involved in tai chi. But the focus of the exercise remains consistent: combining concentration, stretching, balance and grace.

Therapeutic touch

Advocates of therapeutic touch subscribe to the notion that your body is its own form of energy, surrounded by a field of energy. Disturbances to the surrounding energy field can lead to illness.

Some practitioners of therapeutic touch move their hands over a person's body in the belief that they can get rid of the disturbance and transfer healing energy from their hands to the individual who's ill. The benefits of therapeutic touch aren't supported by solid research. More study is needed.

Alternative Systems

Some alternative practices derive from whole systems that combine treatments. They tend to eschew traditional medications and surgery and take a variety of approaches to healing.

Homeopathy

Developed in Germany more than 150 years ago, homeopathy is a controversial treatment based on two beliefs — the law of similars and the law of infinitesimals.

Law of similars

The law of similars is the idea that any substance — plant, animal or mineral — that can produce certain symptoms in a healthy person can, when given in very small doses, cure similar symptoms that occur in an ill person.

Law of infinitesimals

The word *infinitesimal* means "too small to be measured." Homeopathy claims that the more dilute a substance, as long as it has been prepared by a series of shakings called succession, the more potent the medicine. This idea is called the law of infinitesimals.

Many practitioners of conventional medicine dismiss homeopathy as ineffective. Conventional doctors generally find it difficult to believe that homeopathic substances, which often are diluted in distilled water or alcohol to the point where there may be no active molecules left, could be beneficial.

Still, homeopathy has a body of randomized, controlled studies behind it. Many of them have looked at whether the effects of homeopathic treatments can be attributed to the placebo effect. One analysis of more than 100 randomized, controlled studies concluded that the data weren't compatible with the idea that the clinical effects of homeopathy were due strictly to the placebo effect. Most doctors remain skeptical of both the studies and practice of homeopathy.

Ayurveda

Ayurveda may be the oldest system of medicine still practiced today. Hindu in origin, *ayurveda* means "the science of life." It begins with the premise that people differ from one another physically and psychologically, so treatments must take those differences into account.

According to ayurveda, people are made up of three types of energy (doshas). In most people one dosha is dominant. The different combinations of doshas create different metabolic types. Each dosha represents a pair of elements.

- *Vata (space and air), the energy of movement.* People dominated by vata are alert, creative and physically active.
- *Pitta (fire and water), the energy of digestion and metabolism.* People with this primary dosha have larger appetites, warmer bodies and more stable temperaments than those dominated by vata.
- *Kapha (water and earth), the energy of lubrication.* People dominated by kapha gain weight easily, tend to be less physically active and generally have oily skin. They're usually calm, patient and forgiving.

According to ayurveda theory, when the energies get out of balance, such as through diet or stress, illness results. Ayurveda is best known for prevention of illness by promoting balance through nutrition, exercise, herbs, meditation and other treatments.

Naturopathy

Based on their belief in the healing power of nature, early naturopaths recommended soaking in hot springs, walking barefoot through streams and using other water-related activities to treat illness.

Today's naturopaths employ a combination of therapies, including nutrition, herbs, acupuncture and massage. They also use techniques from homeopathy, ayurveda, Chinese medicine and conventional treatments. The main emphasis of naturopathy is on prevention of illness through a healthy lifestyle, including fresh air, clean water and exercise. ■

Is It for You?

When considering unconventional treatments, it's important to keep an open, albeit skeptical, mind. Steer a middle course between uncritical acceptance and outright rejection. Do your homework. Find out all that you can about the treatment and provider. Weigh the benefits and risks. Then base your decision on the outcome.

Some complementary and alternative treatments are less expensive than conventional health care. Others are very costly. Most unconventional procedures aren't covered by health insurance. Find out what the treatment you're considering will cost you. Get it in writing, if possible. Then check with your insurance company to see if it's covered.

If you decide to undergo unconventional treatments, opt for complementary over alternative. There's a big difference between flying to another country for an unproven cancer treatment and augmenting your chemotherapy with meditation or acupuncture. The former can do more harm than good.

Complementary medicine can help you manage stress and relieve some symptoms. But if you become ill, rely on conventional medicine for diagnosis and treatment recommendations. Be sure to tell your medical doctor about all of the treatments you get, conventional and unconventional.

Finally, work in partnership with your health care providers — conventional and unconventional. Take appropriate responsibility for your own health by keeping up with health information and making important lifestyle changes. Eating well, exercising, not smoking, taking safety precautions — such as using your car's seat belt — and managing stress will go a long way toward helping you live a longer, healthier life.

Glossary

The language of medicine is rich with specialized words. This wealth of vocabulary is a mixed blessing. Your doctor can use precise terminology to describe conditions, signs and symptoms to you and his or her colleagues, yet in some cases that same terminology can be confusing, worrisome or incomprehensible to the uninitiated listener.

Whenever possible, we've tried to use language familiar to the layperson to enhance the readability and utility of this book. In most cases, when a medical term is introduced, we define it, give the common term for it and put the medical term in parentheses. This glossary includes many of those terms, along with a wide range of other commonly used medical terms.

Given the limitations of space, this glossary doesn't include most of the conditions discussed in the book. Those are defined in entries devoted to them in the text and can be found by using the index. In addition, you can find drug terms in Chapter 40, "Medications Guide," and testing procedures in Chapter 39, "Diagnostic Tests."

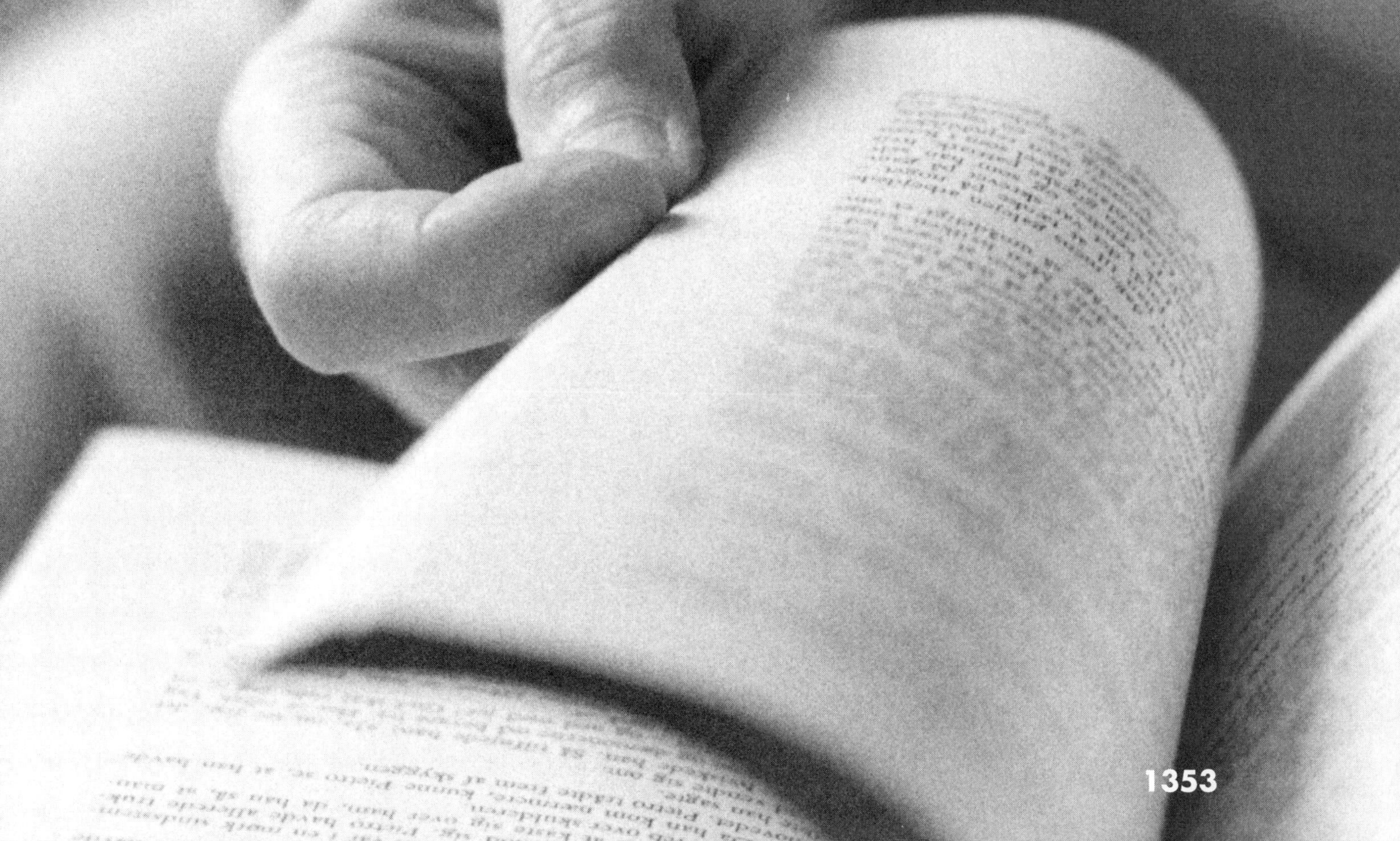

A

ablation. Elimination or removal.

abortion. The ending of a pregnancy by expulsion or extraction of the fetus from the womb before it can survive outside the womb, usually before the 20th week after conception.

abrasion. An area rubbed bare of skin or mucous membrane. Or, the normal wear of tooth enamel by chewing.

abruptio placentae. *See* placental abruption.

abscess. A localized formation of pus in a cavity, caused by the disintegration or displacement of tissue due to bacterial infection.

acetylcholine (ACH). A chemical in the body that carries electric messages between nerves and muscles; a neurotransmitter.

acetylsalicylic acid. Aspirin.

acuity. The sharpness or clarity with which you can see something. Someone with normal visual acuity is said to have 20/20 vision, which means that he or she can see objects clearly from 20 feet away that most people with normal sight are able to see clearly from 20 feet away.

acute. A term used to describe disorders, signs or symptoms that occur abruptly or that run a short course; the opposite of chronic.

addiction. Physical or emotional dependence on a substance — most often alcohol or another drug. Usually causes the user to require increasing amounts of the substance to achieve the same effect.

adenocarcinoma. A form of cancer arising from glands or glandular tissue.

adhesion. Tissue joining two surfaces, as in a healing wound.

adjunct therapy. Additional therapy used in the treatment of cancers. If surgical removal of the tumor is the primary therapy, then chemotherapy or radiation therapy is considered adjunct therapy.

adrenal glands. Endocrine glands that produce a range of hormones, including adrenaline (epinephrine), norepinephrine and corticosteroids.

adrenaline. A naturally occurring hormone that increases heart rate and blood pressure and affects other body functions. Also called epinephrine.

advance directive. A legal document that specifies the types of medical care you do or don't want to receive if you lose mental capacity or are unable to communicate your wishes.

adventitia. The outer layer of an organ.

aerobic. Requiring the presence of oxygen. Aerobic exercise, for example, is performed at an intensity level that allows oxygen intake from breathing to keep up with the body's use of oxygen in the chemical reaction that releases energy in muscles. *See also* anaerobic.

afterbirth. The placenta and membranes discharged from the uterus after childbirth.

agnosia. Loss of ability to interpret stimuli, usually classified according to the sense or senses affected.

agraphia. Loss of ability to write.

albumin. A protein found in animal and plant tissues. Its presence in the urine is one sign of kidney disease.

aldosterone. An adrenal hormone that affects the body's handling of sodium, chloride and potassium.

allergen. Any substance that produces an allergic reaction. Common allergens include cat dander, dust mites, pollen and certain foods.

allergic reaction. An exaggerated immune system response to an allergen. The reaction results from the release of histamine or histamine-like substances in affected cells. Sign and symptoms include rashes, nasal congestion, asthma and, occasionally, shock. *See also* histamine.

alveoli. Microscopic air sacs in the lungs where gases are exchanged. Or, tooth sockets.

amanita mushrooms. A group of mushrooms, most members of which are highly poisonous when eaten.

amaurosis fugax. Temporary visual loss in one eye, usually due to inadequate blood flow to the eye.

ambulatory. Able to walk.

amino acid. A nitrogen-containing component of protein. The body produces many amino acids. Those it needs but can't synthesize are known as essential amino acids and must be obtained through the diet.

amnesia. Loss of memory.

amniotic fluid. The protective liquid surrounding the fetus in the womb.

amputation. The act of cutting off or removing a limb or other body part.

amylase. A digestive enzyme made by the pancreas and salivary glands.

anaerobic. Able to live without oxygen, as do certain bacteria. Or, exercise in which the activity level is vigorous enough that the body uses oxygen faster than it can take it in, limiting the length of time the activity can be continued. *See also* aerobic.

analgesic. An agent that reduces pain.

anaphylaxis. An immediate and sometimes life-threatening allergic hypersensitivity reaction. Signs and symptoms include shock, breathing difficulty, itching, hives, convulsions and coma. *See also* shock.

androgen. A hormone such as testosterone or androsterone that's responsible for the development and maintenance of masculine physical characteristics. Produced in the testicles in males. Also produced in small amounts in females.

anemia. A condition characterized by a reduced number of red blood cells or a reduced amount of hemoglobin or blood.

anesthesia. Partial or complete loss of feeling or sensation. May be brought about by various anesthetics. Sometimes accompanied by loss of consciousness. Local anesthesia is confined to a particular region of the body. General anesthesia affects the whole body.

anesthetics. Substances used to induce anesthesia.

aneurysm. The localized enlargement of a blood vessel, usually an artery, that forms a bulge or sac.

angina pectoris. Episodic pain in the chest caused by a temporary decrease in blood flow to the heart.

angioedema. Allergic swelling of mucous membranes, tissues beneath the skin or in an internal organ.

angiogram. An X-ray picture produced by angiography.

angiography. A method for taking X-ray images of blood vessels after injecting contrast dye into a blood vessel.

angioplasty. A procedure for dilating a narrowed or blocked part of a blood vessel.

annulus. The ring around a heart valve where the valve leaflet merges with the heart muscle.

anorexia nervosa. An eating disorder characterized by a lack of appetite for food and caused by an emotional disturbance. It most often affects females in their teens and twenties and can result in severe loss of weight and even death.

anosmia. Loss of the sense of smell.

anterior chamber. The space in the eye between the iris and cornea filled with a fluid called aqueous humor.

antibodies. Immune system proteins that counteract or eliminate foreign substances known as antigens.

anticoagulant. A medication that keeps blood from clotting. Also called a blood thinner.

antidote. A substance that neutralizes the effects of a poison.

antiemetic. A medication that prevents or alleviates nausea and vomiting.

antigens. Substances foreign to the body that cause antibodies to form.

antihypertensives. Medications used to control high blood pressure.

anus. The outlet of the rectum, through which fecal waste passes.

aorta. The largest artery in the body. It carries blood from the heart's left ventricle and distributes it throughout the body.

aortic valve. The valve between the left ventricle and aorta. A normal aortic valve has three leaflets.

Apgar score. A rating given to a newborn at 1 and 5 minutes after birth, based on skin color, heart rate, muscle tone, respiration and reflexes. Zero to 2 points is given for each sign. Scores close to 10, the highest rating, are desirable.

aphasia. Loss of ability to speak or to understand speech because of brain damage.

aplastic. Arrested development of tissue or an organ.

apnea, sleep. Temporary cessation of breathing during sleep.

aqueous humor. A clear fluid that fills the anterior chamber of the eye. It nourishes the cornea and lens and helps maintain the internal pressure of the eye.

areola. The circular, pigmented area around the nipple of the breast.

arrhythmia. An abnormal heartbeat.

arteriole. A tiny artery that joins a larger artery to a capillary.

arteriosclerosis. A condition in which the walls of arteries become hard and thick, sometimes interfering with blood circulation.

arteritis. Inflammation of arteries.

artery. A blood vessel that carries blood from the heart to other tissues of the body.

arthritis. Inflammation of a joint.

arthroplasty. Surgical replacement or repair of a joint.

ascites. The accumulation of fluid in the abdominal cavity.

asphyxia. Suffocation caused by insufficient oxygen intake.

aspiration. Removal of fluids by suction, as from the nose, throat or lungs. Or, the inhalation into the lungs of fluids, such as water in drowning and stomach contents in vomiting.

asthma. A condition characterized by narrowing of the bronchial tubes, causing wheezing, coughing and difficulty breathing.

astigmatism. A focusing problem that occurs when your cornea is not curved evenly in all directions. Typically, what you see is distorted more in one direction than in others.

asymptomatic. Without symptoms.

ataxia. Incoordination of voluntary muscle movements.

atherectomy. A method for shaving or removing, with a specially designed catheter, atherosclerotic plaques from inside arteries.

atherosclerosis. A condition in which plaques accumulate in the lining of the arteries, resulting in narrower, less flexible pathways for the blood.

atopic dermatitis. *See* eczema.

atresia. Congenital absence of an opening, duct or canal in the body, as in the intestines or esophagus.

atria. Cavities or chambers, such as the upper chambers of the heart, that receive blood from veins and pass it to the ventricles. Singular form is atrium.

atrioventricular. Involving both atria and ventricles.

atrioventricular block. A blocking of the electric signal between the atria and ventricles. Varies in severity from first, second to third degree (complete heart block).

atrioventricular (AV) node. A cluster of cells that slows the flow of electric signals as they pass from the atria to the ventricles.

atrophy. Shrinking (wasting) of tissue or an organ due to disease or lack of use.

aura. A sensation felt before the onset of a convulsion or migraine.

auscultation. The act of listening to the sounds of various organs.

autograft. A surgical operation in which one of your body parts is used to repair another part, as when a pulmonary valve replaces the aortic valve.

autoimmune disease. A disease that occurs when antibodies react against the body's own tissues.

autoimmune response. A reaction by the body to one or some of its own tissues it perceives as foreign substances, resulting in production of antibodies against those tissues.

autologous transfusion. A transfusion of one's own blood previously donated in anticipation of surgery.

autonomic nervous system. The portion of the nervous system that regulates involuntary body functions.

autopsy. An examination of tissues and organs of the body after death.

avulsion. Forced tearing away of a body part or structure, such as a limb or tooth.

B

bacteria. Single-celled microorganisms, some of which cause disease and some of which are beneficial to biologic processes.

barrel chest. An altered shape of the chest cage, as seen in some people with emphysema.

basal cell carcinoma. The most common form of skin cancer, often associated with sun exposure. This tumor can be locally invasive but rarely spreads (metastasizes).

B cell. A type of lymphocyte that works as part of the immune system by producing antibodies to fight infection.

benign. Harmless, not progressive or recurrent, noncancerous.

bile. Bitter-tasting fluid produced by the liver and temporarily stored in the gallbladder before discharge into the small intestine. Bile facilitates the digestion of fats in the small intestine.

bilirubin. Orange or yellowish pigment that's the result of the breakdown of red blood cells. Excess bilirubin in the blood produces jaundice.

biofeedback. A behavior-training program that teaches a person how to control autonomic reactions such as heart rate, blood pressure, skin temperature and muscular tension.

bioprosthesis. A prosthetic valve made of pig or bovine tissue.

biopsy. To take a sample of tissue for laboratory examination.

birth defect. Any of various congenital disorders, from a minor cosmetic irregularity to a life-threatening disorder.

bisexual. A person who is sexually attracted to people of both sexes.

bladder. A membranous sac that holds secretions, most commonly the sac that collects urine before its elimination.

blepharitis. An inflammation along the edge of the eyelid that can cause irritation and itching.

blood pressure. The force placed on the inner walls of the arteries. *See also* diastole and systole.

bone marrow. Soft material found inside bone cavities where blood cells are formed.

bone marrow transplant. A procedure in which a patient's bone marrow is destroyed by chemotherapy or radiation or both and replaced with either donated bone marrow or the patient's own marrow that was collected and stored before chemotherapy or radiation.

bowel. The small or large intestine. The large intestine is sometimes called the colon.

bradycardia. A slow heartbeat.

brainstem. The portion of the brain that connects with the spinal cord. The stem consists of the medulla oblongata, pons and midbrain.

brand name drugs. Drugs carrying a trademark name designated by their manufacturer.

Braxton Hicks contractions. Irregular uterine contractions that occur during pregnancy. Sometimes, they're referred to as false labor.

breech presentation. Positioning of the fetus during labor with feet or buttocks toward the cervix.

bronchial tubes. The two main breathing tubes leading from the windpipe (trachea) to the lungs. Also called bronchi.

bronchiectasis. Abnormal enlargement of the bronchial tubes caused by chronic infection.

bronchiole. One of the subdivisions of a bronchial tube.

bronchitis. Inflammation of the bronchial tubes.

bronchodilator. Medicine used to open (dilate) the airways.

bronchogenic. Arising from a bronchial tube.

bronchoscopy. A procedure in which an instrument is passed into the airway to look at the lung structures or obtain specimens.

bruises. Injuries in which blood vessels are broken and blood escapes beneath the skin, producing a discolored area.

bruit. Sound produced by the flow of blood through a narrowed vessel.

bundle branch block. A condition in which portions of the heart's conduction system become defective and unable to conduct electric signals normally. You can have right or left bundle branch block.

bursa. A fluid-filled sac near or involving a joint or bony prominence that helps to reduce friction between a tendon and bone or between bone and skin.

bypass. *See* cardiopulmonary bypass; coronary artery bypass graft.

C

cachexia. Malnutrition and wasting due to chronic illness.

Caesarean section. Surgical removal of a baby from the womb through an incision in the abdomen and the wall of the uterus.

cafe au lait spots. Coffee-colored areas of pigmentation.

caffeine. A stimulant found naturally in coffee, tea, chocolate and cocoa. It may be added to soft drinks, over-the-counter drugs and other products.

calcitonin. A hormone, produced by the thyroid gland, that affects the amount of calcium in the blood.

calcium. A mineral important for strong teeth and bones and for muscle and nerve function. Dairy products are good sources of calcium.

calculus. An accumulation of mineral salts in various parts of the body or on the teeth.

callus. An area of thickened skin.

calorie. The amount of heat needed to raise the temperature of 1 gram of water by 1 degree Celsius.

cancer. A group of diseases characterized by abnormal growth of cells, resulting in the formation of malignant tumors in various parts of the body. *See also* benign; malignant

candida. A species of yeast-like fungi.

canines. The four teeth situated between a premolar and an incisor. Also called cuspids.

capillaries. Minute blood vessels connecting the smallest arteries to the smallest veins.

caput succedaneum. Swelling of a baby's scalp during labor.

carbohydrates. Compounds composed of starches or sugars and found primarily in breads, cereals, fruits and vegetables.

carcinogens. Cancer-causing agents.

carcinoid tumor. A specific type of tumor that arises in the intestines or a bronchial tube. It typically produces a chemical called serotonin, which can cause flushing, low blood pressure and diarrhea.

carcinoma. A form of cancer made up of epithelial cells. Epithelial cells line body cavities, cover internal organs and line the internal portions of organs.

cardiac. Pertaining to the heart.

cardiac arrest. Sudden cessation of heartbeats.

cardiac catheterization. A procedure in which a catheter is introduced into a blood vessel and guided into the heart in order to measure blood flow and evaluate structural defects.

cardiac cycle. The period from the beginning of one heartbeat to the beginning of the next.

cardiac output. The amount of blood the heart pumps through the circulatory system in 1 minute.

cardiomyopathy. A heart muscle disease that impairs the ability of the heart to pump.

cardiopulmonary. Pertaining to the heart and lungs.

cardiopulmonary bypass. A method by which a machine takes over the function of the heart and lungs during heart surgery.

cardiopulmonary resuscitation (CPR). A technique for reviving a person whose heart and breathing have stopped.

cardiovascular. Pertaining to the heart and blood vessels.

cardiovascular system. The circulatory system, including the heart, arteries, veins and lymphatic system.

cardioversion. Electric shock applied to the chest to convert an abnormal heartbeat to normal.

caries. Decayed areas of tooth or bone due to bacteria. Also known as cavities.

carotid arteries. The principal arteries of the neck that carry blood to the head and brain.

carrier. One who carries and may transmit an infectious agent or genetic defect but doesn't experience the signs and symptoms of conditions caused by that agent or defect.

cartilage. Dense, fibrous connective tissue located throughout the body, including the joints, nose and ears.

catabolism. The breakdown of body tissues as a source of calories.

cataract. A clouding of the normally clear lens of the eye.

catheter. A small, flexible tube that's inserted into a body part to inject or remove liquid.

catheterization. A procedure in which a catheter is inserted into the body.

cc. Cubic centimeter, a unit of volume measurement. Thirty cubic centimeters (30 cc) equals 1 ounce.

CCU. Coronary (cardiac) care unit.

Centers for Disease Control and Prevention (CDC). A division of the Department of Health and Human Services. One of its responsibilities is the study of infectious diseases.

cephalhematoma. A bruised area beneath the outer layer of the skull, usually in a newborn.

cephalopelvic disproportion. A circumstance in which a baby's head is too large to pass through the mother's pelvis.

cerclage. A surgical procedure in which stitches (sutures) are made around the cervix in an attempt to prevent premature birth.

cerebellum. The portion of the brain responsible for balance and coordination.

cerebral embolism. A blood clot that travels through arteries from the site where it formed and blocks blood flow in the brain.

cerebral hemorrhage. Bleeding in the brain.

cerebral vascular accident. *See* stroke.

cerebrovascular. Pertaining to the blood vessels of the brain.

cerebrum. The largest portion of the brain, containing the two hemispheres. It's responsible for speech, memory, vision, personality and muscle control in certain parts of your body.

cervical cap. A contraceptive device that fits tightly over the cervix to help prevent sperm from entering the uterus.

cervical incompetence. A condition in which the cervix begins to open before pregnancy has come to term, causing miscarriage or preterm labor.

cervix. The neck of an organ, such as the neck of the uterus.

chalazion. A relatively painless swelling on the eyelid caused by blockage of a small oil gland.

chancre. A destructive, painless sore on the skin or mucous membranes, usually caused by syphilis.

chemotherapy. The use of medications that have a direct effect on a disease-causing organism or abnormal cells. Widely used in the treatment of cancer.

Cheyne-Stokes respiration. A pattern of breathing with varying depths of respiration and brief periods of apnea.

chloasma. A mild darkening of the facial skin. Often called the mask of pregnancy.

cholesterol. A fat-like substance synthesized in the liver and found in the blood, brain, liver and bile and as deposits in the walls of blood vessels. Essential to the production of sex hormones. Found in foods of animal sources and thought to contribute to heart disease in people who eat large quantities of it over a long period of time.

chordae tendineae. Strong chords that stretch from the edges of the tricuspid and mitral valves to the heart muscle and restrict how far the valve leaflets swing when they close.

chorionic villus sampling. A procedure in which a small sample of cells is removed from the placenta where it joins the uterus. Used to test for chromosome abnormalities such as Down syndrome.

choroid. A thin layer of arteries and veins sandwiched between the retina and sclera of the eye. The choroid plays an important role in nourishing the retina.

chromosome. One of 46 rod-shaped structures in the nucleus of each cell. Carries hereditary information.

chronic. Referring to long-lasting diseases or conditions.

chronic obstructive pulmonary disease (COPD). The overall term for a group of chronic conditions that result in obstruction of lung airways. Usually refers to chronic bronchitis and emphysema. Chronic bronchial asthma, cystic fibrosis, bronchiolitis and bronchiectasis also are sometimes classified as COPD.

chyme. The mixture of partly digested food and digestive secretions found in the stomach.

cilia. The eyelashes. Or, smaller hair-like projections lining the bronchial tubes and upper respiratory tract.

circumcision. Removal of the foreskin from the penis.

claudication. Activity-induced muscle pain produced by inadequate arterial blood flow.

clinical. Pertaining to information gathered from working with patients, as distinct from laboratory findings.

clinical trial. An experiment designed to test the effectiveness and possible side effects of a treatment in humans. The trial is designed using scientific methods and sometimes compares standard therapy or a placebo with the test therapy.

clitoris. The small, erectile organ of the external female genitals.

clot. Coagulated blood.

coagulate. To solidify or change from a liquid to a semisolid, as when blood clots.

coccyx. The tailbone.

cochlea. The snail-shaped tube of the inner ear that's the receptor for sound vibrations.

cognitive. Pertaining to the mental process of thought, including perception, reasoning, intuition and memory.

coitus. Sexual intercourse between a male and female in which the male inserts his penis into the female's vagina.

colic. Pain in the abdomen produced by intermittent spasms of the intestines. In infants it may be manifested by episodes of crying, a distended abdomen and legs drawn up to the chest.

collagen. Fibrous protein found in connective tissues such as skin, ligaments and cartilage.

collateral vessels. Small branches of arteries and veins that develop to bypass narrowed or blocked segments.

colon. The large intestine, extending from the end of the small intestine to the anus. It's responsible for extracting water from undigested food particles and storing the waste, which is eliminated in bowel movements.

colorectal. Pertaining to the colon and rectum.

colostomy. A surgical procedure in which a section of colon is pulled through an opening (stoma) created in the abdominal wall, allowing for the passage of stool into a small bag securely fastened over the opening.

colostrum. The thin, lemon-colored liquid produced by a mother's breasts in the first day or so after giving birth. Its antibodies are beneficial to the infant.

coma. An abnormal state of deep unconsciousness due to illness or accident.

compensatory pause. In the heart, a slight delay that occurs after a premature contraction before the next heartbeat.

complex carbohydrates. Substances, such as starch, composed of several sugars linked together.

computerized tomography (CT). An X-ray technique that uses a computer to construct images of the body.

conception. Fertilization of an egg (ova) by a sperm.

concussion. A temporary disturbance of brain function due to a head injury.

condom. A sheath that fits over an erect penis to catch semen during ejaculation.

conduction system. Special muscle fibers that conduct electric impulses throughout the muscle of the heart.

cones. Light-sensitive cells of the retina that provide your central vision and allow you to see fine detail and color.

congenital. Present at birth. Usually used in reference to an abnormality.

congestion. The presence of excessive blood or fluid, such as mucus, in an organ or tissue.

congestive heart failure. A condition in which the heart is unable to pump enough blood to meet the needs of the body. Characterized by fluid collecting in parts of the body, such as the legs, lungs and liver. Also called heart failure.

conjunctiva. A thin, moist, clear membrane that covers the exposed front portion of the sclera and lines the inside of your eyelids.

conjunctivitis. An inflammation of the conjunctiva, giving your eye a reddish or pinkish coloration.

constipation. The difficult passage of hard, dry stools.

contraception. Measures taken to prevent pregnancy.

contraction. The shortening and thickening of a muscle fiber or a muscle in action.

contracture. Permanent tightness or shortening of a muscle due to disease or injury.

contrast agent. A liquid dye, opaque to X-rays, that's taken into the gastrointestinal tract or injected into a blood vessel or the fluid-filled space around the spinal cord to permit X-ray visualization of structures of the body that couldn't otherwise be seen by X-ray.

contusions. Bruises.

convulsion. A sudden attack commonly characterized by a loss of consciousness and severe, sustained, rhythmic contractions of some or all voluntary muscles. Convulsions are most often a manifestation of a seizure disorder (epilepsy).

cord compression. A condition that prevents proper blood flow through the umbilical cord. Or, pressure on the spinal cord.

cornea. A domed layer of clear tissue at the front of the eye. It helps focus light entering the eye.

coronary. Pertaining to arteries that supply blood to the heart muscle.

coronary angiography. A diagnostic test in which dye is injected into a coronary artery and then an X-ray is taken to detect disease or blockage.

coronary arteries. The arteries that supply blood to the heart muscle.

coronary artery bypass graft. An operation that reroutes the blood supply by bypassing blocked or narrowed coronary arteries.

coronary artery disease. Narrowing or blockage of one or more of the coronary arteries, resulting in decreased blood supply (ischemia) to the heart muscle. Also called ischemic heart disease.

coronary insufficiency. An inability of the coronary arteries to provide enough oxygen to meet the needs of the heart muscle.

coronary occlusion. An obstruction in a coronary artery, interrupting blood flow to the heart muscle.

coronary sinus. The main vein that drains blood into the right atrium from the heart muscle.

corpus luteum. A small, hormone-producing structure that develops in the ovary where an egg had previously matured (the empty follicle).

corticosteroids. Hormones produced by the cortex of the adrenal glands. Or, a class of such hormones used as medications.

cortisol. A hormone produced by the adrenal glands.

cranium. The portion of the skull that houses the brain.

creatinine. A substance excreted in urine that's measured to help evaluate kidney function.

Crohn's disease. A chronic inflammatory disease of the digestive tract, especially the small intestine.

crowning. The appearance of the top of a baby's head at the vaginal opening during labor.

curettage. Scraping of a cavity, such as the uterus.

cusp. A segment of a heart valve.

cuspids. *See* canines.

cyanosis. Bluish discoloration of the skin due to a lack of oxygen in the blood.

cyanotic heart disease. Birth defects of the heart that permit oxygen-depleted (blue) blood to circulate in the body without passing through the lungs.

cyst. A closed sac or cavity filled with a fluid, gas or semisolid substance.

cystic fibrosis. A genetic disorder affecting the respiratory and digestive systems. Most commonly found among whites of Northern European descent.

cystitis. An inflammation of the urinary bladder, usually from a bacterial infection.

cystoscopy. A procedure in which a small instrument (cystoscope) is passed through the urethra to allow for direct examination of the urethra, bladder and, in men, prostate gland.

cytology. The study of cells often used to identify the presence of cancer.

D

debility. A state of physical weakness.

debulking. The surgical removal of the major portion of a tumor mass when a tumor can't be completely removed.

decubitus ulcer. An open sore that forms in the skin because of prolonged pressure. Also called a bedsore.

deep vein thrombosis. A blood clot in the deep veins of the leg.

defibrillation. Electric shock applied to the heart to return an irregular heartbeat to normal.

dehydration. The result of excessive loss of body fluids or inadequate fluid consumption.

delirium. A state of mental confusion, sometimes characterized by disordered speech and often accompanied by hallucinations.

delusion. A firmly held belief with no basis in reality.

dementia. Mental deterioration due to organic causes.

dentin. The tissue of a tooth beneath the enamel and enclosing the pulp cavity.

deoxyribonucleic acid (DNA). A substance found in the nucleus of cells that carries hereditary information.

depression. A feeling of extreme sadness and discouragement. Signs and symptoms include disruption of sleeping and eating patterns and lack of energy.

dermatitis. Inflammation of the skin, often characterized by itching and redness.

dermatochalasis. An age-related drooping of the eyelid skin. The upper eyelid may sag over your eyelashes and interfere with your vision.

dermis. The layer of skin beneath the epidermis.

detoxification. The process of cleansing the body of a drug or toxin, such as alcohol.

dextrose. A simple sugar that's found in the blood. It's also a main component of honey and corn syrup. Also called glucose.

diabetes mellitus. A disorder characterized by high levels of sugar (glucose) in the blood. Diabetes mellitus may be caused by a failure of the pancreas to produce sufficient insulin or by resistance of the body to the action of insulin. Also called diabetes.

diabetic ketoacidosis. A serious condition that may develop in people with diabetes. Owing to insufficient insulin, the body begins breaking down fat, producing an increased level of acids (ketones) in the blood.

diabetic retinopathy. A complication of diabetes that damages the tiny blood vessels that nourish the retina. Diabetic retinopathy is brought on by high blood sugar levels. If untreated, it can lead to blindness.

diagnosis. Identification of a disease or disorder by a doctor.

dialysis. A technique for removing waste and toxins from the blood. Used primarily when the kidneys fail or in cases of overdose of a drug. Includes hemodialysis and peritoneal dialysis.

diaphragm. The muscle that separates the abdomen from the chest. Or, a contraceptive device that fits over the cervix to help prevent sperm from entering the uterus.

diastole. The period during the heart cycle in which the muscle relaxes, followed by contraction of the heart muscle (systole).

diastolic pressure. The lowest blood pressure reached during the relaxation of the heart. Recorded as the second number in a blood pressure measurement.

digestion. The breakdown of food in the digestive system so that its nutrients can be absorbed by the body and its undigestible parts can be excreted as waste.

digit. A finger or toe.

dilatation and curettage (D and C). Dilating the cervix and scraping the lining of the uterus (endometrium) with an instrument.

dilate. To expand or open a structure such as the pupil of the eye or a passageway such as an artery.

diplopia. Double vision.

disk. A plate-like structure such as the cartilage cushion found between every two vertebrae.

dislocation. Displacement of a bone from its normal position at a joint.

diuretics. Drugs that increase the flow of urine. They're often used to treat conditions involving excess body fluid, such as high blood pressure and congestive heart failure. Also called water pills.

diverticulosis. Pouch-like bulges in the wall of the intestine.

DNA. *See* deoxyribonucleic acid.

dominant. A mode of inheritance in which a gene for a particular trait is required from only one parent for that trait to appear in his or her offspring. *See also* recessive.

Down syndrome. The most common type of chromosome abnormality, caused by an extra chromosome 21 (trisomy 21). This abnormality results in varying degrees of mental retardation and other birth defects.

drusen. Clumps of waste deposit that form under the retinal pigment epithelium. They appear as yellow dots behind the retina in the back of the eye. An early sign of macular degeneration.

DTaP vaccine. The immunization that protects against diphtheria, tetanus and whooping cough (pertussis).

duodenum. The section of the small intestine closest to the stomach.

dura mater. The tough outer membrane covering the spinal cord and brain.

dysphagia. Difficulty swallowing or an inability to swallow.

dysplasia. Abnormal development of tissue.

dyspnea. Shortness of breath.

dystocia. Difficult labor usually due to an abnormal position or size of the fetus.

E

echocardiography. A test in which pulses of sound are sent into the chest. The echoes returning from the heart produce images that are recorded as echocardiograms.

eclampsia. A serious complication of pregnancy manifested by convulsions and loss of consciousness, including coma.

ect-, ecto-. Prefixes meaning outside.

ectopic. Abnormal placement, such as a pregnancy that occurs outside the uterus (tubal pregnancy).

ectropion. A condition that develops when the eyelid sags outward from the eye.

eczema. An acute or chronic inflammatory condition of the skin characterized by itching and scaling. Also called atopic dermatitis or dermatitis.

edema. Swelling of body tissues due to accumulation of excess fluid.

effusion. An accumulation of fluid in body cavities or joints.

ejaculation. The ejection of semen that occurs during male orgasm.

ejection fraction. The portion of blood that's pumped out of a filled ventricle. Normal is 50 percent or more.

electrocardiogram (ECG). A recording of the electric activity of the heart.

embolism. A blood clot, air bubble, fat deposit or other foreign substance that moves from the site where it formed and blocks a blood vessel.

embryo. The human organism from the time of implantation in the uterus to about the 10th to 12th week after conception.

emetic. A substance that induces vomiting.

emission. The discharge of fluid.

emphysema. A disease in which the walls of the air sacs (alveoli) of the lungs are weakened or destroyed. This results in lungs that can't empty air normally and can't transfer oxygen efficiently into the bloodstream.

en-, endo-. Prefixes meaning inside or within.

endarterectomy. The surgical removal of material from inside an artery, such as an atherosclerotic plaque.

endocarditis. An inflammation of the membrane that lines the chambers and valves of the heart, usually caused by infection.

endocardium. The thin, inner membrane that lines the cavities of the heart. *See also* epicardium and myocardium.

endocrine gland. An organ or tissue that releases a substance to be used elsewhere in the body.

endoscope. An illuminated optical instrument used to visualize the inside of a hollow organ or cavity.

endothelium. A layer of cells on the inner surface of blood vessels.

endotracheal tube. A tube inserted into the windpipe (trachea) to allow breathing with a ventilator.

enema. Introduction of fluid into the rectum and colon to induce a bowel movement or to introduce a contrast agent for a diagnostic procedure.

entropion. A condition that develops when the eyelid turns in toward the eye.

enzyme. A complex protein that acts as a catalyst for chemical reactions.

epicardium. The thin membrane that covers the surface of the heart muscle. *See also* endocardium and myocardium.

epidemiology. The study of disease in human populations.

epidermis. The outer layer of skin.

epiglottis. The flap of cartilage that covers the voice box (larynx).

epinephrine. *See* adrenaline.

episiotomy. A surgical incision to enlarge the vaginal opening during childbirth.

erection. The swelling and stiffening of the penis during sexual arousal.

erythema. An area of reddened skin due to dilated capillaries.

erythrocytes. Red blood cells, which transport oxygen.

esophagus. The muscular tube that connects the throat (pharynx) with the stomach.

estrogen. A hormone produced primarily in females that contributes to the development and maintenance of feminine physical characteristics, cyclic changes such as menstruation, and changes related to pregnancy. The hormone is also produced in small quantities in males.

ethanol. Grain or ethyl alcohol.

eustachian tube. The tube connecting the middle ear to the throat (pharynx).

excisional biopsy. Tissue removal (biopsy) in which an attempt is made to extract an abnormal growth in its entirety.

expiration. Letting a breath out; exhalation.

extrasystole. A premature heartbeat.

F

faint. A brief loss of consciousness resulting from insufficient blood to the brain.

fallopian tubes. Tubes located on each side of a woman's uterus that convey eggs from the ovaries to the cavity of the uterus.

false labor. Irregular uterine pains and contractions that may occur during pregnancy. Also called Braxton Hicks contractions.

familial hypercholesterolemia. An inherited form of high blood cholesterol levels.

farsightedness. A focusing problem in which you can see faraway objects clearly, but nearby objects appear blurry. Also called hyperopia.

fats. Organic compounds composed of fatty acids. Fats are either saturated or unsaturated. Unsaturated fats are further classified as either monounsaturated or polyunsaturated.

febrile. Feverish.

feces. Body waste such as food residue discharged from the bowels.

femur. The thighbone.

fertility. The ability to reproduce.

fertilization. The process of conception in which a sperm penetrates an egg (ovum), usually in the fallopian tube.

fetal distress. A situation in which a fetus is in potential jeopardy. Indications include a change in fetal activity or heartbeat and meconium-stained amniotic fluid.

fetus. The human being from about the 10th to 12th week after conception until delivery.

fiber. A food substance that resists chemical digestion and passes through the system essentially unchanged.

fibrillation. Quivering or uncontrollable contraction of muscles. Fibrillation in the cardiac muscle causes an irregular heartbeat.

fibrocystic breasts. A benign condition of the breasts characterized by lumps that vary with the menstrual cycle. Also called benign breast disease.

fibroid. A benign tumor of connective and muscular tissue, usually of the uterus. Also called fibroma.

fibula. The smaller of the two bones that run from the knee to the ankle.

flaccid. Soft, limp, without tone.

flatulence. Excessive gas in the stomach and intestines.

floater. A small bit of debris floating in the vitreous that can look like a spot, hair or string before your eye. What you're seeing is the shadow that this material casts on your retina.

fluoride. An element found in nature that helps prevent tooth decay and possibly strengthens bone.

fluoroscopy. Use of X-rays to produce images on a screen rather than on X-ray film.

flutter. Very rapid, regular beating of a heart chamber.

follicle. A small, tubular gland or sac in the skin or ovary. Or, an aggregation of cells in a lymph node.

follicle-stimulating hormone. A hormone that stimulates the development of eggs (ova) in the ovaries.

fontanel. A soft spot atop an infant's head where the bones of the skull have yet to join.

forceps. A surgical instrument used for grasping or compressing tissue.

foreskin. The skin covering the end of an uncircumcised penis. Also called the prepuce.

fovea. A small depression in the center of the macula that contains only cone cells and provides your sharpest vision.

fracture. To break or crack a bone. Or, a break or crack in a bone.

fraternal twins. Twins developing from two separate, fertilized eggs (ova). Also called nonidentical twins.

fructose. A sugar found in fruit, corn syrup and honey.

fundal height. The distance from the top of the pregnant uterus to the pubic bone. This measurement is used in estimating fetal age.

fungus. An organism of plant origin that lacks chlorophyll. Some fungi cause disease.

G

gallbladder. A sac, located under the liver, that stores bile secreted from the liver and releases it into the small intestine during digestion.

gametes. The cells of reproduction — sperm (spermatozoa) and eggs (ova).

gamma globulin. A protein found in the blood that helps fight infection.

ganglion. A mass of nerve tissue made up mostly of nerve cell bodies. Or, a cyst in a tendon sheath.

gangrene. Death and decay of body tissue, usually due to a lack of blood supply. The tissue shrinks and turns black.

gastric. Pertaining to the stomach.

gastroenteritis. An inflammatory condition of the stomach and intestines leading to nausea, vomiting, abdominal pain and diarrhea. Usually of bacterial or viral origin.

gastrointestinal tract. The stomach and intestines.

gene. A structure, within a chromosome, that's responsible for inheritance of a particular characteristic.

general anesthesia. A state of unconsciousness induced by a medication that eliminates sensation.

generalized. Overall, not limited to one area.

generic drug. The nontrademark name of a drug.

genetic. Associated with genes and heredity.

genetic engineering. The manufacture, alteration or repair of genetic material by artificial means.

genetic marker. An identifiable substance that's associated with a normal or an abnormal gene.

genital herpes. A viral infection spread by sexual contact and marked by inflammation and blisters in the infected area.

genitals. Internal and external reproductive organs.

genome. The entire collection of genes of an organism.

geriatrics. The branch of medicine that specializes in the care of diseases and problems related to aging.

germ. A microorganism. Some may cause disease.

German measles. *See* rubella.

gestation. The period of time from conception to birth.

gestational diabetes. Diabetes that develops during pregnancy, resulting in improper regulation of sugar (glucose) levels in the blood.

gigantism. A disorder caused by an overproduction of growth hormone by the pituitary gland. It results in excessive body height and size. Also known as giantism.

gland. Any organ or tissue that releases a substance to be used elsewhere in the body. Endocrine glands release hormones directly into the bloodstream.

glaucoma. A group of eye conditions resulting in abnormally high pressure inside the eyeball. This pressure causes extensive damage to the optic nerve and loss of peripheral vision.

globulin. A category of blood proteins from which antibodies are formed.

globus. A sensation of a lump in your throat in the absence of a physical abnormality. May be related to stress.

glomeruli. Microscopic clusters of blood vessels in the kidneys. Responsible for filtering waste from the blood.

glucagon. A pancreatic hormone that releases the body's stored sugar (glycogen) from the liver into the blood.

glucose. Blood sugar. Also known as dextrose.

gluten. Plant proteins found in grains such as wheat, rye, oats and barley.

glycogen. Stored sugar (glucose) in the liver.

goiter. An enlargement of the thyroid gland.

gonadotropin. A hormone that stimulates the gonads (ovaries and testicles).

gonads. *See* ovaries; testicles.

gonorrhea. A bacterial disease spread by sexual contact.

gout. A condition in which excess uric acid leads to arthritis and kidney stones.

grading. The process of assigning a number to a tumor based on pathologic evidence of its aggressiveness.

grand mal. A term used to describe a generalized convulsion accompanied by a loss of consciousness.

granulocytes. White blood cells (leukocytes) manufactured in the bone marrow and containing granules. They digest and destroy bacteria.

groin. The lower abdominal area where the trunk and thighs meet.

H

halitosis. Bad breath.

hallucination. A false perception with no basis in reality. May be seen, heard or smelled.

hamstrings. The muscles at the back of the thigh. The tendons of the hamstring muscles can be felt at the back of the knee.

handicapped. Impaired physically or mentally in a manner that interferes with normal activities.

hardening of the arteries. *See* arteriosclerosis.

HDL cholesterol. High-density lipoprotein cholesterol. A type of cholesterol thought to help protect against atherosclerosis. The "good" cholesterol.

heart attack. A myocardial infarction. Death of an area of heart muscle caused by blockage of one or more of the coronary arteries that results in sudden interruption of blood to a part of the heart.

heart block. *See* atrioventricular block.

heartburn. A burning sensation beneath the breastbone (sternum) resulting from regurgitation of gastric juices (reflux) from the stomach into the esophagus.

heart catheterization. A diagnostic test in which a catheter is placed into the heart.

heart failure. *See* congestive heart failure.

heart murmur. An abnormal sound heard during the heartbeat. The condition can be a sign of a diseased heart valve or other abnormality.

heart rate. The number of contractions of the heart in 1 minute.

Heimlich maneuver. Abdominal thrusts applied manually to dislodge an object blocking the airway.

hemangioma. A benign tumor of dilated blood vessels.

hematemesis. Vomiting of blood.

hematoma. A blood-filled swelling beneath the skin or in an organ, due to injury to a blood vessel.

hematuria. Blood or blood clots in the urine.

hemiplegia. Paralysis of one side of the body.

hemochromatosis. A defect in iron metabolism with buildup of iron in the body.

hemodialysis. A mechanical technique for removing chemical waste and toxins from the blood. Also called dialysis.

hemoglobin. An iron-containing protein found in the red blood cells. Hemoglobin transports oxygen to body tissues.

hemophilia. An inherited bleeding disorder in which blood clotting is abnormal.

hemoptysis. Coughing or spitting up of blood that comes from bleeding in the voice box (larynx), windpipe (trachea) or lungs.

hemorrhage. Internal or external bleeding.

hemorrhoid. A swollen vein in and around the anus that may bleed.

heparin. A substance that interferes with blood clotting.

hepatic. Pertaining to the liver.

hepatitis. Inflammation of the liver.

heredity. The transmission of genetic traits from parent to child.

hernia. Protrusion of an organ or structure into surrounding tissues. Commonly called a rupture.

heterosexual. A person who is sexually attracted to those of the opposite sex.

hiccup. An involuntary spasm of the diaphragm, followed quickly by shutting of the glottis, resulting in a sharp, sudden intake of breath.

high blood pressure. A condition in which the blood is pumped through the body under increased pressure. Also called hypertension.

hirsutism. Excessive growth of body or facial hair.

histamine. A body chemical in tissues that stimulates production of gastric acid for digestion. Or, the active agent of allergic reactions that result when excessive amounts of histamine are released to combat a perceived invader (allergen). The affected site becomes swollen and congested, resulting in hives, asthma or hay fever.

histology. The study of the microscopic appearance of tissues.

HIV. Human immunodeficiency virus. The virus that causes AIDS and related conditions.

hives. Eruption of welts on the skin. Thought to result from the release of histamine and other chemicals into the bloodstream.

Hodgkin's disease. A form of malignant lymphoma.

homograft. A surgical procedure in which a body part is replaced or repaired using sterilized human tissue, as when the aortic valve is replaced.

homosexual. A person who is sexually attracted to those of the same sex as himself or herself.

hormone. A substance secreted by an endocrine gland and carried through the bloodstream to regulate various body functions.

human immunodeficiency virus (HIV). The virus that causes AIDS and related conditions.

humerus. The bone of the upper arm.

humoral. Pertaining to body fluids.

hydramnios. An excess of amniotic fluid.
hydrocephalus. Increased size of the fluid-filled cavities (ventricles) of the brain.
hydrogenation. The process of changing an unsaturated fat to a more solid, saturated one.
hymen. A membrane partially covering the opening to the vagina.
hymenoptera. The order of insects that includes bees, wasps and ants.
hyper-. A prefix meaning excessive or increased.
hyperactivity. A condition of behavior characterized by constant overactivity, distractibility, impulsiveness, an inability to concentrate and aggressiveness.
hypercholesterolemia. An elevated level of cholesterol in the blood.
hyperglycemia. Excess sugar (glucose) in the bloodstream.
hyperlipidemia. Excess fats (lipids) in the bloodstream.
hyperopia. *See* farsightedness.
hyperplasia. Excess number of cells in tissue.
hypertension. *See* high blood pressure.
hypertrophic cardiomyopathy. An overgrowth of heart muscle that may impede blood flow into and out of the heart.
hyperventilation. Rapid or deep breathing in excess of that needed to supply oxygen to the body.
hypo-. A prefix meaning inadequate or insufficient.
hypochondria. Excessive concern about health.
hypoglycemia. A condition in which sugar (glucose) in the bloodstream falls below normal levels.
hypotension. Low blood pressure.
hypothalamus. A portion of the brain partly responsible for basic functions such as appetite, sleep, body temperature and procreation.
hypoxia. Decreased concentration of oxygen in the blood.

I

iatrogenic disease. A disorder or disease that's a side effect of a prescribed treatment.
identical twins. Twins arising from a single fertilized egg (ovum).
idiopathic. Pertaining to a condition or disease of unknown cause.
ileostomy. A surgical procedure in which a section of the small intestine is brought out through an opening (stoma) created in the abdominal wall, allowing for the passage of stool into a small bag securely fastened over the opening.
ileum. The lower portion of the small intestine.
ilium. The upper portion of the hipbone.
immobilize. To make a limb or other body part immovable in order to aid healing.
immune system. The system that protects the body from invasion by foreign substances such as bacteria, viruses, parasites and fungi.
immunity. Resistance to a disease, particularly an infectious one.
immunization. The introduction of antigens into the body in very small quantities in order to stimulate the development of immunity.
immunoglobulin. A protein that can act as an antibody.
immunosuppressive medications. Drugs that suppress the immune system.
impacted. Pressed firmly together so as to be immovable.
impotence. The inability of a man to achieve or keep an erection and engage in sexual intercourse.
incision. A cut made with a knife.
incisors. The eight front teeth, four in the upper jaw and four in the lower jaw.
incontinence. An inability to control the release of urine or feces.
indigestion. Incomplete or abnormal digestion.
infarct. An area of tissue that dies because of blockage of its blood supply.
infection. A condition in which the body or a part of it is invaded by a microorganism.
infectious. Disease-causing.
inferior vena cava. The large vein returning blood from the legs and abdomen to the heart.
infertility. An inability to reproduce.
inflammation. Body tissue's reaction to injury from infection, physical injury or irritation, resulting in swelling, pain, heat and redness.
inguinal. Pertaining to the groin area.
inoperable. Unsuitable for treatment by surgery.
inotropic medications. Drugs that increase the strength of heart contractions.
insemination. Insertion of semen into the vagina. May result in fertilization of an egg (ovum).
insomnia. The inability to sleep.
inspiration. Taking in a breath; inhalation.
insulin. The pancreatic hormone that enables the body to regulate the amount of sugar (glucose) in the bloodstream. *See also* diabetes mellitus.
insulin reaction. A condition in people who take insulin, resulting in low blood sugar (hypoglycemia) due to excess insulin or reduced carbohydrate intake.
intermittent claudication. Discomfort in the leg muscles brought on by walking and relieved by rest. Produced by inadequate blood flow.
interstitial cystitis. A chronic inflammation of the bladder wall, leading to frequent, painful urination.
intestines. The portion of the digestive tract extending from the stomach to the anus. Responsible for much of the absorption of nutrients. *See also* colon, duodenum, ileum and jejunum.
intolerance. An inability to tolerate pain, a drug therapy or substances such as sugar (glucose) and lactose.
intracranial. Within the skull.
intraocular pressure. Pressure inside the eyeball that's maintained by the aqueous humor. Elevated intraocular pressure can signal glaucoma.

intravenous. Within or into a vein.

intravenous (IV) catheter. A hollow tube inserted into a vein for administration of fluids or medications.

intrinsic factor. A substance found in the gastric juices that allows for the absorption of vitamin B-12 from the intestines.

in vitro fertilization. The process by which an egg (ovum) is fertilized outside the body and transferred into a woman's uterus.

involuntary. Can't be controlled through will.

iris. The colored part of the eye. The iris contains a ring of muscle fibers that can expand or contract the size of the pupil.

ischemia. Deficiency of blood within an organ or part of an organ. Often refers to the situation in which an artery is narrowed or blocked and can't deliver sufficient blood to the organ it supplies.

isometric. Contracting a muscle against resistance without changing its length.

isotonic. Muscular work that produces motion of a body part.

isotope. A form of a chemical element that has similar structure but a different mass. Some isotopes are radioactive.

-itis. A suffix meaning inflammation.

IUD. Intrauterine device. A contraceptive device, made of plastic or metal, that's inserted into the uterus.

J

jaundice. Yellowing of the eyes and skin caused by excess bilirubin. This excess results from blockage of bile passages or from the liver's inability to metabolize bilirubin.

jejunum. The portion of the small intestine located between the duodenum and ileum.

joint. The point of juncture between two or more bones where movement occurs.

jugular veins. The veins, one on each side of the neck, that carry blood from the brain and head to the heart.

K

Kegel exercises. Exercises done to strengthen the muscles that control urinary incontinence in females.

keloid. An abnormally thick scar that can form after surgery or an injury.

keratin. A protein found in hair, nails and the outer layers of skin.

ketoacidosis. A complication of type 1 diabetes (formerly called juvenile or insulin-dependent diabetes) that results from too little insulin. It can cause loss of consciousness (diabetic coma) and death.

ketones. Acidic substances produced when the body must use fat for energy.

kidneys. The two bean-shaped organs located in the back portion of the upper abdomen, one on each side of the spine. Responsible for the formation and excretion of urine and the regulation of the water, electrolyte and acid-alkaline content of blood.

Korotkof sounds. Sounds heard when blood pressure is taken.

kyphosis. Excessive curvature of the spine, resulting in humpback, hunchback or rounding of the shoulders. May result from osteoarthritis, rheumatoid arthritis, osteoporosis, rickets, a compression fracture, a congenital abnormality or other diseases and conditions.

L

labia. Two sets of lip-like genital organs in females. The labia majora are two folds of skin and fatty tissue that protect the vulva. The labia minora are smaller folds inside the labia majora.

labor. The process of uterine muscle contractions that opens the cervix and moves the baby through the birth canal.

labyrinth. The portion of the inner ear responsible for balance.

laceration. A wound caused by tearing of tissue.

lacrimal glands. The tear-producing glands. Located under each brow bone, just above your eye.

lactation. The production and secretion of milk from the breasts.

lactose. Sugar found naturally in milk.

Lamaze method. A program of physical and emotional preparation of mothers for childbirth.

laparoscopy. Examination of the inside of the abdominal cavity by means of a laparoscope, a viewing instrument inserted through a small incision.

larynx. The voice box. It's composed of cartilage housing the vocal cords and the muscles and ligaments used to produce sound.

LDL cholesterol. Low-density lipoprotein cholesterol. Necessary for body functions, but in excessive amounts it tends to accumulate in artery walls. The "bad" cholesterol.

leaflet. The part of a heart valve that opens and closes so that blood flows in one direction.

lens. A clear, elliptical structure located behind the iris and pupil. It works with the cornea to focus light entering the eye. The ability of the lens to thin or thicken allows it to change its focusing power.

lesion. An area of tissue either injured (as in a wound, abscess or sore) or altered (as in a tumor, mole or cyst).

leukemia. A malignant disease of the blood-forming organs. It results in the uncontrolled production of abnormal white blood cells.

leukocytes. White blood cells. They fight infection.

libido. Sexual drive.

ligament. Strong, fibrous connective tissue resembling a band or sheet that connects one bone to another.

ligature. A synthetic or natural filament for tying off blood vessels during surgery to keep the vessels from bleeding. The procedure itself is called ligation.

lightening. The repositioning of a baby lower in the pelvis that usually occurs several weeks before the onset of labor.

lipids. Fats or fat-like substances in the blood, such as cholesterol.

lipoproteins. Proteins combined with lipids to make them dissolve in blood.

liposuction. The process of removing fat deposits from beneath the skin by using a suction device.

lithiasis. The formation of calculi deposits such as gallstones and kidney stones.

liver. The largest internal organ in the body. It's the site of many metabolic functions, including secreting bile, neutralizing poisons, synthesizing proteins and storing glycogen and certain minerals and vitamins.

lobe. A well-defined portion of an organ.

localized. Limited to a discrete area, as in an infection or disease. *See also* generalized; systemic.

lordosis. An exaggerated curvature of the lower portion of the spine, causing swayback.

lower esophageal sphincter. A circular band of muscle where the esophagus joins the stomach.

low vision. Any eye problem that can't be corrected by standard eyeglasses, contact lenses or surgery. It's often the result of eye diseases such as macular degeneration, glaucoma and diabetic retinopathy.

lumbar. Pertaining to the lower back.

lungs. The two cone-shaped, spongy organs of respiration located around the bronchial tubes and their branches.

lung scan. An imaging procedure used to assess blood flow through the lungs.

lymph. Clear fluid present in lymphatic vessels.

lymphatic vessels. Structures throughout the lymphatic system that contain and convey lymph.

lymph nodes. Small (from pinhead-sized to olive-sized) structures found throughout the body that produce white blood cells called lymphocytes and monocytes. These white blood cells help protect the body from invasion by bacteria and other organisms.

lymphocytes. Disease-fighting white blood cells made in the lymph nodes and distributed throughout the body by way of lymphatic fluid and blood.

lymphoma. A type of cancer that begins in lymphatic tissue and may spread to other areas of the body.

M

maceration. Softening and breaking apart of tissue due to soaking it in liquid.

macrophages. Cells found throughout the body, particularly in the spleen, that have the ability to ingest other substances, such as worn-out red blood cells.

macula. A dark reddish patch at the center of your retina that's densely packed with cone cells. The macula is essential to your central vision and allows you to see fine detail.

macular degeneration. A condition that occurs when tissue in the macula deteriorates.

magnetic resonance imaging (MRI). An imaging procedure that uses strong magnetic fields to visualize body structures.

malabsorption. Inadequate absorption of nutrients from the small intestine. Signs and symptoms of malabsorption include loose, fatty stools, diarrhea, weight loss, weakness and anemia.

malaise. A general feeling of illness, discomfort and uneasiness, often a symptom of infection.

male factor infertility. Infertility caused by abnormalities of the semen or sperm.

malignant. A term used to describe cancerous tumors that can grow uncontrollably and spread to other areas of the body (metastasize).

malnutrition. Deficiency of nourishment in the body due to a lack of healthful food or improper digestion and distribution of nutrients.

malpresentation. Abnormal position of the fetus during labor, making normal vaginal delivery difficult or impossible.

mammary gland. A compound gland of the breast that secretes milk.

mandible. The lower jaw.

mania. A mental disorder characterized by an intense feeling of elation and excitability, often accompanied by increased activity.

mastectomy. The surgical removal of a breast.

masticate. Chew.

mastoid process. A round, honeycombed bone mass located behind the ear.

maxilla. The upper jaw.

meconium stool. A newborn's first bowel movements, composed of intestinal secretions and amniotic fluid, usually dark green.

medulla. The center of an organ, gland or bone.

melanin. Pigment that provides dark color to hair, skin and the choroid of the eye.

melanoma. A pigmented tumor of the skin and, in rare cases, of the mucous membranes. A malignant melanoma tumor may be invasive and spread to lymph nodes and other sites more frequently than do other skin cancers.

membrane. A thin, soft layer of tissue that lines, separates or covers an organ or structure.

meninges. The membranes that cover the spinal cord and brain.

meningitis. Inflammation of the membranes that cover the brain or spinal cord, usually caused by infection.

menopause. The gradual cessation of menstrual cycles, at the end of which a woman is no longer able to become pregnant.

menstruation. The monthly shedding of blood and tissue from the lining of the uterus during a woman's reproductive years.

mesentery. A fold in the abdominal lining that connects the intestines to the back of the abdominal wall and contains the arteries and veins that supply the intestines.

metabolism. The process in living things by which food is transformed into forms that can be used by organisms, energy is derived and tissues are broken down into waste products.

metastasis. The spreading of a disease from one part of the body to another, usually by movement of cells (as in cancer), or infection through the lymphatic system or bloodstream.

microbes. One-celled organisms such as bacteria, many of which cause disease.

micturition. Urination.

milia. Pinpoint-sized white spots on a newborn's nose and cheeks. The spots eventually disappear and need no treatment.

miosis. Pupil contraction. Abnormal contraction is often a sign of a disease or disorder.

miscarriage. The premature, spontaneous termination of a pregnancy before the fetus can survive outside the womb. Also called spontaneous abortion.

mitosis. A type of cell division in which new cells have the same number of chromosomes as the parent cell.

mitral valve. The heart valve that allows blood to move into the left ventricle from the left atrium and prevents reverse flow.

mitral valve prolapse. A bulging of the leaflets of the mitral valve into the left atrium during the heart's contraction.

mm HG. Millimeters of mercury. The unit of measurement used in taking blood pressure.

molars. The 12 grinding or chewing teeth, located at the back of both jaws.

mongolian spots. A type of birthmark with large, blue-gray spots resembling bruises. More common in dark-skinned babies, these marks usually disappear later in childhood. Also called blue spot or mongolian macula.

mono-. A prefix meaning one.

monoclonal. Derived from a single cell or clone of cells.

monocytes. Disease-fighting white blood cells made in the lymph nodes and distributed throughout the body by way of lymphatic fluid and the bloodstream.

motility. The ability to move.

motor development. The increasing ability to use muscles.

mucous membranes. Thin, moist membranes that line passages and cavities in contact with air, such as the nose, mouth and eyes.

multiple myeloma. A type of blood cancer that begins in bone marrow. Multiple myeloma may cause bone pain, anemia and hypercalcemia.

murmur. A sound made by turbulent blood moving through the chambers and valves of the heart or through the blood vessels near the heart. May signify a structural defect in the heart or valves.

muscle. Tissue that produces movement by its ability to contract.

musculoskeletal. Pertaining to the muscles and the skeleton.

mutation. A disorder leading to a change that may result from alterations of genetic material.

myalgia. Muscle tenderness or pain.

myelin. A white, fat-like substance that forms a sheath around some nerve fibers.

myelodysplastic disorders. Disturbances of the cells that form a type of white blood cell.

myocardial infarction. Heart attack. Death of an area of heart muscle due to a lack of blood supply.

myocarditis. Inflammation of the heart muscle.

myocardium. The heart muscle. *See also* endocardium and epicardium.

myopathy. Any disease of the muscle.

myopia. *See* nearsightedness.

N

narcosis. A state of stupor, often induced by drugs or other agents.

nares. The nostrils.

natal. Pertaining to birth.

nausea. A sensation of stomach sickness, often followed by vomiting.

nearsightedness. A focusing problem in which you can see nearby objects clearly, but faraway objects appear blurry. Also called myopia.

nebulizer. A device used to spray medicine or humidity into the lungs. Also called an atomizer.

necrosis. Changes due to the death of cells or organs.

neonatal. Pertaining to a newborn up to age 4 weeks old.

neoplasm. New and abnormal growth that may be benign or malignant. A tumor.

neovascularization. The abnormal formation and growth of blood vessels, such as that which occurs under the retina when you have wet macular degeneration, and in the vitreous when you have proliferative diabetic retinopathy.

nephrectomy. The surgical removal of a kidney.

nephritis. Inflammation of a kidney.

nephrons. Structures of the kidney that remove waste and form urine.

nerve. A bundle of fibers that connects the brain and spinal cord with various parts of the body and through which impulses pass.

neuralgia. A sharp pain along the course of a nerve or in its area of distribution.
neural tube. A structure in early fetal life that develops into the brain, spinal cord, spinal nerves and spine.
neural tube defect. A birth defect resulting in improper development of the brain or spinal cord.
neurofibromatosis. A genetic condition that affects the nervous system, muscles, bones and skin.
neurogenic bladder. Loss of normal bladder function due to damage of the nervous system.
neurogenic bowel. Loss of normal bowel function due to damage of the nervous system.
neuromuscular. Pertaining to the nerves and muscles.
neuron. A nerve cell.
neuropathy. Disease of the nerves.
neurotransmitters. Nerve cell chemicals that act as messengers in the brain and nervous system.
nicotine. An addictive chemical found in tobacco.
node. A small, round or egg-shaped tissue or structure.
nonsteroidal anti-inflammatory drugs (NSAIDs). Non-cortisone-based medications used to reduce inflammation.
noradrenaline. A naturally occurring hormone that increases heart rate and blood pressure and affects other body functions. Also called norepinephrine.
norepinephrine. *See* adrenaline; noradrenaline.
nucleus. The center portion of most plant and animal cells. Essential for cell growth, nourishment and reproduction.
nutrients. Substances in food that provide nourishment for the body.
nutrition. A combination of processes by which the body receives and uses substances necessary for daily function, energy, growth and repair.
nystagmus. A repetitive, abnormal movement of the eyeballs.

O

obesity. Above normal body weight, usually defined as more than 20 percent above what's considered healthy for people of your age, height and bone structure.
occipital. Pertaining to the back of the head.
occipital lobe. An area at the back of the brain that receives and processes visual information.
occlusion. Closure of a passage such as ducts or blood vessels. In dentistry, the alignment of upper and lower teeth when the jaws are closed.
occult. Obscure; concealed.
ocular. Pertaining to the eye.
olfactory. Pertaining to the sense of smell.
-oma. Suffix meaning tumor.
oncogenes. Genes present in normal cells that, upon exposure to cancer-inducing factors, may lead to development of tumors.
oncology. The study of tumors.
opportunistic infection. An infection caused by microorganisms that usually aren't harmful in healthy people but can be extremely dangerous in people with suppressed immune systems.
optic disk. The location where the optic nerve forms at the back of the eyeball. It's visible on the retina as a yellowish circle.
optic nerve. A bundle of nerve fibers that carries the visual information gathered by your retina to the visual cortex of your brain.
orbit. The socket that protects and cradles your eyeball. It's formed by a structure of bone that includes the cheekbone, forehead bone, temple bone and bridge of your nose.
orgasm. The climax of sexual intercourse or stimulation of sexual organs. In males, it's associated with the ejaculation of semen, and in females, with contractions of the vagina.
orthopnea. Difficulty breathing except in an upright position.
orthostatic hypotension. A drop in blood pressure upon standing. May cause lightheadedness or fainting.
-osis. Suffix meaning diseased state.
osseous. Pertaining to bones.
osteogenic. Derived from bone.
osteopathy. Any bone disease.
ostomy. A surgically created opening in which a portion of the urinary tract or bowel is brought to the abdominal surface. A generic word for all types of ostomies, such as colostomy and ileostomy.
ova. The female cells of reproduction. After fertilization by a sperm, an egg (ovum) is capable of developing into an embryo, a fetus and then a baby.
ovaries. Gonadal organs in the female that produce eggs (ova) for reproduction and the female sex hormones estrogen and progesterone.
over-the-counter (OTC). A term used to describe medications sold without a prescription.
ovulation. The monthly discharging of an egg (ovum) from an ovary. It occurs approximately 14 days before the onset of the next menstrual period.
oxytocin. The pituitary hormone in adult females that stimulates the release of breast milk.

P

pacemaker. A group of cells located in the atrium of the heart that regulate the heart's rate and rhythm. Or, an electric device used to simulate the natural process by generating electric impulses. Termed an artificial cardiac pacemaker, this device can be placed outside or inside the chest.
palate. The hard roof of the mouth.
palliative. Treatment undertaken not to cure but to improve a problem or condition.

pallor. Paleness.
palpation. A method of examining by touch.
palpitation. A sensation felt as a result of a fluttering or rapid, forceful beating of the heart.
palsy. Paralysis.
pancreas. A gland that produces enzymes essential to the digestion of food. It contains the islets of Langerhans, which secrete insulin into the blood.
papilla. A nipple-like protuberance.
Pap test. A test to detect cancer of the cervix. Named for Dr. G. Papanicolaou.
paralysis. An inability to move a part of the body. Partial paralysis is known as paresis.
paranoia. A mental disorder characterized by suspicion, delusions of persecution and jealousy.
paraparesis. Weakness below the waist, including the legs.
paraplegia. Paralysis below the waist, including both legs.
parasite. An organism that lives on or within another organism at the expense of the host.
parathyroid glands. Endocrine glands located beneath the thyroid gland that help regulate the level of calcium in the blood.
parenteral. A term that describes methods of administering medication, fluid or nutrition other than swallowing, including intravenous (IV), subcutaneous and intramuscular.
parietal lobe. An area of the brain that lies in front of the occipital lobe. Important in processing information from the sense of touch and bringing together sensory information.
paroxysm. A sudden attack, such as a spasm or convulsion. Or, recurrence of symptoms of a disease.
paroxysmal nocturnal dyspnea. Episodic shortness of breath at night.
patella. The kneecap.
pathogen. A disease-producing microorganism.
pathology. The study of the cause and nature of diseases.
patient-controlled analgesia pump. A small pump activated by a patient to inject pain medication as needed. It limits the amount of pain medication allowed within any given period.
pectoral. Pertaining to the chest.
pelvic floor muscles. A group of muscles at the base of the pelvis. They help support the bladder, urethra, rectum and, in women, the vagina and uterus.
pelvic inflammatory disease. An inflammation or infection of the internal female genital organs.
pelvis. The basin-shaped bone structure connecting the spine with the legs.
penis. The male organ for urination and sexual intercourse.
pepsin. The main enzyme in the digestive juices of the stomach.
peptic. Pertaining to digestion or the enzyme pepsin.
percussion. A method of examination by tapping the fingertips over various areas of the body to determine the position, size and consistency of a structure beneath the skin.
percutaneous transluminal coronary angioplasty. A procedure that uses balloon catheters to reopen narrowed coronary arteries. Also called balloon angioplasty or percutaneous coronary intervention.
perforation. The process of making a hole, or the hole itself.
pericardiectomy. Removal of the pericardium.
pericarditis. Inflammation of the pericardium.
pericardium. The membranous sac enclosing the heart.
perinatal. Referring to the time just before, during and immediately after birth.
perineum. The external area between the vulva and anus in a woman or between the scrotum and anus in a man.
periodontal. Pertaining to the area immediately around a tooth.
periosteum. Leather-like tissue that encases bone.
peristalsis. The wave-like motion of muscles, particularly in the digestive system, that forces food or food residue through the digestive tract.
peritoneum. The membrane lining the abdominal cavity.
peritonitis. Inflammation or infection of the peritoneum.
pernicious. Destructive, sometimes fatal. Pernicious anemia is a particular form of anemia caused by an inability to absorb vitamin B-12 from the intestinal tract.
perspiration. Sweat. The salty fluid excreted from the sweat glands of the skin.
pessary. A device inserted into the vagina to support the uterus or to prevent conception.
petechiae. Small hemorrhages that appear in the skin and mucous membranes.
petit mal. A term used to describe a mild form of epileptic attack, characterized by a blank stare and temporary cessation of activity.
pH. A measure of the acidity or alkalinity of a substance.
pharmacology. The study of drugs and their effects.
pharynx. Upper portion of the throat. The passageway for air from the nose to the voice box (larynx) and for food from the mouth to the esophagus.
phenylketonuria. A congenital condition in which the body lacks a specific enzyme. This causes abnormal metabolism that may result in brain damage.
phlebitis. Inflammation of a vein.
phlegm. Thick mucus, especially from the sinuses or respiratory tract.
phobia. A persistent, irrational fear.
phototherapy. Treatment by exposure to light.
pica. An uncommon urge to eat nonfood material such as dirt, baking powder or frost from a freezer.

pigment. Coloring matter.
pineal body. A small, cone-shaped gland in the brain, the function of which is unclear.
pinna. The exterior, easily visible part of the ear.
pituitary gland. An endocrine gland that produces a range of hormones to help control the body's long-term growth, day-to-day functioning and reproductive capabilities. Sometimes called the master gland.
placebo. A nondrug substance that has no specific pharmacologic activity against illness. Sometimes called a sugar pill.
placenta. The spongy uterine structure, developed during pregnancy, through which the fetus takes nourishment and discards waste by way of the umbilical cord. The placenta is shed after delivery, at which point it's known as the afterbirth.
placental abruption. Separation of the placenta from the uterine wall.
placenta previa. An abnormal location of the placenta in which it partially or completely covers the cervical opening.
plague. A term previously used to describe any deadly contagious epidemic disease. Now used primarily to describe infection by *Yersinia pestis* that causes bubonic plague and pneumonic plague.
plaque. A film or deposit of bacteria and other material on the surface of a tooth that may lead to tooth decay or periodontal disease. Or, one of many fatty deposits that accumulate in the lining of the arteries, resulting in narrower, less flexible pathways for the blood.
plasma. The fluid part of the blood and lymph.
platelets. Microscopic-sized disks found in blood. Also known as thrombocytes, platelets are necessary for the clotting of blood.
pleura. The membrane that covers both lungs and lines the chest cavity.
point of focus. The location within the eyeball where visual information is most sharply focused by the cornea and lens. The best sight occurs when the point of focus is directly on the retina.
poly-. A prefix meaning multiple or more than normal.
polyp. A protruding growth, often on a stalk.
positron emission tomography (PET). An imaging technique used for measuring blood flow and the metabolism of body tissues, including the heart and brain.
postpartum. Pertaining to the time after childbirth.
preeclampsia. A condition that can occur during pregnancy. It's marked by pregnancy-induced high blood pressure, protein in the urine and swelling. Also called toxemia.
premolars. Eight teeth in the adult mouth having two points.
prepuce. The foreskin over the glans of an uncircumcised penis.
presbyopia. A problem that occurs when your lens loses its elasticity and ability to thicken or thin. This condition makes it difficult for you to focus on nearby objects.
primary care physician. The doctor responsible for providing or coordinating your general health care.
primary tumor. The site of origin of a cancerous tumor. If the cancer metastasizes to another site, it's called a secondary tumor.
progesterone. A female sex hormone responsible for, among other things, the thickening of the uterine lining in preparation for conception and implantation of a fertilized egg (ovum).
prognosis. A prediction of the course or outcome of a disease.
prolactin. A pituitary hormone that stimulates the breasts to produce milk.
prolapse. Displacement of an organ or a structure, such as the uterus or bladder, by dropping down or protruding.
prophylaxis. A term that refers to prevention of disease or its spread by following certain rules or taking specific precautions.
prostaglandins. A group of extremely active substances that affect many organs. Certain prostaglandins have a role in stimulating the uterine contractions of labor.
prostate gland. A gland located at the base of the bladder in males.
prostate-specific antigen (PSA). A protein, produced by the prostate gland, that can be measured in blood. PSA can be increased by a variety of abnormal conditions in the prostate, including but not limited to prostate cancer.
prosthesis. An artificial substitute for a missing body part, such as an arm or leg.
protein. Complex nitrogen-containing compounds composed of amino acids. Essential for the growth and repair of tissue.
prothrombin. A component of circulating blood that interacts with calcium salts to form thrombin, a step in the process of blood clotting.
prothrombin time. A test that measures the activity of certain clotting factors. It's often used to determine whether a person is receiving the correct dose of an anticoagulant.
pruritus. Itching.
psychogenic. Originating in the mind. Or, pertaining to the development of the mind.
psychomotor. Pertaining to voluntary physical movement.
psychosis. A mental disturbance of serious magnitude that's characterized by a loss of contact with reality. Delusions and hallucinations are often present.
psychosomatic. Pertaining to the relationship of the mind and body. Psychosomatic illnesses are those in which a physical disorder is caused or aggravated by emotional factors.
ptosis. A condition that causes the upper eyelid to droop over your eye and partially block your vision.

ptyalin. An enzyme in saliva that helps to break down starch into sugars.

puberty. A period of rapid change in boys and girls during which sex characteristics mature. In girls (usually between 9 and 16 years) it's marked by the beginning of menstruation (menarche), and in boys (usually between 9 and 14 years) it's marked by discharge of semen and deepening of the voice.

pudendal block. A local anesthetic injection used to ease the pain of the last part of labor and for an episiotomy.

pulmonary. Pertaining to the lungs.

pulmonary artery. A blood vessel that carries oxygen-depleted blood from the right ventricle of the heart to the lungs.

pulmonary embolism. A condition in which a clot or other substance lodges in a lung artery.

pulmonary function test. A test used to measure the ability of the lungs to exchange air.

pulmonary valve. The valve between the right ventricle and the pulmonary artery.

pulmonary veins. Those blood vessels that carry newly oxygenated blood from the lungs back to the heart.

pupil. The dark area in the center of your iris through which light passes into your eye.

purpura. A condition characterized by hemorrhages of tiny blood vessels causing patches on the skin or on mucous membranes. The patches begin as red, change to purple and then to brownish-yellow before disappearing.

purulent. Forming or containing pus.

pus. Thick, whitish-yellow fluid containing leukocytes and bacteria, formed at the site of certain kinds of infections.

pyloric stenosis. An obstruction at the outlet of the stomach.

pylorus. The opening at the stomach outlet into the duodenum.

pyrexia. Fever.

Q

quadriparesis. Weakness of all four limbs.

quadriplegia. Complete paralysis of all four limbs.

quickening. The first perception of fetal movements, usually between 16 and 20 weeks of pregnancy.

R

radial pulse. The pulse felt at the wrist.

radiation therapy. The use of high-energy waves to treat disease such as cancer. Sources of radiation include X-ray, cobalt and radium.

radius. The smaller of the two bones in the lower arm. It connects to the base of the thumb.

radon. A radioactive gas found in nature. A byproduct of disintegrating radium.

rales. Abnormal breathing sounds, sometimes indicating fluid in the air sacs (alveoli) of the lungs.

rash. Eruption on the skin, usually temporary.

Raynaud's disease. Changes in skin color due to spasm of small blood vessels, especially with exposure to cold.

recessive. A mode of inheritance in which a gene for a particular trait must be inherited from both parents in order for that trait to appear in their offspring. *See also* dominant.

rectum. The lowest portion of the large intestine. Stores stool until it's expelled.

reflex. An involuntary response to a stimulus.

reflux. Backflow or regurgitation.

refraction. The bending of light waves by the cornea and lens as light passes into the eyeball. Refraction allows images to be sharply focused and clear.

refractory. A temporary condition that resists treatment or a nerve or muscle that resists stimulation.

regurgitation. Backflow.

rejection. Refusal to accept, as with a transplanted organ.

relapse. Recurrence of disease after apparent recovery.

remission. Abatement of signs and symptoms.

REM sleep. Rapid eye movement sleep. The period of sleep when dreaming occurs and the eyes move cyclically even though closed.

renal. Pertaining to the kidneys.

renal failure. The inability of the kidneys to excrete wastes, concentrate urine and maintain electrolyte balance.

renin. A hormone released by the kidneys that affects blood pressure.

reperfusion. Resumption of blood flow.

resection. The surgical removal of an organ or tissue.

resident physician. A medical doctor or dentist participating in a postgraduate specialty training program.

respiration. Breathing.

resuscitation. The restoration of breathing or a heartbeat after cardiac arrest.

retina. A thin layer of tissue on the inside back wall of your eyeball that receives and organizes visual information. The retina is connected to the brain by the optic nerve.

retinal detachment. Separation of the retina from the choroid. If untreated this condition almost always leads to visual loss.

retinal pigment epithelium. A layer of tissue forming the outermost surface of the retina. Deterioration of the retinal pigment epithelium plays an important role in macular degeneration.

retinopathy. An abnormality of the retina that may cause deterioration of eyesight.

rheumatic fever. An inflammatory illness that may follow streptococcal infection and damage the heart.

Rh factor. Rhesus factor. A protein found in the blood serum of people who are Rh positive.

rhinovirus. A large subgroup of viruses that cause the common cold.

right heart failure. Decreased function of the right ventricle, resulting in swelling in the legs and abdominal organs, especially the liver. *See* congestive heart failure.

risk factors. Conditions that increase chances of a disease developing. Such factors can be chemical, physiological, behavioral, psychological, genetic or environmental, among others.

rods. Light-sensitive cells of the retina that provide your peripheral vision and allow you to see in dim light. Or, rod-shaped bacteria.

root canal. The space in the root of the tooth that contains nerves.

roughage. Indigestible fiber of fruits, vegetables and cereals that aids in the evacuation of waste.

rubella. A highly contagious viral disease marked by a red, eruptive rash. Also called German measles.

rupture. The tearing or bursting of tissue or an organ.

S

sacroiliac joint. The juncture between the sacrum and ilium. Not a true joint because this point has no movement.

sacrum. The triangular bone at the base of the spine just above the coccyx. Composed of five fused vertebrae and part of the bony pelvis.

saline. Salt (sodium chloride) solution.

saliva. Fluid secreted by the salivary glands that moistens food and begins the process of digestion.

saphenous vein. A large vein in the leg.

sarcoma. A malignant tumor originating in connective tissue or bone.

scabies. A skin disorder caused by a mite. Characterized by redness, itching and swelling of the involved area.

scapula. The shoulder blade.

Schlemm's canal. An open channel behind the trabecular meshwork that allows aqueous humor to drain from the eye.

sciatic nerve. The largest nerve in the body, formed by the motor and sensory nerves to and from the legs and feet. It begins at the base of the spinal cord as a number of roots and passes through the pelvis, down the back of each thigh to the heel.

sclera. A tough, white, leathery coating that forms the circular eyeball shape and protects the internal structures of the eye. Also known as the white of your eye.

sclerosis. The hardening or thickening of an organ or tissue, usually due to abnormal or excessive growth of fibrous tissue.

scrotum. The skin sac that holds the testicles.

sebaceous glands. Oil glands of the skin.

sebum. A fatty substance secreted by the sebaceous glands to lubricate the skin.

secretion. The process of producing materials by glands. Also, the substance produced.

seizure. A sudden attack, often including convulsions. If recurrent, often referred to as a seizure disorder or as epilepsy.

semen. Thick, whitish fluid containing reproductive cells (spermatozoa) and other fluids, discharged through the male urethra at ejaculation.

seminal vesicles. Sac-like structures located behind the bladder in the male, which secrete fluid that's part of the composition of semen.

seminoma. A type of malignant tumor of the testicle.

sepsis. The state of being infected with disease-causing microorganisms in the bloodstream.

septal defect. A hole in the wall of the heart separating the two atria or the two ventricles.

septicemia. Another term for sepsis.

septum. A wall dividing two cavities or compartments of the body.

serum. Watery fluid left after coagulation of the blood to form a clot. Serum containing antibodies to a specific disease may be injected into a person to give temporary resistance to that disease. This is called passive immunity. *See also* vaccine.

shock. A clinical condition in which the body reacts to injury or severe pain by dilation or relaxation of blood vessels, producing what can be called circulatory failure. Signs and symptoms include rapid pulse and breathing, very low blood pressure, pallor, clammy skin and, sometimes, unconsciousness.

shunt. A passage that diverts blood flow from one main route to another. Often constructed artificially.

sickle cell disease. A group of inherited diseases that lead to abnormal red blood cells and anemia.

sick sinus syndrome. A failure of the sinus node to properly regulate the heartbeat. It may result in periods of either fast or slow heartbeat.

side effects. Unwanted changes produced by medication or other treatment, ranging from trivial and transient (minor headache or dry mouth) to more serious (asthma, gastrointestinal bleeding).

silent ischemia. An insufficient supply of blood and oxygen to the heart muscle without signs and symptoms.

sinuses. Empty spaces or cavities within bone structure. Most commonly, the several sets of cavities adjacent to and connected to the nose by small openings.

sinus node. The heart's natural pacemaker.

sodium. A mineral that's essential in maintaining the fluid balance of the body. Table salt (sodium chloride) is nearly half sodium.

somatostatin. A hormone that helps regulate the body's production and release of the pancreatic hormones insulin and glucagon. It's also found in other tissues of the body, where it may have other functions.

sonogram. *See* ultrasound scan.

spasm. An involuntary movement produced by a muscular contraction.

speculum. A device used to examine a body opening such as the nose or vagina.

spermatozoa. The male cells of reproduction. When one such cell combines with an egg (ovum), fertilization has occurred. Produced by the testicles and transmitted in semen. Also referred to as sperm.

spermicide. A birth control agent used to kill sperm cells by contact.

sphincter. A circular muscle at an opening that can contract and expand to close and open it. The body has several sphincter muscles, including those at the anus, bladder, stomach and esophagus.

sphygmomanometer. A device used to measure blood pressure.

spina bifida. A birth defect in the spinal column through which the spinal cord may protrude.

spinal canal. The space that contains the spinal cord and is protected by vertebrae of the backbone.

spinal column. The bony assemblage of vertebrae; spine.

spinal cord. A lengthy, cord-like bundle of nerves that links nerves in the trunk and extremities with the brain.

spleen. The organ, located to the left and just in front of the stomach, that stores and at times manufactures blood cells.

spontaneous abortion. A miscarriage.

sprain. Ligament damage, usually in the ankles and knees.

sputum. The fluid produced by coughing. If certain disorders or infections are suspected, the sputum may be examined in a laboratory.

squamous cell carcinoma. A malignant tumor arising from cells known as squamous epithelium.

stable angina. A predictable pattern of cardiac pain caused by ischemia.

staging. The process of categorizing the extent or spread of cancer for the purpose of planning treatment.

stenosis. The abnormal narrowing or closure of an opening or passageway in the body.

stenosis, aortic. Narrowing of the valve opening between the left ventricle and aorta.

stenosis, mitral. Narrowing of the valve opening between the left atrium and ventricle.

stent. A device, implanted during surgery, that helps keep tissues in place, as when a tubular, mesh-like material is placed inside a blood vessel to keep it open.

sterilization. The process by which all microorganisms, such as bacteria, viruses and parasites, are removed from a substance or item, such as surgical instruments, to prevent infection. Or, the process, usually surgical, of rendering a man or woman incapable of reproduction.

sternum. The breastbone, in the upper central portion of the chest and abutted by the ends of the clavicle and the ribs.

steroids. *See* corticosteroids.

stethoscope. A device for listening to sounds produced in the body.

stillborn. A term that refers to a fetus dead at birth.

stomach. The sac-like organ to which food is delivered by the esophagus.

stomatitis. Inflammation of the mucous membranes of the mouth. May occur as a complication of chemotherapy or radiation therapy.

stool. Body waste, such as food residue, evacuated from the large bowel.

strain. Muscular injury produced by abuse or overuse of a muscle.

strep throat. Streptococcal infection of the throat.

striae. Streaks or stripes.

stroke. A condition produced by obstruction of an artery that blocks the flow of blood to a portion of the brain or by bleeding into the brain.

stupor. A state of reduced consciousness in which responsiveness and feeling are lessened.

sty. A painful, red lump, resembling a boil or pimple, on the eyelid. It's caused by a bacterial infection.

subacute. A term used to distinguish the intermediate duration of a disease that's neither chronic nor characteristically of brief duration.

subcutaneous. Beneath the skin.

sucrose. The simple sugar processed from sugar cane and sugar beets.

sudden infant death syndrome (SIDS). The sudden, unexplained death of an infant.

sunblock. An over-the-counter preparation applied to the skin to limit damage from the rays of the sun.

superior vena cava. The large vein returning blood from your head and arms to your heart.

supine. Lying on the back.

suppository. A pharmaceutical preparation in a solid form, intended to be inserted into a passage such as the rectum or vagina.

suppuration. The formation and discharge of pus from an injury or infection.

suture. The process of joining two surfaces by stitching. Or, the surgical stitch itself.

synapse. The junction between two nerve cells (neurons).

syncope. Fainting.

syndrome. A collection of signs and symptoms that characterize an ailment.

synovial fluid. The clear, fluid lubricant in a joint.

syringe. An instrument for injecting or withdrawing fluids.

systemic. Affecting or pertaining to several areas of the body rather than one of its parts.

systole. The period during the heart cycle in which the heart muscle contracts, followed by relaxation (diastole).

systolic pressure. The highest blood pressure produced by the contraction of the heart. Recorded as the first number in a blood pressure measurement.

T

tachycardia. An abnormally rapid heart rate.

tachypnea. Rapid breathing.

tamponade. Compression of an organ, such as pericardial tamponade, in which pericardial fluid compresses the heart.

tartar. Plaque deposits on the teeth.

Tay-Sachs disease. A recessive genetic disorder, common among Ashkenazi Jews, in which the enzyme needed to break down certain lipids is absent.

T cell. A type of white blood cell (lymphocyte) that's part of the body's immune system.

temporal lobes. Areas located on each side of the brain that are important in processing memory.

temporomandibular joint (TMJ). The joint between the lower jaw and the temporal bone of the skull.

tendon. Cord-like tissue that connects muscles to bones.

testicles. The male gonads that produce sperm for reproduction and the male sex hormone testosterone. Also called testes.

testosterone. A male sex hormone produced in the testicles.

thalassemia. Inherited anemias found predominantly among people of Mediterranean descent.

thoracic. Having to do with the chest (thorax).

thorax. The chest.

thrills. Vibrations due to abnormal blood flow.

thrombin. An enzyme that's part of the process of blood coagulation.

thrombocyte. Blood platelet, essential to the clotting process.

thrombolysis. The dissolution of blood clots.

thrombophlebitis. Clotting of blood and inflammation in a vein.

thrombus. A blood clot.

thrush. A fungal infection of the mouth.

thymus. A gland located in the upper chest that produces T cells, which are essential to developing the body's immune response.

thyroid gland. An endocrine gland that helps control the body's rate of function and contributes to maintaining a balance between the calcium in the blood and bones through production of the hormones thyroxine and calcitonin.

thyroxine. A thyroid hormone that controls the pace of chemical activity (metabolism) in the body.

TIA. *See* transient ischemic attack.

tibia. The shinbone. The larger of the two bones in the lower leg.

tic. An involuntary muscle spasm, usually of the face, head, neck or shoulder. A twitch.

tincture. A medication that's an alcoholic solution of a vegetable or animal extract or a chemical substance.

tissue. A collection of similar cells that, taken together, form a body structure.

tocolytic medications. Medications used to inhibit labor.

tonsils. Two masses of lymph tissues, located on either side of the back of the throat, that help filter out unwanted bacteria.

topical. Pertaining to the surface of the body.

tourniquet. A device tightened over an extremity to stop bleeding.

toxemia. A condition in which toxins circulate throughout the body via the blood. *See also* preeclampsia.

toxic. Poisonous.

toxin. A poisonous substance.

toxoid. A biologic toxin treated so that it's no longer dangerous but upon injection into the body will induce antibodies to form. For example, tetanus toxoid.

toxoplasmosis. An infectious disease caused by a microscopic parasite found in infected cat feces and undercooked meat.

trabecular meshwork. A sieve-like system of spongy tissue through which aqueous humor passes before draining from the eye through Schlemm's canal.

trachea. The tube that connects the throat to bronchial tubes in the lungs. Also called the windpipe.

traction. A treatment of some fractures and dislocations involving mechanical pulling on a body part.

tranquilizer. A medication used to reduce tension and anxiety.

transducer. A device that translates pressure, temperature, pulse or sound into an electric signal.

transfusion. The delivery of blood or a blood component into the bloodstream.

transient ischemic attack (TIA). A disorder caused by temporary lack of circulation to a part of the brain. It differs from a stroke in that the signs and symptoms generally disappear completely within 24 hours.

transplantation. The surgical transfer of an organ or tissue from one position or person to another.

transvaginal. Through the vagina, such as a transvaginal ultrasound.

tremor. An involuntary shaking that can result from a disease or a nervous disorder, as a side effect of a medication or from some other cause.

triceps. A muscle in the arm that upon contraction extends the arm at the elbow.

tricuspid valve. The heart valve between the right atrium and right ventricle.

trigeminal nerve. The nerve that delivers sensory stimuli to the brain from the face, teeth and tongue.

triglyceride. A form of fat that the body makes from sugar, alcohol or excess calories.

trimester. One of the three periods of pregnancy, each lasting about 3 months.

truncal obesity. Fat deposited in the thorax and abdomen instead of the hips and thighs.
truss. A device worn externally to hold a hernia or organ in place.
tubal ligation. A sterilization procedure in the female in which the fallopian tubes are tied and cut.
tubules. Small tubes or canals, such as those located in the kidneys.
tumor. An abnormal growth of tissue. The tumor may be malignant or benign.
tumor markers. Substances circulating in the blood that are produced by tumors. The level of the tumor marker may reflect the activity or extent of the tumor.
tympanic membrane. The eardrum.

U

ulcer. An open sore on the skin or a mucous membrane.
ulcerative colitis. A disease characterized by inflammation of the lining of the colon and rectum.
ulna. The larger of the two bones in the forearm.
ultrasound scan. A technique that uses very high frequency sound waves to produce images of the inside of the body. Also known as ultrasonography.
umbilical cord. The structure that transports nutrients and oxygen from the placenta to the fetus and carries away fetal waste.
umbilical hernia. A bulge caused by stretched tissue around the umbilicus.
umbilicus. The navel. The scar formed by removal of the umbilical cord from the newborn following birth.
undescended testicle. Failure of a testicle to enter the scrotum.
unicuspid. A heart valve with one leaflet.
unstable angina. New or increasing chest pain caused by decreased blood flow to the heart.
urea. The principal waste product in urine. A nitrogen-containing product of protein metabolism. Its concentration in blood may be used as a measure of kidney function.
uremia. The buildup of urea in the bloodstream.
ureter. The tube that delivers urine from the kidney to the bladder.
urethra. The tube draining the bladder to outside of the body. In males, this canal is also the passage for semen.
uric acid. A waste byproduct of metabolism. When too little is excreted or too much is produced, the buildup can lead to the development of gout.
urination. The act of voiding fluid wastes (urine).
urine. Fluid waste produced in the kidneys, stored in the bladder and released through the urethra.
urticaria. *See* hives.
uterus. The female organ in which the fetus develops. Also called the womb.
uvula. The pendulous tissue at the back of the palate.

V

vaccination. Injection of a vaccine to create immunity.
vaccine. Weakened or killed microorganisms or viruses of a specific disease introduced into the body in order to stimulate immunity.
vagina. The passage connecting the female external genitalia with the uterus. Also called the birth canal.
vaginitis. Infection of the vagina.
vagus nerve. The nerve that serves the esophagus, voice box (larynx), stomach, intestines, lungs and heart.
variant angina. Chest pain caused by a spasm of the coronary arteries.
varicose veins. Dilated and distended veins due to defective valves in the veins.
vascular. Pertaining to blood vessels.
vas deferens. One of the two ducts that transport sperm to the urethra.
vasectomy. A sterilization procedure in the male involving tying and cutting the vas deferens to prevent sperm from entering the semen.
vasodilators. Medications that widen or dilate blood vessels.
vasopressors. Drugs that elevate blood pressure.
vasovagal syncope. Simple faint.
vegans. People who don't eat food of animal origin.
vein. A blood vessel that returns blood to the heart.
venous. Pertaining to veins.
ventilation. The exchange of air in and out of the lungs.
ventilator. A machine that assists or controls breathing; a respirator.
ventricles. The two main pumping chambers of the heart. The left ventricle pumps blood to the body, and the right ventricle pumps blood to the lungs. Or, the fluid-filled cavities of the brain.
venule. A small vein.
verruca. A wart.
vertebra. Any one of the 33 bones that make up the spine.
vertigo. Dizziness accompanied by the illusion of motion.
vesicle. A small sac containing a liquid.
viral. Pertaining to or caused by a virus.
virulent. Highly poisonous or infectious.
virus. Microscopic infectious agents that reproduce only in host cells.
viscera. The internal organs, especially those within the abdominal cavity.
visual field. The area in front of you that you can see at a given moment without moving your eyes. It's made up of the your central and peripheral vision.
vital signs. Respiration, heart rate and body temperature.
vitamins. Organic substances essential for most metabolic functions of the body.
vitreous. A clear, gelatinous substance that fills the vitreous cavity. It helps maintain the shape of the eyeball and its internal pressure. Also called vitreous humor.

vitreous cavity. A chamber inside the eyeball extending from the back of the lens to the retina. It's filled with vitreous.

vomit. The ejection of partially digested matter from the stomach through the mouth. Or, the matter itself.

vulva. The external female genitals, including the clitoris and labia.

W

wart. A harmless growth on the skin, produced by a virus.

wen. A cyst that develops in a sebaceous gland.

wheezing. A whistling sound produced during breathing.

withdrawal. The experience of stopping the use of a substance to which you're addicted, such as medications, illegal drugs or alcohol. Signs and symptoms may be physiologic, psychologic or both.

womb. *See* uterus.

X

X-rays. Electromagnetic waves that penetrate most solid matter. Used in X-ray machines to produce images of internal structures of the body. Or, the photographs made using this diagnostic technique. Also called roentgen ray.

Z

zygote. The egg (ovum) after it's fertilized by a sperm.

Resources

It has been said that we live in an Information Age. Never before have Americans been bombarded with so much data, including sometimes seemingly conflicting information on how to stay healthy, cope with illness, control health care costs and deal with an increasingly complex health care system. This book is devoted to providing answers to a wide range of health and medical questions, but no single volume can address all of the issues that may interest you and other readers. So we offer you this sampling of organizations that may provide additional information. We neither promote nor endorse these organizations. (Addresses, telephone numbers and Web site addresses are subject to change.)

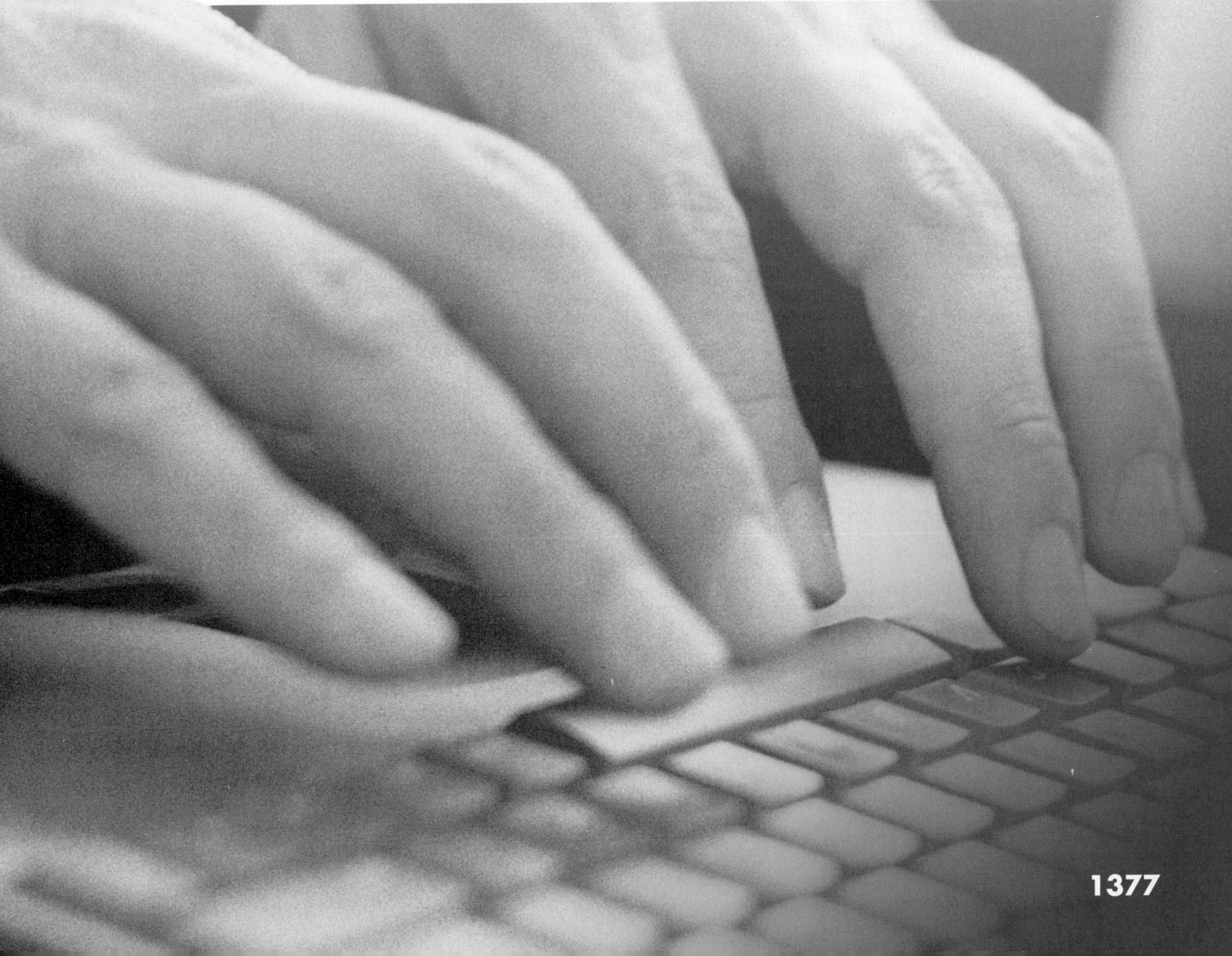

Acoustic Neuroma Association
600 Peachtree Parkway, Suite 108
Cumming, GA 30041-6899
770-205-8211
www.anausa.org

Aerobics and Fitness Association of America
15250 Ventura Blvd., Suite 200
Sherman Oaks, CA 91403-3297
877-968-7263 or 818-905-0040
www.afaa.com

Agency for Healthcare Research and Quality
P.O. Box 8547
Silver Spring, MD 20907-8547
800-358-9295 or 301-594-1364
www.ahrq.gov

Al-Anon Family Group Headquarters
1600 Corporate Landing Parkway
Virginia Beach, VA 23454-5617
888-425-2666 or 757-563-1600
www.al-anon.alateen.org

Alcoholics Anonymous
475 Riverside Drive, 11th Floor
New York, NY 10115
212-870-3400 (check local listings nationwide)
www.aa.org

Alexander Graham Bell Association for the Deaf and Hard of Hearing
3417 Volta Place N.W.
Washington, DC 20007
202-337-5220
www.agbell.org

Alliance for Retired Americans
888 16th St. N.W., Suite 520
Washington, DC 20006
888-373-6497 or 202-974-8222
www.retiredamericans.org

Alzheimer's Association
919 N. Michigan Ave., Suite 1100
Chicago, IL 60611-1676
800-272-3900 or 312-335-8700
www.alz.org

Alzheimer's Disease Education and Referral Center
P.O. Box 8250
Silver Spring, MD 20907-8250
800-438-4380 or 301-495-3311
www.alzheimers.org

American Academy of Allergy, Asthma and Immunology
611 E. Wells St.
Milwaukee, WI 53202
800-822-2762 or 414-272-6071
www.aaaai.org

American Academy of Child and Adolescent Psychiatry
3615 Wisconsin Ave. N.W.
Washington, DC 20016-3007
202-966-7300
www.aacap.org

American Academy of Dermatology
930 E. Woodfield Road
Schaumburg, IL 60173-4927
847-330-0230
www.aad.org

American Academy of Family Physicians
11400 Tomahawk Creek Parkway
Leawood, KS 66211-2672
800-274-2237 or 913-906-6000
www.aafp.org

American Academy of Ophthalmology
655 Beach St.
San Francisco, CA 94120-7424
415-561-8500
www.aao.org

American Academy of Orthopaedic Surgeons
6330 N. River Road
Rosemont, IL 60018-4262
847-823-7186
www.aaos.org

American Academy of Otolaryngology — Head and Neck Surgery
1 Prince St.
Alexandria, VA 22314-3357
703-836-4444
www.entnet.org

American Academy of Pediatrics
141 Northwest Point Blvd.
Elk Grove Village, IL 60007-1098
847-434-4000
www.aap.org

American Association of Endodontists
211 E. Chicago Ave., Suite 1100
Chicago, IL 60611-2691
800-872-3636 or 312-266-7255
www.aae.org

American Association of Homes and Services for the Aging
2519 Connecticut Ave. N.W.
Washington, DC 20008-1520
202-783-2242
www.aahsa.org

American Association of Kidney Patients
3505 E. Frontage Road, Suite 315
Tampa, FL 33607
800-749-2257 or 813-636-8100
www.aakp.org

American Association of Neurological Surgeons
5550 Meadowbrook Court
Rolling Meadows, IL 60008-3852
888-566-2267 or 847-378-0500
www.neurosurgery.org

American Association of Poison Control Centers
3201 New Mexico Ave., Suite 310
Washington, DC 20016
202-362-7217
www.aapcc.org

American Association of Retired Persons
601 E St. N.W.
Washington, DC 20049
800-424-3410 or 202-434-2277
www.aarp.org

American Board of Medical Specialties
1007 Church St., Suite 404
Evanston, IL 60201-5913
866-275-2267 or 847-491-9091
www.abms.org

American Board of Oral and Maxillofacial Pathology
1 Urban Centre, Suite 690
4830 W. Kennedy Blvd.
Tampa, FL 33609-2571
813-286-2444
www.abomp.org

American Board of Orthodontics
401 N. Lindbergh Blvd., Suite 308
St. Louis, MO 63141
314-432-6130
www.americanboardortho.com

American Board of Pathology
1 Urban Centre, Suite 690
4830 W. Kennedy Blvd.
Tampa, FL 33609-2571
813-286-2444
www.abpath.org

American Board of Periodontology
4157 Mountain Road, PBN 249
Pasadena, MD 21122
410-437-3749
www.perio.org

American Brain Tumor Association
2720 River Road, Suite 146
Des Plaines, IL 60618-4117
800-886-2282 or 847-827-9910
www.abta.org

American Cancer Society
1599 Clifton Road N.E.
Atlanta, GA 30329-4250
800-227-2345 or 404-320-3333
www.cancer.org

American Chronic Pain Association
P.O. Box 850
Rocklin, CA 95677
800-533-3231 or 916-632-0922
www.theacpa.org

American College of Cardiology
9111 Old Georgetown Road
Bethesda, MD 20814-1699
800-253-4636, extension 694, or 301-897-5400
www.acc.org

American College of Emergency Physicians
1125 Executive Circle
Irving, TX 75038-2522
800-798-1822 or 972-550-0911
www.acep.org

American College of Gastroenterology
4900 B S. 31st St.
Arlington, VA 22206-1656
703-820-7400
www.acg.gi.org

American College of Obstetricians and Gynecologists
Resource Center
409 12th St. S.W.
Washington, DC 20090-6920
202-638-5577
www.acog.org

American College of Radiology
1891 Preston White Drive
Reston, VA 20191-4397
800-227-5463 or 703-648-8900
www.acr.org

American College of Rheumatology
1800 Century Place, Suite 250
Atlanta, GA 30345
404-633-3777
www.rheumatology.org

American College of Surgeons
633 N. St. Clair St., 24th Floor
Chicago, IL 60611-3211
312-202-5000
www.facs.org

American Council of the Blind
1155 15th St. N.W., Suite 1004
Washington, DC 20005
800-424-8666 or 202-467-5081
www.acb.org

American Dental Association
211 E. Chicago Ave.
Chicago, IL 60611
312-440-2500
www.ada.org

American Diabetes Association
1701 N. Beauregard St.
Alexandria, VA 22311
800-342-2383 or 703-549-1500
www.diabetes.org

American Dietetic Association
216 W. Jackson Blvd.
Chicago, IL 60606-6995
800-877-1600 or 312-899-0040
www.eatright.org

American Foundation for Suicide Prevention
120 Wall St., 22nd Floor
New York, NY 10005
888-333-2377 or 212-363-3500
www.afsp.org

American Foundation for Urologic Disease
1128 N. Charles St.
Baltimore, MD 21201-5559
410-468-1800
www.afud.org

American Geriatrics Society
Empire State Building, Suite 801
350 Fifth Ave.
New York, NY 10018
212-308-1414
www.americangeriatrics.org

American Health Care Association
1201 L St. N.W.
Washington, DC 20005
202-842-4444
www.ahca.org

American Hearing Research Foundation
8 S. Michigan Ave., Suite 814
Chicago, IL 60603-4539
312-726-9670
www.american-hearing.org

American Heart Association
7272 Greenville Ave.
Dallas, TX 75231-5129
800-242-8721 or 214-373-6300
www.americanheart.org

American Hospital Association
1 N. Franklin St.
Chicago, IL 60606-3421
312-422-3000
www.aha.org

American Lung Association
61 Broadway, Sixth Floor
New York, NY 10006
212-315-8700
www.lungusa.org

American Medical Association
515 N. State St.
Chicago, IL 60610
312-464-5000
www.ama-assn.org

American Music Therapy Association
8455 Colesville Road, Suite 1000
Silver Spring, MD 20910
301-589-3300
www.musictherapy.org

American Nurses Association
600 Maryland Ave. S.W., Suite 100 W.
Washington, DC 20024
800-274-4262 or 202-651-7000
www.nursingworld.org

American Occupational Therapy Association
4720 Montgomery Lane
Bethesda, MD 20824-1220
301-652-2682
www.aota.org

American Osteopathic Association
142 E. Ontario St.
Chicago, IL 60611
800-621-1773 or 312-202-8000
www.aoa-net.org

American Parkinson Disease Association
1250 Hylan Blvd., Suite 4B
Staten Island, NY 10305-1946
800-223-2732 or 718-981-8001
www.apdaparkinson.org

American Psychiatric Association
1400 K St. N.W.
Washington, DC 20005
888-357-7924 or 202-682-6220
www.psych.org

American Psychological Association
750 First St. N.E.
Washington, DC 20002-4242
800-374-2721 or 202-336-5510
www.apa.org

American Public Health Association
800 I St. N.W.
Washington, DC 20001-3710
202-777-2742
www.apha.org

American Red Cross
8111 Gatehouse Road
Falls Church, VA 22042
877-272-7337
www.redcross.org

American Self-Help Group Clearinghouse
100 E. Hanover Ave., Suite 202
Cedar Knolls, NJ 07927-2020
973-326-6789
www.selfhelpgroups.org

American Social Health Association Health Line
P.O. Box 13827
Research Triangle Park, NC 27709
919-361-8400
www.ashastd.org

American Society for Reproductive Medicine
1209 Montgomery Highway
Birmingham, AL 35216-2809
205-978-5000
www.asrm.org

American Society of Anesthesiologists
520 N. Northwest Highway
Park Ridge, IL 60068-2573
847-825-5586
www.asahq.org

American Speech-Language-Hearing Association
10801 Rockville Pike
Rockville, MD 20852
800-638-8255 or 301-897-5700
www.asha.org

American Stroke Association
7272 Greenville Ave.
Dallas, TX 75231
888-478-7653
www.strokeassociation.org

American Tinnitus Association
65 S.W. Yamhill St., Suite 200
Portland, OR 97204
800-634-8978 or 503-248-9985
www.ata.org

American Trauma Society
8903 Presidential Parkway, Suite 512
Upper Marlboro, MD 20772-2656
800-556-7890 or 301-420-4189
www.amtrauma.org

American Veterinary Medical Association
1931 N. Meacham Road, Suite 100
Schaumburg, IL 60173
847-925-8070
www.avma.org

Amyotrophic Lateral Sclerosis Association
27001 Agoura Road, Suite 156
Calabasas Hills, CA 91301-5104
800-782-4747 or 818-880-9007
www.alsa.org

Associated Services for the Blind
919 Walnut St.
Philadelphia, PA 19107
215-627-0600
www.asb.org

Association for Macular Diseases
210 E. 64th St., Eighth Floor
New York, NY 10021
212-605-3777
www.macula.org

Asthma and Allergy Foundation of America
1233 20th St. N.W., Suite 402
Washington, DC 20036
800-727-8462 or 202-466-7643
www.aafa.org

Benign Essential Blepharospasm Research Foundation
P.O. Box 12468
Beaumont, TX 77726-2468
409-832-0788
www.blepharospasm.org

Better Hearing Institute
515 King St., Suite 420
Alexandria, VA 22314
888-432-7435 or 703-684-3391
www.betterhearing.org

Cancer Care
275 Seventh Ave.
New York, NY 10001
800-813-4673 or 212-712-8080
www.cancercare.org

Center for Nutrition Policy and Promotion
Department of Agriculture
3101 Park Center Drive, Room 1034
Alexandria, VA 22302-1594
703-305-7600
www.usda.gov/cnpp

Centers for Disease Control and Prevention
1600 Clifton Road
Atlanta, GA 30333
800-311-3435 or 404-639-3534
www.cdc.gov

Centers for Medicare and Medicaid Services
7500 Security Blvd.
Baltimore, MD 21244-1850
410-786-3000
www.cms.hhs.gov

Christopher and Dana Reeve Paralysis Resource Center
636 Morris Ave.
Short Hills, NJ 07078
800-539-7309 or 973-467-8270
www.paralysis.org

Christopher Reeve Paralysis Foundation
500 Morris Ave.
Springfield, NJ 07081
800-225-0292
www.christopherreeve.org

Clearinghouse on Disability Information
Office of Special Education and Rehabilitative Services
Switzer Building, Room 3132
330 C St. S.W.
Washington, DC 20202-2524
202-205-8241
www.ed.gov/offices/OSERS

Crohn's and Colitis Foundation of America
386 Park Ave. S., 17th Floor
New York, NY 10016-8804
800-932-2423 or 212-685-3440
www.ccfa.org

Cystic Fibrosis Foundation
6931 Arlington Road
Bethesda, MD 20814
800-344-4823 or 301-951-4422
www.cff.org

Department of Health and Human Services
200 Independence Ave. S.W.
Washington, DC 20201
877-696-6775 or 202-619-0257
www.hhs.gov

Depression and Related Affective Disorders Association
Meyer 3-181
600 N. Wolfe St.
Baltimore, MD 21287-7381
410-955-4647 or 202-955-5800
www.drada.org

Diabetes Exercise and Sports Association
P.O. Box 1935
Litchfield Park, AZ 85340
800-898-4322
www.diabetes-exercise.org

Digestive Disease National Coalition
507 Capitol Court N.E., Suite 200
Washington, DC 20002
202-544-7497
www.ddnc.org

Easter Seals
230 W. Monroe, Suite 1800
Chicago, IL 60606
800-221-6827 or 312-726-6200
www.easter-seals.org

Epilepsy Foundation of America
4351 Garden City Drive, Suite 500
Landover, MD 20785-7223
800-332-1000 or 301-459-3700
www.epilepsyfoundation.org

Eye Bank Association of America
1015 18th St. N.W., Suite 1010
Washington, DC 20036
202-775-4999
www.restoresight.org

Family Caregiver Alliance
690 Market St., Suite 600
San Francisco, CA 94104
415-434-3388
www.caregiver.org

Federal Consumer Information Center
Department WWW
31451 United Ave.
Pueblo, CO 81009
888-878-3256 or 719-948-4000
www.pueblo.gsa.gov

Food and Drug Administration
5600 Fishers Lane
Rockville, MD 20857
888-463-6332 or 301-827-4573
www.fda.gov

Food and Nutrition Service
Department of Agriculture
3101 Park Center Drive
Alexandria, VA 22302
703-305-2281
www.fns.usda.gov

Foundation Fighting Blindness
11435 Cronhill Drive
Owings Mills, MD 21117-2220
888-394-3937 or 410-568-0150
www.blindness.org

Gastro-Intestinal Research Foundation
70 E. Lake St., Suite 1015
Chicago, IL 60601-5907
312-332-1350
www.girf.org

Guiding Eyes for the Blind
611 Granite Springs Road
Yorktown Heights, NY 10598
800-942-0149 or 914-245-4024
www.guidingeyes.org

Guillain-Barre Syndrome Foundation International
P.O. Box 262
Wynnewood, PA 19096
610-667-0131
www.gbsfi.org

Health Insurance Association of America
555 13th St. N.W.
Washington, DC 20004
208-824-1600
www.hiaa.org

Health On The Net Foundation
Medical Informatics Division
University Hospital of Geneva
24, rue Micheli-du-Crest
1211 Geneva 14
Switzerland
www.hon.ch

Health Resources and Services Administration
Parklawn Building
5600 Fishers Lane
Rockville, MD 20857
301-443-3376
www.hrsa.gov

Hospice Education Institute
3 Unity Square
P.O. Box 98
Machiasport, ME 04655-0098
800-544-2213 or 207-255-8800
www.hospiceworld.org

Hospice Foundation of America
2991 S St. N.W.
Washington, DC 20009
800-854-3402 or 202-638-54219
www.hospicefoundation.org

Huntington's Disease Society of America
158 W. 29th St., Seventh Floor
New York, NY 10001-5300
800-345-4372 or 212-242-1968
www.hdsa.org

International Association for Medical Assistance to Travellers
417 Center St.
Lewiston, NY 14092
716-754-4883
www.iamat.org

International Hearing Society
16880 Middlebelt Road, Suite 4
Livonia, MI 48154
800-521-5247 or 734-522-7200
www.ihsinfo.org

Intestinal Disease Foundation
Landmarks Building, Suite 525
1 Station Square Drive
Pittsburgh, PA 15219-1138
877-587-9606 or 412-261-5888
www.intestinalfoundation.org

Juvenile Diabetes Research Foundation International
120 Wall St., 19th Floor
New York, NY 10005-4001
800-533-2873 or 212-785-9500
www.jdrf.org

Laurent Clerc National Deaf Education Center
800 Florida Ave. N.E.
Washington, DC 20002
202-651-5051
www.clerccenter.gallaudet.edu

Leukemia and Lymphoma Society
1311 Mamaroneck Ave.
White Plains, NY 10605
877-464-3400 or 914-949-5213
www.leukemia-lymphoma.org

Lighthouse International
111 E. 59th St.
New York, NY 10022-1202
800-829-0500 or 212-821-9200
www.lighthouse.org

Living Bank
4545 Post Oak Place, Suite 315
Houston, TX 77027
800-528-2971 or 713-528-2971
www.livingbank.org

Lupus Foundation of America
1300 Piccard Drive, Suite 200
Rockville, MD 20850-4303
301-670-9292
www.lupus.org

March of Dimes Birth Defects Foundation
1275 Mamaroneck Ave.
White Plains, NY 10605
888-663-4637 or 914-428-7100
www.modimes.org

MayoClinic.com
Mayo Clinic Health Information
200 1st St. S.W.
Rochester, MN 55905
www.MayoClinic.com

Mended Hearts
7272 Greenville Ave.
Dallas, TX 75231-4596
888-432-7899 or 214-706-1442
www.mendedhearts.org

Midwest Bioethics Center
1021-1025 Jefferson St.
Kansas City, MO 64105
800-344-3829 or 816-221-1100
www.midbio.org

Myasthenia Gravis Foundation National Office
5841 Cedar Lake Road, Suite 204
Minneapolis, MN 55416
800-541-5454 or 952-545-9438
www.myasthenia.org

National Alliance for the Mentally Ill
Colonial Place 3
2107 Wilson Blvd., Suite 300
Arlington, VA 22201-3042
800-950-6264 or 703-524-7600
www.nami.org

National Alliance of Breast Cancer Organizations
9 E. 37th St., 10th Floor
New York, NY 10016
888-806-2226 or 212-889-0606
www.nabco.org

National Alopecia Areata Foundation
14 Mitchell Blvd.
San Rafael, CA 94903
415-472-3780
www.naaf.org

National Aphasia Association
29 John St., Suite 1103
New York, NY 10038
800-922-4622
www.aphasia.org

National Association for Home Care
228 Seventh St. S.E.
Washington, DC 20003
202-547-7424
www.nahc.org

National Association for Visually Handicapped
22 W. 21st St., Sixth Floor
New York, NY 10010
800-677-9965 or 212-889-3141
www.navh.org

National Association of the Deaf
814 Thayer Ave.
Silver Spring, MD 20910-4500
301-587-1788
www.nad.org

National Ataxia Foundation
2600 Fernbrook Lane, Suite 119
Minneapolis, MN 55447
763-553-0020
www.ataxia.org

National Brain Tumor Foundation
414 13th St., Suite 700
Oakland, CA 94612-2603
800-934-2873 or 510-839-9777
www.braintumor.org

National Cancer Institute
National Institutes of Health
6116 Executive Blvd., MSC 8322
Bethesda, MD 20892-8322
800-422-6237
www.cancer.gov

National Center for Complementary and Alternative Medicine
National Institutes of Health
P.O. Box 7923
Gaithersburg, MD 20898
888-644-6226 or 301-519-3153
www.nccam.nih.gov

National Chronic Pain Outreach Association
P.O. Box 274
Millboro, VA 24460-9606
540-862-9437

National Clearinghouse for Alcohol and Drug Information
P.O. Box 2345
Rockville, MD 20847-2345
800-729-6686 or 301-468-2600
www.health.org

National Clearinghouse on Child Abuse and Neglect Information
300 C St. S.W.
Washington, DC 20447
800-394-3366 or 703-385-7565
www.calib.com/nccanch

National Clearinghouse on Families and Youth
P.O. Box 13505
Silver Spring, MD 20911-3505
301-608-8098
www.ncfy.com

National Coalition for Cancer Survivorship
1010 Wayne Ave., Suite 770
Silver Spring, MD 20910
301-650-9127
www.canceradvocacy.org

National Council on Alcoholism and Drug Dependence
20 Exchange Place, Suite 2902
New York, NY 10005-3201
800-622-2255 or 212-269-7797
www.ncadd.org

National Depressive and Manic-Depressive Association
730 N. Franklin St., Suite 501
Chicago, IL 60610-7204
800-826-3632 or 312-642-0049
www.ndmda.org

National Diabetes Information Clearinghouse
National Institutes of Health
1 Information Way
Bethesda, MD 20892-3560
800-860-8747 or 301-654-3327
www.niddk.nih.gov/health/diabetes/diabetes.htm

National Digestive Diseases Information Clearinghouse
National Institutes of Health
2 Information Way
Bethesda, MD 20892-3570
800-891-5389 or 301-654-3810
www.niddk.nih.gov/health/digest/digest.htm

National Down Syndrome Society
666 Broadway, Eighth Floor
New York, NY 10012-2317
800-221-4602 or 212-460-9330
www.ndss.org

National Eye Institute
National Institutes of Health
2020 Vision Place
Bethesda, MD 20892-3655
301-496-5248
www.nei.nih.gov

National Federation of the Blind
1800 Johnson St.
Baltimore, MD 21230
410-659-9314
www.nfb.org

National Headache Foundation
428 W. St. James Place, Second Floor
Chicago, IL 60614-2750
888-643-5552 or 773-388-6399
www.headaches.org

National Health Information Center
P.O. Box 1133
Washington, DC 20013-1133
800-336-4797 or 301-565-4167
www.health.gov

National Heart, Lung and Blood Institute
National Institutes of Health
P.O. Box 30105
Bethesda, MD 20824-0105
800-575-9355 or 301-592-8573
www.nhlbi.nih.gov

National Hemophilia Foundation
116 W. 32nd St., 11th Floor
New York, NY 10001
800-424-2634 or 212-328-3700
www.hemophilia.org

National Herpes Resource Center
American Social Health Association
P.O. Box 13827
Research Triangle Park, NC 27709
919-361-8400
www.ashastd.org

National Hospice and Palliative Care Organization
1700 Diagonal Road, Suite 625
Alexandria, VA 22314
703-837-1500
www.nhpco.org

National Human Genome Research Institute
National Institutes of Health
Building 31, Room 4B09
31 Center Drive, MSC 2152
9000 Rockville Pike
Bethesda, MD 20892-2152
301-402-0911
www.genome.gov

National Information Center for Children and Youth With Disabilities
P.O. Box 1492
Washington, DC 20013
800-695-0285
www.nichcy.org

National Institute for Occupational Safety and Health
4676 Columbia Parkway, MSC 13
Cincinnati, OH 45226
800-356-4674 or 513-533-8466
www.cdc.gov/niosh

National Institute of Allergy and Infectious Diseases
National Institutes of Health
Building 31, Room 7A50
31 Center Drive, MSC 2520
Bethesda, MD 20892-2520
301-496-5717
www.niaid.nih.gov

National Institute of Arthritis and Musculoskeletal and Skin Diseases
National Institutes of Health
Building 31, Room 4C05
31 Center Drive, MSC 2350
Bethesda, MD 20892-2350
877-226-4267 or 301-496-8190
www.niams.nih.gov

National Institute of Child Health and Human Development
National Institutes of Health
Building 31, Room 2A32
31 Center Drive, MSC 2425
Bethesda, MD 20892-2425
800-370-2943 or 301-496-5133
www.nichd.nih.gov

National Institute of Diabetes and Digestive and Kidney Diseases
National Institutes of Health
Building 31, Room 9A04
31 Center Drive, MSC 2560
Bethesda, MD 20892-2560
301-496-3583
www.niddk.nih.gov

National Institute of Environmental Health Sciences
National Institutes of Health
111 Alexander Drive
Research Triangle Park, NC 27709
919-541-3345
www.niehs.nih.gov

National Institute of General Medical Sciences
National Institutes of Health
45 Center Drive, MSC 6200
Bethesda, MD 20892-6200
301-496-7301
www.nigms.nih.gov

National Institute of Mental Health
National Institutes of Health
6001 Executive Blvd., MSC 9663
Bethesda, MD 20892-9663
301-443-4513
www.nimh.nih.gov

National Institute on Aging
National Institutes of Health
Building 31, Room 5C27
31 Center Drive, MSC 2292
Bethesda, MD 2089-2292
301-496-1752
www.nia.nih.gov

National Institute on Alcohol Abuse and Alcoholism
National Institutes of Health
Willco Building
6000 Executive Blvd., MSC 7003
Bethesda, MD 20892-7003
301-443-3860
www.niaaa.nih.gov

National Institute on Deafness and Other Communication Disorders
National Institutes of Health
31 Center Drive, MSC 2320
Bethesda, MD 20892-2320
800-241-1004 or 301-496-7243
www.nidcd.nih.gov

National Institute on Drug Abuse
National Institutes of Health
6001 Executive Blvd., MSC 9561
Bethesda, MD 20892-9561
301-443-1124
www.drugabuse.gov

National Institutes of Health
31 Center Drive, MSC 2320
Bethesda, MD 20892-2320
800-241-1004 or 301-496-4000
www.nih.gov

National Kidney and Urologic Diseases Information Clearinghouse
National Institutes of Health
3 Information Way
Bethesda, MD 20892-3580
800-891-5390 or 301-654-4415
www.niddk.nih.gov/health/kidney/kidney.htm

National Kidney Foundation
30 E. 33rd St., Suite 1100
New York, NY 10016
800-622-9010 or 212-889-2210
www.kidney.org

National Library of Medicine
8600 Rockville Pike
Bethesda, MD 20894
888-346-3656 or 594-5983
www.nlm.nih.gov

National Mental Health Association
2001 N. Beauregard St., 12th Floor
Alexandria, VA 22311
800-969-6642 or 703-684-7722
www.nmha.org

National Neurofibromatosis Foundation
95 Pine St., 16th Floor
New York, NY 10005
800-323-7938 or 212-344-6633
www.nf.org

National Oral Health Information Clearinghouse
National Institutes of Health
1 NOHIC Way
Bethesda, MD 20892-3500
301-402-7364
www.nohic.nidcr.nih.gov

National Organization for Rare Disorders
55 Kenosia Ave.
P.O. Box 1968
Danbury, CT 06813-1968
800-999-6673 or 203-744-0100
www.rarediseases.org

National Osteoporosis Foundation
1232 22nd St. N.W.
Washington, DC 20037-1292
800-223-9994 or 202-223-2226
www.nof.org

National Parkinson Foundation
Bob Hope Parkinson Research Center
Bob Hope Road
1501 N.W. Ninth Ave.
Miami, FL 33136-1494
800-327-4545 or 305-547-6666
www.parkinson.org

National Prevention Information Network
Centers for Disease Control and Prevention
P.O. Box 6003
Rockville, MD 20849-6003
800-458-5231 or 301-562-1098
www.cdcnpin.org

National Psoriasis Foundation
6600 S.W. 92nd Ave., Suite 300
Portland, OR 97223-7195
800-723-9166 or 503-244-7404
www.psoriasis.org

National Rehabilitation Information Center
4200 Forbes Blvd., Suite 202
Lanham, MD 20706
800-346-2742 or 301-459-5900
www.naric.com

National Resource Center on Homelessness and Mental Illness
Policy Research Associates
345 Delaware Ave.
Delmar, NY 12054
800-444-7415 or 518-439-7415
www.nrchmi.com

National Sleep Foundation
1552 K St. N.W., Suite 500
Washington, DC 20005
202-347-3471, extension 205
www.sleepfoundation.org

National Spinal Cord Injury Association
6701 Democracy Blvd., Suite 300-9
Bethesda, MD 20817
800-962-9629 or 301-588-6959
www.spinalcord.org

National Stroke Association
9707 E. Easter Lane
Englewood, CO 80112-3747
800-787-6537 or 303-649-9299
www.stroke.org

National Sudden Infant Death Syndrome
Resource Center
2070 Chain Bridge Road, Suite 450
Vienna, VA 22182
703-821-8955
www.sidscenter.org

National Women's Health Information Center
8550 Arlington Blvd., Suite 300
Fairfax, VA 22031
800-994-9662 or 703-560-6618
www.4woman.org

Neurological Institute of Neurological Disorders and Stroke
National Institutes of Health
P.O. Box 5801
Bethesda, MD 20824
800-352-9424
www.ninds.nih.gov

Office of Research on Women's Health
National Institutes of Health
Building 1, Room 201
9000 Rockville Pike
Bethesda, MD 20892-0161
301-402-1770
www4.od.nih.gov/orwh

Office on Smoking and Health
Centers for Disease Control and Prevention
Publications, MS K-50
4770 Buford Highway N.E.
Atlanta, GA 30341-3717
800-232-1311 or 770-488-5705
www.cdc.gov/tobacco

Oldways Preservation and Exchange Trust
266 Beacon St.
Boston, MA 02116
617-421-5500
www.oldwayspt.org

Osteoporosis and Related Bone Diseases National Resource Center
National Institutes of Health
1232 22nd St. N.W.
Washington, DC 20037-1292
800-624-2663 or 202-223-0344
www.osteo.org

Paget Foundation
120 Wall St., Suite 1602
New York, NY 10005-4001
800-237-2438 or 212-509-5335
www.paget.org

Parkinson's Disease Foundation
William Black Medical Building
Columbia-Presbyterian Medical Center
710 W. 168th St.
New York, NY 10032-9982
800-457-6676 or 212-923-4700
www.pdf.org

President's Council on Physical Fitness and Sports
Department W
200 Independence Ave. S.W., Room 738-H
Washington, DC 20201-0004
202-690-9000
www.fitness.gov

Prevent Blindness America
500 E. Remington Road
Schaumburg, IL 60173
800-331-2020 or 847-843-2020
www.preventblindness.org

Scleroderma Foundation
12 Kent Way, Suite 101
Byfield, MA 01922
800-722-4673 or 978-463-5843
www.scleroderma.org

Sickle Cell Disease Association of America
200 Corporate Point, Suite 495
Culver City, CA 90230-8727
800-421-8453 or 310-216-6363
www.sicklecelldisease.org

Sjogren's Syndrome Foundation
8120 Woodmont Ave., Suite 530
Bethesda, MD 20814
800-475-6473 or 301-718-0300
www.sjogrens.org

Skin Cancer Foundation
245 Fifth Ave., Suite 1403
New York, NY 10016
800-754-6490 or 212-725-5176
www.skincancer.org

Society for Healthcare Consumer Advocacy
1 N. Franklin St.
Chicago, IL 60606
312-422-3726
www.shca-aha.org

Spina Bifida Association of America
4590 MacArthur Blvd. N.W., Suite 250
Washington, DC 20007-4226
800-621-3141 or 202-944-3285
www.sbaa.org

Stuttering Foundation of America
3100 Walnut Grove Road, Suite 603
P.O. Box 11749
Memphis, TN 38111-0749
800-992-9392 or 901-452-7343
www.stutteringhelp.org

Substance Abuse and Mental Health Services Administration
5600 Fishers Lane
Rockville, MD 20857
301-443-4795
www.samhsa.gov

Thyroid Foundation of America
410 Stuart St.
Boston, MA 02116
800-832-8321 or 617-534-1500
www.allthyroid.org

Tourette Syndrome Association
42-40 Bell Blvd.
Bayside, NY 11361
718-224-2999
www.tsa-usa.org

Transplant Recipients International Organization
2117 L St. N.W., Suite 353
Washington, DC 20037
800-874-6386 or 202-293-0980
www.trioweb.org

Tuberous Sclerosis Alliance
801 Roeder Road, Suite 750
Silver Spring, MD 20910
800-225-6872 or 301-562-9890
www.tsalliance.org

United Ostomy Association
19772 MacArthur Blvd., Suite 200
Irvine, CA 92612-2405
800-826-0826 or 949-660-8624
www.uoa.org

United Seniors Health Council
409 3rd St. S.W., Suite 200
Washington, DC 20024
202-479-6973
www.unitedseniorshealth.org

Us Too! International
Prostate Cancer Education and Support
5003 Fairview Ave.
Downers Grove, IL 60515
800-808-7866 or 630-795-1002
www.ustoo.org

Vision Community Services
23A Elm St.
Watertown, MA 02472
617-926- 4232
www.mablind.org

Visiting Nurse Associations of America
11 Beacon St., Suite 910
Boston, MA 02108
617-523-4042
www.vnaa.org

Weight-Control Information Network
National Institutes of Health
1 WIN Way
Bethesda, MD 20892-3665
877-946-4627 or 202-828-1025
www.niddk.nih.gov/health/nutrit/nutrit.htm

Women's Sports Foundation
Eisenhower Park
East Meadow, NY 11554
800-227-3988 or 516-542-4700
www.womenssportsfoundation.org

World Health Organization
2 United Nations Plaza
DC-2 Building, Rooms 0956 to 0976
New York, NY 10017
212-963-3952
www.who.int

Y-Me
National Organization for Breast Cancer Information and Support
212 W. Van Buren, Suite 500
Chicago, IL 60607
800-221-2141 or 312-986-8338
www.y-me.org
■

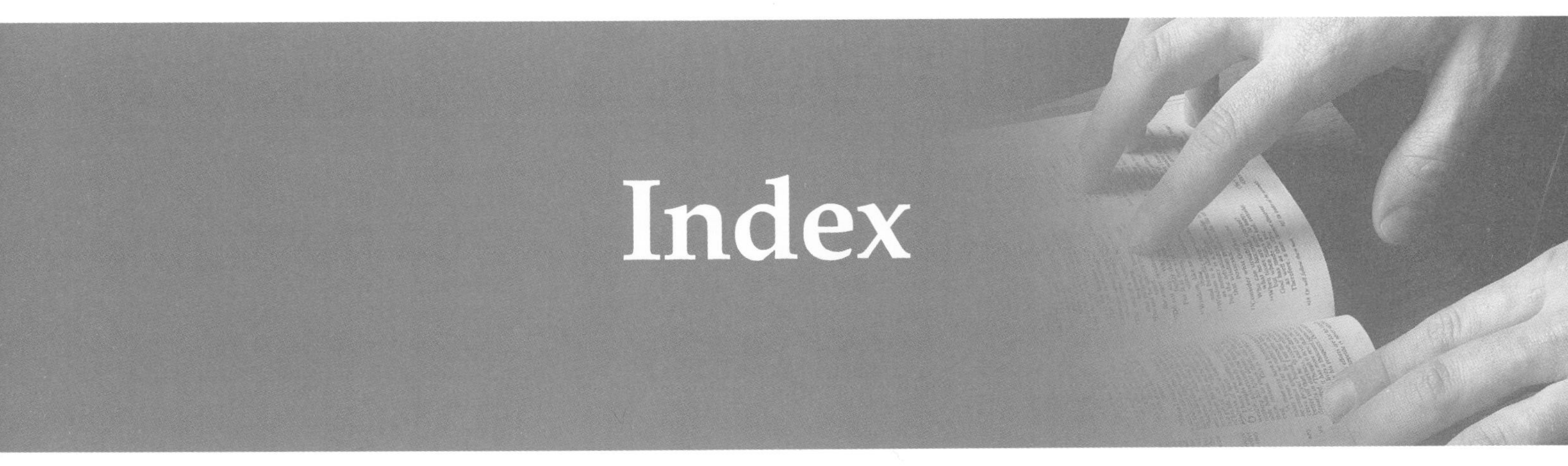

Index

A

Page numbers in ***italics*** indicate illustrations.

Page numbers in ***italics*** indicate illustrations.

B

Page numbers in ***italics*** indicate illustrations.

Page numbers in ***italics*** indicate illustrations.

C

Page numbers in ***italics*** indicate illustrations.

Page numbers in *italics* indicate illustrations.

D

Page numbers in ***italics*** indicate illustrations.

E

Page numbers in *italics* indicate illustrations.

F

G

Page numbers in *italics* indicate illustrations.

H

Page numbers in ***italics*** indicate illustrations.

Page numbers in *italics* indicate illustrations.

I

Page numbers in *italics* indicate illustrations.

J

K

L

M

Page numbers in *italics* indicate illustrations.

Page numbers in ***italics*** indicate illustrations.

N

Page numbers in ***italics*** indicate illustrations.

O

Page numbers in *italics* indicate illustrations.

P

Q

R

S

Page numbers in ***italics*** indicate illustrations.

Page numbers in *italics* indicate illustrations.

T

U

V

W

Page numbers in *italics* indicate illustrations.

X

Y

Z